D1483119

Clinical Practice

Principles and Practice of Ophthalmology

SECTION EDITORS

Daniel M. Albert, M.D.

Thaddeus P. Dryja, M.D.

Frederick A. Jakobiec, M.D., D.Sc.(Med.)

Simmons Lessell, M.D.

Joseph F. Rizzo III, M.D.

Richard M. Robb, M.D.

David S. Walton, M.D.

Clinical Practice

Principles and Practice of Ophthalmology

Volume 4

DANIEL M. ALBERT, M.D.
Frederick A. Davis Professor and Chairman,
Department of Ophthalmology,
University of Wisconsin Medical School,
Madison, Wisconsin

FREDERICK A. JAKOBIEC, M.D., D.Sc.(Med.)
Henry Willard Williams Professor of Ophthalmology,
Professor of Pathology, and Chairman,
Department of Ophthalmology,
Harvard Medical School;
Chief, Department of Ophthalmology, and
Surgeon in Ophthalmology,
Massachusetts Eye and Ear Infirmary,
Boston, Massachusetts

NANCY L. ROBINSON, A.B.
Managing Editor

W.B. SAUNDERS COMPANY
A Division of Harcourt Brace & Company
Philadelphia London Toronto Montreal Sydney Tokyo

W.B. SAUNDERS COMPANY
A Division of Harcourt Brace & Company

The Curtis Center
Independence Square West
Philadelphia, Pennsylvania 19106

Library of Congress Cataloging-in-Publication Data

Principles and practice of ophthalmology : clinical practice / [edited by] Daniel M. Albert, Frederick A. Jakobiec.

p. cm.

ISBN 0–7216–3418–4 (5 v. set)

1. Ophthalmology. I. Albert, Daniel M. II. Jakobiec, Frederick A.

[DNLM: 1. Eye Diseases. 2. Ophthalmology. WW 140 P957 1994] RE46.P743 1994

617.7—dc20
DNLM/DLC 93–7247

PRINCIPLES AND PRACTICE OF OPHTHALMOLOGY: CLINICAL PRACTICE

ISBN Volume 4 0–7216–6603–5
5-Volume Set 0–7216–3418–4

Printed in the United States of America.

Last digit is the print number: 9 8 7 6 5 4 3 2 1

Contributors

Daniel M. Albert, MD
Frederick A. Davis Professor and Chairman, Department of Ophthalmology, University of Wisconsin Medical School, Madison, Wisconsin

R. Rand Allingham, MD
Assistant Professor of Ophthalmology, University of Texas Southwestern Medical Center; Active Attending Ophthalmologist and Assistant Surgeon, Parkland Memorial Hospital and Zale Lipshy University Hospital, Dallas, Texas

Don C. Bienfang, MD
Assistant Professor of Ophthalmology, Harvard Medical School; Surgeon, Brigham and Women's Hospital, Boston, Massachusetts

William P. Boger III, MD
Clinical Instructor, Children's Hospital, Harvard Medical School; Associate in Ophthalmology, Children's Hospital, Boston; Active Staff, Emerson Hospital, Concord, Massachusetts

Mark S. Borchert, MD
Assistant Professor of Ophthalmology, University of Southern California School of Medicine; Staff, Children's Hospital Los Angeles, Los Angeles, California

Alfred Brini, MD
Professor Emeritus, Université Louis Pasteur, Department of Ophthalmology, Strasbourg, France

Stephen C. Cannon, MD, PhD
Fellow in Neurology, Harvard Medical School and Massachusetts General Hospital, Boston, Massachusetts

Louis R. Caplan, MD
Professor and Chairman, Neurology Department, Tufts University School of Medicine; Neurologist-in-Chief, New England Medical Center, Boston, Massachusetts

David G. Cogan, MD
Professor Emeritus, Harvard Medical School, Boston, Massachusetts; Senior Staff Officer, National Eye Institute, Bethesda, Maryland

M. Ronan Conlon, MB, BCh
Fellow, Oculoplastics, Orbital Reconstructive Surgery, and Oncology, University of Iowa Hospitals and Clinics, Department of Ophthalmology, Iowa City, Iowa

James R. Coppeto, MD
Attending, St. Mary's Hospital, Waterbury, Connecticut

James J. Corbett, MD
Professor and Chairman of Neurology and Professor of Ophthalmology, University of Mississippi Medical School; Consultant, Veterans Administration Hospital, Mississippi Methodist Rehabilitation Hospital, and University of Mississippi Medical Center, Jackson, Mississippi

Thaddeus P. Dryja, MD
Professor of Ophthalmology, Harvard Medical School; Surgeon, Massachusetts Eye and Ear Infirmary, Boston, Massachusetts

Steven E. Feldon, MD
Professor of Ophthalmology and Neurological Surgery, University of Southern California School of Medicine; Chief of Staff, Estelle Doheny Eye Hospital, Los Angeles, California

Anthony J. Fraioli, MD
Clinical Instructor in Ophthalmology, Harvard Medical School; Associate Surgeon in Ophthalmology, Massachusetts Eye and Ear Infirmary, Boston, Massachusetts

Stephen J. Fricker, ScD, MD
Associate Professor of Ophthalmology, Harvard Medical School; Surgeon, Massachusetts Eye and Ear Infirmary, Boston, Massachusetts

Anne B. Fulton, MD
Associate Professor of Ophthalmology, Harvard Medical School; Senior Associate in Ophthalmology, Children's Hospital, Boston, Massachusetts

John W. Gittinger, Jr., MD
Professor of Surgery and Neurology, University of Massachusetts Medical School; Chief of Ophthalmology, University of Massachusetts Medical Center, Worcester, Massachusetts

Joel S. Glaser, MD
Professor, Departments of Ophthalmology, Neurology, and Neurological Surgery, Bascom Palmer Eye Institute, University of Miami School of Medicine, Miami, Florida

G. Michael Halmagyi, MD
Clinical Associate Professor, University of Sydney Faculty of Medicine; Staff Neurologist and Head of Eye and Ear Research Unit, Royal Prince Alfred Hospital, Sydney, Australia

Thomas R. Hedges III, MD
Associate Professor of Ophthalmology and Neurology, Tufts University School of Medicine; Associate Ophthalmologist, New England Medical Center; Director of Neuro-Ophthalmology, New England Eye Center, Boston, Massachusetts

Robert S. Hepler, MD
Professor of Ophthalmology, UCLA School of Medicine, Los Angeles, California (on leave of absence); Clinical Professor of Ophthalmology, King Saud University, College of Medicine, Riyadh, Saudi Arabia; Medical Director, King Khaled Eye Specialist Hospital, Riyadh, Kingdom of Saudi Arabia

David G. Hunter, MD, PhD
Assistant Professor, Strabismus and Pediatric Ophthalmology, The Wilmer Ophthalmological Institute, The Johns Hopkins University School of Medicine, Baltimore, Maryland

Frederick A. Jakobiec, MD, DSc(Med)
Henry Willard Williams Professor of Ophthalmology, Professor of Pathology, and Chairman, Department of Ophthalmology, Harvard Medical School; Chief, Department of Ophthalmology, and Surgeon in Ophthalmology, Massachusetts Eye and Ear Infirmary, Boston, Massachusetts

Carl Cordes Johnson, MD, FACS
Associate Clinical Professor (retired), Harvard Medical School; Formerly Associate Chief of Ophthalmology, Massachusetts Eye and Ear Infirmary, Boston, Massachusetts

Barrett Katz, MD
The Wayne and Gladys Valley Professor, and Vice Chairman, Department of Ophthalmology, California Pacific Medical Center and The Smith-Kettelwell Eye Research Institute, San Francisco, California

James R. Keane, MD
Professor of Neurology, University of Southern California; Staff Physician, Los Angeles County Hospital and USC Medical Center, Los Angeles, California

Ramsay S. Kurban, MD
Fellow in Dermatology, Harvard Medical School, Department of Dermatology, Massachusetts General Hospital, Boston, Massachusetts

Simmons Lessell, MD
Professor of Ophthalmology, Harvard Medical School; Director, Neuro-Ophthalmology, Massachusetts Eye and Ear Infirmary, Boston, Massachusetts

Elbert H. Magoon, MD
Clinical Associate Professor at Northeast Ohio University College of Medicine; Attending, Aultman Hospital and Timken Mercy Medical Center, Canton, Ohio

Craig A. McKeown, MD
Assistant Professor of Ophthalmology, Harvard Medical School; Director of Pediatric Ophthalmology and Ocular Motility, Massachusetts Eye and Ear Infirmary, Boston, Massachusetts

Marsel Mesulam, MD
Professor of Neurology, Harvard Medical School; Senior Neurologist and Director, Division of Neuroscience and Behavioral Neurology, Beth Israel Hospital, Boston, Massachusetts

Martin C. Mihm, Jr., MD
Professor of Pathology, Harvard Medical School; Chief of Dermatic Pathology Unit, Massachusetts General Hospital; Adjunct Professor in Pathology, Vanderbilt University; Consultant in Pathology, Children's Hospital (Boston), Boston VA Hospital, New England Deaconness Hospital, Harvard Community Health Plan, Beth Israel Hospital; Associate, Brigham and Women's Hospital, Boston, Massachusetts

Shizuo Mukai, MD
Assistant Professor in Ophthalmology, Harvard Medical School; Assistant Surgeon, Massachusetts Eye and Ear Infirmary, Boston, Massachusetts

Nancy J. Newman, MD
Assistant Professor of Ophthalmology and Neurology and Instructor in Neurosurgery, Emory University School of Medicine; Director, Neuro-Ophthalmology, Emory Eye Center, Atlanta, Georgia; Lecturer in Ophthalmology, Harvard Medical School, Boston, Massachusetts

Robert A. Petersen, MD, DrMedSci
Assistant Professor of Ophthalmology, Harvard Medical School; Senior Associate in Ophthalmology, Children's Hospital; Associate Surgeon, Massachusetts Eye and Ear Infirmary; Associate Surgeon in Ophthalmology, Brigham and Women's Hospital and Beth Israel Hospital, Boston, Massachusetts

Amy A. Pruitt, MD
Assistant Professor of Neurology, University of Pennsylvania School of Medicine; Staff Neurologist, Hospital of the University of Pennsylvania, Philadelphia, Pennsylvania

Joseph F. Rizzo III, MD
Assistant Professor of Ophthalmology, Harvard Medical School; Assistant Surgeon, Active Staff, Massachusetts Eye and Ear Infirmary, Boston, Massachusetts

Richard M. Robb, MD
Associate Professor of Ophthalmology, Harvard Medical School; Ophthalmologist-in-Chief, Children's Hospital, Boston, Massachusetts

Jack Rootman, MD, FRCS(C)
Professor of Ophthalmology and Pathology, University of British Columbia; Active Staff, Vancouver General Hospital and B.C. Children's Hospital; Consulting, Shaughnessy Hospital and B.C. Cancer Agency, Vancouver, B.C., Canada

Alfredo A. Sadun, MD, PhD
Professor of Ophthalmology and Director of Resident Training, University of Southern California School of Medicine; Attending, Doheny Eye Institute, Norris Cancer Hospital, LAC Hospital, and University Hospital, Los Angeles, California

José A. Sahel, MD
Professeur des Universitées, Université Louis Pasteur; Clinique Ophtalmologique, Hôpitaux Universitaires, Strasbourg, France

Maria A. Saornil, MD
Associate Professor of Ophthalmology, Valladolid Medical School, University of Valladolid; Oncology and Pathology Unit, Instituto de Oftalmobiologia Aplicada, University of Valladolid, Valladolid, Spain

Lois Hodgson Smith, MD, PhD
Assistant Professor of Ophthalmology, Harvard Medical School; Associate in Ophthalmology, Children's Hospital, Massachusetts Eye and Ear Infirmary, and Beth Israel Hospital, Boston, Massachusetts

Barbara W. Streeten, MD
Professor of Ophthalmology and Pathology, State University of New York Health Science Center at Syracuse; Attending Ophthalmologist, University Hospital, Syracuse, New York

Michael Wall, MD
Associate Professor of Neurology and Ophthalmology, University of Iowa School of Medicine; Staff, University of Iowa Hospitals and Clinics and Veterans Administration Medical Center, Iowa City, Iowa

David S. Walton, MD
Associate Clinical Professor of Ophthalmology, Harvard Medical School; Surgeon, Massachusetts Eye and Ear Infirmary; Assistant Pediatrician, Massachusetts General Hospital; Consultant in Ophthalmology, Children's Hospital Medical Center, Boston, Massachusetts

Michel Weber, MD
Assistant, Clinique Ophtalmologique, Hôpitaux Universitaires, Strasbourg, France

Jayne S. Weiss, MD
Associate Professor of Ophthalmology and Director of Cornea and External Diseases, University of Massachusetts Medical Center; Instructor of Ophthalmology, Tufts Medical School, Boston, Massachusetts

Christopher T. Westfall, MD, FACS
Chairman, Department of Ophthalmology and Chief of Oculoplastic Surgery Service, Wilford Hall U.S. Air Force Medical Center, San Antonio, Texas; Chief Consultant in Ophthalmology to the Air Force Surgeon General

Valerie A. White, MD, FRCP(C)
Assistant Professor of Pathology and Ophthalmology, University of British Columbia; Pathologist, Vancouver General Hospital; Consultant Pathologist, British Columbia's Children's Hospital and British Columbia Cancer Agency, Vancouver, British Columbia, Canada

Shirley H. Wray, MD, PhD, FRCP
Associate Professor of Neurology, Harvard Medical School; Director, Unit for Neurovisual Disorders, Department of Neurology, and Neurologist, Massachusetts General Hospital, Boston, Massachusetts

To Ellie

D.M.A.

Preface

"INCIPIT." The medievel scribe would write this Latin word, meaning *so it begins,* to signal the start of the book he was transcribing. It was a dramatic word that conveyed promise of instruction and delight. In more modern times INCIPIT has been replaced by the PREFACE. It may be the first thing the reader sees, but it is, in fact, the last thing the author writes before the book goes to press. I appreciate the opportunity to make some personal comments regarding **Principles and Practice of Ophthalmology.**

One of the most exciting things about writing and editing a book in a learned field is that it puts the authors and editors in touch with those who have gone before. Each author shares with those who have labored in past years and in past centuries the tasks of assessing the knowledge that exists in his or her field, of determining what is important, and of trying to convey it to his or her peers. In the course of the work the author experiences the same anticipation, angst, and ennui of those who have gone before. He or she can well envision the various moments of triumph and despair that all authors and editors must feel as they organize, review, and revise the accumulating manuscripts and reassure, cajole, and make demands of their fellow editors, authors, and publisher.

This feeling of solidarity with early writers becomes even more profound when one is a collector and reviewer of books, and conversant with the history of one's field. In Ecclesiastes it is stated, "of the making of books, there is no end" (12:12). Indeed, there are more books than any other human artifact on earth. There is, however, a beginning to the "making of books" in any given field. The first ophthalmology book to be published was Benvenuto Grassi's *De Oculis* in Florence in 1474. Firmin Didot in his famous *Bibliographical Encyclopedia* wrote that Grassus, an Italian physician of the School of Solerno, lived in the 12th century and was the author of two books, *Ferrara Quarto* (1474) and the *Venetian Folio* (1497). Eye care in the 15th century was in the hands of itinerant barber-surgeons and quacks, and a treatise by a learned physician was a remarkable occurrence. The next book on the eye to appear was an anonymous pamphlet written for the layperson in 1538 and entitled *Ein Newes Hochnutzliches Büchlin von Erkantnus der Kranckheyten der Augen.* Like **Principles and Practice of Ophthalmology,** the *Büchlin* stated its intention to provide highly useful knowledge of eye diseases, the anatomy of the eye, and various remedies. It was illustrated with a full-page woodcut of the anatomy of the eye (Fig. 1). At the conclusion of the book, the publisher, Vogtherr, promised to bring more and better information to light shortly, and indeed, the next year he published a small book by Leonhart Fuchs (1501–1566) entitled *Alle Kranckheyt der Augen.*

Fuchs, a fervent Hippocratist, was Professor first of Philosophy and then of Medicine at Ingolstadt, Physician of the Margrave Georg of Brandenburg, and finally Professor at Tübingen for 31 years. Like the earlier *Büchlin,* his work begins with an anatomic woodcut (Fig. 2), then lists in tabular form various eye conditions, including strabismus, paralysis, amblyopia, and nictalops. The work uses a distinctly Greco-Roman terminology, presenting information on the parts of the eye and their affections, including conjunctivitis, ophthalmia, carcinoma, and "glaucoma." The book concludes with a remedy collection similar to that found in the *Büchlin.* Most significant in the association of Leonhart Fuchs with this book is the fact that a properly trained and

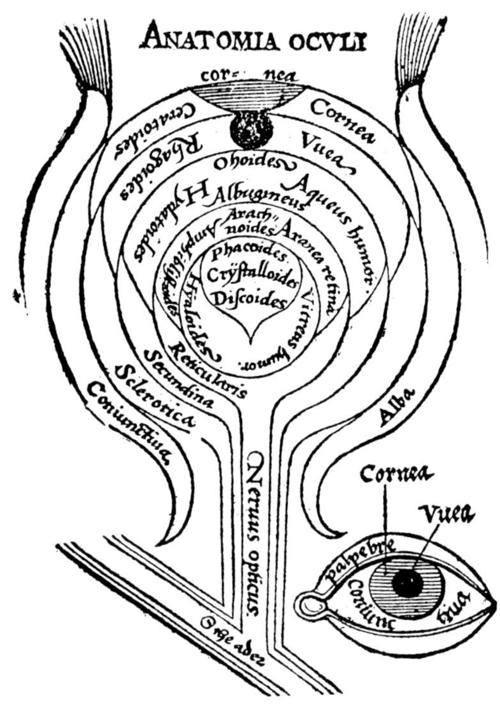

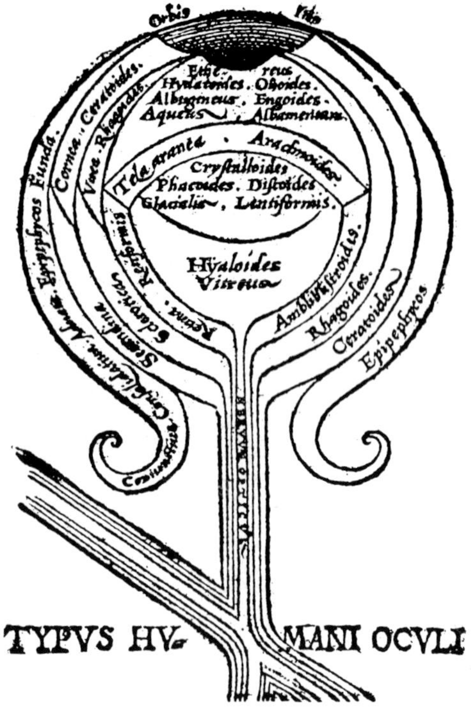

well-recognized physician addressed the subject of ophthalmology.

Julius Hirschberg, the ophthalmic historian, noted that Fuch's *Alle Kranckheyt,* along with the anonymous *Büchlin,* apparently influenced Georg Bartisch in his writing of *Das ist Augendienst.* This latter work, published in 1583, marked the founding of modern ophthalmology. Bartisch (1535–1606) was an itinerant barber-surgeon but nonetheless a thoughtful and skillful surgeon, whose many innovations included the first procedure for extirpation of the globe for ocular cancer. Bartisch proposed standards for the individual who practices eye surgery, noting that rigorous training and concentration of effort were needed to practice this specialty successfully.

By the late 16th century, eye surgery and the treatment of eye disease began to move into the realm of the more formally trained and respected surgeon. This is evidenced by Jacques Guillemeau's *Traité des Maladies de l'Oeil,* published in 1585. Guillemeau (1550–1612) was a pupil of the surgical giant Ambroise Paré, and his book was an epitome of the existing knowledge on the subject.

The transition from couching of cataracts to the modern method of treating cataracts by extraction of the lens, as introduced by Jacques Daviel in 1753, further defined the skill and training necessary for the care of the eyes. The initiation of ophthalmology as a separate specialty within the realm of medicine and surgery was signaled by the publication of George Joseph Beer's two-volume *Lehre von den Augenkrankheiten* in 1813–1817. Beer (1763–1821) founded the first eye hospital in 1786 in Vienna, and his students became famous ophthalmic surgeons and professors throughout Europe.

In England, it was not only the demands of cataract surgery but also the great pandemic of trachoma following the Napoleonic wars that led to the establishment of ophthalmology as a recognized specialty. Benjamin Travers (1783–1858) published the earliest treatise in English on diseases of the eye, *A Synopsis of the Diseases of the Eye,* in 1820. In the United States, acceptance of ophthalmology as a specialty had to await the description of the ophthalmoscope by Helmholtz in 1851, and the additional need of special skills that using the early primitive "Augenspiegel" required.

As the complexity of ophthalmology increased and as subspecialization began to develop in the 19th century, multiauthored books began to appear. This culminated in the appearance in 1874 of the first volume of the Graefe-Saemisch *Handbuch.* The final volume of this great collective work, of which Alfred Carl Graefe (1830–1899) and Edwin Theodor Saemisch (1833–1909) were editors, appeared in 1880. The definitive second edition, which for more than a quarter of a century remained the most comprehensive and authoritative work in the field, appeared in 15 volumes between 1899 and 1918. The great French counterpart to the Graefe-Saemisch *Handbuch* was the *Encyclopédie Française d'Ophtalmologie,* which appeared in 9 volumes (1903–1910), edited by Octave Doin, and filled a similar role for the French-speaking ophthalmologist.

In 1896, the first of 4 volumes of Norris and Oliver's *System of Diseases of the Eye* was published in the United States. The senior editor, Dr. William Fisher Norris (1839–1901), was the first Clinical Professor of Diseases of the Eye at the University of Pennsylvania. Charles A. Oliver (1853–1911) was his student. Norris considered the *System* to be his monumental work. For each section he chose an outstanding authority in the field, having in the end more than 60 American, British, Dutch, French, and German ophthalmologists as contributors. Almost 6 years of combined labor on the part of the editors was needed for completion of the work. In 1913, Casey A. Wood (1856–1942) introduced the first of his 18 volumes of the *American Encyclopedia and Dictionary of Ophthalmology.* The final volume appeared in 1921. Drawn largely from the Graef-Saemisch *Handbuch* and the *Encyclopédie Française d'Ophtalmologie,* Wood's *Encyclopedia* provided information on the whole of ophthalmology through a strictly alphabetic sequence of subject headings.

The book from which the present work draws inspiration is Duke-Elder's *Textbook of Ophthalmology* (7 volumes; 1932) and particularly the second edition of this work entitled *System of Ophthalmology* (15 volumes, published between 1958 and 1976). The *System of Ophthalmology* was written by Sir Stewart Duke-Elder (1898–1978) in conjunction with his colleagues at the Institute of Ophthalmology in London. In 1976, when the last of his 15 volumes appeared, Duke-Elder wrote in the Preface:

> The writing of these two series, the *Textbook* and the *System,* has occupied all my available time for half a century. I cannot deny that its completion brings me relief on the recovery of my freedom, but at the same time it has left some sadness for I have enjoyed writing it. As

> Edward Gibbon said on having written the last line of *The Decline and Fall of the Roman Empire:* "A sober melancholy has spread over my mind by the idea that I have taken everlasting leave of an old and agreeable companion."

Duke-Elder adds a final line that I hope will be more apropos to the present editors and contributors. "At the same time the prayer of Sir Francis Drake on the eve of the attack of the Spanish Armada is apposite: 'Give us to know that it is not the beginning but the continuing of the same until it is entirely finished which yieldeth the true glory.'" The void that developed as the Duke-Elder series became outdated has been partially filled by many fine books, notably Thomas Duane's excellent 5-volume *Clinical Ophthalmology.*

Inspiration to undertake a major work such as this is derived not only from the past books but from teachers and role models as well. For me, this includes Francis Heed Adler, Harold G. Scheie, William C. Frayer, David G. Cogan, Ludwig von Sallmann, Alan S. Rabson, Lorenz E. Zimmerman, Frederick C. Blodi, Claes H. Dohlman, and Matthew D. Davis.

Whereas the inspiration for the present text was derived from Duke-Elder's *Textbook* and *System* and from teachers and role models, learning how to write and organize a book came for me from Adler's *Textbook of Ophthalmology,* published by W. B. Saunders. This popular textbook for medical students and general practitioners was first produced by Dr. Sanford Gifford (1892–1945) in 1938. Francis Heed Adler (1895–1987), after writing the 6th edition, published in 1962, invited Harold G. Scheie (1909–1989); his successor as Chairman of Ophthalmology at the University of Pennsylvania, and myself to take over authorship. We completely rewrote this book and noted in the Preface to the 8th edition, published in 1969: "This book aims to provide the medical student and the practicing physician with a concise and profusely illustrated current text, organized in a convenient and useable manner, on the eye and its disorders. It is hoped that the beginning, or even practicing, ophthalmologist may find it of value."

In 1969 it was apparent that even for the intended audience, contributions by individuals expert in the subspecialties of ophthalmology were required. The book was published in Spanish and Chinese editions and was popular enough to warrant an updated 9th edition, which appeared in 1977. One of the high points of this work was interacting with John Dusseau, the Editor-in-Chief for the W. B. Saunders Company. As a 10th edition was contemplated, I became increasingly convinced that what was needed in current ophthalmology was a new, comprehensive, well-illustrated set of texts intended for the practicing ophthalmologist and written by outstanding authorities in the field. I envisioned a work that in one series of volumes would provide all of the basic clinical and scientific information required by practicing ophthalmologists in their everyday work. For more detailed or specialized information, this work should direct the practitioner to the pertinent journal articles or more specialized publications. As time progressed, a plan for this work took shape and received support from the W. B. Saunders Company.

Memories of the formative stages of the **Principles and Practice of Ophthalmology** remain vivid: Proposing the project to Fred Jakobiec in the cafeteria of the Massachusetts Eye and Ear Infirmary in early 1989. Having dinner with Lew Reines, President and Chief Executive Officer, and Richard Zorab, Senior Medical Editor, at the Four Seasons Hotel in May 1989, where we agreed upon the scope of the work. My excitement as I walked across the Public Garden and down Charles Street back to the Infirmary, contemplating the work we were to undertake. Finalizing the outline for the book in Henry Allen's well-stocked "faculty lounge" in a dormitory at Colby College during the Lancaster Course. Meeting with members of the Harvard Faculty in the somber setting of the rare-book room to recruit the Section Editors. Persuading Nancy Robinson, my able assistant since 1969, to take on the job of Managing Editor. The receipt of our first manuscript from Dr. David Cogan.

We considered making this work a departmental undertaking, utilizing the faculty and alumni of various Harvard programs. However, the broad scope of the series required recruitment of outstanding authors from many institutions. Once the Section Editors were in place, there was never any doubt in my mind that this work would succeed. The Section Editors proved a hard-working and dedicated group, and their choice of authors reflects their good judgment and persuasive abilities. I believe that you will appreciate the scope of knowledge and the erudition.

The editorship of this book provided me not only with an insight into the knowledge and thinking of some of the finest minds in ophthalmology but also with an insight into their lives. What an overwhelmingly busy group of people! Work was completed not through intimidation with deadlines but by virtue of their love of ophthalmology and their desire to share their knowledge and experience. The talent, commitment, persistence, and good humor of the authors are truly what made this book a reality.

It was our intent to present a work that was at once scholarly and pragmatic, that dealt effectively with the complexities and subtleties of modern ophthalmology, but that did not overwhelm the reader. We have worked toward a series of volumes that contained the relevant basic science information to sustain and complement the clinical facts. We wanted a well-illustrated set that went beyond the illustrations in any textbook or system previously published, in terms of quantity and quality and usefulness of the pictures.

In specific terms, in editing the book we tried to identify and eliminate errors in accuracy. We worked to provide as uniform a literary style as is possible in light of the numerous contributors. We attempted to make as consistent as possible the level of detail presented in the many sections and chapters. Related to this, we sought to maintain the length according to our agreed-upon plan. We tried, as far as possible, to eliminate repetition and at the same time to prevent gaps in information. We worked to direct the location of information into a logical and convenient arrangement. We attempted to separate the basic science chapters to the major extent into the separate **Basic Sciences** volume, but at the same time to integrate basic science information with clinical detail in other sections as needed. These tasks were made challenging by the size of the work, the number of authors, and the limited options for change as material was received close to publishing deadlines. We believe that these efforts have succeeded in providing ophthalmologists and visual scientists with a useful resource in their practices. We shall know in succeeding years the level of this success and hope to have the opportunity to improve all these aspects as the book is updated and published in future editions. Bacon wrote: "Reading maketh a full man, conference a ready man, and writing an exact man." He should have added: *Editing maketh a humble man.*

I am personally grateful to a number of individuals for making this book a reality. Nancy Robinson leads the list. Her intelligent, gracious, and unceasing effort as Managing Editor was essential to its successful completion. Mr. Lewis Reines, President of the W. B. Saunders Company, has a profound knowledge of publishing and books that makes him a worthy successor to John Dusseau. Richard Zorab, the Senior Medical Editor, and Hazel N. Hacker, the Developmental Editor, are thoroughly professional and supportive individuals with whom it was a pleasure to work. Many of the black-and-white illustrations were drawn by Laurel Cook Lhowe and Marcia Williams; Kit Johnson provided many of the anterior segment photographs. Archival materials were retrieved with the aid of Richard Wolfe, Curator of Rare Books at the Francis A. Countway Library of Medicine, and Chris Nims and Kathleen Kennedy of the Howe Library at the Massachusetts Eye and Ear Infirmary.

The most exciting aspect of writing and editing a work of this type is that it puts one in touch with the present-day ophthalmologists and visual scientists as well as physicians training to be ophthalmologists in the future. We hope that this book will establish its own tradition of excellence and usefulness and that it will win it a place in the lives of ophthalmologists today and in the future.

"EXPLICIT," scribes wrote at the end of every book. EXPLICIT means *it has been unfolded.* Olmert notes in *The Smithsonian Book of Books,* "the unrolling or unfolding of knowledge is a powerful act because it shifts responsibility from writer to reader. . . . Great books endure because they help us interpret our lives. It's a personal quest, this grappling with the world and ourselves, and we need all the help we can get." We hope that this work will provide such help to the professional lives of ophthalmologists and visual scientists.

DANIEL M. ALBERT, M.D.
MADISON, WISCONSIN

To my beloved family, both living and elsewhere;
To my cherished teachers and trainees, both past and present;
To my incomparable patients, both cured and uncured;
And to my supportive colleagues and friends, all insufficiently celebrated in my preface.

F.A.J.

Preface

Because of the pellucid beauty of the organ and tissues it studies, ophthalmology affords many pleasures and allurements. Although it might be more of a confessional than a verifiable statement, I have always believed that many individuals are also attracted to ophthalmology with the inchoate fantasy (later found to be erroneous) that it is an encapsulated and somewhat secessionist medical specialty one can totally master; this may indeed be an expression of the ophthalmic temperament's constitutive tropism toward control. Ophthalmology, furthermore, has long been a discipline that has generated exquisite teaching aids; most of the diseases and tissues we contend with are amenable to photographic documentation and elegant analysis by modern imaging and angiographic techniques. The quest for mastery in ophthalmology is marked by the periodic appearance of comprehensive textbooks, an example of which is the present enterprise.

If one person certainly could not do it today, is it possible for multiple authors to create a *Summa Ophthalmologica?* In my professional lifetime the most bruited effort was Duke-Elder's *System of Ophthalmology,* which encompassed 15 volumes, appearing ad seriatim from 1958 to 1976. As a resident-in-training, I remember anticipating the arrival of each new volume, and of devouring it from cover to cover because of the spectacular tour d'horizon that was provided. Early in my career, I was privileged to become involved with the orbit section of Duane's 5-volume *Clinical Ophthalmology* and subsequently with the anatomy, embryology, and teratology section of his 3-volume *Biomedical Foundations of Ophthalmology,* both of which were intended to supersede Duke-Elder. Now, having acquired more experience and maturity, I am aware that it is impossible for an ophthalmic diorama to rival the timelessness of Thomas Aquinas' *Summa Theologica,* Immanuel Kant's *Kritiken*, or Bertrand Russell's *Principia Mathematica,* all of which self-reflexively proceed from deductions based on a priori axioms. Ophthalmology is a contingent, empirical, and nonoracular discipline, and its intellectual artifacts necessarily reflect the imperfections and messiness of human inductive knowledge. At their best, the present and predecessor efforts to produce comprehensive ophthalmic textbooks are temporary codifications, inventories, and snapshots of an ever-unfolding field, much as sequential photograph albums reveal the fructifying growth and evolution of families over generations.

Why, then, was the present project undertaken, and what are its distinctive features? Dan Albert and I began jointly planning this work in early 1989, shortly after I arrived in Boston from New York City to become Chief of Ophthalmology at the Massachusetts Eye and Ear Infirmary and Chairman of the Department of Ophthalmology at the Harvard Medical School. We felt the time was right for a new gesamtwerk for ophthalmology, fraught as it might be with the limitations alluded to previously. We believed that the Harvard environment would be especially conducive to producing an outstanding work of scholarship. Initially the **Principles and Practice of Ophthalmology** textbook carried the subtitle "The Harvard System"; this was reflected in the contract signed with the publisher as well as in the stationery that was used throughout the project in correspondence with the contributors. Whereas it is true that all of the section editors and the vast majority of the 440 contributors are by design either present or past faculty or trainees of the Harvard Medical School, the Massachusetts Eye and Ear Infirmary, or the Schepens Eye Research Institute (now formally affiliated with the Harvard Department of Ophthalmology), it quickly became apparent that there was no single "Harvard" or systematic way of thinking about the various topics covered in these volumes. Even within the Harvard Department there are manifold approaches to basic science and clinical problems. Therefore, we were led to abandon the subtitle. Nonetheless, I personally am unabashedly proud that the high quality and erudition of the chapters derive from the intellectual formation that many contributors received from their association with the greater Harvard ophthalmic environment; well represented within this cadre are recent residents and fellows.

Of the 6 volumes, the longest **(Basic Sciences)** deals with the basic sciences of ophthalmology in ten sections. It is in this realm that one will expect the most rapid changes in subject matter in the immediate years ahead; on the other hand, this may be the most fecund and valuable of all the volumes, because there has not been a recent effort to synthesize the burgeoning of knowledge that has attended the revolutions in morphologic investigations, pharmacology, cell biology, immunology, and, lately, molecular genetics. Not every topic in the visual basic sciences could be covered: For example, an extensive and conventional repetition of the facts of embryology and anatomy has not been essayed, since there already exist serviceable references for these comparatively static subjects. The focus instead was on investigations that had been particularly rewarding and luminous over the past 10 years. My advice to readers is to approach each chapter in this volume as if it were an article in the *Scientific American* and to derive both knowledge and pleasure from these lapidary syntheses.

The 5 clinical volumes have been organized along the lines of standard anatomic and tissue-topographic demarcations. Additionally, there are systematic approaches to some established and newly emerging nodal points of knowledge: neuroophthalmology; the eye and systemic disease; pediatric ophthalmology; ocular oncology; ophthalmic pathology; trauma; diagnostic imaging; optical principles and applications; and psychological, social, and legal aspects of ophthalmology. Efforts were made to reduce unnecessary duplication from section to section in the coverage of various subjects; however, when it was felt that it would be profitable to have the same disease or topic covered from several perspectives, this was permitted. We are aware that, despite the length of our present undertaking, the end result is one of comprehensiveness but not exhaustiveness. It should be remembered that there already exist many published and revised multivolume treatises on subjects covered herein. What we have aimed for is to provide the generalist with a digestible up-to-date overview of ophthalmology and also to provide the superspecialist with readily accessible introductions to topics outside of his or her intensive areas of expertise.

Another distinctive feature of the present volumes is the prodigious number of illustrations, totaling well over 6000 if one includes tables, diagrams, and graphs. About half of these are in color, which enhances the aesthetic and teaching value of the entire project. The bibliographies are often daunting and will serve as pathfinders into the larger universe of their subjects. I would particularly like to thank Ms. Kit Johnson of the Infirmary for providing many of the color illustrations for diseases of the eyelids, conjunctiva, and anterior segment of the eye. For voluptuaries of ophthalmology, these and the fundus illustrations should provide a sumptuous feast.

It staggers the mind to contemplate the quotidian and oppressive amount of effort expended on this project—the incalculable atomistic acts of assemblage, the gently hectoring telephone calls, the background acquisition and scope of the basic science and clinical knowledge, the multiple textual revisions, the amassing of bibliographies and illustrations, and so on—and indeed the formidable cost of producing each of the individual chapters, much of which was borne by the authors themselves. Even as we are hopeful that these volumes will make a major positive impression on American and international ophthalmology, modesty in the face of our challenging task rather than arrogance has inspired the lofty goals that sustained the creation of the **Principles and Practice of Ophthalmology.** Still, I have no doubt that many of the chapters contained in these volumes are the most incandescent, scholarly, and useful summary presentations of their subjects that have been crafted up to now. In a many-authored textbook there will be some unevenness, the result of the idiosyncrasies of the contributors as well as the state of development of their subject matter. My own criterion for the success of this enterprise is a simple one: that 50 percent or more of the chapters will have achieved the status of being the best overviews and introductions for their subjects. Regarding topics that should have been covered but were somehow missed or that were surveyed inadequately, the chief editors, the section editors, the authors, and the publisher will look forward to hearing from readers and reviewers about any constructive criticisms on how to improve the textbook in its next edition. We are also exploring various mechanisms for issuing supplemental chapters to rectify some of these perceived and real deficiencies before the next edition.

Based on my familiarity with ophthalmic texts, I think the present work is the largest ophthalmic publication ever to appear *all at once as a complete set.* The W. B. Saunders Company is consequently to be congratulated for having maintained the highest standards of production in terms of copy editing, printing, paper quality, indexing, and reproduction of color and black-and-white illustrations. Mr. Richard Zorab, Senior Medical Editor, was a tireless and relatively humane flogger of myself and the other contributors to meet realistic deadlines; Mrs. Hazel N. Hacker was our highly expert Developmental Editor, and Mrs. Linda R. Garber kept the movement of manuscripts and galleys on schedule with minimal breakage. Ms. Nancy Robinson was a compassionate, patient, and effective intradepartmental Managing Editor. I particularly applaud the ability of the publisher to keep the price of the 6 volumes, with all their color illustrations, at a respectable level so that they are within the reach of trainees, basic scientists, and clinicians in an era of highly competitive National Institutes of Health funding and when ophthalmic reimbursements are being ratcheted down.

It is my compressed personal philosophy that we live to feel, think, and act and that the highest emanations of these faculties are enthusiasm, creativity, and love. This textbook is a manifestation of all six of these capacities, served up in superabundance. May the response of the ophthalmic community be commensurate with the spiritual and intellectual largesse lavished by the contributors on these volumes. Finally, although I somewhat iconoclastically do not fully subscribe to the notion of role models (because I believe that each person should construct his or her unique identity and excellence by cultivating one's intrinsic gifts while at the same time selectively interiorizing the finest qualities of many exemplars), I would like to thank my many professional friends and colleagues who have played salutary roles in the parturition of my own career, and who have taught me and/or supported me to this point in my professional life so that I could participate in this magnificent and bracing academic adventure: Dean S. James Adelstein, Dr. Henry Allen, Dr. Myles Behrens, Mr. Alexander Bernhard, Dr. Frederick Blodi, Dr. Sheldon Buckler, Dr. Alston Callahan, Dr. Charles J. Campbell, Dr. H. Dwight Cavanaugh, Mr. Melville Chapin, Dr.

David Cogan, Dr. D. Jackson Coleman, Dr. Brian Curtin, Dr. Donald D'Amico, Dr. Arthur Gerard DeVoe, Dr. Jack Dodick, Dr. Claes Dohlman, Dr. Anthony Donn, Dr. Thomas Duane, Dr. Howard Eggers, Dr. Robert Ellsworth, Dr. Andrew Ferry, Dr. Ben Fine, Dr. Ramon L. Font, Dr. Max Forbes, Dr. Ephraim Friedman, Mr. J. Frank Gerrity, Dr. Gabriel Godman, Dr. Evangelos Gragoudas, Dr. W. Richard Green, Dr. Winston Harrison, the late Dr. Paul Henkind, Dr. George M. Howard, Dr. Takeo Iwamoto, Dr. Ira Snow Jones, Mrs. Diane Kaneb, Dr. Donald West King, Dr. Daniel M. Knowles, Dr. Raphael Lattes, Dr. Simmons Lessell, Dr. Harvey Lincoff, Mr. Martin Lipton, Dr. Richard Lisman, Mr. Richard MacKinnon, Dr. Ian McLean, Dr. Julian Manski, Dr. Norman Medow, Mr. August Meyer, Dr. George (Bud) Merriam, Jr., Dr. Karl Perzin, Dr. Kathryn Stein Pokorny, Dr. Elio Raviola, the late Dr. Algernon B. Reese, Mr. William Renchard, Dr. Rene Rodriguez-Sains, Dr. Evan Sacks, Dr. Charles Schepens, Dr. James Schutz, the late Dr. Sigmund Schutz, Dr. Jesse Sigelman, Mr. F. Curtis Smith, Dr. William Spencer, Ms. Cathleen Douglas Stone, Dr. R. David Sudarsky, Dr. Myron Tannenbaum, Dr. Elise Torczynski, Dean Daniel Tosteson, Dr. Arnold Turtz, Dr. Robert Uretz, the late Dr. Sigmund Wilens, Dr. Marianne Wolff, Dr. Myron Yanoff, and Dr. Lorenz E. Zimmerman.

I hope that this textbook will touch the lives of those who read it as much as these individuals have influenced my own.

Ad Astra Per Aspera!

FREDERICK A. JAKOBIEC, M.D., D.SC.(MED.)
BOSTON, MASSACHUSETTS

Contents

VOLUME 1

VOLUME 2

SECTION IV

Retina and Vitreous, 683

Edited by EVANGELOS S. GRAGOUDAS and DONALD J. D'AMICO

VOLUME 3

SECTION VII

Glaucoma, 1289

Edited by R. RAND ALLINGHAM, A. ROBERT BELLOWS, and CLAUDIA U. RICHTER

VOLUME 4

SECTION X

Ophthalmic Pathology, 2099

Edited by DANIEL M. ALBERT, THADDEUS P. DRYJA, and FREDERICK A. JAKOBIEC

SECTION XI

Neuroophthalmology, 2387

Edited by JOSEPH F. RIZZO III and SIMMONS LESSELL

VOLUME 5

SECTION XIII

The Eye and Systemic Disease, 2847

Edited by MARIANA D. MEAD and LLOYD M. AIELLO

SECTION XIV

Ocular Oncology, 3195

Edited by DANIEL M. ALBERT and ROBERT A. PETERSEN

SECTION XV

Trauma, 3357

Edited by BRADFORD J. SHINGLETON and JOHN W. SHORE

SECTION XVI

Diagnostic Imaging, 3503

Edited by ALFRED L. WEBER and RICHARD L. DALLOW

SECTION XVII

Clinical Application of Optical Principles, 3601

Edited by PERRY ROSENTHAL

SECTION XVIII

Psychologic, Social, and Legal Aspects, 3697

Edited by FRANCES E. NASON and A. VAN C. LANCKTON

SECTION X

Ophthalmic Pathology

Edited by
DANIEL M. ALBERT, THADDEUS P. DRYJA,
and FREDERICK A. JAKOBIEC

Chapter 180

Principles of Pathology

DANIEL M. ALBERT

DEFINITION

The word *pathology* is derived from two Greek words: the word for suffering (pathos) and the word for reason or study (logos). Pathology in the modern sense is defined as the branch of medicine that encompasses the essential nature of disease, especially of the structural and functional changes in tissues that cause or are caused by disease. Whereas historically the stress in pathology was on morphologic changes associated with disease, in modern pathology the distinction between structure and function no longer exists. The study of disease goes beyond the anatomic alterations caused by the disease and the disturbances in physiologic function; it includes biochemical disorders, genetic abnormalities, and immunologic dysfunctions. The understanding of a disease encompasses the following factors: etiology, pathogenesis, morphology of the lesion, effects of the lesion on function, secondary changes, symptoms and signs, course and prognosis, complications, treatment, and the dangers of treatment.[1]

HISTORICAL HIGHLIGHTS OF OPHTHALMIC PATHOLOGY

Pathology had its beginning as a systematized science with the publication of the text *De Sedibus et Causis Morborum (On the Seats and Causes of Disease)* by Morgagni in 1761.[2] Morgagni (1682 to 1771) was a professor of anatomy at Padua, and his book consisted of a number of letters written to a young friend that contain early accounts of changes in a variety of organs that he noted at autopsy. An early and important work in English on pathology was that by Baillie (1761 to 1823) entitled *Morbid Anatomy of Some of the Most Important Parts of the Human Body*.[3] This work, however, contained nothing on the eye. This was remedied by Wardrop (1782 to 1869) who, in 1808, published the first volume of his *Essays on the Morbid Anatomy of the Human Eye*, which was the first textbook on ophthalmic pathology.[4]

Major contributions to ophthalmic pathology in the years subsequent to Wardrop's text continued to come primarily from ophthalmologists. Undoubtedly, it built on the concepts and contributions of such outstanding pathologists as Virchow (1821 to 1902), whose *Cellular Pathology* in 1858 stated the concept of cellular pathology clearly and completely.[5] Among the giants of ophthalmic pathology are Fuchs (1851 to 1930), Greeff (1862 to 1938), Morax (1866 to 1935), Parsons (1868 to 1957), Verhoeff (1874 to 1968), and Friedenwald (1897 to 1955).[6] Although the list is too numerous to mention completely in this chapter, three senior living ophthalmic pathologists continue to play major roles: Ashton in England and Cogan and Zimmerman in the United States.

CELLULAR INJURY AND CELLULAR RESPONSE

Definition and Causes

As Virchow first pointed out in his *Cellular Pathology* in 1858, virtually all forms of injury to the tissues of the eye and adnexa and other structures begin with molecular or structural alterations in the component cells.[5] These cells normally have a well-defined range of structure and function, which are determined by genetic constraints, metabolic flexibility, and the influence of neighboring cells. Within these limits, the cell is said to be in a homeostatic *steady state*. A number of external or internal endogenous stresses or stimuli may occur that alter the steady state. When a cell is exposed to such an injury, it usually reacts in ways that will reestablish its equilibrium. To achieve this, the cell may alter its structure, its function, or both.

Cellular reactions to injury usually involve a number of adaptations in which a new, but altered, steady state is reached, permitting the cell to survive. The cellular response is usually reversible. For example, a photoreceptor cell in a detached retina undergoing resultant degeneration returns to its previous state if the retina is reattached. Occasionally, the response to injury is irreversible. This may be the case in an acquired ptosis, in which muscle cells enlarge and achieve a new equilibrium. This adoptive response is termed *hypertrophy*. Conversely, the ciliary muscle in a presbyopic individual with an inflexible lens capsule may undergo an adaptive response in which there is a decrease in the size and function of cells termed *atrophy*.

Cotran, Kumar, and Robbins define *cell injury* as a sequence of events that occurs if the limits of adaptive capability are exceeded or when no adaptive response is possible.[7] They state: "*Adaptation, reversible injury,* and *cell death,* then, should be considered states along a continuum of progressive encroachment on the cell's normal function and structure."

Whether an injury induces adaptation, a reversible response, or cell death is determined by the nature and severity of the injury and the intrinsic genetic, metabolic, and other variable properties of the cell itself.

Types of Cellular Injury

Most causes of reversible cell injury and cell death can be grouped into several broad categories. These categories include hypoxia, physical agents, chemical agents and drugs, infectious agents, immunologic reactions, genetic derangements, and nutritional imbalances and are described further in Table 180–1.

Morphology of Injured Cells

A summary of the principal components of the cell and the range of changes seen following injury are summarized in Table 180–2. The earliest manifestation of most forms of injury to cells is *cellular swelling,* which is caused by an impairment of cell volume regulation by the plasma membrane.[8] This is recognized microscopically by enlargement, pallor, and increased turgor of the cells. Continued accumulation of water results in the appearance of clear vacuoles within the cytoplasm. This pattern of reversible injury is sometimes called *hydropic change* or *vacuolar degeneration.* Less commonly in ophthalmic pathology, *fatty change* and *hyaline degeneration* may be indicators of reversible cell injury. Fatty change refers to the intracellular accumulation of neutral fat within cells and represents an increase in intracellular lipids. Hyaline, which means glassy or transparent, is used to denote elements in tissues that appear by light microscopy to be smudged, usually eosinophilic, with a loss of fine detail. Hyaline change may occur within cells or between cells.

Cellular Adaptation

ATROPHY

Atrophy refers to a decrease in the size of a cell or a group of cells due to a loss of cell substance. Atrophy is also applied to an organ or tissue. In simple atrophy, the part becomes smaller because its component cells become smaller. In numerical atrophy, the part shrinks because its component cells become less numerous. The following are major causes of atrophy:[7] (1) decreased work load; (2) loss of innervation; (3) diminished blood supply; (4) inadequate nutrition; (5) loss of endocrine stimulation; and (6) aging. Atrophy usually implies diminished function, but atrophic cells are not dead.

Table 180–1. MAJOR CAUSES OF REVERSIBLE CELL INJURY AND CELL DEATH

1. *Hypoxia:*	May occur on the basis of ischemia, inadequate oxygenation of blood, or loss of oxygen-carrying capacity
2. *Physical agents:*	Includes mechanical trauma, burns, freezing, radiation, and electric shock
3. *Chemical agents and drugs:*	Includes poisons, pollutants, industrial toxins, alcohol, narcotics, and therapeutic drugs
4. *Infectious agents:*	Primarily viruses, rickettsiae, bacteria, fungi, and parasites
5. *Immunologic reactions:*	Ranges from anaphylactic reaction to foreign protein and autoimmune diseases
6. *Genetic derangements:*	May result in a lack or abnormality of an enzyme vital to cell metabolism
7. *Nutritional imbalances:*	Range from protein-caloric deficiencies to nutritional excess

Data from Cotran RS, Kumar V, and Robbins SL: Robbins Pathologic Basis of Disease, 4th ed. Philadelphia, WB Saunders, 1989.

HYPERTROPHY AND HYPERPLASIA

Hypertrophy is an increase in the size of cells resulting in an increase in the size of the related part of the body. It occurs in tissues whose cells rarely divide, with muscle being the classic example. *Hyperplasia* is an enlargement in a tissue or organ caused by an increase in the number of constituent cells, with or without an alteration in their size. In hypertrophy and hyperplasia, although there is an increase in size of the organ, tissue, or cell involved, the cells are basically normal.

METAPLASIA

Metaplasia is a reversible change in both cell proliferation and differentiation, in which one adult cell type (epithelial or mesenchymal) is substituted for another. In ocular tissues, this occurs usually as a late stage of ocular injury and most commonly involves pigment epithelium or lens epithelium.

DYSPLASIA

Although not an adaptive process, *dysplasia* is closely related to hyperplasia and is sometimes referred to as "atypical hyperplasia." It is defined by Howes[9] as a "disturbance in cell growth involving both a cell proliferation and an abnormal or disorderly differentiation." It is used to describe two separate processes. One is abnormal developmental organization of a tissue or organ, as is seen in retinal dysplasia. Its more common usage in pathology, however, is to describe epithelial or less commonly mesenchymal cells that have undergone proliferation and atypical cytologic alterations involving cell size, shape, and organization. In this sense, it is applied to the entity of epithelial dysplasia seen in stratified squamous epithelium.

CALCIFICATION

Calcification is the deposition of calcium salts and is a common process that occurs in a variety of pathologic conditions.[10] It is divided into two forms: (1) dystrophic calcification in which calcium is deposited in abnormal tissue, and (2) metastatic calcification in which calcium salts are seen in previously normal tissues as a result of some derangement in calcium metabolism.

IRREVERSIBLE CELL DAMAGE AND CELL DEATH

When a cell cannot adapt to injury, it may survive for a time but then will die. Such cells exhibit a sequence

Table 180–2. CELLULAR REACTION TO INJURY

Organelle	Definition and Function	Change
Nucleus	The usually central spheroid body within a cell surrounded by a nuclear membrane and containing the chromatin, nucleolus, and nucleoplasm	Clumping and condensation of chromatin along nuclear membrane and nucleoli is common. In severe injury the nucleus shrinks and its chromatin is compressed *(pyknosis)*. The pyknotic nucleus may break into fragments *(karyorrhexis)*. Less often the nucleus swells and becomes rarified *(karyolysis)*. The nuclear shape may become irregular with folds and invaginations, and nuclear membrane is dilated.
Nucleolus	Rounded body present in the nucleus of most cells; the site of synthesis of ribosomal RNA	With many types of injuries, electron-dense spherules appear; the normal constituent network of strands collapses and is segregated into fibrillar, granular, amorphous, and electron-dense zones.
Cell sap	The protoplasm of the cell exclusive of that of the nucleus; the site of many chemical activities of the cell	May become swollen with increased uptake of water or shrunken with water loss. Often contains free or disrupted ribosomes. The quality of glycogen varies widely. Droplets of fat are common.
Cell membrane	The membrane surrounding the cell, formed by two dense layers separated by a middle lucent layer, composed of structural lipids and proteins	Shows folds and projections; pinocytic activity is increased; microvilli are usually shrunken or lost but may be swollen or disrupted. Tight junctions, desmosomes, and gap junctions
Cytoskeleton	A reinforcement in the cytoplasm including microfilaments, intermediate filaments, and microtubules that are assembled and disassembled as the activity of the cell changes	The number and distribution of filaments may be abnormal; tangles of filaments may occur or there may be failure to assemble filaments or microtubules.
Mitochondria	Elongated, spherical organelles that serve as the main source of cell energy by converting adenosine diphosphate (ADP) to adenosine triphosphate (ATP)	Often are few and widely separated but may increase in number. Size and shape may be abnormal, and the folded inner membrane (cristae) may be distorted.
Endoplasmic reticulum	Membrane-bound tubules and cisterns that may have ribosomes on the outer surface (rough) or lack ribosomes (smooth). The ribosome is a site of protein synthesis.	Smooth or rough membranes may proliferate or may be reduced in quantity; the pattern is often distorted. Dilatation is common. Ribosomes may lose their orderly arrangement and may become detached or malformed.
Golgi apparatus	A system of membrane-bound, flattened vesicles that form a temporary "way station" for secretory materials passing from the rough endoplasmic reticulum	May increase in size and become more numerous or may shrink and disappear. The golgi are often dilated and may be filled with retained materials.
Pinocytotic vesicles	Fluid-filled vesicles formed by invaginations of the cell membrane	Increased in many types of injured cells
Phagosomes	Vesicles formed from the cell membrane in the process of phagocytosis	May be much increased; cells normally showing no phagocytic activity may ingest cellular debris or even entire cells
Autophagosomes	A membrane budding from the endoplasmic reticulum containing elements of the cell's own cytoplasm, often with one or more organelles	Autophagocytosis often augmented
Lysosomes	A heterogeneous group of "dense bodies," some of which contain acid hyaluronidase or "lytic" enzymes. "Secondary" lysosomes are digestive vacuoles containing material taken in from outside the cell.	Many injurious agents damage lysosomes, releasing their contents that damage cells and tissues.
Secretory granules	Particles that contribute to the cell's secretion	May be abnormal in size, shape, and number
Microbodies	Membrane-bound particles originating in the endoplasmic reticulum containing enzymes and other substances	Common in some types of injured cells

Adapted and expanded from Ritchie AC: Boyd's Textbook of Pathology, 9th ed. Philadelphia, Lea & Febiger, 1990.

of changes recognizable by light and electron microscopy referred to as *necrosis*. Necrosis, then, is the sum of the morphologic changes that follow cell death in a vital tissue or organ.[11] The changes of necrosis are induced by enzymatic digestion of the cell and denaturation of proteins. There are five characteristic histologic types of necrosis: coagulation necrosis, liquefaction necrosis, fat necrosis, caseous necrosis, and gangrenous necrosis. Recognition of the type of necrosis is important because it gives insight into the cause of cell injury (Table 180–3).

INFLAMMATION AND REPAIR

Inflammation is defined as the local reaction of vascularized living tissue to injury. The inflammatory reaction at first consists primarily of alterations in the blood vessels, resulting in the accumulation of fluid and blood cells. Inflammation is essentially protective, making possible the closely related process of repair. *Repair* in turn involves the replacement of injured tissue by additional parenchymal cells *(regeneration)*, combined with the elaboration of fibroblastic scar tissue *(scarring)*. However, inflammation may also be destructive and damaging, as is seen for example in the eye in corneal injuries, retinal diseases, and uveitis. With regard to the cause of inflammation, almost anything that causes injury to living tissue can cause inflammation. The inflammatory process is generally divided into *acute inflammation*, which is primarily an exudative response, and *chronic inflammation*, which is both exudative and proliferative.

Acute Inflammation

The "arena" of the inflammatory response is usually thought of as vascularized connective tissue (Fig. 180–1), although in the eye avascular tissues, notably the cornea may be the initial site of inflammation. Participating in the inflammatory response are the various components shown in Figure 180–1. The circulating cells involved are neutrophils, monocytes, eosinophils, lymphocytes, basophils, and platelets. Also involved are cells within the connective tissue: the mast cells, fibroblasts, macrophages, and lymphocytes. Elements of the connective tissue matrix including endothelium, basement membrane, elastic fibers, collagen fibers, and proteoglycans are also important. An understanding of certain fundamental terms describing the movement and composition of fluid in cells (Table 180–4) is needed for appreciating the changes of inflammation.

Acute inflammation usually begins within minutes of injury and generally lasts for a few days or 1 wk before resolving. The principal features of the acute inflammatory response are vasodilatation and increased blood flow, increased microvessel permeability, and exudation of plasma and leukocytes. This leads to an accumulation of leukocytes. The sequence of leukocyte emigration can be divided into three stages: (1) The leukocytes move through the vessels at the site of the injury, and they pass out of the central column and assume positions in contact with the endothelium *(margination)*. (2) The white blood cells then adhere in large numbers to the microvessels *(adhesion)*. (3) At points in the interendothelial junction, motile white blood cells squeeze through and escape to the peripheral tissues *(emigration)*. Initially neutrophils predominate but disintegrate after 24 to 48 hr and are replaced by monocytes. Neutrophils and monocytes then move toward chemical signals that emanate from the area of the injury *(chemotaxis)*.[12] The sequence of leukocytic events is shown schematically in Figure 180–2. This is followed by phagocytosis, intracellular degradation, and extracellular release of leukocyte products.

Table 180–3. TYPES OF NECROSIS

	Histologic Features	Cause
Coagulation necrosis	Cell converted to acidophilic, opaque "tombstone" with loss of nucleus but preservation of cellular shape	Denaturization of structural proteins and enzymatic proteins that block proteolysis of cell; most commonly from sudden, severe ischemia
Liquefaction necrosis	Tissue converted to cystic structure filled with debris and fluid	Actions of hydrolytic enzymes with digestion of dead cells, occurring with autolysis and heterolysis. Characteristic of ischemic process in brain tissue as well as in bacterial lesions
Fat necrosis	Foci of vague outlines of necrotic fat cells, the lipid contents having been lipolysed, with a surrounding inflammatory reaction	Lipases are activated and released and destroy fat cells, causing enzymatic necrosis of fat. Classically seen in acute pancreatic necrosis; occurs occasionally in orbital fat
Caseous necrosis	Typical appearance of cheesy material composed of soft, friable, gray-white debris. Microscopically, there is an amorphous appearance with cell outlines preserved.	A combination of coagulation and liquefactive necrosis. Seen in the center of tuberculous infections and attributed to the capsule of *Mycobacterium tuberculosis*
Gangrenous necrosis	A term usually used in clinical practice rather than to describe a distinctive pattern of cell death. Histologic picture is a combination of coagulative necrosis and liquefaction necrosis	Ischemic cell death and coagulative necrosis with superimposed liquefactive action of bacteria and leukocytes. Classically applied to a limb that has lost blood supply and has secondary bacterial infection

Data from Cotran RS, Kumar V, Robbins SL: Robbins Pathologic Basis of Disease. Philadelphia, WB Saunders, 1989.

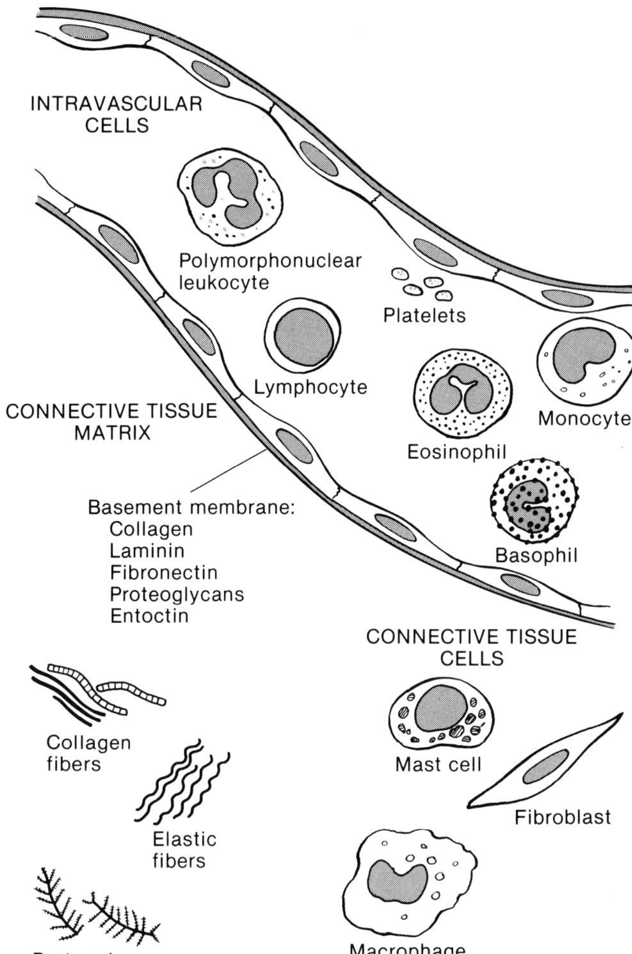

Figure 180–1. Components of the inflammatory response. The circulating cells involved are neutrophils, monocytes, eosinophils, lymphocytes, basophils, and platelets. Cells within the connective tissue that participate are the mast cell, fibroblast, macrophage, and lymphocyte. Involved elements of the connective tissue matrix are endothelium, basement membrane, elastic fibers, collagen fibers, and proteoglycans.

PHAGOCYTOSIS

The process of phagocytosis is illustrated in Figure 180–3. The functions of phagocytosis are to kill infectious organisms and remove debris of necrotic tissue. *Phagocytosis* involves recognition and attachment of the bacteria or extraneous matter to the phagocyte surface; *engulfment* or ingestion of the particles into phagosomes; and *degradation* of particles or killing of microorganisms within the phagolysosomes. A further important occurrence is the release of leukocyte products both within the phagolysosomes and also into the extracellular space. The most important of these leukocyte products are lysosomal enzymes; oxygen-derived active metabolites; and products of arachidonic acid metabolism, including prostaglandins and leukotrienes. These products, which are summarized in Table 180–5, serve as important chemical mediators of inflammation.[12]

Table 180–4. TERMS OF IMPORTANCE IN ACUTE INFLAMMATION

Exudation:	Leakage of fluid, proteins, and blood cells from the vascular system into the interstitial tissue
Exudate:	Inflammatory extravascular fluid with high protein concentration resulting from a disturbance in normal permeability of small blood vessels
Transudate:	Ultrafiltrate of blood plasma resulting from hydrostatic imbalance with lower specific growth
Edema:	Excess fluid (exudate or transudate) in interstitial tissue
Pus:	A *purulent exudate* containing a high concentration of leukocytes and lysosomal enzymes

Data from Cotran RS, Kumar V, Robbins SL: Robbins Pathologic Basis of Disease. Philadelphia, WB Saunders, 1989.

ROLE OF LYMPHATICS IN ACUTE INFLAMMATION

The lymphatics may also drain bacterial or chemical agents away from the primary site of inflammation. This may result in lymph node enlargement. In ophthalmic pathology this is an important process with regard to the lid, but the globe and orbit lack lymphatics.

MONONUCLEAR PHAGOCYTES

Most macrophages that occur in inflammatory reactions come from the blood monocytes.[14] Other mononuclear phagocytes occur in the bone marrow as stem cells, monoblasts, and promonocytes, and in tissues. This latter group of macrophages in tissue includes histiocytes in connective tissue, fixed and free macro-

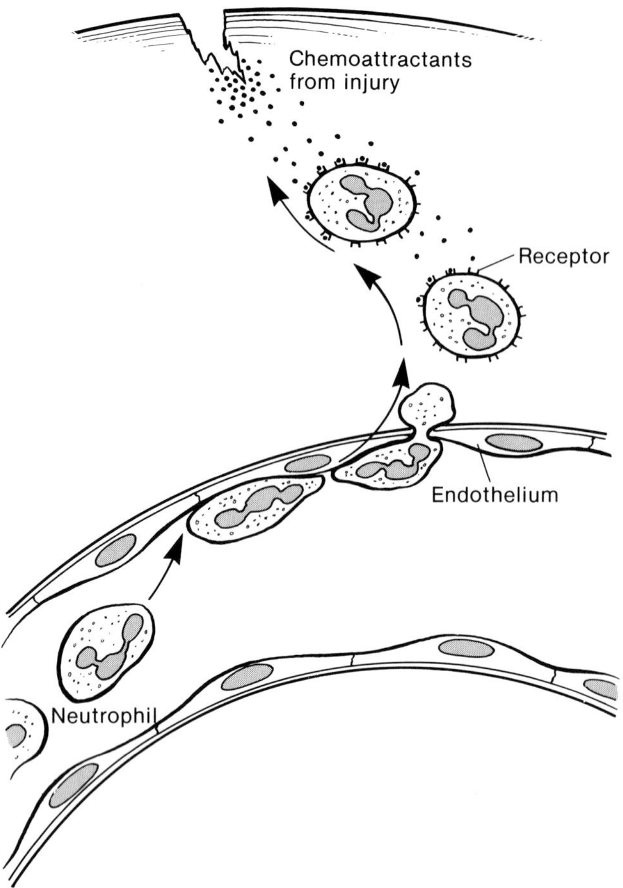

Figure 180–2. Leukocytic events in inflammation. Schematic depiction of the sequence of events of leukocytic emigration illustrating margination, adhesion, and chemotaxis.

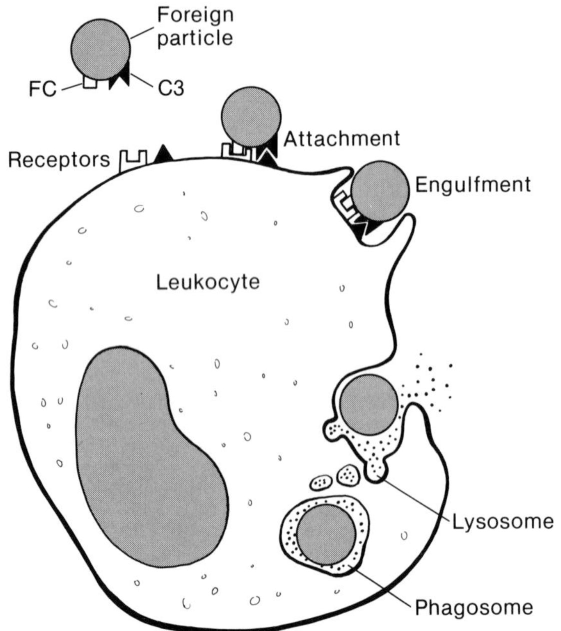

Figure 180–3. Phagocytosis. Schematic depiction illustrating recognition, attachment, engulfment, and degradation. Note the presence of the lysosome and phagosome.

Table 180–5. CHEMICAL MEDIATORS OF INFLAMMATION

Mediators	Action
Plasma Proteases	
Kinin system	Causes contraction of smooth muscle and dilatation of blood vessels through the release of bradykinin
Complement system	Increased vascular permeability, chemotaxis to promote phagocytosis, and lysis of target organisms
Clotting system	Converts fibrogen to fibrin; fibrinopeptides formed cause increased vascular permeability and chemotactic activity for leukocytes
Preformed Cell Mediators	
Histamine	Stored in mast cells and basophils and causes vasodilatation and increased permeability
Serotonin	Present in mast cells and platelets and causes vasodilatation and increased permeability
Lysosomal components	With release from leukocytes, these cause vascular leakage chemotaxis and immobilization of neutrophils
Newly Synthesized Cell Mediators	
Prostaglandins	"Autocoids" (local short-range hormones) cause vasodilatation, hemostasis, and thrombosis
Leukotrienes	Powerful chemotactic agents that cause aggregation of leukocytes, vasoconstriction, and increased vascular permeability
Platelet stimulating factor	Derived from basophils; causes aggregation of platelets and vasoconstriction. Also causes the release of histamine and serotonin and synthesis of prostaglandins and leukotrienes
Cytokines	Most important cytokine mediators of inflammation are interleukin 1 and tumor necrosis factor. Major action is on endothelium, stimulating increased adhesion of white blood cells; also induces vasodilatation (through PGI2) and makes endothelial surface thrombogenic

phages in the lymph nodes and the spleen, microglial cells in nervous tissue, Langerhans' cells in the skin, and dendritic cells in the lymphoid tissue. The last two cell types are not phagocytic. In addition to serving as "scavenger cells," phagocytes are involved in all phases of healing, or progression of the inflammatory response, as well as having a basic role in specific immunity.[14, 15]

OUTCOMES OF ACUTE INFLAMMATION

Acute inflammation may subside either with complete resolution or the area of inflammation may heal by scarring. Alternatively, in infections with pyogenic organisms, the outcome may be abscess formation, or the inflammation may persist and the character of the inflammation may change and progress to chronic inflammation.

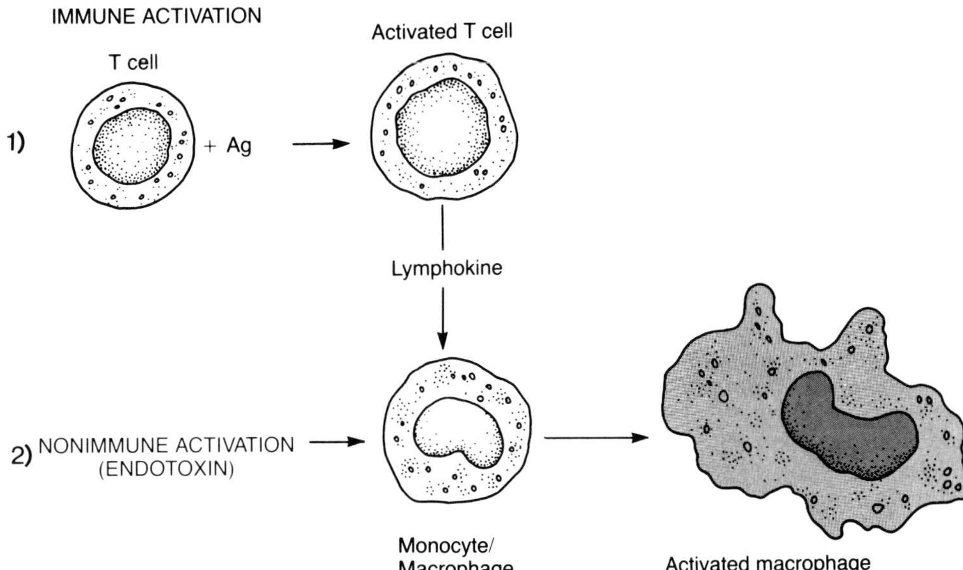

Figure 180–4. Macrophages. (From Cotran RS, Kumar V, Robbins SL: Robbins Pathologic Basis of Disease. Philadelphia, WB Saunders, 1989.)

Chronic Inflammation

Most chronic inflammations begin as acute inflammation that persists or occurs repeatedly. In addition, chronic inflammation may not have an apparent initial neutrophilic response but may commence with lymphocytes and macrophages as often occurs in uveitis. The characteristic histologic appearance of chronic inflammation consists of an infiltration of macrophages, lymphocytes, and plasma cells associated with a proliferation of fibroblasts and often fine vessels. Macrophages are derived from monocytes, which transform within the extravascular tissue into these larger cells[16] as shown in Figure 180–4. Macrophages accumulate in three ways: continuous migration from the circulation *(recruitment);* local mitotic *division;* and by *prolonged survival.* The other types of cells found in chronic inflammation are lymphocytes, plasma cells, eosinophils, and mast cells.

Granulomatous Inflammation

A *granuloma* is a nodule, usually less than 2 mm in diameter, composed of macrophages. These may be modified macrophages called *epithelioid cells* or multinucleated giant cells. The lesions are usually surrounded by lymphocytes. The term *granulomatous inflammation* refers to inflammation in which granulomas are present and usually occurs in response to certain infectious agents.

Epithelioid cells are modified macrophages whose abundant pink cytoplasm gives an appearance superficially resembling epithelium. They are derived from blood monocytes. The *giant cells* are of the *Langerhans* (Fig. 180–5) or *foreign body type* (Fig. 180–6) and are formed for the most part by the fusion of epithelioid cells. In the Langerhans' cell, the nuclei are usually arranged around the periphery. Foreign body giant cells may contain foreign material and have scattered nuclei. Lymphocytes, plasma cells, and fibroblasts are seen, and neutrophils are occasionally present as well.

The balance and organization of granulomas give them several distinctive appearances that may help to suggest their etiology. Among the specific types encountered in ophthalmic pathology are the *sarcoidal* or *tuberculois* (Fig. 180–7) as is seen in sarcoid or rheumatoid arthritis; the *zonular* pattern (Fig. 180–8), as is seen in lens-induced uveitis; and the diffuse pattern (Fig. 180–9), as is seen in sympathetic ophthalmia.

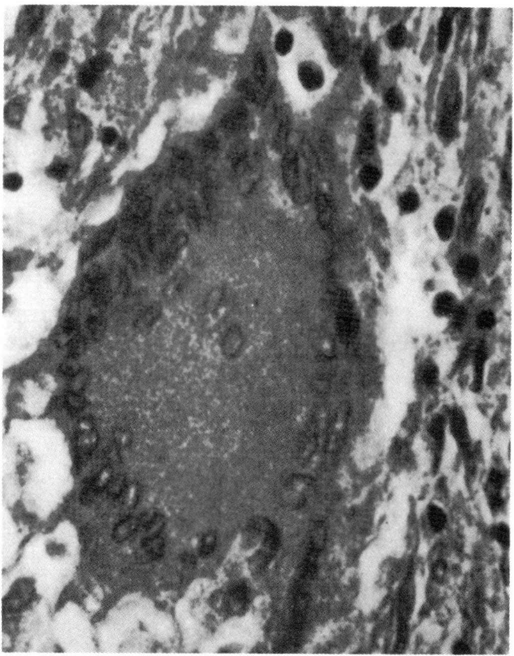

Figure 180–5. Giant cells. (From Cotran RS, Kumar V, Robbins SL: Robbins Pathologic Basis of Disease. Philadelphia, WB Saunders, 1989.)

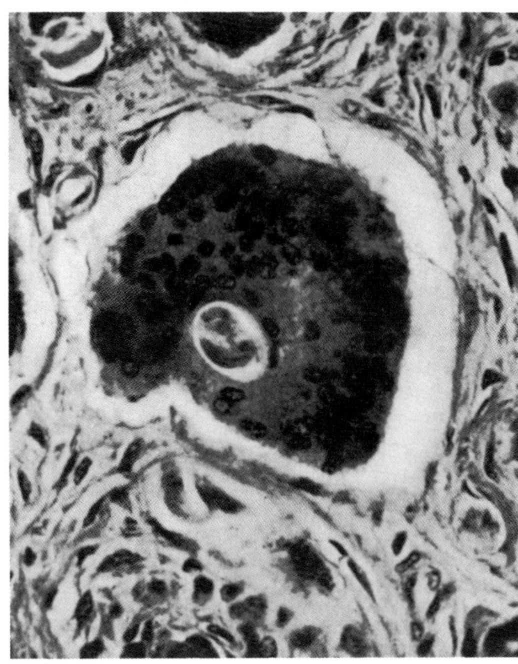

Figure 180–6. Foreign body giant cell. (From Cotran RS, Kumar V, Robbins SL: Robbins Pathologic Basis of Disease. Philadelphia, WB Saunders, 1989.)

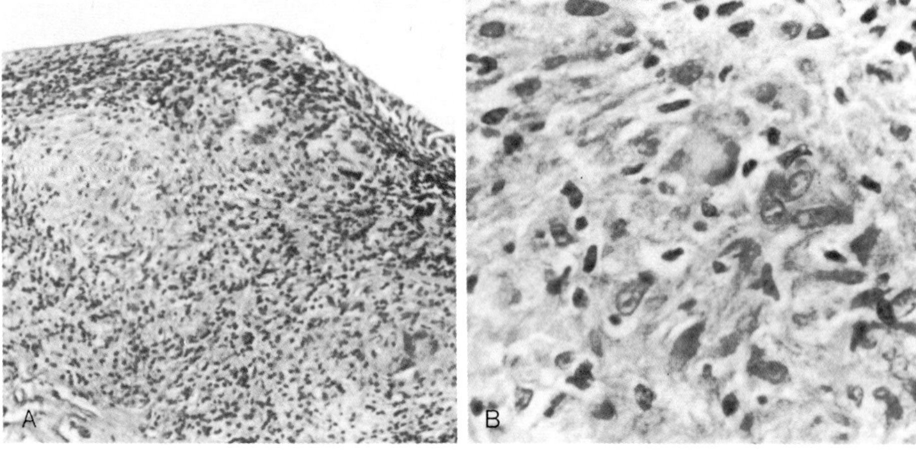

Figure 180–7. *A,* Conjunctival biopsy specimen showing noncaseating granulomas typical of sarcoid. ×180. *B,* Epithelioid cells of sarcoid nodule. ×720. (From Spencer WH: Ophthalmic Pathology: An Atlas and Textbook, Vol 1, 3rd ed. Philadelphia, WB Saunders, 1985, p 38.)

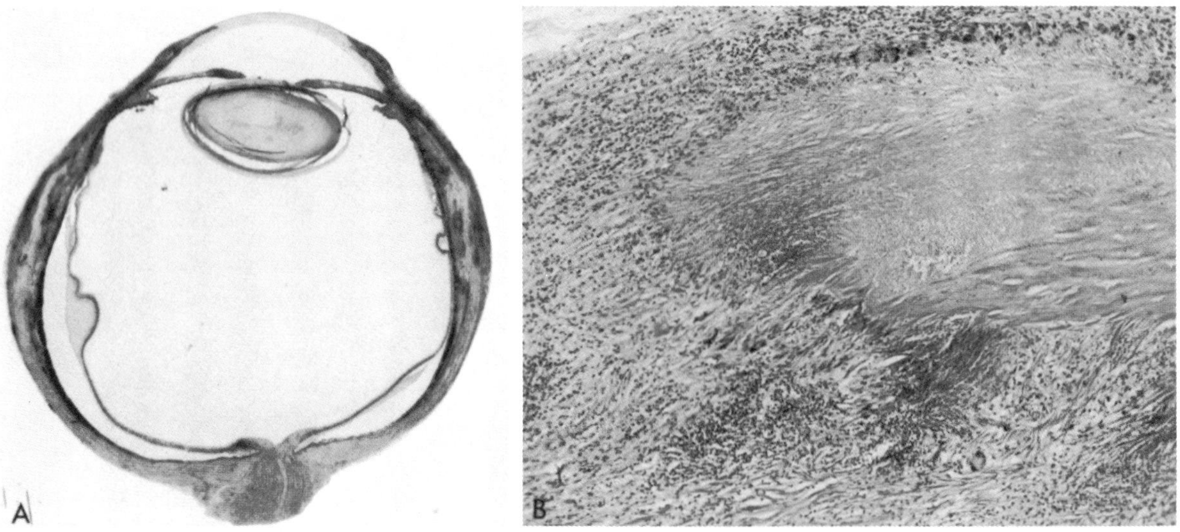

Figure 180–8. Nodular scleritis. *A,* Fusiform thickening of preequatorial sclera, limbus, and peripheral cornea. H&E, ×5. AFIP Acc. 50814. *B,* Nodular scleritis. A discrete sequestrum of scleral collagen lies at the center of a zone of necrotizing granulomatous inflammation. H&E, ×115. AFIP Neg. 57-1163. (From Spencer WH: Ophthalmic Pathology: An Atlas and Textbook, Vol 1, 3rd ed. Philadelphia, WB Saunders, 1985, p 408.)

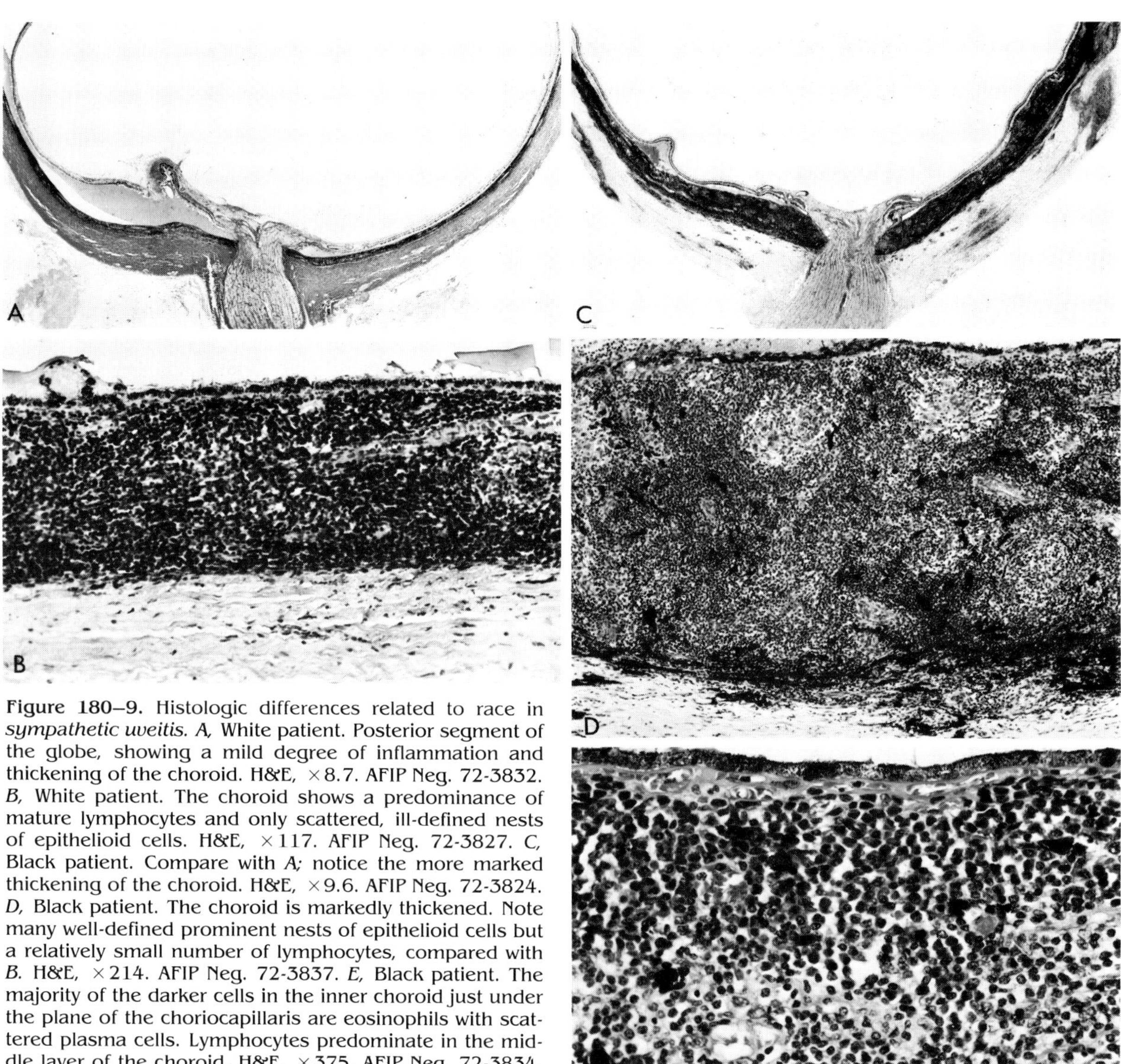

Figure 180–9. Histologic differences related to race in *sympathetic uveitis. A,* White patient. Posterior segment of the globe, showing a mild degree of inflammation and thickening of the choroid. H&E, ×8.7. AFIP Neg. 72-3832. *B,* White patient. The choroid shows a predominance of mature lymphocytes and only scattered, ill-defined nests of epithelioid cells. H&E, ×117. AFIP Neg. 72-3827. *C,* Black patient. Compare with *A;* notice the more marked thickening of the choroid. H&E, ×9.6. AFIP Neg. 72-3824. *D,* Black patient. The choroid is markedly thickened. Note many well-defined prominent nests of epithelioid cells but a relatively small number of lymphocytes, compared with *B.* H&E, ×214. AFIP Neg. 72-3837. *E,* Black patient. The majority of the darker cells in the inner choroid just under the plane of the choriocapillaris are eosinophils with scattered plasma cells. Lymphocytes predominate in the middle layer of the choroid. H&E, ×375. AFIP Neg. 72-3834. (From Marak GE Jr, Font RL, Zimmerman LE: Histologic variations related to race in sympathetic ophthalmia. Am J Ophthalmol 78:935–939, 1974.)

Experimental studies indicate that poorly digestible irritants or T cell–mediated immunity with production of gamma interferon is necessary for granuloma formation.[17]

Wound Healing

Following inflammation, repair may occur by *regeneration* of the injured tissue or by *replacement* usually by connective tissue. Certain cells such as surface epithelium, lymphoid tissue, and hematopoietic tissues consist of "labile cells" that proliferate continuously and are capable of regeneration. "Stable cells" such as the parenchymal cells of glands, fibroblasts, smooth muscle cells, osteoblasts, and chondroblasts have a more limited capacity for regeneration. "Permanent cells" such as central nervous system nerve cells and skeletal muscle cells are incapable of mitotic division in postnatal life. In ocular injuries, while regeneration contributes to some extent, the predominant method of repair is usually replacement by connective tissue, which is a process called *wound healing.*

Wound healing starts early in inflammation with phagocytosis and digestion by macrophages of the remaining necrotic debris in the area of injury. At about the same time, there is a proliferation of capillaries and small blood vessels together with fibroblasts. This new tissue because of its velvety granular appearance is called *granulation tissue* and is characteristic of healing inflammation. The fibroblasts actively synthesize collagen and proteoglycans. Some large fibroblasts develop features of smooth muscle cells and are called myofibroblasts.[18]

In the granulation tissue as healing proceeds, the amount of collagen increases and the blood vessels, fibroblasts, and other cells are resorbed. A variety of types of collagen are involved in the wound healing.[19] Eventually, broad bundles of collagen replace the fine collagen formed early, and together with spindle-shaped fibroblasts, elastic tissue, extracellular matrix, and residual vessels form the final scar.

If the edges of the wound are closely approximated, as is the case in the surgical incision, the healing is referred to surgically as *"primary intention"* or "primary union." If the edges of the wound cannot be brought together and there is significant loss of cells and tissue, granulation tissue grows into the wound from its margin and base and the wound is said to heal by *"secondary intention"* or "secondary union."

The healing of specialized tissue is a complex topic.[1] Surface epithelium can fill in a small defect by spreading out from the edges. In larger defects, mitoses occur within the expanding margins of the epithelium. Endothelium heals in a manner similar to surface epithelium, with the endothelial cells at the edge spreading across the defect and mitosis occurring behind the advancing edge. Bone heals in a manner analogous to fibrous tissue. The clot between the bone edges is converted here by osteoblasts into a mass of immature bone called callus. This is remodeled by osteoclasts and replaced by orderly haversian bone. Striated and smooth muscle, as noted, can proliferate but heal primarily by scarring. Cartilage may regenerate or heal by replacement and connective tissue or by ossification.

The underlying mechanisms involved in healing and repair are extremely complicated and are well summarized by Cotran, Kumar, and Robbins.[7] A simplified summary of the effects of major polypeptide growth factors is presented in Table 180–6.

Two abnormal variants of healing should be recognized. A *pyogenic granuloma* (Fig. 180–10) is an overexuberant growth of granulation tissue that extends

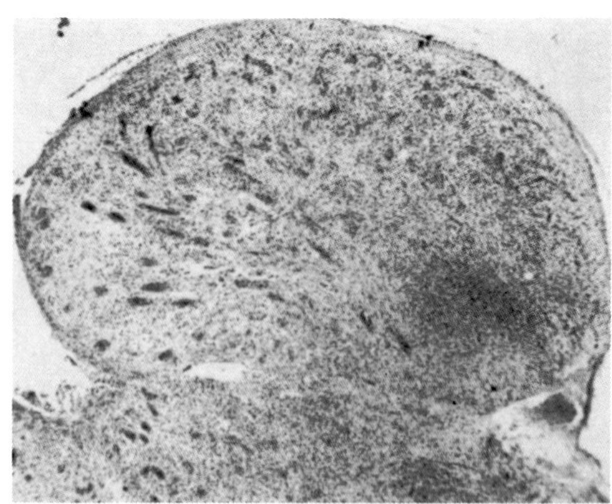

Figure 180–10. Pyogenic granuloma. Smooth-surfaced, elevated mass protrudes through a defect in the palpebral conjunctival epithelium. The mass consists of loosely coherent acute and chronic inflammatory cells interspersed with vascular channels (inflammatory granulation tissue). H&E, ×50. AFIP Acc. 28901. (From Spencer WH: Ophthalmic Pathology: An Atlas and Textbook, Vol 1, 3rd ed. Philadelphia, WB Saunders, 1985, p 153.)

through a break in the epithelium. Despite the name "pyogenic," this lesion does not involve pus. With age, the pyogenic granuloma either thickens into a lesion resembling a capillary hemangioma or is reduced to a fibrous nodule. Keloids (Fig. 180–11) are scars in skin in which there is an excessive production of collagenous tissue. These disfiguring lesions extend above the surface of the skin and are similar in histologic appearance but more severe than hypertrophic scars. They are common particularly in women and in black patients.

Table 180–6. MAJOR POLYPEPTIDE FACTOR

	Action
Epidermal growth factor (EGF)	Causes cell division in a variety of epithelial cells and fibroblasts
Platelet-derived growth factor (PDGF)	Stimulates proliferation and migration of fibroblasts, smooth muscle cells, and monocytes
Fibroblastic growth factors (FGF)	Induces angiogenesis
Transforming growth factor α (TGF α)	Stimulates cell division in epithelial cells and fibroblasts
Transforming growth factor β (TGF β)	Stimulates fibrogenesis; deactivates macrophages; inhibits growth of most cell types in culture. *Inhibits* most cell types in vivo
Interleukin 1 (IL-1)	Participates in fibroplasia and connective tissue remodeling
Tumor necrosis factor (TNF)	Stimulates angiogenesis and plays role in fibroplasia and connective tissue remodeling

Data from Cotran RS, Kumar V, and Robbins SL: Robbins Pathologic Basis of Disease. Philadelphia, WB Saunders, 1989.

IMMUNOLOGIC DISORDERS

Immunology is considered in detail in Section V (see Chaps. 59 to 65 of *Principles and Practice of Ophthalmology: Basic Sciences*). The reader is referred to that section for a detailed discussion of the subject. A brief summary of some basic principles of immunology and key terms are given here to provide an understanding of the relevant topics included in ophthalmic pathology.

Identification of Cells of the Immune System by the Pathologist

With advances in immunohistochemical technique, the pathologist is increasingly called upon to make certain distinctions and determinations regarding specimens in the orbit and adnexa in patients with diseases of immunity. Specifically, these include: (1) distinguishing monoclonal from polyclonal lymphoid proliferations; (2) defining the stages of B-cell maturation; (3) identifying markers of differentiation in non-Hodgkin's lymphoma; and (4) distinguishing lymphoid malignancies from poorly differentiated epithelial or mesenchymal tumors.[20]

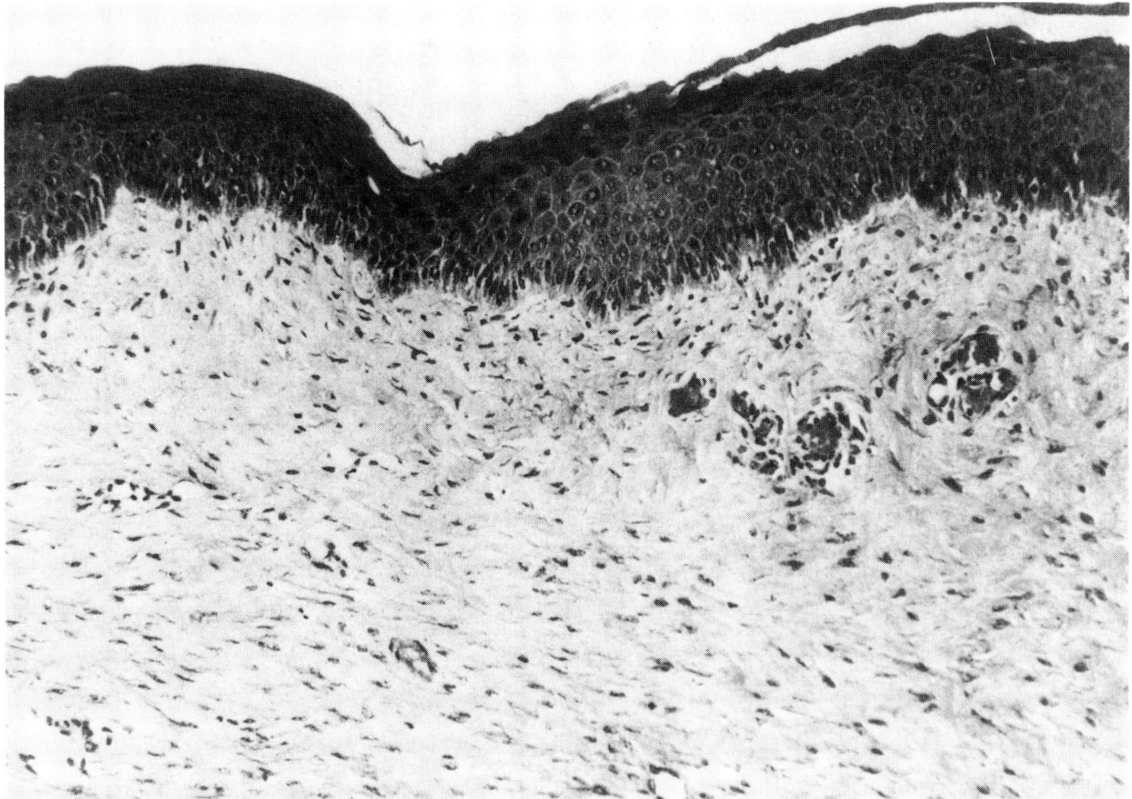

Figure 180–11. Keloids. (From Weiner MJ, Albert DM: Congenital corneal keloid. Doc Ophthalmol 67:192, 1989.)

Major Cellular Participants of the Immune System

LYMPHOCYTES

T and B lymphocytes constitute the principal cellular components of adaptive immune responses. The source of T lymphocytes is from stem cells in the bone marrow. Following migration to the thymus, these cells become differentiated into mature T cells. These T cells are then found in the blood and also in peripheral lymphoid tissues. T cells participate both in cellular immune reactions (e.g., cytotoxic [killer] T cells) and in regulatory functions (e.g., helper-inducer cells).

B lymphocytes are found in the bone marrow, blood, and lymphoid tissues. These cells express surface immunoglobulin. Outside of the blood B cells become plasma cells, and the immunoglobulin secreted by them is identical to the specificity of the surface immunoglobulin of the precursor lymphocyte. By immunophenotyping, it is possible to distinguish between neoplastic (clonal) and reactive (polyclonal) proliferations of B cells.

MACROPHAGES

As noted in the previous discussion on inflammation, macrophages for the most part have their origin in the blood monocyte and are part of the mononuclear phagocyte system (MPS). Their function in the immune response includes: (1) processing and presenting antigen to immunocompetent T cells[14]; (2) producing interleukin 1 (IL-1) and other soluble factors[21]; (3) acting as effector cells in the delayed hypersensitivity reaction and other forms of cell-mediated immunity; and (4) secreting proteolytic enzymes and toxic metabolites.

LYMPHOKINE-ACTIVATED KILLER CELLS (LAK CELLS)

These cells histologically resemble large lymphocytes with granules in their cytoplasm. LAK cells share cell-surface antigens with T cells and macrophages but are nevertheless considered to be distinct from these latter cells. LAK cells lyse tumor cells and virus-infected cells without previous sensitization. The mechanism of action appears to be both direct interaction with the target cells as well as antibody-dependent cellular cytotoxicity.

DENDRITIC AND LANGERHANS' CELLS

Dendritic cells are present in lymphoid tissue, and Langerhans cells are related cells within the epidermis. These cells take up and process antigenic signals and present this information to lymphoid cells. As noted, macrophages also have antigen-presenting capability, but dendritic histocytic cells and Langerhans' cells are not phagocytic.

Identification of Lymphocytes in Immune-Mediated Diseases and Lymphomas

Numerous monoclonal antibodies are available for detection of immune cell antigens. A summary of some of these are presented in Table 180–7. It is important to note that lymphoid antigens are best preserved for histologic examination by avoiding primary fixation in buffered formalin, B_5, or other common fixatives. Snap-freezing fresh tissue followed by lyophilization or acetone fixation are good methods of preserving the antigenicity of lymphoid markers.[22, 23]

However, even in formalin-fixed, paraffin-embedded tissue, many antibodies are available for diagnostic purposes.[20] Leukocyte common antibodies identify leukocyte common antigen (LCA), which is a glycoprotein found on the cell membrane of a variety of cells derived from bone marrow, including granulocytes, thymocytes, macrophages, and immature erythroid cells. This is useful in identifying undifferentiated tumor cells that are related to the hematopoietic lineage rather than being of epithelial or sarcomatous derivation. Additional antibodies delineate B cells from T cells. Other antibodies are capable of recognizing stages of lymphoid differentiation as indicated in Table 180–7. These antibodies are used most effectively as a panel.

Table 180–7. SOME IMMUNE CELL ANTIGENS DETECTED BY MONOCLONAL ANTIBODIES

Antigen Designation*	Comments
Primary T Cell–Associated	
CD2	Receptor for sheep erythrocytes; present on all T cells (peripheral and intrathymic) and NK cells
CD3	Present on all peripheral T cells; asociated with the T-cell antigen receptor
CD4	Present on 60% of peripheral T cells and some monocytes; a marker for T helper-inducer cells
CD5	Present on all T lymphocytes, peripheral and intrathymic
CD7	Present on all T lymphocytes
CD8	Present on 30% of peripheral T cells; marker for cytotoxic cells
CD25	Receptor for interleukin 2; present on activated T cells, B cells, and monocytes
Primary B Cell–Associated	
CD19	Present on B cells, from pre-B stage to mature B cells; absent from plasma cells
CD20	Appears on pre-B cells after CD19; otherwise similar to CD19 in distribution
CD10	Common acute lymphoblastic leukemia antigen (CALLA); present on pre-B cells
Primary Monocyte- or Macrophage-Associated	
CD13	Present on blood monocytes and granulocytes
CD33	Present on myeloid stem cells and mature monocytes
CD11b	Present on monocytes, granulocytes, and some NK cells; receptor for complement (C3b)
Primarily NK Cell–Associated	
CD16	Present on all NK cells and granulocytes; low-affinity receptor for Fc portion of IgG
Present on All Leukocytes	
CD45	
CD11a	

From Cotran RS, Kumar V, and Robbins SL: Robbins Pathologic Basis of Disease. Philadelphia, WB Saunders, 1989.

*The antigens are designated by the prefix CD (cluster designation) (based on Third International Workshop on Human Leukocyte Differentiation Antigens as reported by Shaw S: Immunol Today 8:1, 1987).

Immune Mechanisms Resulting in Tissue Injury

Most immunologic reactions are part of the body's defense against disease and have beneficial effects. The pathologist, however, is often confronted with examples of harmful immunologic reactions in which tissue is damaged by reactions to exogenous antigens, as well as by reactions to antigens that are intrinsic to the body. Immunologic tissue injuries (hypersensitivity reactions) are distinguished according to the immune mechanism involved, and four major types are summarized in Table 180–8.

DISEASES OF BLOOD VESSELS

Arteriosclerosis

The term *arteriosclerosis,* which literally means hardening of the arteries, at present is generally used to describe a group of vascular diseases that are characterized by thickening and loss of elasticity of the wall of the artery. The three forms of this disease are *atherosclerosis; Mönckeberg's medial calcific sclerosis;* and *arteriolosclerosis.*

ATHEROSCLEROSIS

Atherosclerosis is a common lesion that affects large- and medium-sized arteries. Three precursor lesions of atherosclerosis are described: fatty streaks, granulomatous elevations, and mural thrombi.[1] Some of these lesions may progress to full-blown atheroma, the characteristic lesion of this disease. The atheroma is a focal plaque which thickens the intima.

On microscopic examination there is a fatty amorphous core that often has cholesterol crystals with surrounding fibrosis and intimal cell proliferation. A mild inflammatory reaction with lymphocytes and macrophages is commonly seen. Atheromata frequently become calcified, and thrombi develop on the surface. The enlarging atheroma erodes the media and compromises the lumen of the artery.

Table 180–8. IMMUNOLOGICALLY MEDIATED INJURY

Type	Mechanism	Examples of Resulting Disorders
Anaphylactic or reaginic type	Fixation of IgE to mast cells and basophils with release of vasoactive amines	Hay fever, types of asthma, urticaria, and eczema
Cytotoxic type	IgG, IgM bound to surface of cell with lysis, phagocytosis, or cellular cytotoxicity	Hemolytic anemia, transfusion reaction, glomerulonephritis
Immune complex disease	Antigen-antibody complexes with activation of complement attracts neutrophils and macrophages causing the release of lysosomal enzymes	Systemic lupus erythematosus, Arthus reaction, serum sickness
Cell-mediated injury (delayed hypersensitivity)	Activated T lymphocytes secrete lymphokines with the proliferation of sensitized T cells	Contact sensitivity, tuberculosis

Ischemia is the most common and severe of the complications, but emboli and aneurysms may also occur. The pathogenesis is thought to involve repeated local injury to the intima with a complex interaction between local factors, plasma lipids, and thrombosis. A number of risk factors exist, including age, sex (more severe in men than women younger than 50 yr of age), hyperlipidemia, obesity, diabetes mellitus, hypertension, smoking, and lack of exercise.

MÖNCKEBERG'S MEDIAL CALCIFIC SCLEROSIS

This disorder begins in middle age and affects small- to medium-sized arteries of the muscular type. The basic defect is degeneration and calcification of the media of these arteries. The vessels that are most severely affected include the femoral, tibial, radial, and ulnar arteries; it is commonly seen in vessels removed for temporal artery biopsy. Mönckeberg's sclerosis often occurs in individuals with atherosclerosis but the two disorders are distinct anatomically, clinically, and presumably etiologically.[7] Mönckeberg's sclerosis generally causes no symptoms and has little clinical significance.

ARTERIOLOSCLEROSIS

Arteriolosclerosis is the term used to describe at least two entities: *hyaline arteriolosclerosis* and *hyperplastic arteriolosclerosis*. Both occur in arterioles and small muscular arteries, and both are related to hypertension but may involve other causes as well. In hyaline arteriolosclerosis the media of the affected vessel is hyalinized, showing on microscopy a homogeneous eosinophilic appearance. In addition to its association with hypertension, this is also seen as part of the microangiopathy characteristic of diabetes mellitus. It is presumed that the effects of hypertension or diabetes on the endothelium result in leakage and accumulation of hyaline. Damage results from compromise of the arteriolar lumen with impairment of blood supply. Hyperplastic arteriolosclerosis is a characteristic change seen with acute and severe elevations of blood pressure. The histopathologic change is that of intimal hyperplasia, having a concentric laminated "onion skin" appearance and resulting in narrowing of the lumen.

Inflammatory Diseases of Blood Vessels: The Vasculitides

Inflammation of blood vessels is termed *vasculitis* or *angiitis*. Inflammation of arteries is called *arteritis*, and inflammation of the arterioles is called *arteriolitis*. Finally, inflammation of lymphatics is called *lymphangitis*.

Many classifications of vasculitis exist. A useful one is division into those immunologically mediated, infectious, and secondary as given in Table 180–9. Of particular interest to ophthalmologists are temporal arteritis, Wegener's granulomatosis, Takayasu's arteritis, sarcoidal angiitis, and Eales' disease. These diseases together with diabetic microangiopathy and hypertensive retinopathy are discussed in detail elsewhere but are mentioned briefly here.

Temporal Arteritis (Giant Cell Arteritis, Cranial Arteritis)

This is a disease affecting primarily elderly individuals and is characterized by focal granulomatous inflamma-

Table 180–9. CLASSIFICATION OF VASCULITIDES

- Probably immunologically mediated
  - Polyarteritis nodosa
  - Hypersensitivity vasculitis
  - Overlap syndromes
  - Special forms of vasculitis
    - Allergic granulomatosis
    - Allergic vasculitis
    - Eales' disease
    - Erythema elevatum diutinum
    - Henoch-Schönlein purpura
    - Isolated vasculitis of the central nervous system
    - Mucocutaneous lymph node syndrome
    - Purpura pigmentosa chronica
    - Sarcoidal angiitis
    - Serum sickness
    - Wegener's syndrome
- Infectious vasculitis
- Secondary vasculitis
  - Acute inflammation
  - Fibrosis
  - Hypertension

From Ritchie AC: Boyd's Textbook of Pathology, 9th ed. Philadelphia, Lea & Febiger, 1990. Reprinted by permission.

tion of medium- and small-sized arteries, and especially the cranial vessels. Approximately half of patients have symptoms of headache, tenderness over the artery, visual loss, diplopia, jaw pain, or polymyalgia rheumatica syndrome. A positive result on a temporal artery biopsy (Fig. 180–12) is diagnostic, although up to 40 percent of biopsies of the temporal artery may have negative results in patients with the disease.[24] The classic histologic finding is a granulomatous lesion, usually with giant cells, in proximity to the internal elastic membrane.

Wegener's Granulomatosis

This disease consists of acute necrotizing granulomas of the upper and lower respiratory tract, necrotizing glomerulitis, and focal necrotizing vasculitis, which may involve the eye and adnexa.[25]

Takayasu's Arteritis

This disease, also called pulseless disease, was originally reported by the Japanese ophthalmologist Takayasu in 1908.[26] He described the loss of vision and a wreathlike vascular anastomosis around the optic disc. The histopathologic findings are a granulomatous vasculitis of medium and larger arteries. The aortic arch is involved in about one third of cases. The ocular and central nervous system signs occur as a result of narrowing of the major arteries arising from the arch of the aorta, which compromises blood flow to the neck and head as well as to the arms.[27]

Sarcoidal Angiitis

Sarcoidal angiitis is seen primarily in the lungs but can also affect the eyes. Histopathologic changes consist of infiltrates of lymphocytes and macrophages in vessels, as well the presence of sarcoidal granulomata. There may be narrowing and occlusion of involved vessels. In a study of 202 patients, posterior segment disease occurred in 25.3 percent and included chorioretinitis and periphlebitis.[28]

Eales' Disease

This is a poorly understood retinal vasculitis that affects primarily males and results in hemorrhage of the retina and vitreous. Typically, the disease affects the veins in the peripheral fundus in one or more sectors, but there are marked variations in the severity and distribution.[29] The histopathologic findings are primarily phlebitis and periphlebitis with some involvement of the smaller arterioles.[30]

Diabetic Microangiopathy

Diabetic retinopathy is classified into two subgroups: (1) background and nonproliferative retinopathy, and (2) proliferative retinopathy.[31] In background retinopathy, basement membrane thickening occurs that is identical to the thickening seen in diabetic microangiopathy in general. There is insudation of blood-borne constituents through abnormally permeable endothelium. Pericyte degeneration occurs, followed by the development of capillary microaneurysms. Microaneurysms may develop thromboses and become occluded. Microvascular obstructions and nonperfusion of capillaries occur, and arteriolar hyalinization is seen.

Proliferative retinopathy occurs in response to severe ischemia and hypoxia of the retina and is thought to be due to a retinally derived angiogenic factor that induces neovascularization. The new vessels usually extend from the larger veins and are surrounded by areas of capillary closure. They may also arise from the region near the optic disc. The new capillaries are incompletely formed and poorly supported. Initially, they proliferate within the potential space between the inner limiting membrane of the retina and the posterior face of the vitreous but subsequently extend into the vitreous cavity. Bleeding is common as the vessels are stretched by vitreous contraction. The neovascularization is followed by the development of a fibrous component, resulting in a neovascular membrane called retinitis proliferans. The fibrous component adds to the traction on the underlying retina and often causes retinal detachment.

Hypertensive Retinopathy

Hypertensive changes in the retinal arterioles cause diminution in their diameter.[31] In acute severe hypertension, as is seen in toxemia of pregnancy or as occurs at the onset of malignant hypertension, these changes initially appear clinically as focal spasms. The narrowing usually occurs in chronic hypertension in a more diffuse and slowly progressive manner. Sclerotic changes of the retinal arterioles involve a hyaline or "onion skin" thickening of the arteriolar wall with a narrowing of the diameter of the lumen.

PIGMENTED CELLS IN THE SKIN AND EYE AND DISTURBANCES OF PIGMENTATION

Dermal melanocytes are cells within the epidermis that are responsible for the production of melanin, which is a brown pigment. Uveal melanocytes probably represent a counterpart of the dermal melanocyte. Although similarities exist and often the same terms are used, there are important variations between dermal and ocular pigmented lesions. It must also be borne in mind that, unlike the skin, the eye contains a second

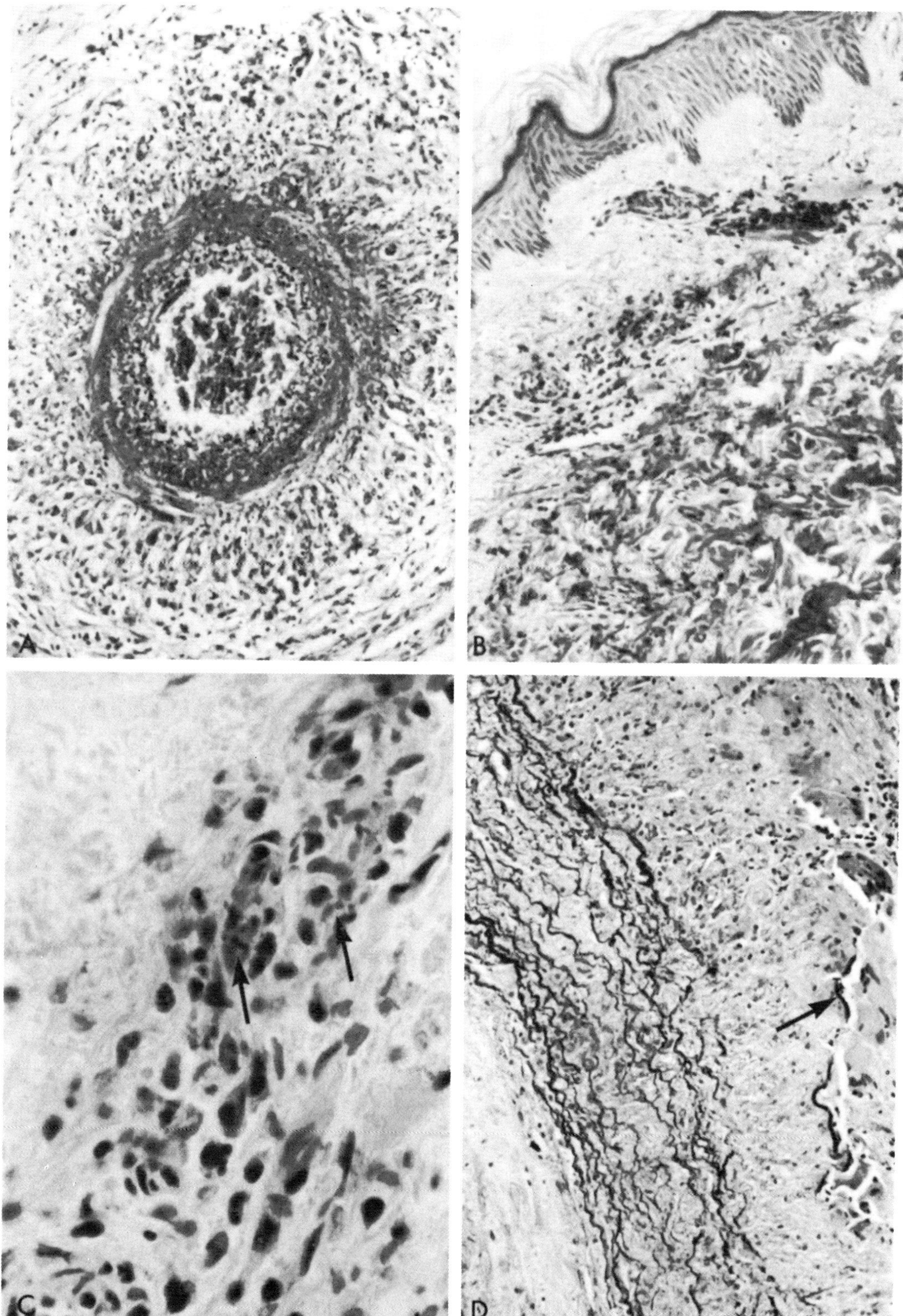

Figure 180–12. *A,* Artery from a case of periarteritis nodosa. The inner vessel wall shows a fibrinoid necrosis, and numerous inflammatory cells are seen both in the vessel wall and the adjacent connective tissue. ×160. *B,* Leukocytoclastic angiitis in skin. The superficial small blood vessels are obscured by inflammatory cells. ×40. *C,* At higher power, these vessels are distorted by an infiltration of neutrophils in their walls *(arrows).* ×400. *D,* Portion of temporal artery. The lumen is toward the bottom left. A subintimal fibrosis and inflammation of the vessel wall are evident. In this elastic stain, the elastic lamina *(arrow)* is fragmented, and a giant cell reaction is seen adjacent to the fragmented elastic membrane, as is found in many cases of temporal arteritis. ×40. (From Spencer WH: Ophthalmic Pathology: An Atlas and Textbook, Vol 1, 3rd ed. Philadelphia, WB Saunders, 1985, p 80.)

population of pigmented cells called the pigment epithelium.

Albinism

Albinism is a hereditary disorder in which the melanocytes are unable to synthesize melanin.[32] Two clinical variants exist: (1) ocular albinism, and (2) oculocutaneous albinism. Ocular albinism is inherited as an X-linked recessive trait, and the inability to synthesize melanin is limited to the eye. In oculocutaneous albinism the hair, skin, and eyes lack pigmentation. Biochemically, albinism may be either of the "tyrosinase-negative" or "tyrosinase-positive" type. A number of ocular disturbances may be present in addition to the lack of pigment, including developmental abnormalities of the macula, astigmatism, and myopia.

Vitiligo

In contrast to albinism, in which melanocytes are present but no melanin is produced, vitiligo is a disease characterized by the loss of melanocytes.[33] The loss may be either partial or complete, and various patterns are seen in the skin. Theories of pathogenesis include autoimmunity, neurohumoral factors, and destruction of melanocytes by toxic metabolites of melanin synthesis. In addition to involvement in the skin, the uveal tract and pigment epithelium of the eye may be involved.

Freckle

A freckle or ephelis is a lesion in which the melanocytes are normal in number but are hypertrophic. In the skin, freckles are due primarily to an increased amount of melanin pigment within the basal keratinocytes. Such lesions are common in light-skinned individuals after exposure to the sun.

Lentigo

Lentigo (plural: lentigenes) is a hyperplasia of melanocytes that in the skin produces a hyperpigmented basal cell layer in the epidermis. Lentigo has a characteristic linear pattern. These lesions may occur on the conjunctiva or other mucous membranes. They are common and benign and occur at all ages, but most often in infancy and childhood.

Nevi

Nevi of the uveal tract may consist of any of a spectrum of cells ranging from dendritic cells closely resembling normal uveal melanocytes through plumper cells with vesicular-appearing nuclei to polygonal cells typical of melanocytoma and balloon cells with accumulated fat. Nevi of the skin, in contrast to lentigenes, consist of round to oval-shaped cells arranged in nests that differ significantly from the dendritic melanocytes from which they arose. A variety of clinical and histologic types of nevi are seen.[34] The clinical and histologic types of cutaneous nevi are summarized in Table 180–10. The most common nevus is the *noncongenital nevocellular nevus* or *common acquired nevus*. These nevi develop during childhood or the teenage years. The lesion initially consists of nests of cells that grow along the dermoepidermal junction *(junctional nevus)*. The nevus evolves in time to consist of both epidermal nests and dermal nests of cells *(compound nevus)*. Older lesions lose their epidermal components and show only dermal nests *(dermal nevus)*. An important feature of benign nevi is their maturation with downward growth. Deeper cells within the dermis tend to be nonpigmented and arranged in cords or may be spindle-shaped and resemble neural tissue.

Malignant Melanomas

Malignant melanomas of the uveal tract consist of a spectrum of cells ranging from thin spindle-shaped cells (spindle A cells) to epithelioid cells and were given their definitive classification by Callender.[35] Uveal melanoma is discussed in detail elsewhere.

The Callender classification does not apply to conjunctival and cutaneous melanomas. Melanoma cells are larger than nevus cells and grow as irregular nests or as individual cells in nodules that extend through all the layers of the epidermis and dermis. Typically, these cells have large nuclei with chromatin clumping at the periphery of the nuclear membrane and distinct eosinophilic nucleoli. In contrast to prognostic indicators in uveal melanomas, the concept of radial and vertical growth is a key factor in judging the malignant potential of cutaneous lesions.[36, 37] During the stage of radial growth the melanoma tends to extend horizontally within the epidermal and superficial dermal layers, and these lesions have a low incidence of metastases. Eventually the melanoma may assume a vertical growth

Table 180–10. CLINICAL AND HISTOLOGIC TYPES OF CUTANEOUS NEVI

Type	Comment
Common acquired nevus	Flat brown lesion, slightly raised centrally
Junctional nevus	Most of the nevus cells along the dermoepidermal junction
Compound nevus	Contains both epidermal and dermal nests
Dermal nevus	Contains only dermal nests
Congenital nevocellular nevus	Usually large with numerous hairs
Blue nevus	Nevus cells extend deep into the dermis giving a blue-gray color
Compound nevus of Spitz	Usually seen in childhood; composed of spindle and epithelioid nevus cells
Halo nevus	Surrounded by a zone of hypopigmentation
Dysplastic nevus ("BK mole")	Shows atypia; may progress to dysplasia and malignancy

component, and the probability of metastasis may be predicted by measuring in millimeters the depth of invasion of this vertical growth phase below the granular cell layer of the overlying epidermis.[38, 39]

SKIN

Composition of the Skin

Skin consists of the surface epidermis and the underlying dermis. There is an irregular border between these two components, with dermal papillae projecting upward into the epidermis and ridges of epidermis separating the papillae *(Rete's ridges).*

Histologic Structure of the Epidermis

The epidermis consists of two types of cells: *dendritic cells* and *keratinocytes.* The dendritic cells include the melanocytes lodged between the basal cells, the *Langerhans' cells,* in the upper epidermis; and certain *"indeterminate cells"* that lack the melanosomes and Langerhans' granules (Fig. 180–13).

The predominant cell type is the *keratinocyte,* which is characterized by intercellular bridges and considerable cytoplasm. In most normal skin the keratinocytes differentiate into four distinguishable layers: (1) the *basal cell layer;* (2) the *squamous cell layer;* (3) the *granular layer;* and (4) the *horny layer.* The basal cell layer, squamous cell layer, and granular cell layer (i.e., the nucleated epidermis) are collectively termed the stratum malpighii.

The *basal cell layer* consists of a single layer of columnar cells that have a basophilic cytoplasm and a dark-staining nuclei. The cells are connected to each other by intercellular bridges or desmosomes and are attached to the underlying tissue by a periodic acid-Schiff (PAS)–positive subepidermal basement zone. In the normal epidermis, mitotic activity occurs primarily in the basal cell layer.

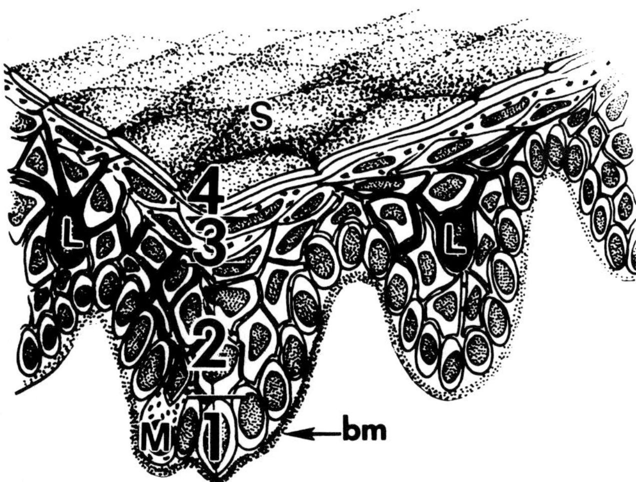

Figure 180–13. Cells composing normal epidermis. Keratinocytes that undergo progressive upward maturation from ovoid cells of the basal layer cell (1) that rest on the basement membrane (bm), to more polyhedral stratum spinosum cells (2), then to flattened stratum granulosum (granular) cells (3), and finally to anucleate cells of the epidermal surface(s), the stratum corneum (4). Dendritic melanocytes (M) and Langerhans cells (L) are interspersed in relatively low numbers within the epidermal layer. (From Cotran RS, Kumar V, Robbins SL: Robbins Pathologic Basis of Disease. Philadelphia, WB Saunders, 1989, p 1278.)

Above the *basal cell layer* is the squamous cell layer that consists of a mosaic of polygonal cells generally 5 to 10 layers thick. The cells are interconnected by intercellular bridges.

The *granular cell layer* is superficial to the squamous cell layer and consists of somewhat flattened cells containing keratohyaline granules that form the interfibrillary substance cementing the keratin fibrils. In this zone the dissolution of the nucleus and other cell organelles begins. The thickness of the granular layer is proportional to the thickness of the horny layer and is usually one to three layers thick in the area of the lids.

The *horny layer* is the product of completely keratinized anucleate cells and stains eosinophilic on routine sections. Mucous membranes such as the conjunctiva normally lack the granular and horny layers.

The major component of the connective tissue of the dermis is collagen, including the fine reticulum fibers. Amorphous ground substance fills the spaces between collagen fibers and bundles. Interepidermal nerve endings are represented by the Merkel cell-neurite complexes. Eccrine glands are tubular glands that excrete sweat and serve primarily in the regulation of heat. Apocrine glands, represented in the lid by the glands of Moll, are primarily scent glands that function by decapitation secretion. Sebaceous glands are holocrine glands that form their secretion by the decomposition of their cells. These occur both in association with hair structures as well as independently. The hair follicle consists of five components: the dermal hair papilla, the hair matrix, the hair, the inner root sheath, and the outer root sheath (Fig. 180–14). The dermal blood vessels consist of a subdermal plexus of small arteries and veins. The interconnected arterioles arising from the arteries extend into the dermis and give rise to capillary loops. The descending portion of the capillaries connect to venules that empty into the subdermal plexus of the veins. Under normal conditions, lymph vessels are extremely difficult to recognize in sections of the skin. Both smooth and striated muscle are intimately associated with the skin surrounding the eye.

Disorders in the Development of the Epidermis

Acanthosis refers to an increase in the thickness of the stratum malpighii. *Dyskeratosis* refers to premature keratinization of individual keratinocytes. Lever[33] describes two types of dyskeratosis—one occurring in certain acantholytic diseases and the other occurring in certain epidermal neoplasias. *Hyperkeratosis* denotes an increased thickness of the horny layer. *Parakeratosis* refers to the retention of nuclei in the horny layer and is associated with a diminished granular layer. Although

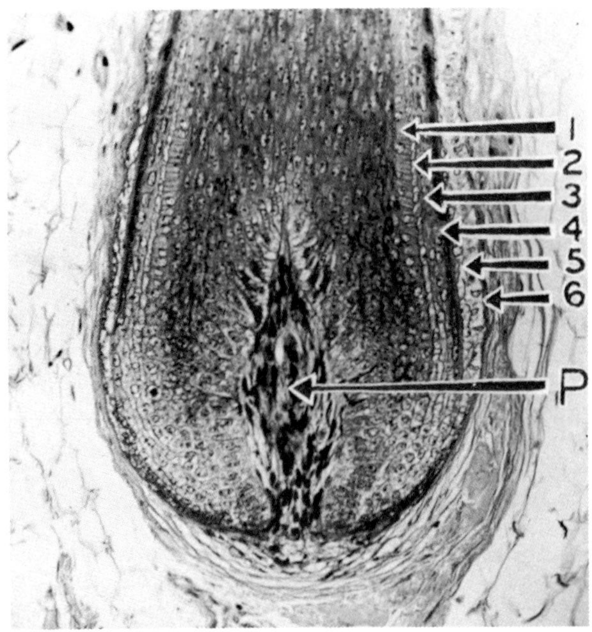

Figure 180–14. Hair follicle. The dermal hair papilla (P), composed of connective tissue, protrudes into the hair bulb. The various linings of the hair can be recognized. They are from the inside to the outside: (1) the hair cuticle; (2) the inner root sheath cuticle; (3) the Huxley layer; (4) the Henle layer (which stains dark because of the presence of trichohyaline granules); (5) the outer root sheath; and (6) the glassy or vitreous layer (×200). (From Lever WF, Schaumberg-Lever G: Histopathology of the Skin, 6th ed. Philadelphia, JB Lippincott, 1983, p 26.)

parakeratosis was previously interpreted as representing excessively rapid cell proliferation, it is now considered primarily to be a defect in cellular differentiation.[33] *Acantholysis* is a loss of coherence between the epithelial cells as a result of degeneration of the intercellular bridges and is seen in pemphigus and certain other disorders.

Infectious Diseases of the Skin

The lids and skin surrounding the eyes may be infected by a variety of viruses, bacteria, fungi, and parasites. These are discussed in detail elsewhere. Among the most serious are herpes simplex, herpex zoster, and fungal infections. The viral exanthems sometimes require the attention of the ophthalmologist. *Verrucae* or warts are caused by papilloma viruses and are characterized histologically by undulant epidermal hyperplasia with a zone of cytoplasmic vacuolization involving the superficial epidermal layers. On electron microscopy the pale zones correlate with the presence of numerous intranuclear viral particles.

Molluscum contagiosum is a 2- to 4-mm umbilicated papule that is caused by a poxvirus. Histologically there is a distinctive cup-shaped epidermal hyperplasia, and the cells above the basal cell layer have intracytoplasmic inclusion bodies *("molluscum bodies")*.

There are other dermatologic infections and infestations that the ophthalmologist and ophthalmic pathologist must recognize. *Impetigo* is a staphylococcal or streptococcal infection that is seen most commonly in children. Of considerable importance is the erythematous plaque seen in *Lyme disease* as a result of the spirochete transmitted by the tick *Ixodes dammini*, a parasite of white-tailed deer and field mice. Pediculosis may confront the ophthalmologist, particularly in the case of the pubic louse, and these parasites or their eggs may require to be identified in the pathology laboratory.

Inflammatory Dermatoses

ACUTE INFLAMMATORY DERMATOSES

Among the thousands of specific inflammatory dermatoses that have been described, several are of particular significance to ophthalmic pathology, including urticaria, contact dermatitis, ectopic dermatitis, drug-related eczematous dermatitis, photoeczematous eruption, primary irritant dermatitis, erythema multiforme, and erythema nodosum. Important features of these are summarized in Table 180–11.

CHRONIC INFLAMMATORY DERMATOSES

Among the diseases included in this category that are of significance to the ophthalmologist are *lupus erythematosus* and *psoriasis.*

LUPUS ERYTHEMATOSUS

Lupus erythematosus occurs in two forms: discoid lupus erythematosus (DLE) and systemic lupus erythematosus (SLE). The disease is discussed in Chapter 235.

DLE lesions are localized to the skin, and patients do not progress to the systemic form. Over one third of the patients with SLE, however, exhibit lesions that are clinically and histologically identical to those of the discoid form.[34] The typical cutaneous lesions consist initially of sharply defined erythematous scaling patches, which in time may appear as atrophic scarring. Histologically, the major changes are:[33]

1. Thinning and atrophy of the epidermal layer with loss of the normal rete ridge pattern
2. Hyperkeratosis with keratotic plugging
3. Hydropic degeneration of the basal cells
4. A patchy lymphoid cell infiltrate
5. Edema and vasodilatation in the epidermis

PAS stain demonstrates a thickening of the epidermal basement membrane, and direct immunofluorescence shows a band of immunoglobulin and complement along the dermoepidermal junction.[40]

PSORIASIS

Psoriasis is a chronic disorder that affects between 1 and 2 percent of individuals in the United States.[34] It is characterized by well-demarcated papules and plaques covered with whitish scales. The lids are commonly involved, although typically the scalp, lumbosacral region, and extensor surfaces of the extremities are most severely affected. The histologic picture consists of marked acanthosis with absence of the stratum granulosum and severe parakeratosis associated with elongation of the rete ridges and elongation and edema of the papillae. Microabscesses are often present.

Table 180–11. IMPORTANT INFLAMMATORY DERMATOSES

Type	Pathogenesis	Clinical Features	Histology
Urticaria	Antigen-related mast cell degranulation or direct effect of chemical exposure	Pruritic wheals	Dermal edema separates collagen bundles; perivenular mononuclear infiltrates
Contact dermatitis	Delayed hypersensitivity resulting from topically applied chemicals	Itching and burning	Edema fluid in the epidermis
Atopic dermatitis	Unknown	Erythematous plaques	Edema fluid in the epidermis
Drug-related eczematous dermatitis	Systemic drug	Eruption related to drug administration	Edema fluid in the epidermis with eosinophils present
Photoeczematous eruption	Ultraviolet light	Eruption on exposed skin	Edema fluid in the epidermis with deeper infiltrate
Primary irritant	Repeated rubbing or other trauma	Eruption at site of trauma	Edema fluid in the epidermis
Erythema multiforme	Cytotoxic reaction pattern associated with infections, drug administration, malignancy, or collagen vascular disease	"Target lesion" is a red macule or papule with a pale center; associated with macules, papules, vesicles, and bullae	Degenerating and necrotic epithelium with infiltrating lymphoid cells and microvascular injury
Erythema nodosum	Panniculitis associated with infection, drug administration, malignancy, chronic inflammatory diseases, but often of unknown cause	Acute panniculitis developing flat, bruise-like lesion	Edema and neutrophilic infiltration later followed by lymphocytic and granulomatous inflammation

BLISTERING (BULLOUS) DISEASES

Pemphigus

Vesicles and blisters are a primary feature of *pemphigus* and *bullous pemphigoid.* Pemphigus is a relatively rare autoimmune bullous disorder for which four clinical and pathologic varieties are described.[41]

Of these, *pemphigus vulgaris* accounts for more than 80 percent of the cases. All forms of pemphigus bullae rupture easily, leaving denuded areas covered with dried serum. The cardinal histopathologic lesion is a loss of coherence between the epidermal cells (acantholysis), with disappearance of intercellular bridges, and detachment of epithelial cells, which assume a rounded shape. This is accompanied by dermal inflammation with infiltration of lymphocytes, histiocytes, and eosinophils. Hashimoto and Lever[42] concluded that dissolution of the intercellular cement substance is the primary event in the formation of bullae. Serum from patients with pemphigus has been demonstrated to contain antibodies to intercellular cement substances of skin and mucous membranes.[43]

Bullous Pemphigoid

This disease occurs in older patients and involves cutaneous lesions and bullae of mucosal surfaces. The disease usually has a more benign course than pemphigus. The principal histopathologic change is detachment of the epidermis from the dermis, resulting in subepidermal, nonacantholytic bullae.[43] Bullae arise both on noninflamed skin and within areas of erythema. Dermal changes, therefore, are minor in noninflammatory bullae and consist of a perivascular infiltrate of lymphocytes and eosinophils.

NEUROPATHOLOGY

Neural Constituents of the Eye

The retina and optic nerve developed embryologically as an ectopic portion of the primitive forebrain and retain their similarity to other components of the central nervous system. The four major components of the retina and optic nerve are: (1) neurons, (2) neuroglia, (3) microglia, and (4) vascular connective tissue. The inner layers of the retina maintain a lamination comparable to that of the gray matter of the cortex. The optic nerve demonstrates a similar compartmentalization by pia and absence of sheaths of Schwann as in the white matter of the brain. The optic nerves differ from tracts in the brain in having a relatively abundant connective tissue septa that allows for pathologic reactions not shared by the intracranial portions of the central nervous system.[44]

Neurons and Their Response to Injury

Neurons are the cells that are specialized to act as communicating units of the nervous system. There is great histologic variation among the many types of neurons. Most have a cell body, a dendrite, and an axon. The cell body contains cytoplasm with clumps of rough-surfaced endoplasmic reticulum, free ribosomes (Nissl's substance), and the nucleus. Also included in the neuronal cytoplasm are microtubules, synaptic vesicles, and neurofilaments.[45] In the course of disease or injury a variety of changes may occur to the neurons. Four major types of reaction are: (1) atrophy and degeneration; (2) intraneuronal body formation; (3) intraneuronal storage; (4) chromatolysis or axonal reaction; and (5) axonal degeneration.[46] These are summarized in Table 180–12. An example of infarctions and ischemic necrosis of the retina is shown in Figure 180–15.

Neuroglial Cells and Their Response to Injury

The neuroglial cells consist of *ependymal cells, astrocytes, oligodendrocytes,* and according to some authors, the *microglia.*[46] The ependymal cells line the cerebral ventricles and the central canal of the spinal cord. Astrocytes are present in the retina, disc, and optic nerve of the eye. Astrocytes have a complex function that appears to include physical and biochemical support of the neurons, insulation of the receptive surface of the neurons, and participation with capillary endothelial cells in the maintenance of the blood-retina and the blood-brain barriers.[47] With ordinary staining methods, astrocytes are recognized as round or oval cells with pale nuclei that are smaller in size than a neuron. With special stains (e.g., Cajal's gold sublimate), astrocytes are seen to have large coarse processes that form a framework for other neural cells (Fig. 180–16). Astrocytes are subdivided into protoplasmic and fibrous types according to their shape. Protoplasmic astrocytes occur mostly in gray matter, and the fibrous type occurs mainly in white matter. The retina and optic nerve astrocytes are the counterparts of fibroblasts in the rest of the body. They usually respond to injury and disease by becoming larger and by laying down more cell processes and proliferating. This form of reactive astrocytosis is usually referred to as *"gliosis."* The hypertrophic astrocytes present in the early stages of glial reaction are

Table 180–12. REACTION OF NEURONS TO INJURY

Atrophy and Degeneration
1. Swelling, fragmentation, and dissolution of cell bodies and processes; neurons may initially appear swollen with lipoidal vacuoles in their cytoplasm and subsequently become shrunken and ill-defined
2. Glial reaction is variable
3. Transsynaptic degeneration may occur

Intraneuronal Body Formation
1. Various degenerative diseases are associated with neurofibrillary tangles or other intracytoplasmic neuronal bodies

Intraneuronal Storage
1. In inborn errors of metabolism, biochemical or ultrastructural stored substances in neurons may reveal the diagnosis

Chromatolysis (Axonal Reaction)
1. Following injury to the axon, the cell body loses Nissl's substance and becomes rounded and pale-staining (chromatolysis)

Axonal Degeneration
1. There is rapid dissolution of the distal segment and a more gradual degeneration of the proximal segment and often the cell body (wallerian degeneration). Local dilatations of axons (spheroids) may occur following damage, especially around the edge of infarcts. In demyelinating diseases, the myelin becomes swollen and cavuolated and is taken.

Adapted from Morris JH: The nervous system. *In* Cotran RS, Kumar V, Robbins SL: Robbins Pathologic Basis of Disease, 4th ed. Philadelphia, WB Saunders, 1989.

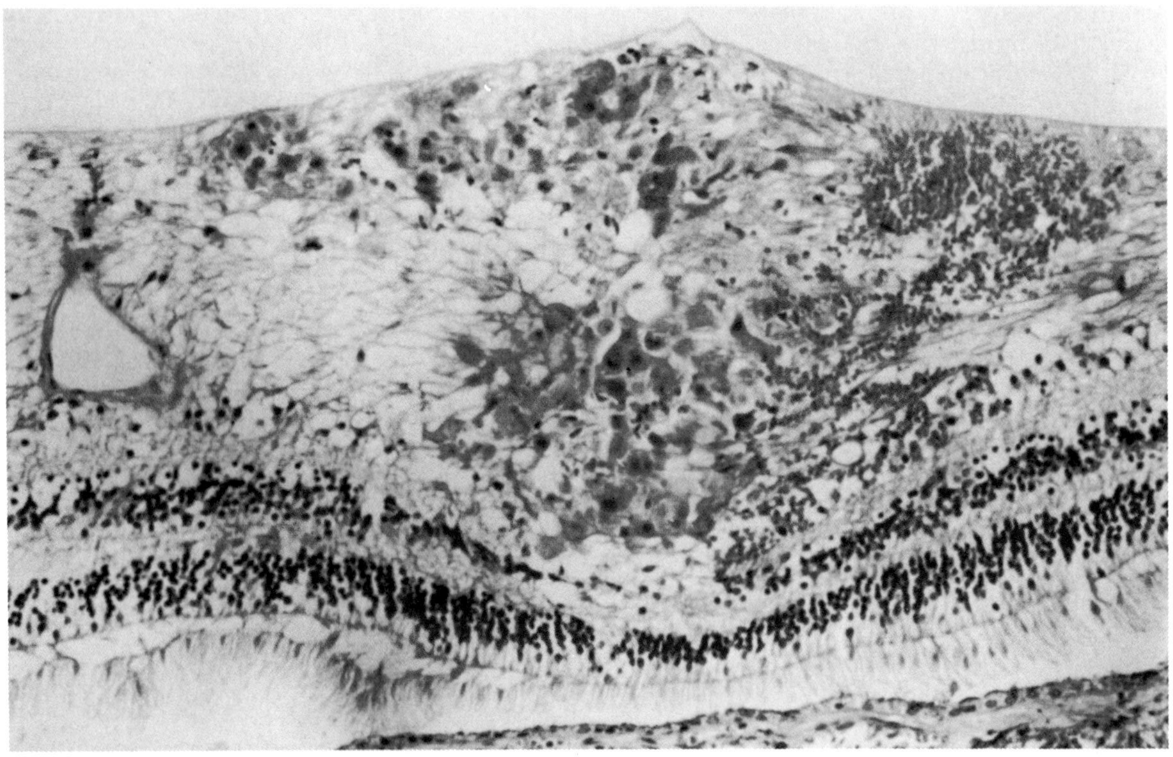

Figure 180–15. Infarctions and ischemic necrosis of the retina. (From Spencer WH [ed]: Ophthalmic Pathology: An Atlas and Textbook, 3rd ed, vol. 1. Philadelphia, WB Saunders, 1985, p 96.)

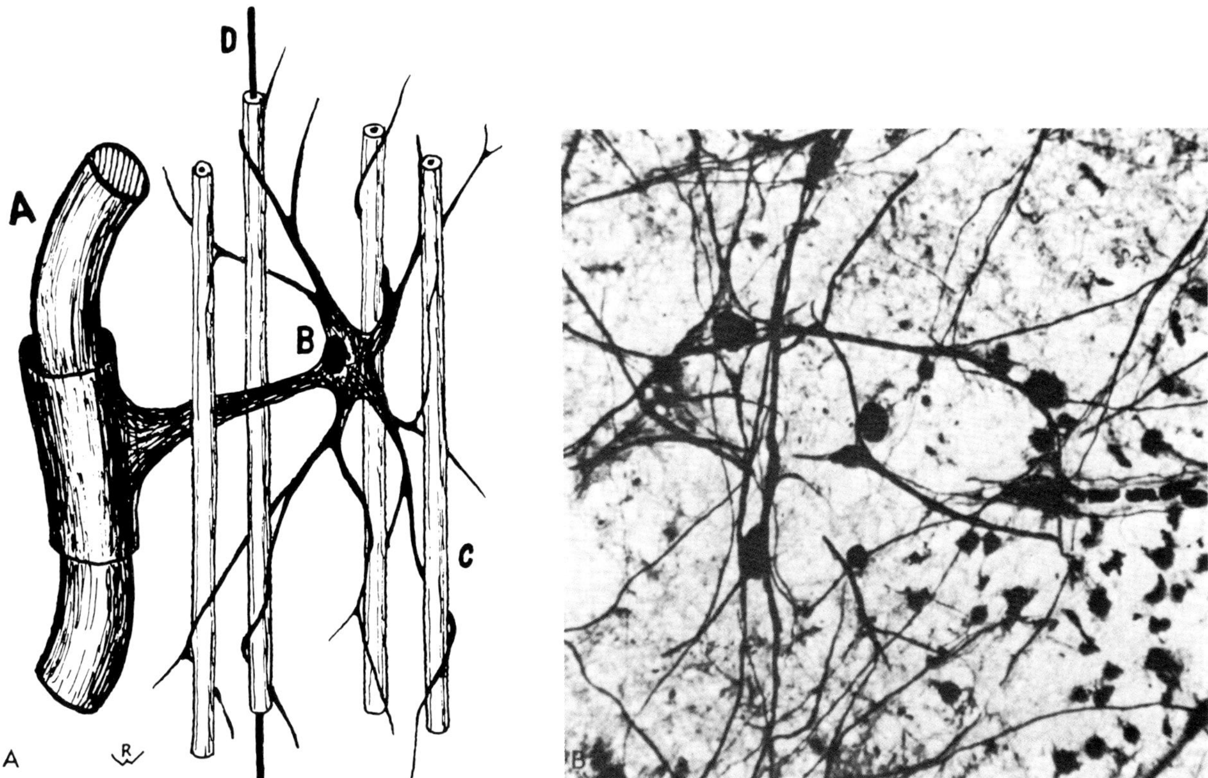

Figure 180–16. *A*, Schematic representation of astrocyte *(B)*, with one of its major processes forming a cuff about a small blood vessel *(A)* and other processes wrapped around nerve fibers (C and *D*). *B*, Astrocytes of an inner plexiform layer of retina (note astrocytic processes in relation to capillaries on right side of field.) (Courtesy of J. R. Wolter, M.D.) (From Spencer WH [ed]: Ophthalmic Pathology: An Atlas and Textbook, 3rd ed, vol. 1. Philadelphia, WB Saunders, 1985, p 98.)

called *gemistocytic astrocytes*. When gliosis occurs, the affected tissue consists almost entirely of cellular processes of astrocytes rather than collagen or an equivalent extracellular fibrous protein. In severe acute degenerations of the retina, the neuroglia are destroyed along with the neurons. In addition, the astrocytes in the optic pilae degenerate readily and seldom proliferate. In chronic progressive gliosis and in pilocystic astrocytomas, eosinophilic opaque bodies form in the astrocytic processes and are known as *Rosenthal's fibers*. In addition, spherical basophilic PAS-positive structures known as *corpora amylacea* accumulate with age in astrocytic processes and are commonly seen in the optic disc and optic nerve.

Oligodendrocytes are the counterpart of Schwann cells of the peripheral nervous system and are seen in myelinated areas of the central nervous system, including the optic nerve. With routine staining methods the nuclei alone are seen and are small, round, and deeply staining, resembling lymphocytes. With special stains (e.g., Hortega's silver carbonate), their processes can be visualized; they are delicate and unbranched. In the optic nerve, the oligodendrocytes are arranged in rows parallel to the axis cylinders. The principal function of oligodendrocytes is the production and maintenance of myelin in the central nervous system, and accordingly diseases affecting these cells appear as disorders of myelin and myelination. Examples of these are acquired demyelinating disease and the leukodystrophies. Oligodendrocytes respond to direct injury by swelling; their cytoplasm becomes pale, and a perinuclear halo is apparent.

Microglia and Their Response to Injury

Microglia have long been considered to be the "histiocytes of the nervous system," and recent work indicates that they are part of the mononuclear-phagocyte (reticuloendothelium) system and are derived from mesoderm. With routine stains their small, elongated nuclei can be seen, but with special stains (e.g., Hortega's silver carbonate) their short, branching processes are also observed. Following tissue injury, they appear to be able to function as macrophages. Particularly in an area of infarction, they become filled with lipid and have a prominent foamy appearance; such microglia are called *Gitter's cells*.

APPLICATION AND IMPACT OF THE POLYMERASE CHAIN REACTION IN DIAGNOSTIC PATHOLOGY

Since its development by scientists at Cetus in 1985, the polymerase chain reaction (PCR) has revolutionized the way in which DNA analysis is performed in both research and clinical laboratories.[48, 49] PCR is essentially an in vitro enzymatic amplification of a specific DNA segment, allowing for the synthesis of millions of copies of that DNA segment. Advances in the reagents, instruments, and protocols for carrying out PCR have made this technique accessible to the pathology laboratory.[50] This accessibility has been referred to as "democratizing the DNA sequence"[51] or enabling "the practice of molecular biology without a permit."[52]

Principle of the PCR

The PCR amplifies one segment of DNA in a complex mixture. In order to accomplish this, it is necessary to know at least some of the DNA sequence flanking the region to be assayed before amplification can be carried out. The method replaces techniques that originally required cloned genes for performance.

The PCR consists of a three-step cycle: *denaturation, primer binding,* and *DNA synthesis.* In the *first step* the sample is heated to between 94° and 98°C to denature the native double-stranded DNA (Fig. 180–17). At these temperatures the hydrogen bonds break, yielding single-stranded DNA. The *second step* (primer binding or annealing) is carried out at a reduced temperature of 37° to 65°C. Here two short oligonucleotide primers (usually 20 to 25 nucleosides long) hybridize to one of the two separated strands. These short DNA primers are selected with the knowledge of the DNA sequence flanking the region to be assayed so that they will encompass the desired genetic material. The primers hybridize in such a manner that extension from each 3-hydroxyl end is directed toward the other (see Fig. 180–17). The primers thus define the two ends of the DNA segment of interest. The specificity of the PCR depends on the precision of the DNA-DNA annealing reaction. The two primers must, of course, not bind to one another. Furthermore, their sites of hybridization must be sufficiently far apart so that they will allow subsequent synthesis of new products.

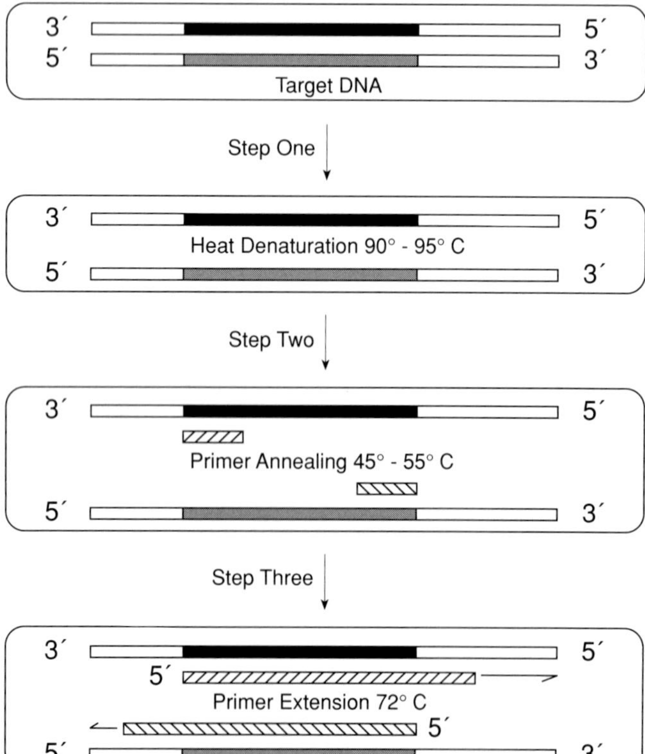

Figure 180–17. Polymerase chain reaction. (From Blanco R: The polymerase chain reaction and its future applications in the clinical laboratory. Deaconess Hosp Clin Lab Bull 6:1–2, 1991.)

In the final step of the reaction, the annealed primers are extended on the template strand with a DNA polymerase. This step utilizes a thermostable DNA polymerase Taq DNA polymerase isolated from the thermophilic bacterium *Thermus aquaticus.*[53] The enzyme catalyses this reaction at a maximum temperature of 72°C in the presence of excess deoxyribonucleoside triphosphates. If the newly synthesized strand extends to or beyond the region complementary to the other primer, it acts as a template for new primer-extension reaction. Thus as the set of cycles continues, each doubles the number of desired molecules in the reaction, and the result is an exponential amplification of a specific sequence of DNA, the ends of which are bounded by the selected primers.

The usefulness of the PCR is in the geometric expansion of a number of "short products" that contain only the DNA segment of interest. The primer-extension products of the original target DNA templates "the long products," which contain three prime ends of various lengths that expand only arithmetically. After about 30 cycles, the primers and deoxyribonucleoside triphosphates are progressively exhausted, the Taq polymerase is saturated with product, and the reaction reaches a plateau. At this point the reaction mixture consists almost entirely of the DNA segment of interest.

It should be noted that (1) because the primers become incorporated into the PCR product, and (2) because mismatches between the primer and the initial genomic template can be tolerated, it is possible to introduce via the primers new sequence information, such as sequences that encode a monoclonal antibody epitope.[53]

Diagnostic Applications of the PCR

The first diagnostic application of PCR was in the prenatal diagnosis of sickle cell anemia. This was accomplished through the amplification of β-globin sequences.[54] Normal and mutant alleles in this disease could be identified, and this technique was soon applied to β-thalassemia and to the analysis of human leukocyte antigen (HLA) polymorphisms. Using a "reverse dot blot" method, the cystic fibrosis gene can be identified. In the area of cancer research PCR has been useful in the identification of chromosomal abnormalities; specific mutations; oncogenes; and tumor suppressor genes, including the retinoblastoma gene. Certain cancers are associated with RNA or DNA tumor viruses, and PCR has been used to detect these viruses, including human papilloma virus in squamous cell carcinoma of the conjunctiva. The detection of specific pathogenic sequences by PCR is becoming increasingly important in the diagnosis of infectious disease, particularly when the pathogen is difficult to culture, as well as in immunologic diseases.[55] A summary of diagnostic applications of the PCR is included in Table 180–13.

Limitations of the PCR

As noted, the principal disadvantage of the PCR technique is the necessity to have prior knowledge of some of the DNA sequence flanking the region to be assayed. The second major problem arises from the sensitivity to the technique: The PCR technique carries a major risk of false-positive reactions caused by contamination or "carry-overs" from previously amplified DNA. This requires the most meticulous laboratory technique as well as the inclusion of established positive and negative controls.

Table 180–13. DIAGNOSTIC APPLICATIONS OF THE PCR

Infectious Agents that Can Be Detected by Means of the PCR
HIV-1, HIV-2, and double infection
HTLV-1 and associated myelopathy or tropical spastic paresis
CMV
Hepadnavirus
Papillomavirus in urine
Cutaneous herpes simplex virus
Human parvovirus B19
Hepatitis B virus in serum
Slow virus in the brain (BK and JC)
Mycoplasma pneumoniae
Enterotoxigenic *Escherichia coli*
Legionella pneumophila
Trypanosoma cruzi
Toxoplasma gondii
Genetic Diseases that Can Be Detected by Means of the PCR
Sickle cell anemia
Beta-thalassemia and hemoglobin H disease
Phenylketonuria
Diabetes (insulin-gene mutation)
Cystic fibrosis (allele linked)
Hemophilia A (allele linked)
Hemophilia B (gene mutation)
Hemophilia B (allele linked)
Clotting factor VIII mutation
Alpha$_1$-antitrypsin deficiency (allele linked)
Leber's hereditary optic neuropathy (mitochondrial mutation)
Apolipoprotein mutations
Duchenne's muscular dystrophy
Lesch-Nyhan syndrome
Huntington's disease (allele linked)
Residual leukemia (Philadelphia chromosome)
Lymphoma dissemination
Diseases Whose Pathogenesis Has Been Clarified by PCR
Diabetes mellitus
Pemphigus vulgaris
Myasthenia gravis and multiple sclerosis
Oncogene-linked cancers (e.g., Philadelphia chromosome)
Association of Virus and Cancer Shown by PCR
HTLV-1 and leukemia
HTLV-11
Papillomavirus and cervical cancer
Papillomavirus and corneal lesions
Hepatitis B virus and hepatocellular carcinoma
Detection of minimal residual disease after antineoplastic treatment

Adapted from Blanco R: The polymerase chain reaction and its future applications in the clinical laboratory. Deaconess Hosp Clin Lab Bull 6:1–2, 1991.

TECHNIQUES OF EXAMINING THE EYE FOR PATHOLOGY

Gross Examination of the Eye

The human eye has a spherical shape and measures approximately 25 mm anteriorly and posteriorly; 24 mm transversely; and 24 mm vertically. The cornea superimposes a more sharply curved sphere onto the sclera and has a horizontal diameter of approximately 12 mm and a vertical diameter of 11 mm. Through an examination of the major landmarks on the external surface of the globe, the right eye can be differentiated from the left (Fig. 180–18).[56] Useful features in orienting the globe are the prominence of the nasal long posterior ciliary artery compared with the temporal. These vessels are also useful in determining the horizontal plane. Furthermore, the entry of the ciliary nerves on either side of the optic nerve is useful in verifying the horizontal meridian.

The tendinous insertion of the superior oblique muscle into the upper temporal quadrant and the fleshy inferior oblique attachment near the horizontal meridian on the

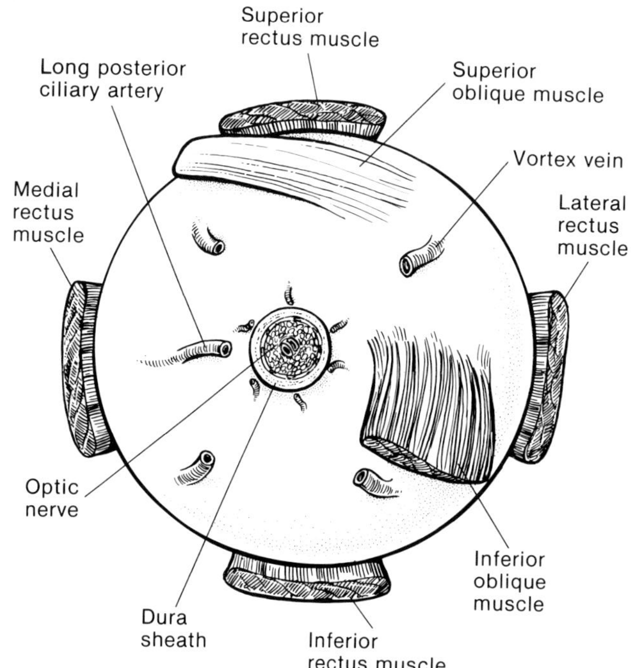

Figure 180–18. Anatomic landmarks seen on the posterior surface of the globe that are useful in orienting the globe at the time of gross examination.

Table 180–14. HISTOLOGIC STAINS USED IN OCULAR PATHOLOGY

Staining Techniques	Substances, Cellular Components, and Tissues that are Stained	Staining Characteristics
Paraffin Sections Fixed in 10% Neutral Buffer Formalin		
Hematoxylin	Nucleic acids within cellular nuclei	Blue
Eosin	Cytoplasmic organelles	Varying shades of pink
Periodic acid–Schiff	Mucopolysaccharides and glycoproteins (e.g., glycogen, ocular basement membranes)	Rose to purplish red
Masson trichrome	Collagen (e.g., sclera or cornea)	Blue
	Smooth muscle (e.g., ciliary muscle)	Red
Alcian blue	Mucopolysaccharides (e.g., vitreous, mucin), pretreatment with hyaluronidase eliminates hyaluronic acid, chondroitin 4 sulfate, and chondroitin 6 sulfate	Blue
Perl's iron	Iron (hemosiderin) (e.g., iron foreign bodies, blood products)	Blue
Alizarin red	Calcium	Dark red
Von Kossa	Calcium	Black
Luxol fast blue	Myelin (e.g., optic nerve)	Blue
Weigert	Myelin	Black
Bodian, Cajal, Golgi	Neurons	Black
Sudan black B	Lipid (e.g., meibomian [sebaceous] gland secretions)	Black
Oil red O	Lipid	Red
Congo red	Amyloid (e.g., lattice corneal dystrophy)	Pale red
Thioflavine T	Amyloid	Flourescence (white)
Crystal violet	Amyloid	Purplish violet
Phosphotungstic acid hematoxylin (PTAH)	Delineation of cross-striations in skeletal muscle, fibrin, and glial fibers	Blue
Verhoeff's modified elastin stain	Elastic fibers	Blue-black
Brown and Brenn stain	Gram-positive bacteria	Blue
	Gram-negative bacteria	Red
Kinyouns acid fast, Fite, Ziehl-Neelson	Acid-fast bacilli	Red
Grocott's modification of Gomori's methanamine silver	Fungi	Delineated in black
Gomori's reticulum technic	Reticulum fibers	Black
Mayer's mucicarmine rhodanine	Mucin and capsule of *Crytococcus*	Rose to red
	Copper	Bright red to yellow red
Cresyl violet	Nerve cells and glia	Blue
Fontana Masson	Argentaffin cells and melanin	Black
Melanin bleach	Bleaches out melanin that may obscure nuclear detail and mitotic figures	Melanin is bleached
Plastic Embedded Sections Fixed in Glutaraldehyde, Paraformaldehyde, or Osmium Tetroxide for Electron Microscopy		
Thick Sections		
Toluidine blue	Membranes of cell organelles and cell walls	Varying shades of blue
Methylene blue		
Mallory blue		
Thin Sections		
Uranyl acetate and lead citrate		Varying shades of gray and black

Adapted from Apple DJ, Rabb MF: Ocular Pathology: Clinical Applications and Self-Assessment. St. Louis, CV Mosby, 1985 and Sheehan DC and Hrapchak B: Theory and Practice of Histotechnology, 2nd ed. St Louis, CV Mosby, 1980.

temporal side are also useful guides in determining the superior and inferior halves of the globe, as well as right versus left. Additional identification may be obtained from the rectus muscles, with the medial rectus muscle attaching approximately 5.5 mm from the limbus; the inferior rectus attaching 6.5 mm from the limbus; the lateral rectus attaching approximately 7 mm from the limbus; and the superior rectus attaching approximately 7.7 mm from the limbus. The upper vortex veins exit from the sclera approximately 7 mm on the nasal side and 8 mm posterior on the temporal side. The lower vortex veins exit approximately 6 mm posterior to the equator on either side of the vertical meridian. A technique for gross sectioning is shown in Figure 180–19.

Histologic Stains

For routine examination, paraffin sections stained with hemotoxylin and eosin are usually obtained. A number of additional stains have particular affinities for tissue, organisms, or minerals and are extremely useful.[51] These are summarized in Table 180–14. Plastic embedding is used primarily for electron microscopic examination but can also be deployed for light microscopy (see Table 180–14). Immunohistochemical stains have become of extreme importance in diagnostic work, and these are discussed elsewhere.

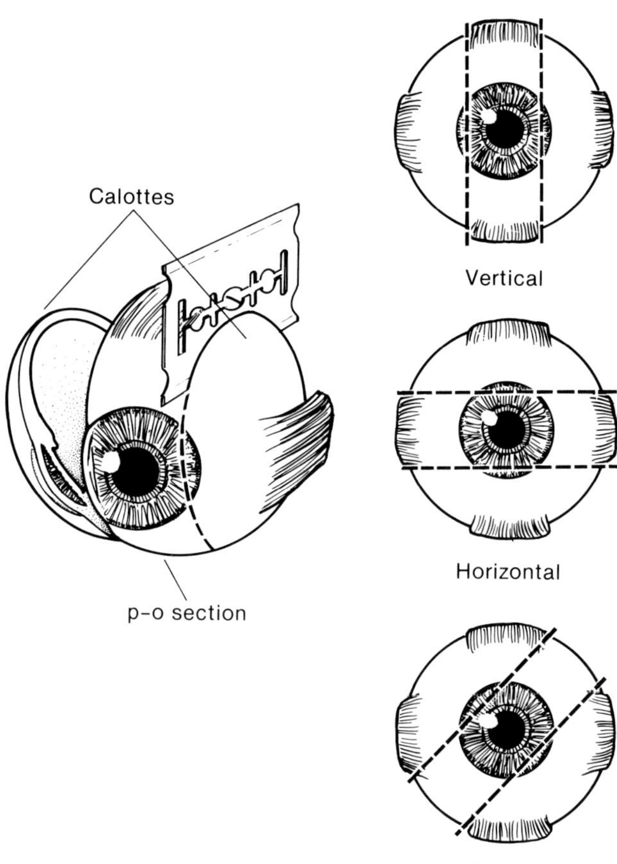

Figure 180–19. The eye is examined and oriented so that the pathologist is aware of the orientation and location of pathology. If routine examination is done, the eye is opened in a horizontal plane so that the pupil-optic nerve (P-O) section will contain the macula. If a tumor or site of pathology exists, the eye is cut so that the pupil-optic nerve section includes the pathology. If there is pathology as well in the caps or calottes, these may be submitted for sectioning.

Limitations of Histopathologic Diagnosis

Although histologic study continues to be one of the most effective methods of diagnosis in ophthalmology, it must be remembered that these have their limitations. Frequently, the principal determination of a histologic study will be to confirm previous clinical observations to rule out possible diseases. Occasionally, the histologic picture will be merely suggestive of the diagnosis and will sometimes be entirely nonspecific.

REFERENCES

1. Ritchie AC: Boyd's Textbook of Pathology, 9th ed. Philadelphia, Lea & Febiger, 1990.
2. Morgagni G: The Seats and Causes of Diseases Investigated by Anatomy, vols. 1 to 5. [Translated from Latin] London, Benjamin Alexander, A Millar, T Cadell, Johnson, and Payne, 1769.
3. Baillie M: The morbid anatomy of some of the most important parts of the human body. London, J Johnson & G Nicol, 1973.
4. Wardrop J: Essays on the Morbid Anatomy of the Human Eye, vols. 1 and 2. Edinburgh, G Ramsay & Co, 1808 to 1818.
5. Virchow RLK: Die Cellulorpathologic in ihrer Begrudung auf physiologische und pathologische Geweselehre. Berlin, A Hirschwald, 1858.
6. Ashton N: The evolution of ocular pathology. *In* Albert DM, Puliafito CA (eds): Foundations of Ophthalmic Pathology. New York, Appleton-Century-Crofts, 1979, pp 1–18.
7. Cotran RS, Kumar V, Robbins SL: Robbins Pathologic Basis of Disease, 4th ed. Philadelphia, WB Saunders, 1989.
8. Reimer KA, Ideker RE: Myocardial ischemia and infarction. Hum Pathol 18:462, 1987.
9. Howes EL Jr: Basic mechanisms in pathology. *In* Spencer WH (ed): Ophthalmic Pathology: An Atlas and Textbook, 3rd ed, vol. 1. Philadelphia, WB Saunders, 1985.
10. Schoen FJ, Harasaki H, Kim KM, et al: Biomaterial-associated calcification: Pathology, mechanisms and strategies of prevention. J Biomed Material Res 22:A1, 1988.
11. Majino G, et al: Cellular death and necrosis: Chemical, physical and morphological changes in rat liver. Virchows Arch 333:421, 1960.
12. Becker EL, Ward P: Chemotaxis. *In* Parker CW (ed): Clinical Immunology. Philadelphia, WB Saunders, 1980, p 272.
13. Harlan JM: Consequences of leukocyte vessel wall interactions in inflammatory and immune reactions. Semin Thromb Hemost 13:434, 1987.
14. Johnston RB Jr: Monocytes and macrophages. N Engl J Med 318:747, 1988.
15. Unanue ER, Allen PM: The basis for the immunoregulatory role of macrophages and other accessory cells. Science 236:551, 1987.
16. Ryan G, Manjo G: Inflammation: A Scope Publication. Upjohn Co.
17. Unanue ER, Benacerraf B: Immunological events in experimentally induced granulomas. Am J Pathol 71:349, 1973.
18. Schoefl GI: Studies of inflammation. III: Growing capillaries: Their structure and permeability. Virchows Arch Pathol Anat 337:97, 1963.
19. Fleischmajer R, Perlish JS, Timpl R, et al: Biology, chemistry and pathology of collagen. Ann N Y Acad Sci 460:1, 1985.

20. Linder J: Monoclonal antibodies marking paraffin-embedded lymphocytes. *In* DeLellis RA (ed): Advances in Immunohistochemistry. New York, Raven Press, 1988, pp 261–300.
21. Nathan CF: Secretory products of macrophages. J Clin Invest 79:319, 1987.
22. Stein H, Gatter KC, Heryet A, et al: Freeze-dried paraffin-embedded human tissue for antigen labelling with monoclonal antibodies. Lancet 2:71–73, 1984.
23. Tanaka M, Tanaka H, Ishikawa E: Immunohistochemical demonstration of surface antigen of human lymphocytes with monoclonal antibody in acetone-fixed paraffin-embedded sections. J Histochem Cytochem 32:452–454, 1984.
24. Allsop CJ, Gallagher PJ: Temporal artery biopsy in giant cell arteritis: A reappraisal. Am J Surg Pathol 5:317, 1981.
25. Fauci AS, Haynes BF, Katz P, Wolff SP: Wegener's granulomatosis: Prospective clinical and therapeutic experience with 85 patients for 21 years. Ann Intern Med 98:76, 1983.
26. Takayasu H: Case report of a peculiar abnormality of the retinal central vessels. Acta Soc Ophthalmol Jpn 12:554–556, 1908.
27. Lupi-Herrara E, Sanchez Torres G, Marcushamer J, Mispireta J, et al: Takayasu's arteritis: Study of 107 cases. Am Heart J 93:94, 1977.
28. Obenauf CD, Shaw HE, Snydor CF, Klintworth GK: Sarcoidosis and its ophthalmic manifestations. Am J Ophthalmol 86:648–655, 1978.
29. Donders PC: Eales' disease. Doc Ophthalmol 12:1–21, 1958.
30. Ashton N: Pathogenesis and aetiology of Eales's disease. Acta XIX Concilium Ophthalmologicum 2:828–840, 1962.
31. Albert DM, Dryja TP: The eye. *In* Cotran RS, Kumar V, Robbins SL: Robbins Pathologic Basis of Disease, 4th ed. Philadelphia, WB Saunders, 1989, pp 1451–1468.
32. Kinnear PE: Albinism. Surv Ophthalmol 30:75, 1985.
33. Lever WF, Schaumburgh-Lever G: Histopathology of the Skin, 5th ed. Philadelphia, JB Lippincott, 1975.
34. Murphy GF, Mihm MC Jr: The skin. *In* Cotran RS, Kumar V, Robbins SL: Robbins Pathologic Basis of Disease, 4th ed. Philadelphia, WB Saunders, 1989, pp 1277–1313.
35. Callender GR: Malignant melanotic tumors of the eye: A study of histologic types in 111 cases. Trans Am Acad Ophthalmol Otolaryngol 36:131–142, 1931.
36. Mihm MC: The clinical diagnosis, classification and histogenetic concepts of the early stages of cutaneous malignant melanomas. N Engl J Med 284:1078, 1971.
37. Murphy GF, Murphy G, Lopansri S, Mihm MC, et al: Capsule dermatopathology: Clinicopathologic types of malignant melanoma: Relevance to biologic behavior and diagnostic surgical approach. J Dermatol Surg Oncol 11:673, 1985.
38. Clark WH, Elder DE, Guerry D IV, et al: A study of tumor progression: The precursor lesion of superficial spreading and nodular melanoma. Hum Pathol 15:1147, 1985.
39. Breslow A: Thickness, cross-sectioned areas and depth of invasion in the prognosis of cutaneous melanoma. Ann Surg 182:572, 1970.
40. Harrist TJ, Mihm MC: The specificity and usefulness of the lupus band test. Arthritis Rheum 23:479, 1980.
41. Ahmed AR: Clinical features of pemphigus. *In* Ahmed AR (ed): Clinics in Dermatology—Pemphigus. Philadelphia, JB Lippincott, 1983, p 13.
42. Hashimoto K, Lever WF: An electron microscopic study of pemphigus vulgaris of the mouth with special reference to the intercellular cement. J Invest Dermatol 48:540, 1967.
43. Lever WF: Pemphigus. Medicine 32:1, 1953.
44. Cogan DG: Neurology of the Visual System. Springfield, IL, Charles C Thomas, 1966.
45. Peters A, et al: The Fine Structure of the Nervous System: The Neurons and Supporting Cells. Philadelphia, WB Saunders, 1976.
46. Morris JH: The nervous system. *In* Cotran RS, Kumar V, Robbins SL: Robbins Pathologic Basis of Disease, 4th ed. Philadelphia, WB Saunders, 1989.
47. Janzer RC, Raff MC: Astrocytes induce blood-brain barrier properties in endothelial cells. Nature 325:253, 1987.
48. Saiki RK, Scharf S, Faloona F, et al: Enzymatic amplification of beta-globulin genomic sequences and restriction site analysis for diagnosis of sickle cell anemia. Science 250:1350, 1985.
49. Mullis KB, Faloona F: Specific synthesis of DNA in vitro via polymerase catalyzed chain reaction. Methods Enzymol 155:335, 1987.
50. Blanco R: The polymerase chain reaction and its future applications in the clinical laboratory. Deaconess Hosp Clin Lab Bull 6:1–2, 1991.
51. Appenzeller T: Research news: Democratizing the DNA sequence. Science 247:1030–1032, 1990.
52. Erlich HA, Gelfand D, Sinsky JJ: Recent advances in the polymerase chain reaction. Science 252:1643–1651, 1991.
53. Brock TD, Freeze H: Thermus aquaticus gen. n. and sp. n., a nonsporulating extreme thermophile. J Bacteriol 98:289, 1969.
54. Martin GA, et al: Cell 63:843, 1990.
55. Embury SH, Scharf SJ, Saiki RK, et al: Rapid prenatal diagnosis of sickle cell anemia by a new method of DNA analysis. N Engl J Med 316:656, 1987.
56. Lew AM: The polymerase chain reaction and related techniques. Curr Opin Immunol 3:242–246, 1991.
57. Apple DJ, Rabb MF: Ocular Pathology: Clinical Applications and Self-Assessment. St. Louis, CV Mosby, 1985.

Chapter 181

Conjunctival and Corneal Pathology

JAYNE S. WEISS

CONJUNCTIVAL PATHOLOGY

Conjunctiva is an easily accessible tissue source for diagnostic biopsy. In a histopathologic review of 2455 conjunctival biopsies, the most common lesions in order of decreasing frequency were pterygium, nevus, dysplasia, nonspecific nongranulomatous inflammation, and epithelial inclusion cysts. The most common conjunctival malignancies in order of decreasing frequency were squamous cell carcinoma, melanoma, and sebaceous cell carcinoma.[1] Major sources of conjunctival pathology are addressed in this section.

Congenital and Developmental Malformations

Congenital and developmental conjunctival malformations include cryptophthalmos, epitarsus, vascular hamartomas (proliferation of tissue elements usually found in the involved area), and choristomas (tissue elements not usually found in the involved area). Failure of development of the embryonic lid fold leads to cryptophthalmos, in which orbital margins and globe are covered by the smooth facial skin. The lids, cilia, palpebral fissure, conjunctiva, and cornea may be absent. Epitarsus is an abnormal fold of tarsal conjunctiva with conjunctival epithelium lining its front and back surfaces. Temporary lid sutures may be needed to correct resultant ectropion.

The vascular hamartomas include arterial, venous, and lymphatic abnormalities. Telangiectasias of the conjunctiva are abnormally dilated or tortuous conjunctival capillaries. The lesion may be isolated or may be associated with ataxia telangiectasia (Louis-Bar syndrome), hereditary hemorrhagic telangiectasias (Rendu-Osler-Weber disease), or anorexia nervosa/bulimia.[2] Conjunctival varicosities result from venous dilatation, which may be associated with similar lesions of the orbit.

Both capillary hemangiomas and lymphangiomas may manifest early in life. The hemangiomas are composed of capillary and endothelial cell proliferation (Fig. 181–1). Lymphangiomas contain channels lined by endothelial cells and devoid of pericytes. Conjunctival lymphangiomas are usually associated with lymphangiomas of the eyelid or orbit.

Lymphangiectasias are wormlike dilatations of the lymphatics (Fig. 181–2). They may wax and wane in size, depending on the amount of fluid accumulation. The X-linked recessive disease congenital conjunctival lymphedema (Nonne-Milroy-Meige disease) occurs when congenital lymphatic dysplasia results in edema of the extremities and commonly the conjunctiva. In lymphangiectasia hemorrhagica conjunctiva, blood cells fill the lymphatics because of an abnormal connection between conjunctival blood vessels and lymphatic channels.

Dermoids, dermolipomas, and dermoid cysts are choristomas of the conjunctiva. Limbal dermoids usually occur inferotemporally and may contain connective tissue, pilosebaceous material, and fat cells (Fig. 181–3). Dermolipomas that also contain connective tissue appear yellow because of fat components. Dermoid cysts are lined by nonkeratinizing conjunctival epithelium with pilosebaceous structures in their wall.

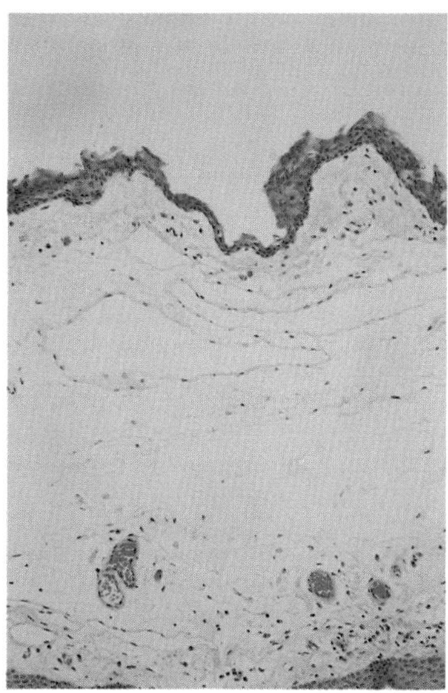

Figure 181–2. Lymphangiectasia with localized dilatation of conjunctival lymphatics. H&E, ×10.

Infectious and Noninfectious Conjunctivitis

Conjunctivitis is one of the most common conjunctival abnormalities. Classification of the type of inflammatory cell infiltration can help to elucidate the etiology of conjunctivitis (Table 181–1). Neutrophils are most characteristic of bacterial infections; basophils and eosinophils are more frequently encountered in allergic responses; and mononuclear cells are more characteristic of viral infections. Multinucleated cells may be found in conjunctival inflammation associated with *Chlamydia* infection, tuberculosis, rubella, herpes infection, sarcoid, or foreign bodies.

True inflammatory membranes or pseudomembranes may be present. True inflammatory membranes consist of fibrin-cellular debris, which is attached to the underlying epithelium. When the debris is removed, the epithelium also detaches, leaving a bleeding surface. These true membranes occur in epidemic keratoconjunctivitis and in pneumococcal, *Staphylococcus aureus*,

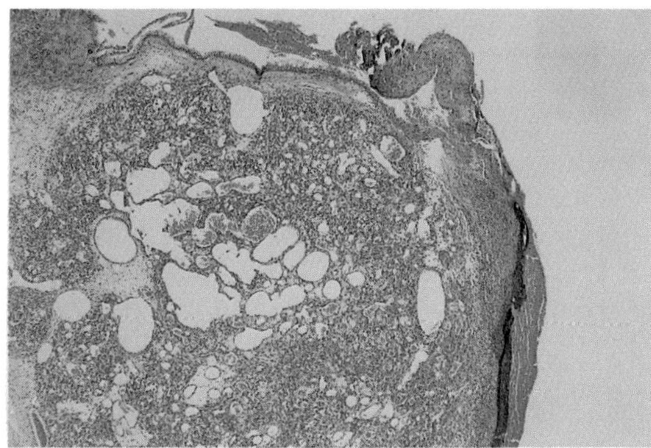

Figure 181–1. Conjunctival hemangioma demonstrating multiple vascular channels lined by endothelial cells. H&E, ×2.5.

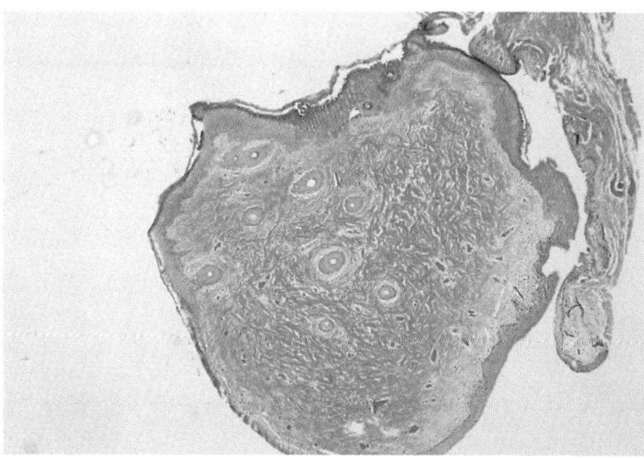

Figure 181–3. Conjunctival dermoid demonstrating pilosebaceous elements in a dense connective tissue matrix. H&E, ×2.5.

Table 181–1. TYPES OF INFLAMMATORY CELLS

Cell Type	Etiology
Neutrophil	Bacterial
Eosinophil	Allergic
Basophil	
Lymphocyte	Viral
Multinucleated	Chlamydia Tuberculosis Rubella Herpes Sarcoid Foreign body

and *Corynebacterium diphtheriae* infections. A pseudomembrane can easily be removed because the fibrin-cellular debris is not attached to the underlying epithelium. Pseudomembranes occur in chemical burns, vernal conjunctivitis, pharyngeal conjunctival fever, and *Streptococcus hemolyticus* infection. Both true inflammatory membranes and pseudomembranes may occur in epidemic keratoconjunctivitis, *C. diphtheriae* infection, ligneous conjunctivitis, and Stevens-Johnson syndrome.

Conjunctival edema, hyperemia, and membrane formation are the most prominent findings in acute conjunctivitis. With chronicity, papillary or follicular formation may result. In papillary hypertrophy, folds of conjunctiva containing a blood vessel core are surrounded by hyperplastic epithelium. Subepithelial tissue may contain chronic inflammatory cells. Papillae are frequently encountered in bacterial infections and allergic responses.

Follicular hypertrophy is a result of lymphoid hyperplasia in the conjunctiva (Fig. 181–4). These follicles lack the central vascular core. They may be associated with allergy, viral and chlamydial infections, and drug toxicity.

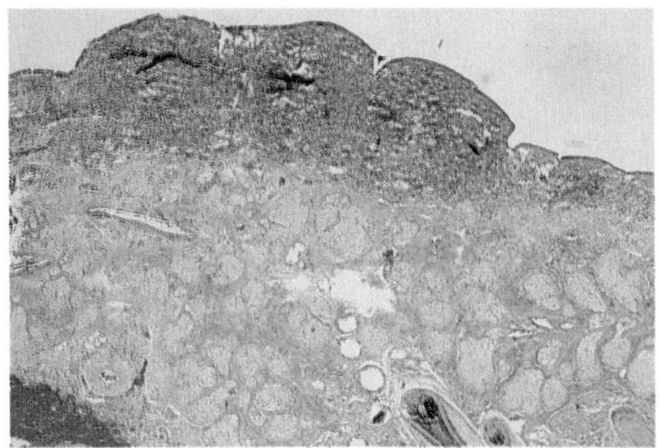

Figure 181–4. Follicle demonstrating areas of localized lymphoid hyperplasia within the conjunctival epithelium. H&E, ×2.5.

Bacterial, viral, chlamydial, fungal, and parasitic organisms can cause conjunctivitis. Bacterial conjunctivitis is frequently a self-limited condition. However, gonococcal conjunctivitis results in a hyperacute condition that can be easily diagnosed by gram-negative intracellular diplococci seen on Gram's stain. Viral conjunctivitis usually results in follicular conjunctival reaction. Cytomegalovirus infection of the conjunctiva is reported in AIDS, with cytomegalic cells surrounding and invading the walls of the conjunctival vessels.[3] Cells from conjunctival scrapings of patients with AIDS reveal human T-cell lymphotrophic virus type III antigens by indirect immunofluorescence.[4]

Chlamydiae are obligate intracellular parasites resembling gram-negative basophilic coccoid spheroid bacteria. These organisms are responsible for trachoma, adult and neonatal inclusion conjunctivitis, lymphogranuloma venereum, and ornithosis. The severity of trachoma has been graded by MacCallan[5] depending on the maturity of follicles and the presence of conjunctival scarring. In stage I, immature follicles on the upper tarsal plate are noted without scarring. Conjunctival epithelial cells may demonstrate the perinuclear inclusions described by Halberstaedter and Prowazeck. By stage II, follicles have become mature, but scarring is still not present. Leber's cells, macrophages with phagocytized debris, are noted. During stage III, mature follicles and conjunctival scarring are present. Herbert's pits appear at the peripheral cornea. Linear conjunctival scarring may result in the horizontal Arlt's line. By stage IV, scarring is prominent, although tarsal follicles are no longer noted.

Inclusion conjunctivitis occurs in newborns by transmission of *Chlamydia trachomatis* through the birth canal. In adults, sexual transmission of the infection can result in a follicular conjunctival reaction. Specialized stains and immunofluorescence have been used to detect the organism.[6] Lymphogranuloma venereum may cause a granulomatous or a follicular conjunctivitis.

Fungal organisms may infect the conjunctiva. Conjunctival rhinosporidiosis can be transmitted through contaminated soil. The organism, which can be detected by histopathologic examination, may manifest an atrophic and an endosporulating phase.[7, 8] Chronic conjunctival reaction can result from degeneration of the *Onchocerca volvulus* microfilariae. Other ocular signs, including uveitis, choroiditis, and neuritis, are usually associated.[9]

Parinaud's oculoglandular syndrome is a granulomatous inflammatory conjunctivitis associated with prominent preauricular lymph nodes. It can result from many causes, including cat-scratch disease,[10, 11] tuberculosis, syphilis, tularemia, and sarcoid, and infection with *Leptothrix*, rickettsiae, viruses, and fungi.

Noninfectious conjunctivitis includes inflammations caused by physical trauma, chemical insult, or allergic reactions. Vernal conjunctivitis is a bilateral recurrent allergic conjunctivitis that usually affects young adults during the spring season. Tarsal conjunctiva is invaded by chronic inflammatory cells and eosinophils, resulting in cobblestone giant papillae. Chronic inflammatory cell infiltration causes hyperplasia of limbal tissue. Eosinophilic concretions in these limbal nodules are called Horner-Trantas dots. Immunopathologic study reveals an anaphylactic response.[12] Contact lens wearers with giant papillary conjunctivitis complain of decreased lens tolerance, itching, or mucus accumulation. On histopathologic examination, the tarsal conjunctiva demonstrates giant papillary formation reminiscent of vernal conjunctivitis.[13]

An allergic response to an antigen can result in a conjunctival nodule called a *phlyctenule*. This raised lesion consists of lymphocytes, histiocytes, and plasma cells. Acutely, polymorphonuclear leukocytes may also be found.[14]

Ligneous conjunctivitis is a rare recurrent bilateral inflammation usually found in girls. On histopathologic examination, the conjunctival epithelium is thickened and dyskeratotic. True and pseudomembrane formation are noted. The subepithelium contains chronic inflammatory cells, fibrin, and eosinophilic debris.

Conjunctival Degenerations

Degenerations of the conjunctiva result from aging, exposure, and deposition of foreign material. These include xerosis, pinguecula, pterygium, and amyloidosis. Prolonged drying causes xerosis, which is epidermalization with keratin formation. This may result from abnormal lid movement, tear hyposecretion, or mucus deficiency from either goblet cell loss, conjunctival scarring, or lipid deficiency. Xerosis may also be associated with anorexia nervosa/bulimia.[2, 15] Pinguecula occurs when subepithelial connective tissue undergoes basophilic degeneration, hyalinization, and elastosis.[16] In Gaucher's disease, pinguecula demonstrates yellowish discoloration. Gaucher's cells and elastosis are noted on histologic examination.[17] In pterygia, the abnormal tissue invades the epithelium with breakdown of Bowman's layer. Subepithelial amyloid deposition may occur in systemic amyloidosis but more commonly is an isolated conjunctival deposit. The well-characterized staining features of amyloid include metachromasia, dichroism to green light, fluorescence with thioflavine-T, and staining and birefringence with Congo red. Foreign body–type reaction with epithelioid cells may be present.

Local application of silver-containing compounds may lead to argyrosis, with grayish discoloration of the conjunctiva. Silver granules are deposited in the epithelial basement membrane and the subepithelial stroma. Phenothiazines, mercury, gold, atabrine, and epinephrine may also deposit in the conjunctiva.[18]

Conjunctival Abnormalities Associated With Systemic Diseases

Systemic diseases, including metabolic, rheumatologic, collagen vascular, and dermatologic, may have conjunctival manifestations. Derangement in systemic metabolism may result in abnormal conjunctival deposits in cystinosis, alkaptonuria, dysproteinemias and paraproteinemias, mucopolysaccharidosis, mucolipidosis, Addison's disease, porphyria, jaundice, and hypercalcemia. Water-soluble cystine crystals are present in the subepithelial conjunctival connective tissue in cystinosis. Because these crystals dissolve in aqueous solutions, the conjunctiva must be fixed in absolute alcohol or processed by frozen section.[19] In alkaptonuria, abnormal metabolism of tyrosine-phenylalanine results in accumulation of homogentisic acid in the subepithelial conjunctival connective tissue.[20] The ultrastructure of these dark-brown extracellular pigment granules resembles melanin. In multiple myeloma, alterations of serum proteins can result in precipitation of these substances in the conjunctival stroma.[21] Conjunctival biopsy samples may demonstrate ultrastructural abnormalities in lysosomal storage disease before clinical signs manifest.[22, 23] Diagnosis of mucolipidosis may be established by electron microscopy of the conjunctiva. In mucolipidosis IV, conjunctival epithelial cells contain concentric lamellar bodies (phospholipids) and fine granular material (acid mucopolysaccharide).[24–26] Melanin deposits may be found in the basal conjunctival epithelium in Addison's disease. In jaundice, bilirubin usually deposits in the conjunctiva and episclera, not the scleral tissue. Diseases with systemic abnormalities of calcium and phosphate metabolism may cause calcium deposition in the conjunctival subepithelium.

Malnutrition may result in keratinization and Bitot's spots caused by vitamin A deficiency. Vascular dilatation can result from vitamin B deficiency. Vitamin C deficiency can result in spontaneous hemorrhages.[27] Graft-versus-host disease occurs in patients who have undergone allogeneic bone marrow transplantation. Conjunctival involvement includes pseudomembrane formation and may be an indication of degree of severity of the systemic involvement.[28]

Patients with sarcoidosis may have conjunctival granulomas, which may or may not be clinically apparent. On histopathologic examination, these demonstrate noncaseating granulomatous inflammatory infiltration with giant cells. Nichols and coworkers reported that in patients with known sarcoidosis, biopsy of an area of conjunctiva without obvious nodules demonstrated granulomatous reaction on histopathologic examination 50 percent of the time.[29]

Patients with rheumatoid arthritis may manifest keratoconjunctivitis sicca and dry mouth, called *Sjögren's syndrome*. Immune deposits are present in the walls of conjunctival blood vessels. These findings may also be noted in other collagen vascular diseases.[30]

Dermatologic diseases with accompanying conjunctival changes include ocular pemphigoid, erythema multiforme, scleroderma, xeroderma pigmentosum, ichthyosis congenita, Dego's disease, acanthosis nigricans, molluscum contagiosum, acne rosacea, atopic dermatitis, dermatitis herpetiformis, epidermolysis bullosa, and erythema nodosum. Ocular pemphigoid (benign mucous membrane pemphigoid, chronic cicatricial conjunctivitis) is a bilateral conjunctival disease with an initial inflammatory stage demonstrating subepithelial vesicles with edema and hyperemia. Subepithelial fibrosis, goblet cell loss, and keratinization may follow, leading to symblepharon formation and xerophthalmia. Conjunctival biopsy specimens from a site without symblepharon frequently demonstrate positive linear direct immunofluorescence.[31, 32] Dermatologic manifestations are noted in 21 percent, and oral mucosa lesions in 50 percent.[33, 34]

In erythema multiforme (Stevens-Johnson syndrome), abnormal vascular proliferation in the skin and mucous membranes may undergo spontaneous regression. Subepithelial conjunctival bullae may heal with scarring, loss of goblet cells, and symblepharon formation.[35]

Bullous pemphigoid and pemphigus vulgaris are respectively associated with subepithelial and intraepithelial bullae. These mucous membrane diseases usually do not involve the eye.

Conjunctival Tumors

Tumors of the conjunctiva include cysts, pseudoneoplasms, and true neoplasms. Dermoids are the second most common congenital conjunctival tumor. Conjunctival cysts may be confused with dermoids clinically. Cysts, however, do not contain adnexal structures, are more often located superomedially than dermoids, and do not have associated osseous defects.[36] Epithelial inclusion cysts may occur postoperatively because of implantation of surface epithelium. The cyst is filled with clear fluid and lined by conjunctival epithelium (Fig. 181–5). Ductal cysts are formed by the accessory lacrimal glands. These are filled with PAS-positive material and lined by a double layer of epithelium.

Epithelial tumors range from the benign, including keratoacanthoma and pseudoepitheliomatous hyperplasia, to the precancerous lesion epithelial dysplasia to frank carcinoma (Table 181–2). The rapid growth of pseudoepitheliomatous hyperplasia may raise suspicion for a neoplastic process. This lesion contains hyperplastic epithelium and chronic nongranulomatous subepithelial inflammation. Keratoacanthoma may also undergo rapid growth. A central keratin core differentiates it from pseudoepitheliomatous hyperplasia. Hereditary benign intraepithelial dyskeratosis is inherited in an autosomal dominant fashion. Bilateral raised horseshoe-

Table 181–2. CONJUNCTIVAL SQUAMOUS LESIONS

Type	Polarity	Epithelial Layers Involved
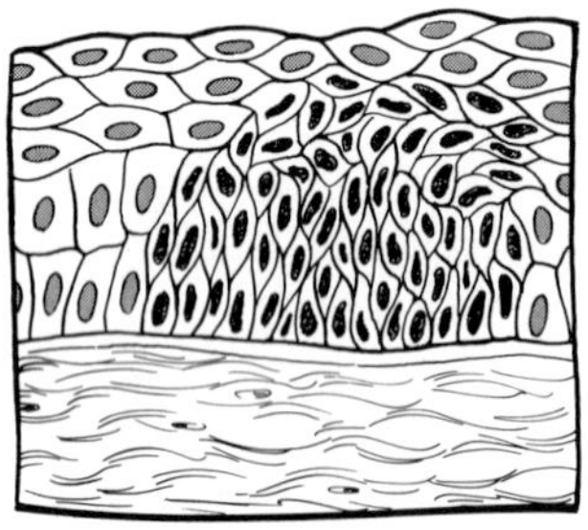 Conjunctival dysplasia	Disturbed	Deep layers of epithelium
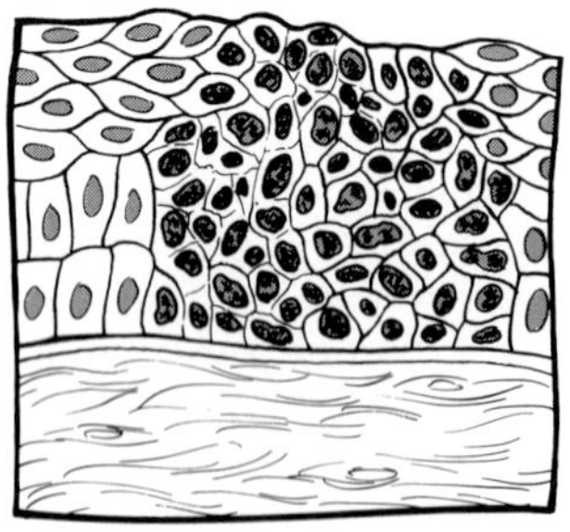 Carcinoma in situ	Disturbed	Entire thickness of epithelium
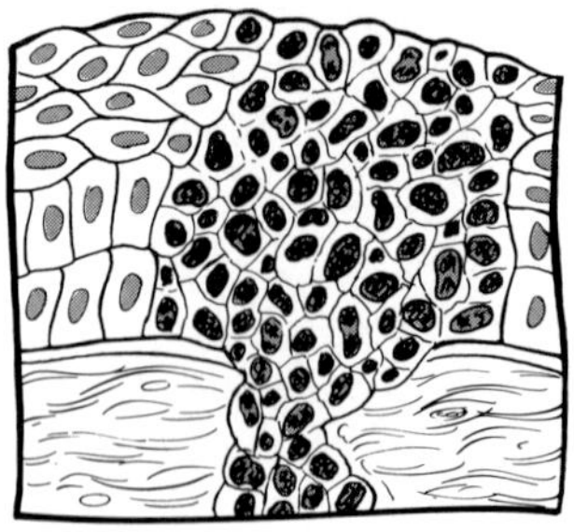 Squamous cell carcinoma	Disturbed	Entire thickness—breaking through basement membrane

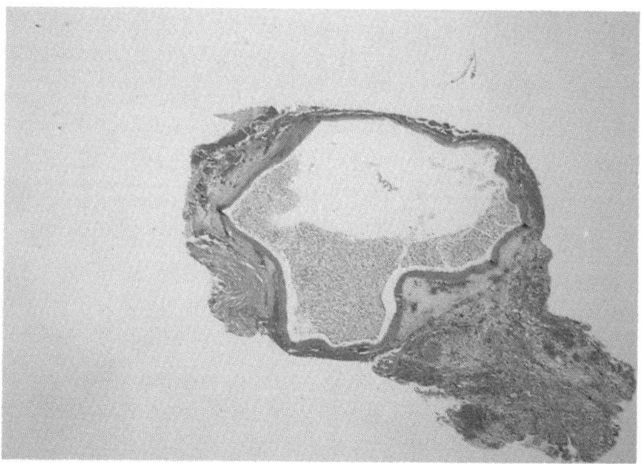

Figure 181–5. Epithelial inclusion cyst—conjunctival cyst filled with keratinizing squamous epithelium surrounding eosinophilic material. H&E, ×1.25.

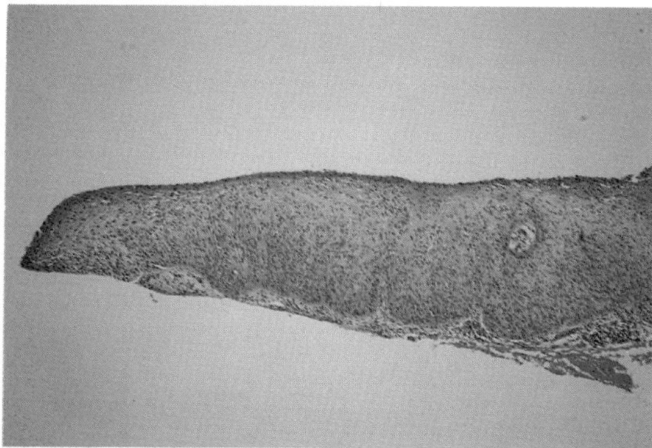

Figure 181–7. Squamous cell carcinoma in situ demonstrating proliferation of atypical squamous cells with loss of polarity confined to the epithelium. The basement epithelium is intact. H&E, ×4.

shaped plaques occur on the conjunctiva. Similar lesions may occur on the oral mucosa. Acanthosis and dyskeratosis cause thickening of the epithelium. Papillomas may be flat, elevated, or polypoid. Histopathologic examination reveals a fibrovascular core surrounded by hyperplastic nonkeratinized squamous epithelium (Fig. 181–6). Inverted follicular keratosis is another benign epithelial tumor.

Clinical examination of conjunctival dysplasia reveals thickening or keratinization (leukoplakia) of the conjunctiva. Histopathologic examination reveals alteration in the polarity of cells with disturbance of cellular maturation. Acanthosis, cellular atypia, and an increase in nuclear:cytoplasmic ratio may be noted. The deeper or basal epithelial layers are usually involved.

Carcinoma in situ may resemble conjunctival dysplasia clinically and histopathologically. However, on histopathologic examination, the entire thickness of the epithelium is involved in carcinoma in situ (Fig. 181–7). In addition, the affected area may be thickened and demonstrate pleomorphism of the epithelium with increased mitotic figures.

Squamous cell carcinoma usually occurs in a juxtalimbal location, with conjunctival thickening, leukoplakia, and vascularization. The abnormality is not confined to the epithelium alone but breaks through the basement membrane to involve the substantia propria and can invade the cornea and sclera. Metastasis is rare, and invasive tendency is low. Conjunctival scraping for cytologic examination can be helpful in identifying dysplasia, carcinoma in situ, and squamous cell carcinoma.[37]

Mucoepidermoid carcinoma is a tumor combining squamous cells and keratin with mucus-secreting cells. Histochemical stains for mucin can confirm the diagnosis. Mucoepidermoid carcinoma is more locally aggressive than squamous cell carcinoma and may demonstrate an early recurrence and an increased incidence of intraocular and orbital invasion.[38]

Kaposi's sarcoma is a malignant vascular tumor that is typically encountered in patients with AIDS. Histopathologically, the tumor is similar to a pyogenic granuloma with vascular proliferation that has undergone malignant transformation. Neoplastic capillary formations are admixed with malignant pleomorphic spindle cells (Fig. 181–8). Tumor cells may stain positive for

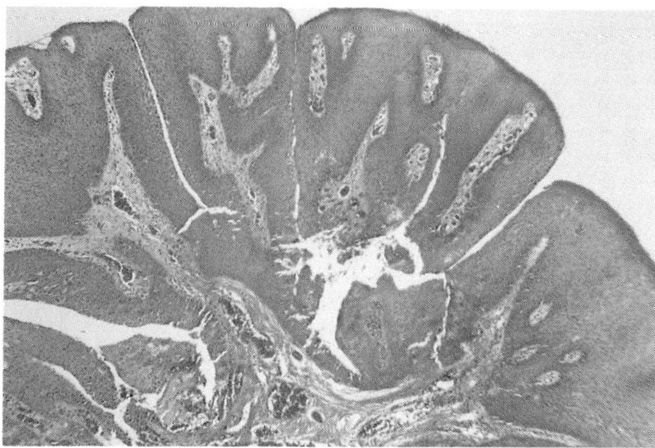

Figure 181–6. Conjunctival papilloma with finger-like projections of acanthotic conjunctival epithelium surround a central fibrovascular core. H&E, ×4.

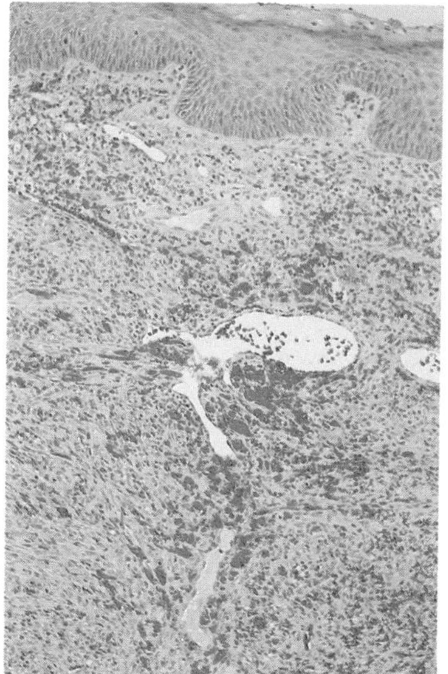

Figure 181–8. Kaposi's sarcoma with proliferation of abnormal capillary formations lined by malignant pleomorphic spindle cells. H&E, ×10.

Factor VIII.[39] Angiosarcoma is a vascular conjunctival tumor that may be associated with a similar orbital lesion. Metastasis may occur in up to 20 percent of cases.[40]

Pigmented lesions may be congenital or acquired, benign or malignant (Table 181–3). Nevi are the most frequent conjunctival tumor. These are divided into five categories, depending on clinical and histopathologic characteristics. These congenital tumors are composed of nevus cells, but pigmentation may not occur until early adulthood. Pigmentation may increase after puberty and result in apparent growth of the tumor. This alone is not evidence of malignant transformation. The nevus cells have a tendency to form nests. Fifty percent of conjunctival nevi also demonstrate cyst formation. Despite the many differentiating characteristics from malignant lesions, more than one-third of surgically excised conjunctival tumors are diagnosed histopathologically as nevi.[41]

Junctional, subepithelial, and compound nevi are clinically indistinguishable. All move with the conjunctiva over the sclera. These lesions are differentiated on the basis of the depth of the nevus cell proliferation. By contrast, the blue nevus and the lesion of melanosis oculi do not move with the conjunctiva. The cells in these lesions are more elongated and spindle shaped and have more prominent branching processes than the other nevus cells.[42] In addition, these cells are found in a deeper subepithelial location. Junctional, subepithelial, and compound nevi are brown, compared with the blue, dark-gray appearance of the blue nevus or melanosis oculi. Nevus of Ota or congenital oculodermal melanocytosis occurs when a blue nevus of the periorbital skin is associated with a conjunctival blue nevus. This condition is more frequent in Asians and blacks.

The malignant potential of the different classes of nevi also varies. Junctional and compound nevi have a low malignant potential, whereas a subepithelial nevus may not have any malignant predisposition. The blue nevus is only considered to have malignant potential if it is very cellular. It is then classified as a cellular blue nevus. Congenital melanocytosis and congenital oculodermal melanocytosis in white patients are associated with an increased chance of uveal malignant melanoma. Only rarely does conjunctival melanoma occur.[43]

Acquired melanosis manifests in middle age as a

Table 181–3. BENIGN PIGMENTED CONJUNCTIVAL LESIONS

Type	Moves with Conjunctiva	Color	Malignant Potential
Junctional nevus	Yes	Brown	Low
Subepithelial nevus	Yes	Brown	Possibly none
Compound nevus	Yes	Brown	Low

Table 181–3. BENIGN PIGMENTED CONJUNCTIVAL LESIONS *Continued*

Type	Moves with Conjunctiva	Color	Malignant Potential
Blue nevus	No	Dark blue/gray	Malignant potential if cellular blue nevus
Melanosis oculi	No	Dark blue/gray	In whites, increased uveal melanoma, rarely conjunctival melanoma
Primary acquired melanosis	Yes (if no associated conjunctival malignancy)	Brown speckled (may wax and wane)	25% for all PAM 75% for PAM with atypia

PAM, primary acquired melanosis.

speckled brown conjunctival pigmentation. The lesion moves with the conjunctiva over the sclera. It may wax and wane, recede, or even enlarge while remaining benign. However, the lesion may become malignant. Benign acquired melanosis may be a clinicopathologic diagnosis because it can frequently resemble a junctional nevus (Fig. 181–9). However, the onset of acquired melanosis is at age 40 to 50 yr, whereas junctional nevi first appear at a much younger age. On histopathologic examination of the acquired melanosis lesion, few to many nevus cells may be found in the junctional area. However, if these cells appear markedly atypical or there is evidence of superficial invasion into the substantia propria, the diagnosis of malignant melanoma must be entertained.[44] Primary acquired melanosis (PAM) with atypia has been noted to evolve to melanoma. This is especially true when epithelioid cells are noted or basilar hyperplasia is not prominent.[45]

According to Zimmerman, 50 percent of conjunctival melanomas arise de novo and 50 percent arise from acquired melanosis or conjunctival nevi.[46, 47] More melanomas arise from junctional or compound nevi than from acquired melanosis. However, the mortality rate from a conjunctival melanoma arising from PAM or de novo is 40 percent, compared with a mortality rate of

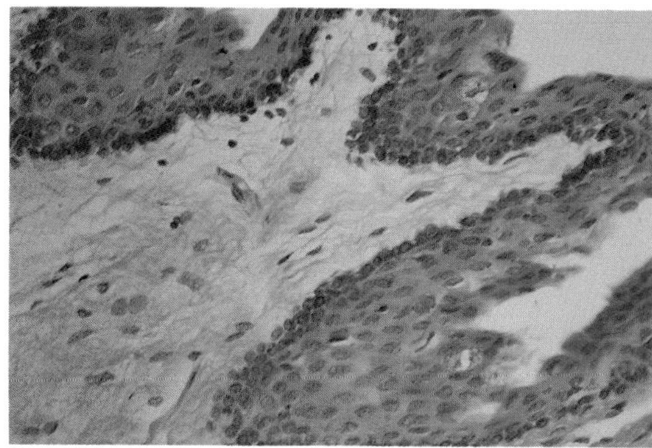

Figure 181–9. Primary acquired melanosis in which benign-appearing pigmented cells are noted in the basal layers of the conjunctival epithelium. H&E, ×25.

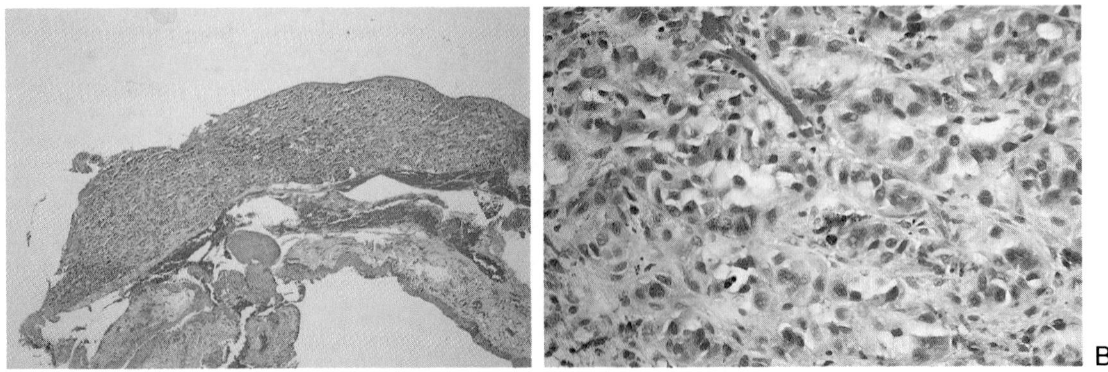

Figure 181–10. *A* and *B*, Conjunctival melanoma with proliferation of pleomorphic cells involving the entire epithelium, with loss of normal polarity, invading through the basement membrane into the substantia propria. *A*, H&E, ×2.5. *B*, H&E, ×25.

20 percent if the origin was a conjunctival nevus.[48] Histopathologic features have prognostic significance for patients' survival (Fig. 181–10 *A* and *B*). Metastasis is increased in invasive melanomas that are greater than 0.8 mm thick. Jakobiec reports that the presence of a pagetoid growth pattern in patients with PAM and conjunctival melanoma is the single most sensitive histologic feature associated with death. Patients with pagetoid growth in the PAM component had a 44 percent mortality rate, compared with a 25 percent mortality rate in all conjunctival melanomas. Other risk factors for death include involvement of the palpebral, caruncular, or forniceal conjunctiva and invasion of the episclera, sclera, or cornea.[49]

CORNEAL PATHOLOGY

Corneal tissue examined in the pathology laboratory usually is obtained from penetrating keratoplasty surgery. Corneal biopsies have become a source of histopathologic material requiring specialized techniques to identify fungal or *Acanthamoeba* organisms. Pseudophakic and aphakic bullous keratopathy are the most common diagnoses for excised corneal buttons.[50] Failure of the active metabolic endothelial pump mechanism results in endothelial decompensation, with fluid accumulation in the stroma and epithelium. Stromal edema may result in separation of the collagen lamella with stromal thickening and loss of transparency, which are noted on clinical examination. Chronic inflammation and scarring may follow. Epithelial edema first occurs intracellularly and then intercellularly. Further progression may lead to bullae formation, separation of the basement membrane from the epithelium, basement membrane disruption and reduplication, and pannus formation (Fig. 181–11). Corneal opacification caused by stromal edema may make clinical examination of the endothelium difficult, although Descemet's membrane folds may still be evident. Histopathologic examination may reveal loss of endothelial cells (Fig. 181–12) and intracellular endothelial edema with vacuolation. Descemet's membrane may be thickened. The endothelium may undergo metaplasia, resulting in posterior collagenous membrane formation (Fig. 181–13). Prolonged edema may result in superficial and deep vascularization.

Congenital Corneal Abnormalities

Abnormalities of the corneal size and shape may occur congenitally. Microcornea is usually autosomal dominant and may be associated with other abnormalities. The horizontal diameter of the cornea is shortened to less than 11 mm, causing steepening of the cornea and shortening of the anterior segment. Megalocornea is usually inherited in a recessive X-linked fashion and is frequently an isolated bilateral abnormality. The corneal diameter is greater than 13 mm. Cornea plana may demonstrate autosomal dominant or autosomal recessive inheritance. It is frequently associated with other ocular abnormalities such as posterior embryotoxin and congenital iris and lens anomalies. The corneal curvature is flattened, so the corneal diameter may appear decreased. Unlike microcornea and megalocornea, corneal plana demonstrates many histopathologic changes, including epithelial keratinization, defects of Bowman's layer, stromal scarring, and vascularization. Corneal opacification may cause reduced visual acuity.

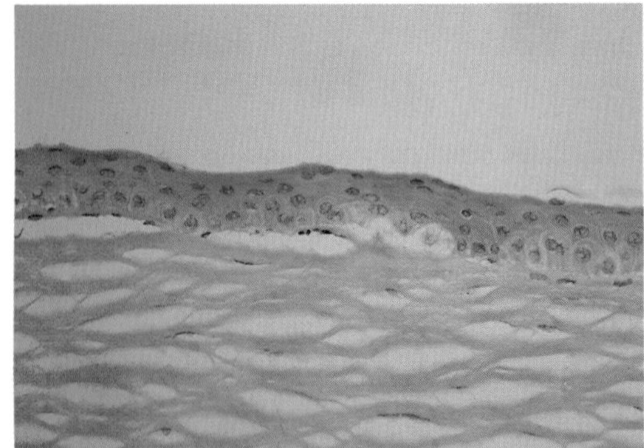

Figure 181–11. Aphakic bullous keratopathy with edema of the basal epithelial cells, intraepithelial and subepithelial cysts in a corneal specimen from a patient with aphakic bullous keratopathy. H&E, ×25.

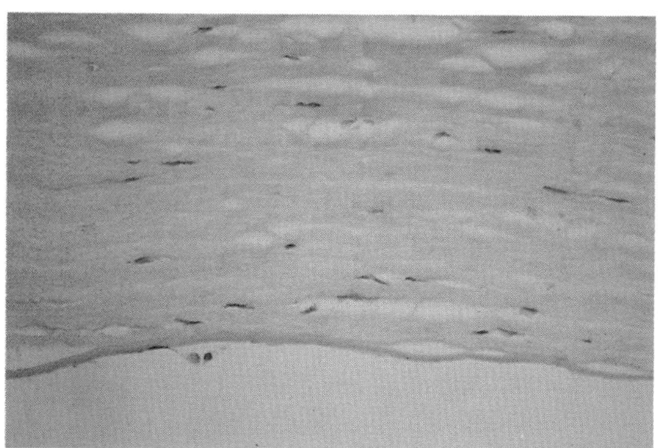

Figure 181–12. Only rare endothelial cells are noted in this corneal specimen from a patient with aphakic bullous keratopathy. H&E, ×25.

Congenital corneal opacities may result from anterior cleavage anomalies and may be associated with abnormalities of the iridocorneal angle and iris. Sclerocornea results in bilateral opacification and vascularization of the cornea so that it resembles the adjacent sclera. The extent of the condition can vary so that the abnormality involves only the peripheral cornea or the entire cornea. Associated anomalies, such as nystagmus, strabismus, aniridia, cornea plana, glaucoma, and microphthalmos, may occur. Electron microscopic examination reveals random orientation of collagen fibers of various diameters. Both congenital hereditary endothelial dystrophy and congenital hereditary stromal dystrophy can result in complete corneal opacification.

Congenital corneal opacities have been divided into three groups: (1) peripheral; (2) central combined with a lens anomaly; and (3) central and peripheral opacities, as well as iris stromal and trabecular meshwork abnormalities.[51]

Peripheral forms of the anterior chamber cleavage syndrome include posterior embryotoxin and Rieger's syndrome. Posterior embryotoxin or Axenfeld's anomaly is noted in 15 to 30 percent of normal eyes.[52] Schwalbe's line is visible on clinical examination because the termination of Descemet's membrane is more central and enlarged. Although usually sporadic, autosomal recessive and dominant inheritance patterns have been reported. When posterior embryotoxin is associated with iris processes inserting into Schwalbe's ring, Axenfeld's anomaly is diagnosed. Fifty percent of patients may develop glaucoma. Rieger's syndrome is generally an autosomal dominant condition. Prominence of the Schwalbe's ring with attached iris strands is associated with iris stromal hypoplasia, pupillary anomalies, and iridocorneal adhesions. Fifty percent of patients may develop glaucoma. Facial, dental, and bony abnormalities may be present.

Peters' anomaly is usually inherited as an autosomal recessive trait. Bilateral central corneal opacification with local absence of Descemet's membrane and endothelium and abnormalities of the deep stroma are noted. Anomalies of the anterior segment include iridolenticular corneal synechiae and anterior polar cataract. Twenty percent of cases are unilateral. In the area of iridolenticular adhesion, Descemet's membrane is absent and Bowman's membrane may also be absent. Von Hippel's internal ulcer is similar to Peters' anomaly, but no lens abnormalities are noted. Because histopathologic evidence may suggest inflammation, the presumed cause is intrauterine infection. Posterior keratoconus is a unilateral sporadic condition characterized by posterior umbilication of the central cornea, causing thinning of the posterior stroma. Descemet's membrane is present but may be thick enough to rupture subsequently. In addition, Bowman's membrane may also be absent.[53]

Forceps injury to the cornea may result in Descemet's breaks due to ocular compression. Corneal edema resolves, and regeneration of Descemet's membrane results in visible vertical folds. Histopathologic examination demonstrates focal thickening of Descemet's membrane, indicating the prior area of rupture.

Keratitis

Keratitis may occur on an infectious or an autoimmune basis. Invasion of inflammatory cells may lead to scarring in nonulcerative keratitis. Destruction of corneal tissue, including epithelium, Bowman's membrane, and stroma, is the characteristic change found in ulcerative keratitis.

Nonulcerative keratitis can involve the superficial epithelium, Bowman's layer, or stroma. Damage and erosion of the superficial epithelial cells may result from direct trauma, toxicity from topical medication, inflammation, or corneal dystrophy. Histopathologic examination demonstrates vacuolation of the epithelium, loss of hemidesmosomes, detachment from the basement membrane, and possible lymphocytic infiltration.[54]

NONULCERATIVE

Dendritic keratitis may be found in infection with herpes simplex or herpes zoster or in type II tyrosinemia. In herpes simplex, which is the most common cause of dendritic keratitis, intranuclear epithelial inclusions may

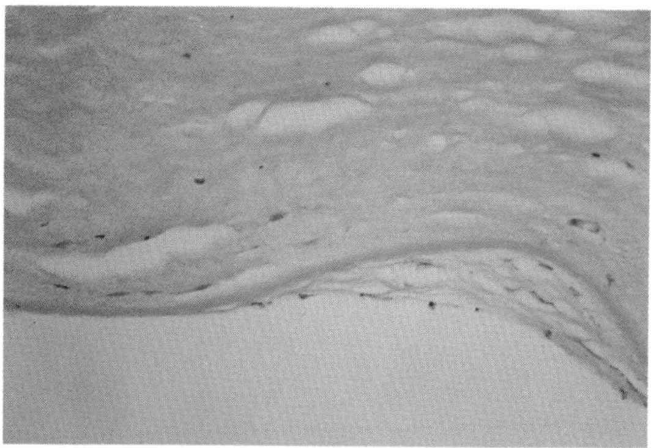

Figure 181–13. Posterior collagenous membrane or retrocorneal membrane noted posterior to Descemet's membrane with paucity of endothelial cells. H&E, ×25.

be noted. Subepithelial keratitis can occur after epidemic keratoconjunctivitis. Adenovirus 3, 4, 6, 8, and 19 may cause subepithelial coarse deposits, with lymphocytic infiltrates noted in Bowman's layer and intranuclear epithelial viral inclusions.[55] Leprosy may cause subepithelial infiltrates, pannus formation, and enlargement of the corneal nerves. In trachoma, Bowman's layer may be replaced by inflammatory infiltrates. Punctate keratitis is seen in superior limbic keratoconjunctivitis, in which the conjunctival epithelium demonstrates dyskeratosis, acanthosis, and inflammatory cell infiltration.

Stromal keratitis can be caused by bacterial, viral, nematode, and protozoal organisms. Congenital syphilis can cause a bilateral deep interstitial keratitis and uveitis in the first or second decade. Resolution of corneal vascularization results in ghost vessels. Acute edema, collagen necrosis, and deep lymphocytic infiltration are noted. Band keratopathy, deep vascularization, thickening of Descemet's membrane, and formation of concentrically laminated Descemet's scrolls may subsequently result.[56] Acquired syphilis occurs unilaterally approximately 10 yr after infection and results in a sectoral interstitial keratitis. Tuberculosis and leprosy are other bacterial causes of interstitial keratitis. Stromal keratitis can result from herpes simplex virus. Modified indirect immunoperoxidase techniques may be used to detect cells infected with this virus.[57]

Interstitial keratitis in Cogan's syndrome is similar histopathologically to syphilitic interstitial keratitis. However, these patients have negative syphilis serologies and concomitant vestibular auditory symptoms.

Onchocerciasis is caused by nematode infestation resulting in superficial punctate keratitis, deep interstitial keratitis, secondary glaucoma, optic neuritis, and chorioretinitis. This major cause of world blindness results from penetration of the *O. volvulus* adult worm through the skin to the ocular tissue. These filarial nematodes are surrounded by lymphocytic and plasma cell infiltration in the cornea.[9, 58]

Ophthalmia nodosa results from ocular implantation of insect or plant hairs, causing nodular conjunctivitis and interstitial keratitis. Caterpillar hairs are a frequent cause of this condition.[59]

Protozoal diseases such as leishmaniasis, trypanosomiasis, nosematosis, and *Acanthamoeba* infection may cause interstitial keratitis. *Acanthamoeba* infection usually occurs in contact lens wearers with poor contact lens hygiene. Epithelial keratitis, patchy stromal infiltrates, and radial keratoneuritis precede the classic ring infiltrate. The organism exists in an active trophozoite or an inactive cyst form. Early diagnosis is imperative for successful treatment of the disease. The organism is notoriously difficult to culture and may not be apparent with commonly used stains. Corneal biopsy may be needed to identify it. Trophozoite and cyst forms can be rapidly stained with calcofluor white stain (Fig. 181–14*A*, *B*, and *C*). With the epifluorescence microscope, the cyst walls stain green and the trophozoites stain red.[60] Corneal biopsy may demonstrate *Acanthamoeba* organisms and chronic inflammatory cell infiltrate. Immunofluorescent stains may aid in identification of the organism.[61–65]

ULCERATIVE

Ulcerative keratitis may be secondary to infection or autoimmune phenomena. In infectious processes, an epithelial defect may allow bacterial or fungal invasion. Proteolytic enzymes cause stromal necrosis and corneal

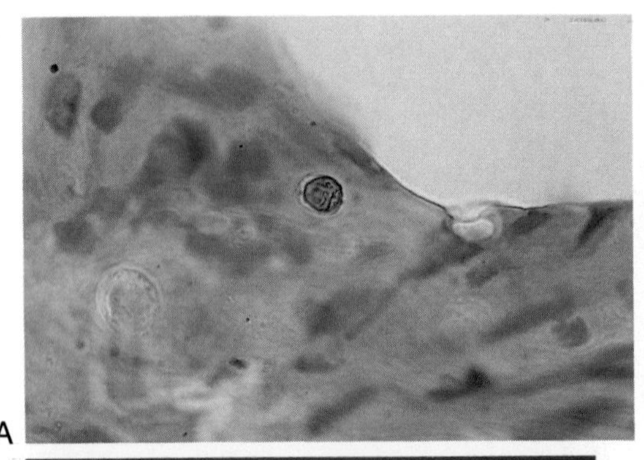

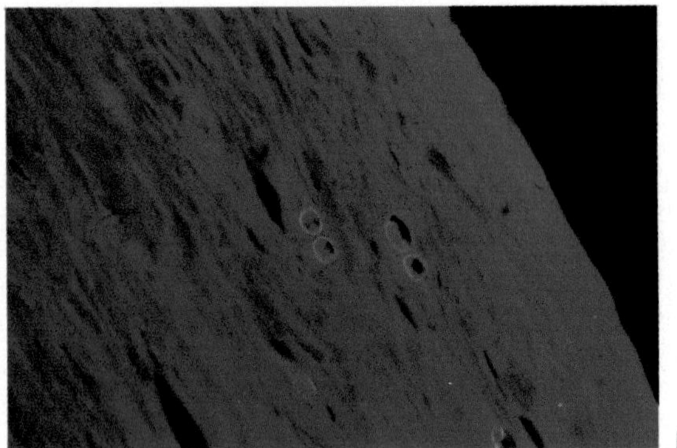

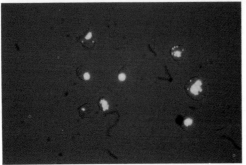

Figure 181–14. *Acanthamoeba castellanii. A,* Many acanthamoeba cysts demonstrated within the corneal scraping. Gram's stain. *B, A. castellanii* cysts within the corneal tissues. Calcofluor white stain. *C, A. castellanii* trophozoites with internalized FITC-labeled latex B. (*A, B,* and *C,* courtesy of Robert E. Silvany, The University of Texas, Southwestern Medical Center at Dallas.)

thinning. If there is inextricable progression of the necrosis, the stroma may completely dissolve so that only Descemet's membrane remains. Intraocular pressure may cause this descemetocele to bulge forward with corneal ectasia. As the necrotic process continues with invasion of polymorphonuclear leukocytes and lymphocytes, corneal perforation may result. If macrophages and fibroblasts become the prominent cellular element, then scarring and vascularization result.

Ulcerative keratopathies without infectious causes include marginal, phlyctenular, and ring ulcers. The limbal marginal ulcer that frequently develops is an allergic reaction to *Staphylococcus* toxin. Histopathologic examination of the marginal ulcer reveals an area of epithelial and stromal necrosis with invasion by lymphocytes and plasma cells. The ring ulcer may develop from circumferential spread of the marginal ulcer or may result from ischemia. Occlusive vasculitis in Wegener's granulomatosis may result in ring ulceration. Histopathologic examination may confirm occlusive vasculitis as well as infiltration by plasma cells, lymphocytes, and neutrophils.[66]

Peripheral marginal degenerations include Terrien's degeneration and Mooren's ulcer. Terrien's is a bilateral thinning of the peripheral cornea that usually begins superiorly and slowly spreads circumferentially. The epithelium remains intact while the stroma thins and is invaded by blood vessels and lipid. Histopathologic examination reveals fibrinoid degeneration and vascularization of the thinned corneal stroma. Lymphocyte and plasmacytic infiltration may be present.[67, 68] Mooren's ulcer is a unilateral progressive marginal guttering that may cause extensive corneal necrosis. On histopathologic examination, the epithelium and Bowman's layer are necrotic, vascularization of the cornea is seen, and only minimal inflammatory cell infiltration is noted.

Infectious ulcerative keratitis may be caused by bacterial, viral, or fungal organisms. Bacterial or fungal invasion frequently occurs after the epithelium has been débrided. However, diphtheria bacillus and *Neisseria gonorrhoeae* can infiltrate and attack the epithelial layers. Initial infiltration by polymorphonuclear leukocytes may be followed by stromal necrosis. Fungal ulceration may occur in an immunocompromised host or after trauma from plant matter. Satellite lesions occur near the central ulceration. Organisms are most readily retrieved from the wall and not the central crater. Fungi can be demonstrated by PAS, Gomori's, methenamine silver, and Gridley's stains. On histopathologic examination, microabscesses around the ulcer are frequently granulomatous. However, there may be evidence of nongranulomatous or acute inflammatory cellular material.

The most common central corneal ulcer is produced by herpes simplex. The virus can cause deep stromal keratitis without ulceration (disciform) or with ulceration (metaherpetic), superficial epithelial keratitis, uveitis, or keratouveitis. Immunologic factors may produce a disciform keratitis because live viral particles are not found in the stroma. Bowman's membrane is degenerated, the stroma is necrotic, and endothelium may be involved. Metaherpetic keratitis is marked by thinning of the stroma, peripheral vascularization, and possible endothelial decompensation. In herpetic infection, viral particles may be found in the corneal epithelium. Multinucleated giant cells may be present in the corneal stroma. Granulomatous reaction to Descemet's membrane may be noted in herpes simplex or herpes zoster infection.[69, 70] Herpes zoster may cause ulcerative keratitis or dendritic keratitis. Intranuclear viral inclusion bodies may be noted.

Corneal Dystrophies

Corneal dystrophies are hereditary diseases with bilateral corneal opacification. These disorders are classified by the layer of corneal involvement and the type of abnormal deposit. Specialized stains allow identification of the corneal dystrophy. Corneal dystrophies involving the epithelial layer include Meesman's dystrophy, Cogan's microcystic dystrophy (map, dot, fingerprint), primary hereditary band keratopathy, and Vogt's anterior crocodile shagreen.

Meesman's (Stocker-Holt) dystrophy is inherited as an autosomal dominant trait and may appear within the first few years of life. Intraepithelial cysts are noted on clinical examination. Light microscopy reveals that the cysts are filled with cellular debris and PAS-staining substance. Further characterization of this peculiar substance by electron microscopy reveals that it is a homogeneous substance derived from tonofilaments. The basement membrane may be thickened, but the underlying corneal tissues are unaffected. It is possible that a disturbance of the cytoplasmic ground substance results in cellular homogenization with cyst formation.[71, 72]

Cogan's microcystic dystrophy may be inherited as an autosomal dominant trait and usually afflicts older women. Three clinical forms—map, dot, or fingerprint—can occur independently or simultaneously. In the dot form, gray central opacities are caused by the presence of intra- and interepithelial microcysts. Fingerprint lesions result from reduplication of the epithelial basement membrane. Map pattern may be caused by multilamination of the basement membrane and collagen formation.[73, 74]

Corneal verticillata (Fleischer-Gruber) is a bilateral whorl-like corneal epithelial opacification found in Fabry's disease. This X-linked recessive hereditary disease manifests a deficiency of the enzyme α-galactosidase, resulting in intracellular accumulation of ceramide trihexoside. This glycolipid accumulates in corneal epithelial vacuoles. The vortex-like pattern of opacification may result from basement membrane reduplication and accentuation of the normal centripetal growth pattern.[75, 76]

Reis-Bücklers dystrophy is a dominantly inherited dystrophy that manifests within the first decade of life with subepithelial opacities. A honeycomb pattern of opacification with scarring eventually leads to visual decrease by the fifth decade. Histopathologic examination of the cornea reveals epithelial thinning, PAS deposition on the focally disrupted basement membrane. Recurrent erosive episodes may result from loss of

Table 181–4. STROMAL CORNEAL DYSTROPHIES

Dystrophy	Hereditary	Abnormal Substance	Histochemistry	Electron Microscopy
Macular	Autosomal recessive	Glycosaminoglycans (keratin sulfate)	Colloidal iron—blue Alcian blue—blue PAS—pink	Membrane-bound vacuoles with fibrillogranular material (peculiar substance)
Lattice	Autosomal dominant	Amyloid	Congo red—orange-red (birefringence and dichroism with Congo red) Thioflavine T—green (fluorescence with thioflavine T) Metachromasia with crystal violet PAS—pink-red Masson's trichrome—red	Nonbranching microfibrils
Granular	Autosomal dominant	Hyalin	Masson's trichrome—bright red PAS—weak pink H & E—pink	Electron-dense rhomboid-shaped rods
Fleck	Autosomal dominant	Glycosaminoglycans Lipid	Colloidal iron—blue Alcian blue—blue Sudan black—black Oil red O—red	Membrane-bound vacuoles with fibrillogranular material +/− electron-dense deposits
Schnyder's	Autosomal dominant	Lipid, triglyceride, and cholesterol	Sudan black—black Oil red O—red	+/− cholesterol crystals
Pre-Descemet's membrane (cornea farinata)	Autosomal dominant	Lipid-like material (lipofuscin?)	Sudan black—black Oil red O—red	Membrane-bound vacuoles with fibrillogranular material and electron-dense deposits

hemidesmosomes and poor epithelial adhesion.[77] Electron microscopy demonstrates peculiar curly material with a 100-nm length in the subepithelial fibrous tissue, which parallels the distribution of attachment proteins.[78]

The classic triad of corneal stromal dystrophies includes macular, granular, and lattice dystrophies (Table 181–4). Congenital hereditary stromal dystrophy, hereditary fleck dystrophy (Francois Neetans), Schnyder's dystrophy, and cornea farinata are also included.

Macular dystrophy is unusual because it is inherited as an autosomal recessive trait, unlike most of the other corneal dystrophies. Visual decrease may result by the fourth decade because of focal stromal opacification with clouding of the intervening corneal stroma. In some patients, an enzymatic defect of keratin sulfate degradation may be present.[79, 80] Basophilic substance is noted in Bowman's layer, in keratocytes, between stromal lamellae, and in the endothelial cells. This substance stains positively for acid mucopolysaccharide with alcian blue stain (Fig. 181–15). Secondary corneal guttata may be present.

Lattice dystrophy is inherited as an autosomal dominant trait and may begin in the first decade. Lattice-shaped lines in the anterior stroma and recurrent erosion may occur. By the fifth decade of life, reduction of visual acuity may necessitate corneal transplantation. On histopathologic examination, amyloid deposits are noted in the stroma, mostly superficially. Focal hypertrophy and atrophy of the epithelium are noted. Electron microscopy shows nonpolarizing, thinned, nonaligned filaments and polarizing normally aligned filaments. The amyloid deposits have characteristic staining properties (Fig. 181–16*A* and *B*).[81, 82] When hereditary systemic amyloidosis is associated with lattice dystrophy, Meretoja's syndrome is present. Unlike the isolated lattice dystrophy, Meretoja's syndrome does not result in recurrent erosions but does affect the peripheral cornea. Amyloid deposits may be noted in Bowman's layer and throughout the stroma.[83]

Granular dystrophy is an autosomal dominant inherited condition and is the most common stromal dystrophy of the cornea. It may occur in the first decade of life, with snowflake stromal axial deposits with clear intervening stroma. Good visual acuity may be maintained until middle age. These hyaline deposits stain well with Masson's trichrome (Fig. 181–17). The depos-

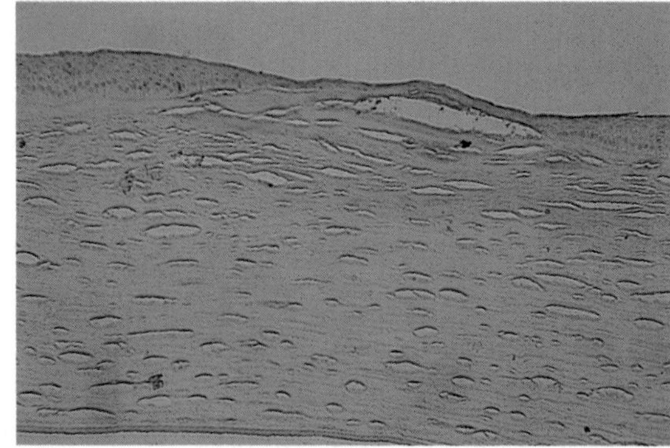

Figure 181–15. Macular dystrophy in which abnormal deposits of acid mucopolysaccharide stain blue with alcian blue stain. Alcian blue, ×10.

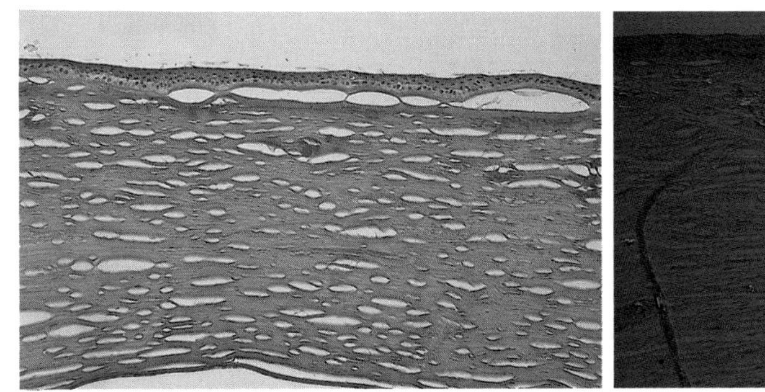
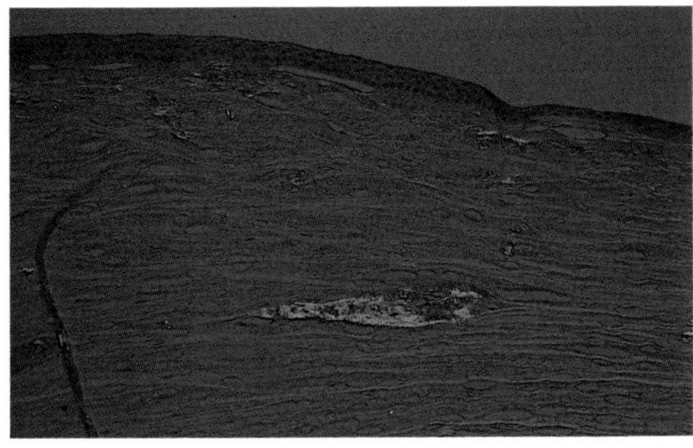

Figure 181–16. Lattice dystrophy. *A*, Amyloid deposits stain dark pink with PAS. PAS, ×10. *B*, Polarization of Congo red–stained section reveals yellow-orange amyloid deposits. Congo red, ×10.

its may be present throughout the stroma but are usually more prominent anteriorly. Intraepithelial rod and trapezoidal crystalline granules may be noted on electron microscopic examination of recurrent cases.[84]

Fleck dystrophy (dystrophy mouchetée of Francois Neetans), is an autosomal dominant inherited dystrophy with bilateral small stromal circular and punctate opacities. Histopathologic examination reveals positive staining for alcian blue, colloidal iron, oil red O, and Sudan stain, demonstrating the presence of mucopolysaccharide and lipid.[85]

Cornea farinata (pre-Descemet's membrane dystrophy) may be an autosomal dominant inherited condition. Bilateral pre-Descemet's opacities appear by the seventh decade and do not interfere with vision. Intracytoplasmic inclusions are filled with PAS-positive material and are noted in the pre-Descemet's keratocytes.[86]

Schnyder's central stromal crystalline dystrophy may be a misnomer because only 50 percent of patients demonstrate the classic corneal cholesterol crystals.[86a–88] This autosomal dominant inherited dystrophy may demonstrate bilateral ringlike central corneal opacities, diffuse corneal haze, anterior stromal crystals, or prominent arcus lipoides. Although many affected patients have systemic hyperlipidemia, Schnyder's dystrophy is thought to be a localized abnormality of cholesterol metabolism resulting in cholesterol deposition in the cornea. The cholesterol deposits have previously been described as affecting only the superficial stroma. However, newer histopathologic studies demonstrate abnormal accumulations of lipid, triglyceride, and cholesterol in the basal epithelium, Bowman's membrane, and throughout the corneal stroma up to Descemet's membrane (Fig. 181–18). Specialized staining techniques using oil red O, which stains esterified cholesterol and triglycerides, and the fluorescent cholesterol probe filipin (Fig. 181–19*A* and *B*), which stains only unesterified cholesterol, reveal that all three substances may be present in these corneas.[89, 90]

Congenital hereditary stromal dystrophy of the cornea may be inherited in an autosomal dominant fashion and manifests nonprogressive bilateral corneal opacification. Histopathologic examination demonstrates abnormal clefting of the stromal lamella.[91, 92]

Polymorphic stromal dystrophy is bilateral and may not have a hereditary component. It may actually be a corneal degeneration. On histopathologic examination, the posterior filamentous opacities stain positive for amyloid.[93]

Corneal endothelial dystrophies include Fuchs' dystrophy, congenital hereditary endothelial dystrophy, and posterior polymorphous dystrophy. Corneal guttata are excrescences in Descemet's membrane of the central cornea. Histopathologically, these appear similar to the Hassal–Henle warts that occur in the corneal periphery as an aging phenomenon. Corneal guttata can be associated with endothelial decompensation. When epithelial involvement occurs because of endothelial decom-

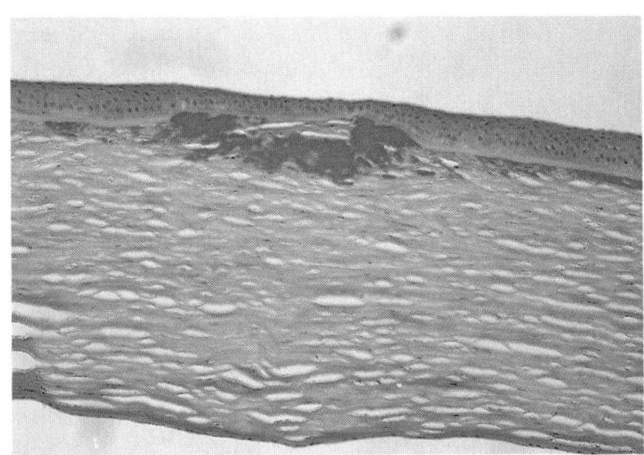
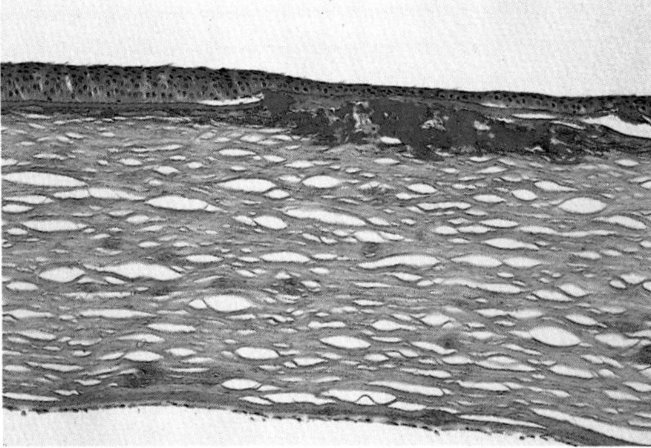

Figure 181–17. Granular dystrophy. *A*, Hyalin deposits stain dark pink with H&E. H&E, ×10. *B*, Hyalin deposits stain bright red with Masson's trichrome stain. Masson's trichrome, ×10.

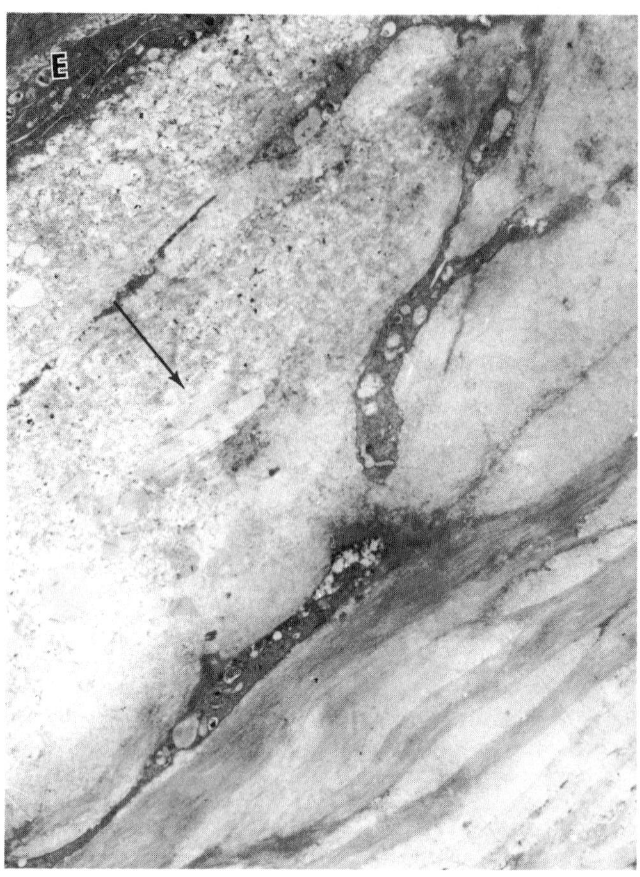

Figure 181–18. Electron micrograph reveals accumulation of cholesterol crystal *(arrow)* and lipid in Bowman's layer in Schnyder's dystrophy. An edge of epithelium (E) is indicated. ×14,200. (Courtesy of Weiss JS, Rodrigues MM, Kruth HS, et al: Panstromal Schnyder's corneal dystrophy: Ultrastructural and histochemical studies. Ophthalmology 99:1072, 1992.)

pensation, the patient has Fuchs' dystrophy. This condition is usually encountered in older women and may occur as an autosomal dominant trait. Histopathologic examination reveals epithelial edema with cyst and bullae formation, thickening of the basement membrane, stromal edema and scarring, thickening of Descemet's membrane, corneal guttata, and loss of endothelial cells.[94, 95] The histopathologic changes in Fuchs' dystrophy may appear identical to those found in aphakic or pseudophakic corneal edema, except for the presence of corneal guttata, which are usually noted in Fuchs' dystrophy.

Congenital hereditary endothelial dystrophy is usually inherited as an autosomal recessive trait, but autosomal

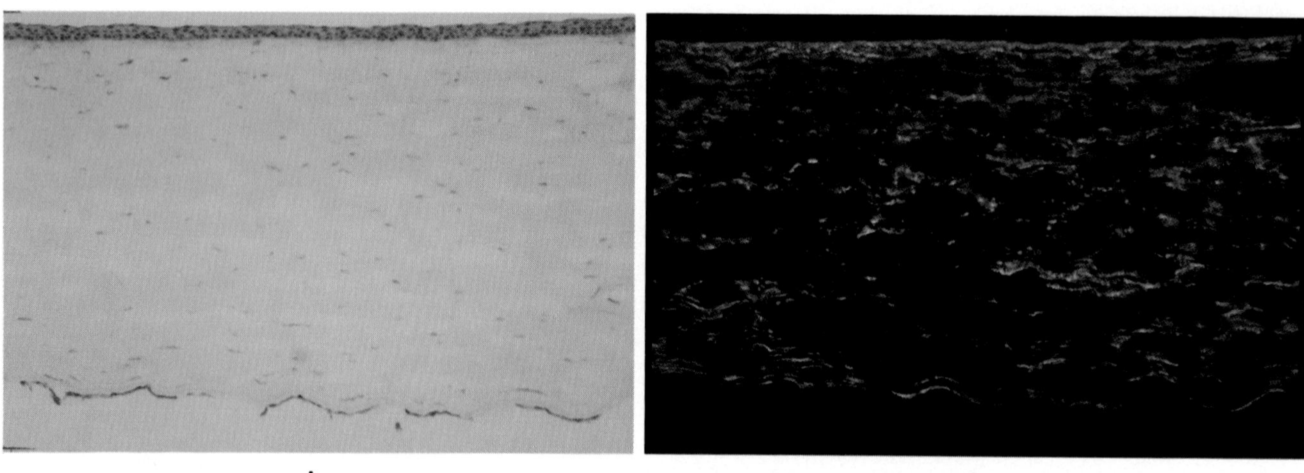

Figure 181–19. Schnyder's cornea stained with filipin and hematoxylin. Heavy deposits of filipin-stained lipid (unesterified cholesterol) are noted throughout the corneal stroma. Fluorescent *(A)* and brightfield *(B)* image of the same microscopic field. ×40. (Courtesy of Weiss JS, Rodrigues MM, Kruth HS, et al: Panstromal Schnyder's corneal dystrophy: Ultrastructural and histochemical studies. Ophthalmology 99:1072, 1992.)

dominant inheritance has been reported. Congenital bilateral corneal opacification and edema may progress. Histopathologic examination reveals loss of endothelial cells and abnormalities of Descemet's membrane. Epithelial and stromal edema is noted.[96]

Schlichting's posterior polymorphous dystrophy may be inherited as an autosomal dominant or autosomal recessive trait. Bilateral opacification and vesicle formation are noted in the area of Descemet's membrane and endothelium, causing minimal decrease in visual acuity. On histopathologic examination, Descemet's membrane is thickened, with metaplasia of the endothelium to epithelium-like cells. Electron microscopy of the endothelial layer reveals atypical cells with cytoplasmic filaments,[97, 98] which are characteristic of epithelial cells.

Corneal dystrophies are usually bilateral corneal opacifications without accompanying systemic findings. The exceptions are Meretoja's syndrome and Schnyder's dystrophy. Hereditary metabolic diseases may also result in bilateral corneal opacification and systemic abnormalities, which result from accumulation of the offending substance.

Corneal clouding may occur at a young age in I-H (Hurler's syndrome), I-S (Scheie's syndrome), and VI (Maroteux-Lamy syndrome) mucopolysaccharidoses. Intracytoplasmic vacuoles containing acid mucopolysaccharide are found throughout the cornea and stain positively with Alcian blue stain.[99, 100]

Fabry's disease and Niemann-Pick disease are two of the sphingolipidoses with corneal findings. Membranous inclusions containing lipids are found in the epithelium, keratocytes, and endothelium of patients with Niemann-Pick disease.[101] Corneal clouding may also occur in mucolipidosis II, III, and IV, with accumulation of acid mucopolysaccharide and glycolipid.[25] Urate crystals may be found in the corneal epithelium and subepithelium in gout. Crystalline deposition in cystinosis and alkaptonuria has already been discussed.

Keratoconus is a bilateral corneal dystrophy that may not be hereditary. Corneal ectasia, frequently asymmetric in severity, leads to irregular astigmatism, corneal scarring, and visual loss. On histopathologic examination, the central cornea is thin, with scarring of Bowman's membrane and the corneal stroma. Healed ruptures of Descemet's membrane may be noted in patients who have undergone previous attacks of hydrops.[102] Iron deposition on the corneal epithelium corresponds to the clinical finding of the Fleischer's ring, which surrounds the cone. Generalized thinning of the entire cornea is called *keratoglobus*.[103]

The iridocorneal endothelial (ICE) syndromes are unilateral disorders characterized by migration of abnormal corneal endothelium resulting in a constellation of corneal edema, angle-closure glaucoma, and iris atrophy. The specific name of the disease entity—*Chandler's syndrome, essential iris atrophy*, or *iris nevus (Cogan-Reese) syndrome*—depends on which is the most prominent abnormality. Electron microscopy reveals posterior collagenous membrane formation posterior to Descemet's membrane and degeneration of the endothelial cells with filopodial cytoplasm projections that are suggestive of endothelial migration. Unlike posterior polymorphous dystrophy, the endothelium in the ICE syndromes does not demonstrate any epithelium-like alterations.[104–106] Corneal endothelial abnormalities with stromal edema are most prominent in Chandler's syndrome.[107]

Corneal Degenerations

Corneal degenerations may be secondary to aging, prior disease, or deposition of foreign substances. One of the most common corneal degenerations is arcus senilis, in which a bilateral ring-shaped perilimbal corneal stromal infiltration is present. Peripheral stromal lipid is deposited between Bowman's membrane and Descemet's membrane, with the highest concentration in the midstroma, decreasing toward Bowman's and Descemet's. A clear zone at the limbal edge corresponds to the end of Bowman's layer. Similar histopathologic changes are noted in arcus juvenilis. Patients who are younger than 50 years and have arcus senilis may have hyperlipidemia. In older patients, arcus senilis is not necessarily associated with abnormal cholesterol metabolism.

Pterygium formation is common in warmer climates with increased sun exposure. Bowman's membrane is replaced by areas of basophilic degeneration that are similar to those in pinguecula.

Calcific band keratopathy, a white stippled opacification composed of calcium granules, involves the interpalpebral epithelium and Bowman's layer. On H&E stain, basophilic granules are noted in the epithelial basement membrane, Bowman's layer, and superficial stroma (Fig. 181–20). Small circular clear areas in the opacity represent corneal nerves passing through Bowman's layer. Band keratopathy is associated with ocular disease, including long-standing glaucoma and uveitis in juvenile rheumatoid arthritis. It may occur after corneal injury. Systemic disorders of calcium metabolism, chronic renal failure, hyperparathyroidism, and gout can result in band keratopathy.

Pannus formation may be an inflammatory or degenerative process. Connective tissue, which usually contains blood vessels, invades beneath the corneal epithe-

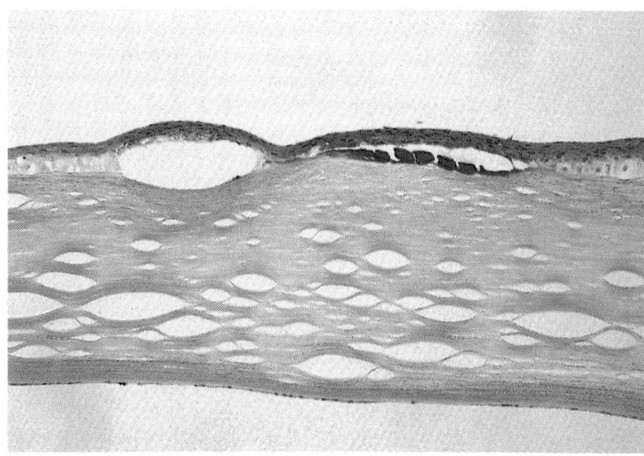

Figure 181–20. Basophilic granules are noted in the area of basement membrane and Bowman's layer in band keratopathy. H&E, ×10.

lium to separate it from Bowman's layer. When pannus is associated with other ocular diseases, fibrous vascular tissue may also be noted. If the pannus results from an inflammatory process, chronic inflammatory cells may invade. In the late stages of both degenerative and inflammatory pannus, scarring may occur.

Vogt's limbal girdle is a bilateral comma-shaped interpalpebral white limbal opacity usually occurring in patients older than 40 yr. Unlike arcus senilis, it affects only the horizontal meridian of the cornea. It does not involve the corneal circumference; it only involves the superficial, not the deep stroma; and it does not spare the limbal margin. Histopathologic changes are similar to those in pinguecula, with fragmentation of elastic fibers as well as basophilic deposition in Bowman's layer and superficial stroma.[108]

Lipid keratopathy may occur after prior ocular injury. Abnormal corneal blood vessels leak yellow-white lipid into the corneal stroma. The lipid may extravasate into the area of pannus between Bowman's layer and the epithelium. Local amyloid deposition may occur in the corneal epithelium, Bowman's layer, vessel wall, and adjacent stroma after ocular disease. Specialized amyloid stains identify this material.[109] Amyloid deposition also occurs in primary amyloidosis, polymorphic stromal dystrophy, and lattice dystrophy.

Spheroidal degeneration has also been called *carotenoid* or *elastotic degeneration, Labrador keratopathy*, and *climatic droplet keratopathy*. The most descriptive name is probably *band-shaped keratopathy* or *noncalcific band keratopathy*, because the yellow corneal spherules occur in a band-shaped area in the superficial cornea near the limbus. This occurs in men older than 50 yr of age and is related to outdoor exposure. Spherical particles resembling oil drops are found in Bowman's layer and superficial stroma. These do not contain lipid. Amorphous hyaline basophilic granules are noted on histopathologic examination.

Salzmann's nodular degeneration usually follows chronic keratitis in older women. An elevated unilateral nodule is noted near areas of previous corneal damage. Histopathologic examination reveals evidence of epithelial hypertrophy and atrophy. Bowman's membrane may be replaced by hyalin-like material.

Corneal degenerations that are primarily epithelial in character include keratitis sicca, filamentary keratitis, neuroparalytic keratopathy, and lagophthalmic keratopathy. Insult to the corneal epithelium by drying in keratitis sicca or from prolonged exposure in lagophthalmos leads to epithelial acanthosis and hypertrophy. Prolongation of these phenomena results in epithelial erosion, keratinization, or epidermalization of the cornea. Exfoliation of degenerated epithelial cells can result in corneal filaments composed of detached epithelium and mucus strands.

Filamentary keratitis can occur in keratoconjunctivitis sicca, superior limbic keratoconjunctivitis, viral infections, diabetes mellitus, psoriasis, ectodermal dysplasia, and prolonged patching. Sjögren's syndrome in patients with rheumatoid arthritis is a major cause of keratoconjunctivitis sicca. After trigeminal denervation, the corneal epithelium may lose the desmosome attachments. Poor epithelial adhesion and recurrent erosion may result. Neurotrophic disease may also occur in diabetic patients. Defective epithelial adhesion is also the underlying problem in recurrent erosion syndrome. Incomplete healing of a deep corneal abrasion may result in desquamation of abnormal epithelium and basement membrane.

Pigment granules from melanin, metallic agents, and medication may deposit in the cornea, leading to discoloration, loss of transparency, and decreased vision. Pigmentation of the limbal basal epithelium may occur spontaneously or after trauma in dark-skinned individuals. Conjunctival pigmented lesions such as nevi, acquired melanosis, and malignant melanoma may secondarily extend from the limbus to the corneal epithelium. Endothelial phagocytosis of pigment may result in Krukenberg's spindle—a vertical pigment line noted in pigmentary glaucoma and pigmentary dispersion syndrome. Endothelial pigment may also be noted after intraocular inflammation, trauma, and surgery and in myopia, aging, and pseudoexfoliation. Extracellular amber granules may deposit in Bowman's layer in the hereditary disease ochronosis.[20]

Blood staining of the cornea may occur after hyphema, particularly if elevation of intraocular pressure has resulted in endothelial damage. Erythrocytic cells penetrate the intact Descemet's membrane and deposit intracellularly and extracellularly. Hemosiderin is also present. Clearing of cornea may take years and begins peripherally.[110]

The most common iron depositions in the cornea are the epithelial iron lines. The Hudson-Stähli line occurs in a horizontal pattern in the inferior third of the cornea, without associated corneal pathology. Fleischer's ring is a circular epithelial iron deposit surrounding the cone of keratoconus. Ferry's line occurs on the corneal margin of a filtering bleb. Stocker's line is proximal to the advancing edge of a pterygium. Retention of an intraocular or intracorneal iron foreign body may result in ocular siderosis. Iron granules may deposit in any layer of the cornea but are usually more prominent in the deeper cornea. Siderosomes are noted within the keratocytes.[111]

Corneal deposits from metallic granules may result from trauma or from topical and systemic administration. Chalcosis causes copper deposition in Descemet's membrane that is identical to that in Wilson's disease. Patients with Wilson's disease may demonstrate the circumferential Kayser-Fleischer ring in Descemet's membrane. Electron-dense granules rich in copper and sulfur may be present in the peripheral and central cornea.[112] Topical administration of Argyrol eye drops can result in argyrosis. Silver deposits are noted in Descemet's membrane.[113, 114] Patients who have rheumatoid arthritis and who receive more than 1 g of gold compounds are at risk for development of ocular chrysiasis. On histopathologic examination, the posterior corneal stroma demonstrates red-blue stippling. After tattooing with gold compounds, corneas demonstrate black amorphous deposition in the superficial stroma.[115]

Systemic administration of amiodarone, chlorpromazine, chloroquine, or indomethacin can result in radial whirling corneal opacities that reverse on cessation of therapy.[116] Topical administration of epinephrine may lead to deposition of adrenaline oxidation products (adrenochrome) in the cornea. These brown-black pigment deposits in the subepithelium stain black with Fontana's stain but not iron stain. Epithelial corneal crystals may be present in multiple myeloma. Immunofluorescent and immunoperoxidase techniques demonstrate the presence of immunoglobulins in these crystals.[117–119] Conjunctival and corneal cystine crystals are deposited in the disease cystinosis.[19]

Corneal Tumors

Tumors of the cornea are unusual and frequently result from juxtalimbal invasion from conjunctival neoplasms such as melanomas. Corneal intraepithelial neoplasia appears as a translucent thickening of the epithelium with the fimbriated borders. The lesion usually occurs at the corneal limbus and is associated with conjunctival pathology. The spectrum of pathology ranges from corneal epithelial dysplasia to frank carcinoma in situ. Histopathologic examination of the débrided epithelium may reveal acantholysis, dyskeratosis, and keratinization. Failure of excision of any adjacent dysplastic conjunctiva may lead to a recurrence of the corneal lesion after débridement.[120–122]

REFERENCES

1. Grossniklaus HE, Green WR, Chan C, et al: Conjunctival lesions in adults: A clinical and histopathologic review. Cornea 6:78, 1987.
2. Gilbert JM, Weiss JS, Sattler AL, et al: Ocular manifestations and impression cytology of anorexia nervosa. Ophthalmology 97:1001, 1990.
3. Brown HH, Glasgow BJ, Holland GN, et al: Cytomegalovirus infection of the conjunctiva in AIDS. Am J Ophthalmol 106:102, 1988.
4. Ablashi DV, Sturzengger S, Hunter EA, et al: Presence of HTLV III in tears and cells from the eyes of AIDS patients. J Exp Pathol 3:693, 1987.
5. MacCallan AF: The epidemiology of trachoma. Br J Ophthalmol 15:369, 1931.
6. Woodland RN, Malam J, Darougar S: A rapid method for staining *Chlamydia psittaci* and *Chlamydia trachomatis*. J Clin Pathol 35:642, 1982.
7. Savino DF, Margo CE: Conjunctival rhinosporidiosis: Light and electron microscopic study. Ophthalmology 90:1482, 1983.
8. Jimenez JF, Young DE, Hough AJ Jr: Rhinosporidiosis. A report of two cases from Arkansas. Am J Clin Pathol 82:611, 1984.
9. Garnar A: Pathology of ocular onchocerciasis: Human and experimental. Trans R Soc Trop Med Hyg 70:374, 1977.
10. Wear DJ, Malaty RH, Zimmerman LR, et al: Cat-scratch disease bacilli in the conjunctiva of patients with oculoglandular syndrome. Ophthalmology 92:1282, 1985.
11. English CK, Wear DJ, Margileth AM, et al: Cat scratch disease: Isolation and culture of the bacterial agent. JAMA 259:1347, 1988.
12. Abu el-Asrar AM, Van den Oord JJ, Geboes K, et al: Immunopathological study of vernal conjunctivitis. Graefes Arch Clin Exp Ophthalmol 227:374, 1989.
13. Allansmith MR: Pathology and treatment of giant papillary conjunctivitis. I: The U.S. perspective. Clin Ther 9:443, 1987.
14. Hassan AM, El-Gammal Y: Histopathological study of phlyctenulosis. Bull Ophthalmol Soc Egypt 61:267, 1961.
15. Rouland JF, Amzallag T, Bale F, et al: Xerophthalmia caused by self-induced deficiency disease. J Fr Ophthalmol 12:173, 1989.
16. Hogan MJ, Alvarado J: Pterygium and pinguecula: Electron microscopic study. Arch Ophthalmol 78:174, 1967.
17. Chu FC, Rodrigues MM, Cogan DG, et al: The pathology of pinguecula in Gaucher's disease. Ophthalmic Paediatr Genet 4:7, 1984.
18. Kincaid MC, Green WR, Hoover RE, et al: Ocular chrysiasis. Arch Ophthalmol 100:1791, 1982.
19. Dodd MJ, Pusin SM, Green RW: Adult cystinosis: A case report. Arch Ophthalmol 96:1054, 1978.
20. Kampik A, Sani JN, Green WR: Ocular ochronosis: Clinical, pathologic, histochemical, and ultrastructural studies. Arch Ophthalmol 98:1441, 1980.
21. Benjamin I, Taylor H, Spindler J: Orbital and conjunctival involvement in multiple myeloma: Report of a case. Am J Clin Pathol 63:811, 1975.
22. Libert J: Diagnosis of lysosomal storage disease by the ultrastructural study of conjunctival biopsies. Pathol Annu 15:37, 1980.
23. Kenyon KR: Ocular manifestations and pathology of systemic mucopolysaccharidosis. Birth Defects 12:133, 1976.
24. Riedel KG, Zwaan J, Kenyon KR, et al: Ocular abnormalities in mucolipidosis IV. Am J Ophthalmol 99:125, 1985.
25. Livni N, Merin S: Mucolipidosis IV: Ultrastructural diagnosis of a recently defined genetic disorder. Arch Pathol Lab Med 102:600, 1978.
26. Traboulsi EI, Green WR, Luckenbach MW: Neuronal ceroid lipofuscinosis: Ocular histopathologic and electron microscopic studies in the later infantile, juvenile, and adult forms. Graefes Arch Clin Exp Ophthalmol 225:391, 1987.
27. Volcker HE, Naumann GOH: Conjunctiva. *In* Naumann GOH, Apple DJ (eds): Pathology of the Eye. New York, Springer-Verlag, 1986.
28. Jabs DA, Wingard G, Green WR, et al: The eye in bone marrow transplantation. III: Conjunctival graft versus host disease. Arch Ophthalmol 107:1343, 1989.
29. Nichols CW, Eagle RC Jr, Yanoff M, et al: Conjunctival biopsy as an aid in the evaluation of the patient with suspected sarcoidosis. Ophthalmology 87:287, 1980.
30. Karpik SJ, Schwartz MM, Dickey LE, et al: Ocular immune reactions in patients dying with systemic lupus erythematosus. Clin Immunol Immunopathol 35:295, 1985.
31. Frith PA, Venning VA, Wojnarowska F, et al: Conjunctival involvement in cicatricial bullous pemphigoid: A clinical and immunopathological study. Br J Ophthalmol 73:52, 1989.
32. Roat MI, Sossi G, Lo CY, et al: Hyperproliferation of conjunctival fibroblasts from patients with cicatricial pemphigoid. Arch Ophthalmol 107:1064, 1989.
33. Mondino BJ, Brown SI: Ocular cicatricial pemphigoid. Ophthalmology 88:95, 1981.
34. Foster CS, Wilson LA, Ekins MB: Immunosuppressive therapy for progressive ocular cicatricial pemphigoid. Ophthalmology 89:340, 1982.
35. Ignat F, Oprescu M: Manifestari Ocular in Sindromol Stevens-Johnson. Rev Chir [Oftalmol] 33:287, 1989.
36. Jakobiec FA, Bonanno PA, Sigelman J: Conjunctival adnexal cysts and dermoids. Arch Ophthalmol 96:104, 1978.
37. Sanderson TL, Pustai W, Shelley L: Cytologic evaluation of ocular lesions. Acta Cytol 24:391, 1980.
38. Brownstein S: Mucoepidermoid carcinoma of the conjunctiva with intraocular invasion. Ophthalmology 88:1226, 1981.
39. Macher AM, Palestine A, Masur H, et al: Multicentric Kaposi's sarcoma of the conjunctiva in a male homosexual with the acquired immunodeficiencies syndrome. Ophthalmology 90:879, 1983.
40. Hufnagel T, Ma L, Kuo TT: Orbital angiosarcoma with subconjunctival presentation: Report of a case and literature review. Ophthalmology 94:72, 1987.
41. Reese AB: Nevus. *In* Reese AB (ed): Tumors of the Eye, 3rd ed. New York, Harper & Row, 1976.
42. Eller W, Bernadino VB Jr: Blue nevi of the conjunctiva. Ophthalmology 90:1469, 1983.
43. Folberg R, Jakobiec FA, Bernadino VB, et al: Benign conjunctival melanocytic lesions: Clinicopathologic features. Ophthalmology 96:436, 1989.

44. Folberg R, McLean IW, Zimmerman LE: Conjunctival melanosis and melanoma. Ophthalmology 91:673, 1984.
45. Folberg R, McLean IW, Zimmerman LE: Primary acquired melanosis of the conjunctiva. Hum Pathol 16:129, 1985.
46. Zimmerman LE: Criteria for management of melanosis. Arch Ophthalmol 76:307, 1966.
47. Zimmerman LE: Discussion of pigmented tumors of the conjunctiva. *In* Boniuk M (ed): Ocular and Adenexal Tumors: New Controversial Aspects. St. Louis, CV Mosby, 1964.
48. Yanoff M, Fine BS: Ocular melanotic tumors. *In* Yanoff M, Fine BS (eds): Ocular Pathology: A Text and Atlas, 2nd ed. New York, Harper & Row, 1982.
49. Jakobiec FA, Folberg R, Iwamoto T, et al: Clinicopathologic characteristics of premalignant and malignant melanocytic lesions of the conjunctiva. Ophthalmology 96:147, 1989.
50. Robin JB, Gindi JJ, Koh K, et al: An update of indications of penetrating keratoplasty. Arch Ophthalmol 104:87, 1986.
51. Waring GO III, Rodrigues MM, Laibson PR: Anterior chamber cleavage syndromes: A stepladder classification. Surv Ophthalmol 20:3, 1975.
52. Hinzpeter EN, Naumann GOH: Cornea and sclera. *In* Naumann GOH, Apple DJ (eds): Pathology of the Eye. New York, Springer-Verlag, 1986.
53. Krachmer JH, Rodrigues MM: Posterior keratoconus. Arch Ophthalmol 96:1867, 1978.
54. Thygeson P: Clinical and laboratory observations of superficial punctate keratitis. Am J Ophthalmol 61:1344, 1966.
55. Dawson CR, Hanna L, Togni B: Adenovirus type 8 infections in the U.S. IV: Observations on the pathogenesis of lesions in severe eye disease. Arch Ophthalmol 87:258, 1972.
56. Scattergood KD, Green WR, Hirst LW: Scrolls of Descemet's membrane in healed syphilitic interstitial keratitis. Ophthalmology 90:1518, 1983.
57. Catalano RA, Webb RM, Smith RS, et al: Modified immunoperoxidase method for rapid diagnosis of herpes simplex keratitis. Am J Clin Pathol 36:102, 1986.
58. Paul EV, Zimmerman LE: Some observations on the ocular pathology of onchocerciasis. Hum Pathol 1:581, 1970.
59. Watson PG, Sevel D: Ophthalmia nodosum. Br J Ophthalmol 50:209, 1966.
60. Sylvany RE, Luckenbach MW, Moore MB: The rapid detection of acanthamoeba in paraffin-embedded sections of corneal tissue with calcofluor white. Arch Ophthalmol 105:1366, 1987.
61. Mathers W, Stevens G Jr, Rodrigues MM: Immunopathology and electron microscopy of acanthamoeba keratitis. Am J Ophthalmol 103:626, 1987.
62. Epstein RJ, Wilson LA, Visvesvera JS: Rapid diagnosis of acanthamoeba keratitis from corneal scrapings using indirect fluorescent antibody staining. Arch Ophthalmol 104:1318, 1986.
63. Wilhelmus KR, Osato MS, Font RL, et al: Rapid diagnosis of acanthamoeba keratitis using calcofluor white. Arch Ophthalmol 104:1309, 1986.
64. Key SN III, Green WR, Willaert E, et al: Keratitis due to *Acanthamoeba castellanii:* A clinicopathologic case report. Arch Ophthalmol 98:475, 1980.
65. Margo CE: Acanthamoeba keratitis. Arch Pathol Lab Med 11:759, 1987.
66. Austin P, Green WR, Sallyer DC, et al: Peripheral corneal degeneration and occlusive vasculitis in Wegener's granulomatosis. Am J Ophthalmol 85:311, 1978.
67. Terrien F: Dystrophie marginale symétrique des deux cornées avec astigmatisme regulier consecutif et guerison par la cauterisation ignée. Arch Ophtalmol (Paris) 20:12, 1900.
68. Brito C, Honrubia F, Elia J: Maladie de Terrien. J Fr Ophtalmol 5:675, 1982.
69. Green WR, Zimmerman LE: Granulomatous reaction to Descemet's membrane. Am J Ophthalmol 64:555, 1967.
70. Hedges TR III, Albert DM: The progression of the ocular abnormalities of herpes zoster: Histopathologic observations of nine cases. Ophthalmology 89:165, 1982.
71. Tremblay M, Dube I: Meesmann's corneal dystrophy: Ultrastructural features. Can J Ophthalmol 17:24, 1982.
72. Fine BS, Yanoff M, Pitts E, et al: Meesmann's epithelial dystrophy of the cornea. Am J Ophthalmol 83:633, 1977.
73. Laibson PR, Krachmer JH: Familial occurrence of dot (microcystic) map, fingerprint dystrophy of the cornea. Invest Ophthalmol 14:397, 1975.
74. Cogan DG, Kuwabara T, Donaldson DD, et al: Microcystic dystrophy of the cornea: A partial explanation for its pathogenesis. Arch Ophthalmol 92:470, 1974.
75. Riegel EM, Pokorny KS, Friedman AH, et al: Ocular pathology of Fabry's disease in a hemizygous male following renal transplantation. Surv Ophthalmol 26:247, 1982.
76. Weingeist TA, Blodi FC: Fabry's disease: Ocular findings in a female carrier: A light and electron microscopic study. Arch Ophthalmol 85:169, 1971.
77. Perry HD, Fine BS, Caldwell DR: Reis-Buckler's dystrophy: A study of 8 cases. Arch Ophthalmol 97:664, 1979.
78. Lohse E, Stock EL, Jones JC, et al: Reis-Buckler's corneal dystrophy: Immunofluorescent and electron microscopic studies. Cornea 8:200, 1989.
79. Klintworth GK: Research into the pathogenesis of macular cornea dystrophy. Trans Op Soc U K 100:186, 1980.
80. Klintworth GK, Smith CF: Abnormalities of proteoglycans and glycoproteins synthesized by corneal organ cultures derived from patients with macular cornea dystrophy. Lab Invest 48:603, 1983.
81. Klintworth GK, Ferry AP, Sugar A, et al: Recurrence of lattice corneal dystrophy type 1 in the corneal grafts of two siblings. Am J Ophthalmol 94:540, 1982.
82. McTigue JW, Fine BS: The human cornea, a light and electron microscopic study of the normal cornea and the stromal lesion in lattice and its alterations in various dystrophies. Trans Am Ophthalmol Soc 65:591, 1967.
83. Donders PC, Blanksma LJ: Meretoja syndrome: Lattice dystrophy of the cornea with hereditary generalized amyloidosis. Ophthalmologica 178:173, 1979.
84. Johnson BL, Brown SI, Zaidman GW: A light and electron microscopic study of recurrent granular dystrophy of the cornea. Am J Ophthalmol 92:49, 1981.
85. Nicholson DH, Green WR, Cross HE, et al: A clinical and histopathological study of Francois-Neetens speckled corneal dystrophy. Am J Ophthalmol 83:554, 1977.
86. Curran RE, Kenyon KR, Green WR: Pre-Descemet membrane corneal dystrophy. Am J Ophthalmol 77:711, 1974.
86a. Weiss JS: Schnyder's dystrophy of the cornea: A Swede-Finn connection. Cornea 11:93, 1992.
87. Weiss JS, Rodrigues M, Rajagopalan S, et al: Atypical Schnyder's crystalline dystrophy of the cornea: A light and electron microscopic study [Abstracts]. Proc Int Soc Eye Research 6:198, 1990.
88. Weiss JS, Rodrigues M, Rajagopalan S, et al: Schnyder's corneal dystrophy: Clinical, ultrastructural, and histochemical studies. Ophthalmology 97(Suppl):141, 1990.
89. Rodrigues MM, Kruth HS, Krachmer JH, et al: Unesterified cholesterol in Schnyder's corneal crystalline dystrophy. Am J Ophthalmol 104:157, 1987.
90. Rodrigues MM, Kruth HS, Krachmer JH, et al: Cholesterol localization in ultrathin frozen sections in Schnyder's corneal dystrophy. Am J Ophthalmol 110:513, 1990.
91. Waring GO III, Rodrigues MM, Laibson PR: Corneal dystrophies. I: Dystrophies of the Bowman's layer, epithelium, and stroma. Surv Ophthalmol 23:71, 1978.
92. Waring GO III, Rodrigues MM, Laibson PR: Corneal dystrophies. II: Endothelial dystrophies. Surv Ophthalmol 23:147, 1978.
93. Mannis MJ, Krachmer JH, Rodrigues MM, et al: Polymorphic amyloid degeneration of the cornea. Arch Ophthalmol 99:1217, 1981.
94. Rosenblum P, Stark WJ, Maumenee IH, et al: Heriditary Fuchs' dystrophy. Am J Ophthalmol 90:455, 1980.
95. Rodrigues MM, Krachmer JH, Hackett J, et al: Fuchs' corneal dystrophy: A clinicopathologic study of the variation in corneal edema. Ophthalmology 93:789, 1986.
96. Stainer GA, Akers PH, Binder PS, et al: Correlative microscopy and tissue culture of congenital hereditary endothelial dystrophy. Am J Ophthalmol 93:456, 1982.
97. Johnson BL, Brown SI: Posterior polymorphous dystrophy: A light and electron microscopic study. Br J Ophthalmol 62:89, 1978.

98. Rodrigues MM, Sun TT, Krachmer JH, et al: Epithelialization of corneal endothelium in posterior polymorphous dystrophy. Invest Ophthalmol Vis Sci 19:832, 1980.
99. Schwartz MF, Werblin TP, Green WR: Occurrence of mucopolysaccharide in corneal grafts in the Maroteaux-Lamy syndrome. Cornea 4:58, 1985.
100. Goldberg MF, Maumenee AE, McKusick VA: Corneal dystrophies associated with abnormalities of mucopolysaccharide metabolism. Arch Opthalmol 74:516, 1965.
101. Palmer M, Green WR, Maumenee IH, et al: Niemann-Pick disease type C: Ocular histopathologic and electron microscopic studies. Arch Ophthalmol 103:817, 1985.
102. Teng CC: Electron microscopic study of the pathology of keratoconus. Am J Ophthalmol 55:18, 1963.
103. Knieper P, Rochels R, Nover A: Zur histologie des keratoglobus. Klin Monatsbl Augenheilkd 177:58, 1980.
104. Rodrigues MM, Stulting RD, Waring GO III: Clinical, electron microscopic, and immunohistochemical study of the corneal endothelium and Descemet's membrane in the iridocorneal endothelial syndrome. Am J Ophthalmol 101:16, 1986.
105. Eagle RC Jr, Shields JA: Iridocorneal endothelial syndrome with contralateral guttate endothelial dystrophy: A light and electron microscopic study. Ophthalmology 84:862, 1987.
106. Rodrigues MM, Jester JV, Richards R, et al: Essential iris atrophy: A clinical immunohistologic and electron microscopic study in an enucleated eye. Ophthalmology 95:69, 1988.
107. Richardson TM: Corneal decompensation in Chandler's syndrome: A scanning and transmission electron microscopic study. Arch Ophthalmol 97:2112, 1979.
108. Vogt A: Weitere ergebnisse der spalt lampenmikroskopie des vorderen bulbusabschnittes I: Hornhaut. Graefes Arch Clin Exp Ophthalmol 106:63, 1921.
109. Hidayat AA, Risco JM: Amyloidosis of corneal stroma in patients with trachoma: A clinicopathologic study of 62 cases. Ophthalmology 96:1203, 1989.
110. McDonnell PJ, Green WR, Stevens RE, et al: Blood staining of the cornea: Light microscopic and ultrastructural features. Ophthalmology 92:1668, 1985.
111. Talamo JH, Topping TM, Maumenee AE, et al: Ultrastructural studies of cornea, iris, and lens in a case of siderosis bulbi. Ophthalmology 92:1675, 1985.
112. Johnson RE, Campbell RJ: Electron microscopic, x-ray energy spectroscopic, and atomic absorption spectroscopic studies of corneal copper deposition and distribution. Lab Invest 46:564, 1982.
113. Karcioglu ZA, Caldwell DR: Corneal argyrosis: Histologic, ultrastructural, and microanalytic study. Can J Ophthalmol 20:257, 1985.
114. Hanna C, Fraunfelder FT, Sanchez J: Ultrastructural studies of argyrosis of the cornea and conjunctiva. Arch Ophthalmol 92:18, 1974.
115. McCormick SA, DiBartolomeo AG, Raju VK, et al: Ocular chrysiasis. Ophthalmology 92:1432, 1985.
116. D'Amico DJ, Kenyon KR, Ruskin JN: Amiodarone keratopathy: Drug-induced lipid storage disorder. Arch Ophthalmol 99:257, 1981.
117. Klintworth GK, Bredehoeft SJ, Reed JW: Analysis of corneal crystalline deposits in multiple myeloma. Am J Ophthalmol 86:303, 1978.
118. Green Ed, Morrison LK, Love PE, et al: A structurally aberrant immunoglobulin paraprotein in a patient with multiple myeloma and corneal crystal deposits. Am J Med 88:304, 1990.
119. Spiegel P, Grossniklaus HE, Reinhart WJ, et al: Unusual presentation of paraproteinemic corneal infiltrates. Cornea 9:81, 1990.
120. Campbell RJ, Bourne WM: Unilateral central corneal epithelial dysplasia. Ophthalmology 88:1231, 1981.
121. Brown HH, Glasgow BJ, Holland EN: Keratinizing corneal intraepithelial neoplasia. Cornea 8:220, 1989.
122. Presyna AP, Monte JS, Satchidnand SK: Unilateral cornea intraepithelial neoplasia: Management of the recurrent lesion. Ann Ophthalmol 22:103, 1990.

Chapter 182

Pathology of the Uveal Tract

JOSÉ A. SAHEL, MICHEL WEBER,
M. RONAN CONLON, and DANIEL M. ALBERT

CONGENITAL AND DEVELOPMENTAL ABNORMALITIES

Persistent Pupillary Membrane

Failure of reabsorption of the anterior portion of the tunica vasculosa lentis during fetal development results in a relatively common condition known as persistent pupillary membrane. One can see both complete and incomplete failure of reabsorption of the tunica vasculosa lentis, the former condition being extremely rare. The persistent pupillary membranes extend from the minor circle of the iris to either the anterior lens surface or the posterior surface of the cornea.[1] In the latter situation, this can be associated with corneal opacification; however, this condition generally is asymptomatic and is noticed incidentally at slit-lamp examination (Fig. 182–1).

Histopathologic examination of the membrane has shown it to be composed of mesodermal elements without vascularization. Isolated elements of the anterior tunica vasculosa lentis may remain centrally on the lens and appear as tan-colored "chicken tracks."

Persistence of the Tunica Vasculosa Lentis

The tunica vasculosa lentis is a network of vessels surrounding the lens, which is derived posteriorly from the posterior hyaloid system and anteriorly from a vascular arcade formed between the annular vessel and major arterial circle of the iris. It is more common to

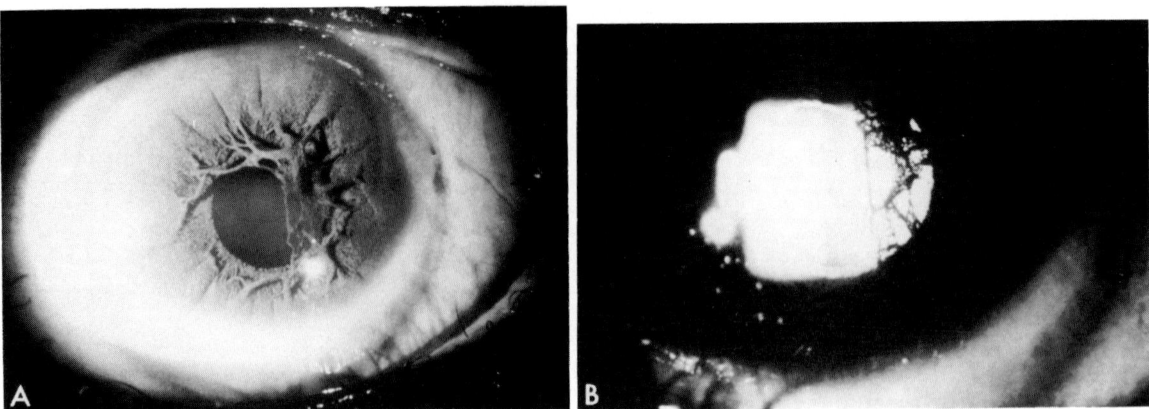

Figure 182–1. Persistent pupillary membrane *(A)*, by direct illumination and *(B)*, by retroillumination. (From Spencer WH [ed]: Ophthalmic Pathology: An Atlas and Textbook, 3rd ed. Philadelphia, WB Saunders, 1986, p 1391.)

see persistence of the posterior aspect of this vascular membrane in association with persistence of the primary vitreous in persistent hyperplasic primary vitreous (PHPV). Isolated persistence of the tunica vasculosa in the absence of PHPV is rare but has been reported in trisomy 13.

Iris Cysts

Cysts of the iris may be primary or secondary. Primary cysts of the iris have been found to be lined by two principle types of epithelium: (1) cornea-like epithelium with goblet cells, believed to be derived from the iris stroma and (2) neuroepithelium from the posterior pigmented epithelium of the iris. The more common type of primary cyst of the iris is lined by neuroepithelium and may occur at the pupillary border, midiris, or peripheral iris in increasing order of frequency.[2] Less commonly, cysts of stromal origin are seen in children. Complications of iris cysts include distortion of the pupillary aperture, pupillary occlusion, dislocation of the cysts, and secondary glaucoma.

The most common causes of secondary cysts of the iris are trauma and miotic therapy. Traumatic cysts are lined by epithelium, not surprisingly similarly to the conjunctiva.

Iris Hypoplasia and Aniridia

Congenital absence of the iris is referred to as aniridia. This condition is rarely seen in its complete form with usually a rudimentary iris stump being visible on gonioscopy (Fig. 182–2). Rather than being a condition seen in isolation, aniridia is part of a group of related ocular disorders characterized by the presence of iris hypoplasia. Multiple congenital ocular anomalies have been reported with aniridia.[3]

An autosomal dominant inheritance pattern is present in as many as two thirds of patients with this condition, the remainder of cases being sporadic.[4] The significance of this hereditary pattern is the association of Wilms' tumor, genitourinary abnormalities, and mental retardation in the sporadic cases with partial deletion of the short arm of chromosome 11, specifically the 11p13 band.

The exact pathogenesis of this condition has not been fully elucidated. This disorder has been characterized by some as a colobomatous disorder as a result of early reports of ocular colobomas in patients with aniridia. Others have proposed a mesodermal theory with failure of development of the rim of the optic cup leading to iris hyoplasia.[5] Finally, the presence of retinal anomalies and absence of iris musculature have lead some to subscribe to the view that this condition is a developmental failure of neuroectoderm (neuroectodermal theory).[3]

The most striking histopathologic feature of this condition is an arrest in the development of the neural crest–derived iris tissue. Other features that may be seen include corneal pannus and localized lenticular opacities. Glaucoma occurs in over 50 percent of these patients, and it is believed to be related to progressive closure to the iris stump over the trabecular meshwork with aging. This progressive closing of the angle may be due to contracture of peripheral iris strands that extend onto the trabecular wall (Fig. 182–3).[6]

Coloboma

Coloboma is the term used to describe a localized defect or notch in tissue. It is derived from the Greek word meaning *mutilated* or *curtailed*. These lesions are typically caused by failure of fusion of the embryonic fissure anywhere along the optic nerve to the inferonasal border of the iris. The normal embryonic fissure begins to close initially at its midpoint and proceeds proximally to the optic disc and distally to the rim of the cup. This process is usually completed in the normal eye by the sixth week of gestation. An arrest in this process is believed to be responsible for the development of a colobomatous defect. Typical iris coloboma refers to colobomas that are located inferonasally, and these may be associated with ciliary body or chorioretinal defects.

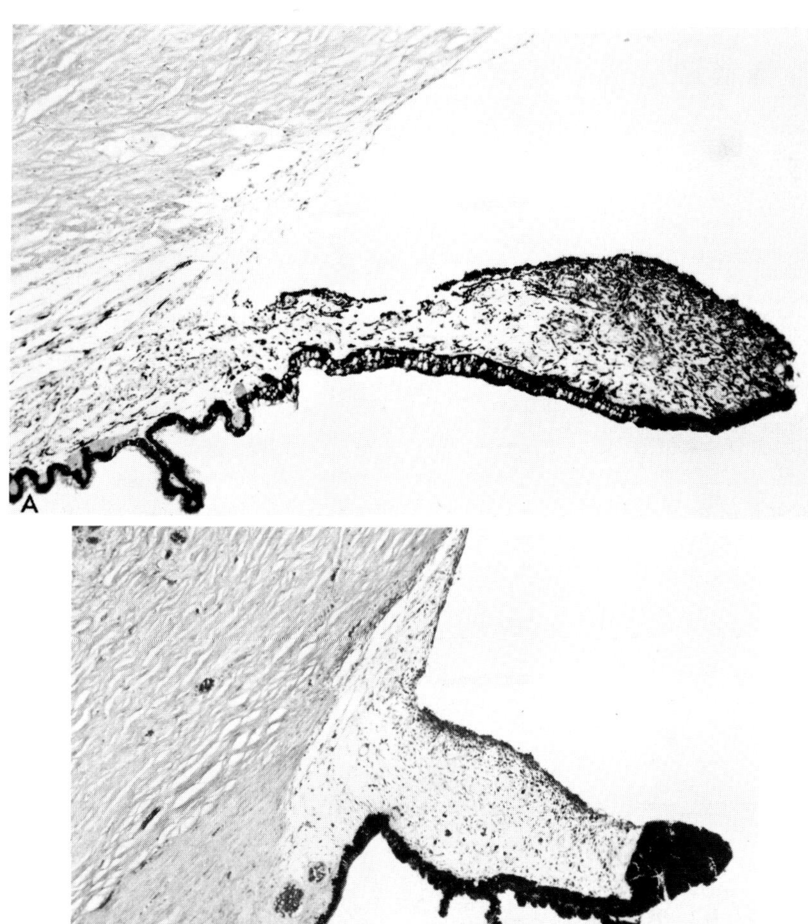

Figure 182–2. Aniridia. *A*, Small stump of iris with no dilator or sphincter muscle. H&E, ×63, AFIP Neg 82-6743. *B*, Area showing iris remnant directly continuous with the trabecular meshwork. H&E, ×58, AFIP Neg 82-5346. (From Spencer WH [ed]: Ophthalmic Pathology: An Atlas and Textbook, 3rd ed. Philadelphia, WB Saunders, 1986, p 1394.)

Defects elsewhere on the iris are considered atypical and are not associated with other colobomatous defects.

Iris colobomas may extend from the pupillary margin to the peripheral cornea, producing a "keyhole" defect (Fig. 182–4), or the defect may be only partial, producing a notch in the pupil margin in the area of the iris coloboma. The lens zonules are often absent, producing a notch in the lens that is sometimes mistakenly referred to as a lens coloboma. Remnants of neural crest tissue may sometimes bridge the colobomatous defect.

A chorioretinal coloboma is caused by failure of the inner layers (neurosensory) and outer layers (retinal pigment epithelium [RPE]) to fuse along the optic fissure. Because an intact retina is required to stimulate the normal development of the underlying choriocapillaris, a chorioretinal defect is created by failure of the retina to fuse. A primitive intercalary membrane of undifferentiated neuroepithelium bridges the gap and may contain retinal vessels. The area often has a white appearance secondary to the absence of the RPE, allowing easy visibility of the underlying sclera. The sclera bridging the defect is often ectatic and bulges posteriorly, forming a posterior staphyloma in the area of the coloboma. In some circumstances, failure of fusion of the outer layers allows the inner layers to evert through the gap and to produce a cystic mass. The presence of a cystic mass in the orbit during development can lead to extreme microophthalmia.

A number of inheritance patterns have been associated with this anomaly. Autosomal dominant inheritance without associated systemic abnormalities is well recognized. Penetrance of this trait is variable, as is the phenotypic expression of the defect. Autosomal recessive inheritance has been postulated in isolated, sporadic colobomas. Ocular colobomas have also been described with a variety of chromosomal disorders and chromosomal syndromes.

Congenital Oculodermal Melanocytosis (Nevus of Ota)

This condition is caused by a failure of migration of melanocytes to their normal resting position in the surface epithelium. As a consequence, an excess of melanocytes may become situated in the sclera, episclera uvea, dermis of the eyelid, orbital soft tissue, optic nerve meninges, and the oral and buccal mucosa.[7–10] When the pigmentary change is confined to the sclera and episclera without involvement of the skin, the term *ocular melanosis* is used to describe this condition.

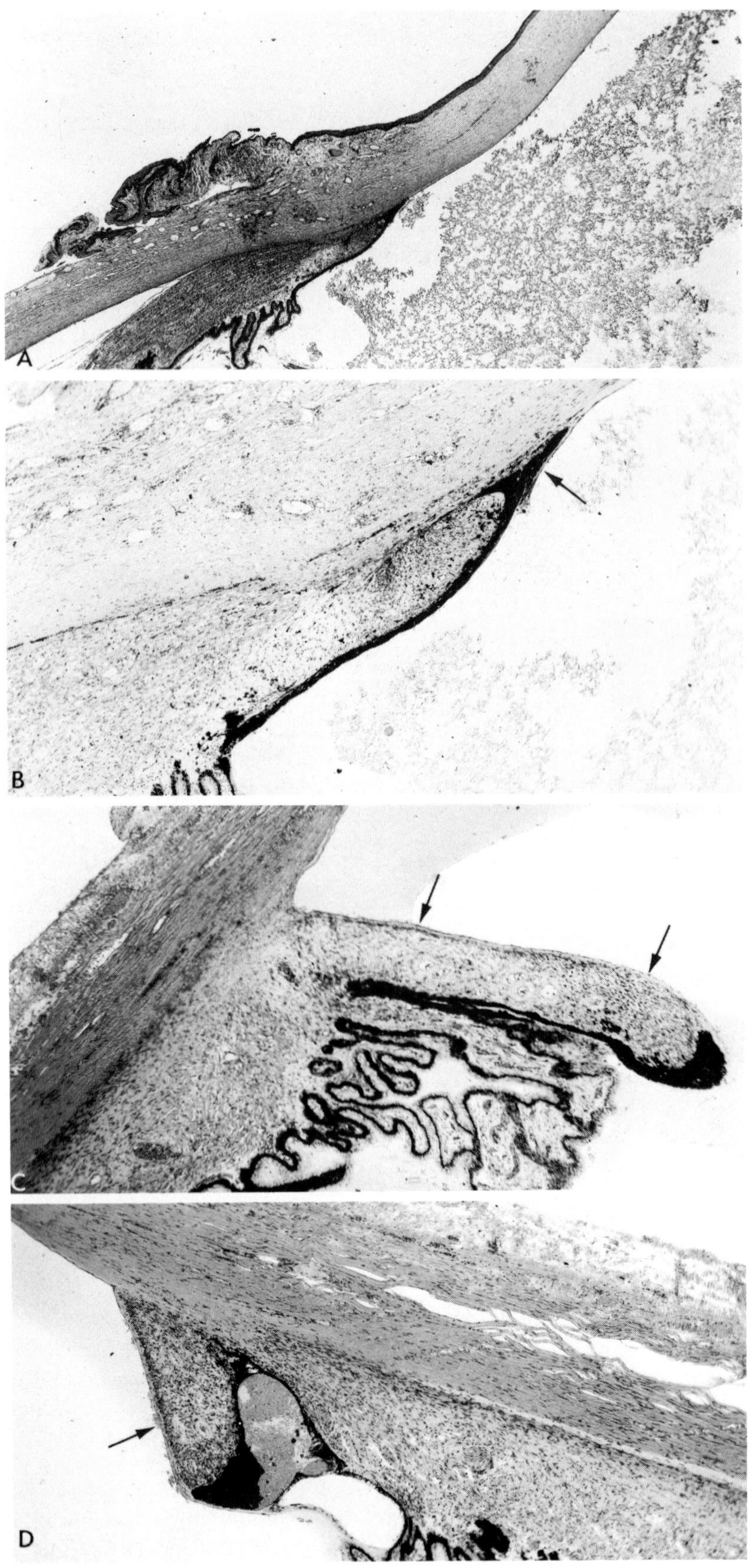

Figure 182–3. Late changes in aniridia. There is development of peripheral anterior synechiae and overgrowth of corneal endothelium with production of basement membrane (*arrows*), endothelialization, and decemetization. H&E. *A*, ×14, AFIP Neg 60-6367; *B*, ×50, AFIP Neg 60-6363; *C*, ×50, AFIP Neg 60-6365; *D*, ×50, AFIP Neg 60-6366. (From Spencer WH [ed]: Ophthalmic Pathology: An Atlas and Textbook, 3rd ed. Philadelphia, WB Saunders, 1986, p 1398.)

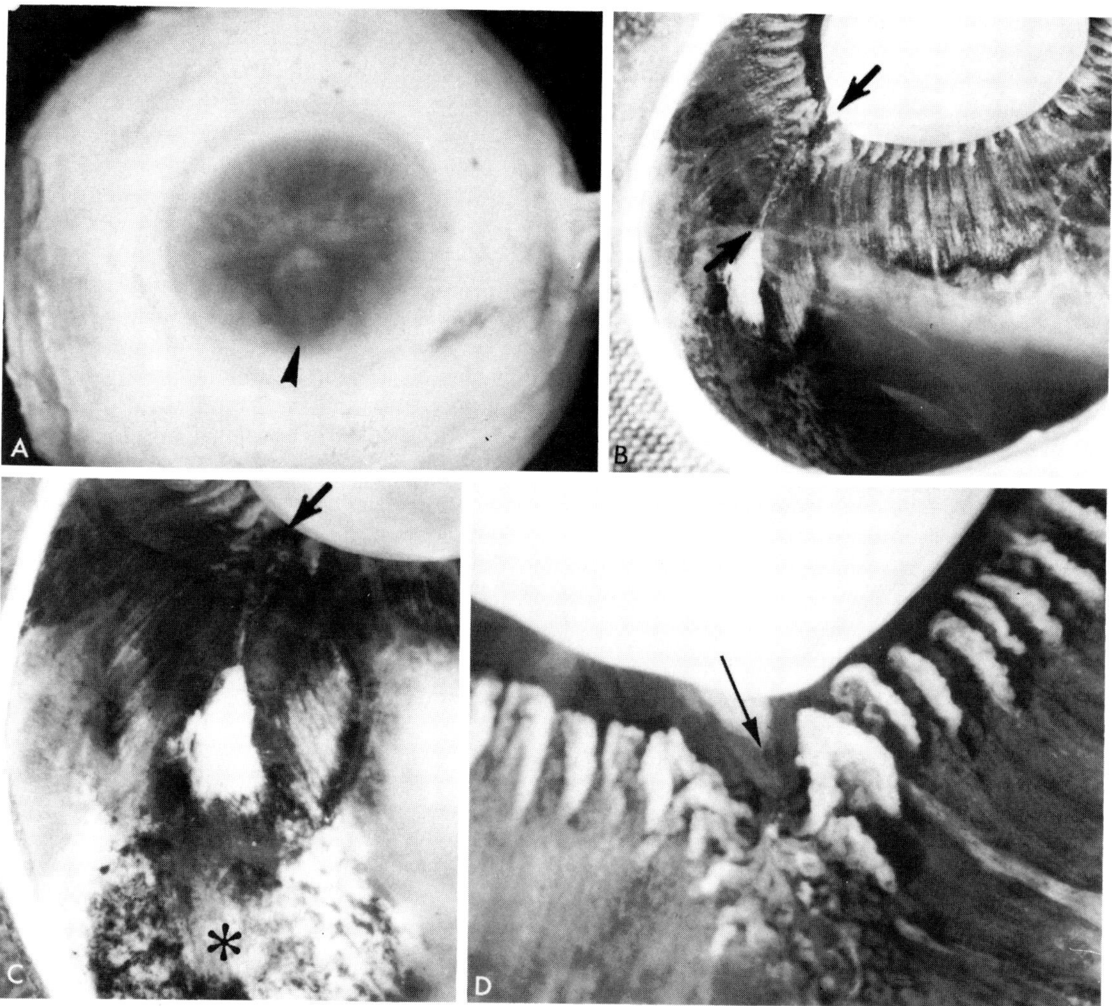

Figure 182–4. Coloboma in iris (*A, arrowhead*), ciliary body (*B, C,* and *D, arrows*), and choroid (*C, asterisk*). EP 53986. (From Spencer WH [ed]: Ophthalmic Pathology: An Atlas and Textbook, 3rd ed. Philadelphia, WB Saunders, 1986, p 1400.)

Clinically, this gives rise to slate-gray or bluish appearance of the sclera as opposed to the dusty brown appearance of primary acquired melanosis or racial melanosis. The conjunctiva should move freely over the discolored sclera. The pigment within the sclera has the distinctive feature of outlining the lymphatics and blood vessels. The diffuse involvement of the uveal tract can give rise to iris heterochromia and a darker appearance to the fundus on the affected side.

Gonder and associates estimated the prevalence of ocular melanocytosis to be 0.038 percent in the white population (5251 patients examined) and no cases of oculodermal melanocytosis were found or identified in the same patient population. In the same study, the prevalence of oculodermal melanocytosis in black patients (6915 patients examined) was found to be 0.014 percent (1 patient), and no black patients were diagnosed with ocular melanocytosis.[11] The prevalence of ocular melanocytosis in the Asian population is higher, with a reported prevalence between 0.4 and 0.84 percent in various studies.[8, 12, 13]

It is generally accepted that white patients with ocular melanocytosis are at an increased risk for developing uveal melanoma. Two studies have calculated ocular melanocytosis to be 30 to 35 times more common in patients with uveal melanoma.[14, 15]

Histologically, the episclera and sclera are not infiltrated by true nevus cells but rather by dentiform melanocytes containing an abundant amount of melanin granules.

UVEITIS

The clinical classification of uveitis is based on the location of uveal involvement (anterior, intermediate, posterior, and panuveitis), the nature (acute or chronic) of the inflammation, the expectation of recurrences, and the etiology, pathogenesis, or both. Among the etiologies, infectious factors, ocular inflammatory syndromes of known or unknown cause, ocular inflammatory disease associated with systemic diseases, and predisposing factors such as genetic (e.g., HLA antigens or allergic predisposition) can be recognized.

Inflammation[16] is tissue response to noxious stimuli, either infectious or noninfectious. The noninfectious stimuli include exogenous factors such as trauma or surgery and endogenous agents such as tissue necrosis or reaction to allergens.

Inflammation may be suppurative or nonsuppurative. Suppurative responses are characterized by polymorphonuclear leukocytic infiltration in the involved tissue. Suppurative inflammation may result from exogenous factors (e.g., corneal ulcer, keratitis, trauma, or surgery) or endogenous factors or conditions (e.g., metastatic bacterial emboli or necrosis of intraocular tumors). Nonsuppurative inflammation may be fibrinous, serous, serosanguineous, or putrefactive. In the eye, an example of a nonsuppurative inflammation is acute anterior uveitis.

Inflammation may be granulomatous or nongranulomatous. Nongranulomatous inflammation is present when the main cellular infiltrate is composed of lymphocytes. In the uveal tract, these are predominantly T lymphocyte subtypes. B lymphocytes and their antibody-producing derivatives, plasma cells with Russell bodies, are present to a lesser extent.

Granulomatous inflammation is characterized by epithelioid cells, which are transformed macrophages with a glassy eosinophilic cytoplasm resulting from abundant vimentin filaments. Epithelioid cell are so named because of their superficial resemblance to epithelium. Their cell membranes interdigitate with neighboring cells. In diffuse granulomatous inflammation, the epithelioid cells are randomly spread among a background infiltrate, including lymphocytes and other inflammatory cells. When the epithelioid cells cluster together, the discrete type of granulomatous inflammation is present.

Granulomas are aggregates of epithelioid cells often surrounded by a rim of lymphocytes. Deposits over the corneal endothelium are called "mutton-fat" or keratic precipitates. Those that seed the iris rim or pupillary margin are termed, respectively, Busacca's or Koeppe's nodules, and may be observed directly by gonioscopy on the ciliary band. Choroidal granulomas may be observed as deep nodules—for example, in tuberculosis—or small superficial dots—for example, in sympathetic ophthalmia.

When the granulomas are minute, uniform in size, and do not undergo necrosis, they are sarcoidal. Langerhans' giant cells, plasma cells, and lymphocytes are present about such histiocytic aggregates. Granulomas that undergo central necrosis or caseation are said to have tuberculoid features. Another discrete type, as seen around rheumatoid nodules or a lens-induced uveitis, is termed zonal.

Exogenous Uveitis

Uveal tract inflammation may occur during corneal diseases such as corneal ulcer or keratitis caused by bacteria, viruses, or fungi or after trauma, including surgery, caused by infectious factors or induced by intraocular lenses.

The data drawn from study of exogenous infectious factors are discussed in Chapter 28. The differences between exogenous infectious uveitis and endogenous infectious uveitis are based on the respective bacteria causing each and the fact that there is usually no breakdown in the hematoocular barrier at the onset of exogenous uveitis.

In eyes with intraocular lens (IOL) implants, an inflammatory reaction of the iris and ciliary body can occur.[17] Minimal inflammatory reaction of the iris to the IOL has been described. Granulomatous reaction to the implanted lens is less frequent, most often seen when the haptics are in contact with the iris and ciliary body. A granulomatous reaction in the iris may be related to suture material. Chronic inflammation of the ciliary body was observed in 18 to 33 percent of eyes upon histopathology but was noted clinically in only 0.35 percent of patients. Granulomatous inflammation could be seen at the erosion site caused by the haptics. Transient and persistent inflammatory reaction may be related to the IOL and surface contaminants; multinucleated giant cells are likely a reaction to a foreign body (an IOL).[17] As reported in the literature, organisms involved in exogenous endophthalmitis are gram-positive bacteria in 56 to 89 percent of all cases, gram-negative bacteria in 7 to 35 percent, and fungi in 2 to 11 percent.[18–20] The gram-positive organisms include *Staphylococcus epidermidis* and *S. aureus*,[21–23] *Streptococcus* α hemolytic,[24] *D*,[24] *suis*,[21, 22] *Pneumoniae*,[20, 24, 25] *Bacillus aureus* (occurring especially in association with a retained intraocular foreign body, this organism produces intraocular gas in anaerobic conditions),[26–29] *Propionibacterium acnes* (anaerobic organisms that induce chronic anterior uveitis months to years after extracapsular cataract surgery),[30, 31] and *Rhodococcus equi*.[32]

The gram-negative organisms are the following: *Pseudomonas aeruginosa*,[20, 24] *Proteus mirabilis*,[24, 33] *Haemophilus influenzae*,[34, 35] *Escherichia coli*,[20] *Neisseria meningitidis* and *N. gonorrhoeae*,[36] *Serratia marcescens*,[37] and *Aeromonas hydrophila*.[18, 38, 39]

Endogenous Uveitis

HYPERSENSITIVITY UVEITIS

Coombs' classification of hypersensitivity reactions provides a useful way to understand the different mechanisms involved in the immune response (I, immediate; II, antibody-dependent cytotoxic; III, immune complex; IV, delayed). Recently, type V (stimulating antibody) was added.[40] There are few examples of diseases that are caused by a single type of hypersensitivity reaction. Ocular inflammations such as sarcoidosis, Behçet's disease, sympathetic ophthalmia, Vogt-Koyanagi-Harada syndrome, and phakoantigenic uveitis involve a complex combination of immune mechanisms. For complex reasons that are not fully understood, immune responses normally directed against antigens can become directed against the patient's own tissues. This autoallergy is mediated by the antibody-producing B lymphocytes and the proliferation of sensitized effector T cells. If these autoreactive B and T cells are not eliminated, blocked, or suppressed, then autoimmune reactions are produced.

Sarcoidosis

Ocular involvement occurs in 25 percent of patients with sarcoidosis[40, 41] and may account for up to 7 percent of uveitis. Uveitis in sarcoidosis may be granulomatous or nongranulomatous, acute or chronic, localized or diffuse.

Anterior uveitis accounts for 66 percent of the ocular inflammation: in half of the patients there is acute inflammation with pain, photophobia, and ciliary injection; the other half are chronic with moderate anterior chamber flare and cells, and mutton-fat keratic precipitates. Iris nodules on the pupillary rim (Koeppe's nodules) (Fig. 182–5*A*) and midiris (Busacca's nodules) (Fig. 182–5*B*) are found in 35 to 41 percent of patients and are associated with a supervening membrane of fibroinflammatory tissue.[42] One fourth of patients with ocular sarcoidosis have posterior uveitis and retinal vasculitis. Periphlebitis is a major feature that may be complicated by minor vascular occlusion and capillary closure. Other than vitreous cellular reaction, the posterior segment lesions include "candle-wax drippings,"[41, 43] retinal neovascularization, and multiple, small choroidal granulomas resembling Dalen-Fuchs nodules. The optic nerve can be involved (disc edema, neovascularization, and granuloma formation).

Histopathologic examination reveals granulomatous noncaseating inflammatory infiltrates often associated with a foreign-body type of giant cells. Acidophilic bodies (asteroid bodies) (Fig. 182–6) and calcified basophilic bodies (Schaumann's bodies) can be found in epithelioid or giant cells. These elements are not specific to sarcoidosis.

Three different types of macrophages in the sarcoid granulomas have been identified.[40] The periphery contains a large number of antigen-presenting interdigitating cells; the center of the granuloma consists of macrophage-derived epithelioid and giant cells. Tissue histiocytes, the third type occasionally seen, are more diffusely distributed in the granuloma and are not restricted to the granuloma. Granulomas can be observed in iris nodules, ciliary or choroidal inflammation, perivenously, and in the optic nerve.

The cause of sarcoidosis remains unknown. An underlying defect of heightened cell-mediated immunity is suspected of being the primary cause of the disease. Hypersensitivity reaction types III and IV and human leukocyte antigen (HLA) predispositions are implicated in this disease.[40] However, an infectious etiology suspected of being Mollicute-like organisms or cell wall–deficient bacteria has been observed in the vitreous of four ocular sarcoidosis cases.[43, 44] The lymphocyte subpopulations in sarcoidal granulomas are composed principally of T4 helper lymphocytes and display the interleukin 2 (IL2) receptors, as do epithelioid cells and giant cells. Few B lymphocytes are present. Rings of suppressor-cytotoxic T8 cells encircle the granuloma, whereas the T4 cells are found throughout the granulomas.[45]

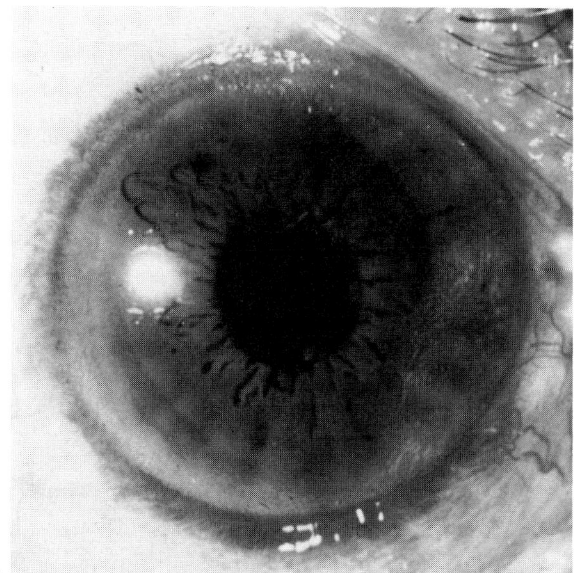
A

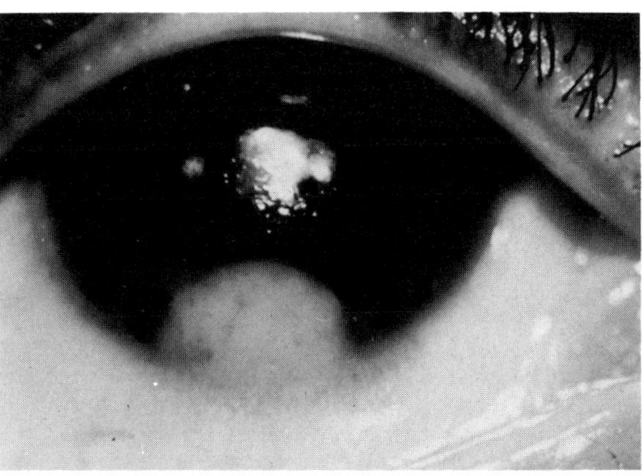
B

Figure 182–5. Sarcoidosis. *A*, Multiple sarcoid nodules (Koeppe's) of pupillary membrane of iris. *B*, Large sarcoid nodule (Busacca's) of peripheral iris and anterior chamber. (From Spencer WH [ed]: Ophthalmic Pathology: An Atlas and Textbook, 3rd ed. Philadelphia, WB Saunders, 1986, p 1968.)

Behçet's Disease

Ocular involvement occurs in 70 percent of patients with Behçet's disease,[40] which causes a suppurative and nongranulomatous uveitis, hemorrhagic infarction of the retina, and retinal detachment.[46] This systemic disorder also includes relapsing episodic aphthosis, genital and other mucocutaneous ulcerations, arthritis, and meningoencephalitis. Ophthalmic manifestations include recurrent uveitis (iridocyclitis, vitritis), retinal vasculitis, and necrotizing retinitis. It is linked to HLA-B51 and is 30 times more prevalent in Japan (where it occurs 1/10,000) than in the United States. Behçet's disease results from an occlusive vasculitis triggered by allergic or viral features such as herpesvirus type 1, which is

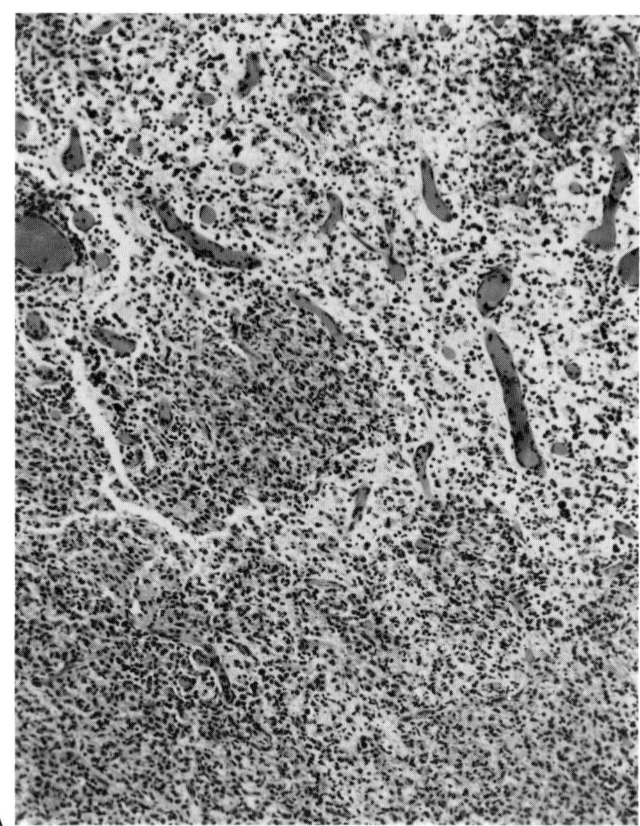

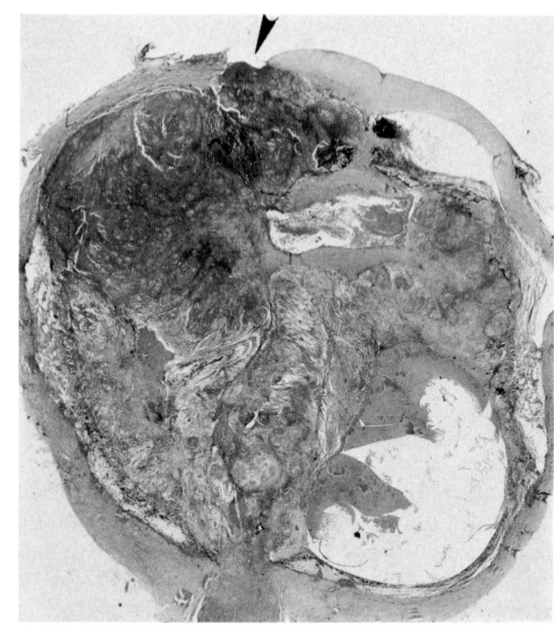

Figure 182–6. Ocular sarcoidosis. *A*, Iris biopsy of large peripheral iris and anterior chamber sarcoid nodule shows epithelioid nodules and new, thin-walled vessels. H&E, ×125. *B*, Section of whole eye, much of which is filled by granulomatous inflammatory tissue. The retina is detached, and granuloma extends through the wound site where the iris lesion was biopsied (*arrowhead*). H&E, ×4. (From Spencer WH [ed]: Ophthalmic Pathology: An Atlas and Textbook, 3rd ed. Philadelphia, WB Saunders, 1986, p 1970.)

more often present in circulating lymphocytes of affected patients than in controls.[47] In affected subjects, relapses apparently are triggered by foods such as English walnuts and chocolate.

Histopathologic examination reveals an obliterative vasculitis, nongranulomatous choroiditis and retinitis, and retinal perivasculitis. In iridocyclitis before steroid therapy, a sterile hypopyon (suppurative infiltrative inflammation with leukocytes) is common (Fig. 182–7).

Pathologic specimens of advanced cases show lymphocytic perivascular infiltration as well as a diffuse infiltration with lymphocytes, plasma cells, and macrophages of the choroid and retina.[213] Neutrophil microabscesses can be observed in the iris stroma with chronic inflammatory cell infiltrates. Iris vessels are infiltrated by lymphocytes and may show rubeosis.[48] At the end-stage, retinal vessels are atrophic amid mild gliosis. As in other retinochoroiditis, extensive destruction of the retinal pigment epithelium is apparent.[46, 213] Immunohistochemical studies show immune complex deposits of IgG, C3, and IgA in episcleral and choroidal veins and an obliterative vasculitis, including arteriolar fibrinoid necrosis, which may initiate vascular thromboses.[49]

The cause of Behçet's disease is obscure, but genetic viral and allergic factors have been all implicated.[50] Behçet's disease is an autoimmune disorder involving type III hypersensitivity and results from immunocomplex-mediated damage to endothelial cells of blood vessels. An abnormal B-cell function with increased numbers of circulating antibodies of all classes is also present. Aberration of T-cell subsets and abnormal polymorphic function have been reported.[51, 52] Autoantibodies are uncommon but have been demonstrated against mucosal antigen and anticardiolipin antibodies, particularly in association with retinal vascular disease.[53, 54]

Sympathetic Ophthalmia

A more detailed discussion of this entity is given in Chapter 33. Sympathetic ophthalmia is a granulomatous inflammation involving the fellow to the injured eye, occurring characteristically a few days to many years after the first eye had been traumatized by a perforating injury in the region of the ciliary body. This disease can also occur after intraocular surgery, such as cataract extraction, evisceration, cyclocryotherapy, and vitrectomy. Less frequently, it has been reported in association with perforated corneal ulcers and choroidal melanomas.

Eighty percent of cases occur within 3 mo of injury. Classically, pain, photophobia, loss of accommodation, and decreased vision are present in the sympathetic eye with symptom exacerbation in the injured eye. This may occur from 5 days[55] to 8 yr[56] after the initial injury.

Granulomatous iridocyclitis and vitritis with mutton-

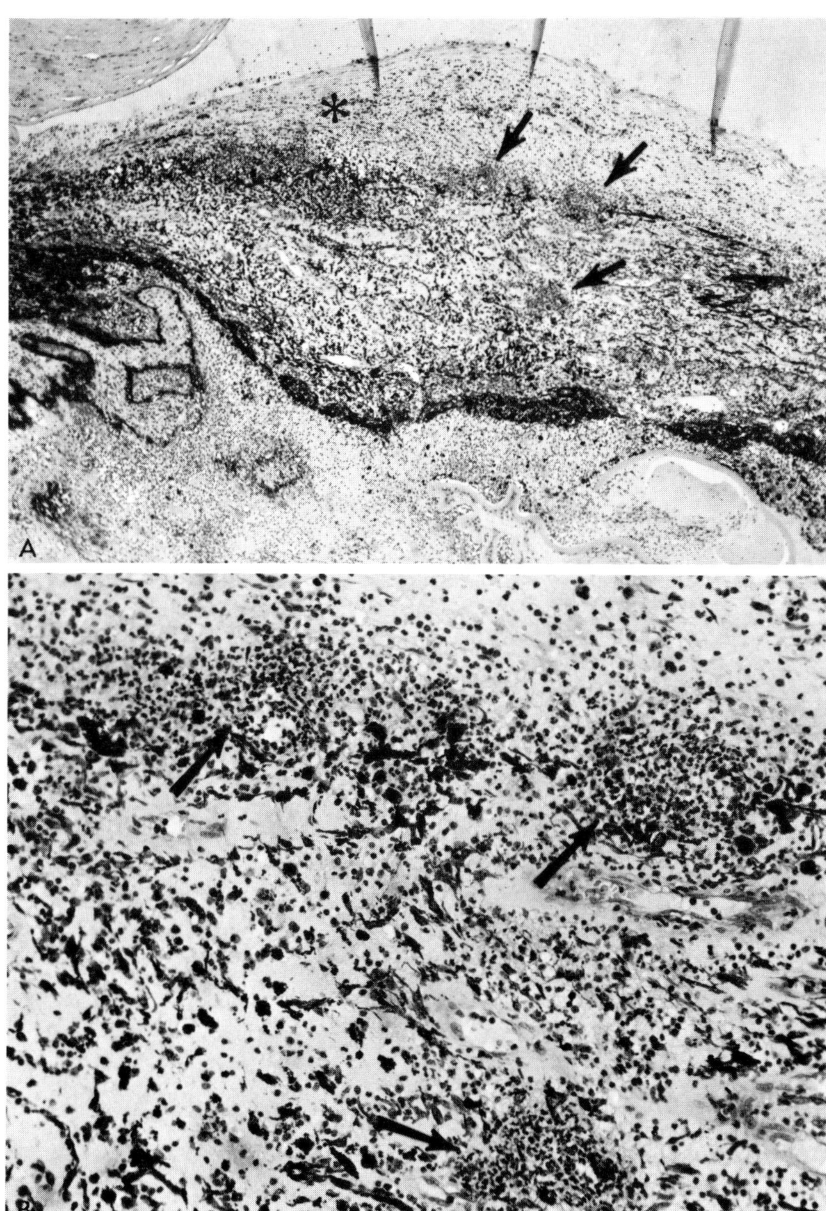

Figure 182–7. Behçet's disease. *A*, Eye with end-stage disease with extensive intraocular inflammation. Dense fibroinflammation and vascular membrane (*asterisk*) is present on the anterior surface of the iris. Neutrophilic microabscesses (*arrows*) are present in the iris. H&E, ×35. *B*, Higher-power view shows intense chronic inflammatory cell infiltrate in the iris and several neutrophilic microabscesses (*arrows*). H&E, ×185, EP 60804. (Courtesy of W. H. Spencer, M.D.)

fat keratic precipitates manifest bilaterally. Thickening of the iris stroma with inflammatory nodules with loss of iris detail, pupillary occlusion, and rubeosis occurs.[57] Clusters of small, depigmented, yellow, millet seed–shaped lesions, known as Dalen-Fuchs nodules, are observable in the fundus although not pathognomonic of sympathetic ophthalmia, since they also occur in sarcoidosis and Vogt-Koyanagi-Harada syndrome.[58]

On histopathologic examination, the injured and sympathetic eyes are similar in that the main feature is diffuse, nonnecrotizing granulomatous inflammation in the uvea. The choroid is markedly thickened and infiltrated by lymphocytes and nests of macrophages, epithelioid, and giant cells (Fig. 182–8). Other classic histopathologic findings include the relative lack of retinal involvement, spacing of the choriocapillaris, and the formation of Dalen-Fuchs nodules consisting mainly of epithelioid cells located between Bruch's membrane and the RPE (Fig. 182–9).

Recently, breaks in Bruch's membrane at the Dalen-Fuchs nodules have been observed.[59] Other histopathologic features reported are retinal perivasculitis, retinitis, and optic atrophy. T lymphocytes are the principal mediators of choroidal infiltrates: relatively higher numbers of T helper-inducer T cells in the early stage and relatively higher suppressor-cytotoxic T cells in the later stage.[60] B lymphocytes and plasma cells are present to a lesser degree but never as conspicuously as in Vogt-Koyanagi-Harada syndrome.[67]

The pathogenesis is probably related to hypersensitivity to uveal pigment, which is induced by antigens, including infectious agents or substances present in the photoreceptor retinal layer acting as possible autoantigens. This hypothesis has been substantiated by the

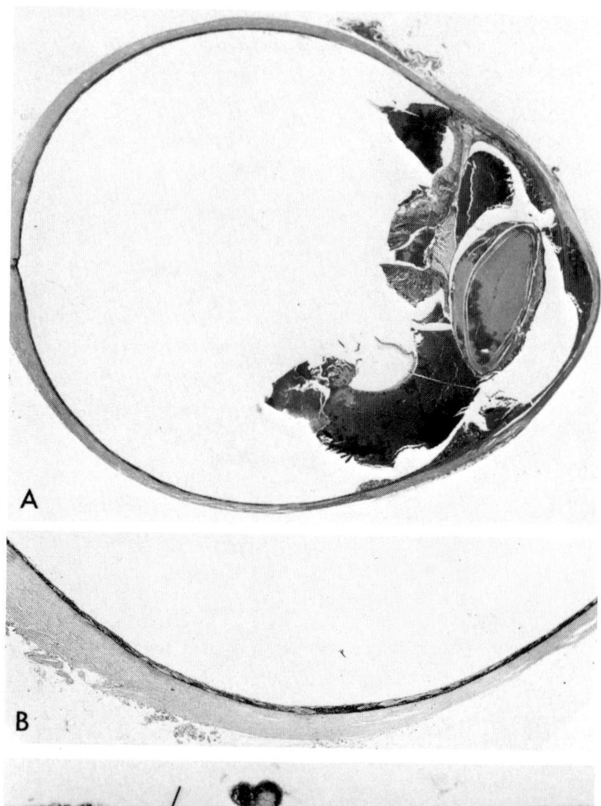

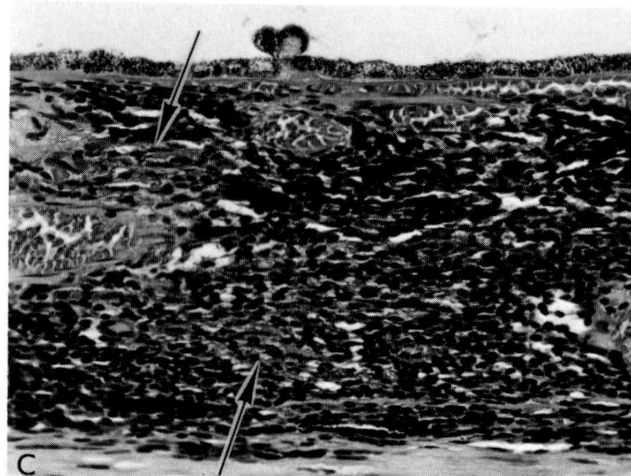

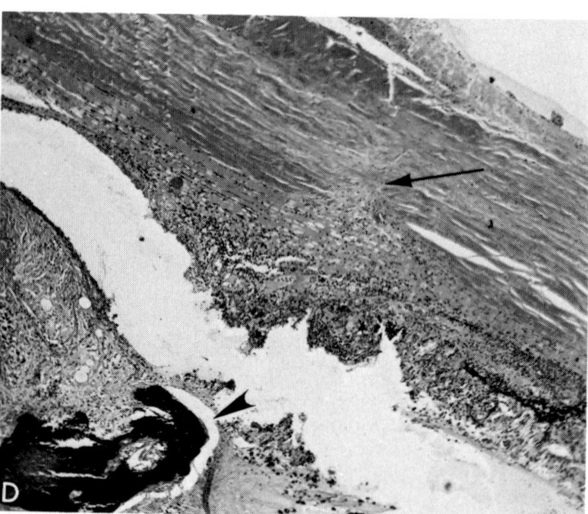

Figure 182–8. Sympathetic ophthalmia with onset 18 yr after contusion and unsuspected scleral rupture. *A*, The original horizontal sections of the globe revealed total detachment of the retina, massive intraocular hemorrhage, and granulomatous choroiditis but no evidence of a penetrating injury. H&E, ×3, AFIP Neg 64-233. *B*, Low-power view showing slightly thickened choroid. H&E, ×13, AFIP Neg 64-1379. *C*, The choroid is thickened by a lymphocytic infiltrate that spares the choriocapillaris and has foci of epithelioid cells (*arrows*). H&E, ×300, AFIP Neg 64-905. *D*, Scar of perforation (*arrow*) in area of ciliary body. Detached retina is degenerated, with calcification (*arrowhead*). H&E, ×50, AFIP Neg 64-1378. (From Stafford WR: Sympathetic ophthalmia. A report of a case with onset 18 yr after contusion with unsuspected scleral rupture. Surv Ophthalmol 10:232–237, 1965.)

production of experimental sympathetic ophthalmia with retinal S antigen. Increased numbers of T lymphocytes[61, 62] in the choroidal infiltrate suggest that the disease is due to cell-mediated immunity against antigens found in the photoreceptors, the RPE, and the choroidal melanocytes. Killer cell autoantibody-mediated cytotoxicity (type II) is another possible mechanism.

Vogt-Koyanagi-Harada Syndrome

Vogt-Koyanagi-Harada syndrome is a unilateral or bilateral granulomatous inflammation of the uveal tract and retina associated with varying degrees of skin and hair depigmentation, alopecia, and meningeal irritation.[63, 64] It accounts for 8 percent of uveitis in Asians compared with 1 percent in non-Asians and Native Americans. In the late stage, bilateral exudative retinal detachment, cerebrospinal fluid pleocytosis, and meningitis occur in a complex known as Harada's syndrome.[65]

The disease is characterized by panuveitis with mutton-fat keratic precipitates, aqueous cells and flare, iris nodules, synechiae, vitreous haze and cells, optic disc swelling, retinal edema, hemorrhages, exudates, nonrhegmatogenous detachment, and choroidal and RPE infiltrates. In a few reported cases, the reported histopathologic findings resemble those seen in sympathetic ophthalmia, with a diffuse lymphocytic infiltrate composed mostly of T cells but with a larger proportion of suppressor-helper cells directed against uveal melanocytes. Unlike sympathetic ophthalmia, choriocapillaris and retinal destruction is reported to be more extensive, although this may be partly the result of late analysis in the course of the disease.[66] Immunopathology data show

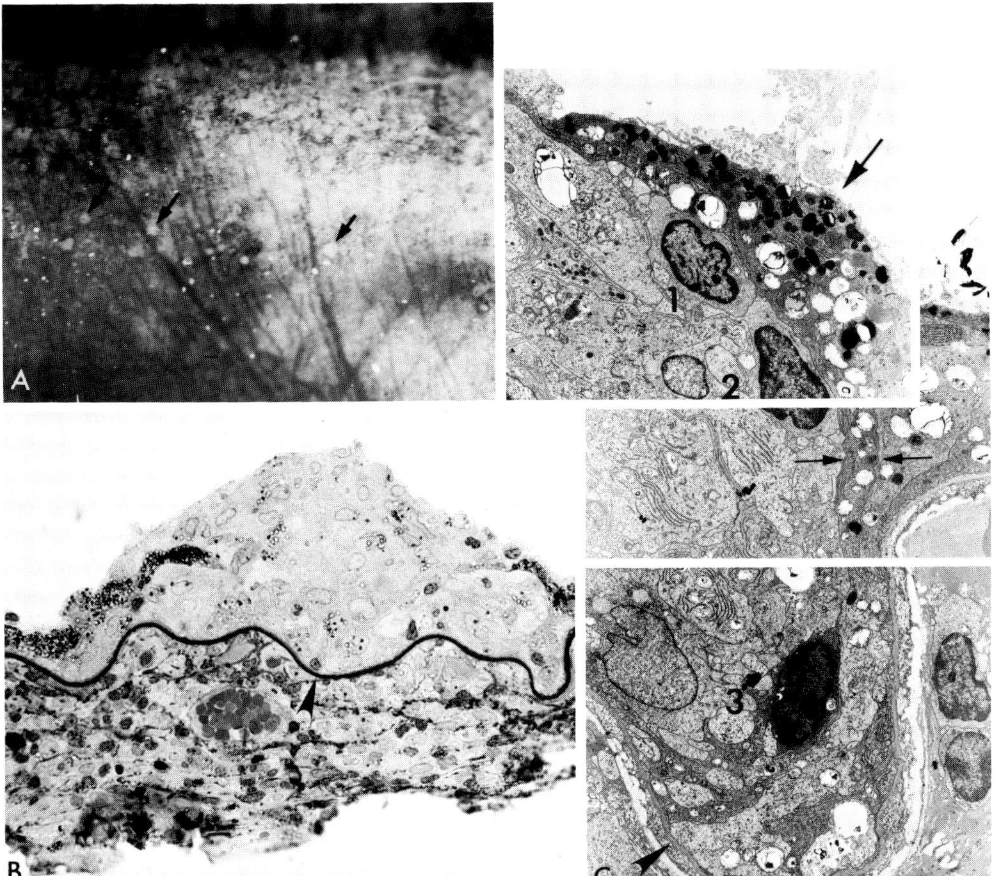

Figure 182–9. Dalen-Fuchs nodules in sympathetic ophthalmia. *A*, Minute, grayish-white Dalen-Fuchs nodules (*arrows*) are numerous on the peripheral pigment epithelium. The ora serrata is above. The sensory retina has been removed to make the nodules more readily visible. *B*, Single Dalen-Fuchs nodule from retinal periphery. Bruch's membrane (*arrowhead*) is continuous and intact here (as well as in serial sections). The underlying choroid shows mild, nongranulomatous mononuclear infiltrate. The nodule is composed of "epithelioid" cells into which adjacent pigment epithelium progressively attenuates. The peripheral area of the nodule to the right is seen in C as a montage of electron micrographs. Toluidine blue, ×350. *C*, Montage showing single pigment epithelial cell (*arrow*) with basement membrane (*arrowhead*). The cell process is thin and elongated (between *arrows*) toward its attachment, forming a broad footplate on its basement membrane. Three adjacent mononuclear cells are labeled *1*, *2*, and *3*. AFIP Acc 1481771. (From Font RL, Fine BS, Messmer E, et al: Light and electron microscopic study of Dalen-Fuch's nodules in sympathetic ophthalmia. Ophthalmology 90:66–75, 1983.)

foci of B lymphocyte aggregation and scattering macrophages in the uvea and retina.[67] Besides granulomatous inflammation, a nongranulomatous inflammation of the optic nerve and arachnoid may be present (Fig. 182–10).

The cause remains unknown. A delayed hypersensitivity reaction to melanin-containing structures may be operative. Cell-mediated immunity to human myelin basic protein,[68] antiganglioside antibodies,[69] anti-outer segments of photoreceptors, and anti-Müller cell antibodies[70] have all been detected in sera of patients with Vogt-Koyanagi-Harada syndrome.

This autoimmune reaction against the melanocytes could be induced by an unknown triggering agent with subsequent alteration of the antigenic-determining sites on the surface of the melanocytes. The intraocular plasma cell and B lymphocytic infiltration, the formation of exudative retinal detachment, and the elevated serum IgD levels confirm to some extent the role played by the humoral immunity in sympathetic ophthalmia.[69, 70]

Phacoanaphylactic Uveitis

This granulomatous inflammation is centered by crystalline material secondary to rupture of the lens capsule. Histopathologic examination reveals a granulomatous inflammation with neutrophil leukocytes centered around the lens proteins (Fig. 182–11). Epithelioid cells and occasional giant multinucleated cells surround the neutrophils, with lymphocytes and plasma cells peripheral to the epithelioid cells. Usually the iris is inflammatory, and the uveal tract is involved with a chronic nongranulomatous inflammation.[71, 72]

INFECTIOUS UVEITIS

Metastatic Bacterial Endophthalmitis

Several distinct clinical forms of metastatic bacterial endophthalmitis can be empirically designated as focal (anterior or posterior), diffuse (anterior or posterior),

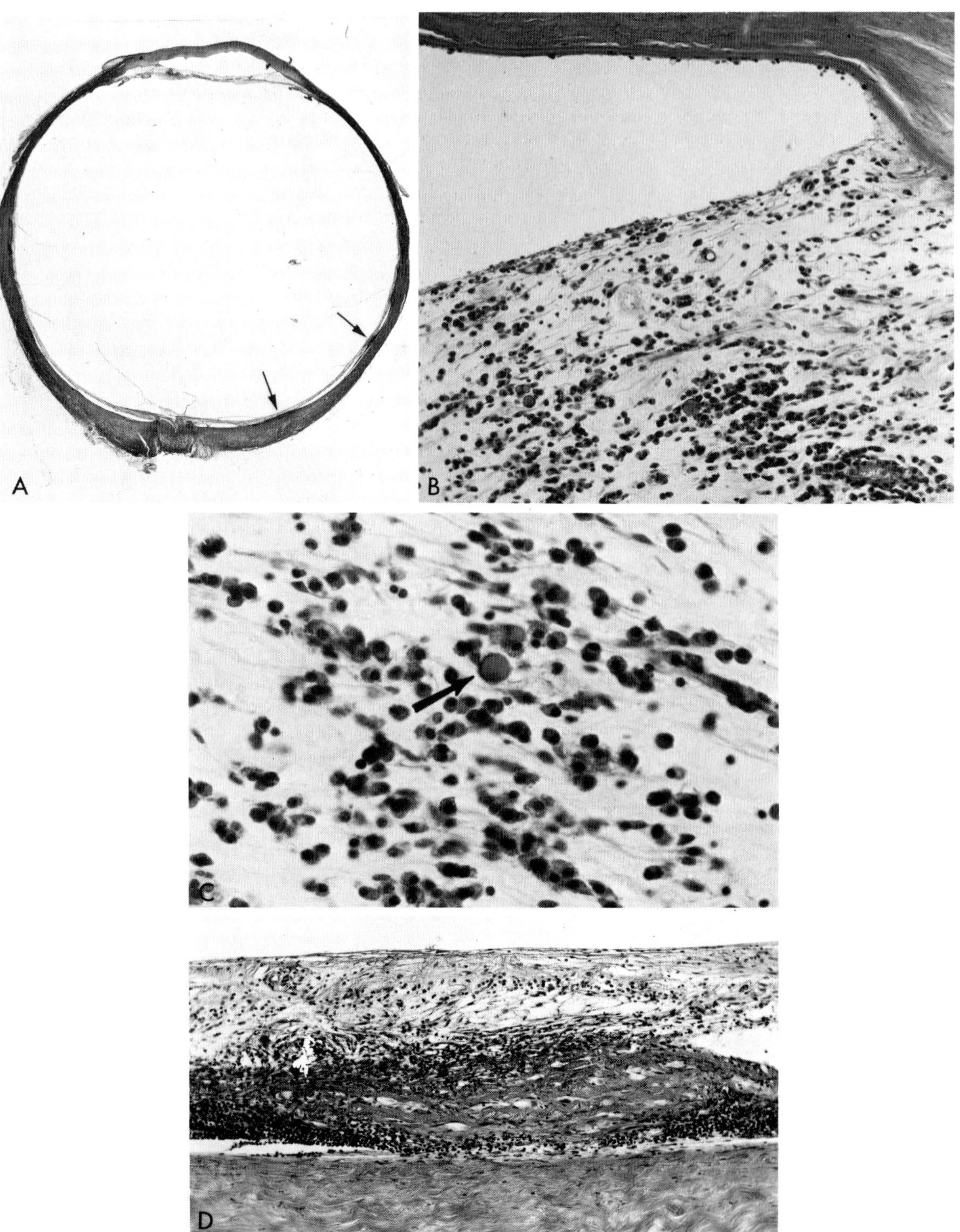

Figure 182–10. Vogt-Koyanagi-Harada (VHK) syndrome. Case of a 19-year-old white man with all the features of VHK except tinnitus. *A*, This eye has broad anterior synechiae and pupillary membrane. Focal areas of chorioretinal scarring are scattered throughout (*arrows*). The retina is attached. H&E, ×4. *B*, The anterior chamber angle is closed by peripheral anterior synechiae, and the iris is diffusely infiltrated by lymphocytes and plasma cells. H&E, ×160. C, At higher power, numerous plasma cells and a plasmacytoid cell (*arrow*) are evident in the iris. *D*, A plaque of proliferated retinal pigment epithelium with basement membrane material containing lymphocytic infiltrates is interposed between the disorganized gliosed retina (*above*) and the atrophic choroid (*below*). H&E, ×115, AFIP Acc 529804. (From Perry HD, Font RL: Clinical and histopathologic observations in severe Vogt-Koyanagi-Harada syndrome. Am J Ophthalmol 83:242–254, 1977. Reprinted with permission from the Ophthalmic Publishing Company.)

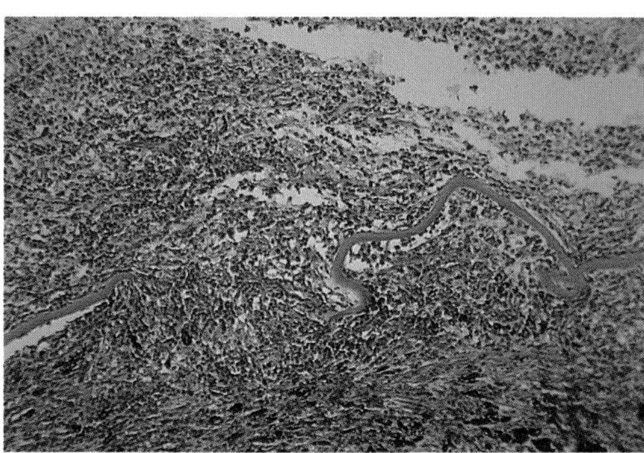

Figure 182–11. Phacolytic endophthalmitis in sympathizing eye enucleated 6 mo after onset of uveitis. H&E, ×35, AFIP Acc 77289.

and panophthalmitis. Focal intraocular inflammation appears to be concentrated in one or a few discrete foci having the appearance of whitish nodules or plaques in the iris, ciliary body, retina, or choroid. In the retina, whitish emboli can be seen in multiple retinal arterioles, with perivascular hemorrhages and inflammatory infiltration (Roth's spot). Anterior diffuse inflammation is characterized by severe generalized signs of inflammation involving the anterior segment; edema, hypopyon, or fibrinous dot in the anterior chamber is typical. Posterior diffuse inflammation is characterized by an intense inflammatory reaction in the vitreous. Panophthalmitis is present if inflammation affects all three layers of the globe.

Histopathologic examination reveals focal inflammation with bacteria and inflammatory cells occluding the lumina of vessels and infiltrating the surrounding tissue. In Roth's spots, the white center may contain organisms, although most are sterile and consist of white blood cells and, often, a fibrin thrombus occurring at the site of extravasation of blood. The reason that septic emboli occur more frequently in the retina than in the choroid is unknown. Diffuse inflammation shows numerous bacteria and inflammatory cells with necrosis and hemorrhage of the involved tissues.

During the course of bacteremia, any causative bacteria can produce endophthalmitis. Certain organisms clearly have a propensity to invade the eye from the bloodstream.

Gram-positive organisms, which appear to be decreasing as a causative agents,[73] include *Bacillus cereus* (with brown chocolate exudate in the anterior chamber), *Streptococcus* species, *S. aureus*, *Listeria monocytogenes*, and *Clostridium perfringes*. Gram-negative organisms include *N. meningitidis, H. influenzae, Klebsiella pneumoniae, E. coli, Serratia* species, *Salmonella* species, *Actinobacillus* species, and *P. aeruginosa*.

Tuberculosis

Usual ocular manifestations include iridocyclitis, iris nodules, choroiditis multifocal, and choroidal tuberculomas (Fig. 182–12).[74] The choroidal tuberculomas may follow regression of characteristic ischemic retinal vasculitis (Earle's disease).[75] Acute tuberculous endophthalmitis is rare.

In large tuberculomas, caseation necrosis is present with zonal granulation surrounding the coagulative necrosis. Miliary choroidal tuberculosis causes a multifocal, discrete, sarcoid-like inflammation, but with caseating necrosis affecting the centers of the epithelioid granulomas. Histologic examination shows severe inflammatory cell infiltration by lymphocytes, plasma cells, multinucleated giant cells, and acid-fast bacilli with surrounding granulomas (Fig. 182–13).[76] Resolved cases may show choroidal neovascularization.[77]

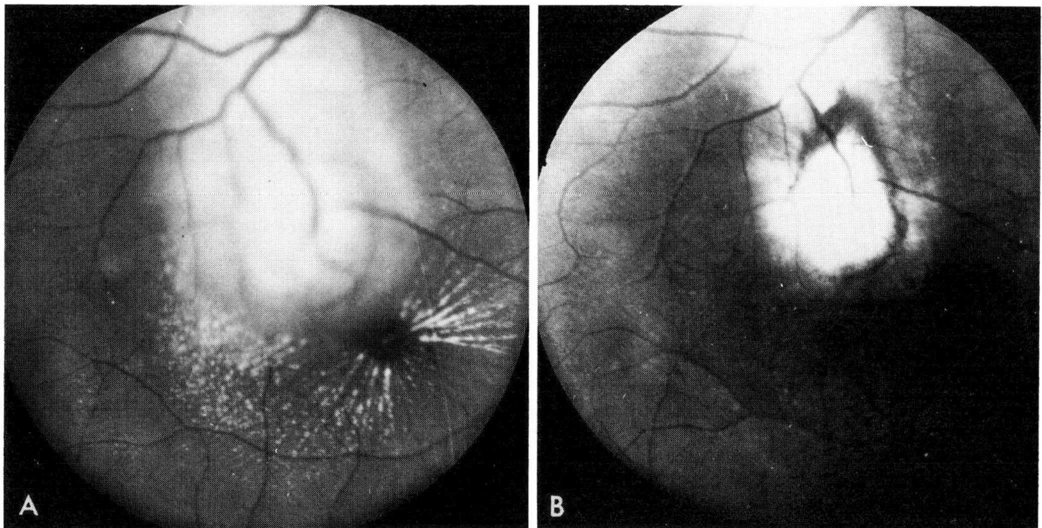

Figure 182–12. Tuberculoma of the choroid in a 22-year-old-man with known active pulmonary tuberculosis. *A,* Raised yellowish choroidal lesion with surrounding serous elevation of the neurosensory retina, intraretinal exudation, and macular star. Retinal vessels are seen over the lesion and appear normal. *B,* Choroidal lesion 2 mo after status shown in *A*. The active lesion is smaller and is now surrounded by an accumulation of pigment epithelium. Beyond the lesion are areas of retinal pigment epithelium degeneration. The area of exudation has diminished, and the macular star is no longer present. Retinal arterialization of the scar has occurred. (From Cangemi FE, Friedman AH, Josephberg R: Tuberculoma of the choroid. Ophthalmology 87:252–258, 1980.)

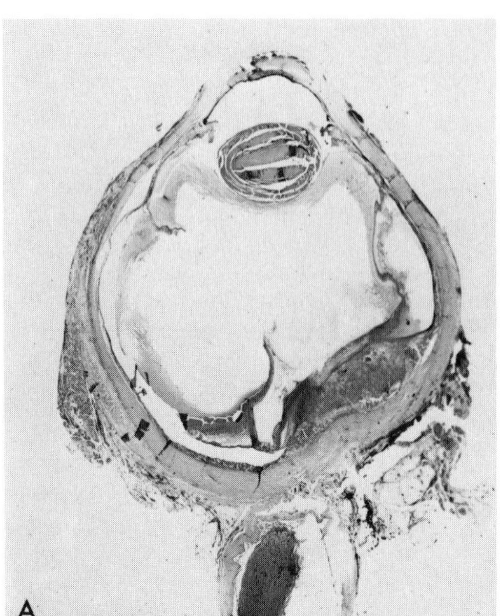

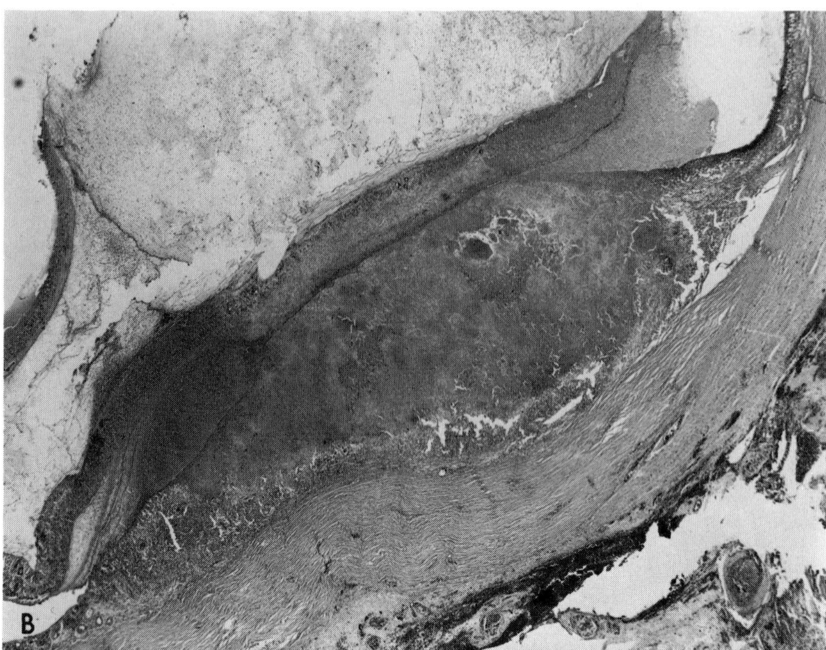

Figure 182–13. Tuberculous granuloma of the choroid with acute panophthalmitis. *A,* Section of left globe showing large choroidal granuloma. H&E, ×3.5, AFIP Neg 66-8899. *B,* Choroidal granuloma with necrosis of the overlying retina and inflammatory reaction in the vitreous. H&E, ×10, AFIP Neg 66-8900.

Leprosy

This disease affects 10 million people living in the tropics of Cancer and Capricorn.[214] It is clinically subdivided into two types with intermediate forms. In lepromatous leprosy, ocular involvement includes the cornea, sclera, and iris; iridocyclitis can be either insidious or acute and exudative. The iris often develops striking white globular bodies enmeshed in the stroma (leprotic pearls). In tuberculoid leprosy, ocular involvement is rare. Lagophthalmos and corneal hypoesthesia can be observed.

In lepromatous leprosy, histopathologic examination reveals granulomatous inflammation occurring with characteristic formation of lepromas. These consist of distended histiocytes with fatty, vacuolated cytoplasm (Virchow's cells) with bacteria (*Mycobacterium leprae*), and pale-staining histiocytes with amorphous cytoplasm (*M. leprae* cells).[78] The lepromas can be observed on the iris and the ciliary body as collections of lymphocytes, fibroblasts, and characteristic large, swollen macrophages with a cytoplasm replete with acid-fast bacilli (foam). Choroidal involvement is rare and consists of chronic inflammatory lesions also containing bacilli (Fig. 182–14).[78] In tuberculoid leprosy, lesions are akin to noncaseating tuberculosis and are characterized by minimal bacteria and a florid granulomatous inflammation. Discrete tubercular or sarcoidal inflammation is present with nodules of varying size.

Syphilis

Ocular pathology may be present in both congenital and acquired syphilis. In the congenital form, ocular involvement consists of interstitial keratitis. Iritis may occur either as roseola in the initial stages of secondary syphilis, with a hyperemic, bright red spot in the middle third of the iris that lasts several days and resolves, or as yellow to brown papules at the pupillary margin or ciliary border. Retinal periphlebitis and juxtapapillary chorioretinitis heal with severe scarring. Chorioretinitis and neuroretinitis are rarely seen in acquired syphilis (Fig. 182–15).

In syphilitic chorioretinitis, chronic granulomas and inflammation are characterized by lymphocytes, epithelioid and plasma cells, and treponemas (*Treponema pallidum*). Choroidal inflammation results in large atrophic patches with the disappearance of external retinal layers and RPE and internal choroidal layers surrounded by a zone of RPE proliferation with chorioretinal adhesions. These follow breaks in Bruch's membrane with ensuing invasion of the choroid by glial elements and pigment epithelium.[79] A neovascular membrane of the choroid is a common complication.[80]

Pneumocystis carinii Choroidopathy

Pneumocystis carinii causes an opportunistic pneumonitis in immunocompromised hosts, including 80 percent of patients with AIDS.[81] It features multiple round-to-oval, pale yellow-white, slightly elevated choroidal lesions one-half disc in diameter that may coalesce and undergo necrosis without surrounding inflammation. Optic disc edema and cotton-wool spots attributed to HIV microangiopathy and cytomegalovirus (CMV) retinitis may be present.

Histopathology reveals dense sheets of pneumocystic organisms infiltrating the choroid, choriocapillaris, and choroidal vessels. An amorphous, foamy, acellular, eo-

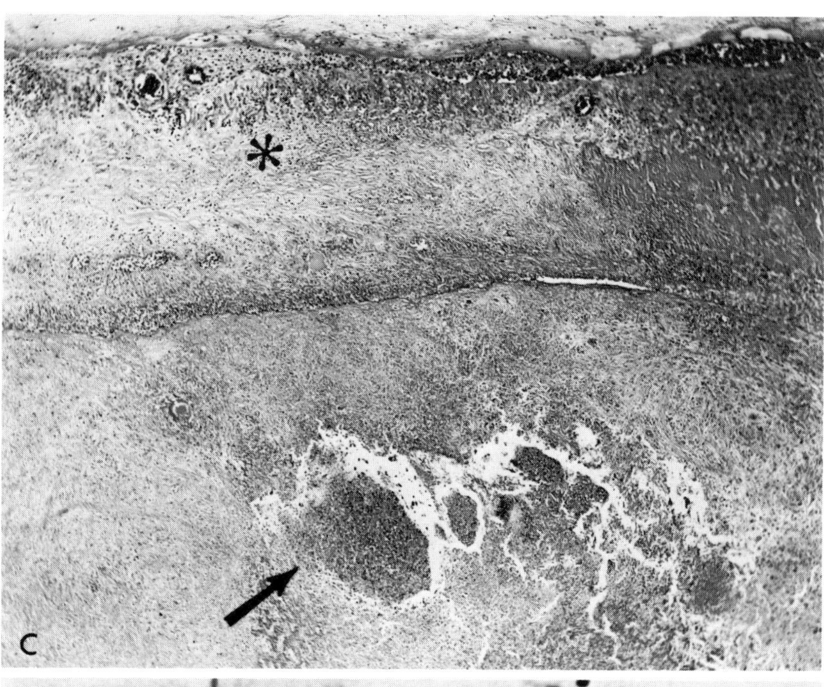

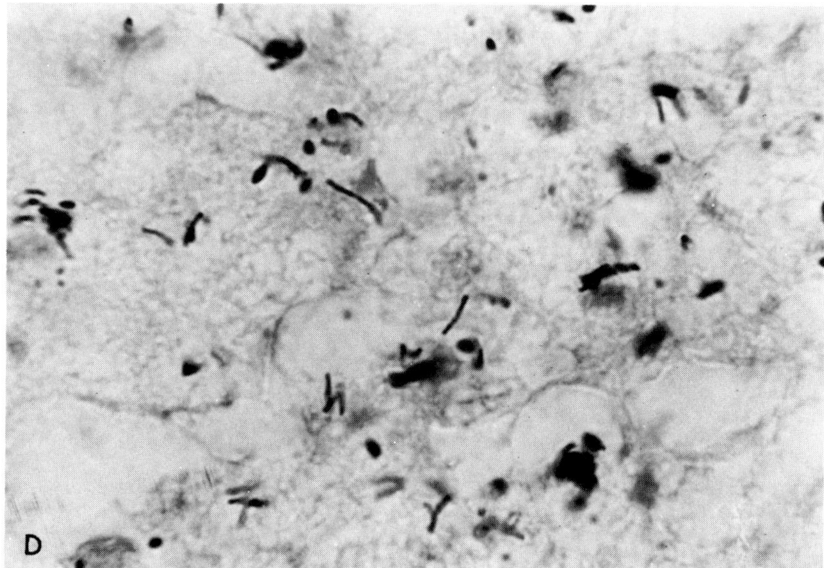

Figure 182–13 *Continued.* *C*, Area of caseous necrosis in choroidal granuloma (*arrow*) and necrotic supradjacent retina (*asterisk*) H&E, ×50, AFIP Neg 66-8901. *D*, Acid-fast bacilli in necrotic retina. Kinyoun's acid-fast stain ×1400, AFIP Neg 66-8904. (From Spencer WH [ed]: Ophthalmic Pathology: An Atlas and Textbook, 3rd ed. Philadelphia, WB Saunders, 1986, p 1818.)

sinophilic infiltrate may be present within the choroidal vessels. Gomori's methenamine silver (GMS) stain is useful for demonstrating these cystic or crescentic organisms.[82]

Nocardiosis

Nocardia steroides is a filamentous, gram-positive aerobic bacteria that may involve the eye either exogenously, following penetrating injury or surgery, or endogenously, mostly in immunosuppressed hosts with pneumonia or meningitis. This organism often involves the choroid, giving rise to a subretinal mass that may simulate a choroidal tumor or a large solid detachment of the RPE.

The choroid is thickened by inflammatory cells composed chiefly of lymphocytes and plasma cells with focal neutrophil microabscesses about focal areas of choriocapillaris (Fig. 182–16).[83] A necrotizing granulomatous inflammation with epithelioid cells and giant cells is present. Focal disruption in Bruch's membrane allows the inflammation to extend to the retina and vitreous. The organisms are well demonstrated by GMS, Gram's, and Ziehl-Neelsen stains.

Lyme Disease

Lyme disease is an infectious disorder caused by *Borrelia burgdorferi*, a spirochete of the tick *Ixodes dammini*. The most common manifestations are rash and arthritis and neurologic and cardiac signs and symptoms. Ocular findings include hemorrhagic conjunctivitis, keratitis, iritis, iridocyclitis, pars planitis, retinal vasculitis, optic neuritis, and Vogt-Koyanagi-Harada syndrome.

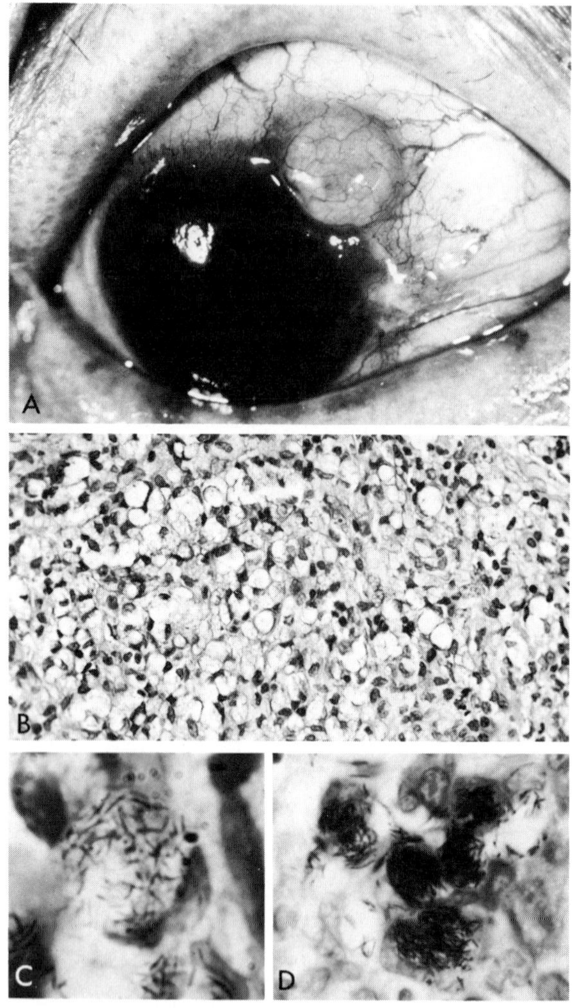

Figure 182–14. Lepromatous leprosy. *A*, Patient with lepromatous uveitis, loss of lashes, and a lepromatous nodule straddling the limbus. AFIP Neg. 65-12701-2. *B*, Nodule consists of large histiocytes. H&E, ×400, AFIP Neg 65-13050. *C* and *D*, These histiocytes contain numerous acid-fast bacilli in a globus configuration. Fite-Faraco stain, ×1050, AFIP Negs 65-12701-1, 67-5086. (Courtesy of James H. Allen, M.D.)

To our knowledge, no clinicopathologic study of ocular involvement in Lyme disease has been reported. However, the pathology of multisystem involvement in this condition includes direct invasion of the tissue by the *Borrelia* organism, small vessel occlusion, and vasculitis as a consequence of plasma cell panvascular infiltration.[84]

VIRAL UVEITIS

Herpes Simplex and Herpes Zoster Viruses

Herpetic uveitis is a frequent complication of herpes keratitis, but it may also occur without keratitis. Rarely, herpes simplex virus (HSV) may cause unilateral or bilateral acute retinal necrosis characterized by panuveitis and dense, pale-yellow, retinal lesions. Following herpetic infection, granulomatous inflammation of the iris is histologically found to consist of lymphocytes, macrophages, plasma cells, and fibrin. Iris edema or necrosis has been reported. In acute retinal necrosis, histopathologic examination reveals full-thickness nec-

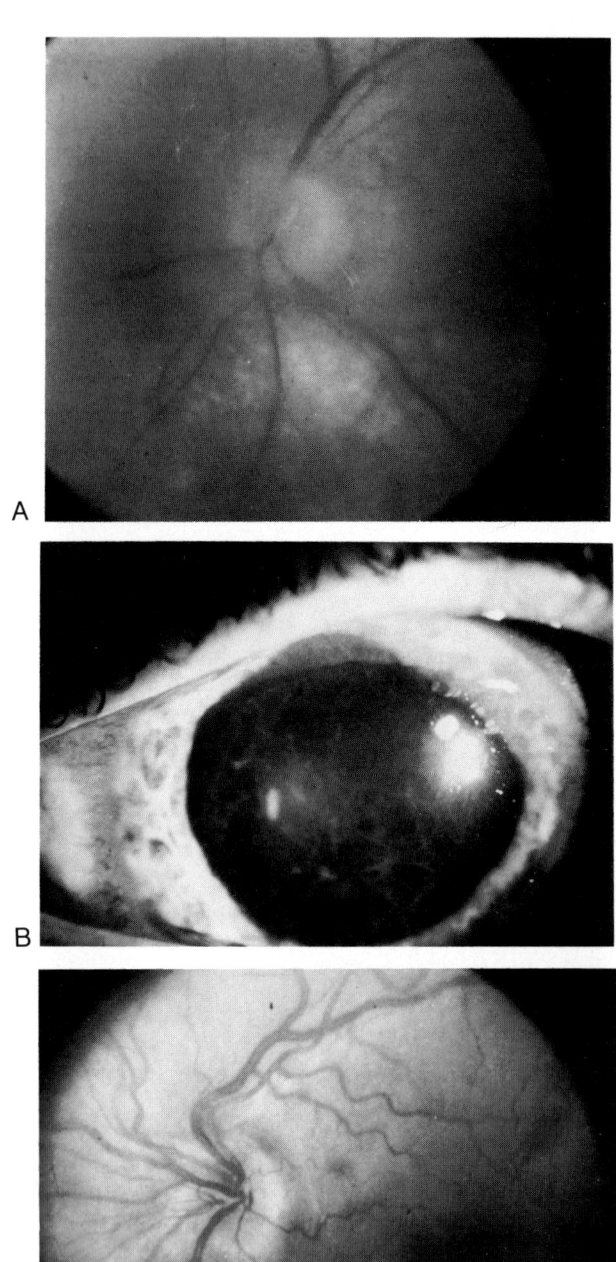

Figure 182–15. *A*, Acquired syphilis with ocular involvement. Vitritis, optic neuritis, and round, yellow-white chorioretinal lesions surrounding the optic disc. *B*, Severe fibrinous and plastic iritis with marked swelling of the iris along its pupillary margin. *C*, Flame-shaped retinal hemorrhages along retinal vessels with generalized edema of the posterio pole. (From Ross WH, Sutton HFS: Acquired syphilitic uveitis. Arch Ophthalmol 98:496–498, 1980. Copyright 1980, American Medical Association.)

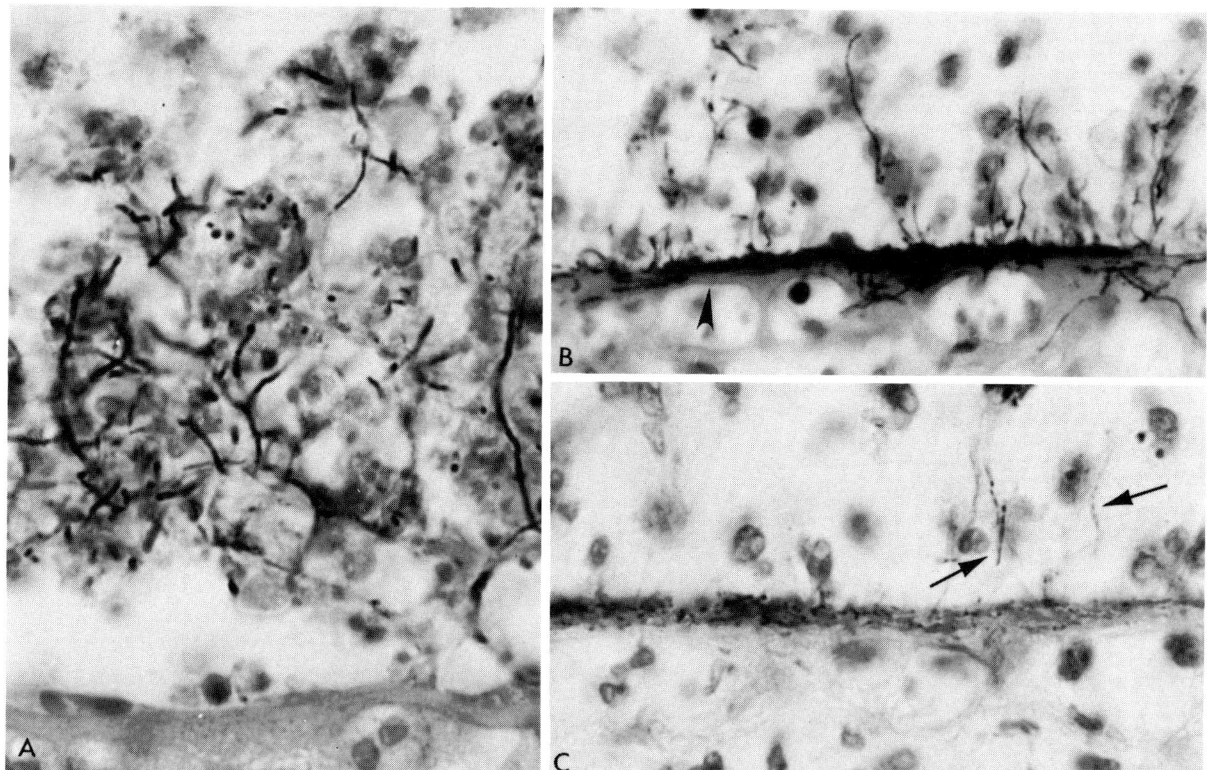

Figure 182–16. Intraocular nocardiosis. *A*, Branching, filamentous, gram-positive organisms growing along Bruch's membrane, the choriocapillaris, and the subretinal space. Brown and Brenn, ×900, AFIP Neg 68-4318. *B*, High-power view of the subretinal space, showing gram-positive organisms branching at approximately 90-degree angles. *Arrowhead*, Bruch's membrane. Brown and Brenn, ×1200, AFIP Neg 68-4432. C, Organisms that are partially acid-fast are predominantly concentrated along Bruch's membrane. Note the beaded appearance of branching filaments (*arrows*). Fite-Faraco stain, cross-modification ×1100, AFIP Neg 68-4433. (From Meyer SL, Font RL, Shaver RP: Intraocular nocardiosis. Report of three cases. Arch Ophthalmol 83:536–541, 1970. Copyright 1970, American Medical Association.)

rotizing retinitis, thrombosing retinal and choroidal arteritis, segmental necrotizing optic neuritis, panuveitis, and vasculitis. Numerous intranuclear inclusion bodies typical of HSV were evident by light and electron microscopy in the retina and RPE. HSV had been suspected as a cause of acute retinal necrosis because of high antibody titers to HSV or HSV antigen in the vitreous.[77–87] Diagnosis may also be based on identification of virus particles morphologically compatible with the herpesvirus family (varicella zoster virus,[88] HSV-1,[88–91] HSV-2, herpesvirus B, cytomegalovirus, Epstein-Barr virus [EBV]) by electron microscopic examination.[89, 90, 92]

Epstein-Barr Virus

Ocular disease has traditionally been described in association with acute EBV infection. It causes various ocular inflammations, including conjunctivitis, episcleritis, keratitis, uveitis, and optic neuritis. Acute, bilateral, severe anterior uveitis, and acute punctate outer retinitis choroiditis with panuveitis have been described.

High anti-EBV IgG antibody titers in the aqueous humor are evidence of anterior uveitis caused by this organism.[93] There is no biopsy evidence helpful in implicating this virus as a direct cause of posterior uveitis. However, serologic evidence can be highly suggestive for an association of EBV with ocular disease.

Cytomegalovirus

Infection with CMV can cause serious disease in the unborn infant and the immunosuppressed patient, particularly in AIDS. Ocular signs in congenital diseases are chorioretinitis and optic atrophy. In acquired infection, the most striking finding is a necrotizing retinitis characterized by multiple, granular, yellow-white areas associated with extensive retinal hemorrhages and vascular sheathing. Often, there is a sharp demarcation line separating the necrotizing retina from the normal retina.

The retina is thickened, and its laminar architecture is markedly disrupted by the presence of many enlarged cells containing prominent Cowdry type A intranuclear eosinophil inclusions with surrounding clear zones, giving the cells an "owl's-eye" appearance. The underlying RPE is typically disrupted, and varying degrees of chronic inflammatory cells are present in the underlying choroid. Intranuclear inclusions may be identified in the RPE, the optic nerve, and vascular endothelial cells of the choroid. Electron microscopy demonstrates viral particles.[94–96]

Congenital Rubella Syndrome

Ocular effects include microphthalmia, corneal opacities, angle dysgenesis with glaucoma, iris hypoplasia, congenital cataract, and nongranulomatous iridocyclitis.

Nongranulomatous iridocyclitis[97] with lymphocytic infiltrate and secondary iris hypoplasia is due to direct viral infection (Fig. 182–17).[98] The ciliary body also can show nongranulomatous inflammation. The salt-and-pepper fundus appearance is due to alternating areas of pigment epithelium hyperpigmentation and hypopigmentation. The retina and the choroid are unaffected.

FUNGAL UVEITIS

Candida albicans

Endogenous *C. albicans* endophthalmitis is an infection caused by a saprophytic organism that tends to occur in immunocompromised hosts. Risk factors for this infection are the prior use of broad-spectrum antibiotics, systemic steroids, major surgery, diabetes mellitus, alcoholism, parenteral alimentation, toxicomania, and AIDS.[99, 100] The ocular presentation is that of retinitis or endophthalmitis, often with whitish vitreous opacities.

Histopathology reveals chronic nongranulomatous inflammation. This arises in the inner choroid from septic foci lodging in the choriocapillaris. Bruch's membrane is usually ruptured, with formation of subretinal, intraretinal, and vitreal abscesses. Other findings include retinal necrosis, vasculitis, and vitreous nodules composed of polymorphonuclear granulocytes within which are found budding yeast forms or pseudomycelium.[101]

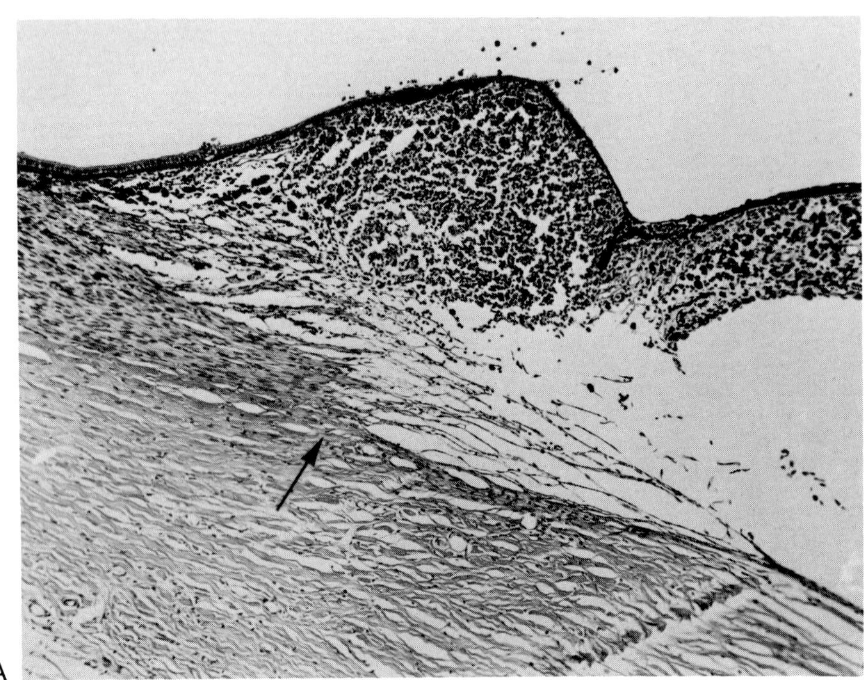

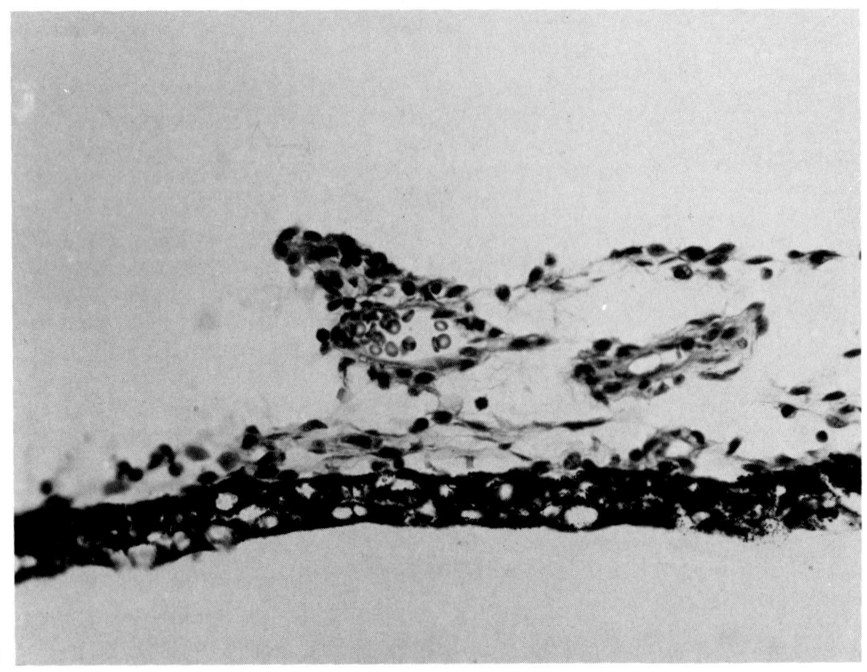

Figure 182–17. *A,* Rubella iridocyclitis. An intense, nongranulomatous inflammatory cell infiltration of the iris and ciliary body is seen. The scleral spur is hypoplastic (*arrow*), and the longitudinal fibers insert directly into the trabecular meshwork. Inflammation in such cases may also contribute to glaucoma. H&E, ×80, AFIP Neg 67-766. *B,* Rubella, iris changes. In addition to nongranulomatous iritis, the iris may show hypoplasia with incomplete development of the stroma and dilator muscle. Such eyes are notorious for failure of or poor pupillary dilatation with mydriatics. H&E, ×305, AFIP Neg 65-3963. (From Zimmerman LE: Histopathologic basis for ocular manifestations of congenital rubella syndrome. The Eighth William Hamlin Wilder Memorial Lecture. Am J Ophthalmol 65:837–862, 1968. Reprinted with permission from the Ophthalmic Publishing Company.)

Histoplasmosis and Presumed Ocular Histoplasmosis

Histoplasmosis is caused by *Histoplasma capsulatum*, a dimorphic fungus endemic to the eastern and central United States. The presumed ocular histoplasmosis syndrome consists of the occurrence of a characteristic multifocal choroiditis, with peripheral punched-out chorioretinal, peripapillary, and macular scars in patients with a positive result on a histoplasmin skin test in the United States[102] or a negative result on a histoplasmin test in Europe.

Histopathologically, one finds a granulomatous choroiditis with hyperplasia of the RPE, breaks in Bruch's membrane, organizing subretinal hemorrhages, and chorioretinal adhesions. Subsequent development of choroidal subretinal neovascularization in macular lesions results in a disciform scar (Fig. 182–18). The organism has never convincingly been observed within these lesions. However, in cases of disseminated histoplasmosis or postoperative endophthalmitis, necrotizing choroidal granulomas containing the yeast form of the dimorphic fungus have been demonstrated.[102]

Cryptococcal Choroiditis

Cryptococcus neoformans spreads from a primary pulmonary focus and has a predilection for the central nervous system (CNS) tissue, including the optic nerve, leptomeninges, and choroid. Such uveitis may precede or follow CNS infection, occurring either from a blood-borne nidus that lodges in the choriocapillaris or as an extension of an intracranial source along the leptomeninges.[103, 104] In patients with HIV infection, *Cryptococcus* is a major cause of neuroophthalmic complications.[105] Chorioretinitis consists of multiple, discrete, slightly elevated, amelanotic retinal or choroidal lesions 500 to 3000 μ in diameter. Retinal perivascular sheathing, vitritis, and anterior uveitis also may occur.

Histopathology reveals a granulomatous inflammation present within the choroid and microabscesses with giant cells centered about the capsule of the organism, occasionally breaking through Bruch's membrane to involve the retina and vitreous.[106] *Cryptococcus* is a budding yeast identifiable by PAS, GMS, or Mayer's muchematein stain; it grows well on blood agar and Sabouraud's medium.

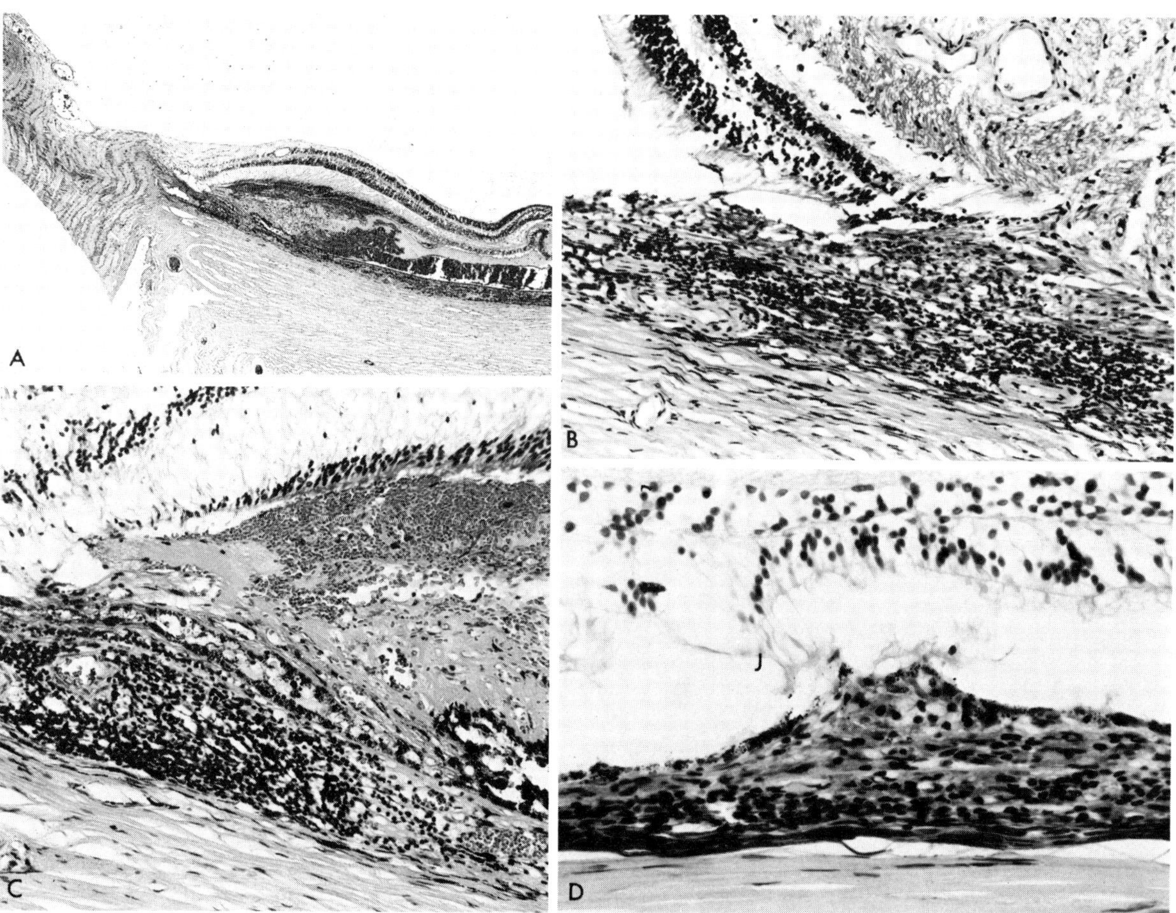

Figure 182–18. Presumed ocular histoplasmosis. Temporal peripapillary area showing an intense granulomatous choroiditis, hyperplasia of the retinal pigment epithelium, and early organization of subretinal hemorrhage. H&E, ×155. (From Spencer WH [ed]: Ophthalmic Pathology: An Atlas and Textbook, 3rd ed. Philadelphia, WB Saunders, 1986, p 1866.)

Aspergillus

Aspergillus fumigatus choroiditis or retinitis occurs through hematogenous spread, mostly in immunocompromised patients.[107] It also can appear as an acute bilateral necrotizing retinitis.[108]

On histopathologic examination, the choroid exhibits extensive infiltration by polymorphonuclear leukocytes, lymphocytes, plasma cells, and macrophages. Thrombosis and necrosis with hyphae extending through vessel walls and accumulating in tissue spaces are typical of *Aspergillus* involvement.[108]

PARASITIC UVEITIS

Toxoplasmosis

Because of an intracellular parasite, *Toxoplasma gondii*, human toxoplasmosis can be acquired congenitally, as an acquired infection in adulthood, or by reactivation of quiescent tissue cysts, such as in immunocompromised and patients with AIDS.

Ocular toxoplasmosis presents as multifocal or focal necrotizing retinochoroiditis. Focal periarterial exudates or plaques simulating arterial emboli may occasionally occur.

On histopathology, necrosis of the infected retina, with *T. gondii* organisms and cysts within the inner retina, is apparent.[109] Pigment epithelium undergoes massive proliferation adjacent to necrotic areas. The underlying choroid is infiltrated by lymphocytes and plasma cells and may itself undergo necrosis with obliteration of the choriocapillaris.[110, 111]

Toxocariasis

Intraocular involvement by *Toxocara canis* is an important cause of childhood blindness. There usually is a history of geophagia or contact with puppies. Ocular involvement can assume several clinical patterns: posterior chorioretinitis, peripheral retinochoroiditis, optic papillitis, endophthalmitis, motile chorioretinal nematodes, or diffuse unilateral subacute neuroretinitis.[112]

Most cases on record are eyes that were enucleated because of suspected retinoblastoma.

In cases of endophthalmitis, there is often a retinal detachment with an identifiable focus of granulomatous inflammation, usually composed of numerous eosinophils forming an eosinophilic abscess. Surrounding the abscess are epithelioid cells, inflammatory granulation tissue infiltrated by eosinophils, lymphocytes, and plasma cells. In the center of the abscess, larvae or the remnants of degenerated larvae can be seen.[113–117]

Onchocerciasis

Infection by *Onchocerca volvulus* closely simulates the tapetoretinal dystrophies. Ocular signs include varying degrees of RPE and retinal atrophy, usually associated with optic disc swelling or pallor and slight swelling of the choroid.

Histopathology reveals that the tiny worm is found along with infiltration of lymphocytes and plasma cells (Fig. 182–19).

SPECIFIC FORMS OF UVEITIS

Anterior Autoimmune Uveitis

The prevalence of abrupt anterior ocular inflammation or uveitis is 0.1 to 0.2 percent, with an incidence of 17/100,000 persons. This is twice the rate of posterior and combined uveitis.

The basis of autoimmune uveitis lies in the complex interplay of regulatory controls that serve as antimicrobial and antineoplastic defenses but attack ocular cells.

Autoimmunity to ocular (S antigen, α-crystallin), articular (type II collagen),[215] proteoglycan, and bacterial remnants (including the cell wall or peptidoglycan)[216] is suspected of being the underlying cause of most uveitis. In each instance, specific bacterial pathogens may infect a distant site, leading to a sterile inflammation in the eye and other organs. Nonviable or "dormant" fastidious bacteria may also act as persistent ocular antigens.

Ocular inflammation may be triggered by an exogenous infection by bacteria, yeast, or viruses sharing an antigenic determinant that is coincidentally similar to a host protein. Molecular mimicry, a process by which an immune response directed against a foreign protein cross-reacts with a normal host protein, may play a role in autoimmunity. Such molecular mimicry occurs between S antigen, interphotoreceptor binding protein, and rhodopsin and *E. coli*, yeast, and hepatitis B proteins.[217] Infection or trauma and ensuing inflammation disrupts the vascular endothelium and increases vascular permeability to more antigens and inflammatory cells. The initial inflammation sets up the preconditions for T-cell activation, the simultaneous presentation to them of MHC class II antigens, surface membrane–bound proteins elaborated by macrophages as well as inflamed RPE and endothelial cells and the retinal antigens released by the initial injury to which sensitization has taken place. This causes further inflammation, and therefore further augments the cycle.

Cell-mediated immunity is more active than humoral immunity. The major cell involved is the activated helper T lymphocyte that releases cytokines, including interleukin 2 (IL2) that attract monocytes, leukocytes, and other inflammatory cells. IL2 released by invading monocyte or macrophage precursors and gamma interferon enhances cytotoxic T cells and augments antibody production by B cells. This allows invasion by inflammatory cells and causes release of more cytokine proteins that regulate development and triggering of lymphocytes. Lymphocytes may interact with vascular endothelium that express major histocompatibility antigens and amplify the immune response. In most cases, no etiologic diagnosis is possible.[217, 219]

In adults, bilateral, nongranulomatous chronic anterior uveitis is associated with systemic conditions such as Reiter's disease, ulcerative colitis, and HLA-B27 arthropathies in one half of cases.

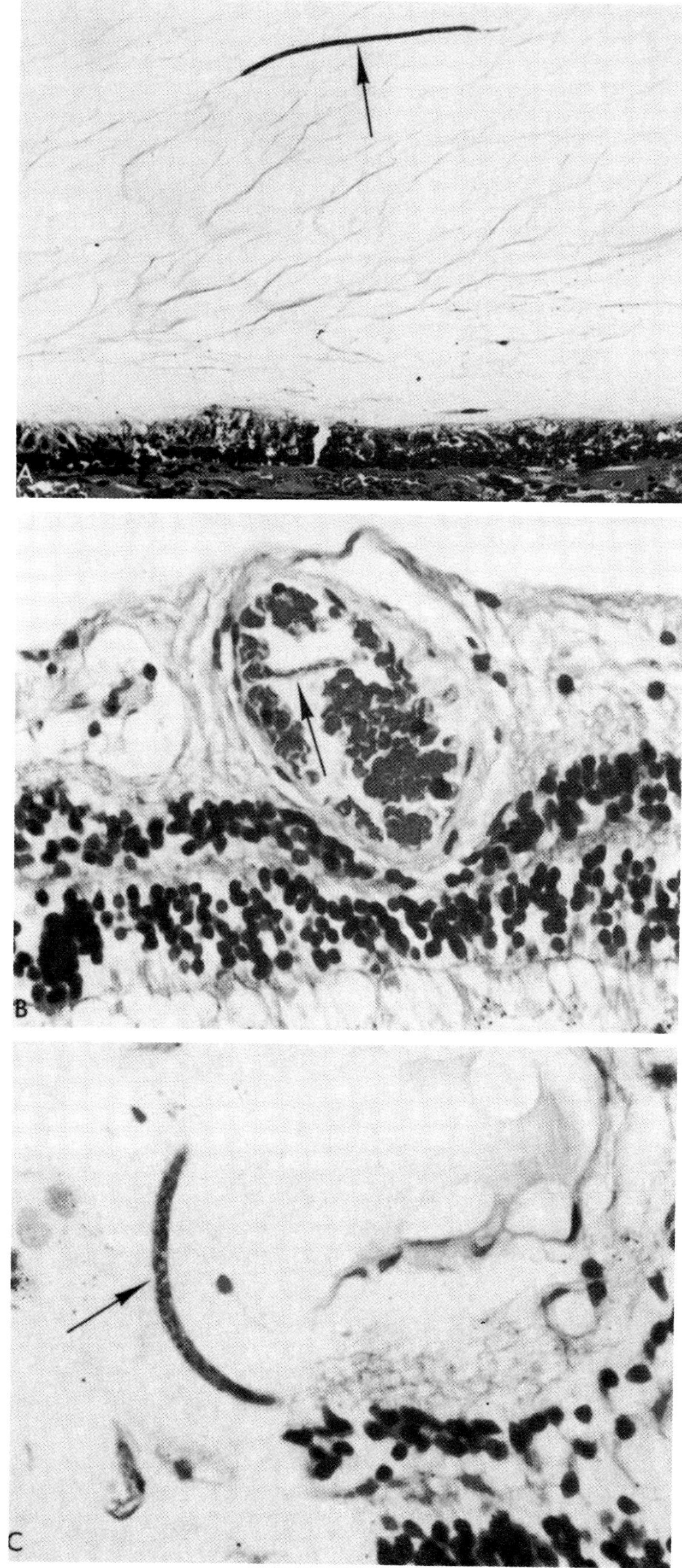

Figure 182–19. Onchocerciasis with microfilariae (*arrows*). *A*, in vitreous, H&E, ×195, AFIP Neg 66-7544; *B*, in retinal vessel, H&E, ×485, AFIP Neg 70-6057; and C, in retina, H&E, ×675, AFIP Neg 70-2055. (From Paul EV, Zimmerman LE: Some observations on the ocular pathology of onchocerciasis. Hum Pathol 1:581–594, 1970.)

Juvenile Rheumatoid Arthritis

Uveitis in children is rare, except for those with juvenile rheumatoid arthritis, who are negative for IgM rheumatoid factor. Up to 20 percent of such children experience recurrent attacks of uveitis. The risk increases for females, with the pauciarticular type, with circulating antinuclear antibodies, and with those who are HLA-DW5– and HLA-DPw2–positive. Of these, as much as 25 percent develop visual impairment from complicated cataract or secondary inflammatory glaucoma.

The iris may show infiltration by plasma cells and Russell bodies. IgM and IgG are present in the anterior chamber aqueous between acute attacks, suggesting that the primary insult results in a leaking blood-ocular barrier. This facilitates sequestering of circulating antigen-antibody complexes and results in recurrence and chronic inflammation.[220] Studies performed late in chronic disease show discrete and multiple areas of granulomatous inflammation involving the ciliary body and choroid, with infiltration extending through emissary canals. No fibrinoid necrosis and scleral inflammation are seen as they are in adult rheumatoid scleritis.[221]

Genitourinary Disease Associations

Tubulointerstitial nephritis that predominantly affects adolescent females may affect the elderly and may account for 2 percent of uveitis seen in a tertiary referral practice.[222, 223] Serologic investigations point to a possible role of *Chlamydia* infection in this disease.[224]

Gastrointestinal Disease Associations

Crohn's disease and ulcerative colitis are uncommon idiopathic chronic inflammatory gout disorders with frequent extraintestinal inflammatory manifestations in eyes, orbit, lungs, joints, and skin. Cell wall–deficient bacterial pathogens that infect leukocytes have been suspected of playing a role in its pathogenesis.[225, 226] Subclinical chronic inflammatory lesions in the ileum related to the uveitis have been identified in HLA-B27–positive patients.[227]

Arthritis

From 10 percent[228] to 20 percent[229] of uveitis sufferers also have arthritis. This includes mostly juvenile rheumatoid arthritis, adult ankylosing spondylitis, or Reiter's syndrome. Other arthropathies such as gout, osteoarthritis, or adult rheumatoid arthritis are not associated with uveitis.

HLA-B27–Positive Ankylosing Spondylitis

People carrying HLA-B27, especially young males, have eight times the risk of noncarriers of developing uveitis and 70 times the risk of acquiring ankylosing spondylitis. Those patients with ankylosing spondylitis have a high risk of developing uveitis regardless of whether or not they are HLA-B27–positive.[230]

HLA determinants are groups of genes on chromosome 6 that function normally as universal surface receptors to signal killer T lymphocytes that a particular cell has been infected by virus (HLA type I). In macrophages they serve to present foreign antigen signals to T lymphocytes to release lymphokines and excite a humoral response with eventual production of antibody (HLA type II).

The molecular mechanisms by which HLA-B27 causes development of autoimmunity and uveitis are uncertain. The A1 portion of HLA-B27, which functions as a receptor for antigen for presentation and activation of T cells, possesses a thiol group (-SH) on a cysteine and lysine residue within its antigen-receiving site.

One theory of its mechanism of initiation of inflammation is that cross-sensitivity occurs because of this molecule. The pathogenic site is known to be identical to part of the amino acid residue sequence, for instance, in *Klebsiella* nitrogenase. Organisms such as *Salmonella*, *Shigella*, *Yersinia*, *Campylobacter*, and other gram-negative bacteria have been implicated in the pathogenesis of uveitis, either as a direct infective cause, by molecular mimicry of HLA-B27 determinants, or by similarity to ocular antigens.[231–233]

HLA-B27–Negative Uveitis

α_1-Antitrypsin phenotype is present in 8.8 percent of patients with uveitis who are HLA-B27–negative but not in those who are HLA-B27–positive. A direct immunochemical mechanism, or linkage to genes on chromosome 14, associated with immunoglobulin synthesis, may be important in this subset of uveitis.[118]

Fuchs' Heterochromic Iridocyclitis

First described in 1902, this disease comprises a unilateral discrete iridocyclitis with heterochromia, cataract, and often glaucoma. Hypochromia is secondary to stromal iris atrophy with loss of stromal pigment. Characteristically, there are no anterior or posterior synechiae. Gonioscopy shows a fine rubeosis of delicate iris vessels bridging the angle that bleed upon paracentesis (Amsler's sign).[119]

Histopathologic examination reveals that lymphocytes (a mixture of IL2 receptor–negative helper and suppressor T cells and B lymphocytes) and plasma cells infiltrate the iris and the ciliary body. There is necrosis of both layers of the iris and ciliary body atrophy. Hyalinization of iris arterioles contributes to their fragility and vascular occlusion, and ischemia within the iris has been individualized. Immunohistochemical analysis of iris biopsy specimens in Fuchs' heterochromic cyclitis failed to show any specific immunohistologic abnormality.[119, 120]

Peripheral Uveitis

Peripheral uveitis is inflammation of the ciliary body, vitreous base, and peripheral retina. It now includes what was formerly Fuchs' cyclitis, chronic cyclitis, and pars planitis, and accounts for 16 percent of all uveitis in a referral practice, mostly affecting children and young adults. Intermediate uveitis or pars planitis is characterized by peripheral vitreoretinal inflammation and prominent fibroglial reactions with adjacent vitreous.

In 80 percent of patients, the condition is bilateral and if initially unilateral, it eventually affects the contralateral eye in 30 percent. The front of the eye remains relatively unaffected, with inflammation beginning about the peripheral pars plana. Cystoid macular edema occurs in 25 to 30 percent. Other complications include cataract, angle-closure glaucoma from peripheral anterior synechiae, retinal and choroidal neovascularization, and vitreous hemorrhage. The cause is unknown, and there is no HLA linkage or familial associations.

The pathologic examination shows that the peripheral "snowbank" consists of an inflammatory exudate composed of activated T lymphocytes with a helper:suppressor ratio of 10:1, and a fibroglial scar (GFAP + vimentin) of Müller cell origin and basement membrane material (type IV collagen and laminin). These cells collect about retinal vessels as well as those of the choroid. Few macrophages, B cells, or natural killer (NK) lymphocyte cells are present within the inflammatory infiltrate. However, B lymphocytes predominate within the aqueous humor and at a focus at the iris-ciliary body junction.

Birdshot Choroidoretinopathy

This is a rare disease (133 reported cases) that affects Caucasians between 40 and 60 yr of age. It is associated with HLA-A29 in more than 95 percent of patients.

Ocular signs include moderate to marked nongranulomatous vitreal inflammation and small, uniform, creamy-colored lesions without hyperpigmentation of the RPE sparing the macula. Cystoid macular edema is often found (in 63 percent of cases) and to a lesser extent, retinal vasculitis and subretinal neovascularization occur.

Inflammation consisting of multiple, scattered focal lesions at the chorioretinal interface, with minimal vasculitis. Choroidoretinal lesions show granulomatous inflammation with lymphocytic infiltrate.

This is an autoimmune inflammatory disease affecting the retina and choroid.[121] Retinal S antigen hypersensitivity is found in 90 percent of the patients studied.[122] There is also a genetic predisposition (HLA-A29).

Acute Placoid Pigment Epitheliopathy

This bilateral disease affects young adults (15 to 40 yr of age) and is characterized by multiple, flat, cream-colored patches at the level of the RPE of the posterior pole. Lesions are often at different stages of healing. Clinically, mild anterior uveitis is often noted. Fluorescein angiography shows early hypofluorescence of the patches followed by hyperfluorescence in the late venous phase. The disease tends to resolve in 2 to 3 mo, leaving some alteration of RPE with return to good visual acuity. Subretinal vascularization is rare. Occasionally, retinal venous vasculitis occurs topographically independent of the choroidal lesions.[123, 141] To our knowledge, no clinicopathology data have been published. A clinicopathologic case report can describe a multifocal posterior uveitis that appears to be Harada's disease rather than acute placoid pigment epitheliopathy.

Most authors suggest that the pigment epitheliopathy is secondary to a multifocal choroidal vasculitis. Each individual placoid lesion seen clinically may represent an area of focal swelling of the RPE cells overlying a nonperfused lobule of choriocapillaris.

The probable histopathology changes are affected RPE cells with cloudy cytoplasm and altered pigment in the acute phase and depigmentation or hyperpigmentation of some RPE cells with little retinal photoreceptor degeneration in the late phase. The viral prodromes that commonly precede acute placoid pigment epitheliopathy suggest that viral or other infectious agents may be the inciting antigens. A possible hypersensitivity mechanism has also been proposed.[124]

Serpiginous Choroiditis

This is a rare, chronic, usually bilateral disorder characterized by irregular areas of RPE loss with variable scarring (pigment clumping and hypopigmentation of the RPE). The process usually begins in the peripapillary region and extends by recurrences in an irregular fashion to the midperiphery. Vision is greatly affected if the process involves the macula. Retinal vasculitis, papillitis, hyalitis, and neovascularization have occasionally been observed.

Histopathologically, diffuse lymphocyte infiltration of the choroid is seen; prominent focal infiltrates are observed at the margins of the RPE. Atrophy of the choriocapillaris, RPE, and photoreceptors appear secondarily. A defect of Bruch's membrane that allows passage of subretinal neovascularization membranes and fibroglial scar into the choroid can occur.

The cause remains unknown. The association of HLA-B7, the recurrent slow progression, and the long duration of serpiginous choroiditis argue for an immunologically mediated mechanism in genetically predisposed persons.

DEGENERATIVE CONDITIONS

Systemic Disease

DIABETES

Although much attention has been given in the ophthalmic literature to the retinal vascular changes in diabetes mellitus, there is convincing evidence that the uveal tract is diffusely involved in this disease process.[125–127] Because of the close anatomic and metabolic relationship between the outer retinal layers and the choroid, investigators have become increasingly interested in anatomic changes at this level in the pathogenesis of diabetic retinopathy.[125, 126]

In light and electron microscopic studies of eyes of patients who had had diabetes mellitus for 14 to 23 yr,

Hidayat and Fine[126] noted marked thickening of the basement membrane of the choriocapillaris and other small choroidal blood vessels, narrowing of vessel lumina in keeping with choroidal dropout and scarring, and leakage of proteinaceous fluid into the choroidal stroma. Another feature of the choroidal vasculopathy they described was the presence of homogeneous PAS nodules that resembled those of diabetic glomerulosclerosis (Kimmelstiel-Wilson disease). Fryczkowski and coworkers,[125] using scanning electron microscopy to study vascular casts in autopsies of 24 former patients with diabetes mellitus, noted the vasculature to have increased tortuosity, areas of dilatation and narrowing, vascular loops and microaneurysms, and areas of choroidal drop-out. Neovascularization of the iris was identified in eyes that were clinically known to have this condition. None of the control eyes used in the study demonstrated the changes similar to those seen in the diabetic eyes.

NEUROFIBROMATOSIS

Neurofibromatoses (NF) are a group of genetic disorders with multiple ophthalmic manifestations and systemic changes. The underlying defect appears to be related to abnormal growth of neural tissue. Although the presentation of this disorder may occur in varying degrees of severity, two distinctive forms are now recognized.

The most common NF type 1 previously known as von Recklinghausen's or peripheral NF, is an autosomal dominant condition that occurs with a frequency of 1/3500 individuals in the general population. NF type 2 is the next most frequently encountered type, which is characterized by bilateral acoustic neuromas; hence the former name, central neurofibromatosis. NF 2 is also dominantly inherited and occurs with a frequency of 1/50,000 persons.

The natural history of these two conditions is distinct, as is the genetic basis. NF 1 has been localized to long arm of chromosome 17 and the NF 2 locus is the long arm of chromosome 22.

Lisch nodules are a feature of NF 1 that are seen in up to 92 percent of patients with this disease.[128] Perry and Font demonstrated histopathologically that these nodules were composed of cells of melanocytic origin, and further studies have shown that the presence or number of nodules does not correlate with the extent of the disease process.[129] In the presence of plexiform neuromas of the upper eyelid, glaucoma is seen in the ipsilateral eye in 50 percent of patients.[130] The uveal tract can often be diffusely thickened by an intermixture of Schwann cells, ganglion cells, melanocytes, and concentric ovoid bodies. Electron microscopic studies by Eagle and coworkers[131] have determined the ovoid bodies to be of Schwann cell origin. Although nevi of the choroid are more common in patients with NF, this has not been shown to place these patients at increased risk for developing uveal melanoma.[132]

AMYLOIDOSIS

Amyloidosis is a diverse group of diseases characterized by the deposition of a fibrillar protein in body tissues. The classification of this disease has previously been made according to a number of factors: genetic (familial or nonfamilial), the presence of underlying disease (primary or secondary), and the site of the disease process (localized or systemic). Increasing knowledge concerning the chemical nature of the fibrillar deposits have led to changes in the nomenclature and classification of the disease. Amyloidosis is now classified as localized or systemic, either of which may be primary or secondary.[133] In primary amyloidosis, the deposit has been found to be derived from immunoglobulin light chain fragments in the serum, whereas in secondary amyloidosis, the amyloid fibrils are derived from an acute phase protein called serum amyloid A.[134, 135]

A wide variety of ocular tissues have been reported to be involved in the various forms of amyloidosis: the cornea,[136] conjunctiva,[137, 138] eyelid,[138] orbit,[139] lacrimal gland,[140, 141] optic nerve,[142] retina,[143] extraocular muscles,[144] vitreous,[145, 146] and uveal tract.[147–149] Deposition of amyloid has been described in both the anterior and posterior uveal tract.

A total of five histologically proven cases of iris involvement in amyloidosis have been reported: four in ocular leprosy[150, 151] and one in primary (nonfamilial) systemic amyloidosis.[149] A scalloped pupillary margin has been reported in some cases of primary familial amyloidosis; however, these eyes have not been examined histopathologically.[152, 153] Other changes involving the iris include the deposition of amyloid on posterior pigment epithelium in a saw-tooth configuration that may be difficult to distinguish histopathologically from pseudoexfoliation. Amyloid deposits have also been identified in the trabecular meshwork in patients with systemic and localized amyloidosis. This finding has clinically frequently been correlated with a history of an elevated pressure.[147, 149]

In cases of posterior uveal tract deposition, the choriocapillaris has been shown to be infiltrated with and without obliteration of the overlying RPE.[147–149] Why the overlying RPE is unaffected in some cases has not yet been fully explained.

CYSTINOSIS

Cystinosis is characterized by the accumulation of the nonprotein cystine in the lysosomes of cells as a result of a defect in the transport system from the lysosome to the cytosol. Two varieties of this disorder are recognized in humans: (1) the benign adult form, which is characterized by the deposition of crystals in the cornea in an otherwise asymptomatic patients, and (2) the nephropathic form, an autosomally recessively inherited storage disease in which crystal formation has been reported in kidneys, bone marrow, liver, reticuloendothelial cells, and ocular tissues, including the cornea, conjunctiva, iris, and the RPE.

Clinically, the nephropathic form manifests in the first year of life with polydipsia, polyuria, and electrolyte imbalances caused by a renal tubular Fanconi syndrome. In the most severe forms, a renal transplant can be required in the first decade of life. The adult benign form, as the name suggests, is limited to deposition of crystals within the cornea and is not associated with any untoward systemic effects.

Histopathologic studies have demonstrated the accumulation of cystine crystals in the cornea, conjunctiva,[154, 155] iris, pigmented and nonpigmented epithelium of the ciliary body, RPE, choroid, and sclera. Ultrastructural studies have shown the crystals to be predominantly needle-shaped in the cornea and hexagonal in configuration in other ocular tissues. Accumulation of the crystals in the RPE has been associated with degeneration of the cells, clinically manifesting as a patchy, peripheral loss of the RPE. Despite the alteration in the RPE, the photoreceptors have been reported to be relatively spared.[156, 157] In addition to the presence of crystals within the choroid, a homogeneous, granular, electron-dense material has been observed that Sanderson and colleagues[156] speculated may represent a noncrystalline form of cystine (Fig. 182–20).

The use of topical cysteamine (0.1%), which contains a free sulphur group that binds cystine, can reverse the deposition of crystals within the cornea.[158] Oral cysteamine has not proved to be effective in the treatment of corneal crystals; however, it has been shown to be of use in improving renal function in young patients.[159]

HOMOCYSTINURIA

Homocystinuria is an autosomally recessive inborn error of metabolism caused by a deficiency of the enzyme cystathionine B-synthetase.[160] This enzyme is responsible for the conversion of the amino acid homocystine to cystathionine, and its absence results in ele-

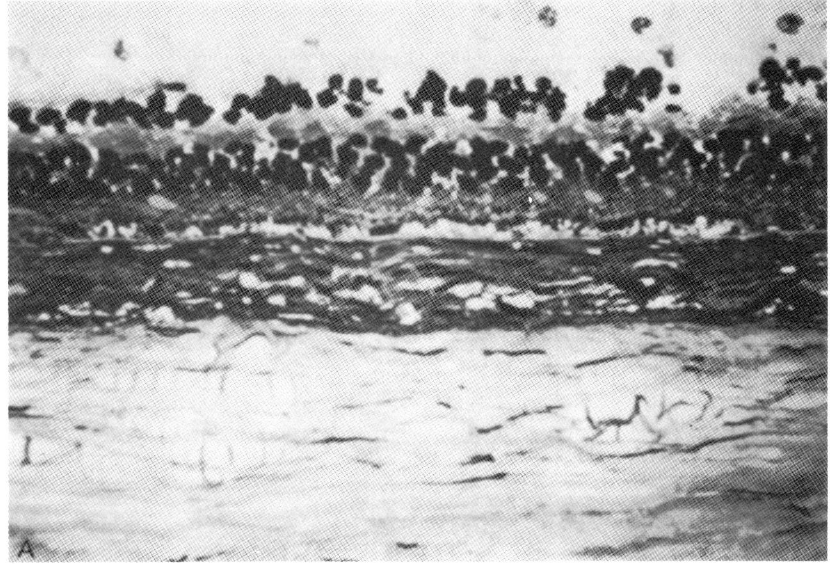

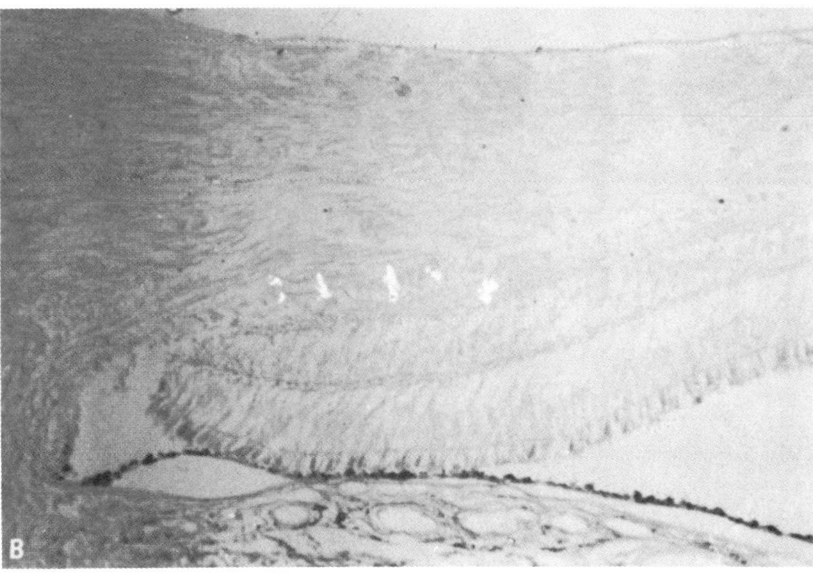

Figure 182–20. Cystinosis. *A*, Cystine crystals in retinal pigment epithelium of a patient who had the childhood form of cystinosis. 1 μ thick, epoxy resin section, ×480. *B*, Polarized light demonstrates crystals in the peripapillary retina of childhood form of cystinosis. Frozen section, unstained, ×50, EP27737. *A*, from Sanderson PA, Kuwabara T, Stark WJ, et al: Cystinosis. A clinical, histopathologic, and ultrastructural study. Arch Ophthalmol 91:270–274, 1974. Copyright 1974, American Medical Association. *B*, from Spencer WH [ed]: Ophthalmic Pathology: An Atlas and Textbook, 3rd ed. Philadelphia, WB Saunders, 1986, p 1196.)

vated plasma levels of homocystine. Many of the structural defects associated with this condition are secondary to an excess of homocystine in the plasma that inhibits the formation of cross-links in collagen. Mental retardation in some degree is estimated to occur in up to as much as 50 percent of patients.[161] These patients are also predisposed to thromboembolic disease secondary to chronic chemical injury to the endothelium. Anesthesia is a recognized precipitator of thromboembolic episodes, and prophylactic anticoagulation should be instituted in these patients prior to surgery.

VASCULAR DISEASES

The choroid is generally considered the vascular sheath of the eye and as such is intimately involved in maintaining homeostasis with the ocular tissues. The choroid vasculature is not an anatomically privileged site and is subject to both local (mechanical) and systemic processes that can affect the vascular supply of tissues of the eye. Interestingly, the response of uveal tract to alterations in its vascular supply may vary from ischemic necrosis to the uncontrolled proliferation of the vessels seen in rubeosis iridis. The following section discusses some of the more common local and systemic processes that can affect the choroidal vasculature, with particular reference to possible histopathologic changes.

Ischemia and Necrosis

Ischemia of the choroid may be related to both localized and systemic factors and may be confined to either the anterior or posterior uveal tract, or a combination of both. Localized ischemia of the iris is a well-documented finding in angle-closure glaucoma, and this event may lead to corectopia following the attack. Histopathologically, acute elevations of the intraocular pressure can lead to ischemic necrosis of the pupillary margin with severe attenuation to absence of the sphincter muscle. Areas of complete atrophy of the iris with hole formation are not an infrequent clinical or histopathologic observation.

Localized ischemia affecting the iris is a not-infrequent sequela to herpes zoster ophthalmicus. Almost any ocular tissue can be involved by the process, and the uveal tract is no exception. Involvement of the iris and the ciliary body is often a complicating factor in many case of herpes zoster ophthalmicus. Frequent histopathologic changes include focal necrosis of the pigment epithelium of the iris, infiltration of the ciliary body by lymphocytes, perineuritis, and a granulomatous choroiditis.[162] In a histopathologic review of 9 cases of herpes zoster ophthalmicus, Hedges and Albert[163] noted that in the early stages of the disease inflammation of the uvea may be limited to a nongranulamatous inflammation of the iris, ciliary body, and choroid. In the same study, some eyes displayed infiltration of the trabecular meshwork with macrophages and inflammatory cells, and the authors speculated this might be a contributing factor to the development of glaucoma, which is a recognized complication of this disease.

Rubeosis Iridis (Fig. 182–21)

A multitude of conditions have been associated with the development of new vessels on the iris surface and are included under the rubric *rubeosis iridis*.

Histopathologically, Henkind[164] noted the following features: (1) neovascularization can start separately on the iris at the pupillary border and in the midperiphery; (2) new vessels initially arise from vessels within the iris stroma and then grow on the iris surface; (3) connective tissue can grow in association with the new vessels and can eventually cover the iris surface; (4) shrinkage of the connective tissue can shrink the new vessels, making them too difficult to observe histopathologically; (5) the anterior surface of the iris eventually loses its convoluted appearance, and the anterior and posterior surface eventually become parallel; (6) contraction of the anterior connective tissue results in drawing of the posterior pigmented epithelium to the surface of the iris in a condition termed ectropion uvea; (7) further shrinkage of the anterior fibrovascular membrane results in bending of the sphincter muscle into a J-shaped configuration (ectropion of the sphincter); (8) new iris vessels have thin walls in contrast to the normally thick-walled vessels of the iris stroma; and (9) loss of the dilator muscle was evident in many cases.

Electron microscopic studies of rubeosis have demonstrated the presence of a confluent layer of myofibroblasts (fibroblasts with smooth muscle differentiation), not detectable clinically, covering the new vessels on the iris surface.[165] This myoblastic proliferation is believed to be responsible for the development of ectropion uvea and synechial closure of the angle, not infrequent complications of this process. Other electron microscopic studies have demonstrated the endothelium of the new capillaries to lack the normal intercellular connections, thus explaining the early leakage in fluorescein angiography.[166, 167]

The origin and extent of the new iris vessels was reviewed by Henkind.[164] The new vessels have connections with branches of the major arterial circle of the iris or with branches of the anterior ciliary arteries. These vessels were shown to drain into either normal iris and ciliary body veins or paralimbally into episcleral veins.

Choroidal Neovascularization

Choroidal neovascularization is a recognized complication of many diseases of the retina and the choroid; however, its role in the pathogenesis of age-related macular degeneration is most recognized. The term is used to describe new blood vessels emanating from the choroid that have "broken" through Bruch's membrane to lie between this membrane and the retinal pigment epithelium. The presence of these abnormal vessels is readily appreciable by fluorescein angiography and is indicated by the leakage of dye.

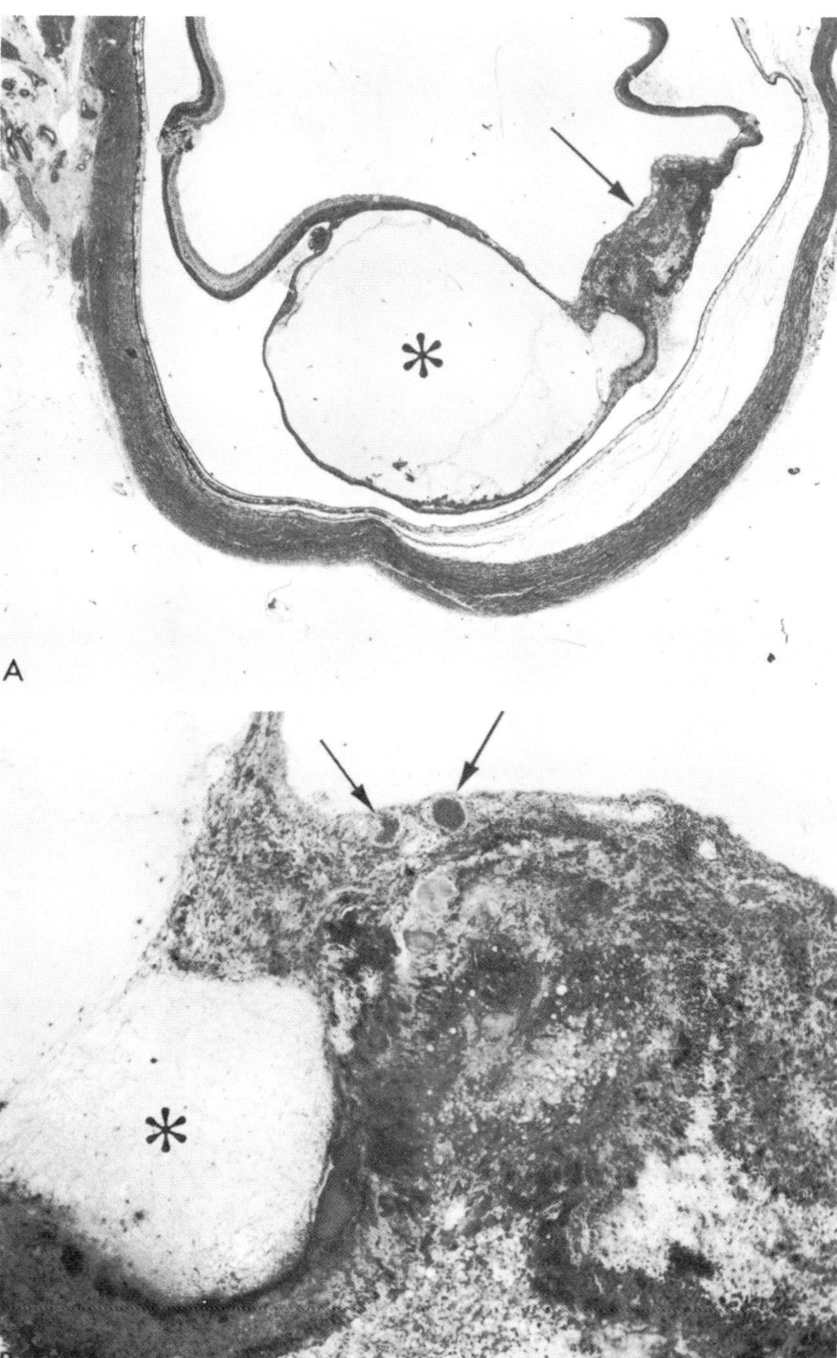

Figure 182–21. Iris neovascularization following central retinal vein occlusion (CRVO). *A,* Open angle with early neovascularization (*arrows*). H&E, ×300 EP 38375. *B,* Rubeosis iridis (*arrows*) with peripheral anterior synechia and endothelialization and decemetization (*arrowhead*) of the false angle. Van de Grift, ×350, EP 41223. (From Green WR, Chan CC, Hutchins GM, Terry JM: Central retinal vein occlusion. A prospective histopathologic study of 29 eyes in 28 cases. Retina 1:27–55, 1981; and Trans Am Ophthalmol Soc 79:371–422, 1981.)

Histopathologic studies have noted thickening and calcification of Bruch's membrane, drusen, RPE clumping, and disruption of the choriocapillaris as common findings in eyes with choroidal neovascular membranes caused by age-related macular degeneration. Of course, the specific histopathologic features are related to the underlying disease process.

The initiating event in the growth of choroidal neovascular membranes through the Bruch's membrane is not fully understood. It has been postulated that focal breaks in Bruch's membrane may be responsible for the subsequent growth of new blood vessels; however, not all eyes with histopathologically identifiable breaks in Bruch's membrane develop choroidal neovascular membranes.[168, 169] Animals studies have implicated lytic factors within the choriocapillaris and inflammation of Bruch's membrane as other possible pathogenic factors in the development of choroidal neovascular membranes.[170, 171]

Aging and Degenerative Conditions

ANGIOID STREAKS (Fig. 182–22)

Angioid streaks are a degenerative condition of Bruch's membrane characterized by bilateral, irregular,

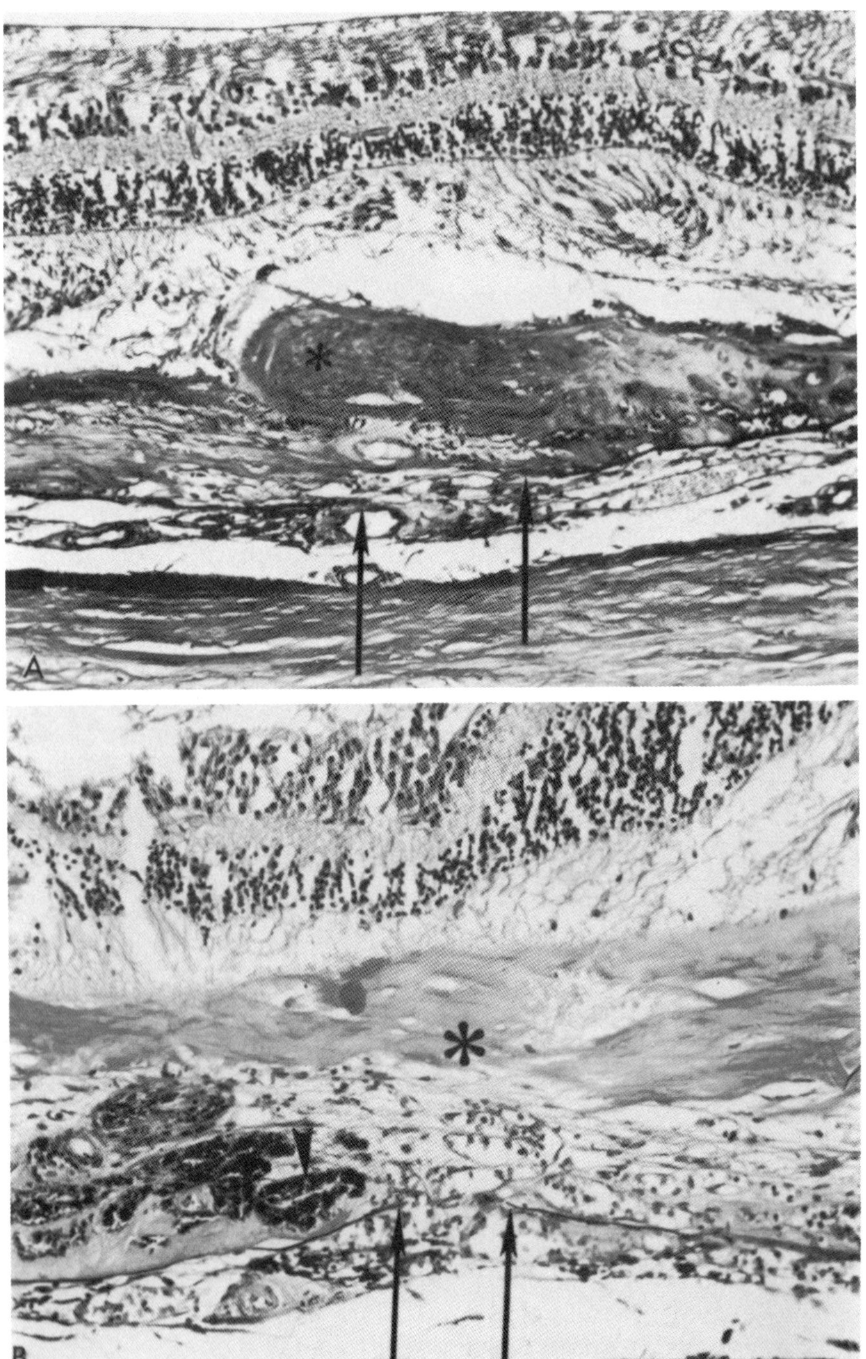

Figure 182–22. Angioid streaks in a patient with pseudoxanthoma elasticum. *A,* Histologic section through macula of right eye. Arrows delimit edges of angioid streak. Fibrovascular disciform scar (*asterisk*) is located between Bruch's membrane and residual retinal pigment epithelium (RPE). RPE is discontinuous over the lesion with prominent photoreceptor loss. H&E, ×130. *B,* Histologic section through macula of left eye. Arrows delimit edges of angioid streak. Tubular configuration of hypertrophic and hyperplastic RPE (*arrowhead*) is present in the midst of dense fibrous scar (*asterisk*). H&E, ×155. (From Spencer WH [ed]: Opthalmic Pathology: An Atlas and Textbook, 3rd ed. Philadelphia, WB Saunders, 1986, p 1027.)

jagged lines radiating from the peripapillary area to the peripheral fundus, deep to and crossing the retinal vessels.[172] They were named by Knapp[173] in recognition of their vessel-like appearance, although it was suggested early[174] and confirmed[175] that the lesions corresponded to breaks in Bruch's membrane. Several studies have confirmed and contributed to an understanding of the natural history of this condition.[176, 177] McKusick thought that this condition belonged to a group of chronic, progressive, accelerated "wear-and-tear" processes.[178] According to Dreyer and Green,[177] the primary alteration is a break in the elastic layer of Bruch's membrane with associated thickening of the RPE basement membrane and thinning of the RPE. Following rupture of Bruch's membrane, "disruption" of the choriocapillaris and RPE atrophy provide a weakened resistance to fibrovascular ingrowth into the retina. Elevation and subsequent hyperplasia of the surrounding RPE may follow. These authors have shown that calcium deposition, particularly in cases of pseudoxanthoma elasticum, is associated with Bruch's membrane alterations. The visual complications of subretinal new vessels have been described in Chapter 66.

Angioid streaks have been described in various systemic conditions such as pseudoxanthoma elasticum, Paget's disease, and sickle cell disease.[179–183]

IRIDOCORNEAL ENDOTHELIAL SYNDROMES

Essential iris atrophy, Chandler's syndrome, and Cogan-Reese iris-nevus syndrome represent a spectrum of the iridocorneal endothelial syndromes. These rare, acquired, unilateral conditions mainly affect young women. They constitute a combination of iris stromal atrophy, iridocorneal and Descemet's membrane abnormalities, and a tendency to secondary glaucoma from trabecular obstruction and angle-closure with pupillary block.

Essential iris atrophy features corectopia, iris atrophy, and hole formation. Metaplastic endothelial cells on the anterior iris surface cause contracture and stretching of the iris stroma. Iris nodules result from areas of effacement of iris stroma and are prominent in the Cogan-Reese iris-nevus syndrome. Chandler's syndrome features broad iridocorneal adhesions. These follow contracture of the abnormal endothelial membrane that migrated from the cornea to the iris over the chamber angle and onto the iris surface. These cells deposit Descemet-like basement membrane in their wake, resulting in obstruction of the outflow tract and unilateral glaucoma with peripheral anterior synechiae.

Histopathologic examination reveals proliferation of corneal endothelial cells that acquire migratory and contractile properties. These ectopic pleomorphic cells are separated from Descemet's membrane by a thick accumulation of collagen. The trabecular meshwork and anterior iris are covered by a multilayered membrane. These cells differ from normal endothelial cells, having increased cytoplasmic filaments, microvilli, filopodia, keratin, and junctional complexes, or desmosomes. A low-grade inflammatory response with mononuclear cells results from iris ischemia and necrosis associated with these cells.[184]

In progressive (or essential) iris atrophy, corectopia develops as "ischemic" iris is drawn toward prominent peripheral anterior synechiae (melt holes) while a "stretch hole" develops on the opposite side of the true pupil.

Chandler's syndrome is a variation with milder iris changes but more florid corneal endothelial disturbance with a multilayered corneal endothelium and a normal Descemet's membrane. Broad-based, peripheral anterior synechiae manifest as an extension of a glassy, cuticular membrane covered by a single layer of endothelial cells. Glaucoma is often mild.

The iris-nevus syndrome variant features melanotic nodules influenced and distorted by the ectopic endothelial membrane.[131, 155, 185–187]

It has been suggested that this disease appears prenatally as a consequence of a corneal endothelium defect, since an abnormal Descemet's membrane is present in the fetal layer.[188] Overgrowth of Descemet's membrane is present in unrelated conditions, including posterior polymorphous dystrophy and following inflammation. The condition behaves as a benign neoplasm of the corneal endothelium.[189]

CHORIORETINAL DYSTROPHIES AND ATROPHIES

Primary choroidal atrophies feature progressive and bilateral loss of choroidal vasculature secondary to a primary defect of the pigment epithelium, retina, or choroidal vessels.

Geographic locations and patterns define the classification. Choroidal vascular atrophy may be maximal about the macula, perimacular area, or the optic disc.[190] Conditions that affect only the choriocapillaris and spare the larger outer choroidal vessels are more common, and except for choroideremia, are benign. They occur during the third and fourth decades of life and generally have an autosomal dominant inheritance. Those that also affect the larger outer choroidal vessels tend to be more fulminant (e.g., gyrate atrophy).

CHORIOCAPILLARIS ATROPHY

Peripapillary regional choroidal dystrophy (peripapillary choroidal sclerosis) is mostly a sporadic or senile change. The pathology is centered on the optic disc. It rarely occurs as an inherited abiotrophy of the choriocapillaris and is correlated with shallow optic disc cupping.[191] It manifests progressive extension by finger-like processes of choroidal atrophy along major vessels about the disc.

Histopathology reveals loss of RPE, choriocapillaris, and photoreceptors with larger vessels intact and breaks in Bruch's membrane sometimes associated with neovascularization. Müller cells in the region of the atrophy deposit an abnormally thickened basement membrane.[192]

CENTRAL AREOLAR CHOROIDAL DYSTROPHY

Central areolar choroidal dystrophy (macular regional choroidal dystrophy; circulate, annular choroidal atrophy; central choroidal sclerosis; central progressive areolar choroidal dystrophy), a rare autosomal dominant choroidal atrophy, involves the macula and manifests in the second to fourth decade of life. Macular changes progress by the fifth decade to show the characteristic lesions, manifesting clinically with a central scotoma. Electroretinogram is normal, but electrooculogram may show a flat response. Fluorescein angiography of the lesion initially shows early hyperfluorescence through defective RPE.[193–195] A similar picture occurs associated with olivopontocerebellar degeneration.

Choroidal sclerosis appears rather as an atrophy of choriocapillaris, RPE, and outer retina.[196] Normal large-caliber choroidal vessels that transverse circumscribed regions without the choriocapillaris give an impression of sclerosis. Within these are discrete zones of total atrophy of the choriocapillaris, RPE, and outer retina.[196, 197]

A similar pathology occurs in age-related maculopathy, in which degeneration and thinning of the RPE, associated with changes in Bruch's membrane, result in atrophy of the underlying choriocapillaris.[198]

DIFFUSE CHOROIDAL ATROPHY WITH CHORIOCAPILLARIS ATROPHY

Diffuse choriocapillaris atrophies include X-linked choroideremia and autosomal dominant diffuse choriocapillaris atrophy. These have distinct fundus and fluorescein angiographic appearances.[199]

Diffuse choroidal atrophy with choriocapillaris atrophy (generalized choroidal sclerosis, diffuse choroidal sclerosis) is a slowly progressing autosomal dominant condition that manifests as decreased visual acuity, night blindness, and visual field constriction between the first and fourth decades.[199]

The fundus is stippled or mottled with pale-yellow atrophy of the retina and choroid, often with a fish-net pattern. This starts in the central area and spreads peripherally. Occasionally, primary peripheral lesions progress centrally. The characteristic lesions include pigment epithelial and choriocapillaris atrophy that spread to involve the entire fundus, with later retinal attenuation and optic atrophy. Fluorescein angiography shows diffuse hyperfluorescence from window defects and later hypofluorescence from the combined choriocapillaris-RPE atrophy (Fig. 182–23).

There is widespread RPE and photoreceptor loss with variable loss of choriocapillaris.[200, 201]

CHOROIDEREMIA

Choroideremia (progressive tapetochoroidal dystrophy) is a slowly progressing, X-linked condition that variably manifests visual-field constriction, decreased visual acuity, and night blindness by the age of 10 yr. This begins in the midperipheral, equatorial, or paramacular regions with pigment stippling or granularity. These early changes are also evident in female carriers, who possess a mosaic of normal and abnormal cells through Barr body inactivation of one X chromosome.

The early manifestation is indistinguishable from central areolar choroidal dystrophy. Later, there is loss of the choriocapillaris and eventually of the larger choroidal vessels. By the age of 40 yr, the disease has progressively encroached on previously spared areas of the

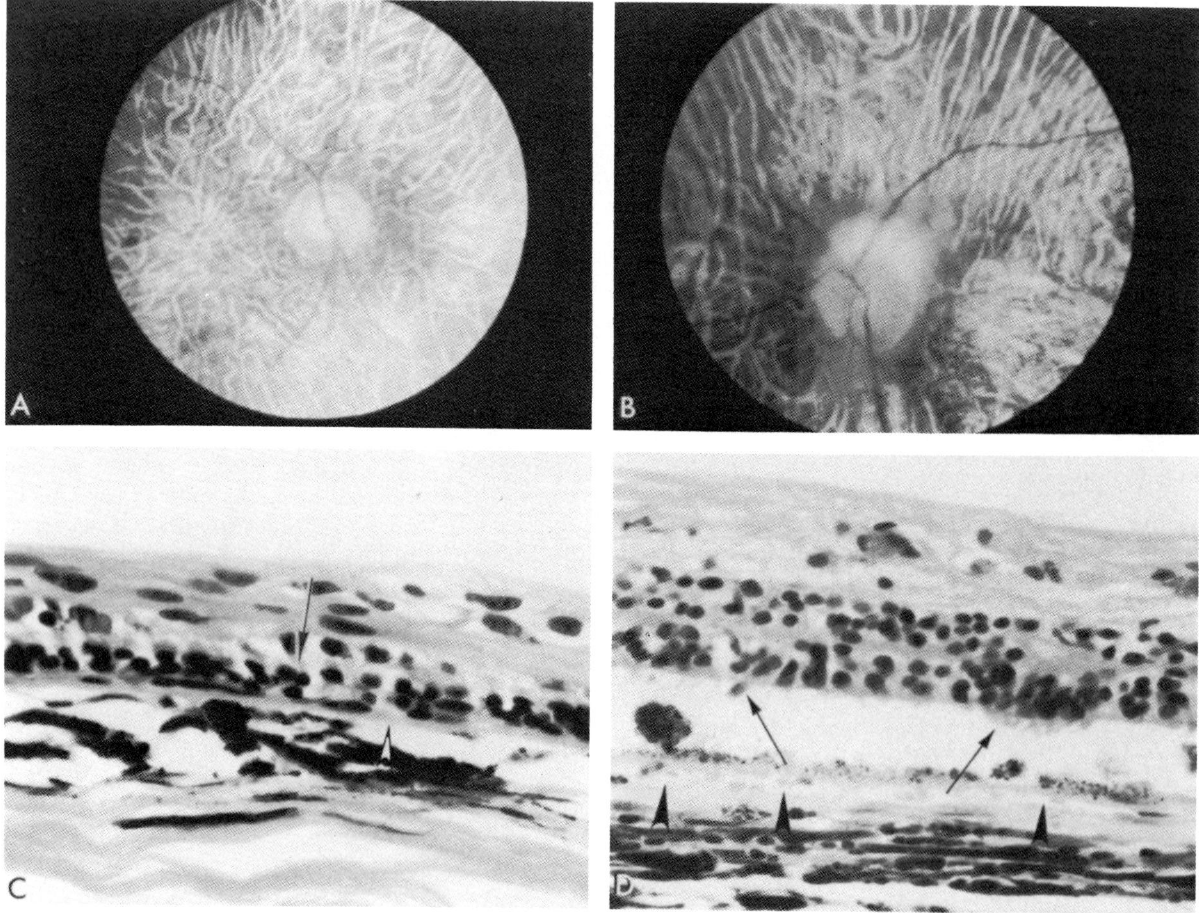

Figure 182–23. Diffuse choroidal atrophy. *A*, Right eye, *B*, Left eye. C, Typical area showing retinal pigment epithelium (RPE) and outer retinal layers. Remaining inner nuclear layer (*arrow*) rests against Bruch's membrane (*arrowhead*). Choroidal vessels are not present, but melanocytes are. H&E, ×700. *D*, Area of less intense changes shows an intact choriocapillaris (*arrowheads*), an intact but hypopigmented RPE, and loss of outer segments of photoreceptors. A few stubby inner segments (*arrows*) remain. Outer nuclear layer is slightly thinned. H&E, ×600, EP 33283. (From Green WR: Pathology of the retina. *In* Frayer WC [ed]: Lancaster Course in Ophthalmic Histopathology, Unit 9. Philadelphia, FA Davis, 1981.)

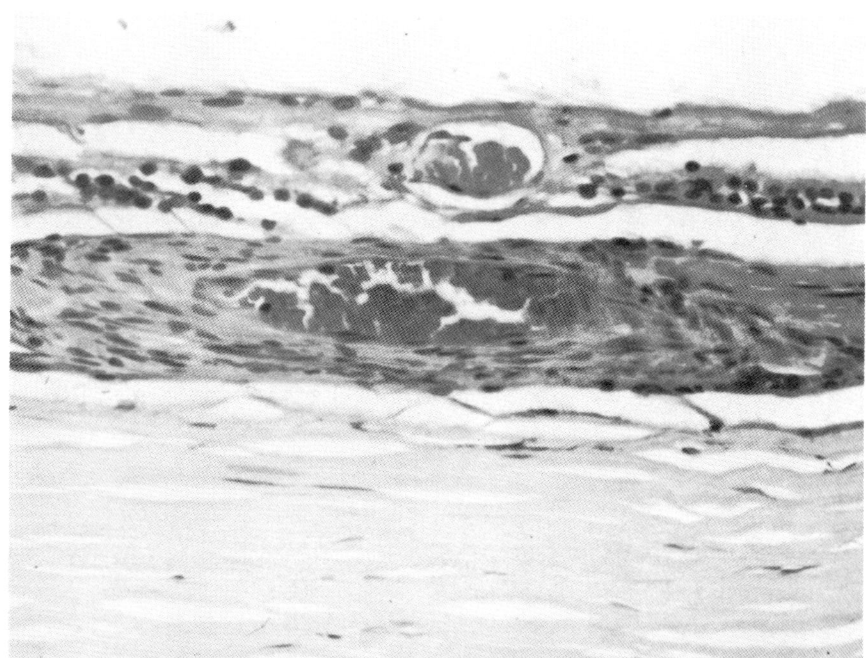

Figure 182–24. Choroideremia. Area where a single choroidal artery remains. Retinal pigment epithelium and outer retinal layers are intact, and inner nuclear layer rests against Bruch's membrane. H&E, ×330. (From Spencer WH [ed]: Ophthalmic Pathology: An Atlas and Textbook, 3rd ed. Philadelphia, WB Saunders, 1986, p 1226.)

fundus, with secondary retinal vessel attenuation and disc pallor. Deterioration to only light perception often occurs in the fifth decade. Fluorescein angiography shows early window defects and hyperfluorescence, with later hypofluorescence in areas of choriocapillaris atrophy.[202, 203]

Changes affect the entire uveal tract and mainly include extensive chorioretinal atrophy. The iris shows thinning and associated loss of the dilator muscle and iris vasculature. The early stippling represents island or RPE loss with overlying absence of photoreceptors and underlying choriocapillaris disturbance. Choroidal vessels in anterior uninvolved pigmented fundus show capillary basement membrane fragmentation (Fig. 182–24).

Within the area marked by choriocapillaris atrophy, there is fragmentation and loss of Bruch's membrane, and graded outer and midretinal atrophy and degeneration. Under this atrophic choroid, chorioretinal adhesions result from RPE cells having phagocytic activity that migrates into the gliotic retina above, with formation of epiretinal membranes.

The primary degeneration may be of the retina, RPE, or choriocapillaris.[203–206] Primary disease of the RPE may explain some observed changes, since it modulates choriocapillaris growth.[207] Posterior clinically involved areas show a total loss of choriocapillaris, a decrease in endothelial fenestrae, and widespread vascular occlusion. These point to a primary lesion of the vascular endothelium.

TOTAL CHOROIDAL ATROPHIES

Gyrate atrophy is an autosomally recessive condition related to defective ornithine metabolism (deficiency of ornithine aminotransferase). The gene is probably located on chromosome 10.[208, 209] This condition manifests clinically between the second and third decades by slowly progressive night blindness and a ring scotoma. Vision decreases to less than 20/200 by the age of 40 yr. Associated features are myopia, visual-field constriction, and development of a posterior subcapsular cataract between the second and third decades. The initial fundal lesions, midperipheral islands of chorioretinal atrophy, may coalesce into a garland. These circumferential, confluent atrophic lesions have sharply scalloped margins that abut and extend into the normal retina. Fluorescein angiography shows loss of choriocapillaris with larger vessels spared. These circumscribed lesions leak from their borders in the late phase of the angiogram.[172, 200, 202, 210] Histopathologic studies have shown focal atrophy of photoreceptors and adjacent RPE hypoplasia at the posterior pole. In the midperiphery, an abrupt transition between the normal zone and the zone of total retinal, RPE, and choroidal atrophy is noticeable. Ultrastructural mitochondrial abnormalities are detected in the photoreceptors, corneal endothelium, and nonpigmented ciliary epithelium.[210, 211] These data suggest a primary photoreceptor abnormality.[211]

REFERENCES

1. Levy WJ: Congenital iris lesions. Br J Ophthalmol 41:120, 1957.
2. Shields JA: Primary cysts of the iris. Trans Am Ophthalmol Soc 79:771, 1981.
3. Nelson LB, Spaeth GL, Nowinski TS: Aniridia. A review. Surv Ophthalmol 28:621, 1984.
4. Falls HF: A gene producing various defects of the anterior segment of the eye with a pedigree of a family. Am J Ophthalmol 32:41, 1949.
5. Mann I: Persistence of capsulopupillary vessels as a factor in the production of abnormalities of the iris and lens. Arch Ophthalmol 11:174, 1934.
6. Grant WM, Walton DS: Progressive changes in the angle in congenital aniridia with the development of glaucoma. Am J Ophthalmol 78:842, 1974.
7. Gupta GP, Gangwar DN: Naevus of Ota. Br J Ophthalmol 49:364, 1965.

8. Mishima Y, Mevorah B: Nevus of Ota and nevus Ito in American Negroes. J Invest Dermatol 44:133, 1961.
9. da Costa Estima A, des Santos Carneiro R: Ota nevus: Presentation of a case. Br J Plast Surg 25:49, 1972.
10. Lever WF, Schamburgh-Lever G: Melanocytic nevi and malignant melanoma. *In* Lever WF, Schamburgh-Lever G (eds): Histopathology of the Skin. Philadelphia, JB Lippincott, 1975.
11. Gonder JR, Ezell PC, Shields JA, et al: A study to determine the prevalence rate of ocular melanocytosis. Ophthalmology 89:950, 1982.
12. Ota M, Tanino H: Nevus fusco-caeruleus ophthalmomaxillans. Tokyo Med J. 63:1243, 1939.
13. Yoshida K: Naevus fusco-caeruleus ophthalmo-maxillaris Ota. Tohoku J Exp Med 55(Suppl):34, 1952.
14. Gonder JR, Shields JA, Albert DM, et al: Uveal malignant melanoma associated with ocular and oculodermal melanocytosis. Ophthalmology 89:953, 1982.
15. Velazquez N, Jones IS: Ocular and oculodermal melanocytosis associated with uveal melanoma. Ophthalmology 91:1472, 1983.
16. Duke-Elder S, Perkins ES: Disease of the uveal tract. *In* Duke-Elder S: System of Ophthalmology. St. Louis, CV Mosby, 1966.
17. Champion R, McDonnell P, Green WR: Intraocular lenses. Surv Ophthalmol 30:1, 1985.
18. Michelson JB: Infectious clinical uveitis. Curr Opin Ophthalmol 1:373, 1990.
19. Schulman JA, Fiscella RG, Peyman GA, et al: Infectious endophthalmitis. Curr Opin Ophthalmol 1:389, 1990.
20. Adenis JP, Denis F: L'Endophthalmie. Poitiers, Ellipses, 1988, p 29.
21. Puliafito CA, Baker AS, Haaf J: Infectious endophthalmitis. Review of 36 cases. Ophthalmology 89:921, 1982.
22. Landers JH, Chapell CW: Bilateral metastatic endophthalmitis. Retina 1:175, 1981.
23. Meyers SM, Wagnild JP, Wallow IHL: Septic choroiditis with serous detachment of the retina in dogs. Invest Ophthalmol Vis Sci 17:1104, 1978.
24. Stern GA, Engel HM, Driebe WT: The treatment of postoperative endophthalmitis. Results of differing approaches to treatment. Am J Ophthalmol 96:62, 1989.
25. Macoul KL: Pneumococcal septicemia presenting as a hypopyon. Arch Ophthalmol 81:144, 1969.
26. Hamady R, Zaltas M, Paton B: *Bacillus*-induced endophthalmitis: A new series of 10 cases and review of the literature. Br J Ophthalmol 74:26, 1990.
27. Affeldt JC, Flynn HW, Forster RK: Microbial endophthalmitis resulting from ocular trauma. Ophthalmology 94:407, 1987.
28. Brinton GS, Topping TM, Hyndiuk RA: Posttraumatic endophthalmitis. Arch Ophthalmol 102:547, 1984.
29. Al-Hemidan A, Byrne-Rhodes KA, Tabbara KF: *Bacillus cereus* panophthalmitis associated with intraocular gas bubble. Br J Ophthalmol 73:25, 1989.
30. Meisler DM, Mandelbaum S: *Propionibacterium*-associated endophthalmitis after extracapsular cataract extraction: Review of reported cases. Ophthalmology 96:54, 1989.
31. Semel J, Nobe J, Bowe B, et al: *Propionibacterium acnes* isolated from explanted intraocular lens in pseudophakic bullous keratopathy. Cornea 8:259, 1989.
32. Hillman D, Garretson B, Piscella R: *Rhodococcus equi* endophthalmitis. Arch Ophthalmol 107:20, 1989.
33. Duker JS, Belmont JB: Late bacterial endophthalmitis following retinal detachment surgery. Retina 9:263, 1989.
34. Pach JM: Traumatic *Haemophilus influenzae* endophthalmitis. Am J Ophthalmol 106:497, 1988.
35. Taylor JR, Cibis GW, Hamtil LW: Endophthalmitis complicating *Haemophilus influenzae* type B meningitis. Arch Ophthalmol 98:324, 1980.
36. Jenson AD, Naidoff MA: Bilateral meningococcal endophthalmitis. Arch Ophthalmol 90:396, 1973.
37. Bigger JF, Melzer G, Mandell A: *Serratia marcescens* endophthalmitis. Am J Ophthalmol 72:1102, 1971.
38. Frieling JS, Rosenburg R, Edelstein M: Endogenous *Aeromonas hydrophilia* endophthalmitis. Arch Ophthalmol 21:117, 1989.
39. Sawush MR, Michels RG, Stark WJ: Endophthalmitis due to *Propionibacterium acnes* sequestered between IOL optic and posterior capsule. Ophthalmic Surg 20:90, 1989.
40. James DG, Graham E, Hamblina A: Immunology of multisystem ocular disease. Surv Ophthalmol 30:155, 1985.
41. James DG, Neville E, Langley DA: Ocular sarcoidosis. Trans Ophthalmol Soc UK 96:133, 1986.
42. Mizuno K, Yakahashi J: Immunology of multisystem ocular disease. Surv Ophthalmol 30:155, 1986.
43. Wirostko E, Johnson L, Wirostko B: Sarcoidosis-associated uveitis. Parasitization of vitreous leucocytes by Mollicute-like organisms. Acta Ophthalmol (Copenh) 67:415, 1989.
44. Garner A: Mollicutes. What are they? Br J Ophthalmol 73:859, 1989.
45. Chan CC, Wetzig R, Palestine A: Immunohistopathology of ocular sarcoidosis. Report of a case and discussion of immunogenesis. Arch Ophthalmol 105:1398, 1987.
46. Green WR, Koo BS: Behçet's disease. A report of the ocular histopathology on one case. Surv Ophthalmol 12:324, 1967.
47. Eglin R, Lehner T, Subak-Sharpe JH: Detection of RNA complementary to herpes simplex virus in mononuclear cells from patients with Behçet's syndrome and recurrent oral ulcers. Lancet 2:1356, 1982.
48. Fenton RH, Easom HA: A histopathologic study of the eye. Arch Ophthalmol 72:71, 1964.
49. Mullaney J, Collum LMT: Ocular vasculitis in Behçet's disease. Int Ophthalmol 7:183, 1985.
50. Shimizu T, Ehrlich GE, Inaba G: Behçet's disease. Semin Arthritis Rheum 8:233, 1979.
51. Adinolfi M, Lehner T: Acute phase proteins and C_9 in patients with Behçet's syndrome and aphthous ulcers. Clin Exp Immunol 25:36, 1976.
52. Sakane T, Konati H, Shinsuke T, et al: Functional aberration of T cells subsets in patients with Behçet's disease. Arthritis Rheum 43:746, 1982.
53. Hull RG, Harris EN, Gharavi AE: Anticardiolipin antibodies: Occurrence in Behçet's disease. Ann Rheum Dis 43:746, 1984.
54. Michelson JB, Chisari FV: Behçet's disease. Surv Ophthalmol 26:190, 1982.
55. Theis O: Gedanken über der Ausbruch der sympathischen Ophthalmie. Klin Monatsbl Augenheilkd 112:185, 1947.
56. Morse PH, Duker JR: Sympathetic ophthalmitis: Report of a case proven pathologically eight years after original injury. Am J Ophthalmol 68:508, 1969.
57. Goto H, Rao Narsing NA: Sympathetic ophthalmia and Vogt-Koyanagi-Harada syndrome. Int Ophthalmol Clin 30(4):279, 1990.
58. Forrester JV, Liversidge J, Dua HS: Comparison of clinical and experimental uveitis. Curr Eye Res 9(Suppl):75, 1990.
59. Chan CC, Benezra D, Rodrigues MM: Immunochemistry and electron microscopy of choroidal infiltrates and Dalen-Fuchs nodules in sympathetic ophthalmia. Ophthalmology 92:580, 1984.
60. Chan CC, Nussenblatt RB, Fujikawa LS: Sympathetic ophthalmia. Immunopathological findings. Ophthalmology 93:690, 1986.
61. Jakobiec FA, Marboe CC, Knowles DM: Human sympathetic ophthalmia: An analysis of the inflammatory infiltrate by hybridoma-monoclonal antibodies, immunochemistry and correlative electron microscopy. Ophthalmology 10:76, 1983.
62. Kaplan HJ, Waldrep JC, Chan WC, et al: Human sympathetic ophthalmia. Immunologic analysis of the vitreous and uvea. Arch Ophthalmol 104:240, 1986.
63. Vogt A: Frühzeitigen Ergrauen der Zilien und Bemerkungen über der sogenannten plötzlichen Eintritt dieser Veränderung. Klin Monatsbl Augenheilkd 4:228, 1906.
64. Koyanagi Y: Dysakusis, Alopecia und Poliosis bei schwerer Uveitis nicht traumatischen Ursprungs. Klin Monatsbl Augenheilkd 82:194, 1929.
65. Harada Y: Beitrag zur kliniischen kenntnis von nichtreitriger Choroiditis (Choroiditis diffusa acta). Acta Soc Ophthalmol Jpn 30:356, 1926.
66. Lubin JR, Albert DM: A clinicopathological study of the Vogt-Koyanagi-Harada syndrome. Int Ophthalmol Clin 22(3):141, 1982.
67. Chan CC, Palestine AG, Kuwabara T: Immunopathological study of Vogt-Koyanagi-Harada syndrome. Am J Ophthalmol 105:607, 1988.
68. Manor RS, Livine E, Cohen S: Cell-mediated immunity to human myelin basic protein in Vogt-Koyanagi-Harada syndrome. Invest Ophthalmol Vis Sci 18:204, 1979.

69. Yokoyama MM, Matsui Y, Kamashiroya HM: Humoral and cellular immunity studies in patients with Vogt-Koyanagi-Harada syndrome and pars planitis. Invest Ophthalmol Vis Sci 20:364, 1981.
70. Chan CC, Nussenblatt RB, Palestine AG, et al: Antiretinal autoantibodies in Vogt-Koyanagi-Harada disease, Behçet's disease and sympathetic ophthalmia. Ophthalmology 92:1025, 1985.
71. Chan CC: Relationship between sympathetic ophthalmia phacocanaphylactic endophthalmitis and Vogt-Koyanagi-Harada disease. Ophthalmology 95:619, 1988.
72. Easom HA, Zimmerman LE: A clinico-pathologic correlation and bilateral phacoanaphylaxis: A clinico-pathologic correlation of sympathogenic and sympathizing eye. Arch Ophthalmol 72:9, 1964.
73. Greenwald MJ, Wohl LG, Sell CH: Metastatic bacterial endophthalmitis: A contemporary reappraisal. Surv Ophthalmol 31:81, 1986.
74. Illingsworth RS, Wright T: Tubercles of the choroid. Br Med J 2:365, 1948.
75. Shah SM, Howard RS, Sarkies NJC: Tuberculosis presenting as retinal vasculitis. J R Soc Med 81:223, 1988.
76. Blodi FL: Ein Tuberkulom der Aderhaut, ein Melanom vortäuschend. Klin Monatsbl Augenheilkd 170:845, 1977.
77. Chung YM, Yeh TS, Sheu SJ, et al: Macular subretinal neovascularization in choroidal tuberculosis. Ann Ophthalmol 21:225, 1989.
78. Prendergast JJ: Ocular leprosy in the United States. Arch Ophthalmol 23:112, 1940.
79. Blodi FC, Hervouet F: Syphilitic chorioretinitis: A histologic study. Arch Ophthalmol 79:294, 1968.
80. Halperin LS, Lewis H, Blumenkranz MS, et al: Choroidal neovascular membrane and other chorioretinal complications of acquired syphilis. Am J Ophthalmol 108:554, 1989.
81. Freeman WR, Gross JG, Labelle J, et al: *Pneumocystis carinii* choroidopathy: A new clinical entity. Arch Ophthalmol 107:863, 1989.
82. Rao NA, Zimmerman PL, Boyer D, et al: A clinical, histopathologic, and electron microscopic study of *Pneumocystis carinii* choroiditis. Am J Ophthalmol 107:218, 1989.
83. Font RL: Intraocular nocardiosis with multiple detachments of the retinal pigment epithelium. Presented at the Verhoeff Society Meeting, Washington, DC, 1990.
84. Winterkorn JM: Lyme disease: Neurologic and ophthalmic manifestations. Surv Ophthalmol 35:191, 1990.
85. Matsuo T, Nakayama T, Tsuji T, et al: Immunological studies of uveitis. 2. Immune complex containing retinal S antigen in patient with chronic intractable uveitis. Jpn J Ophthalmol 30:480, 1986.
86. Lewis ML, Culbertson WW, Post JD, et al: Herpes simplex virus type 1. A cause of the acute retinal necrosis syndrome. Ophthalmology 96:875, 1989.
87. Culbertson WW, Blumenkranz MS, Pepose JS, et al: Varicella zoster virus is a cause of the acute retinal necrosis syndrome. Ophthalmology 93:559, 1986.
88. Culbertson WW, Blumenkranz MS, Haines H, et al: The acute retinal necrosis syndrome. Part 2: Histopathology and etiology. Ophthalmology 89:1317, 1982.
89. Nanda M, Curtin VT, Hilliard JK, et al: Ocular histopathologic findings in a case of human herpes B virus infection. Arch Ophthalmol 108:713, 1990.
90. De Venecia G, Zu Rhein GM, Pratt MV, et al: Cytomegalic inclusion retinitis in an adult. Arch Ophthalmol 86:44, 1971.
91. Freeman WR, Thomas EL, Rao NA, et al: Demonstration of herpes group virus in acute retinal necrosis syndrome. Am J Ophthalmol 102:701, 1986.
92. Walker EA: Guillain-Barré syndrome and pan-uveitis. Scott Med J 35:22, 1990.
93. Usui M, Sakai J: Three cases of EB virus–associated uveitis. Int Ophthalmol 14:371, 1990.
94. Friedman AH: The retinal lesions of the acquired immune deficiency syndrome. Trans Am Ophthalmol Soc 82:447, 1984.
95. Winward KE, Hamed LM, Glaser JS: The spectrum of optic nerve disease in human immunodeficiency virus infection. Am J Ophthalmol 107:373, 1989.
96. Jensen OA, Gerstoft J, Thomsen HK, et al: Cytomegalovirus retinitis in the acquired immunodeficiency syndrome (AIDS): Light-microscopical, ultrastructural and immunohistochemical examination of a case. Acta Ophthalmol (Copenh) 62:1, 1984.
97. Zimmerman LE: Histopathologic basis for ocular manifestations of congenital rubella syndrome. Am J Ophthalmol 65:837, 1968.
98. Yanoff M, Schaffer DB, Scheie HG: Rubella ocular syndrome: Clinical significance of viral and pathologic studies. Trans Am Acad Ophthalmol Otolaryngol 72:896, 1968.
99. Nahata MC, Davidorf FH, Caldwell JH, et al: *Candida* endophthalmitis associated with total parenteral nutrition. JPEN J Parenter Enteral Nutr 5:150, 1981.
100. Hogeweg M, deJong PT: *Candida* endophthalmitis in heroin addicts. Doc Ophthalmol 55:63, 1983.
101. Aguilar GL, Blumenkranz MS, Egbert PR, et al: *Candida* endophthalmitis after intravenous drug abuse. Arch Ophthalmol 97:96, 1979.
102. Pulido JS, Folberg R, Carter KD, et al: *Histoplasma capsulatum* endophthalmitis after cataract extraction. Ophthalmology 97:217, 1990.
103. Stone SP, Bendig J, Hakim J, et al: Cryptococcal meningitis presenting as uveitis. Br J Ophthalmol 72:167, 1988.
104. Schulman JA, Leveque C, Coats M, et al: Fatal disseminated cryptococcosis following intraocular involvement. Br J Ophthalmol 72:171, 1988.
105. Jabs DA, Green WR, Fox R, et al: Ocular manifestations of acquired immune deficiency syndrome. Ophthalmology 96:1092, 1989.
106. Hiss PW, Shields JA, Augsburger JJ: Solitary retinovitreal abscess as the initial manifestation of cryptococcosis. Ophthalmology 95:162, 1988.
107. Weiss JN, Hutchkins RK, Balogh K: Simultaneous *Aspergillus* endophthalmitis and cytomegalovirus retinitis after kidney transplantation. Retina 8:193, 1988.
108. Bodoia RD, Kinyoun JL, Lou QL, et al: *Aspergillus* necrotizing retinitis: A clinico-pathologic study and review. Retina 9:226, 1989.
109. Grossniklaus HE, Specht CS, Allaire G, et al: *Toxoplasma gondii* retinochoroiditis and optic neuritis in acquired immune deficiency syndrome: Report of a case. Ophthalmology 97:1342, 1990.
110. Parke DW II, Font RL: Diffuse toxoplasmic retinochoroiditis in a patient with AIDS. Arch Ophthalmol 104:571, 1986.
111. Rao NA, Font RL: Toxoplasmic retinochoroiditis: Electron-microscopic and immunofluorescence studies of formalin-fixed tissue. Arch Ophthalmol 95:273, 1977.
112. Shields JA: Ocular toxocariasis: A review. Surv Ophthalmol 28:361, 1984.
113. Ashton N: Larval granulomatosis of the retina due to *Toxocara*. Br J Ophthalmol 44:129, 1960.
114. Irvine WC, Irvine ARJ: Nematode endophthalmitis: *Toxocara canis*—Report of one case. Am J Ophthalmol 47:185, 1959.
115. Tabbara KF: Other parasitic infections. *In* Tabbara KF, Hyndiuk RA (eds): Infections of the Eye. Boston, Little, Brown, & Co, 1986.
116. Wilder HC: Nematode endophthalmitis. Trans Am Acad Ophthalmol 55:99, 1950.
117. Wilkinson CP: Ocular toxocariasis. *In* Ryan SJ (ed): Retina, 11th ed. St. Louis, CV Mosby, 1989.
118. Fearnley IR, Spalton DJ, Ward AM, et al: alpha$_1$-Antitrypsin phenotypes in acute anterior uveitis. Br J Ophthalmol 72:636, 1988.
119. Schwab IR: Fuchs' heterochromic iridocyclitis. Int Ophthalmol Clin 30(4):252, 1990.
120. Wetzig RP, Chan CC, Nussenblatt RB, et al: Clinical and immunopathological studies of pars planitis in a family. Br J Ophthalmol 72:5, 1988.
121. Priem HA, Oosterhuis JA: Birdshot chorioretinopathy: Clinical characteristics and evolution. Br J Ophthalmol 72:646, 1988.
122. Nussenblatt RB, Mittal KK, Ryan S, et al: Birdshot retinochoroidopathy associated with HLA-A29 antigen and immune responsiveness to retinal S-antigen. Am J Ophthalmol 94:147, 1982.
123. Kirkham TH, Ffytche TJ, Sanders MD: Placoid pigment epitheliopathy with retinal vasculitis and papillitis. Br J Ophthalmol 56:875, 1972.
124. Charteris DG, Lee WR: Multifocal posterior uveitis: Clinical and pathological findings. Br J Ophthalmol 74:688, 1990.
125. Fryczkowski AW, Hodes BL, Walker J: Diabetic choroidal and

iris vasculature—scanning electron microscopy findings. Int Ophthalmol 13:269, 1989.
126. Hidayat AA, Fine BS: Light and electron microscopic observations of seven cases. Ophthalmology 92:512, 1985.
127. Yanoff M: Ocular pathology and diabetes. Am J Ophthalmol 67:21, 1969.
128. Lewis RA, Riccardi VM: von Recklinghausen neurofibromatosis. Incidence of iris hamartoma. Ophthalmology 88:348, 1981.
129. Perry HD, Font RL: Iris nodules in von Recklinghausen neurofibromatosis: Electron microscopic confirmation of their melanocytic origin. Arch Ophthalmol 100:1635, 1982.
130. Grant WM, Walton DS: Distinctive gonioscopic findings in glaucoma due to neurofibromatosis. Arch Ophthalmol 79:127, 1968.
131. Eagle RCJ, Font RL, Yanoff M, et al: Proliferative endotheliopathy with iris abnormalities: The iridocorneal endothelial syndrome. Arch Ophthalmol 97:2104, 1979.
132. Wiznia RA, Freedman JK, Mancini AD: Malignant melanoma of choroid in neurofibromatosis. Am J Ophthalmol 86:684, 1978.
133. Husby G, Sletten K: Chemical and clinical classification of amyloidosis. Scand J Immunol 23:253, 1986.
134. Glenner GG: Amyloid deposits and amyloidosis. The β-fibrilloses. (First of two parts). N Engl J Med 302:1283, 1980.
135. Glenner GG: Amyloid deposits and amyloidosis. The β-fibrilloses (Second of two parts.) N Engl J Med 302:1333, 1980.
136. Ramsey MS, Fine BS, Cohen SW: Localized corneal amyloidosis: Case report with electron microscopic observations. Am J Ophthalmol 73:560, 1972.
137. Richlin JJ, Kuwabara T: Amyloid disease of the eyelid and conjunctiva. Arch Ophthalmol 67:138, 1962.
138. Smith ME, Zimmerman LE: Amyloidosis of the eyelid and conjunctiva. Arch Ophthalmol 75:42, 1966.
139. Nehen J: Primary localized orbital amyloidosis. Acta Ophthalmol 57:287, 1979.
140. Conlon MR, Chapman WB, Burt WL, et al: Primary localized amyloidosis of the lacrimal glands. Ophthalmology 98:1556, 1991.
141. Levine MR, Buckman G: Primary localized orbital amyloidosis. Ann Ophthalmol 18:165, 1986.
142. Macoul KL, Winter FC: External ophthalmoplegia secondary to systemic amyloidosis. Arch Ophthalmol 79:182, 1968.
143. Falls HF, Jackson J, Carey JH, et al: Ocular manifestations of hereditary primary systemic amyloidosis. Arch Ophthalmol 54:660, 1955.
144. Witschel H, Mobius W: Ocular changes in generalized amyloidosis (author's transl). Klin Monatsbl Augenheilkd 165:610, 1974.
145. Kantarjian AD, DeJong RN: Familial amyloidosis with nervous system involvement. Neurology 3:399, 1953.
146. Hamburg A: Unusual cause of vitreous opacities: Primary familial amyloidosis. Ophthalmologica 162:173, 1971.
147. Paton D, Duke JR: Primary familial amyloidosis: Ocular manifestations with histopathological observations. Am J Ophthalmol 61:736, 1966.
148. Tso MOM, Bettman JWJ: Occlusion of the choriocapillaris in primary nonfamilial amyloidosis. Arch Ophthalmol 86:281, 1971.
149. Schwartz MF, Green WR, Michels RG, et al: An usual case of ocular involvement in primary systemic nonfamilial amyloidosis. Ophthalmology 89:394, 1982.
150. Rodrigues M, Zimmerman LE: Secondary amyloidosis in ocular leprosy. Arch Ophthalmol 85:277, 1971.
151. Ratnakar KS, Mohan M: Amyloidosis of the iris. Can J Ophthalmol 11:277, 1976.
152. Lesell S, Wolf PA, Benson MD, et al: Scalloped pupils in familial amyloidosis. N Engl J Med 293:914, 1975.
153. Andrade C: A peculiar form of peripheral neuropathy familial atypical generalized amyloidosis with specialized involvement of the peripheral nerves. Brain 75:408, 1952.
154. Wong VG, Kuwabara T, Brubaker R, et al: Intralysomal cystine crystals in cystinosis. Invest Ophthalmol 9:83, 1970.
155. Patel A, Kenyon KR, Hirst LW, et al: Clinicopathologic features of Chandler's syndrome. Surv Ophthalmol 27:327, 1983.
156. Sanderson PO, Kuwabara T, Stark W, et al: Cystinosis: A clinical, histopathologic, and ultrastructural study. Arch Ophthalmol 91:270, 1974.
157. Wong VG, Lietman PS, Seegmiller JE: Alterations of pigment epithelium in cystinosis. Arch Ophthalmol 77:361, 1967.
158. Kaiser-Kupfer MI, Fujikawa L, Kuwabara T, et al: Removal of corneal crystals by topical cysteamine in nephropathic cystinosis. N Engl J Med 316:775, 1987.
159. Gahl WA, Reed GF, Thoene JG, et al: Cysteamine therapy for children with nephropathic cystinosis. N Engl J Med 316:971, 1987.
160. Skovby F: Homocysteinuria: Clinical, biochemical, and genetic aspects of cystathionine beta-synthetase and its deficiency in man. Acta Paediatr Scand [Suppl] 321:1, 1985.
161. Mudd HJ, Skovby F, Levy HL, et al: The natural history of homocysteinuria due to cystathionine β-synthetase deficiency. Am J Hum Genet 37:1, 1985.
162. Naumann GOH, Gass JDM, Font RL: Histopathology of herpes zoster ophthalmicus. Am J Ophthalmol 65:110, 1968.
163. Hedges TRI, Albert DM: The progression of the ocular abnormalities of herpes zoster. Histopathological observations of nine cases. Ophthalmol 89:165, 1982.
164. Henkind P: Ocular neovascularization. The Krill memorial lecture. Am J Ophthalmol 13:287, 1978.
165. John T, Sassani JW, Eagle RCJ: The myofibroblastic component of rubeosis iridis. Ophthalmology 90:721, 1983.
166. Tamura T: Electron microscopic study on the small blood vessels in rubeosis iridis diabetica. Acta Soc Ophthalmol Jpn 72:2340, 1969.
167. Goldberg MF, Tso MOM: Rubeosis iridis and glaucoma associated with sickle cell retinopathy: A light and microscopic study. Am Acad Ophthalmol Otolaryngol 85:1028, 1978.
168. Sarks SH: New vessel formation beneath the retinal pigment epithelium in senile eyes. Br J Ophthalmol 57:951, 1973.
169. Foos RY, Trese MT: Chorioretinal juncture: Vascularization of Bruch's membrane in peripheral fundus. Arch Ophthalmol 100:1492, 1982.
170. Heriot WJ, Henkind P, Bellhorn BW, et al: Choroidal neovascularization can digest Bruch's membrane: A prior break is not essential. Ophthalmology 91:1603, 1984.
171. Penfold PL, Killingsworth MC, Starks SH: An ultrastructural study of the rate of leukocytes and fibroblasts in the breakdown of Bruch's membrane. Aust N Z J Ophthalmol 12:23, 1984.
172. Gass JDM: Stereoscopic Atlas of Macular Disease, 3rd ed. St. Louis, CV Mosby, 1987.
173. Knapp P: Ein seltner Augenspiegelbefund: Sclerosis chorioideae circinata. Klin Monatsbl Augenheilkd 45:171, 1907.
174. Kofler A: Beitraege zur Kenntnis der Angioid streaks (Knapp). Arch Augenheilkd 82:134, 1917.
175. Hagedoorn A: Angioid streaks. Arch Ophthalmol 21:746, 1939.
176. Verhoeff FA: Histological findings in a case of angioid streaks. Br J Ophthalmol 32:531, 1948.
177. Dreyer R, Green WR: The pathology of angioid streaks: A study of twenty-one cases. Trans Am Acad Ophthalmol Otolaryngol 31:158, 1978.
178. McKusick VA: Heritable Disorders of Connective Tissue, 4th ed. St. Louis, CV Mosby, 1972.
179. Paton D: The Relation of Angioid Streaks to Systemic Disease. Springfield, IL, Charles C Thomas, 1972.
180. Nagpal KC, Asdourian G, Goldbaum M, et al: Angioid streaks and sickle haemoglobinopathies. Br J Ophthalmol 60:31, 1976.
181. Connor PJJ, Juergens JL, Perry HO: Pseudoxanthoma elasticum and angioid streaks: A review of 106 cases. Am J Med 30:537, 1961.
182. Grand MG, Isserman MJ, Miller CW: Angioid streaks associated with pseudoxanthoma elasticum in a 13-year-old patient. Ophthalmology 94:197, 1987.
183. Mansour AM: Systemic associations of angioid streaks. Int Ophthalmol Clin 31:61, 1991.
184. Rodrigues MM, Jester JV, Richards R, et al: Essential iris atrophy. A clinical, immunohistologic, and electron microscopic study in an enucleated eye. Ophthalmology 95:69, 1988.
185. Shields MB: Progressive essential iris atrophy, Chandler's syndrome, and the iris nevus (Cogan-Reese) syndrome: A spectrum of disease. Surv Ophthalmol 24:3, 1979.
186. Yanoff M: Iridocorneal endothelial syndrome: Unification of a disease spectrum. [Editorial] Surv Ophthalmol 24:1, 1979.
187. Alvarado JA, Murphy CG, Maglio M, et al: Pathogenesis of Chandler's syndrome, essential iris atrophy, and the Cogan-Reese syndrome. I. Alterations of the corneal endothelium. Invest Ophthalmol Vis Sci 27:853, 1986.

188. Alvarado JA, Murphy CG, Juster RP, et al: Pathogenesis of Chandler's syndrome, essential iris atrophy, and the Cogan-Reese syndrome. II. Estimated age at disease onset. Invest Ophthalmol Vis Sci 27:873, 1986.
189. Eagle RCJ, Shields JA: Iridocorneal endothelial syndrome with contralateral guttate endothelial dystrophy: A light and electron microscopic study. Ophthalmology 94:862, 1987.
190. Krill AE, Archer D: Classification of the choroidal atrophies. Am J Ophthalmol 72:562, 1971.
191. Jonas JB, Nguyen XN, Gusek GC, et al: Parapapillary chorioretinal atrophy in normal and glaucoma eyes. I: Morphometric data. Invest Ophthalmol Vis Sci 30:908, 1989.
192. Weiter J, Fine BS: A histologic study of regional choroidal dystrophy. Am J Ophthalmol 83:741, 1977.
193. Schocket SS, Ballin N: Circinate choroidal sclerosis. Trans Am Acad Ophthalmol Otolaryngol 74:527, 1970.
194. Knapp P: Ein seltener Augenspiegelbefund (sclerosis chorioideae circinata). Klin Monatsbl Augenheilkd 45:171, 1907.
195. Chopdar A: Annular choroidal sclerosis. Br J Ophthalmol 60:512, 1976.
196. Ashton NE: Central areolar choroidal sclerosis. Br J Ophthalmol 60:140, 1953.
197. Ferry AP, Llovera I, Shafer DM: Central areolar choroidal dystrophy. Arch Ophthalmol 88:39, 1972.
198. Sarks SH: Senile choroidal sclerosis. Br J Ophthalmol 57:98, 1973.
199. Hayasaka S, Shoji K, Kanno C, et al: Differential diagnosis of diffuse choroidal atrophies. Diffuse choriocapillaris atrophy, choroideremia, and gyrate atrophy of the choroid and retina. Retina 5:30, 1985.
200. Sierra JM, Ogden TE, Van Boemal GB: Inherited Retinal Disease. A Diagnostic Guide. Part II. Abnormalities of Choroidal Vessels. St. Louis, CV Mosby, 1989.
201. Carr RE, Mittl RN, Noble KG: Choroidal abiotrophies. Trans Am Acad Ophthalmol Otolaryngol 79:1975.
202. McCulloch CL: Choroideremia and other choroidal atrophies. *In* Newsome DA (ed): Retinal Dystrophies and Degenerations. New York, Raven Press, 1988.
203. Rodrigues MM, Ballintine EJ, Wiggert BN, et al: Choroideremia: A clinical, electron microscopic, and biochemical report. Ophthalmology 91:873, 1984.
204. Cameron JD, Fine BS, Shapiro I: Histopathologic observations in choroideremia with emphasis on vascular changes of the uveal tract. Ophthalmology 94:187, 1987.
205. Flannery JG, Bird AC, Farber DB, et al: A histopathologic study of a choroideremia carrier. Invest Ophthalmol Vis Sci 31:229, 1990.
206. Nussbaum RL, Lewis RA, Lesko JG: Choroideremia is linked to the fragment length polymorphism DXYS1 at Xq13-21. Am J Hum Genet 37:473, 1985.
207. Henkind P, Gartner S: The relationship between retinal pigment epithelium and the choriocapillaris. Trans Ophthalmol Soc UK 103:444, 1983.
208. Hotta Y, Inana G: Gene transfer and expression of human ornithine aminotransferase. Invest Ophthalmol Vis Sci 30:1024, 1989.
209. Vannas SK, Simell O, Sipila I: Gyrate atrophy of the choroid and retina. The ocular disease progresses in juvenile patients despite normal or near-normal plasma ornithine concentration. Ophthalmology 94:1428, 1987.
210. Inana G, Hotta Y, Zintz C, et al: Expression defect of ornithine aminotransferase gene in gyrate atrophy. Invest Ophthalmol Vis Sci 29:1001, 1988.
211. Wilson DJ, Weleber RG, Green WR: Ocular clinicopathologic study of gyrate atrophy. Am J Ophthalmol 111:24, 1991.
212. McLendon BF, Bron AJ, Mitchell CJ: *Streptococcus* suis type II (Group R) as a cause of endophthalmitis. Br J Ophthalmol 62:729–731, 1978.
213. Michelson JB, Friedlaender MH: Behçet's disease. Int Ophthalmol 30:271–278, 1990.
214. Guinto RS, Binford CH: Leprosy. VA Med Bull (MB10) Washington DC May 25, 1965.
215. Petty RE, Johnston W, McCormick AQ, et al: Uveitis and arthritis induced by adjuvant: Clinical, immunologic and histologic characteristics. J Rheumatol 16(4):499–505, 1989.
216. Fox A: Role of bacterial debris in inflammatory diseases of the joint and eye. APMIS 98:957–968, 1990.
217. Hooks JJ, Detrick B: Immunologic uveitis. Curr Opinion 1:396–401, 1990.
218. Darrell RW, Wagener HP, Kurland LT: Epidemiology of uveitis: Incidence and prevalence in a small urban community. Arch Ophthalmol 68:502–514, 1962.
219. Opremcak EM, Cowans AB, Orosz CG, et al: Enumeration of autoreactive helper T lymphocytes in uveitis. Invest Ophthalmol Vis Sci 32:2561–2567, 1991.
220. Rahi AHS, Kanski JJ, Fielder A: Immunoglobulins and antinuclear factor in aqueous humour from patients with juvenile "rheumatoid" arthritis (Still's disease). Trans Ophthalmol Soc UK 97:217–222, 1977.
221. Hinzpeter EN, Naumann G, Bartelheimer HK: Ocular histopathology in Still's disease. Ophthalmol Res 2:16–24, 1971.
222. Rosenbaum JT: Bilateral anterior uveitis and interstitial nephritis. Am J Ophthalmol 105:534–537, 1988.
223. Salu P, Stempels N, Vanden Houte K, et al: Acute tubulointerstitial nephritis and uveitis syndrome in the elderly. Br J Ophthalmol 74:53–55, 1990.
224. Stupp R, Mihatsch MJ, Matter L, et al: Acute tubulo-interstitial nephritis with uveitis (TINU syndrome) in a patient with serologic evidence for *Chlamydia* infection. Klin Wochenschr 68:971–975, 1990.
225. Johnson LA, Wirostko E, Wirostko WJ: Crohn's disease uveitis: Parasitization of vitreous leukocytes by mollicute-like organisms. Am J Clin Pathol 91(3):259–264, 1989.
226. Wirostko E, Johnson L, Wirostko B: Ulcerative colitis associated chronic uveitis: Parasitization of intraocular leukocytes by mollicute-like organisms: Sympathetic Ophthalmia. J Submicrosc Cytol Pathol 22(2):231–239, 1990.
227. Mielants H, Veys EM, Verbraeken H, et al: HLA-B27 positive idiopathic acute anterior uveitis: A unique manifestation of subclinical gut inflammation. J Rheumatol 17:841–842, 1990.
228. Kimura SJ, Hogan MJ, O'Conner GR, et al: Uveitis and joint disease: A review of 191 cases. Trans Am Ophthalmol Soc 64:291–310, 1966.
229. VanMetre TE Jr, Brown WH, Knox DL, et al: The relationship between nongranulomatous uveitis and arthritis. J Allergy 36:211–215, 1965.
230. Linssen A, Rothova A, Valkenburg HA: The lifetime cumulative incidence of acute anterior uveitis in a normal population and its relation to ankylosing spondylitis and histocompatibility antigen HLA-B27. Invest Ophthalmol Vis Sci 32:2568–2578, 1991.
231. Wakefield D, Stahlberg TH, Toivanen A, et al: Serologic evidence of *Yersinia* infection in patients with anterior uveitis. Arch Ophthalmol 108:219–221, 1990.
232. Saari KM, Kauranen O: Ocular inflammation in Reiter's syndrome associated with *Campylobacter jejuni* enteritis. Am J Ophthalmol 90:572–573, 1980.
233. Welsh J, Avakian H, Ebringer A: Uveitis, vitreous humor and *Klebsiella:* Cross reactivity studies with radioimmunoassay. Br J Ophthalmol 65:323–328, 1981.
234. Spencer WH (ed): Ophthalmic Pathology: An Atlas and Textbook, 3rd ed. Philadelphia, WB Saunders, 1986, pp 1328–1338.

Chapter 183

Pathology of the Lens*

BARBARA W. STREETEN

The lens is a simple structure histologically, its remarkable complexity hidden at the molecular and functional levels. It has the unique ability to remain transparent for 7 decades or more in spite of continuous growth and metabolism in a closed avascular system. This is accomplished without the help of a nucleus or even a standard complement of organelles in most of its cells. Functionally the lens falls short of perfection by failing to provide us with a lifetime of accommodation, a defect probably inherent in the design of the system, abetted by the processes of aging. Most of serious lens pathology, however, results from insults deriving from an aging or imperfect host and a less than benign environment, expressed in various forms of cataract. Fortunately, our understanding of lens susceptibility to disease and genetic defects is increasing rapidly and should be a major beneficiary in this era of molecular biology.

EMBRYONIC DEVELOPMENT AND MATURATION OF THE LENS

Embryonic-Fetal Period of Development

For its size and complexity of function, the lens is unique in deriving entirely from one germinal cell layer, the surface ectoderm. Early in the fourth week of gestation (Table 183–1), lens development begins as a placodal thickening of the single cell–layered surface ectoderm, induced by the close approach of the optic vesicle (Fig. 183–1).[1, 2] When the optic vesicle invaginates to form the optic cup, the lens placode develops a central pit and buds down into the optic cup as the lens vesicle. Late in the fourth week the lens vesicle separates completely from the surface ectoderm (primitive epidermis). In the fifth week its cavity begins to fill up with primary lens fibers, formed by elongation of the posterior lens epithelial cells (see Fig. 183–1*D*). The nuclei of these new lens fiber cells migrate forward to the level of the equator, and from this time on, lens nuclei are absent behind the equator except in cataract formation.

In the eighth week the secondary lens fibers form by mitosis and migration of new lens epithelial cells from the preequatorial (germinative) zone of the epithelium. As each cuboidal cell approaches the equator, its nucleus becomes progressively more oval, and the cell elongates. One cytoplasmic arm extends anteriorly under the epithelial layer, and a posterior arm creeps along the posterior capsule. Both ends of this new hexagonal flat lens fiber grow toward the poles, where they join new fibers from other areas at the sutures. A curved bow of lens nuclei marks this entry of new cells into the cortex and will identify active lens fiber formation throughout life (Fig. 183–2). At the end of this bow, the lens fiber nuclei rapidly disappear through a program of self-destruction of unknown mechanism.[3] Lysosomes are also lost at about this time, although most other organelles are preserved in small numbers.

The earliest lens sutures are a horizontal anterior line and a vertical posterior line. As the embryonic period ends and the fetal period begins in the third month, the secondary lens fibers enlarge the circumference that must be spanned. The resulting sutures become more complex, forming an upright Y anteriorly and an inverted Y posteriorly in this fetal nucleus (Fig. 183–3). The Y pattern results from the fact that the anterior and posterior arms of the fiber have different lengths.[4] Fibers reaching the center of the lens at one end do not go quite as far at the other end, terminating on one of the extensions of the main suture. Sutures created postnatally have increasingly more complex stellate branches as the lens expands in girth, causing many fibers to meet before they reach the center of the lens.

The lens capsule is detectable ultrastructurally at the lens vesicle stage, but by light microscopy this basement membrane surrounding the lens is not detectable until the fifth week, using periodic acid–Schiff staining.

From the fifth to the end of the sixth week a complex vascular system, the tunica vasculosa lentis, develops around the lens, supplying its nutrition during the next few months of rapid growth. This system arises from ramifications of the hyaloid artery posteriorly, joining branches from the annular vessel at the edge of the optic cup anteriorly. The posterior portion of this system and the matrix it produces constitute the primary vitreous (Fig. 183–4).

During the fourth and fifth months gradual atrophy of the tunica vasculosa lentis occurs. The anterior portion has a longer functional life, forming the major circle of the iris and the pupillary membrane. By the eighth month, only atrophic remnants of the hyaloid artery remain, and the pupillary membrane has atrophied back to its last arcade, forming the minor circle of the iris.

At the end of the third or early fourth fetal month, zonular fibrils can be seen passing from the ciliary

*Funded in part by Research Grant EY01602 from the National Eye Institute, National Institutes of Health.

Table 183–1. CHRONOLOGY OF LENS DEVELOPMENT

Gestational Age	Crown Rump	Lens Events	Associated Ocular Events
Early fourth week	4 mm	Development of lens placode	Invagination of optic cup
	5 mm	Lens pit forms	
Late fourth week	6 mm	Lens vesicle completed	Hyaloid artery into fetal fissure
			Annular vessel anterior to cup
Late fourth–early fifth week	7–9 mm	Separation of lens vesicle	Optic cup invagination complete
Fifth week	10 mm	Primary lens fibers elongate	Fetal fissure closure begins
			Hyaloid system and tunica vasculosa lentis forming
End of fifth week	13 mm	Lens capsule seen	Nerve fibers reach optic stalk
End of sixth week	18 mm	Primary lens fibers complete	Fetal fissure closed. Lid folds arising
Eighth week	26 mm	Secondary lens fibers begin	Slitlike anterior chamber present
End of eighth week	30 mm	Y-sutures forming	Cornea, anterior chamber well formed
Third month	31–70 mm	Fetal period begins	Optic cup grows forward. Major iris circle and pupillary membrane form
End of third month	65–70 mm	Zonular fibers visible	Ciliary processes developing. Secondary vitreous begins
Fourth to fifth month	71–150 mm	Full zonular system	Tunica vasculosa lentis atrophies
Eighth month		Hyaloid artery tail in Cloquet's canal	Hyaloid artery detaches from disc
			Pupillary membrane atrophied
Birth		Fetal nucleus close to anterior capsule	

Collated from data in Barber[1] and Mann.[2]

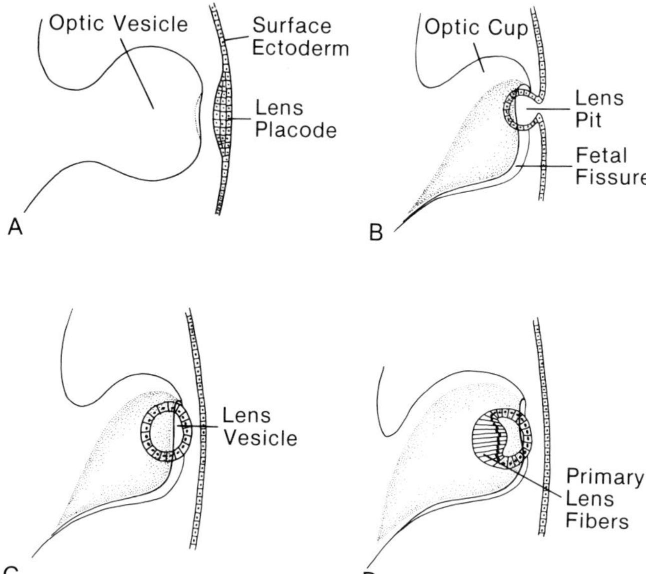

Figure 183–1. Diagram of lens development in the fourth and fifth weeks of gestation. (Modified from Barber AN: Embryology of The Human Eye. St. Louis, CV Mosby, 1955.)

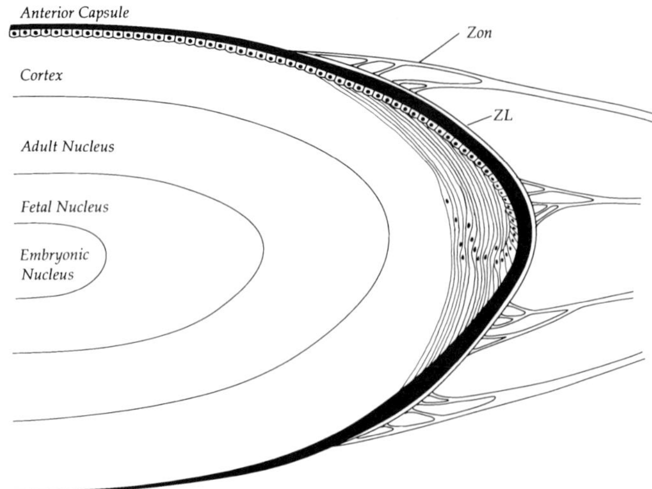

Figure 183–2. Schematic view of a cross section through the young adult lens. Equatorial lens epithelial cells are elongating to form secondary lens fibers. A "bow" of nuclei identifies these new fibers throughout life. Approximate sites of the biomicroscopic lens nuclei are shown. (Zon, zonular bundles; ZL, zonular lamella.)

epithelium toward the lens. These noncollagenous fibrils were once referred to as the "tertiary vitreous" owing to a misconception of their nature. By the sixth month a delicate but complete zonular system is present, inserting on the anterior and posterior lens capsule and covering the surface of the ciliary epithelium except for the anterior portion of the ciliary processes.

Both primary and secondary (definitive) vitreous are collagenous and important for lens pathology because

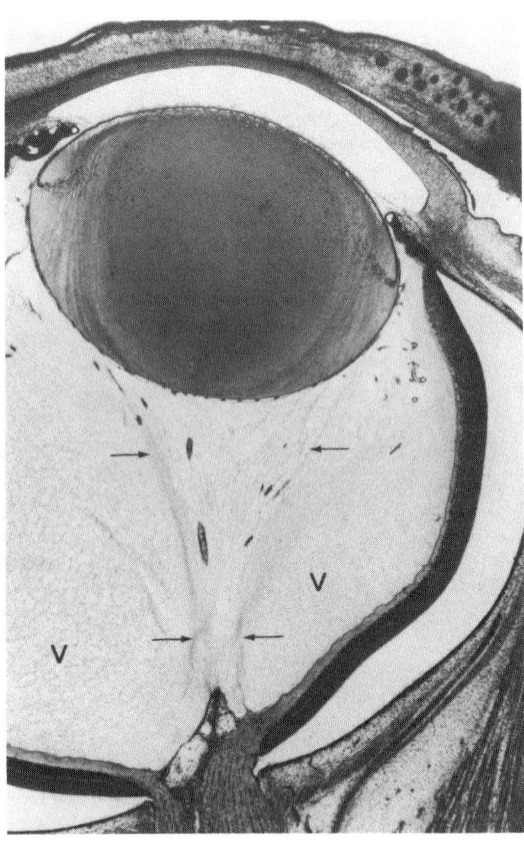

Figure 183–4. Relation of the lens to the primary and secondary vitreous at the end of the third month. The secondary vitreous (V) compresses the vascular primary vitreous into a central funnel (between *arrows*). Tiny capillaries of the tunica vasculosa lentis partially surround the lens. (From Naumann GOH, et al: Pathologie des Auges. Berlin, Springer-Verlag, 1980.)

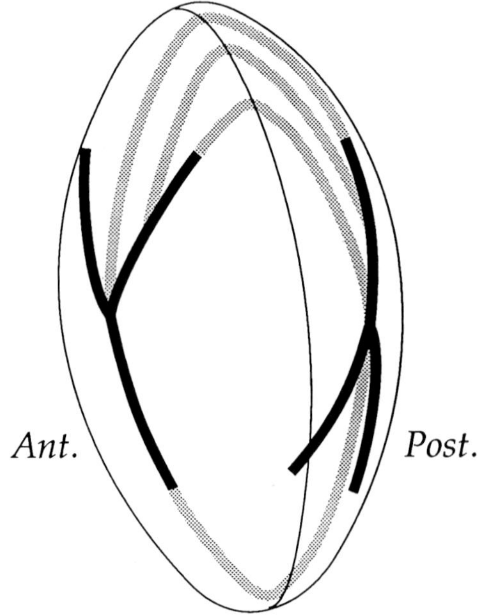

Figure 183–3. Diagram of Y-suture formation in the fetal nucleus. Each lens fiber *(shaded stripes)* has a longer course from the equator to either the anterior upright or the posterior inverted Y-suture. (Modified from Hogan MJ, Alvarado JA, Weddell JE: Histology of the Human Eye: An Atlas and Textbook. Philadelphia, WB Saunders, 1971.)

of their close attachment to the lens throughout development. The onset of secondary vitreous secretion from the inner layer of the optic cup in the third month (see Table 183–1) pushes the vascularized primary vitreous centrally into a funnel-shaped space called Cloquet's canal (see Fig. 183–4). The primary vitreous does not atrophy completely until the sixth fetal month, a prolonged period during which many pathologic events can interfere with its regression. The fibrils on the surface of the secondary vitreous condense to form the anterior hyaloid membrane, firmly attached to the lens capsule at the edge of the posterior equator at Wieger's "ligament" (ligamentum hyaloideocapsulare).[1]

Structure of the Mature Lens

In the young adult the lens is a biconvex structure of about 8 mm in equatorial diameter and 3.5 mm in thickness, less rounded than the newborn lens, which is similar in thickness but only about 6 mm in diameter. Expansion has been greater in the equatorial direction, molded by zonular tension on the capsule and the malleable young lens fibers. In the young eye the lens capsule is 7 to 8 μm in thickness at both the anterior pole and the equator, but only 2 μm at the posterior pole.[6] The preequatorial regions are significantly thicker where the zonules insert, reaching 12 to 15 μm anteriorly and 18 to 22 μm posteriorly. By age 35 most of these capsular thicknesses have doubled, but the anterior preequatorial has thickened only to 21 μm, and the posterior to 23 μm. With aging the equatorial and posterior capsular regions thin to almost their original dimensions.

The lens capsule is the basement membrane of the lens epithelial cells, carbohydrate-rich and thus intensely positive with the PAS stain. It appears very homogenous by light microscopy (Fig. 183–5) but has a faintly fibrillar and laminated ultrastructure (Fig. 183–6). The primary components of the capsule are type IV collagen, the glycoprotein adhesion protein laminin, and the proteoglycan heparan sulfate.[7,8] The capsule's fibrillar structure is achieved by networks of type IV collagen tetramers, linked together by small globular components (NC 1-domains) at the ends of the four extended arms (see Fig. 183–6, *upper inset*).

Beginning in the second decade,[9,10] inclusions of 50-nm banded fibers and fibrogranular aggregates resembling zonular fibrils appear in the anterior capsule, particularly in the preequatorial region (see Fig. 183–6, *lower inset*). The superficial capsule is more loosely fibrillar, especially under the inserting zonular fibers, as they form a layer covering the equatorial and preequatorial region, called the zonular lamella (Figs. 183–2 and 183–7).[11]

The lens epithelium is composed of regular low cuboidal cells, 14 μm wide and 8 μm high, with round nuclei (Fig. 183–8) before elongating at the equator. Their lateral cell membranes have extensive interdigitations, with desmosomal junctions, and contain the usual organelles in small numbers. Strands of occludens tight junctions are present irregularly at their apical borders, with occasional macula adherens junctions above them.[12] Rare gap junctions are seen at the epithelial cell-fiber interface. Mitoses occur predominantly in the preequatorial region.

The lens cortical fibers display an obvious lamellar pattern, easily seen by light microscopy (Fig. 183–9). Most of the fibers have a granular cytoplasm with few organelles and are linked by gap junctions (Fig. 183–10*A*). The epithelial and superficial fiber cells have a finely filamentous cytoskeleton with prominent arrays of peripheral actin bundles, possibly related to their frequent changes in shape.[14] The fibers are hexagonal in cross section (see Fig. 183–8) and joined together along their lengths by ball-and-socket interdigitations (see Fig. 183–10*B*).[13,15] Intersecting low ridges and grooves are prominent interconnecting sites in the deeper cortical and nuclear fibers, where they become covered by microvilli in senescence (see Fig. 183–10*C*).[13] A very high content of water-soluble protein is present in the fibers, predominantly as the α, β, and γ lens crystallins.[16]

CONGENITAL ABNORMALITIES OF THE LENS

Abnormalities of Lens Embryogenesis

APHAKIA AND PSEUDOPHAKIA

Primary aphakia with complete failure of lens formation is rare, usually accompanied by other severe ocular defects.[17] Indeed, there is experimental evidence that the vitreous cannot develop in the absence of at least the primordium of a lens, precluding any possibility of a normal globe.[18] Several cases have been reported in association with microphthalmia following maternal rubella[19–20] and in trisomy 13.[21] Rarely, duplication of the lens has been seen.[22]

More commonly a small or incompletely formed lens gives a false impression of aphakia, or pseudophakia, sometimes referred to as "secondary" aphakia. The primary lens fibers can degenerate, leaving a peripheral white ring of cataractous secondary lens fibers (Soemmerring's ring), with collapsed anterior and posterior capsules adherent to each other centrally. Because the soft, young lens fibers can completely liquefy and become absorbed, pseudophakia may be difficult to appreciate even histologically, but with the periodic acid–

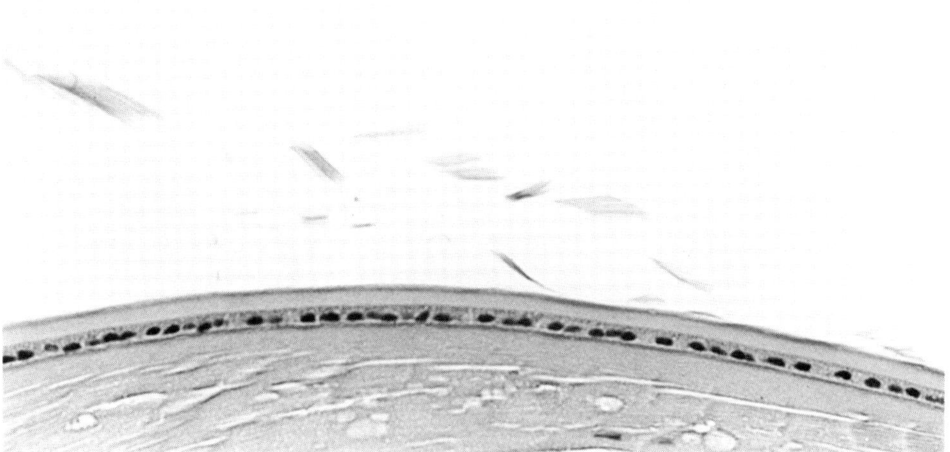

Figure 183–5. Peripheral anterior lens capsule showing ribbons of inserting zonular fibers, cuboidal epithelial cells, and underlying lens fibers. H&E, ×320.

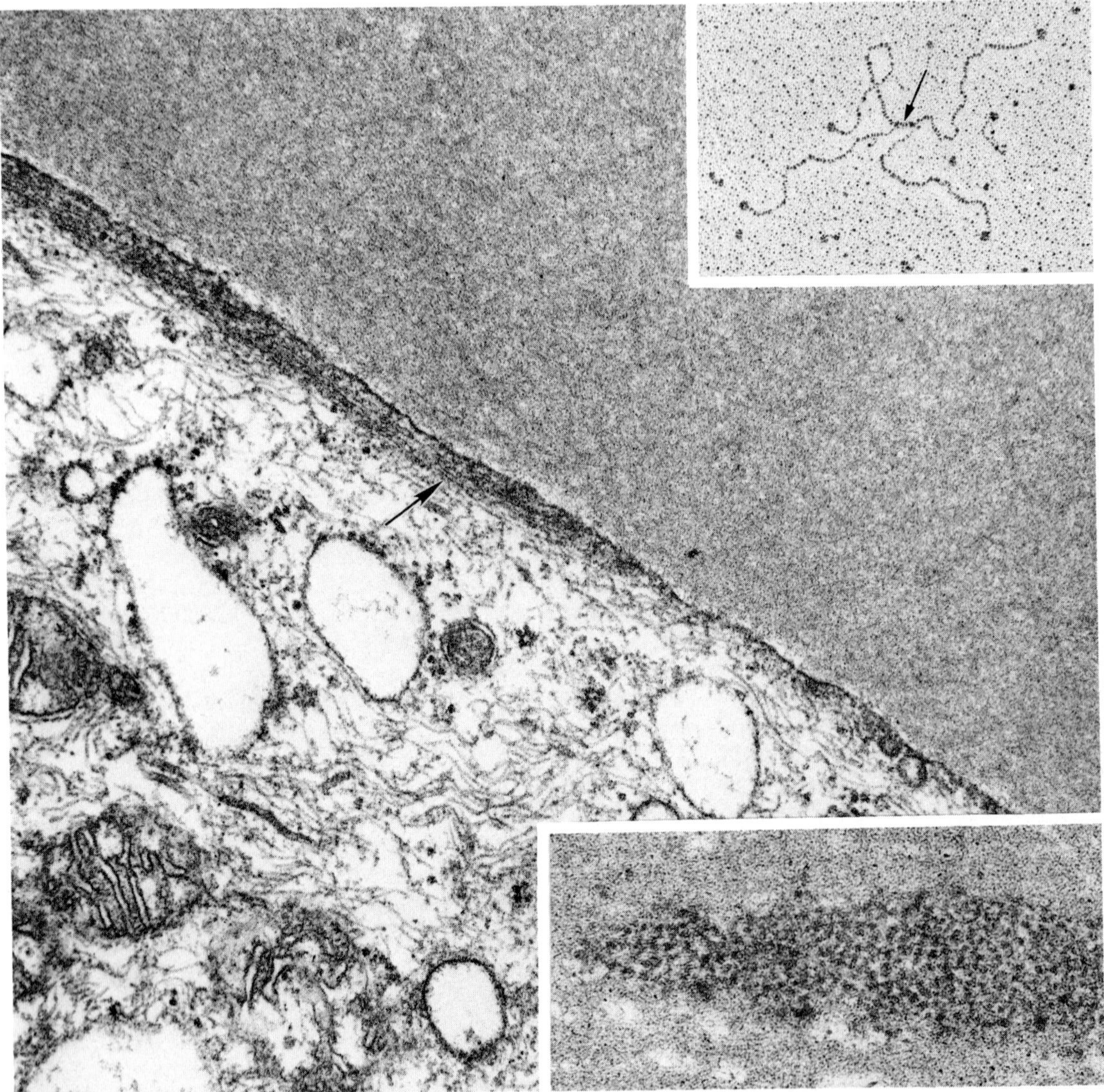

Figure 183–6. Faintly fibrillar architecture of the human lens capsule. Actin filaments *(arrow)* at edge of lens epithelial cell. ×62,500. *Upper Inset,* Typical tetramer of collagen IV from bovine lens capsule. The four molecules are linked together in the center by their carboxy terminal ends (7S region) *(arrow)*. Round globules at the other ends of each molecule (NC 1–domains) are thought to link adjacent tetramers into networks. Rotary shadowed, ×108,000. *Lower Inset,* Fibrillar inclusion from mid lens capsule. ×70,000.

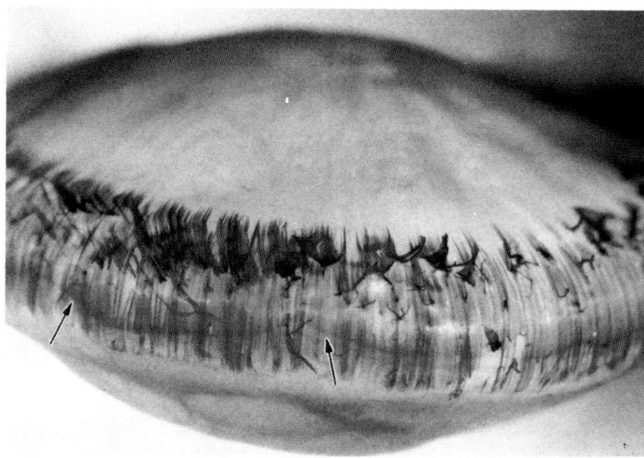

Figure 183–7. An intact lens showing a layer of anterior inserting and meridional zonules around its equator. The posterior zonules have been torn away with the vitreous, making visible an undulating line of nuclei marking the posterior limit of the lens epithelial cells *(arrows)*. Gomori's hematoxylin.

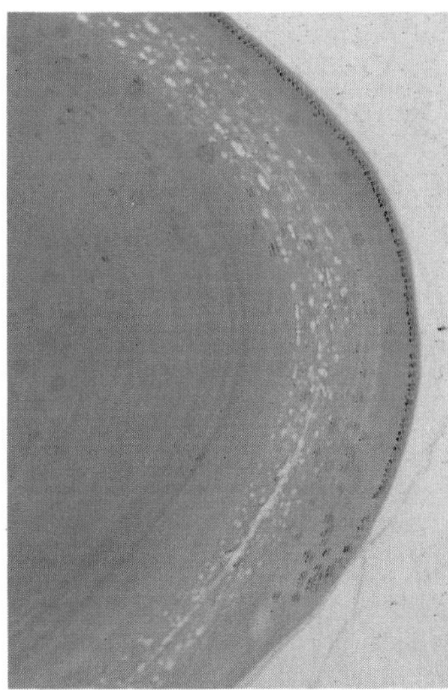

Figure 183–9. Lamellar structure of the lens cortex clearly seen in a lens with early vacuolar fiber swelling. H&E, ×33.

Schiff stain, a two-layer empty lens capsule will be found lying in some relation to the lens space. The lens contents and fossa can be largely replaced by bone or adipose tissue (Fig. 183–11), the latter reported primarily in eyes with persistent hyperplastic primary vitreous (PHPV) and, possibly, a hallmark of this anomaly.[23] Rarely a lens may be extruded or completely digested during some intrauterine disease process, causing a true secondary aphakia.

IMPERFECT OR DELAYED LENS-CORNEAL SEPARATION

A commoner vulnerable stage occurs during separation of the developing lens from the cornea. This defect could theoretically occur any time between the fourth and eighth weeks when programmed ingrowth of corneal stromal and endothelial mesenchyme completes corneal formation. If defective, this process can result in a cataractous lens adherent to a malformed or ectatic cornea, rarely as a cystic structure (Fig. 183–12). If separation is simply delayed, or if a slender attachment to the cornea remains, an anterior polar opacity of the lens frequently results (Fig. 183–13), associated with a variety of abnormalities in central corneal development. These lens sequelae have been described most often in Peters' anomaly,[24, 25] posterior keratoconus,[26–28] and midline clefting syndromes.[29] In bilateral posterior keratoconus, some patients have also shown abnormalities of the urinary tract, stunting of growth, and midline facial clefting defects.[28]

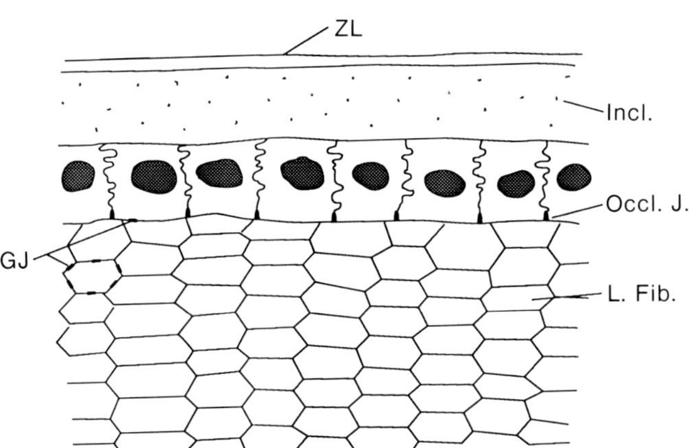

Figure 183–8. Diagram of the midperipheral lens cut coronally, showing hexagonal outline of the lens fibers (L. Fib.). Many gap junctions (GJ) connect the fibers to each other and occasionally to the overlying epithelium. A few tight junctions (Occl. J.) connect the apices of epithelial cells. (Incl., fibrillar capsular inclusions; ZL, zonular lamella.)

COLOBOMA OF THE LENS

Coloboma refers to focal absence of a tissue layer, typically occurring from failure in complete closure of the fetal fissure. Coloboma of the lens is not a true coloboma, but instead a notch in the equator due to an absence of zonular fibers from an underlying colobomatous ciliary body. This absence results in a lack of tension on the lens capsule in that region. No lens tissue is missing, and the notched equator is actually thicker and more rounded than normal. The defect is usually in the inferior nasal quadrant ("typical" coloboma area) and may be associated with iris or other colobomas along the old fissure pathway. Lens notches, however, can occur wherever zonules are absent or deficient, so they can appear elsewhere and have different etiologies, such as zonular rupture during early surgery for congenital glaucoma (Fig. 183–14). Flattening of the inferior lens rather than notching occurs from larger areas of deficient zonular fibers over extensive colobomas of the ciliary body (Fig. 183–15), or in some lens-dislocating diseases. Minor indentations of the lens equator between inserting zonules are sometimes seen in normal young lenses clinically and in gross specimens.

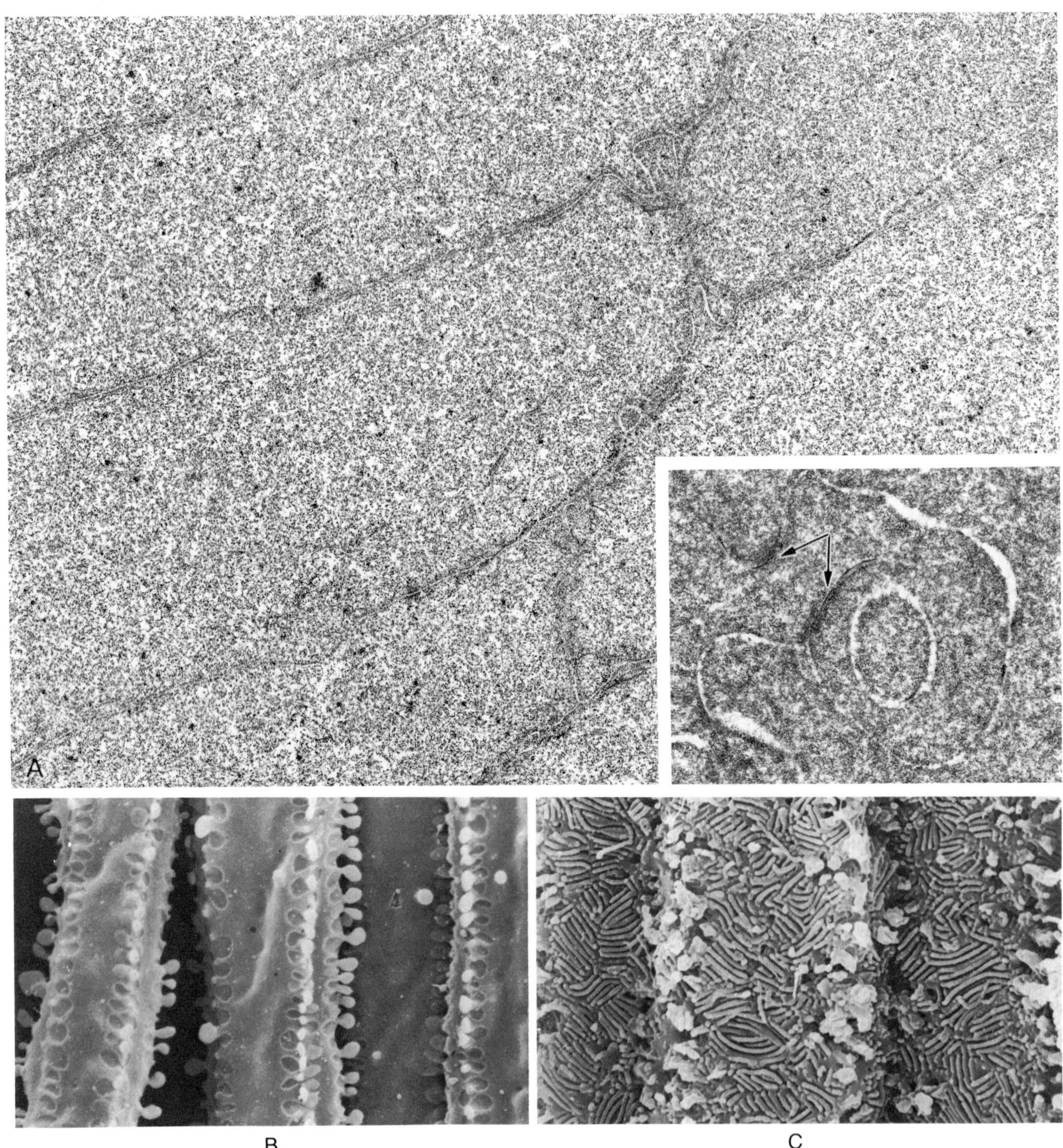

Figure 183–10. Cortical lens fibers. *A,* Longitudinal section of midcortical lens fibers showing granular cytoplasm and a few irregular interdigitations. ×11,600. *Inset,* Gap junctions at ball-and-socket interdigitations *(arrows).* ×26,160. *B,* Scanning electron micrograph along the length of three lens fibers, showing large numbers of ball-and-socket interdigitations at the edges. ×8,000. *C,* Deep cortical fibers in senescence, showing many microvilli covering the flat surfaces, and irregular lateral interdigitations. ×8,000. (*B* and *C* courtesy of Dr. J. Kuszak.)

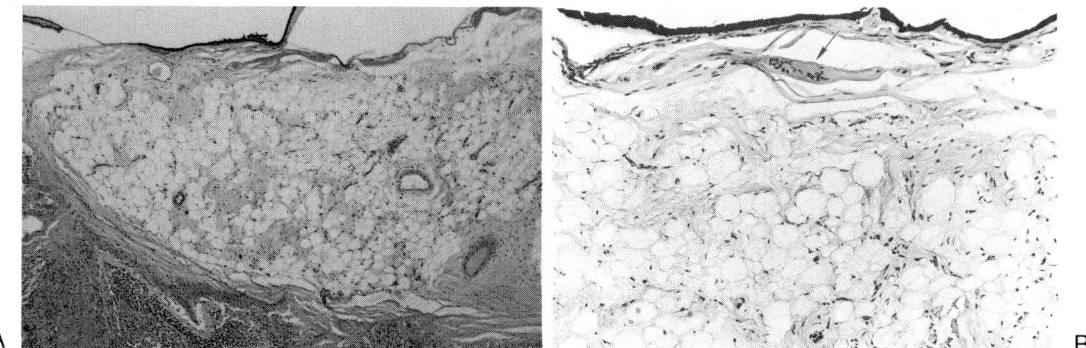

Figure 183–11. Fatty metaplasia in the lens space. *A,* Fat cells fill the lens space between the remnant of iris anteriorly and detached retina posteriorly, in an eye with persistent hyperplastic primary vitreous. Fragment of residual lens capsule just visible behind iris. PAS, ×20. *B,* Fragment of a lens capsule *(arrow)*, cortical material, and nuclei indicate that the lens was at least partially formed. H&E, ×165.

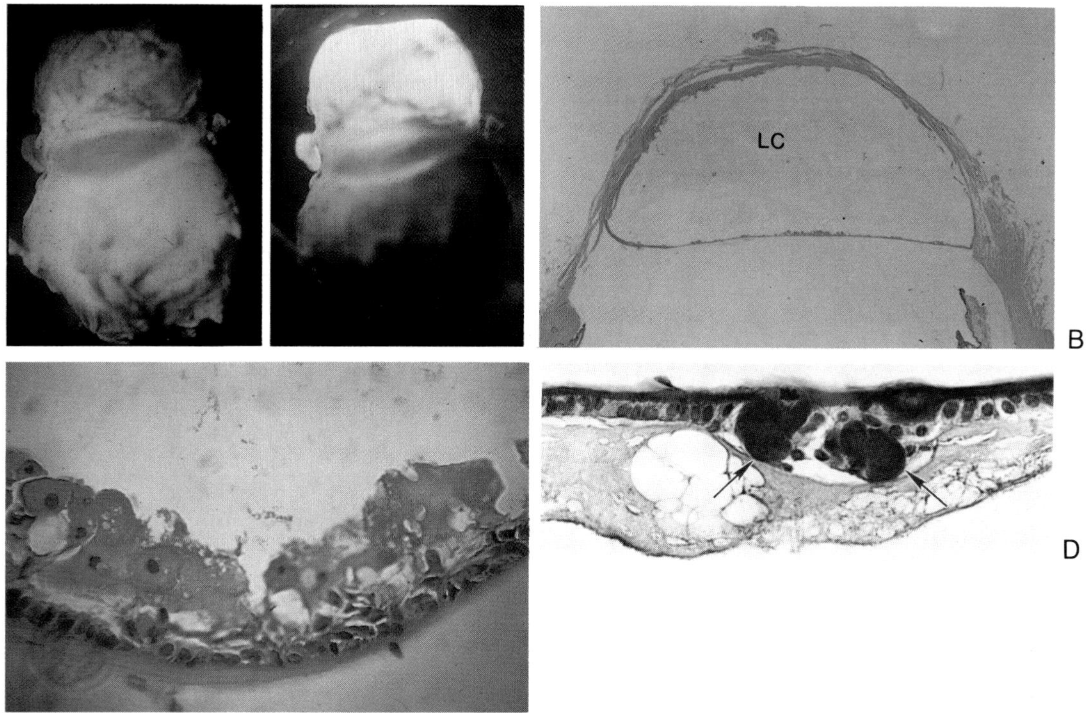

Figure 183–12. Congenital cystic lens. *A,* Superior three fourths of the cornea is ectatic, containing a large lens cyst. Right side is transilluminated. *B,* Huge lens cyst (LC) densely adherent to the malformed cornea. H&E. *C,* Lens epithelium and capsule form the wall of the cyst with two to three layers of nucleated bladder cells (abortive lens fibers) on the inner surface. H&E, ×32. *D,* Many PAS-positive nodules of aberrant lens capsule *(arrows)* and focally disorganized lens epithelial cells. PAS, ×380.

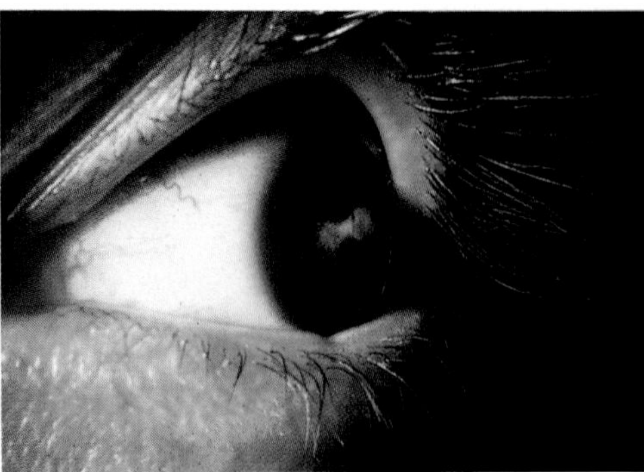

Figure 183–13. Small, anterior, polar white cataract attached by a stalk to an opacity of the central cornea in Peter's syndrome. Iris strands are adherent to the periphery of the corneal opacity. Note small notch in central lower lid. (Courtesy of Dr. Gabriel Marin.)

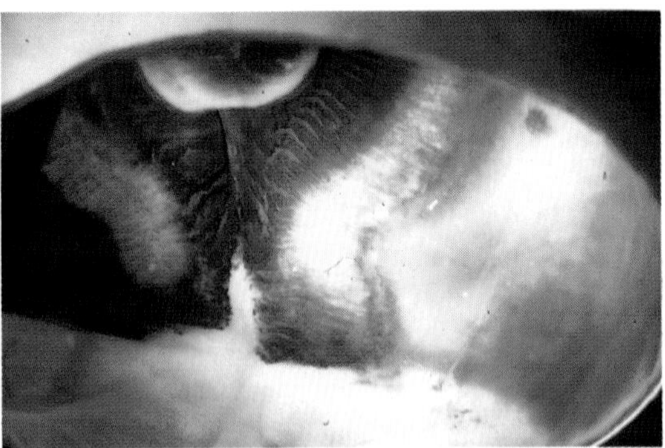

Figure 183–15. Flattening of the anterior lens overlying a coloboma of the ciliary body that opens into a very large, white coloboma posteriorly. The lens shows peripheral, white, cortical cataract and dense brunescent nuclear sclerosis.

PHAKOMATOUS CHORISTOMA

Tumors of the lens do not occur in the human, but lens anlagen have been reported to develop aberrantly in the lower lid nasally as a phakomatous choristoma.[30, 31] This firm, nodular lesion is noted in the early postnatal period. Cuboidal epithelial cells resembling lens epithelium are seen in strands, small aggregates, and cystic structures lying in a dense fibrous stroma (Fig. 183–16). Focally they are surrounded by thick basement membrane, like lens capsule. The aggregates often contain large, pink clumps resembling cortical lens fibers, and by electron microscopy show lens fiber-like granular cell processes with prominent interdigitating plasma membranes.[31] It has been suggested that this tumor derives from abnormal migration of primordial lens epithelial cells, perhaps displaced to the fetal fissure area during formation of the early lens placode.

Abnormalities of Lens Size and Shape

MICROPHAKIA AND SPHEROPHAKIA

Isolated and Zonule-Related. The small newborn lens is relatively more rounded or spherophakic than that of the adult, so aberrations in size and shape must be quite extreme to be noted at birth, usually requiring visibility of the lens edge in the pupil. Microphakia and spherophakia may be isolated idiopathic anomalies[32] or may be associated with a number of other ocular defects, such as microphthalmia. Severely cataractous lenses in the newborn, as in trisomy 13 and rubella, are often spherophakic, microspherophakic, or both.[33] Lenses are typically both microphakic and spherophakic when their zonular fibers are deficient in number, strength, or both and fail to exert sufficient traction on the capsule. This configuration is often accompanied by ectopia lentis in the hereditary lens-dislocating diseases (see later section). High degrees of microphakia without zonular disease imply some defect in lens growth.

Lowe's Syndrome. A microphakic lens that is, by contrast, strikingly thin is characteristic of Lowe's ocu-

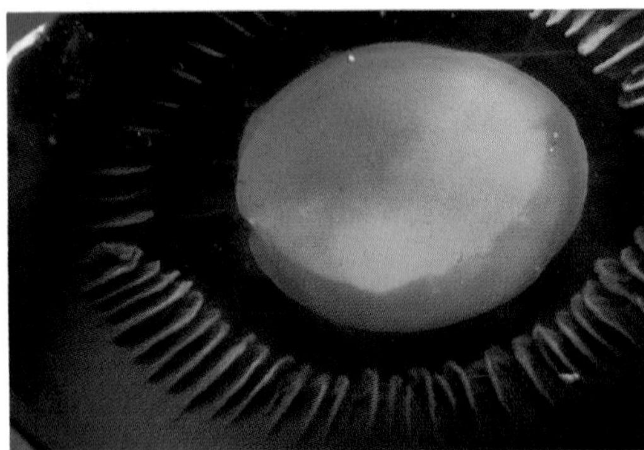

Figure 183–14. Small notch in peripheral lens at 9 o'clock, due to the absence of zonular fibers from the single collapsed ciliary process. History of goniotomy for congenital glaucoma.

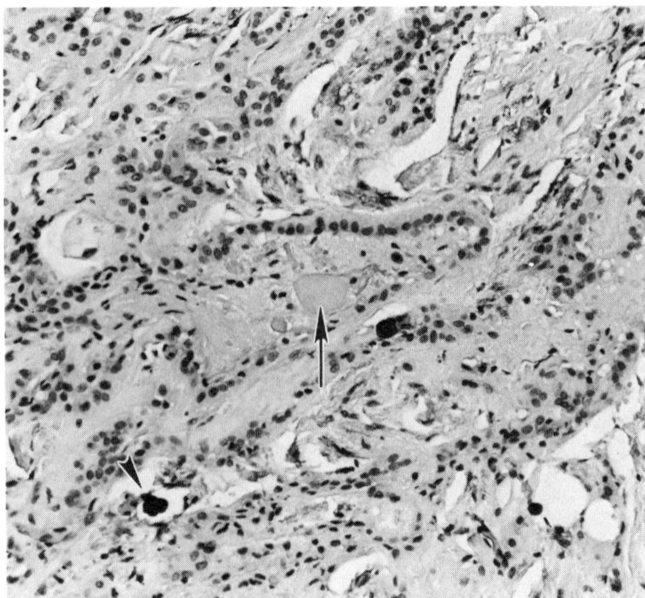

Figure 183–16. Phakomatous choristoma of the lower lid. Nodular and diffuse proliferation of cuboidal lens epithelial cells, occasionally enclosing globules of cortical differentiation *(arrow)*, surrounded by dense fibrous tissue. Focal calcium nodules are also present *(arrowhead)*. H&E, ×165. (Courtesy of Dr. Pearl Rosenbloom.)

locerebrorenal syndrome. This syndrome consists of a small, discoid cataractous lens, acidosis, and aminoaciduria with decreased ability of the kidneys to make ammonia, associated with renal rickets, hypotonia, mental retardation, congenital cataract, and glaucoma in 50 percent of cases.[34] Lowe's syndrome is transmitted as an X-linked recessive trait, owing to a defect on the long arm of the X-chromosome (Xq24–26 region).[35] Female carriers have characteristic white, punctate cortical opacities and subcapsular plaquelike opacities, especially posteriorly.[36, 37] The combination of congenital cataract and glaucoma is unusual in genetically transmitted disease of either type (although quite common in congenital rubella syndrome) and should suggest the possibility of Lowe's syndrome.

The most unique feature of the lens pathology, a small discoid lens without demarcation into nucleus and cortex, was established early.[33, 38] Initially there may be a posterior bulge (posterior lenticonus) due to a defective capsule. The lens equator is unusually thin and pointed (Fig. 183–17*A*). PAS-positive, irregular nodular excrescences protrude inward from the capsule,[33] similar to those reported in trisomy 21,[39] Miller's syndrome (congenital aniridia, Wilms' tumor, and hamartomas),[40] and median cleft face syndrome (see Fig. 183–12*D*).[29] These discoid lenses are almost completely cataractous, with many globular balloon cells and fibrous subcapsular plaques of metaplastic epithelial cells (see Fig. 183–17*B*), as recently reviewed.[41] Many of the fibers have retained nuclei, also seen in the cataracts of rubella,[38] Leigh's disease,[42] and trisomy 13.[43] The occasional Soemmerring's ring configuration suggested to Tripathi and colleagues[41] that failure to form primary lens fibers or subsequent degeneration of these fibers was the primary cause of flatness of the lenses, lacking differentiation into cortex and nucleus. In association with poor subsequent fiber formation, this may indicate that the genetic defect directly affects the lens cells, rather than that the cataract results from the metabolic derangements. The punctate cataracts in carriers may be due to random X-chromosome inactivation in the embryonic cells of female heterozygotes, according to the Lyon hypothesis.[44]

The cause of the glaucoma is not certain. The anterior chamber angle is infantile, with the iris root and meridional ciliary muscle inserting more anteriorly on the trabecular meshwork than is usual for the age.[33, 38] Another speculation is that traction on the zonule by the small lens prevents development of the angle. Since the glaucoma is usually well established before 3 yr of age, the eyes are often buphthalmic.

ANTERIOR LENTICONUS

Lenticonus is a conelike bulging of the superficial lens cortex and capsule in the central region, either anterior or posterior, and more rarely in both directions. A broader spherical bulge is referred to as lentiglobus. These are seldom recognized at birth but may present in the first or second decades as myopia, progressive in unusual spurts, with an "oil-droplet" fundus reflex from the cone.

Alport's Syndrome. Alport's syndrome is a characteristic and important prototype of a genetic basement membrane disease, commonly associated with anterior lenticonus (Fig. 183–18). This bilateral disease was first definitively described by Alport as an acute hemorrhagic nephropathy with deafness in 1927,[45] with the lenticonus recognized later.[46] It is most often transmitted as an X-linked dominant trait, affecting homozygous males severely, with some expression in female heterozygotes. In some families it is equally severe in males and females. Autosomal dominant and recessive transmission are also described.[47] The tissues affected seemed at first an unlikely assortment, with deafness and acute hemorrhagic nephropathy,[45] anterior lenticonus,[46] anterior polar and cortical cataracts,[48] albipunctatus-like spots in the fundus,[49] and, more rarely, vesicles on Descemet's membrane like those in posterior polymorphous corneal dystrophy.[50, 51]

In the common X-linked form, Alport's syndrome clearly affects the composition of basement membranes, first recognized by the absence of the normal Goodpasture basement membrane antigen in affected males.[52] In several kindreds mutations have now been reported on the newly recognized α5-chain of type IV collagen, coded for on the X chromosome (Xq22 region),[53] in the same region to which the Alport gene has been localized. These and probably other collagen IV defects appear to cause the basement membranes of the affected tissues to be more fragile than usual.

By light microscopy the chief pathology in lenses from the Alport syndrome has been thinning of the anterior capsule over the lenticonus.[54–57] In an ultrastructural

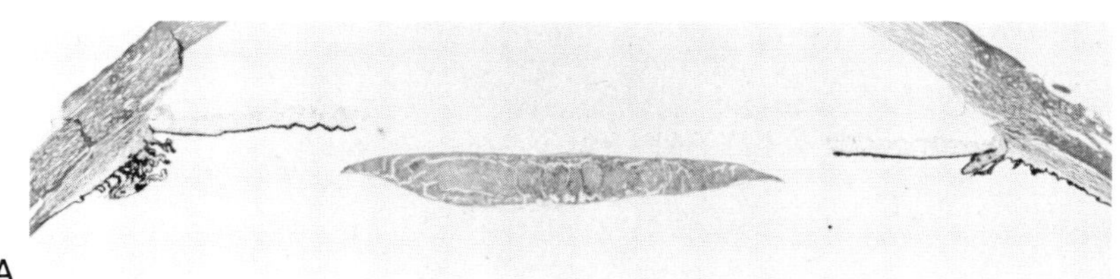

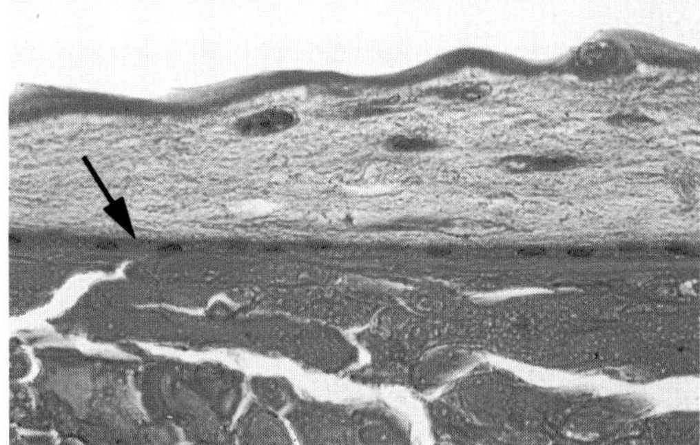

Figure 183–17. Lowe's syndrome. *A,* Small discoid lens showing sharply pointed ends, and no differentiation into cortex and nucleus. PAS. *B,* Anterior subcapsular fibrous cataract sequestered from the cataractous cortex by a complete layer of lens epithelial cells *(arrow).* Scanty basement membrane around some of the metaplastic epithelial cells in the fibrous cataract. PAS, ×800. (*A* and *B* courtesy of Dr. Ramesh Tripathi.)

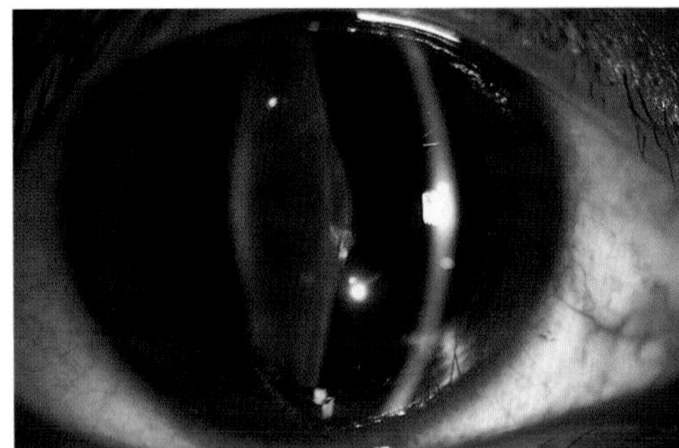

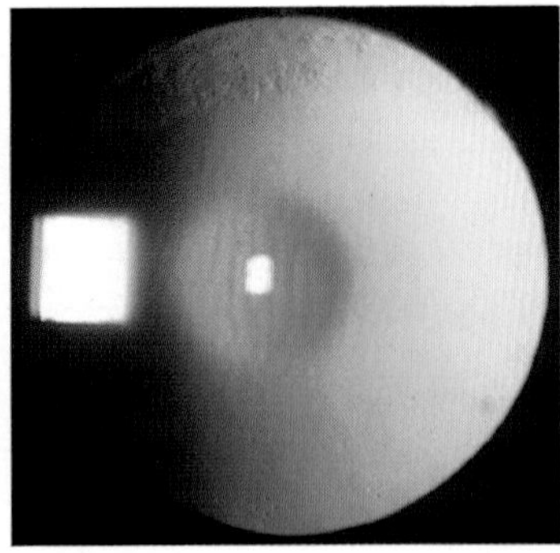

Figure 183–18. Anterior lenticonus in Alport's syndrome. *A,* Forward coning of the central lens capsule seen in slit-beam section. *B,* Cone by retroillumination resembles an oil droplet. (From Teekhasaenee C, Nimmanit S, Wutthiphan S, et al: Posterior polymorphous dystrophy and Alport syndrome. Ophthalmology 98:1207, 1991.)

study, the capsule in the center of the cone was 4 μm in thickness, and the edge 12 μm, compared with a normal thickness of 18 μm at age 30 (Fig. 183–19*A*).[57] The outer third of the capsule was looser and much more fibrillar than normal. The inner two thirds was remarkable for innumerable dehiscences at intervals of 2 to 6 μm in the center of the capsule, varying from 0.09 to 2 μm in width, extending straight outward and also forming a honeycomb network within the capsule (see Fig. 183–19*B*). The dehiscences contained filaments of unknown type measuring 3 to 7 nm. Ruptured lens epithelial cells were prolapsed into some of the larger breaks. Intact epithelial cells under the cone showed many degenerate changes, including mitochrondrial swelling and irregularly shaped nuclei, with focal spindle cells, multilayering, and pyknosis.

This evidence of capsular fragility may explain the spontaneous ruptures of lenticonus described clinically.[51, 55, 58] Ultrastructure of the kidney shows both thinning and laminar thickening of the glomerular basement membranes, with breaks and fraying[51, 57, 59] (see Fig. 183–19*C*), presumably leading to the episodes of hematuria. In severely affected individuals, death occurs from hypertension and renal failure. The course can be ameliorated by kidney transplantation, thus an ophthalmologist making a diagnosis of anterior lenticonus must refer these patients for careful medical evaluation.

POSTERIOR LENTICONUS

Posterior lenticonus may be bilateral or unilateral, with a slight female preponderance, and is occasionally familial.[60–65] A bilateral familial anterior and posterior lenticonus has been described.[63] Posterior lenticonus gives a central oil-droplet reflex on ophthalmoscopy, like the anterior form, because of light refraction by the cone. In females it is apt to occur sporadically, usually unilaterally and without other anomalies, although it can be associated with microphthalmia and other local and systemic abnormalities. The bulging posterior capsule is also thin in posterior lenticonus,[65] but its ultrastructure has not been examined.

In the normal infantile lens after fixation a posterior concavity (reverse lenticonus) is almost invariably seen. The cause of this artifactual deformity is unknown but may have some relation to the artifactual fold of oral retina (Lange's fold) displaced anteriorly in the same eyes. Both might result from contraction of the thick anterior vitreous gel and zonules in the infant, as the eye dehydrates during fixation.

Congenital Cataracts

A large proportion of lens pathology is concerned with cataractogenesis, as most abnormalities affecting the lens cause an opacification of this transparent structure—which is a definition of the clinical term "cataract." Much less is known about the pathogenesis of congenital cataracts, particularly the nonprogressive ones unique to the embryonic–early fetal period. The spectrum of possible etiologies of congenital cataract is almost as wide as that in the adult and includes disease primary in the fetus or secondary to maternal factors, such as genetic abnormalities, metabolic disease, infection, drugs, trauma, tumors, and idiopathic cause, which is still the largest group. Almost all types can be hereditary, from small nuclear opacities to total cataract.

Congenital cataracts are very common, noted by Francois in 1 of every 250 newborns (0.4 percent).[66] From 8 to 25 percent have been reported to be familial, with autosomal dominant transmission most frequent.[67] Research in lens development and hereditary cataracts in animals suggests that some cases are related to mutations in the crystallin genes, which vary considerably in timing and intensity of expression during embryogenesis.[68] Autosomal dominant transmission of balanced translocations between chromosomes 2 and 14 has been linked in one family to anterior polar cataracts,[69] and balanced translocation between chromosomes 3 and 4 to an infantile rapidly progressive mature cataract.[70] Linkage analysis has identified a posterior polar cataract locus on chromosome 16.[71] These preliminary reports raise expectations for rapid progress in the molecular biology of hereditary cataractogenesis within the next decade.

The pathology of congenital cataracts is reasonably classified at this stage of knowledge by geographic localization of the opacity, which may point immediately to an etiologic group, or to important metabolic diseases for investigation. The common association with other

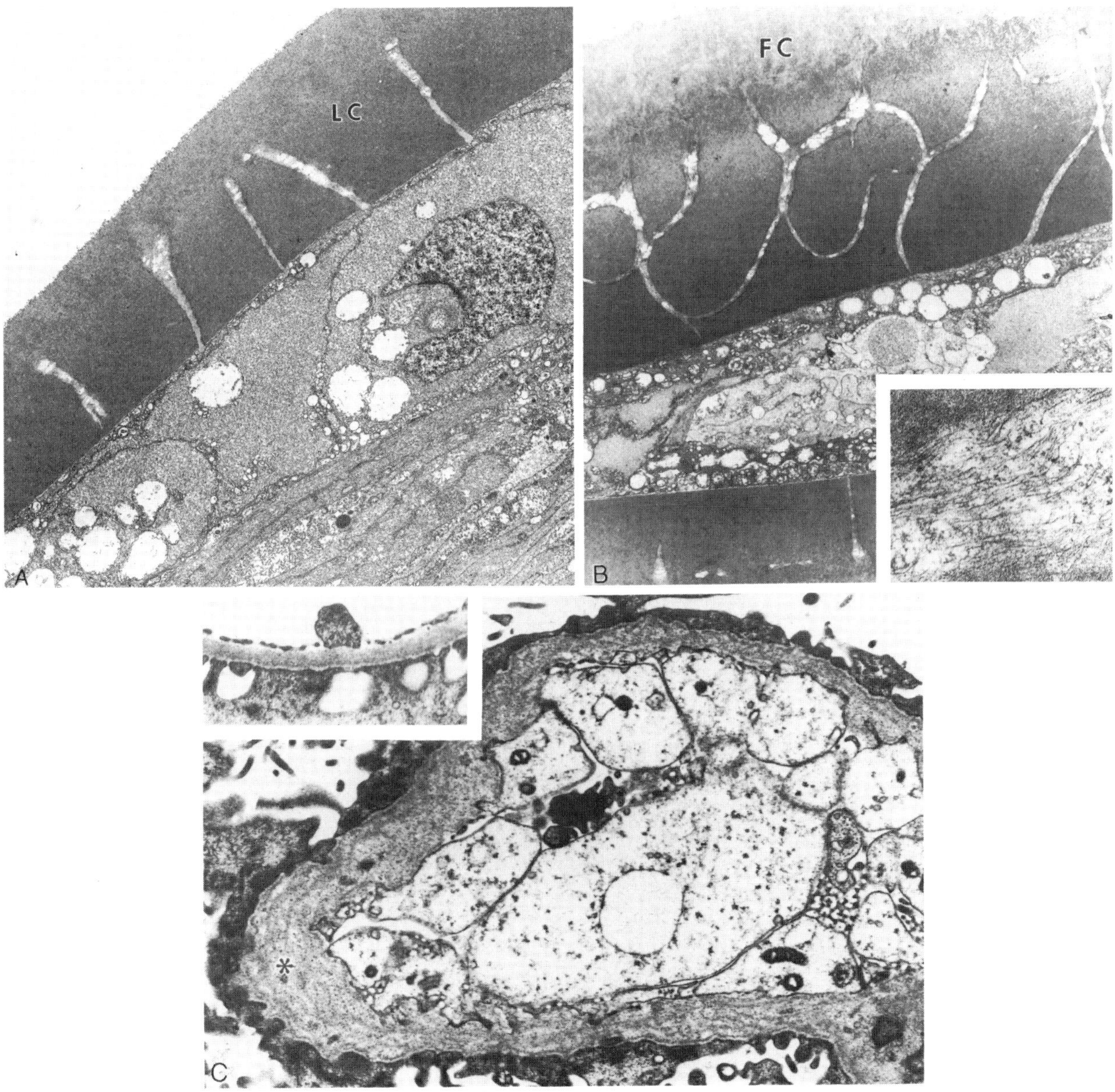

Figure 183–19. Alport's syndrome. *A,* Marked thinning of the anterior lens capsule (LC), with multiple breaks in anterior capsulectomy specimen. Inner capsule splits are partially filled with necrotic cellular debris. ×12,300. *B,* The capsular breaks form a honeycomb when cut obliquely. Outer capsule (FC) is abnormally fibrillar. ×5,940. *Inset,* Fine 4- to 7-nm fibrils and granular material lie within the capsular breaks. ×67,500. *C,* Laminar splitting of the glomerular basement membrane enclosing granular aggregates *(asterisk)* in same patient 5 years earlier. ×17,400. *Inset,* Normal homogeneous, thin basement membrane. ×15,200. (From Streeten BW, Robinson MR, Wallace RN, et al: Lens capsule abnormalities in Alport's syndrome. Arch Ophthalmol 105:1693, 1987. Copyright 1987, American Medical Association.)

ocular or systemic abnormalities can also assist in categorizing the process.

ANTERIOR POLAR CATARACT

Small anterior polar opacities may occur anywhere over the pupillary region at the site of an abnormal pupillary membrane or other vascular attachment, sometimes traceable to the minor circle of the iris. Histopathology of these small foci shows subcapsular proliferation of metaplastic epithelial cells as spindle cells. A true anterior polar cataract may also be small but has histopathologic evidence of superficial cortical fiber loss, besides formation of a fibrous subcapsular scar deriving from the lens epithelial cells.

Uveitis and trauma commonly cause anterior subcapsular cataracts in the adult and also may play a role in the fetus. The frequency of anterior polar cataract in delayed lens separation from the cornea and other anterior mesenchymal defects (see Fig. 183–13) indicates that genetic or programming mishaps are additional etiologic factors in the fetus; nevertheless there is often no identifiable cause. The pathogenesis of congenital anterior polar cataract follows a predictable course, with sequestration of the cataract plaque by new epithelium growing under it (see Fig. 183–17*B*). This process is

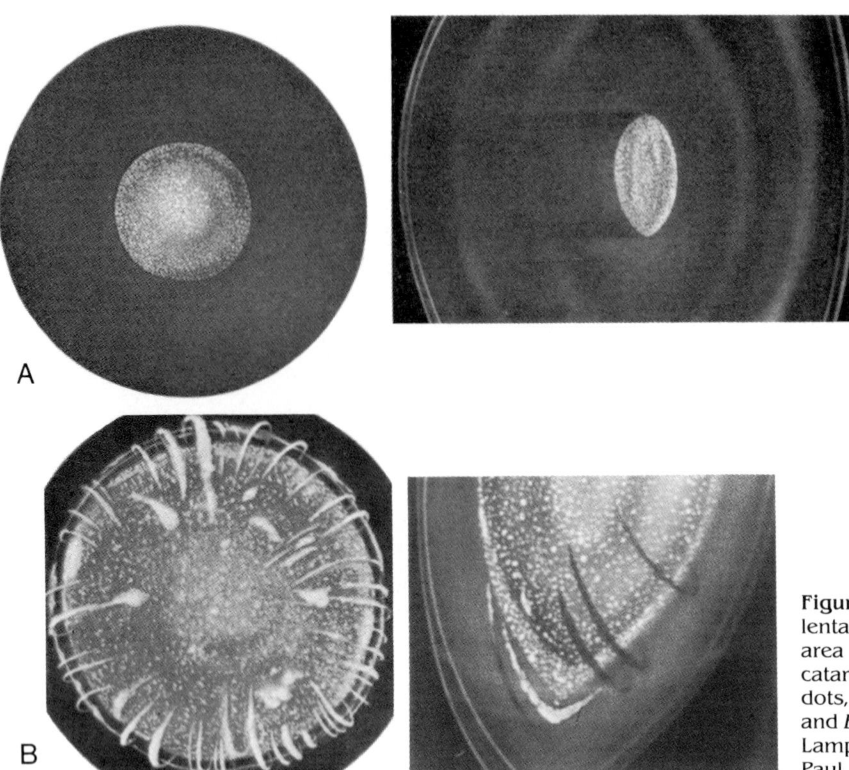

Figure 183–20. Fetal cataracts. *A*, Cataracta pulverulenta occupying the embryonic and inner fetal nuclear area (see slit beam section on right). *B*, Fetal zonular cataract involving the whole fetal-embryonic lens with dots, cloudy opacification, and peripheral "riders." (*A* and *B* from Berliner ML: Biomicroscopy of the Eye. Slit Lamp Microscopy of the Living Eye. Vol. II. New York, Paul B. Hoeber, Inc., Harper and Brothers, 1949.)

identical to that in the adult and will be described in that section. The congenital plaque is somewhat more likely to be limited to the polar area and to be elevated. It may also be reduplicated with one or two underlying twin opacities, thought to represent successive ingrowth of clear lens fibers between the plaque and the injured lens fibers, perhaps indicating recurrent injury.

POSTERIOR POLAR CATARACT

A remnant of the posterior tunica vasculosa lentis known as Mittendorf's dot can mark the site of the former hyaloid artery on the lens capsule or the closely adherent anterior hyaloid membrane. It consists of a small amount of fibrous tissue, with residual vascular basement membrane if there is an attached hyaloid artery tail.[72] Collagenized plaque cataracts at the posterior pole occur but are much less common than they are anteriorly, and they are also rare in the adult.

NUCLEAR CATARACT

Embryonal and Y-Sutural Cataracts. In prenatal life the lens forms two nuclear areas, the embryonic and the fetal (see Fig. 183–2). The two bean-shaped zones of relucency between the Y-sutures in the adult lens by biomicroscopy constitute the embryonic nucleus, which can become opacified from an injurious event in the first 2 months of gestation. Anterior axial embryonic cataracts include opacities in this area but more commonly on the Y-sutures, estimated by some to occur in at least 20 percent of the population.[66, 73a] These clusters of white, dotlike opacities appear on or close to one or both Y-sutures. Denser Y-sutural cataracts can develop somewhat later and have a more stellate form. These opacities are usually of no visual significance but point to minor disturbances during the fetal period. Often they show dominant inheritance, with concordance in identical twins. Their pathogenesis is unknown, probably representing the vulnerability of young lens fibers to edema and opacification at their sutural ends, a weakness that continues throughout life.

Fetal Nuclear Cataracts. The entire fetal nucleus or portions of it may be involved in a cataract, which can take many forms, even within families having these autosomal dominantly inherited cataracts. In the beautiful cataracta pulverulenta centralis (Coppock's cataract), the fetal nuclear and embryonal areas are filled with dotlike opacities, sometimes polychromatic (Fig. 183–20),[73a, 74, 75] with varying degrees of opacification in the two areas. The cataract is 1 to 2.5 mm in diameter. Linkage with the Duffy blood group locus is evidence that the defective gene for this cataract resides on the long arm of chromosome 1.[76] Histopathology of these cataracts is rare. In a fetal nuclear cataract 2.5 mm in diameter (Fig. 183–21*A*), the embryonal nuclear area had irregular, pale eosinophilic staining with marked loss of its lamellar architecture (see Fig. 183–21*B*). The peripheral fetal nuclear zone retained a more lamellar architecture with myriads of small vacuolar spaces containing fine basophilic dot opacities (see Fig. 183–21*C*). A few longer curved vacuoles containing blue dots followed the lamellae peripherally.

A more common larger fetal cataract 4 to 5.5 mm in diameter involves most of the embryonic-fetal region and almost always has short segments of opaque lamellar

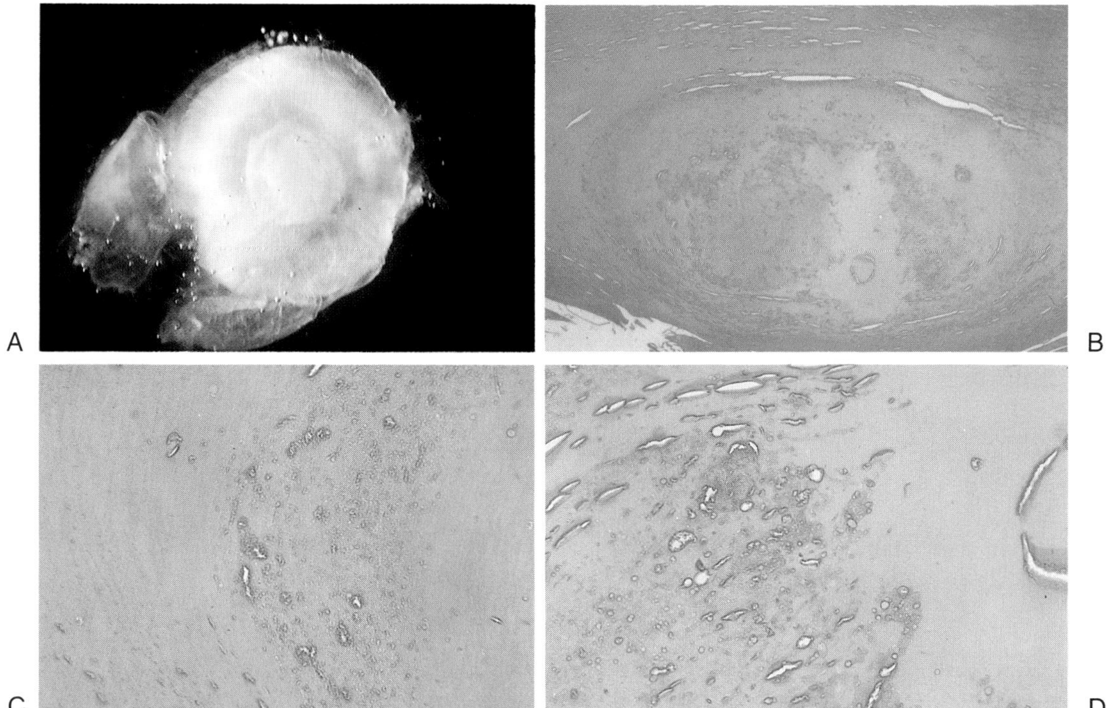

Figure 183–21. Congenital fetal nuclear cataract. *A,* 2.5-mm fetal nuclear cataract in an 8-mm lens of a 22-year-old woman. Dense ring around an opaque center. The posterior capsule ruptured during intracapsular cataract extraction. *B,* Oval demarcated area occupying the lower half of the figure is the fetal nuclear cataract. H&E, ×13. *C,* Fine and confluent vacuoles compose the dense peripheral ring around the cataract. H&E, ×66. *D,* Embryonic central region of cataract has distorted homogeneous and vacuolar architecture, with crystal-like spaces. No retained nuclei. H&E, ×66.

"riders" (see Fig. 183–20*B*). This form is classified as a congenital zonular cataract because it affects a whole zone or region of the lens. While these fetal cataracts are stationary, the larger ones may require surgery in infancy because they occupy so much of the central visual axis.

Zonular Cataract. A zonular or lamellar cataract similar to the fetal types previously described can develop at any age, whenever a layer, or "lamella," of newly forming fibers at the surface of the lens is injured and becomes opaque, or a sector or zone becomes opacified. As new transparent fibers are added peripherally, the opaque injured fibers become gradually more deeply embedded in the lens as a lamella or zone of cataract (Fig. 183–22). If the opacity exceeds 5.75 mm in diameter it is presumed to have developed postnatally, as the newborn lens has a maximal diameter of 6 mm.[67]

A diffuse lamellar cataract can be produced by hypocalcemia with or without tetany in a mother or infant. Not all of the newly forming fibers appear to be affected equally, so the cataract occurs in groups of linear spokes rather than a complete ring opacity. The low calcium in the aqueous results in loss of intracellular calcium, increasing membrane permeability. Cellular hydration and loss of other ions can produce permanent injury and opacification. Histologically there is fiber swelling with globular breakdown and membrane debris between them,[73a] resembling the changes in any focal area of adult cataract. The implication of a lamellar cataract at any age is that the injurious stimulus was limited in time, due to factors such as trauma, metabolic episodes, or unknown developmental changes.

Rubella Cataract. A special kind of nuclear cataract is produced by infection with the rubella virus in the first trimester. The embryopathic potential of this virus was recognized by Gregg, who reported its cataractogenic effects in 1941.[77] Many other reports followed during the severe rubella epidemics around the world from 1940 to 1965. These studies established the severe bilateral ocular effects, including microphthalmia, pigmentary retinopathy, cataract, and glaucoma. Besides ocular disease, the congenital rubella syndrome can

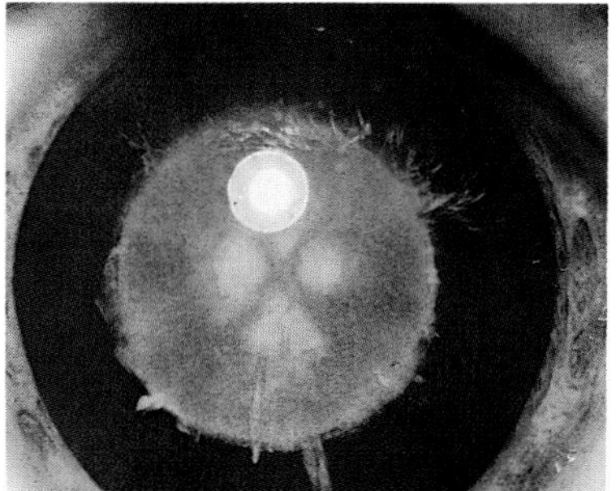

Figure 183–22. Congenital zonular cataract in patient aged 19 years, surrounded by completely transparent fibers. A few "riders" at the periphery of the opacity. Etiology unknown. (From Donaldson DD: Congenital lamellar cataract. Arch Ophthalmol 74:426, 1965. Copyright 1965, American Medical Association.)

A

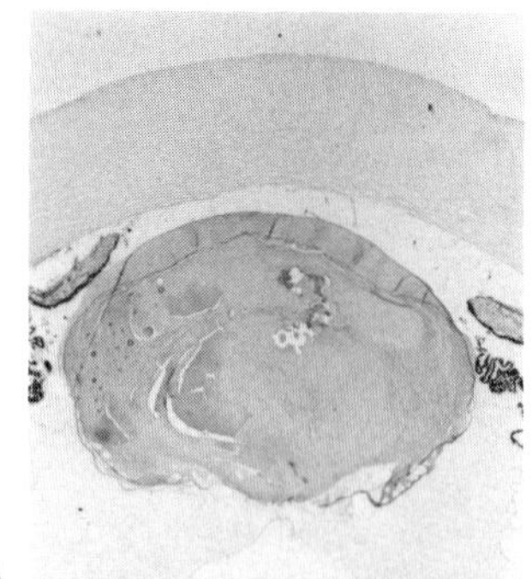

B

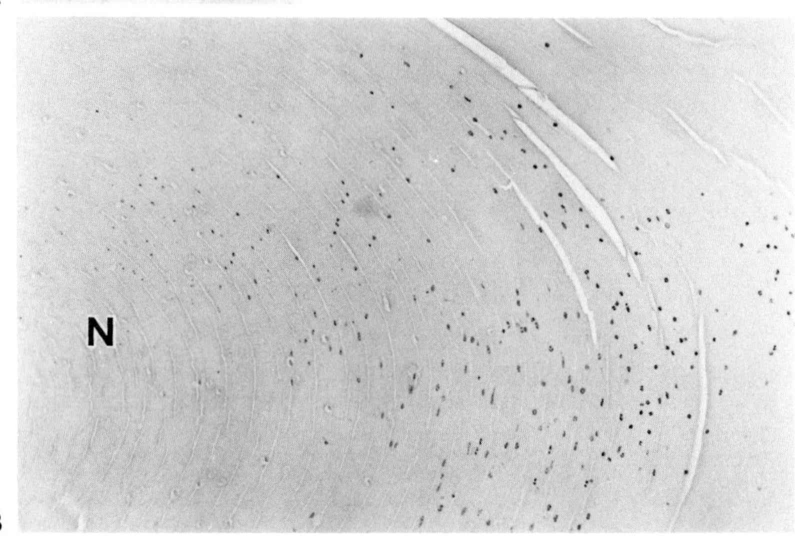

Figure 183–23. Rubella cataract. *A,* Spherophakia and microphakia in a rubella cataract. H&E, ×16. *B,* Retained nuclear remnants in the fetal nuclear area (N) on the left, with larger remnants in newer fibers on the right, indicating a prolonged cataractogenic effect. H&E, ×165.

include cardiovascular defects, particularly patent ductus arteriosus, mental retardation, deafness, growth stunting, hepatosplenomegaly, and thrombocytopenia. Since the virus can pass the placental barrier, maternal infection with rubella during the first 4 wk of pregnancy results in 50 percent of fetuses becoming infected, but for the whole first trimester only 20 percent are infected, highlighting the chiefly embryopathic effect of the virus.[78, 79]

Since infection occurs when both primary and secondary lens fibers are forming during the first trimester, the opacity may involve a variable portion of the central region in the newborn lens. It is a uniform dense nuclear opacity (Fig. 183–23*A*), unlike most congenital nuclear cataracts, or it may progress to a total cataract. The lenses are apt to be microspherophakic (see Fig. 183–23*B*). The histopathologic hallmark is retention of cell nuclei with varying degrees of nuclear pyknosis and karyorrhexis in fibers of the embryonic–early fetal lens (see Fig. 183–23*C*), indicating a failure to completely mature. Retained nuclei in the central lens dating infection to the first trimester are important but not completely specific for rubella, as they can be seen in Lowe's syndrome,[33] trisomy 13,[43] and Leigh's syndrome.[42] The affected central lens may become condensed and homogeneous, like an adult nuclear sclerosed cataract, and float in a bag of liquefied cortex, as in an adult morgagnian cataract.

Mature cataracts can develop by the time of birth or later, as the cells contain infective virus beyond the first trimester. Virus is shed and can be cultured from the lens for many years after birth, posing the hazard of endophthalmitis by intraocular spread at the time of lens extraction or of infection of unvaccinated health care personnel.[80] The lens can be completely absorbed spontaneously, leaving only the capsule.[19, 20, 81]

It is of interest that maternal infection with varicella can also cause congenital cataract,[82] as can other herpesviruses and Toxoplasma, but no unusual clinical or histopathologic appearances have been described.

Other Late Fetal and Developmental Cataracts

CORONARY-CERULEAN CATARACTS

Several characteristic lens opacities detectable bilaterally at birth or in early childhood are named by their shape or color, such as the coronary club-shaped opacities found around the peripheral lens, often associated with cerulean (blue) dots (Fig. 183–24). These may be present in a narrow zonular or more diffuse distribution and are essentially stationary, with only a very small increase in number during adult life.[82] Cogan and Kuwabara[39] studied peripheral opacities in Down's syndrome lenses, which they hypothesized were of this clinical type. Wartlike excrescences of capsular basement membrane projected between the epithelial cells, as discussed earlier in other syndromes (Fig. 183–

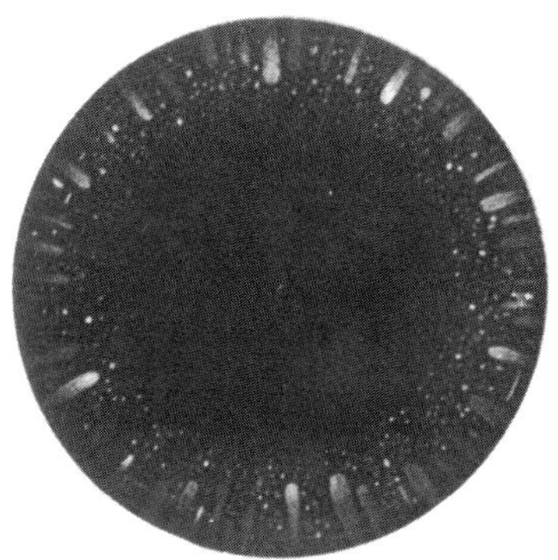

Figure 183–24. Peripheral spokes and club-forms of a classic coronary cataract, associated with cerulean dot opacities. (From Berliner ML: Biomicroscopy of the Eye. Slit-Lamp Microscopy of the Living Eye. Vol. II. New York, Paul B. Hoeber, Inc., Harper and Brothers, 1949.)

25*A*).[29, 33, 40] There were also nodules of aberrant epithelial cells partially surrounded by PAS-positive basement membrane incorporating granular debris, directly under the equatorial capsule (see Fig. 183–25*B*). With further growth these nodules appeared to separate from the capsule, becoming displaced into the cortex and degenerating into granular foci. This pathogenesis of a cortical opacity from aberrant cell growth within the epithelium was surprising and offered a new view of how such opacities could slowly increase in number with age. Robb and Marchevsky,[83] however, did not find such nodules in Down's syndrome lenses, although 5 of 21 patients had 50- to 150-μ elliptical granular foci between the lamellae, which may represent cerulean opacities. The lenses were not seen clinically in either study, so the pathogenesis of these interesting cataracts remains uncertain.

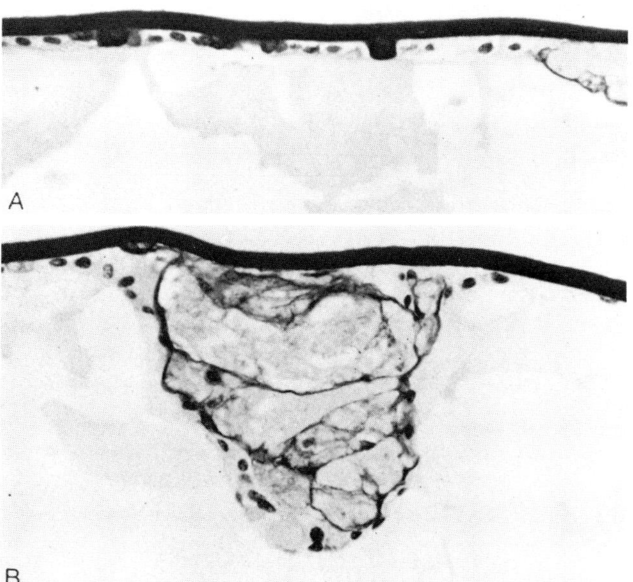

Figure 183–25. Cataract in Down's syndrome. *A,* Capsular nodular excrescences between the epithelial cells. PAS, orig. mag. ×400. *B,* Nodular proliferation of epithelial cells, partly surrounded by PAS-positive membrane and enclosing granular material of unknown type. PAS, orig. mag. ×250. (From Cogan DG, Kuwabara T: Pathology of cataracts in mongoloid idiocy. Docum Ophthalmol 16:73, 1962.)

CRYSTALLINE CATARACTS

Crystalline cataracts are rare bilateral, congenital opacities that have a very different pattern, with dark spokes and refractile crystals radiating outward from the center of the lens with no apparent relation to the normal lamellar architecture.[73b] The more common coralliform pattern has blunted rays emanating from the center of the lens into the juvenile nucleus but not reaching the lens capsule (Fig. 183–26 *A*). Several pathologic studies have shown the rays to be composed of rectangular or rhomboid crystals containing tyrosine and cysteine, surrounded by degenerate lens fibers.

In a recent study of this cataract,[84] large polygonal crystals (see Fig. 183–26*B*) were noted on scanning electron microscopy and, on transmission electron microscopy, were seen to be surrounded by multiple membranes (see Fig. 183–26*C*). Electron probe analysis showed that the crystals contained carbon, nitrogen, oxygen, and sulfur, suggesting the presence of cystine. Biochemically there was a higher concentration than normal of water-soluble β2 and γ2 crystallins. It was hypothesized that free sulfhydryl groups had become cysteinized, preventing formation of normal disulfide bonds and insolubilization of the protein. The 5-year-old patient had shown an increasing number of these crystals with decreasing vision. Interestingly she also had the "uncombable hair syndrome," with shiny, very blonde, wiry hair like spun glass (see Fig. 183–26*D*), showing histologic abnormalities of hair formation typical of that syndrome. These two conditions are usually inherited separately as autosomal dominant traits, but both might have abnormal disulfide bonding.

CHONDRODYSPLASIA PUNCTATA

Two syndromes of chondrodysplasia punctata, frequently called congenital stippled epiphyses,[85–89] have shown early cataracts of a mixed pattern. The lenses are generally small, sometimes appearing subluxed (Fig. 183–27), and have rather bizarre anterior subcapsular cataracts, extensive cortical cataracts, and, rarely, posterior lenticonus.[88] This group of diseases includes an autosomal dominant form (Conradi-Hünermann syndrome) and a lethal autosomal recessive form (Zellweger's syndrome).[87] Other tissues affected are the central nervous system, kidney, cartilage, bone, muscle, and liver. Growth is retarded, and contractures occur. These diseases appear to be due to enzyme deficiencies related to mitochondrial function. The embryonic and inner fetal nucleus of the lens has been normal in all cases examined by histopathology, but the later lens cells show erratic direction of growth and balloon cell formation,[88] suggesting that the metabolic defect began to affect secondary lens fiber formation in the fifth month of gestation. In the only ultrastructural lens study, there was proliferation of mitochondria in the epithelium, with many nonlipid cytoplasmic inclusions in the epithelial cells.[85]

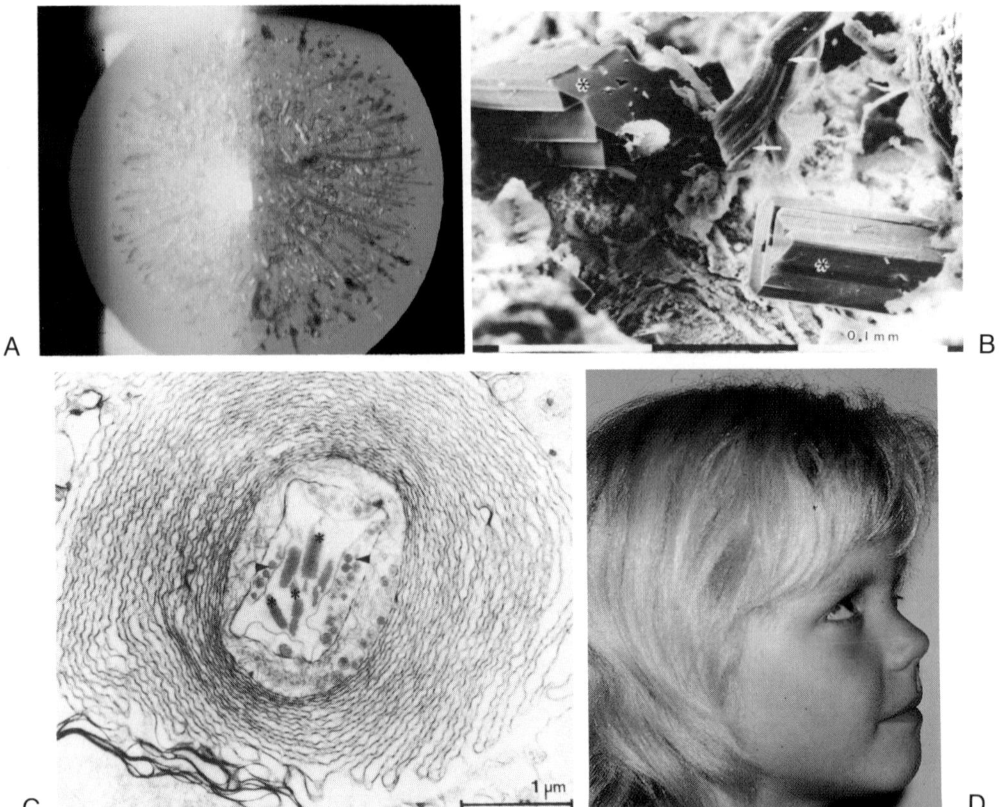

Figure 183–26. Crystalline cataract. *A,* The cataract shows a spokelike pattern of opacification radiating outward from the center of the lens with polychromatic refractility. *B,* Polygonal crystals *(asterisks)* in lens cortex from an extracapsular cataract extraction. Surrounded by lens fibers *(arrows)* and cataractous debris. SEM. BAR = 0.1 mm. *C,* Polygonal crystalline plates *(asterisks)* and circular bodies *(arrowheads)* surrounded by multiple folded membranes. TEM. BAR = 1 μ. (*A–D,* From deJong PT, Bleeker-Wagemakers EM, Vrensen GF, et al: Crystalline cataract and uncombable hair. Ophthalmology 97:1181, 1990. Courtesy of Dr. deJong.) *D,* Patient's hair is very pale, and wiry like spun glass, owing to the "uncombable hair syndrome."

HALLERMANN-STREIFF SYNDROME

Hallermann-Streiff syndrome (mandibulooculofacial dysmorphia) is a multisystem disease showing hypoplasia of the mandible with a "birdlike facies," microphthalmia, microcornea, congenital cataract, and often glaucoma.[90] Some patients have more generalized defects with dwarfism, dental deformities, and hypotrichosis. This disease is almost certainly genetic, but its etiology and nature are unknown. Although all cases have been sporadic, the disease has been reported in monozygotic twins. Mature cataracts may develop in the first few weeks of life and have been observed to undergo capsular rupture and complete absorption.[91] Reports of pathologic examinations have been few[90–92] but have shown a very similar chronic uveitis with extensive anterior synechiae, some degree of cyclitic membrane incorporating any lens remnants, and sometimes a granulomatous reaction to residual lens capsule.[91, 92] These findings imply an immunologic component of the phacoanaphylactic type in the cataract absorption. How common this is, and whether inflammation has any relation to the cataractogenesis itself, are unknown. Abnormal fraying of collagen has been noted in the sclera of one case with nanophthalmia and uveal effusion.[93]

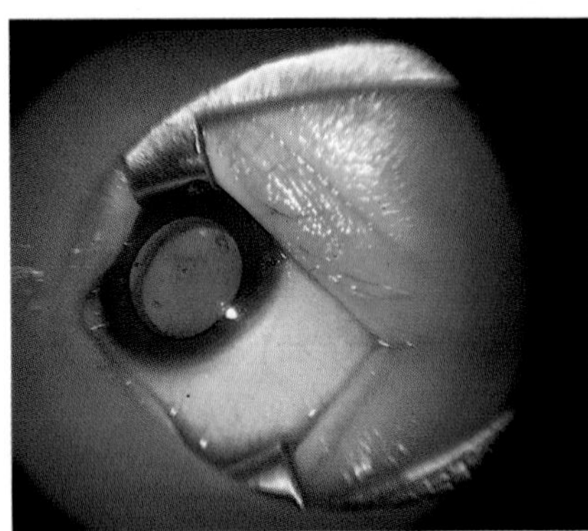

Figure 183–27. Edge of microphakic lens visible in the pupil of a patient with Conradi's stippled epiphyses syndrome. (Courtesy of Dr. Sylvia Norton.)

TRANSIENT NEONATAL LENS VACUOLES

Neonatal lens vacuoles have been seen primarily in premature infants, developing between the eighth and fourteenth postnatal days and persisting for several weeks to as long as 9 months before disappearing completely.[94–96] They occur bilaterally and symmetrically in the posterior subcapsular cortex near the Y-sutures. The vacuoles can develop into very large, multilocular cystlike separations of the outer cortical fibers (Fig. 183–

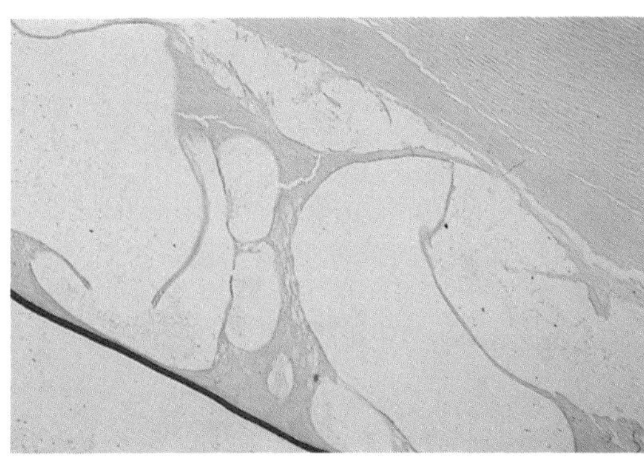

Figure 183–28. Vacuoles and large cystlike separations of the posterior cortical lens fibers in a premature infant. PAS, ×230. (Courtesy of Dr. Myron Yanoff.)

28).[96] In the surrounding fibers there are both intracellular and extracellular smaller vacuoles containing fine granular material with small, dense lipoidal particles at their edges. Lesser changes in the anterior subcapsular fibers may sometimes be seen as well. Their etiology is unknown.

PERSISTENT HYPERPLASTIC PRIMARY VITREOUS

Persistent hyperplastic primary vitreous (PHPV) is an uncommon, usually unilateral abnormality in which there is persistence of a plaque of primary vitreous behind the lens, supplied by a patent hyaloid artery (Fig. 183–29*A*). The ciliary processes are drawn inward

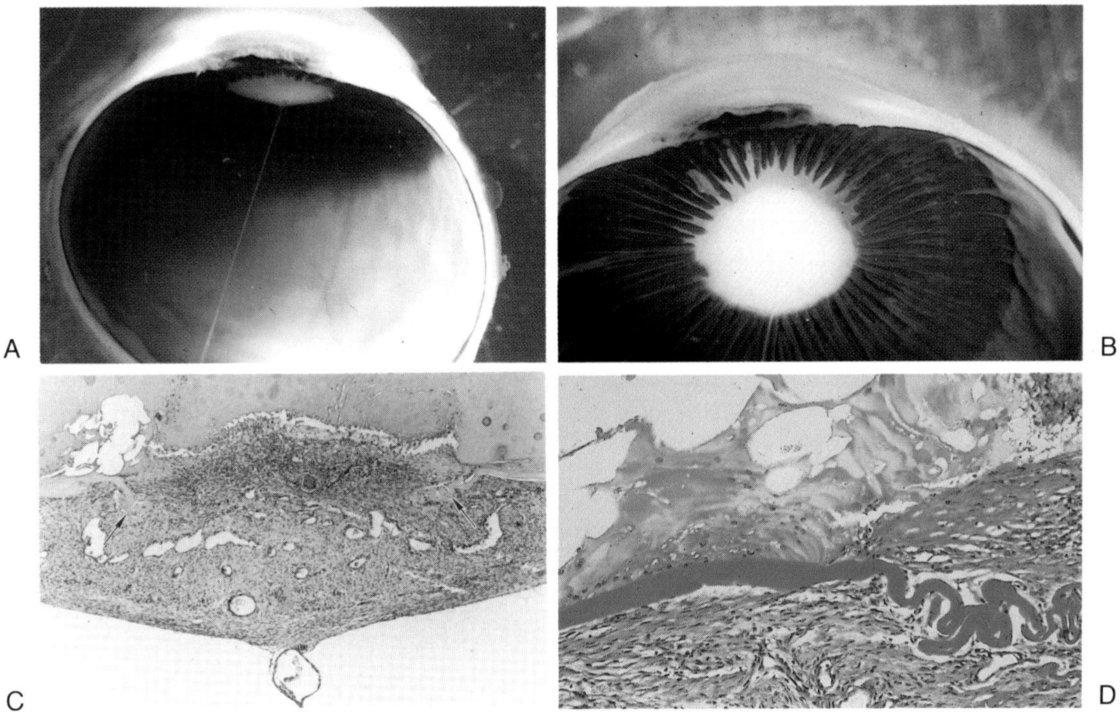

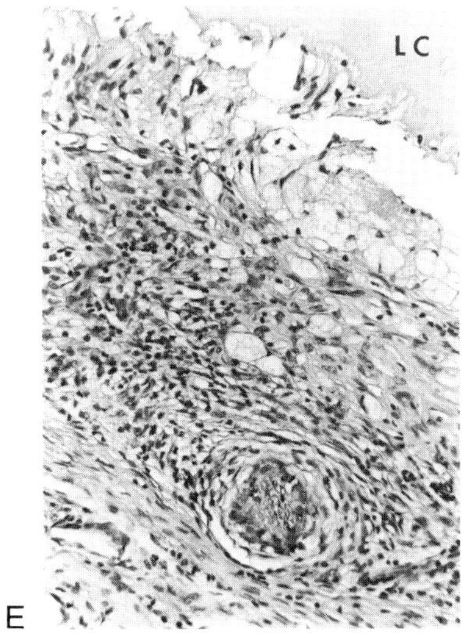

Figure 183–29. Persistent hyperplastic primary vitreous. *A,* Persistent hyaloid artery passing from the optic disc to a plaque of persistent hyperplastic primary vitreous (PHPV) in a 3-month-old infant. *B,* Ciliary processes pulled inward to the white plaque of PHPV, with the hyaloid artery inserting centrally. *C,* PHPV plaque shows thin collagen bundles, small fibroblasts, and thin-walled blood vessels deriving from hyaloid artery below. H&E, ×65. *D,* Ruptured redundant lens capsule in PHPV. PAS, ×100. *E,* Granulomatous inflammatory reaction with large giant cell below, and inflammatory cells among the fraying cataractous lens fibers. (LC, lens cortex.) H&E, ×300. (*D* and *E,* From Caudill JW, Streeten BW, Tso MOM: Phacoanaphylactoid reaction in persistent hyperplastic primary vitreous. Ophthalmology 92:1153, 1985.)

by their attachment to the plaque (see Fig. 183–29*B*), often lying against the posterior lens, so they are visible in the pupil. The eye and cornea are slightly smaller (microphthalmic) than on the normal side. Both of these signs are important in the differential diagnosis from retinoblastoma. PHPV was first looked upon as a persistence of the tunica vasculosa lentis. Its present name was given by Reese[97] when its closer relation to development of the primary vitreous was recognized.

The lens is initially clear in PHPV, becoming cataractous later in most eyes. By histopathology the lens epithelium is frequently seen to extend posteriorly as a cuboidal cell layer rather than as migrating spindle cells. The central posterior capsule is very thin to focally absent in the majority of cases. It lies directly on the PHPV, which is a hypercellular plaque of small spindle cells in a collagenous matrix with thin-walled vessels (see Fig. 183–29*C*). Cataract develops first in the defective posterior capsular area, typically during the first few postnatal months. The lens may become intumescent with shallowing of the anterior chamber, and a pupillary block or angle-closure glaucoma can ensue. Redundancy of the posterior capsular ends often suggests that intumescence and an acute capsular rupture have occurred (see Fig. 183–29*D*). A granulomatous inflammatory reaction with only a few polymorphonuclear leukocytes and lymphocytes has occasionally been observed among the degenerating posterior cortical fibers and in the PHPV plaque itself[98, 99] (see Fig. 183–29*E*). This reaction was suggested to be a type of phacoanaphylaxis in which the paucity of polymorphonuclear leukocytes and eosinophils was due to low levels of complement-fixing antibody to lens protein in this congenital disease.[99] In one case the inflammation and capsular rupture had clearly developed in utero.[99]

In some eyes with PHPV the lens cortex is completely replaced by fat cells (see Fig. 183–11), probably derived from adipose differentiation in the mesenchyme of the primitive vitreous plaque, and postulated to be a hallmark of PHPV when present.[23]

METABOLIC SUGAR CATARACTS

Metabolic sugar cataracts are discussed later, in the section on cataracts in abnormalities of carbohydrate metabolism.

CATARACTOGENESIS IN THE ADULT

No classification of adult cataracts will be completely satisfactory until the etiologies are known, but each has its usefulness for different purposes. Knowing the time of onset is helpful for assessing the cause and even possible complications of surgery. The terms congenital and developmental cataract encompass lens opacities noted at birth and during infancy. Juvenile cataract implies onset during the period of childhood through adolescence. Presenile cataract refers to an onset that occurs at any time from early adult life to age 60 years, with the term senile used thereafter. Cataracts developing in the juvenile period are due primarily to ocular disease, trauma, or the use of drugs such as corticosteroids, but several important types of cataracts indicate an early phase or carrier state of genetic disease. Some presenile cataracts with onset in the fourth to sixth decades may have a similar genetic basis. Histopathology and ultrastructure are seldom suggestive of a specific cause, showing changes common to all subcapsular, cortical, and nuclear cataracts.

Anterior Subcapsular Cataract

Anterior subcapsular cataracts in the adult typically follow uveitis, trauma, or both (Fig. 183–30). They may be multifocal, depending on the type of trauma, extent of posterior synechiae, or location of other injury. Causes can be bizarre, such as assiduous use of a mail-order vibrator on the lids to erase wrinkles (Fig. 183–31*A*) and injury by an electric shock from a high-power line, showing a stellate sutural pattern in both. Just as in the congenital anterior polar plaque (see previous section), there is initial necrosis of lens epithelium and superficial lens fibers, followed by reactive proliferation and metaplasia of the adjacent cuboidal lens epithelium to spindle cells. These metaplastic cells invade the injured area, sometimes in a stellate pattern following the sutures (see Fig. 183–31*B*), and produce a multilayered hypercellular plaque (see Fig. 183–31*C*). The plaque is slowly filled with collagen, the reactive cells decrease in number, and the plaque is converted to a fibrous scar. Eventually this scar and any remaining damaged tissues are isolated by growth of a new epithelial layer under the plaque, continuous with the adjacent original epithelial layer (Fig. 183–32). The early fibroblast-like proliferative epithelial cells show a few desmosomal junctions and produce little matrix other than pericellular basement membrane (Fig. 183–33*A*). Later there are also profuse collagen fibrils 28 to 70 nm in diameter, elastic microfibrils (see Fig. 183–33*B*), multilaminar basement membrane, and acid mucopolysaccharides.[100, 101] By immunostaining, collagens I, III, and IV and fibronectin have been demonstrated in this matrix.[102]

Multiple, small (0.2 to 0.3 μm) anterior subcapsular cataracts, referred to as *glaukomflecken,*[103] can occur

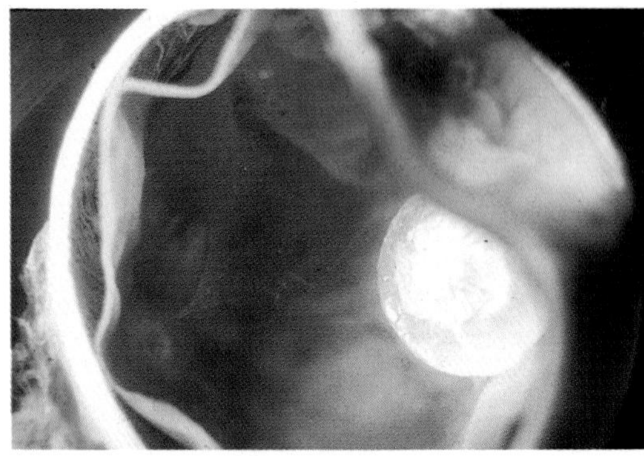

Figure 183–30. Large, white, anterior subcapsular cataract following severe contusive trauma with chronic uveitis.

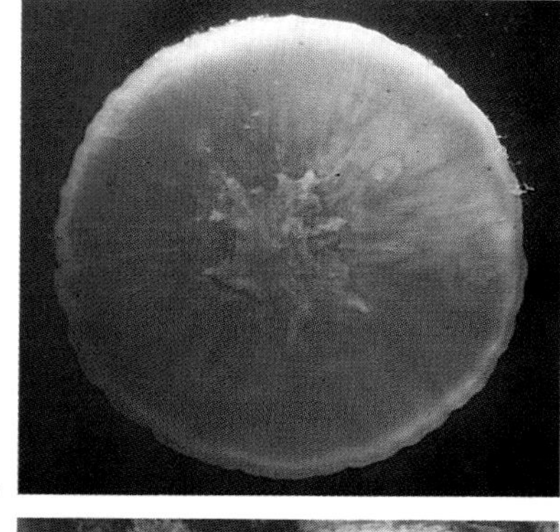

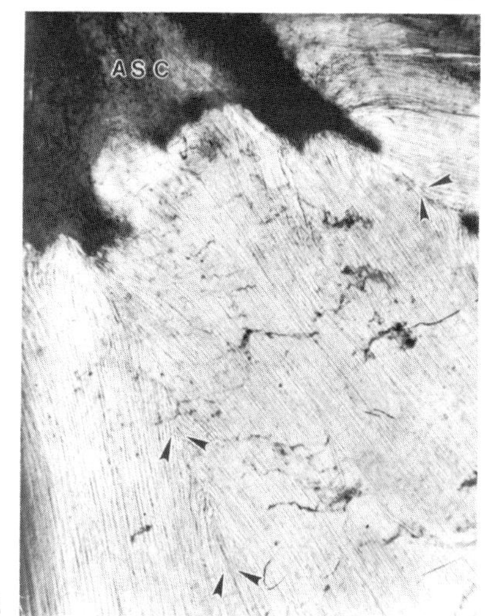

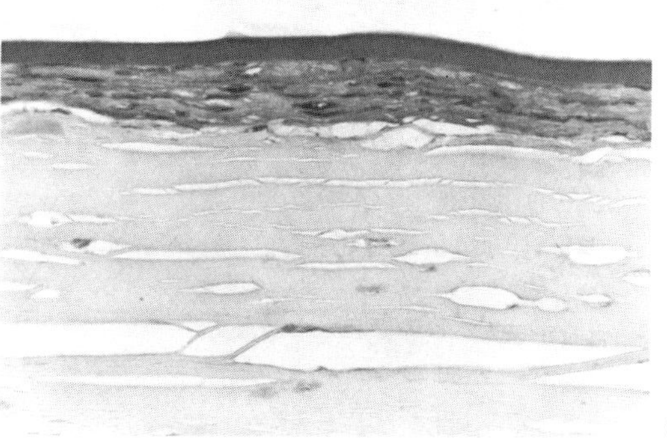

Figure 183–31. Vibration cataract. *A,* Early stellate, anterior subcapsular cataract following use of a vibrating lid massager by a 37-year-old woman. *B,* Edge of the cataract (ASC) in a whole-lens preparation shows that the stellate prolongations are oriented along the sutures *(arrowheads).* Hematoxylin, ×12. *C,* Reactive proliferation of metaplastic lens epithelial cells as multilayered spindle cells. H&E, ×140.

under the central anterior capsule following acute attacks of glaucoma, possibly as a result of anoxia from iris pressure or reduced aqueous perfusion. The course of these opacities through an early diffuse phase, later breaking up into discrete geographic opacities or disappearing completely, has been described by Jones.[104] With time, the opacities that remain are displaced into the lens by new clear fibers. Acutely there is focal necrosis of the lens epithelium histologically.[105] The opacities that do not regress presumably had focal necrosis of the underlying lens fibers as well, stimulating small epithelial cell fibrous scars.

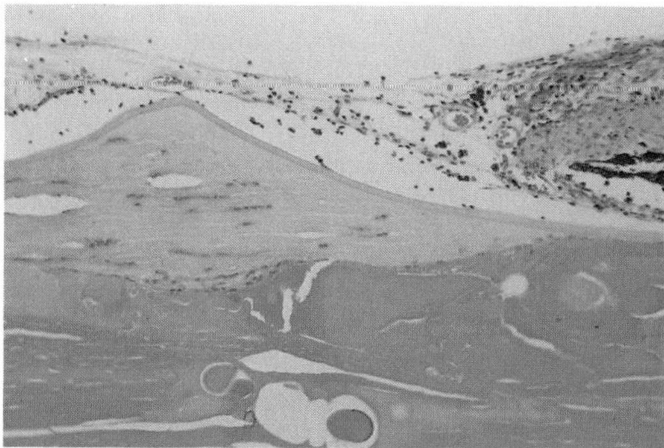

Figure 183–32. Mature anterior subcapsular plaque, almost completely collagenized, with a new layer of cuboidal lens epithelial cells separating plaque from the lens cortex. Note the pupillary membrane, posterior synechiae, and chronic inflammatory cells. In a 49-year-old diabetic with a chronic corneal ulcer. H&E, ×33.

Posterior Subcapsular Cataract

Posterior subcapsular cataract (PSC) is in many ways the most interesting of the adult cataracts because it is the one most likely to occur in the presenile period and to be related to disturbances of cellular metabolic activity, such as chronic exposure to corticosteroids, external beam irradiation, or associated with ocular diseases such as retinitis pigmentosa and other genetic diseases. PSC is also very frequent in the senile period and causes the most rapid loss of central vision because of its position in the central visual axis. The clinical appearance varies from a just visible granularity of the subcapsular posterior pole to a large granular-vacuolar plaque (Fig. 183–34). The cellular dynamics of the process, as followed in flat preparations of the superficial lens capsule, appear to be similar in all types of PSC, although the reasons for the aberrant cell behavior undoubtedly differ for specific cataracts.

The earliest microscopic change found in experimental and human PSC is a disorganization of the normally highly regular meridional rows of lens epithelial cell nuclei at the equator (Fig. 183–35),[106–107] where the cells are preparing to enter the cortex as new lens fibers. An increasing number of these cells fail to mature into lens fibers but instead become nomadic spindle cells migrating back to the posterior pole. This process begins segmentally, often in the inferior nasal quadrant in senile cataracts. Nucleated migratory cells have been noted in the posterior pole very early in experimental radiation

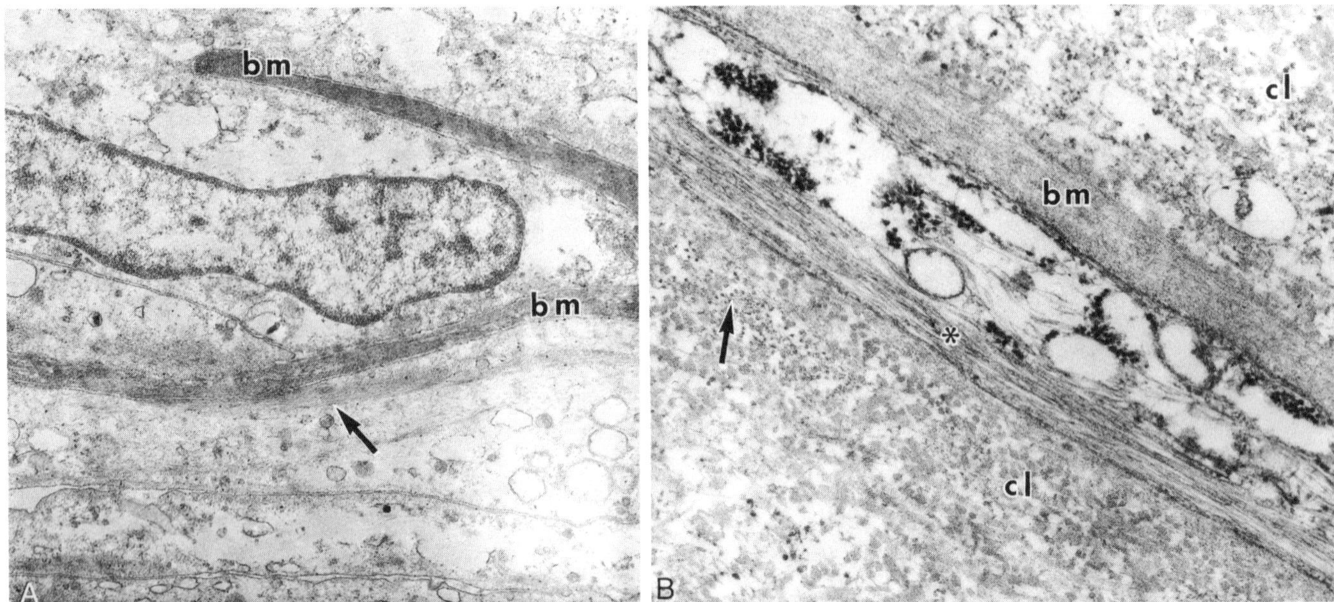

Figure 183–33. Matrix of anterior subcapsular cataracts. *A,* Young plaque from patient in Figure 183–31 showing six vacuolated spindled lens epithelial cells producing no matrix except basement membrane (bm) around two cells. Large actin bundle *(arrow)* in one cell. ×19,000. *B,* Mature congenital plaque in a 6-year-old patient with profuse collagen fibrils (cl) 28 to 70 nm in diameter and elastic microfibrils *(arrow).* Basement membrane (bm) produced by these fibroblast-like cells is primarily on the outer capsular side of the cell. ×59,000. Profuse actin and intermediate filaments are oriented along the opposite side of the cell *(asterisk).* ×59,000.

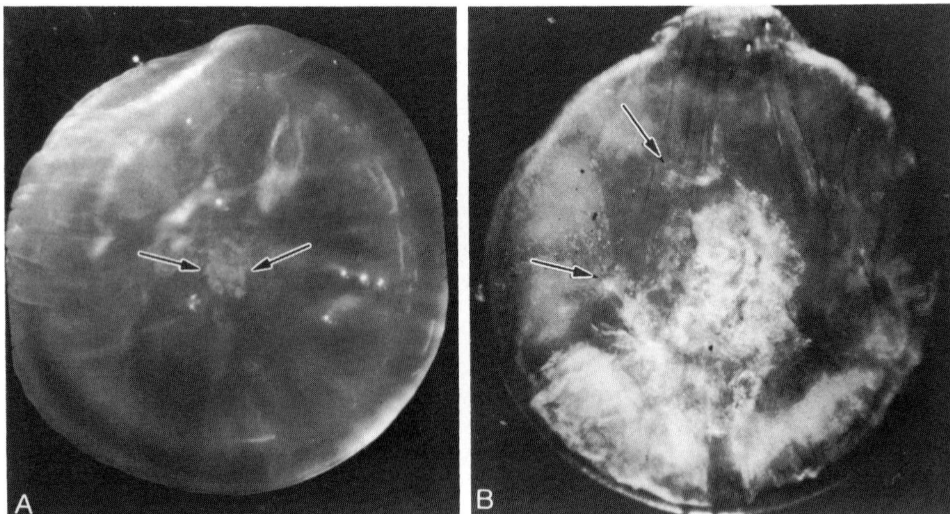

Figure 183–34. Posterior subcapsular cataract. *A,* Small, round, steroid-induced cataract with early nuclear sclerosis. *B,* Large subcapsular cataract showing stellate borders *(arrows),* and dense inferior cortical cataract below. Cryoprobe bleb above.

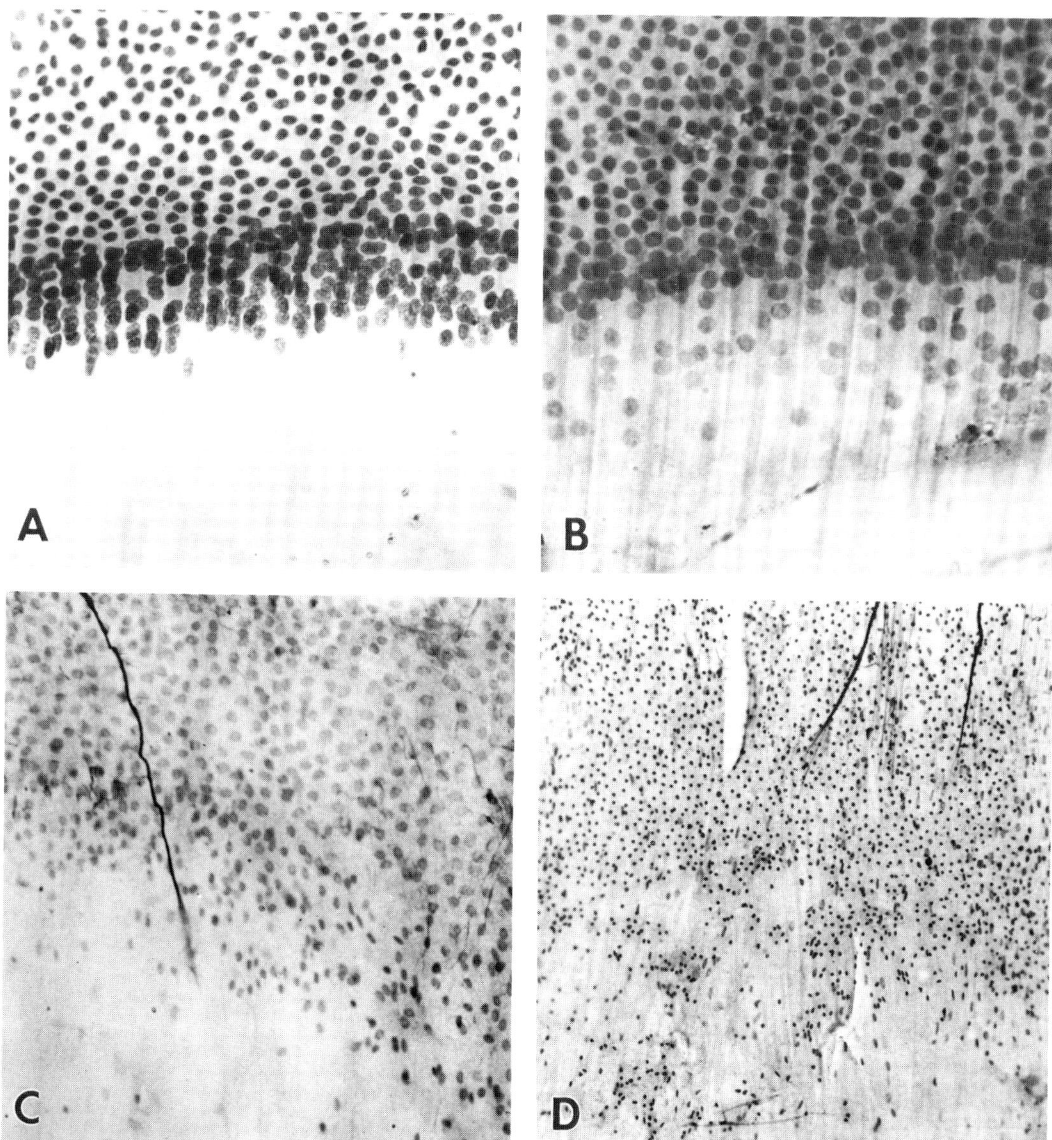

Figure 183–35. The meridional nuclear rows in caractogenesis. *A,* Parallel rows of lens epithelial cell nuclei at the equator in a young adult. *B,* Mild loss of regularity in a nuclear sclerosed cataract. *C,* Disruption of regular meridional rows with posterior migration of lens epithelial cells toward the posterior pole, in posterior subcapsular cataract. *D,* Complete loss of lens epithelial cell organization and differentiation at the equator, with many posteriorly migrating cells in an advanced corticosteroid-induced cataract. Dark strings are zonular fibers. Lens whole mounts. Hematoxylin, ×140 *(A);* ×140 *(B).* ×140 *(C);* ×70 *(D).* (From Streeten BW, Eshaghian J: Human posterior subcapsular cataract. A gross and flat preparation study. Arch Ophthalmol 96:1653, 1978. Copyright 1978, American Medical Association.)

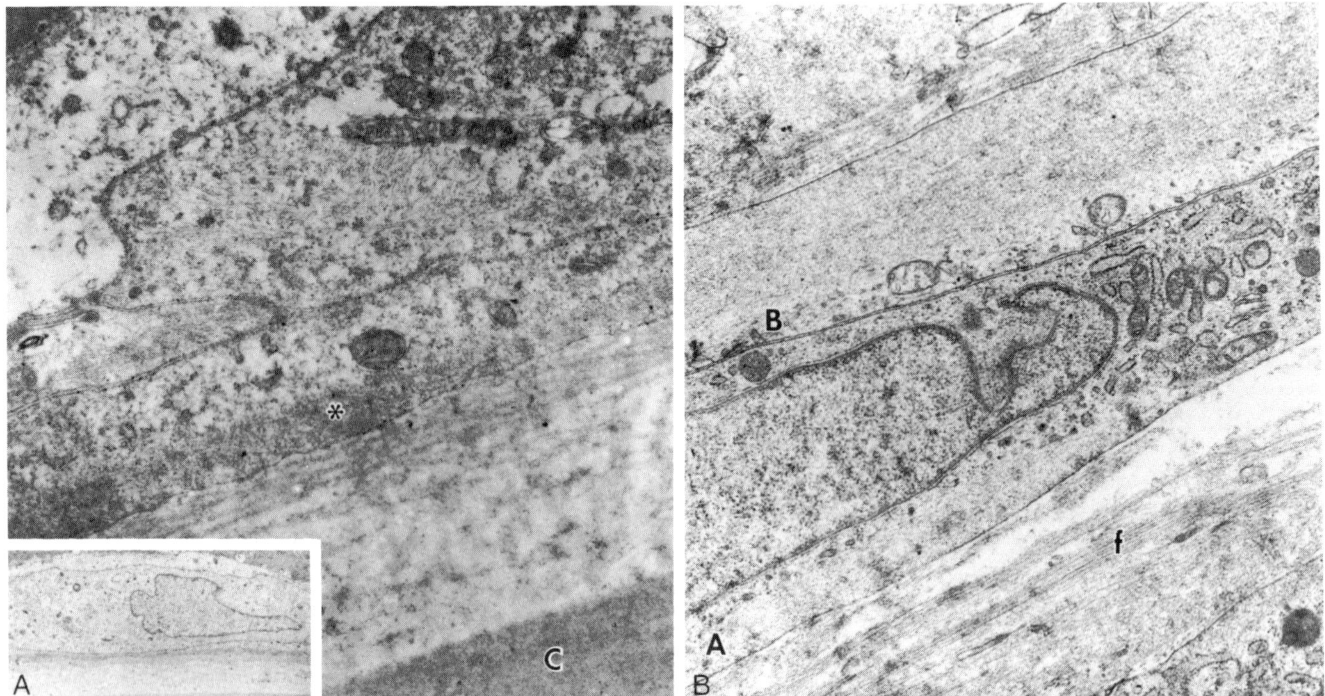

Figure 183–36. Ultrastructure of posteriorly migrating cells. *A,* Migrating lens epithelial cells have irregularly spindled nuclei (*inset,* ×4,400), larger mitochondria than those in the equatorial cells, prominent actin filaments *(asterisk),* and secretion of new multilaminar basement membrane between the cells and the capsule proper (C). ×30,000. *B,* Three active migratory cells in the cataractous area. Scanty extracellular matrix consists of fine filaments (f) and cellular debris. Migratory cell B has granular cytoplasm like a normal lens fiber. Cell B has granular cytoplasm. ×29,500. (From Eshaghian J, Streeten BW: Human posterior subcapsular cataract. An ultrastructural study of the posteriorly migrating cells. Arch Ophthalmol 98:134, 1980. Copyright 1980, American Medical Association.)

PSC, before the first visible subcapsular granular dots,[108] indicating that initiation begins in the equatorial epithelial cells. For most other PSCs, it is not clear what inhibits equatorial cell differentiation into lens fibers, or whether the cells are actively stimulated to migrate posteriorly.

In conventional sections, the counterpart of the meridional row change is an absence of the equatorial nuclear bow, and the presence of nuclei out of place under the posterior capsule along the pathway to the posterior pole. Ultrastructurally these migratory cells have peripheral actin bundles and become more fibroblast-like as they progress to the posterior pole, showing many mitochondria (Fig. 183–36*A*), short segments of rough endoplasmic reticulum, and Golgi and lysosome-like bodies (see Fig. 183–36*B*).[109, 110] Multiple layers of migratory cells are arranged in a ring around the larger PSCs (Fig. 183–37), where they often round up as nucleated Wedl[111] (balloon) cells (Fig. 183–38*A*). Balloon cells show some differentiation, resembling lens fibers ultrastructurally, with granular cytoplasm, scant organelles, and ball-and-socket junctions (see Fig. 183–

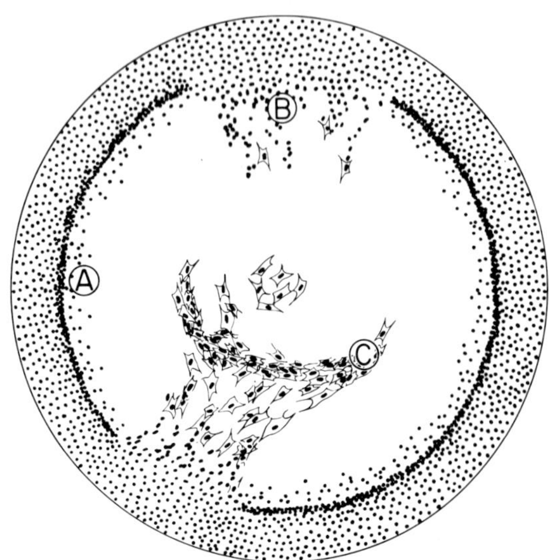

Figure 183–37. Diagram of the cellular changes in posterior subcapsular cataract. The pattern of regular meridional rows (A) is disrupted by posterior migration of the lens epithelial cells (B), becoming larger and more spindled and fibroblast-like as they extend into the posterior pole, surrounding the liquefying posterior subcapsular cataract in a ring (C). (From Eshaghian J, Streeten BW: Human posterior subcapsular cataract. An ultrastructural study of the posteriorly migrating cells. Arch Ophthalmol 98:134, 1980. Copyright 1980, American Medical Association.)

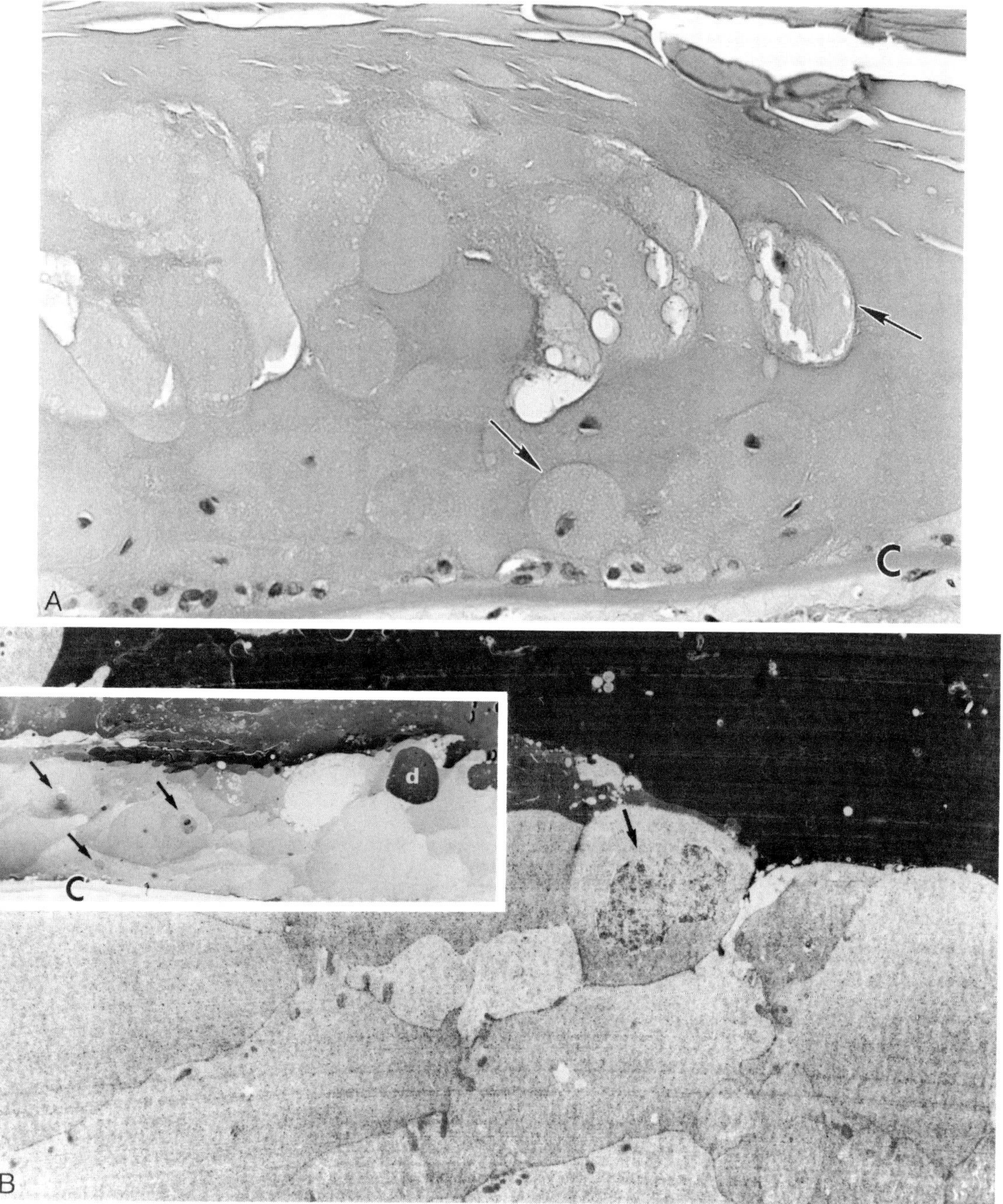

Figure 183–38. Balloon cells in posterior subcapsular cataract. *A*, Aggregation of migratory cells under the capsule (C) rounding up as nucleated balloon cells at the edge of a large posterior subcapsular cataract. H&E, ×150. *B*, Nucleated lens fiber-like cell *(arrow)* making some interdigitated connections with more normal lens fibers, at the border of a completely cataractous dark cortex above. ×4,400. *Inset*, Several bladder cells *(arrows)* from same area. (C, capsule; d, dense cataractous cortex.) Toluidine blue, ×280.

Illustration continued on following page

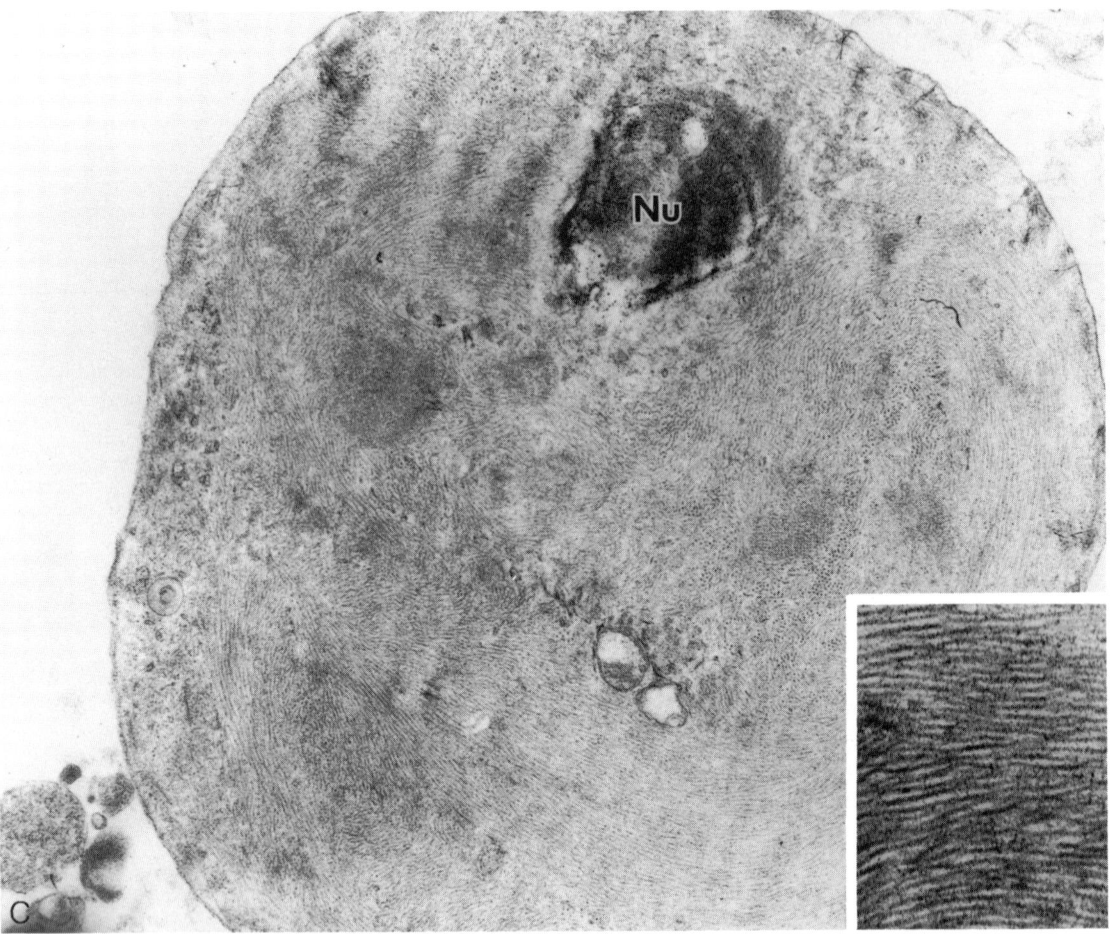

Figure 183–38 *Continued C,* Rounded, degenerate migratory cell with a karyorrhectic nucleus (Nu) and a large number of cytoplasmic filaments. ×19,000. *Inset,* Higher power of the 10-nm intermediate filaments. ×86,000. (*B* and *C* from Eshaghian J, Streeten BW: Human posterior subcapsular cataract. An ultrastructural study of the posteriorly migrating cells. Arch Ophthalmol 98:134, 1980. Copyright 1980, American Medical Association.)

38*B*), making the term "abortive lens fibers" appropriate.[110] Other balloon cells are round, degenerating migratory cells containing large numbers of intermediate filaments (see Fig. 183–38*C*).

The migratory cells growing into the degenerate cortex at the edge of the PSC produce minimal extracellular matrix with no banded collagen or basement membrane (see Fig. 183–36*B*), in sharp contrast with lens cell behavior in anterior subcapsular cataract, and the rare posterior polar cataract. Quite early the whole disclike center of the PSC becomes liquefied, with degeneration of both migratory cells and adjacent lens fibers (Fig. 183–39). The capsule is very thin over this liquefied area and often ruptures during intracapsular cataract extraction.

Progression can be quite rapid in this cataract, possibly aided by lysosomal enzymes from the degenerating nucleated cells. Cortical and nuclear cataract may be added as the PSC progresses, as well as involvement of equatorial cells from other sectors.

Cortical Cataract

The earliest type of cortical cataract in older patients is often a spokelike opacification of lens fibers in the equatorial region, especially common in the inferonasal and inferior quadrants (Fig. 183–40*A*). Since all lens fibers have arms extending both anteriorly and posteriorly, these opacities can usually be followed in both directions (see Fig. 183–40*B*). Extensions of the wedgelike opacities toward the midline have been called "cuneiform" cataracts. By slit-lamp examination the opaque fibers are often interspersed with clear "water clefts," indicating breakdown of fibers with extracellular fluid accumulation. By histopathology, water clefts are areas where the cortical lamellae are separated by swollen, degenerate lens fiber debris appearing as anuclear, pink, globular aggregates (morgagnian globules), surrounded by paler pink, granular material (Fig. 183–41). Very little evidence of new fiber formation (bow activity) is present at the equator.

By electron microscopy these intercellular spaces contain varying-sized globules of cortical material and cell membrane remnants (Fig. 183–42). The degenerate cell membranes often form crystalloid patterns of circles and loops.

As this process spreads throughout the lens, calcium may be deposited in the cellular debris as basophilic hydroxyapatite granules, or foci of large colorless calcium oxalate crystals (Fig. 183–43).[112, 113] The lens epithelial cells often show focal proliferation during this

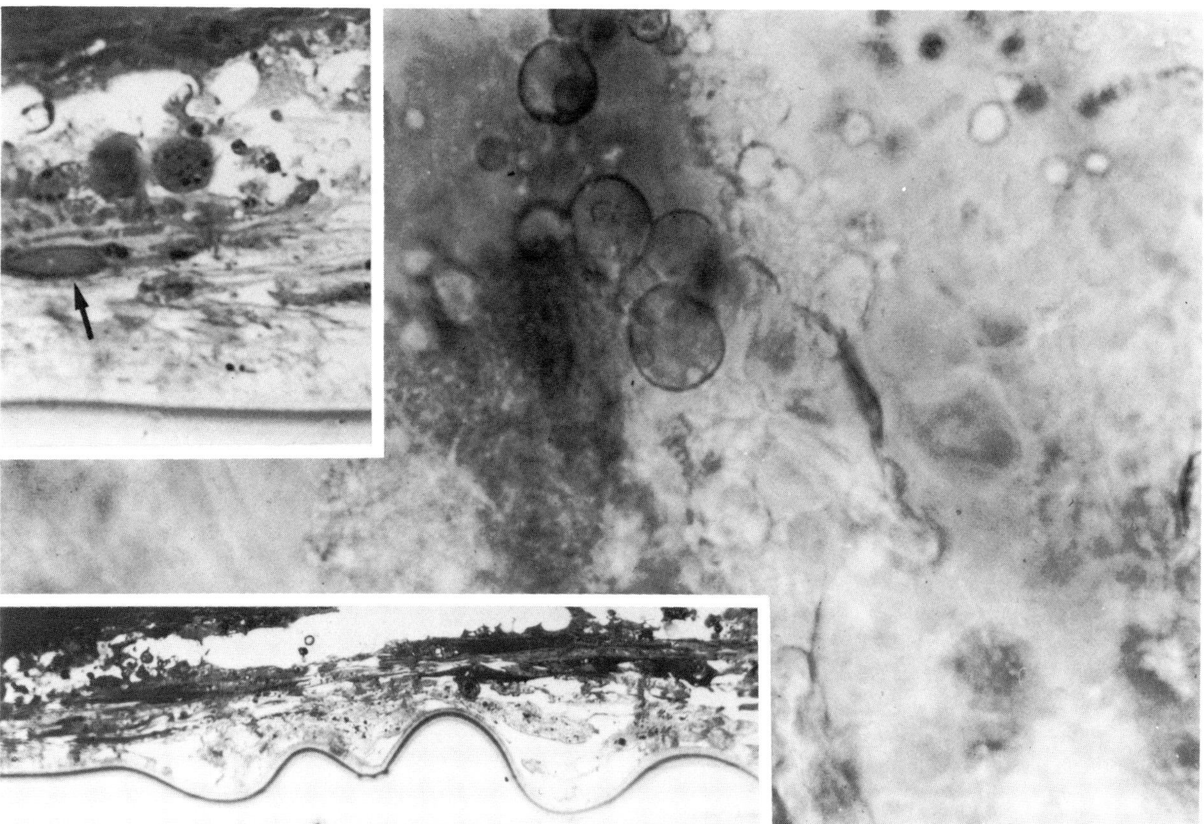

Figure 183–39. Liquefying posterior subcapsular cataract consisting mostly of globular and granular debris. *Lower Inset,* Capsular wrinkling over this fluid cataractous area. *Upper Inset,* Nucleus of a migratory cell *(arrow)* growing into the cataractous debris. Toluidine blue. Main figure is from a fresh unfixed cataract. ×700. *Insets,* 1-μm toluidine blue sections: lower, ×400; upper, ×800. (From Eshaghian J, Streeten BW: Human posterior subcapsular cataract. An ultrastructural study of the posteriorly migrating cells. Arch Ophthalmol 98:134, 1980. Copyright 1980, American Medical Association.)

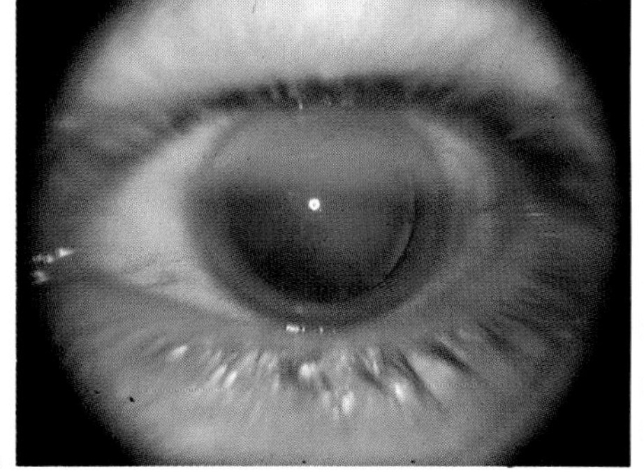

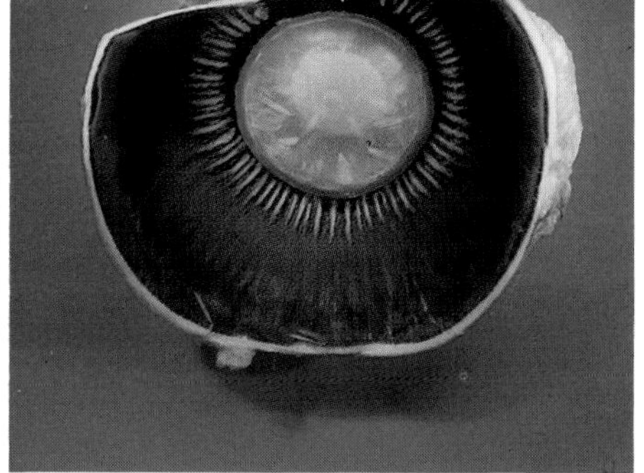

Figure 183–40. Cortical cataract. *A,* Inferior nasal cortical spoking with early nuclear sclerosis. *B,* Scattered, white, cortical spoke opacities extending around the equator both anteriorly and posteriorly, seen from the vitreal side. Some nuclear sclerosis is present.

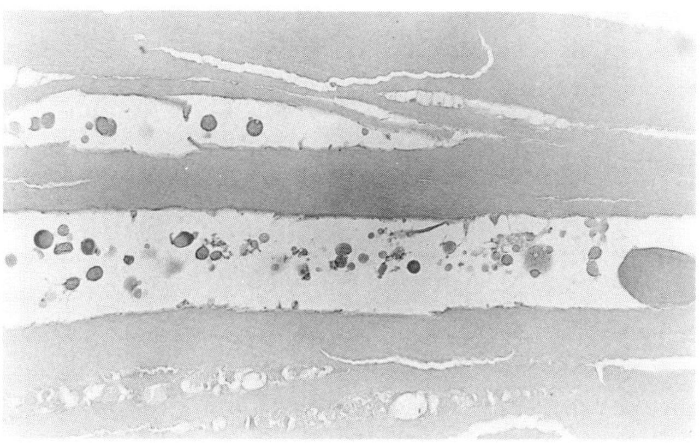

Figure 183–41. Fluid and morgagnian globules in water clefts separating the lens fiber lamellae. Early clefts developing below. H&E, ×230.

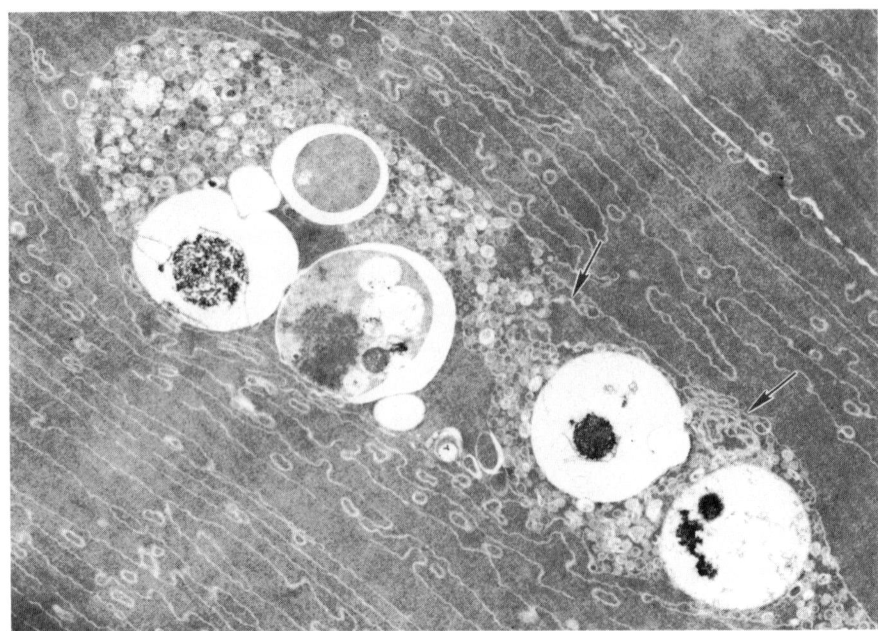

Figure 183–42. Cortical cataract showing a vacuolar-globular (morgagnian) degeneration of lens fibers, and a replicative pattern of degenerate cell membranes. These "crystalloid arrays" appear to derive directly from cell membranes *(arrows).* ×12,600.

cataractogenesis, but a gradual cellular degeneration and dropout occurs. When the whole lens is involved in this process and clinically appears opaque and white, the cataract is said to be mature. At any point in the late maturing process there can be an osmotic effect from the increase in molecules due to breakdown of proteins, resulting in a swollen or "intumescent" lens (Fig. 183–44). When all the fibers have liquefied, the lens will be a bag of fluid lenticular material except for the hard, amber-colored or dark-brown (brunescent) nucleus in the older adult (Fig. 183–45). This floating nucleus and some wrinkling of the anterior capsule may be visible clinically, indicating a "hypermature" cataract that will have virtually no remaining epithelium and a very thin capsule. Such a lens is obviously difficult to control at the time of cataract surgery and may rupture spontaneously with mild trauma. A phacolytic glaucoma due to egress of soluble lens proteins can develop in this hypermature phase (see later section on phacolytic glaucoma). If the capsule ruptures, a phacoanaphylactic inflammatory reaction can be induced by the remaining cortex and nucleus (see later section on phacoanaphylactic endophthalmitis).

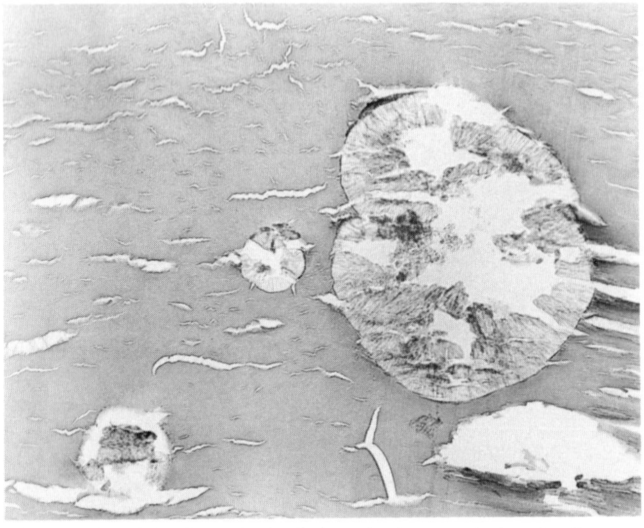

Nuclear Sclerosed Cataract

The commonest aging cataract results from sclerosis of the lens nucleus. Both *nucleus* and *sclerosis* are hard to define in this context because they are clinical terms, not conforming strictly to anatomic boundaries or pathologic criteria. The process is a slow one, merging imperceptibly with the changes of aging. There is increasing involvement of the central lens fibers so that the "nucleus" increases in size and density with time, causing an acquired myopia by its increased index of refraction. Pari passu there is a color change from the lemon-yellow

Figure 183–43. Three foci of sharply demarcated pale sheaves of calcium oxalate crystals in an old cataractous lens. H&E, ×140.

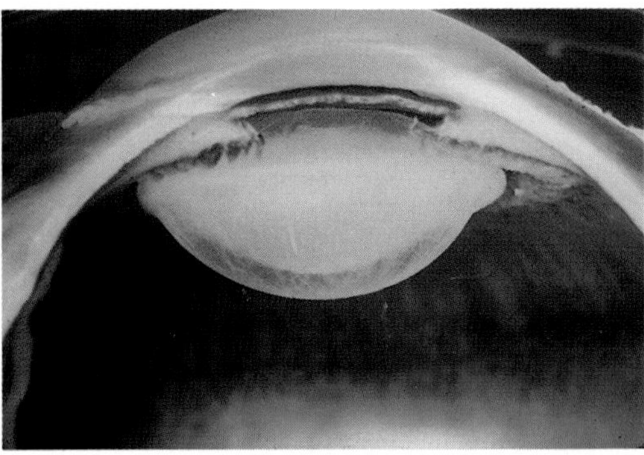

Figure 183–44. Severely intumescent lens with clear fluid distention of the posterior capsule. Patient terminally ill with Creutzfeldt-Jakob disease, acquired from corneal transplantation. Separation of the posterior cortical fibers resembles that in neonatal transient vacuoles.

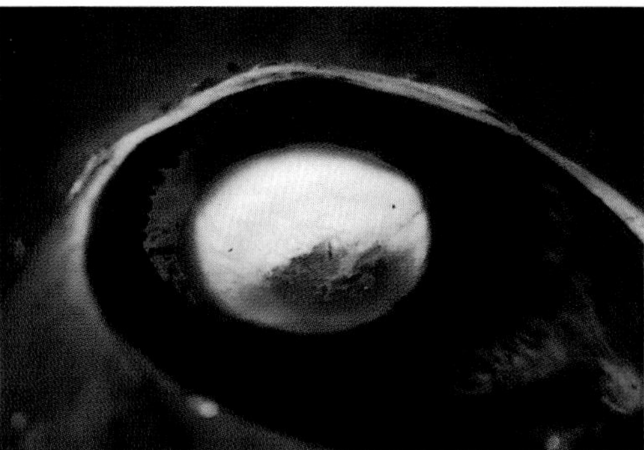

Figure 183–45. Hypermature milky cataract in which a dense brunescent nucleus lies inferiorly.

of the still transparent older nucleus to an amber and eventually a dark-brown (brunescent) region that may occupy most of the lens (Fig. 183–46). Sclerosis refers to the undoubted increase in hardness of the central lens, but the exact nature of this change and its pathogenesis are unclear, as discussed elsewhere (see Chapters 39 to 41).

By light microscopy the sclerotic central lens no longer shows separation into lamellae but instead appears homogeneous, with only rare foci of globular fiber breakdown. The area of homogeneity increases in width and thickness, corresponding with the color changes seen clinically and on gross examination. It tends to crack away from the cortex so the extent of this hard region is more easily appreciated (Fig. 183–47). This "cracking away" of the nucleus is the histologic counterpart of nuclear separation achievable in cataract surgery. By electron microscopy the cytoplasm of the fibers appears very dense, with poor definition of plasma membranes and cell junctions.

Mechanisms in Senile Cataractogenesis

In senile and, especially, nuclear cataractogenesis, large intracellular protein aggregates appear to develop from conformational changes in lens fiber proteins, followed by oxidative reactions, with abnormal disulfide and other covalent linkages causing the fibers to lose their transparency.[114] More recently, emphasis has been given to light scattering by abnormalities of the lens cell membranes themselves, which would also result in loss of transparency. Changes in the membranes, in turn, lead to increased permeability of the cells, with hydration and swelling of fibers. Damage to the lens cell membranes by photooxidation of proteins has been extensively studied as a primary cause of membrane damage and accompanying color changes, whether due to chronic ultraviolet ray exposure or enhanced by photosensitizers in the diet or drugs.[115–117] Oxidative damage could be contributed to by decreasing natural antioxidants in the lens, such as glutathione,[118] inositol, and ascorbic acid. Aging, diet, and other disease all could play roles in deficiency of antioxidants (for further discussion see Chapters 39 to 41).

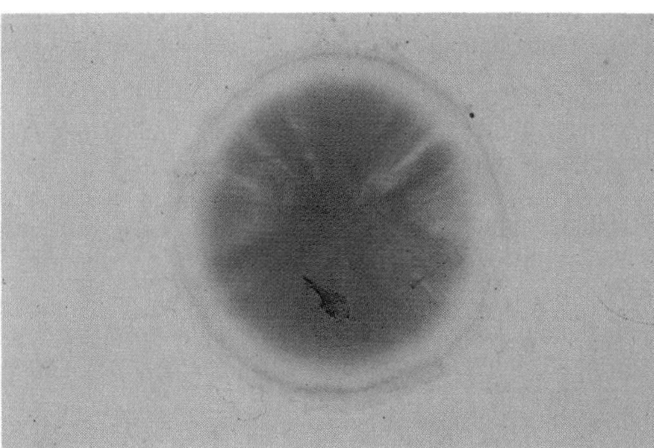

Figure 183–46. Brunescent cataract removed intercapsularly. The brown "nucleus" occupies almost the entire lens.

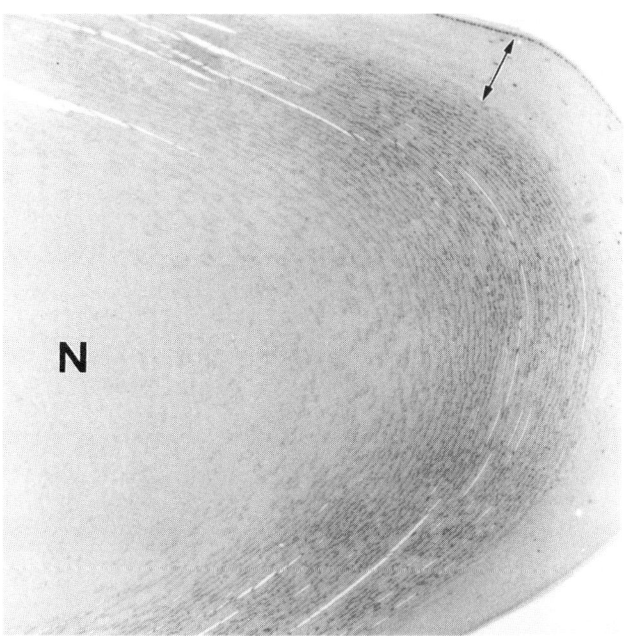

Figure 183–47. Advanced nuclear sclerosis showing a marked anteroposterior thickening of the lens, with an enlarging homogeneous nuclear region (N) that tends to crack away from the softer cortex *(double arrow)*. H&E, ×42.

CATARACT DUE TO PENETRATING AND NONPENETRATING TRAUMA AND TUMORS

Both penetrating and nonpenetrating trauma to the lens can lead to cataract formation (Fig. 183–48). Penetrating trauma from exogenous injury or ocular surgery usually results in rapidly progressive cataract (see Fig. 183–48*A*), with lens fiber swelling, fragmentation, and opacification. The lens capsule has some elasticity and usually flaps outward, preventing closure of the rupture. Aqueous and inflammatory mediators enter the lens, and a small number of macrophages may be found among the fraying fibers. Few other inflammatory cells

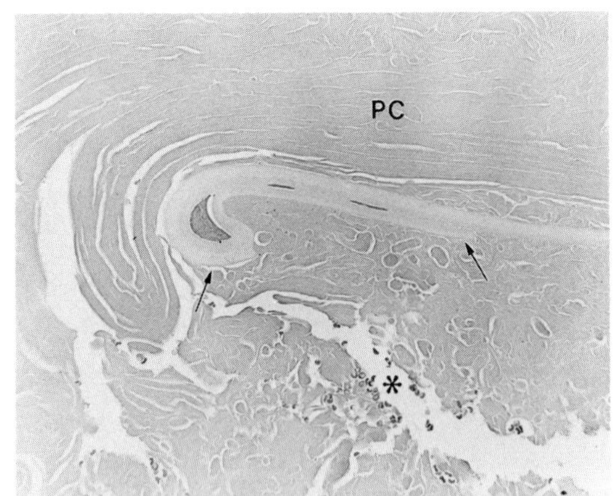

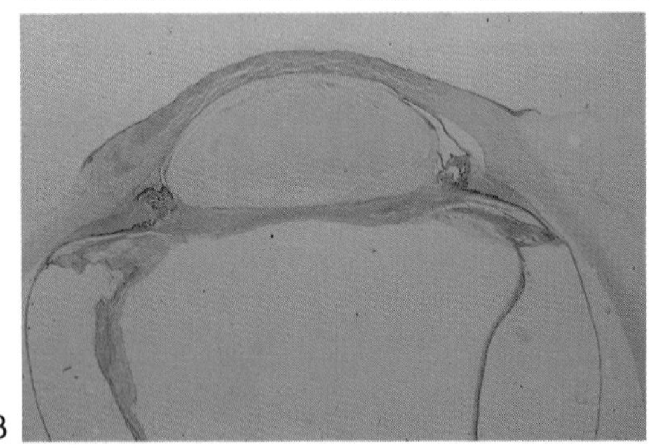

Figure 183–48. Direct and indirect injury to the lens capsule. *A,* Perforation of the posterolateral lens capsule 5 days previously. The capsule has flapped back on itself *(arrows),* and the extruded cortex shows advanced globular degeneration. Only a few red cells are present *(asterisk).* The posterior cortex (PC) still within the lens shows much less cataractous change. H&E, ×135. *B,* Enormously swollen intumescent lens and iris remnant fill the anterior chamber, pushed forward by cyclitic membrane 5 months after a perforating limbal-ciliary body wound. This 18-month-old child fell on one of his toys, but the lens capsule was not perforated.

are present unless infection or an immunologic reaction supervenes. Following injury within the first decade, all of the lens contents may be absorbed. When the capsular break is central, a Soemmerring ring cataract[119] can form (Fig. 183–49) as the anterior and posterior capsules fuse at the edges of the dehiscence, isolating a peripheral

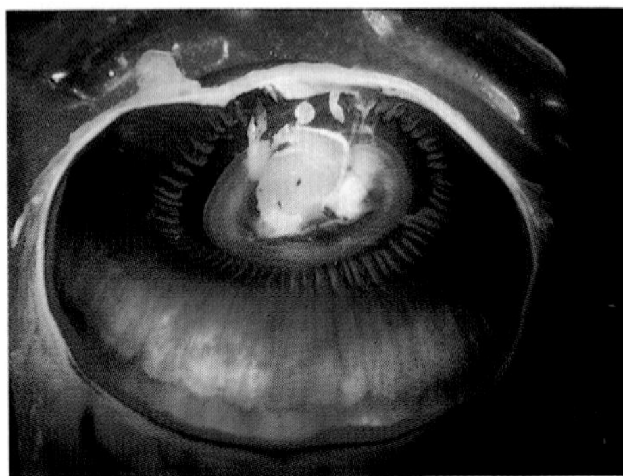

Figure 183–49. Yellowish Soemmerring's ring of cataractous equatorial lens material after surgery for a traumatic cataract at age 15. Further surgery was performed for contusion-angle glaucoma.

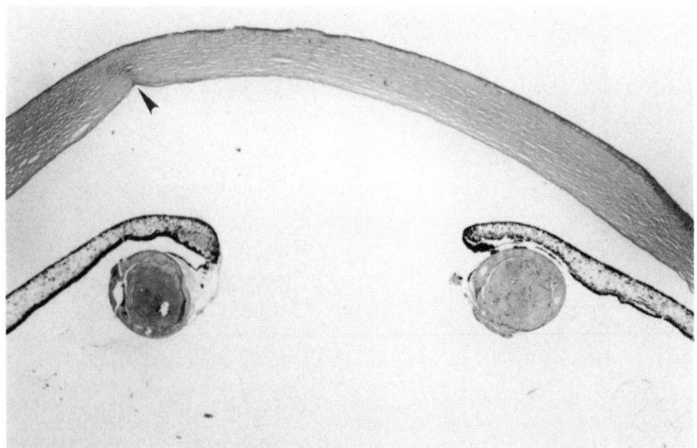

Figure 183–50. Soemmerring's ring cataract, following a perforating corneal wound paracentrally *(arrowhead).* H&E, ×16.

circle of yellow-white cataractous lens cortex (Fig. 183–50). This complete or incomplete ring can remain forever and can even dislocate as an intact structure.

If the capsular penetration is small and quickly sealed by a capsular flap and fibrin, or by adherence to the overlying iris, a localized nonprogressive opacity can result but is uncommon. Even without capsular perforation, contusive trauma associated with hemorrhage and inflammation can result in intumescence and mature cataract within months (see Fig. 183–48*B*).

Nonpenetrating concussive injury can infrequently cause a rupture of the lens capsule, especially if there is an advanced cataract with thin capsule. More commonly a petaliform ("foliaform" or "rosette-shaped") contusion cataract forms in the anterior or posterior cortex or both (Fig. 183–51), as extensively illustrated by Duke-Elder and MacFaul.[120a] They suggest that the concussive force of the iris striking the lens may injure the lens fiber cells joining sutures at that moment, increasing their permeability and resulting in small fluid vacuoles at their tips. The dramatic feathery opacification around the sutures emphasizes again the vulnerability of lens fibers at these sites. The anterior rosette is said to be commoner after contusive injury, and the posterior after penetrating injury. These traumatic cataracts may be transitory, or they can remain as stellate lamellar cataracts if the lens fibers are damaged sufficiently. The ultrastructure of this petaliform cataract does not appear to have been investigated but is unlikely to be unique. A circular imprint of iris melanin pigment adhering to the capsule at the pupil can also result from severe contusive injury, called a Vossius ring opacity.[120a]

Direct trauma to the lens from an adjacent tumor is an infrequent cause of cataract but can complicate anterior segment tumors, such as medulloepitheliomas of the ciliary body and anteriorly located retinoblastomas. In adults, slowly growing tumors of the ciliary body or iris, benign or malignant, may present with focal cataracts, progressing to diffuse involvement. Liquefaction and absorption of the focal cataractous lens fibers can occur, and subcapsular fibrous cataracts develop at the pressure sites, producing marked deformity of the lens (Fig. 183–52).

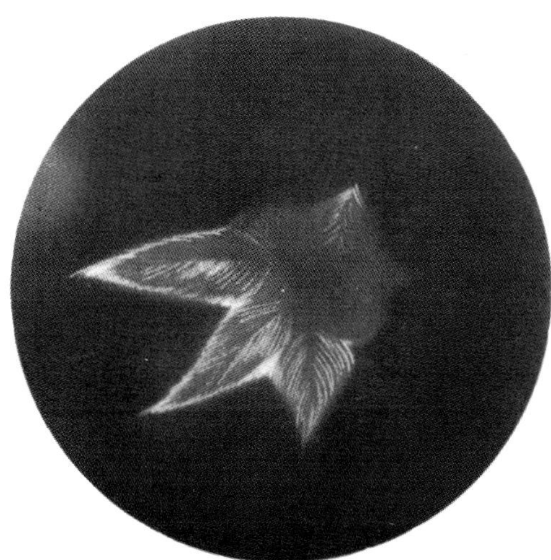

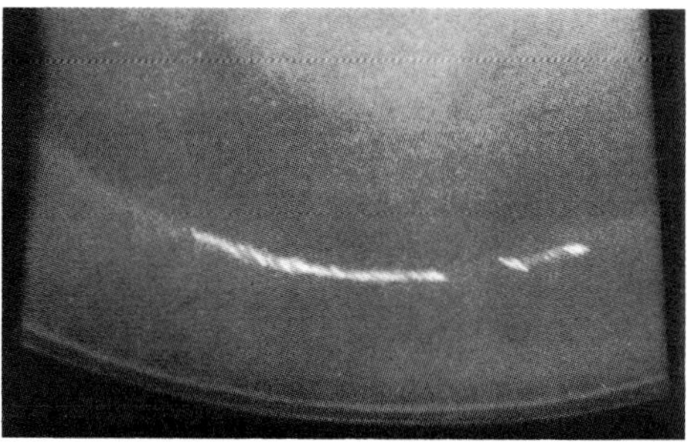

Figure 183–51. Partial petaliform contusion cataract has a feathery exaggeration of the sutural pattern, following edema and permanent injury to the sutural ends of the lens fibers, 12 years after injury. Slit beam localization shows that the injury occurred during early formation of the adult nucleus. (From Berliner ML: Biomicroscopy of the Eye. Slit Lamp Microscopy of the Living Eye. Vol. II. New York, Paul B. Hoeber, Inc., Harper and Brothers, 1949.)

LENS REACTIONS FOLLOWING EXTRACAPSULAR CATARACT EXTRACTION

The pathology of cataract surgery and intraocular prosthetic lens implantation is a large subject affecting many intraocular tissues and will not be dealt with here, except for the reactions of the lens cells themselves in extracapsular cataract extraction. Such reactions were familiar to the early surgeons using extracapsular procedures both planned and unplanned[121, 122a] and continue to be the commonest complication of this surgery.[123–130] The problems arise from continued viability of the lens epithelium remaining on a capsule after removal of the cortex and nucleus, and its ability to proliferate in several patterns.

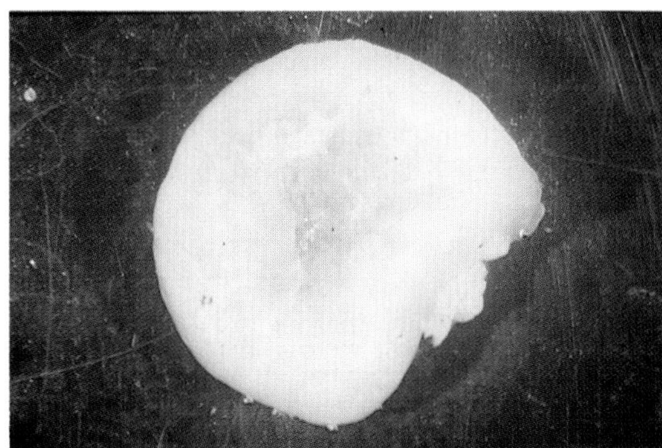

Figure 183–52. Mature cataract from a 63-year-old woman showed this peculiar deformity after intracapsular removal. An adjacent slowly growing malignant melanoma of the ciliary body had caused a focal cataract that was absorbed, and replaced by nubbins of subcapsular fibrous cataract.

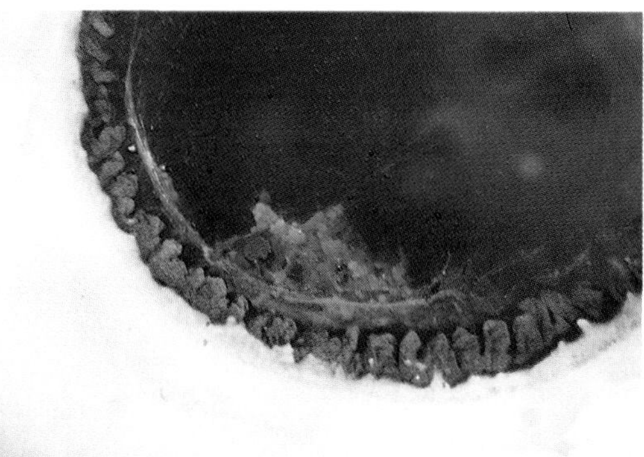

Figure 183–53. Multiple, small, round Elschnig's pearls proliferating from the anterior capsular edge inferiorly after an abortive intracapsular cataract extraction.

If the edges of the anterior capsule adhere to the posterior capsule after capsulectomy, a closed space will be reestablished in which the remaining epithelial cells may continue to form cataractous material, predominantly nucleated bladder cells. The resulting Soemmerring's ring is usually not a problem, lying out of sight behind the iris unless it dislocates and requires removal.

When there is a space between the anterior and the posterior capsule or dehiscences in the anterior capsule the epithelial cells are prone to migrate outward, forming large abortive lens fibers called Elschnig's pearls[121, 122a to d, 129] (Fig. 183–53). Clinically the pearls look like translucent fish eggs, which can fill the pupil or remain hidden behind the iris. By histopathology each fish egg is a nucleated bladder cell 5 to 120 μm (Fig. 183–54), identical to those proliferating within the capsule in Soemmerring's ring but lying outside, usually without a basement membrane. By scanning electron microscopy these cells often show spindle processes at one end, and surface microvilli.[129, 130]

A problem of greater importance than Elschnig's pearls is the opacification of the posterior capsule that

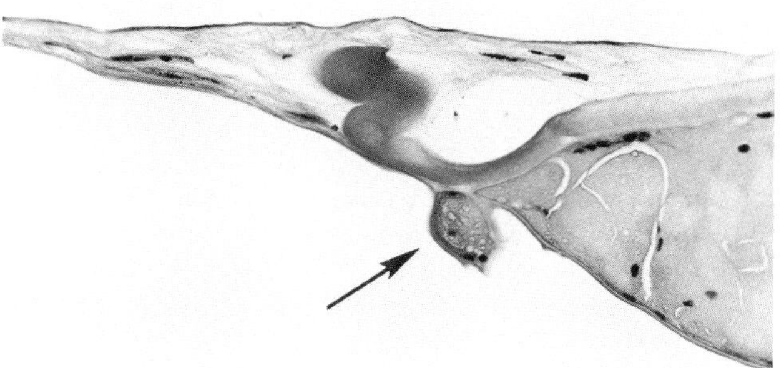

Figure 183–54. Single Elschnig's pearl *(arrow)* at the edge of an anterior capsular break, now sealed by fibrous scar. H&E, × 135.

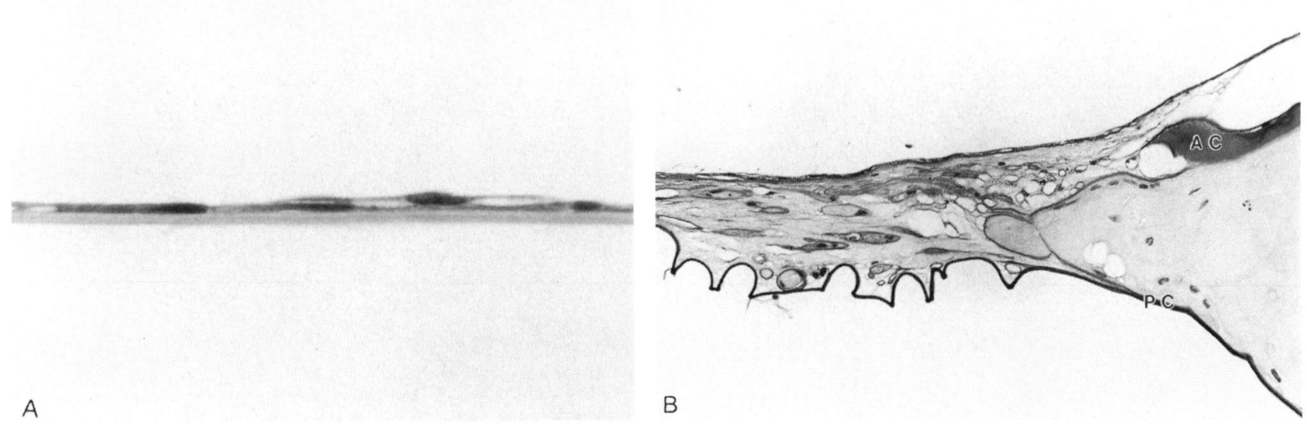

Figure 183–55. Lens cell proliferation on posterior capsule. *A*, Two layers of lens epithelial cells proliferating on central posterior capsule, with no evidence of matrix. H&E, ×660. *B*, Abundant collagen secretion by lens epithelial cells, like that in an anterior subcapsular cataract, from edge of a lens cortical remnant. Contraction of the collagen has thrown the posterior capsule into deep wrinkles. (AC, anterior capsule; PC, posterior capsule.) PAS, ×330.

occurs in high frequency after extracapsular extraction (formerly called "secondary" or "after-cataract").[122a] It is estimated that 50 percent of patients will have visually significant opacification of the posterior capsule in 3 to 5 yr after surgery[125] and that children and young adults are even more susceptible to this proliferative process.[123] In response to unknown stimuli, the remaining epithelial cells migrate across the capsule primarily as a few layers of spindle cells (Fig. 183–55*A*), showing myofibroblastic characteristics ultrastructurally.[127] These cells have the capacity to produce a matrix of fibrous and basement membrane collagens and other extracellular molecules like those in an anterior subcapsular cataract. They can also stimulate contraction of even small quantities of this collagen matrix, wrinkling the posterior capsule (see Fig. 183–55*B*), with resultant distortion of vision and glare. It is not clear why these cells grow predominantly as spindle cells over most of the capsule yet sometimes as lens fiber–like pearls near the anterior capsule.

CATARACT FROM DEPOSITION OF HEAVY METALS IN THE LENS

Chalcosis Lentis

A "sunflower" cataract due to copper deposition (chalcosis lentis) has long been one of the hallmarks of Wilson's disease, although it occurs in fewer than 20 percent of these patients.[131] In this autosomal recessively inherited disease there is reduced copper binding to ceruloplasmin in the liver with excessive deposition in tissues, especially the liver, causing cirrhosis, and in the basal ganglia of the brain. Plasma levels of both copper and ceruloplasmin are low. The cataract is a greenish or greenish-brown surface opacity in the central lens that may be disclike, with short stellate processes rather than a full flower-petal pattern (Fig. 183–56*A*). A similar pattern may be noted in the posterior lens capsule. Light and electron microscopy show that the copper is in the inner portion of the capsule, in small granular aggregates mostly confined to the central region, increasing in size as they are carried outward, similar to their distribution in Descemet's membrane. The underlying epithelial cells and cortical lens fibers appear normal.[132] The copper can be selectively stained with rhodanine or rubeanic acid (see Fig. 183–56*B*). What component of the lens cell basement membrane binds the copper is unknown. It gradually disappears by treatment with the chelator penicillamine, along with the Kayser-Fleischer ring in Descemet's membrane.[133]

Similar deposits in the lens capsule have been described in patients with elevated serum copper levels associated with monoclonal gammopathies of multiple myeloma,[134–136] and pulmonary carcinoma.[137] A localized increase in copper ions resulting from an intraocular foreign body will also lead to deposits in the capsule. The migration of these deposits outward in the capsule after removal of the foreign body has been used to estimate the normal rate of lens capsule formation per year.[138]

Other Metal Deposits

Mercury that gains entry to the aqueous from exogenous sources, such as topical medications containing mercurial preservatives (e.g., phenylmercuric nitrate),[139, 140] or from occupational exposure[141] also accumulates in the lens capsule basement membrane,[139] as will silver in argyrosis[142] and gold in chrysiasis.[143]

Iron usually remains within the epithelial cells that take it up, rather than appearing in the basement membrane. In siderosis or hemosiderosis the lens epithelium takes on a yellow-brown or rusty appearance,[120b] from minute dots of intracellular iron, identifiable by Perls' or other iron stains (Fig. 183–57). Focal rusty-brown nodules of subcapsular cataract may develop. When the foreign body is in the lens there may be progression to a mature cataract, with diffusion of ionizable iron throughout the lens fibers. The iron

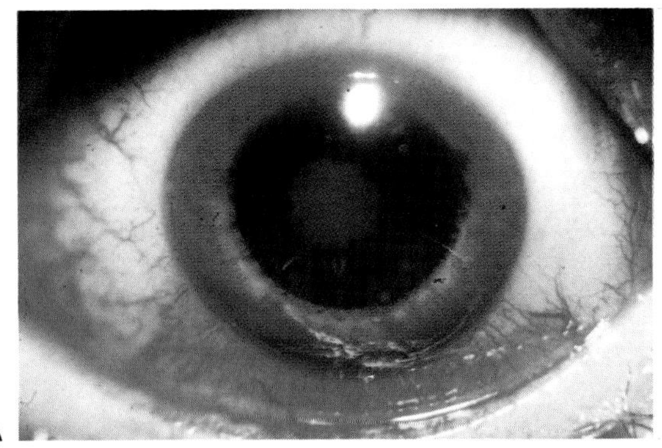

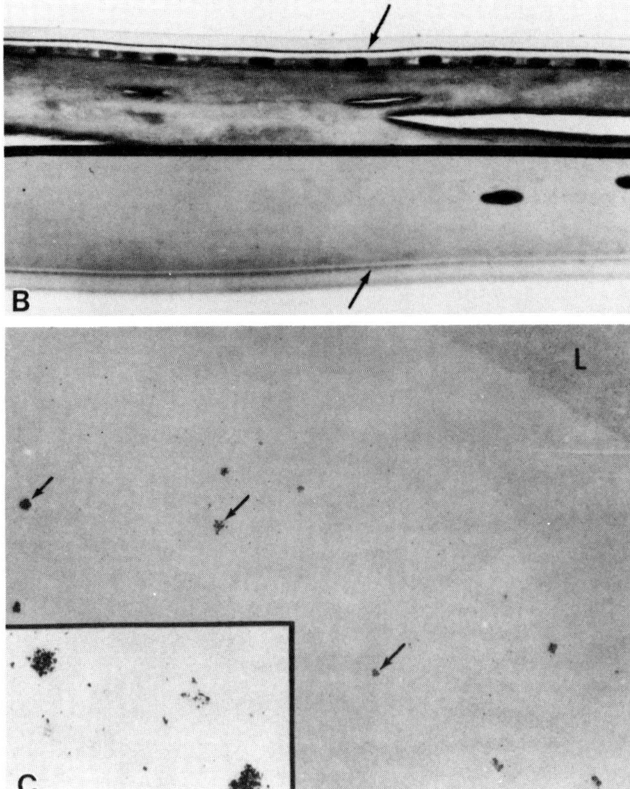

Figure 183–56. Wilson's disease. *A,* Dark brown peripheral Kaiser-Fleischer corneal ring. Anterior lens capsule has an irregular, faintly brownish disc-like opacity, with a few petaliform faintly brownish disc-like opacity, with a few petaliform lateral processes. *B,* The upper figure shows a dense line of copper in the inner third of the anterior lens capsule *(arrow)*. Rhodanine ×470. The lower figure shows a similar but fainter line in the posterior capsule *(arrow)*. Rhodanine ×580. *C,* Fine deposits of copper in the posterior lens capsule *(arrows)*. L = capsule. ×28,000. *Inset,* Deposits are aggregates of granules. ×74,000. (Courtesy of Dr. Mark O. M. Tso. AFIP Negatives 74-6778-3 and 74-6778-8. From Tso MOM, Fine BS, Thorpe HE: Kaiser-Fleischer ring and associated cataract in Wilson's disease. Am J Ophthalmol 79:479, 1975. Reprinted with permission from the Ophthalmic Publishing Company.)

appears to bind to enzymes within these cells, becoming insoluble and incorporated in phagolysosomes, with eventual cellular degeneration.

CATARACTS IN HEREDITARY SYSTEMIC DISEASE

Diseases of Carbohydrate Metabolism

GALACTOSEMIA

Galactosemic cataract is a major one to recognize in the newborn period because of its association with mental retardation, preventable to at least some extent by early restriction of galactose intake. This autosomal recessive disease is present in the homozygous state in about 1 per 40,000 live births, owing to a gene abnormality on chromosome 9.[144] Cataract and the systemic effects are due to a defective galactose-1-phosphate uridyl transferase, one of four enzymes that catalyze the conversion of galactose to glucose-1-phosphate (Fig. 183–58).[144–146] Because of this deficiency, galactose and galactose-1-phosphate accumulate in tissues, stimulating the enzyme aldose reductase to convert these sugars to the sugar alcohol galactitol (dulcitol). As in diabetes mellitus, the normal cell membranes are impermeable to this sugar alcohol, which exerts an osmotic effect within the cells, drawing in water, with swelling and eventual rupture of the cell membranes. Osmotically significant increases in galactitol and galactose-1-phos-

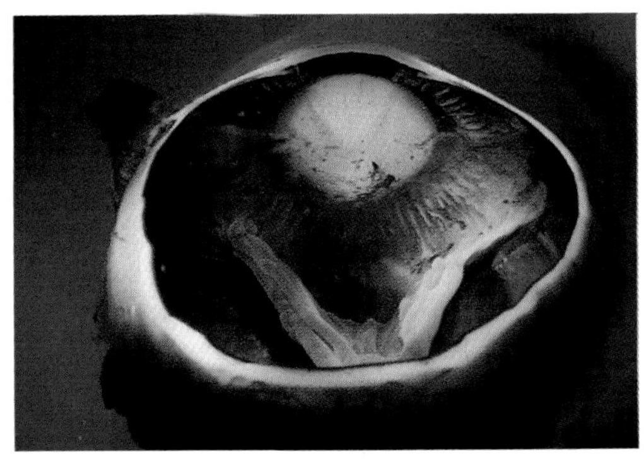

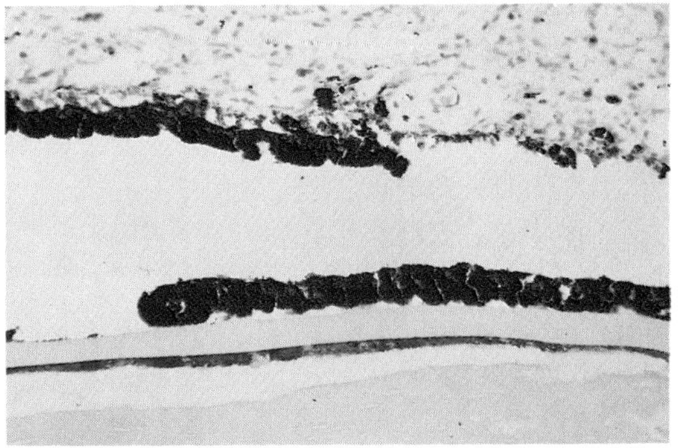

Figure 183–57. Siderosis bulbi. *A,* Mature cataract and siderosis secondary to intraocular iron-containing foreign body. Ciliary processes and detached retina both have a prominent rusty color. *B,* Lens epithelial cells containing abundant blue-staining iron shown by Perls' stain in hemosiderosis oculi. Iron is also seen in the iris dilator muscle and stroma. ×66.

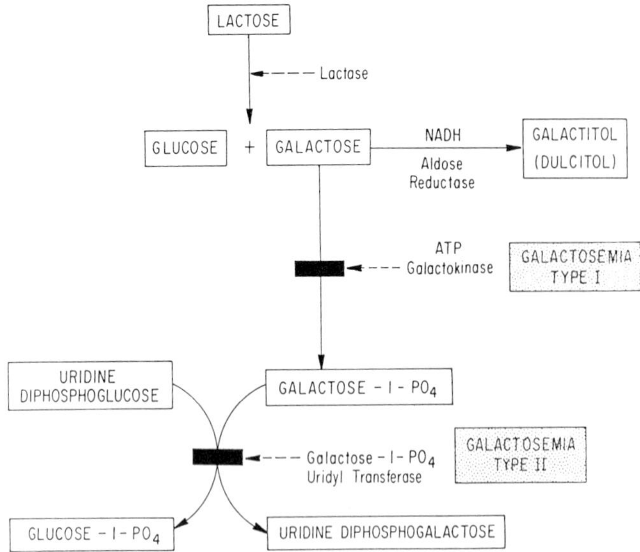

Figure 183–58. Galactose metabolic pathway showing the enzyme defect in two types of hereditary galactosemia. (From Klintworth GK, Landers MB III: The Eye: Structure and Function in Disease. © 1976, the Williams & Wilkins Co., Baltimore.)

phate have been found in a lens from a galactosemic fetus.[147]

The galactosemic infant shows no cataract or abnormality at birth but has a persistent failure to thrive, with vomiting, edema, and hepatosplenomegaly. Bilateral cataracts and early retardation may not be recognized until 1 to 2 mo of age. An "oil-droplet" appearance is seen in the central lens, as the nuclear fibers begin to swell, sometimes surrounded by zonular opacities. This early nuclear edema can disappear completely with rapid dietary restriction. In the lens of a 5-month-old fetus aborted after the diagnosis of galactosemia by amniocentesis, Vannas and colleagues[148] reported intracellular edema and mitochondrial swelling in the anterior lens epithelial cells, with lesser changes in the posterior lens fiber cells, not found in age-matched control abortuses. The enzyme deficiency thus appears to affect lens metabolism in intrauterine life, making an early postnatal diagnosis a matter of urgency. The rat model of galactosemia has similar clinical and pathologic changes,[149] preventable by administration of aldose reductase inhibitors by oral or topical routes.[150] Heterozygotes do not appear to be at risk for cataract.[151]

Cataracts of nuclear, zonular, and posterior cortical types have also been reported with deficiency of the enzyme galactokinase,[152–154] the first enzyme in the galactose metabolic pathway (see Fig. 183–58). The mechanism of cataractogenesis is the same as that in the usual galactosemia, with accumulation of galactose and galactitol. The disease is also inherited as an autosomal recessive trait, in about the same incidence as the galactose-uridyl transferase defect. Bilateral cataracts occur in the first year of life, but systemic disease is usually absent, possibly because of the low accumulation of galactose-1-phosphate with decreased activation of the aldose reductase pathway. Heterozygotes are at increased risk for cataracts in the first year of life.[155]

DIABETES MELLITUS

Diabetes mellitus is a disease whose complex genetic and multifactorial etiology is beyond the scope of this short discussion. The usual cataract in these patients does not differ from senile cataract in its morphology but occurs 20 to 30 yr earlier than in normoglycemic patients. In juvenile diabetic patients a rare "snowflake" cataract may also develop, with superficial whitish vacuoles and snowflake opacities in the subcapsular region, rapidly progressing to a mature cataract. The pathogenesis of this more unique cataract has not been explained. The occurrence of a reversible swelling or early intumescent change in lenses of diabetic patients, causing "fluctuating myopia," is an important effect of significant hyperglycemia and may be the first sign of the disease. It is thought that accumulation in diabetic patients of the sugar alcohol sorbitol, an end product of glucose reduction by aldose reductase, exerts an osmotic effect in the lens cells, like galactitol in galactosemia. Pirie and Van Heyningen found that lenses from diabetic patients without cataracts had increased sugars and sugar alcohols, not detected in normal control subjects although present in cataractous lenses from both groups.[156] Some have questioned whether the level of sugar alcohols has osmotic significance in adult cataracts.[157]

Besides the role of sugar alcohols in these cataracts, current research is focusing increasingly on the stress hyperglycemia places on antioxidant pathways in the lens. The glycosylation of proteins, especially the crystallins, can cause oxidation of sulfhydryl groups, with abnormal cross-linking and aggregation of proteins.[158] Aldose reductase inhibitors can function additionally as free-radical–trapping agents, as well as increasing the availability of NADPH+, a cofactor for the antioxidant glutathione reductase. Reduced glutathione activity might be of importance also in glucose-6-phosphate dehydrogenase deficiency, another disease of carbohydrate metabolism that has been linked to cataractogenesis.[159]

Lysosomal Storage Diseases

These diseases result from deficiency of the lysosomal enzymes necessary for cellular metabolic functions and are transmitted as autosomal or X-linked recessive traits. They show lysosomal inclusions of characteristic though not necessarily diagnostic types in epithelial cells and/or fibroblasts and endothelial cells. When the inclusions occur in lens epithelial cells they are frequently responsible for a subtle anterior lens opacification, with or without changes in the posterior subcapsular-sutural area.

FABRY'S DISEASE

This X-linked recessive disease leads to the intracellular accumulation of neutral glycosphingolipids, especially trihexosyl ceramide in many ocular and systemic epithelial and endothelial cells, resulting from a defect in the lysosomal hydrolase α-galactosidase A.[160] This

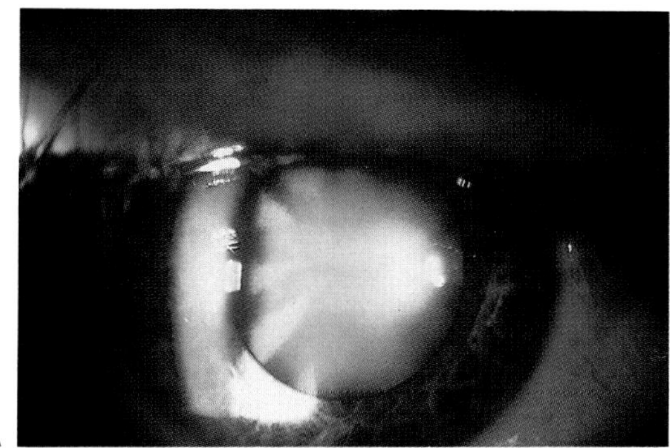
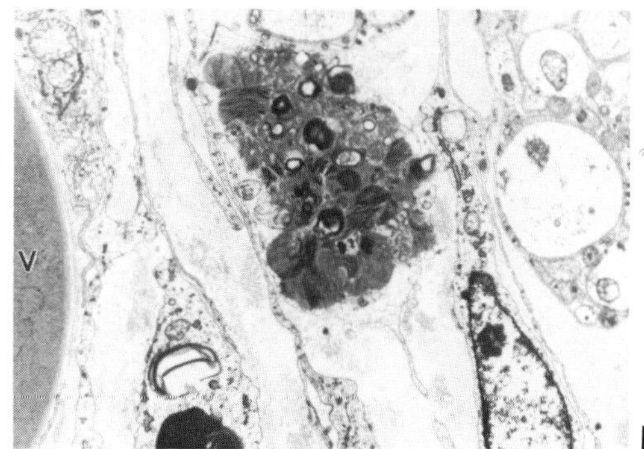

Figure 183–59. Fabry's disease. *A*, Broad wedges of anterior cortical stellate cataract in a male with Fabry's disease. *B*, Typical aggregate of laminated dense cytoplasmic inclusions in a vessel wall cell of the conjunctiva in Fabry's disease. (V, vessel.) (Courtesy of Dr. Alan Friedman.)

potentially fatal disease can cause renal failure and cardiovascular, gastrointestinal, and central nervous system disturbances as well as telangiectatic skin lesions (angiokeratomas), paresthesias, acral pain, and reduced sweating.

Corneal epithelial cell involvement produces the classic "vortex dystrophy" with which all other whorl-like corneal superficial opacities are compared. In 35 percent of hemizygotes (males) in one large series, the lens had granular fine or denser wedgelike opacities in the superficial capsular region anteriorly (Fig. 183–59*A*), and in 37 percent there were very fine, stellate sutural opacities under the capsule posteriorly.[161] In both cornea and anterior lens, the opacities are due to cytoplasmic aggregates of laminated dense material in lysosomal vacuoles of epithelial cells, which can be identified in conjunctival biopsies (see Fig. 183–59*B*),[162, 163] and are stainable by Sudan black B in paraffin sections. No inclusions have been seen in lens fiber cells, most of which lack lysosomes, so the posterior sutural opacities are unexplained. Female heterozygotes seldom show lens opacities, only 14 percent having posterior opacities in the aforementioned series, whereas 90 percent had vortex corneal deposits.[161] Examining the corneas in female members can be useful for identifying families at risk for this disease.

NIEMANN-PICK DISEASE TYPE A

Niemann-Pick disease type A is the only other sphingolipid storage disease having lens changes, consisting of subtle, brownish, anterior capsular opacification and later many small, white opacities posteriorly.[164] It is due to deficiency of sphingomyelinase, causing sphingomyelin to accumulate as laminated membranous inclusions in many cells, presumably including the lens epithelium. A cherry-red spot in the fovea is usually present in this disease.

MANNOSIDOSIS

Mannosidosis is a lysosomal storage disorder with a Hurler-like phenotype and mental retardation, due to α-mannosidase deficiency. It is transmitted as an autosomal recessive trait in two forms—a type I, with early fatality, and a less severe type II.[165, 166] Cataracts in the severe form resemble those in Fabry's disease, with posterior cortical spoke-shaped opacities. Type II has punctate cortical opacities. Conjunctival fibroblasts are a good biopsy source, showing the fibrogranular complex carbohydrate storage material in distended lysosomes.

MUCOLIPIDOSIS I

Mucolipidosis I also has a Hurler-like phenotype, due to deficiency of an acid neuraminidase enzyme.[167] Because this enzyme is necessary for sialic acid turnover in both mucopolysaccharides and gangliosides, there is considerable variability in the tissues affected. The only cataracts are posterior spokelike sutural opacities similar to those in Fabry's disease and mannosidosis. The lysosomal contents are clear, as in mucopolysaccharidoses, with few electron-dense lipid lamellae. Conjunctival epithelium, fibroblasts, and endothelial cells all contain this material, so conjunctival biopsies can be useful.

Myotonic Dystrophy

Cataract formation in myotonic dystrophy is an important feature of the syndrome, whose chief characteristic is slowness of contracted muscles to relax. Associated with it are ptosis, facial muscle weakness, frontal baldness and testicular atrophy in males, cardiac muscle conduction defects, atrophy of distal muscles of the limbs, and possible mental impairment.[168] Myotonic dystrophy is transmitted as an autosomal dominant disease, due to a defective gene on the long arm of chromosome 19, that encodes for a member of the protein kinase family.[169, 170] An unstable trinucleotide (triplet) repeat in the DNA of the gene leads to an increasing accumulation of these repeats. The gene thus is enlarged in subsequent generations, paralleling an increasing severity of the disease. Cataracts occur in almost all adults with myotonic dystrophy. Early the lens shows iridescent crystals in a zone deep to the anterior and posterior capsules, exhibiting especially green and red colors. A posterior subcapsular stellate cataract may then develop, followed by cortical vacuoles and clefts of a nonspecific type and finally complete opacification.

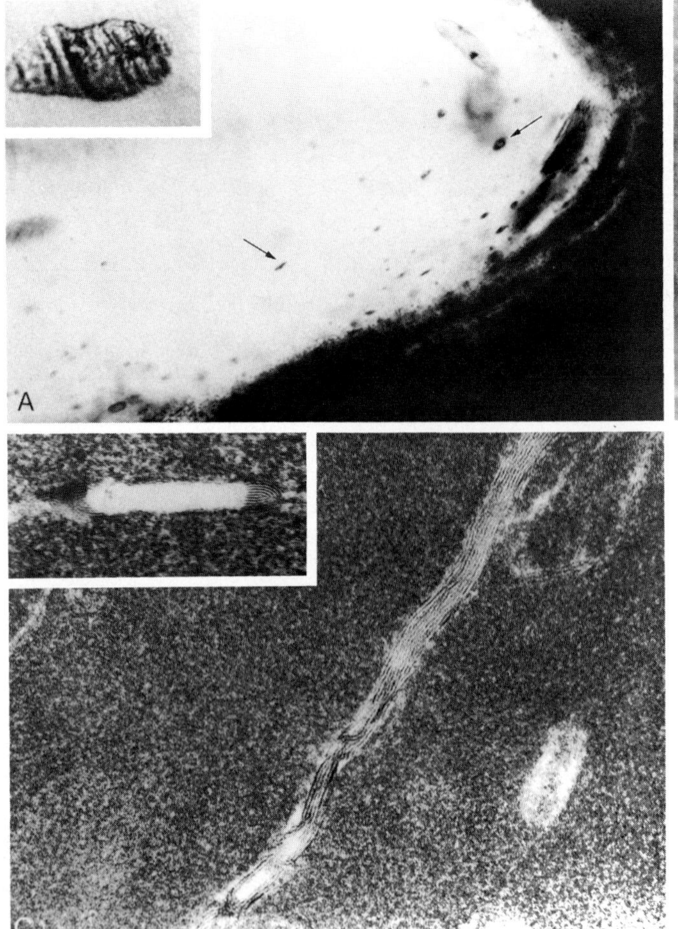

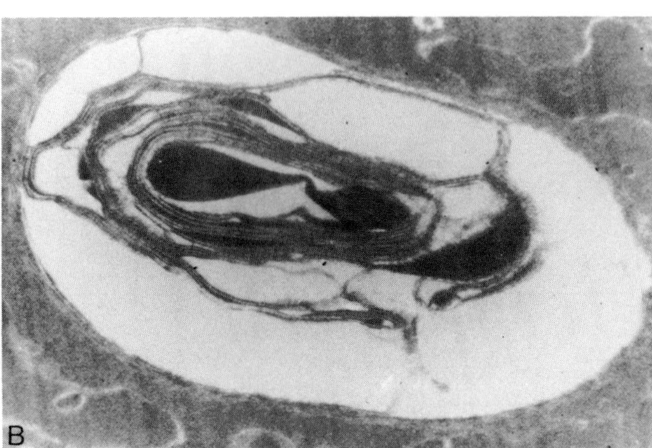

Figure 183–60. Myotonic dystrophy. *A,* Cross section through edge of lens with small "rice grain" diffuse cortical opacities (*arrows*). *Inset,* Spiral birefringence in one of the opacities under polarized light. ×110. *B,* Ultrastructural appearance of a typical small opacity, consisting of whorls of fine concentric membranes with enclosed dense material. ×12,500. *C,* Myelin figure-like splitting of lens fiber cell membranes. ×142,200. *Inset,* ×162,700. (From Dark AJ, Streeten BW: Ultrastructural study of cataract in myotonia dystrophica. Am J Ophthalmol 84:666, 1977. Reprinted with permission from the Ophthalmic Publishing Company.)

The iridescent crystals, when examined grossly, are 6 to 35 μm long, like small grains of rice, and show spiral birefringence (Fig. 183–60*A*).[171, 172] Ultrastructurally these bodies consist of vacuoles containing whorls of multilaminated electron-dense material whose laminae vary from 2 to 70 nm in width (see Fig. 183–60*B*). Other smaller linear aggregates of electron-dense membrane-like forms are frequent throughout the lens. Similar changes have been observed in extraocular[173] and other muscles, and in red cells in myotonic dystrophy. These changes are not specific, however, and can be seen to some extent among degenerating lens fibers in many nonmyotonic cataracts. The lens epithelial cells have changes commonly associated with chronic injury, such as cytoplasmic lipid droplets, mitochondrial vacuolization, and extension of cell processes into the preequatorial lens capsule with an increased number of capsular inclusions.

Hypoparathyroidism and Other Hypocalcemias

Hypocalcemia appears to underlie the cataract seen in hypoparathyroidism of all types, whether it develops after thyroid surgery or in patients unresponsive to the renal effects of parathyroid hormone (pseudohypoparathyroidism) or is of idiopathic etiology.[122c] Patients with pseudopseudohyperparathyroidism do not develop cataracts, as they have neither hypocalcemia nor hyperphosphatemia. Unlike the acute zonular cataract of tetany in childhood, the cataracts in these adult hypoparathyroidisms take many years to develop, such as an average of 11 years in postoperative hypoparathyroidism. They are commonest in the idiopathic type, in which Pohjola[174] found cataract reported in 58 percent of 118 cases. The lens opacities are usually small, white dots but can aggregate into larger flakes, often interspersed with angular iridescent crystals like those in myotonic dystrophy. An intumescent mature cataract can develop rapidly, especially after thyroid surgery. The histopathology is not specific,[122c] and no ultrastructure has been reported.

PRIMARY AND SECONDARY CATARACTOGENESIS IN HEREDITARY DISEASE

There are dozens of other syndromes of known or suspected genetic etiology in which some form of cataract has been described in an apparently related association, although seldom with characteristics specific to that syndrome. Extensive bibliographies of these associations are available,[175, 176a] and new examples are reported yearly. The commonest lens opacity in these often autosomal dominant hereditary diseases is the posterior subcapsular cataract. What is often difficult to determine is whether the cataract is due to the genetic defect or is secondary to local ocular changes. Discoveries such as expression of crystallins in nonocular cells are promising new avenues for understanding these associations.[68, 68a]

In a group of patients with pigmentary retinopathy, with and without involvement of other systems, Heckenlively[177] found posterior subcapsular cataracts (PSCs) in 41 percent. The highest frequency was in autosomal dominant retinitis pigmentosa (49 percent), and the lowest in the cone-rod degenerations (27 percent). He concluded that this relatively low frequency meant that the cataract was secondary rather than due to the genetic defect in these hereditary retinal degenerations. The highest frequency may actually be in gyrate atrophy, a retinal dystrophy not represented in his study, in which all patients may develop PSCs.[178]

Retinitis Pigmentosa

As indicated earlier, the pathogenesis of PSC in almost all these diseases is unclear. For example, in many kindreds with autosomal dominant retinitis pigmentosa the retinal defect has been traced to point mutations in the rhodopsin gene on the long arm of chromosome 3.[179] The affected patients often have PSCs, yet the rhodopsin gene is thought to be expressed exclusively in rod photoreceptors (Dr. Dryja, Verhoeff Society, 1991). Cataractogenesis here would appear to be a secondary phenomenon, possibly due to factors deriving from the degenerating retina. One such factor might be soluble toxic aldehydes from peroxidation of degenerating rod outer segment lipids, as postulated in the cataractogenesis accompanying hereditary retinal degeneration in the RCS rat.[180] Anterior subcapsular as well as posterior subcapsular cataracts have been reported in retinitis pigmentosa, without significant ultrastructural differences from other types.[181, 182]

Refsum's Disease

Either a direct or an indirect effect could be represented in Refsum's disease, in which about one third of cases have PSC along with pigmentary retinopathy, night blindness, cerebellar ataxia, peripheral neuropathy, skin lesions, and cardiac deposition of lipids.[176b] This complex syndrome is an autosomal recessive disorder due to absence of the peroxisomal α-hydroxylose necessary for oxidation and degradation of dietary phytanic acid. Accumulation of this branched-chain fatty acid results in lipid deposits in many organs and cells, including the ciliary pigment epithelium, which may also show cystic changes.[183, 184] Deposits have not been specifically mentioned in lens cells, but it is possible that they could express the defect.

Gyrate Atrophy of the Choroid and Retina

The association of PSC with autosomal dominant gyrate atrophy of the choroid and retina[178, 185] has more evidence for a direct effect. The mitochondrial enzyme ornithine aminotransferase, which is defective in this X-linked recessive disease, is expressed in normal lens epithelium[186] and presumably has a function in lens metabolism. The cataract has an early onset in the first decade, causing an opacification in the posterior axial region and spreading along the posterior sutures. Ultrastructurally there are posteriorly migrated epithelial cells, balloon cells, and overlying degeneration and liquefaction of lens fibers in the posterior pole and sutural areas.[178] The inner capsule shows a more unique general thickening by loose lamellar layers of basement membrane, seen to a much lesser extent in senile subcapsular cataracts,[107] and in retinitis pigmentosa.[182]

Stickler's Syndrome

The category of secondary effect seems very likely for the cataracts in the autosomal dominant Stickler syndrome (progressive arthroophthalmopathy).[187] The distinctive cataracts are more apt to be cortical wedges and flecks than PSCs and appear quite early. As one of the "empty vitreous" syndromes, Stickler's syndrome has a severe vitreoretinopathy and shows genetic linkage to the type II collagen molecule,[188] the main collagen of the vitreous. Since the lens does not contain type II collagen, the cataracts are likely to be secondary to the abnormal vitreous or accompanying retinal pathology, as high myopia and retinal detachment are common in this syndrome.

Neurofibromatosis Type II

A statistical linkage of PSC with neurofibromatosis type II and bilateral acoustic neuromas has been reported.[189] Given the young age of the patients and the absence of other intraocular disease, the cataracts may be due in some way to expression in the lens cells of the defective neurofibromatosis gene located on the long arm of chromosome 22. As noted by Kaiser-Kupfer and associates[189] the gene for β-2 lens crystallin is in the same area on this chromosome.

Cerebrotendinous Xanthomatosis

The autosomal recessive disease cerebrotendinous xanthomatosis has an incidence of cataract approaching 70 percent usually beginning in the second decade.[190, 191] Xanthomas occur at about the same time, affecting all tendons but especially thickening the Achilles tendon. Progressive cerebellar ataxia and dementia follow slowly. The disease appears to result from lack of a mitochondrial 26-hydroxylase, with incomplete degradation of cholestanol, a normal product of cholesterol metabolism. Cholesterol and cholestanol accumulate in almost every tissue, including the central nervous system, with elevated levels in the plasma. The cataracts are nuclear and cortical, sometimes described as zonular, with irregular white dots and whorls. Microscopy has shown cortical vacuoles with dispersed granular debris but no cholesterol crystals in either lens or iris.[191] This disease should be considered in all juvenile cataracts, as treatment with chenodeoxycholic acid is useful.[192]

CATARACT ASSOCIATED WITH DERMATOLOGIC DISEASE

Cataracts are frequently associated with diffuse dermatologic disease of genetic origin, such as the Rothman and Werner types of ectodermal dysplasia.[193, 194] It is tempting to attribute this association to the embryologic derivation of the lens from surface ectoderm, but the nature of these defects is currently unknown. Cataracts are also frequent with incontinentia pigmenti (Bloch-Sulzberger syndrome),[195] possibly secondary to the retinal detachment with massive gliosis that occurs in this condition. Patients with congenital ichthyosis, especially the X-linked type, may have associated congenital cataracts.[195] Atopic dermatitis is also suspected of having an association with cataract, but cataracts of all types have been attributed to this entity. Bilateral anterior subcapsular cataracts with onset between 15 and 30 years of age[195] may represent a true association.

CATARACT INDUCED BY DRUGS

Many drugs have been associated with the development of cataract, representing interference with lens metabolism by a number of different routes, which can only be touched upon here. The most significant ones today are the corticosteroids, owing to their frequent usage and the severe effect on central vision of the resulting PSC. In rheumatoid arthritis, 30 to 40 percent of patients receiving 10 mg of prednisone for 2 yr develop PSCs, and almost all will develop them if high doses are continued for 4 yr.[196] This effect is not related to patient age or specific disease, although it may occur earlier in young patients. As previously shown (see Fig. 183–35*D*), the meridional rows of the equatorial lens epithelial cells are markedly disorganized in these "steroid" cataracts. This abnormality of growth may be related to the presence of glucocorticoid receptors on lens cells, in addition to the evidence that they metabolize cortisol in vitro, suggesting that these agents could have a regulatory effect on growth and differentiation of lens cells.[197]

The topical miotic drugs, especially the anticholinesterases (echothiophate iodide, diisopropyl fluorophosphate), have been frequently indicted in cataractogenesis. In primates the early subcapsular vacuoles and opacities correlate with widened intercellular spaces, especially near sutures, some showing membranous debris ultrastructurally.[198] The superficial lens fibers are also swollen, indicating increased permeability, which appears to underlie the toxic effects of these drugs.

Intravitreally injected drugs, such as antibiotics, that have retinal toxicity are usually cataractogenic as well. Many drugs used for their antimitotic effects are also cataractogenic. Busulfan (Myleran), a radiomimetic drug, causes a typical PSC with posteriorly migrated epithelial cells.[199]

Two drugs introduced briefly for lowering cholesterol and for weight reduction were severely cataractogenic. Triparanol (MER-29) blocked the reduction of 24-dehydrocholesterol to cholesterol, leading to feathery radial cortical cataracts with accumulation of lipid complexes between the fibers.[200] Dinitrophenol, advanced for weight reduction, produced a toxic cataract that was difficult to reproduce in animals but was thought to result from interference with oxidative phosphorylation.[122d] As an example of the psychotropic group of drugs, phenothiazide (chlorpromazine) produces a very different anterior polar stellate cataract with deposition of a melanin-like pigment in the anterior subcapsular lens, the exact site not known, associated with skin, corneal, and conjunctival pigmentation.[201] Other photosensitizing drugs, such as psoralens, have the potential for seriously enhancing actinic photooxidation of lens fiber proteins.

CATARACT INDUCED BY RADIATION

The sources of electromagnetic radiation energy most important in damage to the lens are ionizing radiation (x-rays, gamma rays, and neutrons), emission of infrared or ultraviolet rays from various hot bodies, and microwave and shortwave diathermy radiation (Fig. 183–61).[202–204]

Ionizing radiation is one of the most potent cataractogenic agents known, and the lens is its most sensitive

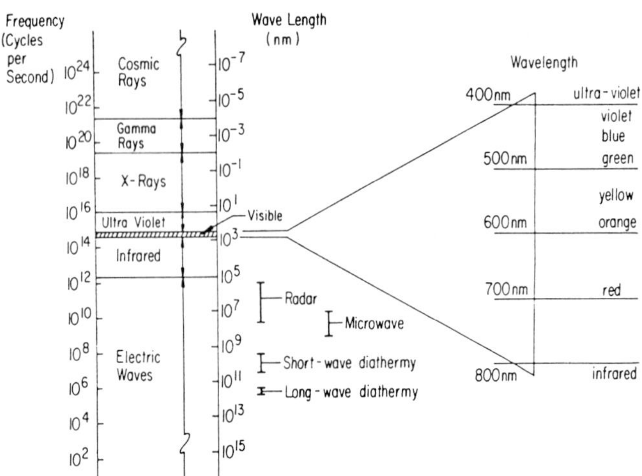

Figure 183–61. Electromagnetic spectrum. (From Klintworth GK, Landers MB III: The Eye: Structure and Function in Disease. © 1976, the Williams & Wilkins Co., Baltimore.)

target within the adult eye. Its damage is dose related and cumulative, and the pathologic effects are similar with all types. The first effect is on nuclei of cells in mitosis, which in the lens reside in the preequatorial zone of lens epithelium and are probably more susceptible in young eyes. During a delay period dependent on the dose and period of delivery there is an arrest of mitosis. When cell division resumes, there is considerable cellular pleomorphism and cell death, even affecting some of the previously resting cells when they attempt mitosis. Cells at the equatorial bow that should be forming new lens fibers become edematous, and many will migrate posteriorly to form a subcapsular cataract at the posterior pole,[106, 108] whose pathology does not differ from others of that type (see previous section on posterior subcapsular cataract). The minimum cataractogenic dose has been considered to be about 500 rad, but under some circumstances it may be as low as 200 rad.[202a] Damage to the DNA and cell membranes by free radical formation and oxidative reactions is a basic factor in this cataractogenesis.[204]

An important question long considered is whether actinic radiation by short-wavelength ultraviolet A and B rays is cataractogenic from usual daily doses, or whether it could be when combined with dietary or other deficiency of antioxidants.[116, 117] Such an effect would be due primarily to heat denaturation of lens proteins. At present there is mainly statistical evidence for this theory, from the incidence of cataract in different environments.

Lasers (light amplification by stimulated emission of radiation) as sources of intense, coherent, monochromatic radiation within the ultraviolet-infrared spectrum have found widespread use therapeutically in the eye because of their ability to produce controlled burns from absorption of the focused light beam. Lasers can cause cataracts when focused on the lens or from inadvertent heat transfer through the iris.[205] The resulting globular-granular lens fiber degeneration has no distinctive characteristics.

Microwave irradiation induces PSCs in experimental animals and humans when given in high or repeated dosages,[206, 207] but its potential for lens damage in small chronic dosage is unclear, as recently reviewed.[204] The mechanism of cataractogenesis is due in part to heat denaturation of antioxidants and probable thermoelastic expansion of the tissues.

CATARACT IN UVEITIS

As discussed earlier, secondary cataractogenesis is very common, owing to trauma, tumors, degenerative processes, retinal and corneal processes, and especially uveitis. In general, anterior inflammation and other injurious processes lead to anterior cataract, and posterior ones to posterior cataract. Concomitant long-term therapy with steroids may induce, in addition, a PSC, and glaucoma medications may be responsible for vacuolar-cortical cataract. Posterior synechiae are very commonly associated with underlying anterior subcapsular fibrous cataract.

These generalizations have many important exceptions. In Fuchs' heterochromic iridocyclitis,[208a, 209] a syndrome with mild iridocyclitis and cataract with or without glaucoma, the lens is usually completely free from posterior synechiae. Cataract is apt to occur quite early in this disease but is a posterior subcapsular type, suggesting that its etiology may be more related to the basic cause of the inflammation than to its localization.

It is likely that many factors are related to cataract development in uveitis, including the presence of inflammatory mediators, increasing lens cell permeability, nonphysiologic changes in the aqueous or vitreous, decreases in lens antioxidants, synechiae and membranes interfering with lens cell metabolism, and direct involvement of lens cells by an infectious or toxic agent.

INFLAMMATIONS OF THE LENS

Infectious Phakitis

The lens is not immune to infectious phakitis from bacterial or fungal agents or to viral infection, although only intrauterine direct viral infection, such as by rubella, is well documented. Parasitic infestation of the lens by intraocular worms has been reported rarely, usually attributed to a filaria.[208b] The lens capsule appears to be a barrier to invasion by most agents. The usual mechanism of infection is by penetrating trauma to the lens, but the capsule may also be digested by proteolytic enzymes released from bacteria and leukocytes. A lens abscess can result (Fig. 183–62), with eventual complete necrosis and absorption of the cortex, and the nucleus as well in younger eyes.

Lens-Induced Inflammations

The concept that the lens is responsible for inducing specific intraocular inflammations is widely accepted. Understanding these reactions depends on knowledge, still incomplete, of which lens proteins or protein fragments are immunogenic and what the tolerance level is for them in normal and pathologic eyes. The minor degree of inflammation following extracapsular cataract extractions and protein leakage in phacolytic glaucoma

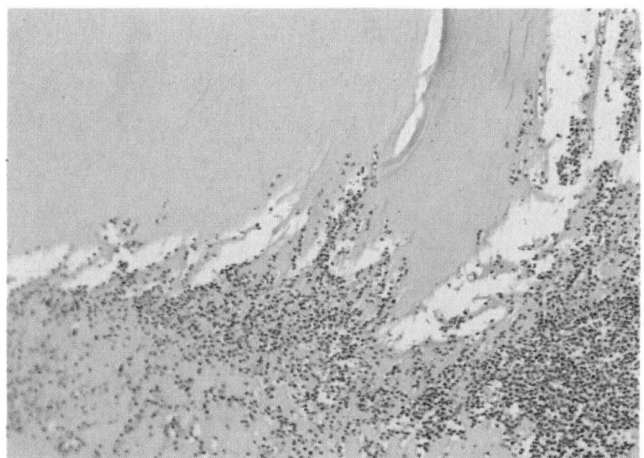

Figure 183–62. Lens abscess among the fraying lens cortical fibers from a metastatic bacterial endophthalmitis. H&E, ×33.

indicates that lens material enjoys considerable immunologic tolerance, in spite of limited exposure to cells of the immune system. Yet circulating antibodies to lens proteins have been found in patients with uveitis, and even in normal individuals as reviewed by Rahi and Garner.[211] Still largely unexplored is the possibility of a genetic basis for individual heightened reactivity to lens antigens.

PHACOLYTIC GLAUCOMA

In the presence of a hypermature cataract with advanced liquefaction of the cortex (Fig. 183–63*A*), an acute elevation of intraocular pressure can occur with aqueous flare, cells and white particles sometimes giving the appearance of hypopyon, in a process called phacolytic glaucoma.[212] Macrophages are the only inflammatory cells in this reaction, phagocytosing fine eosinophilic material similar to the liquefied cortex still within the capsule. Macrophages apparently swollen with denatured lens protein that leaked through the capsule are seen on the anterior lens and iris surface, in the iris stroma, the chamber angle, and trabecular meshwork (see Fig. 183–63*B*). These macrophages can be recognized in diagnostic anterior chamber aspirates.[213]

The cause of the glaucoma has been an intriguing question, with most favoring the predominant role of macrophages in clogging the trabecular spaces or macrophages and increased protein.[212] Epstein, Jedziniak, and Grant[214] found high molecular weight protein aggregates (greater than 150×10^6) in the aqueous and liquefying cortex in phacolytic glaucoma, not present in immature cataractous lenses, and also showed that this quantity of high molecular weight protein was sufficient to obstruct aqueous outflow.[215] The size of the aggregates and perhaps their type must be of special significance, as macrophages containing such material have been noted in the aqueous of young patients in the second week after needling of cataracts, but were not associated

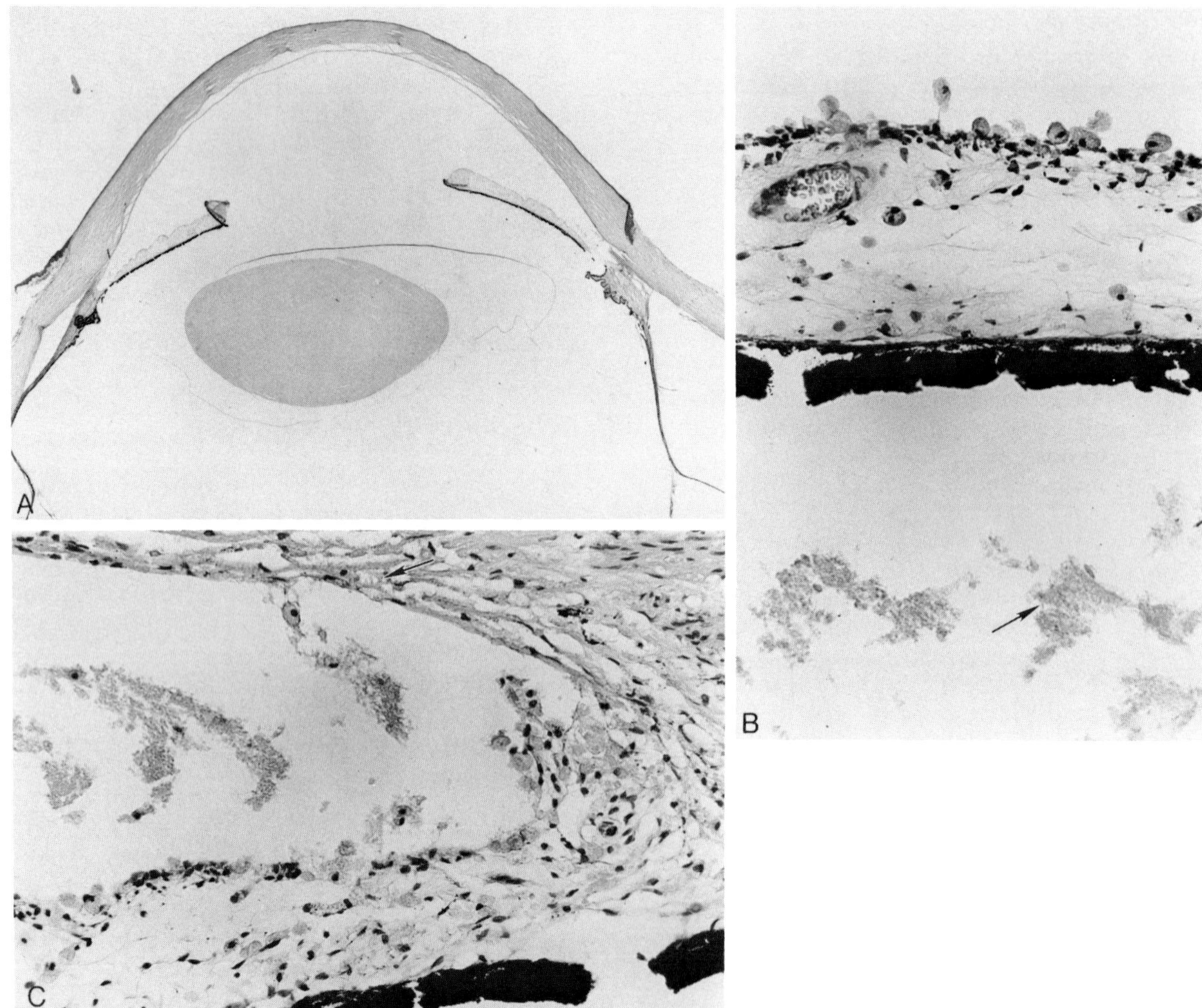

Figure 183–63. Phacolytic glaucoma. *A,* Morgagnian cataract with thin, though intact, capsule and remaining lens nucleus in an elderly patient with phacolytic glaucoma. Some granular material just visible within the lens capsule and angle of the anterior chamber. *B,* Macrophages containing granular lens material in phacolytic glaucoma. Aggregates of lens protein are present in the posterior chamber *(arrow).* H&E. ×310. *C,* Lens protein aggregates in angle and trabecular spaces *(arrow),* being phagocytosed by macrophages. H&E, ×310.

with glaucoma.[216] Gamma crystallin appears to be especially chemotactic for macrophages, even in normal lenses, and is much less chemotactic for polymorphonuclear leukocytes.[217]

In one study of 125 eyes removed for phacolytic glaucoma, 24 percent had histopathologic evidence of contusion angle deformity,[218] and many had a history of trauma. Since there is often a long delay in removal of traumatic cataracts, the degree of protein breakdown in these lenses may be unusually advanced, favoring both protein leakage from the capsule and high molecular weight protein aggregation.

PHACOANAPHYLACTIC ENDOPHTHALMITIS

The severe inflammatory reaction in phacoanaphylactic endophthalmitis stands in dramatic contrast with that in phacolytic glaucoma, in which the immune system is not involved. Verhoeff and Lemoine's choice of the term "phakoanaphylactica" in 1922[219] recognized the autoallergic nature of this inflammation, but they could not know that both B- and T-cell components of the immune system are involved in this lens reaction, rather than just the IgE and complement of anaphylaxis.

The lens capsule is always found to be ruptured in phacoanaphylactic endophthalmitis. Usually the rupture has an obvious origin from external or surgical traumatic perforation (Fig. 183–64*A*), but it may follow spontaneous rupture of the capsule or rare causes, such as capsular dissolution by tumor.[220] Phacoanaphylaxis can also be a bilateral disease, affecting a previously normal lens in the second eye. It has been reported in about 25 percent of eyes removed for sympathetic uveitis, with histopathologic confirmation in either the exciting or the sympathizing eye, or both.[221, 222] Explanation of the capsular rupture in the second eye is only conjectural, but it might be spontaneous, secondary to a hypermature

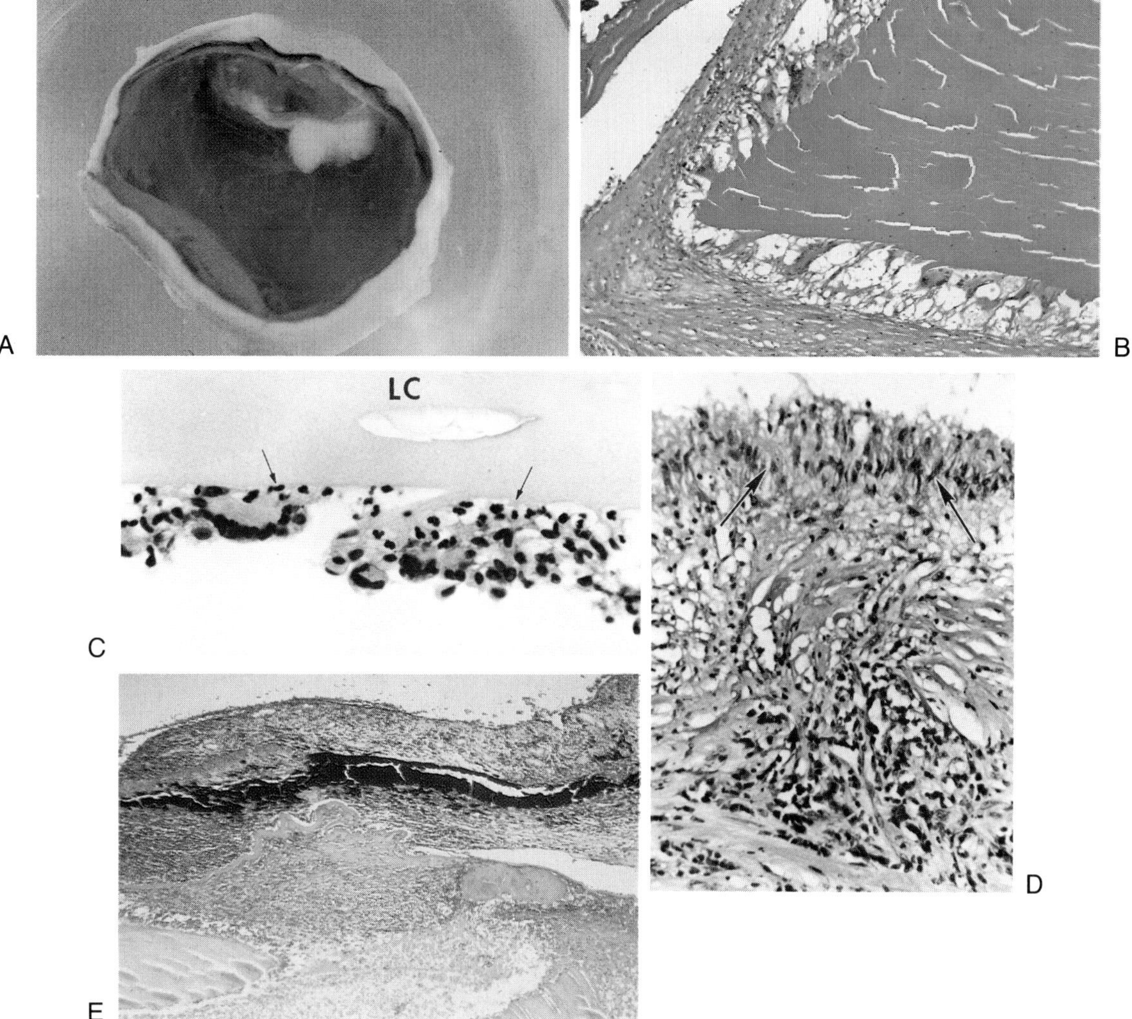

Figure 183–64. Phacoanaphylactic endophthalmitis. *A,* Suppurative and granulomatous reaction surrounding lens capsule. Nucleus has slipped out of capsule and lies over the pars plana on the left. *B,* Granulomatous inflammation around a lens remnant. H&E, ×33. *C,* Inner zone of reaction showing polymorphonuclear cells *(arrows)* closely attached to fraying cortex (LC) with surrounding giant cells. H&E, ×520. *D,* Second zone is a ring of marginated epithelioid cells *(arrows)* and granulation tissue with lymphocytes and plasma cells in the outermost third ring of the zonal reaction. H&E, ×240. *E,* Severe iritis overlying the site of spontaneous lens capsule rupture, producing phacoanaphylaxis. H&E, ×33.

cataract complicating the sympathetic inflammation, or due to direct attack on the capsule by sensitized leukocytes. A less severe granulomatous lens reaction has been described in some eyes with ruptured lens capsule due to PHPV[95, 96] (see earlier section on persistent hyperplastic primary vitreous).

Phacoanaphylactic endophthalmitis is usually a severe granulomatous inflammation with mutton-fat keratic precipitates. Fibrin and pupillary membrane may obscure the lens involvement, so it is often an unexpected diagnosis, made by the pathologist after enucleation. In some suspected cases, however, the diagnosis can be made by finding lens material or giant cells in aspirates of aqueous or vitreous.[213]

The histopathologic reaction is a classic granulomatous one, with a zonal distribution (see Fig. 183–64*B*). The innermost zone shows polymorphonuclear leukocytes adjacent to the fraying and necrotic lens fibers (see Fig. 183–64*C*). In an outer, second zone are marginating epithelioid cells, giant cells, and granulation tissue (see Fig. 183–64*D*). The most peripheral, third zone has lymphocytes, plasma cells, and sometimes eosinophils. This third zone will lie in whatever tissue is closest to the inciting lens material. Since this is usually the iris, the presence of a heavy lymphocytic and plasma cell iris infiltrate adjacent to the lens capsule is suggestive of a phacoanaphylactic reaction (see Fig. 183–64*D*). The finding of even a few inflammatory cells within the lens is clear evidence that the capsule is ruptured somewhere, and further sections must be made to find the rupture site, which is often quite small.

The presence of polymorphonuclear leukocytes as the forward troops among the swollen and disintegrating lens fibers suggests that they have been attracted by complement-fixing immune complexes of lens antigens and specific antibodies, and that their enzymes are involved in the lens fiber necrosis (type III hypersensitivity). Besides this evidence of humoral hypersensitivity, and the plentiful plasma cells (B cells), the characteristic granulomatous response indicates T-cell activation, resulting in a typical complex immunologic disease process.

Experimental evidence strongly supports the possibility of a mixed immunologic response to lens antigens in this process. Marak and associates[223, 224] produced an experimental lens-induced granulomatous endophthalmitis (ELGE) in the rat by rupturing the lens capsule of animals previously sensitized to lens proteins. The disease could be passively transferred by serum from sensitized rats. Deficiency of C3 during sensitization gave a much lower rate of ELGE induction, showing that B cells and type III hypersensitivity were involved. Rahe, Misra, and Morgan[225] and Marak and colleagues[224] hypothesize that tolerance for len proteins at the T-cell level may be bypassed or overwhelmed in this disease, or that suppressor T-cell function is reduced. The infrequency of the disease and its sometime association with another uncommon immunologic disease, sympathetic uveitis, suggest an additional genetic factor in susceptibility to this disease.

The term "phacotoxic" endophthalmitis was suggested by Irvine and Irvine[226] for a nongranulomatous inflammation appearing to be centered around an intact lens but having a primarily plasma cell and lymphocytic response. There has been no proof of a relation to the lens in these cases. No further comment can be made about the spectrum of lens-induced inflammations until specific lens antigens have been investigated for an ability to produce differing inflammatory responses.

LENS-INDUCED GLAUCOMA

Besides the infrequent occurrence of phacolytic glaucoma due to blockage of aqueous outflow by lens proteins and macrophages from a hypermature lens, the lens may be an indirect cause of glaucoma when inflammatory posterior synechiae completely obstruct the pupil. A relative pupillary block is a frequent development in elderly patients with shallow anterior chambers, as the lens thickens during cataractogenesis, causing a narrow-angle glaucoma. The same process may occur earlier in patients with high hyperopia and small eyes, during growth of a normal-sized lens. It is a more predictable occurrence in eyes with microphthalmia, or nanophthalmia (globes with anteroposterior diameters of 19.5 mm or less). An intumescent lens complicating a traumatic injury is a frequent cause of glaucoma. Subluxed or dislocated lenses may also cause pupillary block, most frequently when luxated into the anterior chamber.

EXFOLIATION OF THE LENS CAPSULE

Glass Blower's Capsular Delamination ("True" Exfoliation)

Delamination, or peeling, of the central anterior lens capsule in sheetlike lamellae was described by Elschnig in glass blowers in 1922.[227] The tanks of molten glass they worked with reached temperatures up to 1500°C, giving off thermal radiation rich in infrared rays, with much less ultraviolet. Capsular peeling and a frequent PSC were thought to require several decades of such exposure.[202b] Fortunately this occupational thermal injury has been virtually eliminated by the use of protective goggles.

By histopathology the peeling capsule showed a splitting of the outer layers, involving in some cases up to a third of the capsule thickness. The separated lamellae retained their PAS positivity.[228] Ultrastructurally there was a simple splitting between the looser superficial capsular layers and the deeper more laminated ones.[229] This process was originally called capsular exfoliation, later renamed "true" exfoliation by Dvorak-Theobald to distinguish it from "pseudoexfoliation," a name which she also coined.[230]

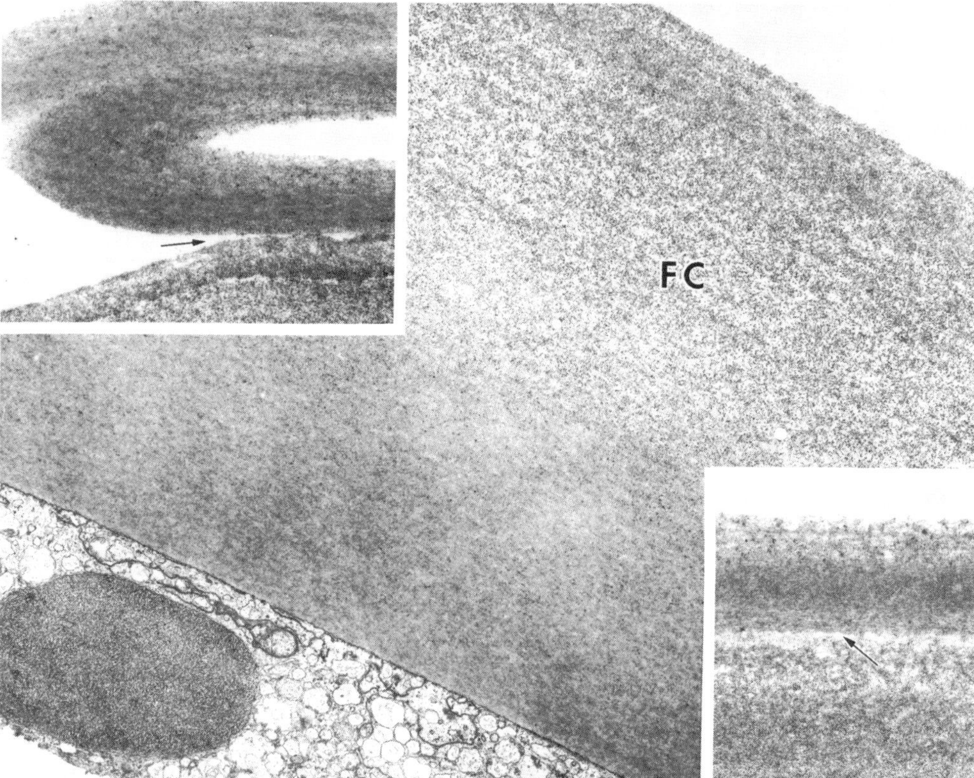

Figure 183–65. Spontaneous peeling of the lens capsule. Inner third of a peeling lens capsule appears normal, but outer half is rarefied and coarsely fibrillar (FC), with superficial layers of varying density. ×7,640. *Upper Inset,* A thick superficial layer has separated *(arrow)* and lies folded on the lens capsule. ×7,320. *Lower Inset,* Another thick lamella shows early splitting *(arrow)* in an adjacent area. ×8,480.

Idiopathic Capsular Peeling (Exfoliation)

Peeling of the anterior lens capsule into delicate membranes, long strands, or blebs has been reported in elderly persons several times in recent years.[231–233] Where examined, the peeled lamellae had normal PAS positivity, as in glass blower's delamination. In a specimen the author studied ultrastructurally, the splitting occurred superficially within an abnormal coarsely fibrillar area involving the outer two thirds of the lens capsule (Fig. 183–65). The opposite lens in one reported patient had exfoliative material on its surface,[232] so it is possible that isolated capsular peeling, in at least some cases, is related to the pseudoexfoliation syndrome.

Pseudoexfoliation of the Lens Capsule (Senile Exfoliation, Fibrillopathia Epitheliocapsularis, Exfoliation Syndrome, Basement Membrane Exfoliation Syndrome, Pseudoexfoliative Fibrillopathy)

Pseudoexfoliation of the lens capsule, a much commoner process than the isolated capsular peeling described earlier, was first noted in 1917 by Lindberg in Finland and was later reported in more complete detail by Vogt.[234] It was named for the accumulation of small, white aggregates visible clinically on the lens capsule, pupillary edge, and other anterior segment structures, thought by Dvorak-Theobald[230] to be deposited on the structures rather than exfoliating from them. Peeling of the superficial lens capsule has, however, been shown ultrastructurally in recent years,[235–237] and the search for a more felicitous and definitive name continues. This disease has a significant association (40 to 60 percent) with open-angle glaucoma ("capsular glaucoma"). Cataract is seen in about 40 percent of affected eyes.[238] Pseudoexfoliation has been found in all racial groups, although it is almost absent in the Eskimo, with a frequency varying in most areas from 4 to 6 percent in patients older than 60 years of age, as reviewed by Forsius.[239] Much higher frequencies are reported among northern Scandinavians, Saudi Arabians, Navaho Indians, and Australian aborigines, varying from 8 to 35 percent in individuals in these populations older than 70 years of age. Distribution is approximately equal in males and females. It is unilateral in about 50 percent of cases, and the condition progressed to bilaterality in 13 percent of patients in one long-term study.[238]

The earliest clinical sign of pseudoexfoliation appears to be a subtle, grayish opacification of the anterior capsule out to the level of the anterior zonular insertion, sometimes showing radial striations correlating with the folds on the posterior iris.[240, 241] Erosions develop in the paracentral (intermediate) region of this opacified cap-

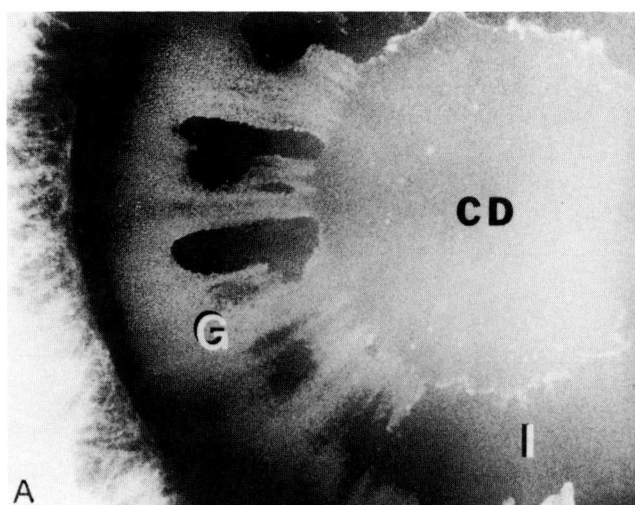

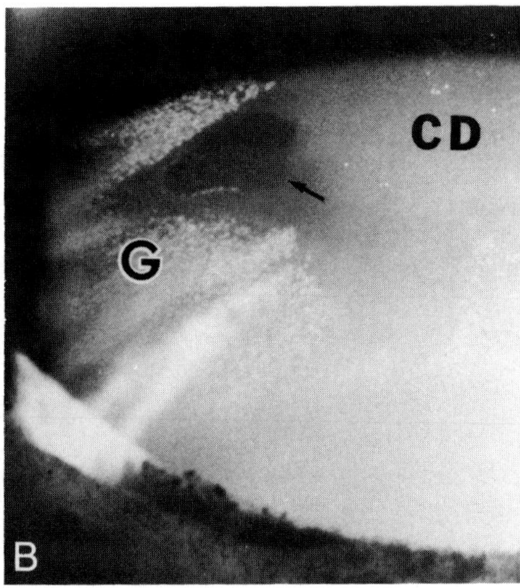

Figure 183–66. *A,* Typical pseudoexfoliation of the lens capsule with peripheral white granular zone (G), large eroded intermediate zone (I), and central disc (CD), with edges peeling inward. *B,* Prominent peripheral granulations in another pseudoexfoliative lens. Early intermediate zone erosion *(arrow).* (From Dark AJ, Streeten BW: Precapsular film on the aging lens capsule. Precursor of pseudoexfoliation? Br J Ophthalmol 74:717, 1990.)

sule, and tiny, whitish vegetations appear anterior to the zonular insertion (Fig. 183–66). Eventually a disc of mild opacification is left centrally with edges peeling inward, and a lateral margin peeling outward. White dandruff-like material is also seen on this central disc, the zonular fibers, anterior hyaloid membrane, pupillary and anterior iris, trabecula, and infrequently the cornea, and by cycloscopy[242] on the ciliary processes.

By histopathology, as recently reviewed,[243, 244] pseudoexfoliative material on all surfaces appears as bushlike eosinophilic excrescences (Fig. 183–67*A*). The iris pigment epithelium has a saw-tooth, clumped appearance and sheds its pigment easily (see Fig. 183–67*B*), and aggregates may appear on both iris surfaces (see Fig. 183–67*C*). The lens capsule shows a change unique to this disease in the preequatorial germinative zone, where a layer of abnormal fibrogranular material with the same staining characteristics as the vegetations is added to the deep capsule.[245, 246] It appears first in patches (see Fig. 183–67*A, middle*),[247] becoming a thick confluent layer as the disease advances. Ultrastructurally in all sites the aggregates of this fibrillopathy are composed of fibers 15 to 40 nm in diameter, appearing to be composites of finer subunits (Fig. 183–68). Cross-banding at 20 to 25 nm and 45 to 50 nm extends beyond the margins of the fibers, seen more clearly in thinner (type A) fibers (see Fig. 183–68*A*) but obscured by granular material in thicker (type B) fibers (see Fig. 183–68*B*).[248]

Additional sites of pseudoexfoliative material have been reported in the stroma and vascular walls of the iris, sometimes completely occluding these vessels, and throughout the trabecular tissues (see reviews).[243, 244, 249] Extrabulbar sites were first noted in the conjunctiva,[250] later in the walls of posterior ciliary arteries,[251] in multiple skin sites[248] (Fig. 183–69), skin sites[248] (Fig. 183–69), orbital tissues,[252] and most recently in several visceral organs (lung, heart, liver, kidney, and gall-bladder), and meninges.[252a, 252b] These localizations are strong evidence that pseudoexfoliation is a systemic disease, whose extent has not yet been fully explored. Since the fibrillopathy has been shown in the conjunctiva of some glaucoma patients without lens exfoliation in either eye,[253] its true frequency is currently indeterminate.

The nature of this fibrillopathy and its causation are still unclear. The abnormal material shows histochemical and immunopositivity for elastic system microfibrils, like the ocular zonular fibers.[254–256] Epitopes are present for other proteins characteristic of elastic tissue—amyloid P protein, elastin, and the adhesion protein vitronectin,[257–259] and digestion studies show chondroitin sulfate and hyalonate.[260] Positive immunoreactions for the basement membrane components heparan sulfate,[261] laminin,[262] and nidogen/entactin have been reported, and several extrinsic components have been seen in some basement membranes, including chondroitin sulfate, fibronectin and amyloid P protein.[263]

It is suggested that pseudoexfoliative material is an amyloid,[264] an abnormal basement membrane,[251] degenerated zonules,[265, 266] or an abnormality of matrix synthesis with aberrant expression particularly for elastic components.[267] In the skin and conjunctiva it is closely associated with elastotic degenerative material, suggesting that it might be a type of elastosis involving primarily the microfibrils.[248, 267] An abnormal matrix or serum molecule has not been ruled out in this disease.

A hereditary basis for pseudoexfoliation has been strongly suspected, although transmission across generations has been documented infrequently. The disease has been reported in identical twins.[268] Environmental factors have also been considered, especially cumulative exposure to actinic radiation,[269] as well as slow virus infection or other immunologic process.[270]

The most important known complication of pseudoexfoliative fibrillopathy is an open-angle glaucoma, usually occurring in the same eye as the pseudoexfoliative aggregates. In the United States, 20 percent of patients have glaucoma or ocular hypertension when first seen, and 15 percent develop elevated pressure within 10

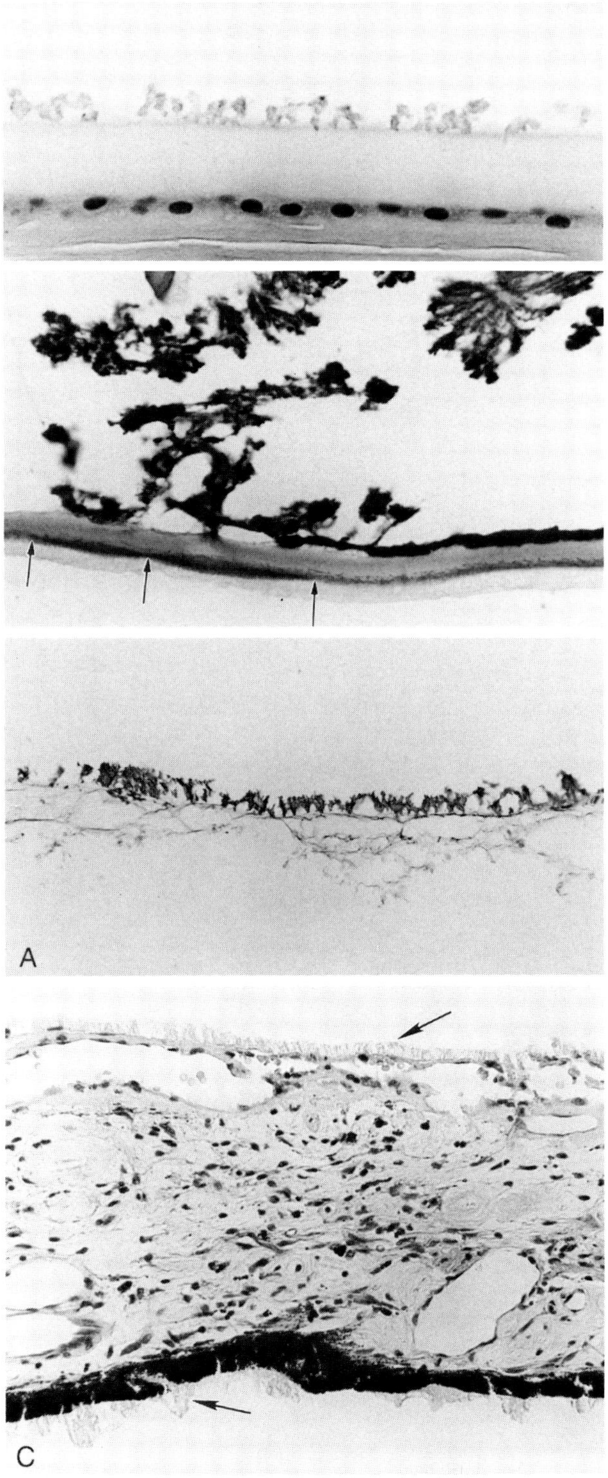

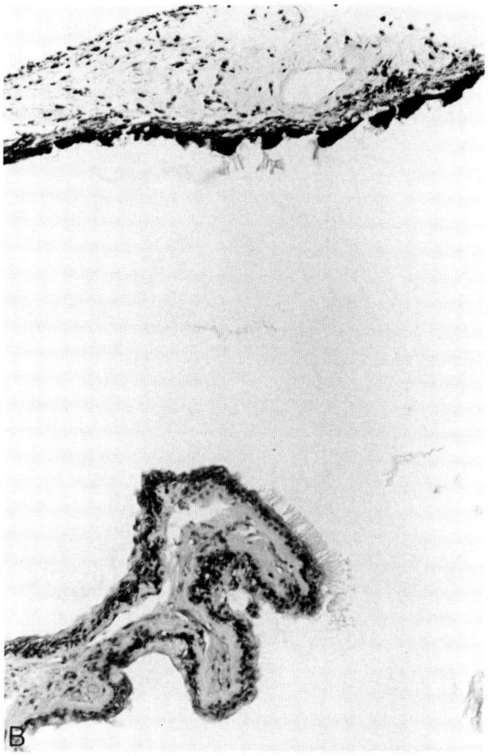

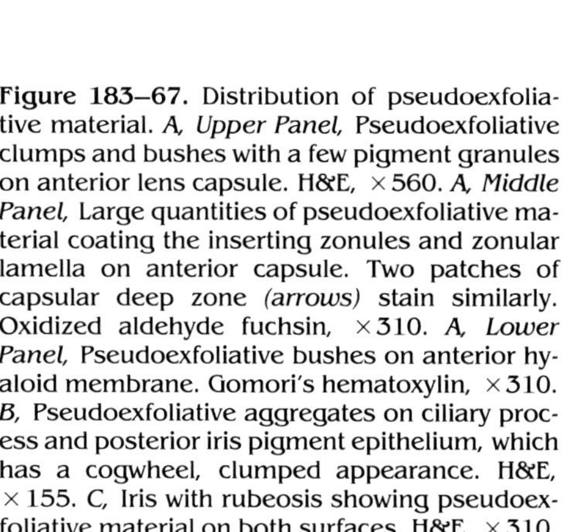

Figure 183–67. Distribution of pseudoexfoliative material. *A, Upper Panel,* Pseudoexfoliative clumps and bushes with a few pigment granules on anterior lens capsule. H&E, ×560. *A, Middle Panel,* Large quantities of pseudoexfoliative material coating the inserting zonules and zonular lamella on anterior capsule. Two patches of capsular deep zone *(arrows)* stain similarly. Oxidized aldehyde fuchsin, ×310. *A, Lower Panel,* Pseudoexfoliative bushes on anterior hyaloid membrane. Gomori's hematoxylin, ×310. *B,* Pseudoexfoliative aggregates on ciliary process and posterior iris pigment epithelium, which has a cogwheel, clumped appearance. H&E, ×155. *C,* Iris with rubeosis showing pseudoexfoliative material on both surfaces. H&E, ×310.

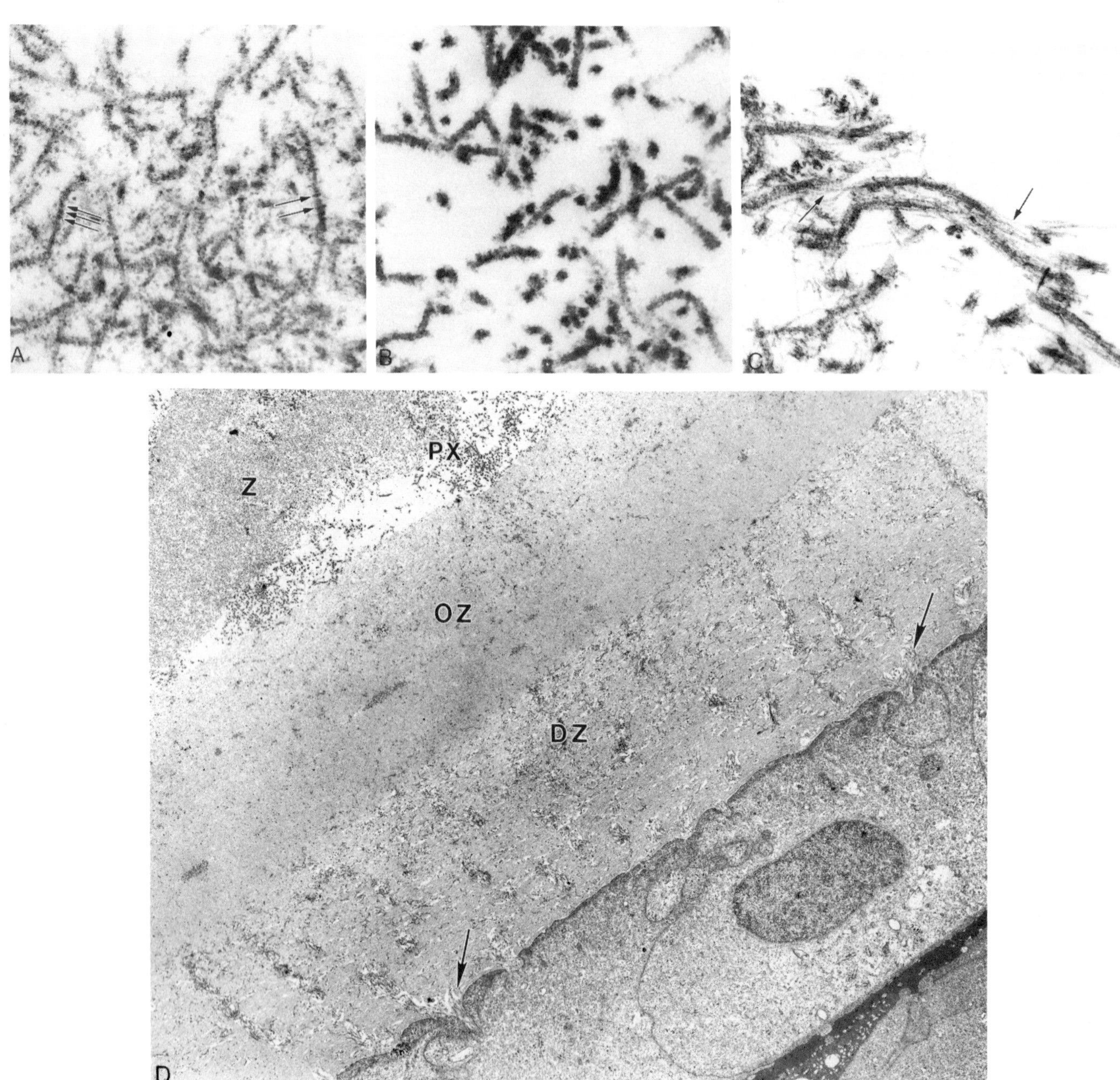

Figure 183–68. Ultrastructure of pseudoexfoliative fibrillopathy on the lens capsule. *A,* Typical thin pseudoexfoliative fibers showing both 50-nm *(double arrows)* and 25-nm *(triple arrows)* banding. ×62,500. *B,* Thicker, fuzzy fibers with banding obscured. ×62,500. *C,* High-power view of pseudoexfoliative fibers shows that they are composed of several subunits bound together by denser material. Microperiodicity visible in some fibrils *(arrow).* ×76,300. *D,* Midperipheral lens capsule has two zones, an outer more normal zone (OZ) and a deep zone (DZ) with sprays of abnormal fibrils extending out from pits in the epithelium *(arrows).* Pseudoexfoliative fibers (PX) under zonule (Z). ×6,540.

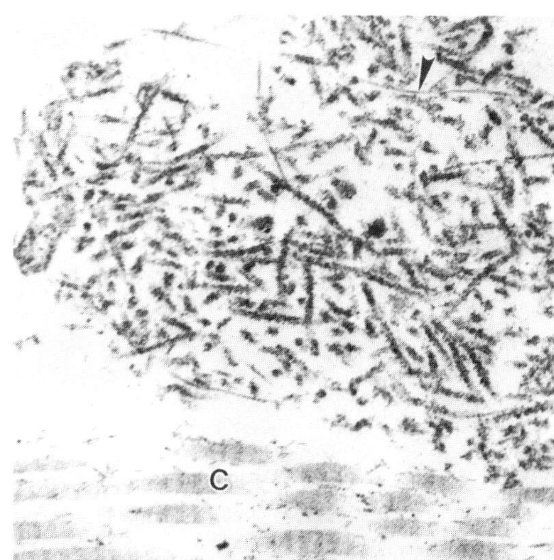

Figure 183–69. Pseudoexfoliative fibrillopathy in the retroauricular skin. Elastic microfibrils *(arrowhead)* course through the nodule. Collagen fibers below (C). ×47,500.

years.[271] Patients with pseudoexfoliative disease are not steroid "responders," unlike patients with chronic open-angle glaucoma. The glaucoma thus appears to be secondary, due to accumulation of pseudoexfoliative material and uveal pigment in the outflow pathways. The material may also be synthesized or processed by the trabecular endothelial cells.

DISLOCATION OF THE LENS

The lens is described as dislocated or luxated when it lies completely outside the lens patellar fossa, in the anterior chamber, the vitreous, or directly on the retina. Zonular and vitreal attachments to the lens capsule must be completely severed for posterior luxation, but a few attachments may still be present in an anteriorly luxated lens, especially if it is a small lens, which can pop back and forth with dilatation of the pupil. The lens is said to be subluxed or partially dislocated when it is still within the lens space, with some zonular fibers and/or Wieger's vitreal ligament attached to restrict completely free movement.

Traumatic Dislocation

The commonest cause of lens subluxation-luxation in most large series has been trauma,[272, 273] although the frequency varies from 22 to 50 percent in different samples (Table 183–2). It usually follows penetrating wounds or severe contusive injury and is often associated with cataract and rhegmatogenous retinal detachment (Fig. 183–70). The site of zonular breakage is not known but presumably would be at their lens attachments, as in intracapsular cataract extraction (Fig. 183–71).[274] The glaucoma liable to occur in these traumatic dislocations is usually due to hemorrhage early and to contusion angle deformity (angle recession) or synechiae later. In many eyes with dislocated lenses and glaucoma, injury appears to cause an earlier onset of primary open-angle

Table 183–2. CAUSES OF LENS DISLOCATION

Cause	
Trauma, Perforating and Nonperforating	
Secondary to Ocular Processes ("Consecutive")	
Staphylomas, ectasias	
Buphthalmias	
High myopia	
Hypermature cataract	
Syphilis, chronic uveitis	
Perforated corneal ulcer	
Displacement by tumors or contracting scars	
Unknown Etiology, Possibly Hereditary	
Pseudoexfoliation syndrome	
Primary Hereditary Systemic Disease	**Hereditary**
Marfan's syndrome, inherited	AD
Marfan variants	AD
Congenital contractual arachnodactyly	
Asymmetric Marfan's syndrome	
Homocystinuria	AR
Weill-Marchesani (brachymorphia-spherophakia)	AR, AD
Dominant spherophakia (McGavic type)	AD
Simple ectopia lentis et pupillae	AR
Hyperlysinemia	AR
Sulfite oxidase deficiency	AR
Primary Hereditary Systemic Disease, Infrequently Associated with Ectopia Lentis	
Aniridia with microcornea	Oxycephaly
Conradi's syndrome	Pfaundler syndrome
Crouzon's disease	Pierre Robin syndrome
Dominantly inherited blepharoptosis, high myopia and ectopia lentis	Proportional dwarfism and ectopia lentis
Ehler-Danlos syndrome	Refsum's syndrome
Familial pseudomarfanism	Retinitis pigmentosa
Kniest syndrome	Sprengel's deformity
Mandibulofacial dysostosis	Sturge-Weber syndrome
Megalophthalmos	Wildervanck's syndrome

AD, Autosomal dominant; AR, autosomal recessive.

glaucoma. The lens may be displaced more slowly by masses in the vicinity, such as iris or ciliary body cysts or tumors (see Fig. 183–58).

Inflammation and Lens Dislocation

There is little evidence for inflammation as a frequent cause of lens dislocation, perhaps because zonular fibers are not susceptible to collagenase and have limited

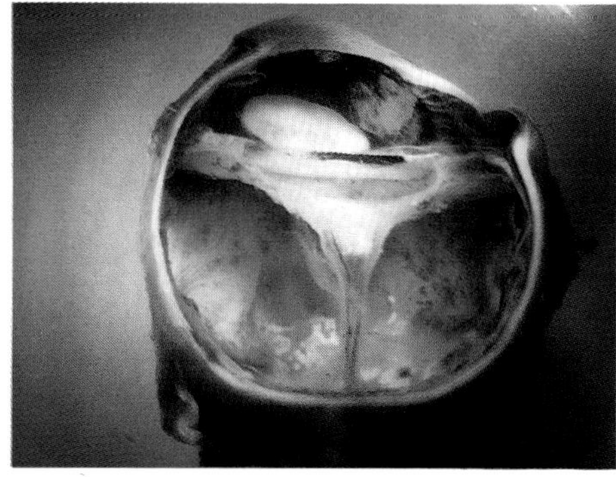

Figure 183–70. Cataractous lens lying free on an organized anterior hyaloid (cyclitic) membrane following old contusion injury. No zonular fibers remain. The retina is completely detached, and the choroid shows evidence of old postcontusion pigmentary degeneration. A small staphyloma is seen at the temporal equator.

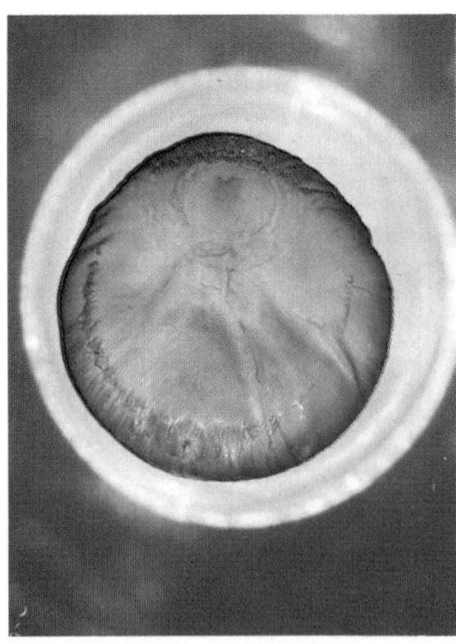

Figure 183–71. A lens removed by intracapsular cataract extraction (cryoprobe mark superiorly). The only zonules remaining are some tips at the anterior insertion and a few meridionals around the equator. Gomori's hematoxylin stain.

susceptibility to the elastase commonly released in inflammation but instead are most susceptible to tryptic enzymes.[275] Two studies reported a high frequency of positive serology for syphilis in patients with traumatic dislocated lenses,[276, 277] which was not confirmed in another well-controlled study.[278] The issue remains unresolved.

Pseudoexfoliative Disease and Lens Dislocation

Pseudoexfoliative disease is an important cause of lens subluxation, occurring spontaneously in as many as 5 percent of these patients,[279, 280] although it is often occult until the time of cataract extraction. Iridodonesis, usually a subtle sign of subluxation, may be absent because the iris is relatively immobile from deposits of pseudoexfoliative material in its stroma and muscle, or because of posterior synechiae to the midzone of the lens.[281] In some cases a tremulousness of the lens may be seen during movement (phacodonesis). The zonules tend to break in midstream or at the ciliary body, so their stublike broken ends wave during movement[280] and are extensively infiltrated with pseudoexfoliative material (Fig. 183–72). Their fragility is reflected in a higher frequency of zonular dehiscences and lens subluxation, with a five times higher frequency of vitreous loss during extracapsular cataract extraction.[282–284]

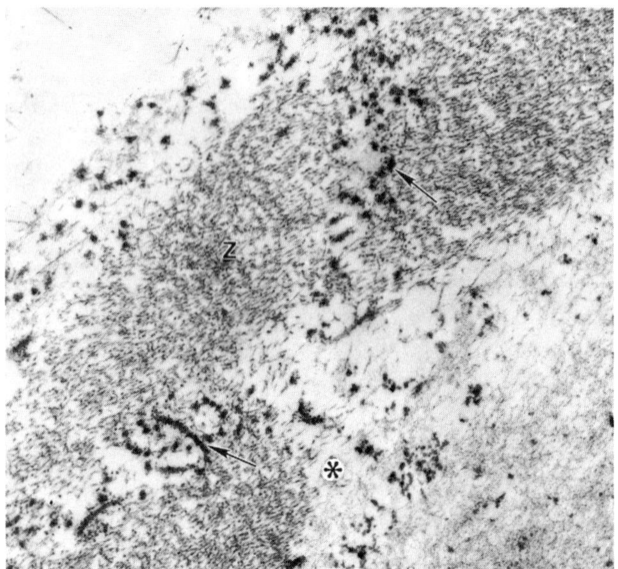

Figure 183–72. Zonular bundles (Z) infiltrated with pseudoexfoliative fibers *(arrows)* as they insert on the lens capsule *(asterisk)*. ×50,000.

HEREDITARY LENS-DISLOCATING DISEASES

In the absence of significant trauma, bilateral dislocation of the lens, with or without systemic or other ocular signs, is always presumptively due to a genetic abnormality, either inherited or from a new mutation. A limited number of systemic diseases has been associated with lens dislocation with any frequency, most of them diseases of connective tissue (see Table 183–2). In a representative sample of 310 children requiring surgery for lens dislocation, Seetner and Crawford[285] found that 16 had Marfan's syndrome, 7 idiopathic ectopia lentis, 4 homocystinuria, 2 ectopia lentis et pupillae, and 1 a hereditary condition of unknown type. Recognition of dislocation at any age requires further investigation to rule out heritable syndromes that can be fatal or have significant morbidity if not treated appropriately. Treatment may be only partially effective, such as dietary restriction in homocystinuria, and repair of an enlarging aorta before development of dissecting aneurysm in Marfan's syndrome, but is nevertheless worthwhile. Because of overlapping signs and a paucity of specific tests, there are difficulties in diagnosing many of the connective tissue syndromes. Molecular biology is rapidly changing this picture, allowing identification of specific gene defects so that more meaningful characterization of the abnormalities will become possible.

Nature of the Zonular Apparatus

Since the common denominator in this group of predominantly connective tissue diseases is lens dislocation, it is reasonable to expect that the defect in many will specifically involve the zonular apparatus. The zonule is made up of highly oriented 10-nm fibrils with a microperiod of 10 to 12 nm and a macroperiod of 45 to 55 nm (Fig. 183–73*A*), aggregated into fibers and bundles.[286] By rotary shadowing the fibrils are visualized as beads held together by multiple filaments (see Fig. 183–73*B*), showing evidence of a capacity to stretch.[287]

The zonular fibrils are composed of cysteine-rich glycoprotein[288, 289] whose chief component appears to be fibrillin.[290] They demonstrate a marked morphologic and biochemical similarity to the microfibrils that are the basic unit of the elastic system, called oxytalan when

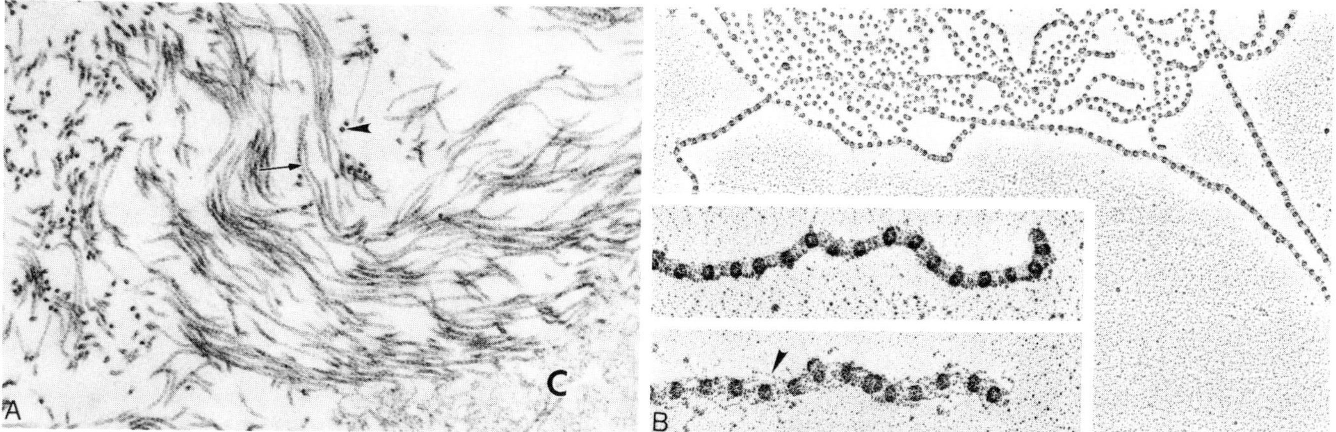

Figure 183–73. Zonular anatomy. *A,* Zonular fibrils inserting on the anterior lens capsule (C). A microperiodicity of 10 to 12 nm is seen *(arrow)* and a tubular cross section *(arrowhead).* ×68,000. *B,* Rotary shadowing of zonular fibrils showing a loose clump with a "string of beads" appearance. ×38,000. *Upper Inset,* An individual fibril composed of regularly spaced 29-nm beads. ×108,000. *Lower Inset,* Partially disrupted fibrils show that the beads are held together by multiple thin filaments with a faint microperiodicity *(arrowhead).* ×108,000.

occurring in nonelasticized bundles. These two fibril types are also cross-reactive antigenically,[290, 291] confirming that zonular fibrils are part of the systemic elastic system and offering a basis for understanding lens dislocation in diseases of connective tissues. It is anticipated that other defects will be found in components related to the zonular system, such as adhesion molecules between the fibrils or at their attachment sites.

Simple (Isolated) Ectopia Lentis

Simple ectopia lentis is usually transmitted as an autosomal dominant disease, most often present at birth with upward and temporal displacement of the lenses.[292] Genetic linkage analysis in these families has shown localization of the defect to the region of the fibrillin gene on chromosome 15, the gene harboring mutations in Marfan's syndrome.[292] As in many types of congenital dislocation, the lenses are small and spherical (microphakic and spherophakic). In some families a delayed onset of simple ectopia lentis has been described, presenting in even the sixth and seventh decades with a tendency to downward dislocation.[293] Two scanning electron microscopic studies of lenses from simple ectopia lentis[294, 295] have shown small spherical lenses with marked deficiency of zonular fibers, and poor aggregation of those present. In each study, a few abnormally thick fibrils of zonular or other type were seen focally on the lens.

Ectopia Lentis et Pupillae

Ectopia lentis et pupillae is inherited as an autosomal recessive trait.[296, 297] In two studies surveying 198 cases of ectopia lentis in schools for the blind, 81 to 93 percent of patients with no evidence of systemic disease had simple ectopia lentis, and 7 to 19 percent showed ectopia lentis et pupillae.[298, 299] The pupils are oval or slitlike, showing more than the normal 0.5 mm nasal and downward eccentricity (Fig. 183–74), and are often asymmetric. They are usually displaced in a direction opposite that of the lens, that is, toward the site of the most defective zonular fibers. The irides often have an atrophic appearance and may dilate poorly. A study of 16 patients from 8 families found ectopia lentis present in 93 percent, marked iris transillumination in 66 percent, and cataract in 34 percent.[296]

The cataracts are nuclear and cortical and can progress rapidly to maturity. Rarely the lens was microspherophakic. Axial myopia (average AP diameter of 26 mm) was common, with occasional retinal detachment. Progression of the ectopia was uncommon. The ectopia in both tissues has been attributed to a defective neuroectodermal layer, resulting in failure of the iris pigment epithelial cells to develop normal dilator muscle, presumably accompanied by poor secretion of zonular fibrils.

Marfan's Syndrome

Marfan's syndrome is the most frequent cause of heritable lens dislocation, with a prevalence of 4 to 6 per 100,000, transmitted as an autosomal dominant

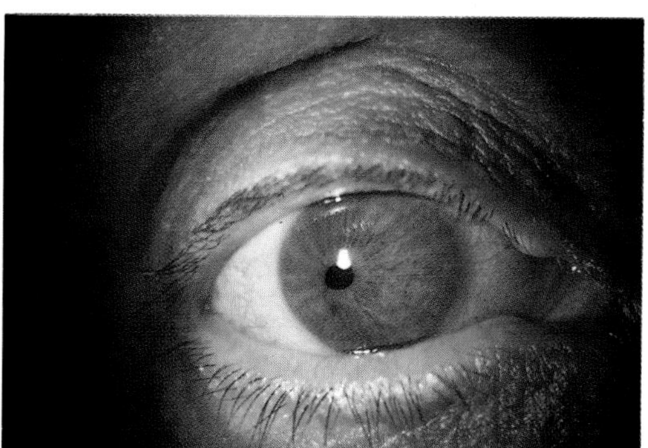

Figure 183–74. Ectopia lentis et pupillae in a 70-year-old man. (Courtesy of Dr. Sylvia Norton.)

trait.[300, 301] Of 196 patients with ectopia lentis seen in the Heredity Clinic at Johns Hopkins Hospital, 72 percent had Marfan's syndrome, 22 percent homocystinuria, and 5 percent Weill-Marchesani syndrome. Sixty percent of patients with Marfan's syndrome diagnosed by rigorous criteria have ectopia lentis, which along with a positive family history constituted the best corroborating features of Marfan's syndrome. The typical marfanoid habitus, with disproportionate growth of extremities, especially the lower ones, arachnodactyly, joint laxity, pectus excavatum, scoliosis, and increasing dilatation of the ascending aorta with aortic insufficiency, is the other cardinal feature of the syndrome. Death frequently results from dissecting aneurysm of the aorta.

Lens subluxation or dislocation may be present at birth and progress slowly in an upward or up and out direction, or remain stationary.[301] The zonules may appear intact and stretched across the pupillary space or focally attenuated, broken or absent. The irides often transilluminate peripherally. High axial myopia is usual in these large eyes, sometimes with staphylomata, bluish sclerae, and large corneas with a greater radius of curvature than usual. Retinal detachment is frequent in the larger eyes (mean axial length of 28.47 mm, versus 24.90 mm in eyes without detachment), even without cataract surgery. Glaucoma may be present, often correlated with an incompletely developed angle showing prominent iris processes.

Histopathologically,[302–306] the eyes from patients with Marfan's syndrome have shown marked enlargement, poor development of the iris dilator muscle, and hypopigmentation of the iris pigment epithelium, with elongation of the ciliary body and processes. The subluxed lenses from a patient with Marfan's syndrome may be approximately normal in size or small, showing a flatter curvature of the lower half and a posterior bulge (Fig. 183–75*A*) due to weakness or absence of the inferior zonules, reducing traction on the capsule. By scanning electron microscopy[306–308] the zonular bundles are thin and scanty. In one study the zonular fibrils and superficial capsular fibrils were substantially larger than normal.[307] Ultrastructure in an 8-year-old and a 14-week-old infant both of whom died of cardiac complications consistent with Marfan's syndrome showed no abnormality of the zonular fiber structure.[306]

In a study of three extracted Marfan lenses[308] the zonular bundles were thin and poorly aggregated (see Fig. 183–75*B*). In the youngest patient (16 years old), the zonular fibrils were normal except for a slightly wider diameter with prominent microperiodicity. The two older patients (34 and 38 years old) had, on the contrary, thinner, very tightly aggregated zonular fibrils with poorly visible microperiodicity (see Fig. 183–75*C*). It is possible that further changes can occur with age, or that the young patient represented a different genetic defect.

A major breakthrough in the understanding of the etiology of Marfan's syndrome has been the finding that positivity to fibrillin antibody is reduced or even absent on dermal elastic system microfibrils of most patients with Marfan's syndrome, or in cultures of their dermal fibroblasts.[309, 310] Patients with Marfan's syndrome in many kindreds have now been shown to have one of several point mutations in chromosome 15, band 21,[311, 312] which is the site of the fibrillin gene.[313] Other fibrillin-related genes reside on different chromosomes and may be defective in Marfan's syndrome variants which do not appear to be associated with ectopia lentis.[312] These localizations can now be utilized in clinical diagnostic tests for Marfan's syndrome.

Homocystinuria

Homocystinuria is one of several hereditary diseases with some phenotypic similarities to the Marfan's syndrome but very different associated signs and metabolic abnormalities.[314–317] It is transmitted as an autosomal recessive disease, with a prevalence of 1:200,000 newborns in most countries, although 1:60,000 in Ireland. The patients have fair skin with a malar flush, pale coarse hair, poor peripheral circulation, a 50 percent incidence of mental retardation, and often a marfanoid habitus, with arachnodactyly, pectus deformities, and osteoporosis. They are subject to major thromboembolic episodes, both arterial and venous, throughout the body, especially following anesthesia. Lens dislocation and subluxation are not present at birth but occur progressively thereafter in a downward direction. More than 90 percent have dislocated lenses by the third decade.

The disease is most often caused by a virtual absence of cystathionine β-synthetase, the enzyme that catalyzes the conversion of homocysteine to cystathionine (Fig. 183–76).[316, 318] Two different forms of this enzyme deficiency occur, determined by the response to pyridoxine (vitamin B_6), precursor of the co-enzyme for cystathionine β-synthetase. In the pyridoxine-responsive type, the defective enzyme has a marked reduction in binding to its co-enzyme. In both types, the levels of methionine, homocystine, and homocysteine are elevated in the serum and excreted excessively in the urine. Methylation enzyme defects can also occur in this pathway. The pathogenesis of thromboembolism and defective zonules is still uncertain, but the high level of precursors could activate clotting by several mechanisms.[318, 319] The deficiency of cystathionine β-synthetase may decrease the availability of cysteine for incorporation into the high cysteine-containing zonule, which could result in reduced sulfhydryl cross-links and fragmentation. An implication is that continual renewal of some components is necessary for zonular integrity.

The lens is often spherophakic, with a crenated border (Fig. 183–77*A*), and may dislocate into the anterior chamber, occluding the pupil and producing glaucoma, sometimes with cataract. The globe is elongated, and retinal detachment is frequent, usually following lens surgery. As the disease progresses the zonules rupture in midstream, forming a "fringe" of broken opaque zonular fibers retracted around the lens.[320]

By histopathology the ciliary body has a thin fusiform profile owing to poor development of the circular muscle, and is covered by a thick PAS-positive layer (see Fig. 183–77*B*). Ultrastructurally this layer consists of multilaminar basement membrane of the ciliary nonpig-

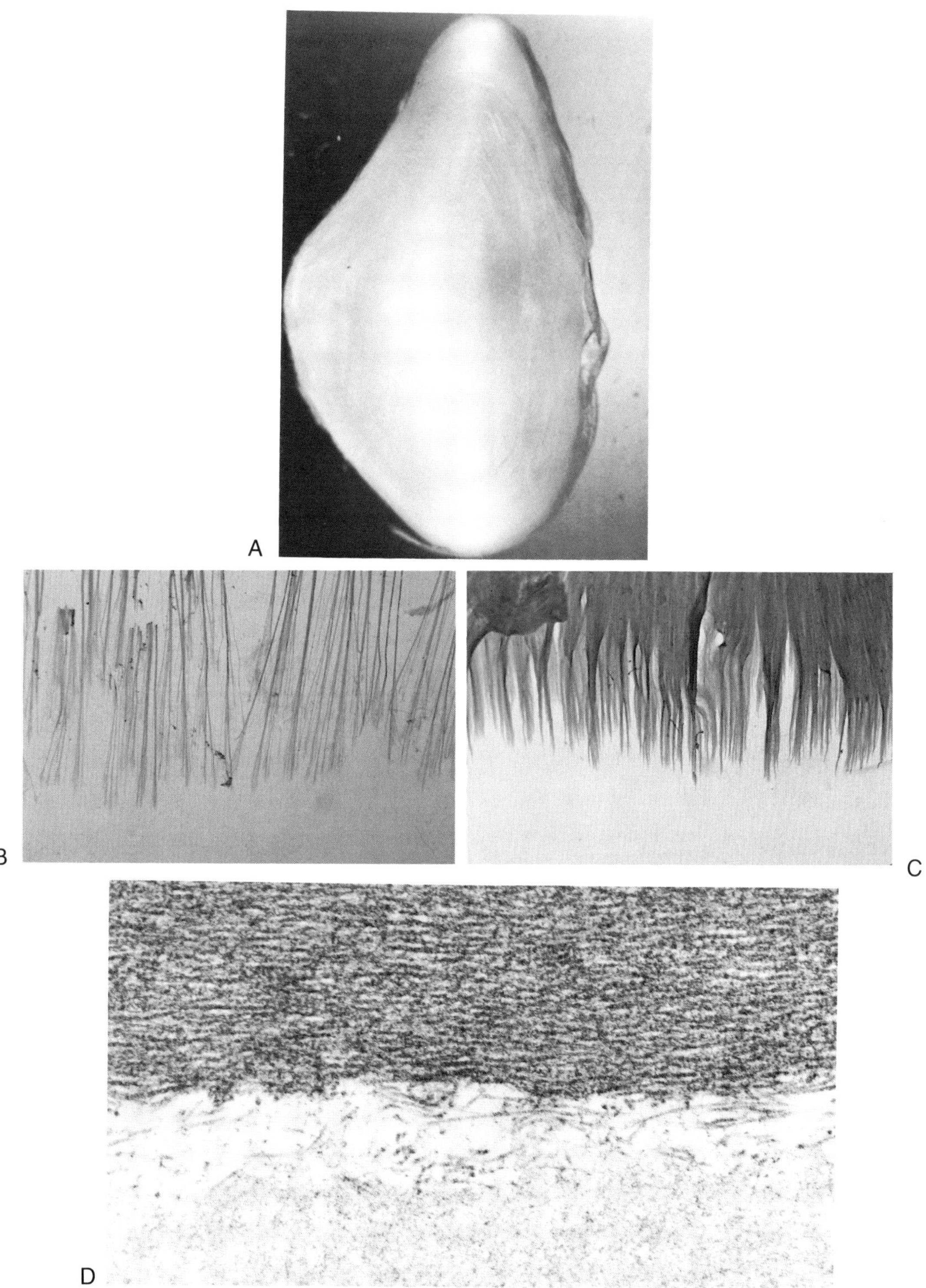

Figure 183–75. Marfan's syndrome. *A,* Side view of an intracapsularly extracted Marfan lens showing the flatter inferior curvature and bulging of the lower part of the posterior pole from reduced zonular traction. *B,* Scanty thin zonular bundles inserting on the anterior lens capsule. Capsule *(below)* is unstained. Immunostained with fibrillin antibody. ×500. *C,* Normal thick anterior zonular insertion in control patient stained identically. ×500. *D,* Tightly aggregated straight zonular fibrils with poorly visualized microperiodicity and a somewhat fuzzy outline inserting on the anterior lens capsule. ×68,000.

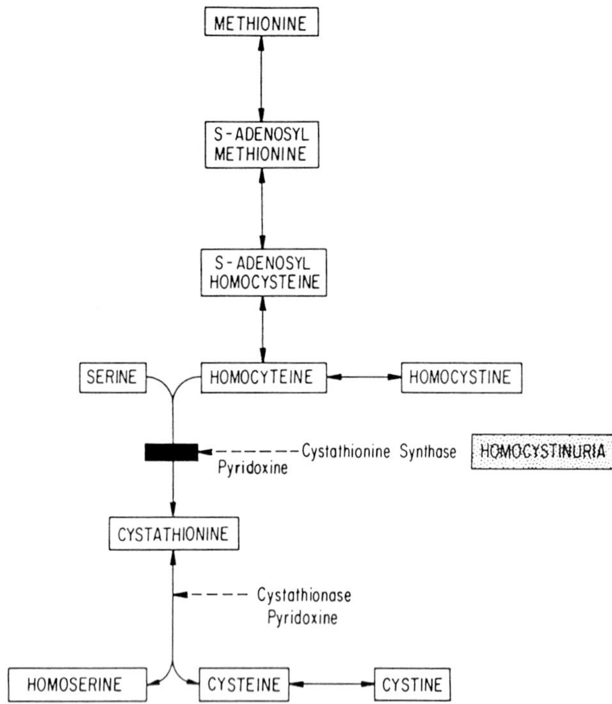

Figure 183–76. Metabolic pathway in cystine metabolism showing the enzyme defects in two types of hereditary homocystinuria. (From Klintworth GK, Landers MB III: The Eye: Structure and Function in Disease. Baltimore, Williams & Wilkins, 1976.)

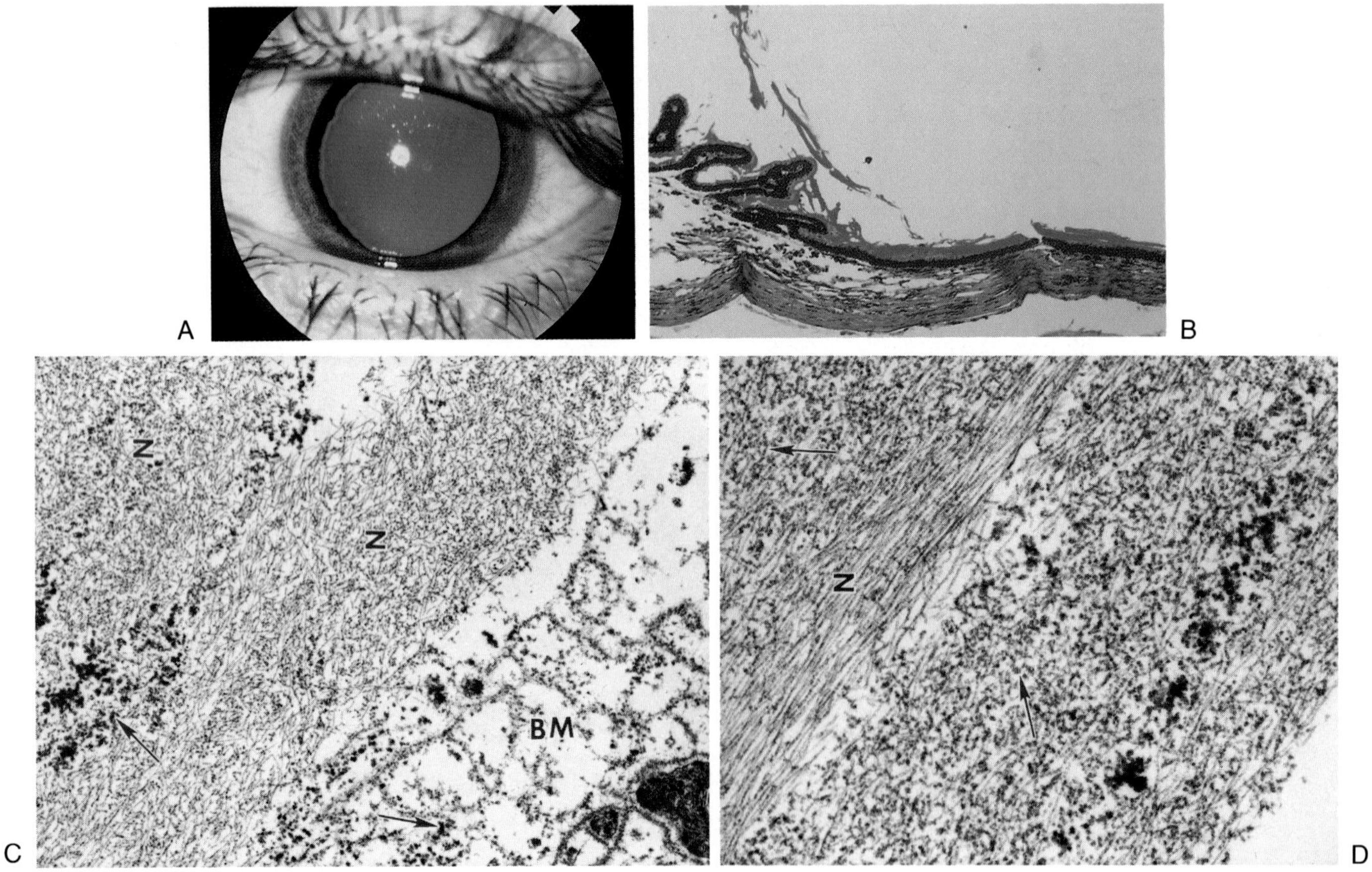

Figure 183–77. Homocystinuria. *A,* Subluxed lens in a patient with homocystinuria. Note scalloped border of lens. (Courtesy of Dr. John Hoepner.) *B,* Thick layer of PAS-positive material lying on the ciliary body, with thick free zonular bundles, in a young patient with homocystinuria. PAS, ×140. *C,* The zonular fibrils (Z) appear short and matted and intermingled with large, coarse granules *(arrow),* also present in the multilaminar basement membrane (BM) of the ciliary epithelium. ×30,200. *D,* Normal zonular bundle (Z) passing through degenerate short zonular fragments and dense granules *(arrows).* ×50,800.

ment epithelium and a thicker layer of nonoriented zonular fibrils (see Fig. 183–77*C*).[321, 322] The fibrils are fragmented into thin short lengths, increasingly intermingled with osmiophilic dense granules, which are also present in the basement membrane. In young eyes some normally formed zonular fibrils are still evident (see Fig. 183–77*D*), passing through the zonular fragments and dense granules. The latter may represent a breakdown product that cannot be further metabolized. By scanning electron microscopy the zonular bundles inserting on the lens show an "abnormal porous sponge-like appearance,"[320] undoubtedly due to the short, disoriented fibrils of which they are composed. The ciliary nonpigment epithelium shows progressive degenerative vacuolization and marked enfolding of the epithelial surface. Progressive degeneration of the peripheral retina and its pigment epithelium also occurs.[318]

Weill-Marchesani Syndrome

In almost all respects the signs of the Weill-Marchesani syndrome (spherophakia-brachymorphism)[323–328] are the reverse of those in Marfan's syndrome. Inheritance usually appears to be autosomal recessive, with expression in some heterozygotes, but consanguinity in several kindreds makes genetic evaluation difficult. Transmission as a possible autosomal dominant trait is also recorded.[327, 328]

The patients are short in stature, with short, broad hands and feet, limited joint mobility, a well-developed muscular appearance, thick skin, and brachycephaly. The lenses are small and spherophakic, with up to 15 to 20 diopters of lenticular myopia occurring progressively in most patients. Both microcornea and megalocornea have been described. There is a high incidence of subluxation, usually downward but sometimes central, with tilting and eventual dislocation. Clinically the zonular bundles may appear taut or lax and abnormally elongated. Episodes of pupillary block glaucoma are frequent, almost inevitable,[326] as the small lens comes forward to occlude the pupil. Relief of the pupillary block by mydriatics and worsening by miotics led to the term "inverse juvenile glaucoma."[329]

There has been no histopathologic examination of an eye or a lens from a patient with autosomal recessively inherited Weill-Marchesani syndrome, nor one conforming in all respects to the criteria for this syndrome. It is not certain how the McGavic type should be classified, as discussed below, so it is being described separately.

Dominant Spherophakia (McGavic Type)

A kindred with this syndrome was reported by McGavic[330, 331] as dominantly inherited Weill-Marchesani syndrome in 1959, with a follow-up in 1966. In this three-generational family, a father, six of his 12 offspring, and four grandchildren of both sexes had spherophakia, ectopia lentis, and secondary glaucoma, with signs of brachymorphism in most of the kindred. There was also a high frequency of coronary thrombosis. McKusick[332] examined this family and concluded that the disease was not Weill-Marchesani syndrome but ectopia lentis in a family of generally short stature, since unaffected members were equally short. Kloepfer and Rosenthal[333] have noted in recessive Weill-Marchesani kindreds that short stature and spadelike hands occur in 92 percent of heterozygotes, so the short stature of parents may not be normal for those families. However, the clear autosomal dominant transmission and mild skeletomuscular signs in the McGavic kindred suggest that this family has a different defect from that originally described, and one not necessarily associated with a Weill-Marchesani phenotype, as two of the four affected persons in the third generation were not of short stature and had little evidence of brachymorphism. Genetic studies are clearly needed in the Weill-Marchesani syndromes.

In the McGavic type of ectopia lentis, the zonular bundles were very long, thick, and redundant at surgery. By both histopathology and electron microscopy the changes in the zonule and ciliary body resembled those in homocystinuria,[334] although there was no biochemical evidence of homocystinuria. The PAS-positive mat over the ciliary nonpigment epithelium (Fig. 183–78*A*) is much thicker than that in homocystinuria, with greater accumulation of large, dense granules (see Fig. 183–78*B*). There are enormous quantities of well-formed zonular fibrils at their posterior attachments to the ciliary pars plana epithelium (see Fig. 183–78*C*). These quickly become mixed with dense granules and lose most evidence of a fibrillar nature. The marked proliferation and degeneration of the ciliary nonpigment epithelium resemble those in homocystinuria. These patients were 4 to 5 decades older than those with homocystinuria, which may correlate with the more advanced degeneration. The similarity of these two genetically very different diseases is striking and must hold important clues to the pathogenesis of each.

Sulfite Oxidase Deficiency

A further interesting linkage of lens dislocation with diseases of sulfur metabolism was the recognition of two patients with lens dislocation and sulfite oxidase deficiency,[335, 336] and two with combined sulfite oxidase deficiency and xanthine oxidase deficiency,[337, 338] transmitted as autosomal recessive traits. The symptoms developed in the first year of life, with poor feeding, severe neurologic abnormalities, seizures, myoclonus, and severe mental retardation. Dislocated lenses were noted after delays of several months to 4 yr. Lens dislocation has now been reported in 7 of 15 patients with the combined enzyme deficiency.[339] This deficiency has been shown to result from a defect in the molybdenum cofactor common to both enzymes, and is now called molybdenum cofactor deficiency.[339]

Sulfite oxidase is an enzyme in the mitochondrial intermembrane space,[337, 340] necessary for the final degradation of sulfur-containing amino acids by oxidizing sulfite to sulfate. All patients lacked sulfite oxidase and

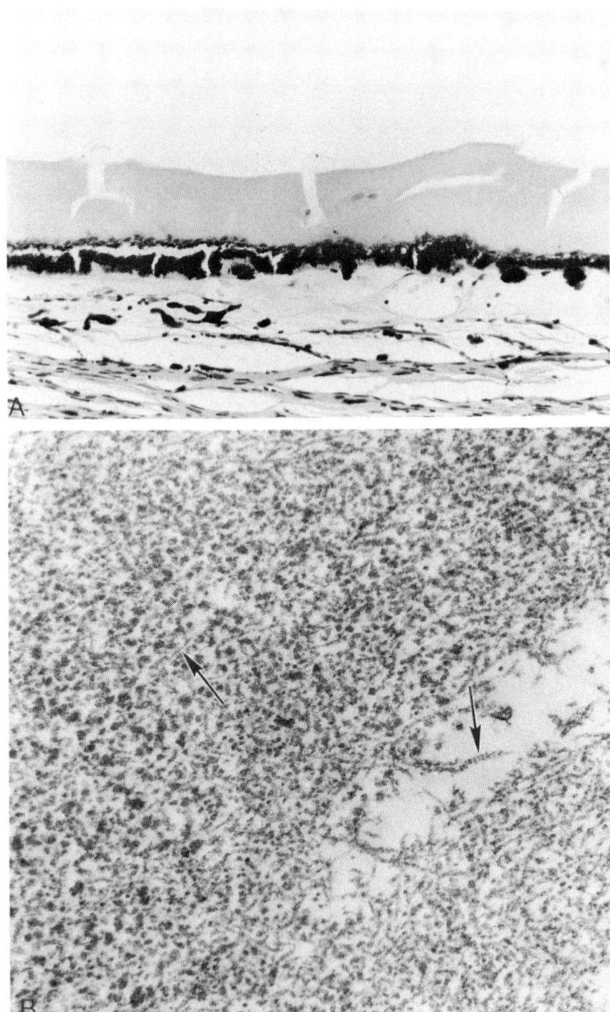

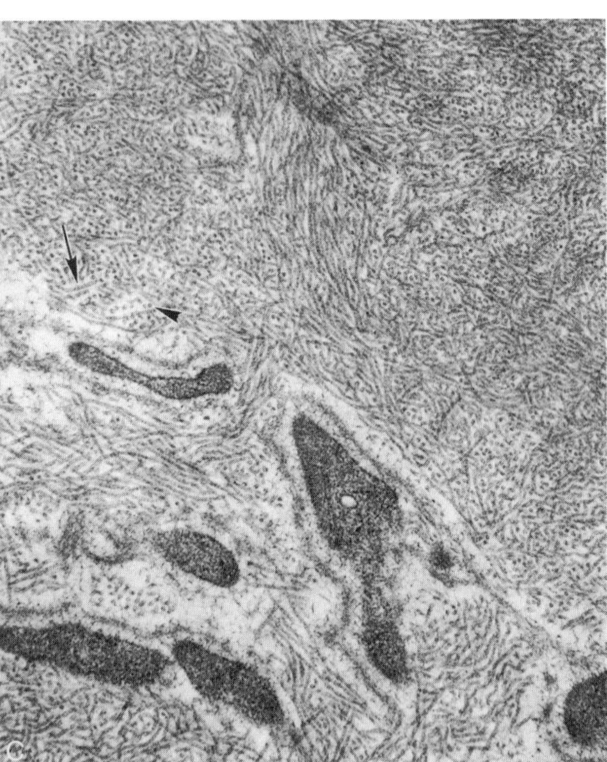

Figure 183–78. Dominant spherophakia, McGavic type. *A*, Thick PAS-positive layer over the ciliary body pars plana. H&E, ×280. *B*, Degenerating zonular fibrils mixed with electron dense irregular granules similar to those in homocystinuria. A few recognizable banded zonular fibrils are still present *(arrows)*. ×55,000. *C*, Profusion of normal-appearing zonular microfibrils on the pars plana epithelium, showing well-defined microperiodicity *(arrow)* and tubular cross section *(arrowhead)*. ×56,200.

had excretion of sulfite, thiosulfate, and *S*-sulfo-cysteine in large quantities in the urine. The excess sulfite can destroy disulfide bonds and react with free sulfhydryl groups as well. This toxic effect may be relevant to the lens dislocation as disulfide linkages are important for intramolecular bonds in fibrillin, and prossibly for intermolecular linkages. Since lens dislocation can occur with isolated sulfite oxidase deficiency, the frequently accompanying xanthine oxidase deficiency is not thought to be related to the ectopia.[341] The ocular pathology showed hypoplasia of the ciliary body, decrease in retinal ganglion cells, absence of myelin in the optic nerve, and ectopia lentis not specifically described.[342]

Hyperlysinemia

Hyperlysinemia is a rare defect of amino acid metabolism inherited as an autosomal recessive trait. Of the seven reported cases,[343] one showed bilateral superior subluxation of the lenses with a right lateral rectus muscle palsy, and another had bilateral spherophakia. Four patients had severe mental retardation, muscle hypertonia, convulsions, and strabismus. Two patients had no other associated signs. Because of the high frequency of consanguinity in these cases, and marked variation in phenotype, it cannot be certain that all the signs derived from a single gene defect. Hyperlysinemia results from deficiency of a lysine degradative enzyme, lysine-ketoglutarate reductase, which can be demonstrated in fibroblast skin cultures. How the chemical defect correlates with the disease, particularly the lens subluxation, is unknown.

Infrequent Causes of Hereditary Lens Dislocation

Many other disease processes, hereditary and nonhereditary, have occasionally been found in association with lens dislocation (see Table 183–2). The infrequency of association suggests that in some cases other causes may actually be responsible. Alternatively, the diagnosis of the underlying disease could be in error because of the many shared phenotypic characteristics among diseases of the connective tissue matrix. New variants of the commoner phenotype are also possibilities.

REFERENCES

1. Barber AN: Embryology of The Human Eye. St. Louis, CV Mosby, 1955.
2. Mann I: The Development of the Human Eye, 3rd ed. New York, Grune & Stratton, 1964.
3. Kuwabara T, Imaizumi M: Denucleation process of the lens. Invest Ophthalmol Vis Sci 13:973, 1974.
4. Hogan MJ, Alvarado JA, Weddell JE: Histology of the Human Eye: An Atlas and Textbook. Philadelphia, WB Saunders, 1971.
5. Apple DJ, Hamming NA, Gieser DK: Differential diagnosis of leukocoria. *In* Peyman GA, Apple DJ, Sanders DR (eds): Intraocular Tumors. New York, Appleton-Century-Crofts, 1977, p 240.
6. Salzmann M: The Anatomy and Histology of the Human Eyeball. [Translation by Brown EVL]. Chicago, University of Chicago Press, 1912, p 165.
7. Mohan PS, Spiro RG: Macromolecular organization of basement membranes. Characterization and comparison of glomerular basement membrane and lens capsule components by immunochemical and lectin affinity procedures. J Biol Chem 261:4328, 1986.
8. Yurchenco PD, Schittny JC: Molecular architecture of basement membranes. FASEB 4:1577, 1990.
9. Dark AJ, Streeten BW, Jones D: Accumulation of fibrillar protein in the aging human lens capsule. Arch Ophthalmol 82:815, 1969.
10. Seland JH: Ultrastructural changes in the normal human lens capsule from birth to old age. Acta Ophthalmol 52:688, 1974.
11. Berger E: Beitrage zur anatomie der zonula zinnii. Graefes Arch Clin Exp Ophthalmol 28:28, 1882.
12. Maisel H, Harding CV, Alcala JR, et al: The Morphology of the Lens. *In* Bloemendahl H (ed): Molecular and Cellular Biology of the Eye Lens. New York, John Wiley & Sons, 1981.
13. Kuszak JR, Ennesser CA, Umlas J, et al: The ultrastructure of fiber cells in primate lenses: A model for studying membrane senescence. J Ultrastruct Mol Struct Res 100:60, 1988.
14. Rafferty MS, Goosens W: Cytoplasmic filaments in the crystalline lens of various species: Functional correlations. Exp Eye Res 26:177, 1978.
15. Kuwabara T: The maturation of the lens cell: A morphologic study. Exp Eye Res 20:427, 1975.
16. deJong WW: Evolution of lens and crystallins. *In* Bloemendahl H (ed): Molecular and Cellular Biology of the Eye Lens. New York, John Wiley & Sons, 1981.
17. Mann I: Developmental Abnormalities of the Eye, 2nd ed. Philadelphia, JB Lippincott, 1957.
18. Coulombre AJ: Experimental embryology of the vertebrate eye. Invest Ophthalmol 4:411, 1965.
19. Wolter JR, Hall RC, Mason RCH: Unilateral primary congenital aphakia after German measles. Am J Ophthalmol 58:1011, 1964.
20. Vermeij-Keers C: Primary congenital aphakia and the rubella syndrome. Teratology 11:257, 1975.
21. Manschot WA: Primary congenital aphakia. Arch Ophthalmol 69:571, 1963.
22. Grey RHB, Ricci MSC: Congenital duplication of the lens. Br J Ophthalmol 60:693, 1976.
23. Font RL, Yanoff M, Zimmerman LE: Intraocular adipose tissue and persistent hyperplastic primary vitreous. Arch Ophthalmol 82:43, 1969.
24. Tripathi RC, Tripathi BJ, Gaster RN: Clinicopathologic study of Peter's anomaly. *In* The Cornea in Health and Disease. Roy Soc Med Int Congress and Symposium Series No. 40. London, Academic Press, 1981, p 1147.
25. Norton SW, Streeten BW: Corneal rupture in the neonate: Management and pathology. *In* Cavanagh HD (ed): Cornea. New York, Raven Press, 1988.
26. Greene PB: Keratoconus posticus circumscriptus: Report of a case. Arch Ophthalmol 34:432, 1945.
27. Karlin DB, Wise GN: Keratoconus posticus. Am J Ophthalmol 52:119, 1961.
28. Streeten BW, Karpik AG, Spitzer KH: Posterior keratoconus associated with systemic abnormalities. Arch Ophthalmol 101:616, 1983.
29. Kinsey JA, Streeten BW: Ocular abnormalities in the median cleft face syndrome. Am J Ophthalmol 83:261, 1977.
30. Zimmerman LE: Phakomatous choristoma of the eyelid: A tumor of lenticular anlage. Am J Ophthalmol 71:169, 1971.
31. McMahon RT, Font RL, McLean IW: Phakomatous choristoma of eyelid: Electron microscopic confirmation of lenticular derivation. Arch Ophthalmol 94:1778, 1976.
32. Johnson VP, Grayson M, Christian JC, et al: Dominant microspherophakia. Arch Ophthalmol 85:534, 1971.
33. Zimmerman LE, Font RL: Congenital malformations of the eye. JAMA 196:684, 1966.
34. Lowe CU, Terrey M, MacLachlan EA: Organic-aciduria, decreased renal ammonia production, hydrophthalmos and mental retardation: A clinical entity. Am J Dis Child 83:164, 1952.
35. Wadelius C, Fagerholm P, Pettersson U, et al: Lowe oculocerebrorenal syndrome: DNA-based linkage of the gene to Xq24-q26, using tightly linked flanking markers and the correlation to lens examination in carrier diagnosis. Am J Hum Genet 44:241, 1989.
36. Gardner RJ, Brown N: Lowe syndrome: Identification of carriers by lens examination. J Med Genet 13:449, 1976.
37. Cibis GW, Waeltermann JM, Whitcraft CT, et al: Lenticular opacities in carriers of Lowe's syndrome. Ophthalmology 93:1041, 1986.
38. Curtin VT, Joyce EE, Ballin H: Ocular pathology of the oculo-cerebral-renal syndrome of Lowe. Am J Ophthalmol 64:533, 1964.
39. Cogan DG, Kuwabara T: Pathology of cataracts in mongoloid idiocy. Doc Ophthalmol 16:73, 1962.
40. Haicken BH, Miller DR: Simultaneous occurrence of congenital aniridia, hamartoma and Wilms tumor. J Pediatr 78:497, 1971.
41. Tripathi RC, Cibis GW, Tripathi BJ: Pathogenesis of cataracts in patients with Lowe's syndrome. Ophthalmology 93:1046, 1986.
42. Borit A: Leigh's necrotizing encephalomyelopathy: neuroophthalmologic abnormalities. Arch Ophthalmol 85:438, 1971.
43. Hoepner JA, Yanoff M: Ocular anomalies in trisomy 13–15: An analysis of 13 eyes with two new findings. Am J Ophthalmol 24:729, 1972.
44. Lyon MF: Sex chromatin and gene action in the mammalian X-chromosome. Am J Hum Genet 14:135, 1962.
45. Alport AC: Hereditary familial congenital hemorrhagic nephritis. Br Med J 1:504, 1927.
46. Arnott EJ, Crawford MA, Toghill PJ: Anterior lenticonus and Alport's syndrome. Br J Ophthalmol 50:390, 1966.
47. Finegold J, Bois E, Chompret A, et al: Genetic heterogeneity of Alport syndrome. Kidney Int 27:672, 1985.
48. Sohar E: Renal disease, inner ear deafness and ocular changes. Arch Intern Med 97:627, 1956.
49. Peterson WS, Albert DM: Fundus changes in the hereditary nephropathies. Ophthalmology 78:762, 1974.
50. Sabates R, Krachmer JH, Weingeist TA: Ocular findings in Alport's syndrome. Ophthalmologica 186:204, 1983.
51. Teekhasaenee C, Nimmanit S, Wutthiphan S, et al: Posterior polymorphous dystrophy and Alport syndrome. Ophthalmology 98:1207, 1991.
52. Keraj K, Kim Y, Vernier RL, et al: Absence of Goodpasture's antigen in male patients with familial nephritis. Am J Kidney Dis 11:626, 1983.
53. Barker DF, Hostikka SL, Zhou J, et al: Identification of mutations in the COL IV A5 collagen gene in Alport syndrome. Science 248:1224, 1990.
54. Brownell RD, Wolter JR: Anterior lenticonus in familial hemorrhagic nephritis. Arch Ophthalmol 71:481, 1964.
55. Gregg JB, Becker SF: Concomitant progressive deafness, chronic nephritis and ocular lens disease. Arch Ophthalmol 69:293, 1963.
56. Govan JAA: Ocular manifestation of Alport's syndrome: An hereditary disorder of basement membranes? Br J Ophthalmol 67:493, 1983.
57. Streeten BW, Robinson MR, Wallace RN, et al: Lens capsule abnormalities in Alport's syndrome. Arch Ophthalmol 105:1693, 1987.
58. Ehrlich LH: Spontaneous rupture of the lens capsule in anterior lenticonus. Am J Ophthalmol 29:1274, 1946.
59. Hinglais N, Grunfeld J-P, Bois E: Characteristic ultrastructural

lesion of the glomerular basement membrane in progressive hereditary nephritis (Alport's syndrome). Lab Invest 27:473, 1972.
60. Howitt D, Hornblass A: Posterior lenticonus. Am J Ophthalmol 66:1133, 1968.
61. Crouch ER, Parks MM: Management of posterior lenticonus complicated by unilateral cataract. Am J Ophthalmol 85:503, 1978.
62. Reccio R, Magli A, Pignalosa B, et al: Rare association of hyperglycinuria and lenticonus in two members of the same family. Ophthalmologica 178:131, 1979.
63. Kepoor S: Familial anterior and posterior lenticonus. Ophthalmologica 178:186, 1979.
64. Pollard ZF: Familial bilateral posterior lenticonus. Arch Ophthalmol 101:1238, 1983.
65. Makley T: Posterior lenticonus: Report of a case with histologic findings. Am J Ophthalmol 39:308, 1955.
66. Francois J: Congenital Cataracts. Assen, The Netherlands, van Gorcum, 1963, pp 1–3.
67. Merin S: Congenital cataracts. *In* Renie WA (ed): Goldberg's Genetic and Metabolic Eye Disease, 2nd ed. Boston, Little, Brown, 1986.
68. Clayton R: Developmental genetics of the lens. *In* Maisel H (ed): The Ocular Lens: Structure, Functions, and Pathology. New York, Marcel Dekker, 1985.
68a. Piatigorsky J: Molecular biology: Recent studies on enzyme/crystallins and on α-crystallin gene expression. Exp Eye Res 50:725–727, 1990.
69. Moross T, Vaithilingam SS, Styles S, et al: Autosomal dominant anterior polar cataracts associated with a familial 2:14 translocation. J Med Genet 211:52, 1984.
70. Reese PD, Tuck-Muller CM, Maumenee IH: Autosomal dominant congenital cataract associated with chromosomal translocation [t(3;4)(p26.2′5)]. Arch Ophthalmol 105:1382, 1987.
71. Richard J, Maumenee IH, Rowe S, et al: Congenital cataract possibly linked to haptoglobin. Birth Defects 20:570, 1984.
72. Yanoff M, Fine BS (eds): Ocular Pathology: A Text and Atlas, 2nd ed. New York, Harper & Row, 1982, p 588.
73a. Duke-Elder S (ed): System of Ophthalmology, vol. III, part 2, Normal and Abnormal Development: Congenital Deformities. St. Louis, CV Mosby, 1964, pp 731–742.
73b. Duke-Elder S (ed): System of Ophthalmology, vol. III, part 2, Normal and Abnormal Development: Congenital Deformities. St. Louis, CV Mosby, 1964, pp 745–748.
74. Rosen E: Coppock cataract and cataracta pulverulenta centralis. Br J Ophthalmol 29:641, 1955.
75. Berliner ML: Biomicroscopy of the Eye: Slit-Lamp Microscopy of the Living Eye, vol. II. New York, Paul B. Hoeber, Inc, Harper & Bros., 1949, p 1097.
76. Renwick JH, Lawler SD: Probable linkage between a congenital cataract locus and the Duffy blood group locus. Ann Hum Genet 27:67, 1963.
77. Gregg HM: Congenital cataract following German measles in the mother. Trans Ophthalmol Soc Austr 3:35, 1941.
78. Yanoff M, Schaffer DB, Scheie HG: Rubellar ocular syndrome—clinical significance of viral and pathologic studies. Trans Am Acad Ophthalmol Otolaryngol 72:896, 1968.
79. Zimmerman LE: Histopathologic basis for ocular manifestations of congenital rubella syndrome. Am J Ophthalmol 65:837, 1968.
80. Rawls WE, Phillips CA, Melnick JL, et al: Persistent virus infection in congenital rubella. Arch Ophthalmol 77:430, 1967.
81. Boger WP III, Peterson RA, Robb RM: Spontaneous absorption of the lens in the congenital rubella syndrome. Arch Ophthalmol 99:433, 1981.
82. Cotlier E: Congenital varicella cataract. Am J Ophthalmol 86:627, 1978.
83. Robb RM, Marchevsky A: Pathology of the lens in Down's syndrome. Arch Ophthalmol 96:1039, 1978.
84. deJong PTVM, Bleeker-Wagemakers EM, Vrenson GFJM, et al: Crystalline cataract and uncombable hair. Ophthalmology 97:1181, 1990.
85. Allansmith M, Senz E: Chondrodystrophia congenita punctata (Conradi's disease): Review of the literature and report. Am J Dis Child 100:109, 1960.
86. Ryan H: Cataracts of dysplasia epiphysalis punctata. Br J Ophthalmol 54:197, 1970.
87. Hammond A: Dysplasia epiphysalis punctata with ocular anomalies. Br J Ophthalmol 54:755, 1970.
88. Levine RE, Snyder AA, Sugarman GI: Ocular involvement in chondrodysplasia punctata. Am J Ophthalmol 77:850, 1976.
89. Kretzer FL, Hittner HM, Mehta R: Ocular manifestations of Conradi and Zellweger syndromes. Metab Pediatr Ophthalmol 5:1, 1981.
90. Donders PC: Hallermann-Streiff syndrome. Doc Ophthalmol 44:161, 1977.
91. Wolter JR, Jones DH: Spontaneous cataract absorption in Hallermann-Streiff syndrome. Ophthalmologica 150:401, 1965.
92. Makley T: Hallermann-Streiff syndrome: Case presented at the Verhoeff Ophthalmic Pathology Meeting, 1988.
93. Stewart DH III, Streeten BW, Brockhurst RJ, et al: Abnormal scleral collagen in nanophthalmos: An ultrastructural study. Arch Ophthalmol 109:1017, 1991.
94. McCormick AQ: The transient cataracts in premature infants: A new clinical entity. Am J Ophthalmol 3:202, 1968.
95. Alden ER, Kaliva RA, Hodson WA: Transient cataracts in low-birth-weight infants. J Pediatr 82:314, 1973.
96. Yanoff M, Fine BS, Schaffer DB: Histopathology of transient neonatal lens vacuoles: A light and electron microscopic study. Am J Ophthalmol 76:363, 1973.
97. Reese AB: Persistent hyperplastic primary vitreous. Am J Ophthalmol 40:317, 1955.
98. Haddah R, Font RL, Reeser T: Persistent hyperplastic primary vitreous: A clinicopathologic study of 62 cases and review of the literature. Surv Ophthalmol 23:123, 1978.
99. Caudill JW, Streeten BW, Tso MOM: Phacoanaphylactoid reaction in persistent hyperplastic primary vitreous. Ophthalmology 92:1153, 1985.
100. Henkind P, Prose P: Anterior polar-cataract: Electron microscopic evidence of collagen. Am J Ophthalmol 63:768, 1967.
101. Font RL, Brownstein S: A light and electron microscopic study of anterior subcapsular cataracts. Am J Ophthalmol 78:972, 1974.
102. Peng Y, Sawaguchi S, Yue B, et al: Morphologic and immunohistochemical studies of anterior subcapsular cataract. Invest Ophthalmol Vis Sci 31(Suppl):445, 1990.
103. Vogt A: Neue Falle von Linsenkapselglaukome (Glaucoma Capsulare). Klin Monatsbl f Augenh 84:1, 1930.
104. Jones B: Dots in lens with glaucoma. Cataracta glaucomatosa and its role in the diagnosis of the acute glaucomas. Trans Ophthalmol Soc UK 79:753, 1959.
105. Anderson DR: Pathology of the glaucomas. Br J Ophthalmol 56:146, 1972.
106. Worgul BV, Rothstein H: Radiation cataract and mitosis. Ophthalmic Res 7:21, 1975.
107. Streeten BW, Eshaghian J: Human posterior subcapsular cataract. A gross and flat preparation study. Arch Ophthalmol 96:1653, 1978.
108. Worgul BV, Merriam GR Jr, Szechter A, et al: Lens epithelium and radiation cataract. I. Preliminary studies. Arch Ophthalmol 94:996, 1976.
109. Greiner JV, Chylack LT: Posterior subcapsular cataracts: Histopathologic study of steroid-associated cataracts. Arch Ophthalmol 97:135, 1979.
110. Eshaghian J, Streeten BW: Human posterior subcapsular cataract. An ultrastructural study of the posteriorly migrating cells. Arch Ophthalmol 98:134, 1980.
111. Wedl C: Atlas der Pathologischen Histologie des Auges. Leipzig, Germany, Georg. Wigand Verlag, 1860.
112. Zimmerman LE, Johnson FB: Calcium oxalate crystals within ocular tissues. Arch Ophthalmol 60:372, 1958.
113. Johnson FB, Karuna P: Histochemical identification of calcium oxalate. Arch Pathol 74:347, 1962.
114. Harding JJ: Changes in lens proteins in cataract. *In* Bloemendahl H (ed): Molecular and Cellular Biology of the Eye Lens. New York, John Wiley & Sons, 1981.
115. Lerman S: Evaluation of risk factors in human cataractogenesis. Dev Ophthalmol 21:120, 1991.
116. Brilliant LB, Grasset MC, Pokhrel RP, et al: Association among

cataract prevalence, sunlight hours, and altitude in the Himalayas. Am J Epidemiol 118:250, 1983.

117. Bochow TW, West SK, Azar A, et al: Ultraviolet light exposure and risk of posterior subcapsular cataract. Arch Ophthalmol 107:369, 1989.
118. Reddy VN: Glutathione and its function in the lens—An overview. Exp Eye Res 50:771, 1990.
119. Soemmerring DW: Beobachtungen uber der organischen Veranderungen in Auge nach Staaroperationen. (Frankfurt, 1828). Cited by Duke-Elder S *in* Duke-Elder S (ed): System of Ophthalmology, vol. XI, Diseases of the Lens and Vitreous: Glaucoma and Hypotony. St. Louis, CV Mosby, 1969, p 238.

120a. Duke-Elder S, MacFaul PA (eds): System of Ophthalmology. XIV: Injuries. Part I. Mechanical Injuries. St. Louis, CV Mosby, 1972, pp 121–141.

120b. Duke-Elder S, MacFaul PA (eds): System of Ophthalmology, XIV, Injuries. Part I. Mechanical Injuries. St. Louis, CV Mosby, 1972, pp 525–536.

121. Elschnig A: Klinisch-anatomischen Beitrag zur Kenntris des Nachstaares. Klin Monatsbl Augenheilkd 49:444, 1911.

122a. Duke-Elder S (ed): System of Ophthalmology. XI: Diseases of the Lens and Vitreous: Glaucoma and Hypotony. St. Louis, CV Mosby, 1969, pp 233–243.

122b. Duke-Elder S (ed): System of Ophthalmology. XI: Diseases of the Lens and Vitreous: Glaucoma and Hypotony. St. Louis, CV Mosby, 1969, pp 183–188.

122c. Duke-Elder S (ed): System of Ophthalmology. XI: Diseases of the Lens and Vitreous: Glaucoma and Hypotony. St. Louis, CV Mosby, 1969, pp 175–180.

122d. Duke-Elder S (ed): System of Ophthalmology. XI: Diseases of the Lens and Vitreous: Glaucoma and Hypotony. St. Louis, CV Mosby, 1969, pp 109–111.

123. Hiles DA, Watson BA: Complications of implant surgery in children. Am Intraocular Implant Soc J 5:24, 1979.
124. Hiles DA, Johnson BL: The role of the crystalline lens epithelium in post-pseudophakos membrane formation. Am Intraocular Implant Soc J 6:141, 1980.
125. Wilhelmus KR, Emery JM: Posterior capsule opacification following phacoemulsification. Ophthalmic Surg 11:264, 1980.
126. McDonnell PJ, Green WR, Maumenee AE, Iliff WJ: Pathology of intraocular lenses in 33 eyes examined postmortem. Ophthalmology 90:386, 1983.
127. McDonnell PJ, Zarbin MA, Green WR: Posterior capsule opacification in pseudophakic eyes. Ophthalmology 90:1548, 1983.
128. Apple DJ, Mamalis N, Loftfield K, et al: Complications of intraocular lenses: A historical and histopathological review. Surv Ophthalmol 29:1, 1984.
129. Kappelhof JP, Vrensen GFJM, de Jong PT, et al: An ultrastructural study of Elschnig's pearls in the pseudophakic eye. Am J Ophthalmol 101:58, 1986.
130. Jongebloed WL, Dijk F, Kruis J: Soemmerring's ring, an aspect of secondary cataract: A morphological description by SEM. Doc Ophthalmol 70:165, 1988.
131. Walshe JM: The eye in Wilson's disease. *In* Bergsma D, Bron AJ, Cotlier E (eds): The Eye and Inborn Errors of Metabolism. New York, Alan R. Liss, 1976, pp 187–189.
132. Tso MOM, Fine BS, Thorpe HE: Kayser-Fleischer ring and associated cataract in Wilson's disease. Am J Ophthalmol 79:479, 1975.
133. Cairns JE, Williams HP, Walshe JM: "Sunflower cataract" in Wilson's disease. Br Med J 3:95, 1969.
134. Goodman SI, Rodgerson DO, Kauffman J: Hypercupremia in a patient with multiple myeloma. J Lab Clin Med 70:57, 1967.
135. Ellis PP: Ocular deposition of copper in hypercupremia. Am J Ophthalmol 68:423, 1969.
136. Lewis RA, Falls HF, Troyer DO: Ocular manifestations of hypercupremia associated with multiple myeloma. Arch Ophthalmol 93:1050, 1975.
137. Martin NF, Kincaid MC, Stark WJ, et al: Ocular copper deposition associated with pulmonary carcinoma, IgG monoclonal gammopathy and hypercupremia: A clinicopathologic correlation. Ophthalmology 90:110, 1983.
138. Seland JH: Production of human lens capsule illustrated by a case of chronic lenticular chalcosis. Acta Ophthalmol 54:301, 1976.
139. Garron LK, Wood IS, Spencer WH, et al: A clinical pathologic study of mercurialentis medicamentosus. Trans Am Ophthalmol Soc 74:295, 1976.
140. Kennedy RE, Rosa PD, Landers PH: Atypical band keratopathy in glaucoma patients. Trans Am Ophthalmol Soc 69:124, 1971.
141. Kark RAP, Poskanzer DC, Bullock JO, et al: Mercury poisoning and its treatment with *N*-acetyl-D, L-penicillamine. N Engl J Med 285:10, 1971.
142. Friedman B, Rotth A: Argyrosis corneae. Am J Ophthalmol 13:1050, 1930.
143. Roberts WH, Wolter JR: Ocular chrysiasis. Arch Ophthalmol 56:48, 1956.
144. Mets MB: The eye and the chromosome. *In* Renie WA (ed): Goldberg's Genetic and Metabolic Eye Disease, 2nd ed. Boston, Little, Brown, 1986.
145. Francois J: Ocular manifestations of inborn errors of carbohydrate and lipid metabolism. I: Classical galactosaemia. Bibl Ophthalmol 84:2, 1975.
146. Klintworth GK, Landers MB III: The Eye: Structure and Function in Disease. Baltimore, Paul B. Hoeber, Inc, Williams & Wilkins, 1976.
147. Gitzelmann R, Curtius HC, Schneller I: Galactitol and galactose-1-phosphate in the lens of a galactosaemic infant. Exp Eye Res 6:1, 1967.
148. Vannas A, Hogan MJ, Golbusms WI: Lens changes in a galactosemic fetus. Am J Ophthalmol 80:726, 1975.
149. Kinoshita JH: Cataracts in galactosemia. Invest Ophthalmol 4:786, 1965.
150. Hu TS, Datiles M, Kinoshita JH: Reversal of galactose cataracts with sorbinil in rats. Invest Ophthalmol Vis Sci 24:640, 1983.
151. Huang SS, Huang PC: Biochemical diagnosis of genetic and metabolic eye diseases. *In* Renie WA (ed): Goldberg's Genetic and Metabolic Eye Disease. Boston, Little, Brown, 1986.
152. Monteleone JA, Beutler E, Monteleone PL, et al: Cataracts, galactosuria and hypergalactosemia due to galactokinase deficiency in a child. Am J Med 50:403, 1971.
153. Beutler F, Matsumatos F, Kuhl W, et al: Galactokinase deficiency as a cause of cataracts. N Engl J Med 288:1203, 1973.
154. Francois J: Ocular manifestations of inborn errors of carbohydrate and lipid metabolism. II: Galactokinase deficiency. Bibl Ophthalmol 84:11, 1975.
155. Beutler E, Matsumoto F: Galactokinase and cataracts. Lancet 1:1161, 1978.
156. Pirie A, Van Heyningen R: The effect of diabetes on the content of sorbitol, glucose, fructose and inositol in the human lens. Exp Eye Res 3:124, 1964.
157. Gabbay KH: Hyperglycemia, polyol metabolism, and complications of diabetes mellitus. Annu Rev Med 26:521, 1975.
158. Stevens VJ, Rouzer CA, Mornier UA, et al: Diabetic cataract formation: Potential role of glycosylation of lens crystallins. Proc Natl Acad Sci USA 75:2918, 1978.
159. Orzalesi M, Sorcinelli R, Guiso G: Increased incidence of cataracts in male subjects deficient in glucose-6-phosphate dehydrogenase. Arch Ophthalmol 99:69, 1981.
160. Johnson DL, Desnick RJ: Molecular pathology of Fabry's disease: Physical and kinetic properties of α-galactosidase A in cultured human endothelial cells. Biochim Biophys Acta 538:195, 1972.
161. Sher NA, Letson RD, Desnick RJ: The ocular manifestations in Fabry's disease. Arch Ophthalmol 97:671, 1979.
162. Weingeist TA, Blodi FC: Fabry's disease: ocular findings in a female carrier: A light and electron microscopic study. Arch Ophthalmol 85:169, 1971.
163. Font RL, Fine BS: Ocular pathology in Fabry's disease. Histochemical and electron microscopic observations. Am J Ophthalmol 73:418, 1972.
164. Walton DS, Robb RM, Crocker AC: Ocular manifestations of group A Niemann-Pick disease. Am J Ophthalmol 85:174, 1978.
165. Orbisser AI, Murphree AL, Garcia CA, et al: Ocular findings in mannosidosis. Am J Ophthalmol 82:465, 1976.
166. Letson RD, Desnick RJ: Punctate lenticular opacities in type II mannosidosis. Am J Ophthalmol 85:218, 1978.
167. Cibis GW, Harris DJ, Chapman AL, et al: Mucolipidosis I. Arch Ophthalmol 101:933, 1983.

168. Burian HM, Burns CA: Ocular changes in myotonic dystrophy. Am J Ophthalmol 63:22, 1967.
169. Buxton J, Shelbourne P, Davies J, et al: Detection of an unstable fragment of DNA specific to individuals with myotonic dystrophy. Nature 355:547–548, 1992.
170. Caskey CT, Pizzuti A, Fu YH, et al: Triple repeat mutations in human disease. Science 256:784–789, 1992.
171. Dark AJ, Streeten BW: Ultrastructural study of cataract in myotonia dystrophica. Am J Ophthalmol 84:666, 1977.
172. Eshaghian J, March WF, Goosens W, et al: Ultrastructure of cataract in myotonic dystrophy. Invest Ophthalmol Vis Sci 17:289, 1978.
173. Kuwabara T, Lessell S: Electron microscopic study of extraocular muscles in myotonic dystrophy. Am J Ophthalmol 82:303, 1976.
174. Pohjola S: Ocular manifestations of idiopathic hypoparathyroidism. Acta Ophthalmol 40:255, 1962.
175. Garner A, Klintworth GK: The causes, types and morphology of cataracts. *In* Pathobiology of Ocular Disease: A Dynamic Approach. Part B, 2nd ed. New York, Marcel Dekker, 1993 (in press).
176a. Nelson LB, Calhoun JH, Huley RD: Pediatric Ophthalmology, 3rd ed. Philadelphia, WB Saunders, 1991, pp 8–13.
176b. Nelson LB, Calhoun JH, Huley RD: Pediatric Ophthalmology, 3rd ed. Philadelphia, WB Saunders, 1991, pp 451–452.
177. Heckenlively J: The frequency of posterior subcapsular cataract in the hereditary retinal degenerations. Am J Ophthalmol 93:733, 1982.
178. Kaiser-Kupfer M, Kuwabara T, Uga S: Cataract in gyrate atrophy: Clinical and morphologic studies. Invest Ophthalmol Vis Sci 24:432, 1983.
179. Dryja TP, McGee TL, Reichel E, et al: A point mutation of the rhodopsin gene in one form of retinitis pigmentosa. Nature 343:364, 1990.
180. Hess HH, O'Keefe TL, Kuwabara T, Westney IV: Numbers of cortical vitreous cells and onset of cataracts in Royal College of Surgeons rats. Invest Ophthalmol Vis Sci 32:200, 1991.
181. Dilley KJ, Bron AJ, Habgood JO: Anterior polar and posterior subcapsular cataract in a patient with retinitis pigmentosa: A light microscopic and ultrastructural study. Exp Eye Res 22:155, 1976.
182. Eshaghian J, Rafferty NS, Goossens W: Ultrastructure of human cataract in retinitis pigmentosa. Arch Ophthalmol 98:2227, 1980.
183. Levy IS: Refsum's syndrome. Trans Ophthalmol Soc UK 90:181, 1970.
184. Toussaint D, Danis P: An ocular pathologic study of Refsum's syndrome. Am J Ophthalmol 72:342, 1971.
185. Takki KK, Milton RC: The natural history of gyrate atrophy of the choroid and retina. Ophthalmology 88:292, 1981.
186. Mito T, Shiono T, Ishiguru S, et al: Immunocytochemical localization of ornithine aminotransferase in human ocular tissues. Arch Ophthalmol 107:1372, 1989.
187. Seery CM, Pruett RC, Liberfarb RM, Cohen BZ: Distinctive cataract in the Stickler syndrome. Am J Ophthalmol 110:143, 1990.
188. Francomano CA, Liberfarb RM, Hirose T, et al: The Stickler syndrome is closely linked to Col2A1, the structural gene for type II collagen. Pathol Immunol Res 7:104, 1988.
189. Kaiser-Kupfer MI, Freidlin V, Datiles MB, et al: The association of posterior lens capsular opacities with bilateral acoustic neuromas in patients with neurofibromatosis type 2. Arch Ophthalmol 107:541, 1989.
190. Bjorkhem I, Skrede S: Familial diseases with storage of sterols other than cholesterol. Cerebrotendinous xanthomatosis and phytosterolemia. *In* Scriver CR, et al (eds): Metabolic Basis of Inherited Disease, 6th ed. New York, McGraw-Hill, 1989.
191. Seland JH, Slagsvold JE: The ultrastructure of lens and iris in cerebrotendinous xanthomatosis. Acta Ophthalmol 55:201, 1977.
192. Salen G, Meriwether TW, Nicolau G: Chenodeoxycholic acid inhibits increased cholesterol and cholestanol synthesis in patients with cerebrotendinous xanthomatosis. Biochem Med 14:57, 1975.
193. Cole HV, Gifford HK, Simmons JT, et al: Congenital cataracts in sisters with congenital ectodermal dysplasia. JAMA 129:723, 1945.
194. Petrohelos MA: Werner's syndrome: A survey of three cases, with a review of the literature. Am J Ophthalmol 56:941, 1963.
195. Worobec-Victor SM, Bain MAB: Oculocutaneous genetic diseases. *In* Renie WA (ed): Goldberg's Genetic and Metabolic Eye Disease, 2nd ed. Boston, Little, Brown, 1986.
196. Williamson J, Paterson RWW, McGavin DDM, et al: Posterior subcapsular cataracts and glaucoma associated with long-term oral corticosteroid therapy in patients with rheumatoid arthritis and related conditions. Br J Ophthalmol 53:361, 1969.
197. Weinstein BI, Kandaloft N, Ritch R, et al: 5-Alpha-dihydrocortisol in human aqueous humor and metabolism of cortisol by human lenses in vitro. Invest Ophthalmol Vis Sci 32:2130, 1991.
198. Philipson B, Kaufman PL, Fagerholm P, et al: Echothiophate cataracts in monkeys: Electron microscopy and microradiography. Arch Ophthalmol 97:340, 1979.
199. Hamming NA, Apple DJ, Goldberg MF: Histopathology and ultrastructure of busulfan-induced cataract. Graefes Arch Clin Exp Ophthalmol 200:139, 1976.
200. Von Sallmann L, Grimes P, Collins E: Triparanol-induced cataract in rats. Arch Ophthalmol 70:522, 1963.
201. Siddall JR: The ocular toxic findings with prolonged and high dosage chlorpromazine intake. Arch Ophthalmol 74:460, 1965.
202a. Duke-Elder S, MacFaul PA (eds): System of Ophthalmology, vol. XIV, Radiational Injuries, part 2, Nonmechanical Injury. St. Louis, CV Mosby, 1972, pp 837–1010.
202b. Duke-Elder S, MacFaul PA (eds): System of Ophthalmology, vol. XIV, Radiational Injuries, Part 2, Nonmechanical Injury. St. Louis, CV Mosby, 1972, pp 878–885.
203. Cogan DG, Donaldson DD, Reese AB: Clinical and pathological characteristics of radiation cataract. Arch Ophthalmol 47:55, 1952.
204. Lipman RM, Tripathi BJ, Tripathi RC: Cataracts induced by microwave and ionizing radiation. Surv Ophthalmol 33:200, 1988.
205. McCanna R, Chandra SR, Stevens TS, et al: Argon-laser–induced cataract as a complication of retinal photocoagulation. Arch Ophthalmol 100:1071, 1982.
206. Hirsch SE, Appleton B, Fine BS, Brown PVK: Effects of repeated microwave irradiations on the albino rabbit eye. Invest Ophthalmol Vis Sci 16:315, 1977.
207. Appleton B, McCrossan GC: Microwave lens effects in humans. Arch Ophthalmol 88:259, 1972.
208a. Duke-Elder S (ed): System of Ophthalmology. IX: Diseases of the Uveal Tract. St. Louis, CV Mosby, 1966, pp 594–602.
208b. Duke-Elder S (ed): System of Ophthalmology. IX: Diseases of the Uveal Tract. St. Louis, CV Mosby, 1966, pp 456–457.
209. Lowenfeld IE, Thompson HS: Fuchs heterochromic cystitis. A critical review of the literature. I: Clinical characteristics of the syndrome. Surv Ophthalmol 17:394, 1973; II: Etiology and mechanisms. Surv Ophthalmol 18:2, 1973.
210. O'Connor GR: Heterochromic iridocyclitis (Doyne lecture). Trans Ophthalmol Soc UK 104:219, 1985.
211. Rahi AHS, Garner A: Immunopathology of the Eye. Oxford, Blackwell Scientific Publications, 1976.
212. Flocks M, Littwin CS, Zimmerman LE: Phacolytic glaucoma: A clinicopathologic study of 138 cases of glaucoma associated with hypermature cataract. Arch Ophthalmol 54:37, 1955.
213. Green RW: Diagnostic cytopathology of ocular fluid specimens. Ophthalmology 91:726, 1984.
214. Epstein DL, Jedziniak JA, Grant WM: Identification of heavy-molecular-weight soluble protein in aqueous humor in human phacolytic glaucoma. Invest Ophthalmol Vis Sci 17:398, 1978.
215. Epstein DL, Jedziniak JA, Grant WM: Obstruction of aqueous outflow by lens particles and by heavy-molecular-weight soluble lens proteins. Invest Ophthalmol Vis Sci 17:272, 1978.
216. Yanoff M, Scheie HG: Cytology of human lens aspirate. Its relationship to phacolytic glaucoma and phacoanaphylactic endophthalmitis. Arch Ophthalmol 80:166, 1968.
217. Rosenbaum JT, Samples JR, Seymour B, et al: Chemotactic activity of lens proteins and the pathogenesis of phacolytic glaucoma. Arch Ophthalmol 105:1582, 1987.
218. Smith ME, Zimmerman LE: Contusive angle recession in phacolytic glaucoma. Arch Ophthalmol 74:799, 1965.
219. Verhoeff FH, Lemoine AN: Endophthalmitis phacoanaphylactica. Am J Ophthalmol 5:700, 1922.
220. Carrillo R, Streeten BW: Malignant teratoid medulloepithelioma in an adult. Arch Ophthalmol 97:695, 1979.

221. Blodi F: Sympathetic uveitis an allergic phenomenon. Trans Am Acad Ophthalmol Otolaryngol 63:642, 1959.
222. Easom HA, Zimmerman LE: Sympathetic ophthalmia and bilateral phacoanaphylaxis: A clinicopathologic correlation of the sympathogenic and sympathizing eyes. Arch Ophthalmol 72:9, 1964.
223. Marak GE Jr, Font RL, Alepa FFP: Experimental lens–induced granulomatous endophthalmitis: passive transfer with serum. Ophthalmic Res 8:117, 1976.
224. Marak GE Jr, Font RL, Alepa FFP: Immunopathogenicity of lens crystallins in the production of lens-induced granulomatous endophthalmitis. Ophthalmic Res 10:30, 1978.
225. Rahi AHS, Misra RH, Morgan G: Immunopathology of the lens. III: Humoral and cellular immune responses to autologous lens antigens and their roles in ocular inflammation. Br J Ophthalmol 61:164, 1977.
226. Irvine SR, Irvine AR Jr: Lens-induced uveitis and glaucoma. Part II. The "phacotoxic" reaction. Am J Ophthalmol 35:370, 1952.
227. Elschnig A: Detachment of the zonular lamella in glassblowers. Klin Mbl Augenheilk 69:732, 1922.
228. Callahan A, Klein BA: Thermal detachment of the anterior lamella of the anterior lens capsule: A clinical and histologic study. Arch Ophthalmol 59:73, 1958.
229. Burde RM, Bresnick G, Uhrhammer J: True exfoliation of the lens capsule: an electron microscopic study. Arch Ophthalmol 82:651, 1969.
230. Dvorak-Theobald GD: Pseudoexfoliation of lens capsule: Relation to "true" exfoliation of the lens capsule as reported in the literature and role in production of glaucoma capsulare. Am J Ophthalmol 37:1, 1954.
231. Brodnick JD, Tate GW: Capsular delamination (true exfoliation) of the lens: Report of a case. Arch Ophthalmol 97:1693, 1979.
232. Cashwell LF Jr, Hollerman IL, Weaver RG, et al: Idiopathic true exfoliation of the lens capsule. Ophthalmology 96:348, 1989.
233. Johnson G, Minassian D, Franken S: Alterations of the anterior lens capsule associated with climatic keratopathy. Br J Ophthalmol 73:229, 1989.
234. Vogt A: Ein neues Splatlampenbild des Pupillengebieties: Hellblauer Pupillinsaufilz Hautchenbildung auf der Lindsevorderkapsel. Klin Monatsbl Augenheilk 75:1, 1925; Graefes Arch Ophthalmol 111:91, 1923.
235. Ghosh M, Speakman JS: Inclusions in human lens capsule and their relationship to senile exfoliation. Am J Ophthalmol 7:413, 1972.
236. Davanger M: The pseudoexfoliation syndrome: A scanning electron microscopic study. I. The anterior lens surface. Acta Ophthalmol 53:809, 1975.
237. Dark AJ, Streeten BW, Cornwall CC: Pseudoexfoliative disease of the lens: a study in electron microscopy and histochemistry. Br J Ophthalmol 61:462, 1977.
238. Roth M, Epstein DL: Exfoliation syndrome. Am J Ophthalmol 89:477, 1980.
239. Forsius H: Exfoliation syndrome in various ethnic populations. Acta Ophthalmol 184 (Suppl):71, 1988.
240. Bartholemew RS: Pseudo-capsular exfoliation in the Bantu of South Africa. I: Early or pregranular stage. Br J Ophthalmol 55:693, 1971.
241. Dark AJ, Streeten BW: Precapsular film on the aging human lens: Precursor of pseudoexfoliation? Br J Ophthalmol 74:717, 1990.
242. Mizuno K, Murois S: Cycloscopy of pseudoexfoliation. Am J Ophthalmol 87:513, 1979.
243. Dark AJ, Streeten BW: Pseudoexfoliation syndrome. *In* Garner A, Klintworth GK (eds): Pathobiology of Ocular Disease, A Dynamic Approach, Part B, 2nd ed. New York, Marcel Dekker, 1992, pp 1303–1320 (in press).
244. Morrison JC, Green WR: Light microscopy of the exfoliation syndrome. Acta Ophthalmol 184 (Suppl):5, 1988.
245. Bertelson TI, Drablos PA, Flood PR: The so-called senile exfoliation (pseudoexfoliation) of the lens capsule, a product of lens epithelium. Acta Ophthalmol 42:1096, 1964.
246. Ashton N, Shakib M, Collyer R, et al.: Electron microscopic study of pseudo-exfoliation of the lens capsule. I: Lens capsule and zonule fibers. Invest Ophthalmol 4:141, 1965.
247. Bertelsen TI, Seland JH: Flat whole-mount preparations of the lens capsule in fibrillopathia epitheliocapsularis. Acta Ophthalmol 49:938, 1972.
248. Streeten BW, Dark AJ, Wallace RN, et al: Pseudoexfoliative fibrillopathy in the skin of patients with ocular pseudoexfoliation. Arch Ophthalmol 110:490, 1990.
249. Seland JH: The ultrastructural changes in the exfoliation syndrome. Acta Ophthalmol Suppl 184:28, 1988.
250. Ringvold A: On the occurrence of pseudo-exfoliation material in extra-bulbar tissue from patients with pseudo-exfoliation syndrome of the eye. Acta Ophthalmol 51:411, 1973.
251. Eagle RG, Font RL, Fine BW: The basement membrane exfoliation syndrome. Arch Ophthalmol 97:510, 1979.
252. Schlötzer-Schrehardt U, Küchle M, Naumann GOH: Electron microscopic identification of pseudoexfoliative material in extrabulbar tissue. Arch Ophthalmol 109:565, 1991.
252a. Schlötzer-Schrehardt UM, Koca MR, Naumann GOH, Volkholz H: Pseudoexfoliation syndrome: Ocular manifestation of a systemic disorder? Arch Ophthalmol 110:1752–1756, 1992.
252b. Streeten BW, Li ZY, Wallace RN, et al: Pseudoexfoliative fibrillopathy in visceral organs of a patient with pseudoexfoliation syndrome. Arch Ophthalmol 110:1757, 1992.
253. Prince AM, Streeten BW, Ritch R, et al: Preclinical diagnosis of pseudoexfoliation syndrome. Arch Ophthalmol 105:1076, 1987.
254. Streeten BW, Dark AJ, Barnes CW: Pseudo-exfoliative material and oxytalan fibers. Exp Eye Res 38:523, 1984.
255. Garner A, Alexander RA: Pseudoexfoliative disease: Histochemical evidence of an affinity with zonular fibers. Br J Ophthalmol 68:574, 1984.
256. Streeten BW, Gibson SA, Dark AJ: Pseudoexfoliative material contains an elastic microfibrillar-associated glycoprotein. Trans Am Ophthalmol Soc 84:304, 1986.
257. Li Z-Y, Streeten BW, Yohai N: Amyloid P protein in pseudoexfoliative fibrillopathy. Curr Eye Res 8:217, 1989.
258. Li Z-Y, Streeten BW, Wallace RN: Association of elastin with pseudoexfoliative material: an immunoelectron microscopic study. Curr Eye Res 7:1163, 1988.
259. Li Z-Y, Streeten BW, Wallace RN: Vitronectin localizes to pseudoexfoliative fibers in ocular and conjunctival sites by immunoelectron microscopy. Invest Ophthalmol Vis Sci 32 (Suppl):777, 1991.
260. Streeten BW, Gibson SA: Digestion studies of pseudoexfoliative material on the lens capsule. Invest Ophthalmol Vis Sci 25 (Suppl):150, 1984.
261. Harnisch JP, Barrach HS, Hassell JR, Sinha PK: Identification of a basement membrane proteoglycan in exfoliation material. Graefes Arch Clin Exp Ophthalmol 215:273, 1981.
262. Konstas AG, Marshall GE, Lee WR: Immunogold localization of laminin in normal and exfoliative iris. Br J Ophthalmol 74:450, 1990.
263. Schlötzer-Schrehardt U, Küchle M, Naumann GOH: Immunohistochemical localization of basement membrane components in pseudoexfoliation material on the lens capsule. Curr Eye Res 11:343–355, 1992.
264. Ringvold A, Husby G: Pseudoexfoliative material—An amyloid-like substance. Exp Eye Res 17:289, 1973.
265. Roh YB, Ishibashi T, Ito N, Inomata H: Alteration of microfibrils in the conjunctiva of patients with exfoliation syndrome. Arch Ophthalmol 105:978, 1987.
266. Chijiiwa T, Araki H, Ishibashi T, Inomata H: Degeneration of zonular fibrils in a case of exfoliation glaucoma. Ophthalmologica 199:16, 1989.
267. Streeten BW, Brookman L, Ritch RN, et al: Pseudoexfoliative fibrillopathy in the conjunctiva: A relation to elastic fibers and elastin. Ophthalmology 94:1439, 1987.
268. Teikari JM: Genetic factors in simple and capsular open angle glaucoma in population based twin study. Acta Ophthalmol 65:715, 1987.
269. Taylor HR: The environment and the lens. Br J Ophthalmol 64:303, 1980.
270. Ringvold A: Exfoliation syndrome: Immunological aspects. Acta Ophthalmol Suppl 184:66, 1988.
271. Yanoff M: Intraocular pressure in exfoliation syndrome. Acta Ophthalmol Suppl 184:59, 1988.

272. Nirankari MS, Chaddah R: Displaced lens. Am J Ophthalmol 63:1719, 1967.
273. Jaffe NS, Jaffe MS, Jaffe GF: Cataract Surgery and Its Complications. St. Louis, CV Mosby, 1990, p 303.
274. Streeten BW, Robinson JP: Posterior zonules and lens extraction. Arch Ophthalmol 96:132, 1978.
275. Raviola G: The fine structure of the ciliary zonule and ciliary epithelium with special regard to the organization and insertion of the zonular fibrils. Invest Ophthalmol Vis Sci 10:851, 1971.
276. Smith JL, Singh JA, Moore MB Jr, et al: Seronegative ocular and neurosyphilis. Am J Ophthalmol 59:753, 1965.
277. Jarret WH II: Dislocation of the lens. Arch Ophthalmol 78:289, 1967.
278. Rosenbaum LJ, Podos SM: Traumatic ectopia lentis. Some relationships to syphilis and glaucoma. Am J Ophthalmol 64:1095, 1967.
279. Gifford H Jr: A clinical and pathologic study of exfoliation of the lens capsule. Am J Ophthalmol 46:508, 1958.
280. Bartholomew RS: Lens displacement associated with pseudocapsular exfoliation. Br J Ophthalmol 54:744, 1970.
281. Dark AJ: Cataract extraction complicated by capsular glaucoma. Br J Ophthalmol 63:465, 1979.
282. Guzek JP, Holm M, Cotter J: Risk factors for intraoperative complications in 1000 extracapsular cataract cases. Ophthalmology 94:461, 1987.
283. Skuta GL: Zonular dialysis during extracapsular cataract extraction in pseudoexfoliation syndrome. Arch Ophthalmol 105:632, 1987.
284. Naumann GOH: Exfoliation syndrome as a risk factor for vitreous loss in extracapsular cataract surgery. Acta Ophthalmol Suppl 184:129, 1988.
285. Seetner AA, Crawford JS: Surgical correction of lens dislocation in children. Am J Ophthalmol 91:106, 1981.
286. Streeten BW: The zonular apparatus. *In* Tasman W, Jaeger EA (eds): Biomedical Foundations of Ophthalmology, Anatomy Section. 2nd ed. New York, Harper & Row, 1992.
287. Wallace RN, Streeten BW, Hanna RB: Rotary shadowing of elastic system microfibrils in the ocular zonule, vitreous, and ligamentum nuchae. Curr Eye Res 10:99, 1991.
288. Buddecke E, Wollensak J: Zur Biochemie der Zonulafaser des Rinderanges. Z Naturforsch 21:337, 1966.
289. Streeten BW, Gibson SA: Identification of extractable proteins from the bovine ocular zonule: major zonular antigens of 32kD and 250kD. Curr Eye Res 7:139, 1988.
290. Sakai LY, Keene DR, Engvall E: Fibrillin, a new 350kD glycoprotein, is a component of extracellular microfibrils. J Cell Biol 103:2499, 1986.
291. Streeten BW, Licari PA, Marucci AA, et al: Immunohistochemical comparison of ocular zonules and the microfibrils of elastic tissue. Invest Ophthalmol Vis Sci 21:130, 1981.
292. Francois J: Heredity in Ophthalmology. St. Louis, CV Mosby, 1961, pp 161–164.
292a. Tsipouras P, DelMastro R, Safarazi M, et al: Genetic linkage of the Marfan syndrome, ectopia lentis, and congenital contractural arachnodactyly to the fibrillin genes on chromosomes 15 and 5. N Engl J Med 326:905, 1992.
293. Waardenburg PJ, Franceschetti A, Klein D: Genetics and Ophthalmology. Assen, the Netherlands, Royal Von Gorcum, 1961, pp 954–957.
294. Seland JH: The lenticular attachment of the zonular apparatus in congenital simple ectopia lentis. Acta Ophthalmol 51:520, 1973.
295. Farnsworth PM, Burke PA, Blanco J, et al: Ultrastructural abnormalities in a microspherical ectopic lens. Exp Eye Res 27:399, 1978.
296. Goldberg MF: Clinical manifestations of ectopia lentis et pupillae in 16 patients. Ophthalmology 95:1080, 1988.
297. Luebbers JA, Goldberg MF, Herbst R, et al: Iris transillumination and variable expression in ectopia lentis et pupillae. Am J Ophthalmol 83:647, 1977.
298. Clark CC: Ectopia lentis: A pathologic and clinical study. Arch Ophthalmol 21:124, 1939.
299. Lund A, Stontaft F: Congenital ectopia lentis. Acta Ophthalmol 29:33, 1950.
300. Pyeritz RE, McKusick VA: The Marfan syndrome: Diagnosis and management. N Engl J Med 300:772, 1979.
301. Maumenee IH: The eye in the Marfan syndrome. Trans Am Ophthalmol Soc 79:684, 1981.
302. Dvorak-Theobald G: Histologic eye findings in arachnodactyly. Am J Ophthalmol 24:1132, 1941.
303. Lutman FC, Heel JB: Inheritance of arachnodactyly, ectopia lentis and other congenital anomalies (Marfan's syndrome) in the E. family. Arch Ophthalmol 41:276, 1949.
304. Reeh MJ, Lehman WL: Marfan's syndrome: Arachnodactyly with ectopia lentis. Trans Am Acad Ophthalmol Otolaryngol 58:212, 1954.
305. Wachtel JG: The ocular pathology of Marfan's syndrome. Arch Ophthalmol 76:512, 1966.
306. Ramsey MS, Fine BS, Shields JA, et al: The Marfan syndrome: A histopathologic study of ocular findings. Am J Ophthalmol 76:102, 1973.
307. Farnsworth PM, Burke PA, Dotto ME, et al: Ultrastructural abnormalities in a Marfan's syndrome lens. Arch Ophthalmol 95:1601, 1977.
308. Streeten BW, Li Z-Y, Wallace RN, et al: The ocular zonule in Marfans's syndrome. Invest Ophthalmol Vis Sci Suppl 31:102, 1990.
309. Hollister DW, Godfrey M, Sakai LY, et al: Immunohistologic abnormalities of the microfibrillar-fiber system in the Marfan syndrome. N Engl J Med 323:152, 1990.
310. Godfrey M, Menashe V, Weleber RG, et al: Cosegregation of elastin-associated microfibrillar abnormalities with the Marfan phenotype in families. Am J Hum Genet 46:652, 1990.
311. Dietz H, Cutting GR, Pyeritz RE, et al: Marfan syndrome caused by a recurrent de novo missense mutation in the fibrillin gene. Nature 352:337, 1991.
312. Lee B, Godfrey M, Vitale E, et al: Linkage of Marfan syndrome and a phenotypically related disorder to two different fibrillin genes. Nature 352:330, 1991.
313. Magenis RE, Meslen CL, Smith L, et al: Localization of the fibrillin (FBN) gene to chromosome 15 and band 21.1. Genomics 11:346, 1991.
314. Carson MAJ, Neill DN: Metabolic abnormalities detected in a survey of mentally backward individuals in Northern Ireland. Arch Dis Child 37:505, 1962.
315. Gerritsen T, Vaughn JG, Waisman HA: The identification of homocystine in the urine. Biochem Biophys Res Commun 9:493, 1962.
316. Mudd SH, Finkelstein JD, Irreverre F, et al: Homocystinuria: an enzymatic defect. Science 143:1443, 1964.
317. Mudd SH, Skovby F, Levy HL, et al: The natural history of homocystinuria due to cystathionine β-synthase deficiency. Am J Hum Genet 37:1, 1985.
318. Spaeth GL: The usefulness of pyridoxine in the treatment of homocystinuria: A review of postulated mechanisms of action and a new hypothesis. Birth Defects 12:347, 1976.
319. Nelson LB, Maumenee IH: Ectopia lentis. Surv Ophthalmol 27:143, 1982.
320. Ramsey MS, Dickson DH: Lens fringe in homocystinuria. Br J Ophthalmol 59:338, 1975.
321. Henkind P, Ashton N: Ocular pathology in homocystinuria. Trans Ophthalmol Soc UK 85:21, 1965.
322. Ramsey MS, Yanoff M, Fine BS: The ocular histopathology of homocystinuria. Am J Ophthalmol 74:377, 1972.
323. Weill E: Ectopie du cristallen et malformations générales. Ann d'Oculist 169:21, 1932.
324. Marchesani O: Brachydaktylic und angeborene Kugellinse als Systemerkrankung. Klin Monatsbl Augenheilkd 103:392, 1939.
325. Jensen AD, Cross HE, Paton D: Ocular complications in the Weill-Marchesani syndrome. Am J Ophthalmol 77:261, 1974.
326. Jones RF: The syndrome of Marchesani. Br J Ophthalmol 45:377, 1961.
327. Probert LA: Spherophakia with brachydactyly. Am J Ophthalmol 36:1571, 1953.
328. Young ID, Fielder AR, Caseg TA: Weill-Marchesani syndrome in mother and son. Clin Genet 30:475, 1986.
329. Urbanek J: Glaucoma juvenile inversum. Z Augenheilkd 77:171, 1930.

330. McGavic JS: Marchesani's syndrome. Am J Ophthalmol 47:413, 1959.
331. McGavic JS: Weill-Marchesani syndrome, brachymorphism and ectopia lentis. Am J Ophthalmol 62:820, 1966.
332. McKusick VA: Heritable Disorders of Connective Tissue, 4th ed. St. Louis, CV Mosby, 1972, p 61.
333. Kloepfer HW, Rosenthal JW: Possible genetic carriers in the spherophakia-brachymorphia syndrome. Am J Hum Genet 7:398, 1975.
334. Yanoff M, Fine BS: Ocular Pathology: A Text and Atlas, 3rd ed. Philadelphia, JB Lippincott, 1989, p 379.
335. Irreverre F, Mudd SH, Heiser WD, et al: Sulfite oxidase deficiency: studies of a patient with mental retardation, dislocated ocular lenses, and abnormal urinary excretion of S-sulfo-cysteine, sulfite and thiosulfate. Biochem Med 1:187, 1967.
336. Shih VE, Abrams IF, Johnson JL, et al: Sulfite oxidase deficiency: Biochemical and clinical investigations of a hereditary metabolic disorder in sulfur metabolism. N Engl J Med 297:1022, 1977.
337. Duran M, Beemer FA, Heider CVD, et al: Combined deficiency of xanthine oxidase and sulfite oxidase: A defect of molybdenum metabolism or transport. J Inherited Metab Dis 1:175, 1978.
338. Beemer FA, Deileman JW: Combined deficiency of xanthine oxidase and sulfite oxidase: ophthalmological findings in a 3-week-old girl. Metab Pediatr Ophthalmol 4:49, 1980.
339. Johnson JL, Wadman SK: Molybdenum cofactor deficiency. *In* Scriver CR, et al (eds): The Metabolic Basis of Inherited Disease. Vol I, 6th ed. New York, McGraw-Hill, 1989, p 1463.
340. Johnson JL, Rajagoplan KV: The oxidation of sulfite in animal systems. Excerpta Medica. Sulfur in Biology. Ciba Foundation Symp 72:119, 1980.
341. Mudd SH, Levy HL, Skovby F: Disorders of transsulfuration. *In* Scriver CR, et al (eds): The Metabolic Basis of Inherited Disease, Vol I, 7th ed. New York, McGraw-Hill, 1933.
342. Smith RS: Ocular pathology in sulfite oxidase deficiency. Invest Ophthalmol Vis Sci 17 (Suppl):247, 1978.
343. Smith TH, Holland ME, Woody MC: Ocular manifestations of familial hyperlysinemia. Trans Am Acad Ophthalmol Otolaryngol 75:355, 1971.

Chapter 184

Pathology of the Retina and Vitreous

JOSÉ A. SAHEL, ALFRED BRINI, and DANIEL M. ALBERT

RETINOPATHY OF PREMATURITY

Retinopathy of prematurity (ROP)[1–7] (formerly termed *retrolental fibroplasia*)[13] is classically defined as an oxygen-induced vitreoretinal disease of premature infants. ROP was the leading cause of infant blindness between 1940 and the early 1950s and continues to occur with disturbing frequency. Terry[8] first defined the clinical aspects of the condition, but it was another decade before its true nature was recognized as a result of studies by Campbell,[9] Ashton and colleagues,[10] and Patz and coworkers.[11] ROP occurs bilaterally, almost exclusively in infants with an immature, incomplete retinal vascular system, and particularly in premature infants who weighed less than 1.5 kg at birth and who received oxygen therapy. The recent rise in the incidence of ROP is accounted for by the increasing survival rate of very small (600-g) premature infants who require a minimal oxygen level to avoid neurologic and pulmonary complications of prematurity.

Retinal Angiogenesis and Immaturity

Immaturity of the retinal vascular tree is currently thought to be the underlying cause of its vulnerability to injury on exposure to oxygen.[9–14] The peripheral retinal vasculature is formed in the hypoxic environment in utero from the fourth month of gestation to after birth.[14–18] Angiogenesis in the inner retina proceeds from the optic nerve to the periphery, the temporal retina being fully vascularized only after birth because of the nasal location of the optic disc. Foos[4–6] described the vasculogenic wave as a mixed cellular type including an "anterior vanguard," containing spindle-shaped cells derived from mesenchymal cells from the adventitia of the hyaloid system or, according to Cogan and Kuwabara[19] and Friedenwald and colleagues,[20] from the glia. Flower and associates,[21] however, doubted the concept of a vanguard-derived primitive vasculature in higher animals. Foos also described a posterior "rear guard," containing primitive endothelial cells, which aggregate into cords. These subsequently lumenize, forming the primordial capillary network by selective atrophy or hypertrophy of subpopulations (Fig. 184–1).[6, 22]

The stimuli inducing this process are oxygen tension,[23] a relative hypoxia generated by developmental thickening and neuronal differentiation, or other metabolic and hemodynamic factors. The most important feature of retinal angiogenesis is that by the eighth month of gestation, the temporal peripheral retina remains avascular.[6, 7, 18, 24–26]

In addition, biochemical abnormalities linked to retinal immaturity have been implicated, including diminution of superoxide dismutase activity, low levels of interstitial retinal binding protein, and consequently an insufficient transfer of the antioxidant vitamin E to the inner retina.[7] The inner retina and the spindle cells present at birth thus are extremely sensitive to free radicals induced by oxygen or other factors, such as light or medications.[7, 12, 16–18, 27]

Retinal immaturity and oxygen toxicity vary from one

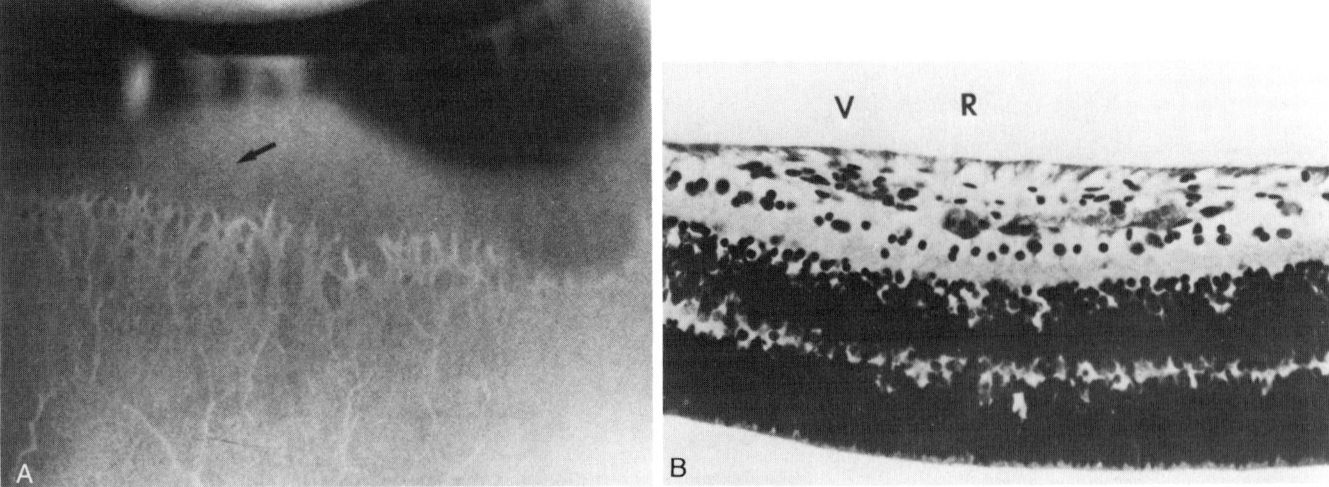

Figure 184–1. *A*, Developing retinal vasculature in inferior fundus of right eye from a 775-g stillborn infant, showing an irregular fimbriated line that represents advancing vasoformative tissue. Peripheral neovascularized retina is more transparent and in phases shows slight microcystic change *(arrow)*. ×15. *B*, Microscopic appearance of vasoformative tissue, which consists of a vanguard (V) containing a few layers of spindle-shaped cells in the nerve fiber layer and a rear guard (R) containing primitive endothelial cells. Posteriorly, primordial capillaries have formed. H&E, ×540. (From Foos RY: Retinopathy of prematurity: Pathologic correlation of clinical stages. Retina 7:260, 1987.)

infant to another, ranging from the historic oxygen-induced retrolental fibroplasia in the early 1950s to acute ROP, frequently observed today in very small premature infants receiving "safe" levels of oxygen. In these babies, the previously defined safe oxygen dose (an ambient concentration of not more than 40 percent, corresponding to a partial pressure in the arterial blood of 160 mmHg) is now considered unsafe. In addition, occasional cases of oxygen-induced peripheral ROP in full-term babies have been reported. Such occurrences

Table 184–1. CLINICOPATHOLOGIC CORRELATES IN THE INTERNATIONAL CLASSIFICATION STAGING OF ROP[6, 22, 25–27]

Stages	Clinical Features	Pathologic Correlates
1	Demarcation line (white: separating vascularized from nonvascularized retina)	Demarcation line: thickening of the normal angiogenesis wave, comprising two zones: (1) anterior vanguard zone: numerous spindle cells with extensive gap junctions; (2) rear guard zone (clinically undetectable): differentiating endothelial cells forming new, dilated capillaries (see Fig. 184–2)
2	Ridge (elevated, pink)	Posterior extension of the demarcation line: further hyperplasia of the surface, vanguard tissue. Posterior proliferation of the endothelial cells of the rear guard tissue: progenitors of new, dilated capillaries, leaking fluorescein (see Fig. 184–3)
Regression	Small tufts of new vessels on retina leaking fluorescence, with no residual scar common at these stages	
3	Extraretinal fibrovascular proliferation	Anterior and posterior growth of fibrovascular proliferative tissue into the vitreous (scaffold); commonly placoid in the region of the ridge; less frequently mounded or pedunculated Common to stages 3 and 4: vitreous synchisis and condensation (related to proliferation?) providing the scaffold for proliferative vitreoretinopathy, retinal buckling, folding
4	Subtotal retinal detachment, exudative or tractional (1) extrafoveal: concave traction; (2) including fovea: fold from the disc to periphery (zone III). Often temporal drawing of nasal retina: meridional fold	Traction consecutive to proliferative vitreoretinopathy: glial proliferation, sheets of myofibroblasts proliferating in intravitreal strands along the collapsed and condensed vitreous scaffold; exudation from vascular tufts (see Fig. 184–5)
Plus disease	Vascular dilatation	
5	Total retinal detachment, funnel-shaped	Fibrous traction. Anterior folding and drawing of the retina (see Fig. 184–6)
Arrested disease	White linear scars or folds	

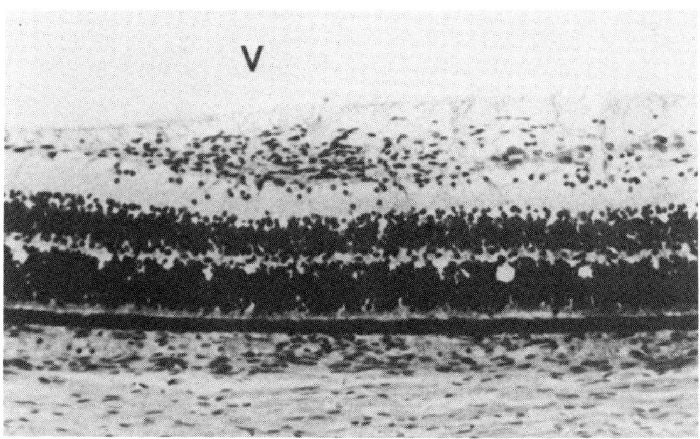

Figure 184–2. Retinopathy of prematurity stage 1 (985-g infant) showing thickening of retina, which is related to proliferation of spindle cells in vanguard (V). H&E, ×300. (From Foos RY: Retinopathy of prematurity: Pathologic correlation of clinical stages. Retina 7:260, 1987.)

may be viewed either as isolated forms of exudative peripheral proliferative retinopathy or the result of oxygen sensitivity or other insults to a barely mature retinal temporal vasculature.[12, 25]

Pathogenesis

Current models and theories of ROP pathogenesis are discussed in detail in Chapter 224 in connection with their therapeutic implications. In the classic theories based on kitten, young mouse, and puppy models, hyperoxia induces a vasoobliterative phase with functional constriction of the immature retinal blood vessels followed by structural obliteration.[10–14] The more immature the retina is, then the higher the hypoxic phase and the longer it lasts, and the less reversible this vascular destruction becomes. If the hyperoxia is sufficiently prolonged, on cessation of oxygen exposure the peripheral retina remains ischemic. A proliferative phase ensues, with intense fibrovascular proliferation beginning at the junction of the vascular and avascular zones and continuing through the internal limiting membrane into the vitreous.

Kretzer and associates[16] and Hittner and colleagues[17] from results obtained from their electron microscopic studies of human premature whole-eye donations, ascribed a key role to the development of extensive gap junctions between the spindle cells of the vanguard after oxygen and free-radical injuries. This process interferes with the normal maturation of the retinal vasculature and induces neovascularizations from the existing premature capillaries of the rear guard.[16–18] In both theories, additional retinal vascularization and subsequent changes in the overlying vitreous are the key causes of folding, buckling, and rolling of the peripheral retina, with the vitreous providing a scaffold for fibrovascular proliferation.[7, 16–18] At this stage, the pathogeneses of ROP and other proliferative vitreoretinopathies become similar.

Clinicopathologic Correlations of the International Classification of ROP Stages

The international classification of the clinical stages of acute ROP, which was established in 1984, was followed by 1987 by a classification of retinal detachments and other changes in this disease (see Chaps. 57 and 224).[1, 2] Several investigators[6, 22, 26, 27] have provided clear, clinically fruitful clinicopathologic correlations of ROP stages (Table 184–1; Figs. 184–2 to 184–6).

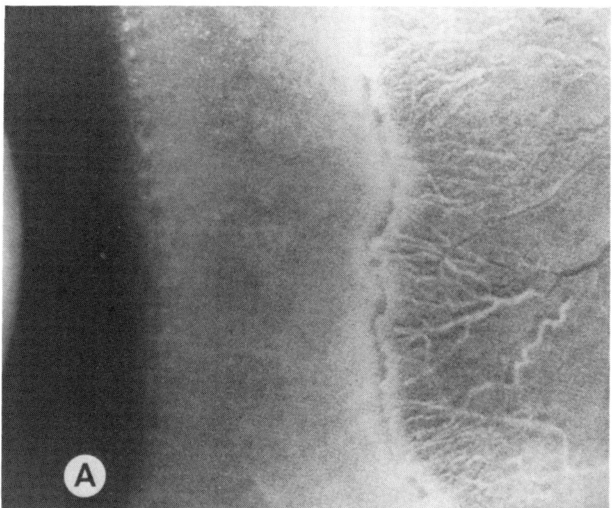

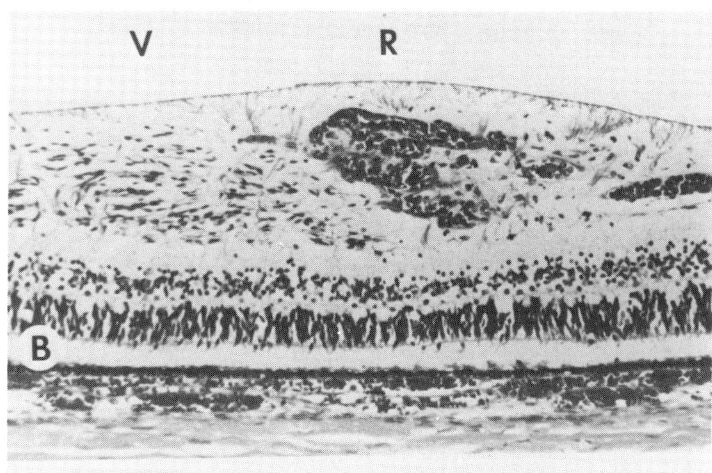

Figure 184–3. Retinopathy of prematurity, stage 2 (29-wk infant) with conspicuous hyperemia. *A,* Photomicrograph shows moderately elevated ridge (red), marked hyperemia, and tortuosity of retinal vessels posterior to ridge and vitreous haze. ×15. *B,* Photomicrograph of ridge shows the posterior aspect of a markedly thickened and extensive vanguard zone (V) and conspicuous vasodilation of rear guard zone (R), which has been characterized clinically as an arteriovenous shunt. H&E, ×250. (From Foos RY: Retinopathy of prematurity: Pathologic correlation of clinical stages. Retina 7:260, 1987.)

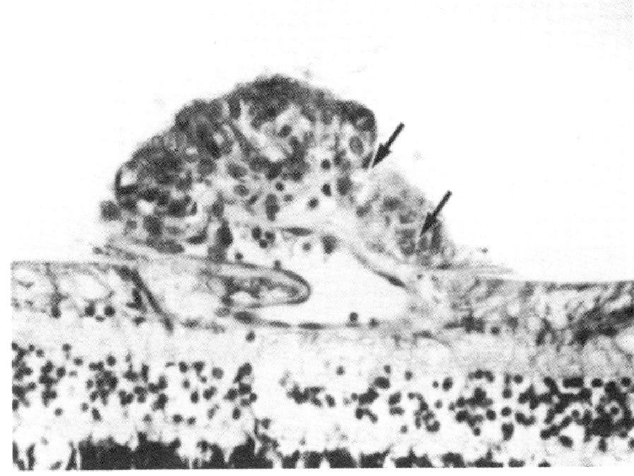

Figure 184–4. Retinopathy of prematurity (820-g infant) stage 3, polypoid extraretina vascularization. Microsection shows a small polyp on retina surface with a central feeder vessel *(asterisk)*, many plump endothelial cells, and a few patent capillaries *(arrows)*. H&E, ×540. (From Foos RY: Chronic retinopathy of prematurity. Ophthalmology 95:563, 1985.)

PERSISTENT HYPERPLASTIC PRIMARY VITREOUS

The vitreous has three components: the primary, the secondary, and the tertiary vitreous.[28–31] The primary vitreous forms during the first months of fetal life in the space between the lens and the retina. It consists of mesodermally derived tissue, including the hyaloid vessels and its branches, and a fibrillar meshwork of uncertain origin. Remnants of the primitive hyaloid system often persist in small infants anteriorly (Mittendorf's dot behind the lens posterior pole), posteriorly (Bergmeister's papilla at the optic disc), or more extensively (hyaloid vessel).

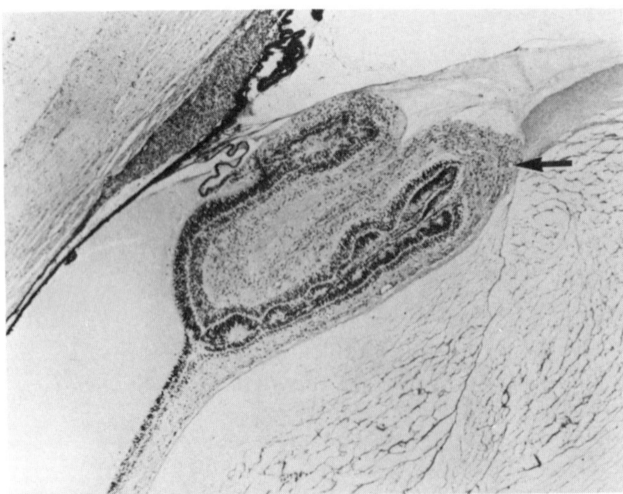

Figure 184–5. Retinopathy of prematurity stage 5 (6-month-old infant, birth weight of 820 g) showing microscopic features of peripheral retina, which is folded and rolled like a scroll. Extraretinal vascularization is notable only at the summit of some of the folds *(arrow)*. Posteriorly, the foreshortened retina is detached and serous exudate is present in retroretinal space and overlying the vitreous body. Epiretinal and retroretinal membranes are lacking. H&E, ×60. (From Foos RY: Chronic retinopathy of prematurity. Ophthalmology 92:563, 1985.)

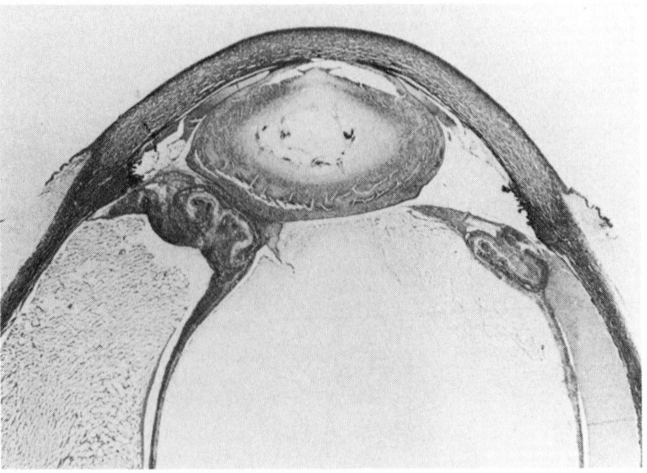

Figure 184–6. Retinopathy of prematurity stage 5 (6-month-old infant, birth weight of 820 g), showing folding and rolling and peripheral retina with foreshortening and detachment of the retina. Retrolental region shows only condensed vitreous with slight serous exudate. Picroanaline blue, ×13. (From Foos RY: Chronic retinopathy of prematurity. Ophthalmology 92:563, 1985.)

The secondary vitreous, or definitive adult vitreous, forms during the second month of embryonic development. It is composed of 99 percent water bound with collagen and hyaluronic acid. The tertiary vitreous, developed during the fourth month of gestation, forms the zonules of Zinn, which suspend the lens.

Persistent hyperplastic primary vitreous is almost always observed clinically in its anterior form.[32–34] A plaque of fibrovascular tissue typically adheres to the posterior part of the lens and extends to elongated ciliary processes (Fig. 184–7). Fat, smooth muscle, and cartilage may be seen in the retrolental mass.[35, 36] Multiple malformation may be associated, including retinal dysplasia, microphthalmia, cataract, and anterior segment dysgenesis.

Spitznas and colleagues[34] confirmed the fibrovascular nature of the tissue mass in an ultrastructural study of tissue excised from four infants with anterior persistent hyperplastic primary vitreous. The investigators showed that the hyaloid artery is surrounded by glial cells at its point of entry into the posterior pole of the retrolental mass, and the anterior surface is covered with lens remnants showing sings of early disturbance of lens

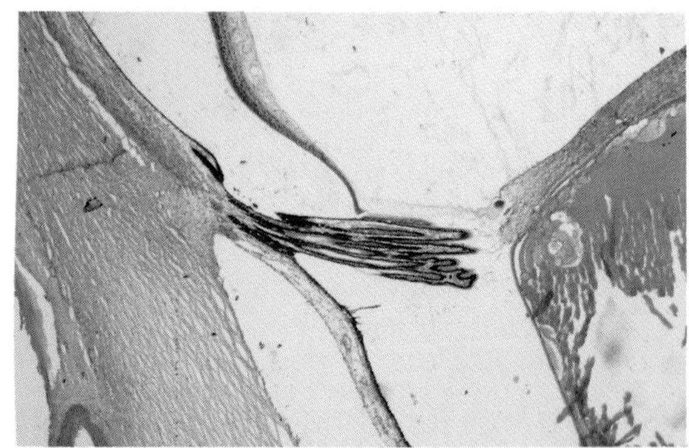

Figure 184–7. Persistent hyperplastic primary vitreous attraction of ciliary processes by fibrovascular scar. H&E, ×4.

development, particularly absence of the posterior lens capsule. They concluded that the developmental defect in persistent hyperplastic primary vitreous may involve not only the vitreous but also the hyaloid vascular system and parts of the lens. These findings are still unconfirmed.[37]

RETINAL DYSPLASIA, DEGENERATIONS, AND DYSTROPHIES

Retinal Dysplasia

Retinal dysplasia is a congenital condition characterized by abnormal proliferation and folding of the developing retina (the inner layer of the optic cup), with resultant tubular or rosette-like configurations of retina.[38] Retinal dysplasia appears as the consequence of chromosomal abnormalities (i.e., trisomy 13) or intrauterine trauma or infection.

The abortive cellular elements of the photoreceptor layer are arranged into tubules forming rosettes around a central lumen (Fig. 184–8). Depending on the degree of differentiation and maturation of the dysplastic retina, the rosettes are bordered by one, two, or three layers. Although Reese and Blodi[39] described retinal dysplasia as a bilateral syndrome occurring in conjunction with multiple systemic malformations, most investigators after Hunter and Zimmerman[40] considered retinal dysplasia to be a retinal lesion encountered in various situations rather than a clinical syndrome.[41]

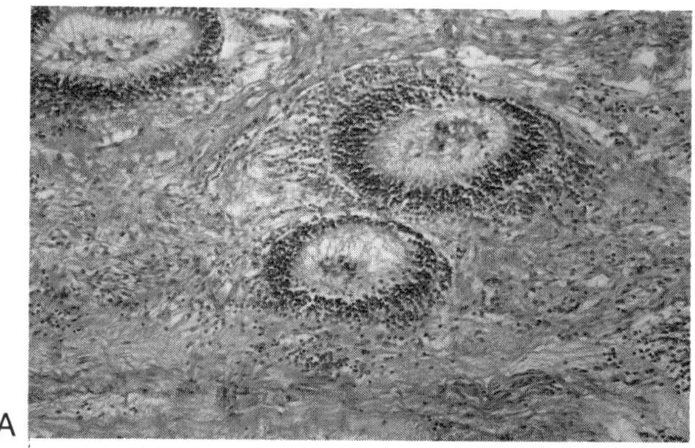

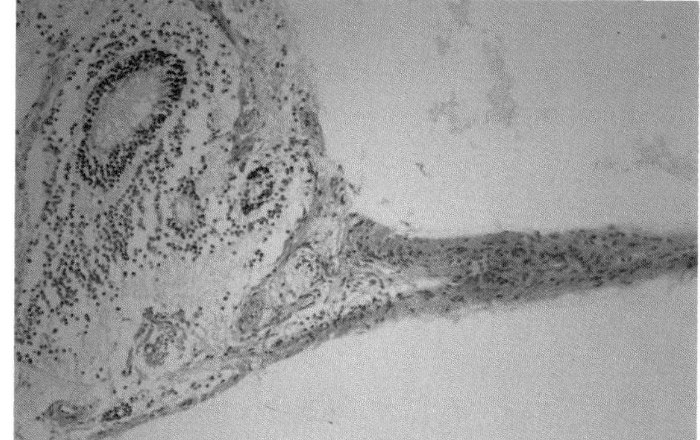

Figure 184–8. *A*, Retinal dysplasia associated with hydrocephaly showing rosette formation. H&E, ×40. *B*, Remnant of hyaline artery and area of dysplasia in retina.

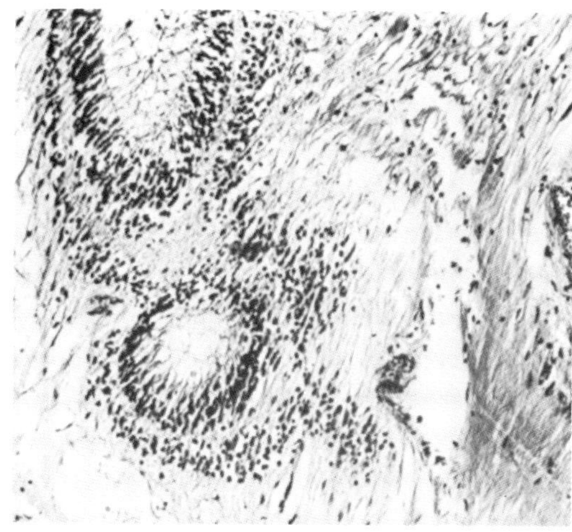

Figure 184–9. High-power photomicrograph of retina. Marked folding of the retina has produced structures bearing some resemblance to dysplastic rosettes. Severe gliosis is present. H&E, ×40. (From Blair NP, Albert DM, Liberfarb RM, Hirose T: Hereditary progressive arthro-ophthalmopathy of Stickler. Am J Ophthalmol 88:876, 1979. Reprinted with permission from the Ophthalmic Publishing Company.)

Hereditary Vitreoretinal Degenerations

It should be emphasized that for most hereditary vitreoretinal conditions, histopathologic data from the early stages are scarce.

Wagner-Jansen-Stickler Vitreoretinal Dystrophy. This disease is characterized by an optically empty vitreous cavity containing thick retrolenticular, transvitreal, and preretinal membranes and strands, particularly adherent to the retina. These abnormal elements correspond to dense cortical vitreous and demonstrate areas of glial ingrowth, lattice-like retinal degeneration, and increased lobe size (Fig. 184–9).[42–45]

Goldmann-Favre Vitreoretinal Degeneration.[28–46] This is a rare autosomal recessive condition characterized by night blindness, constriction of the peripheral visual field, nonrecordable electroretinograms, and peripheral pigmentary changes similar to retinitis pigmentosa. An optically empty vitreous cavity except for condensed veils is a striking finding on clinical examination. Macular retinoschisis, frequently peripheral retinoschisis, and secondary cataract are also seen. In the histopathologic findings in one case, described by Peyman and colleagues in 1977,[47] a full-thickness eye-wall biopsy specimen showed changes restricted to the inner retina and photoreceptors (i.e., absence of photoreceptor outer segments) that suggested primary degeneration of the neural retina.

Familial Exudative Vitreoretinopathy. In 1969, Criswick and Schepens[48] observed this autosomal dominant condition in six patients from two families. The condition clinically simulates most stages of ROP, but a history of prematurity or oxygen administration is absent (see Chap. 57). A few histopathologic reports mention the posterior attachment of a prominent, acellular, amorphous vitreous membrane. This membrane, along with a fibrocellular component, induces retinal traction, folding, and detachment. Whether the vascular abnor-

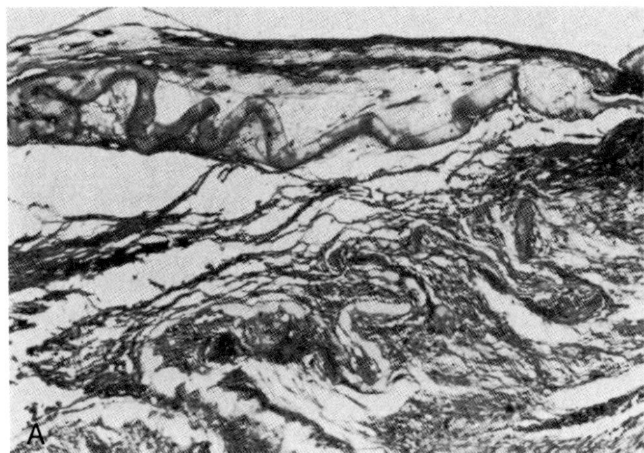

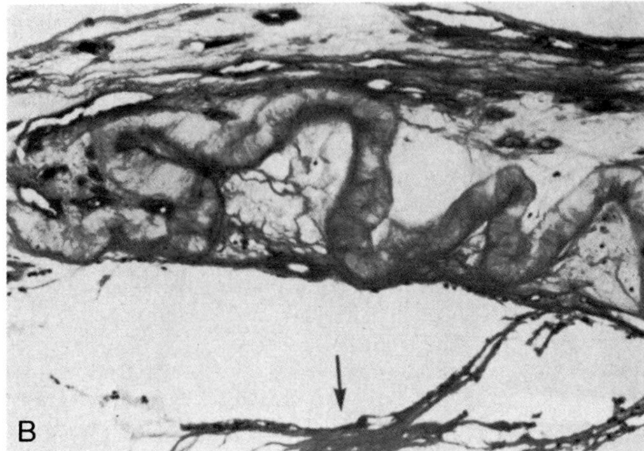

Figure 184–10. *A*, Detached gliotic retina showing dense amorphous folded band on retinal surface with condensed, organized vitreous-like material internal to it. H&E, ×200. *B*, Higher-power view of folded band on retinal surface *(arrow)* showing organized material in it as well as macrophages and fibroblasts. H&E, ×500. (From Brockhurst RJ, Albert DM, Zakov ZN: Pathologic findings in familial exudative vitreoretinopathy. Arch Ophthalmol 99:2143, 1981. Copyright 1981, American Medical Association.)

malities are primary or secondary remains undetermined (Fig. 184–10).[49, 50]

Congenital Retinoschisis. This X-linked bilateral disorder results from retinal splitting in the nerve fiber layer, involving the macular and inferior temporal retina. Vitreous abnormalities (e.g., condensation with adherence to the splitting retina, liquefaction, and cavitation) may have a key pathogenetic role.[51, 52]

Lattice Degeneration. Lattice degeneration is a common finding at autopsy (6 percent in the study by Straatsma and Allen[53]). The relationship between these lesions and retinal breaks and detachment and their management is discussed elsewhere (see Chap. 93). Retinal thinning after degeneration of retinal neurons is associated with cleavage and liquefaction of the overlying vitreous. In contrast, the vitreous is condensed and strongly attached at the margins of the lesion, with subsequent glial proliferation. Fibrosis and occlusion of retinal vessels in the degenerated area, intermixed with atrophy and hyperpigmentation of the retinal pigment epithelium (RPE), account for the most characteristic features.[38, 54, 55]

Snowflake Degeneration. This is a bilateral, peripheral, autosomal dominant degeneration. It is characterized by the presence of retinal yellow-white spots, fibrillary vitreous condensation and subsequent retinal vascular sheathing, irregular equatorial pigmentation, and more prominent vitreous abnormalities (strands).[56] To the best of our knowledge, histopathologic data are unavailable.

Autosomal Dominant Vitreoretinochoroidopathy. This recently described condition shares histologic features with retinitis pigmentosa (e.g., multifocal loss of photoreceptors and altered pigment epithelial cells) and vitreoretinal degenerations (e.g., extensive preretinal membranes).[57]

Retinitis Pigmentosa. Various systemic and ocular diseases result in retinal degeneration, characterized by photoreceptor loss. Retinitis pigmentosa comprises several types of bilateral progressive pigmentary retinopathy, classified primarily according to the mode of inheritance. Very few histopathologic studies have used well-preserved eyes in the early stages of retinitis pigmentosa. Insight into pathogenesis has been gained mainly from animal model studies,[58] biochemistry, and genetics.[59]

A review of available pathologic data was provided by several studies,[60–62] most of which suggested a primary defect in the photoreceptor layer and secondary changes in the RPE layer, glial cells, inner retina, and choriocapillaris (Fig. 184–11). Nevertheless, it should be emphasized that because primary defects in the pigment epithelial layer were demonstrated in animal models of inherited retinal degenerations, such as a defect of phagocytosis in RCS rats, similar abnormalities can be expected in some human subtypes of inherited retinal degeneration. Therefore, despite striking similarities in most reports of advanced cases, distinguishing between primary and secondary lesions in late cases and drawing implications from one subtype to another can be deceptive. The most common findings include loss, shortening, and disorganization of the photoreceptors (usually rods in focal areas); atrophy, hypoplasia, degeneration, depigmentation, or proliferation; and aggregation of the RPE with increased phagosomal material and lipofuscin content. In addition, glial proliferation (from Müller's cells) forming epiretinal membranes occurs and is often associated with marked optic disc gliosis. Proliferation accounts for the clinical pallor and retinal blood vessel attenuation. Variations in geographic and cellular-type repartition of these "elementary lesions" are correlated with the various clinical features.[58, 60–62]

Hereditary Macular Dystrophies

Hereditary macular dystrophies include rare conditions sharing bilateral, slowly progressive retinal involvement restricted to the posterior pole, with early onset and often a positive family history.

Stargardt's Disease and Fundus Flavimaculatus. These two disorders, the most common hereditary macular dystrophies, are no longer considered separate entities

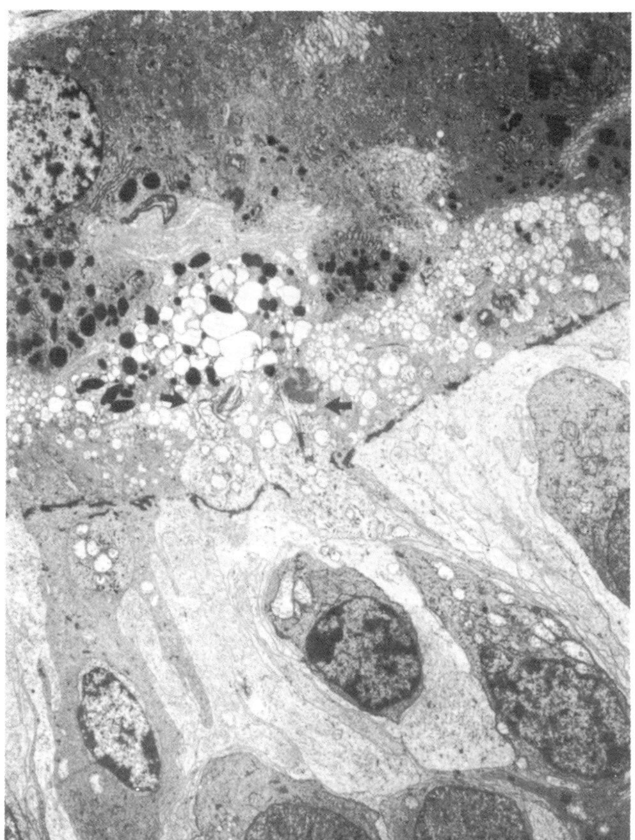

Figure 184–11. The postequatorial retina includes regions in which the subretinal space is reduced, leaving the remaining photoreceptor inner segments in direct apposition to the apical membrane of the retinal pigment epithelium. The last vestiges of two photoreceptor outer segments are observed *(arrows)*. ×3330. (From Flannery JG, Farber D, Bird AC, Bok D: Degenerative changes in a retina affected with autosomal dominant retinitis pigmentosa. Invest Ophthalmol Vis Sci 30:191, 1989.)

because some patients with features of Stargardt's disease (i.e., pigmentary maculopathy surrounded by rare yellow to white flecks) develop features of fundus flavimaculatus (i.e., yellowish-white flecks disseminated throughout and beyond the posterior pole). Conversely, Stargardt's disease is considered by some to be a variant of fundus flavimaculatus with early macular involvement. The transmission is autosomal recessive with conservation of the phenotypic expression in the same family. Histopathologic examinations place the major abnormality at the RPE level. Pathologic findings vary considerably, however, and some reports emphasize increased accumulation of lipofuscin and melanolipofuscin in pigmented cells (Fig. 184–12).[63–65]

It should be noted that McDonnell and colleagues,[66] in their ultrastructural study of a case of "pure" fundus flavimaculatus, found no lipofuscin or PAS-positive material. Rather, the main abnormality was an accumulation of a tubulovesicular membranous material. Therefore, it is likely that this disease group reflects more than one process and that the macular degeneration may represent a different pathologic entity from fundus flavimaculatus.[65, 67]

Best's Vitelliform Macular Dystrophy. Histopathologic studies show an accumulation of lipofuscin in RPE cells, particularly in the foveal area; deposition of heterogenous material from degenerating pigment epithelial cells; and secondary degeneration of photoreceptor cells, with a subretinal collection of outer segment debris and phagocytic cells (Fig. 184–13).[67–69]

Dominant drusen of Bruch's membrane[70] were studied by Gass and colleagues,[71] who observed nodular thickening of the basement membrane of the RPE. This implies that these drusen differ from age-related drusen. In contrast, on histopathologic examination of two cases, Sorsby's pseudoinflammatory macular dystrophy showed features similar to disciform scars in age-related macular degeneration (e.g., ruptures in Bruch's membrane, subretinal neovascular tissue, and gliosis of the outer retina).[72]

VITREOUS DETACHMENT

Vitreous aging and detachment are widely recognized as crucial factors in the pathogenesis of retinal detachment, whether rhegmatogenous or tractional, as well as in the development of idiopathic vitreoretinal macular disorders.

Vitreous body aging is initially characterized by the formation of thickening fibers and the progression of central liquefaction (syneresis). Vitreous liquefaction is accelerated in myopic eyes and by inflammation (e.g.,

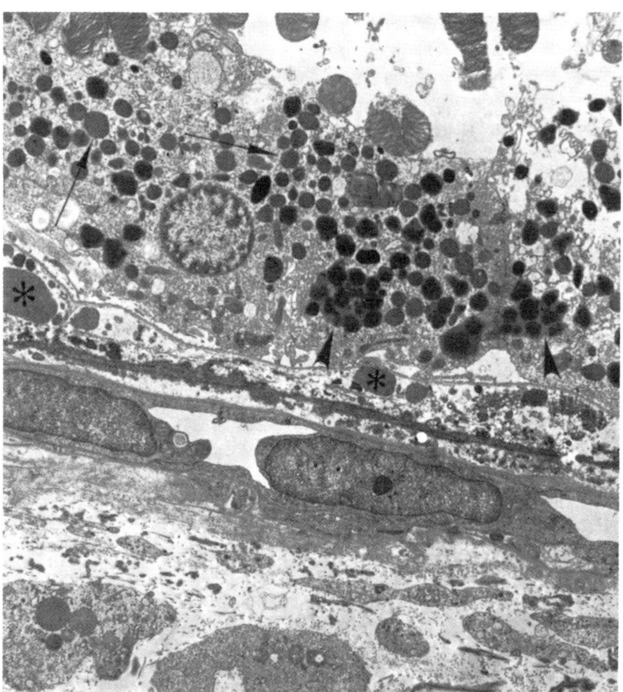

Figure 184–12. Transmission electron micrograph of an enlarged retinal pigment epithelial cell shows intracytoplasmic accumulation of lipofuscin *(arrows)* and complex melanolipofuscin conglomerates *(arrowheads)*, which appear to be membrane bound. Beneath the retinal pigment epithelial basal lamina, lightly osmiophilic granular collections *(asterisks)* are similar in appearance to intracytoplasmic lipofuscin. Original magnification, ×4000. (From Lopez PF, Maumenee IH, delaCruz A, Green WR: Autosomal dominant fundus flavimaculatus: Clinicopathologic correlation. Published courtesy of Ophthalmology 97:798, 1990.)

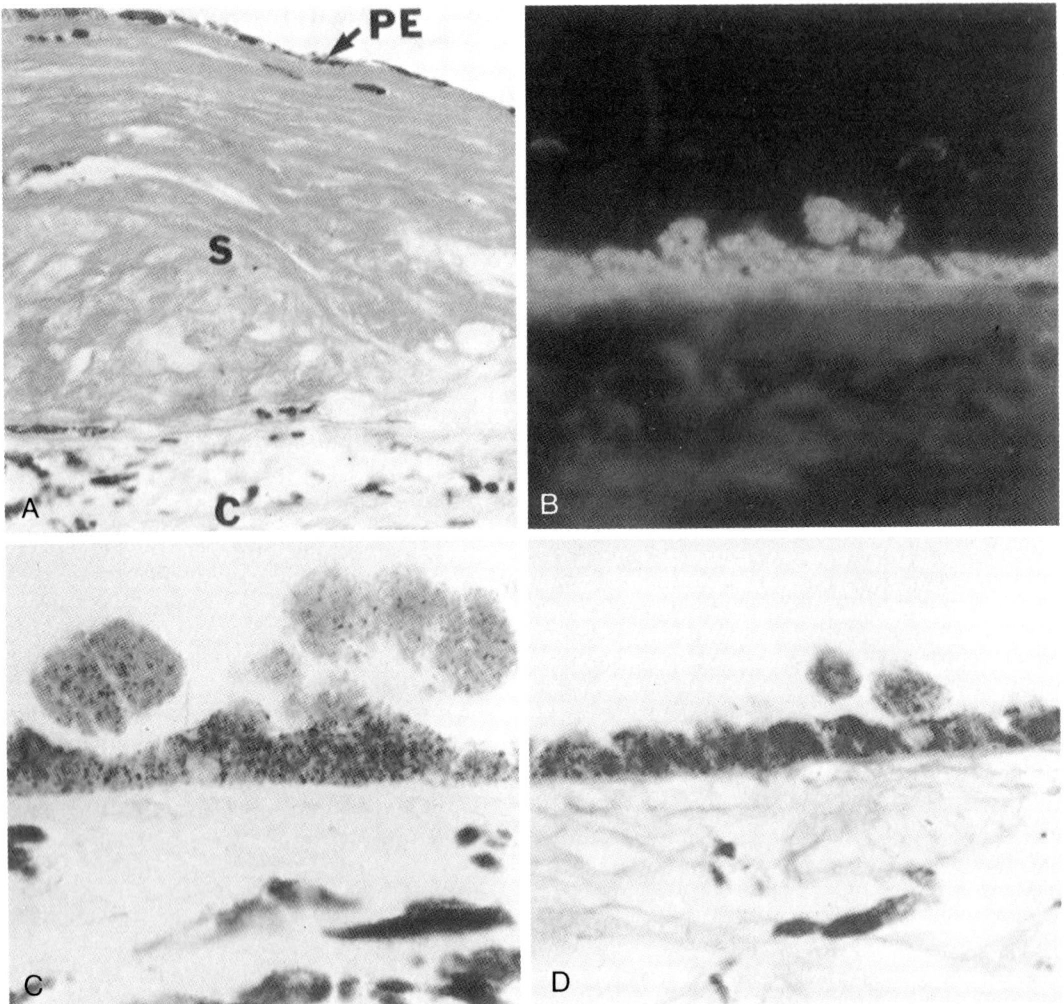

Figure 184–13. *A*, Neovascularized scar (S) was present beneath pigment epithelium (PE) and choroid (C) in macula of left eye of donor. Masson's trichrome. *B*, Photomicrograph of unstained frozen section taken with epifluorescent illumination. Pigment epithelium is filled with autofluorescent material that stained with Sudan black *(C)* and was PAS positive *(D)*. Cells within subretinal space were filled with similar material. (From O'Gorman S, Flaherty WA, Fishman GA, Berson EL: Histopathologic findings in Best's vitelliform macular dystrophy. Arch Ophthalmol 106:1261, 1988. Copyright 1988, American Medical Association.)

uveitis and trauma). The biochemical and ultrastructural events underlying vitreous syneresis are discussed in *Principles and Practice of Ophthalmology: Basic Sciences,* Chapter 55. Foos[73] detected 25 percent vitreous liquefaction in autopsy studies of eyes from subjects in their third decade. Posterior vitreous detachment (PVD) was detected in at least one eye in 10 percent of subjects younger than 50 yr, 27 percent of subjects between 60 and 69, and 63 percent older than 70. In the same study, a significant correlation was found between the degree of vitreous syneresis and the prevalence of PVD. Both phenomena are age related.[73, 74] According to Eisner,[75, 76] PVD occurs acutely as a consequence of posterior cortical vitreous tearing. The liquefied vitreous gel empties through the premacular gap in the retrovitreal space, inducing vitreous collapse and PVD.[77, 78] Eisner suggests differentiating this type of rhegmatogenous vitreous detachment from vitreous detachments occurring without identifiable cortical vitreous breaks, as in proliferative diabetic retinopathy. This view is not unanimously accepted.[54]

Complications of PVD

As the vitreous separates from the retina, complications may be induced either by traction on preexisting vitreoretinal adhesions with subsequent intravitreal or retrovitreal hemorrhage and retinal tearing, or by incomplete separation of the cortical vitreous.

In the case of traction or retrocortical adhesions, peripheral retinal breaks may evolve to retinal detachment (discussed later). The pathogenesis of macular holes and their relationship to PVD are still debated. In 1987, Gass proposed that posterior vitreous alterations occurring before the development of PVD are the cause of macular holes.[79, 80] He suggested that contraction of prefoveal vitreous induces traction detachment of the fovea at early stages. Prolonged traction causes development of macular holes, with formation of an operculum. PVD occurs later, with the operculum remaining adherent anteriorly to the posterior hyaloid membrane. Histopathologic study of tissue removed on vitrectomy for impending idiopathic macular holes confirmed the

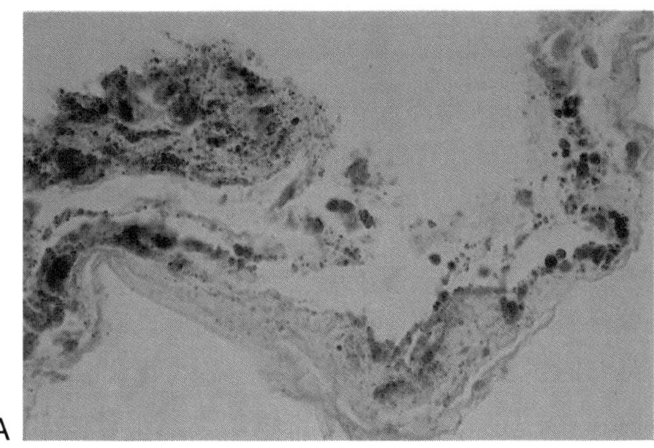

A

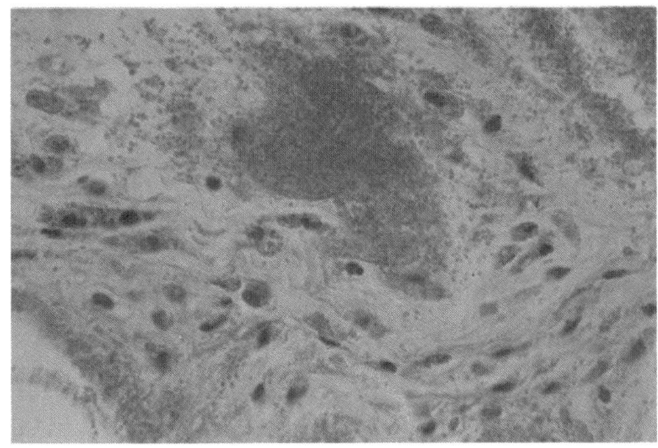

B

Figure 184–14. *A*, Epiretinal membrane; predominance of retinal pigment epithelium–derived pigmented cells in epiretinal membrane. H&E, ×10. *B*, Epiretinal membrane: fibroblast-like partially pigmented cells with collagen formation. H&E, ×40.

presence of indigenous vitreous collagen on the posterior retina.[81, 82] At the base of the hole, nodular proliferation of the RPE overlays eosinophilic material, which is visible as yellow deposits.[79]

The pathogenesis of idiopathic epiretinal macular membranes is discussed in detail in Chapter 74. The once widely mentioned finding of PVD in such cases now is questioned in view of the frequent perioperative finding of a large, empty intravitreal space mistaken for the retroretinal space.[83] Contraction of the thin layer of cortical vitreous tissue remaining in front of the macula is implicated in the development of premacular idiopathic membrane.[84] However, Smiddy and colleagues[82] found PVD in 101 eyes of their series of surgically excised idiopathic macular pucker. Almost all nonneuronal cell types in the macular region have been implicated and detected in epiretinal membranes, including hyalocytes,[85] glial cells,[86, 87] and RPE cells (Fig. 184–14).[84–88] New collagen is present in these membranes. The RPE cells predominate in most series.[84, 88–91] The pathogenetic significance of this finding is not yet understood; it may represent migration of RPE cells through subclinical or self-healed retinal breaks, transretinal migration of RPE cells, and even transformation of glial cells. Myofibroblastic differentiation of migrating and proliferating cells is a common finding, accounting for membrane retraction.[84] In cases of vitreomacular traction syndrome, surgically excised specimens contain new collagen, predominantly fibrous astrocytes, and some myofibroblasts. Cell migration to the vitreoretinal junction is thought to be either a consequence of incomplete PVD or a preexisting event causing vitreoretinal adhesion and limiting PVD.[91]

Therefore, it should be emphasized that despite the reservations expressed about the role of PVD in the pathogenesis of some vitreomacular diseases, its role in vitreoretinal disorders should not be overlooked and should be reevaluated.[92–97]

VITREOUS OPACITIES

Asteroid Hyalosis

Asteroid hyalosis is a common degenerative process usually occurring unilaterally in patients older than 60 yr. Asteroid bodies are attached to the collagenous vitreous frame and may arise from vitreous fibril degeneration.[98] Asteroid bodies consist of an amorphous basophilic PAS-positive substance that stains positively with lipid and acid mucopolysaccharide stains (Fig. 184–15). Birefringent crystals are embedded in this substance. These characteristics[99] support Verhoeff's suggestion that asteroid hyalosis represents a calcium-containing lipid (probably phospholipid).[100]

Cholesterosis Bulbi

After intravitreal hemorrhage, cholesterol crystals may accumulate and move freely inside the vitreous cavity. Histologically, cholesterol crystals are dissolved by routine alcohol dehydration and appear as empty slitlike spaces. Other sequelae of vitreous hemorrhages include hemosiderosis, ghost cells, hemoglobin spherulosis,[101] and macrophages containing blood breakdown products.

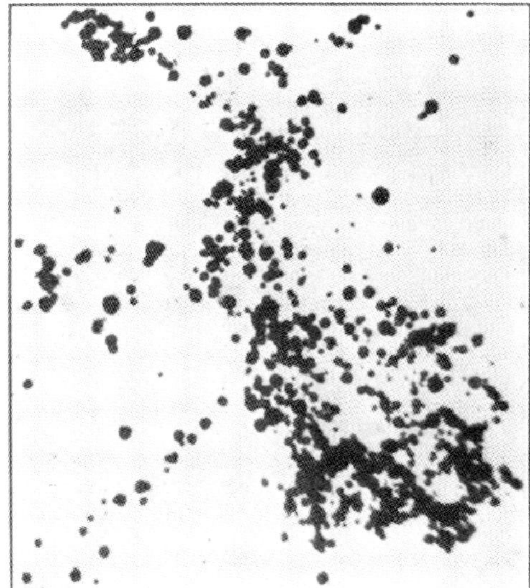

Figure 184–15. Group of asteroid opacities as seen by transmitted light. (From Verhoeff FH: Microscopic findings in a case of asteroid hyalitis. Am J Ophthalmol 4:155, 1921. Reprinted with permission from the Ophthalmic Publishing Company.)

Systemic Primary Amyloid

Systemic primary amyloid can induce early bilateral vitreous opacification. Excised vitreous shows the usual staining reactions characteristic of amyloid. Doft and colleagues[102] showed immunocytochemically that the major amyloid constituent resembles prealbumin.

RETINAL DETACHMENT

Retinal detachment is a separation between the RPE and the neuroepithelium at the embyronic cavity between the two layers of the optic vesicle.

Retinal Attachment

Attachment of the neurosensory retina to the RPE, except at the optic disc and ora serrata, is dependent on various mechanisms: intraocular pressure, vitreous support and pressure, gravity, interdigitation of photoreceptor outer segments and RPE apical microvilli, interphotoreceptor matrix and adhesion molecules, the subretinal space, and RPE-dependent active transport of fluids, ions, and molecules from the subretinal space to the choroid.[103–106]

Mechanisms of Detachment

The weak attachment of the neurosensory retina to the RPE can be altered by three principal mechanisms, resulting in retinal detachment.[38–54]

Rhegmatogenous Retinal Detachment. The most common type of retinal detachment results from accumulation of vitreous fluid beneath the neural retina through a tear or a hole. This breach in the neuroepithelial continuity is most often secondary to degenerative retinal changes linked to vitreous alterations with vitreous traction. These various vitreoretinal abnormalities range from the equatorial lattice-type paravascular vitreoretinal adhesions to less worrisome lesions such as degenerative retinoschisis, white without pressure or peripheral cystoid degeneration. When vitreous adheres to the internal limiting membrane, vitreous traction may lead to hole formation.

The main changes following retinal detachment involve the outer layers of the sensory retina, presumably as a consequence of separation from the blood supply and interruption of the normal shedding of photoreceptor outer segments by the RPE. Earlier changes detected experimentally in owl monkeys are disruption and disorganization of outer segments with separation of phagosomes from the RPE. The RPE undergoes degenerative hyperplasia at the posterior limit of the detached retina. After 3 mo, this hyperplasia may generate a demarcation line showing fibrous metaplasia histologically. Proliferation of the RPE at the ora serrata results in large, pigmented plaque (ringschwiele).

Cystic changes appear in the neurosensory retina, preferentially in the outer layers. In long-standing inferior detachments, intraretinal macrocystoid spaces may develop in the equatorial area (Fig. 184–16).[107–109]

After successful retinal reattachment surgery, the rare eyes investigated in two postmortem studies showed photoreceptor atrophy in 26 percent and 26.5 percent of eyes, respectively, and unexpectedly high incidence of epiretinal membranes (75 and 60 percent), macular pucker (20 percent), and cystoid macular edema (10 and 20 percent) (Fig. 184–17).[110, 111] Studies such as these shed light on causes of clinically unexplained reduced vision after successful retinal reattachment surgery and on the exact incidence and role of epiretinal proliferations.

Tractional Retinal Detachment. The neuroepithelium may be pulled by intravitreal membranes as a result of trauma (spontaneous or surgical), with vitreous incarceration in the wound or proliferative retinopathies such as diabetic retinopathy, sickle cell disease, ROP, and proliferative vitreoretinopathy following rhegmatogenous retinal detachment. In these entities, secondary retinal holes can occur. Therefore, intrication of both types is common.

Exudative, Transudative, or Hemorrhagic Retinal Detachment. These types of detachments result from accumulation of subretinal fluid from the choroidal or retinal vessels. This situation can occur in many diseases, including choroidal melanomas (and other tumors), inflammatory conditions (Harada's disease, scleritis, sym-

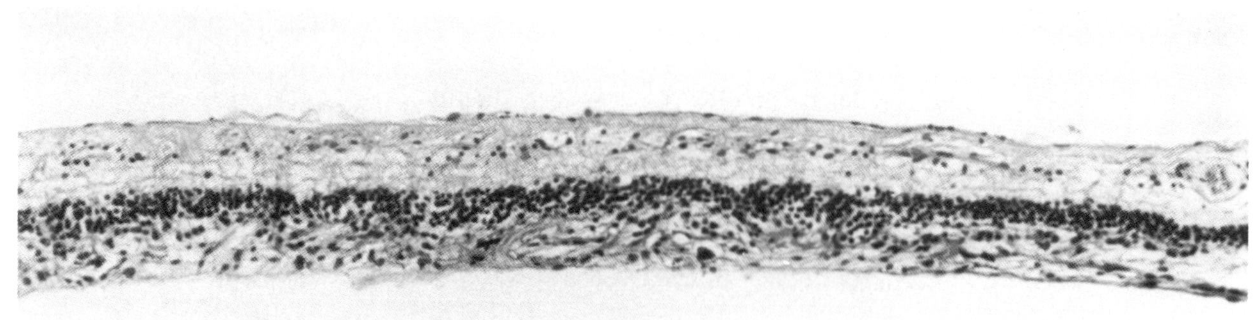

Figure 184–16. Midperipheral retina. Patient had total retinal detachment. Postoperative visual acuity was 20/200. Note absence of photoreceptors and atrophy of outer plexiform and outer nuclear layers. H&E, original magnification ×100. (From Barr CC: The histopathology of successful retinal reattachment. Retina 10:189, 1990.)

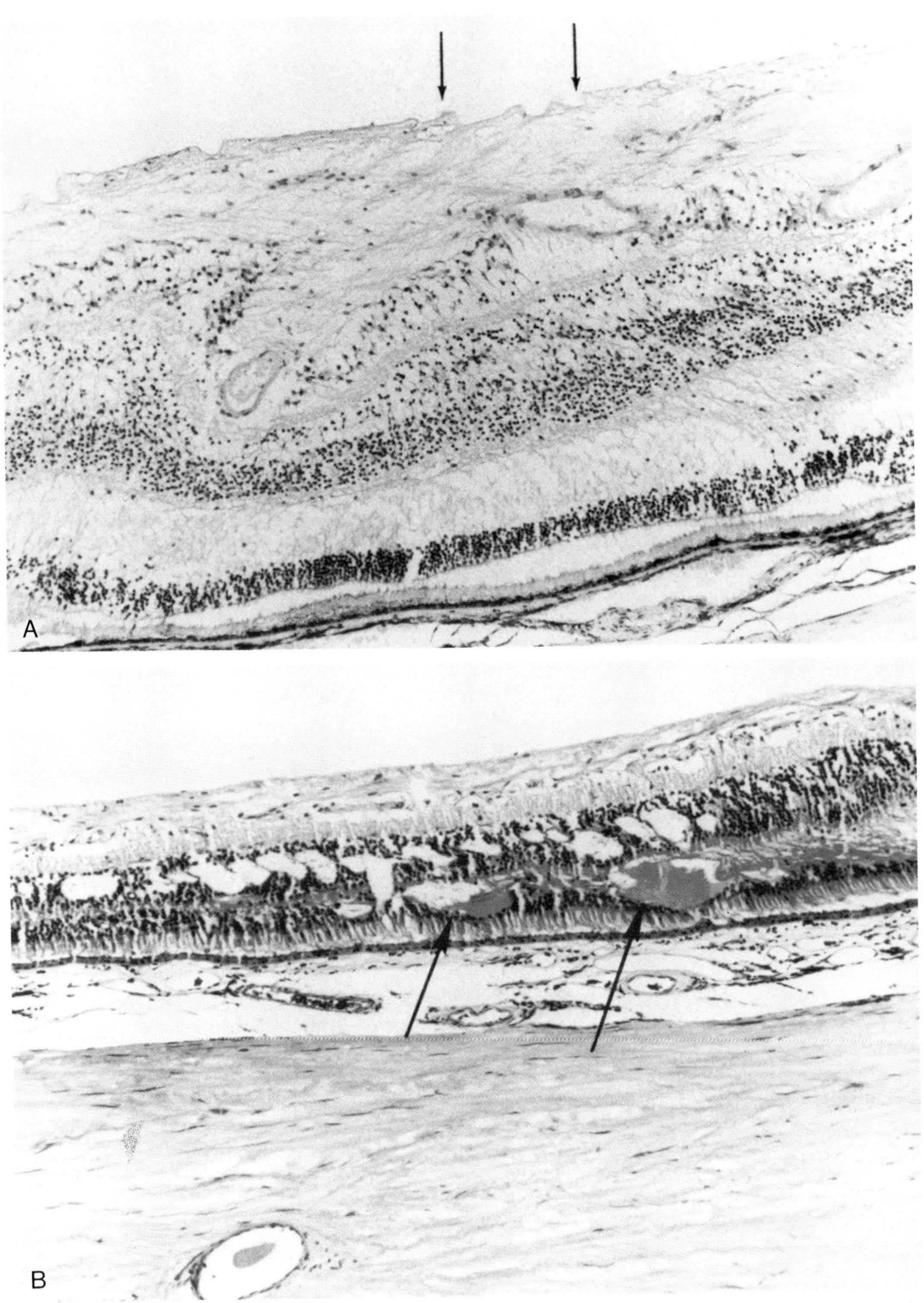

Figure 184–17. *A*, Macular area demonstrating retinal folding and edema from epiretinal membrane *(arrows)*. Final visual acuity was 5/200. H&E, original magnification × 100. *B*, Macular area. Visual acuity was 20/25. Note cystoid spaces in the outer plexiform layer and the outer nuclear layer as indicated by arrows. H&E, original magnification × 100. (From Barr CC: The histopathology of successful retinal reattachment. Retina 10:189, 1990.)

pathetic ophthalmia), and vascular disease (hypertension, eclampsia).

Proliferative Vitreoretinopathy

Proliferative vitreoretinopathy (PVR), a major cause of failure of retinal detachment surgery, is found on histopathologic examination to be the migration and proliferation of retinal, subretinal, and intravitreal cells on both surfaces of the neural retina as well as on the vitreous base and posterior surface. The growth and subsequent contraction of the cellular membranes are the causes of traction retinal detachments. Formerly described as massive vitreous retraction or massive periretinal retraction, PVR is now recognized as a separate entity.[112–120] Understanding the pathogenesis and mechanisms of this major challenge in vitreoretinal surgery will contribute further to better prevention and treatment.

The first cellular event is the release and dispersion of RPE cells into the vitreous cavity during retinal tearing, separation, cryotherapy, and scleral depression.[121–125] These RPE cells migrate inferiorly in the vitreous cavity and attach preferentially to the inferior retina. Migration and chemotaxis of RPE cells to collagen and sodium hyaluronate are mediated by fibronectin and platelet-derived growth factor, both normal serum components that may enter the vitreous cavity as a consequence of cryotherapy-induced breakdown of the normal blood-ocular barrier. The interaction of RPE cells with the extracellular matrix components (collagen and in some cases fibrin) presumably induces morphologic change from an epithelial to a fibroblastic type, then active engagement and dragging of vitreous fibrils (5 mm/24 hr) with subsequent contraction of the vitreous gel. Production of a chemoattractant to astrocytes and a growth factor follows. This factor appears to be transforming growth factor beta, a chemoattractant to fibroblasts (as well as fibronectin and platelet-derived growth factor). In addition, monocytes stimulate fibroblast proliferation and production of collagen and fibronectin.

Although RPE cells obviously are a major factor in the formation of PVR membranes, the glial and monocytic cell types as well as the normal (type I) and newly formed (types II and III) collagen fibrils have a key role in membrane development and contraction. Many fibroblasts and fibroblast-like cells of these membranes assume a myofibroblastic morphology with cytoplasmic strands of contractile intermediate filaments, such as the myofibroblasts involved in wound contraction during the normal healing process. This finding, as well as a recent demonstration of the very early proliferative response (days 2 to 4) of every nonneuronal cell type to retinal detachment,[126] supports the view that PVR may simply be an exaggerated and mislocated healing process with devastating consequences.[127, 128]

Although the proportions of cellular types may vary from one case to another,[95, 96, 129, 130] collagen development and dragging as well as myofibroblastic properties appear to be the common denominator of PVR membranes that accounts for their contraction. Cellular invasion, proliferation, and membrane contraction may occur at various locations on the posterior vitreous surface, producing a taut transvitreal membrane close to the equator and extending from the vitreous base and the anterior cortex to the pars plana, ciliary processes, or iris. This membrane causes an anterior PVR with consecutive circumferential retinal folds, peripheral radial folding, reopening of retinal breaks,[131] and on the inner retinal surface distortion and "star folding" (Fig. 184–18).[38, 54, 132]

The subretinal space is another site of membrane formation where subretinal proteins cause the induction of early (1 wk) RPE migration and attachment to the retina. This is followed by proliferation of fibrocytes, macrophages, fibrous astrocytes, and myofibrocytes associated with fibrin and collagen deposition. Simple subretinal membranes with little extracellular material currently are distinguished from taut subretinal membranes with a prominent contractile RPE and collagen types I to IV components.[133–136] The role of these membranes in retinal detachment surgery failure is still disputed.[54, 133–137]

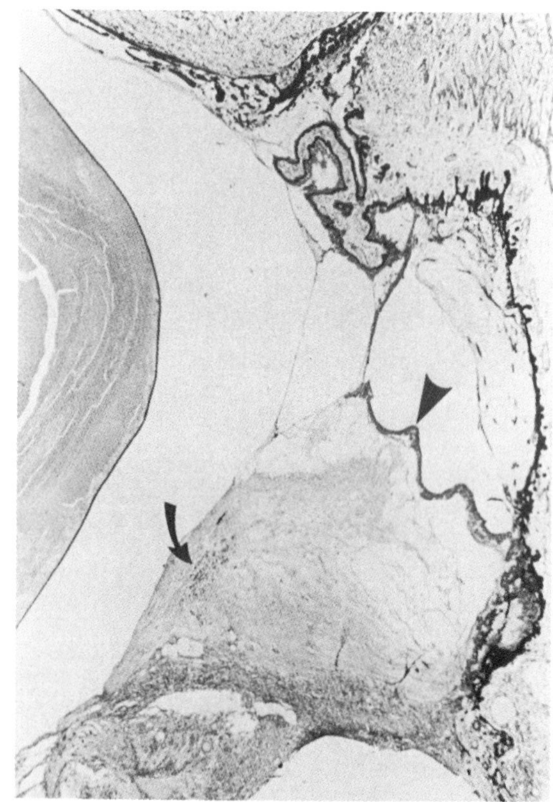

Figure 184–18. Densely organized vitreous at vitreous base in anterior proliferative vitreoretinopathy tissue is tightly adherent to the retina surface, where prominent glial proliferation is noted. Most of the organized vitreous contains proliferated metaplastic pigment epithelial cells *(arrow)* embedded in fibrous extracellular matrix. Attachments to pars plana and pars plicata have caused tractional separation of nonpigmented and pigmented neuroepithelial layers *(arrowhead)*. PAS, ×7.88 (From Elner SG, Elner VM, Diaz-Rohena R, et al: Anterior PVR. II: Clinicopathologic, light microscopic and ultrastructural findings. *In* Freeman HM, Tolentino FI [eds]: Proliferative Vitreoretinopathy (PVR). New York, Springer-Verlag, 1989.)

The international classification of PVR and its recent updates are well correlated with the previously mentioned clinicopathologic studies pioneered by Machemer and colleagues in the 1970s.[112–121]

AGE-RELATED MACULAR DEGENERATION

Age-related macular degeneration (AMD) is considered the leading cause of legal blindness both in people older than 65 yr and in the general population in developed countries.[138, 139] However, the exact definition, etiology, and classification have not been clearly formulated. For instance, most reports include drusen in their descriptions of clinicopathologic correlations without reference to visual loss, because drusen appear both as precursors to and integral features of all stages.[140] However, in the Framingham study, visual impairment was required to consider an eye with drusen or pigment changes as having AMD.[138] Moreover, drusen appear as a ubiquitous and often asymptomatic feature of retinal aging.

Except for drusen and pigment changes, the main lesions of AMD are associated with central visual loss, including serous detachment of the RPE (5 to 10 percent), geographic atrophy of the RPE and choriocapillaris (5 percent), and complications of subretinal neovascularization (more than 80 percent). Nevertheless, it should be emphasized that clinicopathologic studies detected such alterations in many asymptomatic eyes from the elderly at autopsy and showed a clear correlation of their severity with age.[141, 142] It is apparent that visual loss in AMD is the end-point of a continuum in chorioretinal senescence beginning at the RPE level and leading to photoreceptor degeneration and death. For these reasons, it will be difficult in the following discussion to separate age-related alterations from lesions that are an integral part of AMD.

Etiopathology

Among the numerous functions and malfunctions attributed to the RPE (e.g., glial, epithelial, physical, and macrophagic), the main mechanism implicated in macular aging is impairment of the interaction between the RPE and the outer segment of the photoreceptors. Biologic renewal of the outer segments implies continuous phagocytosis by the RPE of the altered discs. Age-related limitations of the biochemical pathways responsible for molecular degradation of this phagocytized material induce a progressive abnormal accumulation of waste material within the RPE. This material, principally lipofuscin, interferes with the normal cell metabolism and leads to the formation of deposits at various levels of Bruch's membrane and the deposition of drusen, a characteristic feature of retinal aging.[143–146]

A thorough discussion of the current theories of the mechanisms of aging (i.e., the biologic clock, biologic renewal, and the wear-and-tear theories and their intricacies) is found in Chapter 56. Further insights into the role of molecular biology, free radicals, lipoperoxidation, light toxicity, and dietary agents are expected in the near future.[79, 143, 144, 147–150]

Histopathology

Aging of the RPE is correlated histopathologically with an increase in size and content of lipofuscin parallel to a decrease of the number of melanin granules. The bases of RPE cells lose their digitations, and the cells become less cuboidal and regular in shape.[77, 151–153] The cells are separated from their basal membrane by membranous debris and basal laminar deposits. Degeneration of RPE cells can occur in several patterns, including lipoidal degeneration and apoptosis, while neighboring cells phagocytize the pigment released by degenerating cells and migrate in an attempt to maintain cell-to-cell contact. Pigment changes and atrophy result from exhaustion of these compensating processes (Fig. 184–19).[154]

On ultrastructural examination, Bruch's membrane is an acellular membrane composed of five layers (i.e., basal membrane of the RPE, inner collagen layer, elastic layer, outer collagen layer, and the basement membrane of the choriocapillaris). All are progressively altered with increasing age.[155] Debris starts accumulating in Bruch's membrane in the inner collagen layer during the second decade of life and later on in the elastic layer, the outer collagen layer, and the choriocapillaris.[156] Early light microscopy studies have shown thickening, increased basophilia, and calcifications of Bruch's membrane[157–159] corresponding at the ultrastructural level to accumulation of coated membrane-bound bodies containing granular and vesicular material, and mem-

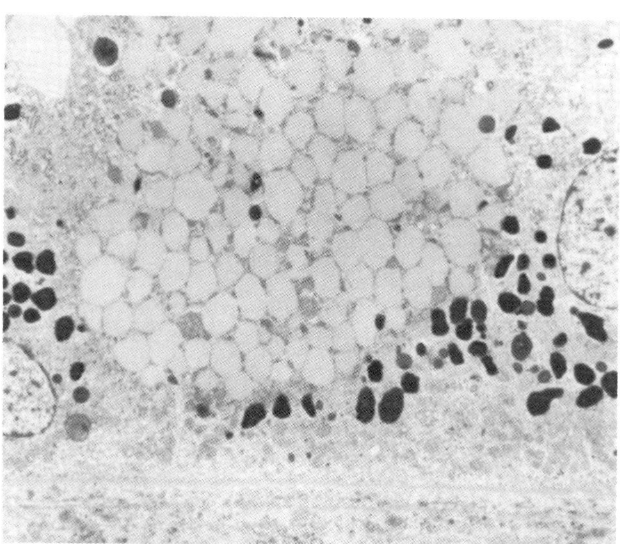

Figure 184–19. A single retinal epithelial pigment cell with marked accumulation of lipid inclusions in an eye of a 40-year-old woman who had systemic lupus erythematosus and who had an orbital exenteration because of a squamous cell carcinoma of the lid. EP 4227, paraphenylenediamine, ×3790. (From Green WR: Clinicopathologic studies of senile macular degeneration. *In* Nicholson DH [ed]: Ocular Pathology Update. New York, Masson, 1980, pp 115–144.)

branous debris along with a segment of long-spacing collagen.[157–159] Progressive mineralization of Bruch's membrane, particularly the elastic layer, accounts for loss of elasticity and increased fragility.

During the seventh decade of life, as demonstrated by Sarks and colleagues,[152, 153] a fine granular material accumulates between the RPE and its basement membrane. These basal laminar deposits are a major feature of age-related RPE impairment and are considered an abnormal secretory product elaborated by RPE cells, with subsequent deposition of collagen and fibronectin and later formation more internally of a hyalinized PAS-positive deposit (Fig. 184–20).[153–160]

Drusen are localized deposits of extracellular material between the basement membrane of the RPE and the inner collagen layer of Bruch's membrane. They are classified clinically and pathologically into several subtypes: hard, soft, diffuse, basal, nodular, mixed, and

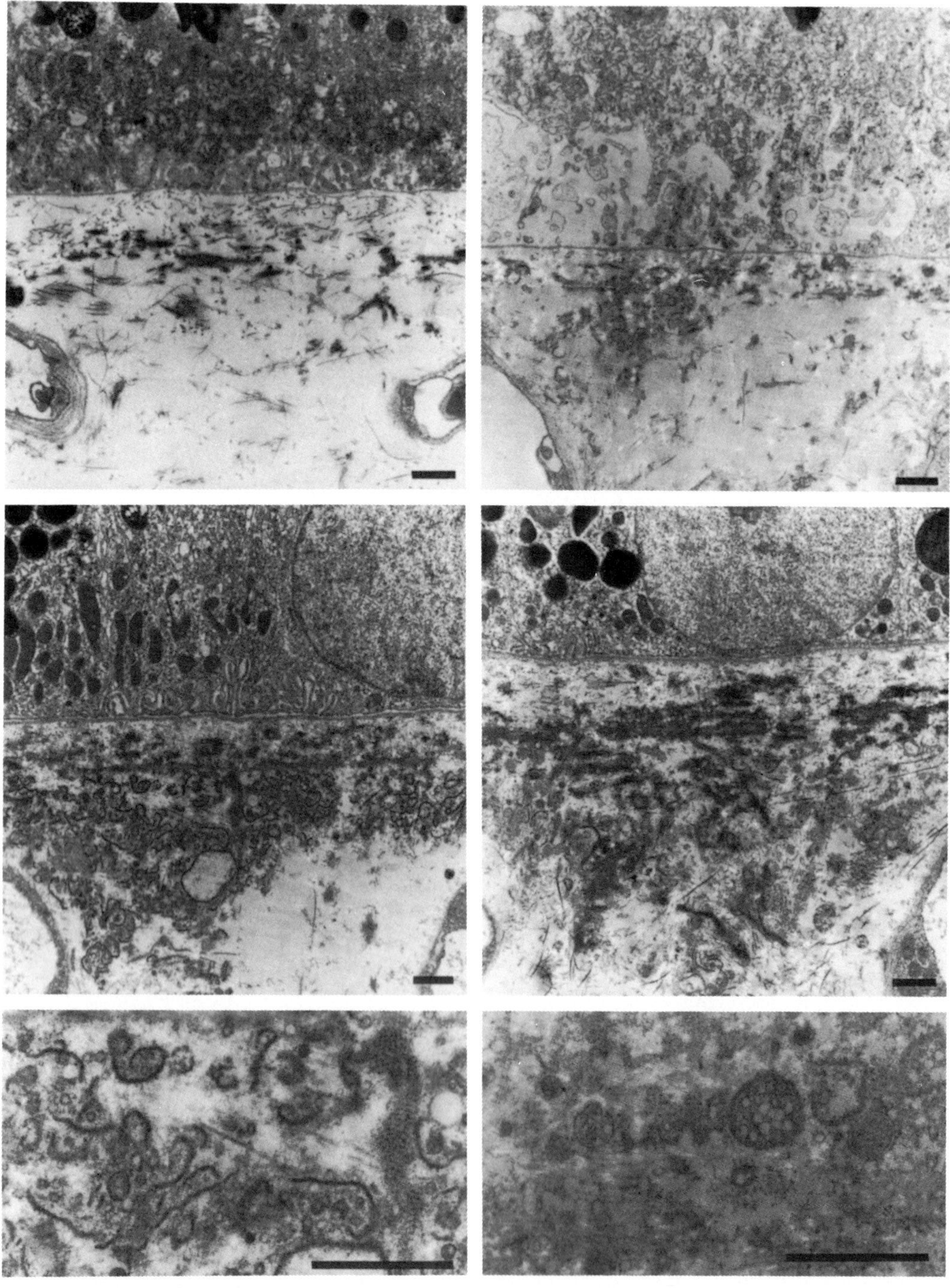

Figure 184–20. Electron micrographs of Bruch's membrane from eyes of a 1-year-old donor *(top left)*; a 17-year-old donor *(top right)*; a 47-year-old donor *(center left)*; and a 73-year-old donor *(center right)*. Deterioration of the normal ultrastructure of Bruch's membrane is demonstrated and typified by the accumulation of membranous debris in the inner and outer collagenous layers. *Bottom,* Characteristic particles of debris are shown at higher magnification. Bar = 1 μm. (From Pauleikhoff D, Harper CA, Marshall J, Bird AC: Aging changes in Bruch's membrane: A histochemical and morphologic study. Ophthalmology 97:171, 1990.)

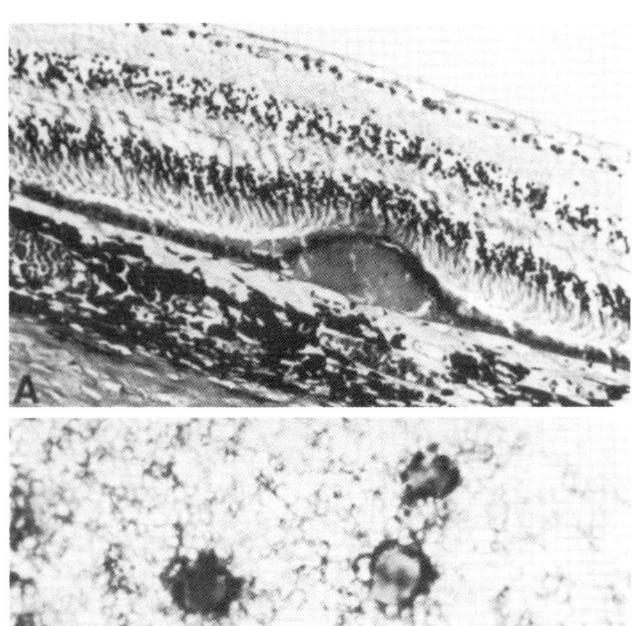

Figure 184–21. *A,* A druse in macular area with an intact and normal appearing overlying retinal pigment epithelium (RPE). H&E, ×100. *B,* Flat preparation of RPE showing three drusen with loss of overlying pigment and surrounding hypertrophic RPE. (EP 30977, PAS, ×100.) (From Green WR: Clinicopathologic studies of senile macular degeneration. *In* Nicholson DH [ed]: Ocular Pathology Update. New York, Masson, 1980, pp 115–144.)

calcified regressing drusen. Hard drusen are correlated histopathologically with the accumulation of a hyaline PAS-positive material in the collagenous zones of Bruch's membrane (Fig. 184–21). Data from ultrastructural studies[146, 153, 161, 162] support the hypothesis that hard drusen develop either by extrusion of the basal portion of RPE cells (apoptosis) with its content of membranous debris (e.g., bristle-coated vesicles, tubelike structures) or by lipidization and lipoid degeneration of single cells.[163, 164] Soft (serous) drusen consist of amorphous material that stains lightly with PAS and contains ultrastructurally membranous debris located between the thickened basement membrane of the RPE and the other layers of Bruch's membrane (Fig. 184–22).[165] The actual difference between soft drusen and serous detachments of RPE may be only a matter of size. Moreover, some investigators consider these drusen to be merely an "intra-Bruch's membrane separation" as a consequence of an ill-defined localized accentuation of the continuous layer of membranous debris called *diffuse drusen*[166, 167] or *basal linear deposits*.[152, 153] Therefore, soft drusen, like basal linear deposits, reflect a diffuse and severe dysfunction of the RPE that is likely to predispose to vascularization.

In contrast, hard drusen are considered representative of a more localized degenerative process, akin to dominant drusen. A correlation between hard drusen, reticular degeneration of the RPE, and geographic atrophy has been reported.[153]

Other types of drusen have been described; most represent either mixed or evolving patterns (e.g., mixed [soft] drusen and calcified drusen). Some degree of confusion exists about the terminology of drusen as a result of disagreement among pathologists regarding the precise definition of certain terms and the clinicopathologic correlations that they denote.

Visual loss in AMD results from photoreceptor degeneration and death as a consequence of geographic atrophy of the RPE and choriocapillaris or the complications of subretinal neovascularization.

Choroidal Alterations and Atrophic Form (Geographic or Areolar Atrophy)

Atrophy of the choriocapillaris is a common finding in AMD, as shown by Kornzweig[168] and confirmed by others.[169] The extremely high rate of oxidative metabolism of photoreceptors is impaired, with subsequent photoreceptor degeneration and death in the areas of RPE atrophy.[143] Sclerosis of the choriocapillaris underlying RPE atrophy in a lobular pattern, with thickening of the intercapillary septae and ultimately total choriocapillaris atrophy, has often been interpreted as an argument for a vascular pathogenesis of AMD. How-

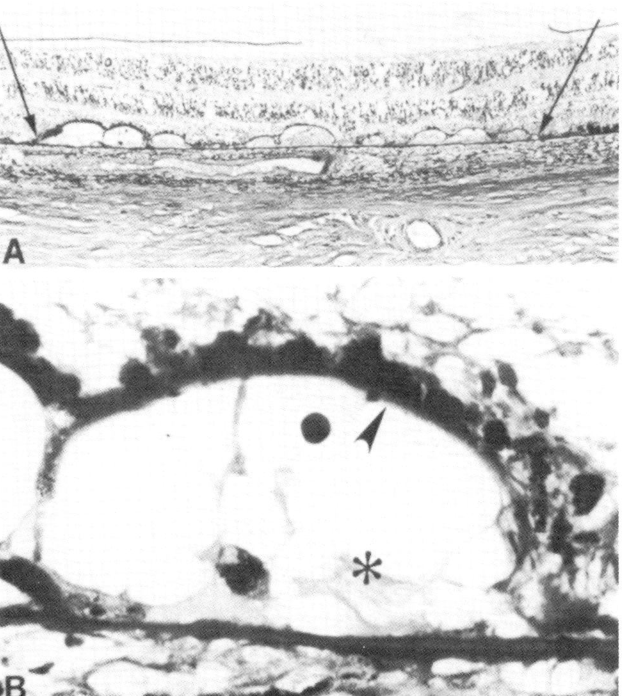

Figure 184–22. *A,* Druse with RPE and photoreceptor atrophy (between *arrows*). PAS × 40. *B,* Higher power view of druse with separation of the inner thickened portion of Bruch's membrane *(arrow)*. Some of the drusen material appears to have been washed out (*). PAS ×465 EP 34138. (From Green WR, Key SN III: Senile macular degeneration: A histopathologic study. Trans Am Ophthalmol Soc 75:180–254, 1977.)

ever, Green and Key[166] emphasized that such choroidal ischemia should have induced retinal lesions reaching to the inner nuclear layer,[170] whereas retinal lesions in AMD are limited at early stages to the RPE and photoreceptor layer. Moreover, Henkind and Gartner[171] have shown experimentally that destruction of the RPE induces *secondary* atrophy of the choriocapillaris. Geographic atrophy also can follow serous detachment of RPE or can coexist with subretinal neovascularization.

The pathogenesis of subretinal neovascularization is still disputed. Histopathologic findings include (1) breaks in Bruch's membrane either secondary to thickening and increased fragility or produced by the neovascular ingrowth; (2) a granulomatous inflammatory pattern with macrophages, lymphocytes, and fibroblasts; (3) basal laminar deposits and soft drusen; and (4) RPE depigmentation, hypertrophy and hyperplasia, and folding.[152, 153, 166, 172, 173]

The interpretation of these findings as primary, secondary, or coincidental is still speculative. The subretinal capillaries are fenestrated, like their choroidal precursors, and induce subretinal transudates, exudates, and hemorrhage. Cystoid macular edema may be produced by subfoveolar new vessels.[79] RPE tears, which are actually intra-Bruch's membrane tears, most often are related to subretinal neovascularization.[79, 166, 174] Disciform scars with a thickened vascular component and proliferation of the RPE are associated with photoreceptor atrophy, cystoid macular degeneration, and often choroidoretinal anastomosis (Fig. 184–23).[152, 166, 175]

CHOROIDORETINAL MANIFESTATIONS OF TRAUMA

Direct Injury to Ocular or Periocular Tissue

Traumatic Retinopathy. Usually occurring after severe direct blunt ocular trauma, this condition is often termed *commotio retinae* or *Berlin's edema*, in recognition of its first description by Berlin in 1873.[176] The main feature of commotio retinae is whitening of the outer retina involving either the macular area only or extending to the peripheral retina. This clinical picture is sometimes asymptomatic but may be associated with transient or permanent visual loss. The histopathologic features underlying the gray-white retinal opacity and its visual consequences were better understood after the studies by Berlin,[176] Blight and Hart,[177] Sipperly and colleagues,[178] Cogan,[179] and Hart and associates[180] all attributed this deep retinal opacity to extra- or intracellular edema (Fig. 184–24). Histologic findings in animal models have correlated this opacity with fragmentation of the photoreceptor outer segments and early damage to the photoreceptor cells. This disruption is followed after 24 hr by phagocytosis of fragmented outer segments by RPE cells. After 48 hr, the RPE cells begin to migrate into the neural retina, and with severe trauma these cells may be found throughout the entire retinal tissue. Disappearance of photoreceptor outer segments, in conjunction with RPE hyperplasia and migration, may result in direct apposition of multilayered RPE cells to photoreceptor inner segments and in diffuse thinning of the entire outer retina.[177, 178] In the peripheral retina, such a clinicopathologic picture simulates retinitis pigmentosa.[179] In their animal model of traumatic retinop-

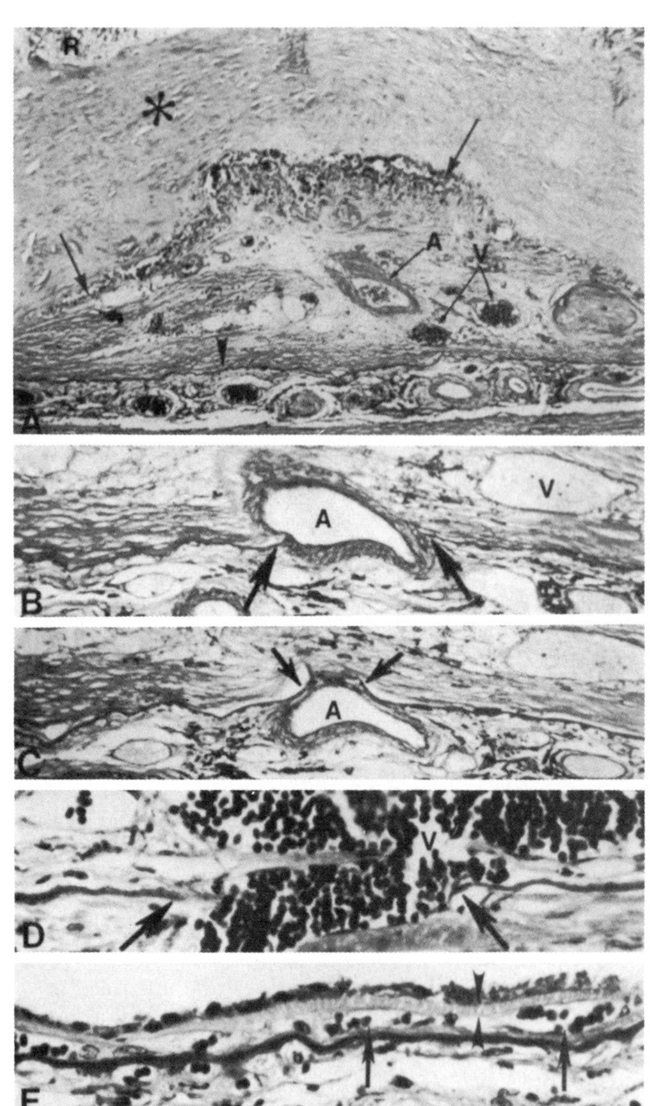

Figure 184–23. Long-standing disciform scar with artery and vein from choroid. *A,* Disciform scar with neovascularized component *(asterisk)* located between retina (R) and detached and thickened inner aspect of Bruch's membrane *(arrows)*. The retinal pigment epithelium has degenerated and is no longer present. The intra-Bruch's membrane component of the scar is vascularized, located between the detached and thickened portion of Bruch's membrane *(arrows)* and the remainder of Bruch's membrane *(arrowhead)* and contains a thick-walled artery (A) and thin-walled veins (V), which were traced into the choroid. EP 42880, PAS, ×10. *B,* Level showing artery (A) traversing break in Bruch's membrane (between *arrows*). Vein (V) is located in the intra-Bruch's component of the scar. PAS, ×100. *C,* Level showing artery (A) within choroid just beneath discontinuity of Bruch's membrane (between *arrows*). PAS, ×160. *D,* Level showing choroidal vein (V) traversing break in Bruch's membrane (between *arrows*). PAS, ×160. *E,* Area showing choroid neovascularization *(arrows)* extending beyond the disciform scar. The retinal pigment epithelium is intact. Thickening of the inner aspect of Bruch's membrane (between *arrowheads*) and capillary-like vessels are present between the thickened area and the remainder of Bruch's membrane. PAS, ×160.

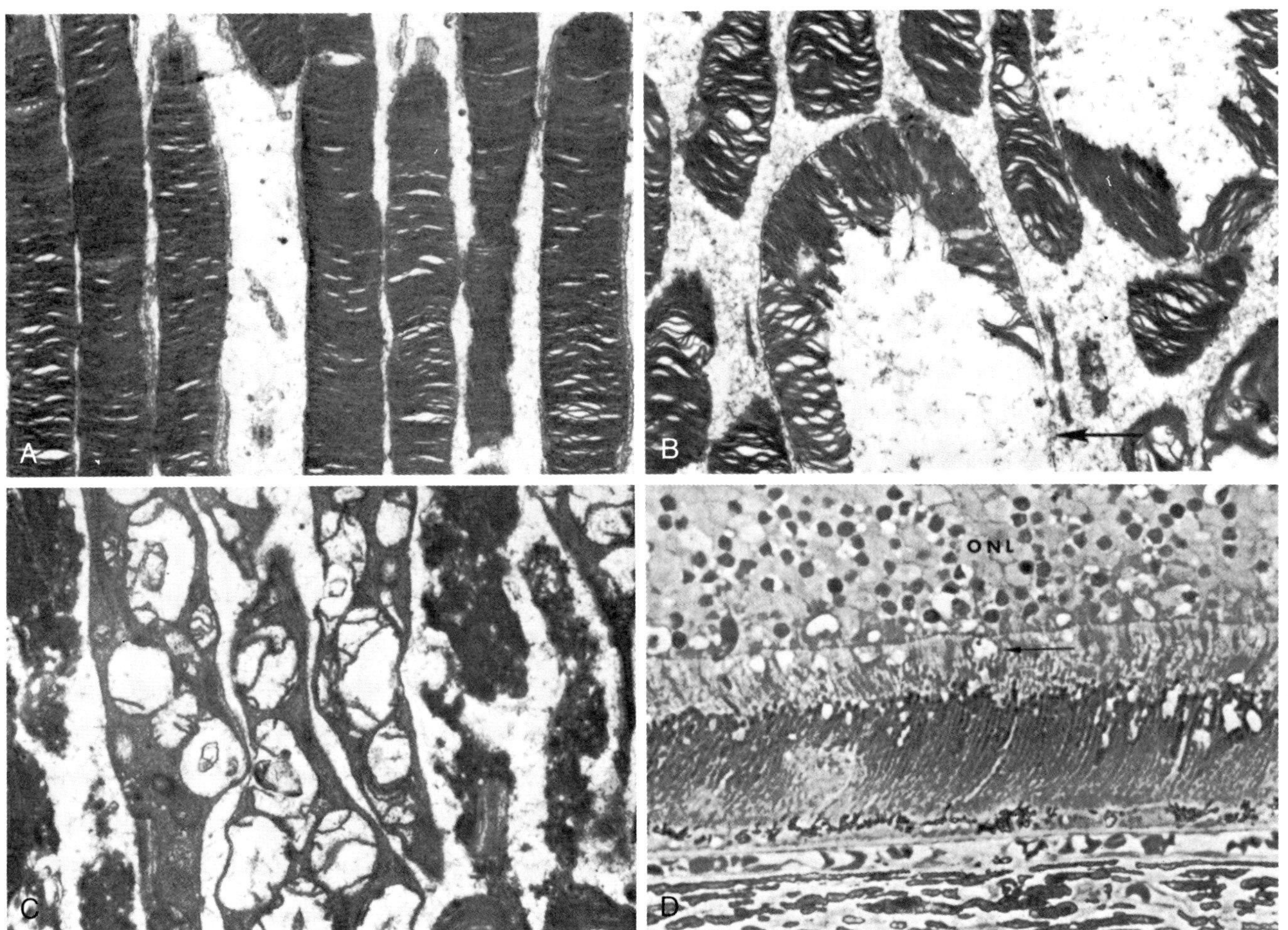

Figure 184–24. *A*, Electron micrographs of normal photoreceptor outer segments of owl monkey. ×9000. *B*, Compared with damaged outer segments *(bottom)* 4 hr after trauma. Note marked disruption of lamellar pattern and frank ruptures of plasma membrane *(arrow)*. ×12,000. *C*, Electron micrograph of inner segments of photoreceptors 21 hr after trauma shows marked disruption of mitochondria. ×12,000. *D*, Photomicrograph 40 hr after trauma. Note vacuolation of inner segment layer of photoreceptors *(arrow)* and marked number of pyknotic nuclei in outer nuclear layer (ONL). Paraphenylenediamine, ×140. (From Sipperly JO, Quigley HA, Gass JDM: Traumatic retinopathy in primates: The explanation of commotio retinae. Arch Ophthalmol 96:2267, 1978. Copyright 1978, American Medical Association.)

athy, Blight and Hart described, in addition to photoreceptor outer segment disruption, transient damage to the RPE cell membranes associated with intracellular edema.[177]

Traumatic Retinal Holes, Tears, Dialysis, and Detachment. The effects of direct or indirect trauma on the vitreoretinal interface may result in various types of retinal damage, including subretinal, intraretinal, or intravitreous hemorrhage; macular hole caused by vitreoretinal traumatic separation;[181] retinal dialysis, giant tears, or horseshoe-shaped tears with opercula, which can be classified according to associated vitreoretinal relationships; and avulsion of the vitreous base.[182, 183]

Indirect Ocular Injury

Purtscher's Retinopathy. First described in 1912, this retinopathy is characterized by peripapillary retinal hemorrhages and multiple patches of superficial whitening occurring after severe head trauma.[184] However, similar fundus findings are encountered after fat emboli and a rapid increase of nontraumatic intravascular pressure most often caused by strenuous activities. These ophthalmoscopic features are associated with fluorescein leakage from the retinal arterioles, capillaries, and venules, as well as with arteriolar obstruction. Pathogenetic hypotheses include trauma-related acute endothelial damage predisposing the retinal vessels to intravascular coagulopathy or granulocytic aggregation, as well as air or fat embolism following chest compression or long bone fracture, respectively.[79, 185] These presumptive mechanisms are supported by histopathologic and experimental studies that are compatible with retinal arteriolar occlusion.[186, 187]

Shaken Baby Syndrome. Various ophthalmic findings involving mainly the retina are present in association with neurologic and neurovegetative symptoms.[79, 188] The clinical picture is similar to Purtscher's retinopathy or retinal central vein occlusion.[79] Histopathologic findings include intraretinal hemorrhage as well as submeningeal bleeding around the optic nerve (Fig. 184–25).[79, 189]

Choroid Rupture. Most posttraumatic choroid ruptures involve only Bruch's membrane and the underlying choriocapillaris. Direct ruptures occur anteriorly at the site of impact. Indirect ruptures occur as a consequence

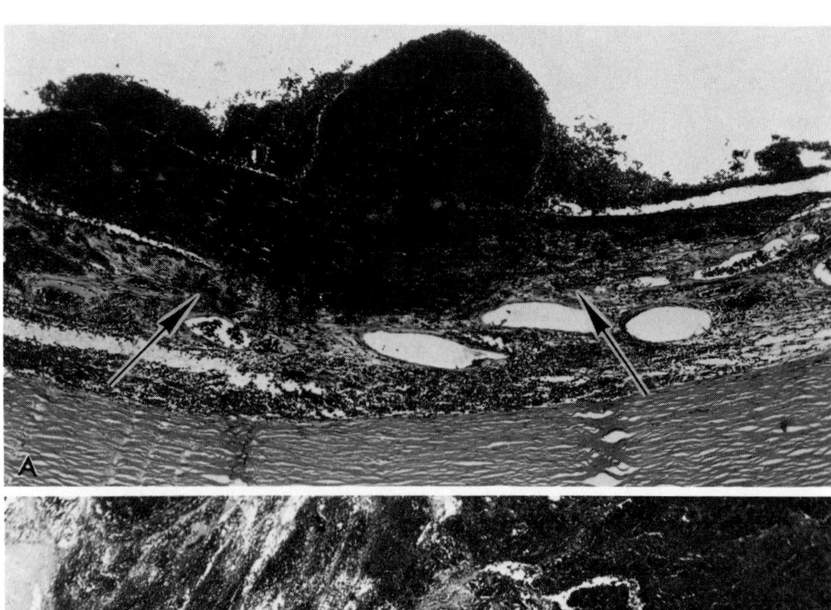

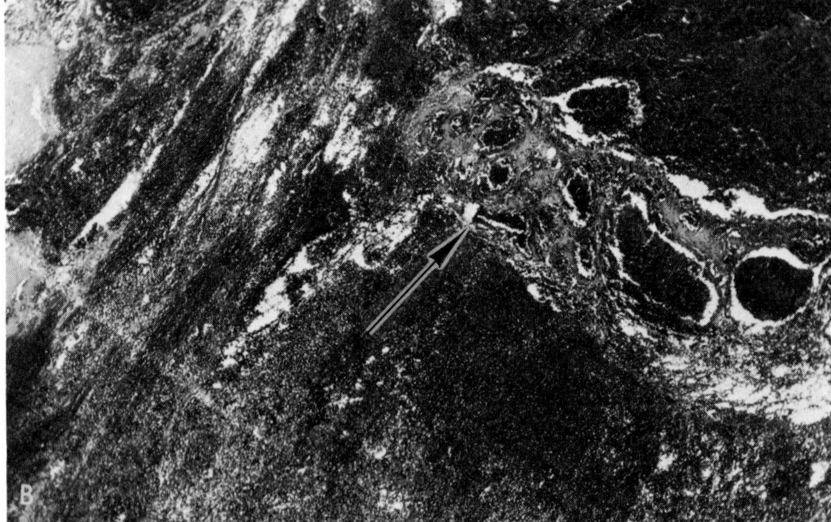

Figure 184–25. Examples of recent indirect choroid ruptures. *A*, There is discontinuity of retinal pigment epithelium and Bruch's membrane (between *arrows*), with hemorrhage extending into the subretinal space. H&E, ×40, EP 55725. *B*, Area shows one margin *(arrow)* of choroid rupture. H&E, ×30, EP 46627. (From Spencer WH [ed]: Ophthalmic Pathology: An Atlas and Textbook, vol. 3. Philadelphia, WB Saunders, 1986, p 1792.)

of coexisting lateral forces and the stabilizing effect of the optic nerve on adjacent structures and are generally posterior and display crescent shapes concentric to the optic nerve.[185, 190, 191] Histopathologic findings at early stages include acute subretinal hemorrhage often associated with serous detachment of the macula and juxtapapillary region (Fig. 184–26).[79, 191] As early as 6 to 14 days after injury, hemorrhage is followed by fibroblastic proliferation, after 3 to 4 wk resulting in the formation of mature scar tissue. RPE hyperplasia at the margins of the rupture is part of the healing process as well as choroid neovascularization. The latter most often regresses spontaneously without sequelae. However, in some instances subretinal or intravitreal new vessels may persist or develop at later stages and induce visual loss as a consequence of bleeding or exudation. Chorioretinal anastomoses also were reported by Goldberg.[192] The role of Bruch's membrane breaks in the induction of choroid neovascularization is still debated.[79, 190]

Intraocular Foreign Bodies. These substances may be organic, such as vegetable or hair, or inorganic, such as lead, iron, copper, or gold. Intraocular iron may become oxidized and produce localized siderosis if the foreign body lodges in the sclera, or siderosis bulbi when the foreign body is intravitreally diffuse.[193, 194] The iron concentrates mainly in intraocular epithelial cells (e.g., iris and ciliary body epithelium, RPE, and inner limiting membrane neurosensory retina).[195] Accumulation of intracellular iron leads to inner retinal and RPE degeneration followed by full-thickness retinal degeneration and secondary gliosis (Fig. 184–27). A similar clinical picture is encountered after long-standing intraocular hemorrhage (hemosiderosis bulbi) (Fig. 184–28).[79, 196] Chalcosis differs because staining is primarily in the "glass membranes" of the eye, as is also seen in Wilson's disease.[197–199] Chalcosis is also marked by an inflamma-

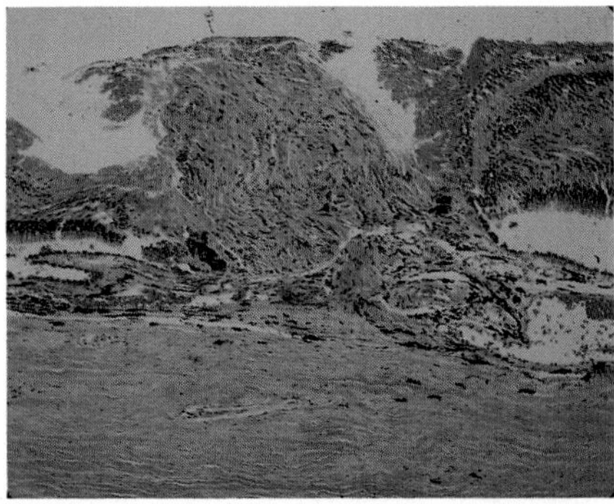

Figure 184–26. Choroid rupture. Retinal hemorrhage and scar formation.

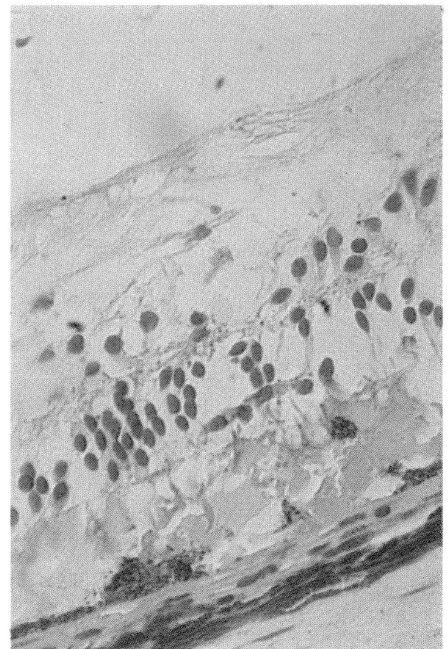
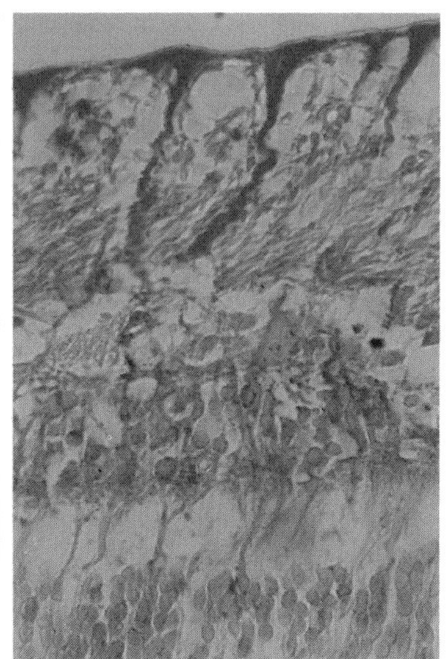

Figure 184–27. *A,* Retinal degeneration and thinning following siderosis. H&E, ×40. *B,* Iron stain showing deposits in the retina. ×63.

tory reaction involving leukocytes, macrophages, and Müller's cells.

RETINAL RADIATION AND DRUG TOXICITY

The literature on retinal radiation and drug toxicity has increased dramatically during the past two decades as better understanding has been gained of the role and side effects of radiation in the treatment of ocular tumors and the lengthening list of potentially retinotoxic drugs used in therapy and industry.

Photic retinopathy is a general term that describes various types of light-related damage to retinal cells resulting from photochemical, photodynamic, photocoagulative, or even mechanical processes. Solar retinopathy is characterized by focal loss of photoreceptor cell nuclei and other segments in the foveal area associated with focal necrosis, thinning, and depigmentation of foveal RPE cells.[79, 200–204]

Chloroquine retinopathy is correlated histopathologically with degeneration of RPE cells, subretinal pigment clumping, and photoreceptor cell elements.[205] Electron microscopy has disclosed inclusions in the ganglion cell layer; experimental studies have demonstrated chloroquine deposition in ganglion cells, photoreceptors, and RPE cells.[206, 207]

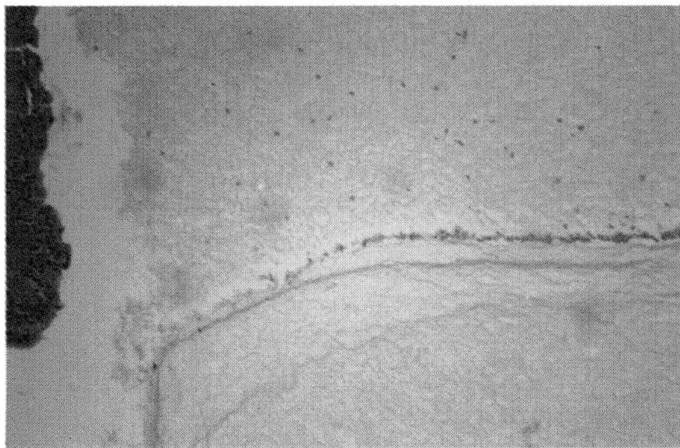

Figure 184–28. Retrohyaloidal hemorrhage. H&E, ×4.

RETINAL VASCULAR DISEASE

Hypertensive Retinopathy

After Liebreich's[208] early recognition of hypertensive fundus changes and the accumulation of abundant literature on this topic during the ensuing 150 years, hypertensive retinopathy, optic neuropathy, and choroidopathy remain the focus of vivid controversy. In keeping with Hayreh and colleagues' suggestion,[209] it is useful in some ways to classify hypertensive retinal lesions into vascular and extravascular, although such a separation is artificial. Almost every attempt to classify hypertensive fundus changes, particularly those seen ophthalmoscopically, has been controversial.[209–211] Tso and coworkers,[211, 212] after reviewing experimental and clinical data, proposed to divide hypertensive retinopathy into vasoconstrictive, exudative, sclerotic, and complications of the sclerotic phase and delineated the mechanisms underlying these phases. The vasoconstrictive phase is characterized by reversible stimulation of the vascular tone of muscular retinal arteries as an autoregulatory mechanism. Further or prolonged blood pressure elevation results in definitive narrowing of the vascular lumen at the precapillary level.

Disruption of the blood-retinal barrier characterizes the exudative phase as a consequence of poorly understood vascular endothelial necrosis or disruption.[213] Transudation of plasma into the vessel wall and around degenerated pericytes and arteriolar muscle cells occurs, inducing further vascular lumen narrowing. Disruption of the blood-retinal barrier at the RPE and endothelial levels, along with intraluminal elevated pressure, induces leakage with consecutive retinal hemorrhage of various shapes and locations. This is accompanied by edema and exudates predominantly in the macular region. Cotton-wool spots are nonspecific features of inner retinal ischemia also encountered in AIDS, collagen diseases, blood dyscrasias and malignancies, central retinal vein occlusion, and diabetic retinopathy. Cotton-wool spots result from the interruption of axonal orthograde and retrograde energy-dependent organelle trans-

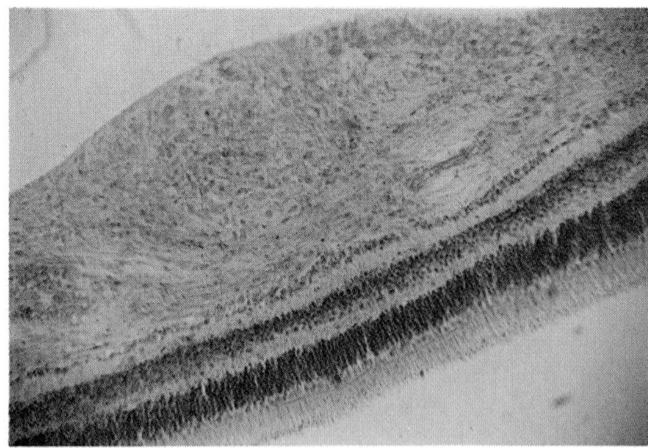

Figure 184–29. Cotton-wool spot thickening in the gangion cell layer. H&E, ×10.

port in the ganglion cell axons, with accumulation of mitochondria and lamellar dense bodies in swollen interrupted nerve fibers (Fig. 184–29).

Loss of autoregulation may result from fibrinoid necrosis or hyalin degeneration leading to dilatation. Hyperplasia of the vascular tunica media occurs with chronic mild pressure elevation (Fig. 184–30). Chronic, poorly controlled hypertension leads to a sclerotic phase. Sclerotic vessels are not specific to hypertensive retinopathy but are commonly encountered in the normal population and appear to be the result of aging-related factors. Other progressive vascular changes of hypertensive retinopathy include narrowing of arteries; arteriovenous crossing abnormalities ranging from mild nicking to branch venous occlusion (Fig. 184–31); arteriosclerosis ranging from mild to severe (copper or silver wiring); arterial tortuosity; and arterial branching.[197, 211, 213–215]

Vascular lumen narrowing and obstruction by intimal arteriosclerotic changes predispose to thrombosis and aggravation of ischemia. Remodeling of the vascular bed with reopening of capillaries and development of collaterals is usually not sufficient to reverse the ischemic retinal damage and its sensory consequences. Furthermore, the vascular response includes formation of telangiectases and neovascularization, which further aggravate the increase of vascular permeability with its edematous, exudative, and hemorrhagic consequences. In considering the natural history of hypertensive retinopathy, the concurrent effects of hypertensive choroidopathy and neuropathy must be taken into account. Moreover, the sequence of events as related earlier is not unanimously accepted. Hayreh and colleagues[209] emphasized that the earlier lesions observed in experimental hypertension in monkeys are focal intraretinal periarteriolar transudates followed almost simultaneously by diffuse or cystoid macular edema, acute focal RPE lesions, and optic disc edema (a feature of optic hypertensive neuropathy). The lesions appearing subsequently are cotton-wool spots, characteristic of localized inner retinal ischemia, and later retinal lipid deposits followed by arteriolar changes.[209] Controversy about the staging, natural history, and pathogenesis of hypertensive retinopathy is unresolved.

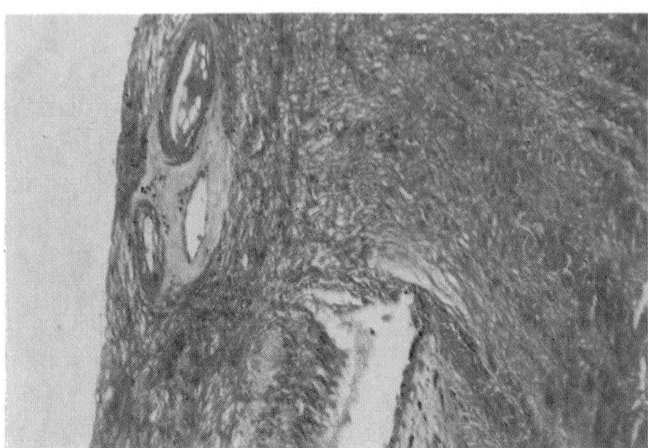

Figure 184–30. Hyperplasia of vascular tunica with narrowing of the vascular lumen.

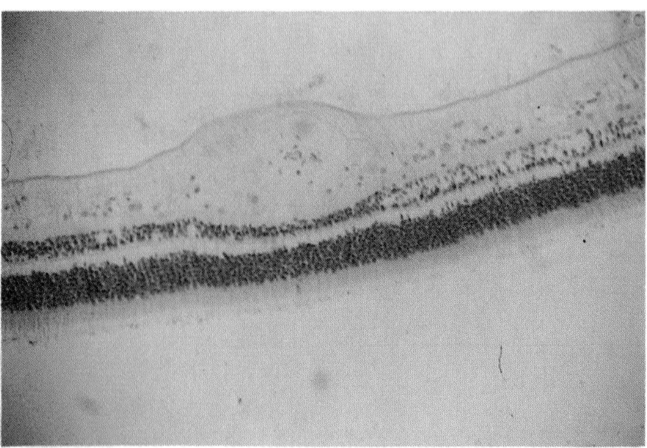

Figure 184–31. Branch vein occlusion in a hypertensive patient. H&E, ×4.

Diabetic Retinopathy

The clinical classification, predisposing factors, and data collected from epidemiologic studies of diabetic retinopathy are reviewed in *Basic Sciences,* Chapter 111 and *Clinical Practice* Chapters 55 and 56. This chapter presents the main anatomic lesions of diabetic retinopathy with their clinical correlates and presumed pathogenesis.[215–220]

Clinically, diabetic retinal lesions are usually divided into background (intraretinal vascular changes) and proliferative phases, initially incipient and later preretinal. The pathologic process can be studied as a microangiopathy characterized by capillary microaneurysm formation, dilatation and hyperpermeability with exudates, hemorrhages, and edema; capillary occlusion resulting in microinfarctions; shunts and neovascularization within and at the retinal inner surface and optic nerve; and vitreous hemorrhage, traction, and tractional retinal detachment.

Capillary Basement Membrane Thickening. This is the earliest change in the retinal, cerebral, and renal capillaries observed in diabetic humans and in animal models.[221] Various biochemical processes (e.g., sorbitol and aldose-reductase pathway, altered basement membrane collagen, critical protein glycosylation, and decrease in heparan sulfate proteoglycan production) take part in the pathogenesis of this early change. The structural and functional role of basement membrane thickening in the alteration of the capillary retinal bed, the breakdown of the blood-retinal barrier, the regulation of pericytes, and endothelial cell proliferation are not fully understood.[218, 219]

Loss of Capillary Pericytes.[222–227] In the early 1960s, Cogan and colleagues first demonstrated loss of capillary pericytes using an original technique of trypsin digestion of formalin-fixed retinal specimens.[227] In the retina of normal young adults, the pericyte:endothelial cell ratio is 1:1. Pericyte drop-out is detected by the presence of balloon-like spaces or pericyte "ghosts" in digest preparations. Loss of intramural pericytes is considered a specific characteristic of diabetic retinopathy and is not detectable in the other organs involved in diabetic vascular complications. Explanations for such a specificity remain putative (e.g., selective presence of the sorbitol pathway in retinal pericytes). The loss of pericytes has an important impact on the regulation of microvascular blood flow, the formation of microaneurysms, and the inhibition of endothelial cell proliferation.[224–226]

Microaneurysms. Microaneurysms are the earliest ophthalmoscopically detectable change in diabetic retinopathy, although more of them are observed microscopically or by fluorescein angiography. They commonly are considered to be the result of pericyte loss with focal weakening of the microvessel wall and focal dilatation.[227] Most microaneurysms appear in the posterior retina in areas of ischemia. This has led some investigators[220] to speculate that microaneurysms might represent an early intraretinal microvascular anomaly produced by bidimensional endothelial cell proliferation, probably as a consequence of loss of inhibition by the normal basal membrane and pericytes.[218, 224] The line between so-called background and proliferative appears at the early stage of microaneurysms to be rather theoretical. Whether induced by localized weakening of the vascular wall or by early vascular proliferation, microaneurysms cause a breakdown of the inner blood-retinal barrier and predispose to edema, exudates, and hemorrhage. Some microaneurysms may not hyperfluoresce on fluorescein angiography because of occlusion by their increased basement membrane elaboration.

In conjunction with or secondary to microaneurysm formation, arteriolar-venular shunts with capillary dilatation, decrease in capillary blood flow, and capillary atrophy occur consecutively.[228, 229] Other related abnormalities are capillary acellularity, intraluminal basement membrane thickening, and swelling of the arteriolar wall (as in hypertensive retinopathy). As a result, a significant part of the microvascular bed is destroyed, providing a basis for retinal ischemia.[220, 229]

The breakdown of the blood-retinal barrier is a functional event that occurs early in diabetic retinopathy and is produced by various intricate mechanisms at the inner and outer levels of the blood-retina barriers. These include microaneurysms, vascular dilatation, increased intraluminal and transmural pressures, opening of the tight junctions between endothelial cells, and endothelial fenestration. The RPE is also involved by the metabolic alterations and biochemical processes described earlier, including alterations in the aldose-reductase–dependent pathways. Increased infolding of the basal plasmic membrane of RPE cells also contributes to early breakdown of the blood-retina barrier.[230]

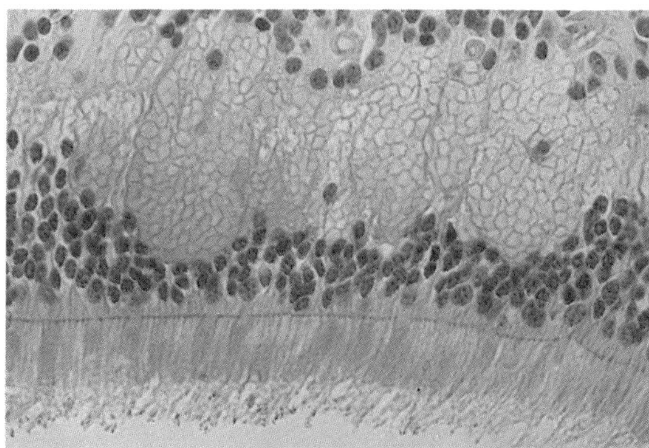

Figure 184–32. Intraretinal hemorrhage with thickening of the outer plexiform layer in diabetic retinopathy. H&E, ×40.

Intraretinal Hemorrhages. Intraretinal hemorrhages may assume various shapes according to retinal location. Dot and blot hemorrhages spread from the inner nuclear layer into the outer plexiform layer. Flame hemorrhages are located between the axons of the nerve fiber layer. Larger hemorrhages may involve several or all retinal layers, the latter often appearing globular. Localized hemorrhages probably originate from aneurysms or altered capillaries. Larger hemorrhages are often significant features of severe "background" retinopathy and may break into the vitreous space (Fig. 184–32).

Edema. Macular edema is the main cause of visual loss in patients with background retinopathy. Macular edema usually is classified into focal and diffuse edema, whether cystoid or not. Extravascular fluid leakage results from the structural and functional alterations described earlier at the capillary level. Some studies have shown that moderate amounts of fluid initially accumulate in Müller's cells.[231–234] Further accumulation leads to excessive ballooning and degeneration of Müller's cells and formation of multiple cystoid spaces in the outer plexiform and inner nuclear layers (Fig. 184–33). The lesions at this stage are often irreversible and may evolve toward macular retinoschisis or hole (Fig. 184–34).

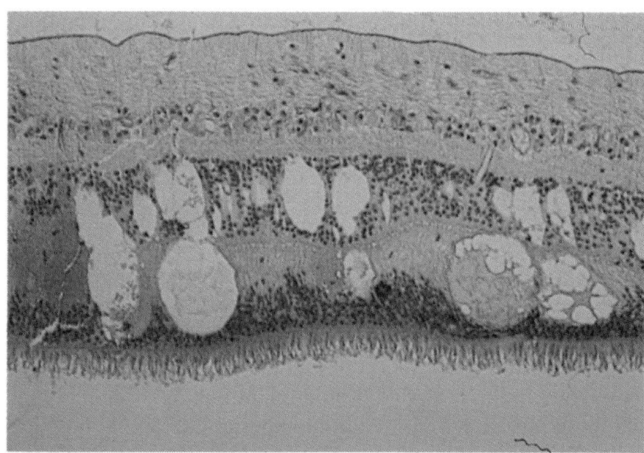

Figure 184–33. Cystoid retinal edema in diabetic retinopathy. H&E, ×40.

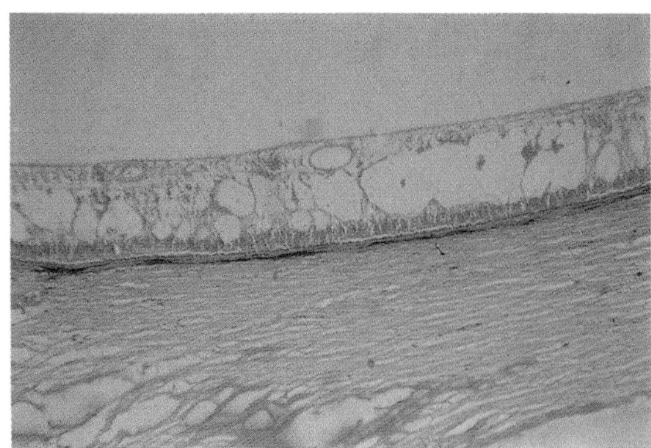

Figure 184–34. Cystoid retinal degeneration following long-standing cystoid macular edema in diabetic retinopathy. H&E, ×10.

In focal edema, the leakage diffuses from foci of microaneurysms in a circinate pattern. The aqueous content of the exudate pools and is progressively resorbed in the outer plexiform layer. The insoluble lipoproteins form hard exudates that accumulate at some distance from the leaking zone in complete or partial rings, separating the edematous zone from the surrounding nonedematous retina. If the leak is appropriately treated by photocoagulation, the edema is transported through the RPE and adjacent capillaries. However, the exudates cannot follow this path and are progressively removed by macrophages. These can be observed histopathologically as lipid-laden macrophages and are particularly numerous in the outer plexiform layer.[79, 196, 229] Cystoid macular edema is uncommon in focal circinate retinopathy.

In contrast, diffuse macular edema often is associated with macular cystoid pooling. Diffuse leakage through a dilated capillary bed and an altered outer blood-retinal barrier are often bilateral. Lipid accumulation is theoretically unlikely in this process because large molecules remain intravascular. The imbalance between the intracapillary hydrostatic and tissue osmotic pressures on one hand and the plasmatic osmotic and tissue hydrostatic pressures on the other may be enhanced by capillary dilatation to compensate for capillary occlusion and widening of intercapillary spaces. For this reason, diffuse macular edema and macular ischemia may coexist and contribute to central visual loss.

An intermediate or preproliferative stage between background and proliferative retinopathy is characterized by the addition or exacerbation of the following changes: (1) larger, darker hemorrhages; (2) intraretinal microvascular anomalies (i.e., irregular segmental dilatations of the capillary bed that developed as new vessels originating from the venous side of the microvascular bed and produced at the border of areas of arteriolar nonperfusion);[235] (3) multiple cotton-wool spots reflecting acute extensive hypoxia;[236] and (4) venous dilatation and beading. All of these "transitional" findings related to increasing retinal ischemia contribute to poor visual prognosis, because in the macular region irreversible and untractable visual loss ensues. These changes are probably not just forerunners but actually part of the proliferative phase.

Proliferative Diabetic Retinopathy. Proliferative diabetic retinopathy is thought of as a vision-threatening response to retinal ischemia.[237–239] The presence of acidic and basic fibroblast growth factor and synthesis has been demonstrated using immunocytochemistry and in situ hybridization in many retinal cell types. Insulin-like growth factor also has been implicated. Loss of inhibition of new vessel formation by pericytes and normal basement membrane and putatively by the RPE suggests an imbalance between neovascularization promoting and inhibiting factors in the onset of proliferative diabetic retinopathy.[217–219, 224, 240]

New vessels initially proliferate intraretinally from the venous side of the microcirculation. After having broken through the inner limiting membrane, they spread parallel to the inner retinal surface. As they grow toward the vitreous, they become densely attached to the posterior hyaloid if it is not detached.[241] Because of their lack of tight junctions and the presence of fenestrations between endothelial cells, these new vessels are extremely leaky. In parallel or as a consequence of the neovascular network leakage and proteolytic activity, vitreous syneresis and collapse occur. Vitreous retraction is limited by the strong neovascular tufts that are accompanied by a fibroglial component (originating from Müller's cells or astrocytes, hyalocytes, pericytes, RPE) forming preretinal membranes adherent to the retinal surface and the posterior hyaloid (Fig. 184–35).[196, 197, 220, 242] Traction on this fibrous tissue may provoke bleeding, retinal traction, or rhegmatogenous detachment, all causes of severe visual loss. Other sites

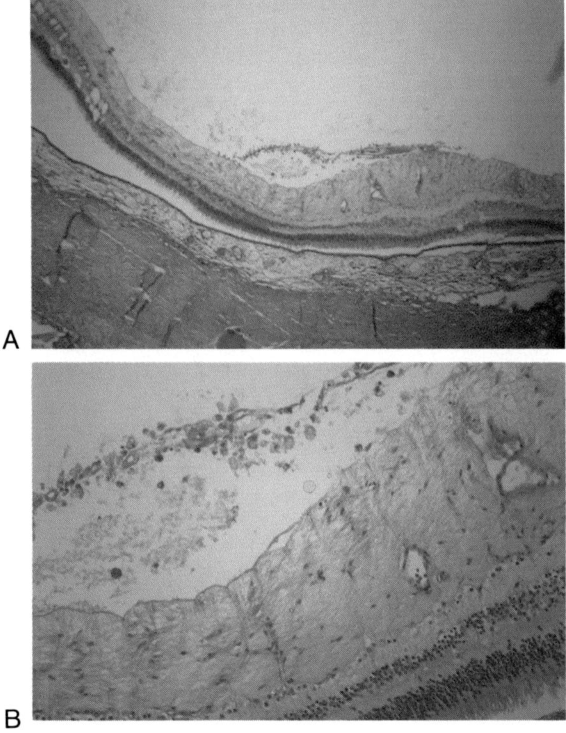

Figure 184–35. *A,* Cystoid retinal edema and intraretinal gliosis in the ganglion cell layer with preretinal proliferation. H&E, ×10. *B,* Thickening of the inner retina secondary to gliosis. Preretinal proliferation. H&E, ×40.

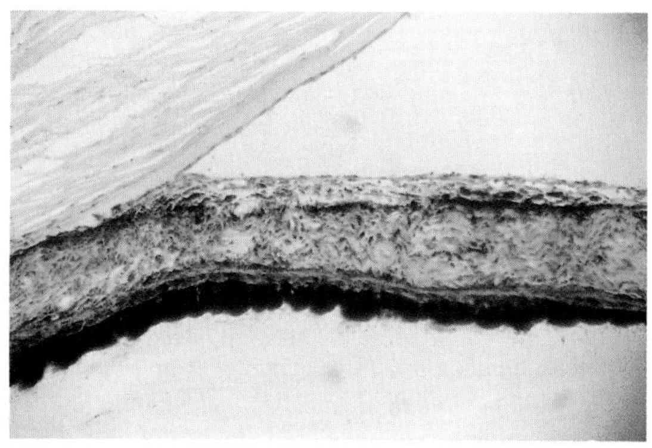

Figure 184–36. Proliferative diabetic retinopathy. Angle-closure with synechiae rubeosis iridis. H&E, ×10.

of neovascularization include the optic nerve and the iris (rubeosis iridis) (Fig. 184–36).

Coats' Disease

Coats' disease is characterized by vascular alterations, intraretinal exudates, and massive subretinal exudation or hemorrhage with cholesterol clefts and lipid-laden macrophages (Fig. 184–37*A*). Vascular changes include peripheral telangiectases (Fig. 184–37*B*), arteriovenous anastomosis, aneurysms of various sizes, and obliterative changes such as sheathing, sclerosis, perivasculitis, and fibrin deposition (Fig. 184–37*C*).[243] Occlusion of the vascular lumen can result from endothelial swelling or proliferation and thickening of the wall by intramural fibrillar deposits.

Intraretinal exudation usually occurs within the outer retina and is often associated with hemorrhage leading to the accumulation of fibrin, PAS-positive deposits, cholesterol clefts, and lipid-laden macrophages (Fig. 184–37*D*). The retina is usually detached, with subretinal exudates containing albumin, cholesterol clefts, macrophages, epithelioid cells, and ghost or foamy cells (Fig. 184–37*E*). The latter are derived from the RPE or histiocytes and glial cells. At later stages, the subretinal space is replaced by connective tissue, with fibrosis and fibrous metaplasia of RPE cells.[243–250]

RETINOBLASTOMA

Retinoblastoma is the most common malignant eye tumor of childhood and the second most common primary intraocular malignancy of the eye. Approximately 1 per cent of all deaths due to cancer before 15 yr of age have been attributed to retinoblastoma.[251, 252] The cell of origin has been a topic of debate since the Scottish surgeon Wardrop first recognized retinoblastoma as a discrete tumor, distinct from "fungus haematodes" or soft cancers that arose from the breast and limbs.[253, 254] His astute observations, published in 1809, were based on dissections and made without benefit of the microscope and convinced him that the tumor arose from the retina. Various pathologists of the 19th century, including Robin and Langenbeck,[255] confirmed these observations. Virchow named it a "glioma of the retina,"[256, 257] supporting glial cells as the cell of origin of the tumor. Flexner[258] and later Wintersteiner[259] suggested the use of the term *neuroepithelioma,* believing that the tumor was of neuroepithelial origin, and regarded rosettes that bear their names as an attempt to form photoreceptors. Verhoeff[258–260] concluded that the tumor was derived from undifferentiated embryonic retinal cells called *retinoblasts,* comparable to the neuroblasts originating from the medullary epithelium, and proposed the term *retinoblastoma.*[261–263] The American Ophthalmological Society adopted this term in 1926.[264] The term *retinoblastoma* for undifferentiated tumors had been proposed by Mawas in France in 1922–1924.[264] Zimmerman proposed to restrict the name *retinocytoma* to differentiated tumors displaying benign features under thorough histologic sampling, for which Gallie and colleagues prefer the term *retinoma.*[264, 265] The most widely held concept of histogenesis of retinoblastoma holds that it generally arises from a multipotential precursor cell that could develop into almost any type of inner or outer retinal cell. This heterogeneity of the histopathologic, ultrastructural, and immunohistochemical features of retinoblastoma has been described.[264, 266–268]

By light microscopy, undifferentiated retinoblastoma is composed of small round cells with a large hyperchromatic nucleus of various shapes and scanty cytoplasm (Fig. 184–38). Differentiated areas are found within many, most commonly as rosettes, first described by Flexner and Wintersteiner in the 1890s.[258, 259] These structures consist of clusters of cuboidal or short columnar cells around a central lumen (Fig. 184–39). The nuclei are displaced away from the lumen, which by light microscopy appears to have a limiting membrane resembling the external limiting membrane of the retina. Photoreceptor-like elements protrude through the membrane, and some taper into fine filaments.[260, 264] The lumen of these rosettes contains hyaluronidase-resistant acid mucopolysaccharides similar to that found between normal photoreceptors and the pigment epithelium.[269] Homer Wright–type rosettes are seen less frequently than Flexner-Wintersteiner–type rosettes. These are composed of radial arrangements of cells around a central tangle of fibrils[270] and are identical to the rosettes found in neuroblastomas and medulloblastomas.

An additional differentiated structure is the fleurette, first described by Tso and coworkers.[271] These are thought to represent a higher degree of photoreceptor differentiation. The term was applied to denote the fleur-de-lis–like arrangement of the apparently abortive photoreceptor structures (Fig. 184–40) characterized by larger cells with abundant eosinophilic cytoplasm and less hyperchromatic nuclei than the surrounding areas. Tso and colleagues suggest that tumors containing such benign components might be less radioresponsive.[272] A few tumors are exclusively composed of benign-appearing cells exhibiting photoreceptor differentiation with almost no mitoses. These tumors represent the retinomas or retinocytoma[265] and may be the most benign end of the spectrum of malignant possibilities induced by the genetic mechanisms of retinoblastoma formation.

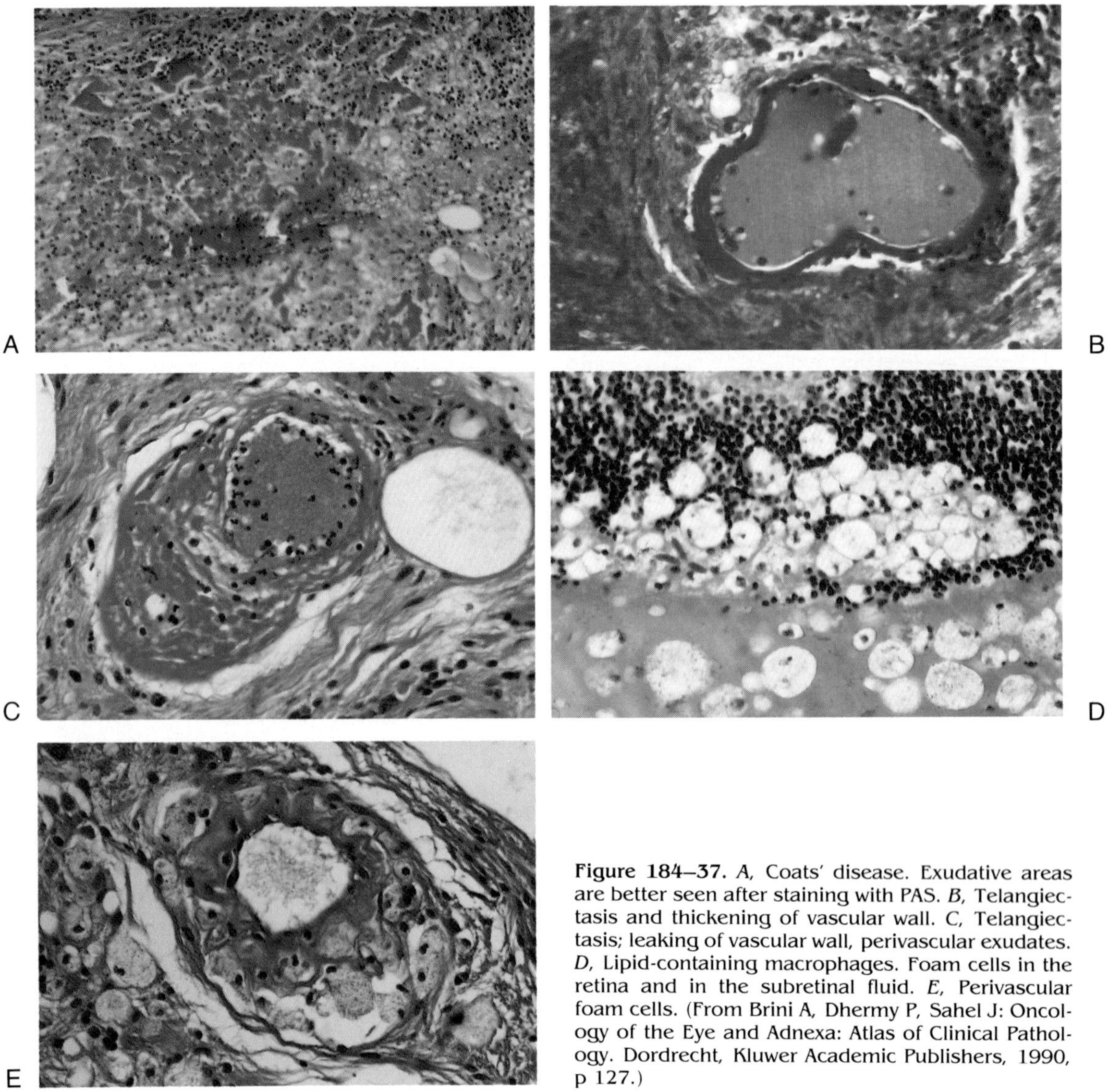

Figure 184–37. *A,* Coats' disease. Exudative areas are better seen after staining with PAS. *B,* Telangiectasis and thickening of vascular wall. *C,* Telangiectasis; leaking of vascular wall, perivascular exudates. *D,* Lipid-containing macrophages. Foam cells in the retina and in the subretinal fluid. *E,* Perivascular foam cells. (From Brini A, Dhermy P, Sahel J: Oncology of the Eye and Adnexa: Atlas of Clinical Pathology. Dordrecht, Kluwer Academic Publishers, 1990, p 127.)

Malignant transformation of this variant has been reported, however.[273]

Exophytic and endophytic growth patterns are classically described. Although both types of growth patterns can often be seen in the same tumor on histologic examination, this distinction is still clinically relevant.

An *exophytic* pattern denotes growth primarily in the subretinal space, giving rise to a retinal detachment. Tumor cells may then infiltrate through Bruch's membrane into the choroid[274] and subsequently invade either blood vessels or ciliary nerves or vessels.

An *endophytic* pattern describes growth into the vitreous space, and the tumor is seen ophthalmoscopically as one or more masses on the surface of the retina. In contrast to the exophytic pattern, retinal vessels are not visible above the tumor. Tumor cells may be seen as spheroid masses floating in the vitreous and anterior chamber, simulating endophthalmitis or iridocyclitis. (Fig. 184–41). Secondary deposits or seeding of tumor cells into other areas of the retina may be confused with multicentric tumors.

In widespread retinoblastoma with necrosis, the diagnosis may be confused by the degree of inflammation present (Fig. 184–42). Areas of tumor necrosis are common in large tumors. Common findings include collars of viable tumor cells in uniform thickness sur-

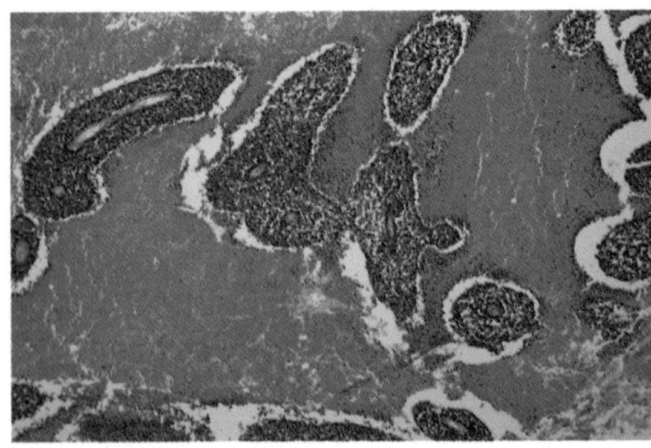

Figure 184–38. Undifferentiated retinoblastoma with large areas of necrosis. H&E, ×4.

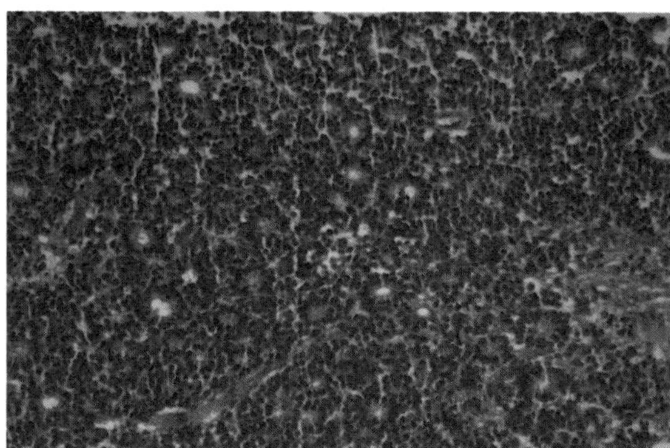

Figure 184–39. Flexner-Wintersteiner rosettes. The aspect under low power has been compared to a flower bud. They differ from Homer Wright rosettes, which present a fibrillar center and are less distinctive. (From Brini A, Dhermy P, Sahel J: Oncology of the Eye and Adnexa: Atlas of Clinical Pathology. Dordrecht, Kluwer Academic Publishers, 1990, p 123.)

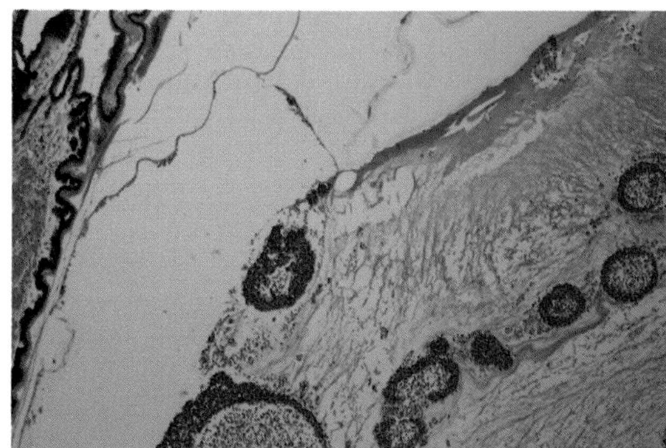

Figure 184–41. Histopathologic aspect of the spherical intravitreous floaters that are easily recognizable with the slit lamp and pathognomonic. (From Brini A, Dhermy P, Sahel J: Oncology of the Eye and Adnexa: Atlas of Clinical Pathology. Dordrecht, Kluwer Academic Publishers, 1990, p 121.)

rounding the remaining blood vessels, often designated inappropriately as "pseudorosettes"; beyond these collars, ischemic areas of necrosis are prominent. Areas of intra- and extracellular calcification are often present. In other areas of necrosis, large numbers of lymphocytes are observed, and hyperplasia of the vascular endothelium is seen, possibly including the lumen of vessels in some areas.[275–277] Precipitated DNA tumor cells are occasionally evident both surrounding and within the wall of the vessels and other structures at a distance from the tumor.[278] It should be noted that areas of photoreceptor cell differentiation are devoid of necrosis. Probably related to necrosis, numerous inflammatory cells may be present, and in some cases, secondary endophthalmitis may occur.[264, 279, 280] Rubeosis iridis accompanied by ectropion uveae may develop, with resultant glaucoma or hyphema.[280]

Ultrastructural early investigations of retinoblastoma served primarily to expand the previous light microscopic descriptions of the tumor.[266, 281–285] More noteworthy contributions gave evidence of the presence of photoreceptor cell elements in retinoblastoma,[260, 271, 272, 286] and a strong resemblance of retinoblastoma to human fetal retina has been demonstrated.[287, 288]

Retinoblastoma cells have been examined in some detail using transmission electron microscopy.[289] Photoreceptor cell elements occur within Flexner-Wintersteiner rosettes, and fleurettes represent photoreceptor cell differentiation. Triple membrane structures involving both the nuclear and cytoplasmic membranes are extremely common in retinoblastoma and fetal retina. Cytomembranes that structurally resemble a nuclear envelope annulate lamellae occur in a high percentage of tumor cells. Cilia are plentiful and appear in longitudinal, oblique, and transverse planes. In the latter planes, nine double tubules with no central pairs are seen. This "9 + 0" pattern is characteristic of the photoreceptor cell. Microtubules can be identified in most retinoblastoma cells, most commonly in the Golgi's area, but may be diffusely distributed throughout the cytoplasm. These cytoplasmic components have an outside diameter of 15 to 27 nm, a wall thickness of approximately 5 nm, and an indefinite length. The microtubules are often clumped together and on occasion may appear in the nucleus. The tubular structures in rod fibers observed by Fine[290] and by Sheffield[291] behave in a similar manner. Bristle-coated vesicles are found free in the cytoplasm, budding from the cell membrane, and in the intercellular spaces. These are

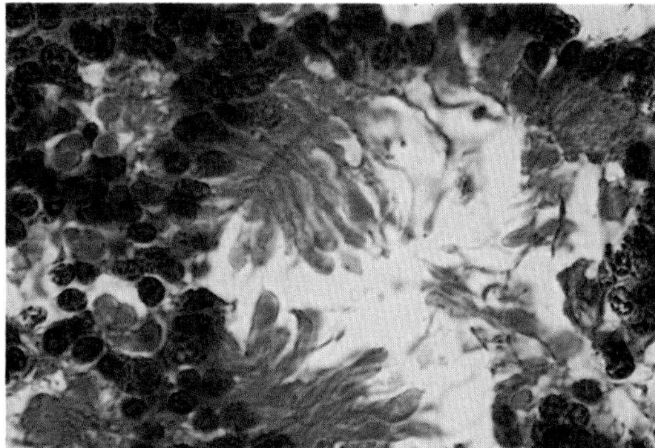

Figure 184–40. Clusters of well-differentiated visual cells (Tso's "fleurettes"). The outer segments of the photoreceptors converge toward large cavities. (From Brini A, Dhermy P, Sahel J: Oncology of the Eye and Adnexa: Atlas of Clinical Pathology. Dordrecht, Kluwer Academic Publishers, 1990, p 123.)

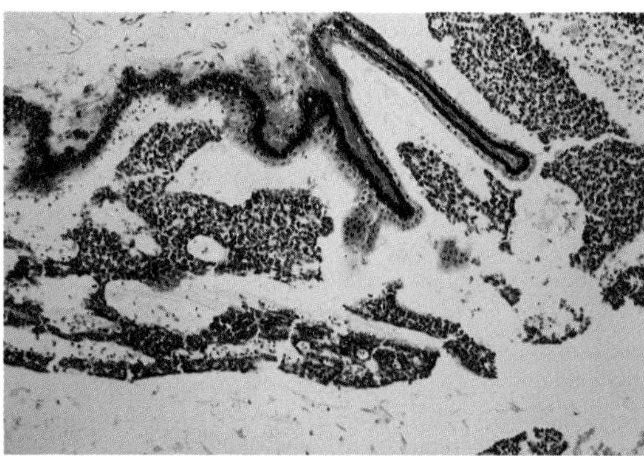

Figure 184–42. Histopathology of this diffuse variety in the area of the ciliary body. It is worth noting that the invasion of the optic nerve is also possible in this type. (From Brini A, Dhermy P, Sahel J: Oncology of the Eye and Adnexa: Atlas of Clinical Pathology. Dordrecht, Kluwer Academic Publishers, 1990, p 119.)

believed to form at the cell surface by a pinocytic invagination of the apical membrane and subsequently to move toward and fuse with multivesicular bodies that serve to transport protein. Occasional retinoblastoma cells contain numerous dense-core granules structurally similar to those in cells of sympathetic innervation. Zonula adherens–like cell attachments occur and are similar to the junctions between normal photoreceptor cells. Giant cells have occasionally been demonstrated in retinoblastoma. Their significance is not clearly understood.[292]

Scanning electron microscopy of the surface morphology of retinoblastoma has been described.[289, 293]

Two distinct populations of retinoblastoma cells have been observed, one with abundant distinctive surface characteristics and the second relatively featureless. The first type of cell exhibits surface projections that are continuous with the plasma membrane and of various lengths (microvilli), spherical extensions of the cell surface representing transient extrusions of cytoplasms (zeiotic blebs), and ruffle-like structures (lamellipodia) on the free margin of the cell. Long, slender projections (filopodia) also develop. The second population of cells are spherical and smooth and are thought to represent cells in mitosis.

Most immunohistochemical studies aim at determining whether retinoblastomas derive from a common progenitor cell capable of differentiation into either glial or neuronal cells or from neuron-committed cells.[294–297] Variables in these studies include tissue fixation, staining procedures, specific areas taken into consideration, tumor cell differentiation, antigen expressivity, and age of tumor. Consequently, caution is required when interpreting most immunohistochemical results.[298–302] A related controversy surrounds the interpretation of proliferating glial cells, seen occasionally. Whether they represent tumor cells or reactive stroma has not been fully resolved.

Neuronal Markers

Many studies have demonstrated neuron-specific enolase (NSE) tumor cell lines.[300, 303–305] NSE has been detected in undifferentiated areas, well-differentiated areas, well-differentiated Flexner-Wintersteiner rosettes, and fleurettes.[300, 304] Synaptophysin, a neural membrane glycoprotein of presynaptic vesicles, was detected immunohistochemically in 45 of 54 formalin-fixed and paraffin-embedded retinoblastoma specimens.[306]

As described, strong evidence supports the presence of photoreceptor cell elements in retinoblastoma. Since the compelling preliminary studies by Felberg and Donoso,[307] many antigens attributed to photoreceptor cells in the retina have been under scrutiny.[308] Rhodopsin monoclonal antibodies have been demonstrated in fleurettes and Flexner-Wintersteiner rosettes. S antigen (arrestin) monoclonal and polyclonal antibodies have been detected[309] in the same differentiated structures, in diffuse areas of differentiated retinoblastoma, in trilateral retinoblastoma, and in cell lines. S antigen could not be identified in undifferentiated retinoblastomas. Donoso and colleagues further demonstrated that monoclonal antibodies to rhodopsin and S antigen bound to the same areas.[295, 310] They also mention a personal observation of retinoblastoma staining positively for α-transducin. This can be related to Bogenmann and coworkers' finding of transcripts for the L-transducin, as well as to the red or green cone cell photopigment in retinoblastoma cell lines.[311, 312] Genes to rod cell marker genes were not expressed, leading these researchers to suggest a cone lineage.

In the lumen of Flexner-Wintersteiner rosettes, Rodrigues and associates noted interphotoreceptor cell binding protein (IRBP), which is secreted by the rod photoreceptor cells into the extracellular matrix. The amount of IRBP in tumor samples correlated with the degree of tumor differentiation.[313–315]

Bridges and colleagues investigated retinoid binding proteins in fresh tumors and in cell lines[316] using a combination of Western blot, Northern blot, and radiolabeled ligand-binding techniques.[317] They found expression to be variable in tumor cells. The only retinoid-binding protein that was consistently expressed by both types of cells was IRPB, which was present at a level similar to that in a normal retina at 22 wk of gestation, suggesting that these findings are consistent with the embryonic origin of the cells. These investigators suggest that the tumor did not arise earlier than the 22-wk stage, but this remains speculative.

Tarlton and Easty tested a panel of 18 monoclonal antibodies against six retinoblastomas and compared the reactivity of the tumor with adult and fetal retina. They found that the closest normal cell type is a 13- to 16-wk outer retinal cell. They noted, however, that the tumor expressed antigens detected in both inner and outer layers.[318] Because of the potential of the precursor cell to differentiate into photoreceptor cells as well as "inner" retinal cells, they speculated a tumor origin from a primitive multipotential cell type that predominated before the eighth week of gestation and declined in parallel with later retinal development.

Conclusions are difficult to draw from such contradictory data. Tissue culture studies were first attempted to determine the cell or origin and differentiation patterns of retinoblastoma.[319–321] Obviously, both *plasticity* and multipotentiality were demonstrated, thus contradicting many studies providing evidence for a neuronal nature and differentiation.

Natural History

Complete spontaneous regression of retinoblastoma is an unusual but well-documented entity. Twenty-two histopathologic reports of 39 such tumors have been published.[275, 322–329] It is usually characterized by a severe inflammatory reaction followed by phthisis bulbi. Most researchers ascribe this to complete intraocular ischemic necrosis of the tumor after a central retinal vessel obstruction.[275, 330] Histopathologic study demonstrates dense calcification, necrotic tissue, fossilized tumor cells, massive proliferation of the RPE, inflammatory reaction, and various degrees of ossification (Fig. 184–43*A*

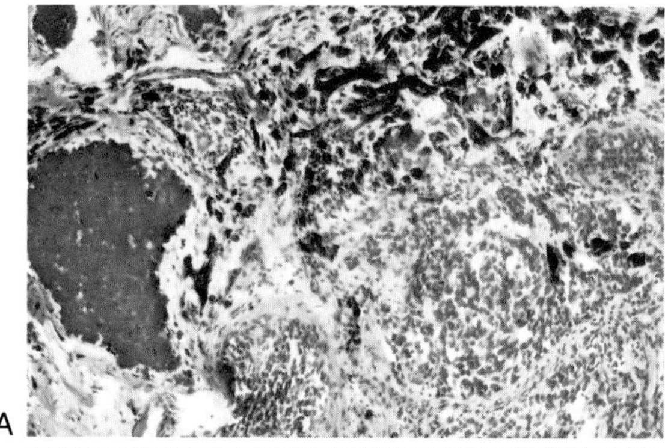
A

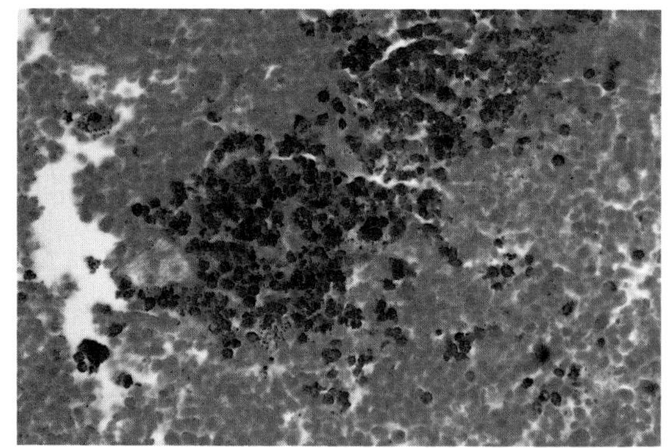
B

Figure 184–43. *A*, Phthisis bulbi. Tumor cells surrounded by an area of necrotic tissue. It is remarkable that this can happen in phthisis bulbi but never in microphthalmia. *B*, Histopathology of regressive retinoblastoma. Tumor cells and areas of calcification. (From Brini A, Dhermy P, Sahel J: Oncology of the Eye and Adnexa: Atlas of Clinical Pathology. Dordrecht, Kluwer Academic Publishers, 1990, pp 118–119.)

and *B*). The constant finding of extensive calcification of these tumors led Verhoeff to speculate that necrosis may result from calcification.[277] He proposed the therapeutic value of hypervitaminosis D, a hypothesis that recently found some support in vitro and in animal studies.[331] Marcus and colleagues emphasize that a reliable distinction has not been made between spontaneous necrosis and retinomas-retinocytomas in nonphthisical eyes.[332] These investigators concur with Zimmerman and others who view such tumors as benign variants of retinoblastoma.[264] Each of these lesions differs from the patterns of tumor observed after irradiation[332] (i.e., formation of a glial scar with complete destruction of the tumor and associated atrophy of surrounding choroid and vessels after treatment).

The pattern in which retinoblastoma is spread both within and outside the eye is well recognized and documented.[264, 328, 333, 334] Retinoblastoma is generally a friable neoplasm that may grow in all directions. Poor cohesion may be related to the apparently defective or absent zonulae adherens or filopodia, which normally contribute to cell-to-cell attachment. Tumor cells commonly seed *anteriorly*, in the vitreous and aqueous. Cells may be deposited on the surface of the iris and in the anterior chamber angle, giving rise to a secondary glaucoma or pseudohypopyon.[335] Clusters of tumor cells may collect on the inner surface of the retina and grow as separate foci, particularly in the peripheral retina and at the ora serrata. These secondary lesions may be mistaken for additional primary sites of tumor development. Intravitreal clusters of cells as well as a major portion of the tumor at the inner retinal surface are helpful in distinguishing secondary tumors from other primaries.[264]

Another common pattern of spread is *posteriorly* into the subretinal space. The significance of minimal choroid invasion is still disputed. Massive invasion of the choroid, however, is usually correlated with a high risk of scleral, orbital, and hematogenous spread. Invasion of the optic nerve may occur at the base of the optic cup, in the area of the central vessels, or into the subarachnoid space adjacent to the optic nerve (Fig. 184–44).

Tumor cells may disseminate hematogenously through the choroidal vessels or through vessels in proximity to the subarachnoid space.[336] Infiltrative spread through the optic nerve[336] or subarachnoid space gives access to the orbital tissues and bones and to brain invasion. Retinoblastoma may also reach the orbit through the emissaria. In a similar manner, tumor may grow through paracentesis sites and spread subconjunctivally.[337] In advanced cases, retinoblastoma may massively penetrate through the sclera and grow extensively into the orbit. Metastases to the preauricular and cervical lymph nodes usually follow such massive extraocular metastases.[338] Recurrence of retinoblastoma in the orbit after enucleation is the consequence of subclinical orbital involvement escaping recognition or from residual tumor in the remaining optic nerve.

Metastases to bone and brain from retinoblastoma are generally undifferentiated and do not show evidence of rosette and fleurette formation. Histopathologically, they may resemble Ewing's sarcoma, neuroblastoma, or other small round cell tumors of childhood. In such cases, immunohistochemistry, tissue culture, and electron microscopy may be of diagnostic value.[264, 293, 339] This lack of differentiation is helpful to distinguish such lesions from midbrain tumors in trilateral retinoblastoma. The most common sites of distant metastasis of retinoblastoma are the central nervous system, skull, distal bones, lymph nodes, and spinal cord.[340] Involvement of bones beyond the skull has been reported in approximately 50 per cent of patients dying of the tumor.

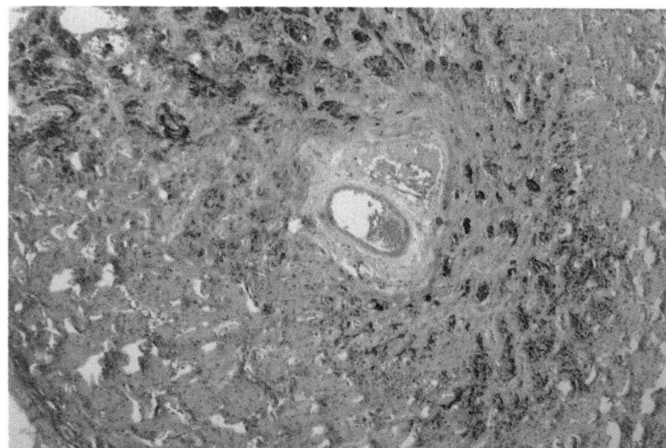

Figure 184–44. If the invasion of the optic nerve (seen here on a perpendicular section) extends farther than the surgical margin, the risk of extension to the orbit and distant metastases is great. (From Brini A, Dhermy P, Sahel J: Oncology of the Eye and Adnexa: Atlas of Clinical Pathology. Dordrecht, Kluwer Academic Publishers, 1990, p 121.)

Most metastases are detected within the first 2 yr after diagnosis; some, however, have appeared years after the last evidence of tumor activity in the retina is noted.[341, 342] In such cases, a new primary tumor should be considered.

Differential Diagnosis

With regard to the clinical differential diagnosis,[343] it is convenient to consider the following three situations:

1. Lesions that appear as a large retrolental mass giving rise to leukocoria. Advanced cicatricial *ROP* is usually seen in very low birth weight infants exposed to oxygen and rarely causes confusion. *Persistent hyperplastic primary vitreous* is almost always unilateral in a microphthalmic eye with characteristically prominent attracted ciliary processes. *Retinal dysplasia* usually appears as a bilateral mass at birth; it can be encountered in trisomy 13 or in *Norrie's disease* (Fig. 184–45*A* and *B*), Warburg's syndrome, and incontinentia pigmenti but can also be isolated and localized. *Larval granulomatosis* such as *ocular toxocariasis* may present either as solitary subretinal granuloma with vitreoretinal strands or as chronic endophthalmitis with opaque vitreous. Ophthalmoscopic and other clinical findings are often sufficient to differentiate retinoblastoma from these "pseudogliomas." *Coats' disease* is unilateral and presents as an exudative retinal detachment with telangiectatic vessels, subretinal exudates, and cholesterol crystals. Calcification and vitreous seeding are absent. Massive retinal gliosis may occur after extensive retinal hemorrhage. *Medulloepitheliomas* differ clearly by a later age of onset, anterior development, and a frequent cystic structure. Retinal detachments with or without proliferative vitreoretinopathy are easy to differentiate.

2. Lesions resembling small endophytic tumors. These include retinal *hamartomas, astrocytomas* as seen in tuberous sclerosis and neurofibromatosis, isolated retinal astrocytomas, *myelinated nerve fibers, retinochoroiditis,* and *metastatic endophthalmitis.*

3. Lesions simulating small exophytic retinoblastoma. These include *Coats' disease, toxocariasis, choroiditis* or *exudative retinitis, choroid hemangioma, angiomatosis retinae,* and *RPE proliferation.*

One of the most difficult confusing diagnostic situations is chronic granulomatous uveitis with hypopyon and diffuse infiltrating retinoblastoma.

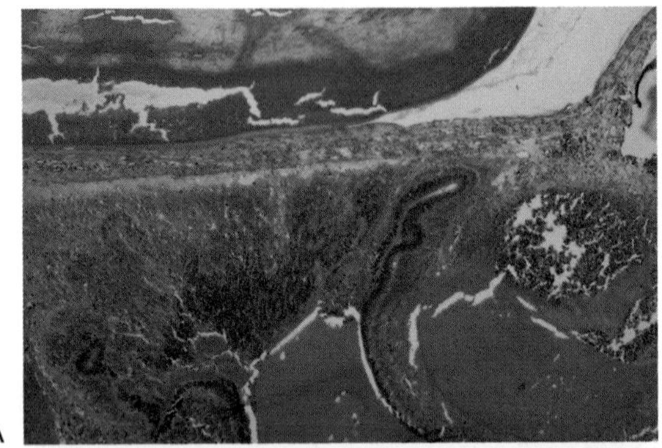

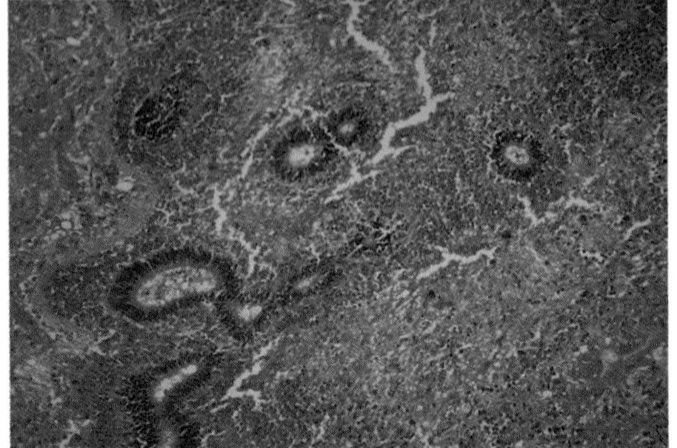

Figure 184–45. Norrie's disease—retinal detachment with dysplasia (the lens is at the top of the picture). Retinal folds; pseudorosettes with quasinormal retinal layers. The pseudocystic cavity on the right *(arrow)* is the result of hemorrhage, a frequent complication of this disease. (From Brini A, Dhermy P, Sahel J: Oncology of the Eye and Adnexa: Atlas of Clinical Pathology. Dordrecht, Kluwer Academic Publishers, 1990, p 123.)

Staging and Prognosis

RETINAL INVOLVEMENT IN LEUKEMIA

Ocular manifestations of leukemia are common, although some of them may not be detected clinically[344] unless the fundus is examined carefully. Duke-Elder asserted that at some stage of the disease, 90 percent of patients display fundus abnormalities.[345] Prevalence figures vary from 28 percent,[346] to 50 percent,[347] to approximately 80 percent.[344] The latter study showed no variation of this percentage between 1923 and 1980 and little difference between acute (82 percent) and chronic (75 percent) leukemia.

The eye may be involved in leukemia through scleral mechanisms such as (1) direct invasion by neoplastic cells whether definite (leukemic infiltrates) or putative (white-centered ocular hemorrhages); (2) hematologic abnormalities associated with leukemia (e.g., anemia, thrombocytopenia); (3) complications of hyperviscosity (i.e., microaneurysms, closure of capillaries, ischemia, neovascularization); and (4) opportunistic infections.

More prospective studies of patients examined at the time of diagnosis are needed to determine accurately the prevalence of ocular changes. Guyer and colleagues[348] found ocular abnormalities in 42 percent of 117 consecutive patients with acute leukemia (51 acute lymphocytic, 66 acute myelogenous). They found an association between thrombocytopenia and retinal hemorrhages in all patients; a lower hematocrit level was counted in patients with acute lymphocytic leukemia and retinal hemorrhages. Anemia was correlated with the finding of a white-centered hemorrhage in patients with nonlymphocytic leukemia.[348]

Retinal infiltrates appear as gray-white nodules or various sizes of streaks along the vessels (Fig. 184–46)[347, 349–351] and are reportedly associated with an elevated leukocyte count, a high proportion of blast cells, and an unfavorable prognosis. Some investigators em-

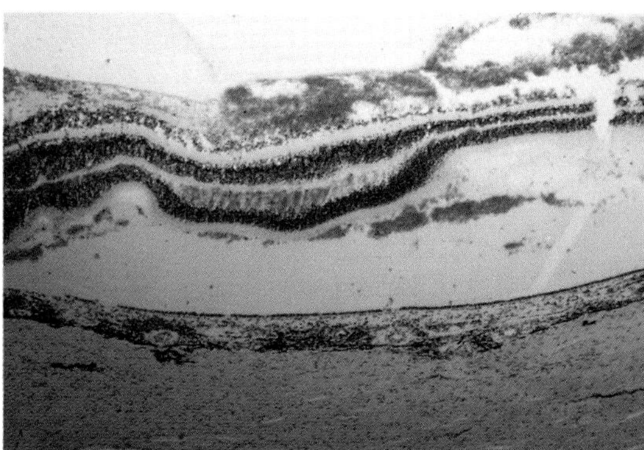

Figure 184–46. Retinal involvement in leukemia.

phasize that ocular leukemic infiltration (Fig. 184–47) detected in autopsy series could be related to the peripheral leukocyte count during the final hours of life.[352] Choroid infiltrates (Fig. 184–48) are more common but are often undetectable clinically except when signaled by the occurrence of RPE alterations (atrophy, hypertrophy, or hyperplasia) or of serous detachment of the RPE or of the sensory retina.[347, 353–356] Vitreous infiltration is less usual than in reticulum cell sarcoma.

LYMPHOMA

Except for the so-called reticulum cell sarcoma, vitreoretinal involvement by tumor cells in Hodgkin's or non-Hodgkin's lymphoma has rarely been documented pathologically.[357–367] Therefore, when hemorrhages or exudate is seen, other mechanisms of retinal involvement should be suspected. Nonetheless, it must be borne in mind that actual retinal infiltrates by tumor cells may occasionally occur.

Diffuse large cell lymphomas are often referred to as *reticulum cell sarcomas* or *histiocytic lymphomas* and *microgliomatosis*.[363–366] Immunohistochemical and in vitro lymphocyte function studies have demonstrated that these tumors are composed of transformed B and T lymphocytes.[367] The misnomer *reticulum cell sarcoma* continues to be used because of the lack of fully accepted definitive classification of non-Hodgkin's lymphomas and the relative paucity of information on intraocular involvement by lymphomas. *Large cell lymphoma* is the preferred term. This tumor occurs most frequently between 37 and 82 yr, with a mean age of diagnosis of 61 yr. Once a rare diagnosis, more than 120 cases have been reported in the past decade.[328, 347, 348, 368–381] Published case reports and pathology societies' presentations have declined, leading to a lack of accumulation of epidemiologic data. It appears, however, that there is no clear sexual or racial predisposition. Eighty percent of reported cases appeared bilaterally but were frequently asymmetric. The mean interval between diagnosis and death was 39 mo.[371]

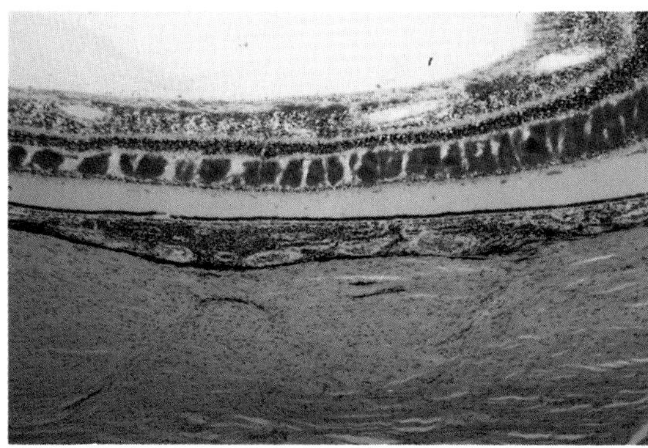

Figure 184–47. Retinal involvement in leukemia.

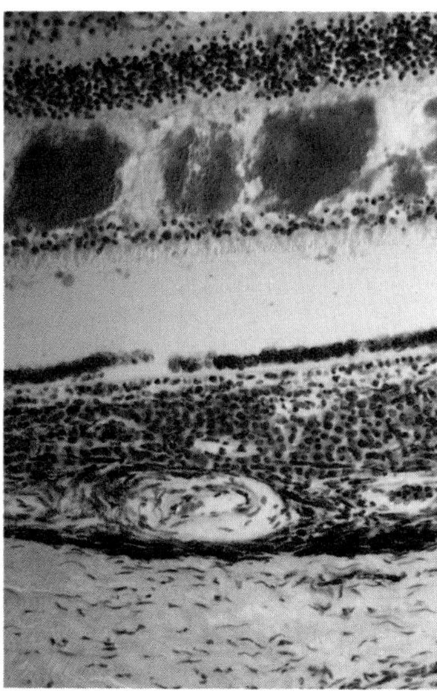

Figure 184–48. Retinal hemorrhages and diffuse leukemic infiltrate of the choroid. The apparent separation of the retina is due to artifact. (From Brini A, Dhermy P, Sahel J: Oncology of the Eye and Adnexa: Atlas of Clinical Pathology. Dordrecht, Kluwer Academic Publishers, 1990, p 131.)

Pathology. Vitreous samples are routinely processed with a Millipore filter and stained with Papanicolaou's stain.[363, 375] The tumor cells typically are large pleomorphic cells with scant cytoplasm and round, oval, or indented nuclei with prominent, eccentrically located nucleoli.[364, 381–383] Characteristic finger-like outpouchings are seen in some nuclei.

On cytopathologic examination, the presence of an intense inflammatory element may be confusing, and finding only normal-appearing lymphocytes in an aspirate does not rule out the diagnosis. Immunocytochemical identification of a monoclonal strain of B cells suggests neoplasia.[384, 385] Electron microscopy may demonstrate intranuclear inclusions, cytoplasmic crystalloids, and occasional pseudopodial extensions and cytosomes, as well as autophagic vacuoles.[386] When a high level of clinical suspicion exists, some practitioners advocate the use of retinochoroid biopsy, arguing that the uvea is more densely infiltrated through the vitreous.[279] Studies of enucleated eyes showed that tumor cells have a perivascular pattern in the retina and brain, whereas uveal involvement consists of diffuse infiltration usually occurring as placoid masses of closely packed cells. The cells characteristically form a mass between the RPE and Bruch's membrane.[364] This uveal infiltration differs from lymphoid uveal infiltrates with low-grade small

Text continued on page 2273

Table 184–2. PHAKOMATOSES

Condition	Etiology	Onset	Skin	CNS	Systemic	Eye	Comments
Retinal and cerebellar angiomatosis (von Hippel-Lindau disease) Blood vessel hamartomas Hemangioblastoma (blood vessels and stromal cells)	Autosomal dominant with incomplete penetrance Gene maps to the short arm of chromosome 3	Ocular symptoms usually begin in early adulthood (third decade of life) Cerebellar hemangioblastomas—average age of onset of symptoms in mid-30s Renal cell carcinoma usually becomes symptomatic in the fifth decade of life		Cerebellar hemangioblastomas present in up to 60% of cases (symptoms: headache, vertigo, vomiting, signs of cerebellar dysfunction) Hemangioblastomas of medulla oblongata and spinal cord less commonly seen	Renal cell carcinoma in approximately 25% of cases Pheochromocytoma in 3–10% of cases (often bilateral) Renal, pancreatic, hepatic, epididymal cysts Adenomas of the kidneys and epididymis	Retinal capillary hemangiomas in 40–60% of cases (bilateral in 50% of cases) Affected patients frequently develop hemorrhage and exudates in the vicinity of the tumor secondary to the incompetent vascular endothelium of the hemangioma Exudative retinal detachments may occur, resulting in rubeosis iridis, neovascular glaucoma, and ultimately phthisis bulbi	von Hippel's disease—retinal involvement only von Hippel-Lindau disease—retinal and CNS involvement Cerebellar hemangioblastomas and renal cell carcinomas are most common causes of death
Neurofibro-matosis (NF) NF 1: peripheral variant (von Recklinghausen's disease) NF 2: central variant (bilateral acoustic neurofibromatosis) Neural tissue hamartomas predominate: Schwann's cells of peripheral and sensory nerves; glial cells of CNS	Autosomal dominant with complete penetrance and variable expressivity NF 1: gene located on the long arm of chomosome 17 (gene *has* been isolated) NF 2: gene located on the long arm of chromosome 22	NF 1: findings may be present from birth or in early childhood; usually becomes clinically apparent at time of puberty; skin findings may worsen with pregnancy Lisch's nodules seen in 90% by age 6 yr NF 2: bilateral acoustic neuromas usually become symptomatic in second or third decade of life	NF 1: Café-au-lait spots Fibroma molluscum Plexiform neurofibromas Elephantiasis neurofibroma Axillary/inguinal freckling NF 2: characteristically without cutaneous involvement; may be a few café-au-lait spots	NF 1: nerve root or spinal cord neurofibromas less common but greater than intracranial or spinal cord gliomas and meningiomas Optic nerve and chiasmal gliomas frequently seen Learning disorder or mild intellectual deficit present in a significant number of cases NF 2: bilateral acoustic neuromas frequently greater than CNS and spinal cord gliomas and meningiomas and neurofibromas of nerve roots	Skeletal: rapidly progressive kyphoscoliosis; pseudoarthroses Hamartomas of the gastrointestinal tract and other organs Pheochromocytomas (10 times more frequent than in general population) Reported associations with other neuroendocrine and malignant tumors	NF 1: Lid: plexiform neurofibromas Orbit: defects in bony orbital wall Cornea: thickened corneal nerves Conjunctiva: neurofibromas Iris: Hamartomas Lisch's nodules (90–100% of cases) Trabecular meshwork, uveal tract (choroid): hamartomas Glaucoma: frequently ipsilateral to upper lid involvement with neurofibroma Optic nerve: gliomas in 15%	Malignant change can be superimposed on the hamartomas: fibrosarcoma, neurofibrosarcoma, malignant schwannoma Absence of greater wing of the sphenoid associated with pulsating exophthalmos Melanocytic nevi Glial hamartomas In severe forms of NF: may be shortened life expectancy related to CNS or malignant tumors, mental retardation, or severe seizures

						Retina: astrocytic hamartoma PSC NF 2: presenile posterior subcapsular cataracts (40% cases) less common-> optic nerve sheath meningiomas/ gliomas	Approximately 25% of patients diagnosed with optic nerve glioma will have NF
Arteriovenous (AV) communication of the retinal and midbrain (Wyburn-Mason syndrome)	Not regarded as hereditary	Adolescence to early adulthood; usually becomes symptomatic before age 30	Vascular facial nevi in up to 50% of patients, usually ipsilateral to affected eye	AV communication of the midbrain may cause cerebral or subarachnoid hemorrhage or increased intracranial pressure Signs of midbrain lesion, hemiplegia/ hemiparesis, cerebellar dysfunction, Parinaud's syndrome Mental changes affecting intelligence and memory Seizures in only 5% of patients	Associated AV communications of the lungs and spinal cord have been reported (rare)	Retinal AV communication (retinal AV aneurysm) unilateral, usually nonprogressive Pulsating exophthalmos, proptosis Visual loss: secondary to retinal or vitreous hemorrhage, vascular leakage in the macular region, or nerve fiber loss secondary to mechanical compression of the optic nerve or anterior visual pathway Ptosis or partial ophthalmoplegia secondary to third-nerve involvement in the midbrain	Morbidity/early mortality in some cases secondary to tendency of intracranial AV communications to bleed, leading to subarachnoid hemorrhage, neurologic deficits, and in some instances death

Table continued on following page

Table 184–2. PHAKOMATOSES *Continued*

Condition	Etiology	Onset	Skin	CNS	Systemic	Eye	Comments
Ataxia telangiectasia (Louis-Bar syndrome) Hamartoma Telangiectasia (histopathology: dilated, tortuous capillaries)	Autosomal recessive A gene for the syndrome has been localized to chromosome region 11q22–23 (may be more than one gene responsible for the disease)	Cerebellar ataxia: onset in infancy, becomes apparent when child begins walking Telangiectasia: onset between 3 and 7 yr of age	Cutaneous telangiectasia (malar area, nose, ears, palate, periorbital region); with increasing age—antecubital and popliteal regions and dorsal aspect of hands/feet Cutaneous infections (impetigo/warts) Seborrheic dermatitis	Cerebellar ataxia (progressive) Choreoathetosis, dysarthria, drooling, slowing of responses Histopathology: marked loss of Purkinje's cells and, to a lesser extent, granule and basket cells of cerebellar cortex Mental retardation in some cases, generally not apparent until adolescence	Hypoplasia of the thymus gland Immunologic problems: functional and numerical deficiency of T cells ± Low IgG level (50%) Low or undetectable IgA Low IgE (75%) Recurrent infections (usually sinopulmonary) in 85% cases Glucose intolerance and insulin resistance Increased frequency of chromosome abnormalities as well as increased susceptibility to chromosome breakage from X-irradiation Increased frequency of T-cell lymphoproliferative disorders	Bilateral bulbar conjunctival telangiectasia in all cases Abnormal extraocular movements common: halting and irregular conjugate gaze (oculomotor apraxia), abnormality of voluntary saccades Fixation nystagmus in 87% of cases, may also be nystagmus in lateral and vertical gaze	Ataxia telangiectasia = oculo-cutaneous telangiectasia + progressive cerebellar ataxia + frequent sinopulmonary infections Cause of death in over half of affected patients is recurrent sinopulmonary infections; many of the remainder develop malignancies, frequently lymphomas or leukemias
Tuberous sclerosis (Bourneville's disease) Tuber = potato shape of the tumor	Autosomal dominant with high penetrance and variable expressivity Gene located on the distal portion of the long arm of chromosome 9	First and second decades (usually first 3 yr) Seizures; onset usually in infancy Adenoma sebaceum; onset usually age 2–4 yr	Adenoma sebaceum in about 85% of cases; angiofibromas—papular rash on the malar region of the face and chin Ash leaf spots (in about 80% of cases), hypopigmented macules (best seen with Wood's light) Shagreen patches (25–30% of cases)—areas of fibromatous infiltration of the skin	Benign periventricular astrocytic hamartomas and "tuber"-like areas of sclerosis in the brain Associated mental retardation (50–60%) may be severe Seizures (80–90%); infantile spasms greater than grand mal Intracranial calcifications (about 50% of cases) in third and fourth ventricles ("brain stones")	Visceral tumors Rhabdomyomas (heart, muscle) Renal cysts and hamartomas Lung hamartomas Bone lesions—pseudocysts and sclerotic patches	Retinal astrocytic hamartomas (53% of cases) May be single or multiple; may be bilateral: flat or raised; classic appearance "mulberry" nodules (may be calcified); glial tumors of the optic disc, so-called giant drusen	Institutional care may be required for severe mental retardation or seizures Complete form: death 5 to 15 yr of age secondary to complications of seizures, gliomas, or intercurrent disease If CNS involvement is slight, life expectancy is normal

Encephalotrigeminal angiomatosis (Sturge-Weber syndrome) Blood vessel hamartoma Cavernous hemangioma	No definite hereditary pattern	Facial angioma present at birth Onset of seizures generally in infancy	Face: facial angioma (nevus flammeus)—dilated, telangiectatic cutaneous capillaries lined by single layer of endothelial cells—most commonly unilateral, often in distribution of V_1 or V_2	Leptomeningeal hemangioma ipsilateral to the facial angioma, usually located in the parietal-occipital region Mental retardation associated with intracranial angioma in over 50% of cases; maldevelopment/atrophy of brain in the vicinity of the lesion Seizures: jacksonian type (begin in infancy) classically contralateral to the facial angioma; become generalized with increasing age; may be associated with hemiparesis or hemiplegia Unilateral calcification of cerebral blood vessels and cortical gyri in vicinity of the leptomeningeal angioma, commonly seen "railroad track" sign		Choroid: cavernous hemangioma, in 40–50% on histopathologic examination, usually ipsilateral to facial nevus flammeus Lids: (common) cavernous hemangioma, ipsilateral to the facial angioma Retina: degenerative changes in some cases secondary to underlying choroidal hemangioma; cystoid degeneration of outer retina; subretinal serous fluid Glaucoma: (30% of patients) may be associated buphthalmos, usually unilateral, ipsilateral to facial lesion Iris: heterochromia of iris in some cases	Glaucoma usually occurs if upper lid has facial hemangioma Cause of glaucoma: may be secondary to incomplete cleavage of anterior chamber angle (in some cases); in cases with normal-appearing angle, possibly secondary to elevated episcleral venous pressure due to presence of an episcleral hemangioma May occasionally be progressive mental deterioration and intractable seizures in association with leptomeningeal hemangioma

CNS, central nervous system.

Table 184–3. OTHER FINDINGS IN THE PHAKOMATOSES

	Tuberous Sclerosis	Neurofibromatosis	Retinal and Cerebellar Angiomatosis	Encephalotrigeminal Angiomatosis	Ataxia Telangiectasia	Arteriovenous Communication of Retina and Midbrain
Hamartoma	Mixed, glial, and vascular (astrocytic hamartomas)	Neural tissue and Schwann's cells or glial cells	Blood vessels + stroma = hemangioblastoma	Cavernous hemangiomas	Dilated, telangiectatic capillaries	Direct AV communications without intervening capillaries
Site	Retina, brain, viscera	Eye, CNS, skin, GI, bone	Retina, CNS (cerebellum)	Face/eyelids, choroid, leptomeninges	Conjunctiva, skin (cerebellar atrophy)	Retina, midbrain
Inheritance	Autosomal dominant (variable expressivity)	Autosomal dominant (variable expressivity)	Autosomal dominant (irregular penetrance)	No definite hereditary pattern	Autosomal recessive	Not regarded as hereditary
Onset	Seizures in infancy; adenoma sebaceum in childhood	Usually puberty, pregnancy, occasionally infancy/childhood	Early adulthood for ocular symptoms	Facial angioma at birth	Cerebellar ataxia in infancy; telangiectasia at age 3–7 yr	Adolescence, early adulthood
Key ocular findings or problems	Astrocytic hamartoma, "giant drusen" of optic nerve	NF 1: Lisch's nodules, optic nerve gliomas, hamartomas of uveal tract, glaucoma NF 2: presenile posterior subcapsular cataracts, optic nerve sheath meningiomas	Retinal capillary hemangioma Secondary problems: exudative retinal detachment, rubeosis, neovascular glaucoma, phthisis bulbi	Choroid hemangioma, glaucoma, secondary retinal changes due to the presence of the choroid hemangioma	Conjunctival telangiectasis, abnormalities of extraocular movements ("oculomotor apraxia")	Retinal AV malformations, pulsating exophthalmos, visual loss in some cases, ptosis/partial ophthalmoplegia
Key systemic findings Mental retardation Seizures Intracranial calcifications	+ (may be severe) + + (periventricular)	+ (usually mild)		+ (common) + + (cerebral blood vessels and cortical gyri)		(5% of cases)
Malignancies or clinically important systemic tumors	Malignant astrocytomas, cardiac rhabdomyomas, renal and pulmonary hamartomas	Fibrosarcomas, neurofibromas, malignant schwannoma	Cerebellar hemangioblastomas, renal cell carcinomas, pheochromocytomas		Lymphoreticular malignancies, recurrent sinopulmonary infections	AV communications of the midbrain

AV, arteriovenous; CNS, central nervous sytem; GI, gastrointestinal; NF, neurofibromatosis.

lymphoplasmocytic lymphomas that do not involve the retina and vitreous and were formerly termed *reactive lymphoid hyperplasis*.[387, 388]

RETINAL METASTASES

In contrast to the uvea, metastases to the retina are rare. Leys and colleagues reported two cases and compiled a review of the literature. This survey found 11 cases of retinal metastasis from carcinoma and 11 cases from skin melanoma.[389] It is likely, however, that the actual incidence is higher because (1) prospective autopsy series should demonstrate foci of metastatic cells, as indicated by Fishman and associates,[390] who found two cases with retinal metastases in a series of 15 consecutive skin melanomas; (2) the use of diagnostic vitreous aspiration or vitrectomy should improve detection of these cases;[391–393] and (3) the length of survival of patients with carcinomas is increasing.

The primary tumor is usually a carcinoma of the lung, breast, stomach, retrosigmoid, or uterus or a skin melanoma.[390, 391, 393–410] Tumor cells gain access to the retina by the internal carotid artery,[397] possibly accounting for the frequent association with brain metastases.[396] Uveal metastases, which represent the most common intraocular malignancy, are frequent (see Chap. 266), and vitreous invasion may be associated with retinal metastases after infiltration of the superficial retina and retinal vessels.[393, 397, 410]

In some patients with a known primary malignancy and metastases, tissue diagnosis may not be necessary. In other instances, vitreous surgery or aspiration[389, 392, 393, 406, 411–413] is necessary and will facilitate the planning and treatment. A modified Papanicolaou stain and cytologic analysis by an experienced pathologist using immunocytochemistry techniques or electron microscopy may be required.

Phakomatoses are discussed in detail in Chapter 270. Tables 184–2 and 184–3 describe phakomatoses.

REFERENCES

1. Committee for the Classification of Retinopathy of Prematurity: An international classification of retinopathy of prematurity. Arch Ophthalmol 102:1130, 1984.
2. Committee for the Classification of Retinopathy of Prematurity: An international classification of retinopathy of prematurity. The classification of retinal detachment. Arch Ophthalmol 105:906, 1987.
3. Flynn JT: Acute proliferation retrolental fibroplasia: Evolution of the lesion. Graefes Arch Clin Exp Ophthalmol 195:101, 1975.
4. Foos RY: Acute retrolental fibroplasia. Graefes Arch Clin Exp Ophthalmol 195:87, 1975.
5. Foos RY: Chronic retinopathy of prematurity. Ophthalmology 92:563, 1985.
6. Foos RY: Retinopathy of prematurity. Retina 7:260, 1987.
7. BenSira I, Nissenkorn I, Kremer I: Retinopathy of prematurity [Review]. Surv Ophthalmol 33:1, 1988.
8. Terry TL: Extreme prematurity and fibroplastic overgrowth of persistent vascular sheath behind each crystalline lens. Am J Ophthalmol 25:203, 1942.
9. Campbell K: Intensive oxygen therapy as a possible cause of retrolental fibroplasia: A clinical approach. Med J Aust 2:48, 1951.
10. Ashton N, Ward B, Serpell G: Role of oxygen in the genesis of retrolental fibroplasia: A preliminary report. Br J Ophthalmol 37:513, 1953.
11. Patz A, Hoeck LE, De LaCruz E: Studies on the effect of high oxygen administration in retrolental fibroplasia: A nursery observation. Am J Ophthalmol 35:1248, 1952.
12. Lucey JL, Dangman B: A re-examination of the role of oxygen in retrolental fibroplasia. Pediatrics 73:82, 1984.
13. Patz A: Retrolental fibroplasia. Surv Ophthalmol 14:1, 1969.
14. Ashton N: Oxygen and the growth and development of retinal vessels: In vivo and in vitro studies. Am J Ophthalmol 62:412, 1966.
15. Bougle D, Vert P, Reichart E, et al: Retinal superoxide dismutase activity in newborn kittens exposed to normogaric hyperoxia: Effect of Vitamin E. Retinopathy of Prematurity Conference Syllabus, vol. 1. December 4–6, 1981, pp 227–242.
16. Kretzer FL, McPherson AR, Hittner HM: An interpretation of retinopathy in terms of spindle cells relationship to vitamin E prophylaxis and cryotherapy. Graefes Arch Clin Exp Ophthalmol 224:205, 1986.
17. Hittner HM, Godio LB, Sper ME, et al: Retrolental fibroplasia: Further clinical evidence and ultrastructural support for efficacy of vitamin E in the preterm infant. Pediatrics 71:423, 1983.
18. Kretzer FL, Hittner HM: Human retinal development: Relationship to the pathogenesis of retinopathy of prematurity. *In* McPherson AR, Hittner HM, Kretzer FL (eds): Retinopathy of Prematurity: Current Concepts and Controversies. Toronto, BC Decker, 1986, pp 27–52.
19. Cogan DG, Kuwabara T: Accessory cells in vessels of the perinatal human retina. Arch Ophthalmol 104:747, 1986.
20. Friedenwald JS, Owens WC, Owens EU: Retrolental fibroplasia in premature infants. III: The pathology of the disease. Trans Am Ophthalmol Soc 49:207, 1952.
21. Flower RW, McLeod DS, Lutty GA, et al: Postnatal retinal vascular development of the puppy. Invest Ophthalmol Vis Sci 26:957, 1985.
22. Garner A: The pathology of retinopathy of prematurity. *In* Silverman WA, Flynn JT (eds): Retinopathy of Prematurity. Boston, Blackwell Scientific, 1985, pp 19–52.
23. Michaelson IC: The mode of development of the vascular system of the retina, with some observations on its significance for certain retinal diseases. Trans Ophthalmol Soc UK 68:157, 1948.
24. Cogan DG: Development and senescence of the human retinal vasculature. Trans Ophthalmol Soc UK 83:465, 1963.
25. Patz A, Palmer EA: Retinopathy of prematurity. *In* Ryan SJ (ed): Retina. St. Louis, CV Mosby, 1977, pp 509–530.
26. Flynn JT, O'Grady GE, Herrera J, et al: Retrolental fibroplasia. I: Clinical observations. Arch Ophthalmol 95:217, 1977.
27. Kushner BJ, Essner D, Cohen I, Flynn JT: Retrolental fibroplasia. II: Pathology correlation. Arch Ophthalmol 95:29, 1977.
28. Goldmann H: Biomicroscopie du corps vitré et du fond d'oeil. Rapp Soc Fr Ophtalmol. Paris, Masson & Cie, 1957, p 164.
29. Hogan MJ, Alvarado JA, Weddell JE: Histology of the human eye. Philadelphia, WB Saunders, 1971.
30. Spencer WH: Vitreous. *In* Spencer WH (ed): Ophthalmic Pathology, 3rd ed, vol. 2. Philadelphia, WB Saunders, 1985.
31. Naumann GOH: Pathologie des Auges. Berlin, Springer Verlag, 1980, pp 646–647.
32. Reese AB: Persistent hyperplastic primary vitreous. Am J Ophthalmol 33:1, 1955.
33. Pruett R, Schepens CL: Posterior hyperplastic primary vitreous. Am J Ophthalmol 69:535, 1970.
34. Spitznas M, Koch F, Pohl S: Ultrastructural pathology of anterior persistent hyperplastic primary vitreous. Graefes Arch Clin Exp Ophthalmol 228:487, 1990.
35. Font RL, Yanoff Y, Zimmerman LE: Intraocular adipose tissue and hyperplastic primary vitreous. Arch Ophthalmol 82:43, 1969.
36. Haddad R, Font RL, Reeser F: Persistent hyperplastic primary vitreous clinicopathologic study of 62 cases and review of the literature. Surv Ophthalmol 23:123, 1978.
37. Witschel H: Letter to the editor. Graefes Arch Clin Exp Ophthalmol 229:297, 1991.
38. Green WR: Retina. *In* Spencer WH (ed): Ophthalmic Pathology, 3rd ed, vol. 2. Philadelphia, WB Saunders, 1985.
39. Reese AB, Blodi FC: Retinal dysplasia. Am J Ophthalmol 33:23, 1950.

40. Hunter WS, Zimmerman LE: Unilateral retinal dysplasia. Arch Ophthalmol 74:23, 1965.
41. Lahav M, Albert DM, Wyand S: Clinical and histopathologic classification of retinal dysplasia. Am J Ophthalmol 75:648, 1973.
42. Wagner H: Ein bisher unbekanntes Erbleiden des Auges (Degeneratio hyaloideo-retinalis hereditaria), beobachtet im Kanton Zurich). Klin Monatsbl Augenheilkd 100:840, 1938.
43. Manschot WA: Pathology of hereditary conditions related to retinal detachment. Ophthalmologica 162:223, 1971.
44. Blair NP, Albert DM, Lieberfarb RM, Hirose T: Hereditary progressive arthro-ophthalmopathy of Stickler. Am J Ophthalmol 88:876, 1979.
45. Hirose T, Lee KY, Schepens CL: Wagner's hereditary vitreoretinal degeneration and retinal detachment. Arch Ophthalmol 89:176, 1973.
46. Favre M: A propos de deux cas de dégénérescence hyaloidéorétinienne. Ophthalmologica 135:604, 1958.
47. Peyman GA, Fishman GA, Sanders DR, Vlchek J: Histopathology of Goldmann-Favre syndrome obtained by full-thickness eye wall biopsy. Ann Ophthalmol 9:479, 1977.
48. Criswick VG, Schepens CL: Familial exudative vitreoretinopathy. Am J Ophthalmol 68:578, 1969.
49. Brockhurst RJ, Albert DM, Zakov ZN: Pathologic findings in familial exudative vitreoretinopathy. Arch Ophthalmol 99:2143, 1981.
50. Van Nouhuys CE: Dominant exudative vitreoretinopathy and other vascular developmental disorders of the peripheral retina. Doc Ophthalmol 54:1, 1982.
51. Yanoff M, Kestesz-Rahn EH, Zimmerman LE: Histopathology of juvenile retinoschisis. Arch Ophthalmol 79:49, 1968.
52. Manschot WA: Pathology of hereditary juvenile retinoschisis. Arch Ophthalmol 88:131, 1972.
53. Straatsma BR, Allen RA: Lattice degeneration of the retina. Trans Am Ophthalmol Otolaryngol 66:600, 1962.
54. Michels RG, Wilkinson CP, Rice TA: Retinal Detachment. St. Louis, CV Mosby, 1990.
55. Byer NE: Lattice degeneration of retina. Surv Ophthalmol 23:213, 1979.
56. Hirose T, Lee KY, Schepens CL: Snowflake degeneration in hereditary vitreoretinal degeneration. Am J Ophthalmol 77:143, 1974.
57. Goldberg MF, Lee FL, Tso MOM, Fishr an GA: Histopathologic study of autosomal dominant vitreoretinochoroidopathy: Peripheral annular pigmentary dystrophy of retina. Ophthalmology 96:1736, 1989.
58. Tso MOM: Retinal Diseases. Philadelphia, JB Lippincott, 1988.
59. Dryja TP, McGee TL, Reichel E, et al: A point mutation of the rhodopsin gene in one form of retinitis pigmentosa. Nature 343:364, 1990.
60. Marshall J, Heckenlively J: Pathologic mechanisms in retinitis pigmentosa. *In* Heckenlively J (ed): Retinitis Pigmentosa. Philadelphia, JB Lippincott, 1988.
61. Szamier RB, Berson EL, Klein R, Meyer S: Sex-linked retinitis pigmentosa: Ultrastructure of photoreceptors and pigment epithelium. Invest Ophthalmol Vis Sci 18:145, 1979.
62. Flannery JG, Farber DB, Bird AC, Bor D: Degenerative changes in a retina affected with autosomal dominant retinitis pigmentosa. Invest Ophthalmol Vis Sci 30:191, 1989.
63. Eagle RC Jr, Lucier AC, Bernadino VB Jr, et al: Retinal pigment epithelial abnormalities in fundus flavimaculatus. Ophthalmology 87:1189, 1980.
64. Klein BA, Krill AE: Fundus flavimaculatus: Clinical, functional and histopathologic observations. Am J Ophthalmol 64:3, 1967.
65. Lopez PF, Maumenee IH, Delacruz Z, Green WR: Autosomal dominant fundus flavimaculatus: Clinicopathologic correlation. Ophthalmology 97:798, 1990.
66. McDonnell PJ, Kivlin JD, Maumenee IH, et al: Fundus flavimaculatus with maculopathy: A clinicopathologic study. Ophthalmology 93:116, 1986.
67. Noble KG: Pathology of the hereditary macular dystrophies. Semin Ophthalmol 2:110, 1987.
68. Weingeist TA, Kobrin JL, Watzke RC: Histopathology of Best's macular dystrophy. Arch Ophthalmol 100:1108, 1982.
69. O'Gorman S, Flaherty JG, Fishman GA, Berson EL: Histopathologic findings in Best's vitelliform macular dystrophy. Arch Ophthalmol 106:1261, 1988.
70. Deutman AF, Jansen MA: Dominantly inherited drusen of Bruch's membrane. Br J Ophthalmol 54:373, 1970.
71. Gass JDM, Jallow S, Davis B: Adult vitelliform macular detachment occurring in patients with basal laminar drusen. Am J Ophthalmol 99:445, 1985.
72. Ashton N, Sorsby A: Fundus dystrophy with unusual features: A histological study. Br J Ophthalmol 35:751, 1951.
73. Foos RY: Posterior vitreous detachment. Trans Am Acad Ophthalmol Otolaryngol 76:480, 1972.
74. O'Malley P: The pattern of vitreous detachment: A study of 800 autopsy eyes. *In* Irvine AR, O'Malley C (eds): Advances in Vitreous Surgery. Springfield, IL, Charles C Thomas, 1976.
75. Eisner G: Biomicroscopy of the Peripheral Fundus: An Atlas and Textbook. New York, Springer Verlag, 1973.
76. Eisner G: Clinical anatomy of the vitreous. *In* Jakobiec FA (ed): Ocular Anatomy, Embryology, and Teratology. New York, Harper & Row, 1982, pp 391, 1122.
77. Sebag J: Aging of the vitreous. Eye 1:254, 1987.
78. Foos RY, Whielter NC: Vitreoretinal juncture synechisis, senilis and posterior vitreous detachment. Ophthalmology 89:1502, 1982.
79. Gass JDM: Stereoscopic Atlas of Macular Diseases: Diagnosis and Treatment, 3rd ed. St. Louis, CV Mosby, 1987, pp 2–18, 43–219, 552–577, 581–600, 684–693.
80. Gass JDM: Idiopathic senile macular hole: Its early stages and pathogenesis. Arch Ophthalmol 106:629, 1988.
81. Smiddy WE, Michels RG, DeBustros S, et al: Histopathology of tissue during vitrectomy for impending idiopathic macular holes. Am J Ophthalmol 108:360, 1989.
82. Smiddy WE, Maguire AM, Green WR, et al: Idiopathic epiretinal membranes, ultrastructural characteristics, clinicopathologic correlation. Ophthalmology 96:811, 1989.
83. Kishi S, Shimizu K: Posterior precortical vitreous pocket. Arch Ophthalmol 108:979, 1990.
84. Jaffe NS: Macular retinopathy after separation of the vitreoretinal adherence. Arch Ophthalmol 78:585, 1967.
85. Green WR, Kenyon KR, Michels G, et al: Ultrastructure of epiretinal membranes causing macular pucker after retinal reattachment surgery. Trans Ophthalmol Soc UK 99:63, 1979.
86. Foos RY: Vitreoretinal juncture—Simple epiretinal membranes. Graefes Arch Clin Exp Ophthalmol 189:231, 1974.
87. Foos RY: Vitreoretinal juncture. Epiretinal membranes and vitreous. Invest Ophthalmol Vis Sci 16:416, 1977.
88. Maguire AM, Smiddy WE, Nanda SK, et al: Clinicopathologic correlation of recurrent epiretinal membranes after previous surgical removal. Retina 10:213, 1990.
89. Grierson I, Hiscott PS, Hitchins CA, et al: Which cells are involved in the formation of epiretinal membranes. Semin Ophthalmol 2:99, 1987.
90. Hiscott PS, Grierson I, McLeon D: Retinal pigment epithelial cells in epiretinal membranes: An immunohistochemical study. Br J Ophthalmol 68:708, 1984.
91. Smiddy WE, Green WR, Michels RG, et al: Ultrastructural characteristics of vitreoretinal traction syndrome. Am J Ophthalmol 107:177, 1989.
92. Smiddy WE, Michels RG, Green WR: Morphology, pathology and surgery of idiopathic vitreoretinal macular disorders. Retina 10:288, 1990.
93. Zarbin MA, Michels RG, Green WR: Epiretinal membrane contracture associated with macular prolapse. Am J Ophthalmol 110:610, 1990.
94. Guyer DR, Green WR, de Bustros S, Fine SL: Histopathologic features of idiopathic macular holes and cysts. Ophthalmology 97:1045, 1990.
95. Johnson RN, Gass JDM: Idiopathic macular holes: Observations, stages of formation, and implications for surgical intervention. Ophthalmology 95:924, 1988.
96. Kampik A, Green WR, Michels RG, Nase PK: Ultrastructural features of progressive idiopathic epiretinal membrane removed by vitreous surgery. Am J Ophthalmol 90:797, 1980.
97. Kampik A, Kenyon KR, Michels RG, et al: Epiretinal and vitreous membranes, comparative study of 56 cases. Arch Ophthalmol 99:1445, 1981.
98. Rodman HI, Johnson FB, Zimmerman LE: New histopathological and histochemical observation concerning asteroid hyalitis. Arch Ophthalmol 66:552, 1961.

99. Miller H, Miller B, Rabinowitz H: Asteroid bodies—An ultrastructural study. Invest Ophthalmol Vis Sci 24:133, 1983.
100. Verhoeff FH: Microscopic findings in a case of asteroid hyalitis. Am J Ophthalmol 4:155, 1921.
101. Grossniklaus HE, Frank KE, Farhi DC, et al: Hemoglobin spherulosis in the vitreous cavity. Arch Ophthalmol 106:961, 1988.
102. Doft BH, Rubinow A, Cohen AS: Immunocytochemical demonstration of prealbumin in the vitreous in heredofamilial amyloidosis. Am J Ophthalmol 97:296, 1984.
103. Michael F: Mechanisms of normal retinal adhesion. *In* Glaser BM, Michels RG (eds): Retina, vol. 3. St. Louis, CV Mosby, 1989, p 71.
104. Zauberman H, Berman ER: Measurement of adhesive forces between the sensory retina and the pigment epithelium. Exp Eye Res 8:276, 1969.
105. Zauberman H, de Guillebon H: Retinal traction in vivo and postmortem. Arch Ophthalmol 87:549, 1972.
106. Hollyfield JG, Varner HH, Rayborn MF, Osterfeld AM: Retinal attachment to the pigment epithelium: Linkage through an extracellular sheath surrounding photoreceptor. Retina 9:59, 1989.
107. Kroll AJ, Machemer R: Experimental retinal detachment in the owl monkey. II: Histology of retina and pigment epithelium. Am J Ophthalmol 66:410, 1968.
108. Kroll AJ, Machemer R: Experimental retinal detachment in the owl monkey: Photoreceptor protein renewal in early retinal reattachment. Am J Ophthalmol 72:356, 1971.
109. Marcus DF, Aaberg TM: Intraretinal macrocysts in retinal detachment. Arch Ophthalmol 97:1273, 1979.
110. Wilson DJ, Green WR: Histopathologic study of the effect of retinal detachment surgery on 49 eyes obtained postmortem. Am J Ophthalmol 103:179, 1987.
111. Barr CC: The histopathology of successful retinal reattachment. Retina 10:189, 1990.
112. Machemer R, Laqua H: Pigment epithelial proliferation and retinal detachment (massive periretinal proliferation). Am J Ophthalmol 80:1, 1975.
113. Guerin CJ, Anderson DH, Fariss RN, Fisher SK: Retinal reattachment of the primate macula. Invest Ophthalmol Vis Sci 30:1708, 1989.
114. Machemer R: Pathogenesis and classification of massive periretinal proliferation. Br J Ophthalmol 62:737, 1978.
115. Laqua H, Machemer R: Glial cell proliferation in retinal detachment (massive periretinal proliferation). Am J Ophthalmol 80:602, 1975.
116. Laqua H, Machemer R: Clinical pathological correlation in massive periretinal proliferation. Am J Ophthalmol 80:913, 1975.
117. Machemer R, VanHorn D, Aaberg TM: Pigment epithelial proliferation in human retinal detachment with massive periretinal proliferation. Am J Ophthalmol 85:181, 1977.
118. Machemer R: Experimental retinal detachment in the owl monkey. II: Histology of retina and pigment epithelium. Am J Ophthalmol 66:410, 1968.
119. The Retina Society Terminology Committee: The classification of retinal detachment with proliferative vitreoretinopathy. Ophthalmology 90:121, 1983.
120. The Retina Society Terminology Committee: An updated classification of retinal detachment with proliferation vitreoretinopathy. Am J Ophthalmol 112:159, 1991.
121. Mandelcorn MS, Machemer R, Finberg R, et al: Proliferation and metaplasia of intravitreal retinal pigment epithelium cell autotransplants. Am J Ophthalmol 80:227, 1975.
122. Glaser BM, Cardin A, Biscoe B: Proliferative vitreoretinopathy: The mechanism of development of vitreoretinal traction. Ophthalmology 94:320, 1987.
123. Glaser BM, Lemor M: Pathobiology of proliferative vitreoretinopathy. *In* Glaser BM, Michels RG (eds): Retina, vol. 3. St. Louis, CV Mosby, 1989, pp 369–383.
124. Campochiaro PA, Kaden IH, Vidaurri-Leal J, Glaser BM: Cryotherapy and intravitreal dispersion of viable retinal pigment epithelial cells. Arch Ophthalmol 103:434, 1985.
125. Singh AK, Michels RG, Glaser BM: Scleral indentation following cryotherapy and repeat cryotherapy enhances release of viable retinal pigment epithelial cells. Retina 6:176, 1986.
126. Fisher SK, Erickson PA, Lewis GP, Anderson DH: Intraretinal proliferation induced by retinal detachment. Invest Ophthalmol Vis Sci 32:1739, 1991.
127. VanHorn DL, Aaberg TM, Machemer R, Fenzl R: Glial cell proliferation in human retinal detachment with massive retinal periretinal proliferation. Am J Ophthalmol 84:383, 1977.
128. Fisher SK, Anderson DH: Cellular effects of detachment on the retina and the retinal pigment epithelium. *In* Glaser BM, Michels RG (eds): Retina, vol. 3. St. Louis, CV Mosby, 1989, pp 259–281.
129. Clarkson JG, Green WR, Massaf D: A histopathologic review of 168 cases of preretinal membrane. Am J Ophthalmol 84:1, 1977.
130. Kenyon KR, Michels RG: Ultrastructure of epiretinal membranes removed by pars plana vitreoretinal surgery. Am J Ophthalmol 83:815, 1977.
131. Elner SG, Elner VM, Diaz-Rohena R, et al: Anterior PVR. II: Clinicopathologic, light microscopic, and ultrastructural findings. *In* Freeman HM, Tolentino FI (eds): Proliferative Vitreoretinopathy (PVR). New York, Springer Verlag, 1988, pp 34–45.
132. Lindsey PS, Michels RG, Luckenbach M, Green WR: Ultrastructural epiretinal membrane causing retinal starfold. Ophthalmology 90:578, 1983.
133. Wilkes SR, Mansour AM, Green WR: Proliferative vitreoretinopathy: Histopathology of retroretinal membranes. Retina 7:94, 1987.
134. Trese MT, Chandler DB, Machemer R: Subretinal strands: Ultrastructural features. Graefes Arch Clin Exp Ophthalmol 223:35, 1985.
135. Hiscott P, Grierson I: Subretinal membranes of proliferative vitreoretinopathy. Br J Ophthalmol 75:53, 1991.
136. Lewis H, Aaberg TM, Abrams GW, et al: Subretinal membranes in proliferative vitreoretinopathy. Ophthalmology 96:1403, 1989.
137. Schwartz D, De La Cruz Z, Green WR, et al: Proliferative vitreoretinopathy: Ultrastructural study of 20 retroretinal membranes removed by vitreous surgery. Retina 8:275, 1988.
138. Leibowitz H, Krueger DE, Maunder LR, et al: The Framingham Eye Study Monograph: An ophthalmological and epidemiological study of cataract, glaucoma, diabetic retinopathy, macular degeneration, and visual acuity in a general population of 2631 adults, 1973–1975. Surv Ophthalmol 24(Suppl):335, 1980.
139. Sorsby A: The incidence and causes of blindness in England and Wales 1963–1968, Ministry of Health Reports on Public Health and Medical Subjects, No. 128. London, Her Majesty's Stationery Office, 1972.
140. Bressler BB, Bressler SB, Fine SL: Age-related macular degeneration. Surv Ophthalmol 32:375, 1988.
141. Feeney-Burns L, Burns RP, Gao CL: Age-related macular changes in humans over 90 years old. Am J Ophthalmol 109:265, 1990.
142. Weale RA: Retinal senescence. *In* Osborne NN, Chader CJ (eds): Progress in Retinal Research. Elmsford, NY, Pergamon Press, 1985, pp 53–73.
143. Young RW: Pathophysiology of age-related macular degeneration. Surv Ophthalmol 31:291, 1987.
144. Young RW: Solar radiation and age-related macular degeneration. Surv Ophthalmol 32:252, 1988.
145. Boulton M, Marshall J: Retinal pigment epithelial detachments in the elderly. Trans Ophthalmol Soc UK 105:674, 1986.
146. Hogan MJ: Role of the retinal pigment epithelium in macular disease. Trans Am Acad Ophthalmol Otolaryngol 76:64, 1972.
147. Merry BJ: Biological mechanisms of ageing. Eye 1:163, 1987.
148. Franceschetti A, François J, Babel J: Dégénérescence maculaire sénile. *In* Les hérédodégénérescences Choriorétiniennes. Paris, Masson, 1963, pp 518–538.
149. Gass JDM: Drusen and disciform macular detachment and degeneration. Arch Ophthalmol 90:206, 1973.
150. Young RW: Visual cells and the concept of renewal. Invest Ophthalmol Vis Sci 16:700, 1976.
151. Marshall J: The ageing retina: Physiology or pathology. Eye 1:282, 1987.
152. Sarks SH: Ageing and degeneration in the macular region: A clinicopathological study. Br J Ophthalmol 60:324, 1976.
153. Sarks JP, Sarks SH, Killingsworth MC: Evolution of geographic atrophy of the retinal pigment epithelium. Eye 2:552, 1988.

154. Sarks SH: Age-related macular degeneration. *In* Ryan SJ, Schachat AP, Murphy RP, Patz A (eds): Retina. Medical Retina, vol. 2. St. Louis, CV Mosby, 1989, pp 149–173.
155. Hogan MJ, Alvarado JA, Weddell JE: Histology of the Human Eye. Philadelphia, WB Saunders, 1971, p 498.
156. Feeney-Burns L, Ellersieck MR: Age-related changes in ultrastructure of Bruch's membrane. Am J Ophthalmol 100:686, 1985.
157. Spencer WH: Symposium: Macular diseases. Pathogenesis: Light microscopy. Trans Am Acad Ophthalmol Otolaryngol 69:662, 1965.
158. Hogan MJ: Bruch's membrane and disease of the macula: Role of elastic tissue and collagen. Trans Ophthalmol Soc UK 87:113, 1967.
159. Hogan MJ, Alvarado J: Studies on the human macula. IV: Aging changes in Bruch's membrane. Arch Ophthalmol 77:410, 1967.
160. Sarks SH, Sarks JP: Age-related macular degeneration: Atrophic form. *In* Ryan SJ (ed): Retina, vol. 2. St. Louis, CV Mosby, 1989, p 149.
161. Sarks SH, Van Driel D, Maxwell L, Killingsworth M: Softening of drusen and subretinal neovascularization. Trans Ophthalmol Soc UK 100:414, 1980.
162. Burns RP, Reeney-Burns L: Clinico-morphologic correlations of drusen of Bruch's membrane. Trans Am Ophthalmol Soc 78:206, 1980.
163. Fine BS: Lipoidal degeneration of the retinal pigment epithelium. Am J Ophthalmol 91:469, 1981.
164. El Baba F, Green WR, Fleischmann J, et al: Clinicopathological correlation of lipidization and detachment of retinal pigment epithelium. Am J Ophthalmol 101:576, 1986.
165. Frank RN, Green WR, Pollack IP: Senile macular degeneration. Clinicopathologic correlations of a case in the predisciform stage. Am J Ophthalmol 75:587, 1973.
166. Green WR, Key SN: Senile macular degeneration: A histopathological study. Trans Am Ophthalmol Soc 75:180, 1977.
167. Green WR, MacDonnell PJ, Yeo JH: Pathologic features of senile macular degeneration. Ophthalmology 92:615, 1985.
168. Kornzweig AL: The eye in old patients. V: Diseases of the macula: A clinicopathological study. Am J Ophthalmol 60:835, 1965.
169. Verhoeff FH, Grossman HP: Pathogenesis of disciform degeneration of macula. Arch Ophthalmol 18:561, 1937.
170. Okun E: Gross and microscopic pathology in autopsy eyes. II: Perichorioretinal atrophy. Am J Ophthalmol 50:574, 1960.
171. Henkind P, Gartner S: The relationship between retinal pigment epithelium and choriocapillaris. Trans Ophthalmol Soc UK 103:444, 1983.
172. Sarks SH: New vessel formation beneath the retinal pigment epithelium in senile eyes. Br J Ophthalmol 57:951, 1973.
173. Kenyon KR, Maumenee AE, Ryan SJ, et al: Diffuse drusen and associated complications. Am J Ophthalmol 100:119, 1985.
174. Hoskin A, Bird AC, Sehmi K: Tears of detached retinal pigment epithelium. Br J Ophthalmol 65:417, 1981.
175. Green WR, Gass JDM: Senile disciform degeneration of the macula: Retinal arterialization of the fibrous plaque demonstrated clinically and histopathologically. Arch Ophthalmol 86:487, 1971.
176. Berlin R: Zur sogenannten commotio retinae. Klin Monatsbl Augenheilkd 1:42, 1873.
177. Blight R, Hart JCD: Structural changes in the outer retinal layers following blunt mechanical non-perforating trauma to the globe. Br J Ophthalmol 61:573, 1977.
178. Sipperly JO, Quigley HA, Gass JDM: Traumatic retinopathy in primates: The explanation of commotio retinae. Arch Ophthalmol 96:2267, 1978.
179. Cogan DG: Pseudoretinitis pigmentosa: Report of two traumatic cases of recent origin. Arch Ophthalmol 81:45, 1969.
180. Hart JCD, Blight R, Cooper R: Electrophysiological and pathological investigation of concussional injury. Trans Ophthalmol Soc UK 95:326, 1975.
181. Margherio RR, Schepens CL: Macular breaks: Diagnosis, etiology and observations. Am J Ophthalmol 74:219, 1972.
182. Cox MS, Schepens CL, Freeman HM: Retinal detachment due to ocular contusion. Arch Ophthalmol 76:678, 1966.
183. Goffstein R, Burton TC: Differentiating traumatic from nontraumatic retinal detachment. Ophthalmology 89:361, 1982.
184. Purtscher O: Angiopathia retinae traumatica: Lymphorrhagien des Augengrundes. Graefes Arch Clin Exp Ophthalmol 82:347, 1912.
185. Williams DF, Mieler WF, Williams GA: Posterior segment manifestations of ocular trauma. Retina 10:S35, 1990.
186. Pratt MV, De Venecia G: Purtscher's retinopathy: A clinicohistopathological correlation. Surv Ophthalmol 14:417, 1970.
187. Ashton N, Henkind P: Experimental occlusion of retinal arterioles (graded glass ballotini). Br J Ophthalmol 49:225, 1965.
188. Friendly DS: Ocular manifestations of physical child abuse. Trans Am Acad Ophthalmol Otolaryngol 75:318, 1971.
189. Ober RR: Hemorrhagic retinopathy in infancy: A clinicopathologic report. Pediatr Ophthalmol Strabismus 17:17, 1980.
190. Wyszinski RE, Grossniklaus HE, Frank KE: Indirect choroidal rupture secondary to blunt ocular trauma. Retina 8:237, 1988.
191. Aguilar LP, Green WR: Choroidal rupture: A histopathological study of 47 cases. Retina 4:269, 1984.
192. Goldberg MF: Choroidoretinal vascular anastomoses after blunt trauma to the eye. Am J Ophthalmol 82:892, 1976.
193. Cibis PA, Yamashita T, Rodriguez F: Clinical aspects of ocular siderohemosiderosis. Arch Ophthalmol 62:180, 1959.
194. Burch PG, Albert DM: Transcleral ocular siderosis. Am J Ophthalmol 84:90, 1977.
195. Tawara A: Transformation and cytotoxicity of iron in siderosis bulbi. Invest Ophthalmol Vis Sci 27:226, 1986.
196. Green WR: Pathology of the macula. *In* Spencer WH (ed): Ophthalmic Pathology: An Atlas and Textbook, vol. 2. Philadelphia, WB Saunders, 1985, pp 924–1034.
197. Yanoff M, Fine BS: Ocular Pathology: A Text and Atlas, 3rd ed. Philadelphia, JB Lippincott, 1989.
198. Rosenthal AR, Appleton H: Histochemical localization of intraocular foreign bodies. Am J Ophthalmol 79:613, 1975.
199. Rosenthal AR, Marmor MF, Leuenberger P, et al: Chalcosis: A study of natural history. Ophthalmology 86:1956, 1979.
200. Tso MOM: Photic maculopathy in rhesus monkey: A light and microscopic study. Invest Ophthalmol Vis Sci 12:17, 1973.
201. Tso MOM, Wallow IHL, Powell JO, Zimmerman LE: Recovery of the rod and cone cells after photic injury. Trans Am Acad Ophthalmol Otolaryngol 76:1247, 1972.
202. Tso MOM, La Piana FG: The human fovea after sungazing. Trans Am Acad Ophthalmol Otolaryngol 79:788, 1975.
203. Tso MOM, Woodford BJ: Effect of photic injury on the retinal tissues. Ophthalmology 90:952, 1983.
204. Weiter J: Phototoxic changes in the retina. *In* Miller D (ed): Clinical Light Damage to the Eye. New York, Springer Verlag, 1987, pp 80–125.
205. Wetterholm DH, Winter FC: Histopathology of chloroquine retinal toxicity. Arch Ophthalmol 71:82, 1964.
206. Ramsey MS, Fine BS: Chloroquine toxicity in the human eye: Histopathologic observations by electron microscopy. Am J Ophthalmol 73:229, 1972.
207. Rosenthal AR, Kolb H, Bergsma D, et al: Chloroquine retinopathy in the monkey. Invest Ophthalmol Vis Sci 17:1158, 1978.
208. Liebreich R: Ophthalmoskopischer Befund bei Morbus Brightii. Graefes Arch Clin Exp Ophthalmol 5:265, 1859.
209. Hayreh SS, Servais GE, Virdi PS: Hypertensive retinopathy. Ophthalmologica 198:173, 1989.
210. Walsh JB: Hypertensive retinopathy: Description, classification and prognosis. Ophthalmology 89:1127, 1982.
211. Tso MOM, Abrams GW, Jampol LM: Hypertensive retinopathy choroidopathy and optic neuropathy: A clinical and pathophysiological approach to classification. *In* Singerman LJ, Jampol LM (eds): Retinal and Choroidal Manifestations of Systemic Disease. Baltimore, William & Wilkins, 1991, pp 79–127.
212. Tso MOM, Jampol LM: Pathophysiology of hypertensive retinopathy. Ophthalmology 89:1132, 1982.
213. Garner A, Ashton N, Tripathi R, et al: Pathogenesis of hypertensive retinopathy: An experimental study in the monkey. Br J Ophthalmol 59:3, 1975.
214. Uyama M: Histopathological study on vascular changes especially on involvements in the choroidal vessels in hypertensive retinopathy. Acta Soc Ophthalmol Jpn 79:357, 1975.
215. Kishi S, Tso MOM, Hayreh SS: Fundus lesions in malignant hypertension: A pathologic study of experimental hypertensive choroidopathy. Arch Ophthalmol 103:1189, 1985.

216. Yanoff M: Ocular pathology of diabetes mellitus. Am J Ophthalmol 67:21, 1969.
217. Merimee TJ: Diabetic retinopathy: A syneresis of perspectives. N Engl J Med 322:978, 1990.
218. Frank RN: Etiologic mechanisms in diabetic retinopathy. *In* Ryan SJ (ed): Retina, vol. 2. St. Louis, CV Mosby, 1989, pp 301–326.
219. Frank RN: On the pathogenesis of diabetic retinopathy: A 1990 update. Ophthalmology 98:586, 1991.
220. Garner A: Pathogenesis of diabetic retinopathy. Semin Ophthalmol 2:4, 1987.
221. Yamashita T, Becker B: The basement membrane in the human diabetic. Diabetes 10:167, 1961.
222. Joyce NC, Decamilli P, Boyles J: Pericytes, like vascular smooth muscle cells, are immunohistochemically positive for cyclic GMP-dependent protein kinase. Microvasc Res 28:206, 1984.
223. Joyce NC, Haire MF, Palade GE: Contractile proteins in pericytes. Part I. J Cell Biol 100:1379, 1985.
224. Antonelli-Orlidge A, Saunders KB, Smith SR, D'Amore PA: An activated form of transforming growth factor beta is produced by cocultures of endothelial cells and pericytes. Proc Natl Acad Sci USA 86:4544, 1989.
225. de Venecia G, Davis MD, Engerman R: Clinicopathologic correlations in diabetic retinopathy. Arch Ophthalmol 94:1766, 1976.
226. Bloodworth JMB Jr, Molitor DL: Ultrastructural aspects of human and canine diabetic retinopathy. Invest Ophthalmol 4:1037, 1965.
227. Cogan DG, Toussaint D, Kuwabara T: Retinal vascular patterns. IV: Diabetic retinopathy. Arch Ophthalmol 66:366, 1961.
228. Bresnick GH, Davis MD, Myers FL, et al: Clinicopathological correlations in diabetic retinopathy. II: Clinical and histologic appearances of retinal capillary microaneurysms. Arch Ophthalmol 95:1215, 1977.
229. Bresnick GH: Background diabetic retinopathy. *In* Ryan SJ (ed): Retina, vol. 2. St. Louis, CV Mosby, 1989, pp 327–366.
230. Grimes PA, Laties AM: Early morphological alteration of the pigment epithelium in streptozotocin-induced diabetes: Increased surface area of the basal cell membrane. Exp Eye Res 30:631, 1980.
231. Fine BS, Brucker AJ: Macular edema and cystoid macular edema. Am J Ophthalmol 92:466, 1981.
232. Wolter JR: The histopathology of cystoid macular edema. Graefes Arch Clin Exp Ophthalmol 216:85, 1981.
233. Tso MOM: Pathology of cystoid macular edema. Ophthalmology 89:902, 1982.
234. Schatz H, Patz A: Cystoid maculopathy in diabetes. Arch Ophthalmol 94:761, 1976.
235. Muraoka K, Schimizu K: Intraretinal neovascularization in diabetic retinopathy. Ophthalmology 91:1440, 1984.
236. Ashton N: Studies of the retinal capillaries in relation to diabetic and other retinopathies. Br J Ophthalmol 47:521, 1963.
237. Michaelson IC: The mode of development of the retinal vessels and some observations of its significance in certain retinal diseases. Trans Ophthalmol Soc UK 68:137, 1948.
238. Michaelson IC: Retinal Circulation in Man and Animals. Springfield, IL, Charles C Thomas, 1954.
239. Patz A: Retinal neovascularization: Early contributions of Professor Michaelson and recent observations. Br J Ophthalmol 68:42, 1984.
240. Baird A, Esch F, Gospodarowicz D, Guillemin R: Retina- and eye-derived endothelial cell growth factors: Partial molecular characterization and identity with acidic and basic fibroblast growth factors. Biochemistry 24:7855, 1985.
241. Foos RY, Krieger AE, Forsythe AB, et al: Posterior vitreous detachment in diabetic subjects. Ophthalmology 87:122, 1980.
242. Baudouin C, Fredj-Reygrobellet D, Lapalus P, Gastaud P: Immunohistopathologic finding in proliferative diabetic retinopathy. Am J Ophthalmol 105:383, 1988.
243. Coats G: Ueber retinitis exudativa (retinitis haemorrhagica externa). Graefes Arch Clin Exp Ophthalmol 81:275, 1912.
244. Woods AC, Duke JR: Coats' disease. I: Review of the literature, diagnostic criteria, clinical finding and plasma lipid studies. Br J Ophthalmol 47:385, 1963.
245. Ishikawa T: Fine structure of subretinal fibrous tissue in Coats' disease. Jpn J Ophthalmol 20:63, 1976.
246. Henkind P, Morgan G: Peripheral retinal angioma with exudative retinopathy in adults (Coats' lesion). Br J Ophthalmol 50:2, 1966.
247. Hada K: Clinical and pathological study on Coats' disease. I: Clinical and histopathological observation. Acta Soc Ophthalmol Jpn 77:438, 1973.
248. Givner J: Coats' disease (retinitis exudativa): A clinicopathologic study. Am J Ophthalmol 38:852, 1954.
249. Bonnet M: Le syndrome de Coats. J Fr Ophthalmol 3:57, 1980.
250. Archer D, Krill AE: Leber's miliary aneurysms and optic atrophy. Surv Ophthalmol 15:384, 1971.
251. Devesa SS: The incidence of retinoblastoma. Am J Ophthalmol 80:263, 1975.
252. Miller RW: Fifty-two forms of childhood cancer: United States mortality experience 1960–1966. J Pediatr 75:685, 1969.
253. Albert DM: Historic review of retinoblastoma. Ophthalmology 94:654, 1987.
254. Wardrop J: Observations on the Fungus Haematodes. Edinburgh, Constable, 1809.
255. Dunphy EB: The story of retinoblastoma. Trans Am Acad Ophthalmol Otolaryngol 68:249, 1964.
256. Virchow R: Die Kranklaften Gesswuelste, vol 2. Berlin, August Hirschwald, 1864.
257. Hemmes GD: Untersuchung nach dem Vorkommen von Glioma Retinae bei Verwandted von mit dieser Krankheit Behafteten. Klin Monatsbl Augenheilkd 86:331, 1931.
258. Flexner S: A peculiar glioma (neuroepithelioma) of the retina. Bull Johns Hopkins Hosp 2:115, 1891.
259. Wintersteiner H: Die Neuroepithelioma Retinae. Eine Anatomische und Klinische Studie. Leipzig, Dentisae, 1897, p 14.
260. Tso MOM, Fine BS, Zimmerman LE: The Flexner-Wintersteiner rosette in retinoblastoma. Arch Pathol 88:664, 1969.
261. Herm RL, Heath P: A study of retinoblastoma. Am J Ophthalmol 41:22, 1956.
262. Verhoeff FH: A rare tumor arising from the pars ciliaris retinae (teratoneuroma) of a nature hitherto unrecognized and its relation to the so-called glioma retinae. Trans Am Ophthalmol Soc 10:351, 1904.
263. Verhoeff FH, Jackson E: Minutes of the proceedings: Sixty-second Annual Meeting. Trans Am Ophthalmol Soc 24:38, 1926.
264. Zimmerman LE: Retinoblastoma and retinocytoma. *In* Spencer WH (ed): Ophthalmic Pathology, vol. 2. Philadelphia, WB Saunders, 1985, p 1292.
265. Margo C, Hidayat A, Kopelman J, Zimmerman LE: Retinocytoma: A benign variant of retinoblastoma. Arch Ophthalmol 101:1519, 1983.
266. Allen RA, Latta H, Straatsma BR: Retinoblastoma. Invest Ophthalmol 1:728, 1962.
267. Macklin MT: A study of retinoblastoma in Ohio. Am J Hum Genet 12:1, 1960.
268. Mafee WF, Goldberg MF, Cohen SB, et al: Magnetic resonance imaging versus computed tomography of leukocoric eyes and use of in vitro proton magnetic resonance spectroscopy of retinoblastoma. Ophthalmology 96:965, 1989.
269. Zimmerman LE: Application of histochemical methods for the demonstration of acid mucopolysaccharides to ophthalmic pathology. Trans Am Acad Ophthalomol Otolaryngol 62:697, 1958.
270. Wright JH: Neurocytoma or neuroblastoma: A kind of tumor not generally recognized. J Exp Med 12:556, 1910.
271. Tso MOM, Zimmerman LE, Fine BS: The nature of retinoblastoma. I: Photoreceptor differentiation: A clinical and histopathologic study. Am J Ophthalmol 89:339, 1970.
272. Tso MOM, Zimmerman LE, Fine BS, Ellsworth RM: A cause of radioresistance in retinoblastoma: Photoreceptor differentiation. Trans Am Acad Ophthalmol Otolaryngol 74:959, 1970.
273. Eagle RC, Shields JA, Donoso L, Milner R: Malignant transformation of spontaneously regressed retinoblastoma, retinoma/retinocytoma variant. Ophthalmology 96:1389, 1989.
274. Wolter JR: Retinoblastoma extension into the choroid: Pathological study of the neoplastic process and thoughts about its prognostic significance. Ophthalmic Paediatr Genet 8:151, 1987.
275. Albert DM, Sang DN, Craft JL: Clinical and histopathologic

observations regarding cell death and tumor necrosis in retinoblastoma. Jpn J Ophthalmol 22:358, 1978.
276. Kremer I, Hartmann B, Haviv D, et al: Immunohistochemical diagnosis of a totally necrotic retinoblastoma: A clinicopathological case. J Pediatr Ophthalmol Strabismus 25:90, 1988.
277. Verhoeff FH: Retinoblastoma undergoing spontaneous regression: Calcifying agent suggested in treatment of retinoblastoma. Am J Ophthalmol 62:573, 1966.
278. Mullaney J: DNA in retinoblastoma. Lancet 2:918, 1968.
279. Char DH: Clinical Ocular Oncology. New York, Churchill Livingstone, 1989.
280. Shields JA: Diagnosis and Management of Intraocular Tumors. St. Louis, CV Mosby, 1983.
281. Bierring F, Egeberg J, Jensen OA: A contribution to the ultrastructural study of retinoblastoma. Acta Ophthalmol 45:424, 1967.
282. François J, Hanssens M, Lagasse A: The ultrastructure of retinoblastomata. Ophthalmologica 149:53, 1965.
283. Ikui H, Tominaya Y, Konomi I, Ueono K: Electron microscopic studies on the histogenesis of retinoblastoma. Jpn J Ophthalmol 10:282, 1966.
284. Matsuo N, Takayama T: Electron microscopic observations of visual cells in a case of retinoblastoma. Folia Ophthalmol Jpn 16:574, 1965.
285. Tokunaya T, Nakamura S: Electron microscopic features of retinoblastoma. Acta Soc Ophthalmol Jpn 67:1358, 1963.
286. Tso MOM, Zimmerman LE, Fine BS: The nature of retinoblastoma. II: Photoreceptor differentiation: An electron microscopic study. Am J Ophthalmol 89:350, 1970.
287. Popoff N, Ellsworth RM: The fine structure of retinoblastoma: In vivo and in vitro observations. Lab Invest 25:389, 1971.
288. Popoff N, Ellsworth RM: The fine structure of nuclear alterations in retinoblastoma and the developing human retina: In vivo and in vitro observations. J Ultrastruct Res 29:535, 1969.
289. Albert DM, Sang DN, Craft JL: Ultrastructure of retinoblastoma: Transmission and scanning electron microscopy. *In* Jakobiec FA (ed): Ocular and Adnexal Tumors. Birmingham, Aesculapius, 1978, p 157.
290. Fine BS: Observations on the axoplasm of neural elements in the human retina. Proceedings of the Third European Regional Conference on Electron Microscopy, vol. B. Prague, Publishing House of Czechoslovak Academy of Science, 1964, p 319.
291. Sheffield JB: Microtubules in the outer layer of rabbit retina. J Microsc 5:173, 1966.
292. Howard MA, Dryja TP, Walton DS, Albert DM: Identification and significance of multinucleate cells in retinoblastoma. Arch Ophthalmol 107:1025, 1989.
293. Craft JL, Robinson NL, Roth NA, Albert DM: Scanning electron microscopy of retinoblastoma. Exp Eye Res 27:519, 1978.
294. Bonnin JM, Rubenstein LJ: Immunohistochemistry of central nervous system tumors: Its contributions to neurosurgical diagnosis. J Neurosurg 60:1121, 1984.
295. Donoso LA, Shields CA, Lee E: Immunohistochemistry of retinoblastoma. Ophthalmic Paediatr Genet 10:3, 1989.
296. Molnar ML, Stefansson K, Marton LS, et al: Immunohistochemistry of retinoblastoma in humans. Am J Ophthalmol 97:301, 1984.
297. Sasaki A, Ogawa A, Nakazato Y, Ishido Y: Distribution of neurofilament protein and neuron-specific enolase in peripheral neuronal tumors. Virchows Arch [A] 407:33, 1985.
298. Campbell M, Chader G: Retinoblastoma cells in tissue culture. Ophthalmic Paediatr Genet 9:171, 1988.
299. Garrido CM, Arra A: Studies of ocular retinoblastoma with immunoperoxidase technique. Ophthalmologica 193:242, 1986.
300. Kivela T: Antigenic Properties of Retinoblastoma Tissue. Helsinki, University of Helsinki, 1987.
301. Kivela T, Tarkkanen A: S-100 protein in retinoblastoma revisited. Acta Ophthalmol 64:664, 1986.
302. Roberts DF, Duggan-Keen M, Aherne GES, Long DR: Immunogenetic studies in retinoblastoma. Br J Ophthalmol 70:686, 1986.
303. Abramson DH, Greenfield DS, Ellsworth RM, et al: Neuron-specific enolase and retinoblastoma: Clinicopathologic correlations. Retina 9:148, 1989.
304. Kivela T: Neuron-specific enolase in retinoblastoma: An immunohistochemical study. Acta Ophthalmol 64:19, 1986.
305. Kobayashi M, Sawada T, Mukai N: Immunohistochemical evidence of neuron specific enolase (NSE) in human adenovirus-12 induced retinoblastoma-like tumor cells in vitro. Acta Histochem Cytochem 18:551, 1985.
306. Virtanen I, Kivela T, Bugnoli M, et al: Expression of intermediate filaments and synaptophysin show neuronal properties and lack of glial characteristics in Y79 retinoblastoma cells. Lab Invest 59:649, 1988.
307. Felberg NT, Donoso LA: Surface cytoplasmic antigens in retinoblastoma. Invest Ophthalmol Vis Sci 19:1242, 1980.
308. Vrabec T, Arbizo V, Adamus G, et al: Rod cell-specific antigens in retinoblastoma. Arch Ophthalmol 107:1061, 1989.
309. Donoso LA, Hamm H, Dietzschold B, et al: Rhodopsin and retinoblastoma. Arch Ophthalmol 104:111, 1986.
310. Donoso LA, Rorke LB, Shields JA, et al: S-Antigen immunoreactivity in trilateral retinoblastoma. Am J Ophthalmol 103:57, 1987.
311. Bogenmann E: Retinoblastoma cell differentiation in culture. Int J Cancer 38:833, 1986.
312. Bogenmann E, Lochrie MA, Simon MI: Cone cell specific genes expressed in retinoblastoma. Science 240:76, 1988.
313. Rodrigues MM, Wiggert B, Shields J, et al: Retinoblastoma: Immunohistochemistry and cell differentiation. Ophthalmology 94:378, 1987.
314. Rodriguez MM, Wilson ME, Wiggert B, et al: Retinoblastoma: A clinical, immunohistochemical, and electron microscopic case report. Ophthalmology 93:1010, 1988.
315. He W, Hashimoto H, Tsuneyoshi M, et al: A reassessment of histologic classification and an immunohistochemical study of 88 retinal blastomas. Cancer 70:2901, 1992.
316. Bridges CDB, Fong SL, Landers RA, et al: Interstitial retinal binding protein (IRBP) in retinoblastoma. Neurochem Int 7:875, 1985.
317. Fong SL, Balakier H, Canton M, et al: Retinoid-binding proteins in retinoblastoma tumors. Cancer Res 48:1124, 1988.
318. Tarlton JF, Easty DL: Immunohistological characterisation of retinoblastoma and related ocular tissue. Br J Ophthalmol 74:144, 1990.
319. Herman MM, Perentes E, Katsetos CD, et al: Neuroblastic differentiation potential of the human retinoblastoma cell lines Y-79 and WERI-Rb1 maintained in an organ culture system. Am J Pathol 134:115, 1989.
320. Kyritsis AP, Tsokos M, Triche TJ, Chader GJ: Retinoblastoma: Origin from a primitive neuroectodermal cell? Nature 307:471, 1984.
321. Lemieux N, Leung T, Michaud J, et al: Neuronal and photoreceptor differentiation of retinoblastoma in culture. Ophthalmic Paediatr Genet 11:109, 1990.
322. Boniuk M, Girard LJ: Spontaneous regression of bilateral retinoblastoma. Trans Am Acad Ophthalmol Otolaryngol 73:194, 1969.
323. Boniuk M, Zimmerman LE: Spontaneous regression of retinoblastoma. Int Ophthalmol Clin 2(2):525, 1962.
324. Karsgaard AT: Spontaneous regression of retinoblastoma: A report of 2 cases. Can J Ophthalmol 6:218, 1971.
325. Lindley-Smith JS: Histology and spontaneous regression of retinoblastoma. Trans Ophthalmol Soc UK 94:953, 1974.
326. Morris WE, LaPiana FG: Spontaneous regression of bilateral retinoblastoma with preservation of normal visual acuity. Am J Ophthalmol 6:1192, 1974.
327. Nehen JH: Spontaneous regression of retinoblastoma. Acta Ophthalmol 53:647, 1975.
328. Reese AB: Tumors of the Eye, 3rd ed. New York, Harper & Row, 1976, p 89.
329. Stewart JK, Smith JLS, Arnold EL: Spontaneous regression of retinoblastoma. Br J Ophthalmol 40:449, 1956.
330. Sang DN, Albert DM: Recent advances in the study of retinoblastoma. *In* Peyman GA, Apple DJ, Sanders DR (eds): Intraocular Tumors. New York, Appleton-Century-Crofts, 1977, p 285.
331. Cohen SM, Saulenas AM, Sullivan CR, Albert DM: Further studies of the effect of vitamin D on retinoblastoma: Inhibition with 1,25 dihydroxycholecalciferol. Arch Ophthalmol 106:541, 1988.
332. Marcus DM, Craft JL, Albert DM: Histopathologic verification of Verhoeff's 1918 irradiation cure of retinoblastoma. Ophthalmology 97:221, 1990.

333. Hogan MJ, Zimmerman LE: Ophthalmic Pathology: An Atlas and Textbook, vol. 2. Philadelphia, WB Saunders, 1962, p 433.
334. Yanoff M, Fine BS: Ocular Pathology: A Text and Atlas, 3rd ed. Philadelphia, JB Lippincott, 1989.
335. Haik BG, Dunleavy SA, Cooke C, et al: Retinoblastoma with anterior chamber extension. Ophthalmology 94:367, 1987.
336. Magramm I, Abramson DH, Ellsworth RM: Optic nerve involvement in retinoblastoma. Ophthalmology 96:217, 1989.
337. Stevenson KE, Hungerford J, Garner A: Local extraocular extension of retinoblastoma following intraocular surgery. Br J Ophthalmol 73:739, 1989.
338. Carbajal UM: Metastasis in retinoblastoma. Am J Ophthalmol 48:47, 1959.
339. Albert DM, Lahav M, Lesser RL, Craft JL: Recent observations regarding retinoblastoma. I: Ultrastructure, tissue culture growth, incidence and animal models. Trans Ophthalmol Soc UK 94:909, 1974.
340. Merriam GR: Retinoblastoma: Analysis of 17 autopsies. Arch Ophthalmol 44:71, 1950.
341. Jafek BW, Lindford R, Foos RY: Late recurrent retinoblastoma in the nasal vestibule. Arch Otolaryngol 94:264, 1971.
342. Yttebsorg J, and Arnesen K: Late recurrence of retinoblastoma. Acta Ophthalmol 50:367, 1972.
343. Howard GM, Ellsworth RM: Differential diagnosis of retinoblastoma: A statistical survey of 500 children. II: Factors relating to the diagnosis of retinoblastoma. Am J Ophthalmol 60:618, 1965.
344. Kincaid MC, Green WR: Ocular and orbital involvement in leukemia. Surv Ophthalmol 27:211, 1983.
345. Duke-Elder S: System of Ophthalmology: Diseases of the Uveal Tract, vol. 9. London, Henry Kimpton, 1966, p 775.
346. McCartney ACE, Olver JM, Kingston JE, Hungerford JL: Forty years of retinoblastoma: Into the fifth age. Eye 2(Suppl):S13, 1988.
347. Allen RA, Straatsma BR: Ocular involvement in leukemia and allied disorders. Arch Ophthalmol 66:490, 1961.
348. Guyer DR, Schachat AP, Vitale S, et al: Leukemic retinopathy: Relationship between fundus lesions and hematologic parameters at diagnosis. Ophthalmology 96:860, 1988.
349. Kuwabara T, Aiello L: Leukemic ciliary nodules in the retina. Arch Ophthalmol 72:494, 1964.
350. Robb RM, Ervin LD, Sallen SE: A pathological study of eye involvement in acute leukemia of childhood. Trans Am Ophthalmol Soc 76:90, 1978.
351. Kincaid MC, Green WR, Kelley JS: Acute ocular leukemia. Am J Ophthalmol 87:698, 1979.
352. Leonardy NJ, Rupani M, Dent G, Klintworth GK: Analysis of 135 autopsy eyes for ocular involvement in leukemia. Am J Ophthalmol 109:436, 1990.
353. Burns CA, Blodi FC, Williamson BK: Acute lymphocytic leukemia and central serous retinopathy. Trans Am Acad Ophthalmol Otolaryngol 69:307, 1965.
354. Clayman HM, Flynn JT, Koch K, Israel C: Retinal pigment epithelial abnormalities in leukemic disease. Am J Ophthalmol 74:416, 1972.
355. Gass JDM: Differential Diagnosis of Intraocular Tumors. St. Louis, CV Mosby, 1977.
356. Jakobiec FA, Behrens M: Leukemic retinal pigment epitheliopathy with report of a unilateral case. J Pediatr Ophthalmol Strabismus 12:10, 1975.
357. Gartner J: Mycosis fungoides mit Beteiligung der Aderhaut. Klin Monatsbl Augenheilkd 131:61, 1957.
358. Karp LA, Zimmerman LE, Payne T: Intraocular involvement in Burkitt's lymphoma. Arch Ophthalmol 85:295, 1971.
359. Keltner JL, Fritsch E, Cykiert RC, Albert DM: Mycosis fungoides, intraocular and central nervous system involvement. Arch Ophthalmol 95:645, 1977.
360. Nelson CC, Hertzberg BS, Klintworth GK: Histopathologic study of 716 unselected eyes in patients with cancer at the time of death. Am J Ophthalmol 95:788, 1983.
361. Schachat AP: Leukemias and lymphomas. *In* Ryan SJ (ed): Retina, vol. 1. St. Louis, CV Mosby, 1989, p 775.
362. Fisher D, Mantell BS, Urich H: The clinical diagnosis and treatment of microgliomatosis: Report of a case. J Neurol Psychiatry 81:591, 1969.
363. Fisher ER, Davis ER, Lemmen LJ: Reticulum cell sarcoma of the brain (microglioma). Arch Neurol Psychiatry 81:591, 1959.
364. Mann RB, Jaffee ES, Berard CW: Malignant lymphoma: A conceptual understanding of morphologic diversity. Am J Pathol 94:105, 1979.
365. Russell DS, Rubenstein LJ: Pathology of the Nervous System, 4th ed, vol. 1. Baltimore, Williams & Wilkins, 1977, p 299.
366. Schaumburg HH, Plank CR, Adams RD: The reticulum cell sarcoma microglia group of brain tumors: A consideration of their clinical features and therapy. Brain 95:199, 1972.
367. Portlock CS: The non-Hodgkin's lymphomas. *In* Wyngaarden JB, Mith LH (eds): Cecil's Textbook of Medicine. Philadelphia, WB Saunders, 1988.
368. Barr C, Green WR, Payne JE, et al: Intraocular reticulum cell sarcoma: Clinicopathologic study of four cases and review of the literature. Surv Ophthalmol 19:224, 1975.
369. Cooper EL, Riker JL: Malignant lymphoma of the uveal tract. Am J Ophthalmol 34:1153, 1951.
370. Currey TA, Deutsch AR: Reticulum cell sarcoma of the uvea. South Med J 58:919, 1965.
371. Freeman LN, Schachat AP, Knox DL, et al: Clinical features, laboratory investigation, and survival in ocular reticulum cell sarcoma. Ophthalmology 94:1631, 1987.
372. Givner I: Malignant lymphoma with ocular involvement. Am J Ophthalmol 239:29, 1955.
373. Green WR. The retina. *In* Spencer WH (ed): Ophthalmic Pathology: An Atlas and Textbook, 3rd ed, vol. 2. Philadelphia, WB Saunders, 1986.
374. Klingele TC, Hogan MJ: Ocular reticulum cell sarcoma. Am J Ophthalmol 79:39, 1975.
375. Michels RG, Knox DL, Erozan YS, Green WR: Intraocular reticulum cell sarcoma: Diagnosis by pars plana vitrectomy. Arch Ophthalmol 93:1331, 1975.
376. Mincker DS, Font RL, Zimmerman LE: Uveitis and reticulum cell sarcoma of the brain with bilateral neoplastic seeding of vitreous without retinal or uveal involvement. Am J Ophthalmol 80:433, 1975.
377. Nevins RC Jr, Frey WW, Elliott JH: Primary solitary intraocular reticulum cell sarcoma (microgliomatosis): A clinicopathologic case report. Trans Am Acad Ophthalmol Otolaryngol 72:867, 1968.
378. O'Connor GR: The uvea. Arch Ophthalmol 89:505, 1973.
379. Babel J, Owens G: Sarcome réticulaire intra-oculaire et cérébral. Arch Ophtalmol (Paris) 35:409, 1975.
380. Sullivan SF, Dallow RL: Intraocular reticulum cell sarcoma: Its dramatic response to systemic chemotherapy and its angiogenic potential. Ann Ophthalmol 9:401, 1977.
381. Vogel MH, Font RL, Zimmerman LE, Levine RA: Reticulum cell sarcoma of the retina and uvea: Report of six cases and review of the literature. Am J Ophthalmol 66:205, 1968.
382. Cravioto H: Human and experimental reticulum cell sarcoma (microglia of the nervous system). Acta Neuropathol 4(Suppl):135, 1975.
383. Polack M: Microglioma and/or reticulosarcoma of the nervous system. Acta Neuropathol (Berl) 6(Suppl):115, 1975.
384. Corriveau C, Esterbrook M, Payne D: Lymphoma simulating uveitis (masquerade syndrome). Can J Ophthalmol 21:144, 1986.
385. Kaplan HJ, Meredith TA, Aaberg TM, Keller RH: Reclassification of intraocular reticulum cell sarcoma (histiocytic lymphoma): Immunologic characterization of vitreous cells. Arch Ophthalmol 98:707, 1980.
386. Horvat B, Pena C, Fisher ER: Primary reticulum cell sarcoma (microgliosis) of the brain. Arch Pathol 87:609, 1969.
387. BenEzra D, Sahel JA, Harris NL, et al: Uveal lymphoid infiltrates: Immunohistochemical evidence for a lymphoid neoplasia. Br J Ophthalmol 73:846, 1989.
388. Jakobiec FA, Sacks E, Kronish JW, et al: Multifocal static creamy choroidal infiltrates: An early sign of lymphoid neoplasia. Ophthalmology 94:397, 1987.
389. Leys AM, VanEyck LM, Nuttin BJ, et al: Metastatic carcinoma to the retina: Clinicopathologic findings in two cases. Arch Ophthalmol 108:1448, 1990.
390. Fishman ML, Tomaszewski MM, Kuwabara T: Malignant melanoma of the skin metastatic to the eye: Frequency in autopsy series. Arch Ophthalmol 94:1309, 1976.

391. Char DH, Schwartz A, Miller TR, Abels JS: Ocular metastases from systemic melanoma. Am J Ophthalmol 90:702, 1980.
392. Engel HM, Green WR, Michels RG, et al: Diagnostic vitrectomy. Retina 1:121, 1981.
393. Robertson DM, Wilkinson CP, Murray JL, Gordy DD: Metastatic tumor to the retina and vitreous cavity from primary melanoma of the skin: Treatment with systemic and subconjunctival chemotherapy. Ophthalmology 88:1296, 1981.
394. Adamuk V: Ein fall von metastatischem melanosarcom der uvea. Z Augenheilkd 21:505, 1909.
395. Albert DM, Lahav M, Troczynski E, Bahr R: Black hypopion: Report of two cases. Graefes Arch Clin Exp Ophthalmol 193:81, 1975.
396. Albert DM, Rubenstein RA, Scheie HG: Tumor metastasis to the eye. I: Incidence in 213 adult patients with generalized malignancy. Am J Ophthalmol 63:723, 1967.
397. Albert DM, Zimmerman AW Jr, Zeidman I: Tumor metastasis to the eye. II: Fate of circulating tumor cells to the eye. Am J Ophthalmol 67:733, 1963.
398. Boente R: Metastatische Melanoblastome in der Retina. Klin Monatsbl Augenheilkd 82:732, 1929.
399. DasGubta T, Brasfield R: Metastatic melanoma. Cancer 17:1323, 1964.
400. DeBustros S, Augsburger JJ, Shields JA, et al: Intraocular metastases from cutaneous malignant melanoma. Arch Ophthalmol 103:937, 1985.
401. Font RL, Naumann G, Zimmerman LE: Primary malignant melanoma of the skin metastatic to the eye and orbit. Am J Ophthalmol 63:738, 1967.
402. Letson AD, Davidorf FH: Bilateral retinal metastases from cutaneous malignant melanoma. Arch Ophthalmol 100:605, 1982.
403. Liddicoat JA, Wolter JR, Wilkinson WC: Retinal metastasis of malignant melanoblastoma: A case report. Am J Ophthalmol 48:177, 1959.
404. Osterhuis JA, DeKeiser RJN, De Wolff-Rovendaal D: Ocular and orbital metastases of cutaneous melanoma. Int Ophthalmol 10:175, 1987.
405. Riffenburgh RS: Metastatic malignant melanoma to the retina. Arch Ophthalmol 66:487, 1961.
406. Schachat AP: Tumor involvement of the vitreous cavity. *In* Ryan SJ (ed): Retina, vol. 1. St. Louis, CV Mosby, 1989, p 805.
407. TerDoesschatte G: Über metastatische Sarkom der Auges. Klin Monatsbl Augenheilkd 66:766, 1921.
408. Uhler EM: Metastatic malignant melanoma of the retina. Am J Ophthalmol 23:158, 1940.
409. Wagenmann D: Ein fall von multipler melanosarkomen mit eigenartigen komplikationen beider augen. Dtsch Med Wochenschr 25:262, 1900.
410. Young SE: Retinal metastases. *In* Ryan SJ (ed): Retina, vol. 1. St. Louis, CV Mosby, 1989, p 591.
411. Eide N, Syrdalen P: Intraocular metastasis from cutaneous malignant melanoma. Acta Ophthalmol 68:102, 1990.
412. Piro P, Pappos HR, Erozan YS: Diagnostic vitrectomy in metastatic breast carcinoma in the vitreous. Retina 2:182, 1982.
413. Sahel JA: Vitreous metastasis from cutaneous melanoma. European Ophthalmic Pathology Society/Verhoeff Society Meeting, Nuremberg, May, 1991.

Chapter 185

Pathology of Glaucoma

MARIA A. SAORNIL and R. RAND ALLINGHAM

TISSUE EFFECTS OF ELEVATED INTRAOCULAR PRESSURE

Glaucoma, an ocular condition characterized by increased intraocular pressure, causes ocular damage leading to visual loss. Although the pressure increase can damage several ocular structures, the most important and irreversible damage occurs to the retinal cell axons in the optic disc at the level of the lamina cribrosa.[1–3]

The optic disc slowly becomes pale and excavated owing to loss of nerve fibers (Fig. 185–1). The superior and inferior portions of the lamina cribrosa become posteriorly displaced and ectatic and compress the ganglion cell axons. The disc cupping enlarges vertically more than horizontally in the early stages,[4] followed by degeneration of the temporal disc and its nasal portions. These findings correlate with the sequence of defects that appear in the visual field.

Acquired, pitlike changes with posterior displacement and focal atrophy of neuronal elements have been observed at the inferior portions of the optic nerve head.[5, 6] The changes seem to correlate with visual field loss,[5] appear more often in low-tension glaucoma,[6–8] and may signal abnormal optic nerve susceptibility to the damaging effects of intraocular pressure.[8] Optic nerve head capillaries disappear as nerve fibers disappear, maintaining the usual capillary-to-tissue ratio.[3, 5] Studies of the optic nerve head in human eyes with known glaucoma have shown blockage of axonal transport at the level of the lamina cribrosa.[2, 9, 10]

Schnabel's cavernous degeneration, an uncommon finding, is seen in the retrobulbar portion of the optic nerve and consists of large cystoid or cavernous spaces containing hyaluronic acid.[11] The degeneration is related to acute pressure increases; its pathogenesis may be related to ischemic changes.[12] Recently, changes in the composition of the extracellular matrix of the lamina cribrosa in areas adjacent to the glaucomatous cups have been reported as the possible cause of the disease.[13]

Retinal changes in glaucomatous eyes show nerve fiber and ganglion cell layer degeneration, usually with secondary gliosis (Fig. 185–2).

In long-standing glaucoma, numerous ocular structures may undergo alteration secondary to increased intraocular pressure.[1] The trabecular meshwork shows sclerosis and fibrosis, and Schlemm's canal may be obliterated in the late stages. The cornea may undergo endothelial decompensation with the appearance of

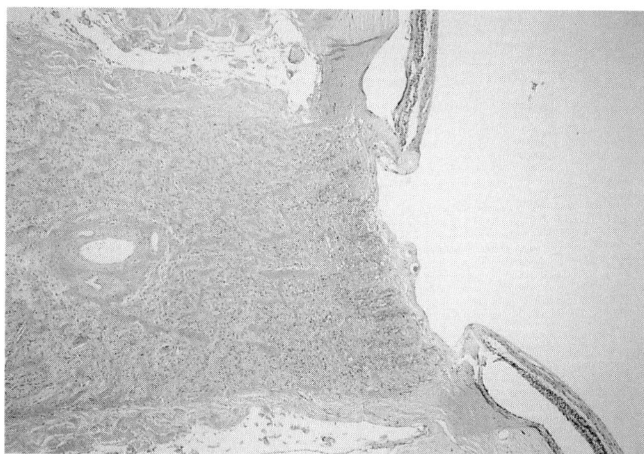

Figure 185–1. Glaucomatous cupping of the optic disc. Loss of prelaminar substance with posterior displacement of the lamina cribrosa. H&E, ×7.88.

chronic edema and its secondary changes: bullous keratopathy, band keratopathy, degenerative pannus, and corneal scarring. The iris stroma becomes atrophic and fibrotic and may show degeneration of the pupillary margin. Atrophy, fibrosis, and hyalinization of the ciliary processes can occur with decreasing stromal cellularity and vascularity. Choroidal atrophy is found in the peripapillary area, in which changes in the retinal pigment epithelium also occur. Scleral staphylomas may develop in young people secondary to long-term elevated intraocular pressure.

OPEN-ANGLE GLAUCOMA

Primary Open-Angle Glaucoma

This is a chronic, slowly progressive, usually bilateral disease with increased resistance to aqueous outflow that results in increased intraocular pressure sufficient to injure the retinal cell axons. The histopathologic findings are controversial. Most of the findings are similar to aging changes, with the exception that they are more severe and appear earlier in glaucomatous eyes.[14–17] Most morphologic findings in primary open-angle glaucoma come from trabeculectomy specimens representing the later stages of the disease. Early changes caused by the disease are not well characterized.

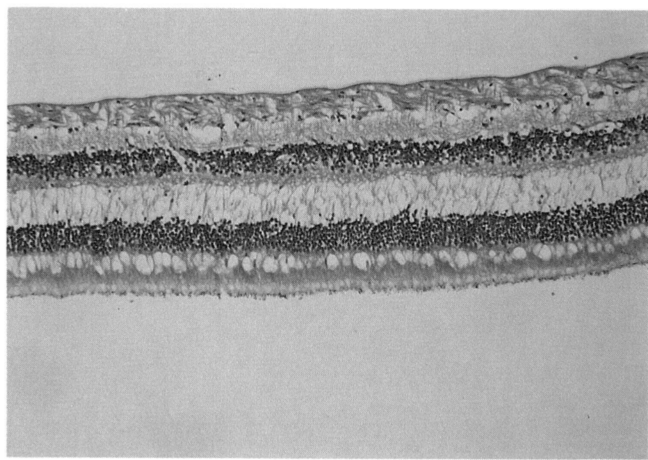

Figure 185–2. Glaucomatous changes in the retina. Attenuation of the nerve fiber layer and ganglion cell layer degeneration with secondary gliosis. H&E, ×31.

Rohen and Witmer[18] first described electron microscopy findings of band-shaped plaques of extracellular material deposited within the cribriform layer of the trabecular meshwork as well as immediately underneath the endothelial lining of Schlemm's canal. Electron-dense plaques have also been observed in the outer wall of Schlemm's canal.[15, 19–22] The relationship of these findings to glaucoma is unclear.[23] Most plaque material originates in the sheath of the elastic-like fiber net beneath the endothelial lining of Schlemm's canal. Cytochemical studies show a number of additional fine fibrils attached to the elastic fiber net.[19, 24] The fibrils are embedded in proteoglycans and seem to be part of the elastic fiber sheath, possibly providing a base for the deposition of additional plaque material.

In the cribriform layer and juxtacanalicular tissue, "matrix vesicles" have been found, indicating cellular degeneration. Some vesicles are lysosomal and contain highly active enzymes that might severely damage the extracellular material of this region.[25]

Alvarado and associates[16] found a greater loss of trabecular cells in primary open-angle glaucoma, a finding later confirmed by other investigators.[26] In some areas, the endothelial lining is absent, and the aqueous humor is in direct contact with the basement membrane.[17] In these areas, an increase of lattice collagen and thickening of the basement membranes with lattice collagen inclusions may occur. Denuded trabecular beams can fuse, obliterating the intertrabecular spaces. Trabecular meshwork cells increase in size and spread to cover the denuded areas. Enlargement of the trabecular cells and thickening and fusion of the lamellae can result in complete obstruction of the uveal and corneoscleral aqueous pathways.[27, 28]

Advanced cases of primary open-angle glaucoma show extreme hyalinization, sclerosis, compaction of the trabecular meshwork, and even obliteration of Schlemm's canal.[1, 17]

Secondary Open-Angle Glaucoma

Secondary open-angle glaucoma, characterized by elevated intraocular pressure in the presence of a well-formed anterior chamber without peripheral anterior synechiae, is caused by blockage of the aqueous outflow by cells and particulate matter in the trabecular meshwork or by membrane formation across the angle. Some cases are transient, but in those that are long-standing, reactive scarring in the trabecular meshwork may maintain the blockage.

Inflammation. Iris and ciliary body inflammation may lead to deposits of proteinaceous exudates, inflammatory products, and cells in the trabecular meshwork that obstruct the aqueous humor passage (Fig. 185–3). In

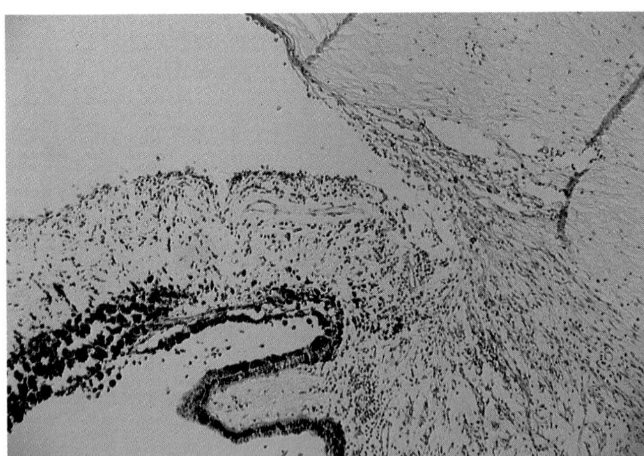

Figure 185–3. Chronic inflammatory infiltrate in iris and ciliary body in an eye with chronic iridocyclitis caused by herpes zoster. Inflammatory cells and pigment granules in the trabecular meshwork. H&E, ×12.

chronic or recurrent uveitis (i.e., Fuchs' heterochromic iridocyclitis) and glaucomatocyclitic crisis (Posner-Schlossman syndrome), reactive scarring can permanently obliterate the intertrabecular spaces or form peripheral anterior synechiae leading to angle-closure.[1, 17, 29–34]

Blood. The presence of blood may produce open-angle glaucoma in several ways. Red blood cells from hemorrhage or macrophages containing degenerated blood cell products (hemolytic glaucoma) may obstruct aqueous outflow (Fig. 185–4).[35] Rigid, degenerating blood cells (ghost cells or erythroclasts) that usually appear after vitreous hemorrhage can migrate to the anterior chamber, obstructing the trabecular spaces more easily than fresh blood owing to their decreased elasticity (ghost cell glaucoma) (Fig. 185–5).[36–39]

Lens. A hypermature cataract may release degenerated cortical material into the anterior chamber, obstructing the trabecular meshwork. This material provokes a phagocytic response, and macrophages, laden with degenerated lens material, can block the angle structures (phacolytic glaucoma).[40, 41] Soluble lens proteins from the hypermature lens have also been demonstrated to cause severe obstruction of aqueous outflow (Fig. 185–6).[41, 42] This cortical material may also be seen on the iris surface and over the posterior retina and optic disc.

Following cataract surgery, lens injury, or neodymium-yttrium-aluminum garnet (Nd.YAG) laser posterior capsulotomy, liberated lens particles and debris may obstruct the trabecular outflow and cause an increase of intraocular pressure.[41, 42] Lens proteins are usually immunologically isolated within the lens capsule. Rupture after extracapsular cataract extraction or trauma may allow sensitization and development of a granulomatous inflammatory reaction composed of mononuclear cells, epithelioid cells, and giant cells, surrounding the damaged area (phacoanaphylactic glaucoma) (Fig. 185–7). Glaucoma may occur as a result of several mechanisms (e.g., lens material in trabecular meshwork, inflammatory reaction).[43, 44]

Pigment. Pigment is often observed in the trabecular meshwork of eyes with normal intraocular pressure. The amount of pigment increases with age or after trauma or inflammation. The pigment granules are located between the trabecular beams, adhering to the trabeculas or within the cytoplasm of the trabecular cells after phagocytosis, and can lead to obstruction to the aqueous outflow (Fig. 185–8).[45]

Pigment-laden macrophages can cause increased intraocular pressure by the same mechanism as in phacolytic or hemolytic glaucoma. Melanomalytic glaucoma can occur secondary to the phagocytosis of melanin derived from necrotic tumor cells of a uveal melanoma by macrophages, which may ultimately obstruct aqueous outflow.[46, 47] A similar response has been observed after severe contusion, or associated with any ocular circumstance with release of pigment.

Pigment-dispersion syndrome is characterized by dispersion of melanin granules into the aqueous humor. Pigment is released from the posterior pigmented iris

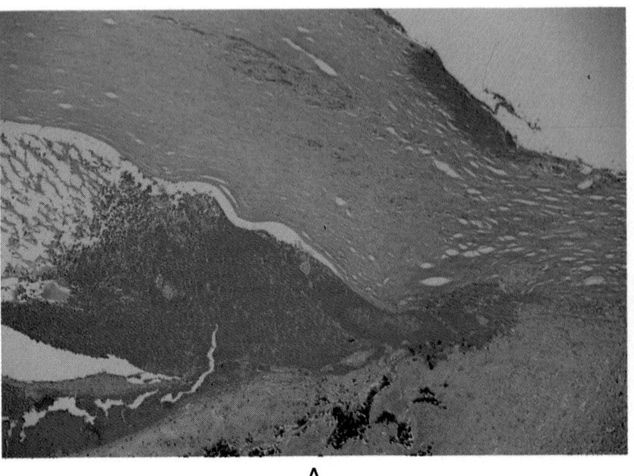

A

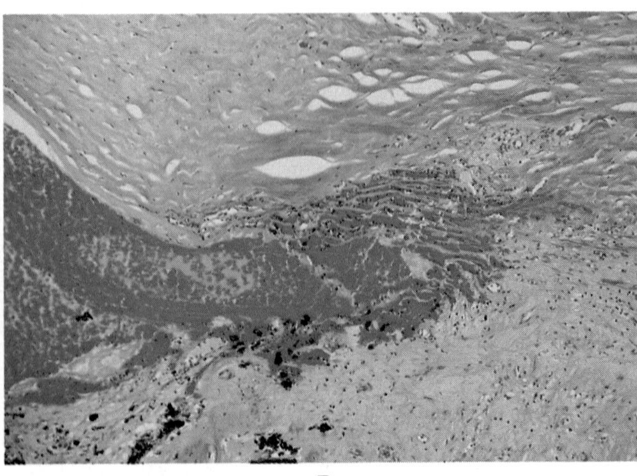

B

Figure 185–4. *A,* Hemorrhage and fibrin in the anterior chamber after hyphema. H&E, ×5. *B,* Red blood cells and degenerated blood cell products filling the trabecular spaces. H&E, ×12.

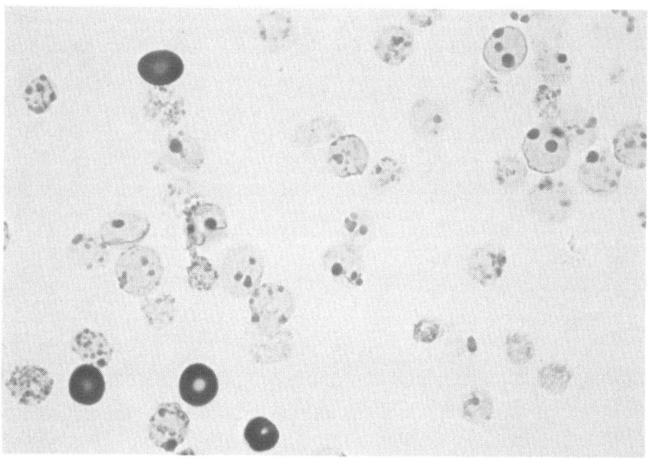

Figure 185–5. Ghost cells. Degenerating blood cells with intact cellular membrane and Heinz bodies. H&E, ×314.

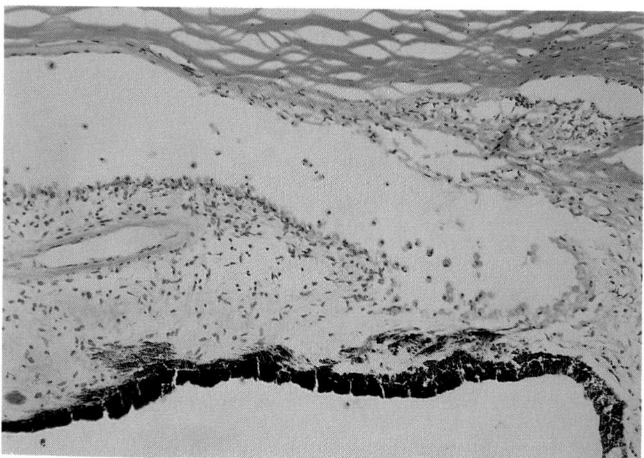

Figure 185–6. Phacolytic glaucoma. Disrupted lens material and macrophages on the iris surface and in angle structures. H&E, ×12.

epithelium presumably owing to contact with lens zonules. When the pigment granules reach the trabecular meshwork, they can be phagocytized by the trabecular endothelium or become trapped within the meshwork. When associated with open-angle glaucoma, it is called pigmentary glaucoma.[48–50]

Electron microscopic studies heve revealed degeneration of endothelial cells of the trabecular meshwork, trapping of cell debris, or breakdown products of pigment-containing cells.[51]

Pseudoexfoliation. This syndrome is characterized by deposits of white, fluffy material over the anterior chamber structures, including the trabecular meshwork (Fig. 185–9). It is often associated with open-angle glaucoma (pseudoexfoliation glaucoma) and pigment dispersion. The associated glaucoma seems to be a form of secondary open-angle glaucoma caused by pseudoexfoliative material. Histologically, the angle is open, and the trabecular meshwork contains pigment granules and accumulations of pseudoexfoliative material that are not phagocytized by the trabecular endothelium and depos-

A

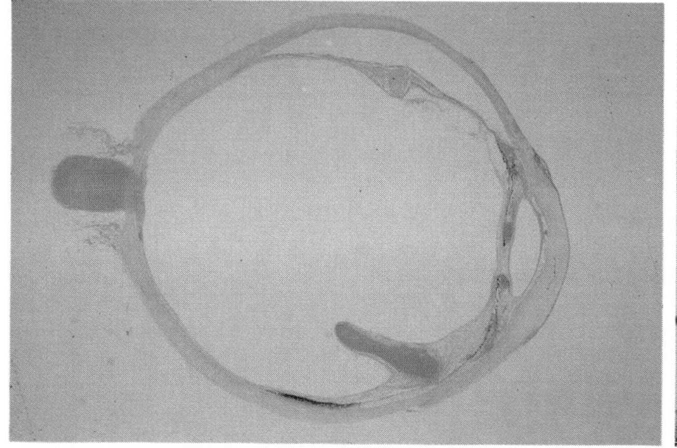

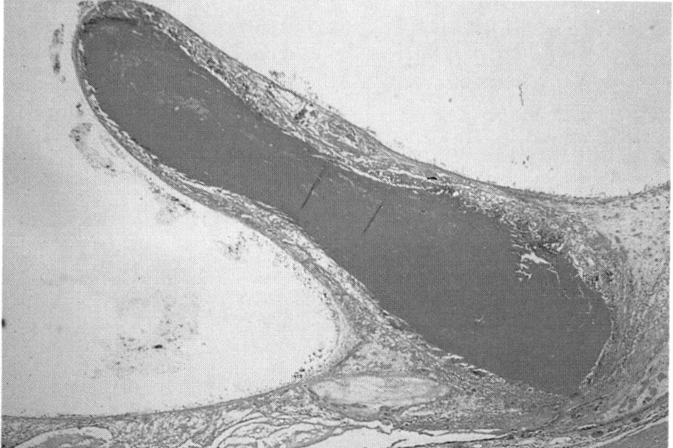

B

C

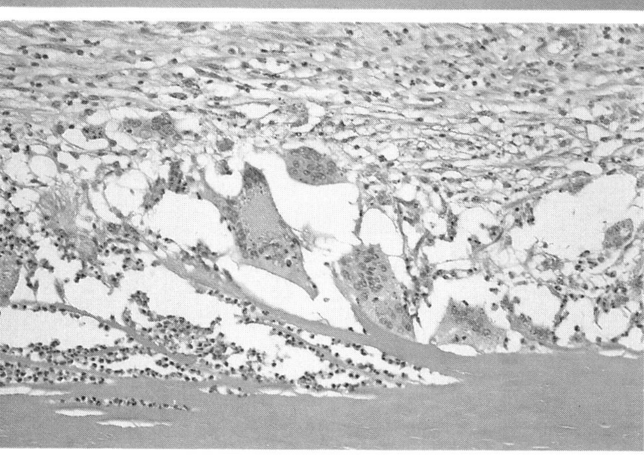

Figure 185–7. Phacoanaphylactic glaucoma. Granulomatous inflammatory reaction with giant cells surrounding lens material. *A*, H&E, ×0.8; *B*, H&E, ×12; *C*, H&E, ×12. (Courtesy of Morton E. Smith, M.D.)

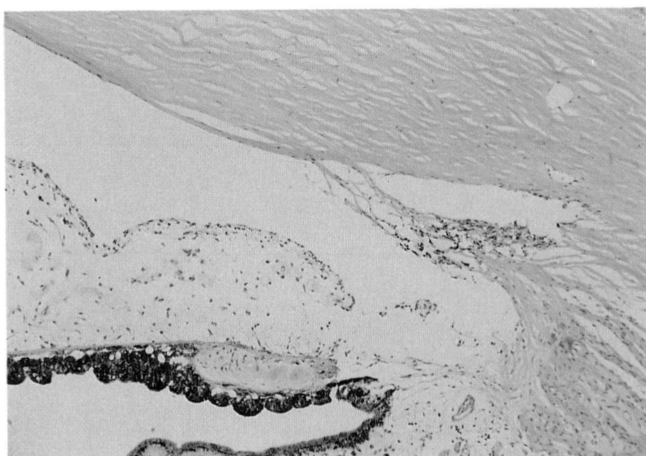

Figure 185–8. Pigment in the trabecular meshwork. H&E, ×12.

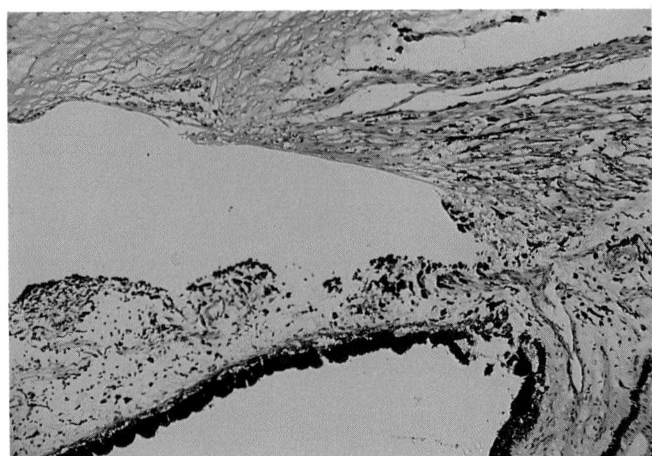

Figure 185–10. Angle recession. Tear in the anterior portion of the ciliary body with posterior displacement of the iris root. H&E, ×12.

its in the intertrabecular spaces, trabecular endothelium, juxtacanalicular tissue, and beneath the endothelium of Schlemm's canal.[52] This material consists of fine fibrils embedded in a homogeneous matrix,[53] which some authors have characterized as a basement membrane material[54] and others as an amyloid-like structure.[53] The exfoliation material appears to be intimately involved with the adventitia of the iris vessels.[55, 56] Electron microscopy has shown deposits of this material on lens capsule, ciliary body, iris, and even conjunctiva,[17] and extensive atrophy of iris pigment epithelium.[57]

Siderosis. Siderosis from retained ocular iron foreign bodies can cause open-angle glaucoma. Breakdown products and iron can accumulate in the trabecular meshwork, producing increased intraocular pressure. The mechanism of this process is unclear.[58]

Contusions. An insult to the ocular anterior segment can damage the trabecular meshwork, the base of the iris (iridodialysis), provoke a tear in the anterior face of the ciliary muscle separating the circular from the meridional fibers (angle recession) (Fig. 185–10), or cause disinsertion of the ciliary muscle at the scleral spur (cyclodialysis) (Fig. 185–11).[59, 60] Scarring in the trabecular meshwork or posterior proliferation of the peripheral corneal endothelium over the angle structures can lead to increased intraocular pressure and glaucoma.

Anterior Chamber Epithelization. Epithelization causes the conjunctival or corneal epithelium to grow over the iris, the angle structures, and the posterior corneal surface and obstruct the trabecular area. This happens as a result of a perforating corneal wound, which permits the epithelium to extend into the anterior chamber. Histologically, a stratified, nonkeratinized epithelium of variable thickness covers the anterior chamber structures.[61, 62]

Anterior Chamber Endothelization. Proliferation of the corneal endothelium over the anterior chamber structures may block the trabecular meshwork. The endothelization is usually one layer thick with an observable basement membrane. The proliferation of the endothelium can occur after trauma or mild inflammation or may be associated with iridocorneal endothelial syndrome (progressive iris atrophy, Chandler's syndrome, Cogan-Reese syndrome, or iris-nevus syndrome) (Fig. 185–12).[63–67]

Fibrovascular Membranes. These membranes may grow over the anterior surface of the iris (rubeosis iridis)

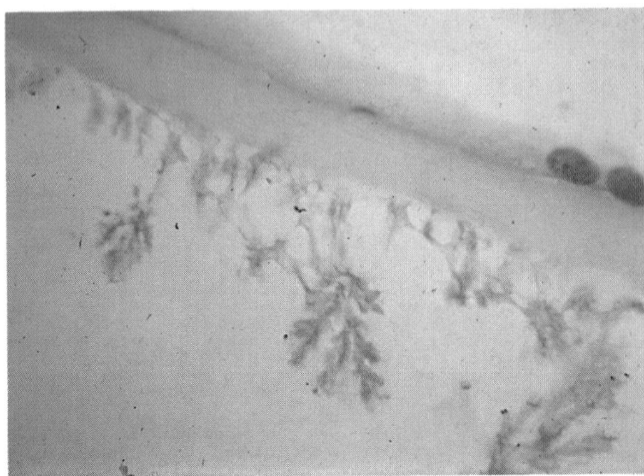

Figure 185–9. Pseudoexfoliation syndrome. Deposits of pseudoexfoliation material on the lens. Fine fibrillar eosinophilic material over the lens capsule. H&E, ×75. (Courtesy of Morton E. Smith, M.D.)

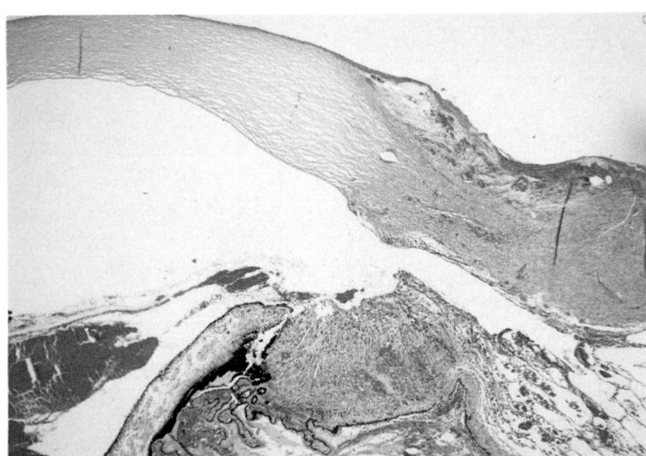

Figure 185–11. Cyclodialysis. Disinsertion of the ciliary muscle from the scleral spur. H&E, ×5.

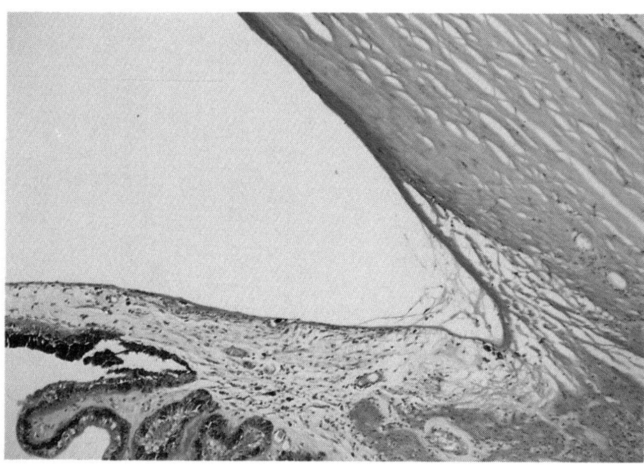

Figure 185–12. Anterior chamber endothelization. Descemet's membrane envelops angle structures. PAS, ×5.

and angle structures in several diseases (e.g., diabetic retinopathy, central retinal vein occlusion, intraocular tumors, long-standing retinal detachment) and cause increased intraocular pressure (neovascular glaucoma). Histopathologically, the neovascular proliferation lies directly over the stromal surface and may arise from iris vessels, usually starting at the pupillary margin. As the proliferation progresses, angle-closure occurs, and membrane contraction can cause irregular pupil dilatation with anterior bowing of the sphincter of the iris and pigment epithelium (ectropion uveae) (Fig. 185–13).[1, 17, 68]

ANGLE-CLOSURE GLAUCOMA

Angle-closure glaucoma is characterized by elevated intraocular pressure caused by the blockage of aqueous outflow due to the apposition of the iris root over the angle structures.

Primary Angle-Closure Glaucoma

This type of glaucoma occurs in eyes with an anatomic predisposition (narrow angle, shallow anterior chamber). It is more frequent in hypertropic eyes in which the sizes of the lens and the anterior chamber are disproportionate. Primary angle-closure glaucoma also occurs in congenitally abnormally small eyes. Greater iris contact with the anterior lens capsule increases resistance to the passage of aqueous humor through the pupil (relative pupillary block). This increase of resistance anteriorly displaces the iris root. When relative pupillary block is greatest, usually when the pupil is mid-dilated, ample closure may occur.

The histopathologic changes in angle-closure glaucoma are the result of a rapid and marked elevation of intraocular pressure. Necrosis of the dilator and sphinc-

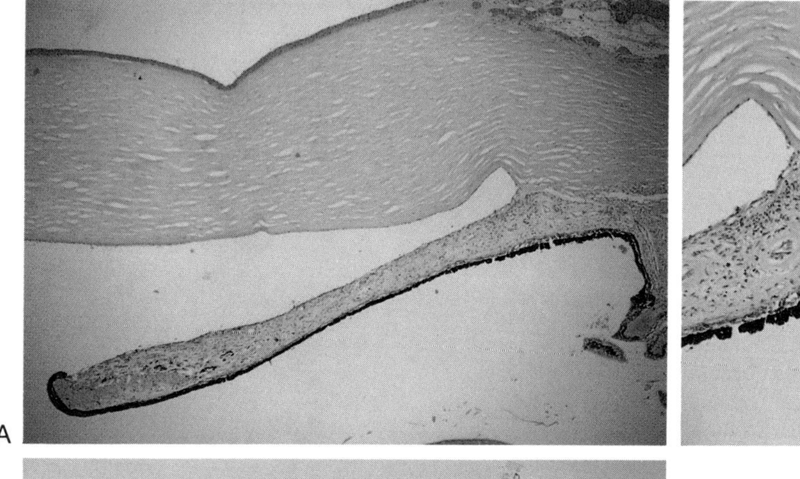

A

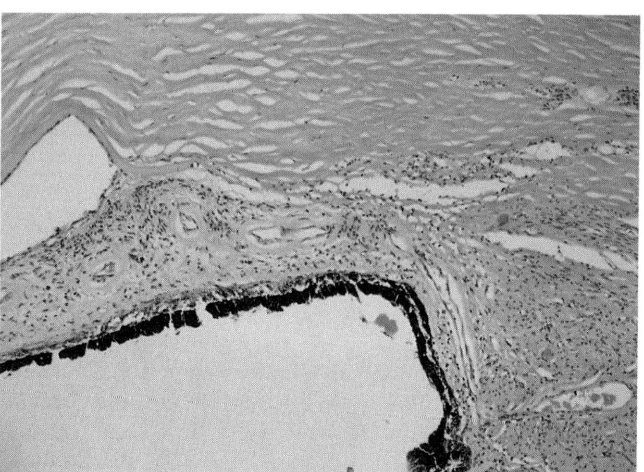

B

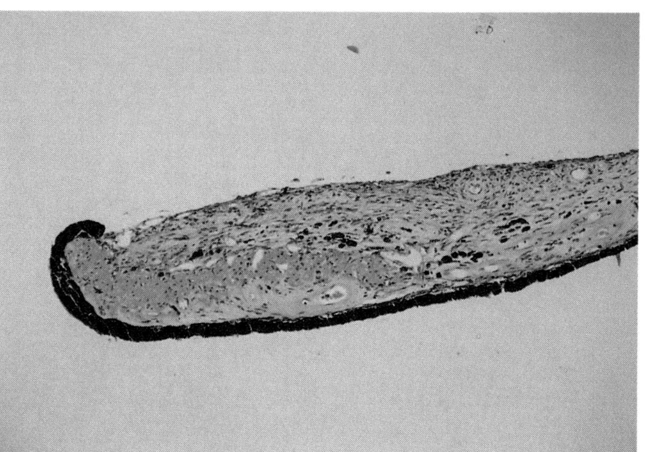

C

Figure 185–13. Neovascular glaucoma. Neovascular membrane over iris surface (*A*, H&E, ×5), producing peripheral synechia (*B*, H&E, ×12) and ectropion uveae (*C*, H&E, ×12).

ter muscles leads to irregularities in pupillary shape. Segmental iris atrophy may be seen, as well as marked general atrophy of the iris stroma. Multiple, small, subcapsular, anterior white lens opacities may be seen (glaukomflecken) that correspond to foci of epithelial cell necrosis with adjacent areas of subcapsular cortical degeneration. The corneal stroma and epithelium become edematous. Venous return can be blocked by the elevated pressure, causing optic disc edema and even central retinal vein occlusion. Prolonged contact of the iris and the trabecular meshwork can lead to the formation of peripheral anterior synechiae, fibrosis, and degeneration of the meshwork.

Secondary Angle-Closure Glaucoma

Blockage of the aqueous flow from the posterior to the anterior chamber may occur in eyes without anatomic predisposition owing to adhesions between the iris and the surrounding structures (trabecular meshwork or peripheral cornea) secondary to other diseases (pupillary block): Iridolenticular block (iris bombé), iridovitreal block in aphakic eyes, or adhesions between the iris and the intraocular lens in pseudophakic eyes. It may also be associated with intraocular inflammation. There are other forms of secondary angle-closure glaucoma without pupillary block. Increased pressure in the posterior segment or ciliochoroidal effusion or edema may anteriorly displace the ciliary body producing blockage of aqueous outflow (i.e., malignant glaucoma or ciliary block glaucoma, intraocular tumors, contraction of retrolental membrane, cyst of iris, and ciliary body).[17]

CONGENITAL GLAUCOMA

Primary congenital glaucoma is present at birth or appears during the first years of life and is associated with angle malformations. It can occur as an isolated condition (trabeculodysgenesis) or can be associated with other systemic (e.g., phakomatoses, Lowe-Terrey-MacLachlan oculocerebrorenal syndrome) or ocular malformations (e.g., dysgenesis of the iris, angle, and peripheral cornea). Secondary congenital glaucoma may be present at birth owing to exposure to intrauterine insult (e.g., rubella).

Primary congenital glaucoma, an abnormal development of the angle structures without evidence of malformation in the surrounding tissues, is the most common form of congenital glaucoma (50 percent of congenital cases). Most cases (60 to 80 percent) are bilateral.[1, 17]

Histopathology shows abnormal anterior attachment of the iris root to the trabecular meshwork, a poorly developed scleral spur and uveal meshwork, abnormal anterior attachment of the longitudinal fibers of the ciliary muscle onto the uveal trabecular bands, thickening of the trabecular beams, and incomplete separation of the angle structures with retained fetal tissue.[1, 69–71]

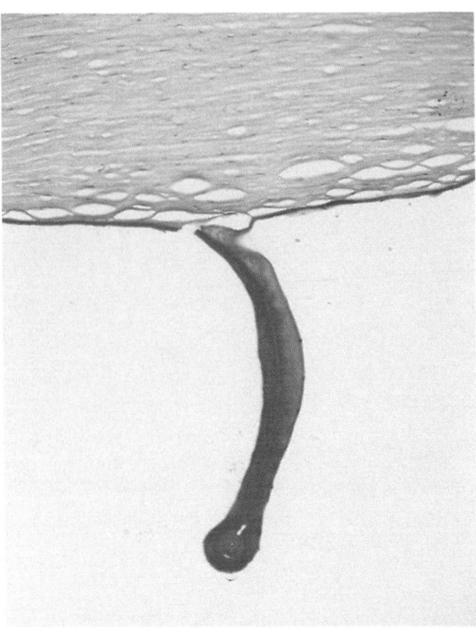

Figure 185–14. Haab's striae. PAS, ×12.

In infants and young children elevated intraocular pressure may cause enlargement of the globe (buphthalmos), limbal tissues (limbal ectasia with deep anterior chamber), and cornea, leading to circumferential or horizontal ruptures of Descemet's membrane (Haab's striae) (Fig. 185–14), corneal clouding, photophobia, blepharospasm, epiphora, and decreased visual acuity. The sclera expands and thins. Cupping occurs early but may regress with early treatment.

Glaucoma may appear frequently in association with developmental or congenital abnormalities (iridocorneal or goniodysgenesis), such as hypoplasia of the iris (aniridia) and iris coloboma, Axenfeld's anomaly, Rieger's syndrome (posterior embryotoxon and iris, facial, and dental anomalies), Peters' anomaly (central corneal defect with absent endothelium and Descemet's membrane), and Marfan's syndrome.

REFERENCES

1. Spencer WH: Glaucoma. *In* Spencer WH: Ophthalmic Pathology, vol 1. Philadelphia, WB Saunders, 1985, pp 480–547.
2. Quigley HA, Addicks EM, Green WR, et al: Optic nerve damage in human glaucoma. II: The site of injury and susceptibility to damage. Arch Ophthalmol 99:635, 1981.
3. Quigley HA: Reappraisal of the mechanisms of glaucomatous optic nerve damage. Eye 1:318, 1987.
4. Kirsch RE, Anderson DR: Identification of the glaucomatous disc. Trans Am Acad Ophthalmol Otolaryngol 77:143, 1973.
5. Radius RL, Maumenee AE, Green WR: Pit-like changes of the optic nerve head in open-angle glaucoma. Br J Ophthalmol 62:389, 1978.
6. Miller KM, Quigley HA: Comparison of the optic disk features in low tension and typical open-angle glaucoma. Ophthalmic Surg 18:882, 1987.
7. Caprioli J, Spaeth GL: Comparison of the optic nerve head in high and low tension glaucoma. Arch Ophthalmol 103:1145, 1985.
8. Javitt JC, Spaeth GL, Katz LJ, et al: Acquired pits of the optic nerve. Increased prevalence in patients with low tension glaucoma. Ophthalmology 97:1038, 1990.

9. Minckler DS, Bunt AM: Pathology of the optic nerve-axonal transport. *In* Nicholson DH (ed): Pathology Update. New York, Masson Co, 1980, pp 145–168.
10. Minckler DS: Histology of the optic nerve damage in ocular hypertension and early glaucoma. Surv Ophthalmol 33:401, 1989.
11. Lampert PW, Vogel MH, Zimmerman LE: Pathology of the optic nerve in experimental acute glaucoma. Invest Ophthalmol 7:199, 1968.
12. Hayreh SS: The pathogenesis of the optic nerve lesions in glaucoma. Trans Am Acad Ophthalmol Otolaryngol 81:197, 1976.
13. Hernandez MR, Andrzejewska WM, Neufeld AH: Changes in the extracellular matrix of the human optic nerve head in primary open-angle glaucoma. Am J Ophthalmol 109:180, 1990.
14. Lutjen-Drecoll E, Shimizu T, Rohrbach M, et al: Quantitative analysis of plaque material in the inner and outer wall of Schlemm's canal in normal and glaucomatous eyes. Exp Eye Res 42:443, 1986.
15. Rohen JW: Why is intraocular pressure elevated in chronic simple glaucoma? Anatomical considerations. Ophthalmology 90:758, 1983.
16. Alvarado J, Murphy C, Juster R: Trabecular meshwork cellularity in POAG and nonglaucomatous normals. Ophthalmology 91:564, 1984.
17. Richt R, Shields B, Krupin T: The Glaucomas. St Louis, Mosby, 1989.
18. Rohen JW, Witmer R: Electron microscopic studies on the trabecular meshwork in glaucoma simplex. Graefes Arch Clin Exp Ophthalmol 183:251, 1972.
19. Rohen JW, Futa R, Lutjen-Drecoll E: The fine structure of the cribriform meshwork in normal and glaucomatous eyes as seen in tangential sections. Invest Ophthalmol Vis Sci 21:574, 1981.
20. Segawa K: Electron microscopic changes of the trabecular tissue in primary open-angle glaucoma. Ann Ophthalmol 11:49, 1979.
21. Rodrigues MM, Spaeth GL, Sivalingam E: Histopathology of 150 trabeculectomy specimens in glaucoma. Trans Ophthalmol Soc UK 96:45, 1976.
22. McMenamin PG, Lee WR: Age-related changes in extracellular materials in the inner wall of Schlemm's canal. Graefes Arch Clin Exp Ophthalmol 212:159, 1980.
23. Alvarado JA, Yun AJ, Murphy CG: Juxtacanalicular tissue in primary open-angle glaucoma and in nonglaucomatous normals. Arch Ophthalmol 104:1517, 1986.
24. Lutjen-Drecoll E, Futa R, Rohen JW: Ultrahistochemical studies on tangential sections of the trabecular meshwork in normal and glaucomatous eyes. Invest Ophthalmol Vis Sci 21:563, 1981.
25. Rohen JW: Presence of matrix vesicles in trabecular meshwork in glaucomatous eyes. Graefes Arch Clin Exp Ophthalmol 218:171, 1982.
26. Grierson I: What is open angle glaucoma? Eye 1:15, 1987.
27. Chaudhry HA, Dueker DK, Simmons RJ, et al: Scanning electron microscopy of trabeculectomy specimens in open-angle glaucoma. Am J Ophthalmol 88:78, 1979.
28. Quigley HA, Addicks EM: Scanning electron microscopy of trabeculectomy specimens from eyes with open angle glaucoma. Am J Ophthalmol 90:854, 1980.
29. Naumann GOH, Apple DJ: Pathology of the Eye. New York, Springer-Verlag, 1986, p 771.
30. Yanoff M, Fine BS: Ocular Pathology. Philadelphia, JB Lippincott, 1989.
31. Wilhelmus KR, Grierson I, Watson PG: Histopathologic and clinical associations of scleritis and glaucoma. Am J Ophthalmol 91:697, 1981.
32. Raitta C, Vannas A: Glaucomatocyclitic crisis. Arch Ophthalmol 95:608, 1977.
33. Kichter PR, Shaffer RN: Interstitial keratitis and glaucoma. Am J Ophthalmol 68:241, 1969.
34. Roth M, Simmons RJ: Glaucoma associated with precipitates on the trabecular meshwork. Ophthalmology 86:1613, 1979.
35. Phelps CD, Watzke RC: Hemolytic glaucoma. Am J Ophthalmol 80:690, 1975.
36. Campbell DG, Simmons RJ, Grant WM: Ghost cells as a cause of glaucoma. Am J Ophthalmol 81:441, 1976.
37. Campbell DG: Ghost cell glaucoma following trauma. Ophthalmology 88:1151, 1981.
38. Lambrou FH, Aiken DG, Woods WD, et al: The production and mechanism of ghost cell glaucoma in the cat and primate. Invest Ophthalmol Vis Sci 26:893, 1985.
39. Cameron JD, Havener VR: Histologic confirmation of ghost cell glaucoma by routine light microscopy. Am J Ophthalmol 96:251, 1983.
40. Flocks M, Littwin CS, Zimmerman LE: Phacolytic glaucoma: A clinicopathological study of one hundred thirty-eight cases of glaucoma associated with hypermature cataract. Arch Ophthalmol 54:37, 1955.
41. Epstein DL: Lens-induced glaucoma. *In* Chandler PA, Grant WM (eds): Glaucoma. Philadelphia, Lea & Febiger, 1979.
42. Epstein DL, Jedziniak JA, Grant WM: Obstruction of aqueous outflow by lens particles and by heavy molecular weight soluble lens proteins. Invest Ophthalmol Vis Sci 17:272, 1978.
43. Perlman EM, Albert DM: Clinically unsuspected phacoanaphylaxis after ocular trauma. Arch Ophthalmol 95:1985, 1977.
44. Zimmerman LE: Lens-induced inflammation in human eyes. *In* Maumenee AE, Silverstein AM (eds): Immunopathology of Uveitis. Baltimore, Williams & Wilkins, 1964.
45. Shimizu T, Hara K, Futa R: Fine structure of trabecular meshwork and iris in pigmentary glaucoma. Graefes Arch Clin Exp Ophthalmol 215:171, 1981.
46. Yanoff M, Scheie HG: Melanomalytic glaucoma. Arch Ophthalmol 84:471, 1970.
47. McMenamin PG, Lee WR: Ultrastructural pathology of melanomalytic glaucoma. Br J Ophthalmol 70:895, 1986.
48. Kupfer C, Kuwara T, Kaiser-Kupfer M: The histopathology of pigmentary dispersion syndrome with glaucoma. Am J Ophthalmol 80:857, 1975.
49. Richter CU, Richardson TM, Grant WM: Pigmentary dispersion syndrome and pigmentary glaucoma: A prospective study of the natural history. Arch Ophthalmol 104:211, 1986.
50. Rodrigues MM, Spaeth GL, Weinreb S, et al: Spectrum of trabecular pigmentation in open-angle glaucoma: A clinico-pathological study. Trans Am Acad Ophthalmol Otolaryngol 81:258, 1976.
51. Richardson TM, Hutchinson BT, Grant WM: The outflow tract in pigmentary glaucoma: A light and electron microscopic study. Arch Ophthalmol 195:1015, 1977.
52. Ringvold A, Vegge T: Electron microscopy of the trabecular meshwork in eyes with exfoliation syndrome. Virch Arch [Pathol Anat] 353:110, 1971.
53. Ringvold A: Pseudoexfoliation material: An amyloid-like substance. Exp Eye Res 17:289, 1973.
54. Sugar HS, Harding C, Barsky D: The exfoliation syndrome. Ann Ophthalmol 8:1165, 1976.
55. Ghosh M, Speakman JS: The ciliary body in senile exfoliation of the lens. Can J Ophthalmol 8:394, 1973.
56. Layden WE, Shaffer RN: Exfoliation syndrome. Am J Ophthalmol 78:835, 1974.
57. Dickson DH, Ramsay MS: Fibrillopathia epitheliocapsularis (pseudoexfoliation): A clinical and electron microscope study. Can J Ophthalmol 10:148, 1975.
58. Burch PG, Albert DM: Transscleral ocular siderosis. Am J Ophthalmol 84:90, 1977.
59. Wolff SM, Zimmerman LE: Chronic secondary glaucoma associated with retrodisplacement of iris root and deepening of the anterior chamber angle secondary to contusion. Am J Ophthalmol 54:547, 1962.
60. Iwamoto T, Witmer R, Landott E: Light and electron microscopy in the absolute glaucoma with pigment dispersion phenomena and contusion angle deformity. Am J Ophthalmol 72:420, 1971.
61. Bernardino VB, Kim JC, Smith TR: Epithelization of the anterior chamber after cataract extraction. Arch Ophthalmol 82:742, 1969.
62. Boruchoff SA, Kenyon KR, Foulks GN, et al: Epithelial cyst of the iris following penetrating keratoplasty. Br J Ophthalmol 64:440, 1980.
63. Alvarado JA, Murphy CG, Juster RP, et al: Pathogenesis of Chandler's syndrome, essential iris atrophy and the Cogan-Reese syndrome. II: Estimated age at disease onset. Invest Ophthalmol Vis Sci 27:873, 1986.
64. Alvarado JA, Murphy CG, Maglio M, et al: Pathogenesis of Chandler's syndrome, essential iris atrophy and the Cogan-Reese

syndrome. I: Alterations of the corneal endothelium. Invest Ophthalmol Vis Sci 27:853, 1986.
65. Eagle RC, Font RL, Yanoff M, et al: Proliferative endotheliopathy with iris abnormalities. The iridocorneal endothelial syndrome. Arch Ophthalmol 97:2104, 1979.
66. Patel A, Kenyon KR, Hirst LW, et al: Clinicopathologic features of Chandler's syndrome. Surv Ophthalmol 27:327, 1983.
67. Rodrigues MM, Jester JV, Richards R, et al: Essential iris atrophy: A clinical, inmmunohistologic and electron microscopic study in an enucleated eye. Ophthalmology 95:69, 1988.
68. Gartner S, Henkind P: Neovascularization of the iris (rubeosis iridis). Surv Ophthalmol 22:291, 1978.
69. Maumenee AE: The pathogenesis of congenital glaucoma: A new theory. Trans Am Ophthalmol Soc 56:507, 1958.
70. Broughton WL, Fine B, Zimmerman LE: A histologic study of congenital glaucoma associated with a chromosomal defect. Arch Ophthalmol 99:481, 1981.
71. Anderson DR: The development of the trabecular meshwork and its abnormality in primary infantile glaucoma. Trans Am Ophthalmol Soc 79:458, 1981.

Chapter 186

Pathology of the Lids

MARIA A. SAORNIL, RAMSAY S. KURBAN,
CHRISTOPHER T. WESTFALL, and MARTIN C. MIHM JR

ANATOMY AND HISTOLOGY

The human eyelid consists of six layers: epidermis, dermis, subcutaneous layer, orbicularis muscle, tarsal plate, and conjunctiva (Fig. 186–1).

The epidermis, the external layer, is a keratinizing squamous epithelium composed of two cell types: keratinocytes and dendritic cells. The former are arranged in four layers, the deepest being the basal cell layer formed by a single row of cells resting on a basement membrane. These cells can contain various amounts of melanin pigment derived from the adjacent dendritic melanocytes. The squamous cell layer (stratum spinosum) consists of polygonal keratinocytes that flatten superficially. The granular layer (stratum granulosum) consists of a row of elongated cells containing basophilic keratohyalin granules. The horny layer (stratum corneum), the most superficial, consists of flat keratinized cells without nuclei. As cells differentiate from the basal to the horny layer, they undergo keratinization. In addition to the keratinocytes, the epidermis contains three types of dendritic cells: clear cell melanocytes, Langerhans' cells, and undetermined dendritic cells.[1]

The dermis, interposed between the epidermis and the underlying orbicularis muscle, is loose and delicate. It contains bundles of collagen, variable amounts of elastic and reticulin fibers, fibroblasts, blood vessels, lymphatics, and small nerve fibers.

The subcutaneous layer contains little adipose tissue and is loosely adherent to the orbicularis muscle. Therefore, swelling, hemorrhage, or acute inflammation is more prominent in the lids than in other locations in the body.

The orbicularis muscle, an elliptical sheet of striated muscle concentric to the eye, functions to close the eye. In the superior part, the tendon of the levator palpebrae passes through the subcutaneous layer into the skin and tarsus. Striated muscle fibers adjacent to the tarsal plate are known as Riolan's muscle. Müller's smooth muscle originates among the fibers of the levator in the upper eyelid and the inferior rectus in the lower eyelid and inserts into the margins of the tarsal plates and also into deep fibers of the orbicularis muscle.

Tarsi are flat semilunar plates composed of dense collagenous tissue. They contribute to lid rigidity and contain the meibomian glands. The inner portion of the tarsus is covered by the palpebral conjunctiva, which adheres closely to the tarsus.

Several epidermal appendages (glands and cilia) are present in the lids. There are two types of sebaceous glands: Zeis', which empty their products into the cilia; and meibomian, situated within the tarsal plates, where they are arranged vertically and parallel to each other and secrete their products into the meibomian ducts that open into the lid margin. There are about 30 meibomian

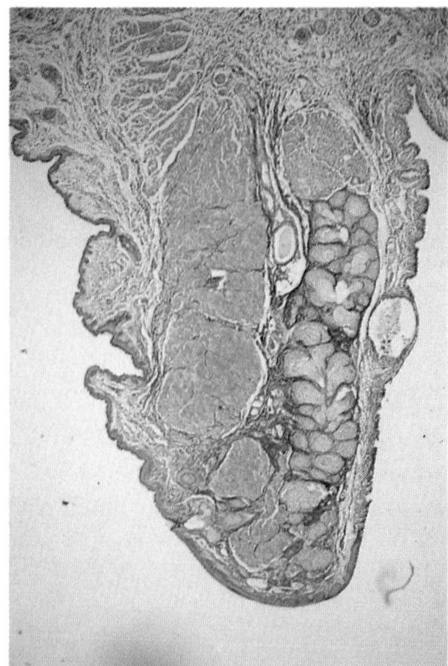

Figure 186–1. Normal eyelid anatomy showing skin, orbicularis muscle, tarsus with meibomian gland, Wolfring's lacrimal gland and conjunctiva. (Masson's Trichromic, ×2.5.)

glands in the upper lid and 20 in the lower. Both Zeis' and meibomian glands undergo holocrine secretion—that is, their acini possess no lumina and extrude secretory products by destruction of their cells.[1]

There are two types of sweat glands: the eccrine (secretion by excretion) and the apocrine Moll's glands (secretion by decapitation). The latter lie near the lid margin and empty their products into the eyelash follicles.

Accessory lacrimal glands with histologic features identical to those in the main lacrimal gland are found in the substantia propria of the conjunctiva. Krause's glands number approximately 42 in the upper fornix and 8 in the lower and are located deep in the subconjunctival tissues at the fornices. Fewer Wolfring's glands (or Ciaccio's glands) are located at the border of the tarsus (two to five in the upper lid and two in the lower); they are larger than Krause's glands.

The vascular supply of the lids is derived from the ophthalmic and lacrimal arteries through their medial and lateral palpebral branches. The veins are more numerous and larger than the arteries and are arranged in dense plexuses in the upper and lower fornices of the conjunctiva. The lymphatics are in pre- and posttarsal plexuses that intercommunicate by channels and drain into the preauricular and submandibular nodes.

BASIC PATHOLOGY TERMINOLOGY OF THE SKIN

Acantholysis. Loss of coherence between epithelial cells, causing vesiculation.

Acanthosis. An increase in the number of layers (thickness) of the epidermis.

Atypia (Anaplasia). Anomalous appearance of the nuclei found in malignant neoplasia: abnormal nucleocytoplasmic ratio, hyperchromatism, abnormal shape, abnormal mitotic figures.

Dyskeratosis. Premature keratinization of individual keratinocytes within the squamous layer.

Dysplasia. Disordered cellular organization often associated with atypia.

Horn Cyst. Aggregates of mature keratin surrounded by basaloid cells, representing immature hair structures. These should be distinguished from horn pearls of squamous cell carcinoma that exhibit incomplete and gradual keratinization.

Hyperkeratosis. Thickening of the keratin layer.

Papillomatosis. Proliferation of subepidermal papillae with epidermal hyperplasia causing the surface of the epidermis to show irregular undulation.

Parakeratosis. Incomplete keratinization characterized by retention of nuclei in the horny layer. This should be distinguished from orthokeratosis, in which no nuclei are observed in the thickened stratum corneum.

Pleomorphism. Variation in size and shape of the tumor cell nuclei, usually associated with variations in cell shape.

INFLAMMATION AND INFECTION

Inflammation

Blepharitis. Blepharitis is diffuse inflammation of the lids; it may be due to either seborrheic dermatitis or a chronic bacterial infection. Clinically, the lid margins may be thickened, erythematous, and ulcerated, with gray scales on the eyelashes. Histologically, blepharitis is a chronic nongranulomatous inflammatory reaction of the lid margins leading to acanthosis and hyperkeratosis of the epidermis.

Hordeolum. Hordeolum occurs as the result of an acute purulent inflammation of either the superficial eccrine or sebaceous glands (external hordeolum or stye) or the meibomian glands (internal hordeolum) of the eyelids. It usually presents as an elevated, superficial, erythematous, painful warm papule. Histologically, polymorphonuclear leukocytes, edema, and vascular congestion are observed.

Chalazion. Chalazion is one of the most common causes of lid swelling or tumor formation. Clinically, it is a hard, painless nodule in the eyelid that results from an obstruction in the sebaceous gland ducts (meibomian and Zeis'). Secreted lipids accumulate and erupt from the gland into the collagen of the tarsus. This lipid material is irritating and provokes a mixed inflammatory reaction including polymorphonuclear leukocytes, lymphocytes, plasma cells, and eosinophils. Mononuclear cells and multinucleate giant histiocytes appear to clear away the lipid material. The result is a chronic lipogranulomatous inflammation in the tarsus arranged in a confluent series of focal granulomas, each centered around a lipid globule from the sebaceous gland (Fig. 186–2).

Viral Infections

Molluscum Contagiosum. This infection is caused by a poxvirus that leads to formation of small, discrete, waxy, skin-colored, dome-shaped papules, usually 2 to 4 mm in diameter with an umbilicated center. Molluscum contagiosum often coexists with follicular conjunc-

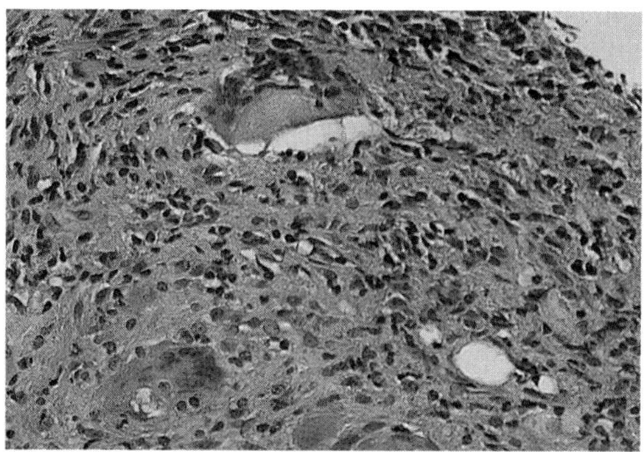

Figure 186–2. Chalazion. Inflammatory response with multinucleated giant cells engulfing lipidized material (lipogranulomatous reaction). H&E, ×50.

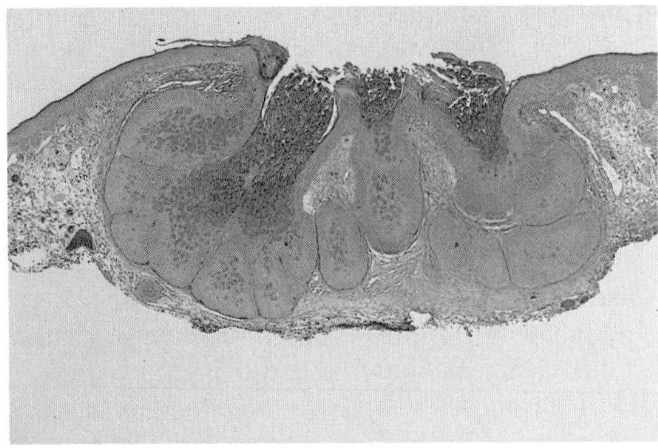

Figure 186–3. Molluscum contagiosum. Epidermal hyperplasia appearing as multiple lobules. Cells show intracytoplasmic inclusion bodies (molluscum bodies) more basophilic at the superficial level, releasing their contents in a central cavity. H&E, ×8.

tivitis caused by the liberation of viral particles into the conjunctival cul-de-sac. Ultimately, the lesions involute spontaneously, at which time there may be mild inflammation.[2] In immunocompromised patients, particularly in those with AIDS, hundreds of lesions of molluscum contagiosum may be seen, showing little tendency to involution.[3]

Microscopically, the epidermis shows acanthosis that grows into the dermis as multiple lobules. Epidermal cells contain large intracytoplasmic inclusion bodies (molluscum bodies) (Fig. 186–3), which form in the lower epidermis and grow as the infected cells move toward the surface, displacing and compressing the nucleus of the cell. At the superficial levels, the molluscum bodies change from eosinophilic to basophilic, and the horny layer disintegrates, releasing the molluscum bodies and filling a central cavity. These changes account for the umbilicated clinical appearance. On electron microscopy, the molluscum bodies are found to contain large numbers of molluscum contagiosum viruses. During spontaneous involution, a mononuclear infiltrate surrounds the lesion and is interpreted as cell-mediated immune rejection by the host.[2]

Verruca Vulgaris. This lesion is papillomatous, circumscribed, firm, and elevated, with a hyperkeratotic surface. It may occur anywhere on the skin and is caused by the human papillomavirus (papovavirus). Histologically, it shows papillomatosis with irregular acanthosis, hyperkeratosis, and parakeratosis. Foci of vacuolated cells containing clumped keratohyalin granules in the upper layers differentiate verruca vulgaris from other papillomas. The vacuolated cells contain round, deeply basophilic bodies surrounded by a clear halo and pale cytoplasm that may represent the viral particles or nuclei infected by virus. Development of squamous cell carcinoma in verruca vulgaris is rare but can occur.[4, 5] As in molluscum contagiosum, involution is associated with mononuclear cell infiltration, suggesting that regression represents a cell-mediated immune response.[6]

Herpes (Simplex, Varicella, and Zoster). This virus, which may affect the lids, begins as vesicles or blisters on an erythematous base. The virus produces profound degeneration of epidermal cells, resulting in marked acantholysis. A smear of the lesion may reveal eosinophilic inclusion bodies in the center of enlarged nuclei, as well as multinucleated epithelial giant cells.[7]

CYSTIC LESIONS

Epidermal Inclusion Cyst, Epidermoid Cyst, and Milia

Epidermoid and epidermal inclusion cysts are identical histologically. They are lined by stratified squamous epithelium, with no epidermal appendages in the wall, and contain keratin debris (Fig. 186–4). The former is present at birth; the latter is acquired and, in the view of the ophthalmic pathologists, caused by traumatic dermal implantation of epidermis. Clinically, these lesions often appear white because of their keratinaceous debris. When they are small, they are called *milia.* They may represent retention cysts, caused by the occlusion of pilosebaceous follicles, sweat pores, or benign keratinizing tumors.[8]

Dermoid Cyst

Dermoid cysts, present at birth, are subcutaneous cysts that usually arise superonasally or temporally in the anterior orbit and represent the result of sequestration of the epidermis along the lines of embryonic closure. Histologically, they are lined by stratified squamous epithelium, and their walls typically have adnexal structures (sebaceous and eccrine sweat glands and hair follicles) that empty their contents into the lumen of the cyst (Fig. 186–5). Rupture of the cyst wall usually provokes an intense foreign body granulomatous reaction.

Sweat Gland Cysts (Hidrocystoma and Ductal or Sudoriferous Cysts)

Sweat gland cysts result from obstruction of a sweat gland duct. They are lined with a double layer of epithelium, the outer myoepithelium and the inner cu-

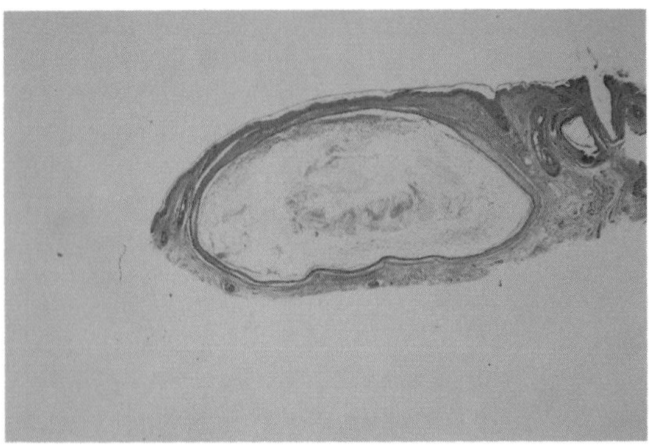

Figure 186–4. Epidermal inclusion cyst lined by stratified squamous epithelium and filled with keratin debris. H&E, ×8.

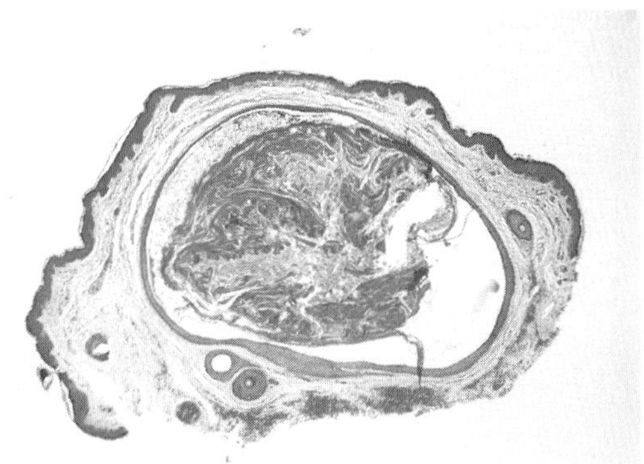

Figure 186–5. Dermoid cyst walled by stratified squamous epithelium with adnexal structures (pilosebaceous apparatus) in association with the cyst wall deep in the dermis. The cyst contains an eosinophilic material mixture of keratin debris and products of the adnexal structures in the wall. H&E, ×8.

boidal epithelium, and are filled with clear fluid (Fig. 186–6). Eccrine hidrocystomas are presumed to arise from the sweat glands throughout the eyelid skin. However, apocrine hidrocystomas are generally restricted to the lid margins because they arise from Moll's glands. Histologically, they have a more columnar inner secretory lining, with eosinophilic cytoplasm and apical decapitation protrusions. Because the contents of the cyst include cytoplasmic debris, the fluid may be more turbid than in eccrine cysts. Apocrine hidrocystomas may also have papillary infoldings into the cyst cavity.[9] They are usually unilateral and solitary; however, multiple and bilateral cases have been reported[10, 11] and can be associated with defects of ectodermally derived structures (i.e., ectodermal dysplasia).[1]

EPITHELIAL TUMORS

Tumors of the epithelium are common and can be divided into three main groups according to their clinical behavior and histologic features: benign, precancerous, and malignant. Benign lesions tend to grow more slowly and ulcerate less frequently than malignant ones. Inflammatory lesions or reactivated epithelial proliferations grow in days or weeks. However, the clinical features of each group often overlap. Furthermore, within each of the categories are lesions that vary in size, color, and duration. They can be of papillary or nodular configuration. Accurate diagnosis depends on histologic examination.[9, 12]

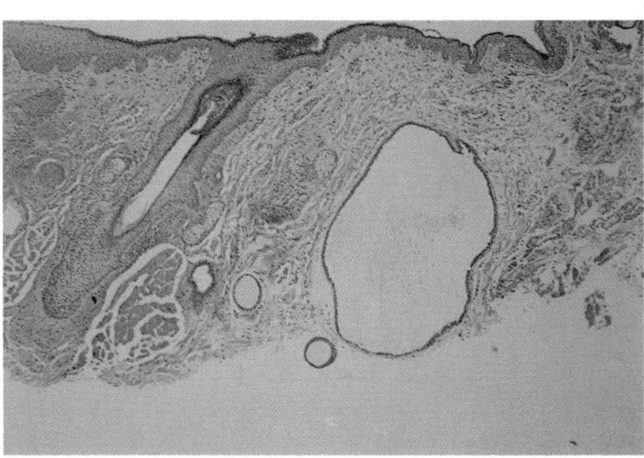

Figure 186–6. Hidrocystoma lined by a double layer of epithelium and filled with clear fluid. H&E, ×12.

Benign

Cutaneous Horn. This tumor typifies the overproduction of keratin by the epidermis; it appears like a filiform extension of solid keratin that projects above the surface of the skin. Histologically, cutaneous horn is characterized by marked hyperkeratosis; different types of lesions can be observed at the base. When removing such lesions, it is essential to obtain a sample of the viable underlying epidermis and dermis to rule out squamous cell carcinoma.[9]

Papilloma. This tumor, one of the most common benign lesions of the eyelid, usually is sessile or pedunculated with a color similar to that of the adjacent skin. Microscopically, the lesions are composed of finger-like projections of vascularized connective tissue, covered by acanthotic epithelium and elongation of the rete ridges and showing areas of hyperkeratosis and focal parakeratosis (Fig. 186–7). Five lesions have similar histology: epidermal nevus, solar keratosis, seborrheic keratosis, verruca vulgaris, and acanthosis nigricans.[7]

Seborrheic Keratosis. This lesion is one of the most common benign proliferations lesions involving the eyelid of middle-aged and older individuals. In Caucasians, the lesions are brownish, waxy, well demarcated, and lobulated, with hyperkeratosis and a verrucous surface. Histologically, seborrheic keratosis is a benign proliferation of basaloid cells. It shows acanthotic epidermis, often containing inclusion cysts (pseudohorn cysts) with some degree of hyperkeratosis and papillomatosis. There are three major types of seborrheic keratoses: acanthotic, in which the most important feature is thickening of the epidermis; hyperkeratotic, characterized by

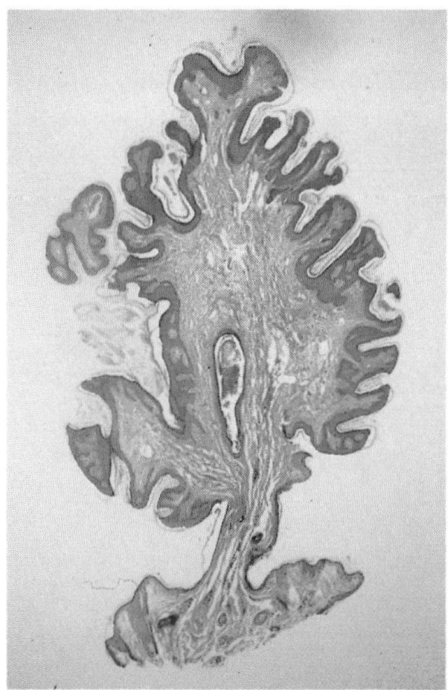

Figure 186–7. Papilloma. Finger-like projections of vascularized connective tissue, covered by acanthotic epithelium, showing hyperkeratosis. H&E, ×4.

marked hyperkeratosis; and reticulated or adenoid, with numerous thin tracts of contiguous epidermal cells extending into the dermis (Fig. 186–8). When irritated, seborrheic keratoses show chronic inflammatory infiltration of the dermis accompanied by squamous proliferation. Distinguishing it from squamous cell carcinoma can be difficult.[13] However, the diagnosis of irritated seborrheic keratosis is made by identifying whorls of squamous cells (squamous eddies) and a palisade of benign basaloid cells in the tumor periphery.

Dermatosis papulosa nigra is a pigmented variant that occurs on the face of black adults and may involve the eyelids.

Inverted Follicular Keratosis. This lesion usually presents as a nodular or wartlike keratotic mass, pink to flesh colored, that surrounds a follicular orifice. It is more common at the lid margin,[14] usually develops in a few months, and tends to recur if incompletely excised.[15] This recurrence may result in an incorrect diagnosis of squamous cell carcinoma. Histologically, inverted follicular keratosis is similar to irritated seborrheic keratosis. Squamous cells collected around a slightly keratinized focus, so-called squamous eddies, are observed. Many pathologists believe it to be a type of irritated seborrheic keratosis.[16]

Pseudoepitheliomatous Hyperplasia. This benign proliferation of the epidermis usually is elevated and has an irregular surface, mimicking either squamous or basal cell carcinoma. These tumors may develop rapidly. They occur in chronic inflammatory processes, at the edges of chronic ulcers or burns, and adjacent to and admixed with certain neoplasms.

Histologic examination shows uneven epidermal cell masses and strands, with irregular proliferation into the dermis, often containing numerous mitotic figures. However, the cells are well differentiated; atypia and dyskeratosis are usually minimal or absent.[17] Nevertheless, pseudoepitheliomatous hyperplasia can be difficult to differentiate from low-grade squamous cell carcinoma.[7]

Keratoacanthoma. Keratoacanthoma occurs mainly on exposed areas of the skin of middle-aged or elderly people. It usually develops in a period of 6 to 8 wk and involutes spontaneously, generally in less than 6 mo. Clinically, it appears as a firm dome-shaped nodule with

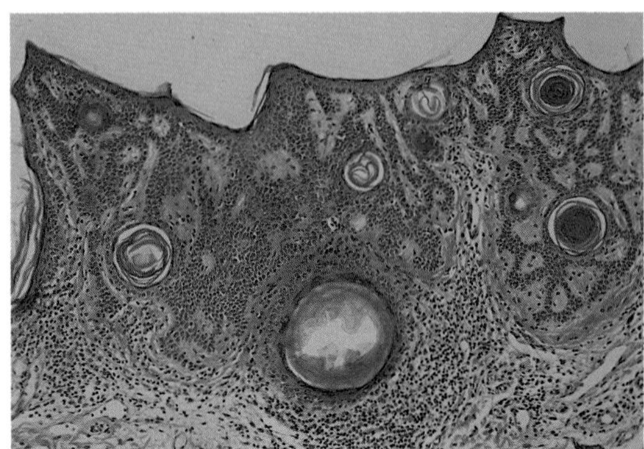

Figure 186–8. Seborrheic keratosis (reticular type). Benign proliferation of basaloid cells with acanthotic epidermis, hyperkeratosis, and papillomatosis, containing horn pseudocyst. H&E, ×32.

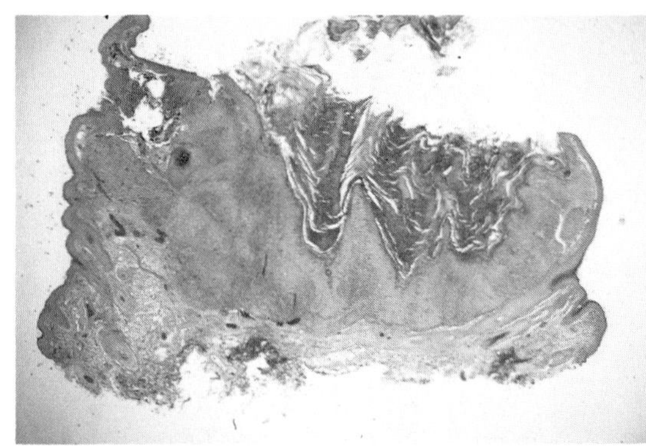

Figure 186–9. Keratoacanthoma. Epidermal hyperplasia, sharply demarcated from the adjacent normal skin, surrounding a central mass of keratin with underlying inflammatory reaction. H&E, ×2.5.

a horn-filled crater in its center. The benign course of this lesion and its probable reactive nature are now well recognized. Histologically, the lesion is cup shaped, with an acanthotic epidermis sharply demarcated from the adjacent normal skin, containing large pale cells with small nuclei, surrounding a central mass of keratin (Fig. 186–9). The epithelial proliferative zones are highlighted by neutrophilic abscesses in which collagen and elastic fibers can be identified. The base of the lesion is frequently uniform and well demarcated from the adjacent dermis by a moderate inflammatory reaction.

Nonmelanocytic Precancerous Lesions

Actinic Keratosis (Solar Keratosis, Senile Keratosis). Actinic keratosis is the most common precancerous cutaneous lesion and occurs on sun-exposed skin of middle-aged individuals. One of the most common sites of involvement is the face, including the eyelids. Clinically, actinic keratoses appear as single or more often multiple scaly keratotic lesions, sometimes showing a nodular horny or warty configuration. If untreated, approximately 13 percent of lesions evolve to squamous cell carcinoma. However, squamous cell carcinoma arising in actinic keratosis is thought to have a relatively favorable prognosis because metastasis has been reported to occur in only 0.5 to 3 percent of patients.[18, 19] Squamous cell carcinoma arising in actinic keratosis has been regarded as a separate, less aggressive entity than squamous cell carcinoma that arises de novo in non–sun-damaged skin.[12] It is our impression, however, that the metastatic potential of squamous cell carcinoma more directly relates to the extent of invasion and degree of differentiation rather than the site of origin. Histologically, the lesions most commonly show hyperkeratosis, parakeratosis, and epidermal atrophy. Hyperplastic variants show papillomatosis and acanthosis. Cellular atypia is found in deeper layers of the epidermis.[7] The atypical cells sometimes form buds that extend downward into the papillary dermis (Fig. 186–10). A hallmark of actinic keratosis is the alternating parakeratosis over-

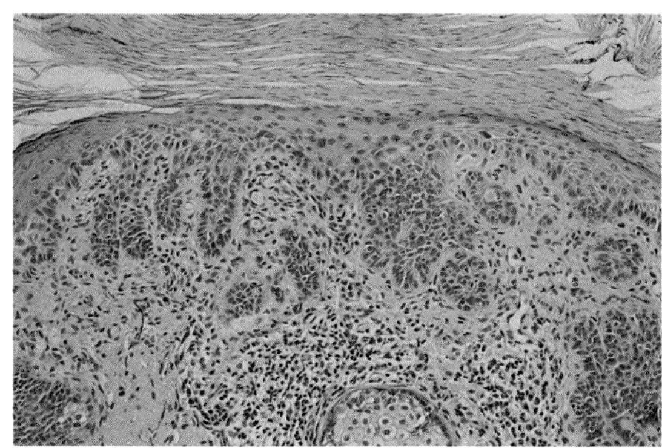

Figure 186–10. Actinic keratosis. Parakeratosis overlying an area composed of atypical keratinocytes. Note the basal crowding of the keratinocytes, loss of epidermal maturation, and the small buds that are extending into the papillary dermis.

lying atypical areas and orthokeratosis overlying intraepidermal appendageal structures.

Carcinoma In Situ (Bowen's Disease). This lesion clinically appears as an erythematous, well-demarcated scaly patch with usually a rectangular, round, or oval shape. It grows slowly. It is usually found in fair-skinned middle-aged individuals. Histologically, these lesions exhibit hyperkeratosis, parakeratosis, acanthosis, dyskeratosis, and loss of the normal polarity. The epidermal cells are replaced by an increased number of atypical cells with hyperchromatic nuclei, showing abnormal mitotic figures. These changes are limited to the epidermis and may extend down the external root sheaths of the hair follicle. The basement membrane remains intact.

Other Precancerous Lesions. The effects of chronic radiation on the skin (radiation dermatitis) include a predisposition to develop squamous cell carcinomas (most commonly), basal cell carcinomas, sebaceous cell carcinomas, or sarcomas.

Xeroderma Pigmentosum. This disease, inherited as autosomal recessive, is characterized by a marked sensitivity of the skin to sunlight. Among other disorders, patients develop malignant tumors including squamous cell carcinoma, basal cell carcinoma, malignant melanoma, sebaceous cell carcinoma, and fibrosarcoma on areas of skin exposed to sun. The main defect has been shown to be an inability to repair damage to DNA after exposure to ultraviolet light.[20, 21]

Malignant

Basal Cell Carcinoma. Basal cell carcinoma is the most common malignancy of the eyelids and accounts for approximately 90 percent of all eyelid malignancies and 20 percent of all eyelid tumors.[22] This tumor is usually seen in elderly fair-skinned people who have had extensive sun exposure. Basal cell carcinoma more frequently develops on the lower lid, followed by the upper lid and medial canthal skin, and is considered to be 20 to 40 times more common than squamous cell carcinoma of the lids.[9]

Basal cell carcinoma begins insidiously, and because it is a tumor of the basal cells located at the bottom of the epidermis, the earliest proliferation initially invades the dermis without epidermal replacement. As the tumor proliferates within the dermis, the overlying epidermis becomes thinned and atrophic but generally does not have the hyperkeratotic surface typical of benign and malignant squamous lesions.[9] Although most of the basal cell carcinomas originate in the epidermis, they can arise deep in the dermis from the basal cells of the hair shafts.

Most basal cell carcinomas are composed of small blue cells having little cytoplasm and, consequently, a high nuclear:cytoplasmic ratio. Peripheral palisading of elongated pseudocolumnar tumor cells and a retraction artifact from the stroma are typical (Fig. 186–11).[9]

The solid variant of basal cell carcinoma is less well differentiated than other types. Other basal cell carcinomas can have glandular (adenoid), sebaceous, or follicular differentiation. No difference exists in the rate of growth between undifferentiated and differentiated tumors. However, some basal cell carcinomas that tend toward squamous differentiation may be more aggressive and locally infiltrating and may metastasize.[23] In such cases, cells with more eosinophilic cytoplasm are present in the middle of the lobules or small islands of basal cells. This variant is often called *metatypical basal cell carcinoma* or less correctly *basosquamous carcinoma.* True basosquamous carcinoma is a collision tumor with juxtaposition of invasive basal cell and squamous cell carcinomas.

Most basal cell carcinomas are nodular, with or without ulceration. The nodular variants appear clinically as firm nodules, often with telangiectatic vessels on the surface. Histologically, the basal cells may grow in large lobules that occasionally become centrally cystic, associated with a clinical cystic appearance. As the lesion enlarges, by growing laterally and radially, the central area may break down, causing ulceration (rodent ulcer).[9] The ulcerative pattern shows histologically a central crater with a raised epithelial margin.

The morphea form of basal cell carcinoma (sclerosing variant) appears clinically as a pale indurated plaque. Histologically, it is characterized by diffuse invasion of the dermis by small cords of cells in dense hyalinized stroma (Fig. 186–12).

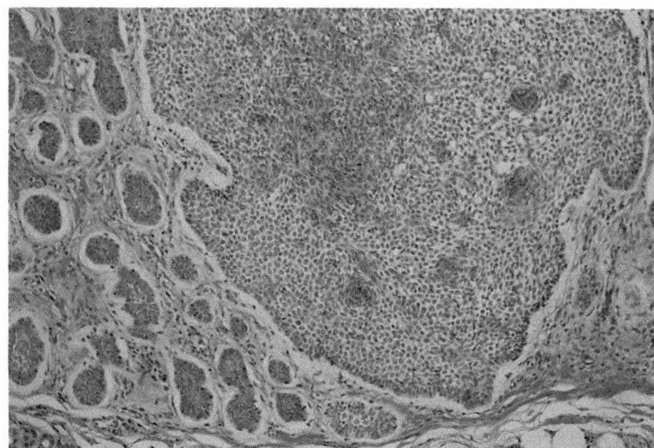

Figure 186–11. Basal cell carcinoma (nodular pattern). Basaloid dermal nests exhibit peripheral palisading and retraction artifact. H&E, ×32.

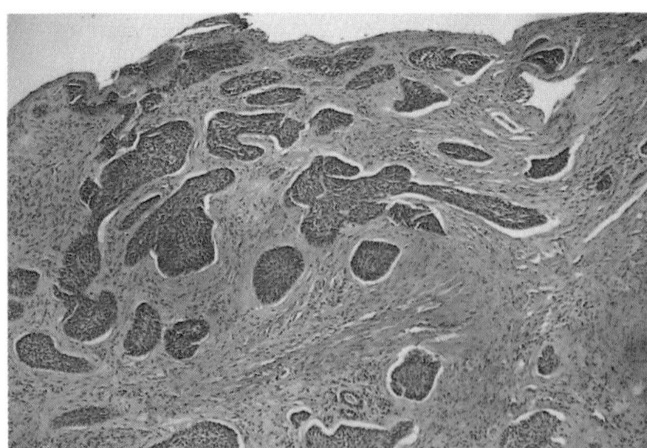

Figure 186–12. Basal cell carcinoma (morphea or sclerosing type). Small cords of cells diffusely invading the dermis in a dense, hyalinized stroma. H&E, ×12.

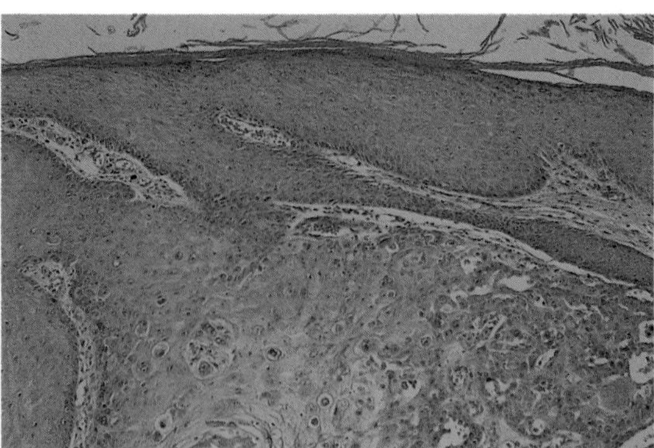

Figure 186–14. Squamous cell carcinoma. Very atypical and pleomorphic keratinocytes are extending from the epidermis and invading into the dermis. Note the individual cell keratinization. H&E, ×25.

The superficial or multicentric pattern exhibits an irregular nodular surface with telangiectatic vessels. Histologically, diffuse multicentric involvement of the epidermis extending into the superficial dermis is apparent (Fig. 186–13). The morphea form and multicentric types are dangerous because the limits of invasiveness often extend beyond the clinically apparent margins of involvement.

Striking blue, brown, or black discoloration of tumor nodules characterizes pigmented basal cell carcinomas. Both the nodular and multicentric types may exhibit this change. Nodular pigmented basal cell carcinomas are often confused with nodular malignant melanoma, whereas multicentric pigmented basal cell carcinomas are confused with superficial spreading melanomas. Increased production of melanin by tumor containing melanocytes with resultant increase of pigmentation of the anaplastic basal cells and melanophages is responsible for this alteration.[7, 24]

Basal cell carcinoma usually is locally infiltrative and rarely metastasizes. If tumor growth is uncontrolled, invasion of vital structures can cause death.

The management of basal cell carcinoma is local excision. For large lesions with diffuse infiltrative growth characteristics, evaluation of frozen sections of the margins or the Mohs' micrographic surgical method may be required for adequate therapy.[25]

Nevoid basal cell carcinoma syndrome consists of multiple basal cell carcinomas that appear early in life. They present as flesh-colored papules associated with cysts of the jaw, bifid rib, anomalies of the vertebrae, and central nervous system tumors. This syndrome is inherited as an autosomal dominant trait.[26]

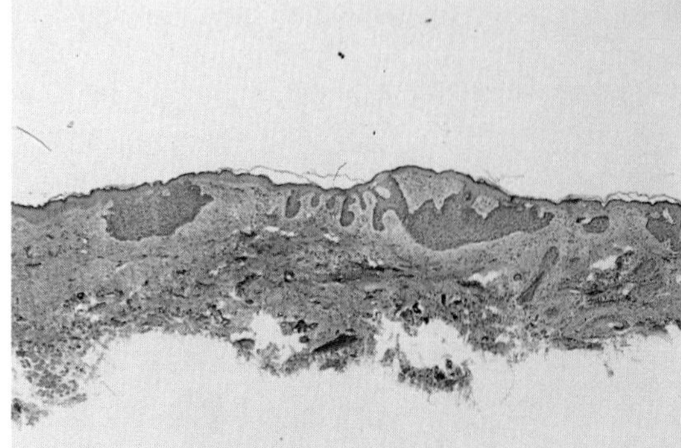

Figure 186–13. Basal cell carcinoma (multicentric or superficial type). Multicentric nests of basal cells extending into the superficial dermis. H&E, ×8.

Squamous Cell Carcinoma. Squamous cell carcinoma typically affects elderly fair-skinned individuals and is almost 40 times less common than eyelid basal cell carcinoma.[27] Squamous cell carcinoma may occur anywhere on the eyelid. However, a tumor of the upper eyelid and outer canthus is more commonly squamous cell carcinoma than basal cell carcinoma. Squamous cell carcinomas usually present as poorly demarcated indurated plaques or nodules that tend to ulcerate.

Squamous cell carcinomas arising in sun-damaged skin often begin with an early intraepidermal phase referred to as *solar, actinic,* or *senile keratosis.* Atypical cells, often bizarre and pleomorphic cells with numerous mitotic figures, eventually replace the full thickness of the epidermis (carcinoma in situ), after which invasion of the dermis occurs (squamous cell carcinoma) (Fig. 186–14). Abnormal keratinization is represented by dyskeratosis and horn pearls. Some atypical epidermal hyperplasias are not necessarily associated with actinic damage, and they, as well as squamous cell carcinoma, may arise de novo. Invasive squamous cell carcinoma is a potentially metastasizing lesion. However, lesions identified early have an excellent prognosis, and local excision is usually curative.

ADNEXAL TUMORS

Benign Sebaceous Gland Tumors

Sebaceous Hyperplasia. This tumor is a greatly enlarged sebaceous gland composed of numerous lobules grouped around a centrally located, wide follicular infundibulum or sebaceous duct. Sebaceous hyperplasia occurs on the face, forehead, cheeks, and eyelids in middle-aged persons and clinically presents as several elevated small, slightly umbilicated papules.

Sebaceous Adenoma. This tumor is a single yellow circumscribed nodule with a predilection for the eyebrow and eyelid. Histologically, it consists of differentiated sebaceous lobules, irregular in size and shape. Cords of benign basaloid cells characteristically divide areas of sebaceous proliferation.

Muir-Torres Syndrome. Patients with this syndrome have sebaceous tumors (hyperplasia, adenomas, and carcinomas) or keratoacanthomas of the eyelids associated with internal malignancy.[28–31]

Sebaceous Gland Carcinoma

Sebaceous gland carcinoma is the second most common malignancy of the eyelids,[32] accounting for 2 to 7 percent of all eyelid tumors and 1 to 5.5 percent of eyelid malignancies. Occurrence in sites other than eyelids is infrequent and exhibits a different clinical behavior.[33] Sebaceous gland carcinoma is observed most commonly in elderly women and in Asians. The preferred sites of involvement are the upper lid, brow, and caruncle.[33–38] Upper and lower lid involvement is common,[34, 39] and involvement of the contralateral eyelid has been reported.[37] The tumor has also been noted to arise in irradiated areas,[40] especially as a second malignancy after irradiation for retinoblastoma.[34, 39]

Sebaceous gland carcinoma may masquerade as less aggressive lesions such as unilateral blepharoconjunctivitis or recurring chalazion. Often misdiagnosed, it usually appears as a slowly enlarging firm yellow mass involving deep structures of the eyelid, causing ulceration only in a late stage.[33, 41, 42]

Histologically, the tumor commonly arises from the meibomian glands and is composed of basophilic cells with hyperchromatic nuclei, small centrally located nucleoli, and foamy cytoplasm with variable degrees of differentiation that stains positive for fat (Fig. 186–15). Sebaceous carcinoma has a strong tendency to spread along the epithelium (pagetoid spread), replacing its entire thickness and enabling it to invade any ocular surface covered by epithelium.[12, 37] The intraepithelial extension is also responsible for the blepharoconjunctivitis that presents months before the tumor is manifested.[38] Some investigators have reported a poorer prognosis in those patients exhibiting pagetoid spread,[43] and it has been postulated that this intraepithelial spread could be responsible for the characteristic multicentricity of the tumor.[44] The tumor also can spread by direct invasion. Four histologic patterns can be found: lobular pattern, with the cells forming well-delineated lobules; comedocarcinoma pattern, in which the lobules are variable in size and characterized by a prominent central necrotic area; papillary pattern, with neoplastic cells that form papillary projections and can mimic a squamous papilloma on the conjunctival surface; and mixed pattern, which can show any combination of patterns.

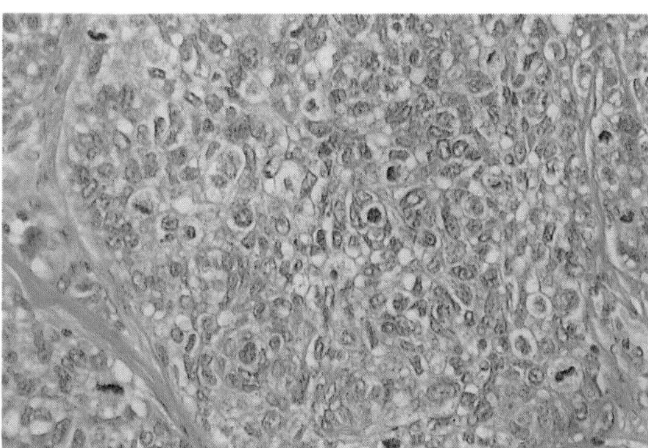

Figure 186–15. Sebaceous cell carcinoma. Basophilic cells with foamy cytoplasm, with hyperchromatic nuclei and numerous mitotic figures. H&E, ×50.

The biologic behavior of the tumor is aggressive, with local extension as well as lymphatic and hematogenous dissemination. Local recurrence is common.[33, 35, 45, 46]

Histologically, sebaceous carcinoma is often misdiagnosed.[38] In obtaining a biopsy sample of this tumor, it is important to preserve fresh tissue for frozen sections and stain for fat because the presence of intracytoplasmic lipid in the tumor cells is essential for the diagnosis. Early diagnosis and adequate treatment with primary wide excision decrease recurrences and improve the prognosis.

Benign Eccrine Gland Tumors

Syringoma. Syringoma is a common sweat gland tumor of the eyelid. It presents in women during puberty or later in life, usually as small skin-colored soft papules. The lesions are frequently numerous and limited to the lower lid. Histologically, syringoma represents an adenoma of intraepidermal eccrine ducts. The numerous small ducts are lined by two rows of cells embedded in a fibrous stroma, some of them with small comma-shaped or tadpole-like configurations. Among the ducts are solid cords of basophilic epithelial cells. Cystic ductal lumina may be filled with keratin.

Chondroid Syringoma (Mixed Tumor of Skin, Pleomorphic Adenoma). These lesions are firm intradermal or subcutaneous nodules that are commonly located on the head and neck and may involve the eyelids. Histologically, they are similar to the pleomorphic adenomas that originate in the lacrimal and salivary glands. The tumors are composed of tubular structures, showing marked variation in size, and are lined by two layers of epithelial cells embedded in an abundant mucoid stroma that may show areas of chondroid differentiation. Chondroid syringomas rarely become malignant, but recurrences from initial incomplete excision may exhibit malignant features.

Clear Cell Hidradenoma (Eccrine Acrospiroma, Clear Cell Myoepithelioma, Nodular Cell Hidradenoma). Clear cell hidradenoma is usually a solitary tumor that clinically appears as an intradermal tumor covered by intact skin. It can occur anywhere on the body, including the eyelids.[47, 47a] Histologically, the tumor is an encapsulated, lobulated mass of epithelial cells containing tubular lumina of variable size and cystic spaces containing eosinophilic material. In solid portions of the tumor, two cell types can be observed: One contains amphophilic cytoplasm with a round nucleus, and the other contains very clear cytoplasm filled with glycogen and a small, dark nucleus. The shapes of the cells vary from polyhedral to cuboidal to spindled. The percentage of clear cells may vary. Although clear cell hidradenomas are benign, malignant variants have been reported.[48]

Malignant Eccrine Gland Tumors

Malignant tumors of eccrine glands can arise in multiple recurrences of benign tumors or de novo. De novo tumors comprise the classic type of eccrine adenocarcinoma and mucinous carcinoma, among others. These lesions can arise anywhere, particularly in the head and neck area.

Eccrine Adenocarcinoma (Infiltrating Signet Ring Cell Carcinoma). This tumor is an unusual type of adnexal tumor involving the skin of the eyelid; it appears as a nodular indurated mass with diffuse infiltrating margins. Microscopic examination shows areas with fairly well-differentiated tubular structures near other undifferentiated areas not identifiable as eccrine sweat gland structure. The atypical cells infiltrate the surrounding tissues and extend into striated muscle. In many areas, the cells are arranged in an Indian-file pattern. Some cells contain single PAS-positive diastase-resistant vacuoles that give them the appearance of a signet ring. They are difficult to differentiate from a metastatic adenocarcinoma, grow slowly, frequently metastasize, show recurrences after excision, and tend to invade the orbit.[1, 49, 50]

Mucinous Adenocarcinoma. This tumor is the rarest type of eccrine carcinoma of the skin,[7] with a predilection for the eyelids of men in mid to late life.[51–56] Clinically, the lesion appears as an elevated nodule or a lobulated mass that is indurated or cystic. Histologic examination reveals large masses or cords of epithelial cells with small ductal structures lying in large pools of mucin separated by thin fibrovascular septa.

Mucinous adenocarcinomas seem to have a more favorable prognosis than other forms of sweat gland carcinomas, with less metastatic potential but a higher recurrence rate.[51] These tumors can be very aggressive locally by invasion of the orbit and adjacent structures.[51, 57]

Apocrine Gland Tumors

Apocrine Adenoma and Apocrine Adenocarcinoma. These extremely rare tumors of the eyelid originate from Moll's gland. Only a few cases of apocrine adenocarcinoma have been reported.[57a, 58, 59] Histologically, the adenoma reveals lobules of mature apocrine cells with central decapitation secretion, often manifested as amorphous material present in the lumen. Well-differentiated apocrine carcinomas resemble the adenoma but also exhibit nuclear pleomorphism and mitoses in the eosinophilic cells. Less well-differentiated apocrine carcinomas almost invariably retain the eosinophilic quality of the apocrine cell but show marked pleomorphism and numerous mitotic figures.

Syringocystadenoma Papilliferum. This tumor represents a proliferation of apocrine gland structures that clinically present as hyperkeratotic or verrucous papules with intermittent discharge, arising de novo or in nevus sebaceous. Histologically, the lesion is characterized by fronds of papillary dermis covered by a double cell lining, the basilar cell being cuboidal in shape and the surface cell having a rectangular appearance topped by decapitation secretion. These structures jut into a cystic space, which may be covered by a hyperkeratotic crust. Numerous plasma cells characteristically infiltrate the stroma.

Oncocytoma. These uncommon tumors arise from the ductal cells of glandular structures and consist of ductal epithelial cells growing in nests with lumina of various sizes. The cells show intense eosinophilia, which on electron microscopic examination is attributed to hypertrophy of the endoplasmic reticulum and accumulation of secretory products and filaments. Atypical mitochondria have also been reported. These lesions occur in the caruncle, lacrimal sac, lacrimal gland, and accessory lacrimal glands of the conjunctiva.[60–62] Only three cases have been reported in the eyelids, and only one of them had a demonstrated origin in Moll's gland.[62–64]

Tumors of Hair Follicle Origin

Benign eyelid tumors of hair follicle origin are uncommon and often misdiagnosed as basal cell carcinoma.[65]

Trichoepithelioma. These tumors present clinically as firm, elevated, skin-colored nodules (solitary or multiple) and tend to involve the face. Microscopically, the characteristic findings are the presence of multiple horn cysts containing keratin surrounded by proliferating basaloid cells in the dermis. Foci of cystic rupture with foreign body giant cell response and calcification are often present. The tumor is surrounded by dense stroma that separates the proliferating cells from the adjacent dermis. This stromal proliferation is distinctly different from basal cell carcinoma, in which the tumor islands infiltrate the normal dermal structures.

Trichofolliculoma. This lesion presents clinically as an asymptomatic, slow-growing, small solitary nodule with a central area of umbilication, representing the aperture of a keratin-filled dilated follicle. Microscopically, a large dilated follicular infundibulum containing keratin and hair-shaft fragments is surrounded by small hair follicles.

Trichilemmoma. Trichilemmoma appears as a small, solitary, slow-growing nodule in middle-aged individuals. It is usually located on the face, most commonly on the nose, followed by the eyelids. Histopathologically, the cells arise from the glycogen-rich outer layer of the hair sheath. They proliferate in lobulated masses and show peripheral palisading overlying a well-developed hyalinized basement membrane. Hair follicles may be present in the lesion. Multiple facial trichilemmomas are a manifestation of Cowden's disease, a disorder associated with multiple hamartomas and breast carcinoma.[66]

Pilomatrixoma (Calcifying Epithelioma of Malherbe). Clinically, this lesion presents as a solitary flesh-colored nodule covered by normal skin. It may be cystic or rock hard on palpation. Most of the lesions appear on the face and upper extremities in young individuals. The upper lid and eyebrow are common sites. Microscopically, the tumor is located in the dermis and is composed of irregular epithelial islands containing basophilic cells (peripheral) and shadow cells (central). Areas of dystrophic calcification are frequently present. Rupture of the lesions is associated with prominent foreign body response.

VASCULAR TUMORS

Capillary Hemangioma

Capillary hemangioma, the most common form of congenital vascular tumor of the eyelid, is a benign condition that appears during the first few weeks of life. Clinically, this lesion is purple-red and elevated, with an irregular surface. Microscopically, the lesions consist of capillaries with a single layer of endothelial cells surrounded by prominent pericytes. Lobules of capillary proliferation are delimited by fibrous septa. Malignant degeneration does not occur. Because most of these lesions involute before the end of the first decade, therapeutic intervention is not usually required.

Cavernous Hemangioma

In contrast to capillary hemangiomas, cavernous hemangiomas appear later in life, tend not to involute, and may require surgical intervention. Clinically, the lesions are blue and may be located deeper than capillary hemangiomas. Histologically, they consist of large vascular channels lined by endothelium, with prominent thick fibrous walls. The presence of smooth muscle cells in these walls always suggests the possibility of a vascular malformation.

Pyogenic Granuloma

The most common acquired vascular lesion of the eyelid is pyogenic granuloma, which usually occurs in response to minor trauma or surgery or in association with chalazion.[67] It appears clinically as a pedunculated reddish mass that grows quickly and tends to bleed easily. Histologically, this tumor is a mass of granulation tissue with prominent capillary proliferation, surface ulceration, and acute inflammation (Fig. 186–16). Local excision is usually curative.

Lymphangioma

Lymphangioma appears as an isolated compressible gray nodule limited to the eyelid or associated with an orbital component. These lesions may be congenital or appear later in life and may become prominent when hemorrhage occurs into the lesion. Histologic findings usually include dilated thin-walled vascular spaces demarcated by endothelial cells and filled with a clear eosinophilic fluid. Valves can be observed in lymphatic channels as delicate thin-walled structures protruding into the lumina.

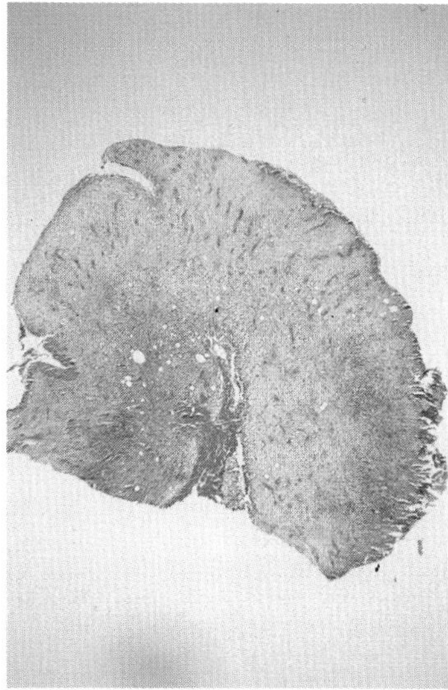

Figure 186–16. Pyogenic granuloma arising from chalazion. Mass of granulation tissue with capillary proliferation, growing around a focus of lipogranulomatous inflammation. H&E, ×2.5.

Kaposi's Sarcoma

Four types of Kaposi's sarcoma have been described.[7] The African or endemic type occurs in children in central to southern Africa. The allograft-associated type was first noted among renal transplant recipients. The epidemic form was first described in the late 1970s among persons with AIDS. Before identification of the epidemic type, the most common form of Kaposi's sarcoma in the United States was found among elderly people, predominantly men of eastern or southern European extraction.[7]

Clinically, Kaposi's sarcoma appears as blue-red or dark-brown plaques and nodules that undergo ulceration in late stages. Kaposi's sarcoma of the skin is seen as an initial presentation in about 30 percent of patients with AIDS.[68] Sixteen percent of patients with AIDS and Kaposi's sarcoma have eyelid involvement.[69] Conjunctival presentation may resemble a hemangioma or a vascular malformation. Seen histologically are neoplastic proliferations of blood vessels, with a predominance of endothelial cells and spindle-cell formations containing vascular slits. Mitoses are common. Red blood cells are noted as cuboidal in shape and in linear or "boxcar" array in the vascular slits. Erythrophagocytosis by tumor cells is common. Hemosiderin deposition is variable. When an inflammatory reaction is present, the lesions can be difficult to differentiate from a pyogenic granuloma.

XANTHELASMA

Xanthelasma is a common lesion that occurs most frequently at the medial aspects of the upper and lower eyelids in middle-aged persons. The lesions are often

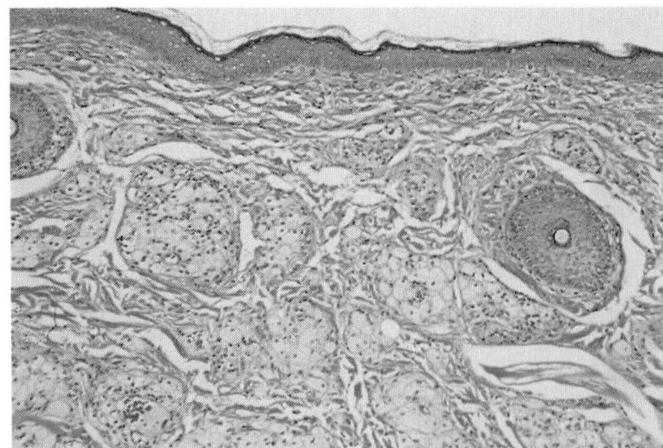

Figure 186–17. Xanthelasma. Clusters of foamy histiocytes containing lipid material in the superficial dermis. H&E, ×32.

bilateral and appear as flat, yellowish soft plaques. Histologically, they are composed of clusters of foamy histiocytes in the superficial dermis; they contain lipid material (Fig. 186–17) and are usually arranged around blood vessels. They commonly occur in persons with normal serum cholesterol levels but can also be associated with elevated levels in about a third of patients. Lesions similar to xanthelasma appear in Erdheim-Chester disease, a multifocal lipogranulomatous condition involving viscera and bones.[70]

MELANOCYTIC DISORDERS AND TUMORS

Melanocytes are dendritic cells originating in the neural crest. After migration from the neural crest, melanocytes localize in the basal layers of the epidermis. On routine histologic sections, melanocytes are seen as cells with elongated nuclei surrounded by a clear space. They produce and secrete melanin, which is transferred through the dendritic process to the neighboring basal and hair follicle cells.[71] Not all melanocytes reach the epidermis during migration; some remain in the dermis, giving rise to dermal melanocytes.

Benign

Benign disorders and tumors composed of epidermal melanocytes include freckles and lentigines; benign tumors derived from dermal melanocytes include mongolian spots, nevus of Ota, nevus of Ito, and blue nevus. Nevus cells or nevomelanocytes are identical to melanocytes but differ in morphologic features, including their arrangement in clusters or "nests," their larger size, and apparent absence of dendrites.[72] Benign tumors composed of nevus cells are called *melanocytic* or *nevocellular nevi.*

Ephelis (Freckle). Ephelides first appear clinically in early childhood as tan-brown macules on sun-exposed skin. Freckles darken and increase in number and size during the summer and lighten in winter. Histologically, the number of melanocytes is normal,[73] but increased melanin is noted in the basal keratinocytes.

Lentigo. Lentigo simplex appears as a dark-brown, often oval macule on sun-protected skin as well as on the palms, soles, and mucous membranes. Solar lentigines are the most common epidermal melanocytic lesions and appear as flat brown macules on sun-exposed skin.[74] Histologic study reveals elongation of the rete ridges, an increased number of melanocytes, and increased melanin in melanocytes and basal keratinocytes.

Nevocellular Nevus. Polygonal nevus cells constitute the primary pathology in this lesion. In acquired lesions, these cells have been categorized into types A, B, and C. Type A is elongated with short, stubby dendrites extending from a cytoplasm exhibiting coarse melanin granules. Type B cells comprise the polygonal to cuboidal cells of the superficial papillary dermal component of the nevus (Fig. 186–18). Their nuclei are usually round and have dotlike nucleoli. These cells may appear in sheets or nests. When in nests, a delicate fibroblast-like cell encloses the cell aggregate. Type C cells are at the base of the type B cells, usually where the nevomelanocytes abut the papillary-reticular dermal junction. They are elongated and fibroblast-like, are associated with a delicate reticulin stroma, and often show mast cell hyperplasia. Nests of type A cells restricted to the lower part of the epidermis form a junctional nevus. In compound nevi, intraepidermal and dermal nevus cell nests with a stromal proliferative reaction are often observed. Dermal nevi show nests and cords of nevus cells in the dermis (see Fig. 186–13).

Congenital melanocytic nevi may have any of the previously described patterns seen in acquired nevocellular nevi and may have one or all of the following histologic arrangements: Nevus cells are seen in a single-cell array between collagen bundles and deep in the lower dermis and subcutis. They may be seen in sebaceous glands, arrector pili muscle bundles, hair follicles, eccrine glands, ducts and nerves,[75] and even in subendothelial deposits in medium-sized arteries and veins.

Blue Nevus. These nevi appear as solitary dome-shaped, smooth blue-black papules. Two histologic types are identified; in both, the epidermis is uninvolved. The common blue nevus is characterized by melanin-filled, spindle-shaped, bipolar dendritic melanocytes irregularly dispersed in the reticular dermis with various degrees of concomitant dermal fibrosis (Fig. 186–19).[76]

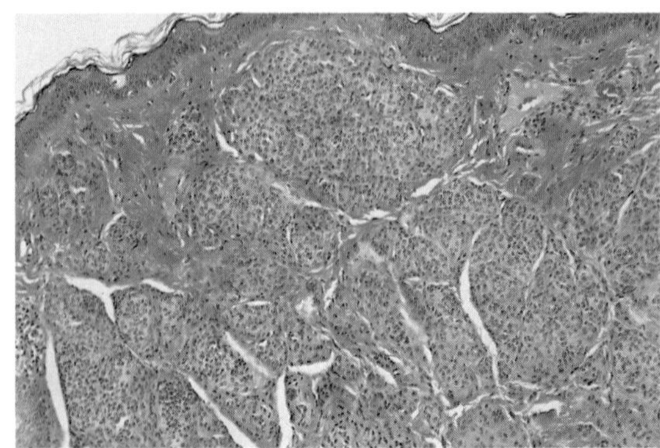

Figure 186–18. Dermal nevus. Polygonal nevus cells are arranged in nets in the dermis. H&E, ×32.

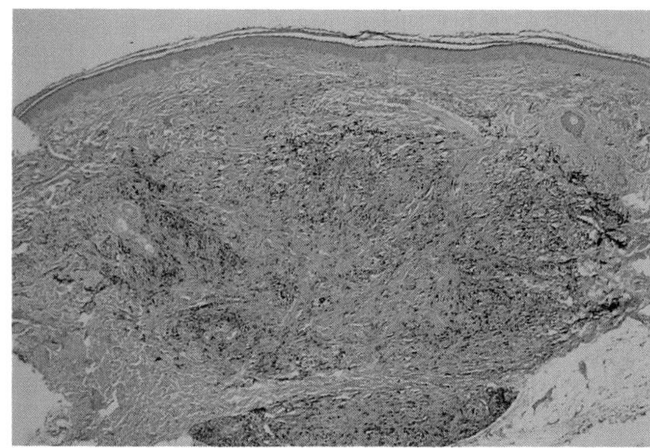

Figure 186–19. Blue nevus. Melanin-filled, spindle-shaped dendritic melanocytes are prominently dispersed in the dermis. H&E, ×10.

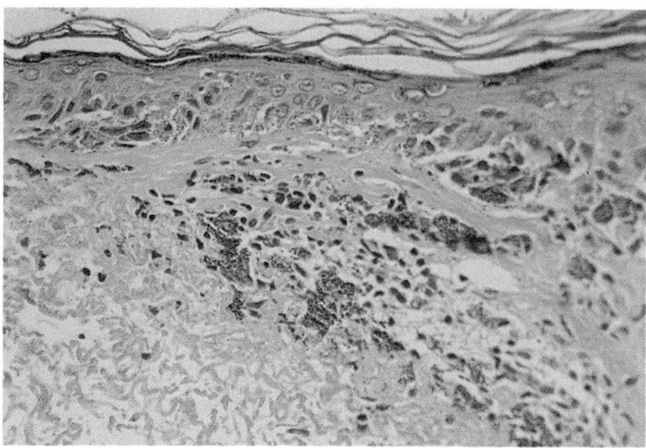

Figure 186–20. Lentigo maligna. Atypical melanocytes with variations in cellular and nuclear size and shape are noted in the lower epidermis. H&E, ×40.

Cellular blue nevi, in addition to having areas identical to those of common blue nevi, have sparsely pigmented clear islands of melanocytes with oval to spindle-shaped nuclei.[76] Although extremely rare, malignant degeneration of blue nevi has been reported.[77]

Nevus of Ota. Clinically, this lesion is a unilateral bluish-gray macular discoloration affecting the periorbital facial skin and occasionally the ipsilateral sclera of the eye.[78] The onset has two peaks: in early childhood and in the teenage years.[79] The primary histopathologic changes are in the upper and middermis, in which fusiform, bipolar, dendritic, heavily-pigmented melanocytes are dispersed. The long axis of these cells is parallel to the skin surface, except around adnexal structures, where the orientation is vertical.[78]

Malignant

Malignant melanocytic tumors include the four major subtypes of cutaneous malignant melanomas—namely, lentigo maligna melanoma, acral lentiginous melanoma, superficial spreading melanoma, and nodular melanoma. In addition, several well-characterized but rare variants of malignant melanoma are recognized, including desmoplastic and neurotropic melanoma,[80, 81] amelanotic melanoma,[82] minimal deviation and borderline melanoma,[83] pedunculated melanoma,[84] balloon cell melanoma,[85] and malignant blue nevus.[77]

Lentigo Maligna and Lentigo Maligna Melanoma. Lentigo maligna melanoma and its preinvasive phase (lentigo maligna) (Fig. 186–20) invariably occur on the face and neck. Lentigo maligna appears as an irregular flat tan-brown patch ranging in size from a few millimeters to several centimeters. The development of a papular darker component usually coincides with the histologic findings of invasion. Initially, melanocytes are only slightly increased in number and appear round, in time followed by diffuse basal proliferation of atypical melanocytes.[86] The histologic spectrum of lentigo maligna varies from a few dispersed atypical melanocytes (corresponding to the clinical tan areas) to large accumulations of normal and abnormal melanocytes in the epidermis in cords, strips, and nests (corresponding to the clinical "flat back" areas).[87] Pleomorphic forms are present with variations in the size and shape of the cells and their nuclei. Multinucleated cells with hyperchromatic nuclei may be present. In lentigo maligna melanoma, the papillary dermis is invaded, and the clinical finding of surface irregularity corresponds to accumulation of a mixture of malignant melanocytes, inflammatory cells, and melanophages in the dermis.[88]

Superficial Spreading Malignant Melanoma. This represents the most common type of malignant melanoma. It appears clinically as a papule or plaque with irregular shades of color including brown, black, gray, white, and even blue. The average size is 2.5 cm, and the trunk and upper extremities are most commonly affected. Histologically, large and usually round, so-called epithelioid, cells are characteristically scattered asymmetrically throughout the epidermis (pagetoid upward migration) (Fig. 186–21).[89] These cells have abundant cytoplasm, finely divided pigment, and large hyperchromatic nuclei. In addition, single-cell infiltration of the papillary dermis occurs, and a marked lymphocytic infiltrate is usually noted in the papillary dermis. As such, the melanoma is identified as being in its radial growth phase and is completely curable by surgical excision. An expansile nodule eventually forms in the papillary dermis, heralding the vertical growth phase and marking the lesion as having metastatic potential.

Nodular Melanoma. This type of malignant melanoma lacks the radial growth phase or extensive intraepider-

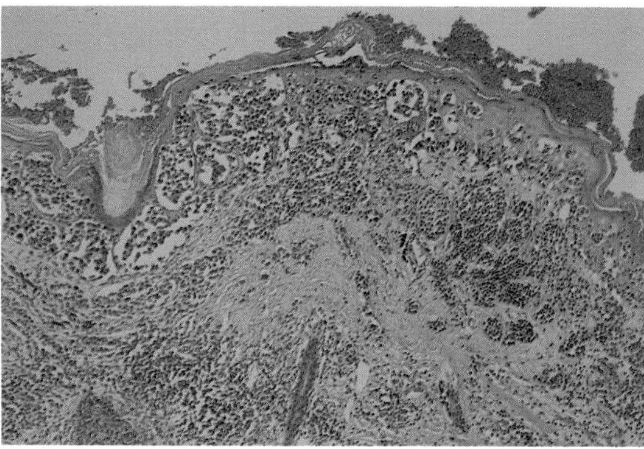

Figure 186–21. Superficial spreading malignant melanoma. Large and atypical melanocytes with hyperchromatic nuclei are scattered through the epidermis. The papillary dermis is infiltrated by similar looking epithelioid cells surrounded by a lymphocytic infiltrate. H&E, ×25.

mal proliferative component characteristic of superficial spreading melanoma. Instead, it represents a pure vertical growth phase disease. The tumor proceeds from an intraepidermal focus to a small, expansile nodule in the papillary dermis that rapidly invades deeper portions. The cells may appear as epithelioid, spindle, nevus-like, or mixed.

Tumor thickness is the single most important factor in predicting survival rates of patients with cutaneous malignant melanoma lacking regional lymph node involvement. The thickness is gauged by measuring the depth of tumor infiltration from the top of the granular layer in the epidermis to the deepest point of penetration of the melanoma.[90] In mucosa, lacking a granular cell layer, the measurement is made from the top of the keratinizing layer to the deepest tumor cell. By convention, when ulceration is present, the measurement is made from the base of the ulcer to the lowest depth of the tumor.[90a]

The anatomic level[88] is identified according to anatomic landmarks in the skin: Level I, all tumor cells are above the basement membrane and confined to the epidermis; level II, the neoplastic cells have broken through the basement membrane and are in the papillary dermis, impinging on the upper part of the reticular dermis; level III, the tumor fills the papillary dermis and reaches the interface between the papillary and reticular dermis; level IV, the tumor penetrates the reticular dermis; and level V, the tumor invades the subcutaneous tissue.[88] In the mucosa, where there is no papillary dermis, the anatomic levels are not applicable.

Clark and colleagues identified six independently significant prognostic factors: mitotic rate per square millimeter, tumor-infiltrating lymphocytes, tumor thickness, anatomic site of the primary melanoma, sex of the patient, and histologic regression.[91]

EYELID MANIFESTATIONS OF SYSTEMIC DISEASE

Systemic diseases often present with cutaneous manifestations. Connective tissue diseases and metabolic disorders are among the most common systemic diseases exhibiting eyelid pathology.

Connective Tissue Diseases

Lupus Erythematosus. Cutaneous lupus erythematosus involves the face in 80 to 90 percent of cases.[92] Lesions may include malar erythema, chronic discoid lesions,[93] nonscarring alopecia, and facial swelling.[94] The discoid lesions are classically well demarcated and atrophic and show telangiectasias, follicular plugging, and hypo- or hyperpigmentation. Histologic findings include hyperkeratosis, hyperkeratotic invaginations into the epidermis, epidermal atrophy, vacuolation along the dermal-epidermal junction with thickening of the basement membrane, and a predominantly perivascular and periappendageal lymphocytic infiltrate.

Dermatomyositis. Cutaneous findings include the "heliotrope" eruption (blue-purple discoloration of the upper eyelid), Gottron's sign (erythema over the knuckles), or Gottron's rash (violaceous papular scaly eruption on the knuckles).[95] The epidermis may be atrophic or normal. Dermal edema with mucin deposition is prominent, and a scant superficial perivenular lymphohistocytic infiltrate is often present. However, the histology may be indistinguishable from lupus erythematosus.

Scleroderma. Systemic scleroderma is a generalized disease involving the skin and other connective tissue–containing organs.[96] A localized cutaneous form of scleroderma, known as *morphea,* may occur. In scleroderma, the skin appears thickened and bound down. Eyelid changes related to scleroderma include stiffness or tightness of the skin and telangiectasia.[97] A violaceous border is often seen around active localized skin lesions. Histologic findings include an atrophic epidermis and thickening of the papillary and reticular dermis with hyalinization of the collagen fibers.[98] The fibrotic process begins at the junction of the dermis and subcutaneous fat, where a linear pattern of collagen deposition may be observed. The affected dermis is hypocellular.

Metabolic Diseases

Amyloidosis. Cutaneous findings in systemic amyloidosis include petechiae and ecchymoses due to infiltration of blood vessels by amyloid. Purpura of the eyelids resulting from rubbing is a frequent and almost diagnostic sign. Other skin findings include smooth, shiny papules, nodules, or plaques distributed in flexural areas, including the eyelids.[99] Localized cutaneous amyloidosis may present as single or multiple nodules (nodular amyloidosis), a pruritic eruption of brown macules on the back and extremities (macular amyloidosis), or persistent, pruritic, hyperkeratotic, discrete papules on the shins (lichen amyloidosus).[99] Histologically, amorphous, often fissured, hyalinized eosinophilic material is present and confined to the papillary dermis in papular lesions. Nodular amyloidosis shows deposition of amyloid in the reticular dermis and even as deep as the subcutis.

Lipoid Proteinosis. This autosomal recessive disorder is characterized by widespread deposition of hyaline material in the skin, oral mucosa, and larynx. Papules, nodules, and infiltrated plaques are noted on the face and extremities. A characteristic finding is waxlike beaded papules along the free margins of the eyelids, which on histologic study reveal hyperkeratosis, acanthosis, and large amounts of an eosinophilic hyaline material replacing the papillary dermis, devoid of significant inflammation. Blood vessel walls are thickened owing to deposition of similar material within and around the basement membrane.[100]

Hemochromatosis. In idiopathic hemochromatosis, 80 percent of patients have cutaneous pigmentation; of these, almost 25 percent show involvement of the eyelids.[101] Histologically, increased melanin is noted in the epidermal basal cell layer; hemosiderin may sometimes be demonstrated extracellularly and within macrophages.[101]

EYELID MANIFESTATIONS OF DERMATOLOGIC DISEASES

As part of the integument, eyelids frequently exhibit the clinical and histologic findings of diseases that predominantly affect the skin. The list of dermatologic diseases with eyelid manifestations would essentially include almost all cutaneous disorders. We have limited the discussion in this section to two disorders with prominent eyelid involvement.

Psoriasis

Psoriasis is a chronic disease manifested by well-demarcated erythematous plaques with overlying silvery scales, characteristically localized to extensor surfaces and sites of trauma. Psoriasis affecting the eyelids may appear as sharply demarcated plaques 1 or 2 cm in diameter. In affected patients, however, trauma can result in lesional development (Koebner's phenomenon). Patients who rub their eyes may have circumferential involvement of the eye, encompassing both lids. Histologic study of fully developed lesions shows parakeratosis with an admixture of neutrophils (Munro's microabscess), hypogranulosis, regular epidermal hyperplasia, occasional spongiform epidermal accumulations of neutrophils, and elongation of the dermal papillae, with thinning of the suprapapillary plates.

Contact Dermatitis

Contact dermatitis, a form of cutaneous inflammation induced by response to a specific sensitizing agent, is believed to be the most common eruption affecting the eyelids and accounts for over 60 percent of eyelid dermatitides.[102] Other cases of eyelid dermatitis may be related to underlying cutaneous disorders such as atopic dermatitis or seborrheic dermatitis. Histologic study of contact dermatitis reveals hyperkeratosis, epidermal hyperplasia, a variable degree of epidermal spongiosis, and a mild to moderate superficial perivascular inflammatory infiltrate containing predominately lymphocytes admixed with eosinophils.

REFERENCES

1. Font RL: Eyelids and lacrimal drainage system. *In* Spencer WH (ed): Ophthalmic Pathology, vol. 3. Philadelphia, WB Saunders, 1986, pp 2141–2336.
2. Steffen C, Markman JA: Spontaneous disappearance of molluscum contagiosum. Arch Dermatol 116:923, 1980.
3. Redfield RR, James WP, Wright DC, et al: Severe molluscum contagiosum in a patient with human T-lymphothropic (HTL-III) disease. J Am Acad Dermatol 13:821, 1985.
4. Shelley WB, Wood MG: Transformation of the common wart into squamous cell carcinoma in a patient with primary lymphedema. Cancer 48:820, 1981.
5. Goette DK: Carcinoma in situ in verruca vulgaris. Int J Dermatol 19:98, 1980.
6. Berman A, Winkelmann RK: Involuting common warts. J Am Acad Dermatol 3:356, 1980.
7. Lever WF, Schaumburg-Lever G: Histopathology of the Skin, 7th ed. Philadelphia, JB Lippincott, 1990.
8. Yanoff M, Fine B: Ocular Pathology. Philadelphia, JB Lippincott, 1989.
9. Jakobiec FA: Tumors of the lids. *In* Anderson RL, Blodi FC, Boniuk M, et al (eds): Symposium on Diseases and Surgery of the Lids, Lacrimal Apparatus and Orbit. Transactions of the New Orleans Academy of Ophthalmology. St. Louis, CV Mosby, 1982, pp 265–307.
10. Sacks E, Jakobiec FA, McMillan R: Multiple bilateral apocrine cystadenomas of the lower lids. Ophthalmology 94:65, 1987.
11. Langer K, Konrad K, Smolle J: Multiple apocrine hidrocystomas on the eyelids. Am J Dermatopathol 11:570, 1989.
12. Font RL, Stone MS, Schanzer MC, et al: Apocrine hidrocystomas of the lids, hypodontia, palmar-plantar hyperkeratosis and onchodystrophy: A new variant of ectodermal dysplasia. Arch Ophthalmol 104:1811, 1986.
13. Ni C, Merriam J, Albert DM: Irritated seborrheic keratosis of eyelids and its differential. Chin Med J 101:555, 1988.
14. Boniuk M, Zimmerman LE: Eyelid tumors with reference to lesions confused with squamous cell carcinoma. II: Inverted follicular keratosis. Arch Ophthalmol 69:698, 1963.
15. Schweitzer JG, Yanoff M: Inverted follicular keratosis: A report of two current cases. Ophthalmology 94:1465, 1987.
16. Lever WF: Inverted follicular keratosis as an irritated seborrheic keratosis. Am J Dermatopathol 5:474, 1983.
17. Winer LH: Pseudoepitheliomatous hyperplasia. Arch Dermatol Syphilol 42:856, 1940.
18. Lund HZ: How often does squamous cell carcinoma of the skin metastasize? Arch Dermatol 92:635, 1965.
19. Moller R, Reymann F, Hou-Jensen K: Metastases in dermatological patients with squamous cell carcinoma. Arch Dermatol 115:703, 1979.
20. Gaasterland DE, Rodrigues MM, Moshell AN: Ocular involvement in xeroderma pigmentosum. Ophthalmology 89:980, 1982.
21. Kraemer KH, Lee MM, Scotto J: Xeroderma pigmentosum. Arch Dermatol 123:241, 1987.
22. Loeffler M, Hornblass A: Characteristics and behavior of eyelid carcinoma (basal cell, squamous cell, sebaceous gland and malignant melanoma). Ophthalmic Surg 21:513, 1990.
23. Borel DM: Cutaneous basosquamous carcinoma: Review of the literature and report of 3 cases. Arch Pathol 95:293, 1973.
24. Resnick KI, Sadun A, Albert DM: Basal cell epithelioma: An unusual case. Ophthalmology 88:1182, 1981.
25. Doxanas MT, Green WR, Iliff CE: Basal cell carcinoma. Am J Ophthalmol 91:726, 1981.
26. Feman S, Apt L, Roth A: The basal nevus syndrome. Am J Ophthalmol 78:222, 1974.
27. Kwitko ML, Boniuk M, Zimmerman LE: Eyelids tumors with reference to lesions confused with squamous cell carcinoma. I: Incidence and errors in diagnosis. Arch Ophthalmol 69:693, 1963.
28. Graham R, McKee P, McGibbon D, et al: Torre-Muir syndrome: An association with isolated sebaceous carcinoma. Cancer 55:2868, 1985.
29. Fahmy A, Burgdorf WHC, Schoosser RH: Muir-Torre syndrome: Report of a case and reevaluation of the dermatopathologic features. Cancer 49:1898, 1982.
30. Tillawi I, Katz R, Pelletiere EV: Solitary tumors of meibomian gland origin and Torre's syndrome. Am J Ophthalmol 104:179, 1987.
31. Jakobiec FA, Zimmerman LE, La Piana F, et al: Unusual eyelid tumors with sebaceous differentiation in the Muir-Torre syndrome. Ophthalmology 95:1543, 1988.
32. Rao NA, Hidayat AA, McLean JW, et al: Sebaceous carcinomas of the ocular adnexa: A clinicopathologic study of 104 cases with five-year follow-up data. Hum Pathol 13:113, 1982.
33. Kass LG, Hornblass A: Sebaceous carcinoma of the ocular adnexa. Surv Ophthalmol 33:477, 1989.
34. Boniuk M, Zimmerman LE: Sebaceous carcinoma of the eyelid, eyebrow, caruncle and orbit. Trans Am Acad Ophthalmol Otolaryngol 72:619, 1968.
35. Ni C, Searl SS, Kuo PK, et al: Sebaceous cell carcinomas of the ocular adnexa. Int Ophthalmol Clin 22:23, 1982.
36. Epstein GA, Putterman AM: Sebaceous adenocarcinoma of the eyelid. Ophthalmic Surg 14:935, 1983.
37. Wolfe JT, Yeatts RP, Wick MR, et al: Sebaceous carcinoma of

the eyelid: Errors in clinical and pathologic diagnosis. Am J Surg Pathol 8:597, 1984.
38. Doxanas MT, Green WR: Sebaceous gland carcinoma: Review of 40 cases. Arch Ophthalmol 102:245, 1984.
39. Lemos KB, Santa Cruz DJ, Baba N: Sebaceous carcinoma of the eyelid following radiation therapy. Am J Surg Pathol 7:305, 1978.
40. Schlernitzaur DA, Font RL: Sebaceous gland carcinoma of the eyelid following radiation therapy for cavernous hemangioma of the face. Arch Ophthalmol 94:1523, 1976.
41. Wagoner MD, Beyer CK, Gonder JR, et al: Common presentations of sebaceous gland carcinoma. Ann Ophthalmol 14:159, 1982.
42. Condon GP, Brownstein S, Codere F: Sebaceous carcinoma of the eyelid masquerading as superior limbic keratoconjunctivitis. Arch Ophthalmol 103:1525, 1985.
43. Russell WG, Page DL, Hough AJ, et al: Sebaceous carcinoma of meibomian gland origin. Am J Clin Pathol 73:504, 1980.
44. Jakobiec FA: Sebaceous carcinoma of the adnexa: Ongoing challenges. Zimmerman Lecture. American Academy of Ophthalmology Annual Meeting, Atlanta, November 1990.
45. Nunery WR, Welsh MG, McCord CD: Recurrence of sebaceous carcinoma of the eyelid after radiation therapy. Am J Ophthalmol 96:10, 1983.
46. Folberg R, Whitaker DC, Tse DT, et al: Recurrent and residual sebaceous carcinoma after Mohs' excision of the primary lesion. Am J Ophthalmol 103:817, 1987.
47. Ferry AP, Haddad HM: Eccrine acrospiroma (porosyringoma) of the eyelid. Arch Ophthalmol 83:591, 1970.
47a. Grossniklaus HE, Knight SH: Eccrine acrospiroma (clear cell hidradenoma) of the eyelid: Immunohistochemical and ultrastructural features. Ophthalmology 98:347, 1991.
48. Headington JT, Niederhuber JE, Beals T: Malignant clear cell acrospiroma. Cancer 41:641, 1978.
49. Grizzard WS, Torczynski E, Edwards WC: Adenocarcinoma of eccrine sweat glands. Arch Ophthalmol 94:2119, 1976.
50. Jakobiec FA, Austin P, Iwamoto T, et al: Primary infiltrating signet-ring carcinoma of the eyelids. Ophthalmology 90:291, 1983.
51. Wright JD, Font RL: Mucinous sweat gland adenocarcinoma of the eyelid. Cancer 44:1757, 1979.
52. Cohen KL, Peiffer RL, Lipper S: Mucinous sweat gland adenocarcinoma of the eyelid. Am J Ophthalmol 92:183, 1981.
53. Lahav M, Albert DM, Bahr R, et al: Eyelid tumors of sweat gland origin. Graefes Arch Clin Exp Ophthalmol 216:301, 1981.
54. Boi S, De Concini M, Detassis C: Mucinous sweat-gland adenocarcinoma of the inner canthus: A case report. Ann Ophthalmol 20:189, 1988.
55. Sanke RF: Primary mucinous adenocarcinoma of the eyelid. Ophthalmic Surg 20:668, 1989.
56. Shuster AR, Maskin SL: Primary mucinous sweat gland carcinoma of the eyelid. Ophthalmic Surg 20:808, 1989.
57. Hold JB, Haines JH, Mamalis N, et al: Mucinous adenocarcinoma of the orbit arising from a stable benign-appearing eyelid nodule. Ophthalmic Surg 21:163, 1990.
57a. Netland PA, Towsend DJ, Albert DM, Jakobiec FA: Hidradenoma papilliferum of the upper eyelid arising from the apocrine gland of Moll. Ophthalmology 97:1593, 1990.
58. Aurora AL, Luxenberg MN: Case report of adenocarcinoma of gland of Moll. Am J Ophthalmol 70:984, 1970.
59. Ni C, Wagoner M, Kieval S, et al: Tumors of the Moll's glands. Br J Ophthalmol 68:502, 1984.
60. Deustch AR, Duckworth JK: Oncocytoma (oxyphilic adenoma) of the caruncle. Am J Ophthalmol 64:459, 1967.
61. Lamping KA, Albert DM, Ni C, et al: Oxyphil cell adenoma: Three case reports. Arch Ophthalmol 102:263, 1984.
62. Biggs SL, Font RL: Oncocytic lesions of the caruncule and other ocular adnexa. Arch Ophthalmol 95:474, 1977.
63. Thaller VT, Collin JR, McCartney AC: Oncocytoma of the eyelid: A case report. Br J Ophthalmol 71:753, 1987.
64. Rodgers IR, Jakobiec FA, Krebs W, et al: Papillary oncocytoma of the eyelid: A previously undescribed tumor of apocrine gland origin. Ophthalmology 95:1071, 1988.
65. Simpson W, Garner A, Collin JR: Benign hair-follicle derived tumors in the differential diagnosis of basal cell carcinoma of the eyelids: A clinicopathological comparison. Br J Ophthalmol 73:347, 1989.
66. Bardenstein DS, McLean IW, Nerney J, et al: Cowden's disease. Ophthalmology 95:1038, 1988.
67. Ferry A: Pyogenic granulomas of the eye and ocular adnexa: A study of 100 cases. Trans Am Ophthalmol Soc 87:327, 1989.
68. Safai B, Johnson KG, Myskowski PL, et al: The natural history of Kaposi's sarcoma in the acquired immunodeficiency syndrome. Ann Intern Med 103:744, 1983.
69. Shuler JD, Holland GN, Miles SA, et al: Kaposi sarcoma of the conjunctiva and eyelids associated with the acquired immunodeficiency syndrome. Arch Ophthalmol 107:858, 1989.
70. Alper MG, Zimmerman LE, LaPiana FG: Orbital manifestations of Erdheim-Chester disease. Trans Am Ophthalmol Soc 81:64, 1983.
71. Urmacher C: Histology of normal skin. Am J Surg Pathol 14:671, 1990.
72. Gottlieb B, Brown AL, Winkelmann RK: Fine structure of the nevus cell. Arch Dermatol 92:81, 1965.
73. Breathnach AS: Melanocyte distribution in forearm epidermis. J Invest Dermatol 29:253, 1957.
74. Rhodes AR: Pigmented birthmarks and precursor melanocytic lesions of cutaneous melanoma identifiable in childhood. Pediatr Clin North Am 30:345, 1983.
75. Rhodes AR, Silverman RA, Harrist TJ, et al: Histologic comparison of congenital and acquired nevomelanocytic nevi. Arch Dermatol 121:1266, 1985.
76. Dorsey CS, Montgomery H: Blue nevus and its distinction from Mongolian spot and nevus of Ota. J Invest Dermatol 19:712, 1954.
77. Goldenhersh MA, Savin RC, Barnhill RL, et al: Malignant blue nevus: Case report and literature review. J Am Acad Dermatol 19:712, 1988.
78. Kopf AW, Weidman AI: Nevus of Ota. Arch Dermatol 85:195, 1962.
79. Hidano A, Kajima H, Ikeda S, et al: Natural history of nevus of Ota. Arch Dermatol 95:187, 1967.
80. Conley J, Lattes R, Orr W: Desmoplastic malignant melanoma (a rare variant of spindle cell melanoma). Cancer 28:914, 1971.
81. Reed RJ, Leonard DD: Neurotropic melanoma: A variant of desmoplastic melanoma. Am J Surg Pathol 3:301, 1979.
82. Gibson LE, Goellner JR: Amelanotic melanoma: Cases studied by Fontana stain, S-100 immunostain, and ultrastructural examination. Mayo Clin Proc 63:777, 1988.
83. Muhlbauer JE, Margolis RJ, Mihm MC, et al: Minimal deviation melanoma: A histologic variant of cutaneous malignant melanoma in its vertical growth phase. J Invest Dermatol 80:635, 1983.
84. Niven J, Lubin J: Pedunculated malignant melanoma. Arch Dermatol 111:755, 1975.
85. Gardner WA, Vazquez MD: Balloon cell melanoma. Arch Pathol 89:470, 1970.
86. McGovern VJ, Mihm MC, Bailly C, et al: The classification of malignant melanoma and its histologic reporting. Cancer 32:1446, 1973.
87. Clark WH, Mihm MC: Lentigo maligna and lentigo maligna melanoma. Am J Pathol 55:39, 1969.
88. Clark WH, From L, Bernardino EA, et al: Histogenesis and biologic behavior of primary human malignant melanoma of skin. Cancer Res 29:705, 1969.
89. Clark WH, Elder DE, Guerry D, et al: A study of tumor progression: The precursor lesions of superficial spreading and nodular melanoma. Hum Pathol 15:1147, 1984.
90. Breslow A: Thickness, cross-sectional areas, and depth of invasion in the prognosis of cutaneous melanoma. Ann Surg 172:902, 1970.
90a. Mihm MC, Googe PB: Problematic pigmented lesions: A case method approach. Philadelphia, Lea & Febiger, 1990.
91. Clark WH, Elder DE, Guerry D, et al: Model predicting survival in stage I melanoma based on tumor progression. J Natl Cancer Inst 81:1893, 1989.
92. Callen JP: Chronic cutaneous lupus erythematosus. Arch Dermatol 118:412, 1982.
93. Donzis PB, Insler MS, Buntin DM, et al: Discoid lupus erythematosus involving the eyelids. Am J Ophthalmol 98:32, 1984.

94. Kearns W, Wood W, Marchese A: Chronic cutaneous lupus involving the eyelid. Ann Ophthalmol 14:1009, 1982.
95. Plotz PH, Dalakas M, Leef RL, et al: Current concepts in the idiopathic inflammatory myopathies: Polymyositis, dermatomyositis and related disorders. Ann Intern Med 11:143, 1989.
96. Krieg T, Meurer M: Systemic scleroderma: Clinical and pathophysiologic aspects. J Am Acad Dermatol 18:457, 1988.
97. West RH, Barnett AJ: Ocular involvement in scleroderma. Br J Dermatol 63:845, 1979.
98. El Baba F, Frangieh GT, Iliff WJ, et al: Morphea of the eyelids. Ophthalmology 89:1285, 1982.
99. Beathnach SM: Amyloid and amyloidosis. J Am Acad Dermatol 18:1, 1988.
100. Jensen AD, Khodadoust AA, Emery JM: Lipoid proteinosis: Report of a case with electron microscopic findings. Arch Ophthalmol 88:273, 1972.
101. Davies G, Dymock I, Harry J, et al: Deposition of melanin and iron in ocular structures in haemochromatosis. Br J Ophthalmol 56:338, 1972.
102. Nethercott JR, Nield G, Holness DL: A review of 79 cases of eyelid dermatitis. J Am Acad Dermatol 21:223, 1989.

Chapter 187

Orbital Pathology

VALERIE A. WHITE and JACK ROOTMAN

The spectrum of diseases occurring in the orbit is vast and, for ophthalmologists and ophthalmic pathologists, is a microcosm of the rest of the body and includes some that are unique to the orbit or have a predilection for it. Several large series of orbital tumors have been compiled to show the relative frequency of the different orbital diseases and their age distribution.[1–4] This chapter is an attempt to provide a reasonably simple and comprehensible classification. The text by Rootman and the chapter by Jakobiec and Font provide excellent descriptions of all aspects of orbital pathology and are not referenced further.[1, 5]

The handling of pathology specimens by both orbital surgeons and pathologists is of utmost importance in obtaining an accurate diagnosis, particularly when dealing with a suspected neoplasm. The proliferation of new histopathologic techniques is so extensive that ophthalmologists cannot be expected to remember what to do in all situations. Therefore, all they have to remember is to discuss the differential diagnosis and handling of tissue with the pathologist before biopsy. Pathologists comply with this request because correct handling brings satisfaction to both clinicians and pathologists. Guidelines are given in later sections for the disposition of tissue in various disorders. Although all of the histopathologic descriptions in this chapter are based on light microscopic examination of H&E-stained slides following fixation, paraffin embedding and sectioning, aspiration biopsy, and cytologic examination of H&E-stained smears have become widely used in the diagnosis of both orbital and intraocular tumors. Some examples are given.[6–12]

CONGENITAL DISORDERS

Congenital Malformations

Various congenital structural malformations of the soft tissues and bones of the orbit occur with histologically normal tissues, and pathologic examination is rarely required. These disorders include orbital asymmetry and craniofacial dysostoses in which the diagnosis is established clinically and radiologically. Primary anomalies of the globe, such as anophthalmia, synophthalmia, congenital cystic eye, and microphthalmia also induce disturbances in growth of normal orbital tissue. Choristomas are foci of normal tissues located in abnormal sites and in the orbit primarily consist of dermoid cysts. These and other congenital cysts are discussed in the following section on all cystic lesions of the orbit. Other much rarer choristomas include ectopic brain and lacrimal gland tissues. Hamartomas are proliferations of disorganized tissues normally encountered in that location. In the orbit, they include capillary hemangiomas and lymphangiomas, which are discussed with vascular lesions, and some of the lesions seen in neurofibromatosis.

NEURAL CHORISTOMAS

Neural choristomas are composed of glial tissue that occasionally contains neurons or meninges. Encephalocele, meningoencephalocele, and meningocele maintain a connection to the intracranial cavity through a defect in the dura and orbital bone, whereas with ectopic brain no such connection is present.[13] Histopathologically, they consist of disorganized glial and fibrous tissue, often demonstrating occasional neurons and foci of calcification. One lesion contained cerebellar tissue, and a cyst with an ependyma-like lining has occasionally been seen.[13, 14]

ECTOPIC LACRIMAL GLAND

The orbital lobe of the lacrimal gland normally extends to the posterior aspect of the globe. More deeply located lobules of ectopic acinar tissue lose their ductal connections, and the buildup of secretions may cause an inflammatory reaction. Rarely, tumors have arisen in ectopic lacrimal gland.[15–17]

HAMARTOMAS

Neurofibromatosis

Neurofibromatosis is a multisystem disorder producing tumors of neural origin as well as bone and skin lesions. It has been associated with a defect on chromosome 17.[18] The orbital tumors occurring in this disorder are discussed in the section on neoplasia.

Cartilaginous Hamartoma

Lesions containing benign cartilage have been reported in the orbit. Some have classified these as tumors rather than hamartomas, but in all instances the histologic appearance has been benign.[19, 20]

Congenital Tumors

Congenital orbital tumors include teratomas, rhabdomyosarcomas, and hemangiopericytomas.[21, 22] The latter two usually present later in life and are described with mesenchymal tumors. Teratomas are defined as tumors containing elements of all three germ layers—ectoderm, mesoderm, and endoderm. They are common in the gonads, mediastinum, and pineal area. More than 50 cases have been reported in the orbit.[23–30] They may present at any time from the fetal stage to adolescence. Most are benign and localized to the orbit. Some, however, are associated with brain involvement and represent extension of a primary intracranial teratoma, usually resulting in death. Cases with brain and orbital involvement have been diagnosed in utero by ultrasonography.[25, 29] Histologically, the tissues are mature and consist of ectoderm represented by keratinizing

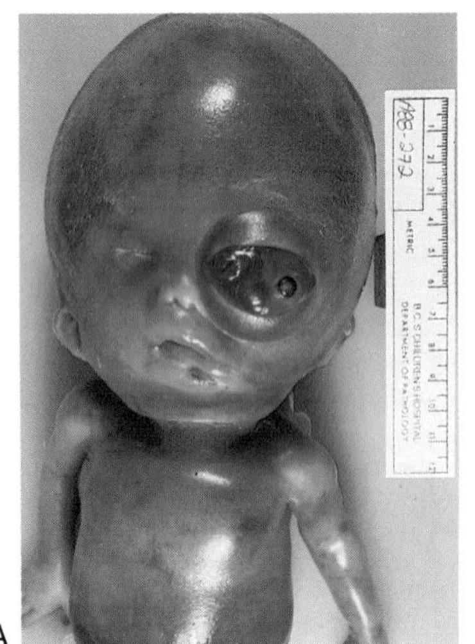

Figure 187–1. Orbital and intracranial teratoma. *A*, Gross photograph of a fetus at 24 weeks of gestation showing orbital and intracranial teratoma diagnosed in utero by ultrasonography. (Courtesy of Dr. Wes Tyson.) *B*, Low-power photomicrograph of orbital teratoma showing compression of the globe by the cystic tumor. H&E, ×1.6. *C*, Sebaceous glandular epithelium. H&E, ×80. *D*, Foci of cartilage and pancreatic glandular tissue. H&E, ×50. *E*, Immature neuroepithelium. H&E, ×50.

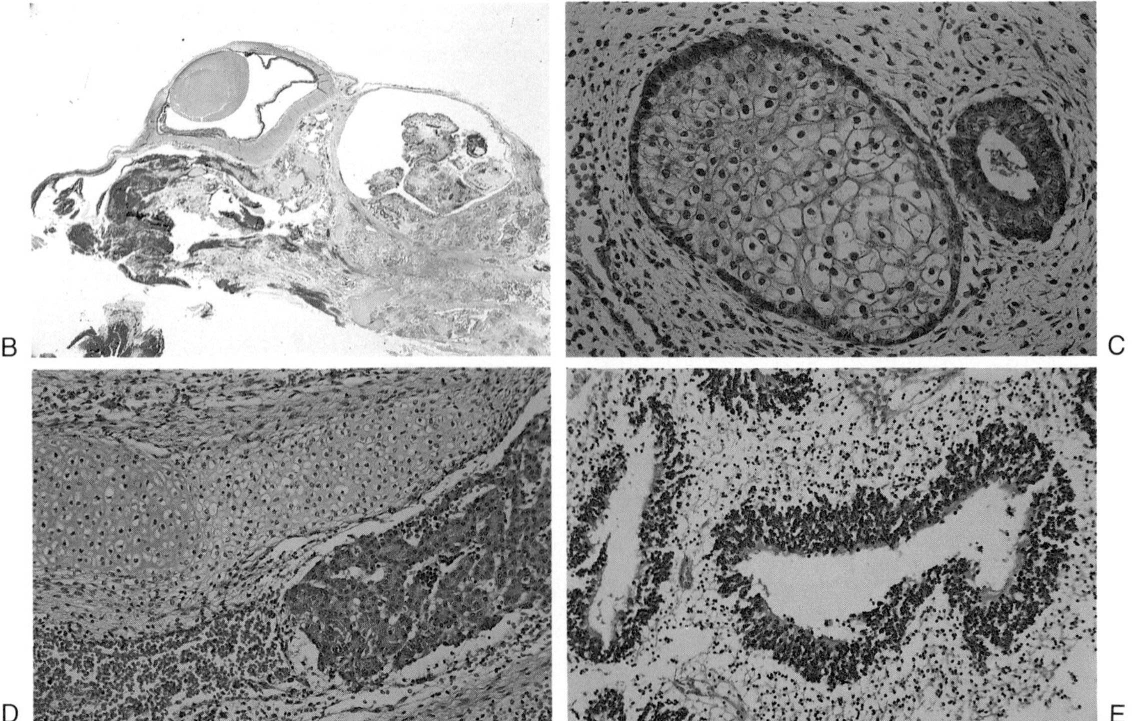

squamous epithelium and adnexal glandular structures; mesoderm by fibrous tissue, cartilage, fat, muscle, and bone; endoderm by gastrointestinal mucosal and glandular tissues; and neuroectoderm by mature brain. When the neural tissue has the appearance of fetal neural tissue, it is said to be immature. This is often seen in cases presenting in fetal life with brain involvement resulting in death (Fig. 187–1).[25, 29] A patient with a teratoma, initially resected, subsequently developed a malignant germ cell tumor.[30]

An allied tumor, usually presenting in the gonads of young children, is the endodermal sinus tumor; several orbital cases have been reported.[31, 32] This is a tumor derived from embryonic tissue that shows extraembryonic differentiation. Histopathologically, a loose network of stroma is lined by flat to cuboidal epithelium. Papillary structures called Schiller-Duval bodies, vascular cores lined by epithelial cells, are present. Anaplasia, mitoses, hemorrhage, and necrosis are frequent. The cells stain strongly for α-fetoprotein. A characteristic feature is numerous PAS-positive, diastase-resistant hyaline globules.

CYSTIC LESIONS

Cystic lesions of the orbit are a heterogeneous group of conditions that may vary greatly in presumed etiology, presentation, and pathologic appearance. They may account for 10 to 30 percent of nonthyroid orbital lesions in large series.[1, 2] We have elected to discuss them under one heading because pathologists recognize these lesions as cystic on study of the specimen, regardless of clinical features. We conducted a retrospective review of 124 cystic lesions of the orbit seen at the Vancouver General Hospital from 1977 to 1989 (Personal observations—VW, JR). The classification was based on the histopathologic appearance of the cyst lining as epithelial or nonepithelial. Cysts with an epithelial lining were further classified according to whether the presumed cause was congenital or acquired (Fig. 187–2). Nonepithelial cysts were classified into hematic, neurogenic, and infectious (Fig. 187–3). Virtually all neurogenic cysts are of congenital origin. Further classification was based on the specific type of lining or cyst wall. It should be stated that in some cases it may be very difficult to determine the exact nature of a cyst, the internal lining having atrophied or ulcerated as a result of pressure or inflammation. In these instances, a description of the lining suffices and the cause is determined by clinical features. None of these lesions was malignant.

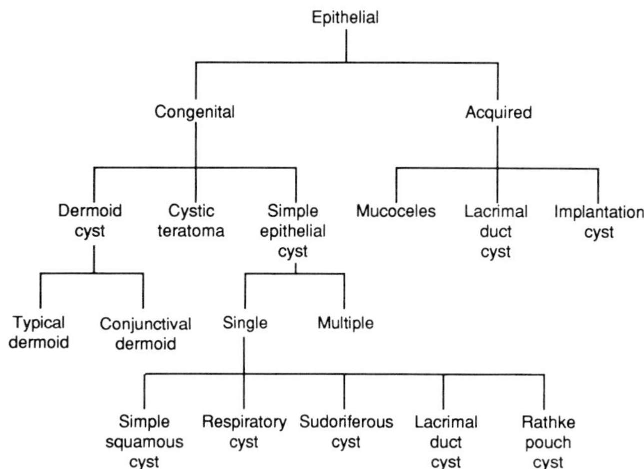

Figure 187–2. Classification of epithelial cysts of the orbit.

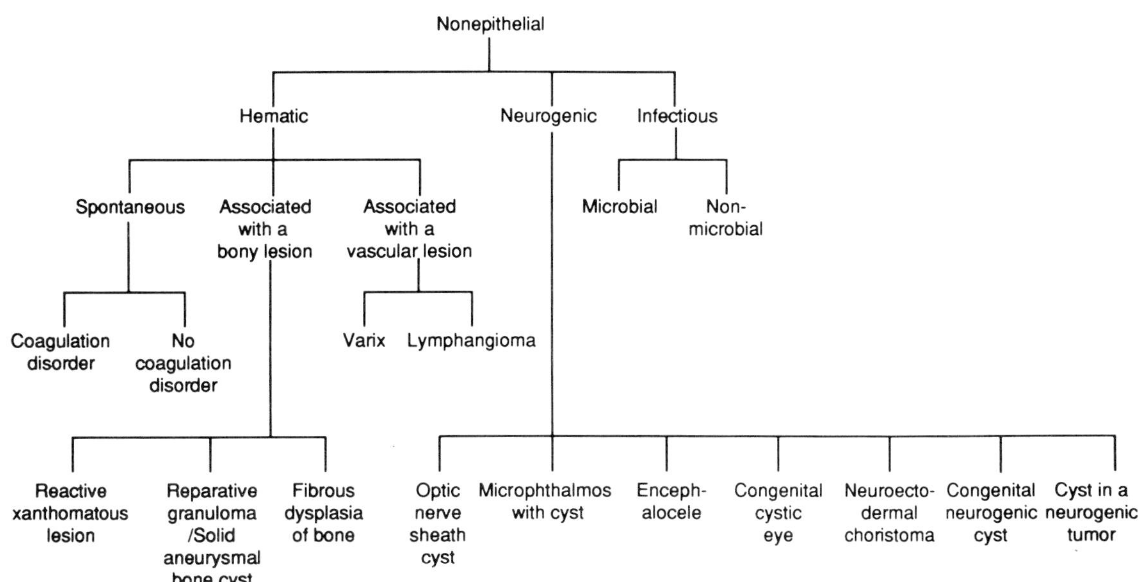

Figure 187–3. Classification of nonepithelial cysts of the orbit.

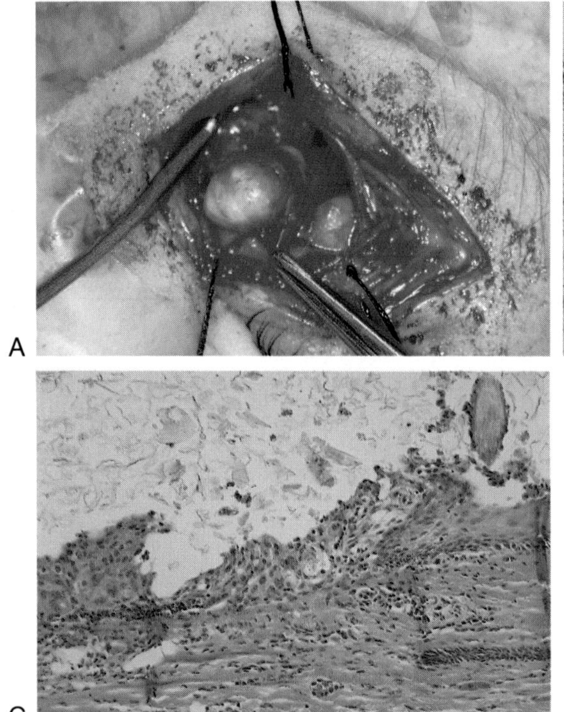

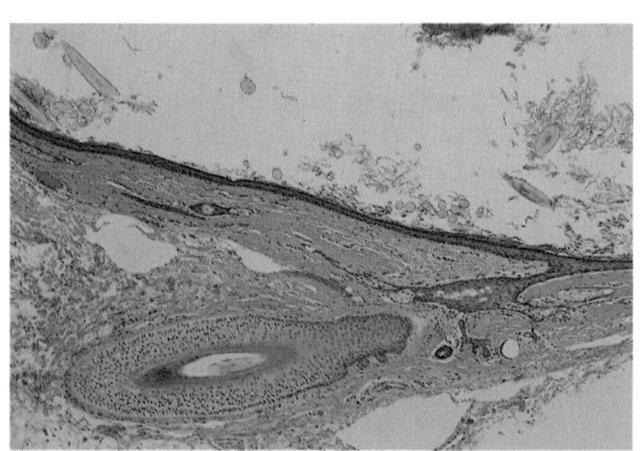

Figure 187–4. Dermoid cyst. *A,* Intraoperative photograph of excision of a dumbbell dermoid, demonstrating the typical gross yellowish appearance. *B,* Dermoid cyst showing stratified keratinizing squamous epithelium with a hair follicle and sebaceous gland in the wall and hairs in the lumen. H&E, ×20. *C,* Ruptured dermoid cyst with replacement of epithelium on the left by foreign body giant cells. H&E, ×50.

Epithelial Cysts

CONGENITAL

Congenital cysts all are distinguished by having an epithelial lining that recapitulates some of the normal orbital and adnexal epithelia. They all are thought to arise from sequestration of normal tissue in abnormal locations during embryonic development and thus are choristomatous cysts.

Dermoid Cysts

Dermoid cysts are the most common congenital epithelial cysts, accounting for 33 percent of cysts in our series and nearly half of orbital lesions seen in childhood, the time when they usually present.[3] They usually occur in the superotemporal orbit in relation to the suture lines of the orbital bones, often with a bony defect. The cyst lining consists of keratinizing stratified squamous epithelium with various adnexal structures embedded in the wall, including sebaceous glands, hair follicles, and eccrine sweat glands (Fig. 187–4). The cyst contents consist of keratin, sebaceous secretions, and hairs that are usually grossly recognizable. A portion of the wall is often replaced by a giant cell foreign body granulomatous response, suggesting previous rupture of the cyst lining.[33] When the oily sebaceous secretions extrude into the surrounding orbital fat, a lipogranulomatous and fibrotic response is initiated and may obscure the original cystic nature of the lesion. Remnants of epithelium and hairs must be looked for to confirm the origin of the inflammation. When only epithelial but no adnexal structures are found in the wall, the lesion is termed an *epidermoid cyst.*

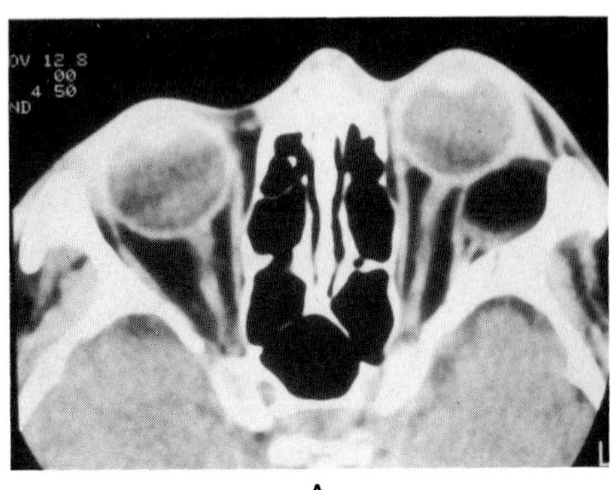

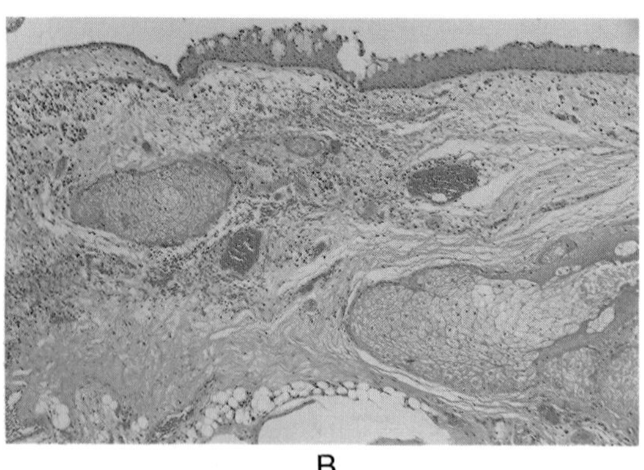

Figure 187–5. Conjunctival dermoid cyst. *A,* Axial computed tomography scan demonstrating a lucent cyst in the lateral portion of the left orbit. Note adjacent excavation of bone and the focal dense area posteriorly. This cyst was entirely intraorbital. *B,* Conjunctival dermoid cyst showing conjunctival epithelium with goblet cells and sebaceous glands in the wall. H&E, ×20.

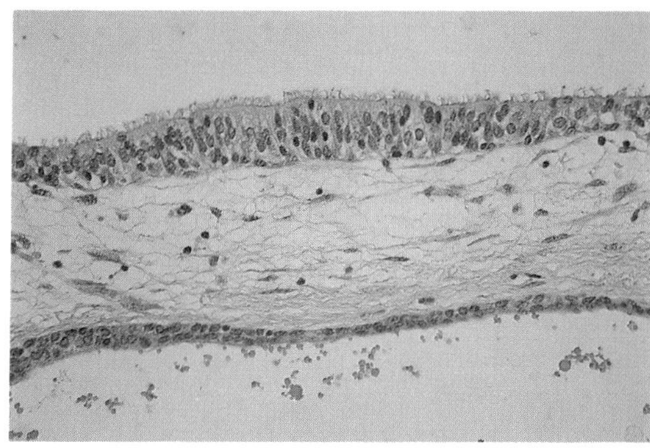

Figure 187–6. Respiratory epithelial cyst. Multiloculated cyst lined by pseudostratified ciliated columnar respiratory epithelium. H&E, ×80.

Conjunctival Dermoid Cysts

Conjunctival dermoid cysts represent sequestrations of conjunctival and caruncular epithelia and as such usually occur in the medial orbit without a bony defect. The cyst lining is composed of a nonkeratinizing stratified squamous or cuboidal epithelium, which may have goblet cells, and the wall contains adnexal structures and occasionally lacrimal gland (Fig. 187–5). The wall sometimes does not have any adnexal structures, making the lesion a simple conjuntival cyst, analogous to an epidermoid cyst. This type of cyst resembles an acquired conjuntival inclusion cyst and can be differentiated only on the basis of lack of historical or clinical evidence of trauma.[34, 35]

Other Epithelial Cysts

These cysts have a lining that may recapitulate the lacrimal duct or apocrine sweat gland epithelium (sudoriferous), or they may show no specific features and be classified as simple.[36] We encountered two cysts lined by pseudostratified ciliated columnar respiratory-type epithelium with no connection to the sinuses (Fig. 187–6). A few have been reported, presumably of a congenital origin.[37] Cysts with mixtures of conjunctival and apocrine epithelia, including oncocytic cells, are also seen.

ACQUIRED

The most common acquired cysts are mucoceles, lacrimal ductal cysts, and implantation cysts.

Mucocele

Mucoceles arise in association with a previous history of chronic sinusitis or fractures involving the sinuses, or they may have no such history. They are most frequently of frontal or ethmoidal sinus origin but may arise from any sinus. They are thought to occur because of poor drainage due to an obstructed ostium, which leads to a buildup of secretions. Over time, the mucocele slowly expands, erodes the sinus wall, and extends into the orbit, where it presents as a cystic mass with displacement of the globe. An alternative explanation for those associated with fractures is implantation of respiratory mucosa into the orbit at the time of trauma; there it slowly expands as a result of continued secretion.[38] Pathologically, these cysts are lined by normal pseudostratified ciliated columnar sinus epithelium with goblet cells. The lining sometimes is atrophic or eroded as a result of pressure. The outer wall of the cyst usually has an extremely dense laminated layer of fibrous connective tissue immediately beneath the epithelium, as well as a minimal to marked chronic inflammatory infiltrate of plasma cells and lymphocytes. It often contains dystrophic calcification (Fig. 187–7). The contents usually consist of a clear to mucoid material containing epithelial debris; they may occasionally be infected and rarely contain fungal hyphae and numerous eosinophils in allergic children.[39, 40] Sinus polyposis may cause erosion of the sinus wall with extension of polyps into the orbit.[41, 42]

Lacrimal Ductal Cysts

Lacrimal ductal cysts occur in the superolateral orbit and are easily observed by everting the upper lid, where they are seen in the conjunctival cul-de-sac. They may be bilateral. Histologically, these cysts are lined by two to three layers of epithelium often containing goblet cells, the inner cuboidal to columnar, the outer flattened basal epithelial cells (Fig. 187–8). The wall may contain

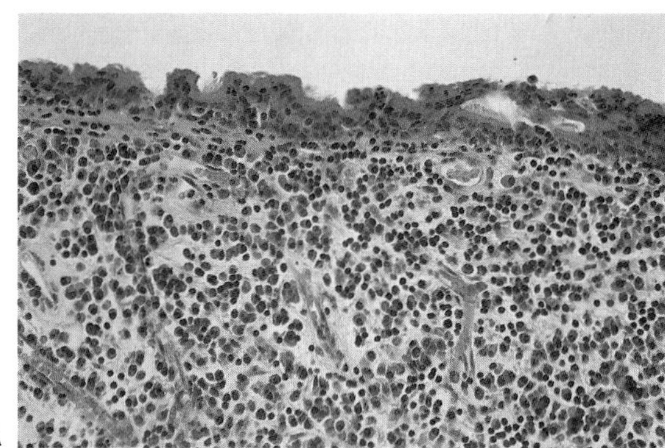

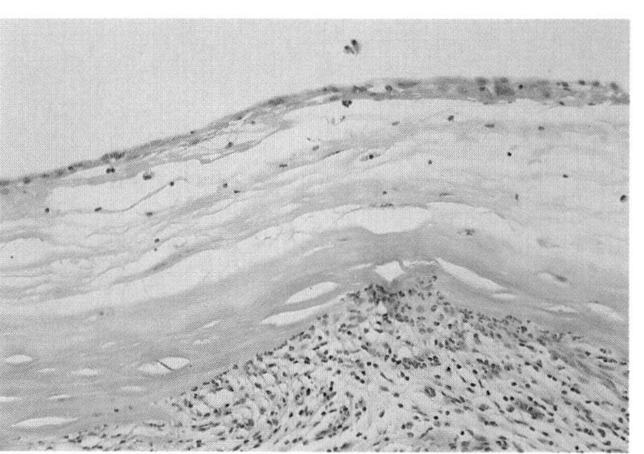

Figure 187–7. Mucocele. *A,* Inflamed mucocele with marked chronic inflammation in the wall and slightly degenerated respiratory epithelium. H&E, ×80. Noninflamed mucocele would resemble the lesion in Figure 187–6; clinical features are necessary to distinguish the two. *B,* Another area with atrophy of the epithelium and dense laminated connective tissue in the wall. H&E, ×50.

A

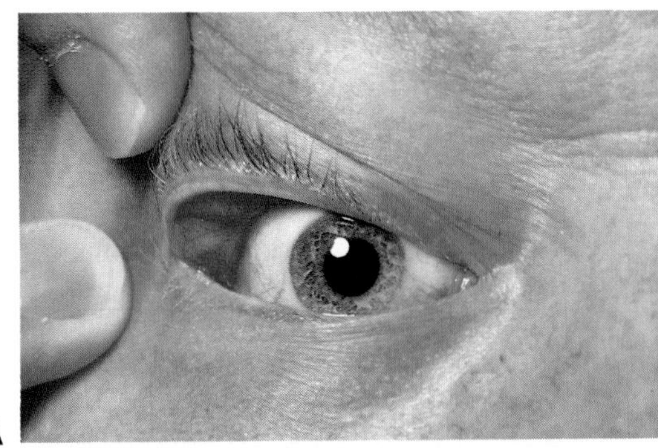

B

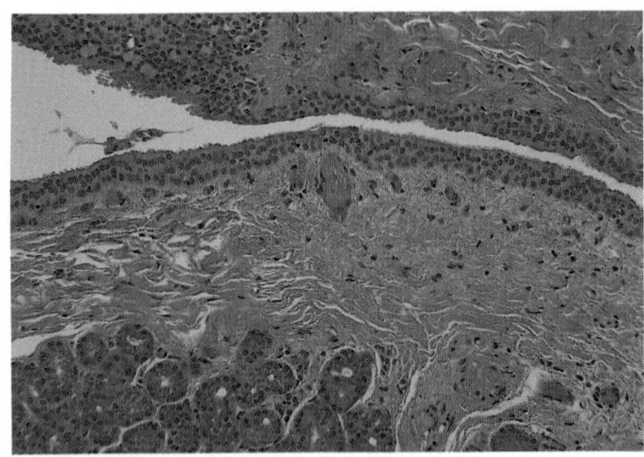

Figure 187–8. Acquired lacrimal ductal cyst. *A,* Clinical photograph of a typical blue domed lacrimal ductal cyst. *B,* Cyst lined by two to three layers of cuboidal to columnar epithelium, with a lacrimal gland in the wall. H&E, ×50.

lacrimal gland acini, and variable inflammation and fibrosis may be present.[43, 44]

Conjunctival Implantation Cysts

Conjunctival implantation cysts lined by conjunctival epithelium are introduced into the orbit as a result of trauma or surgery, particularly muscle surgery. They may occur in any location and become large.

Nonepithelial Cysts

Nonepithelial cysts are a heterogeneous group of cysts distinguished by not having an epithelial lining, and we have divided them into neurogenic, hematic, and infectious lesions.

NEUROGENIC

Neurogenic cysts are often related to primary developmental abnormalities of the globe such as congenital cystic eye and microphthalmos with cyst. They are usually evident at birth as large bluish-red cysts filling the orbit. Other lesions that might be cystic and included in this group are encephaloceles and meningoencephaloceles, which were discussed earlier. We have also encountered a gliotic cyst of the optic nerve in an adult; it contained foci of presumed nonpigmented ciliary body epithelium (Personal observation—VW, JR).

Congenital Cystic Eye

Congenital cystic eye is thought to result from an insult occurring at the fourth week of intrauterine life, preventing normal invagination of the anterior portion of the optic vesicle and giving rise to a cyst lined by dysplastic neuroepithelium with no evidence of the normal ocular structures such as lens, ciliary body, choroid, or retina.[45, 46] Partial invagination of the optic vesicle may allow formation of some very abnormal ocular structures, but the entire cystic eye is severely disorganized.[47–50]

Microphthalmos With Cyst

Microphthalmos with cyst results from failure of closure of the embryonic ocular fissure during the sixth week of gestation, giving rise to a severe colobomatous malformation attended by herniation and proliferation of retinoglial tissue through a scleral defect into the orbit. The eye is markedly microphthalmic and displaced superiorly by the inferiorly located colobomatous cyst, which externally may appear to occupy the entire orbital contents. Pathologically, there is evidence of ocular development with a small globe with cornea, anterior chamber, iris, ciliary body, lens, vitreous cavity, and some choroid. A large defect in the inferior sclera allows protrusion of a cystic structure lined by various combinations of retinal, glial, and undifferentiated neural tissue with disorganized pigment epithelium into the orbit (Fig. 187–9).[46, 51–54] This disorder is usually sporadic but may be inherited as a single anomaly or associated with other congenital malformations.[46, 54]

HEMATIC

Blood-filled cysts have been classified into those occurring in the soft tissues of the orbit and those occurring in bone. The soft tissue lesions occur either in association with a preexisting lymphangioma or varicocele or are spontaneous, one in a patient with a coagulopathy.[55–57] Those in bone occur in association with preexisting fibrous dysplasia, aneurysmal bone cyst, or reparative granuloma, or they just show a xanthomatous infiltrate with no evidence of an underlying lesion. These latter lesions have also been referred to as *cholesterol granulomas.*[58, 59] In these heterogeneous cases, the pathology is that of the underlying lesion, with superimposed recent and old hemorrhage consisting of fresh and degenerating red blood cells, cholesterol clefts surrounded by foreign body giant cell reaction, and hemosiderin-laden macrophages (Fig. 187–10).

INFECTIOUS

Our series had a single case of an infectious cyst due to cysticercosis (Fig. 187–11). This was located within the lateral rectus muscle and was surrounded by an intense granulomatous inflammatory reaction containing many eosinophils. Cysticercosis commonly involves the vitreoretinal space and subconjunctival area, but occa-

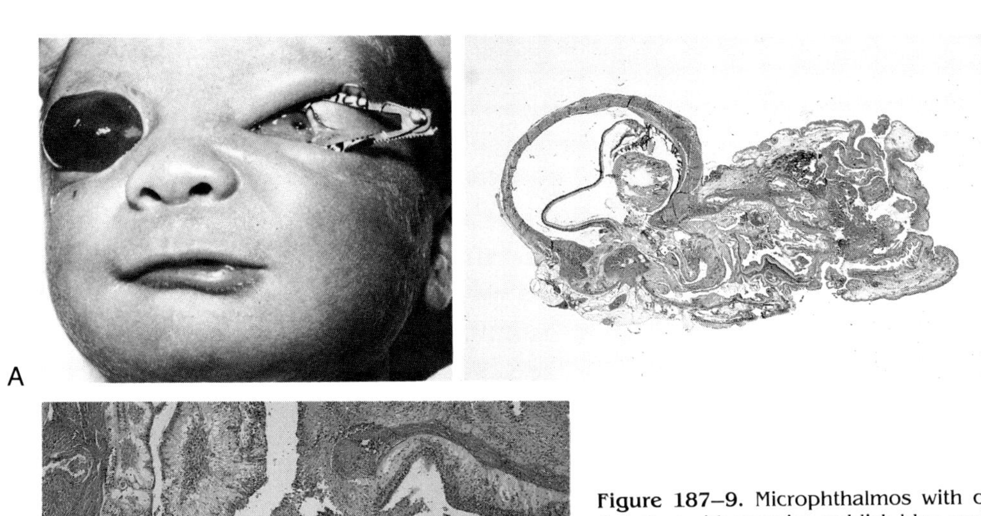

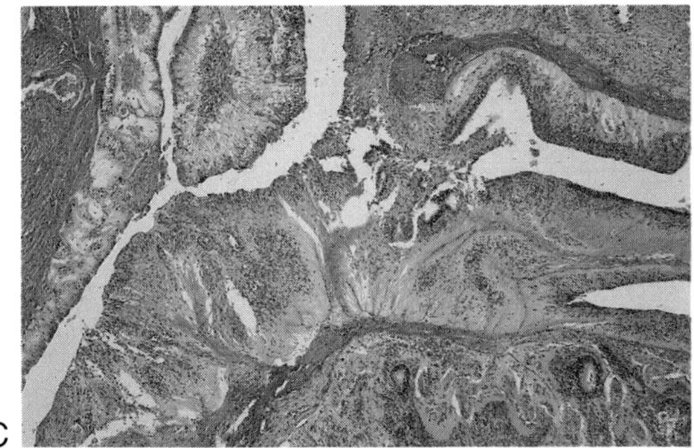

Figure 187–9. Microphthalmos with cyst. *A*, Infant with massive reddish-blue cyst on the right and microphthalmic eye without a cyst on the left. (From Rootman J: Diseases of the Orbit. Philadelphia, JB Lippincott, 1988, p 491.) *B*, Low-power photomicrograph showing a superiorly located microphthalmic globe with a large collapsed cyst. H&E, ×1.4. *C*, Portion of cyst lining showing dysplastic retinal and ciliary epithelium. H&E, ×12.

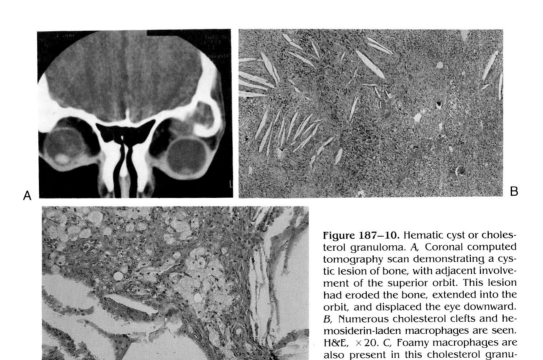

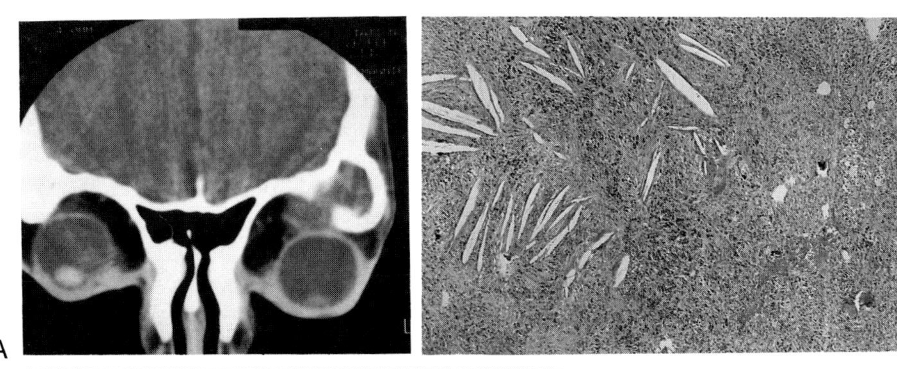

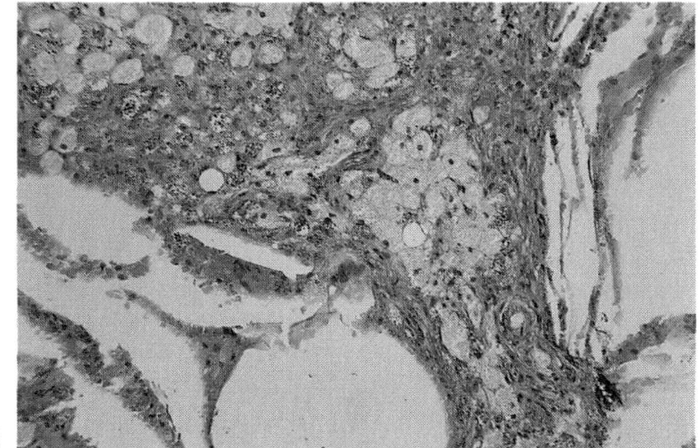

Figure 187–10. Hematic cyst or cholesterol granuloma. *A*, Coronal computed tomography scan demonstrating a cystic lesion of bone, with adjacent involvement of the superior orbit. This lesion had eroded the bone, extended into the orbit, and displaced the eye downward. *B*, Numerous cholesterol clefts and hemosiderin-laden macrophages are seen. H&E, ×20. *C*, Foamy macrophages are also present in this cholesterol granuloma unassociated with an underlying lesion. H&E, ×50.

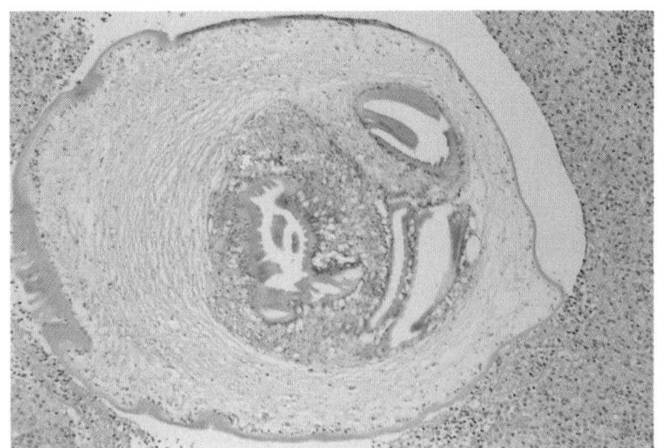
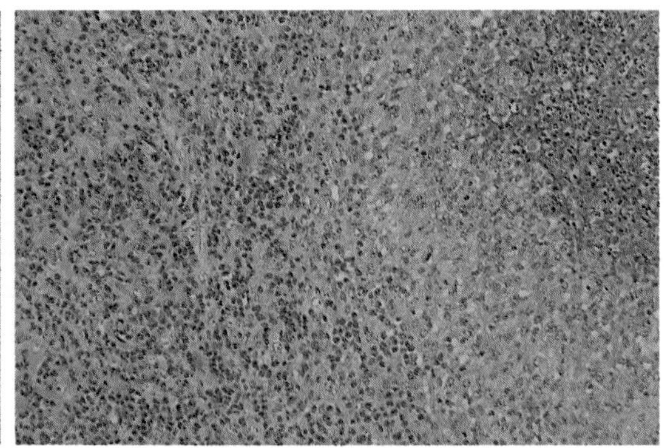

Figure 187–11. Cysticercosis. *A,* Cyst in extraocular muscle caused by larva of *Taenia solium.* H&E, ×20. (From Rootman J: Diseases of the Orbit. Philadelphia, JB Lippincott, 1988, p 160.) *B,* The cyst is surrounded by a granulomatous reaction and numerous eosinophils. H&E, ×50.

sional cases have been reported in the orbit and in the extraocular muscles.[60, 61] Other organisms that may cause cysts in the orbit include *Echinococcus granulosus, Multiceps* species, and *Histoplasma duboisii.*[62–64]

INFLAMMATORY DISEASES

Inflammatory diseases of the orbit can be categorized as infectious and noninfectious. The infections are classified on the basis of specific cause. The noninfectious category is divided into those diseases that have a specific pattern of inflammation on biopsy (e.g., Wegener's granulomatosis) and those that do not. The entire group accounts for approximately 10 percent of orbital disorders in all age groups.[1, 2]

Infections

BACTERIAL

Common Bacterial Infections

Common bacterial infections infrequently require biopsy, the diagnosis being made on clinical examination and microbiologic culture. Infections usually spread from contiguous structures, most commonly the paranasal sinuses, less frequently the teeth, lacrimal sac, eyelids, and fractured orbital bones. Other routes of infection include implantation with foreign bodies, as well as septicemia.[65–67] If biopsy is performed because of uncertainty of diagnosis or at débridement, pathologic examination shows an intense acute neutrophilic inflammatory reaction with some chronic inflammatory cells. Necrotic tissue may be present. Gram's stain should be performed to aid in diagnosis of the class of organism, in case cultures fail to grow.

Tuberculosis

Tuberculosis may rarely affect the orbit, even in North America, spreading from the paranasal sinuses or lacrimal gland or via the blood stream.[68–70] Typical caseating granulomatous inflammation is seen and should lead to the performance of Ziehl-Neelsen stains and tuberculin skin testing. Organisms may be difficult to find, and fluorescent auramine stain should also be used. Rare infections of the orbit with atypical mycobacteria have been reported.[71, 72]

Rhinoscleroma

Rhinoscleroma is an uncommon infection of the upper respiratory tract and is due to *Klebsiella rhinoscleromatis.* It is endemic in Africa, Asia, and South and Central America. Very uncommonly it may involve the orbit, spreading from the adjacent nose or sinuses or via the nasolacrimal duct. It produces a chronic infectious process that evolves through suppurative, granulomatous, and sclerotic stages.[73, 74] Biopsy specimens show the characteristic inflammatory reaction consisting of numerous plasma cells with Russell's bodies, lymphocytes, and foamy macrophages and the Mikulicz's cells containing the bacteria, which are seen on Gram's stain.

Other

Syphilis rarely affects the orbit, producing a periostitis. Diagnosis is by serologic investigation.[75] A case of granuloma inguinale involving soft tissue and bone of the lateral orbit has been described.[76]

FUNGAL

Two fungal infections commonly involve the orbit, usually by invasion from the sinuses. These are the ubiquitous opportunistic organisms *Aspergillus* and *Mucor,* which exist in air and soil, on skin, and as common food molds. They produce one of two clinical syndromes.

The first syndrome is a fulminating infection of the sinuses and orbit extending into the brain in a patient with uncontrolled diabetes or an underlying systemic immunocompromising condition such as leukemia, carcinomatosis, or burns. Biopsy is mandatory to establish the diagnosis and shows necrotic tissue due to invasion of vessels by the fungus, causing infarction. The inflammatory infiltrate may be minimal in pancytopenic patients or may consist of numerous neutrophils. The organism can be tentatively identified by the size of the

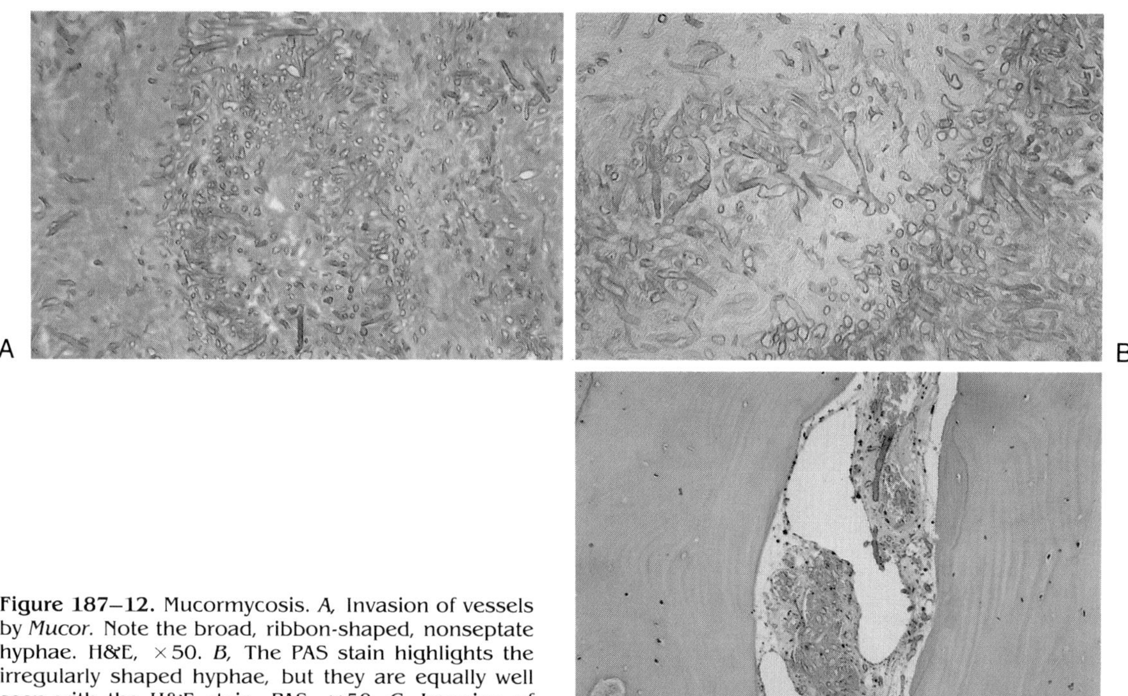

Figure 187–12. Mucormycosis. *A,* Invasion of vessels by *Mucor.* Note the broad, ribbon-shaped, nonseptate hyphae. H&E, ×50. *B,* The PAS stain highlights the irregularly shaped hyphae, but they are equally well seen with the H&E stain. PAS, ×50. *C,* Invasion of bone by *Mucor.* H&E, ×50.

hyphae, the branching pattern, and the presence of septa. *Mucor* shows broad, irregularly shaped nonseptate hyphae measuring from 30 to 50 μ in diameter and branching at right angles (Fig. 187–12). *Aspergillus* species are narrower, measuring 5 to 10 μm in diameter; they are septate, are more regular, and branch at acute angles. All of these features may not be present in a single biopsy specimen. Culture of biopsy material is required for exact speciation. Because this is an emergency situation and these organisms are hematoxophilic, frozen section with H&E staining can be used to speed diagnosis. Both PAS and Grocott's stains should be used on paraffin-embedded tissue when this diagnosis is suspected. Early diagnosis and aggressive therapy are required for survival.[77–82]

The second syndrome is that of a limited infection of the nose, orbit, and sometimes brain in otherwise well patients.[83–85] In these cases, biopsy specimens show well-formed granulomas, often with necrotizing centers surrounded by neutrophils, histiocytes, giant cells, lymphocytes, and plasma cells (Fig. 187–13). The organisms, which may be difficult to find because of partial disruption due to the inflammatory infiltrate, are located in the center of the granulomas, and both special stains should be performed to aid in the search. The more fulminating type of infection is usually caused by *Mucor* and the subacute by *Aspergillus,* but both organisms may cause either syndrome.

Other fungi that may rarely involve the orbit include *Pseudoallescheria boydii* (formerly called *Petriellidium boydii*), *H. duboisii, Sporothrix schenckii,* and *Blastomyces dermatitidis.*[64, 86–90] All require biopsy and culture as outlined earlier for diagnosis. We have seen one case of *P. boydii* infection of the orbit in a leukemic patient who was pancytopenic after chemotherapy (Fig. 187–14).

PARASITIC

The list of parasites that may involve the orbit is lengthy, but examples in North America are few and usually occur in those who have lived or traveled in the Middle East, Africa, Asia, and Central and South America. Again, all of these organisms require excision of the affected tissues and histopathologic examination for diagnosis. General reviews of the tissue appearance and inflammatory reactions of parasites are available.[91, 92] Cysts due to *E. granulosus* are probably the most frequent.[62, 93] Other cystic infections are cysticercosis, produced by the larval stage of the pork tapeworm, *Taenia solium,* and coenurosis, produced by the larval stage of *Multiceps* species.[60, 61, 63, 94] Microfilaria of *Onchocerca volvulus, Loa loa,* and adult worms of *Dirofilaria* species have been seen in the anterior orbit.[95–99] *Trichinella spiralis* may localize in the extraocular muscles. Eggs of *Paragonimus* and of *Schistosoma haematobium* have been reported.[95, 100, 101] Very rarely, infestation with the larvae of certain flies can cause the orbital form of ophthalmomyiasis, producing severe necrotizing damage to the eye and orbital tissues.[102, 103]

Specific Noninfectious Inflammations

The specific noninfectious lesions of the orbit are an important group because recognition of the pattern of inflammation allows for appropriate investigation and treatment of patients. Because the vast majority of this group are granulomatous lesions, it is important that an infectious cause first be ruled out. In a review of 41 granulomatous lesions of the orbit at the Vancouver General Hospital from 1977 to 1989, the most common

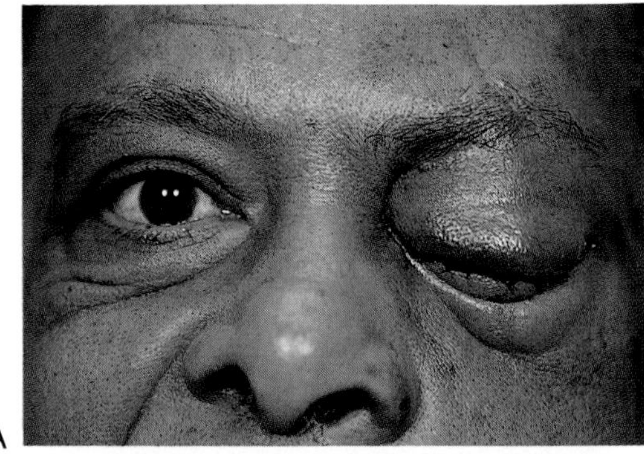

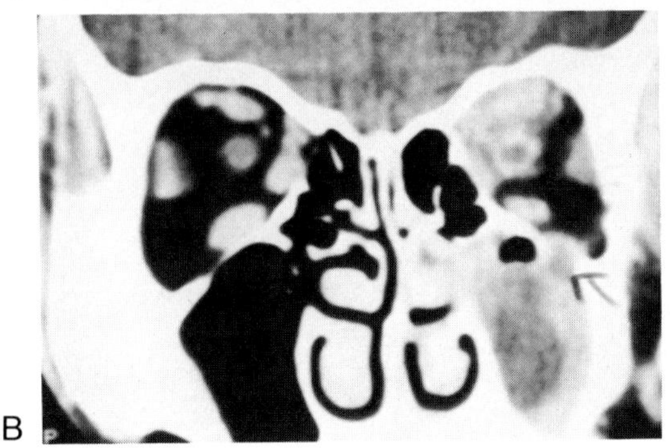

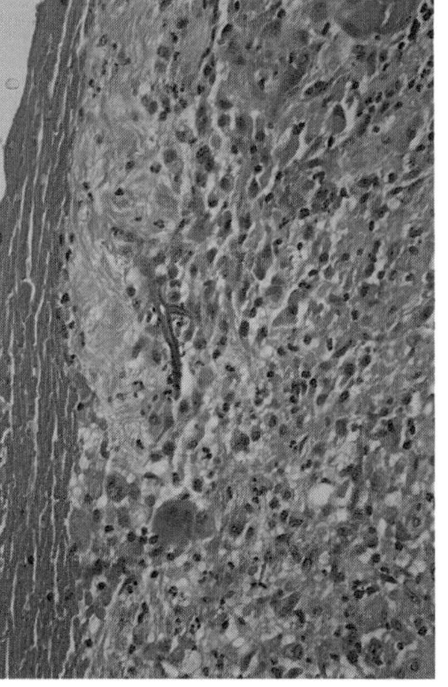

Figure 187–13. Limited orbital mucormycosis. *A,* Clinical photograph of a 56-year-old man who presented with a history of progressive proptosis, lid edema, ptosis, loss of sensation in V1 and V2, and total amaurosis with fixation of the globe. This occurred during a 2-month period following an acute episode of apparent sinusitis. *B,* Computed tomography scan demonstrates an infiltration of the medial orbit, associated with anterior ethmoidal and maxillary sinus involvement, with erosion of adjacent bone. *C,* Biopsy showed nonseptate hyphal fragments surrounded by granulomatous inflammation. H&E, ×80.

lesions were localized or systemic sarcoidosis (discussed under Sarcoidosis and Sarcoid-like Granulomatous Inflammation, although 5 of 13 patients with sarcoid in our series had orbital involvement alone), ruptured dermoid cysts, Wegener's granulomatosis, and fibro-osseous processes (discussed under Neoplasms Arising in Bone).[104]

RUPTURED DERMOID CYSTS

About one fourth of dermoid cysts show histologic evidence of rupture, with portions of the lining replaced by epithelioid and foreign body giant cells (see Fig. 187–4*B*). If the rupture has allowed egress of the cyst contents into the fat, a fibrotic granulomatous response is seen surrounding vacuolated spaces, which presumably contained lipid before tissue processing (Fig. 187–15). Occasional lymphocytes, plasma cells, cholesterol clefts, and hemosiderin-laden macrophages may be noted.

VASCULITIS

Wegener's Granulomatosis

Ocular involvement in Wegener's granulomatosis is frequent, with orbital disease accounting for half of the ocular disease.[105–107] Orbital involvement usually occurs as a result of direct spread from the nose or sinuses, which are always involved. Biopsy is necessary to establish the diagnosis and rule out other disorders that may mimic it. Pathologic interpretation of biopsy samples obtained from head and neck sites is more difficult than from those obtained from the lung, and the classic triad of vasculitis, necrosis, and granulomatous inflammation may not be present.[108, 109] In orbital biopsy specimens, the clue to this diagnosis is a mixed inflammatory infiltrate of neutrophils, lymphocytes, plasma cells, epithelioid histiocytes, giant cells, and occasional eosinophils (Fig. 187–16). The neutrophils are usually in the form of microabcesses, which may be surrounded by poorly formed granulomas or may be superimposed on

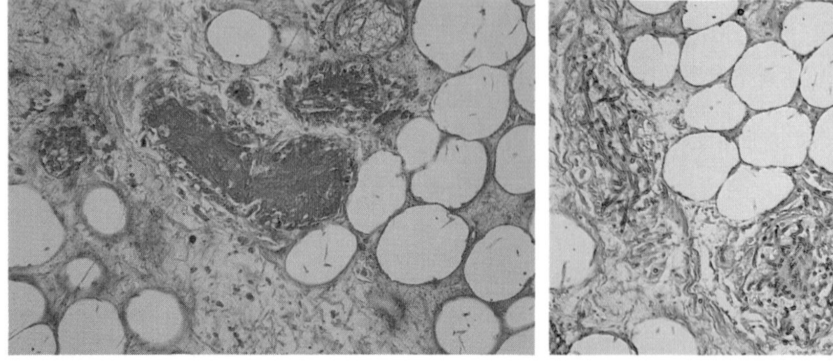

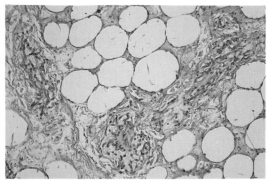

Figure 187–14. *Pseudoallescheria boydii. A,* Invasion of vessels by *P. boydii* with surrounding necrotic orbital tissue and lack of an inflammatory response. H&E, ×80. *B,* Grocott's stain highlights these organisms, which are morphologically similar to *Aspergillus* and can be distinguished only by culture. Grocott, ×80.

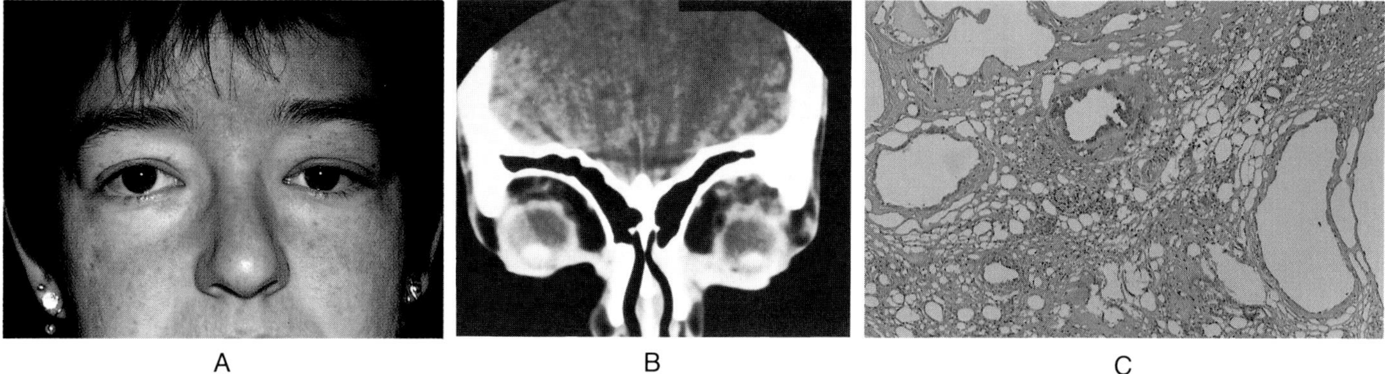

Figure 187–15. Dermoid cyst with massive rupture. *A,* Clinical photograph of a 30-year-old woman with a 3-month history of progressive swelling of the left upper lid and downward displacement of the globe. *B,* Coronal computed tomography scan demonstrates an irregular lesion in the roof of the orbit with focal areas of lucency due to leakage of fat and granulomatous inflammation, associated with a ruptured dermoid cyst. Note irregularity of adjacent bone. *C,* There is extensive infiltration of the orbital tissues by lipid, which is surrounded by foreign body giant cell granulomas and fibrosis. H&E, ×20.

the outline of a vessel that has been destroyed by the inflammation. Infrequently, true fibrinoid necrosis of vessel walls is seen. Small areas of necrosis surrounded by nuclear dust are always present and are presumed to be infarction due to a damaged vessel not seen in the section. Occasionally, in long-standing cases, fibrosis may be significant, resembling a sclerosing orbital lesion.[108] Stains for fungi and acid-fast organisms should always be performed. In some cases, it may be possible to say only that the inflammatory infiltrate is suggestive but not diagnostic, and further investigations should be carried out. Studies now show that the inflammatory infiltrate consists predominantly of T lymphocytes and macrophages, with only a few B lymphocytes and no deposition of immunoglobulin, suggesting cell-mediated immune damage.[110] The demonstration of antineutrophil cytoplasmic antibodies has been found to be a marker for Wegener's granulomatosis.[111] Prompt diagnosis is critical to prevent irreversible damage.[112]

Hypersensitivity Vasculitis

Hypersensitivity vasculitis, sometimes termed *leukocytoclastic vasculitis,* may be seen in the orbit of patients with connective tissue diseases, with Cogan's syndrome, and without an underlying disease.[113] Biopsy shows an

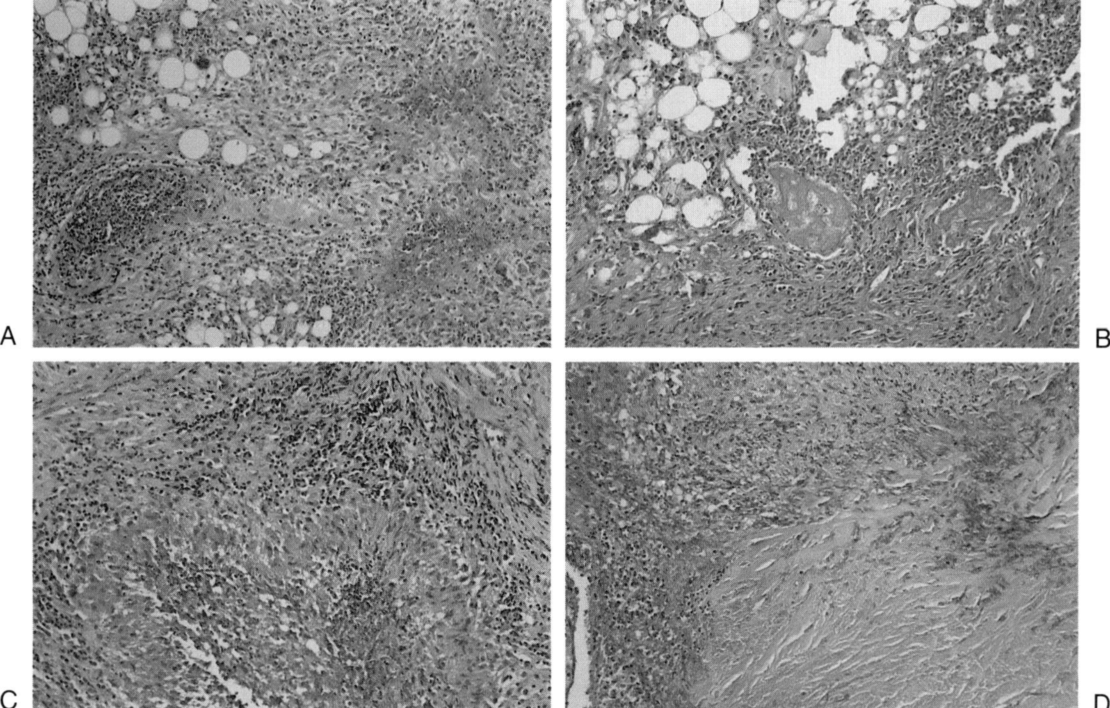

Figure 187–16. Wegener's granulomatosis. *A,* Inflamed and occluded vessel on the left, with two areas of stellate necrosis and neutrophils to the right. Occasional giant cells are present. H&E, ×28. *B,* Thrombosis of small vessels surrounded by mixed inflammatory infiltrate. H&E, ×50. *C,* Fairly well-formed granuloma surrounding a necrotic area. H&E, ×50. *D,* Fibrosis with surrounding mixed inflammation. H&E, ×50.

acute inflammatory infiltrate with nuclear debris or dust surrounding small arterioles, capillaries, and postcapillary venules. Fibrinoid necrosis of the vessel walls is often present.

Other Vasculitides

Very rare reports describe vasculitis involving the orbit in association with the other vasculitides, such as polyarteritis nodosa, Churg-Strauss vasculitis, temporal arteritis, and lymphomatoid granulomatosis (angiocentric lymphoma).[105] A particular vascular inflammation may sometimes be difficult to classify on the basis of biopsy alone, and systemic investigations are necessary to establish the correct diagnosis or to rule out systemic disease.

KIMURA'S DISEASE

Kimura's disease involves the soft tissues of the head and neck region, frequently afflicting regional lymph nodes and parotid and submandibular salivary glands.[114] It is endemic in Asia, where it is often associated with peripheral eosinophilia and elevated serum IgE levels. Several cases with orbital involvement have been described.[115–120] Histopathologic examination shows the presence of a vascular proliferation in which the endothelial cells appear activated and hobnail or histiocytoid endothelial cells may be present. The inflammatory infiltrate consists of reactive germinal centers, which may be infiltrated by eosinophils to the point of producing an abcess; eosinophils usually surround the proliferating vessels. Plasma cells, histiocytes, and mast cells are also present in the paracortical areas. Immunologic studies have shown deposition of IgE in the germinal centers and the presence of surface IgE-positive mast cells.[121] Although two studies support the easy distinction between Kimura's disease and angiolymphoid hyperplasia with eosinophilia, the largest review of ocular cases suggests that this distinction cannot always be made.[114, 118, 121] We have seen one case of Kimura's disease involving the lacrimal gland and cervical lymph nodes in a young Vietnamese male (Fig. 187–17).

NECROBIOTIC XANTHOGRANULOMA WITH PARAPROTEINEMIA

Necrobiotic xanthogranuloma with paraproteinemia is a peculiar disorder characterized clinically by the presence of multiple indurated papules and xanthomatous plaques, which, although they may occur on the skin of the trunk and extremities, have a predilection for the periocular skin, requiring distinction from xanthelasma. Pathologic examination of biopsy specimens shows poorly formed granulomas and sheets of histiocytes, many of which are lipidized, with Touton's and foreign body type giant cells involving the dermis and subcutaneous tissue (Fig. 187–18). Dispersed throughout are tracts of "necrobiotic collagen," often containing giant cells alone. Lymphoid nodules and plasma cells staining for both kappa and lambda light chains may be numerous. Cholesterol clefts may be present. The heterogeneous cellular infiltrate extends into subcutaneous tissue and often the anterior orbit, whereas xanthelasma is confined to the dermis and has a monomorphic infiltrate of foamy histiocytes. Necrobiotic xanthogranulomas are a marker for plasma cell abnormalities, in that although only 3 of 22 patients in one review had overt multiple myeloma, 16 of 22 had a monoclonal gammopathy, 7 had plasmacytosis of the bone marrow, and 2 had a lymphoproliferative disorder. Other laboratory and ophthalmic findings may be present.[122, 123]

A
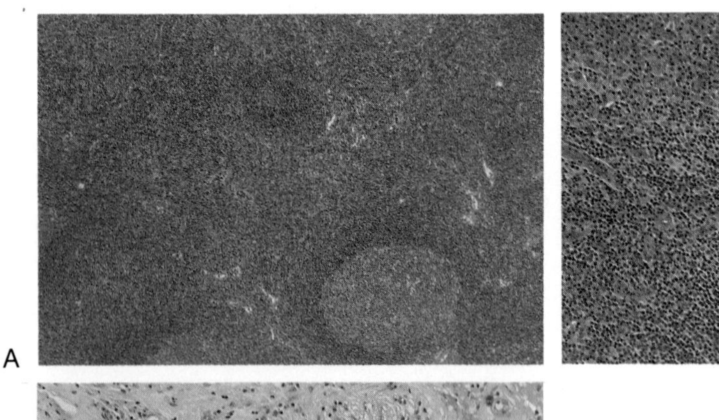

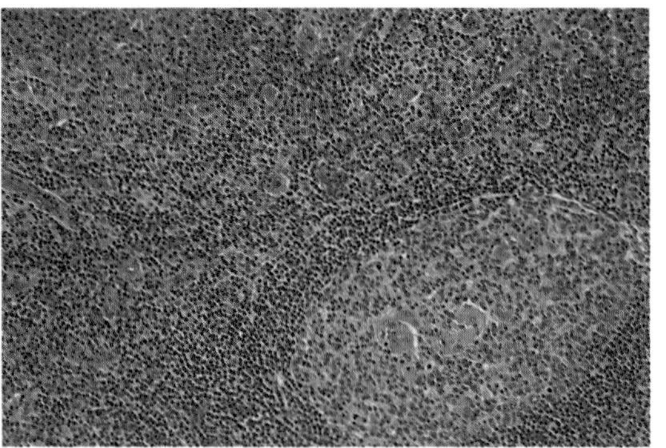
B

C

Figure 187–17. Kimura's disease. *A,* Low-power photomicrograph of cervical lymph node showing reactive germinal centers and proliferating vessels. H&E, ×20. *B,* Reactive germinal center on the lower right surrounded by eosinophils, with a portion of an eosinophilic abscess at upper left. H&E, ×50. C, Involvement of the lacrimal gland with chronic inflammatory infiltrate containing numerous small vessels and occasional eosinophils. H&E, ×50.

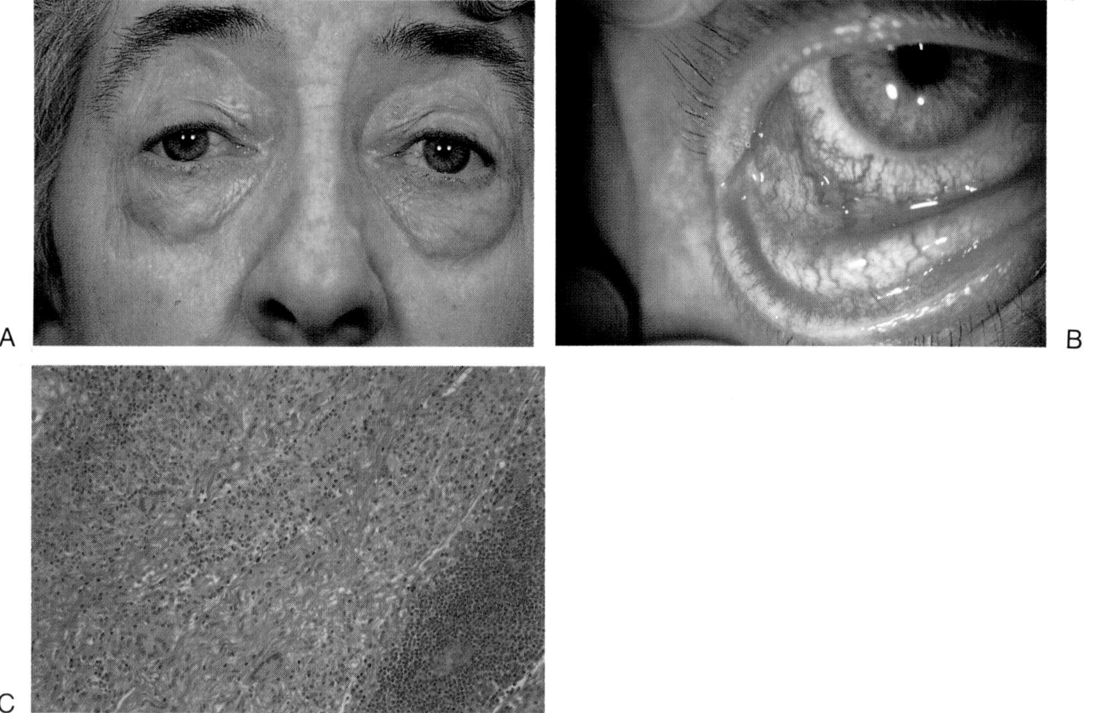

Figure 187–18. Necrobiotic xanthogranuloma with paraproteinemia. *A,* Facial photograph of a 72-year-old woman who presented with progressive ocular irritation and limitation of movement, associated with a waxy yellowish deposition in the upper and lower lids. *B,* Clinical photograph of the fornix demonstrates thickening by a dense yellowish subconjunctival infiltrate and injection of the globe. *C,* Biopsy specimen of the anterior orbital mass shows tracts of collagen with focal necrosis, Touton's giant cells, and chronic inflammation containing plasma cells. H&E, ×50.

PSEUDORHEUMATOID NODULE

Pseudorheumatoid nodule, also called *subcutaneous granuloma annulare,* usually occurs in the subcutaneous tissues of the skin of the scalp, on the extensor surfaces of the extremities, and on the dorsa of hands and feet in patients without a rheumatoid disease. It is histopathologically indistinguishable from that occurring in patients with rheumatic diseases.[124] A few cases have been found to involve the orbit.[125–128] The pathologic picture consists of a palisading granuloma of histiocytes and fibroblasts surrounding a hyaline, eosinophilic necrobiotic area of collagen that may stain positively for acid mucopolysaccharides or fibrin (Fig. 187–19).

FOREIGN BODY GRANULOMAS

Three patients in our series had granulomatous reactions to foreign material, which included bone wax from previous surgery, silicone, and wood. One patient had a nonspecific granulomatous process that could not be further characterized.[104] Foreign body giant cell granulomas often appear extremely irregular and mold themselves to the shape of the foreign material (Fig. 187–20). It is important to examine any biopsy material that shows this type of reaction or that is obtained from patients with a history of trauma by polarized light to locate and attempt to identify the type of foreign material present.

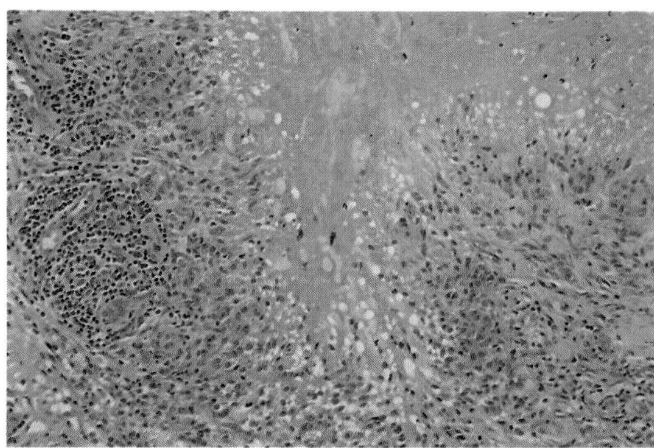

Figure 187–19. Pseudorheumatoid nodule. Palisading granuloma with central "necrobiotic" area. H&E, ×50.

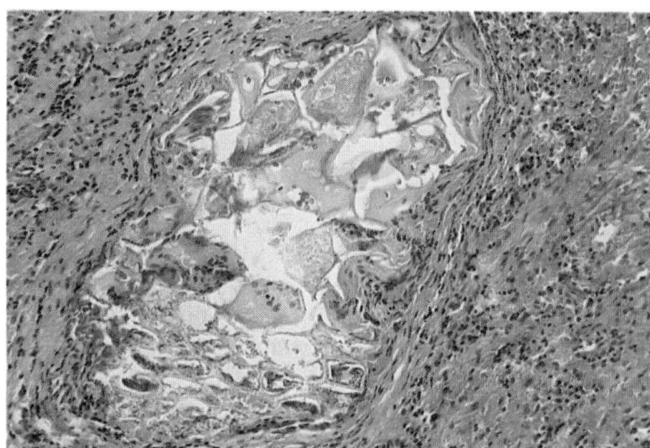

Figure 187–20. Foreign body granulomatous reaction to a fragment of wood that had become embedded in the orbit after trauma. H&E, ×50.

HISTIOCYTOSIS X

Histiocytosis X is a group of histopathologically similar disorders that form a continuum of clinical involvement of single to multiple bony foci, skin, lymph nodes, middle ear, abdominal viscera, and pituitary gland.[129–132] Solitary lesions of the frontal bone of the orbit are common; however, complete investigation of patients is required to evaluate the extent of disease and the treatment needed.[133] Histopathologically, there is a mixture of mono- and binucleated histiocytes with bean-shaped nuclei, prominent nucleoli, and slightly eosinophilic cytoplasm admixed with eosinophils, lymphocytes, plasma cells, and multinucleated histiocytes without much stroma; hemorrhage may be prominent (Fig. 187–21). Ultrastructurally, the pathognomonic organelle is the Langerhans or Birbeck granule, a 40-nm rod or racquet-shaped structure with a central striated line like a zipper.[132–134] Positive immunohistochemical staining for protein S100 is helpful in making the diagnosis.[132, 134]

SINUS HISTIOCYTOSIS WITH MASSIVE LYMPHADENOPATHY

This disease, which usually produces cervical adenopathy in young adults, may involve the orbit in approximately 10 percent of cases.[135] Histopathologic examination shows masses of large histiocytes with small nuclei surrounded by chronic inflammatory cells including lymphocytes and plasma cells. The inflammatory infiltrate is divided into lobules by fibrous tissue, which may be prominent. The histiocytes may show evidence of phagocytosis of lymphocytes and erythrocytes.[135–138] The histiocytes occasionally may show atypical features with large nuclei and prominent nucleoli.[137] Serum gamma globulin levels and erythrocyte sedimentation rate are often elevated.

JUVENILE XANTHOGRANULOMA

Juvenile xanthogranuloma more commonly affects the eyelids and uveal tract in addition to the nonocular skin. A few cases with orbital disease have been reported.[139, 140]

ERDHEIM-CHESTER DISEASE

Two cases of Erdheim-Chester disease have involved the orbit.[141] Both showed a lipogranulomatous process with foamy histiocytes, Touton's giant cells, cholesterol clefts, lymphocytes, and plasma cells. Systemic involvement of bones, heart, lungs, or retroperitoneum was present in the reported cases.

Nonspecific Noninfectious Inflammations

Nonspecific noninfectious inflammations are considered nonspecific because no infectious cause can be identified and the pattern of inflammation does not allow recognition of a specific disease entity. However, because these disorders have been scrutinized closely, they can be recognized clinically, radiologically, and pathologically and antiinflammatory treatment instituted. The major classification divides these disorders into acute, subacute, and chronic processes. The acute and subacute processes have been further categorized according to location.[142–144] Pathologists are seldom called on to diagnose the acute or subacute disorders because biopsy is not usually required. In some instances, biopsy may be performed if the clinical picture is confusing or if there has been no response to treatment or a recurrence. Biopsy specimens show a mixed nonspecific inflammatory infiltrate of neutrophils, lymphocytes, histiocytes, and plasma cells, which may be angiocentric without a true vasculitis (Fig. 187–22). Extraocular muscle involvement has been reported in giant cell polymyositis.[145]

Pathologists are more frequently confronted with the chronic form of nonspecific orbital inflammation because it requires pathologic distinction from a neoplastic process. The major histopathologic feature that differs from the acute or subacute nonspecific inflammatory processes is the presence of a variable degree of fibrosis or desmoplasia. The inflammatory infiltrate again is mixed and moderate or scant in volume. In addition to lymphocytes, plasma cells, and histiocytes, there may be

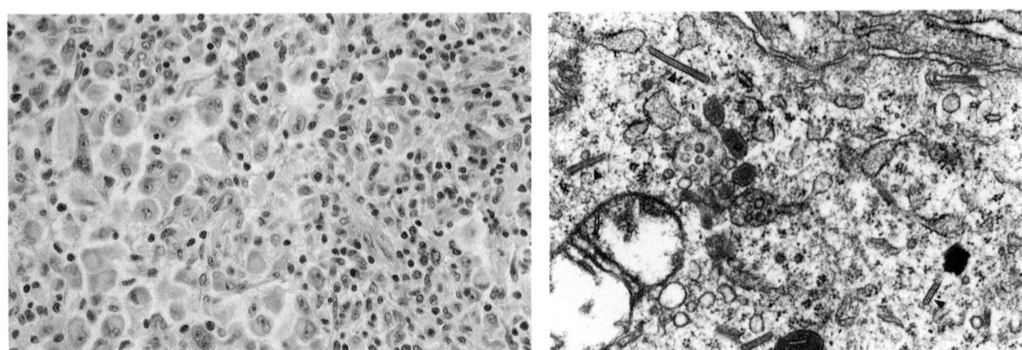

Figure 187–21. Histiocytosis X. *A,* Biopsy sample from a child with an orbital bony and soft tissue mass showing single and multinucleated histiocytes with bean-shaped nuclei, occasional eosinophils, and chronic inflammatory cells. H&E, ×80. *B,* Electron micrograph from the same case showing several rod-shaped Birbeck's or Langerhans' granules in one cell *(arrowheads).* Uranyl acetate, lead citrate, ×58,000.

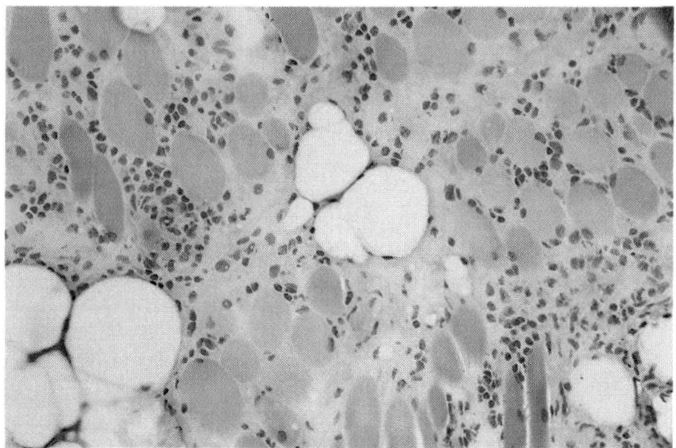

Figure 187–22. Acute myositis. Extraocular muscle surrounded by mixed inflammatory infiltrate. H&E, ×50.

occasional neutrophils, eosinophils, and the formation of lymphoid follicles with germinal centers (Fig. 187–23). Perivascular cuffing with inflammatory cells is frequent, but true vasculitis is not present.[146–149] The pathology is similar to that of retroperitoneal and mediastinal fibrosis and has been associated with these fibrosing disorders in some cases.[150–154] The differential diagnosis includes sclerosing metastases, vasculitis, and granulomatous inflammation. The distinction from a lymphoproliferative process is not a problem in this setting because the inflammatory infiltrate is so polymorphous and the fibroplasia such a major component, both of which are not features of lymphoma. We do not apply the term *pseudotumor,* because it has been used to mean many different entities, preferring instead to describe the actual pathology present.[96] We call this type of lesion *sclerosing orbital inflammation* or *chronic inflammation with fibrosis.*

THYROID ORBITOPATHY

Pathologists are rarely called on to assist in the diagnosis of thyroid or Graves' orbitopathy, because it is usually made clinically, radiologically, and by thyroid hormone testing. However, if the results of these investigations are confusing, biopsy may be undertaken to differentiate between this condition and those that mimic it, such as acute or subacute nonspecific orbital inflammation or a tumor involving an extraocular muscle. The histopathologic findings in thyroid orbitopathy are nonspecific in themselves and therefore must be interpreted in the light of all investigations. The structures primarily affected are the extraocular muscles, most commonly the medial and inferior recti, which show a sparse to moderate inflammatory infiltrate of lymphocytes, plasma cells, and occasional mast cells (Fig. 187–24). In the early stages, this is associated with an often dramatic interstitial deposition of acid mucopolysaccharide, as shown by staining with alcian blue at a pH of 2.5. If biopsy is performed when the disease has been present for a longer time, fibrosis and destruction of the muscles and infiltration by mature fat are seen. Inflammation may affect the orbital fat surrounding the muscle, but involvement of the fat primarily is not present.[155–157] One investigation has shown enlargement and marked variation in size of levator palpebrae superiorus muscle fibers without significant inflammation or fibrosis.[158]

AMYLOID DEPOSITION

Amyloid deposition may be related to systemic or localized disease.[159] When systemic, it may be associated

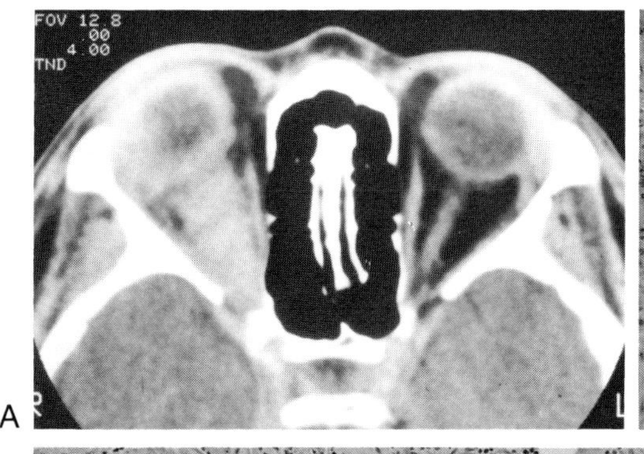

A

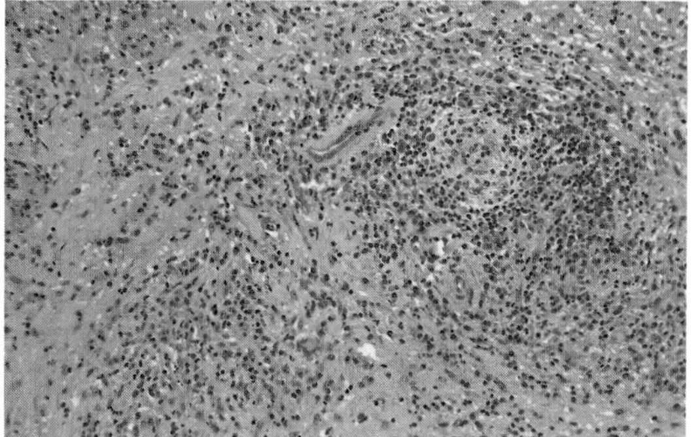

B

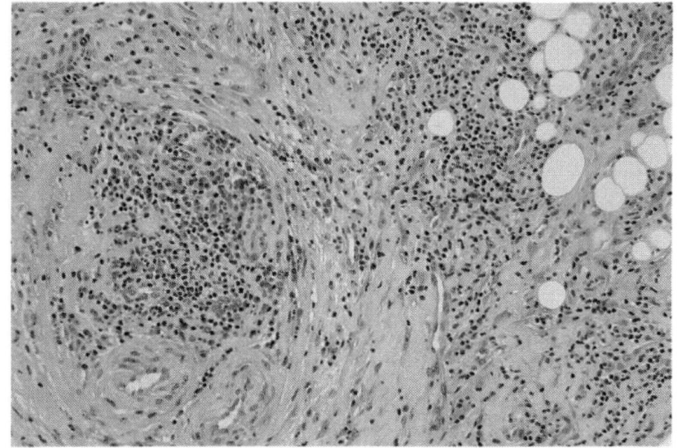

C

Figure 187–23. Sclerosing inflammation. *A,* Axial computed tomography scan of a 42-year-old woman who presented with bilateral swelling of the upper lids with downward displacement of the globes and marked restriction of downward movement on the right side. Note the diffuse infiltrative pattern on the right side. *B,* Sclerosing orbital inflammation with a small germinal center at the upper right, mixed inflammatory infiltrate, and fibrosis. H&E, ×50. *C,* Biopsy sample from another patient showing extension of fibrosis and mixed inflammation into the orbital fat. H&E, ×50.

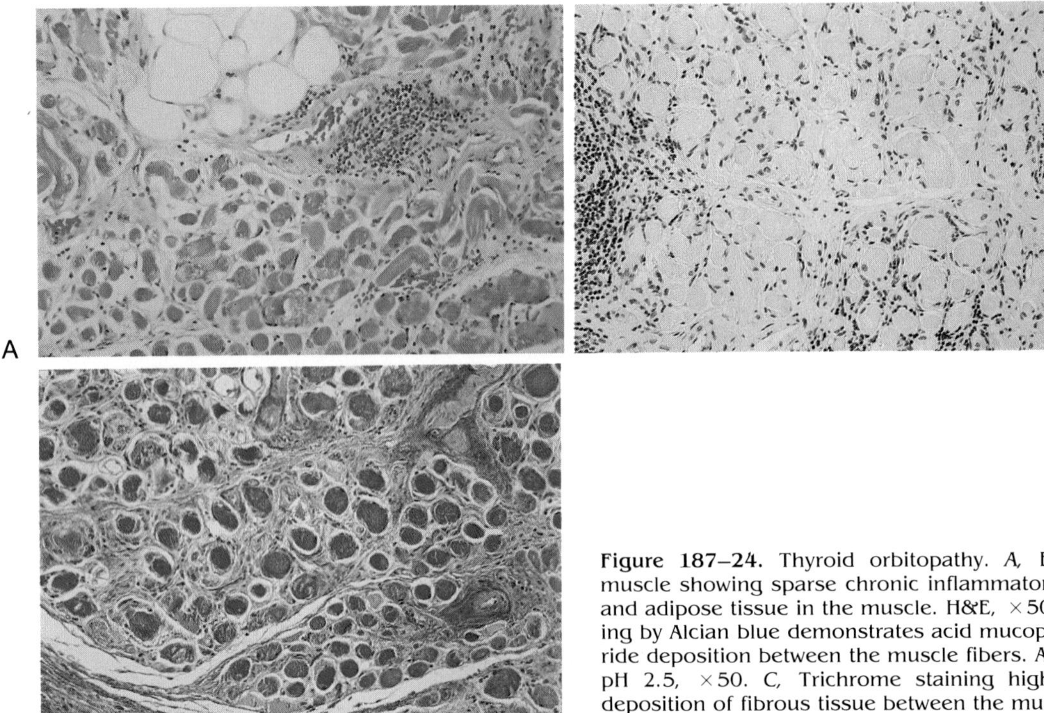

Figure 187–24. Thyroid orbitopathy. *A*, Extraocular muscle showing sparse chronic inflammatory infiltrate and adipose tissue in the muscle. H&E, ×50. *B*, Staining by Alcian blue demonstrates acid mucopolysaccharide deposition between the muscle fibers. Alcian blue, pH 2.5, ×50. *C*, Trichrome staining highlights the deposition of fibrous tissue between the muscle fibers. Masson's trichrome, ×50.

with a plasma cell dyscrasia, a chronic inflammatory condition, or a familial neuropathy. Localized disease may be due to a local lymphoid proliferation, a chronic inflammatory condition, or an organ-limited disease.[160] When amyloid is associated with a plasma cell or lymphoproliferative disease, it has been found to be composed of immunoglobulin light chains. The other groups of amyloid are composed of heterogeneous substances. On H&E staining, amyloid appears as eosinophilic hyaline material, often in round deposits or situated around blood vessels (Fig. 187–25). No matter what the composition of the amyloid, it is orange on Congo red stain and demonstrates red-green dichroism under polarized light.[161] Amyloid may affect many ocular structures and in occasional cases has been found to involve primarily the orbit, including the extraocular muscles and lacrimal gland.[162–168] In the cases of Lucas and colleagues,[166] the amyloid was associated with light chain restriction of

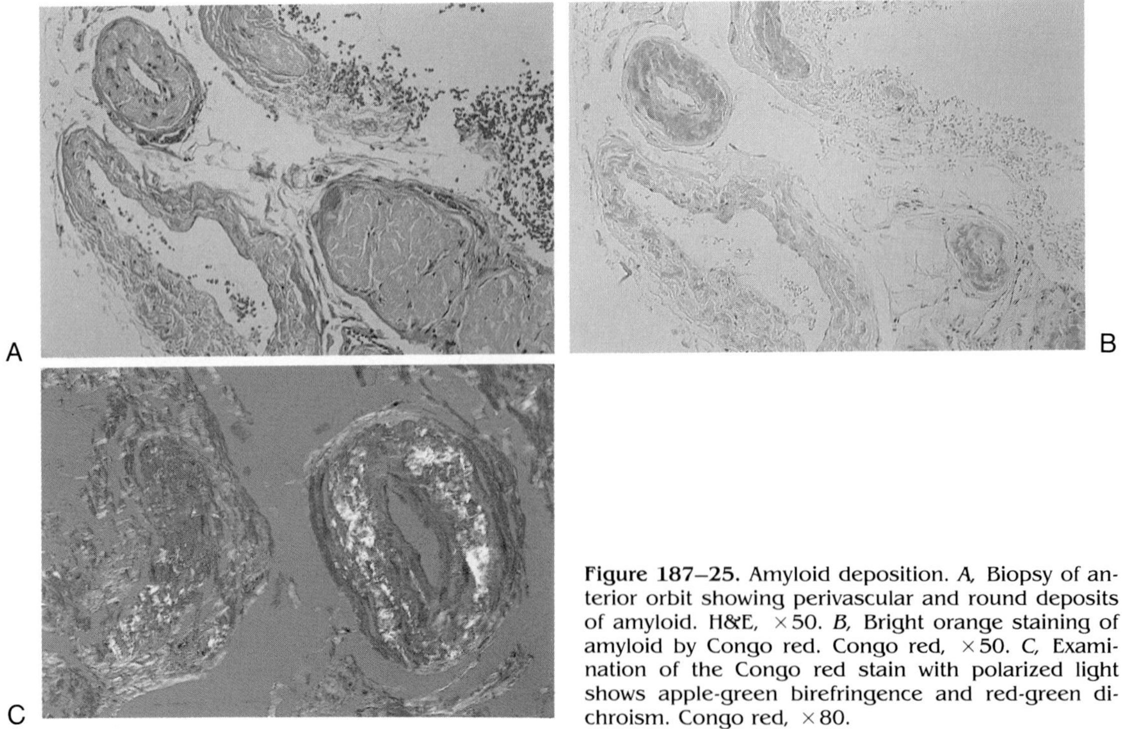

Figure 187–25. Amyloid deposition. *A*, Biopsy of anterior orbit showing perivascular and round deposits of amyloid. H&E, ×50. *B*, Bright orange staining of amyloid by Congo red. Congo red, ×50. *C*, Examination of the Congo red stain with polarized light shows apple-green birefringence and red-green dichroism. Congo red, ×80.

the surrounding lymphocytes and plasma cells, suggesting that this was a monoclonal population even though the infiltrate was not the predominant feature, as would be expected in a lymphoproliferative process.

LYMPHOPROLIFERATIVE AND LEUKEMIC LESIONS

Lymphoproliferative Lesions and Lymphomas

In the past 20 years, lymphomas and the related "benign" lymphoproliferative lesions have been the subject of much confusion, which has affected the classification, the distinction, and the biologic significance of these disorders. This has been especially notable in extranodal lymphoproliferative lesions, including those of the orbit, conjunctiva, and eyelid. Part of this confusion has arisen because of the numerous frequently changing classifications and the rapid explosion in knowledge and technology available to study the immune system, reflected in the many new classifications. Rather than provide intimate details, this section presents pathologic guidelines to help practicing ophthalmologists deal appropriately with patients presenting with lymphoproliferative lesions of the ocular adnexae.

A historical perspective facilitates understanding the current preferred classification, the Working Formulation for Clinical Usage. Before the 1960s, lymphomas were divided into lymphosarcoma and reticulum cell sarcoma. In 1966, Rappaport presented the first reasonable and prognostically useful histopathologic classification of the non-Hodgkin's lymphomas. He categorized the lymphomas into well-differentiated and poorly differentiated lymphocytic, histiocytic, and undifferentiated categories and further subdivided them into nodular and diffuse; this classification is still partially in use.[169] In 1975, Lukes and Collins published their classification based on new technologies that allowed differentiation of lymphomas into B- and T-cell subsets and further subdivision based on the stages of lymphoid progression in the normal lymph node.[170] About the same time, Kiel's classification became popular in Europe.[171] The present classification in general use in North America is the Working Formulation for Non-Hodgkin's Lymphomas, published in 1982. This is an international attempt to synthesize the previous classifications and to present a prognostic classification that can be used when the results of immunophenotyping are not available.[172] The exact details are pertinent to pathologists, but ophthalmologists should know that this classification allows generalization of the specific diagnoses into three grades: low, intermediate, and high, which govern treatment and allow prognostication (Table 187–1).

Ophthalmologists have an important role in ensuring that the specimen from a patient suspected of having a lymphoproliferative lesion is delivered to the pathologist in such a manner that the material can be used in the most appropriate way to allow the largest number of diagnostic investigations to take place. It is no longer appropriate for a specimen to be dropped into formalin or allowed to remain overnight in the operating room refrigerator. A preoperative phone call to the pathologist is essential to discuss any lesion suspected of posing a diagnostic conundrum, particularly a lymphoproliferative lesion. At the Vancouver General Hospital, these lesions are sent to the laboratory immediately after removal, wrapped in sterile saline-dampened Telfa gauze in a hard plastic container. When a specimen is received, a slide is touched to its surface to pick up cells, and an H&E stain is immediately done to confirm a lymphoproliferative process and not another type of lesion. If lymphocytes are present and sufficient material has been received, the specimen will be divided in the following manner to allow the appropriate investigation. A piece is placed in Bouin's or B5 fixative for routine H&E examination and immunophenotyping on fixed tissue (formalin fixation destroys many of the antigens in this category and distorts the nuclear features required for proper classification). A piece is frozen for immunophenotyping on frozen sections and for DNA extraction to detect immunoglobulin or T-cell receptor gene rearrangement.[173, 174] A portion may be submitted in tissue culture media for immunophenotyping in cell suspension and, if the laboratory is equipped, for cytogenetic examination. All of these investigations require a substantial amount of tissue, and not all can be performed on each specimen. The most important factors are that the specimen not be crushed and that it be fixed in Bouin's or B5 fixative, not formalin.

Much of our understanding of the lymphoproliferative lesions involving the ocular adnexae comes from the work of Drs. Jakobiec, Knowles, and their coworkers.[175–181] From their report detailing a series of 108 patients, the following notable conclusions may be drawn: (1) The site of the lymphoproliferative process is paramount, in that 67 percent of patients with eyelid

Table 187–1. WORKING FORMULATION OF NON-HODGKIN'S LYMPHOMAS FOR CLINICAL USE

Low Grade
Small lymphocytic*
Small lymphocytic, plasmacytoid*
Follicular, small cleaved cell*
Follicular, mixed small cleaved and large cell
Intermediate Grade
Follicular, large cell
Diffuse, small cleaved cell*
Diffuse, mixed small and large cell
Diffuse, large cell
High Grade
Large cell, immunoblastic
Lymphoblastic
Small noncleaved, Burkitt's and non-Burkitt's
Miscellaneous
Composite
Mycosis fungoides
Histiocytic
Extramedullary plasmacytoma
Others

*Lymphomas commonly occurring in the orbit.

Data from National Cancer Institute sponsored study of classifications of non-Hodgkin's lymphomas. Cancer 49:2112, 1982.

lesions, 35 percent of patients with orbital lesions, and only 20 percent of patients with conjunctival lesions developed systemic lymphoma during a follow-up of approximately 4 years. (2) The histologic classification of lesions was important in distinguishing those in the small lymphoproliferative categories (hyperplasia, small lymphocytic lymphoma, small cleaved cell lymphoma) from those in all other categories (mixed and large cell) in determining prognosis, where 27 percent versus 46 percent of patients developed systemic lymphoma, respectively. (3) It did not matter whether patients were found to have immunophenotypically polyclonal or monoclonal populations, because equal percentages in each group developed a systemic lymphoma.[175]

These observations mean that even so-called reactive lymphoid hyperplasia in the orbit may imply potential for systemic lymphoma. The essence of this work and that of others is that all patients with a histopathologically verified lymphoproliferative lesion of the ocular adnexae require complete evaluation by a hematooncologist for evidence of systemic disease at the time of diagnosis and at regular follow-up intervals, because approximately one third of these patients have developed or will develop systemic lymphoma.[175, 182, 183] It remains to be seen in ongoing studies whether the new technique of detection of immunoglobulin gene rearrangement will offer better prognostication. Jakobiec and colleagues have found that three of five specimens that were immunophenotypically polyclonal were genotypically monoclonal.[176, 184] We have had a similar experience.

B-CELL LYMPHOMAS

The vast majority of orbital lymphoproliferative lesions are of B-cell origin, although varying numbers of reactive T-cells will be admixed.[175] Most of the lesions are composed of "small" B cells, resembling normal B lymphocytes. In reactive hyperplasia, irregularly and widely spaced germinal centers containing mixtures of small and large lymphocytes, mitotic figures, and tingible body macrophages are surrounded by small lymphocytes, plasma cells, and histiocytes (Fig. 187–26). Some forms of hyperplasia do not contain germinal centers but have a dense mixture of inflammatory cells.

Small lymphocytic lymphomas have a monotonous population of small, almost normal-appearing lymphocytes, some of which may have plasmacytoid features. Multinucleated cells called *polykaryocytes,* deposits of hemosiderin, prominent vessels, and occasional germinal centers may be present (Fig. 187–27). Small cleaved cell lymphomas, which may be follicular or diffuse, have a monotonous population of small cleaved lymphocytes (Fig. 187–28). These are the most common categories encountered in the orbit.

Occasional cases of large cell lymphomas, in which the lymphocyte is about the same size as a histiocyte or endothelial cell, have been described.[175–185] We have encountered two large cell lymphomas of the orbit, one in a patient with AIDS, and a case of Burkitt's lymphoma in this setting has been described (Fig. 187–29).[186, 187] We reported a single case of signet ring morphology in a mixed small cleaved and large cell lymphoma of the orbit, a cellular pattern seen most frequently in adenocarcinomas, so this diagnosis must be ruled out on the basis of immunopathology and electron microscopy (EM).[188]

T-CELL LYMPHOMAS

Involvement of the orbit in T-cell lymphomas is uncommon and usually occurs at the end-stage of mycosis fungoides when there is widespread disease of the skin

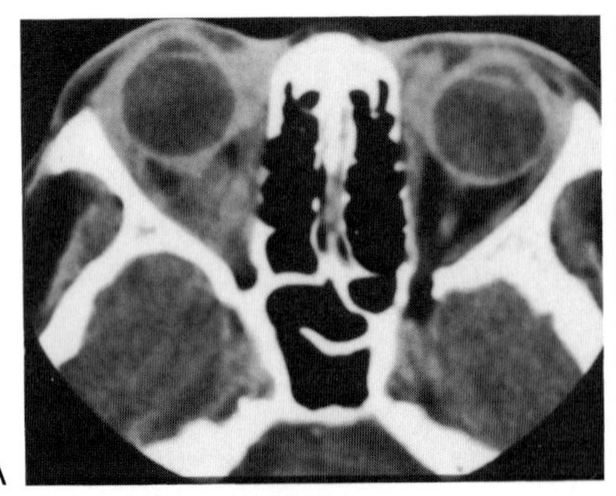

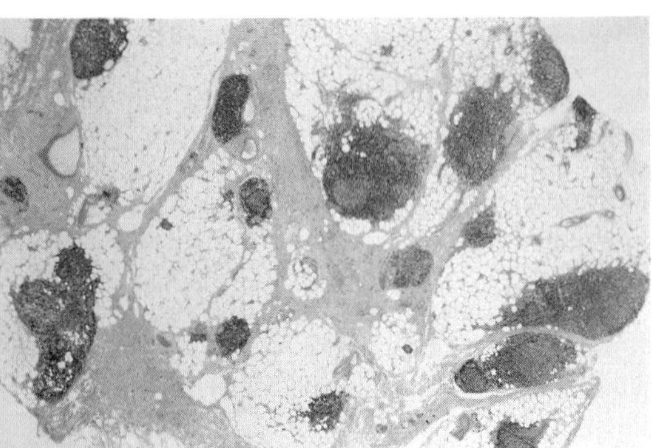

Figure 187–26. Reactive lymphoid hyperplasia. *A,* Computed tomography scan demonstrates an irregular infiltrative mass lesion that obscures the normal orbital fat and was associated with some limitation of inferior rectus function. *B,* Widely and irregularly spaced collections of lymphocytes, some with germinal centers, and fibrosis. H&E, ×5. *C,* Detail of a lymphoid follicle showing a reactive germinal center. H&E, ×20.

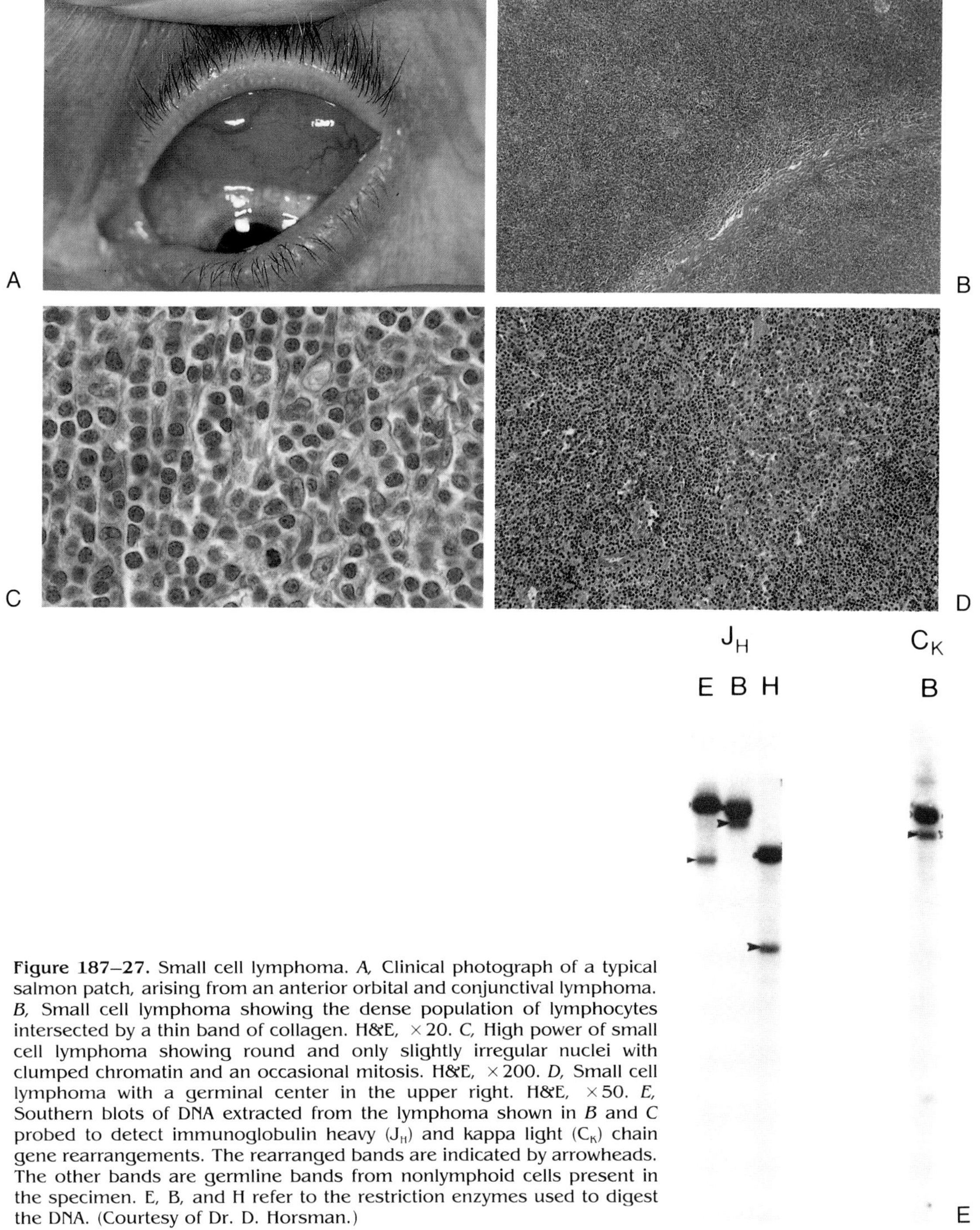

Figure 187–27. Small cell lymphoma. *A,* Clinical photograph of a typical salmon patch, arising from an anterior orbital and conjunctival lymphoma. *B,* Small cell lymphoma showing the dense population of lymphocytes intersected by a thin band of collagen. H&E, ×20. *C,* High power of small cell lymphoma showing round and only slightly irregular nuclei with clumped chromatin and an occasional mitosis. H&E, ×200. *D,* Small cell lymphoma with a germinal center in the upper right. H&E, ×50. *E,* Southern blots of DNA extracted from the lymphoma shown in *B* and *C* probed to detect immunoglobulin heavy (J_H) and kappa light (C_K) chain gene rearrangements. The rearranged bands are indicated by arrowheads. The other bands are germline bands from nonlymphoid cells present in the specimen. E, B, and H refer to the restriction enzymes used to digest the DNA. (Courtesy of Dr. D. Horsman.)

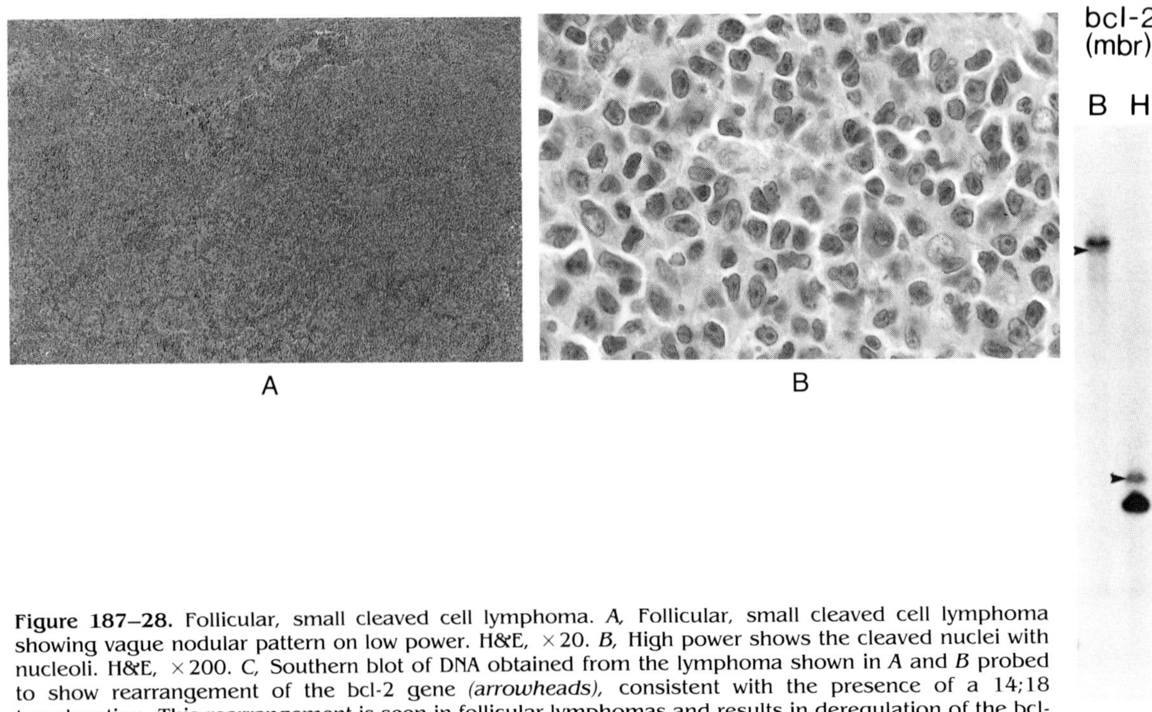

Figure 187–28. Follicular, small cleaved cell lymphoma. *A,* Follicular, small cleaved cell lymphoma showing vague nodular pattern on low power. H&E, ×20. *B,* High power shows the cleaved nuclei with nucleoli. H&E, ×200. *C,* Southern blot of DNA obtained from the lymphoma shown in *A* and *B* probed to show rearrangement of the bcl-2 gene *(arrowheads),* consistent with the presence of a 14;18 translocation. This rearrangement is seen in follicular lymphomas and results in deregulation of the bcl-2 gene. (Courtesy of Dr. D. Horsman.)

and other organs.[189–191] Case reports describing solitary T-cell lymphoma of the orbit and with eyelid and orbital involvement as a presenting sign have been published.[192–194] Histologically, the malignant cells in T-cell disorders often have a markedly convoluted cerebriform nucleus—Sézary's cells—which may suggest the diagnosis. This is not always the case, and confirmation of a T-cell lymphoma depends on immunophenotyping of the biopsy tissue.

Malignant histiocytosis or histiocytic medullary reticulosis infrequently involves the orbit.[131] The histogenesis of the malignant cells is in some dispute, but investigations suggest that in most cases they are T cells.[195–198]

Plasmacytoma

Plasmacytomas could have been categorized as B-cell lymphomas because plasma cells are the end-stage of differentiation of B lymphocytes. However, their pattern of involvement of the orbit and the clinical history are much different and set them apart. Plasma cell tumors may be seen as soft tissue lesions, either polyclonal, reactive, or extramedullary monoclonal plasmacytomas, as a solitary tumor of bone, with or without adjacent soft tissue disease; or orbital bone involvement may be part of the systemic disease multiple myeloma.[199] If a plasma cell tumor is diagnosed on orbital biopsy, a complete physical examination, skeletal survey for osteolytic bone lesions, bone marrow biopsy, serum protein electrophoresis, and immunoelectrophoresis of serum and urine must be undertaken to rule out systemic disease.[200–204]

Histopathologically, plasma cells are easy to recognize because of their oval shape, eccentric nucleus with clumped chromatin, perinuclear halo, and amphophilic cytoplasm (Fig. 187–30). Some of these features may be lost in more poorly differentiated neoplasms. Immunoperoxidase staining for cytoplasmic immunoglobulins on

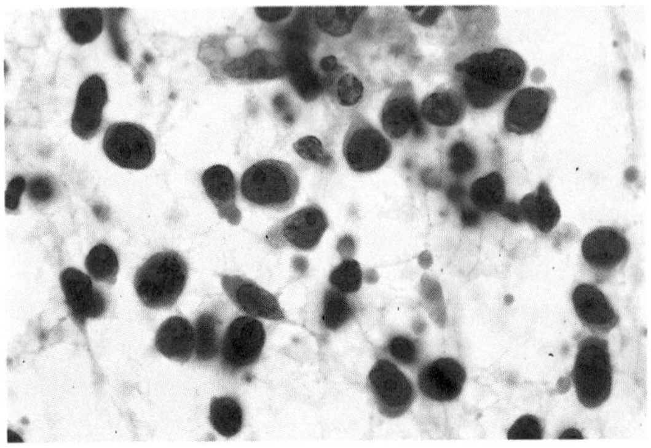

Figure 187–29. Large cell lymphoma. Aspiration biopsy specimen from a large cell lymphoma in the lacrimal gland and cervical lymph nodes. The nuclei are large, vesicular, and pleomorphic, with prominent nucleoli. H&E, ×200.

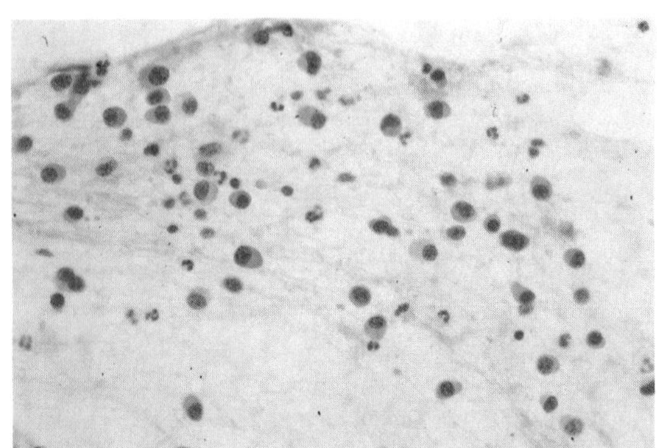

Figure 187–30. Plasmacytoma. Aspiration biopsy sample from a plasmacytoma of the orbit. The cells are oval, with eccentric nuclei and prominent nucleoli. H&E, ×80.

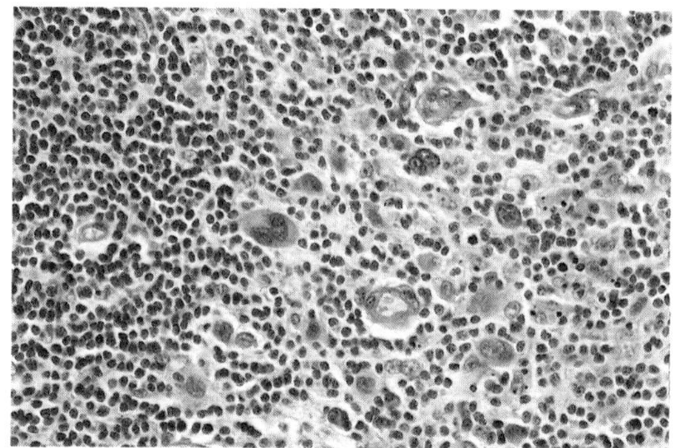

Figure 187–31. Hodgkin's disease. Numerous Reed-Sternberg cells and mononuclear variants are surrounded by nonneoplastic lymphocytes and plasma cells. H&E, ×80.

Bouin's or B5 fixed tissue is most useful in identifying plasma cells and to establish mono- or polyclonality.

Hodgkin's Disease

Involvement of the orbit in Hodgkin's disease is rare; only a few cases have been reported. It usually occurs in the setting of widespread disease.[205] In one case we encountered, although involvement of the orbit was not diagnosed until 29 months after initial presentation with Hodgkin's disease, the asymmetry of the orbit present on old photographs and radiologic evidence of bony excavation suggested that orbital involvement had been present for a much longer time.[206] Histologic diagnosis of Hodgkin's disease rests on the demonstration of Reed-Sternberg cells, the mirror-image binucleate cells with eosinophilic nucleoli, and vesicular nuclei (Fig. 187–31). Rye's classification of lymphocyte-predominant, mixed cellularity, lymphocyte-depleted, and nodular sclerosing types has been in use for many years.[207] A case of nonspecific orbital granuloma in long-standing Hodgkin's disease has been described.[208]

Leukemia

Ocular involvement is common in leukemia but may not always be clinically evident. In a large autopsy series, ocular involvement was present in 80 percent of cases, but orbital involvement was present in only 14 percent of chronic and 7.3 percent of acute leukemias, most of which were not thought to have been clinically evident.[209] Clinical orbital infiltration may be the presenting sign of an acute leukemia or may occur during its course.

The most characteristic association is the chloroma, or granulocytic sarcoma of acute myelogenous leukemia, but a mass can infrequently occur with acute lymphoblastic leukemia, during the blast crisis of chronic myelogenous leukemia, and with chronic lymphocytic leukemias.[210–217] If a patient has been identified as having leukemia, the diagnosis will be easy, but if orbital chloroma is a presenting sign, the main problem lies in suspecting the diagnosis. Grossly, the mass may show a slight greenish tinge due to the presence of myeloperoxidase.

Histopathologic examination shows a mass of undifferentiated cells, which require differentiation from the other "small blue cell tumors" of childhood, the age group in which granulocytic sarcoma is most frequent (Fig. 187–32). To establish the diagnosis of a granulocytic sarcoma, the cytoplasm of the cells must be examined for the presence of eosinophilic granules that contain myeloperoxidase, confirmed by the chloroacetate esterase (Leder's) stain. Ruling out rhabdomyosarcoma, metastatic neuroblastoma, and Ewing's sarcoma is mandatory if there is no evidence of systemic leukemia. Systemic leukemia usually becomes evident at the same time or shortly after a chloroma is diagnosed but in some cases has not appeared for up to 9 months.[216] If the orbital mass occurs in the setting of a lymphoblastic or chronic lymphocytic leukemia, the cells are similar to those described earlier in lymphomas. Examination of bone marrow and peripheral blood is required to help make the correct diagnosis.

NEOPLASMS

Neoplasms account for approximately 20 to 25 percent of orbital diseases and are most common in the seventh to tenth decades.[1] The full range of tumors that occur in the extraorbital soft tissues and bones can occur in the orbit. Excellent references describing soft tissue tumors and EM of tumors are available.[218, 219] The

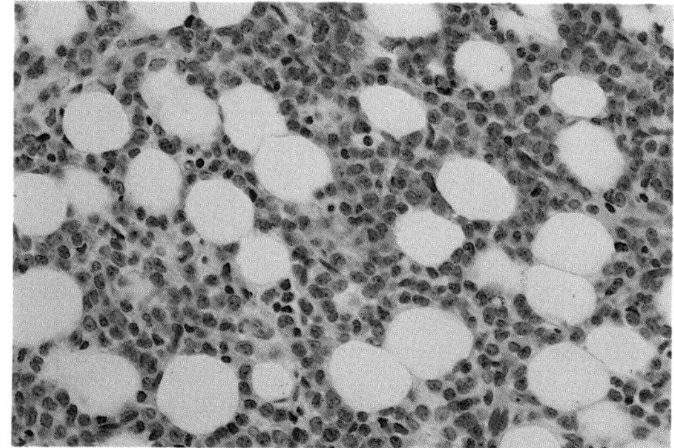

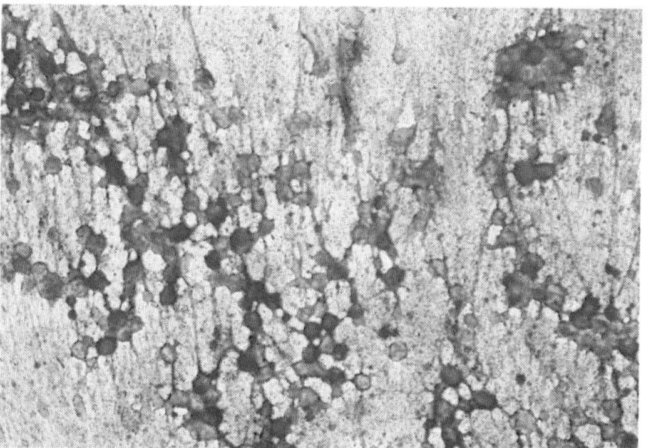

Figure 187–32. Chloroma. *A,* Invasion of orbital fat by cells of myeloid leukemia. H&E, ×80. *B,* Positive chloroacetate esterase stain on a smear of cells from the leukemia in *A.* H&E, ×80.

classification of soft tissue tumors can be confusing, but they are usually named after the type of differentiation present or proposed cell of origin, although it is generally accepted that most malignant tumors arise from an undifferentiated pluripotential cell.

Pathologic analysis is directed at two major aspects: the type of tumor and whether it is malignant. Malignancy is generally determined on routine H&E sections by the assessment of mitoses, anaplasia, and invasive margins in association with the clinical history, whereas typing of the tumor often requires immunohistochemistry, electron microscopy, and more recently cytogenetics. Advances in immunohistochemistry require different fixatives for optimum preservation of antigens, making preoperative consultation with a pathologist mandatory so that appropriate management of the specimen is undertaken. At our institution, fresh tissue from a suspected neoplasm is sent to the laboratory immediately after removal, and a small portion is fixed in 100 percent alcohol for optimum preservation of intermediate filaments, 2.5 percent glutaraldehyde for EM, and the remainder in formalin. If sufficient tissue is available, a fresh sample is submitted for cytogenetic study and a small portion is frozen for future DNA studies. This is particularly important in lesions suspected of being malignant.

Neoplasms With Neurogenic and Neural Crest Differentiation

Neoplasms with neurogenic and neural crest differentiation are grouped together because of their proven or presumed origin from components of peripheral nerve or because they show definite evidence of neural crest or neuroectodermal differentiation. Although most of the structures of the head and neck are thought to be derived from neural crest, they do not retain this differentiation and thus are described in other sections.[220] Peripheral nerve sheath tumors account for the greatest number of tumors in this section; the others are rare.

PERIPHERAL NERVE SHEATH TUMORS

Neurofibromas and schwannomas (or neurilemomas) are the two peripheral nerve sheath tumors that involve the orbit. They are discussed together because of the association with neurofibromatosis and because the features may overlap and precise distinction may not be possible.[221] The spectrum of neurofibromas includes plexiform, diffuse, and isolated forms. Plexiform neurofibromas, which are associated with von Recklinghausen's neurofibromatosis, are hamartomas of peripheral nerves in that the "tumor" is composed of a benign proliferation of cells normally found in the nerve: axons, Schwann's cells, endoneurial cells, and perineurial cells. The tumor is composed of masses of hypertrophied nerves, said to look grossly like a bag of worms and accompanied by an increase in thin-walled blood vessels, which may bleed profusely at the time of surgery (Fig. 187–33). Plexiform neurofibromas lead to marked enlargement of the skin, bone, and soft tissues of the eyelid and orbit, a common site for these lesions.[222–224] Other orbital manifestations of neurofibromatosis include absence of the greater wing of the sphenoid bone, optic nerve gliomas, and meningiomas; other ocular manifestations are common.

Diffuse neurofibromas consist of a diffuse proliferation of bland spindle-shaped cells, which surround and permeate the normal structures without destroying them. Scattered throughout are ovoid bodies, collections of Schwann's cell processes. Although these lesions are said to be uncommon in neurofibromatosis, we have seen them in association with plexiform neurofibromas in many instances.

Isolated neurofibromas consist of circumscribed collections of cells with the EM characteristics of perineurial cells, although axons and Schwann's cells are part of the process; whether they represent entrapped normal cells or a component of the proliferating cells is unclear.[225] They usually arise from the sensory divisions of the trigeminal nerve. On light microscopy, these are similar to the tumors seen in the skin and show a circumscribed tumor composed of spindle-shaped cells with wavy nuclei, often arranged in bundles reminiscent of a nerve (Fig. 187–34). Bodian's stain highlights the axons. Single and multiple isolated tumors may occur but are infrequently associated with neurofibromatosis.[226, 227] Two neurofibromas have been reported in the lacrimal gland.[228]

Amputation neuromas are reactive proliferations of peripheral nerves and fibrous tissue that might be confused histologically with a plexiform neurofibroma. They occur in response to transection of a nerve and are thought to represent an attempt to find the distal segment. Although common elsewhere, they are rare in the orbit, possibly because the involved nerves are small. An amputation neuroma shows a proliferation of disorganized nerves and scarring of adjacent structures, which would be compatible with the history of trauma.[229]

Schwannomas are composed exclusively of Schwann's cells and arise eccentrically from a peripheral nerve. They are encapsulated by perineurium and have two growth patterns (Fig. 187–35). The Antoni A area is highly cellular, with the nuclei often pallisading or forming Verocay's bodies. The nuclei are spindle shaped, with no pleomorphism or mitoses, and the cytoplasm is eosinophilic. The Antoni B areas are myxoid and hypocellular, and the cells are often round or oval. Ancient schwannomas may display areas of hemorrhage, cyst formation, thick-walled blood vessels, xanthoma cells, collagenization, and bizarre nuclei in the absence of mitoses, all thought to represent degenerative changes.[230, 231] EM shows cells with long interdigitating and wrapping processes covered by external lamina, occasional desmosomes, and long spacing collagen.[225] Immunohistochemical staining for protein S100 is helpful in confirming the neural nature of all of these tumors (see Fig. 187–33*D*).

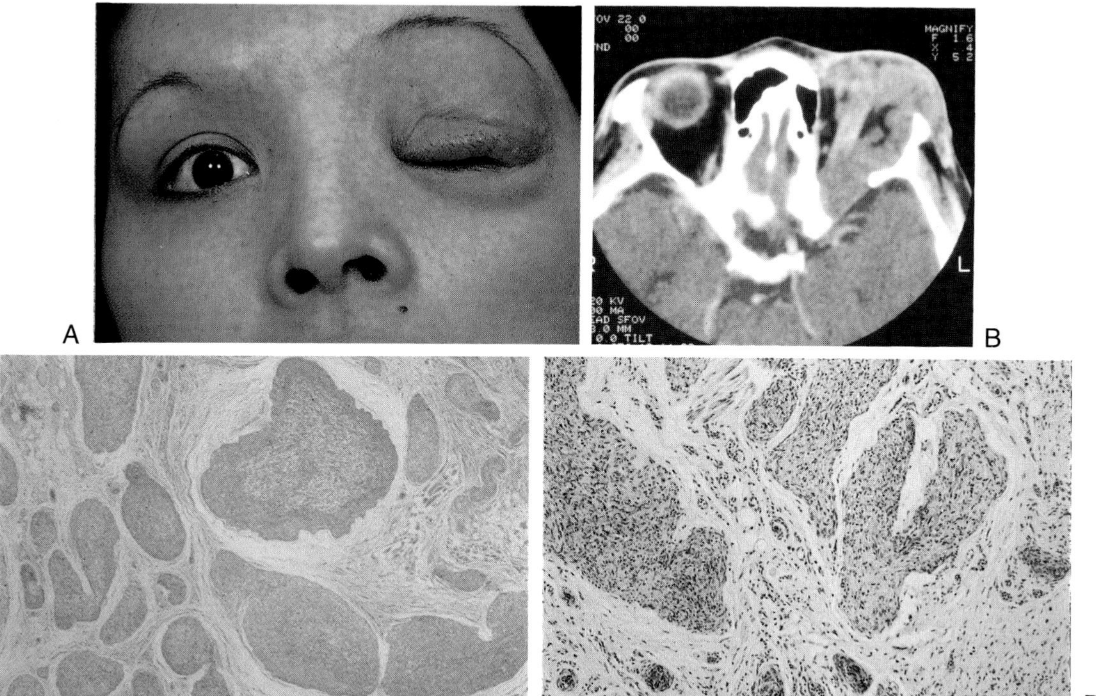

Figure 187–33. Plexiform neurofibroma with von Recklinghausen's disease. *A,* Clinical photograph of a 28-year-old who had a long-standing history of progressive swelling and thickening of the left upper lid. On palpation, this had a typical nodular wormlike feeling. *B,* Axial computed tomography scan of the same patient demonstrates diffuse, irregular involvement of the superior orbit, with enlargement of the superior orbital fissure and absence of part of the sphenoid wing. *C,* Histopathologic examination of some of this tissue shows numerous enlarged nerves responsible for thickening of the eyelid and orbit. H&E, ×5. *D,* Positive staining for protein S100 in the enlarged nerves. Indirect immunoperoxidase, S100, ×20.

Neurofibromas are thought to become malignant more often than schwannomas, but more than half do not arise in association with neurofibromatosis.[232] Malignant peripheral nerve sheath tumors are rare, the largest orbital series of eight cases being reported by Jakobiec and colleagues, with occasional cases by others.[233–235] Most arose in the superomedial orbit from the supraorbital nerve, which was clinically and grossly enlarged, and ultimately spread along this nerve into the middle cranial fossa after many recurrences. A previous plexiform neurofibroma was found in only one case, but a malignant plexiform pattern in which the malignant cells grew to some extent within the confines of the nerve was common. The two basic histologic patterns were spindle cell and epithelioid, but others were present. In all cases, cellular pleomorphism and mitotic figures were prominent so that a diagnosis of malignancy was not difficult. Positive immunoperoxidase staining for protein S100 and EM may be helpful in identifying the neurogenic nature of this tumor, but these specific features are often lost. The greatest aid in diagnosis is recognition of origin from peripheral nerve.

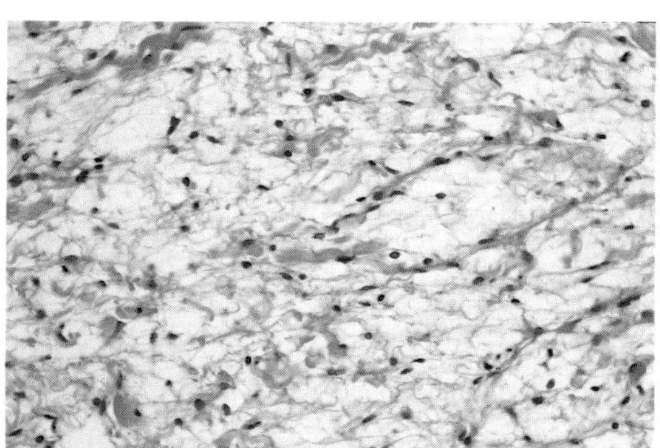

Figure 187–34. Solitary neurofibroma. Solitary neurofibroma with loosely arranged myxoid background containing bland spindle cells. H&E, ×50.

GRANULAR CELL TUMOR

Granular cell tumor, formerly called *granular cell myoblastoma,* is presented here because it is currently thought to arise from Schwann's cells that have assumed a facultative histiocytic role. Several cases have been reported within the soft tissues of the orbit, including one in extraocular muscle.[236–240] It also occurs in conjunctiva, eyelid, lacrimal sac, and caruncle but is most frequent in the skin and tongue. Grossly, it consists of a firm gray mass and histologically shows a proliferation of polyhedral cells with granular eosinophilic cytoplasm that is PAS positive and diastase resistant and stains with immunoperoxidase for protein S100 (Fig. 187–36). EM findings are characteristic, showing cytoplasm full of single membrane-bound granules containing irregularly shaped round and laminated electron-dense material thought to be secondary lysosomes. Groups of cells

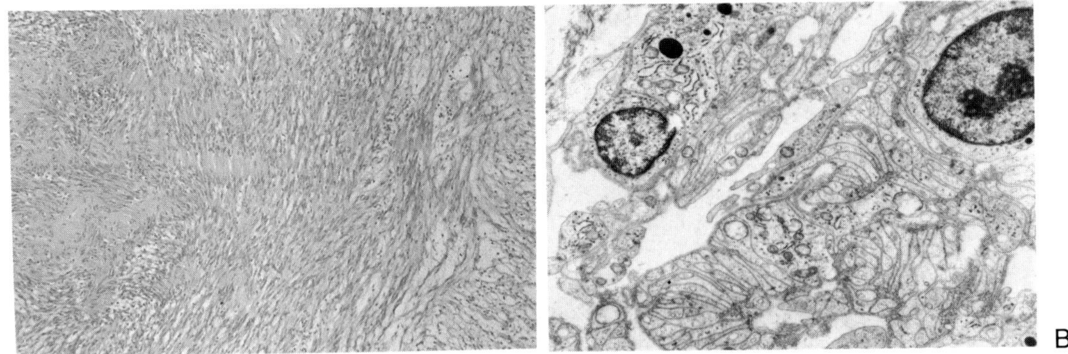

Figure 187–35. Schwannoma (neurilemoma). *A,* Schwannoma showing cellular Antoni A area with Verocay's bodies to the left and hypocellular Antoni B area to the right. H&E, ×20. *B,* Electron micrograph from the schwannoma in *A* shows the long intertwining cell processes covered by external lamina. ×14,000.

surrounded by basal lamina and long spacing collagen may be present.[241]

PRIMARY ORBITAL MELANOMA

Melanoma in the orbit usually arises secondarily from direct or metastatic spread of a choroidal, conjunctival, or cutaneous melanoma or from leptomeningeal melanoma.[242] Primary melanoma of the orbit is a rare condition arising in the setting of oculodermal melanocytosis or nevus of Ota, a developmental anomaly more common in Asians and blacks.[243] At least six cases of orbital melanoma have been reported in this syndrome. Pathologic examination has shown a melanoma similar to a spindle choroidal melanoma, which is associated with increased numbers of nonmalignant spindle melanocytes in the tissues surrounding the melanoma and with a cellular blue nevus in some cases.[243–246]

NEUROEPITHELIAL TUMORS

Neuroepithelial tumors are rare primary tumors that show varied evidence of neuroblastic differentiation and consist of primary neuroblastoma, peripheral neuroepithelioma (also called *peripheral neuroectodermal tumor*), and olfactory neuroblastoma or esthesioneuroblastoma.

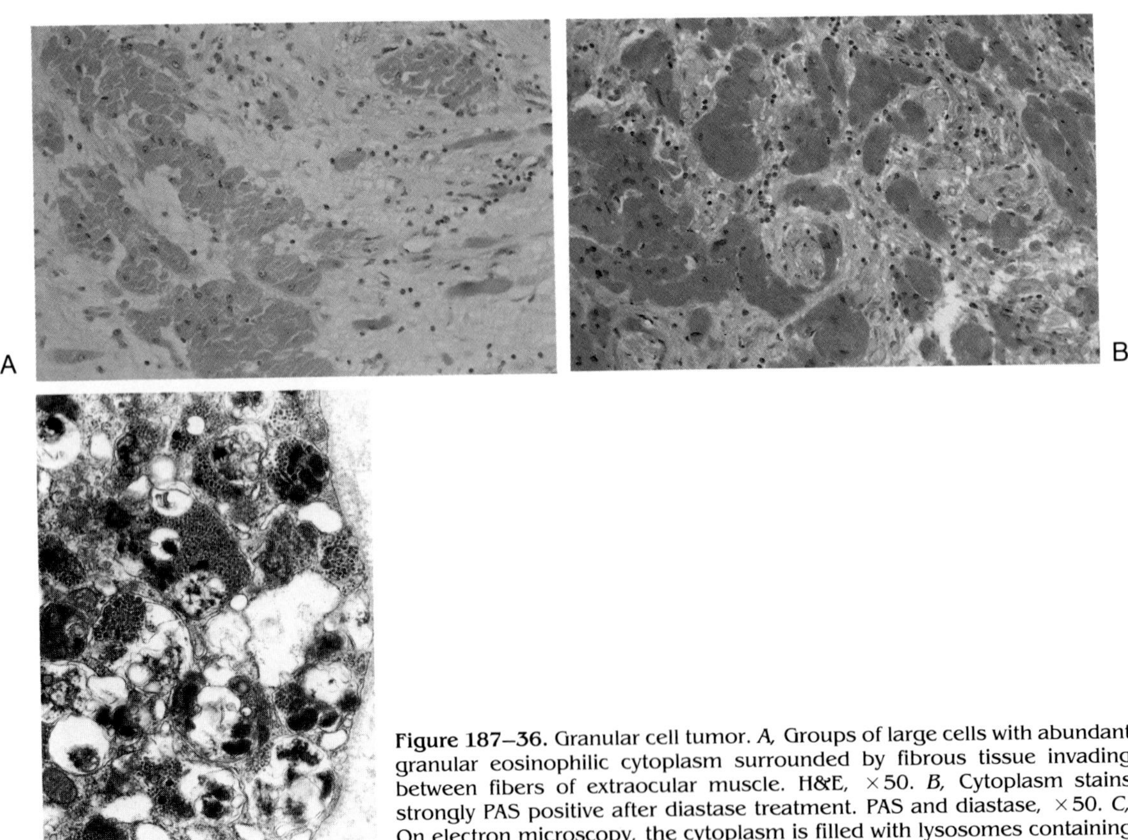

Figure 187–36. Granular cell tumor. *A,* Groups of large cells with abundant granular eosinophilic cytoplasm surrounded by fibrous tissue invading between fibers of extraocular muscle. H&E, ×50. *B,* Cytoplasm stains strongly PAS positive after diastase treatment. PAS and diastase, ×50. *C,* On electron microscopy, the cytoplasm is filled with lysosomes containing material that is irregular in shape and density. The cell is surrounded by external lamina. ×28,000.

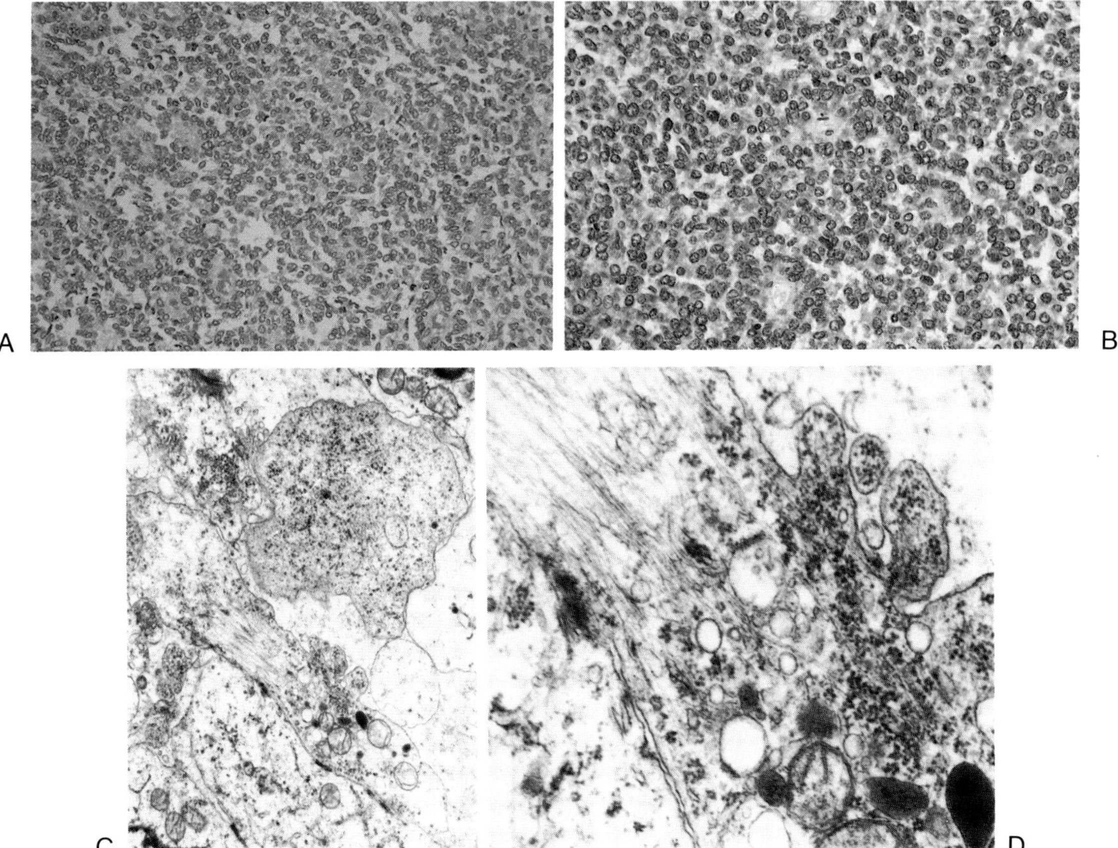

Figure 187–37. Peripheral neuroepithelioma. *A,* Extraorbital peripheral neuroepithelioma showing proliferation of small undifferentiated cells with occasional poorly formed rosettes. This tumor had an 11;22 translocation on cytogenetic examination. H&E, ×50. *B,* Positive staining for neuron-specific enolase. Indirect immunoperoxidase, neuron-specific enolase, ×80. *C,* Electron microscopy from the center of one of the poorly formed rosettes shows numerous cell processes, one of which contains microtubules and dense core granules. ×31,500. *D,* Higher magnification of cell process containing microtubules and dense core granules. ×100,000.

Primary neuroblastoma of the orbit has been reported twice in adults, but like the more frequently occurring tumors in the adrenals of children, it shows small undifferentiated cells, Homer-Wright rosettes, pseudorosettes, and background neuropil. The cells stain positively for neuron-specific enolase (NSE) and show neuritic processes containing dense core granules and microtubules by EM.[247, 248] Peripheral neuroepithelioma is an allied but more poorly differentiated tumor usually occurring in the soft tissues of the extremities of adults, although at least three cases have been reported in the orbit.[249–251] On light microscopy, it shows few rosettes but does stain for NSE (Fig. 187–37). On EM, very occasional cell processes and dense core granules are present.[252, 253] These tumors may be the same as those previously called *extraosseous Ewing's sarcoma,* because cytogenetic investigations have shown a similar translocation (t11;22) in both of these tumors.[254, 255] Olfactory neuroblastomas arise from the sensory nerves of the olfactory plate and involve the orbit secondarily, although patients may present with ophthalmic signs.[256, 257] Histologic features are similar to those of peripheral neuroepithelioma, although some tumors show evidence of olfactory differentiation in the form of specialized rosettes.[258, 259]

PARAGANGLIOMAS AND CARCINOID TUMORS

Paragangliomas occur most frequently in the carotid body, glomus jugulare, and tympanic membrane of the head and neck region, arising from cells thought to have a chemoreceptor function. No normal paraganglion cells have been definitely identified in the orbit, so the origin of these tumors there is unknown. At least 14 orbital cases have been reported in the English literature.[260, 264] These are well-circumscribed vascular masses that histologically show regular cells arranged in nests separated by a myriad of thin-walled blood vessels and fibrous stroma. The cells show little pleomorphism or mitoses and have granular cytoplasm (Fig. 187–38). The granules may be stained by Grimelius's technique and by immunoperoxidase for NSE and chromogranin. EM shows interdigitating cell membranes, intercellular junctions, and dense core granules.[265] One of these tumors was a melanotic paraganglioma showing premelanosomes in addition to neurosecretory granules, emphasizing the pluripotential nature of neural crest tissue.[262]

An allied tumor is the carcinoid, of which one primary orbital and several metastatic cases have been reported.[266–268] These most commonly arise from the neu-

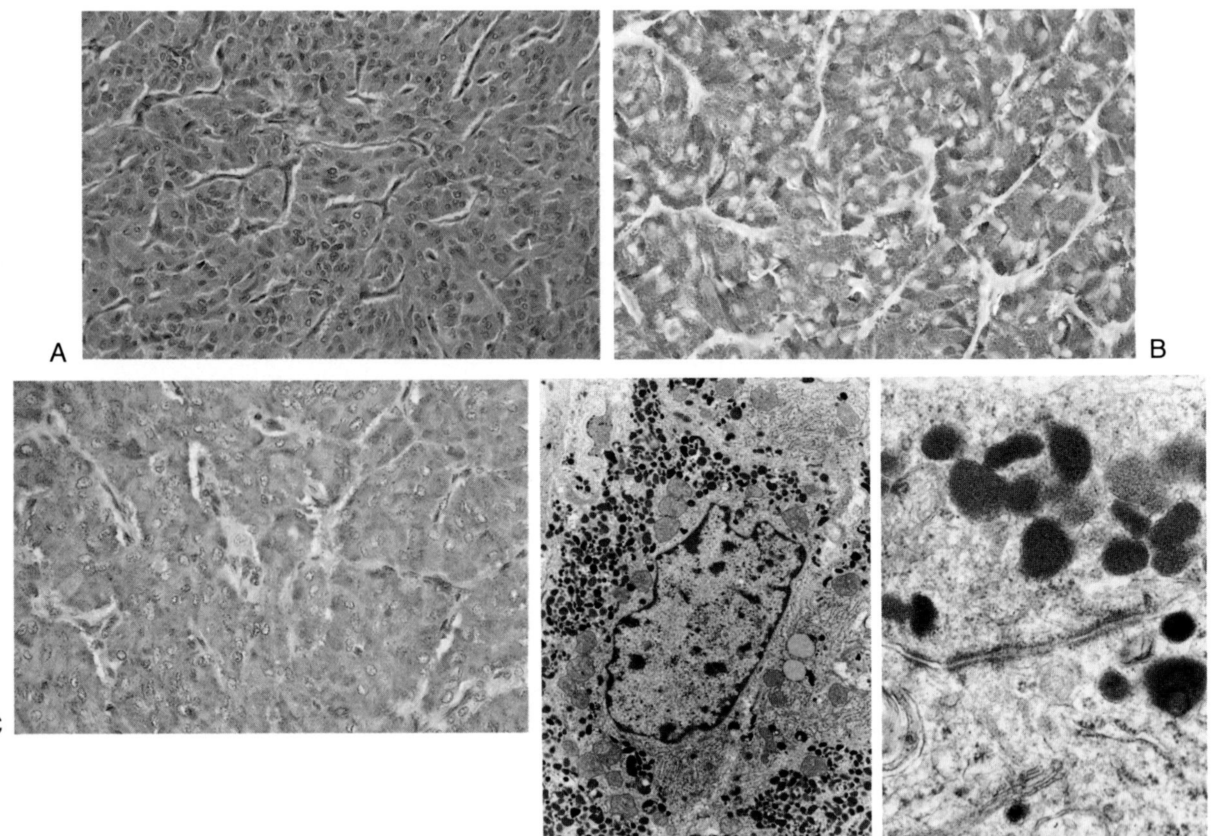

Figure 187–38. Paraganglioma. *A,* Large cells with eosinophilic to amphophilic granular cytoplasm are arranged in nests surrounded by thin-walled blood vessels. H&E, ×50. *B,* Cytoplasm shows strong argyrophilic staining of granules. Grimelius, ×80. *C,* Cytoplasmic granules also stain strongly for chromogranin. Indirect immunoperoxidase, chromogranin, ×80. *D, left,* By electron microscopy, the cytoplasm contains numerous dense core granules. ×6900. *Right,* Higher power shows the irregularly shaped granules and intercellular junctions. ×49,500.

roendocrine cells of the gastrointestinal tract and lung, and again, no normal neuroendocrine cells of the orbit have been described. The cells of this tumor may show solid, trabecular, and tubular patterns without pleomorphism and few mitoses. Cytoplasm is granular and eosinophilic and is positive with Grimelius's stain and for chromogranin. EM shows dense core granules.

RETINAL ANLAGE TUMOR

Also called *melanotic neuroectodermal tumor of infancy,* this uncommon tumor usually occurs in the maxilla, although diverse sites such as the skull, femur, and epididymis have been involved.[269] Primary orbital cases have been described, but they usually involve the orbit secondarily.[270, 271] This tumor shows alveolar structures lined by cuboidal cells resembling pigment epithelial cells surrounding a central area containing small neuroblastic cells, the unit thought to resemble the developing eye. These units are surrounded by a fibrous stroma. The origin is unknown, but displaced anterior neuroepithelium and neural crest have been proposed, although the former is more likely because of the presence of neuroepithelial rather than neural crest melanin.

Neoplasms With Mesenchymal Differentiation

Tumors categorized as neoplasms with mesenchymal differentiation all have mesenchymal features and are further classified on the basis of differentiation toward normal soft tissue structures, such as muscle, fat, or blood vessels.

FIBROBLASTIC TUMORS

Fibroblastic tumors consist of the basic mesenchymal cell; the fibroblast, which contains vimentin intermediate filaments demonstrable by immunohistochemistry and shows abundant rough endoplasmic reticulum (RER); no external lamina; and no desmosomes on EM.

Nodular Fasciitis

Nodular fasciitis, considered to be reactive, commonly occurs on the trunk and upper extremity. Around the eye, it has usually occurred in the conjunctiva and eyelid but has been reported in the deeper orbit.[272, 273] It is noncircumscribed, with a central hypocellular, myxoid, and vascular zone containing chronic inflammatory cells surrounded by a cellular region of plump fibroblasts. The fibroblasts appear reactive rather than atypical but may show normal mitoses and extend into the surrounding tissue, including striated muscle. EM has shown that some of the cells are myofibroblasts, modified fibroblasts showing smooth muscle features of thin filaments and dense bodies, which are common in reparative conditions.[218]

Fibroma and Myxoma

Fibromas are rare benign tumors of fibroblasts that have been reported in the superficial and deep orbit. They are hypocellular and show bundles of regular spindle-shaped cells in a collagenous stroma.[274, 275] Myxomas are a benign fibroblastic proliferation in which the fibroblasts synthesize mucopolysaccharides rather than collagen. The abundant matrix, which stains positively with alcian blue, gives the lesion a hypocellular appearance in which the cells may be stellate as well as spindle shaped. The vascular pattern is not prominent.[276, 277] This lesion must be distinguished from other benign (neurofibroma) and malignant lesions (liposarcoma, malignant fibrous histiocytoma, rhabdomyosarcoma) that may have myxoid areas.

Fibromatosis

The fibromatoses are a group of benign, nonmetastasizing, but locally aggressive fibroblastic proliferations that have been divided into juvenile and adult categories with several entities in each category.[278] Juvenile lesions may be localized or generalized. Several localized cases have been reported in the orbit, usually inferior, of both children and adults, and the orbit has been involved in generalized disease.[279–283] Pathologic examination shows a poorly circumscribed proliferation of uniform fibroblasts arranged in fascicles that are not as cellular as a fibrosarcoma but that may contain variable numbers of normal mitotic figures. Collagen is conspicuous, small blood vessels are present in and around the lesion, and chronic inflammatory cells may be present. EM has shown that most cells have fibroblastic features with occasional myofibroblasts.

Fibrosarcoma

Fibrosarcoma is a rare diagnosis because most fibrosarcomas of the older literature would now be classified as malignant fibrous histiocytomas. True fibrosarcoma has a tendency to occur in children, in whom it has a more favorable prognosis.[284] Few primary orbital cases and one metastasis to choroid and orbit from an infantile limb fibrosarcoma have been reported.[285, 286] Pathologically, a cellular proliferation of regular fibroblasts is arranged in a fascicular or herringbone pattern with little intervening collagen. Mitotic figures are numerous. Fibrosarcoma is much more cellular than fibromatosis but less pleomorphic than malignant fibrous histiocytoma. EM shows the features of fibroblasts only.[287]

FIBROHISTIOCYTIC TUMORS

Fibrohistiocytic tumors constitute a numerically more important group of orbital tumors than the fibroblastic tumors and are distinguished from that group by having a mixture of cell types including fibroblasts, myofibroblasts, histiocytic cells, and undifferentiated mesenchymal cells by light microscopy and EM.[218, 288, 289] Immunohistochemically, they stain for vimentin.

The largest series of orbital fibrous histiocytomas was compiled by Font and Hidayat, who categorized their group of 150 tumors into benign, locally aggressive, and malignant.[290] The benign tumors were well circumscribed and showed small, thin, spindle-shaped cells arranged in a storiform or cartwheeling pattern (Fig. 187–39). Necrosis was absent, and mitoses few. Histiocytic cells, including foamy macrophages and benign giant cells, were occasionally present. Focal areas with irregularly dilated vascular channels often mimicked a hemangiopericytoma pattern. Locally aggressive tumors were similar to benign ones except for showing infiltrating margins and areas of hypercellularity. Mitoses were more frequent than in the benign tumors, but nuclear pleomorphism and necrosis were absent.

The malignant fibrous histiocytomas were larger and had marked nuclear pleomorphism; numerous mitotic figures, including atypical ones; necrosis; multinucleated tumor giant cells; and infiltrating margins (Fig. 187–40). Survival correlated with the histologic classification. Two malignant tumors followed previous orbital radiation, which has been our experience. Other single cases of benign and malignant orbital fibrous histiocytomas, including one angiomatoid variant, some in children, one case metastatic to the orbit, and two cases involving the lacrimal sac, have been reported.[291–303]

MUSCLE TUMORS

Muscle tumors include rhabdomyosarcomas as well as leiomyomas and leiomyosarcomas, tumors of skeletal and smooth muscle, respectively.

Rhabdomyosarcoma

Rhabdomyosarcoma is a malignant soft tissue tumor showing evidence of striated muscle differentiation. It is the most common orbital malignancy of children, although it may be present at birth and occurs in adults.[21, 22, 304–308] The prognosis has improved dramatically during the past 25 years with the institution of radiotherapy and chemotherapy.[308–310] The orbit may be involved secondarily from the adjacent nasopharynx and sinuses.[311, 312] The conjunctiva may infrequently be the site of origin.[313] Because these tumors evolve rapidly, early diagnosis is mandatory and biopsy with proper fixation of tissue is essential. This tumor is one of the "small blue cell tumors of childhood," meaning that the tumor is composed of smallish cells with a high nuclear to cytoplasmic ratio and little cytoplasm with which to identify the cell type. This designation implies a lengthy differential diagnosis, which includes leukemia, lym-

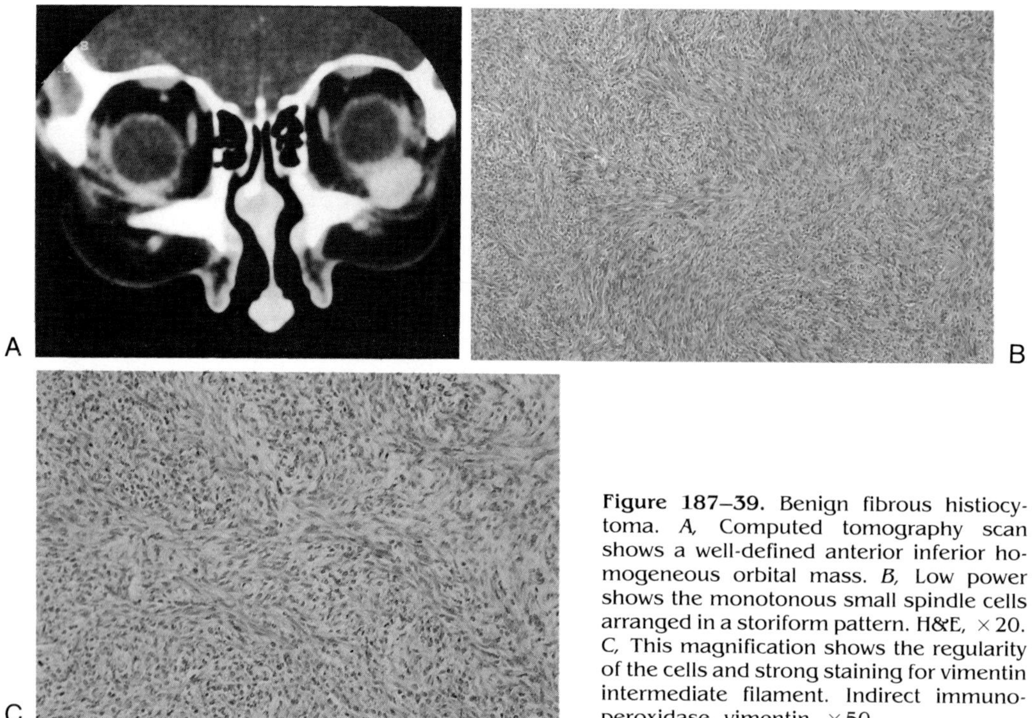

Figure 187–39. Benign fibrous histiocytoma. *A*, Computed tomography scan shows a well-defined anterior inferior homogeneous orbital mass. *B*, Low power shows the monotonous small spindle cells arranged in a storiform pattern. H&E, ×20. *C*, This magnification shows the regularity of the cells and strong staining for vimentin intermediate filament. Indirect immunoperoxidase, vimentin, ×50.

phoma, metastatic neuroblastoma, extraocular spread of retinoblastoma, Ewing's sarcoma, peripheral neuroectodermal tumor, and rhabdoid tumor, in addition to rhabdomyosarcoma, all of which require immunohistochemistry and EM for secure diagnosis and institution of appropriate therapy, which differs markedly. Rhabdomyosarcoma has been divided into three histopathologic types: embryonal, alveolar, and pleomorphic. The embryonal type shows hypercellular areas of small round to spindle-shaped cells that are separated by hypocellular myxoid areas (Fig. 187–41). Very occasional cells may show more abundant eosinophilic cytoplasm in the form of tadpole, racquet, or strap shapes with cross-striations, similar to those seen in normal skeletal muscle, which may be highlighted by trichrome and phosphotungstic acid–hematoxylin (PTAH) histochemical stains. Alveolar rhabdomyosarcoma has cells arranged in spaces similar to the alveoli of the lungs, with the cells at the periphery adherent to the septa and the

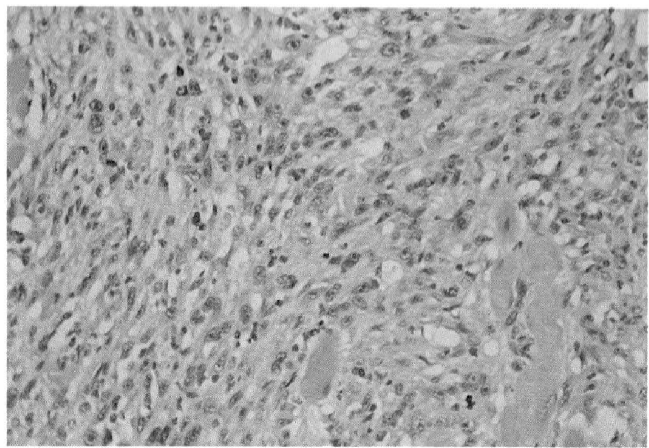

Figure 187–40. Malignant fibrous histiocytoma. This neoplasm shows pleomorphic nuclei, prominent nucleoli, and numerous mitotic figures as it invades an extraocular muscle. H&E, ×50.

degenerative central cells appearing to float (see Fig. 187–41*C*). Tumor giant cells are more frequent in this type, but cells showing cross-striations are infrequent. This type is more common in the inferior orbit and in older children.

Immunohistochemical staining in both types is positive for desmin, the intermediate filament of muscle cells, muscle actin, and infrequently myoglobin, in addition to vimentin, the basic mesenchymal filament.[314–316] EM may show evidence of skeletal muscle features in the form of thick myosin and thin actin filaments in a hexagonal array with focal Z-band formation or more frequently only thick filaments with ribosomes (see Fig. 187–41*D*). Additional nonspecific features include indented nuclei, external lamina, occasional poorly formed junctions, and pinocytotic vesicles.[219, 317] Cytogenetic and molecular genetic investigations have demonstrated characteristic abnormalities in rhabdomyosarcomas that may change the method of diagnosis as the techniques become more available.[318–320] The pleomorphic type is said to occur more commonly in the extremities of adults and is rare in the orbit; however, many of these lesions are reported in the older literature and with newer techniques would be classified as other types of sarcomas.[321]

Leiomyoma and Leiomyosarcoma

Leiomyoma and leiomyosarcoma are smooth muscle tumors that are extremely rare within the orbit.[322–327] Leiomysarcomas have been reported after radiation therapy for retinoblastoma.[328, 329] Leiomyomas are encapsulated and show large bundles of spindle-shaped cells arranged in a whorling pattern with prominent vascularity. Nuclei are cigar shaped, regular, and with-

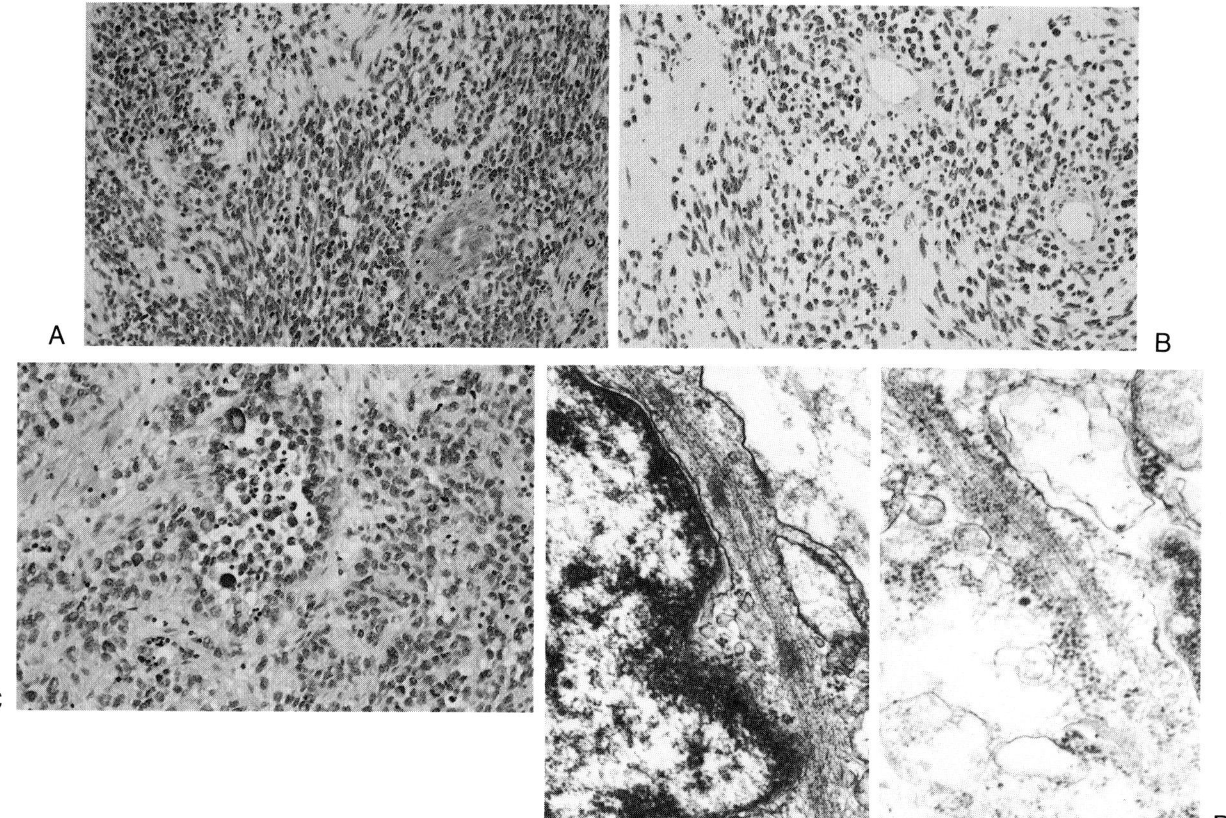

Figure 187–41. Rhabdomyosarcoma. *A*, Embryonal rhabdomyosarcoma with small undifferentiated spindle cells and intervening hypocellular areas. H&E, ×50. *B*, Strong staining for desmin, the intermediate filament of muscle cells. Indirect immunoperoxidase, desmin, ×50. *C*, An extraorbital alveolar rhabdomyosarcoma showing an "alveolar" space with well-preserved cells around the periphery and degenerating cells centrally. A tumor giant cell is present in the upper left of the space. H&E, ×50. *D*, Electron microscopic examination of the rhabdomyosarcoma in *A* and *B* shows infrequent filaments with Z bands, (*left* ×60,000) and beaded thick filaments (right, ×63,000).

out mitoses. Longitudinal cytoplasmic filaments can sometimes be identified with the trichrome stain, and cells are outlined with the reticulin stain.[323, 324, 326, 327] Leiomyosarcomas are unencapsulated, and although they may show the same general arrangement of cells as in a leiomyoma, marked hypercellularity, nuclear pleomorphism, and mitotic figures are present and may be abundant.[322, 325, 326] Evidence of smooth muscle differentiation consists of positive immunohistochemical staining for muscle actin, smooth muscle actin, desmin, and vimentin and on EM by showing that the cytoplasm of virtually all cells contains longitudinally oriented thin filaments with scattered dense bodies, subplasmalemmal densities, pinocytotic vesicles, and external laminae.[314]

ADIPOSE TISSUE TUMORS

Lipomas and liposarcomas are also extremely rare within the orbit despite the large amount of mature fat at this site. Previous high percentages of lipomas in large series probably represented excision of grossly lobulated but otherwise normal orbital fat. Occasional cases of true lipomas have been reported.[330–333] They have been encapsulated or circumscribed and have large components of mature fat. Three lesions were spindle cell lipomas that also contained a component of benign spindle-shaped cells, whereas the other was an angiolipoma containing numerous small vessels.

Liposarcomas are divided into four histologic subtypes: well differentiated, myxoid, round cell, and pleomorphic.[218] Most liposarcomas arise in the retroperitoneum or thigh, where they may grow large. Outcome is dependent on size, site, histologic type, and grade.[218, 334] Only the two more common types having a better prognosis, myxoid and well differentiated, have been described in the orbit.[335–338] These are generally slow-growing masses, which may come to occupy a large portion of the orbit. Diagnosis may be delayed because of the similarity of the tumor to normal orbital fat or benign myxoid tumors. The histopathologic diagnosis in all types rests on the finding of lipoblasts, round cells with their nuclei pushed to one side by a single fat vacuole that occupies the entire cytoplasm. The myxoid type shows occasional lipoblasts dispersed in a myxoid background with a prominent plexiform capillary vascular pattern, which is both helpful and essential to the diagnosis. The well-differentiated type shows lipocytes differing from normal only by a greater irregularity and prominent fibrous bands containing atypical spindle-shaped cells without fat vacuoles. Vascularity is not prominent. This type is the most similar to normal structures. One of our liposarcomas was a rapidly grow-

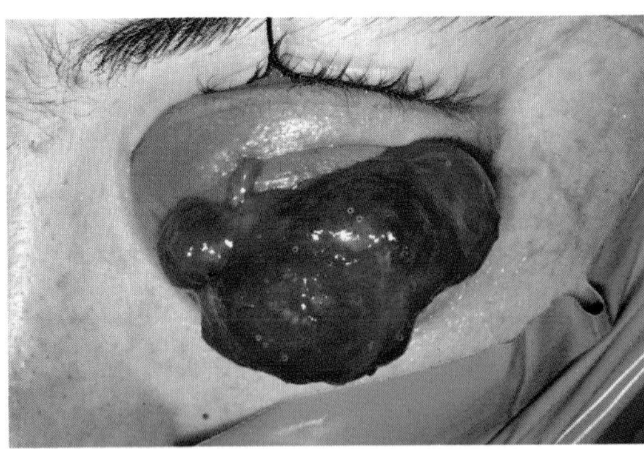

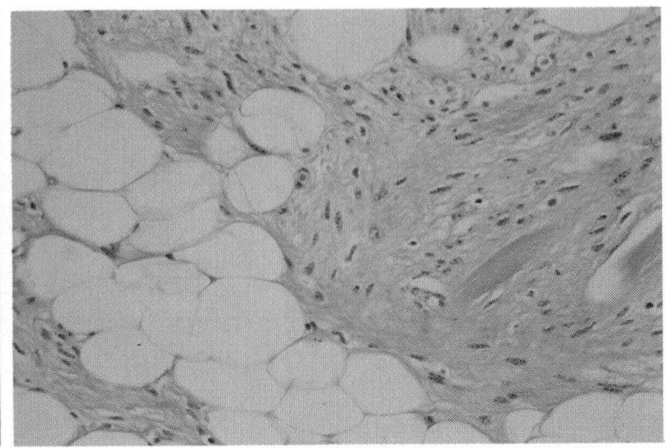

Figure 187–42. Liposarcoma. *A,* This 18-year-old male presented with a 5-month history of progressive infiltration of the left inferior orbit. Surgical photograph taken at the time of a debulking biopsy demonstrates a large, lobulated, fleshy, vascularized mass. *B,* Histopathology shows a well-differentiated liposarcoma with sclerosing areas infiltrating the extraocular muscle. Note the pleomorphic spindle-shaped nuclei that are prominent in the sclerosing area. These tumors may become large but can be deceptively histologically bland. H&E, ×50.

ing tumor in which the anterior and biopsy-sampled component consisted totally of an undifferentiated fibroblastic tumor, which stained positively for protein S100 and was interpreted as a malignant peripheral nerve sheath tumor. Only after exenteration was the correct diagnosis made, when the posterior portion showed well-differentiated liposarcoma with a prominent sclerosing component and the presence of well-differentiated lipoblasts in extraocular muscle (Fig. 187–42). Cases of liposarcoma metastatic to the orbit have been reported.[1, 339]

VASCULAR LESIONS

Vascular lesions are composed of malformations, hamartomas, and neoplasms. We consider the capillary and cavernous hemangiomas and lymphangiomas to be hamartomas rather than benign neoplasms. Particularly with the nonmalignant lesions, the clinical and radiologic examination are of much more importance than the histopathologic examination in establishing a diagnosis, because in some cases no tissue will be excised. Hemangiopericytoma is a true neoplasm with a variable degree of malignancy, whereas angiosarcoma is a highly malignant tumor of blood vesels.

Varix

Varix is a congenitally abnormal orbital vein or veins, which may distend on Valsalva's maneuver and be outlined by injection of contrast media. They may present acutely with thrombosis.[340] Only portions of a lesion may be excised at surgery, and pathologic examination shows a thickened venous wall with intraluminal organizing thrombus in some cases.

Arteriovenous Malformations

Arteriovenous malformations of the orbit may infrequently occur as part of congenital syndromes such as Sturge-Weber or Wyburn-Mason or may be acquired spontaneously or as a result of trauma.[341] Diagnosis rests mainly on arteriography, and these lesions are rarely excised. If tissue is removed, pathologic examination shows a tangled mass of abnormal vessels in which the clear-cut distinction between arteries and veins is lost, with fragmentation of the elastic lamina of arteries and both vessels showing loss of normal muscular layers.[341, 342]

Intravascular Papillary Endothelial Hyperplasia

Intravascular papillary endothelial hyperplasia, which frequently develops in the vessels of the deep dermis or subcutis of the head and neck, has been reported in the orbit and eyelid.[343–345] It occurs within a vein, artery, or preexisting vascular lesion and is considered to represent an exaggerated response to thrombosis of these structures. The lesion is usually well circumscribed by the wall of a vein or artery, the lumen of which shows numerous tufts of fibrin or collagen covered by normal or plump but not atypical endothelial cells, masses of unstructured fibrin, old red blood cells, and hemosiderin (Fig. 187–43). In early stages, numerous endothelial cells are present; these are replaced by collagenous tissue in older lesions. The proliferating endothelial tissue may extend through the wall, a feature that does not imply malignancy.

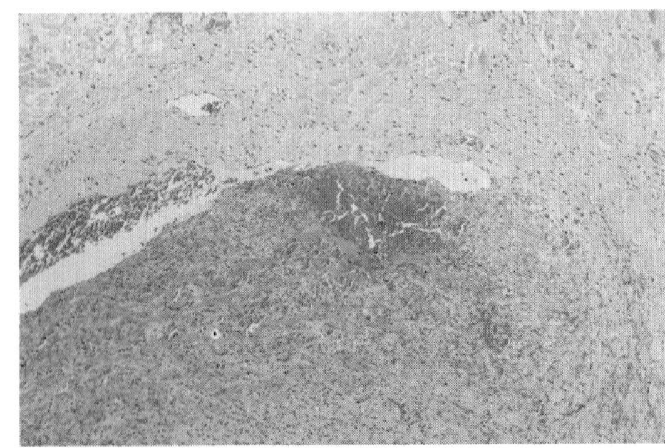

Figure 187–43. Intravascular papillary endothelial hyperplasia. Massive organizing thrombus is present within the lumen of this vein. H&E, ×20.

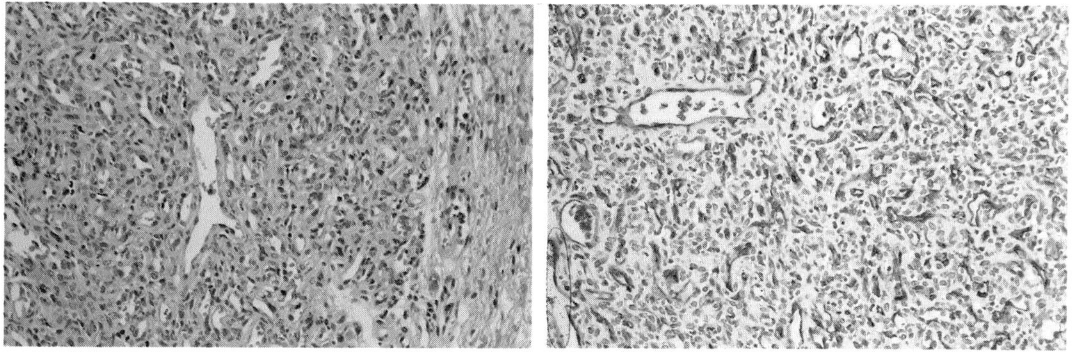

Figure 187–44. Capillary hemangioma. *A,* Cellular capillary hemangioma showing small vessels, some of which contain red blood cells, arranged in lobules surrounded by fibrous tissue. H&E, ×50. *B,* Binding of the lectin *Ulex europaeus*-1 outlines the numerous small vessels in this lesion. Lectin binding, *Ulex europaeus*-1, ×50.

Capillary Hemangioma

Capillary hemangioma commonly involves the ocular adnexae, where it may be superficial, deep, or combined. The superficial lesions, which involve the dermis or conjunctival substantia propria, are called *strawberry nevi* and can be extremely large and disfiguring. These undergo a growth spurt in the first months, after which they may involute with no treatment. In the early stage, these are cellular lesions composed of proliferating capillaries with little intervening stroma, in which the lumina may be difficult to visualize (Fig. 187–44). They have an infiltrative growth pattern and may involve all orbital structures. Later on, the capillaries become dilated and filled with red blood cells, and fibrosis and fat are found between the vessels. The vessels at all stages may be outlined with a reticulin stain, and endothelial cells stain by the immunoperoxidase technique for Factor VIII–related antigen and by lectin binding with *Ulex europaeus*-1.[346]

Cavernous Hemangioma

Cavernous hemangioma is a well-encapsulated, benign, slowly growing vascular lesion occurring in adults. If proptosis, diplopia, or visual field loss is significant, the lesion is removed. Grossly, it is a characteristically plum-colored, bosselated, encapsulated mass that has a spongy appearance on the cut surface (Fig. 187–45). Microscopically, it is well encapsulated by fibrous tissue and shows numerous large vascular channels lined by endothelial cells and surrounded by smooth muscle cells.[347–351] The stroma consists of thick fibrous tissue that may contain bundles of smooth muscle and myxoid foci. The vessels are usually filled with red blood cells. Thrombosis with organization may be present. Tumors may be multiple.

Lymphangioma

Lymphangioma has been called a *choristoma* or *hamartoma,* depending on whether the component vessels are considered to be true lymphatics or dysplastic blood vessels showing some features of lymphatics.[352–356] These poorly circumscribed infiltrating lesions occurring in children and young adults may involve the conjunctiva, eyelid, or deep orbit and often can be only partially removed (Fig. 187–46). Histopathologically, they consist of a myriad of irregularly sized and shaped vascular channels with thin walls embedded in a loose fibrous stroma that contains bundles of smooth muscle and collections of lymphocytes. The vascular channels may be filled with red blood cells or may contain serous fluid, and evidence of old hemorrhage is present in the form of hemosiderin and cholesterol clefts. Thrombosis and

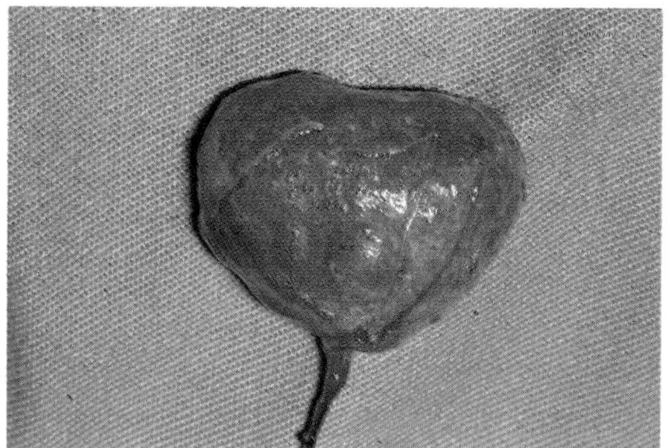

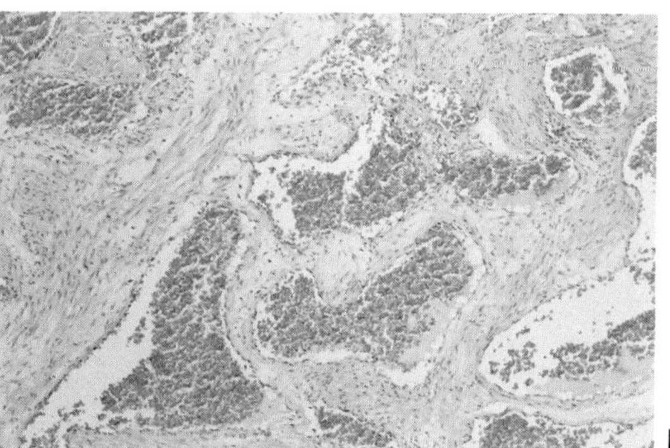

Figure 187–45. Cavernous hemangioma. *A,* Gross surgical photograph of a typical cavernous hemangioma after excision. Note the plum-colored bosselated nature of the lesion with multiple vessels on its surface and a small draining vessel. *B,* Histopathology shows large red blood cell–containing vascular spaces lined by endothelial cells and surrounded by thick fibrous septa with foci of smooth muscle cells. H&E, ×20.

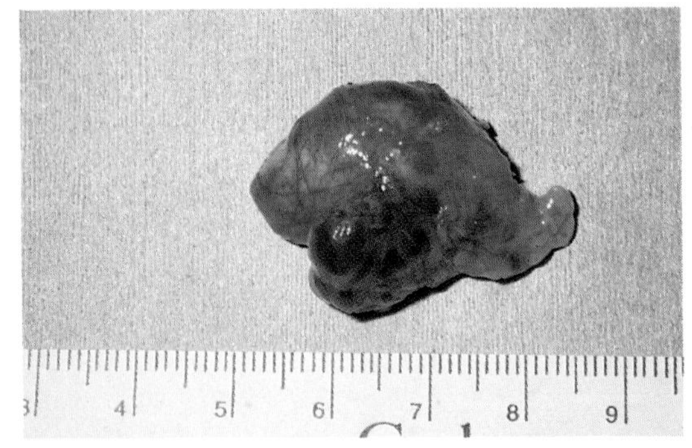

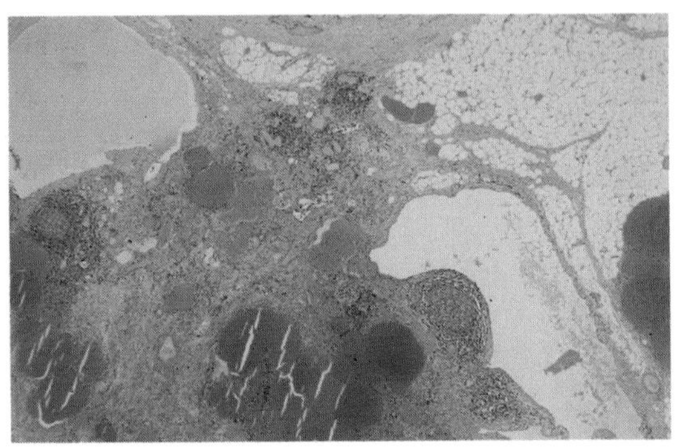

Figure 187–46. Lymphangioma. *A,* Gross surgical specimen of an irregularly lobulated cystic mass removed from the right inferior orbit of an 11-year-old child. Note the multiple saccules of blood and some pale cystic areas, which simply contained xanthochromic fluid. *B,* This lesion contains many irregularly shaped vascular spaces, with the characteristics of blood or lymphatic vessels, embedded in a fibrous stroma containing occasional lymphoid follicles. H&E, ×6.

calcification may be present. EM has shown features of both vascular and lymphatic channels.[351, 353]

Hemangiopericytoma

Hemangiopericytoma is believed to be derived from pericytes and occurs at all ages, as well as at birth.[21, 357] Series of orbital cases have been reported, the largest of 30 patients from the Armed Forces Institute of Pathology.[358–360] The tumors may be grossly encapsulated, although microscopic examination may show invasive margins. The basic pattern consists of the presence of numerous sinusoidal or staghorn-shaped vessels lined by endothelial cells that are surrounded by oval to spindle-shaped cells with clear cytoplasm (Fig. 187–47). Croxatto and colleagues classified their cases into benign, borderline, and malignant based on histopathologic features of increasing cellularity, mitoses, nuclear pleomorphism, hemorrhage, and necrosis. The benign tumors more often showed a totally sinusoidal pattern, whereas the malignant tumors often had mixed sinusoidal and solid patterns.

Vessels may be outlined by a reticulin or immunoperoxidase stain for Factor VIII–related antigen. Reticulin may also surround individual or groups of pericytes (see Fig. 187–47*B*). The pericytes stain for vimentin only.[361] EM shows the vascular channels lined by endothelial cells and surrounded in layers by the pericytes, which display clear cytoplasm with interdigitating processes, occasional thin filaments with dense bodies, and interrupted or complete external lamina.[361, 362] Tumors in all groups recurred and metastasized, although the rate was higher in those classified as borderline or malignant, an experience paralleled by tumors at other sites.[358, 363] Because recurrences and metastases may occur many years after the original tumor, long follow-up is required.[364, 365]

Angiosarcoma

Angiosarcoma is an uncommon, rapidly progressive tumor of endothelial cells often involving the skin and soft tissue.[366] Orbital cases have been reviewed by Hufnagel and colleagues.[367] Pathologically, it shows infiltrating stellate vascular spaces lined by atypical endothelial cells that may assume slitlike spaces and more solid areas. The malignant cells stain for Factor VIII–related antigen and with *Ulex europaeus*-1 lectin, distinguishing it from hemangiopericytoma, in which the neoplastic cells do not stain. EM shows endothelial cells surrounded by basal lamina without pericytes. A case presenting as Tolosa-Hunt syndrome has been described.[368]

TUMORS OF UNCERTAIN HISTOGENESIS

Alveolar Soft Part Sarcoma

Alveolar soft part sarcoma is a rare sarcoma that has a predilection to develop in the buttock and thigh area,

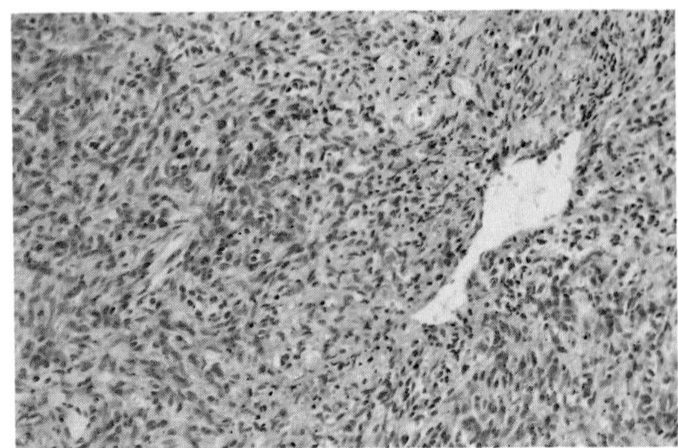

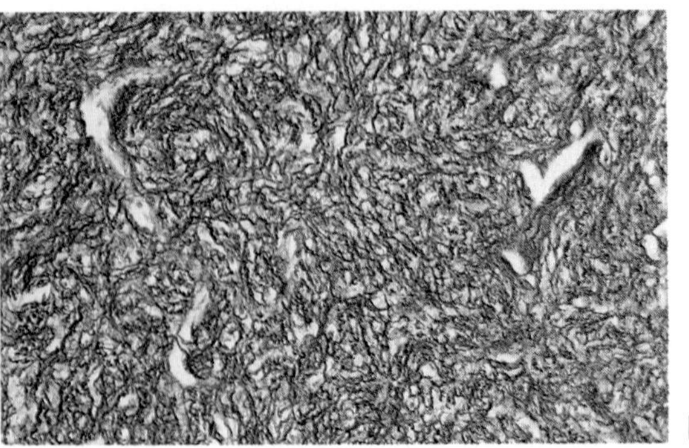

Figure 187–47. Hemangiopericytoma. *A,* Large staghorn vessel surrounded by small, regular, spindle-shaped pericytes. H&E, ×50. *B,* Reticulin stain outlines the large vessels and most of the neoplastic pericytes. Reticulin, ×50.

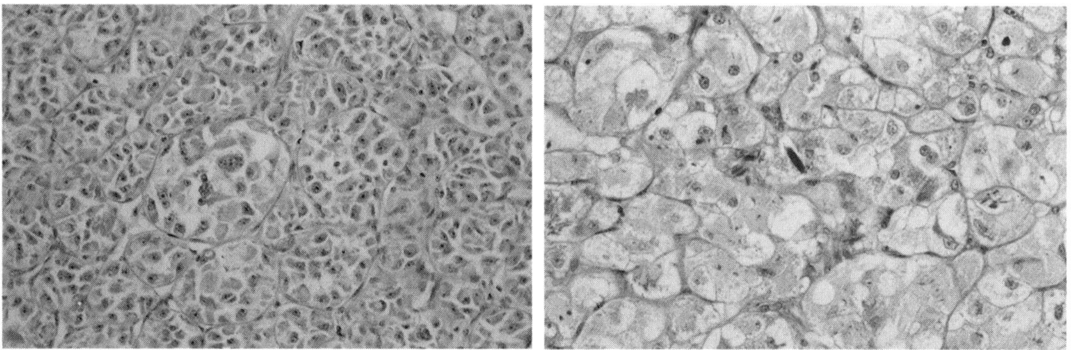

Figure 187–48. Alveolar soft part sarcoma. *A,* Extraorbital example showing cells with prominent nucleoli and abundant eosinophilic cytoplasm arranged in an "alveolar" pattern. H&E, ×50. *B,* PAS stain highlights the characteristic crystals. PAS, ×80.

although the orbit is a site of some preference, with a series of 17 cases having been reported by the Armed Forces Institute of Pathology.[369–371] The tumor occurs in young adults and affects females more often than males. Metastatic disease may develop many years after initial diagnosis. Histopathologically, the tumor has a distinctive arrangement of cells in a pseudoalveolar pattern surrounded by thin fibrovascular septa (Fig. 187–48). The cells are polygonal with vesicular nuclei, prominent nucleoli, and eosinophilic cytoplasm. The characteristic feature, seen in two thirds of cases, is the presence of PAS-positive, diastase-resistant cytoplasmic crystals arranged in bundles or stacks. By EM, these consist of rectangular membrane-bound arrays with a periodicity of 8 to 10 nm. The tumor has been postulated to have many origins, and one group showed that the crystals were composed of renin, although this was later disproved.[372, 373] More recent investigations have supported a skeletal muscle origin.[374–376]

Malignant Rhabdoid Tumor

Malignant rhabdoid tumor, which bears a resemblance to rhabdomyosarcoma, was first noted in the kidney about a decade ago but has since been encountered in other sites, including the orbit.[377, 378] It occurs from infancy to adulthood and often pursues a malignant course. The histopathologic appearance is of a monotonous proliferation of infiltrating cells with mitoses and focal necrosis. The cells show a vesicular nucleus that is often indented by a perinuclear eosinophilic hyaline cytoplasmic mass, which on EM shows a whorled array

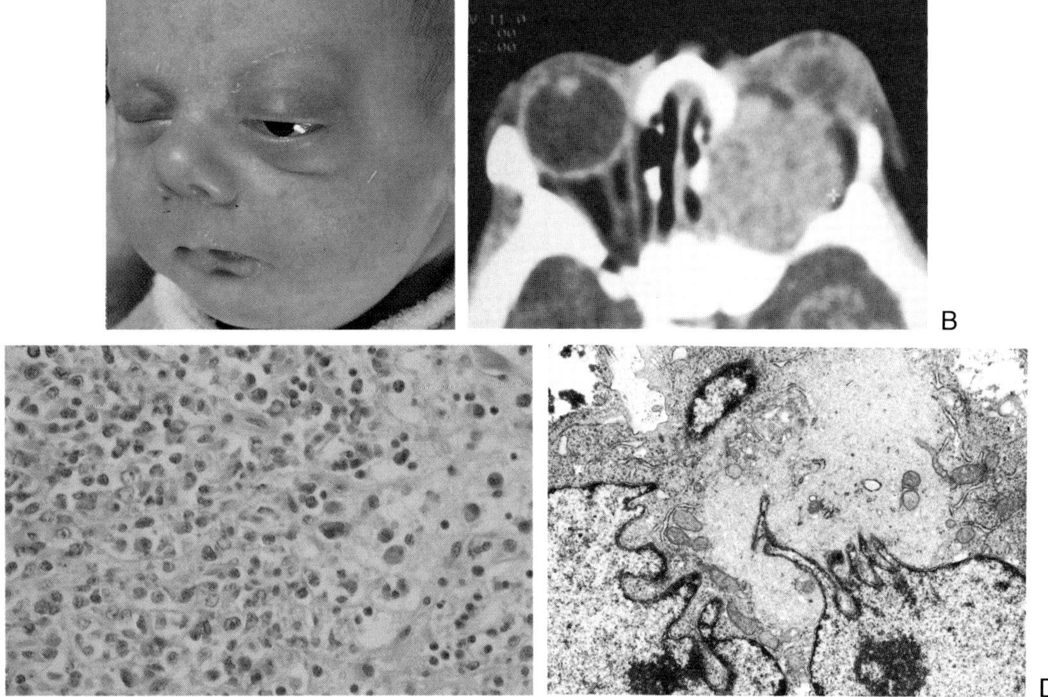

Figure 187–49. Malignant rhabdoid tumor. *A,* A 2-month-old infant who presented with progressive left proptosis, noted almost from the time of birth. On presentation, there was a markedly tense orbit with significant restriction of movement. *B,* Axial computed tomography scan demonstrates a nonhomogeneous irregular lobulated mass, associated with expansion of the orbit. (Courtesy of Rootman J, Damji KF, Dimmick JE: Malignant rhabdoid tumor of the orbit. Ophthalmology 96:1650, 1989.) *C,* Biopsy specimen shows pleomorphic cells, some with bean-shaped nuclei indented by eosinophilic masses in the cytoplasm. H&E, ×80. *D,* Electron microscopy shows pleomorphic nuclei and perinuclear whorls of intermediate filaments in some cells only. The rest of the cells have no specific features. ×15,000.

Table 187–2. MAJOR ORBITAL BONE TUMORS

Lesion	Location	Pathology	References
		Fibroosseous Lesions	
Osteoma	Frontal, ethmoidal sinuses	Mature osteoma shows dense lamellar bone with little fibrous stroma; fibrous osteoma shows more fibrous stroma with osteoblasts	389, 390
Fibrous dysplasia	Frontal, ethmoidal, sphenoidal sinuses, maxilla	Irregular trabeculae of woven bone unlined by osteoblasts; moderately cellular fibrous stroma	391–395
Ossifying fibroma	All; frontal and ethmoidal most common	Cellular fibrous stroma arranged in whorls; bony trabeculae lined by osteoblasts; psammomatoid variant shows round to oval spicules of bone similar to psammoma bodies	396–400
Osteoblastoma	Frontal, ethmoidal	Abundant trabeculae of osteoid and woven bone surrounded by numerous pleomorphic but benign osteoblasts; stroma contains osteoclasts and numerous vessels lined by endothelial cells	401, 402
		Reactive Giant Cell Lesions	
Giant cell reparative granuloma	Most common in mandible; also in maxilla, temporal, sphenoidal, ethmoidal	Small giant cells grouped around hemorrhagic foci and irregularly spaced in a stroma containing oval and spindle-shaped cells with foci of collagen, hemosiderin, and osteoid	403–406
Brown tumor of hyperparathyroidism	Maxilla, ethmoidal, frontal, sphenoidal	Similar histology to giant cell reparative granuloma; can be diagnosed only by finding abnormal serum calcium and phosphate values	407–409
Aneurysmal bone cyst	Sphenoidal, frontal	Blood-filled channels unlined by endothelial cells, surrounded by variably fibrous stroma containing osteoid, giant cells, foci of hemorrhage, and hemosiderin	410–413
Cholesterol granuloma	Most common in frontal; rarely in zygoma, maxilla	Cholesterol clefts surrounded by foreign body giant cells, foci of recent and old hemorrhage, foamy macrophages, lymphocytes, fibrous tissue	58, 59
		Neoplasms	
Osteosarcoma	Maxilla, ethmoidal, frontal; often in patients with germinal mutation of retinoblastoma gene	Trabeculae of osteoid arising directly from a malignant fibroblastic stroma showing hypercellularity, anaplasia, mitoses, and invasion of adjacent structures; malignant chondroblastic areas may be present	414–420
Chondroma	Trochlea	Lobules of hyaline cartilaginous tissue without significant cellular pleomorphism	19, 20
Chondrosarcoma	Maxilla, ethmoidal	Hyaline cartilaginous tissue showing hypercellularity, nuclear pleomorphism, and binucleate cells within lacunae	421
Mesenchymal chondrosarcoma	Bones and soft tissues of orbit	Islands of mature hyaline cartilage embedded in a stroma composed of small spindle-shaped cells similar to hemangiopericytoma	422–425
Ewing's sarcoma	Frontal, maxilla, ethmoidal, sphenoidal	Small undifferentiated cells; PAS positive, diastase sensitive; electron microscopy shows cells with few intercellular junctions and organelles	426–428

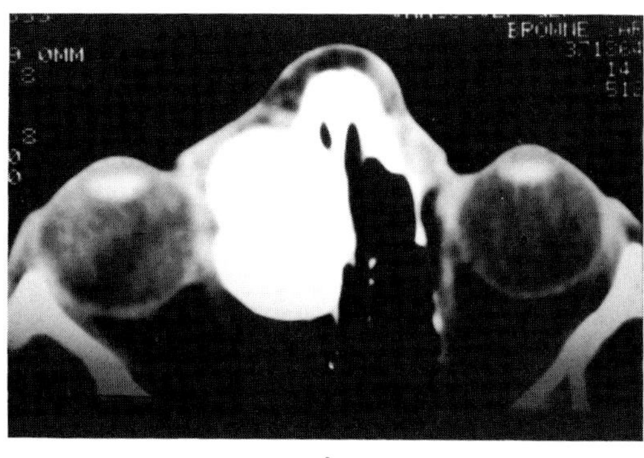

A

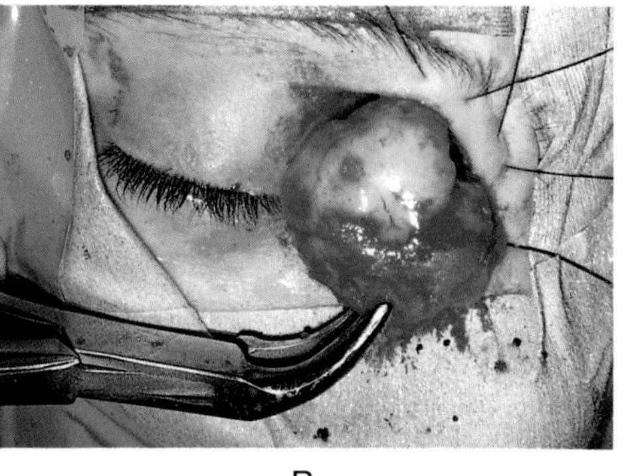

B

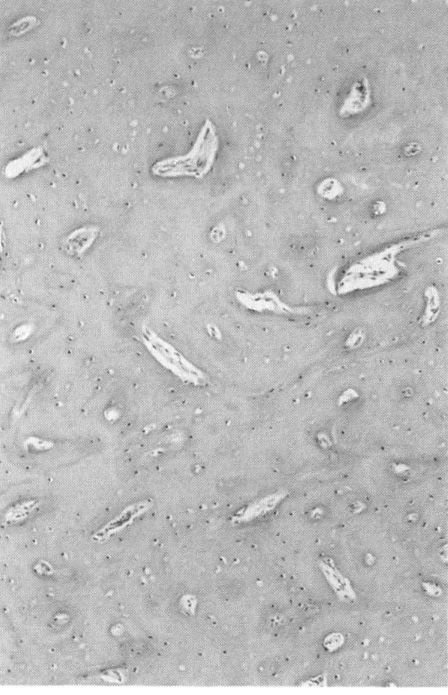

C

Figure 187–50. Osteoma. *A,* Axial computed tomography scan of the orbit of a 17-year-old female who presented with downward, outward displacement of the right globe due to a dense bosselated and lobular mass arising from the ethmoidal sinus. *B,* The clinical photograph demonstrates the large osteoma being extracted through the wound after dissection and removal of adjacent bone. *C,* The lesion is composed of dense bone with only small spaces containing blood vessels. H&E, ×20.

of bundles of intermediate filaments (Fig. 187–49). No features of skeletal muscle or other specific differentiation are found. Immunohistochemically, the tumor stains for vimentin, epithelial membrane antigen, and cytokeratin but does not stain for muscle actin or desmin.[377, 379] These findings suggest a primitive pluripotential tumor.

Other

We have recently diagnosed and treated a case of primary epithelioid sarcoma of the orbit, a tumor that usually arises in the tendon sheaths of the extremities and often pursues an insidious and relentless course with multiple recurrences. This tumor has a nodular growth pattern, often showing central necrosis of the nodules, and therefore requires distinction from a granulomatous process, which it may mimic. Immunohistochemically, it stains for both vimentin and keratin[218] (Personal observation—VW, JR).

Neoplasms Arising in Bone

Neoplasms arising in bone are grouped together because their site of origin dictates a separate differential diagnosis from soft tissue lesions of the orbit. The field of bone pathology is one of the most difficult and in the head is complicated because of the rarity of tumors in this location and because of their slightly different histopathologic characteristics, probably based on the neural crest origin of the facial bones and their lack of enchondral ossification. These factors result in a blurring of distinctive histopathologic appearances within the benign lesions, which are more easily distinguishable when occurring in other bones.[380, 381] For this reason, the lesions are divided into groups in Table 187–2, which gives brief notes about type, location, and histopathologic appearance, as well as references for major tumors occurring in the orbital bones (Figs. 187–50 to 187–56). The malignant lesions are histologically distinct. As with all bone pathology, it is important that the pathologic diagnosis be rendered in accordance with the radiologic interpretation. If there is major disagreement, the diagnosis should be reviewed and consideration given to the possibility that the pathologic specimen is not representative or was taken from the periphery of the lesion. The text by Mirra is the most complete reference on bone tumors occurring throughout the body.[382] The articles by Fu and Perzin and by Blodi discuss tumors specifically located in the facial

Figure 187–51. Fibrous dysplasia. Histopathology shows a fibrous stroma from which arise small spicules of osteoid, often in the shape of a C, without intervening osteoblasts. H&E, ×20.

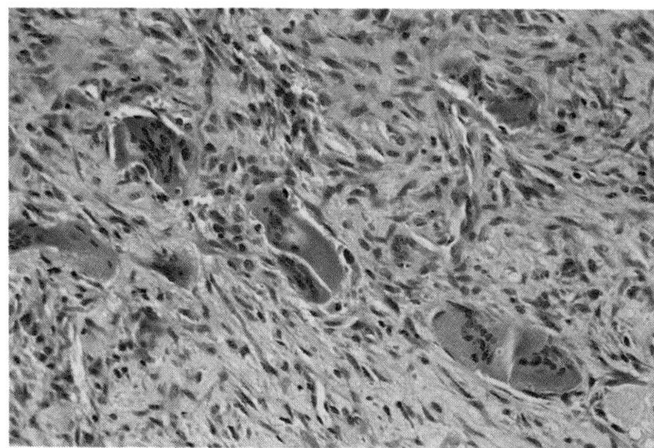

Figure 187–52. Giant cell reparative granuloma. This lesion from a child has a fibrous stroma with irregularly shaped and placed giant cells and foci of hemorrhage. H&E, ×50.

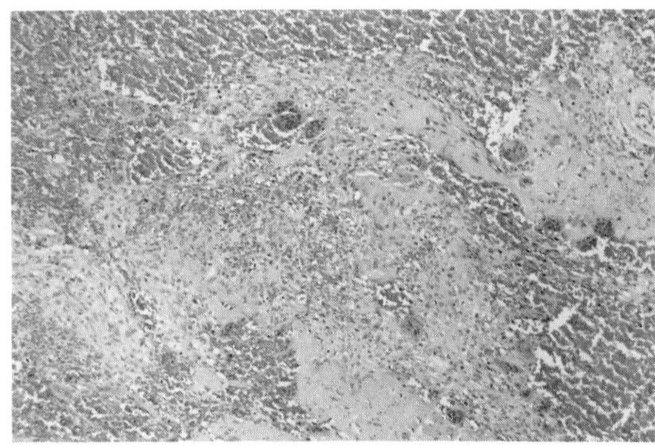

Figure 187–53. Brown tumor of hyperparathyroidism in the frontal bone of an elderly woman. It shows irregular foci of osteoid, surrounded by osteoclasts and osteoblasts, fibrous stroma, recent and old hemorrhage. Hyperparathyroidism was diagnosed only after excision of this tumor, when elevated serum calcium and depressed phosphate levels were found. H&E, ×20.

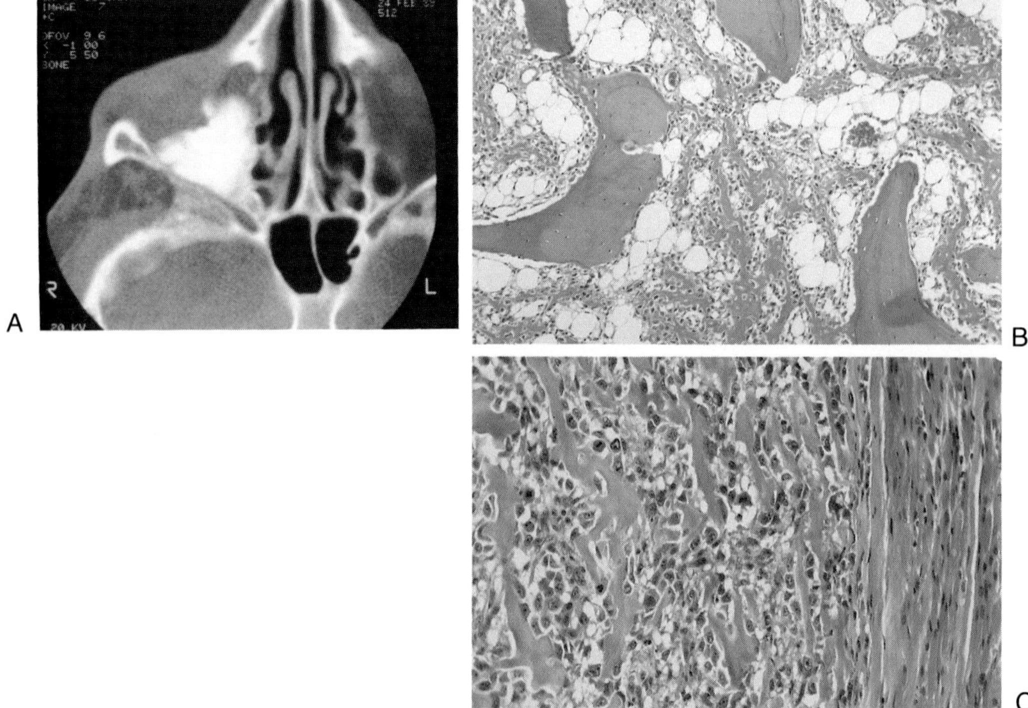

Figure 187–54. Osteosarcoma. *A,* Axial computed tomography scan of an anophthalmic orbit of a 19-year-old male who had undergone enucleation in childhood for a retinoblastoma. Note the irregular ossified mass involving the entire apex of the orbit. *B,* Osteoid surrounded by malignant osteoblasts infiltrates between the normal bone and marrow fat of the orbit. H&E, ×20. *C,* Higher power shows the malignant osteoid infiltrating an extraocular muscle. H&E, ×50.

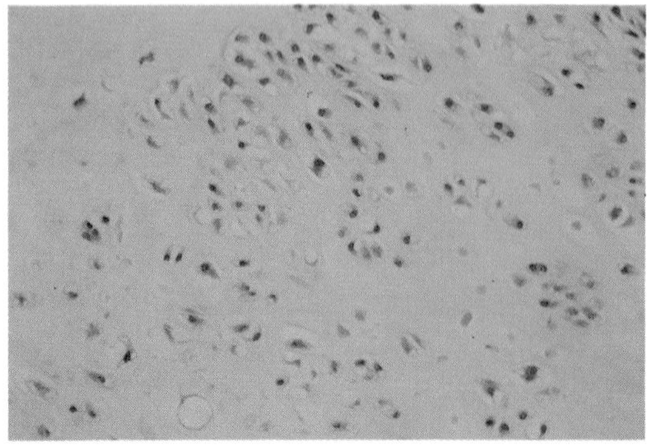

Figure 187–55. Chondrosarcoma. This low-grade chondrosarcoma shows hypercellularity and occasional binucleate chondrocytes in lacunae. H&E, ×50.

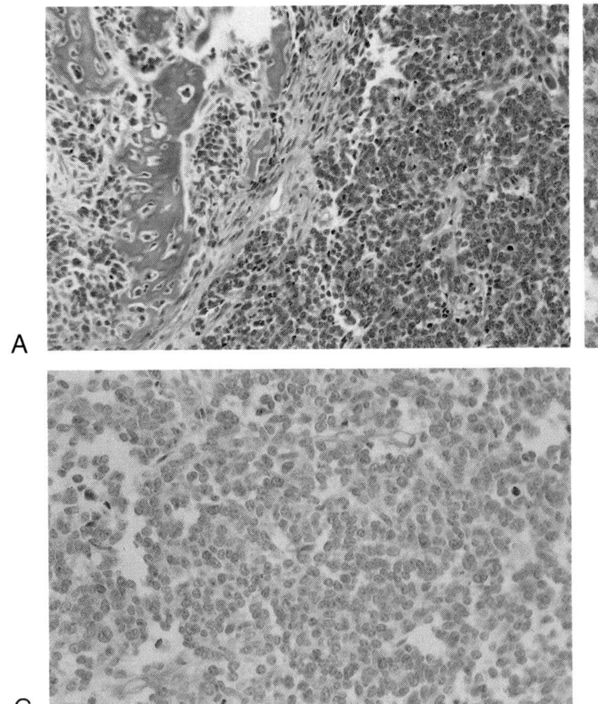

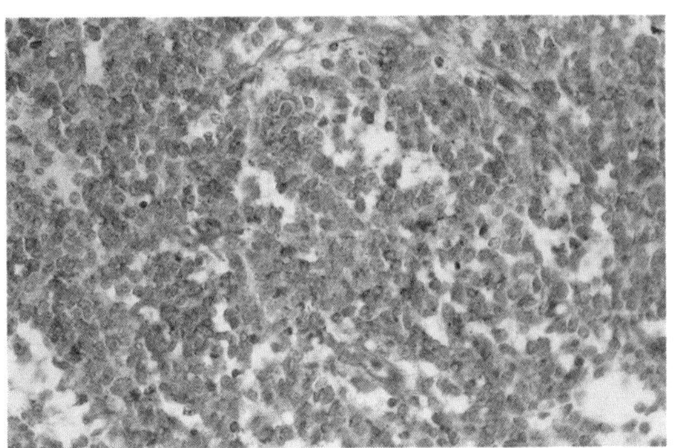

Figure 187–56. Ewing's sarcoma. *A*, This tumor shows small undifferentiated cells infiltrating between the trabeculae of bone. Numerous mitoses are present. H&E, ×50. *B*, The large amount of glycogen normally seen in this tumor is stained by PAS. PAS, ×80. *C*, The glycogen is removed by pretreating the section with diastase. PAS and diastase, ×80.

bones.[383, 384] It must be emphasized that all bone tumors may involve the adjacent soft tissues of the orbit. We have recently seen a case of an osteochondroma of the orbit, a bony neoplasm that rarely occurs in this location. Various other tumors that occur in the soft tissues of the orbit, including myxoma, lipoma, cavernous hemangioma, hemangioendothelioma, fibrous histiocytoma, and lymphoma, have infrequently been reported to occur in the orbital bones.[385–388]

Metastatic Tumors and Tumors Involving the Orbit by Direct Extension

METASTATIC TUMORS

Metastatic tumors account for approximately 10 percent of orbital neoplasia and appear to be increasing in prevalence. Several reviews of metastatic orbital tumors are available.[429–434] The most common primary tumors give rise to the largest number of metastases, with tumors from the breast, lung, gastrointestinal tract, prostate, and kidney, as well as cutaneous melanoma, being the most frequent in adults. Up to 25 percent of metastatic tumors may present before a known primary; therefore, this possibility must always be considered in both the clinical and pathologic differential diagnosis. A distinctive feature is the tendency of some tumors to metastasize to specific sites in the orbit, particularly cutaneous melanoma and breast carcinoma to the extraocular muscles and prostate, renal and thyroid adenocarcinomas and neuroblastoma to bone.[429, 435, 436] Table 187–3 gives brief notes about tumor type, sites of predilection, and pathologic details, as well as references for the major metastatic orbital tumors, listed in approximate order of frequency (Figs. 187–57 to 187–59). Rare metastases have also been reported from ovarian carcinomas and testicular seminomas.[437–439] Metastatic tumors in children are listed separately because the metastases in this age group parallel the common pediatric solid tumors.

TUMORS INVOLVING THE ORBIT BY DIRECT EXTENSION

In addition to metastatic tumors, the orbit is frequently involved by tumors extending from adjacent structures including the nasopharynx and sinuses, skin of the eyelids and face, conjunctiva, globe, intracranial

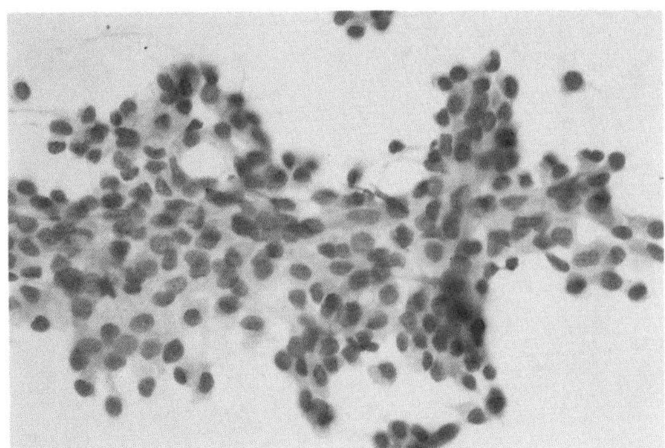

Figure 187–57. Metastatic breast carcinoma. Aspiration biopsy sample of an orbital mass in a patient with previous breast carcinoma shows groups of cohesive malignant epithelial cells with morphology consistent with metastasic adenocarcinoma from the breast. H&E, ×80.

Table 187–3. METASTATIC ORBITAL TUMORS

Tumor	Sites of Metastases	Histology	Histochemistry	Immunohistochemistry	Electron Microscopy	References
			Metastases in Adults			
Breast carcinoma	Soft tissue, EOM, bone	Glandular, cells in single file, histiocytoid	PAS + diastase, alcian blue	Estrogen, progesterone receptors, B72.3, CEA	Extra- and intracellular lumina; mucin secretory vacuoles	435, 436, 440–443
Small cell carcinoma of lung	Soft tissue, bone	Small oval cells in sheets with necrosis; DNA staining of vessels		Keratin, NSE	Dense core granules	444, 445
Adenocarcinoma of colon, stomach, pancreas, lung	Soft tissue, bone	Glandular, mucinous, signet ring or papillary patterns	PAS + diastase, mucicarmine	CEA, keratin	Extra- and intracellular lumina; microvilli with filamentous core rootlets	446–448
Prostatic adenocarcinoma	Bone, soft tissue	Glandular, single cell infiltration	Alcian blue	Prostatic acid phosphatase; prostate-specific antigen	Extracellular gland formation	449–451
Renal adenocarcinoma	Soft tissue, bone	Clear cells in lobules surrounded by vessels; sometimes granular	PAS negative after diastase	Keratin +/− vimentin	Epithelial cells with glycogen and lipid	452–454
Cutaneous melanoma	EOM, soft tissue	Large epithelioid cells; often amelanotic, bizarre cells	Fontana-Masson	S100, HMB-45	Premelanosomes, few junctions, intranuclear cytoplasmic inclusions	435, 436, 455–457
Thyroid carcinoma	Soft tissue, bone	Papillary pattern with ground glass nuclei or follicular		Thyroglobulin in follicular	Papillary shows intranuclear cytoplasmic inclusions; follicular shows epithelial cells with colloid	458
Carcinoid	Soft tissue	Regular cells in lobules, trabeculae	Argyrophil +/− argentaffin	Chromogranin, synaptophysin, serotonin	Epithelial cells with irregular dense core granules	267, 459–461
Squamous carcinoma	Soft tissue	Polygonal groups and single infiltrating cells with eosinophilic cytoplasm		Keratin	Epithelial cells containing tonofilaments joined by desmosomes	433
			Metastases in Children			
Neuroblastoma	Soft tissue, bone	Small undifferentiated cells with occasional rosette formation		NSE	Cells with cytoplasmic extensions containing dense core granules and microtubules	462–464
Ewing's sarcoma	Soft tissue	Small undifferentiated cells	PAS negative after diastase		Cells with poorly formed intercellular junctions, few organelles	463
Wilms' tumor	Soft tissue	Biphasic pattern with tubules and spindle cell stroma				465, 486

CEA, carcinoembryonic antigen; EOM, extraocular muscles; NSE, neuron-specific enolase.

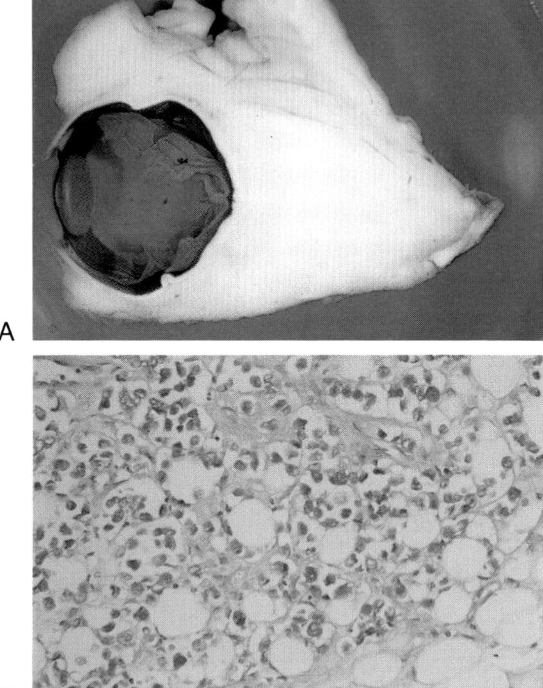

Figure 187–58. Metastatic signet ring carcinoma from the pancreas. *A,* Globe and orbital soft tissue removed at autopsy from an elderly woman who presented with proptosis after the diagnosis of pancreatic carcinoma. *B,* PAS-positive, diastase-resistant, signet ring cells invading the orbital fat. Adenocarcinomas with this morphology are common in the gastrointestinal tract. PAS and diastase, ×50.

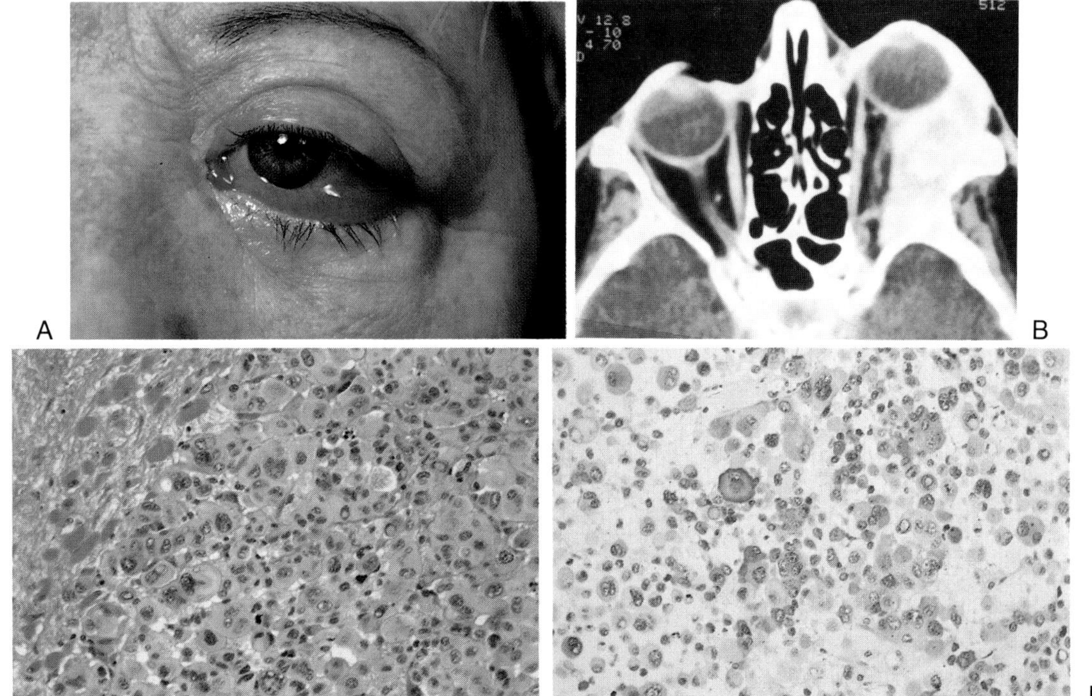

Figure 187–59. Metastatic cutaneous melanoma. *A,* Clinical photograph of a 68-year-old patient who presented with progressive left proptosis and chemosis, associated with marked limitation of movement. *B,* Axial computed tomography scan of the same patient demonstrates a large mass involving the lateral rectus muscle. Note the nonhomogeneity of the lesion with low-density areas due to necrosis. *C,* Pleomorphic amelanotic melanoma that had replaced almost the entire lateral rectus muscle, fibers of which are shown in the upper left. H&E, ×50. *D,* The tumor cells stain moderately with the antimelanoma antibody HMB-45. Indirect immunoperoxidase, ×50.

Table 187–4. TUMORS INVOLVING THE ORBIT BY DIRECT EXTENSION

Extension From	Tumor Types	References
Sinuses—maxillary, ethmoidal, frontal	Epithelial—squamous carcinoma, adenocarcinoma, transitional, adenoid cystic, mucoepidermoid, malignant mixed tumor Nonepithelial—melanoma, rarely sarcomas	467, 468
Nose and nasopharynx	Poorly differentiated squamous carcinoma (lymphoepithelioma), esthesioneuroblastoma, angiofibroma, as well as those tumors occurring in the sinuses	256, 467, 469
Skin of eyelids and surrounding face	Basal cell, squamous and sebaceous carcinomas, cutaneous melanoma, rare sweat gland carcinomas	470–486
Conjunctiva	Squamous, spindle cell squamous, mucoepidermoid and oncocytic carcinomas, conjunctival melanoma	487–490
Globe	Uveal melanoma, retinoblastoma, medulloepithelioma, carcinoma of pigmented and nonpigmented epithelium of ciliary body	491–499
Intracranial cavity and optic nerve	Meningioma, high-grade astrocytoma, chordoma, large pituitary adenoma	500–502
Lacrimal sac	Squamous, transitional and adenocarcinomas arising de novo or in papillomas, melanoma, rare sarcomas	503–505

cavity, optic nerve, and lacrimal sac. Table 187–4 lists the types of tumors that may extend from these sites into the orbit (Figs. 187–60 and 187–61). Many of these tumors are discussed in greater detail in other sections.

INFLAMMATIONS AND NEOPLASMS OF THE LACRIMAL GLAND

Lesions of the lacrimal gland may be congenital, cystic, inflammatory, or neoplastic. The congenital lesions include ectopic lacrimal gland and congenital lacrimal duct cysts. The major cystic lesion, however, is an acquired lacrimal duct cyst, or dacryops, which was discussed under Lacrimal Duct Cysts. The lacrimal gland may be involved by nonspecific inflammation and is the site of two common specific inflammatory processes, namely sarcoidosis and the lymphoepithelial lesion of Sjögren's syndrome. Kimura's disease and Wegener's granulomatosis also occur.[104, 117] Epithelial neoplasms of the lacrimal gland parallel those in the major and minor salivary glands. The lacrimal gland is also frequently involved by lymphomas.

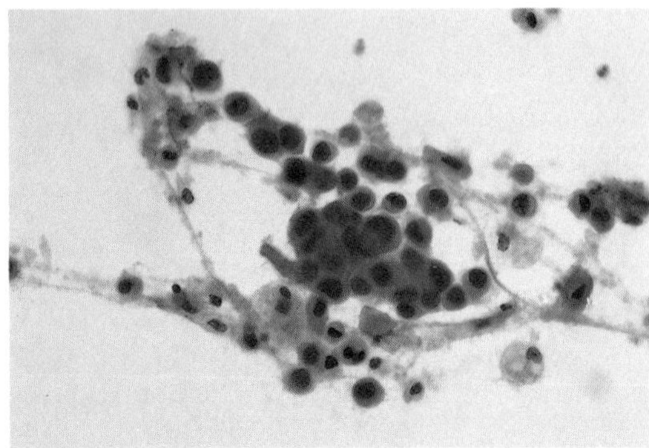

Figure 187–60. Squamous carcinoma from the maxillary sinus. Aspiration biopsy sample of an orbital mass in a patient with squamous carcinoma of the maxillary sinus shows a cluster of malignant epithelial cells with angulated nuclei and orange cytoplasm as seen in squamous carcinoma. H&E, ×80.

Inflammations of the Lacrimal Gland

A similar classification of inflammatory lesions as was used for the soft tissues of the orbit may be applied to the lacrimal gland, with some exceptions. The lacrimal gland may be infected by viral infectious mononucleosis and bacterial organisms, although more unusual infections, including tuberculosis, histoplasmosis, schistosomiasis, and cysticercosis have been described.[87, 94, 100, 101, 506] Stones within the ducts of the palpebral lobe have been reported.[507]

NONSPECIFIC INFLAMMATION

The lacrimal gland may also be the site of a nonspecific inflammatory process that may present as an acute, subacute, or chronic process. If this lesion is sampled by biopsy in the acute phase, a polymorphous inflammatory infiltrate with edema without destruction of the acini is noted. In the subacute or chronic phase, the inflammatory infiltrate consists of lymphocytes and plasma cells, but the striking feature is the decrease or absence of acini with a variable degree of fibrosis (Fig. 187–62).[508, 509]

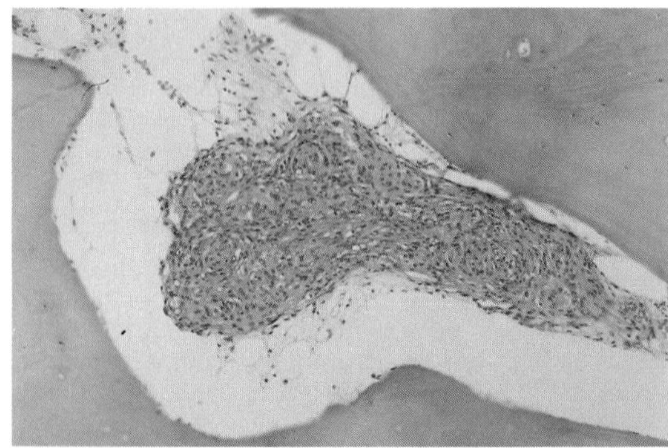

Figure 187–61. Extension of meningioma. Extension of optic nerve meningioma into adjacent orbital bone. H&E, ×20.

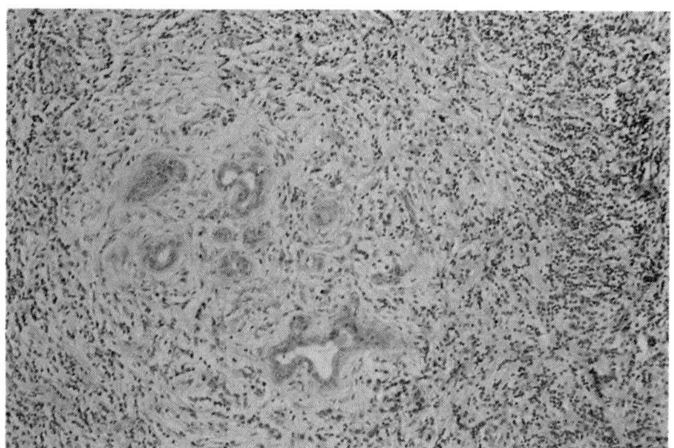

Figure 187–62. Chronic dacryoadenitis. Nonspecific inflammation of the lacrimal gland with loss of acini, preservation of ductules, chronic inflammation, and fibrosis. H&E, ×20.

SPECIFIC INFLAMMATION

Sarcoidosis and Sarcoid-Like Granulomatous Inflammation

Ophthalmic involvement is present in approximately 25 percent of patients with sarcoidosis, and of these, the lacrimal gland is involved clinically in about 25 percent.[510–513] Conversely, in a review of 41 granulomatous lesions of the orbit at the University of British Columbia, 13 were found to show a pattern consisitent with sarcoidosis. Eight involved the lacrimal gland. Only three of these showed evidence of systemic disease after a mean follow-up period of 42 months. The remaining five involved the extralacrimal soft tissue, and three of these had evidence of systemic disease. Thus, although the pathologic recognition of sarcoid-like granulomas in either the lacrimal gland or orbit requires that the patient be investigated and monitored for evidence of systemic disease, this may not always be forthcoming.[104, 514] The extraocular muscles may also be involved.[515] The conjunctiva may be a useful site to sample, producing high yields in some series.[516, 517]

The histopathologic appearance is the same in any site and does not vary much from case to case. It consists of numerous noncaseating granulomas without significant lymphocytic cuffing (Fig. 187–63). Small granulomas are often situated adjacent to blood vessels. Infrequently, the granulomas show central necrosis and moderate lymphocytic inflammation. Giant cells may or may not be frequent and may contain Schaumann's bodies, asteroid bodies, and crystalline inclusions of calcium oxalate.[518] Some cases may have a large amount of fibrosis, making the lesion very firm.

PAS and Ziehl-Neelsen stains should always be performed to rule out fungal and mycobacterial infections. Other granulomatous inflammations, as outlined earlier, should be considered in the pathologic differential diagnosis if the appearance is atypical. It should be emphasized that the inflammation may occasionally be patchy and that if granulomas are not seen on initial sections, deeper sections should be obtained or the paraffin block turned 180 degrees and sectioned from the opposite surface. Immunohistochemical investigations have shown that sarcoid granulomas contain an increased number of T-helper lymphocytes, with helper cells being located centrally and suppressor cells peripherally within the granuloma.[519, 520]

Lymphoepithelial Lesion of Sjögren's Syndrome

The lymphoepithelial lesion of Sjögren's syndrome involves the lacrimal gland or the other major and minor salivary glands and is responsible for keratoconjunctivitis sicca. It may be seen both with and without the associated arthritis and autoimmune features of Sjögren's syndrome.[521] Histopathologically, the lacrimal gland shows an intense chronic inflammatory infiltrate of lymphocytes and plasma cells with the formation of prominent germinal centers (Fig. 187–64). The lymphocytic infiltrate has been found to contain B cells and T-helper cells.[522] The acini of the gland are usually absent, and the remaining ducts may proliferate, producing solid islands of epithelial cells without lumina surrounded by inflammation.[521] Patients with the lymphoepithelial le-

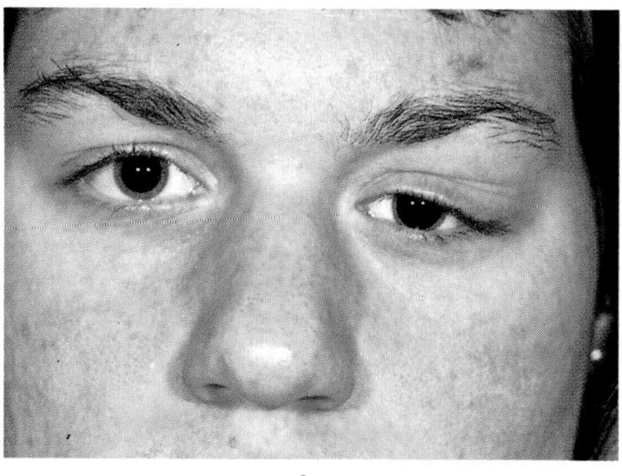

A

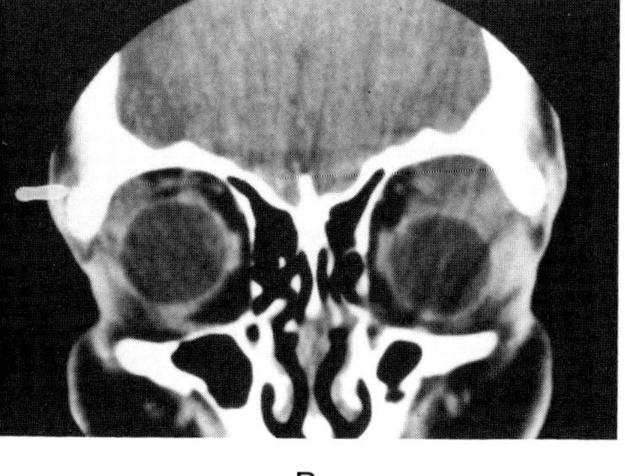

B

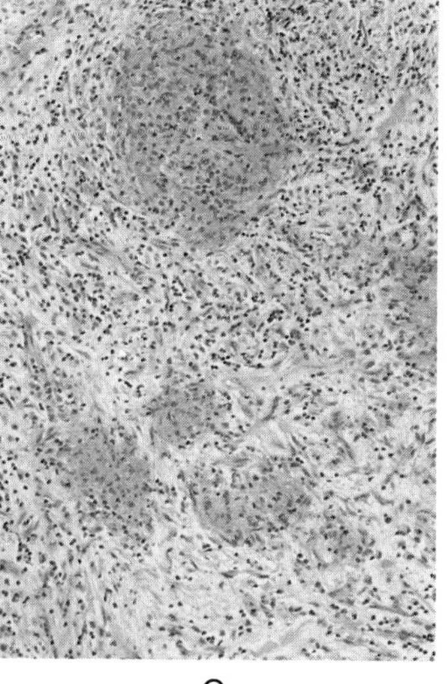

C

Figure 187–63. Localized orbital sarcoid. *A,* This 18-year-old female presented with a 3- to 4-week history of progressive swelling of the left upper lid, with injection and downward displacement of the globe due to a mass lesion of the lacrimal gland. *B,* Coronal computed tomography scans demonstrate bilateral lacrimal enlargement, more on the left than on the right. *C,* Biopsy demonstrates noncaseating granulomas set in a fibrous background with chronic inflammation. No evidence of systemic disease was found. H&E, ×25.

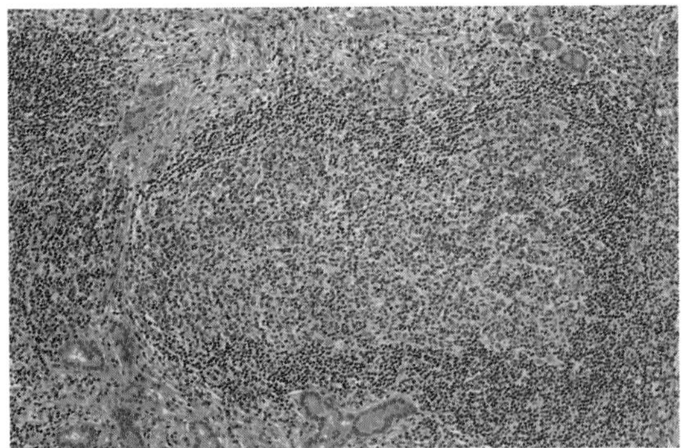

Figure 187–64. Sjögren's syndrome. Large, irregular germinal center in a background of chronic inflammation with loss of the lacrimal acini in a patient with keratoconjunctivitis sicca but not full-blown Sjögren's syndrome. H&E, ×20.

sion involving the salivary glands are at increased risk of developing nodal or extranodal non-Hodgkin's lymphoma.[523] A study has shown that even "benign lymphoepithelial lesions" of both salivary and lacrimal glands have immunoglobulin gene rearrangements in the absence of histologically overt lymphoma, suggesting that clonal expansion occurs in this setting of abnormal immune surveillance and may predispose to lymphoma.[522, 524] Therefore, these patients require careful follow-up to detect the development of lymphoma at an early stage.

Neoplasms of the Lacrimal Gland

Neoplasms account for approximately 50 percent of lacrimal gland masses sampled by biopsy, 50 percent of which are epithelial. Of these, approximately 50 percent are malignant, a higher percentage of malignancies than in the parotid gland.[525–529]

EPITHELIAL NEOPLASMS

Pleomorphic Adenoma

Pleomorphic adenoma, or benign mixed tumor, is the primary benign epithelial lesion of the lacrimal gland; rarely monomorphic adenomas and oncocytomas may occur.[530] Although most tumors occur in the orbital lobe, occasional cases have presented in the palpebral lobe as eyelid masses.[531, 532] They are characteristically bosselated lesions surrounded by a fibrous capsule, often showing nodules of tumor extending through the capsule, and a remnant of the gland with chronic inflammation. When a pleomorphic adenoma is suspected on the basis of clinical and radiographic appearances, the tumor with a rim of surrounding normal tissues should be removed without prior biopsy (Fig. 187–65*A*). This ensures excision of any nodules extending outside the main tumor; recurrences following incomplete removal take the form of multiple scattered nodules.[527]

Histologically, the tumor is biphasic, with epithelial and "stromal" elements (Fig. 187–65*B*). The epithelial portion is composed of small ductules with an inner cuboidal to columnar layer and an outer spindle-shaped layer that often contains clear cells. Squamous metaplasia may be present. The outer layer shows a gradual transition to mesenchymal tissues, which may display myxoid, cartilaginous, bony, or adipose features. Tyrosine crystals, stellate depositions of collagen, and infarction may be present. Ultrastructural examination has shown that ductular cells in pleomorphic adenomas have the characteristics of ductular cells of the normal gland and that the stromal cells retain epithelial features in the form of tonofilaments and desmosomes, although occasional cells show myoepithelial features with thin filaments and dense bodies.[532–534]

Adenoid Cystic Carcinoma

Adenoid cystic carcinoma is the most common of the epithelial malignancies of the lacrimal gland. It may occur from the second decade and has an insidious, progressive course.[527, 535] If the clinical and radiologic features suggest a malignant epithelial neoplasm, biopsy is first undertaken to confirm the diagnosis and plan treatment. Aspiration biopsy may allow diagnosis without open biopsy (Fig. 187–66).[536] Histopathologic examination reveals a tumor that may be arranged in one of several patterns: (1) cribriform (Swiss cheese), (2) basaloid (solid), (3) comedocarcinomatous, (4) tubular,

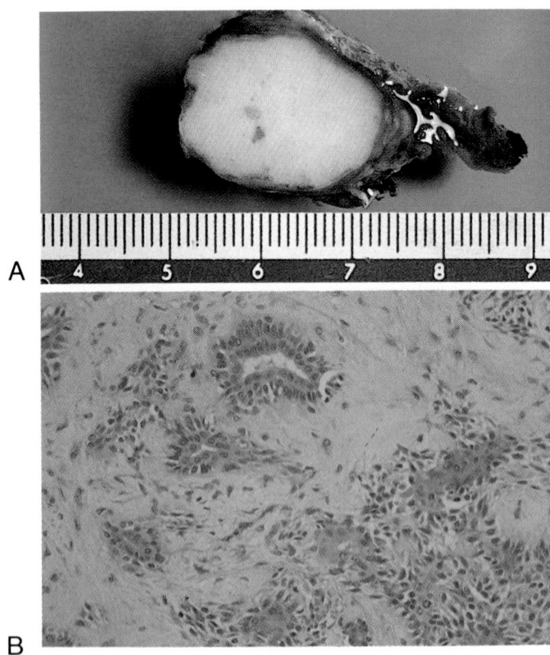

Figure 187–65. Pleomorphic adenoma. *A*, Gross photograph of an excised pleomorphic adenoma, with adjacent lacrimal gland. This whitish lesion has a slightly nodular surface at the site of excrescences through the capsule. *B*, The typical biphasic pattern with ductules lined by two layers of cells merging into the myxoid stroma. H&E, ×50.

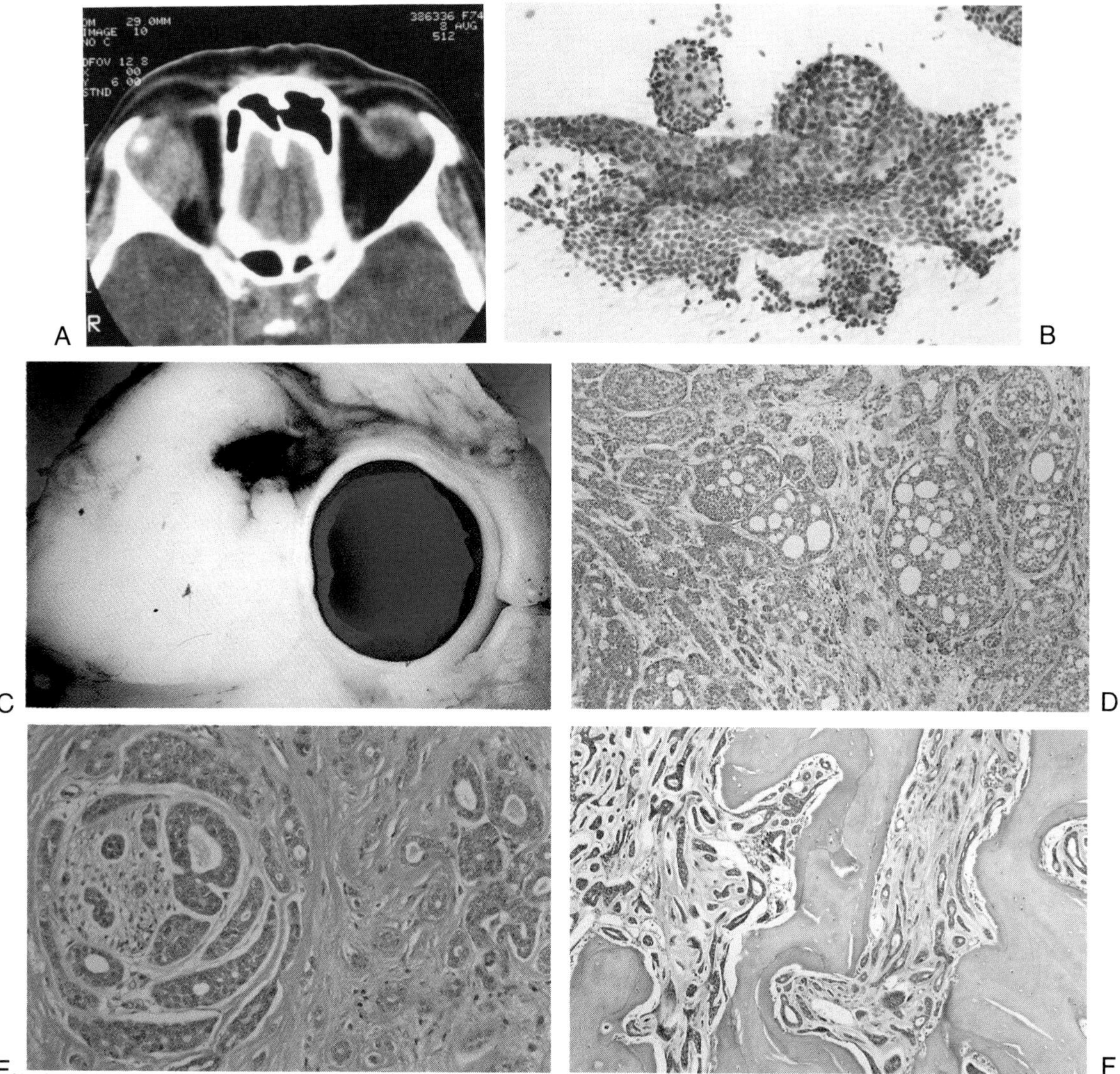

Figure 187–66. Adenoid cystic carcinoma. *A,* This patient presented with a painful lacrimal mass, associated with loss of sensation in the distribution of the zygomatic temporal nerve. The axial computed tomography scan demonstrates a slightly irregular nonhomogeneous right lacrimal gland mass, associated with an area of focal calcification. The adjacent bone appeared to be smooth, even on bone settings. *B,* Aspiration biopsy sample showed round and elongated fragments of tissue, consistent with the cribriform and tubular pattern seen in adenoid cystic carcinoma. H&E, ×50. *C,* Gross photograph of the exenteration specimen showing the huge lacrimal gland mass. The dark area is the site of frozen section biopsy. *D,* Histopathology reveals cribriform and tubular patterns in this field. All other patterns were present. H&E, ×20. *E,* Perineural invasion to the left and tubular and sclerosing pattern to the right. H&E, ×50. *F,* There was extensive involvement of the bone. Note the eosinophilic osteoblastic response on the surface of the bony trabeculae. H&E, ×20.

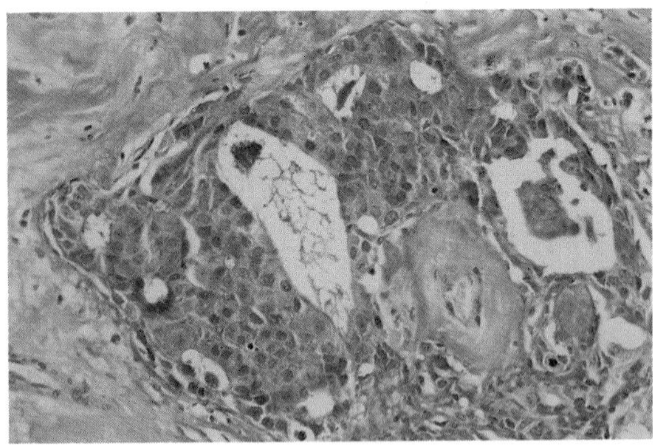

Figure 187–67. Malignant mixed tumor. High-grade adenocarcinoma that occupied almost the entire lacrimal gland in a patient with recent enlargement of a stable lacrimal mass. A small focus of residual pleomorphic adenoma was noted centrally. PAS, ×50.

and (5) sclerosing.[537] In each pattern, the cells are small, with little cytoplasm and inconspicuous nucleoli. Infrequently, the cells form small ductules with true lumina that contain PAS-positive, diastase-resistant mucin, but most of the spaces in the tumor contain material that stains with alcian blue and shows the presence of multilaminated basal lamina on EM.[533]

Perineural and bone involvement are the significant features responsible for this tumor's poor prognosis and are easily identified histologically (Fig. 187–66*E* and *F*). If radical orbitectomy has been performed, it is important to examine all of the bony specimen histologically after decalcification. It has been our experience that even when the bone does not show radiologic evidence of tumor, there may be extensive involvement of the marrow spaces with a slight osteoblastic response that may extend to the resection margins (Fig. 187–66*F*). Some investigators have shown that the basaloid pattern is associated with poorer survival, but all studies do not support this.[537, 538]

Malignant Mixed Tumor

Malignant mixed tumor is the third most common epithelial tumor of the lacrimal gland and is sometimes referred to as *carcinoma ex pleomorphic adenoma.* The term refers to the development of most commonly a poorly differentiated adenocarcinoma or less frequently adenoid cystic carcinoma in a pleomorphic adenoma (Fig. 187–67). Rarely, squamous undifferentiated carcinoma, mixtures of carcinomas, or a spindle cell neoplasm may develop.[529, 539–541] Patients may present after many recurrences of an incompletely excised pleomorphic adenoma, with a rapidly enlarging mass in a preexisting stable lacrimal gland mass or with a suspected carcinoma arising de novo.[529, 539, 542] To classify a tumor as malignant mixed, there should be histologic evidence of residual pleomorphic adenoma in association with a malignant tumor or previous histologically verified pleomorphic adenoma in the case of recurrent tumors.[529, 543]

Other Carcinomas

Other carcinomas include adenocarcinoma arising without an associated pleomorphic adenoma, mucoepidermoid carcinoma, rare oncocytic and squamous cell carcinomas, and a single case of acinic cell carcinoma.[544, 545] The adenocarcinomas usually are poorly differentiated. Mucoepidermoid carcinoma contains a variable mixture of squamous carcinoma and adenocarcinoma with mucus-secreting goblet cells and is much more frequent in the salivary glands, where it is the most common epithelial malignancy (Fig. 187–68). In the salivary glands, the prognosis is more favorable, with better differentiated tumors containing more adenocarcinomatous tissue.[546]

NONEPITHELIAL NEOPLASMS

Nonepithelial neoplasms are largely composed of lymphomas that have the same histopathologic features as those involving the remainder of the orbit and are commonly bilateral. Rare benign and malignant mesenchymal tumors, similar in histology to those discussed earlier, have been reported in and around the lacrimal gland.

Table 187–5 presents a tabular summary of orbital pathology.

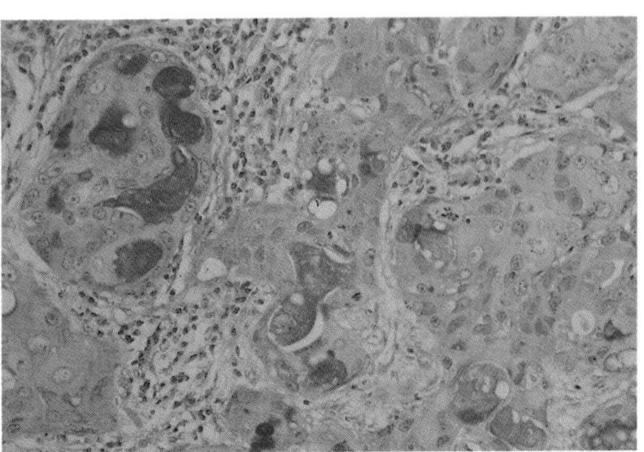

Figure 187–68. Mucoepidermoid carcinoma. High-grade lacrimal mucoepidermoid carcinoma showing poorly differentiated squamous carcinoma containing foci of mucus-producing adenocarcinoma. PAS, ×50.

Table 187–5. TABULAR SUMMARY OF ORBITAL PATHOLOGY

Lesion	Age Range	Summary
Congenital Disorders		
Congenital malformations	Birth to young adulthood	Variety of ectopic lesions and lesions composed of abnormally formed tissues
Congenital tumors	Birth to young adulthood	Most common is teratoma containing tissue of all three germ layers; rarely hemangiopericytomas and rhabdomyosarcomas
Cystic Lesions		
Epithelial Cysts		
Congenital	Childhood to middle age	Includes dermoid, conjunctival dermoid, and cysts lined by other types of epithelium that recapitulate the normal ocular adnexal epithelia; thought to arise from epithelia misplaced during embryonic development
Acquired		
Mucocele	Adulthood	Erosion or displacement of sinus epithelium into orbit due to chronic sinusitis or previous trauma
Lacrimal ductal cyst	Adulthood	Cystic dilatation of lacrimal duct
Implantation cyst	Any age	Implantation of conjunctival epithelium into the orbit as a result of accidental or surgical trauma
Nonepithelial Cysts		
Neurogenic	Birth to young adulthood	Cysts arising as a result of primary developmental abnormalities of the globe; lined by various types of neuroepithelia
Hematic	Childhood to middle age	Repeated hemorrhage into soft or bony tissues or orbit in association with a preexisting lesion, such as a lymphangioma, or occurring spontaneously
Infectious	Young to elderly	Parasitic cysts, most commonly due to *Echinococcus granulosus*
Inflammatory Diseases		
Infections	Childhood to middle age	Includes common bacterial infections, usually associated with sinusitis, fungal infections due to *Mucor* and *Aspergillus* species, and rarely tuberculosis, rhinoscleroma, other fungi and parasites
Specific Noninfectious inflammations		
Ruptured dermoid cysts	Young adulthood to middle age	Egress of oily cyst contents into orbit causes a lipogranulomatous and fibrotic response with destruction of cyst wall
Vasculitis	Young adulthood to middle age	Most common is Wegener's granulomatosis, less commonly hypersensitivity vasculitis and other types
Kimura's disease	Young adulthood to middle age	Vascular proliferation, lymphoid hyperplasia, and eosinophilic inflammation affecting soft tissues of head and neck most commonly in Asians
Necrobiotic xanthogranuloma with paraproteinemia	Middle age	Involvement of periocular skin and anterior orbit by xanthogranulomatous inflammation, Touton's giant cells, and necrosis of collagen; marker for plasma cell disorders
Pseudorheumatoid nodules	Childhood to young adulthood	Palisading granuloma involving subcutaneous tissue, usually in patients without rheumatoid diseases
Foreign body granulomas	Any age	Foreign body giant cell reaction to material implanted during previous trauma
Histiocytosis X	Infancy to middle age	Unifocal or multifocal involvement of bone, soft tissue, skin, or viscera; in the orbit, most commonly is a single bony focus of large histiocytes with bean-shaped nuclei that show Birbeck's or Langerhans' granules by electron microscopy
Other	Young adulthood to elderly	Other rare disorders including sinus histiocytosis with massive lymphadenopathy, juvenile xanthogranuloma, and Erdheim-Chester disease
Nonspecific, noninfectious inflammations	Adolescence to elderly	Classified into acute, subacute, and chronic forms; chronic sampled most frequently and shows fibrosis with chronic inflammation and occasional neutrophils

Table continued on following page

Table 187–5. **TABULAR SUMMARY OF ORBITAL PATHOLOGY** *Continued*

Lesion	Age Range	Summary
Thyroid Orbitopathy	Young adulthood to elderly with peak in middle age	Usually involves extraocular muscles, which show sparse chronic inflammation and infiltration by mucopolysaccharides, fibrous tissue, or fat
Amyloid Deposition	Middle age to elderly	Deposition of eosinophilic material that stains with Congo red; associated with systemic or localized plasma cell or lymphoproliferative disorder or chronic inflammation
Lymphoproliferative lesions and leukemia		
Lymphoproliferative lesions and lymphoma	Middle age to elderly	Lesions composed predominantly of small lymphocytes, sometimes containing other inflammatory cells; demonstration of a monoclonal population or atypical cytologic features required to make a diagnosis of definite lymphoma; lymphomas classified according to Working Formulation; all patients require work-up for systemic lymphoma and continued follow-up
Plasmacytomas	Middle age to elderly	Proliferation of plasma cells involving soft tissue or bone; may be part of systemic multiple myeloma
Hodgkin's Disease	Young adulthood	Rarely involves the orbit, always with prior systemic disease
Leukemia	Childhood to young adulthood	Orbital involvement may be presentation of leukemia or occur in preexisting disease; requires distinction from other childhood malignancies
Neoplasms		
Neoplasms with neurogenic and neural crest differentiation		
Peripheral nerve sheath tumors	Young adulthood to middle age	Includes neurofibromas, schwannomas, and malignant peripheral nerve sheath tumors; may be associated with von Recklinghausen's neurofibromatosis
Granular cell tumor	Young adulthood to middle age	Tumor of uncertain histogenesis postulated to arise from Schwann's cells; composed of cells with granular eosinophilic cytoplasm that contains numerous lysosomes by electron microscopy
Primary orbital melanoma	Middle age	Rare tumor arising in association with oculodermal melanocytosis or cellular blue nevus
Neuroepithelial tumors	Young adulthood to middle age	Tumors composed of small cells showing some evidence of neural differentiation; includes peripheral neuroepithelioma, primary neuroblastoma, and olfactory neuroblastoma
Paraganglioma and carcinoid tumor	Young adulthood to middle age	Neuroendocrine tumors showing neurosecretory granules by electron microscopy; paragangliomas usually primary, whereas carcinoid tumors are most commonly metastatic from the gastrointestinal tract
Retinal anlage tumor	Childhood	Tumor composed of small neuroepithelial and retinal pigment epithelial cells most commonly arising in the maxilla and involving the orbit secondarily
Neoplasms with mesenchymal differentiation		
Fibroblastic tumors	Childhood to elderly	Rare heterogeneous group of benign tumors, reactive to locally aggressive and malignant lesions composed solely of fibroblasts; most fibrosarcomas of older literature now called *malignant fibrous histiocytomas*
Fibrohistiocytic tumors	Childhood to elderly	Includes benign, locally aggressive, and malignant tumors composed of mixtures of fibroblasts, myofibroblasts, and cells with "histiocytic" features; malignant tumors may occur in setting of prior radiation for retinoblastoma and other malignancies
Muscle tumors		
Rhabdomyosarcoma	Childhood to young adulthood	Most common orbital malignancy of childhood composed of small "blue" cells showing skeletal muscle differentiation
Leiomyoma and leiomyosarcoma	Adulthood	Rare benign and malignant tumors showing smooth muscle differentiation
Adipose tissue tumors	Young adulthood to elderly	Rare, usually malignant tumors showing lipoblastic differentiation

Table 187–5. **TABULAR SUMMARY OF ORBITAL PATHOLOGY** *Continued*

Lesion	Age Range	Summary
Vascular lesions		
Varix	Adolescence to middle age	Dilated, tortuous, and abnormal orbital veins, may be thrombosed
Arteriovenous malformation	Childhood	Congenital or acquired malformation of orbital arteries and veins
Intravascular papillary endothelial hyperplasia	Young adulthood to middle age	Exuberant endothelial response to thrombosis of a vessel
Capillary hemangioma	Childhood	Hamartomatous proliferation of capillary-sized blood vessels, most commonly occurring on the facial skin; frequently involutes
Cavernous hemangioma	Adulthood	Hamartomatous proliferation of large blood vessels with thick fibrous walls
Lymphangioma	Childhood to young adulthood	Hamartomatous proliferation of dysplastic blood vessels of all sizes surrounded by lymphoid proliferation and evidence of old hemorrhage
Hemangiopericytoma	Any age	Tumor of pericytes that follows a variable and often protracted course
Angiosarcoma	Middle age	Malignant tumor of endothelial cells usually involving the skin and soft tissue
Tumors of uncertain histogenesis		
Alveolar soft-part sarcoma	Young adulthood	Large cells containing PAS-positive crystals, arranged in a pseudoalveolar pattern
Malignant rhabdoid tumor	Infancy to adulthood	Rare tumor showing monotonous proliferation of cells with eosinophilic cytoplasm; stains for vimentin and epithelial markers
Neoplasms arising in bone	Childhood to elderly	Includes fibroosseous, reactive giant cell, and malignant neoplasms; see Table 187–2
Metastatic tumors and tumors involving the orbit by direct extension		
Metastatic tumors	Childhood to elderly	Includes tumors metastatic from breast, lung, gastrointestinal tract, genitourinary tract, and cutaneous melanoma, most commonly in adults and from neuroblastoma, Ewing's sarcoma, and Wilms' tumor in children; see Table 187–3
Tumors involving the orbit by direct extension	Adulthood	Includes tumors extending into the orbit from the sinonasal tract, eyelid skin, conjunctiva, globe, intracranial cavity, optic nerve, and lacrimal sac; see Table 187–4
Inflammations and Neoplasms of the Lacrimal Gland		
Inflammations of the lacrimal gland		
Nonspecific inflammation	Young adulthood to elderly	Classified into acute, subacute, and chronic forms; chronic most frequently sampled and shows fibrosis, chronic inflammation, and atrophy of acini
Specific inflammation		
Sarcoidosis and sarcoid-like granulomatous inflammation	Young adulthood to elderly	Noncaseating granulomatous inflammation that may be associated with systemic sarcoidosis
Lymphoepithelial lesion of Sjögren's syndrome	Middle age	Intense chronic inflammation containing prominent germinal centers with acinar atrophy and ductular proliferation; not always associated with Sjögren's syndrome
Neoplasms of the lacrimal gland		
Epithelial neoplasms		
Pleomorphic adenoma	Adulthood	Most common benign epithelial neoplasm; shows a biphasic epithelial and "stromal" pattern
Adenoid cystic carcinoma	Young adulthood to elderly	Most common malignant neoplasm, composed of small uniform cells that may assume various histologic patterns; insidious and progressive course is due to perineural and bone involvement

Table continued on following page

Table 187–5. TABULAR SUMMARY OF ORBITAL PATHOLOGY *Continued*

Lesion	Age Range	Summary
Malignant mixed tumor	Adulthood	Adenocarcinoma or adenoid cystic carcinoma arising in a pleomorphic adenoma
Other	Adulthood	Rare epithelial tumors including adenocarcinoma arising de novo, mucoepidermoid carcinoma, oncocytic, acinic cell, and squamous cell carcinomas
Nonepithelial neoplasms	Adulthood	Most common are lymphomas; also other rare mesenchymal neoplasms

REFERENCES

1. Rootman J: Diseases of the Orbit. Philadelphia, JB Lippincott, 1988.
2. Shields JA, Bakewell B, Augsburger JJ, et al: Classification and incidence of space-occupying lesions of the orbit. Arch Ophthalmol 102:1606, 1984.
3. Shields JA, Bakewell B, Augsburger JJ, et al: Space-occupying orbital masses in children. Ophthalmology 93:379, 1986.
4. Henderson JW: Orbital Tumors, 2nd ed. New York, BC Decker, 1980.
5. Jakobiec FA, Font RL: Orbit. *In* Spencer WH (ed): Ophthalmic Pathology, 3rd ed, vol. 3. Philadelphia, WB Saunders, 1986.
6. Zajdela A, Vielh P, Schlienger P, et al: Fine-needle cytology of 292 palpable orbital and eyelid tumors. Am J Clin Pathol 93:100, 1990.
7. Kennerdell JS, Slamovits TL, Dekker A, et al: Orbital fine-needle aspiration biopsy. Am J Ophthalmol 99:547, 1985.
8. Midena E, Segato T, Piermarocchi S, et al: Fine needle aspiration biopsy in ophthalmology. Surv Ophthalmol 29:410, 1985.
9. Liu D: Complications of fine needle aspiration biopsy of the orbit. Ophthalmology 92:1768, 1985.
10. Krohel GB, Tobin DR, Chavis RM: Inaccuracy of fine needle aspiration biopsy. Ophthalmology 92:666, 1985.
11. Augsburger JJ, Shields JA, Folberg R, et al: Fine needle aspiration biopsy in the diagnosis of intraocular cancer. Ophthalmology 92:39, 1985.
12. Czerniak B, Woyke S, Daniel B, et al: Diagnosis of orbital tumors by aspiration biopsy guided by computerized tomography. Cancer 54:2385, 1984.
13. Newman NJ, Miller NR, Green WR: Ectopic brain in the orbit. Ophthalmology 93:268, 1986.
14. Call NB, Baylis HI: Cerebellar heterotopia in the orbit. Arch Ophthalmol 98:717, 1980.
15. Margo CE, Naugle TC, Karcioglu ZA: Ectopic lacrimal gland tissue of the orbit and sclerosing dacryoadenitis. Ophthalmic Surg 16:178, 1985.
16. Mansour AM, Barber JC, Reinecke RD, et al: Ocular choristomas. Surv Ophthalmol 33:339, 1989.
17. Green WR, Zimmerman LE: Ectopic lacrimal gland tissue. Arch Ophthalmol 78:318, 1967.
18. Seizinger BR, Rouleau GA, Ozelius LJ, et al: Genetic linkage of von Recklinghausen neurofibromatosis to the nerve growth factor receptor gene. Cell 49:589, 1987.
19. Bowen JH, Christensen FH, Klintworth GK, et al: A cartilaginous hamartoma of the orbit. Ophthalmology 88:1356, 1981.
20. Jepson CN, Wetzig PC: Pure chondroma of the trochlea: Surv Ophthalmol 11:656, 1966.
21. Isaacs H Jr: Perinatal (congenital and neonatal) neoplasms: A report of 110 cases. Pediatr Pathol 3:165, 1985.
22. Kauffman SL, Stout AP: Congenital mesenchymal tumors. Cancer 18:460, 1965.
23. Weiss AH, Greenwald MJ, Margo CE, et al: Primary and secondary orbital teratomas. J Pediatr Ophthalmol Strabismus 26:44, 1989.
24. Levin ML, Leone CR, Kincaid MC: Congenital orbital teratomas. Am J Ophthalmol 102:476, 1986.
25. Mamalis N, Garland PE, Argyle JC, et al: Congenital orbital teratoma: A review and report of two cases. Surv Ophthalmol 30:41, 1985.
26. Lack EE: Extragonadal germ cell tumors of the head and neck region. Hum Pathol 16:56, 1985.
27. Tuncbay E, Ovul I, Oztop F: Orbito-cranial teratoma. Acta Neurochir 56:73, 1981.
28. Chang DF, Dallow RL, Walton DS: Congenital orbital teratoma: Report of a case with visual preservation. J Pediatr Ophthalmol Strabismus 17:88, 1980.
29. Vinters HV, Murphy J, Wittmann B, et al: Intracranial teratoma: Antenatal diagnosis at 31 weeks' gestation by ultrasound. Acta Neuropathol 58:233, 1982.
30. Garden JW, McManis JC: Congenital orbital-intracranial teratoma with subsequent malignancy: Case report. Br J Ophthalmol 70:111, 1986.
31. Margo CE, Folberg R, Zimmerman LE, et al: Endodermal sinus tumor (yolk sac tumor) of the orbit. Ophthalmology 90:1426, 1983.
32. Katz NNK, Ruymann FB, Margo CE, et al: Endodermal sinus tumor (yolk sac carcinoma) of the orbit. J Pediatr Ophthalmol Strabismus 19:270, 1982.
33. Sherman RP, Rootman J, Lapointe JS: Orbital dermoids: Clinical presentation and management. Br J Ophthalmol 68:642, 1984.
34. Jakobiec FA, Bonanno PA, Sigelman J: Conjunctival adnexal cysts and dermoids. Arch Ophthalmol 96:1404, 1978.
35. Shields JA, Augsburger JJ, Donoso LA: Orbital dermoid cyst of conjunctival origin. Am J Ophthalmol 101:726, 1986.
36. Mims J, Rodrigues M, Calhoun J: Sudoriferous cyst of the orbit. Can J Ophthalmol 12:155, 1977.
37. Newton C, Dutton JJ, Klintworth GK: A respiratory epithelial choristomatous cyst of the orbit. Ophthalmology 92:1754, 1985.
38. James CRH, Lyness R, Wright JE: Respiratory epithelium lined cysts presenting in the orbit without associated mucocele formation. Br J Ophthalmol 70:387, 1986.
39. Kaufman SJ: Orbital mucopyoceles: Two cases and a review. Surv Ophthalmol 25:253, 1981.
40. De Juan E Jr, Green WR, Iliff NT: Allergic periorbital mucopyocele in children. Am J Ophthalmol 96:299, 1983.
41. Jakobiec FA, Trokel S, Iwamoto T: Sino-orbital polyposis. Arch Ophthalmol 97:2353, 1979.
42. Rawlings EF, Olson RJ, Kaufman HE: Polypoid sinusitis mimicking orbital malignancy. Am J Ophthalmol 87:694, 1979.
43. Smith S, Rootman J: Lacrimal ductal cysts: Presentation and management. Surv Ophthalmol 30:245, 1986.
44. Bullock JD, Fleishman JA, Rosset JS: Lacrimal ductal cysts. Ophthalmology 93:1355, 1986.
45. Apple DJ, Rabb MF: Ocular Pathology, 4th ed. St. Louis, Mosby-Year Book, 1991.
46. Waring GO, Roth AM, Rodrigues MM: Clinicopathologic correlation of microphthalmos with cyst. Am J Ophthalmol 82:714, 1976.
47. Pillai AM, Sambasivan R: Congenital cystic eye—A case report with CT scan. Indian J Ophthalmol 35:88, 1987.
48. Wilson RD, Traverse L, Hall JG, et al: Oculocerebrocutaneous syndrome. Am J Ophthalmol 99:142, 1985.
49. Baghdassarian SA, Tabbara KF, Matta CS: Congenital cystic eye. Am J Ophthalmol 76:269, 1973.
50. Helveston EM, Malone E Jr, Lashmet MH: Congenital cystic eye. Arch Ophthalmol 84:622, 1970.
51. Lieb W, Rochels R, Gronemeyer U: Microphthalmos with colobomatous orbital cyst: Clinical, histological, immunohistological, and electronmicroscopic findings. Br J Ophthalmol 74:59, 1990.
52. Awan KJ: Intraocular and extraocular colobomatous cysts in adults. Ophthalmologica 192:76, 1986.

53. Weiss A, Martinez C, Greenwald M: Microphthalmos with cyst: Clinical presentations and computed tomographic findings. J Pediatr Ophthalmol Strabismus 22:6, 1985.
54. Makley TA Jr, Battles M: Microphthalmos with cyst. Surv Ophthalmol 13:200, 1969.
55. Milne HL, Leone CR, Kincaid MC, et al: Chronic hematic cyst of the orbit. Ophthalmology 94:271, 1987.
56. Shapiro A, Tso MOM, Putterman AM, et al: A clinicopathologic study of hematic cysts of the orbit. Am J Ophthalmol 102:237, 1986.
57. Krohel GB, Wright JE: Orbital hemorrhage. Am J Ophthalmol 88:254, 1979.
58. McNab AA, Wright JE: Orbitofrontal cholesterol granuloma. Ophthalmology 97:28, 1990.
59. Parke DW II, Font RL, Boniuk M, et al: "Cholesteatoma" of orbit. Arch Ophthalmol 100:612, 1982.
60. DiLoreto DA, Rootman J, Neigel JM, et al: Infestation of extraocular muscle by *Cystericercus cellulosae*. Br J Ophthalmol 74:751, 1990.
61. Sen DK: Cysticercus cellulose in the lacrimal gland, orbit and eye lid. Acta Ophthalmol 58:144, 1980.
62. Morales AG, Croxatto JO, Crovetto L, et al: Hydatid cysts of the orbit. Ophthalmology 95:1027, 1988.
63. Manschot WA: Coenurus infestation of eye and orbit. Arch Ophthalmol 94:961, 1976.
64. Bansal RK, Suseelan AV, Gugnani HC: Orbital cyst due to *Histoplasma duboisii*. Br J Ophthalmol 61:70, 1977.
65. Hornblass A, Herschorn BJ, Stern K, et al: Orbital abscess. Surv Ophthalmol 29:169, 1984.
66. Krohel GB, Krauss HR, Winnick J: Orbital abscess. Ophthalmology 89:492, 1982.
67. Macy JI, Mandelbaum SH, Minckler DS: Orbital cellulitis. Ophthalmology 87:1309, 1980.
68. Khalil M, Lindley S, Matouk E: Tuberculosis of the orbit. Ophthalmology 92:1624, 1985.
69. Oakhill A, Shah KJ, Thompson AG, et al: Orbital tuberculosis in childhood. Br J Ophthalmol 66:396, 1982.
70. Spoor TC, Harding SA: Orbital tuberculosis. Am J Ophthalmol 91:644, 1981.
71. Smith RE, Salz JJ, Moors R, et al: *Mycobacterium chelonei* and orbital granuloma after tear duct probing. Am J Ophthalmol 89:139, 1980.
72. Levine R: Infection of the orbit by an atypical mycobacterium. Arch Ophthalmol 82:608, 1969.
73. Kestelyn P: Rhinoscleroma with bilateral orbital involvement. Am J Ophthalmol 101:381, 1986.
74. Lubin JR, Jallow SE, Wilson WR, et al: Rhinoscleroma with exophthalmos: A case report. Br J Ophthalmol 65:14, 1981.
75. Cernea P, Marculescu A, Constantin F: L'Osteopériostite syphilitique du sommet de l'orbite. Ann Ocul 201:436, 1968.
76. Endicott JN, Kirconnell WS, Beam D: Granuloma inguinale of the orbit with bony involvement. Arch Otolaryngol 96:457, 1972.
77. Karam F, Chmel H: Rhino-orbital cerebral mucormycosis. Ear Nose Throat J 69:187, 1990.
78. Parfrey N: Improved diagnosis and prognosis of mucormycosis. Medicine 65:113, 1986.
79. O'Keefe M, Haining WM, Young JDH, et al: Orbital mucormycosis with survival. Br J Ophthalmol 70:634, 1986.
80. Ferry AP, Abedi S: Diagnosis and management of rhino-orbitocerebral mycormyocosis (phycomycosis). Ophthalmology 90:1096, 1983.
81. McGill TJ, Simpson G, Healy GB: Fulminant aspergillosis of the nose and paranasal sinuses: A new clinical entity. Laryngoscope 90:748, 1980.
82. Houle TVJ, Ellis PP: Aspergillosis of the orbit with immunosuppressive therapy. Surv Ophthalmol 20:35, 1975.
83. Lowe J, Bradley J: Cerebral and orbital *Aspergillus* infection due to invasive aspergillosis of ethmoid sinus. J Clin Pathol 39:774, 1986.
84. Margo C, Rabinowicz M, Kwon-Chung KJ, et al: Subacute zygomycosis of the orbit. Arch Ophthalmol 101:1580, 1983.
85. Green WR, Font RL, Zimmerman LE: Aspergillosis of the orbit. Arch Ophthalmol 82:302, 1969.
86. Anderson RL, Carroll TF, Harvey JT, et al: *Petriellidium (Allescheria) boydii* orbital and brain abscess treated with intravenous miconazole. Am J Ophthalmol 97:771, 1984.
87. Olurin O, Lucas AO, Oyediran ABO: Orbital histoplasmosis due to *Histoplasma dubiosii*. Am J Ophthalmol 68:14, 1969.
88. Streeten BW, Rabuzzi DD, Jones DB: Sporotrichosis of the orbital margin. Am J Ophthalmol 77:750, 1974.
89. Gordon DM: Ocular sporotrichosis. Arch Ophthalmol 37:56, 1947.
90. Vida L, Moel SA: Systemic North American blastomycosis with orbital involvement. Am J Ophthalmol 77:240, 1974.
91. Gutierrez Y: Diagnostic Pathology of Parasitic Infections with Clinical Correlations. Philadelphia, Lea & Febiger, 1990.
92. Binford CH, Connor DH (eds): Pathology of Tropical and Extraordinary Diseases, vol. 2. Washington DC, Armed Forces Institute of Pathology, 1976.
93. Apple DJ, Fajoni ML, Garland PE, et al: Orbital hydatid cyst. J Pediatr Ophthalmol Strabismus 17:380, 1980.
94. Sen DK: Acute suppurative dacryoadenitis caused by a *Cysticercus cellulosae*. J Pediatr Ophthalmol Strabismus 19:100, 1982.
95. Duke-Elder S, MacFaul PA: The Ocular Adnexa, vol. 13. *In* Duke-Elder S (ed): System of Ophthalmology. London, Henry Kimpton, 1974.
96. Garner A: Pathology of "pseudotumours" of the orbit: A review. J Clin Pathol 26:639, 1973.
97. Font RL, Neafie RC, Perry HD: Subcutaneous dirofilariasis of the eyelid and ocular adnexae. Arch Ophthalmol 98:1079, 1980.
98. Thomas D, Older JJ, Kandawalla NG, et al: The *Dirofilaria* parasite in the orbit. Am J Ophthalmol 82:931, 1976.
99. Brumback GF, Morrison HM, Weatherly NF: Orbital infection with *Dirofilaria*. South Med J 61:188, 1968.
100. Jakobiec FA, Gess L, Zimmerman LE: Granulomatous dacryoadenitis caused by *Schistosoma haematobium*. Arch Ophthalmol 95:278, 1977.
101. Mortada A: Orbital pseudo-tumors and parasitic infections. Bull Ophta Soc Egypt 61:393, 1968.
102. Kersten RC, Shoukrey NM, Tabbara KF: Orbital myiasis. Ophthalmology 93:1228, 1986.
103. Mathur SP, Makhija JM: Invasion of the orbit by maggots. Br J Ophthalmol 51:406, 1967.
104. Satorre J, Antle CM, O'Sullivan R, et al: Orbital lesions with granulomatous inflammation. Can J Ophthalmol 26:174, 1991.
105. Robin JB, Schanzlin DJ, Meisler DM, et al: Ocular involvement in the respiratory vasculitides. Surv Ophthalmol 30:127, 1985.
106. Bullen CL, Liesegang TJ, McDonald TJ, et al: Ocular complications of Wegener's granulomatosis. Ophthalmology 90:279, 1983.
107. Spalton EJ, Graham EM, Page NGR, et al: Ocular changes in limited forms of Wegener's granulomatosis. Br J Ophthalmol 65:553, 1981.
108. Devaney KO, Travis WD, Hoffman G, et al: Interpretation of head and neck biopsies in Wegener's granulomatosis. Am J Surg Pathol 14:555, 1990.
109. Fienberg R: The protracted superficial phenomenon in pathergic (Wegener's) granulomatosis. Hum Pathol 12:458, 1981.
110. Gephardt GN, Shah LF, Tubbs RR, et al: Wegener's granulomatosis. Arch Pathol Lab Med 114:961, 1990.
111. Specks U, Wheatley CL, McDonald TJ, et al: Anticytoplasmic autoantibodies in the diagnosis and follow-up of Wegener's granulomatosis. Mayo Clin Proc 64:28, 1989.
112. Koyama T, Matsuo N, Watanabe Y, et al: Wegener's granulomatosis with destructive ocular manifestations. Am J Ophthalmol 98:736, 1984.
113. Garrity JA, Kennerdell JS, Johnson BL, et al: Cyclophosphamide in the treatment of orbital vasculitis. Am J Ophthalmol 102:97, 1986.
114. Kuo T, Shih L, Chan H: Kimura's disease. Am J Surg Pathol 12:843, 1988.
115. Smith DL, Kincaid MC, Nicolitz E: Angiolymphoid hyperplasia with eosinophilia (Kimura'a disease) of the orbit. Arch Ophthalmol 106:793, 1988.
116. Francis IC, Kappagoda MB, Smith J, et al: Kimura's disease of the orbit. Ophthalmic Plast Reconstr Surg 4:235, 1988.
117. Cook HT, Stafford ND: Angiolymphoid hyperplasia with eosinophilia involving the lacrimal gland: Case report. Br J Ophthalmol 72:710, 1988.
118. Hidayat AA, Cameron JD, Font RL, et al: Angiolymphoid hyperplasia with eosinophilia (Kimura's disease) of the orbit and ocular adnexa. Am J Ophthalmol 96:176, 1983.

119. Bostad L, Pettersen W: Angiolymphoid hyperplasia with eosinophilia involving the orbita. Acta Ophthalmol 60:419, 1982.
120. Amemiya T: Eosinophilic granuloma of the soft tissue in the orbit. Ophthalmologica 182:42, 1981.
121. Hui PK, Ng CS, Kung ITM, et al: Lymphadenopathy of Kimura's disease. Am J Surg Pathol 13:177, 1989.
122. Finan MC, Winkelmann RK: Necrobiotic xanthogranuloma with paraproteinemia. Medicine 65:376, 1986.
123. Robertson DM, Winkelmann RK: Ophthalmic features of necrobiotic xanthogranuloma with paraproteinemia. Am J Ophthalmol 97:173, 1984.
124. Muhlbauer JE: Granuloma annulare. J Am Acad Dermatol 3:217, 1980.
125. Lawton AW, Karesh JW: Periocular granuloma annulare. Surv Ophthalmol 31:285, 1986.
126. Ross MJ, Cohen KL, Peiffer RL Jr, et al: Episcleral and orbital pseudorheumatoid nodules. Arch Ophthalmol 101:418, 1983.
127. Floyd BB, Brown B, Isaacs H, et al: Pseudorheumatoid nodule involving the orbit. Arch Ophthalmol 100:1478, 1982.
128. Rao NA, Font RL: Pseudorheumatoid nodules of the ocular adnexa. Am J Ophthalmol 79:471, 1975.
129. MacCumber MW, Hoffman PN, Wand GS, et al: Ophthalmic involvement in aggressive histiocytosis X. Ophthalmology 97:22, 1990.
130. Moore AT, Pritchard J, Taylor DSI: Histiocytosis X: An ophthalmological review. Br J Ophthalmol 69:7, 1985.
131. Char DH, Ablin A, Beckstead J: Histiocytic disorders of the orbit. Ann Ophthalmol 16:867, 1984.
132. Favara BE, McCarthy RC, Mierau GW: Histiocytosis X. Hum Pathol 14:663, 1983.
133. Jakobiec FA, Trokel SL, Aron-Rosa D, et al: Localized eosinophilic granuloma (Langerhans' cell histiocytosis) of the orbital frontal bone. Arch Ophthalmol 98:1814, 1980.
134. Fartasch M, Vigneswaran N, Diepgen TL, et al: Immunohistochemical and ultrastructural study of histiocytosis X and non-X histiocytoses. J Am Acad Dermatol 23:885, 1990.
135. Foucar E, Rosai J, Dorfman RF: The ophthalmologic manifestations of sinus histiocytosis with massive lymphadenopathy. Am J Ophthalmol 87:354, 1979.
136. Marion JR, Geisinger KR: Sinus histiocytosis with massive lymphadenopathy: Bilateral orbital involvement spanning 17 years. Ann Ophthalmol 21:55, 1989.
137. Friendly DS, Font RL, Rao NA: Orbital involvement in "sinus" histiocytosis. Arch Ophthalmol 95:2006, 1977.
138. Codling BW, Soni KC, Barry DR, et al: Histiocytosis presenting as swelling of orbit and eyelid. Br J Ophthalmol 56:517, 1972.
139. Gaynes PM, Cohen GS: Juvenile xanthogranuloma of the orbit. Am J Ophthalmol 63:755, 1967.
140. Sanders TE: Infantile xanthogranuloma of the orbit. Am J Ophthalmol 61:1299, 1966.
141. Alper MG, Zimmerman LE, La Piana FG: Orbital manifestations of Erdheim-Chester disease. Trans Am Ophthalmol Soc 81:64, 1983.
142. Kennerdell JS, Dresner SC: The nonspecific orbital inflammatory syndromes. Surv Ophthalmol 29:93, 1984.
143. Weinstein GS, Dresner SC, Slamovits TL, et al: Acute and subacute orbital myositis. Am J Ophthalmol 96:209, 1983.
144. Rootman J, Nugent R: The classification and management of acute orbital pseudotumors. Ophthalmology 89:1040, 1982.
145. Kattah JC, Zimmerman LE, Kolsdy MP, et al: Bilateral orbital involvement in fatal giant cell polymyositis. Ophthalmology 97:520, 1990.
146. Mottow-Lippa L, Jakobiec FA, Smith M: Idiopathic inflammatory orbital pseudotumor in childhood. Ophthalmology 88:565, 1981.
147. Weissler MC, Miller E, Fortune MA: Sclerosing orbital pseudotumor: A unique clinicopathologic entity. Ann Otol Rhinol Laryngol 98:496, 1989.
148. Grossniklaus HE, Lass JH, Abramowsky CR, et al: Childhood orbital pseudotumor. Ann Ophthalmol 17:372, 1985.
149. Abramovitz JN, Kasdon KL, Sutula F, et al: Sclerosing orbital pseudotumor. Neurosurgery 12:463, 1983.
150. Osborne BM, Butler JJ, Bloustein P, et al: Idiopathic retroperitoneal fibrosis (sclerosing retroperitonitis). Hum Pathol 18:735, 1987.
151. Richards AB, Skalka HW, Roberts FJ, et al: Pseudotumor of the orbit and retroperitoneal fibrosis. Arch Ophthalmol 98:1617, 1980.
152. DuPont HL, Varco RL, Winchell CP: Chronic fibrous mediastinitis simulating pulmonic stenosis, associated with inflammatory pseudotumor of the orbit. Am J Med 44:447, 1968.
153. Comings DE, Skubi KB, Van Eyes J, et al: Familial multifocal fibrosclerosis. Ann Intern Med 66:884, 1967.
154. Arnott EJ, Greaves DP: Orbital involvement in Riedel's thyroiditis. Br J Ophthalmol 49:1, 1965.
155. Trokel SL, Jakobiec FA: Correlation of CT scanning and pathologic features of ophthalmic Graves' disease. Ophthalmology 88:553, 1981.
156. Sergott RC, Glaser JS: Graves' ophthalmopathy: A clinical and immunologic review. Surv Ophthalmol 26:1, 1981.
157. Kroll AJ, Kuwabara T: Dysthyroid ocular myopathy. Arch Ophthalmol 76:244, 1966.
158. Small RG: Enlargement of levator palpebrae superioris muscle fibres in Graves' ophthalmopathy. Ophthalmology 96:424, 1989.
159. Knowles DM, Jakobiec FA, Rosen M, et al: Amyloidosis of the orbit and adnexae. Surv Ophthalmol 19:367, 1975.
160. Glenner GG: Amyloid deposits and amyloidosis. N Engl J Med 302:1283, 1980.
161. Cohen AS, Connors LH: The pathogenesis and biochemistry of amyloidosis. J Pathol 151:1, 1987.
162. Erie JC, Garrity JA, Norman ME: Orbital amyloidosis involving the extraocular muscles. Arch Ophthalmol 107:1427, 1989.
163. Gonnering RS, Sonneland PR: Ptosis and dermatochalasis as presenting signs in a case of occult primary systemic amyloidosis (AL). Ophthalmic Surg 18:495, 1987.
164. Levine MR, Buckman G: Primary localized orbital amyloidosis. Ann Ophthalmol 18:165, 1986.
165. Liesegang TJ: Amyloid infiltration of the levator palpebrae superioris muscle: Case report. Ann Ophthalmol 15:610, 1983.
166. Lucas DR, Knox F, Davies S: Apparent monoclonal origin of lymphocytes and plasma cells infiltrating ocular adnexal amyloid deposits: Report of 2 cases. Br J Ophthalmol 66:600, 1982.
167. Finlay KR, Rootman J, Dimmick J: Optic neuropathy in primary orbital amyloidosis. Can J Ophthalmol 15:189, 1980.
168. Campos EC, Melato M, Manconi R, et al: Pathology of ocular tissues in amyloidosis. Ophthalmologica 181:31, 1980.
169. Rappaport H: Atlas of Tumor Pathology, Section III, Fascicle 8, Tumors of the Hematopoietic System. Washington DC, Armed Forces Institute of Pathology, 1966.
170. Lukes RJ, Collins RD: New approaches to the classification of the lymphomata. Br J Cancer 31(Suppl II):1, 1975.
171. Lennert K: Malignant Lymphomas Other Than Hodgkin's Disease. New York, Springer-Verlag, 1978.
172. National Cancer Institute sponsored study of classifications of non-Hodgkin's lymphomas: Summary and description of a working formulation for clinical usage. Cancer 49:2112, 1982.
173. Sklar J: What can DNA rearrangements tell us about solid hematolymphoid neoplasms? Am J Surg Pathol 14(Suppl 1):16, 1990.
174. Cossman J, Uppenkamp M, Sundeen J, et al: Molecular genetics and the diagnosis of lymphoma. Arch Pathol Lab Med 112:117, 1988.
175. Knowles DM, Jakobiec FA, McNally L, et al: Lymphoid hyperplasia and malignant lymphoma occurring in the ocular adnexa (orbit, conjunctiva, and eyelids). Hum Pathol 21:959, 1990.
176. Jakobiec FA, Neri A, Knowles DM: Genotypic monoclonality in immunophenotypically polyclonal orbital lymphoid tumors. Ophthalmology 94:980, 1987.
177. McNally L, Jakobiec FA, Knowles DM: Clinical, morphologic, immunophenotypic, and molecular genetic analysis of bilateral ocular adnexal lymphoid neoplasms in 17 patients. Am J Ophthalmol 103:555, 1987.
178. Hornblass A, Jakobiec FA, Reifler DM, et al: Orbital lymphoid tumors located predominantly within extraocular muscles. Ophthalmology 94:688, 1987.
179. Jakobiec FA, Iwamoto T, Patell M, et al: Ocular adnexal monoclonal lymphoid tumors with a favorable prognosis. Ophthalmology 93:1547, 1986.
180. Knowles DM, Jakobiec FA: Ocular adnexal lymphoid neoplasms. Hum Pathol 13:148, 1982.

181. Knowles DM, Jakobiec FA: Orbital lymphoid neoplasms. Cancer 46:576, 1980.
182. White V, Rootman J, Quenville N, et al: Orbital lymphoproliferative and inflammatory lesions. Can J Ophthalmol 22:362, 1987.
183. Ellis JH, Banks PM, Campbell RJ, et al: Lymphoid tumors of the ocular adnexa. Ophthalmology 92:1311, 1985.
184. Neri A, Jakobiec FA, Pellici P, et al: Immunoglobulin and T cell receptor beta chain gene rearrangement analysis of ocular adnexal lymphoid neoplasms: Clinical and biologic implications. Blood 70:1519, 1987.
185. Font RL, Shields J: Large cell lymphoma of the orbit with microvillous projections ("porcupine lymphoma"). Arch Ophthalmol 103:1715, 1985.
186. Antle CM, White VA, Horsman DE, et al: Large cell orbital lymphoma in a patient with acquired immune deficiency syndrome. Ophthalmology 97:1494, 1990.
187. Brooks BL, Downing J, McClure JA, et al: Orbital Burkitt's lymphoma in a homosexual man with acquired immune deficiency. Arch Ophthalmol 102:1533, 1984.
188. Dolman PJ, Rootman J, Quenville NF: Signet-ring cell lymphoma in the orbit: A case report and review. Can J Ophthalmol 21:242, 1986.
189. Lauer SA, Fischer J, Jones J, et al: Orbital T-cell lymphoma in a human T-cell leukemia virus-1 infection. Ophthalmology 95:110, 1988.
190. Whitbeck EG, Spiers ASD, Hussain M: Mycosis fungoides: Subcutaneous and visceral tumors, orbital involvement, and ophthalmoplegia. J Clin Oncol 1:270, 1983.
191. Stenson S, Ramsay DL: Ocular findings in mycosis fungoides. Arch Ophthalmol 99:272, 1981.
192. Henderson JW, Banks PM, Yeatts RP: T-cell lymphoma of the orbit. Mayo Clin Proc 64:940, 1989.
193. Meekins B, Proia AD, Klintworth GK: Cutaneous T-cell lymphoma presenting as a rapidly enlarging ocular adnexal tumor. Ophthalmology 92:1288, 1985.
194. Laroche L, Laroche L, Pavlakis E, et al: Immunological characterization of an ocular adnexal lymphoid T tumor by monoclonal antibodies. Ophthalmologica 187:43, 1983.
195. Robb-Smith AHT: Before our time: Half a century of histiocytic medullary reticulosis: A T-cell teaser? Histopathology 17:279, 1990.
196. Wilson MS, Weiss LM, Gatter KC, et al: Malignant histiocytosis: A reassessment of cases previously reported in 1975 based on paraffin section immunophenotyping studies. Cancer 66:530, 1990.
197. Risdall RJ, Sibley RK, McKenna RW, et al: Malignant histiocytosis. Am J Surg Pathol 4:439, 1980.
198. Warnke RA, Kim H, Dorfman RF: Malignant histiocytosis (histiocytic medullary reticulosis). Cancer 35:215, 1975.
199. Knowling MA, Harwood AR, Bergsagel DE: Comparison of extramedullary plasmacytomas with solitary and multiple plasma cell tumors of bone. J Clin Oncol 1:255, 1983.
200. De Smet M, Rootman J: Orbital manifestations of plasmacytic lymphoproliferations. Ophthalmology 94:995, 1987.
201. Gonnering RS: Bilateral primary extramedullary orbital plasmacytomas. Ophthalmology 94:267, 1987.
202. Mewis-Levin L, Garcia CA, Olson JD: Plasma cell myeloma of the orbit. Ann Ophthalmol 13:477, 1981.
203. Khalil MK, Huang S, Viloria J, et al: Extramedullary plasmacytoma of the orbit: Case report with results of immunocytochemical studies. Can J Ophthalmol 16:39, 1981.
204. Levin SR, Spaulding AG, Wirman JA: Multiple myeloma. Arch Ophthalmol 95:642, 1977.
205. Fratkin JD, Shammas HF, Miller SD: Disseminated Hodgkin's disease with bilateral orbital involvement. Arch Ophthalmol 96:102, 1978.
206. Patel S, Rootman J: Nodular sclerosing Hodgkin's disease of the orbit. Ophthalmology 90:1433, 1983.
207. Lukes RJ, Craver LF, Hall TC, et al: Report of the nomenclature committee. I. Cancer Res 26:1311, 1966.
208. Kielar RA: Orbital granuloma in Hodgkin's disease. Ann Ophthalmol 13:1197, 1981.
209. Kincaid MC, Green WR: Ocular and orbital involvement in leukemia. Surv Ophthalmol 27:211, 1983.
210. Davis JL, Parke DW, Font RL: Granulocytic sarcoma of the orbit. Ophthalmology 92:1758, 1985.
211. Rubinfeld RS, Gootenberg JE, Chavis RM, et al: Early onset acute orbital involvement in childhood acute lymphoblastic leukemia. Ophthalmology 95:116, 1988.
212. Rajantie J, Tarkkanen A, Rapola J, et al: Orbital granulocytic sarcoma as a presenting sign in acute myelogenous leukemia. Ophthalmologica 189:158, 1984.
213. Skinnider LF, Romanchuk KG: Orbital involvement in chronic lymphocytic leukemia. Can J Ophthalmol 19:142, 1984.
214. Cavadar AO, Arcasoy A, Babacan E, et al: Ocular granulocytic sarcoma (chloroma) with acute myelomonocytic leukemia in Turkish children. Cancer 41:1606, 1978.
215. Brownstein S, Thelmo W, Olivier A: Granulocytic sarcoma of the orbit. Can J Ophthalmol 10:174, 1975.
216. Zimmerman LE, Font RL: Ophthalmologic manifestations of granulocytic sarcoma (myeloid sarcoma or chloroma). Am J Ophthalmol 80:975, 1975.
217. Liu PI, Ishimaru T, McGregor DH, et al: Autopsy study of granulocytic sarcoma (chloroma) in patients with myelogenous leukemia, Hiroshima-Nagasaki 1949–1969. Cancer 31:948, 1973.
218. Enzinger FM, Weiss SW: Soft tissue tumors, 2nd ed. St. Louis, CV Mosby, 1988.
219. Dickersin GR: Diagnostic Electron Microscopy: A Text/Atlas. New York, Igaku-Shoin Medical Publishers, 1988.
220. Johnston MC, Noden DM, Hazelton RD, et al: Origins of avian ocular and periocular tissues. Exp Eye Res 29:27, 1979.
221. Qualman SJ, Green WR, Brovall C, et al: Neurofibromatosis and associated neuroectodermal tumors: A congenital neurocristopathy. Pediatr Pathol 5:65, 1986.
222. Van der Meulen J: Orbital neurofibromatosis. Clin Plast Surg 14:123, 1987.
223. Woog JJ, Albert DM, Solt LC, et al: Neurofibromatosis of the eyelid and orbit. Int Ophthalmol Clin 22:157, 1982.
224. Kobrin JL, Blodi FC, Weingeist TA: Ocular and orbital manifestations of neurofibromatosis. Surv Ophthalmol 24:45, 1979.
225. Erlandson RA, Woodruff JM: Peripheral nerve sheath tumors: An electron microscopic study of 43 cases. Cancer 49:273, 1982.
226. Shields JA, Shields CL, Leib WE, et al: Multiple orbital neurofibromas unassociated with von Recklinghausen's disease. Arch Ophthalmol 108:80, 1990.
227. Krohel GB, Rosenberg PN, Wright JE, et al: Localized orbital neurofibromas. Am J Ophthalmol 100:458, 1985.
228. McDonald P, Jakobiec FA, Hornblass A, et al: Benign peripheral nerve sheath tumors (neurofibromas) of the lacrimal gland. Ophthalmology 90:1403, 1983.
229. Messmer EP, Camara J, Boniuk M, et al: Amputation neuroma of the orbit: Report of two cases and review of the literature. Ophthalmology 91:1420, 1984.
230. Konrad EA, Thiel HJ: Schwannoma of the orbit. Ophthalmologica 188:118, 1984.
231. Rootman J, Goldberg C, Robertson W: Primary orbital schwannomas. Br J Ophthalmol 66:194, 1982.
232. Schatz H: Benign orbital neurilemoma: Sarcomatous transformation in von Recklinghausen's disease. Arch Ophthalmol 86:268, 1971.
233. Jakobiec FA, Font FL, Zimmerman LE: Malignant peripheral nerve sheath tumors of the orbit: A clinicopathologic study of eight cases. Trans Am Ophthalmol Soc 83:332, 1985.
234. Lyons CJ, McNab AA, Garner A, et al: Orbital malignant peripheral nerve sheath tumours. Br J Ophthalmol 73:731, 1989.
235. Grinberg MA, Levy NS: Malignant neurilemoma of the supraorbital nerve. Am J Ophthalmol 78:489, 1974.
236. Jaeger MJ, Green WR, Miller NR, et al: Granular cell tumor of the orbit and ocular adnexae. Surv Ophthalmol 31:417, 1987.
237. Dolman PJ, Rootman J, Dolman CL: Infiltrating orbital granular cell tumour: A case report and literature review. Br J Ophthalmol 71:47, 1987.
238. Singleton EM, Nettleship MB: Granular cell tumor of the orbit: A case report. Ann Ophthalmol 15:881, 1983.
239. Moriarty P, Garner A, Wright JE: Case report of granular cell myoblastoma arising within the medial rectus muscle. Br J Ophthalmol 67:17, 1983.
240. Goldstein BG, Font RL, Alper MG: Granular cell tumor of the

orbit: A case report including electron microscopic observations. Ann Ophthalmol 14:231, 1982.
241. Garancis JC, Komorowski RA, Kuzma JF: Granular cell myoblastoma. Cancer 25:542, 1970.
242. Ellis DS, Spencer WH, Stephenson CM: Congenital neurocutaneous melanosis with metastatic orbital malignant melanoma. Ophthalmology 93:1639, 1986.
243. Dutton JJ, Anderson RL, Schelper RL, et al: Orbital malignant melanoma and oculodermal melanocytosis: Report of two cases and review of the literature. Ophthalmology 91:497, 1984.
244. Haim T, Meyer E, Kerner H, et al: Oculodermal melanocytosis (nevus of ota) and orbital malignant melanoma. Ann Ophthalmol 14:1132, 1982.
245. Loffler KU, Witschel H: Primary malignant melanoma of the orbit arising in a cellular blue naevus. Br J Ophthalmol 73:388, 1989.
246. Wilkes TDI, Uthman EO, Thornton CN, et al: Malignant melanoma of the orbit in a black patient with ocular melanocytosis. Arch Ophthalmol 102:904, 1984.
247. Bullock JD, Goldberg SH, Rakes SM, et al: Primary orbital neuroblastoma. Arch Ophthalmol 107:1031, 1989.
248. Jakobiec FA, Klepach GL, Crissman JD, et al: Primary differentiated neuroblastoma of the orbit. Ophthalmology 94:255, 1987.
249. Wilson WB, Roloff J, Wilson HL: Primary peripheral neuroepithelioma of the orbit with intracranial extension. Cancer 62:2595, 1988.
250. Shuangshoti S, Menakanit W, Changwaivit W, et al: Primary intraorbital extraocular primitive neuroectodermal (neuroepithelial) tumour. Br J Ophthalmol 70:543, 1986.
251. Howard GM: Neuroepithelioma of the orbit. Am J Ophthalmol 59:934, 1965.
252. Llombart-Bosch A, Terrier-Lacombe MJ, Peydro-Olaya A, et al: Peripheral neuroectodermal sarcoma of soft tissue (peripheral neuroepithelioma). Hum Pathol 20:273, 1989.
253. Mackay B, Luna MA, Butler JJ: Adult neuroblastoma: Electron microscopic observations in nine cases. Cancer 37:1334, 1976.
254. Whang-Peng J, Triche TJ, Knutsen T, et al: Cytogenetic characterization of selected small round cell tumors of childhood. Cancer Genet Cytogenet 21:185, 1986.
255. Haas OA, Chott A, Ladenstein R, et al: Poorly differentiated, neuron-specific enolase positive round cell tumor with two translocations t(11;22) and t(21;22). Cancer 60:2219, 1987.
256. Rakes SM, Yeatts RP, Campbell RJ: Ophthalmic manifestations of esthesioneuroblastoma. Ophthalmology 92:1749, 1985.
257. Mills SE, Frierson HF Jr: Olfactory neuroblastoma: A clinicopathologic study of 21 cases. Am J Surg Pathol 9:317, 1985.
258. Silva EG, Butler JJ, Mackay B, et al: Neuroblastomas and neuroendocrine carcinomas of the nasal cavity: A proposed new classification. Cancer 50:2388, 1982.
259. Takahashi H, Ohara S, Yamada M, et al: Esthesioneuroepithelioma: A tumor of true olfactory epithelium origin. Acta Neuropathol 75:147, 1987.
260. Archer KF, Hurwitz JJ, Balogh JM, et al: Orbital nonchromaffin paraganglioma: A case report and review of the literature. Ophthalmology 96:1659, 1989.
261. Venkataramana NK, Kolluri VRS, Kumar DVR, et al: Paraganglioma of the orbit with extension to the middle cranial fossa: Case report. Neurosurgery 24:762, 1989.
262. Paulus W, Jellinger K, Brenner H: Melanotic paraganglioma of the orbit: A case report. Acta Neuropathol 79:340, 1989.
263. Amemiya T, Kadoya M: Paraganglioma in the orbit. J Cancer Res Clin Oncol 96:169, 1980.
264. Thacker WC, Duckworth JK: Chemodectoma of the orbit. Cancer 23:1233, 1969.
265. Kliewer KE, Wen D-R, Cancilla PA, et al: Paragangliomas: Assessment of prognosis by histologic, immunohistochemical and ultrastructural techniques. Hum Pathol 20:29, 1989.
266. Zimmerman LE, Stangl R, Riddle PJ: Primary carcinoid tumor of the orbit. Arch Ophthalmol 101:1395, 1983.
267. Riddle PJ, Font RL, Zimmerman LE: Carcinoid tumors of the eye and orbit: A clinicopathologic study of 15 cases with histochemical and electron microscopic observations. Hum Pathol 13:459, 1982.
268. Krohel GB, Perry S, Hepler RS: Acute hypertension with orbital carcinoid tumor. Arch Ophthalmol 100:106, 1982.
269. Johnson RE, Scheithauer BW, Dahlin DC: Melanotic neuroectodermal tumor of infancy: A review of seven cases. Cancer 52:661, 1983.
270. Lamping KA, Albert DM, Lack E, et al: Melanotic neuroectodermal tumor of infancy (retinal anlage tumor). Ophthalmology 92:143, 1985.
271. Prasad KRK, Bhaskaran CS, Reddy SJB, et al: Melanotic neuroectodermal tumor of infancy. Indian J Pathol Microbiol 32:68, 1989.
272. Font RL, Zimmerman LE: Nodular fasciitis of the eye and adnexa: A report of ten cases. Arch Ophthalmol 75:475, 1966.
273. Levitt JM, deVeer JA, Oguzhan MC: Orbital nodular fasciitis. Arch Ophthalmol 81:235, 1969.
274. Herschorn BJ, Jakobiec FA, Hornblass A, et al: Epibulbar subconjunctival fibroma. Ophthalmology 90:1490, 1983.
275. Case TD, Lapiana FG: Benign fibrous tumor of the orbit. Ann Ophthalmol 7:813, 1975.
276. Lieb WE, Goebel HH, Wallenfang T: Myxoma of the orbit: A clinicopathologic report. Arch Clin Exp Ophthalmol 228:28, 1990.
277. Maiuri F, Corriero G, Galicchio B, et al: Myxoma of the skull and orbit. Neurochirurgia 31:136, 1988.
278. Allen PW: The fibromatoses: A clinicopathologic classification based on 140 cases. Am J Surg Pathol 1:255, 1977.
279. Smoot CN, Krohel GB, Smith RS: Adult periorbital fibromatosis. Br J Ophthalmol 73:373, 1989.
280. Waeltermann JM, Huntrakoon M, Beatty EC, et al: Congenital fibromatosis (myofibromatosis) of the orbit: A rare cause of proptosis at birth. Ann Ophthalmol 20:394, 1988.
281. Nasr AM, Blodi FC, Lindahl S: Congenital generalized multicentric myofibromatosis with orbital involvement. Am J Ophthalmol 102:779, 1986.
282. Hidayat AA, Font RL: Juvenile fibromatosis of the periorbital region and eyelid. Arch Ophthalmol 98:280, 1980.
283. Schutz JS, Rabkin MD, Schutz S: Fibromatous tumor (desmoid type) of the orbit. Arch Ophthalmol 97:703, 1979.
284. Chung EB, Enzinger FM: Infantile fibrosarcoma. Cancer 38:729, 1976.
285. Weiner JM, Hidayat AA: Juvenile fibrosarcoma of the orbit and eyelid: A study of five cases. Arch Ophthalmol 101:253, 1983.
286. Rootman J, Carvounis EP, Dolman CL, et al: Congenital fibrosarcoma metastatic to the choroid. Am J Ophthalmol 87:632, 1979.
287. Jakobiec FA, Tannenbaum M: The ultrastructure of orbital fibrosarcoma. Am J Ophthalmol 77:899, 1974.
288. Fletcher CDM: Benign fibrous histiocytoma of subcutaneous and deep soft tissue: A clinicopathologic analysis of 21 cases. Am J Surg Pathol 14:801, 1990.
289. Hoffman MA, Dickerson GR: Malignant fibrous histiocytoma: An ultrastructural study of eleven cases. Hum Pathol 14:913, 1983.
290. Font RL, Hidayat AA: Fibrous histiocytoma of the orbit. Hum Pathol 13:199, 1982.
291. Jakobiec FA, Klapper D, Maher E, et al: Infantile subconjunctival and anterior orbital fibrous histiocytoma. Ophthalmology 95:516, 1988.
292. Larkin DFP, O'Donoghue HN, Mullaney J, et al: Orbital fibrous histiocytoma in an infant. Acta Ophthalmol 66:585, 1988.
293. Betharia SM, Arora R, Kumar S: Malignant fibrous histiocytoma of the orbit. Indian J Ophthal 36:116, 1988.
294. Ros PR, Kursunoglu S, Batlle JF, et al: Malignant fibrous histiocytoma of the orbit. J Clin Neuro Ophthalmol 5:116, 1985.
295. Caballero LR, Rodriguez AC, Sopelana AB: Angiomatoid malignant fibrous histiocytoma of the orbit. Am J Ophthalmol 92:13, 1981.
296. Liu D, McCann P, Kini RK, et al: Malignant fibrous histiocytoma of the orbit in a 3-year old girl. Arch Ophthalmol 105:895, 1987.
297. Krohel GB, Gregor Z: Fibrous histiocytoma. J Pediatr Ophthalmol Strabismus 17:37, 1980.
298. Biedner B, Rothkoff L: Orbital fibrous histiocytoma in an infant. Am J Ophthalmol 85:548, 1978.
299. Rodrigues MM, Furgiuele FP, Weinreb S: Malignant fibrous histiocytoma of the orbit. Arch Ophthalmol 95:2025, 1977.
300. Jakobiec FA, Howard GM, Jones IS, et al: Fibrous histiocytomas of the orbit. Am J Ophthalmol 77:333, 1974.

301. Stewart WB, Newman NM, Cavender JC, et al: Fibrous histiocytoma metastatic to the orbit. Arch Ophthalmol 96:871, 1978.
302. Marback RL, Kincaid MC, Green WR, et al: Fibrous histiocytoma of the lacrimal sac. Am J Ophthalmol 93:511, 1982.
303. Sen DK, Mohan H: Fibroma of the lacrimal sac. J Pediatr Ophthalmol Strabismus 17:410, 1980.
304. Newton WA, Soule EH, Hamoudi AB, et al: Histopathology of childhood sarcomas, intergroup rhabdomyosarcoma studies I and II: Clinicopathologic correlation. J Clin Oncol 6:67, 1988.
305. Bale PM, Parsons RE, Stevens MM: Diagnosis and behavior of juvenile rhabdomyosarcoma. Hum Pathol 14:596, 1983.
306. Harlow PJ, Kaufman FR, Siegel SE, et al: Orbital rhabdomyosarcoma in a neonate. Med Pediatr Oncol 7:123, 1979.
307. Ellenbogen E, Lasky MA: Rhabdomyosarcoma of the orbit in the newborn. Am J Ophthalmol 8:1024, 1975.
308. Wharam M, Beltangady M, Hays D, et al: Localized orbital rhabdomyosarcoma: An interim report of the Intergroup Rhabdomyosarcoma Study Committee. Ophthalmology 94:251, 1987.
309. Abramson DH, Ellsworth RM, Tretter P, et al: The treatment of orbital rhabdomyosarcoma with irradiation and chemotherapy. Ophthalmology 86:1330, 1979.
310. Spaeth EB, Cleveland AF: Rhabdomyosarcoma in infancy and childhood. Am J Ophthalmol 53:463, 1962.
311. Haik BG, Jereb B, Smith ME, et al: Radiation and chemotherapy of parameningeal rhabdomyosarcoma involving the orbit. Ophthalmology 93:1001, 1986.
312. Delbalso AM, Weinstein ZR, Deal JL, et al: Nasopharyngeal rhabdomyosarcoma in an adult with intracranial and intraorbital extension. Ear Nose Throat J 65:420, 1986.
313. Cameron D, Wick MR: Embryonal rhabdomyosarcoma of the conjunctiva. Arch Ophthalmol 104:1203, 1986.
314. Azumi N, Ben-Ezra J, Battifora H: Immunophenotypic diagnosis of leiomyosarcomas and rhabdomyosarcomas with monoclonal antibodies to muscle-specific actin and desmin in formalin-fixed tissue. Mod Pathol 1:469, 1988.
315. Altmannsberger M, Weber K, Droste R, et al: Desmin is a specific marker for rhabdomyosarcomas of human and rat origin. Am J Pathol 118:85, 1985.
316. Kahn HJ, Yeger H, Kassim O, et al: Immunohistochemical and electron microscopic assessment of childhood rhabdomyosarcoma. Cancer 51:1897, 1983.
317. Bundtzen JL, Norback DH: The ultrastructure of poorly differentiated rhabdomyosarcomas. Hum Pathol 13:301, 1982.
318. Scrable H, Witte D, Shimada H, et al: Molecular differential pathology of rhabdomyosarcoma. Genes Chromosomes Cancer 1:23, 1989.
319. Douglass EC, Valentine M, Etcubanas E, et al: A specific chromosomal abnormality in rhabdomyosarcoma. Cytogenet Cell Genet 45:148, 1987.
320. Turc-Carel C, Lizard-Nacol S, Justrabo E, et al: Consistent chromosomal translocation in alveolar rhabdomyosarcoma. Cancer Genet Cytogenet 19:361, 1986.
321. DeJong ASH, Van Kessel-van Vark M, Albus-Lutter Ch.E.: Pleomorphic rhabdomyosarcoma in adults. Hum Pathol 18:298, 1987.
322. Meekins BB, Dutton JJ, Proia AD: Primary orbital leiomyosarcoma: A case report and review of the literature. Arch Ophthalmol 106:82, 1988.
323. Vigstrup J, Glenthoj A: Leiomyoma of the orbit. Acta Ophthalmol 60:992, 1982.
324. Sanborn GE, Valenzuela RE, Green WR: Leiomyoma of the orbit. Am J Ophthalmol 87:371, 1979.
325. Jakobiec FA, Mitchell JP, Chauhan PM, et al: Mesectodermal leiomyosarcoma of the antrum and orbit. Am J Ophthalmol 85:51, 1978.
326. Jakobiec FA, Howard GM, Rosen M, et al: Leiomyoma and leiomyosarcoma of the orbit. Am J Ophthalmol 80:1028, 1975.
327. Jakobiec FA, Jones IS, Tannenbaum M: Leiomyoma: An unusual tumour of the orbit. Br J Ophthalmol 57:825, 1973.
328. Font RL, Jurco S III, Brechner RJ: Postradiation leiomyosarcoma of the orbit complicating bilateral retinoblastoma. Arch Ophthalmol 101:1557, 1983.
329. Folberg R, Cleasby G, Flanagan JA, et al: Orbital leiomyosarcoma after radiation therapy for bilateral retinoblastoma. Arch Ophthalmol 101:1562, 1983.
330. Koganei Y, Ishikawa S, Abe K, et al: Orbital lipoma. Ann Plast Surg 20:173, 1988.
331. Feinfeld RE, Hesse RJ, Scharfenberg JC: Orbital angiolipoma. Arch Ophthalmol 106:1093, 1988.
332. Bartley GB, Yeatts RP, Garrity JA, et al: Spindle cell lipoma of the orbit. Am J Ophthalmol 100:605, 1985.
333. Johnson BL, Linn JG: Spindle cell lipoma of the orbit. Arch Ophthalmol 97:133, 1979.
334. Chang HR, Hajdu SI, Collin C, et al: The prognostic value of histologic subtypes in primary extremity liposarcoma. Cancer 64:1514, 1989.
335. Miller MH, Yokoyama C, Wright JE, et al: An aggressive lipoblastic tumour in the orbit of a child. Histopathology 17:141, 1990.
336. Jakobiec FA, Rini F, Char D, et al: Primary liposarcoma of the orbit: Problems in the diagnosis and management of five cases. Ophthalmol 96:180, 1989.
337. Lane CM, Wright JE, Garner A: Primary myxoid liposarcoma of the orbit. Br J Ophthalmol 72:912, 1988.
338. Naeser P, Mostrom U: Liposarcoma of the orbit: A clinicopathological case report. Br J Ophthalmol 66:190, 1982.
339. Abdalla MI, Ghaly AF, Hosni F: Liposarcoma with orbital metastases: Case report. Br J Ophthalmol 50:426, 1966.
340. Bullock JD, Goldberg SH, Connelly PJ: Orbital varix thrombosis. Ophthalmology 97:251, 1990.
341. Grove AS: The dural shunt syndrome: Pathophysiology and clinical course. Ophthalmology 90:31, 1983.
342. Howard GM, Jakobiec FA, Michelsen WJ: Orbital arteriovenous malformation with secondary capillary angiomatosis treated by embolization with Silastic liquid. Ophthalmology 90:1136, 1983.
343. Font RL, Wheeler TM, Boniuk M: Intravascular papillary endothelial hyperplasia of the orbit and ocular adnexa. Arch Ophthalmol 101:1731, 1983.
344. Weber FL, Babel J: Intravascular papillary endothelial hyperplasia of the orbit. Br J Ophthalmol 65:18, 1981.
345. Sorenson RL, Spencer WH, Stewart WB, et al: Intravascular papillary endothelial hyperplasia of the eyelid. Arch Ophthalmol 101:1728, 1983.
346. Haik BG, Jakobiec FA, Ellsworth RM, et al: Capillary hemangioma of the lids and orbit: An analysis of the clinical features and therapeutic results in 101 cases. Ophthalmology 86:760, 1979.
347. Henderson JW, Farrow GM, Garrity JA: Clinical course of an incompletely removed cavernous hemangioma of the orbit. Ophthalmology 97:625, 1990.
348. Shields JA, Shields CL, Eagle RC: Cavernous hemangioma of the orbit. Arch Ophthalmol 105:853, 1987.
349. Ruchman MC, Flanagan J: Cavernous hemangiomas of the orbit. Ophthalmology 90:1328, 1983.
350. Harris GJ, Jakobiec FA: Cavernous hemangiomas of the orbit. J Neurosurg 51:219, 1979.
351. Iwamoto T, Jakobiec FA: Ultrastructural comparison of capillary and cavernous hemangiomas of the orbit. Arch Ophthalmol 97:1144, 1979.
352. Harris GJ, Sakol PJ, Bonavolonta G, et al: An analysis of thirty cases of orbital lymphangioma. Ophthalmology 97:1583, 1990.
353. Rootman J, Hay E, Graeb D, et al: Orbital-adnexal lymphangiomas: A spectrum of hemodynamically isolated vascular hamartomas. Ophthalmology 93:1558, 1986.
354. Iliff WJ, Green WR: Orbital lymphangiomas. Ophthalmology 86:914, 1979.
355. Reese AB, Howard GM: Unusual manifestations of ocular lymphangioma and lymphangiectasis. Surv Ophthalmol 18:226, 1973.
356. Jones IS: Lymphangiomas of the ocular adnexa: An analysis of 62 cases. Trans Am Ophthalmol Soc 57:642, 1959.
357. Boyle J, Kennedy C, Berry J, et al: Congenital haemangiopericytoma. J R Soc Med 78(Suppl 11):10, 1985.
358. Croxatto JO, Font RL: Hemangiopericytoma of the orbit: A clinicopathologic study of 30 cases. Hum Pathol 13:210, 1982.
359. Henderson JW, Farrow GM: Primary orbital hemangiopericytoma. Arch Ophthalmol 96:666, 1978.
360. Jakobiec FA, Howard GM, Jones IS, et al: Hemangiopericytoma of the orbit. Am J Ophthalmol 78:816, 1974.

361. D'Amore ESG, Manivel JC, Sung JH: Soft-tissue and meningeal hemangiopericytomas. Hum Pathol 21:414, 1990.
362. Nunnery EW, Kahn LB, Reddick RL, et al: Hemangiopericytoma: A light microscopic and ultrastructural study. Cancer 47:906, 1981.
363. Enzinger FM, Smith BH: Hemangiopericytoma: An analysis of 106 cases. Hum Pathol 7:61, 1976.
364. Rice CD, Kersten RC, Mrak RE: An orbital hemangiopericytoma recurrent after 33 years. Arch Ophthalmol 107:552, 1989.
365. Panda A, Dayal Y, Singhal V, et al: Haemangiopericytoma. Br J Ophthalmol 68:124, 1984.
366. Maddox JC, Evans HL: Angiosarcoma of skin and soft tissue: A study of forty-four cases. Cancer 48:1907, 1981.
367. Hufnagel T, Kuo T-T: Orbital angiosarcoma with subconjunctival presentation. Ophthalmology 94:72, 1987.
368. Messmer EP, Font RL, McCrary JA III, et al: Epithelioid angiosarcoma of the orbit presenting as Tolosa-Hunt syndrome. Ophthalmology 90:1414, 1983.
369. Lieberman PH, Brennan MF, Kimmel M, et al: Alveolar soft-part sarcoma: A clinicopathologic study of half a century. Cancer 63:1, 1989.
370. Font RL, Jurco S, Zimmerman LE: Alveolar soft-part sarcoma of the orbit. Hum Pathol 13:569, 1982.
371. Bunt AH, Bensinger RE: Alveolar soft-part sarcoma of the orbit. Ophthalmology 88:1339, 1981.
372. DeSchryver-Kecskemeti K, Kraus FT, Engleman W, et al: Alveolar soft-part sarcoma—A malignant angioreninoma. Am J Surg Pathol 6:5, 1982.
373. Mukai M, Torikata C, Iri H, et al: Alveolar soft-part sarcoma: A review on its histogenesis and further studies based on electron microscopy, immunohistochemistry and biochemistry. Am J Surg Pathol 7:679, 1983.
374. Miettinen M, Ekfors T: Alveolar soft part sarcoma: Immunohistochemical evidence for muscle cell differentiation. Am J Clin Pathol 93:32, 1990.
375. Coira BM, Sachdev R, Moscovic E: Skeletal muscle markers in alveolar soft part sarcoma. Am J Clin Pathol 94:799, 1990.
376. Ordonez NG, Ro JY, Mackay B: Alveolar soft part sarcoma: An ultrastructural and immunocytochemical investigation of its histogenesis. Cancer 63:1721, 1989.
377. Tsuneyoshi M, Daimaru Y, Hashimoto H, et al: Malignant soft tissue neoplasms with the histologic features of renal rhabdoid tumors. Hum Pathol 16:1235, 1985.
378. Rootman J, Damji KF, Dimmick JE: Malignant rhabdoid tumor of the orbit. Ophthalmology 96:1650, 1989.
379. Vogel AM, Gown AM, Caughlan J, et al: Rhabdoid tumors of the kidney contain mesenchymal specific and epithelial specific intermediate filament proteins. Lab Invest 50:232, 1984.
380. deMello DE, Archer CR, Blair JD: Ethmoidal fibro-osseous lesion in a child. Am J Surg Pathol 4:595, 1980.
381. Sanerkin NG, Mott MG, Roylance J: An unusual intraosseous lesion with fibroblastic, osteoclastic, osteoblastic, aneurysmal and fibromyxoid elements: "Solid" variant of aneurysmal bone cyst. Cancer 51:2278, 1983.
382. Mirra JM: Bone Tumors: Clinical, Radiologic and Pathologic Correlations. Philadelphia, Lea & Febiger, 1989.
383. Blodi FC: Pathology of orbital bones. Am J Ophthalmol 81:1, 1976.
384. Fu Y-S, Perzin KH: Non-epithelial tumors of the nasal cavity, paranasal sinuses and nasopharynx: A clinicopathologic study. Cancer 33:1289, 1974.
385. Small ML, Green R, Johnson LC: Lipoma of the frontal bone. Arch Ophthalmol 97:129, 1979.
386. Hornblass A, Zaidman GW: Intraosseous orbital cavernous hemangioma. Ophthalmology 88:1351, 1981.
387. Brackup AH, Haller ML, Danber MM: Hemangioma of the bony orbit. Am J Ophthalmol 90:258, 1980.
388. Friendly DS, Font RL, Milhorat TH: Hemangioendothelioma of frontal bone. Am J Ophthalmol 93:482, 1982.
389. Whitson WE, Orcutt JC, Walkinshaw MD: Orbital osteoma in Gardner's syndrome. Am J Ophthalmol 101:236, 1986.
390. Miller NR, Gray J, Snip R: Giant, mushroom-shaped osteoma of the orbit originating from the maxillary sinus. Am J Ophthalmol 83:587, 1977.
391. Moore AT, Buncic JR, Munro IR: Fibrous dysplasia of the orbit in childhood. Ophthalmology 92:12, 1985.
392. Moore RT: Fibrous dysplasia of the orbit. Surv Ophthalmol 13:321, 1969.
393. Yamaguchi K, Hayasaka S, Yamada T, et al: Orbitocranial fibrous dysplasia. Ophthalmologica 193:225, 1986.
394. Sevel D, James HE, Burns R, et al: McCune-Albright syndrome (fibrous dysplasia) associated with an orbital tumor. Ann Ophthalmol 16:283, 1984.
395. Liakos GM, Walker CB, Carruth JAS: Ocular complications in craniofacial fibrous dysplasia. Br J Ophthalmol 63:611, 1979.
396. Margo CE, Weiss A, Habal MB: Psammomatoid ossifying fibroma. Arch Ophthalmol 104:1347, 1986.
397. Margo CE, Ragsdale BD, Perman KI, et al: Psammomatoid (juvenile) ossifying fibroma of the orbit. Ophthalmology 92:150, 1985.
398. Shields JA, Peyster RG, Handler SD, et al: Massive juvenile ossifying fibroma of maxillary sinus with orbital involvement. Br J Ophthalmol 69:392, 1985.
399. Shields JA, Nelson LB, Brown JF, et al: Clinical, computed tomographic and histopathologic characteristics of juvenile ossifying fibroma with orbital involvement. Am J Ophthalmol 96:650, 1983.
400. Khalil MK, Leib ML: Cemento-ossifying fibroma of the orbit. Can J Ophthalmol 14:195, 1979.
401. Leone CR, Lawton AW, Leone RT: Benign osteoblastoma of the orbit. Ophthalmology 95:1554, 1988.
402. Lowder CY, Berlin AJ, Cox WA, et al: Benign osteoblastoma of the orbit. Ophthalmology 93:1351, 1986.
403. Sebag J, Chapman P, Truman J, et al: Giant cell granuloma of the orbit with intracranial extension. Neurosurgery 16:75, 1985.
404. Hoopes PC, Anderson RL, Blodi FC: Giant cell (reparative) granuloma of the orbit. Ophthalmology 88:1361, 1981.
405. Hirschl S, Katz A: Giant cell reparative granuloma outside the jaw bone. Hum Pathol 5:171, 1974.
406. Sood GC, Malik SRK, Gupta DK, et al: Reparative granuloma of the orbit causing unilateral proptosis. Am J Ophthalmol 63:524, 1967.
407. Parrish CM, O'Day DM: Brown tumor of the orbit. Arch Ophthalmol 104:1199, 1986.
408. Slem G, Varinli S, Koker F: Brown tumor of the orbit. Ann Ophthalmol 15:811, 1983.
409. Naiman J, Green WR, D'Heurle D, et al: Brown tumor of the orbit associated with primary hyperparathyroidism. Am J Ophthalmol 90:565, 1980.
410. Hunter JV, Yokoyama C, Moseley IF, et al: Aneurysmal bone cyst of the sphenoid with orbital involvement. Br J Ophthalmol 74:505, 1990.
411. Johnson TE, Bergin DJ, McCord CD: Aneurysmal bone cyst of the orbit. Ophthalmology 95:86, 1988.
412. Ronner HJ, Jones IS: Aneurysmal bone cyst of the orbit: A review. Ann Ophthalmol 15:626, 1983.
413. Iraci G, Giordano R, Fiore D, et al: Exophthalmos from aneurysmal bone cyst of the orbital roof. Childs Brain 6:206, 1980.
414. Roarty JD, McLean IW, Zimmerman LE: Incidence of second neoplasms in patients with bilateral retinoblastoma. Ophthalmology 95:1583, 1988.
415. Draper GJ, Sanders BM, Kingston JE: Second primary neoplasms in patients with retinoblastoma. Br J Cancer 53:661, 1986.
416. Abramson DH, Ellsworth RM, Kitchin FD, et al: Second nonocular tumors in retinoblastoma survivors: Are they radiation-induced? Ophthalmology 91:1351, 1984.
417. Abramson DH, Ronner HJ, Ellsworth RM: Second tumors in nonirradiated bilateral retinoblastoma. Am J Ophthalmol 87:624, 1979.
418. Dhir SP, Munjal VP, Jain IS, et al: Osteosarcoma of the orbit. J Pediatr Ophthalmol Strabismus 17:312, 1980.
419. Bone RC, Biller HF, Harris BL: Osteogenic sarcoma of the frontal sinus. Ann Otol 82:162, 1973.
420. Bennett JE, Tignor SP, Shafer WG: Osteogenic sarcoma of the facial bones. Am J Surg 116:538, 1968.
421. Fu Y-S, Perzin KH: Non-epithelial tumors of the nasal cavity, paranasal sinuses and nasopharynx: A clinicopathologic study. Cancer 34:453, 1974.
422. Swanson PE, Lillemoe TJ, Manivel JC, et al: Mesenchymal chondrosarcoma. Arch Pathol Lab Med 114:943, 1990.
423. Sevel D: Mesenchymal chondrosarcoma of the orbit. Br J Ophthalmol 58:882, 1974.

424. Guccion JG, Font RL, Enzinger FM, et al: Extraskeletal mesenchymal chondrosarcoma. Arch Pathol 95:336, 1973.
425. Cardenas-Ramirez L, Albores-Saavedra J, de Buen S: Mesenchymal chondrosarcoma of the orbit. Arch Ophthalmol 86:410, 1971.
426. Woodruff G, Thorner P, Skarf B: Primary Ewing's sarcoma of the orbit presenting with visual loss. Br J Ophthalmol 72:786, 1988.
427. Alvarez-Berdecia A, Schut L, Bruce DA: Localized primary intracranial Ewing's sarcoma of the orbital roof. J Neurosurg 50:811, 1979.
428. Beraud R, Fortin P: Sarcome d'Ewing a localisation temporale. Can Med Assoc J 97:338 1967.
429. Goldberg RA, Rootman J, Cline RA: Tumors metastatic to the orbit: A changing picture. Surv Ophthalmol 35:1, 1990.
430. Goldberg RA, Rootman J: Clinical characteristics of metastatic orbital tumors. Ophthalmology 97:620, 1990.
431. Freedman MI, Folk JC: Metastatic tumors to the eye and orbit. Arch Ophthalmol 105:1215, 1987.
432. Reifler DM: Orbital metastasis with enophthalmos. Henry Ford Hosp Med J 33:171, 1985.
433. Font RL, Ferry AP: Carcinoma metastatic to the eye and orbit. III: A clinicopathologic study of 28 cases metastatic to the orbit. Cancer 38:1326, 1976.
434. Ferry AP, Font RL: Carcinoma metastatic to the eye and orbit. I: A clinicopathologic study of 227 cases. Arch Ophthalmol 92:276, 1974.
435. Capone A Jr, Slamovits TL: Discrete metastasis of solid tumors to extraocular muscles. Arch Ophthalmol 108:237, 1990.
436. Weiss R, Grisold W, Jellinger K, et al: Metastasis of solid tumors in extraocular muscles. Acta Neuropathol 65:168, 1984.
437. Malviya VK, Blessed W, Lawrence WD, et al: Retroorbital metastases in ovarian cancer. Gynecol Oncol 35:120, 1989.
438. Ballinger WH, Wesley RE: Seminoma metastatic to the orbit. Ophthalmic Surg 15:120, 1984.
439. Rush JA, Older JJ, Richman AV: Testicular seminoma metastatic to the orbit. Am J Ophthalmol 91:258, 1981.
440. Reifler DM, Davison P: Histochemical analysis of breast carcinoma metastatic to the orbit. Ophthalmology 93:254, 1986.
441. Mottow-Lippa L, Jakobiec FA, Iwamoto T: Pseudoinflammatory metastatic breast carcinoma of the orbit and lids. Ophthalmology 88:575, 1981.
442. Bullock JD, Yanes B: Ophthalmic manifestations of metastatic breast cancer. Ophthalmology 87:961, 1980.
443. Hood CI, Font RL, Zimmerman LE: Metastatic mammary carcinoma in the eyelid with histiocytoid appearance. Cancer 31:793, 1973.
444. Whyte AM: Bronchogenic carcinoma metastasizing to the orbit. J Maxillofac Surg 6:277, 1978.
445. Ferry AP, Naghdi MR: Bronchogenic carcinoma metastatic to the orbit. Arch Ophthalmol 77:214, 1967.
446. Yeo JH, Jakobiec FA, Iwamoto T, et al: Metastatic carcinoma masquerading as scleritis. Ophthalmology 90:184, 1983.
447. Buys R, Abramson DH, Kitchin FD, et al: Simultaneous ocular and orbital involvement from metastatic bronchogenic carcinoma. Ann Ophthalmol 14:1165, 1982.
448. Seretan EL: Metastatic adenocarcinoma from the stomach to the orbit. Arch Ophthalmol 99:1469, 1981.
449. Sher JH, Weinstock SJ: Orbital metastasis of prostatic carcinoma. Can J Ophthalmol 18:248, 1983.
450. Winkler CF, Goodman GK, Eiferman RA, et al: Orbital metastasis from prostatic carcinoma: Identification by an immunoperoxidase technique. Arch Ophthalmol 99:1406, 1981.
451. Wolter JR, Hendrix RC: Osteoblastic prostate carcinoma metastatic to the orbit. Am J Ophthalmol 91:648, 1981.
452. Slamovits TL, Burde RM: Bumpy muscles. Surv Ophthalmol 33:189, 1988.
453. Kindermann WR, Shields JA, Eiferman RA, et al: Metastatic renal cell carcinoma to the eye and adnexae. Ophthalmology 88:1347, 1981.
454. Howard GM, Jakobiec FA, Trokel SL, et al: Pulsating metastatic tumor of the orbit. Am J Ophthalmol 85:767, 1978.
455. Ruusuvaara P, Setala K, Tarkkanen A: Orbital metastasis from cutaneous malignant melanoma. Acta Ophthalmol 67:325, 1989.
456. Orcutt JC, Char DH: Melanoma metastatic to the orbit. Ophthalmology 95:1033, 1988.
457. Font RL, Naumann G, Zimmerman LE: Primary malignant melanoma of the skin metastatic to the eye and orbit. Am J Ophthalmol 63:738, 1967.
458. Hornblass A, Kass LG, Reich R: Thyroid carcinoma metastatic to the orbit. Ophthalmology 94:1004, 1987.
459. Shetlar DJ, Font RL, Ordonez N, et al: A clinicopathologic study of three carcinoid tumors metastatic to the orbit: Immunohistochemical, ultrastructural and DNA flow cytometric studies. Ophthalmology 97:257, 1990.
460. Shields CL, Shields JA, Eagle RC, et al: Orbital metastasis from a carcinoid tumor: Computed tomography, magnetic resonance imaging and electron microscopic findings. Arch Ophthalmol 105:968, 1987.
461. Divine RD, Anderson RL, Ossoinig KC: Metastatic carcinoid unresponsive to radiation therapy presenting as a lacrimal fossa mass. Ophthalmology 89:516, 1982.
462. Musarella MA, Chan HSL, DeBoer G, et al: Ocular involvement in neuroblastoma: Prognostic implications. Ophthalmology 91:936, 1984.
463. Albert DM, Rubenstein RA, Scheie HG: Tumor metastasis to the eye. II: Clinical study in infants and children. Am J Ophthalmol 63:727, 1967.
464. Vanneste JAL: Subacute bilateral malignant exophthalmos due to orbital medulloblastoma metastases. Arch Neurol 40:441, 1983.
465. Fratkin JD, Purcell JJ, Krachmer JH, et al: Wilms' tumor metastatic to the orbit. JAMA 238:1841, 1977.
466. Apple DJ: Wilms' tumor metastatic to the orbit. Arch Ophthalmol 80:480, 1968.
467. Satorre J, Rootman J: Paraorbital sinus and nose neoplasms affecting the orbit and eyelids and their treatment. Curr Opin Ophthalmol 1:542, 1990.
468. Johnson LN, Krohel GB, Yeon EB, et al: Sinus tumors invading the orbit. Ophthalmology 91:209, 1984.
469. Bonavolonta G, Villari G, de Rosa G, et al: Ocular complications of juvenile angiofibroma. Ophthalmologica 181:334, 1980.
470. Amoaku WMK, Bagegni A, Logan WC, et al: Orbital infiltration by eyelid skin carcinoma. Int Ophthalmol 14:285, 1990.
471. Weimar VM, Ceilley RI: Basal-cell carcinoma of a medial canthus with invasion of supraorbital and supratrochlear nerves: Report of a case treated by Mohs' technique. J Dermatol Surg Oncol 5:279, 1979.
472. Csaky KG, Custer P: Perineural invasion of the orbit by squamous cell carcinoma. Ophthalmic Surg 21:218, 1990.
473. Doxanas MT, Iliff WJ, Iliff NT, et al: Squamous cell carcinoma of the eyelids. Ophthalmology 94:538, 1987.
474. Reifler DM, Hornblass A: Squamous cell carcinoma of the eyelid. Surv Ophthalmol 30:349, 1986.
475. Caya JG, Hidayat AA, Weiner JM: A clinicopathologic study of 21 cases of adenoid squamous cell carcinoma of the eyelid and periorbital region. Am J Ophthalmol 99:291, 1985.
476. Folberg R, Whitaker DC, Tse DT, et al: Recurrent and residual sebaceous carcinoma after Mohs' excision of the primary lesion. Am J Ophthalmol 103:817, 1987.
477. Rao NA, Hidayat AA, McLean IW, et al: Sebaceous carcinomas of the ocular adnexa. Hum Pathol 13:113, 1982.
478. Shields JA, Font RL: Meibomian gland carcinoma presenting as a lacrimal gland tumor. Arch Ophthalmol 92:304, 1974.
479. Khalil MK, Duguid WP: Neurotropic malignant melanoma of right temple with orbital metastasis: A clinicopathological case report. Br J Ophthalmol 71:41, 1987.
480. Shields JA, Elder D, Arbizo V, et al: Orbital involvement with desmoplastic melanoma. Br J Ophthalmol 71:279, 1987.
481. Wright JD, Font RL: Mucinous sweat gland adenocarcinoma of eyelid. Cancer 44:1757, 1979.
482. Holds JB, Haines JH, Mamalis N, et al: Mucinous adenocarcinoma of the orbit arising from a stable, benign-appearing eyelid nodule. Ophthalmic Surg 21:163, 1990.
483. Jakobiec FA, Austin P, Iwamoto T, et al: Primary infiltrating signet ring carcinoma of the eyelids. Ophthalmology 90:291, 1983.
484. Khalil M, Brownstein S, Codere F, et al: Eccrine sweat gland

carcinoma of the eyelid with orbital involvement. Arch Ophthalmol 98:2210, 1980.
485. Thomas JW, Fu YS, Levine MR: Primary mucinous sweat gland carcinoma of the eyelid simulating metastatic carcinoma. Am J Ophthalmol 87:29, 1979.
486. Grizzard WS, Torczynski E, Edwards WC: Adenocarcinoma of eccrine sweat glands. Arch Ophthalmol 94:2119, 1976.
487. Iliff WJ, Marback R, Green WR: Invasive squamous cell carcinoma of the conjunctiva. Arch Ophthalmol 93:119, 1975.
488. Rao NA, Font RL: Mucoepidermoid carcinoma of the conjunctiva. Cancer 38:1699, 1976.
489. Gonnering RS, Sonneland PR: Oncocytic carcinoma of the plica semilunaris with orbital extension. Ophthalmic Surg 18:604, 1987.
490. Folberg R, McLean IW, Zimmerman LE: Malignant melanoma of the conjunctiva. Hum Pathol 16:136, 1985.
491. Shields CL, Shields JA, Yarian DL, et al: Intracranial extension of choroidal melanoma via the optic nerve. Br J Ophthalmol 71:172, 1987.
492. Zimmerman LE: Malignant melanoma of the uveal tract. *In* Spencer WH (ed): Ophthalmic Pathology, vol. 3. Philadelphia, WB Saunders, 1986.
493. Kersten RC, Tse DT, Anderson RL, et al: The role of orbital extenteration in choroidal melanoma with extrascleral extension. Ophthalmology 92:436, 1985.
494. Rootman J, Carruthers JDA, Miller RR: Retinoblastoma. Perspect Pediatr Pathol 10:208, 1987.
495. Stannard C, Lipper S, Sealy R, et al: Retinoblastoma: Correlation of invasion of the optic nerve and choroid with prognosis and metastases. Br J Ophthalmol 63:560, 1979.
496. Rootman J, Ellsworth RM, Hofbauer J, et al: Orbital extension of retinoblastoma: A clinicopathological study. Can J Ophthalmol 13:72, 1978.
497. Rootman J, Hofbauer J, Ellsworth RM, et al: Invasion of the optic nerve by retinoblastoma: A clinicopathological study. Can J Ophthalmol 11:106, 1976.
498. Broughton WL, Zimmerman LE: A clinicopathologic study of 56 cases of intraocular medulloepitheliomas. Am J Ophthalmol 85:407, 1978.
499. Grossniklaus HE, Zimmerman LE, Kachmer ML: Pleomorphic adenocarcinoma of the ciliary body. Ophthalmology 97:763, 1990.
500. Marquardt MD, Zimmerman LE: Histopathology of meningiomas and gliomas of the optic nerve. Hum Pathol 13:226, 1982.
501. Font RL, Croxatto JO: Intracellular inclusions in meningothelial meningioma. J Neuropathol Exp Neurol 39:575, 1980.
502. Ferry AP, Haddad HM, Goldman JL: Orbital invasion by an intracranial chordoma. Am J Ophthalmol 92:7, 1981.
503. Ryan SJ, Font RL: Primary epithelial neoplasms of the lacrimal sac. Am J Ophthalmol 76:73, 1973.
504. Lloyd WC III, Leone CR Jr: Malignant melanoma of the lacrimal sac. Arch Ophthalmol 102:104, 1984.
505. Carnevali L, Trimarchi F, Rosso R, et al: Haemangiopericytoma of the lacrimal sac: A case report. Br J Ophthalmol 72:782, 1988.
506. Baghdassarian SA, Zakharia H, Asdourian KK: Report of a case of bilateral caseous tuberculous dacryoadenitis. Am J Ophthalmol 74:744, 1972.
507. Baker RH, Bartley GB: Lacrimal gland ductule stones. Ophthalmology 97:531, 1990.
508. Damato BE, Allan D, Murray SB, et al: Senile atrophy of the human lacrimal gland: The contribution of chronic inflammatory disease. Br J Ophthalmol 68:674, 1984.
509. Amemiya T, Mori H, Koizumi K: Clinical and histocytopathological study of chronic dacryoadenitis. Graefes Arch Clin Exp Ophthalmol 220:229, 1983.
510. Jabs DA, Johns CJ: Ocular involvement in chronic sarcoidosis. Am J Ophthalmol 102:297, 1986.
511. Weinreb RN: Diagnosing sarcoidosis by transconjunctival biopsy of the lacrimal gland. Am J Ophthalmol 97:573, 1984.
512. Obenauf CD, Shaw HE, Sydnor CF, et al: Sarcoidosis and its ophthalmic manifestations. Am J Ophthalmol 86:648, 1978.
513. Siltzbach LE, James DG, Neville E et al: Course and prognosis of sarcoidosis around the world. Am J Med 57:847, 1974.
514. Collison JMT, Miller NR, Green WR: Involvement of orbital tissues by sarcoid. Am J Ophthalmol 102:302, 1986.
515. Stannard K, Spalton DJ: Sarcoidosis with infiltration of the external ocular muscles. Br J Ophthalmol 69:562, 1985.
516. Karcioglu ZA, Brear R: Conjunctival biopsy in sarcoidosis. Am J Ophthalmol 99:68, 1985.
517. Nichols CW, Eagle RC, Yanoff M, et al: Conjunctival biopsy as an aid in the evaluation of the patient with suspected sarcoidosis. Ophthalmology 87:287, 1980.
518. Rosai J: Ackerman's Surgical Pathology, 6th ed, vol. 2. St. Louis, CV Mosby, 1981.
519. van Maarsseven ACMTH, Mullink H, Alons CL, et al: Distribution of T-lymphocyte subsets in different portions of sarcoid granulomas: Immunohistologic analysis with monoclonal antibodies. Hum Pathol 17:493, 1986.
520. Viale G, Codecasa L, Bulgheroni P, et al: T-cell subsets in sarcoidosis. Hum Pathol 17:476, 1986.
521. Font RL, Yanoff M, Zimmerman LE: Benign lymphoepithelial lesion of the lacrimal gland and its relationship to Sjogren's syndrome. Am J Clin Pathol 48:365, 1967.
522. Pepose JS, Akata RF, Pflugfelder SC, et al: Mononuclear cell phenotypes and immunoglobulin gene rearrangements in lacrimal gland biopsies from patients with Sjogren's syndrome. Ophthalmology 97:1599, 1990.
523. McCurley TL, Collins RD, Ball E, et al: Nodal and extranodal lymphoproliferative disorders in Sjogren's syndrome. Hum Pathol 21:482, 1990.
524. Fishleder A, Tubbs R, Hesse B, et al: Uniform detection of immunoglobulin-gene rearrangement in benign lymphoepithelial lesions. N Engl J Med 316:1118, 1987.
525. Shields CL, Shields JA, Eagle RC, et al: Clinicopathologic review of 142 cases of lacrimal gland lesions. Ophthalmology 96:431, 1989.
526. Jakobiec FA, Yeo JH, Trokel SL, et al: Combined clinical and computed tomographic diagnosis of primary lacrimal fossa lesions. Am J Ophthalmol 94:785, 1982.
527. Wright JE: Factors affecting the survival of patients with lacrimal gland tumours. Can J Ophthalmol 17:3, 1982.
528. Ni C, Cheng SC, Dryja TP, et al: Lacrimal gland tumors: A clinicopathological analysis of 160 cases. Int Ophthalmol Clin 22:99, 1981.
529. Perzin KH, Jakobiec FA, Livolsi VA, et al: Lacrimal gland malignant mixed tumors (carcinomas arising in benign mixed tumors). Cancer 45:2593, 1980.
530. Biggs SL, Font RL: Oncocytic lesions of the caruncle and other ocular adnexa. Arch Ophthalmol 95:474, 1977.
531. Parks SL, Glover AT: Benign mixed tumors arising in the palpebral lobe of the lacrimal gland. Ophthalmology 97:526, 1990.
532. Auran J, Jakobiec FA, Krebs W: Benign mixed tumor of the palpebral lobe of the lacrimal gland. Ophthalmology 95:90, 1988.
533. Iwamoto T, Jakobiec FA: A comparative ultrastructural study of the normal lacrimal gland and its epithelial tumors. Hum Pathol 13:236, 1982.
534. Dardick I, van Nostrand AWP, Jeans MTD, et al: Pleomorphic adenoma. I: Ultrastructural organization of "epithelial" regions. II: Ultrastructural organization of "stromal" regions. Hum Pathol 14:780, 1983.
535. Dagher G, Anderson RL, Ossoinig KC, et al: Adenoid cystic carcinoma of the lacrimal gland in a child. Arch Ophthalmol 98:1098, 1980.
536. Malberger E, Gdal-On M: Adenoid cystic carcinoma of the orbit diagnosed by means of aspirative cytology. Ophthalmologica 190:125, 1985.
537. Gamel JW, Font RL: Adenoid cystic carcinoma of the lacrimal gland: The clinical significance of a basaloid histologic pattern. Hum Pathol 13:219, 1982.
538. Lee DA, Campbell RJ, Waller RR, et al: A clinicopathologic study of primary adenoid cystic carcinoma of the lacrimal gland. Ophthalmology 92:128, 1985.
539. Henderson JW, Farrow GM: Primary malignant mixed tumors of the lacrimal gland. Ophthalmology 87:466, 1980.
540. Witschel H, Zimmerman LE: Malignant mixed tumor of the lacrimal gland. Graefes Arch Clin Ophthalmol 216:327, 1981.

541. Konrad EA, Thiel H-J: Adenocarcinoma of the lacrimal gland with sebaceous differentiation. Graefes Arch Clin Exp Ophthalmol 221:81, 1983.
542. Ludwig ME, LiVolsi VA, McMahon RT: Malignant mixed tumor of the lacrimal gland. Am J Surg Pathol 3:457, 1979.
543. Font RL, Patipa M, Rosenbaum PS, et al: Correlation of computed tomographic and histopathologic features in malignant transformation of benign mixed tumor of lacrimal gland. Surv Ophthalmol 34:449, 1990.
544. Wagoner MD, Chuo N, Gonder JR, et al: Mucoepidermoid carcinoma of the lacrimal gland. Ann Ophthalmol 14:383, 1982.
545. De Rosa G, Zeppa P, Tranfa F, et al: Acinic cell carcinoma arising in a lacrimal gland: First case report. Cancer 57:1988 1986.
546. Evans HL: Mucoepidermoid carcinoma of salivary glands: A study of 69 cases with special attention to histologic grading. Am J Clin Pathol 81:696, 1984.

Chapter 188

Pathology of the Optic Nerve

DAVID G. COGAN

DEGENERATION AND ATROPHY

The optic nerve reacts in a stereotypical manner: designated *degeneration* during the active stage and *atrophy* in the end-result. The primary events are loss of axons and of their myelin sheaths, whereas the secondary events are reactive infiltration and gliosis. The histopathologic manifestations vary according to the acuteness or chronicity of the process.

Acute processes of whatever cause show replacement of the myelin by masses of foamy and free-floating macrophages, called "gitter" cells, loaded with neutral fat and cholesterol. Such acute reactions occur with infarction, injuries, and poisons of the optic nerve (Figs. 188–1 and 188–2).

Less acute processes incite a similar but less intense reaction with replacement of the myelin by glia (Fig. 188–3). As the masses of macrophages disappear, lacunas may be left in the optic nerve. These lacunas may appear anywhere along the optic nerve and are nonspecific.[1] Those in front of and behind the lamina cribrosa have been most extensively documented (see Fig. 188–1). Classically associated with glaucomatous optic atrophy, they are collectively known as Schnabel's cavernous atrophy.[2] The "spaces" are of course not empty. They are often filled with hyaluronic acid, staining with Alcian blue or colloidal iron, and are hyaluronidase sensitive, leading some authorities to interpret them as originating in vitreous.[3]

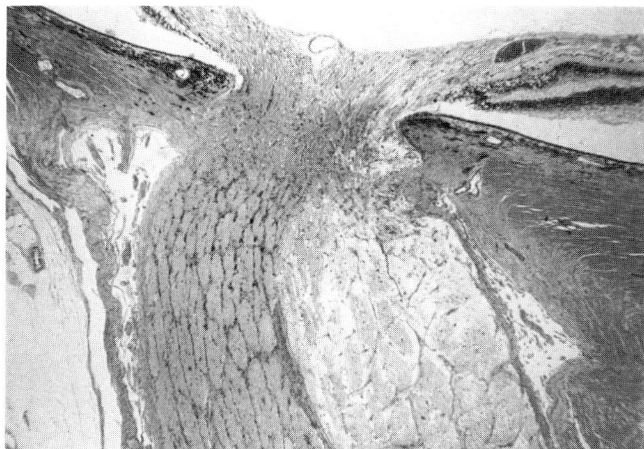

Figure 188–1. Acute degeneration. Right half of the nerve shows severe loss of myelinated tracts and partial destruction of the trabecular framework, which resulted from vascular occlusion of posterior ciliary arteries. This portion of the nerve, in comparison with the intact portion on the left, is somewhat swollen. H&E, ×30.

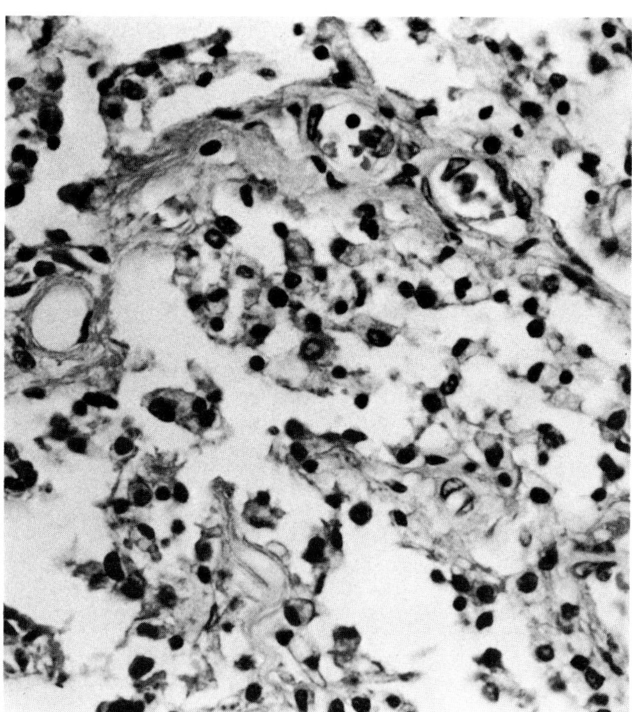

Figure 188–2. Free-floating, fat-laden cells ("gitter cells") in the optic nerve 25 days after ingestion of a fatal dose of methyl alcohol. H&E, ×300.

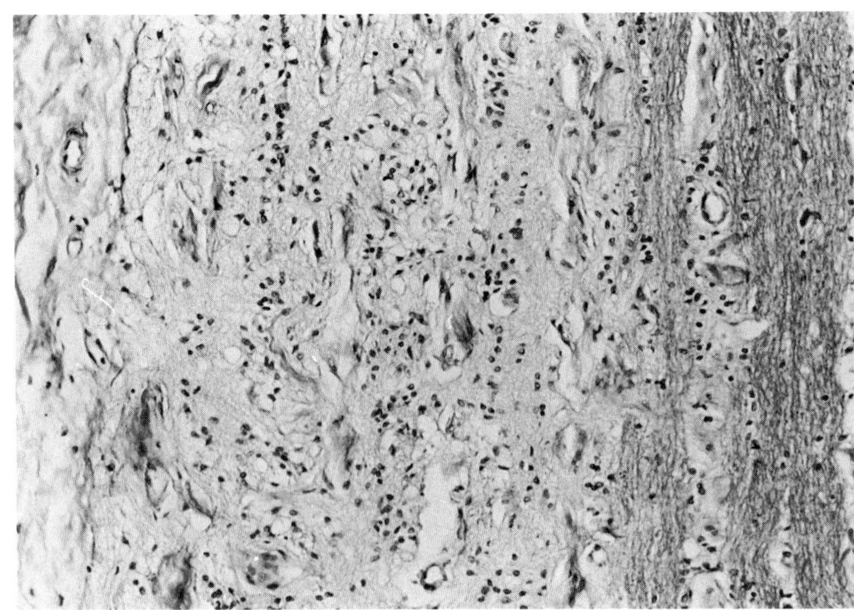

Figure 188–3. Atrophic optic neuropathy after chronic papilledema. The bulk of the nerve is replaced by glial fibers. Residual nerve fibers are evident on the right side of the photograph. Bodian, ×75.

Chronic lesions of the optic nerve, such as those induced by progressive compression of the optic nerve or gradual disappearance of the retinal ganglion cells, show little or no lipid phagocytosis. Instead, there is simply collapse of the optic nerve framework and disorderly arrangement of glial cells (see Fig. 188–3). Electron microscopy shows variable degeneration of the myelinated nerve fibers (Fig. 188–4).

Comparison of degenerative changes in the optic nerve and retina offers a unique opportunity to contrast white matter versus gray matter reactivity. Nowhere else in the nervous system are the two so neatly separate. In the case of infarcts, for instance, the brisk macrophage reaction in the optic nerve and the brain contrasts with that found in the retina, which is practically devoid of reactivity. The contrast of myelin in the nerve and its absence in the retina is responsible for the difference.

PAPILLEDEMA

Papilledema connotes a swollen disc. This is classically associated with increased intracranial pressure. It leads to distention of the meningeal spaces about the nerve (Fig. 188–5) and, in the presence of a firm dura mater, a squeeze on the nerve itself. The back-up pressure results in leakage of serum into the nerve head and congestion of axoplasmic flow anterior to the lamina cribrosa. The swollen nerve head protrudes into the vitreous anteriorly and presses against the retina laterally, presenting a characteristic S-shaped configuration and, often, concentric folds of the outer retinal layers (Fig. 188–6). The angulated, marginal fibers are likely to become necrotic, thus accounting for the bizarre field defects that commonly accompany papilledema. Electron microscopy reveals an accumulation of mitochon-

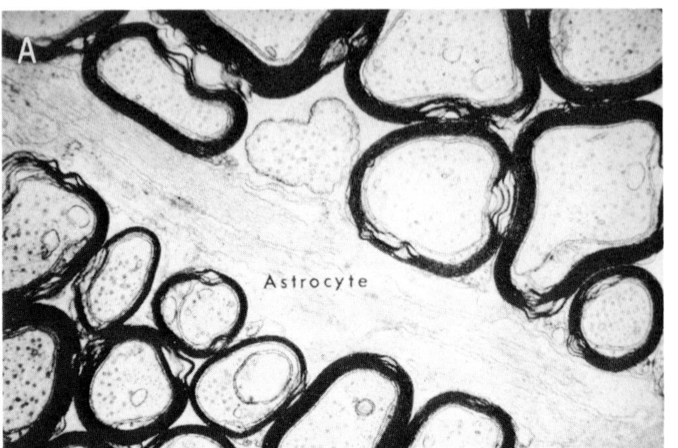

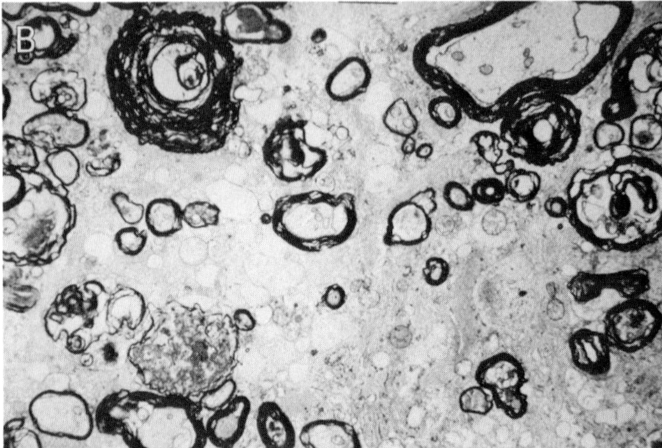

Figure 188–4. *A,* Electron micrograph of normal optic nerve fibers surrounded by myelin sheaths. A single nonmyelinated fiber is present above center. Groups of nerve fibers are separated by astrocytes. ×25,000. *B,* Electron micrograph of degenerating nerve fibers (myelinolysis). ×15,000. (*A* and *B,* Courtesy of T. Kuwabara.)

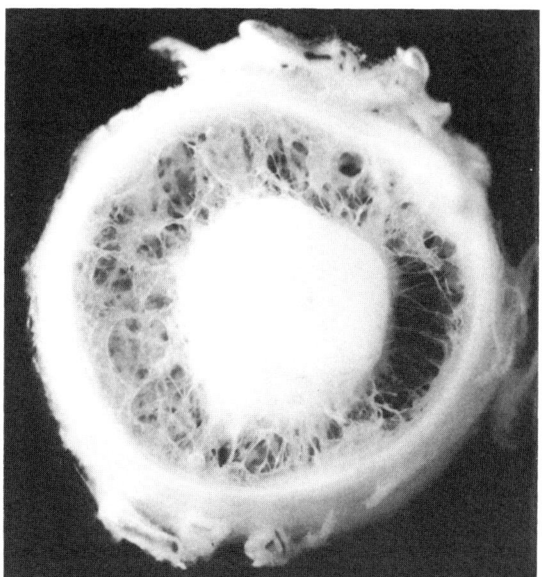

Figure 188–5. Dilatation of the subarachnoid spaces and optic atrophy in a hydrocephalic infant. × 18.

dria and axoplasmic particles in various stages of disintegration (Fig. 188–7).

DRUSEN

Drusen of the optic nerve are hyaline, often calcareous, bodies of various sizes, situated in the prelaminar or nonmyelinated portion of the nerve head. Both eyes are usually affected. Except for an infrequent association with retinitis pigmentosa and a similarity to "mulberry" bodies with tuberous sclerosis, drusen are not known to be associated with other systemic or local conditions. Occasionally, they occur as a dominantly inherited trait. Their pathogenesis is unclear. They have no relationship to drusen of Bruch's membrane, which unfortunately bear the same name.

Large drusen of the nerve head have a characteristic ophthalmoscopic appearance (Fig. 188–8). They appear as translucent, globular bodies protruding from the disc and obscuring its margins. Small drusen embedded in the nerve substance, on the other hand, may present only a subtle elevation of the disc simulating papilledema. Drusen are especially prevalent with small discs and characteristically obscure the physiologic cup. Unless sufficiently large or situated so as to encroach on the vessels, they cause no symptoms. Serious sequelae may result, however, from secondary venous obstruction with consequent papilloretinal hemorrhages, or they may cause optic atrophy through pressure on the adjacent nerve fibers. Fortunately neither occurrence is frequent, and most drusen are discovered fortuitously in asymptomatic patients.

Histopathologically, drusen of the nerve head are laminated, acellular bodies situated exclusively in the prelaminar or nonmyelinated portions of the nerve (Fig. 188–9). Their basophilia varies with the degree of calcification. Just what tissue element gives rise to their formation is unclear, but once formed they continue to enlarge. The lamination suggests that growth occurs by slow accretion. Initially the nerve fibers are simply pushed aside rather than replaced. Rarely are they sufficiently large to occupy the entire nerve head or to cause blindness.

CUPPING

Prolonged pressure within the eye (glaucoma) results in backward bowing of the lamina cribrosa. The vessels are pushed to the nasal side, and the nerve fibers appear to be impaled on the rigid scleral margin (Fig. 188–10).

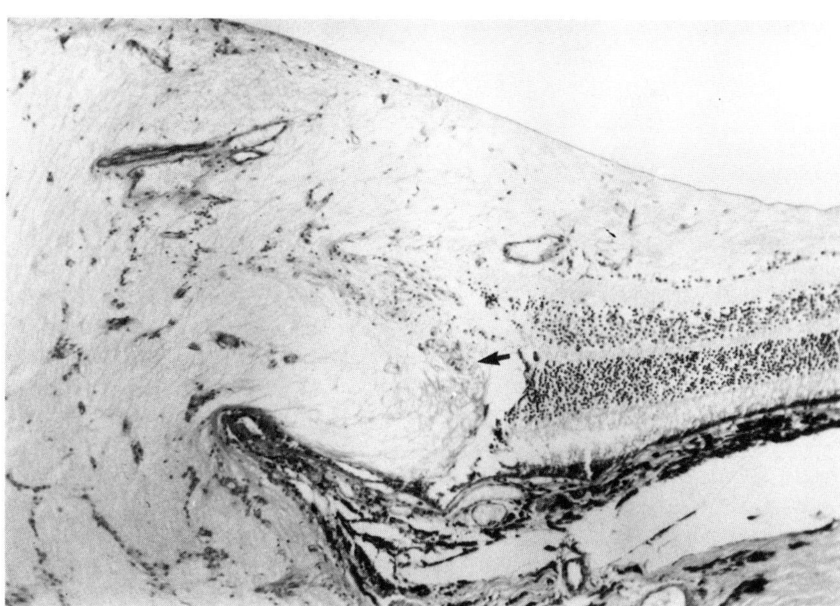

Figure 188–6. Nerve head in papilledema revealing an S-shaped protrusion of the nerve fibers against adjacent retina. A small focus of necrosis *(arrow)* is present at the top of the angulated fibers. H&E, × 200.

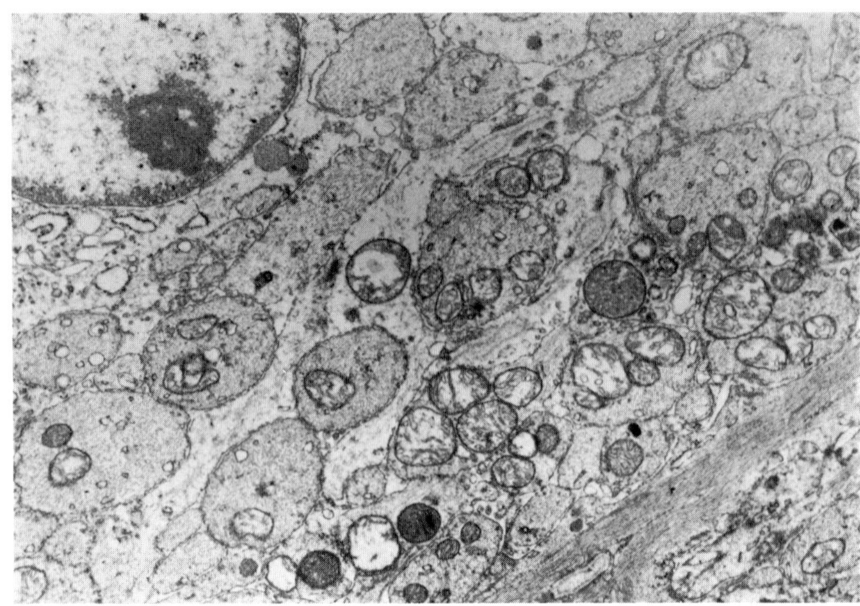

Figure 188–7. Electron micrograph of nerve fibers on the nerve head in papilledema. Note the swollen and partially disintegrating fibers, mitochondria, and other organelles. The nucleus of an astrocyte is present in the upper left corner. ×12,000.

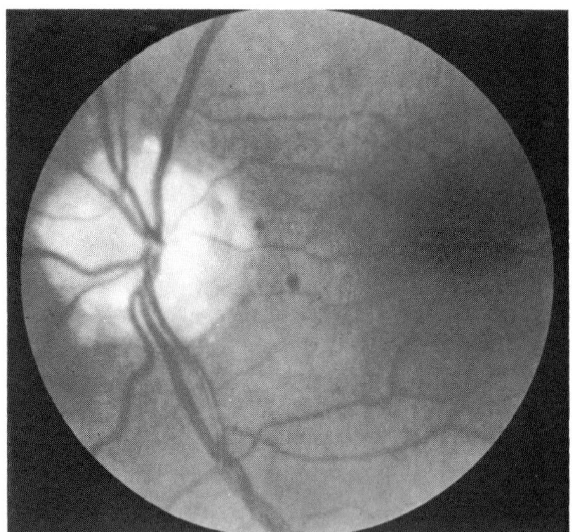

Figure 188–8. Ophthalmoscopic appearance of drusen-forming nodules in the nerve substance. They are especially evident at the margins of the disc.

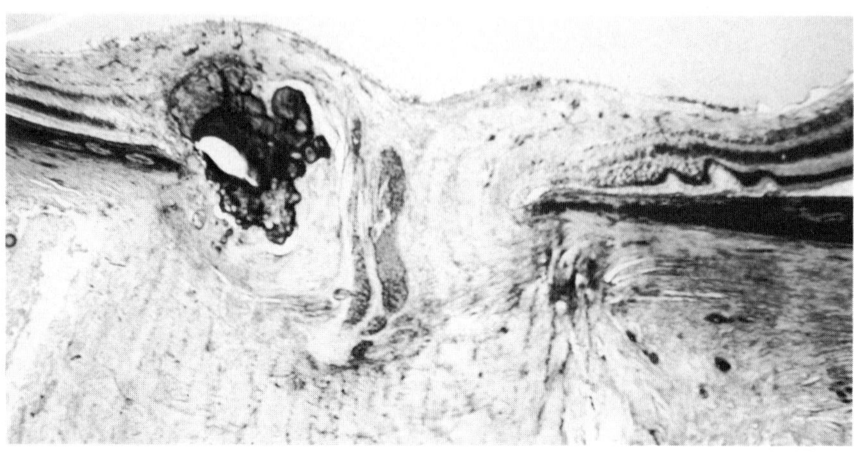

Figure 188–9. Large drusen on nasal half of nerve head. The conspicuous basophilia indicates a degree of calcification. Note a threatened compression of the adjacent vessels. H&E, ×50.

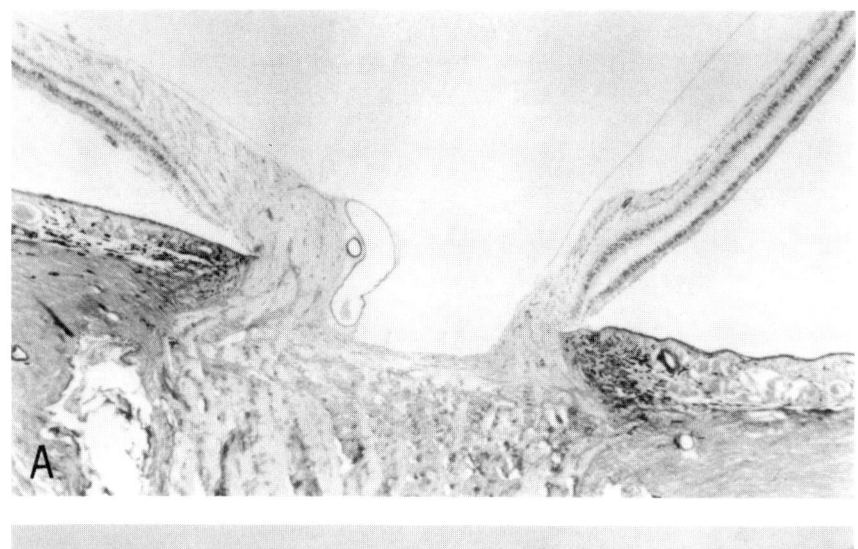

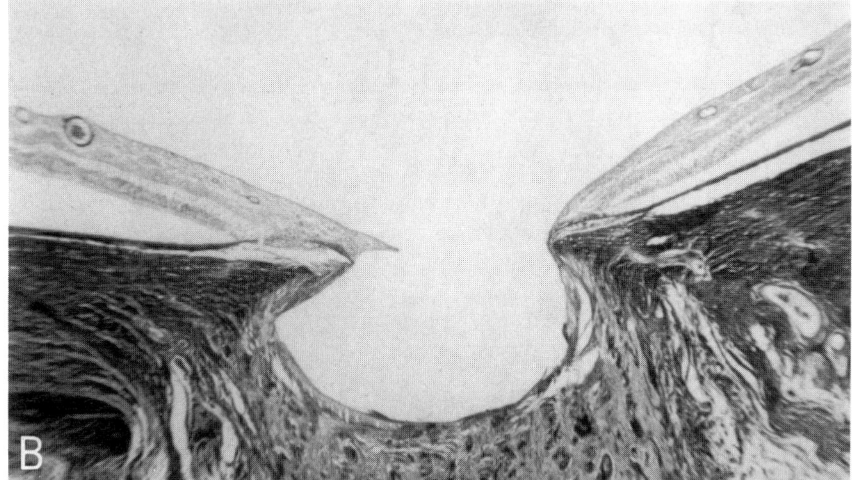

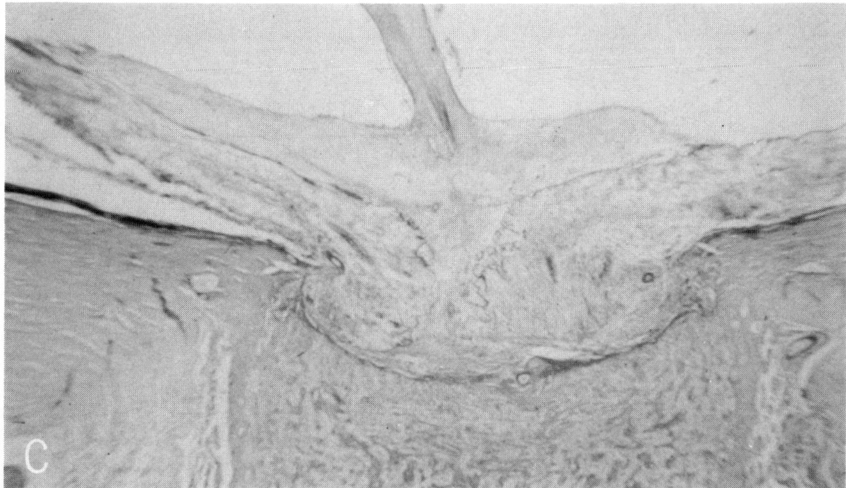

Figure 188–10. Cupping on nerve head. *A,* Cupping confined to temporal half of disc. Note the attenuation of nerve fibers on this side. H&E, ×45. *B,* Total excavation of disc with complete disappearance of nerve fibers at the disc margins. Mallory trichrome, ×40. *C,* Cup filled with retinal and glial tissue. H&E, ×55.

Occasionally, retinal tissue is pulled into the cup or, alternatively, glial tissue fills the cup. Secondary venous occlusion is a frequent eventuality and presents a problem to the pathologist in deciding whether the glaucoma was the result or the cause of the vascular obstruction.

In contrast to the sharply angulated and frequently deep glaucomatous cup, a shelving excavation occurs with optic atrophy due simply to loss of nerve fibers. In contrast to the glaucomatous cup, there is little or no displacement of vessels.

At times, cupping may occur in a normotensive eye. Called low-tension glaucoma, its pathogenesis is obscure. Unconfirmed suppositions postulate an inherently weak lamina cribrosa or insufficient vascular supply.

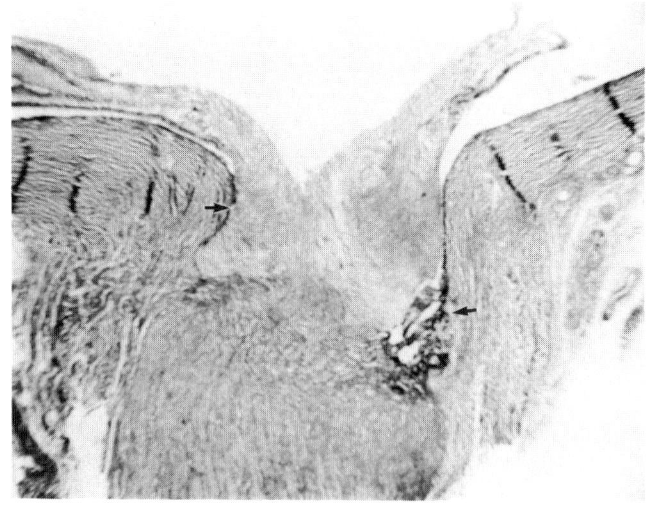

Figure 188–12. Congenital excavation of the disc ("morning-glory" anomaly). The scleral foramen is approximately twice the normal size and is marginated by posterior extension of the pigment epithelium *(arrows)*. H&E, ×30.

CONGENITAL ANOMALIES

Minor congenital anomalies include persistence of the hyaloid system on the disc, vascular loops projecting from the disc, myelination of the nerve fibers extending into the retina, and pigmentation of the disc. With persistence of hyaloid remnants, a vessel may extend forward to the lens and be associated with a retrolenticular, fibrous plaque or may be limited to a gliovascular bud off the disc (Bergmeister's papilla). Myelination of the nerve fibers in the retina is a relatively frequent anomaly in which ophthalmoscopically visible white patches extend from the disc to a variable distance along the paths of retinal nerve fibers. Vascular loops and pigmentation of the disc are curiosities with no recognized clinical or pathologic significance.

Major anomalies of the optic nerve include hypoplasia; colobomatous defects in closure of the embryonic fissure; primary defects in formation of the optic disc; and pits of the nerve head. Optic nerve hypoplasia is simply a small disc with or without visual symptoms (Fig. 188–11). It may be accompanied by radiologic evidence of defects in the septum pellucidum and other midline intracranial structures (De Morsier's syndrome[4, 5]). Colobomatous defects result from failure in closure of the embryonic fissure. Retinal tissue may extend into the fissure, forming a retrobulbar, cystic outpouching from the optic nerve. Occasionally this cystic formation may become larger than the eye and may be the presenting clinical sign. A variant of this colobomatous defect is simply an enlarged optic foramen, the "morning glory" sign[6, 7] in which pigment epithelium and retinal tissue extend deeply into the excavation (Fig. 188–12). Pits of the nerve head are isolated defects of the lamina cribrosa in which the retinal nerve fibers make a loop either into the optic nerve or into the marginal arachnoid space.

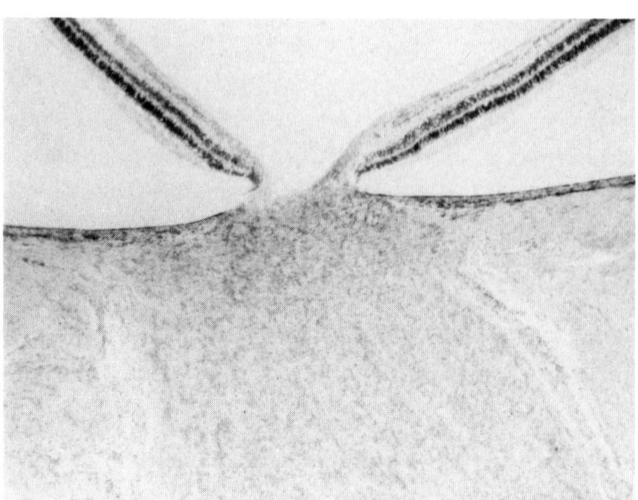

Figure 188–11. Hypoplasia of the nerve head in an infant with multiple congenital anomalies. The disc was estimated to be half the normal diameter. H&E, ×40.

VASCULAR OPTIC NEUROPATHY

Prelaminar vascular optic neuropathy resulting from retinal artery occlusion causes an ischemic collapse of the capillaries in the nerve fiber layer of the nerve head. It is best visualized in retinal digest preparations. The ophthalmoscopic counterpart is pallor of the disc. It is associated with either primary or secondary loss of the ganglion cells in the retina.

Paralaminar and retrolaminar vascular disease results from occlusion or impaired circulation of the posterior ciliary and adjacent choroidal vessels (Fig. 188–13). The ocular manifestation is anterior ischemic optic neuropathy resulting, usually, from atherosclerosis or giant cell arteritis. Anatomically small discs and absence of physiologic cups may be predisposing factors for *nonarteritic* vascular occlusion.[9] The clinical counterpart of anterior ischemic optic neuropathy is swelling of the nerve head with complete or partial blindness.

In the case of *arteritic* neuropathy, the clinical diagnosis is usually confirmed by finding characteristic granulomatous changes in temporal artery biopsies, whence

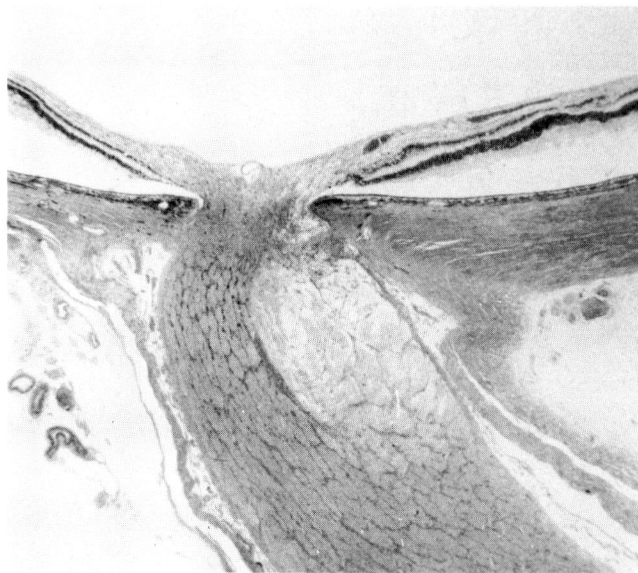

Figure 188–13. Area of necrosis on right side of nerve, which resulted from vascular occlusion of the posterior ciliary arteries. Of note is the localized infarct extending approximately 2 mm behind the lamina cribrosa. This photograph shows the extent of the lesion in a lower magnification of the lesion pictured in Figure 188–1. It represents incipient Schnabel's cavernous atrophy. H&E, ×15.

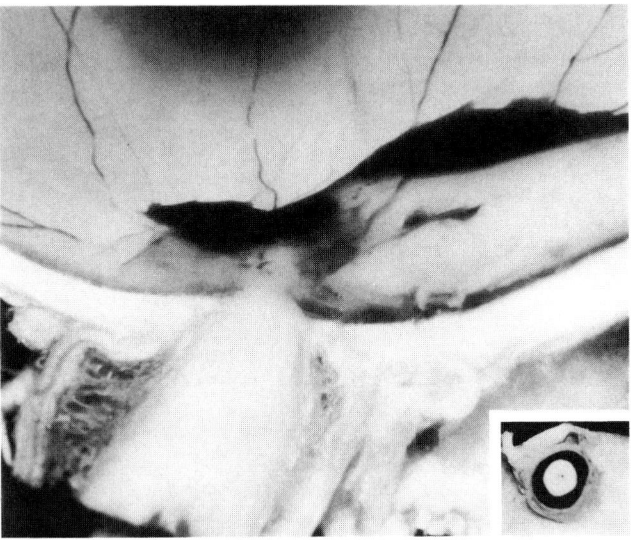

Figure 188–15. Hemorrhage in the subarachnoid space about the optic nerve and in the epipapillary region nerve. The patient had died a few days after rupture of an intracranial aneurysm. Insert shows a cross section of the optic nerve surrounded by blood in the subarachnoid space from another but similar case. Unstained, ×7.

the name temporal arteritis. The histopathologic abnormality consists of fragmentation of elastica, granulomatous infiltration of the vessel wall, and nodular necrosis of the muscularis (Fig. 188–14). Fresh cases also show lipoidal myelinolysis of the optic nerve fibers, whereas late cases show simple collapse of the atrophic nerves

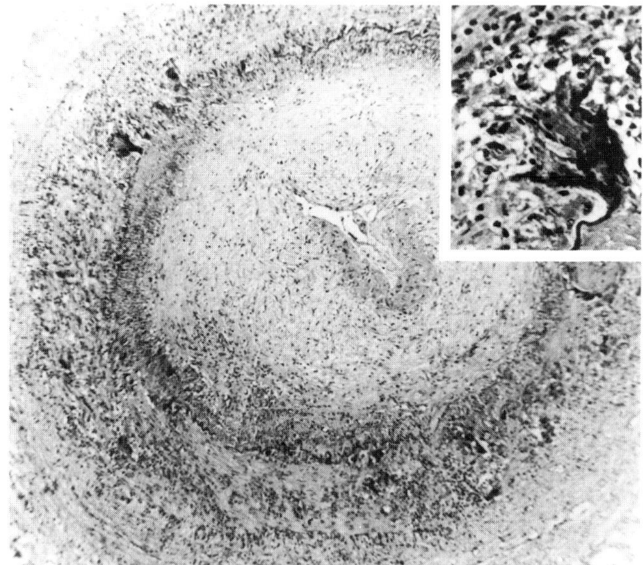

Figure 188–14. Cross section of temporal artery in a case of temporal arteritis. Of note are the massive thickening of the intima, infiltration of the muscularis, fragmentation of the elastica, and multinucleated giant cells. PAS, ×50. Insert shows the fragmentation and associated giant cell reaction. ×300.

and cavitation of the nerve (Schnabel's cavernous optic atrophy[2]).

Posterior ischemic optic neuropathy often masquerades clinically under the erroneous diagnosis of "optic neuritis." Its histopathology has been rarely documented. Lacunar vacuolation may be one of the manifestations.

Hemorrhage into the meningeal sheaths surrounding the optic nerve may be included under the heading of vascular optic neuropathies. The predominant cause is subarachnoid hemorrhage from ruptures of intracranial aneurysms, wherein blood extends from the brain into the meninges about the optic nerve. It is accompanied by swelling and hemorrhage on the nerve head and surrounding retina (Fig. 188–15). Yet it is by no means clear how the blood gets from the optic nerve sheaths into the eye. Rarely is blood found within the nerve itself.

INFLAMMATION

Being in line with the posterior drainage path out of the eye, the optic nerve participates nonspecifically in any intraocular inflammation. On the other hand, several inflammatory diseases are especially likely to affect the optic nerves (Fig. 188–16). These include herpes simplex,[10] Behçet's disease,[11] and sarcoid.[12, 13] Indeed sarcoid of the optic nerve may be the initial manifestation of the systemic disease and then easily confused with a neoplasm.[14] Of the fungal infections, cryptococcosis is especially noteworthy because of its affinity for neural tissue, while inciting surprisingly little reactivity in the optic nerve.

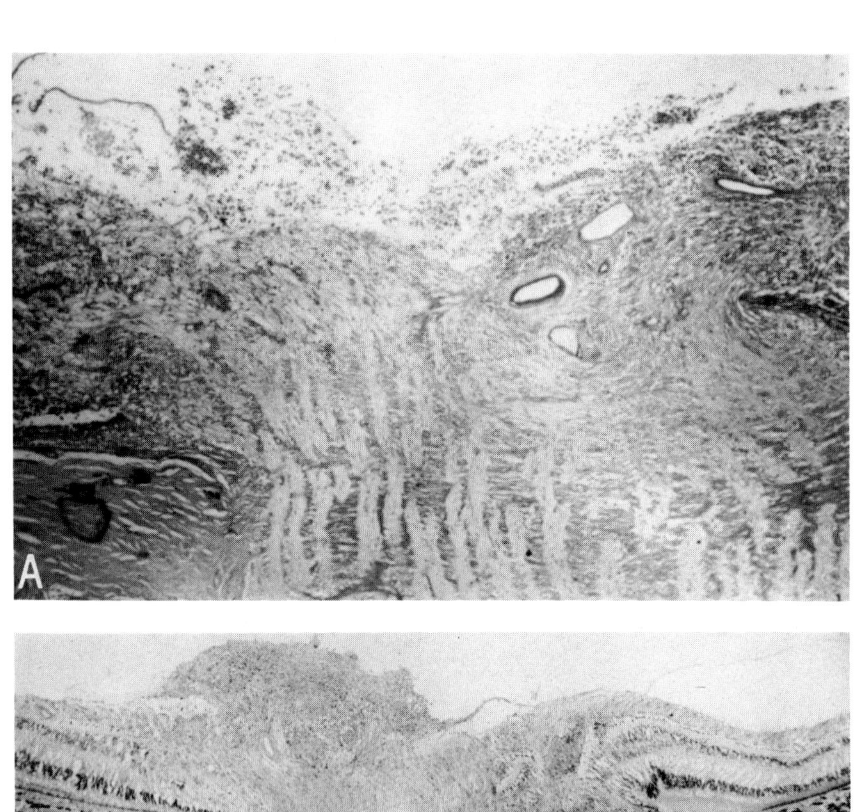

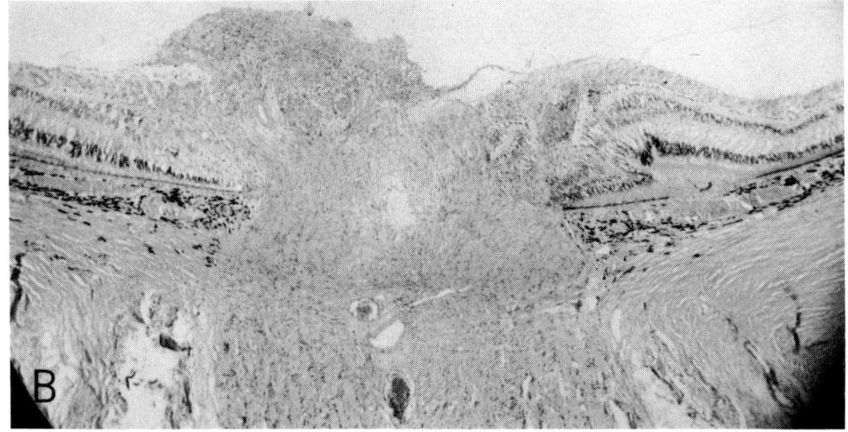

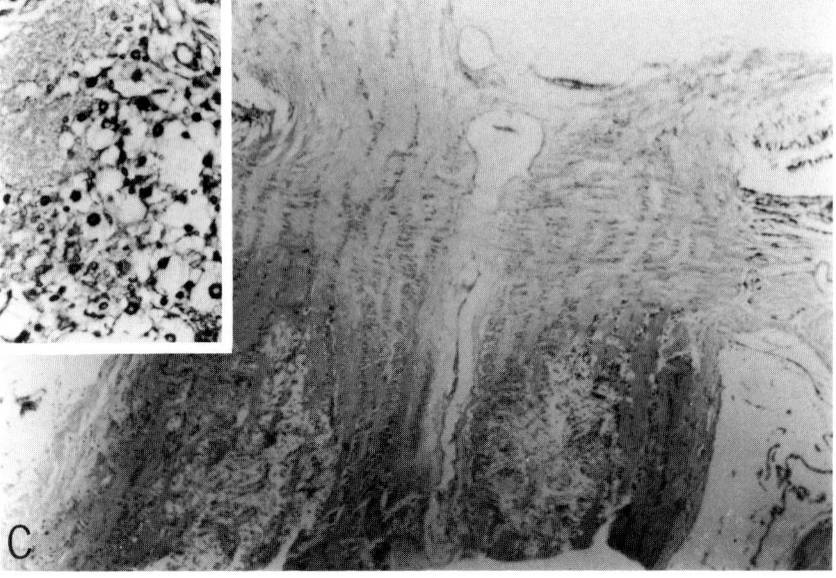

Figure 188–16. Inflammation of nerve head. *A,* Inflammatory cells and debris overlying nerve head in a patient with Behçet's disease. H&E, ×70. *B,* Sarcoid granuloma in and overlying nerve head. H&E, ×40. *C,* Coccidioidomycosis with necrotic foci behind lamina cribrosa. H&E, ×70. Inset shows the yeast in the necrotic areas. Alcian blue, ×300.

HEREDITARY, METABOLIC, AND DEMYELINATIVE OPTIC NEUROPATHY

Dominantly inherited optic atrophy (Kjer type) is the most frequent primary hereditary variety. The recessive form (Behr type) may occur in isolation or may be associated with deafness, diabetes, and neurologic complications. The pathology is simply that of primary optic atrophy, leaving it uncertain as to whether the site of action is in the nerve or in the retinal ganglion cells. A mitochondrial type of X-linked heredity, Leber's optic atrophy,[18] similarly shows nonspecific atrophic changes in the nerve and loss of ganglion cells in the retina.

Optic atrophy also occurs with an array of metabolic diseases associated with pathologic and biochemical changes of the brain (Fig. 188–17). These include Krabbe's disease (globoid leukodystrophy), Canavan's disease (spongy degeneration), Menkes' disease (kinky hair syndrome), adrenoleukodystrophy (associated with adrenal atrophy), Leigh's disease (subacute necrotizing encephalopathy), and nutritional amblyopia (tobacco-alcohol amblyopia). Common to all is loss of the nerve fibers and of their myelin sheaths with replacement by glia (see Fig. 188–17).

Under the ill-defined (and abused) term "optic neuritis" is the optic neuropathy of demyelinative diseases. With multiple sclerosis, plaques and periphlebitis have been found in the optic nerve similar to those found in the brain.[15–17] Some are also associated with lymphocytic ensheathing about the retinal veins. The late stages simply show a loss of nerve fibers (Fig. 188–18).

INJURIES

Injuries to the optic nerve may be of mechanical, chemical, thermal, or radioactive origin. Under the

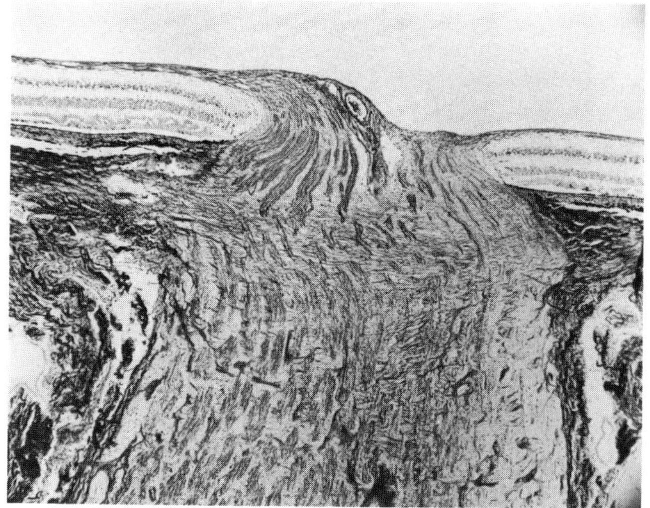

Figure 188–17. Loss of nerve fibers from temporal half of nerve head (right side in photograph) in a patient with juvenile adrenoleukodystrophy. Bodian, ×50.

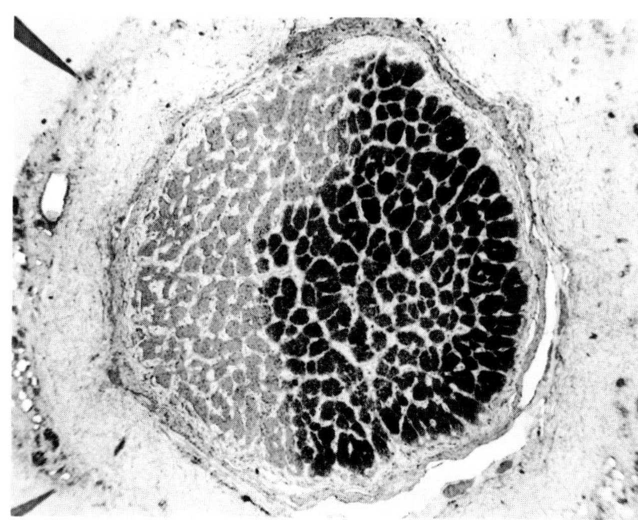

Figure 188–18. Plaque in a patient with long-standing multiple sclerosis and optic atrophy. Of note is the lack of stain in the left half of the nerve. Baker's, ×50.

mechanical category are: (1) The orbital injuries inducing proptosis and avulsion of the optic nerve, and (2) skull injuries with fractures in the region of the optic foramen. These result from transection of the nerve at the orbital apex. The avulsion of the optic nerve produces a chaotic ophthalmoscopic and pathologic picture of papillary exudate and hemorrhage. Fractures or contusions in the region of the optic foramen are a relatively frequent cause of blindness and optic atrophy from injury.

Chemical injuries to the optic nerve are, in general, caused by the same agents that damage the white matter of the brain. These include lead, thallium, chloramphenicol, and ethylene glycol.[19] Most important because of their frequency are the optic neuropathies from the alcohols. Methyl alcohol notoriously causes acute blindness. Ethyl alcohol produces a more insidious visual loss (tobacco-alcohol amblyopia) but may be subacute in spree drinkers. In either case the nerves show, during the active stages, the lipid macrophages characteristic of myelinolysis and later simple optic atrophy. Of the thermal injuries, body burns may result in acute loss of vision after a variable latent period.

Radiation injuries to the optic nerve are real but have been infrequently documented pathologically. Most cases of radiation-induced optic atrophy result from chiasmal damage incidental to pituitary radiation. The visual loss comes on typically several months after the radiation, suggesting a vascular pathogenesis.

TUMORS

Primary tumors of the optic nerve arise from cell types that are native to the nerve. These comprise gliomas, meningiomas, and, rarely hemangiomas, pericytomas, and tumors arising from congenital rests. Secondary tumors are those that extend into the optic nerve from adjacent or distal sites. They include glioblastomas and meningiomas of intracranial origin, retinoblastomas, leukemic infiltration, and various metastases. Melanotic tumors may be primary or secondary. A comprehensive and analytic review of optic nerve tumors was published in 1976.[20] Noteworthy advances since then have been in the fields of neuroimaging,[21, 22] echography,[23] and immunohistology.[24]

Gliomas

Most frequent are the astrocytomas occurring predominantly in children during the first decade of life. Presenting symptoms are proptosis, malalignment of the eyes, blindness, pallor of the disc, and sometimes proliferative tissue on the nerve head. If the tumor has extended into the cranium through the optic foramen to involve the chiasm and opposite optic nerve, diabetes insipidus and other hypothalamic signs are frequent concomitants. X-rays then reveal enlargement of the bony optic foramen and a J-shaped forward extension of the sella turcica. Computed tomography (CT) scans and magnetic resonance imaging (MRI) scans reveal a bulbous or pyriform enlargement of the nerve continuous with the globe or abutting against the apex of the orbit (Fig. 188–19). Specimens reveal similar configuration of the tumor. Somewhat more than 10 percent of the patients with these astrocytomas have neurofibromatosis (von Recklinghausen's disease) with café-au-lait spots of the skin, vitiligo, neurogenic tumors elsewhere, nevi of the iris (Lisch bodies), and occasionally congenital defects of the orbital roof.

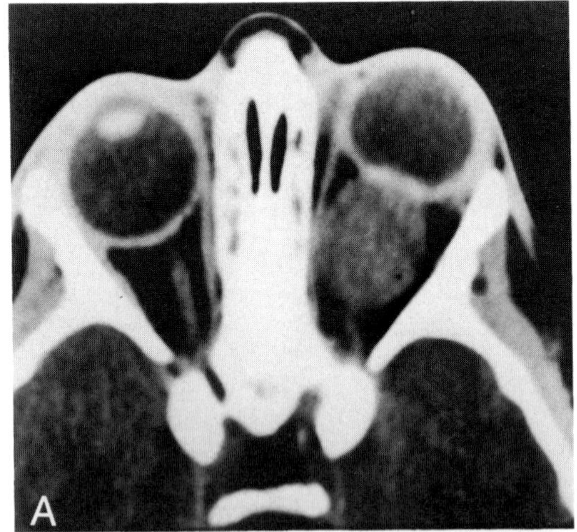

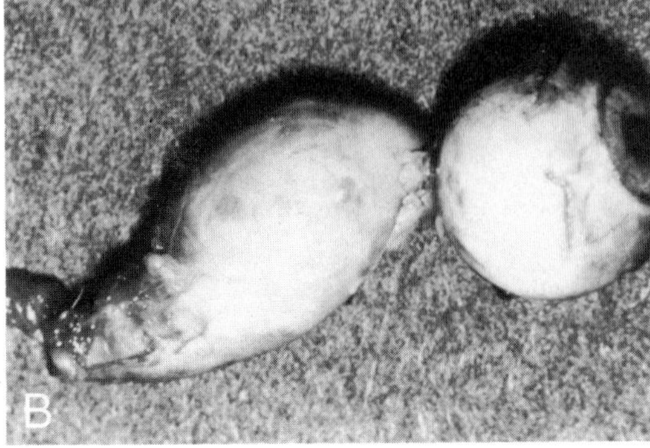

Figure 188–19. Typical manifestation of gliomas in two patients. *A,* CT scan showing pyriform enlargement of the nerve. *B,* Specimen of another but similar case, showing gross appearance of eye and nerve.

Cytologically, these astrocytomas in children have a hairlike appearance by which they are classified as pilocytic astrocytomas (or juvenile type) (Fig. 188–20*A*), but their appearances vary with age, influence of adjacent structures, and presence of mucoid reticulation (see Fig. 188–20*B*).[25] The individual cells are spindle-shaped with elongated nuclei. Rarely, glial giant cells may be present. Eosinophilic hyalinization of some of the fibers forms Rosenthal fibers (see Fig. 188–20*C*). The proliferation of the tumor within the nerve is typically demarcated by the septa, taking on a characteristically departmentalized configuration. Extension into the surrounding meninges, first described by Verhoeff in 1932,[26] is frequent, especially with neurofibromatosis, presenting a random, rather than departmentalized, proliferation of the cells (see Fig. 188–20*D*).[27] Alternatively, the optic nerves have been reported to show a simple hyperplasia of glia with von Recklinghausen's disease.[28] Gliomas arising in the chiasm region show a similar cytology but lack the departmentalization characteristic of the gliomas in the nerve.[25]

Less frequent than the astrocytomas are oligodendrogliomas. They also occur predominantly in children but at a somewhat older age. Oligodendrogliomas consist of uniformly distributed cells with round, darkly staining nuclei surrounded by clear haloes (see Fig. 188–20*E*). The clear cytoplasm may stain for mucin (Alcian blue). Glial fibers are inconspicuous but hyaline and calcareous concretions are relatively frequent.

In adults, benign astrocytomas such as those that occur in juveniles are infrequent.[29] More frequent are aggressive tumors arising intracranially and having cytologic characteristics of glioblastoma multiforme (see Fig. 188–20*F*).[30]

Meningiomas

Meningiomas of the optic nerve may present at any age from childhood to senescence. They may be unilateral or bilateral and are frequently associated with independent meningiomas within the cranium. Visual loss and proptosis are usually the presenting symptoms. Ophthalmoscopically the disc is pale, sometimes associated with proliferative tissue, and frequently with a bypass vein (shunt vessel) on the disc that extends into the choroid. X-rays often reveal a hyperostosis of the optic foramen at the apex of the orbit. CT and MRI scans show a mass contiguous with the optic nerve but, unlike that with gliomas, the tumor is likely to extend through the dura to form an exentric mass. Embedded within the mass is often a "track" corresponding to the position of the optic nerve. As in the case of gliomas, meningiomas are sometimes associated with neurofibromatosis.

Microscopically meningiomas of the optic nerve consist of compact masses of protoplasm-rich cells arranged in whorls (Figs. 188–21*A* and *B*). The nuclei are ellipsoid or round, and the basophilic cytoplasm is prominent.

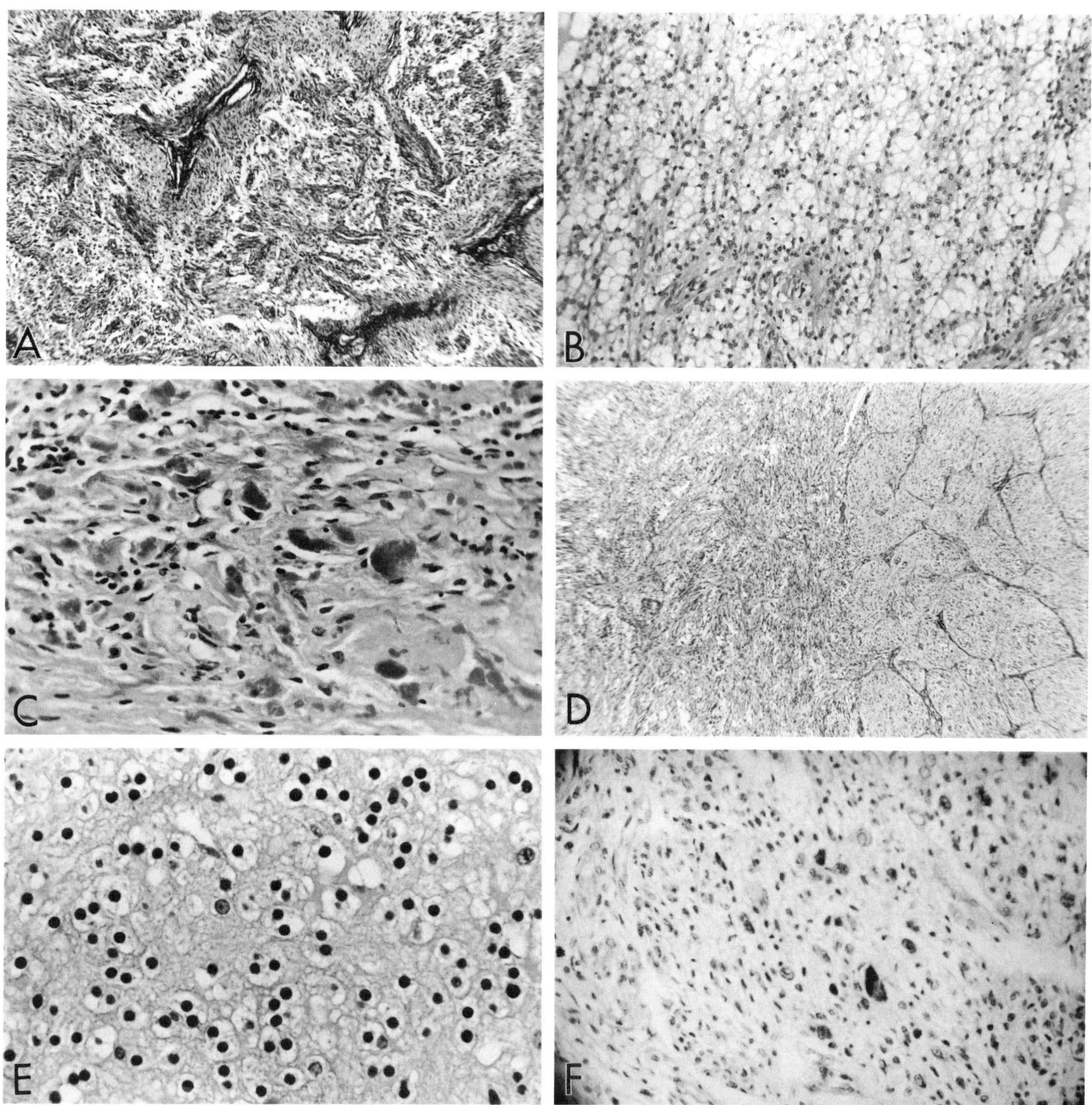

Figure 188–20. Composite photograph showing cytologic appearances of optic nerve gliomas. *A,* Juvenile pilocytic glioma. H&E, ×75. *B,* Mucoid glioma. H&E ×125. *C,* Rosenthal fibers. H&E, ×300. *D,* Extension into meninges. H&E, ×125. *E,* Oligodendroglioma. H&E, ×500. *F,* Pleomorphic glioma (glioblastoma multiforme). H&E, ×300.

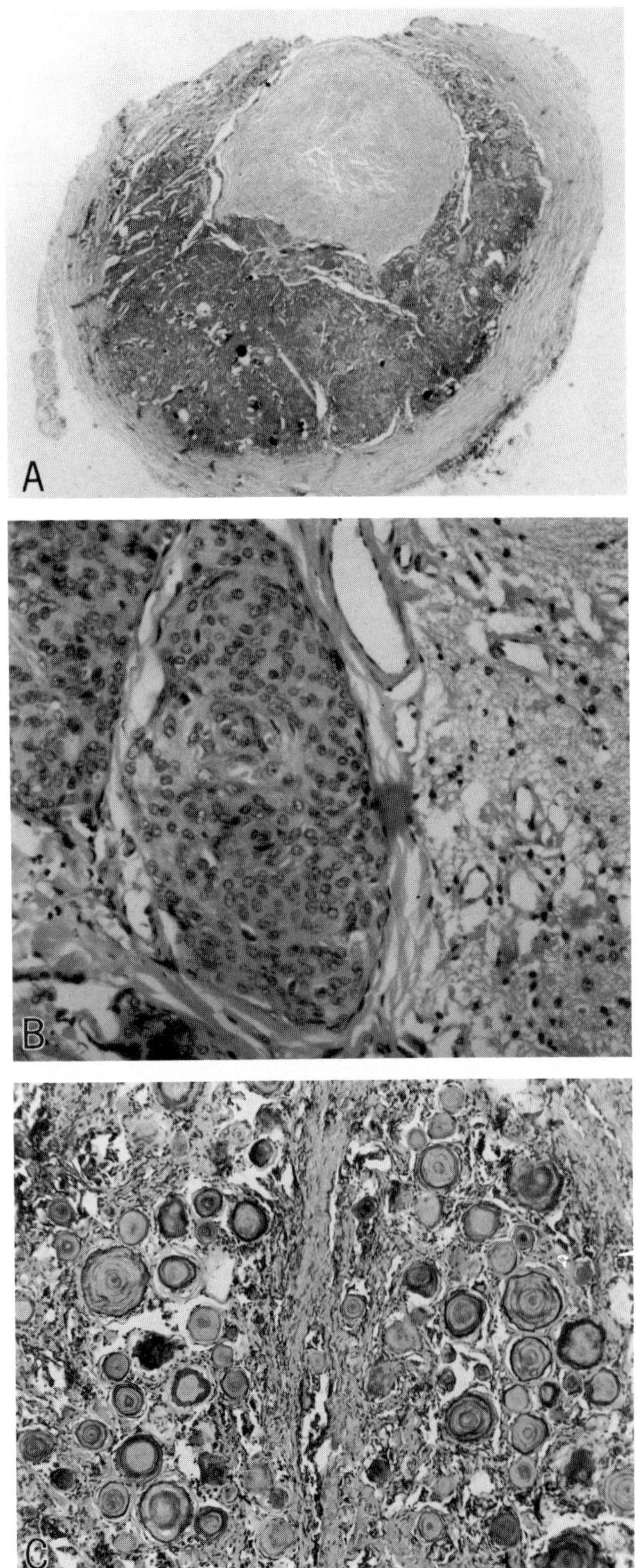

Figure 188–21. Meningioma. *A,* Massive meningioma surrounding an atrophic nerve. H&E, ×20. *B,* Whorl-like cluster abutting the atrophic nerve. H&E, ×250. *C,* Multiple concretions (psammoma bodies) in another case. H&E, ×70.

Laminated and calcareous concretions (psammoma bodies) are frequent, sometimes massive (see Fig. 188–21*C*). They are believed to represent degenerative changes in the whorl-like clusters.

Although typically benign, meningiomas of the optic nerve are invasive and extend into the surrounding orbit.

Leukemic and Lymphomatous Optic Neuropathy

Leukemic or lymphomatous infiltration is a relatively infrequent cause of symptoms but is a common finding in patients dying of leukemia.[31] The neoplastic lymphocytes have a characteristic way of insinuating along the septa of the nerve and into the leptomeninges without necessarily impairing the nerve's function (Fig. 188–22).[32] But visual impairment may eventually supervene, with blindness coming on suddenly, and may be accompanied by vascular occlusive changes in the fundi.

Melanotic Tumors

Melanotic tumors include congenital insinuation of pigment epithelium into the nerve head; benign pigmented tumors of the disc area, called either melanocytomas or magnocellular nevi; and extension of choroidal melanomas into the optic nerve.

Congenital insinuation of pigment epithelium presents ophthalmoscopically as irregularly pigmented masses on the nerve head in partially blind (and usually strabismic) eyes. Microscopically, sheets of incompletely pigmented epithelium interlace a glial mass on the nerve head.

Melanocytomas (magnocellular nevi) occurring in persons of dark complexions present as black masses centering on the disc and radiating into the adjacent retina. Only rarely do they show evidence of growth. Microscopically they consist of large, heavily pigmented, and monotonously uniform cells. Their cell of origin is uncertain, but similar tumors occur in the uvea.

Finally, melanomas arising in the choroid may extend into the optic nerve secondarily.

Other Tumors

Carcinomatous metastases to the optic nerve from primary carcinoma in the lung, stomach, and breast are well documented. Rare cases of hemangiomas, carcinoid, and sarcomas in the optic nerve have also been reported.

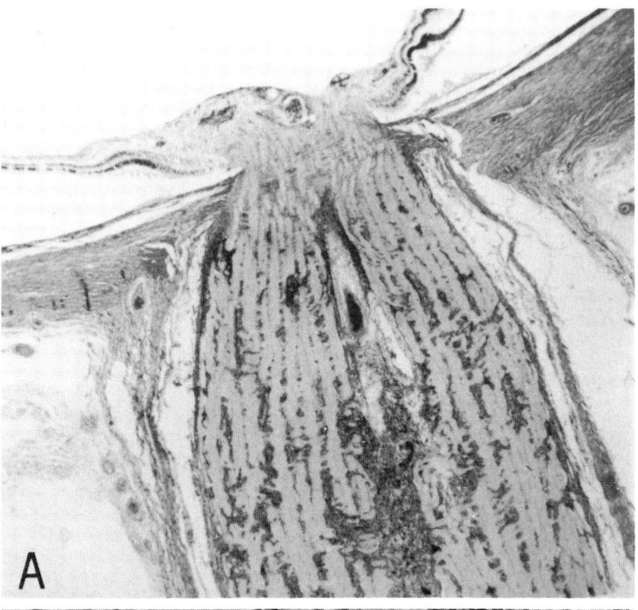

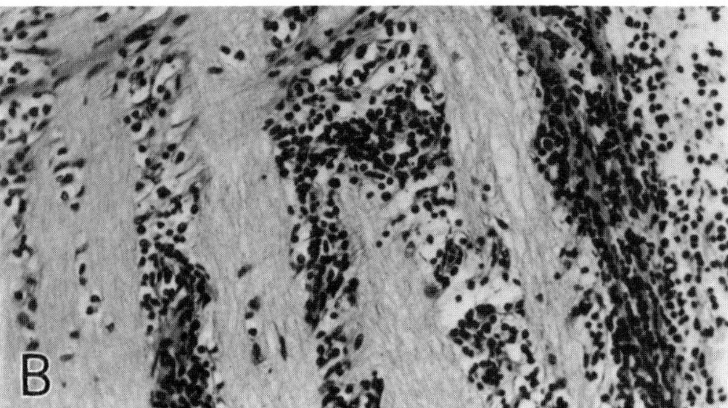

Figure 188–22. Lymphocytic infiltration of optic nerve in leukemia. *A,* H&E, ×30. *B,* H&E, ×125.

REFERENCES

1. Giarelli L, Melato M, Campos E: 14 Cases of cavernous degeneration of the optic nerve. Ophthalmologica 174:316, 1977.
2. Schnabel J: Das glaucomatose Sehnervenleiden. Arch fur Augen 24:273, 1892.
3. Zimmerman LE, De Venecia G, Hamasaki DI: Pathology of the optic nerve in experimental acute glaucoma. Invest Ophthalmol 6:109, 1887.
4. Roessman U: Septo-optic dysplasia (SOD) or DeMorsier syndrome. J Clin Neuro Ophthalmol 9:156, 1989.
5. Barkovich AJ, Fram EK, Norman D: Septo-optic dysplasia:MR imaging. Radiology 171:189, 1989.
6. Kindler P: Morning glory syndrome: Unusual congenital optic disk anomaly. Am J Ophthalmol 69:376, 1970.
7. Manschot WA: Morning glory syndrome: A histopathological study. Br J Ophthalmol 74:56, 1990.
8. Mansour AM, Schoch D, Logani S: Optic disc size in ischemic optic neuropathy. Am J Ophthalmol 106:587, 1988.
9. Beck RW, Savino PJ, Repka MX, et al: Optic disc stricture in anterior ischemic optic neuropathy. Ophthalmology 91:1334, 1984.
10. Johnson BL, Wisotzkey HM: Neuroretinitis associated with herpes simplex encephalitis in an adult. Am J Ophthalmol 83:481, 1977.
11. Fenton RH, Easom HA: Behçet's syndrome: A histopathologic study of the eye. Arch Ophthalmol 72:71, 1884.
12. Gelwan MJ, Kellen RI, Burde RM, Kupersmith MJ: Sarcoidosis of the anterior visual pathway: Successes and failure. J Neurol Neurosurg Psychiatr 51:1473, 1988.
13. Gass JD, Olson CL: Sarcoidosis with optic nerve and retinal involvement. Arch Ophthalmol 94:945, 1976.
14. Jordan DR, Anderson RL, Nerad JA, et al: Optic nerve involvement as the initial manifestation of sarcoidosis. Can J Ophthalmol 23:232, 1988.
15. Arnold AC, Pepose JS, Hepler RS, Foos RY: Retinal periphlebitis and retinitis in multiple sclerosis. I: Pathologic characteristics. Ophthalmology 91:255, 1984.
16. Mogensen PH: Histopathology of the anterior parts of the optic pathway in patients with multiple sclerose. Acta Ophthalmol (Copenh) 68:218, 1990.
17. Sergott RC, Brown MJ: Current concepts on the pathogenesis of optic neuritis associated with multiple sclerosis. Surv Ophthalmol 33:1013, 1989.

18. Singh G, Lott MT, Wallace DC: A mitochondrial DNA mutation as a cause of optic neuropathy. N Engl J Med 320:1300, 1989.
19. Grant WM: Toxicology of the Eye, 3rd ed. Springfield, IL, Charles C Thomas, 1986.
20. Eggers H, Jacobiec FA, Jones IS: Tumor of the optic nerve. Doc Ophthalmol 41:43, 1976.
21. Haik BG: Advanced imaging techniques in ophthalmology. *In* International Ophthalmology Clinic 26(3). Boston, Little, Brown, Company, 1986.
22. Slamovits TL, Gardner TA: Neuroimaging in neuro-ophthalmology. Ophthalmology 96:555, 1989.
23. Atta HR: Imaging of the optic nerve with standardized echography. Eye 2:358, 1988.
24. Kobayashi S, Mouri H, Ikeuch S, Takakura K: Immunohistochemical study on Rosenthal fibers in gliomas using anti-GFAP and anti-ubiquitin antibodies. No To Shinkei 42:59, 1990.
25. Rubinstein LJ: Pathological features of optic nerve and chiasmatic glioma. Neurofibromatosis 1:152, 1988.
26. Verhoeff FH: Tumors of the optic nerve. *In* Penfield W (ed): Cytology and Cellular Pathology of the Nervous System. New York, PB Hoeber, 1932.
27. Stern J, Jakobiec FA, Housepian EM: The architecture of optic nerve gliomas with and without neurofibromatosis. Arch Ophthalmol 98:505, 1980.
28. Spencer WH, Borit A: Diffuse hyperplasia of the optic nerve in von Recklinghausen's disease. Am J Ophthalmol 64:638, 1887.
29. Wulc AE, Bergin DJ, Barnes D, et al: Orbital optic nerve glioma in adult life. Arch Ophthalmol 107:1013, 1989.
30. Hoyt WF, Meshel LG, Lessell S, et al: Malignant optic glioma of adulthood. Brain 96:121, 1973.
31. Guyer DR, Green WR, Schachat AP, et al: Bilateral ischemic optic neuropathy and retinal vascular occlusions associated with lymphoma and sepsis: Clinicopathologic correlation. Ophthalmology 97:882, 1990.
32. Zimmerman LE, Thoreson HT: Sudden loss of vision in acute leukemia. Surv Ophthalmol 64:638, 1887.

Chapter 189

Advanced Diagnostic Techniques—Diagnostic Immunohistochemistry

VALERIE A. WHITE

PRINCIPLES

The purpose of this section is to provide the practicing ophthalmologist with a basic understanding of immunohistochemical procedures as used by the diagnostic surgical pathologist.[1–5] As this technique is used routinely in most laboratories, this enables the ophthalmologist to understand the significance of immunohistochemical stains employed in the diagnosis of a particular case and in the context of an immunopathologic review of cases in a journal article. This section deals only with immunohistochemical procedures and antibodies in general use in the diagnostic laboratory and highlights their use in the diagnosis of neoplasms relevant to the ophthalmologist. At the research level, the same basic techniques are used to identify any number of antigens in any type of tissue.

The basic premise of an immunohistochemical procedure is to localize an antigen of interest in its cell of origin and, in most cases, to view the results at the light microscopic level. The diagnostic usefulness of this premise is that neoplasms derived from or showing differentiation toward a particular cell type retain an antigen that is useful in determining the lineage of that neoplasm. Consequently, the range of antibodies chosen for use in the diagnostic laboratory is aimed at those that will be helpful in distinguishing the derivation of poorly differentiated neoplasms. In addition, immunohistochemical procedures are often routinely used to determine the cell type and immunoglobulin pattern in lymphomas and for the identification of infectious agents (usually viruses) in inflammatory processes.

Antigenicity. Most antigens are proteins; and, in order to be localized at the light microscopic level, the three-dimensional nature of the antigen must be optimally preserved within the constraints of the diagnostic laboratory. This preservation is affected by autolysis, fixation, and embedding. Autolysis is the release of proteolytic enzymes after tissue is removed from blood supply. Thus, it is important that tissues be appropriately fixed as soon as possible after their removal in order both to preserve the antigens and to inactivate these destructive enzymes. If tissue cannot be fixed immediately, it should be refrigerated.

As well as inactivating proteolytic enzymes, the function of fixation is to immobilize antigens at their actual tissue site. Several fixatives are in routine use, and the choice of fixative depends on the antigen or antigens that are required to diagnose a particular neoplasm. This presumption can be based only on clinical information received from the ophthalmologist; thus, in a difficult case, the pathologist always appreciates knowing the differential diagnosis in advance so that tissue may be used optimally. The routine fixative is neutral buffered formalin, an aldehyde, owing to its fast penetration of tissue and its low cost. Most antigens are well preserved by formalin. The other aldehyde in routine use for electron microscopy is glutaraldehyde. This fixative provides optimum preservation of ultrastructure, but because of its extensive cross-linking, it destroys antigenicity for immunohistochemical procedures as performed for light microscopy. Bouin's fixative, a combination of formalin and picric acid, and B5, a combination of mercuric chloride and formalin, are widely used for light microscopy and antigenic preservation, particularly in lymphomas. Alcohol and acetone fix by denaturation and are particularly useful for the preservation of intermediate filaments. Tissue may also be preserved by freezing in liquid nitrogen with subsequent storage at −70°C. This is useful for preservation of all antigens but is not done routinely because of the greater technical expertise required to handle the tissue, limited storage space, and poor morphology. It is used most commonly to preserve cell surface antigens to facilitate the diagnosis of lymphomas. An advantage of freezing some tissue is that DNA can subsequently be extracted and also used in the diagnosis of lymphomas and other tumors. Therefore, when the nature of a tumor is suspected, the appropriate fixative(s) may be chosen. When a tumor is suspected of being a diagnostic dilemma, the routine procedure is to fix tissue in formalin, alcohol, Bouin's fixative, or B5, and glutaraldehyde and to freeze some. This depends on receiving a large enough representative sample and on the sample arriving in the laboratory as soon as possible after surgical removal.

Most tissue is routinely embedded in paraffin wax after fixation; this does not appear to adversely affect antigenicity. Tissue may also be frozen and sectioned after fixation or embedded in a variety of plastics, neither of which method is used routinely.

Antibodies. Two main types of antibodies are in routine use. Polyclonal antibodies are produced by immunization of animals, most commonly rabbits, and by purifying the serum at the time when an appropriate antibody response has occurred.[5] This produces a variety of antibodies to various epitopes on the antigen and of differing affinities. A disadvantage is that this results in a heterogeneous mixture of antibodies that may also contain antibodies to impurities in the immunization agent and naturally occurring antibodies of the animal, which are features that may produce nonspecific staining. A characterized supply lasts only as long as a particular animal. Nevertheless, many of these antibodies are in daily use because of their low cost and proven specificity.

Monoclonal antibodies are produced by the fusion of immunized spleen cells from a mouse with myeloma cells that do not secrete antibody. Following fusion and under appropriate conditions, the myeloma cells produce an endless supply of the mouse antibody, all of an identical nature and all directed toward the same epitope on an antigen. The disadvantage of these antibodies is that they have a lower sensitivity, because only one antibody can bind to the same epitope on an antigen. The production of these antibodies is more complex and time consuming than polyclonal antibodies, thus they are usually more expensive. Mixtures of monoclonal antibodies, each to a different epitope, may be used to enhance sensitivity. These antibodies have come into widespread use in the diagnostic laboratory in the last few years because monoclonal antibodies of high specificity have been produced that can be used on routinely fixed and embedded tissue.

Antigen-Antibody Interaction. This complex noncovalent interaction depends on the tertiary structure of both molecules. The binding is due to hydrogen bonding, electrostatic and Van der Waals forces, and hydrophobicity. In practice, this interaction occurs under relatively simple conditions of buffer and at room temperature.

Detection Systems. A variety of detection systems are available and in routine use. All systems involve the application of a primary antibody to the antigen of interest in appropriately fixed, embedded, sectioned, and subsequently prepared tissue. Because most tissue is embedded in paraffin and the immunohistochemical procedures are carried out in a water-based buffer, the paraffin must be removed with xylene and alcohols. This is not required in frozen tissue. The last step in the procedure is the application of a compound that can be visualized. Some of the methods in use are described.

Direct Method (Fig. 189–1). The primary antibody is labeled with the detectable compound, usually fluorescein. This method is usually used for the detection of immunoglobulin and complement in frozen, unfixed tissue in cicatricial pemphigoid, systemic lupus, and kidney diseases. Observation of the result requires an epifluorescent microscope, and the fluorescent results cannot be viewed together with the light microscopy. Other disadvantages are that the fluorescent label becomes weaker with prolonged exposure to light and that the slides cannot be dehydrated and coverslipped permanently, because this also weakens the fluorescence. Autofluorescence of tissue can cause problems in interpretation.

Indirect Method (Fig. 189–2). Here, as in all of the other systems, the primary antibody directed against the antigen of interest is unlabeled. In this method, after washing, a second antibody directed against the antibody or immunoglobulin of the first animal species is applied, for example, goat anti-rabbit immunoglobulin. The second antibody is labeled, usually with a horseradish peroxidase enzyme. Peroxidase changes a reduced, soluble, colorless compound or chromogen to an oxidized, colored precipitate in the presence of hydrogen peroxide, and this is localized at the site of the antigen-antibody interaction. This is the last step in the staining procedure and produces the visible result that is viewed with an ordinary light microscope. Chromogens com-

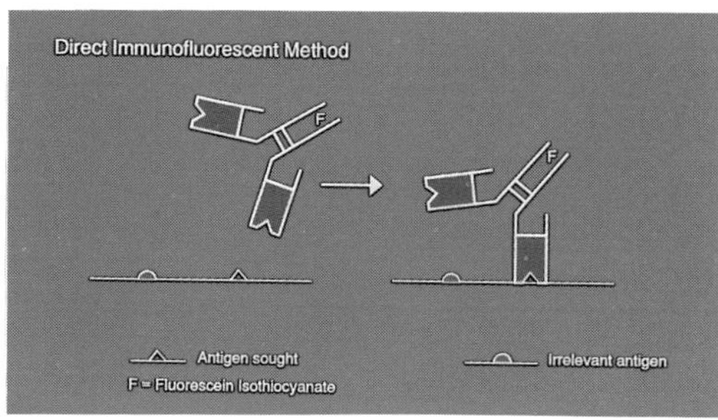

Figure 189–1. Diagrammatic outline of direct immunofluorescent method.

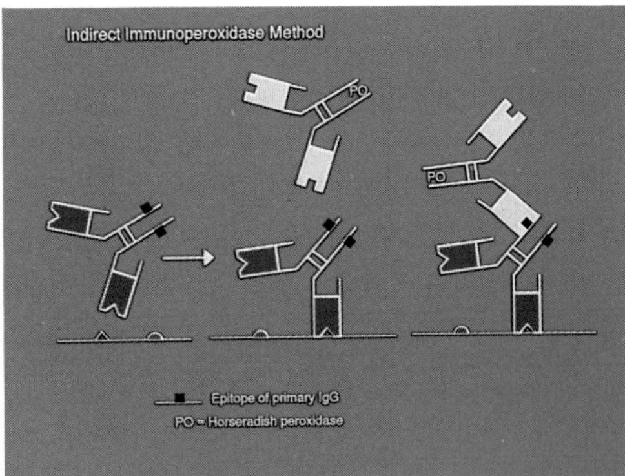

Figure 189–2. Diagrammatic outline of indirect immunoperoxidase method.

monly used are diaminobenzidine, a brown compound, and aminoethylcarbazole, a red compound. It is to be noted that no matter what the primary antibody is, the reaction product always looks the same, except for its distribution. Normal tissue has endogenous peroxidase activity in red blood cells, neutrophils, and other inflammatory cells so that in any method employing peroxidase, the endogenous activity must be blocked before the addition of the primary antibody by the application of hydrogen peroxide.

Peroxidase-Antiperoxidase (PAP) (Fig. 189–3). Three levels of antibody are employed in this method. The first and third antibodies are derived from the same animal species, and the second antibody serves as a bridge between the two, because an antibody has two binding sites. The third antibody is usually labeled with peroxidase, although other enzymes such as alkaline phosphatase and glucose oxidase may be used. The PAP method is in wide use because it is thought to be one of the most sensitive methods owing to the amplification of binding that can occur at each level of antibody. Table 189–1 gives the entire staining procedure for the PAP method.[6, 7]

Avidin-Biotin Peroxidase (ABC) (Fig. 189–4). Avidins are glycoproteins that have a greater affinity for the vitamin biotin than antibodies for antigens. In this method, the second antibody is labeled with biotin. Following this, a complex of many molecules of avidin, biotin, and peroxidase is added that binds to the biotin. The colored product is developed as described earlier.

Other Methods. Protein A from *Staphylococcus aureus* binds to the Fc portion of immunoglobulin and can be labeled with peroxidase or other labels and used as the second step in a two-step procedure. Metals such as gold, silver, nickel, and cobalt can be used to enhance staining. Immunohistochemical techniques are also applied to specimens examined by electron microscopy. This allows subcellular localization of antigens but, owing to the technical expertise required, is usually confined to research applications.[8]

Controls. Owing to nonspecific binding that can occur, all immunohistochemical stains are run with appropriate positive and negative controls. A positive control is a

Table 189–1. GENERAL PROCEDURE FOR IMMUNOPEROXIDASE STAINING OF FIXED TISSUE SECTIONS

1. Cut sections onto poly-L-lysine–coated slides to enhance adherence of sections to slides.
2. Dry at 37°C overnight.
3. Remove paraffin wax from sections by immersing in 3 changes of xylene, 3 of absolute ethanol.
4. Quench endogenous peroxidase in 3% hydrogen peroxide in methanol.
5. Rehydrate in absolute ethanol, 2 changes of 95% ethanol, and immerse in phosphate buffered saline (PBS).
6. Digest sections, if required, in a protease solution.
7. PBS rinse.
8. Block nonspecific binding in 1:1 solution of 10% bovine serum albumin:normal serum from animal species in which the secondary antibody was generated. Tap excess serum from the slide, but do not rinse.
9. Apply appropriate dilution of primary antibody to cover the section on the slide. Dilution, time of incubation, and temperature of incubation will vary. All steps are done in a moist chamber to prevent evaporation.
10. PBS rinse.
11. Apply secondary antibody at appropriate dilution for 30 min.
12. PBS rinse.
13. Add peroxidase-antiperoxidase (PAP) complex at appropriate dilution for 30 min.
14. PBS rinse.
15. Incubate in chromogen in hydrogen peroxide; watch for color development.
16. Rinse under running water.
17. Counterstain with hematoxylin.

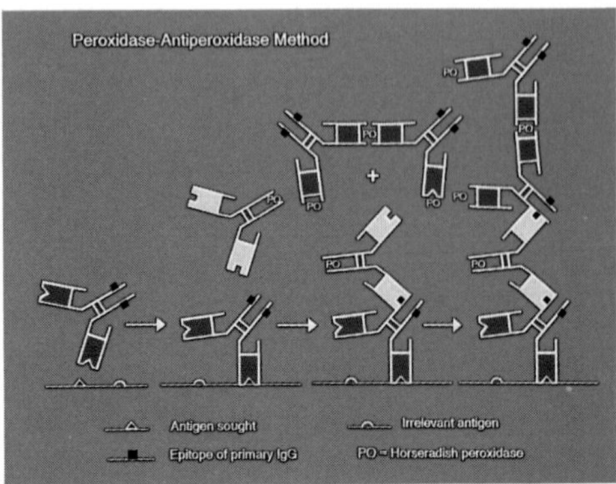

Figure 189–3. Diagrammatic outline of peroxidase-antiperoxidase (PAP) method.

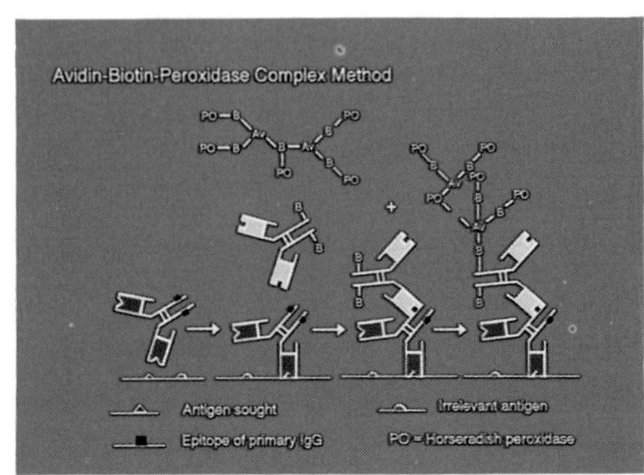

Figure 189–4. Diagrammatic outline of avidin-biotin peroxidase (ABC) method.

specimen that has known reactivity for a particular antigen. It should be a similar type of tissue to the test specimen and should be fixed, embedded, and sectioned in the same manner. In practice, it is difficult to control all of these variables because of the large volume and many different types of specimen being handled, but controls in the same fixative are mandatory. A negative control is a section from the test specimen in which the primary antibody is omitted, but all of the other steps are carried out the same. This control helps to determine whether there is nonspecific binding of the second or third antibody or peroxidase to any of the tissue components. A third control, and probably the best, is the internal positive and negative controls of the test specimen, and these should be looked for before interpreting the stain. For example, if anti-S100 antibody has been applied to look for a melanoma, structures should be looked for within the specimen that normally stain for S100, such as peripheral nerves or dendritic cells. Similarly, structures such as epidermis and connective tissue, known not to contain S100 protein, should be negative. Internal positive and negative controls are not always present in every specimen, such as when the entire specimen consists of a tumor; however, they should be used whenever possible, because they control for all the variables of handling of that particular specimen.

The sensitivity of a detection system refers to the minimum amount of antigen it can detect. Currently PAP and ABC are considered to be the most sensitive detection systems, because of amplification of the final detectable signal that occurs in these methods.[6, 9] In our laboratory, we use the indirect immunoperoxidase method because we have found that it has adequate sensitivity and, because it has only three main steps, the procedure takes a shorter time to perform. Of course, detection of as much of the original antigen in a specimen as possible also depends on optimal handling of the specimen, as described earlier. Specificity refers to whether an antibody binds only to structures known to contain a particular antigen and does not bind to structures known not to contain that antigen. Nonspecific binding can result from similarity of antigenic determinants in different molecules, contaminating antibodies, binding of the secondary or tertiary antibodies to structures in the specimen, endogenous peroxidase activity that has not been fully blocked, and nonspecific binding to the edges of sections, stroma, and necrotic tissue.

Because most diagnostic laboratories purchase their antibodies from commercial sources, they must rely on these sources to properly control their antibody production and screen for the aforementioned problems. However, when using a new antibody for the first time, it is incumbent upon the diagnostic laboratory to test it on a range of known positive and negative controls of different tissue types and fixatives before using it on diagnostic specimens. It should be noted that the onus rests on the pathologist to interpret his or her immunohistochemical stains properly, because commercial antibodies all come with the disclaimer that the antibodies are to be used for research purposes only.

PRACTICE

Immunohistochemical Staining of Normal Tissues. Knowledge of the immunohistochemical staining patterns of normal cells and tissues is vital to an understanding of the use of this technique in the diagnosis of neoplasms. Table 189–2 lists antigens that are commonly stained by routinely used antibodies, and the normal cells and tissues that usually stain. The staining pattern in both normal tissues and neoplasms depends on many variables, including type of tissue, fixation, type of antibody, and procedure; thus results may vary somewhat from one study to another. Table 189–2 and the following tables are an attempt to survey results *usually* obtained.

One of the most diagnostically useful group of antibodies is that to the intermediate filament proteins. These intracellular fibrous proteins are present within almost all cell types and constitute an important part of the cytoskeleton of the cell, "mechanically integrating the cytoplasmic organelles."[37, 38] They are called intermediate because they measure 10 nm in diameter and are intermediate in diameter among thin actin filaments at 6 nm and thicker myosin filaments at 15 nm and microtubules at 25 nm, all of which form part of the cytoskeleton. Biochemical and immunologic characterization distinguished five classes of intermediate filaments and found that they were generally localized in specific types of cells: keratin in epithelial cells, vimentin in nonmyogenic mesenchymal cells, desmin in myogenic mesenchymal cells, neurofilament (NF) in neural cells, and glial fibrillary acidic protein (GFAP) in glial cells.[10, 13, 38] Early investigations of intermediate filament expression in neoplasms suggested that neoplasms derived from or showing differentiation toward a particular type of tissue retained the intermediate filament of that tissue. As these antibodies have been more widely used, it has become evident that the situation in neoplasms is more complex than in the normal adult cell, and the staining patterns are not always as clear-cut. Nevertheless, the restriction of intermediate filament types to specific cell types underlies their use in the diagnosis of neoplasms.

Immunohistochemical Staining of Nonhematopoietic Neoplasms. Antibodies to intermediate filaments are used under the general assumption that carcinomas express keratin proteins; nonmyogenic sarcomas, melanomas, and lymphomas express vimentin; sarcomas of smooth or skeletal muscle express desmin; tumors of glial origin express GFAP; and tumors of neural origin express neurofilament.[1, 10, 39–44] The situation has become confused by the finding of coexpression of two (and sometimes even three) intermediate filaments in some tumors. Coexpression of keratin and vimentin may be seen in renal, ovarian, thyroid, neuroendocrine, breast, and other carcinomas and meningiomas.[1, 18] These neoplasms do not usually present diagnostic problems, and this dual expression is thought to reflect a stage in embryogenesis when dual or triple expression of intermediate filaments is normal.[45] Coexpression of keratin

Table 189–2. IMMUNOHISTOCHEMICAL STAINING OF NORMAL CELLS

Antigen	Cellular Antigen Stained	Normal Cells and Tissues Stained	References
Epithelial Antigens			
Keratin	Intermediate filaments	Epidermis, squamous, columnar, cuboidal, and glandular epithelia, including that of cornea, conjunctiva, lacrimal, sweat, and sebaceous glands	10–14
Epithelial membrane antigen (EMA)	Membrane glycoprotein	Similar to keratin; also present in perineurium and rare lymphoid cells	15–17
Mesenchymal Antigens			
Vimentin	Intermediate filaments	All mesenchymal tissue including fibrous and adipose tissue, smooth muscle, cartilage, bone, vascular endothelium; also melanocytes, Schwann cells, macrophages, lymphocytes, occasional epithelial cells	10, 13, 18
Muscle actin	Actin filaments	Skeletal, smooth and cardiac muscle, smooth muscle of vascular wall and pericytes, myoepithelial cells, cells in capsule of liver, kidney, spleen, and lymph nodes	19, 20
Smooth muscle actin	Actin filaments of smooth muscle	Smooth muscle, smooth muscle of vascular wall, myoepithelial cells	21
Desmin	Intermediate filaments	Skeletal, smooth, cardiac muscle, muscular wall of arteries	10, 19, 20
Myoglobin	Polypeptide containing an oxygen-binding heme group	Skeletal and cardiac muscle	10, 22
Factor VIII-related antigen (factor VIIIR:Ag)	Multimeric glycoprotein required for normal coagulation	Vascular endothelial cells, megakaryocytes, sinusoidal lining cells of spleen; does not stain glomerular endothelia and stains large vessels and lymphatics weakly	24
Ulex Europaeus-1 (UEA)*	Lectin that binds to terminal fucose on blood group antigens	Vascular endothelial cells, some epithelial cells of skin, pancreas, and lung	24, 25
Neural, Neural Crest, and Neuroendocrine Antigens			
Neuron-specific enolase (NSE)	Isoenzyme with restricted distribution	Schwann cells, neurons, smooth muscle, myoepithelial cells, melanocytes, endocrine and neuroendocrine cells	26
Neurofilament	Intermediate filament	Neurons of central and peripheral nervous system	10, 13, 27
Glial fibrillary acidic protein (GFAP)	Intermediate filament	Astrocytes, Schwann cells, ependymal cells, satellite cells of ganglia	10, 27, 28
S100	Soluble, acidic, cytoplasmic, calcium-binding protein	Schwann cells, astrocytes, ependymal cells, adipose tissue, cartilage, melanocytes, some epithelial and myoepithelial cells; Langerhans' cells of skin, interdigitating reticulum cells of lymph nodes	27, 29–32
Chromogranin	Acidic glycoprotein of neurosecretory granule	Adrenal medulla, neuroendocrine cells of gastrointestinal tract, thyroid, and lung, pancreatic islet cells, anterior pituitary, sympathetic ganglia, some neurons and retinal photoreceptors; some epithelial cells of breast, salivary gland ducts, and thymic epithelial cells	33
Synaptophysin	Acidic glycoprotein of presynaptic vesicle	Adrenal medulla, neuroendocrine cells of gastrointestinal tract, pancreas, pituitary, and lung; neurons of brain, spinal cord, and retina	34
Hematolymphoid Antigens			
Leukocyte common antigen	Family of glycoproteins	All leukocytes including bone marrow precursor cells, lymphocytes, granulocytes, monocytes/macrophages, mast cells, Langerhans' cells, dendritic cells; occasionally osteoclasts and mesothelial cells	35
Immunoglobulins	IgM, IgG, IgA, IgD, IgE, κ and λ light chains	Immunoglobulins in cytoplasm of plasma cells in fixed, paraffin-embedded tissue; immunoglobulins on surface of B lymphocytes in fresh, frozen tissue	35
L26	Uncharacterized cell surface antigen	B lymphocytes	36
UCHL1	Subset of leukocyte common antigen	T lymphocytes, myeloid cells	36

*Not an antigen; this is the name of the lectin.

and vimentin is diagnostically useful in some undifferentiated tumors, such as malignant rhabdoid tumors and synovial and epithelioid sarcomas.[46–52] Coexpression of desmin and vimentin is seen in virtually all myogenic sarcomas if properly fixed.[40, 53]

This lack of absolute specificity for a particular antibody is also seen to some degree in all of the antigens listed in Table 189–2. For example, antibody to S100 protein was considered to be specific for neural-supporting cells when it was first used; however, subsequent investigations have revealed its presence in adipose and cartilaginous tissue and tumors. The practical result of these somewhat confusing findings is that the diagnostic pathologist cannot rely entirely on the presence or absence of one particular antibody to make or break a diagnosis. The present practice is for a panel of antibodies to be applied when the light microscopic appearance suggests a range of differential diagnoses in a poorly differentiated neoplasm. The panel should cover the range of differential diagnoses and should contain at least one or two antibodies that should be positive and one or two antibodies that should be negative in each case. In this way the pathologist has support from both positive and negative results and is not caught unawares by a lesion that is spuriously positive or negative for one particular antibody.

The major distinction to be made when the pathologist is confronted with an undifferentiated neoplasm is whether it is a carcinoma, lymphoma, melanoma, or sarcoma. These neoplasms are positive for keratin, leukocyte common antigen (LCA), S100 protein, and vimentin, respectively, and are usually negative with the other antibodies. Therefore, inclusion of several of these antibodies in a panel is extremely useful in the primary categorization of a neoplasm.[10, 39, 40, 54–56] The panel should contain antibodies that cover the range of differential diagnoses suggested by light microscopic examination, including ones that should be negative. Figure 189–5 shows the application of an antibody panel to the diagnosis of a poorly differentiated neoplasm in the liver, which is a common diagnostic problem. It is important that the immunohistochemical results are never interpreted without recourse to the appearance on hematoxylin and eosin (H&E) staining, because this is the starting point that directs all further investigations, including electron microscopy. Furthermore, vastly different neoplasms may have similar immunohistochemical staining profiles. For ease of presentation, in the following tables, a broad range of differential diagnoses is given for each category of light microscopic appearance, but in a particular case only selected antibodies need be applied if light microscopy suggests a more restricted range of diagnoses.

Small Cell Undifferentiated Neoplasms. Most of these neoplasms, with the exception of small cell carcinoma and lymphoma, are more common in children. They are often difficult to distinguish from one another because of a lack of differentiating features on routine H&E stain and immunohistochemistry, and electron microscopy must often be employed for a secure diagnosis. The immunohistochemical staining patterns of these neoplasms are shown in Table 189–3. The diagnosis must also be rendered with knowledge of the site of origin of the tumor, because it may be seen from Table 189–3 that neuroblastoma, retinoblastoma, peripheral neuroepithelioma, and olfactory neuroblastoma have virtually identical immunohistochemical staining patterns, presumably because of their origin from similar types of cells.

Table 189–3. IMMUNOHISTOCHEMICAL STAINING OF SMALL CELL UNDIFFERENTIATED NEOPLASMS

Neoplasm	LCA	Keratin	NSE	NF	Desmin	References
Lymphoma	*	†	†	†	†	54, 56, 57
Leukemia‡	*	†	†	†	†	54, 57, 58
Neuroblastoma	†	†	*	*	†	27, 59, 60
Retinoblastoma	†	†	*	*	†	27, 61–63
Peripheral neuroepithelioma, olfactory neuroblastoma	†	†	*	*	†	27, 42
Rhabdomyosarcoma	†	†	†	†	*	40, 53, 64, 65
Ewing's sarcoma	†	†	†	†	†	60
Wilms' tumor	†	*	†	†	§	42, 46
Small cell carcinoma	†	‖	‖	‖	†	1

*Usually stains for that antigen.
†Usually does not stain.
‡Enzyme histochemistry and other immunohistochemical stains required to distinguish histologically between lymphoma and leukemia.
§May stain if myoid differentiation is present.
‖May or may not stain.

Spindle-Cell Neoplasms. These neoplasms are all sarcomas, except for the spindle cell carcinoma, and have the basic immunohistochemical profile of vimentin positivity and keratin and leukocyte common antigen negativity. Table 189–4 shows the immunohistochemical stains that are required to further differentiate these neoplasms.

Other Neoplasms. These neoplasms are a mixture that usually consists of large polygonal cells, although melanomas and astrocytomas may sometimes have a spindle-like appearance. Table 189–5 shows the immunohistochemical profile of this diverse group of neoplasms. Again, the site of origin is very important because, for example, a tumor arising in the optic nerve is most likely to be a meningioma or astrocytoma, rather than a melanoma. Within this group of neoplasms, the possibility of a metastatic lesion must always be considered. HMB-45 is a recently introduced monoclonal antibody that stains proliferating melanocytes in melanomas, some nevi, and in the fetus. It does not stain resting melanocytes and has only infrequently been reported to stain any other types of tissue; therefore, it is very useful along with the more sensitive, but less specific antibody to S100 protein in the diagnosis of melanomas.[78–81]

Immunohistochemical Staining of Hematopoietic Neoplasms. Table 189–6 shows the use of some immunohistochemical stains in the diagnosis of lymphomas.[35, 36, 54, 57, 92] Leukemias occasionally present as masses that must be distinguished from lymphomas and other neoplasms. They stain positively for LCA, but enzyme histochemistry in addition to other morphologic and clinical features is necessary for diagnosis.

Within the range of lymphoid neoplasms encountered

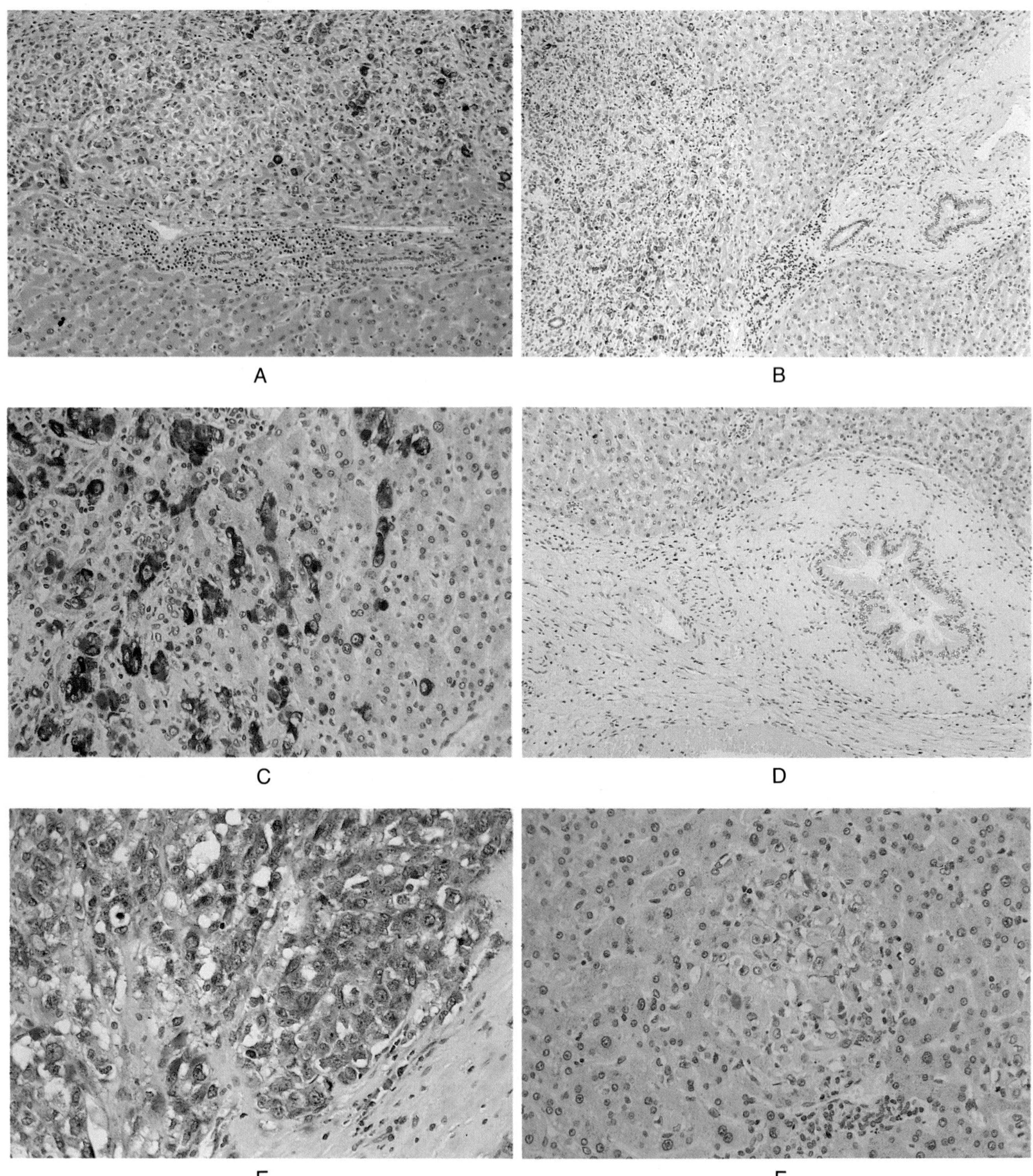

Figure 189–5. *A,* Metastatic neoplasm in the liver. The neoplasm is in the top half of the figure, and the normal liver tissue is in the bottom half. H&E, ×28. *B,* Negative control for immunoperoxidase stains. Primary antibody has been omitted. This is the control for nonspecific binding of the secondary antibody and the peroxidase complex, and it should show no staining. The neoplasm is on the left, and a portal triad is on the right. The brown color is melanin in some tumor cells. ×20. *C,* Staining of the neoplasm by the antimelanoma monoclonal antibody HMB-45. HMB-45, ×50. *D,* Another area with hepatocytes. A portal triad containing a large bile duct and a blood vessel does not stain with this antibody. These structures should not stain, and therefore they represent internal negative controls for this antibody. HMB-45, ×20. *E,* The positive control for HMB-45 is a melanoma with known positive staining. Positive control tests are performed for each antibody used, but only the one for HMB-45 is shown here. This test result must be positive in order to interpret the test specimen. HMB-45, ×50. *F,* Staining of a small nest of tumor cells for S100 protein. Note that the surrounding hepatocytes do not stain. Anti-S100, × 50.

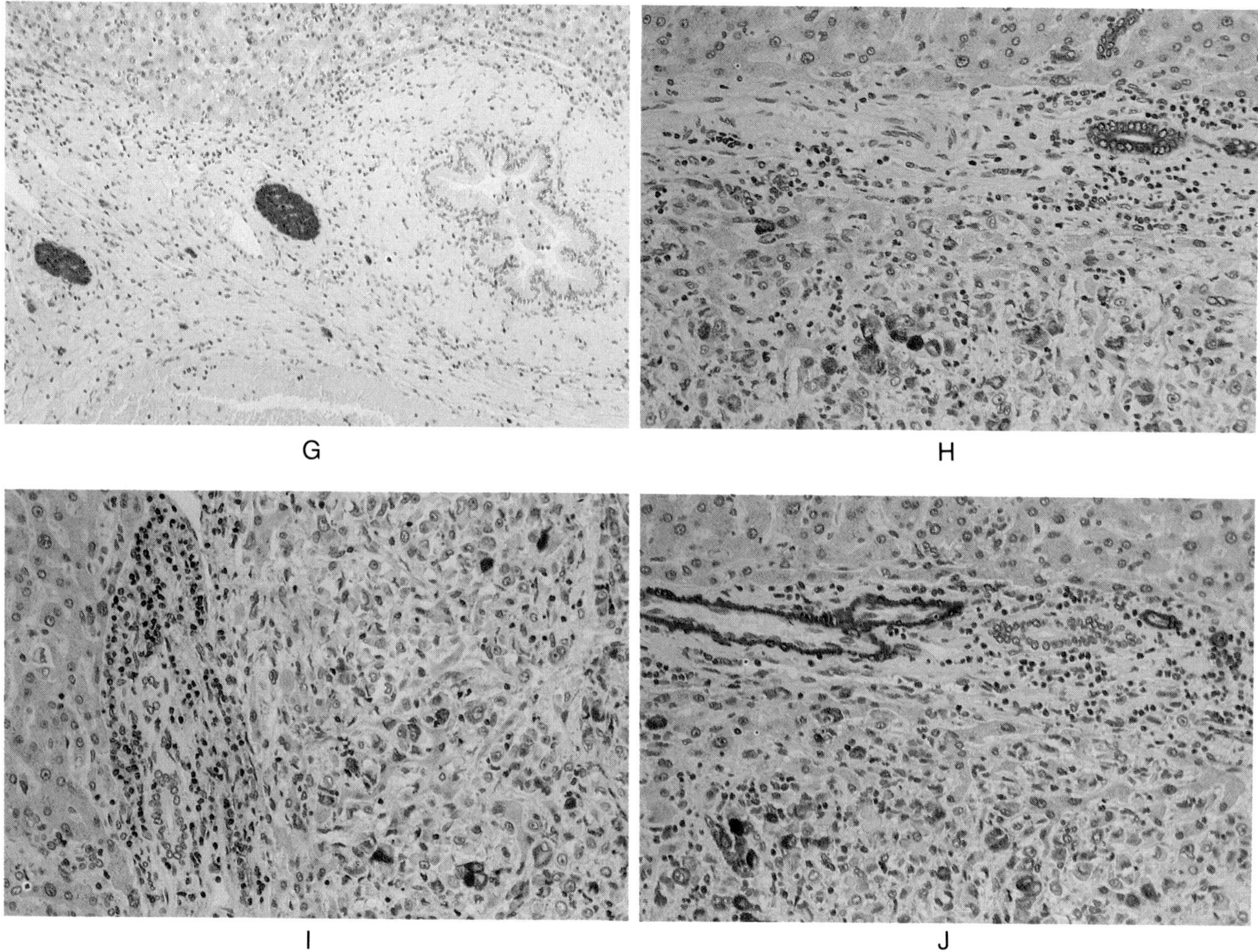

Figure 189–5 *Continued G,* Another area shows staining of peripheral nerves, and this represents an internal positive control for S100 staining. The bile duct epithelium and vessels do not stain and represent internal negative controls. Anti-S100, ×20. *H,* Staining with antibody to keratin intermediate filaments shows staining of bile duct epithelium only (*top right*). Although hepatocytes contain keratin, they stain only with antibodies directed toward keratin of low molecular weight and do not stain with this antibody, which is directed toward keratin of high molecular weight. The tumor cells in the lower part of the field also do not stain. Antikeratin, ×50. *I,* Staining of lymphocytes around a portal triad with an antibody to leukocyte common antigen. The tumor cells, bile duct epithelium, and hepatocytes do not stain. Anti-LCA, ×50. *J,* Staining of the smooth muscle of blood vesels with an antibody to muscle actin. The tumor cells, bile duct epithelium, and hepatocytes do not stain. Anti–muscle actin, ×50. The staining pattern of this panel of antibodies (positive S100 and HMB-45; negative keratin, LCA, and muscle actin) confirms that this neoplasm is a melanoma. The patient had undergone enucleation for a large melanoma of the ciliary body 18 months previously. (*B* to *J,* indirect immunoperoxidase, hematoxylin counterstain.)

Table 189–4. IMMUNOHISTOCHEMICAL STAINING OF SPINDLE-CELL NEOPLASMS*

Neoplasm	Vimentin	Muscle Actin	Smooth Muscle Actin	Desmin	S100	Factor VIIIR:Ag	UEA	Keratin	Myoglobin	References
Fibrous histiocytoma	*	†	†	‡	‡	‡	‡	‡	‡	40, 42, 66, 67
Rhabdomyosarcoma	*	*	‡	*	‡	‡	‡	‡	†	40, 53, 64, 68
Leiomyosarcoma	*	*	*	*	‡	‡	‡	‡	‡	40, 53
Liposarcoma	*	‡	‡	‡	†	‡	‡	‡	‡	31
Hemangiopericytoma	*	‡	‡	‡	‡	‡	‡	‡	‡	41, 59–61
Angiosarcoma	*	‡	‡	‡	‡	†	†	‡	‡	24, 40, 72, 73
Kaposi's sarcoma	*	‡	‡	‡	‡	†	*	‡	‡	24
Schwannoma, neurofibroma	*	‡	‡	‡	*	‡	‡	‡	‡	30–32
Malignant peripheral nerve sheath tumor	*	‡	‡	‡	†	‡	‡	‡	‡	31, 32, 74, 75
Chondrosarcoma	*	‡	‡	‡	†	‡	‡	‡	‡	30
Spindle-cell carcinoma	†	‡	‡	‡	‡	‡	‡	*	‡	1, 76, 77

*Usually stains for that antigen.
†May or may not stain.
‡Usually does not stain.

Talbe 189–5. IMMUNOHISTOCHEMICAL STAINING OF OTHER NEOPLASMS

Neoplasm	Vimentin	Keratin	EMA	S100	NSE	Chromo-granin	Synapto-physin	HMB-45	GFAP	LCA	References
Melanoma-uveal, conjunctival, orbital, metastatic	*	†	†	*	*	†	†	*	†	†	10, 30, 31, 39, 78–82
Carcinoma-metastatic, locally invasive, lacrimal	§	*	*	§	†	†	†	†	§	†	10, 15, 18, 42, 83
Large cell lymphoma	‡	†	†	†	†	†	†	†	†	*	57, 58
Granular cell tumor	*	†	†	*	†	†	†	†	†	†	31, 32, 84
Paraganglioma	*	†	†	‡	*	*	*	†	‡	†	85
Carcinoid tumor	†	*	NA	†	*	*	*	†	†	†	83, 86
Alveolar soft part sarcoma‖	‡	†	†	‡	‡	NA	†	†	†	†	87–89
Malignant rhabdoid tumor	*	*	‡	†	†	†	†	†	†	†	47, 48
Meningioma	*	‡	‡	‡	‡	NA	NA	†	†	†	70, 90
Astrocytoma	*	†	†	‡	‡	†	†	†	*	†	27

*Usually stains for that antigen.
†Usually does not stain.
‡May or may not stain.
§Lacrimal gland neoplasms may stain for vimentin, S100, and GFAP.
‖Some stain for desmin and muscle actin.
NA, Data not available.

Table 189–6. USES OF SOME IMMUNOHISTOCHEMICAL STAINS IN THE DIAGNOSIS OF LYMPHOID PROLIFERATIONS

Antigen	Use and Interpretation
Leukocyte common antigen	Stains almost all lymphomas of all subtypes; negative in virtually all carcinomas, melanomas, sarcomas, germ cell tumors, and neuroepithelial tumors
Immunoglobulins	To confirm B-lymphoid or plasma cell origin of a neoplasm; to demonstrate monoclonality of a B-lymphocytic or plasma cell proliferation and distinguish it from an inflammatory reaction
L26	To confirm B-cell origin of a lymphoma as stains almost all B-cell lymphomas; stains a few high-grade T-cell lymphomas
UCHL1	To confirm T-cell origin of a lymphoma as stains most T-cell lymphomas; stains a few high-grade B-cell lymphomas

by the ophthalmologist the majority are of small B-cell morphology, and a distinction from carcinoma and melanoma is not necessary.[93] Nevertheless, they all stain for LCA. The major problem is in the distinction of a neoplastic proliferation from an inflammatory proliferation. In addition to appropriate morphology, the diagnosis of a neoplastic proliferation has rested on the demonstration of monoclonality, although, as has been amply shown for orbital lymphoid proliferations, this does not always imply that systemic dissemination occurs. Immunohistochemically, monoclonality rests on the demonstration of κ or λ light chain restriction, because one lymphocyte can produce only one type of light chain, and in a neoplastic clone, all lymphocytes are assumed to be derived from one precursor cell.

Unfortunately, this technique, as easy as it sounds, suffers from numerous technical imprecisions and has not been as helpful as was initially envisioned. In fixed, paraffin-embedded tissue, only cytoplasmic immunoglobulin can be stained for reliably by any of the immunohistochemical techniques, and plasma cells and plasmacytoid lymphocytes are the only lymphoid cells with sufficient cytoplasmic immunoglobulin for this demonstration.[35, 57] However, most orbital small lymphocytic proliferations, although containing some, usually reactive, plasma cells, primarily consist of small lymphocytes that have only small quantities of immunoglobulin on the surface membrane of the cell, almost all of which is destroyed by fixation and paraffin embedding. This surface immunoglobulin can be demonstrated in fresh frozen tissue; however, this also has its disadvantages. It requires that a large enough biopsy be taken to be able to freeze a portion and to have enough for routine histology; it requires that the tissue be handled promptly and gently to preserve the immunoglobulin in situ and that the laboratory have the technical expertise to perform immunohistochemical stains on frozen tissue. Figure 189–6 shows the ideal application of immunohistochemical stains to Bouin's fixed and fresh frozen tissue from an orbital lymphoma of small lymphocytic type.

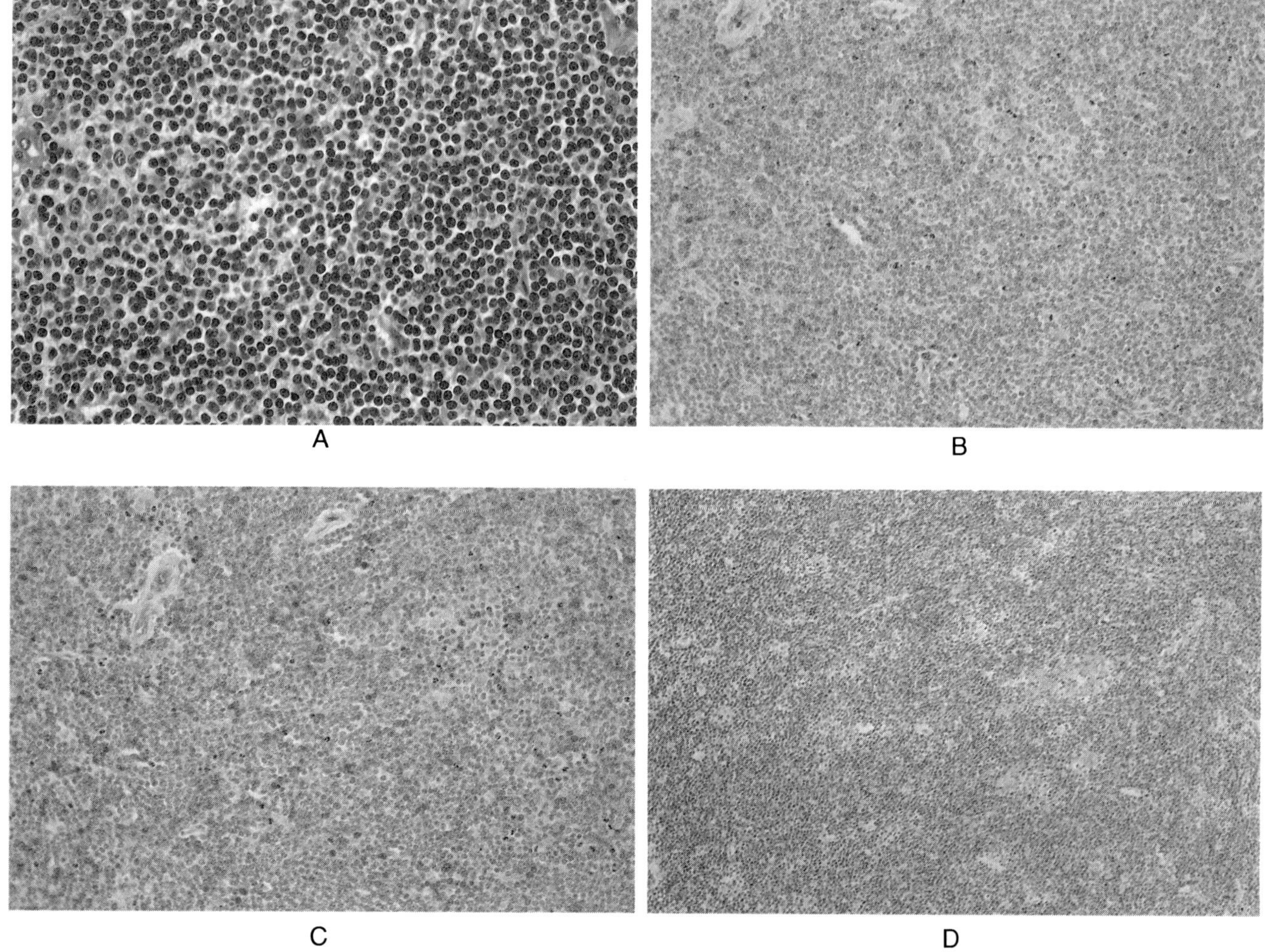

Figure 189–6. *A,* Small lymphocytic lymphoma of the orbit. H&E, ×80. *B,* Staining of Bouin's fixed, paraffin-embedded tissue for immunoglobulin light chains shows randomly dispersed plasma cells. Anti–κ light chains, ×20. *C,* Staining for λ immunoglobulin light chains shows a similar pattern. Anti–λ light chains, ×20. *D,* Staining of the lymphoma by the B-cell antibody L26 shows staining of most of the neoplastic cells with some lack of staining around blood vessels. L26, ×20.

Illustration continued on following page

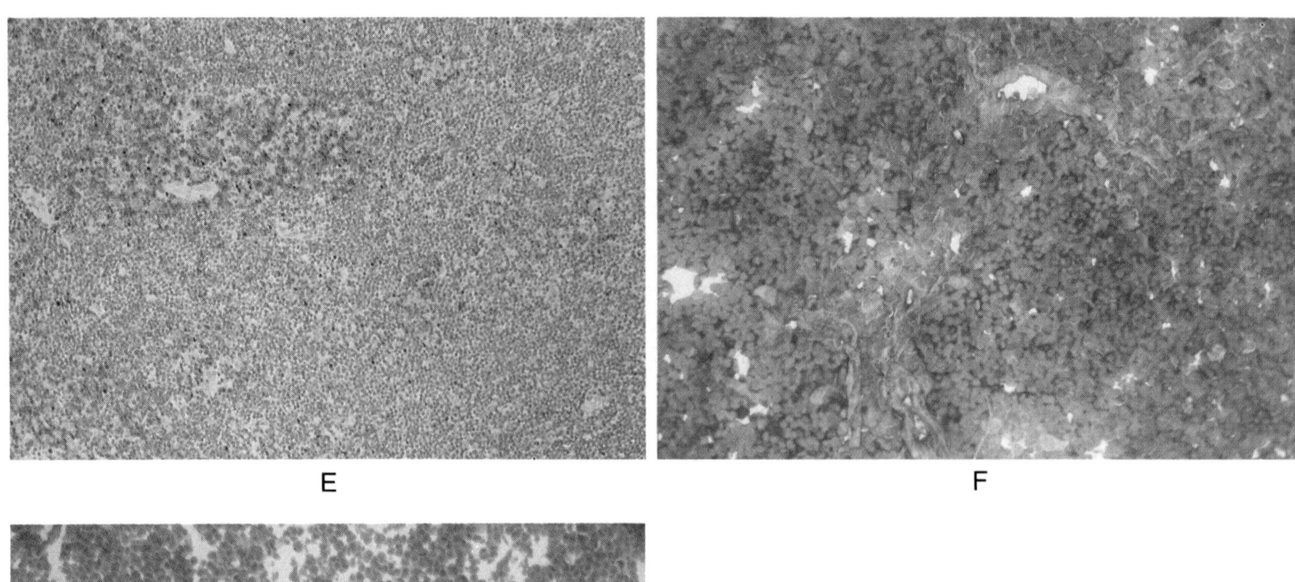

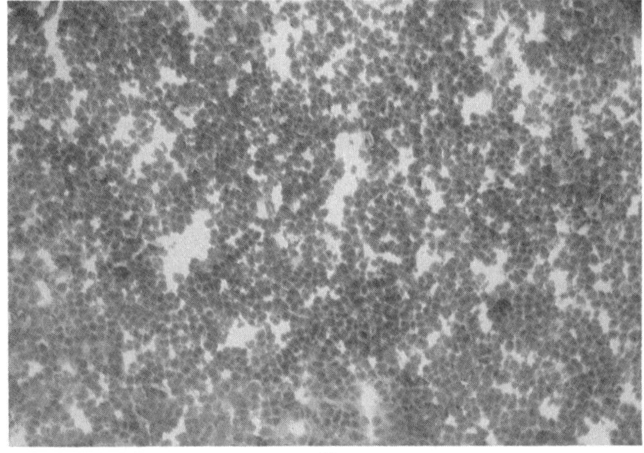

Figure 189–6 *Continued E,* Staining of the lymphoma by the T-cell antibody UCHL-1 shows staining of groups of cells around the vessels. Many B-cell lymphomas have a population of T cells. UCHL-1, ×20. *F,* Staining of fresh frozen lymphoma tissue shows strong surface membrane staining for κ immunoglobulin light chains. Anti–κ light chains, ×50. *G,* Staining of the same tissue for λ immunoglobulin light chains shows almost no evidence of staining. Anti–λ light chains, ×50. This lymphoma shows evidence of a monoclonal population of lymphocytes by the immunoglobulin staining pattern on fresh frozen tissue. It also shows immunoglobulin heavy chain and κ light chain gene rearrangements on DNA analysis. (*B* to *G,* indirect immunoperoxidase, hematoxylin counterstain.)

Even when all of these prerequisites have been attended to, the staining is often less than optimal owing to factors that are difficult to determine, and often a monoclonal population cannot be confirmed by this method. In practice, this may not matter because it has been shown that demonstration of phenotypic monoclonality is not a predictor of patients with an orbital small lymphocytic proliferation who will develop systemic disease.[93, 94] In addition, it has been shown that some phenotypically polyclonal lymphoid proliferations are genotypically monoclonal, following demonstration of immunoglobulin gene rearrangement in DNA extracted from the tumors.[95, 96] Not enough of these lesions have been followed to determine if this is a better predictor of systemic disease, although it is recognized to be much more sensitive than immunohistochemistry in the determination of monoclonality.[97, 98]

L26 and UCHL-1 are two other antibodies that are helpful generally in the diagnosis and typing of lymphomas, recognizing B-cell and T-cell lymphomas, respectively. Because most orbital lymphoid proliferations are of B-cell lineage, this determination is not usually required. These antibodies can also be used to determine the types of lymphocytes present in an inflammatory process.

Immunohistochemistry in Ophthalmic Pathology. All of the aforementioned techniques have been applied to the diagnosis of ophthalmic neoplasms as has been discussed earlier and in Chapter 187. These tools are necessary in the current diagnostic armamentarium.[99–102] Additionally, the same techniques with minor modifications have been used in the diagnosis of cytologic specimens obtained from fine needle aspiration biopsy.[103, 104] Immunohistochemistry has also been successfully applied to study the nature of cell types in inflammatory conditions that affect the eyes, such as cicatricial pemphigoid and ocular rosacea.[105–109]

REFERENCES

1. True LD: Atlas of Diagnostic Immunohistopathology. Philadelphia, JB Lippincott, 1990.
2. Pettigrew NM: Techniques in immunocytochemistry: Application to diagnostic pathology. Arch Pathol Lab Med 113:641, 1989.
3. Rickert RR, Maliniak RM: Intralaboratory quality assurance of immunohistochemical procedures. Arch Pathol Lab Med 113:673, 1989.
4. Swanson PE: Foundations of immunohistochemistry: A practical review. Am J Clin Pathol 90:333, 1988.
5. Roitt I: Essential Immunology, 6th ed. Oxford, Blackwell Scientific Publications, 1988.
6. Sternberger LA, Sternberger NH: The unlabeled antibody

method: Comparison of peroxidase-antiperoxidase with avidin-biotin complex by a new method of quantification. J Histochem Cytochem 34:599, 1986.
7. Sternberger LA, Hardy PH, Cuculis JJ, et al: The unlabeled antibody enzyme method of immunohistochemistry. J Histochem Cytochem 18:315, 1970.
8. Herrera GA: Ultrastructural postembedding immunogold labeling: Applications to diagnostic pathology. Ultrastruct Pathol 13:485, 1989.
9. Hsu S-M, Raine L, Fanger H: Use of avidin-biotin-peroxidase complex (ABC) in immunoperoxidase techniques: A comparison between ABC and unlabeled antibody (PAP) procedures. J Histochem Cytochem 29:577, 1981.
10. Corwin DJ, Gown AM: Review of selected lineage-directed antibodies useful in routinely processed tissues. Arch Pathol Lab Med 113:645, 1989.
11. Cooper D, Schermer A, Sun T-T: Biology of disease: Classification of human epithelia and their neoplasms using monoclonal antibodies to keratins: Strategies, applications and limitations. Lab Invest 52:243, 1985.
12. Sun T-T, Tseng SCG, Huang AJ-W, et al: Monoclonal antibody studies of mammalian epithelial keratins: A review. Ann N Y Acad Sci 455:307, 1985.
13. Gown AM, Vogel AM: Monoclonal antibodies to human intermediate filament proteins. II: Distribution of filament proteins in normal human tissues. Am J Pathol 114:309, 1984.
14. Moll R, Franke WW, Schiller DL, et al: The catalog of human cytokeratins: Patterns of expression in normal epithelia, tumors and cultured cells. Cell 31:11, 1982.
15. Pinkus GS, Etheridge CL, O'Connor EM: Are keratin proteins a better tumor marker than epithelial membrane antigen? A comparative immunohistochemical study of various paraffin-embedded neoplasms using monoclonal and polyclonal antibodies. Am J Clin Pathol 85:269, 1986.
16. Sloane JP, Hughes F, Ormerod MG: An assessment of the value of epithelial membrane antigen and other epithelial markers in solving diagnostic problems in tumour histopathology. Histochem J 15:645, 1983.
17. Sloane JP, Ormerod MG: Distribution of epithelial membrane antigen in normal and neoplastic tissues and its value in diagnostic tumor pathology. Cancer 47:1786, 1981.
18. Azumi N, Battifora H: The distribution of vimentin and keratin in epithelial and nonepithelial neoplasms. Am J Clin Pathol 88:286, 1987.
19. Miettinen M: Antibody specific to muscle actins in the diagnosis and classification of soft tissue tumors. Am J Pathol 130:205, 1988.
20. Tsukada T, McNutt MA, Ross R, et al: HHF35, a muscle actin–specific monoclonal antibody. II: Reactivity in normal, reactive and neoplastic human tissues. Am J Pathol 127:389, 1987.
21. Skalli O, Ropraz P, Trzeciak A, et al: A monoclonal antibody against a smooth muscle actin: a new probe for smooth muscle differentiation. J Cell Biol 103:2787, 1986.
22. Kindblom L-G, Seidal T, Karlsson K: Immuno-histochemical localization of myoglobin in human muscle tissue and embryonal and alveolar rhabdomyosarcoma. Acta Pathol Microbiol Immunol Scand 90:167, 1982.
23. Corson JM, Pinkus GS: Intracellular myoglobin—A specific marker for skeletal muscle differentiation in soft tissue sarcomas. Am J Pathol 103:384, 1981.
24. Ordonez NG, Batsakis JG: Comparison of Ulex europaeus I lectin and factor VIII-related antigen in vascular lesions. Arch Pathol Lab Med 108:129, 1984.
25. Ordonez NG, Brooks T, Thompson S, et al: Use of Ulex europaeus agglutinin I in the identification of lymphatic and blood vessel invasion in previously stained microscopic slides. Am J Surg Pathol 11:543, 1987.
26. Haimoto H, Takahashi Y, Koshikawa T, et al: Immunohistochemical localization of gamma-enolase in normal human tissues other than nervous and neuroendocrine tissues. Lab Invest 52:257, 1985.
27. Perentes E, Rubinstein LJ: Recent applications of immunoperoxidase histochemistry in human neuro-oncology: An update. Arch Pathol Lab Med 111:796, 1987.
28. Achtstatter T, Moll R, Anderson A, et al: Expression of glial filament protein (GFP) in nerve sheaths and non-neural cells re-examined using monoclonal antibodies, with special emphasis on the co-expression of GFP and cytokeratins in epithelial cells of human salivary gland and pleomorphic adenomas. Differentiation 31:206, 1986.
29. Loeffel SC, Gillespie GY, Mirmiran SA, et al: Cellular immunolocalization of S100 protein within fixed tissue sections by monoclonal antibodies. Arch Pathol Lab Med 109:117, 1985.
30. Kahn HJ, Marks A, Thom H, et al: Role of antibody to S100 protein in diagnostic pathology. Am J Clin Pathol 79:341, 1983.
31. Weiss SW, Langloss JM, Enzinger FM: Value of S-100 protein in the diagnosis of soft tissue tumors with particular reference to benign and malignant Schwann cell tumors. Lab Invest 49:299, 1983.
32. Nakajima T, Watanabe S, Sato Y, et al: An immunoperoxidase study of S-100 protein distribution in normal and neoplastic tissues. Am J Surg Pathol 6:715, 1982.
33. Wilson BS, Lloyd RV: Detection of chromogranin in neuroendocrine cells with a monoclonal antibody. Am J Pathol 115:458, 1984.
34. Gould VE, Lee I, Wiedenmann B, et al: Synaptophysin: a novel marker for neurons, certain neuroendocrine cells, and their neoplasms. Hum Pathol 17:979, 1986.
35. Taylor CR: Immunomicroscopy: A diagnostic tool for the surgical pathologist. *In* Bennington JL (ed): Major Problems in Pathology, vol 19. Philadelphia, WB Saunders, 1986.
36. Norton AJ, Isaacson PG: Lymphoma phenotyping in formalin-fixed and paraffin wax-embedded tissues. I: Range of antibodies and staining patterns. Histopathology 14:437, 1989.
37. Steinert PM, Steven AC, Roop DR: The molecular biology of intermediate filaments. Cell 42:411, 1985.
38. Lazarides E: Intermediate filaments as mechanical integrators of cellular space. Nature 283:249, 1980.
39. DeLellis RA, Dayal Y: The role of immunohistochemistry in the diagnosis of poorly differentiated malignant neoplasms. Semin Oncol 14:173, 1987.
40. Altmannsberger M, Dirk T, Osborn M, et al: Immunohistochemistry of cytoskeletal filaments in the diagnosis of soft tissue tumors. Semin Diagn Pathol 3:306, 1986.
41. Du Boulay CEH: Immunohistochemistry of soft tissue tumours: A review. J Pathol 146:77, 1985.
42. Gown AM, Vogel AM: Monoclonal antibodies to human intermediate filament proteins. III: Analysis of tumors. Am J Clin Pathol 84:413, 1985.
43. Virtanen I, Miettinen M, Lehto V-P, et al: Diagnostic application of monoclonal antibodies to intermediate filaments. Ann N Y Acad Sci 455:635, 1985.
44. Osborn M, Weber K: Biology of disease: Tumor diagnosis by intermediate filament typing: A novel tool for surgical pathology. Lab Invest 48:372, 1983.
45. Van Muijen GNP, Ruiter DJ, Warnaar SO: Coexpression of intermediate filament polypeptides in human fetal and adult tissues. Lab Invest 57:359, 1987.
46. Mierau GW, Weeks DA, Beckwith JB: Anaplastic Wilms' tumor and other clinically aggressive childhood renal neoplasms: Ultrastructural and immunocytochemical features. Ultrastruct Pathol 13:225, 1989.
47. Tsuneyoshi M, Daimaru Y, Hashimoto H, et al: Malignant soft tissue neoplasms with the histologic features of renal rhabdoid tumors. Hum Pathol 16:1235, 1985.
48. Vogel AM, Gown AM, Caughlan J, et al: Rhabdoid tumors of the kidney contain mesenchymal specific and epithelial specific intermediate filament proteins. Lab Invest 50:232, 1984.
49. Fisher C: Synovial sarcoma: Ultrastructural and immunohistochemical features of epithelial differentiation in monophasic and biphasic tumors. Hum Pathol 17:996, 1986.
50. Corson JM, Weiss LM, Banks-Schlegel SP, et al: Keratin proteins and carcinoembryonic antigen in synovial sarcomas. Hum Pathol 15:615, 1984.
51. Fisher C: Epithelioid sarcoma: The spectrum of ultrastructural differentiation in seven immunohistochemically defined cases. Hum Pathol 19:265, 1988.
52. Manivel JC, Wick MR, Dehner LP, et al: Epithelioid sarcoma: An immunohistochemical study. Am J Clin Pathol 87:319, 1987.
53. Azumi N, Ben-Ezra J, Battifora H: Immunophenotypic diagnosis

of leiomyosarcomas and rhabdomyosarcomas with monoclonal antibodies to muscle-specific actin and desmin in formalin-fixed tissue. Mod Pathol 1:469, 1988.
54. Gatter KC: Diagnostic immunocytochemistry: Achievements and challenges. J Pathol 159:183, 1989.
55. Michie SA, Spagnolo DV, Dunn KA, et al: A panel approach to the evaluation of the sensitivity and specificity of antibodies for the diagnosis of routinely processed histologically undifferentiated human neoplasms. Am J Clin Pathol 88:457, 1987.
56. Michels S, Swanson PE, Frizzera G, et al: Immunostaining for leukocyte common antigen using an amplified avidin-biotin-peroxidase complex method and paraffin sections. Arch Pathol Lab Med 111:1035, 1987.
57. Norton AJ, Isaacson PG: Lymphoma phenotyping in formalin-fixed and paraffin wax-embedded tissues. II: Profiles of reactivity in the various tumour types. Histopathology 14:557, 1989.
58. Davey FR, Elghetany MT, Kurec AS: Immunophenotyping of hematologic neoplasms in paraffin-embedded tissue sections. Am J Clin Pathol 93(Suppl 1):S17, 1990.
59. Darbyshire PJ, Bourne SP, Allan PM, et al: The use of a panel of monoclonal antibodies in pediatric oncology. Cancer 59:726, 1987.
60. Tsokos M, Linnoila RI, Chandra RS, et al: Neuron-specific enolase in the diagnosis of neuroblastoma and other small, round-cell tumors in children. Hum Pathol 15:575, 1984.
61. Shuangshoti S, Chaiwun B, Kasantikul V: A study of 39 retinoblastomas with particular reference to morphology, cellular differentiation and tumour origin. Histopathology 15:113, 1989.
62. Rodrigues MM, Wiggert B, Shields J, et al: Retinoblastoma: Immunohistochemistry and cell differentiation. Ophthalmology 94:378, 1987.
63. Molnar ML, Stefansson K, Marton LS, et al: Immunohistochemistry of retinoblastomas in humans. Am J Ophthalmol 97:301, 1984.
64. Altmannsberger M, Weber K, Droste R, et al: Desmin is a specific marker for rhabdomyosarcomas of human and rat origin. Am J Pathol 118:85, 1985.
65. Kahn HJ, Yeger H, Kassim O, et al: Immunohistochemical and electron microscopic assessment of childhood rhabdomyosarcoma. Cancer 51:1897, 1983.
66. Hirose T, Kudo E, Hasegawa T, et al: Expression of intermediate filaments in malignant fibrous histiocytomas. Hum Pathol 20:871, 1989.
67. Lawson CW, Fisher C, Gatter KC: An immunohistochemical study of differentiation in malignant fibrous histiocytoma. Histopathology 11:375, 1987.
68. De Jong ASH, Van Kessel-Van Vark M, Albus-Lutter CHE: Pleomorphic rhabdomyosarcoma in adults: immunohistochemistry as a tool for its diagnosis. Hum Pathol 18:298, 1987.
69. d'Amore ESG, Manivel JC, Sung JH: Soft-tissue and meningeal hemangiopericytomas: An immunohistochemical and ultrastructural study. Hum Pathol 21:414, 1990.
70. Winek RR, Scheithauer BW, Wick MR: Meningioma, meningeal hemangiopericytoma (angioblastic meningioma), peripheral hemangiopericytoma, and acoustic schwannoma: A comparative immunohistochemical study. Am J Surg Pathol 13:251, 1989.
71. Bohling T, Paetau A, Ekblom P, et al: Distribution of endothelial and basement membrane markers in angiogenic tumors of the nervous system. Acta Neuropathol 62:67, 1983.
72. Hufnagel T, Ma L, Kuo T-T: Orbital angiosarcoma with subconjunctival presentation. Ophthalmology 94:72, 1987.
73. Miettinen M, Lehto V-P, Virtanen I: Postmastectomy angiosarcoma (Stewart-Treves syndrome): Light-microscopic, immunohistological, and ultrastructural characteristics of two cases. Am J Surg Pathol 7:329, 1983.
74. Wick MR, Swanson PE, Scheithauer BW, et al: Malignant peripheral nerve sheath tumor: An immunohistochemical study of 62 cases. Am J Clin Pathol 87:425, 1987.
75. Stefansson K, Wollmann R, Jerkovic M: S-100 protein in soft-tissue tumors derived from Schwann cells and melanocytes. Am J Pathol 106:261, 1982.
76. Huntington AC, Langloss JM, Hidayat AA: Spindle cell carcinoma of the conjunctiva: An immunohistochemical and ultrastructural study of six cases. Ophthalmology 97:711, 1990.
77. Ellis GL, Langloss JM, Heffner DK, et al: Spindle-cell carcinoma of the aerodigestive tract: An immunohistochemical analysis of 21 cases. Am J Surg Pathol 11:335, 1987.
78. Leong AS-Y, Milios J: An assessment of a melanoma-specific antibody (HMB-45) and other immunohistochemical markers of malignant melanoma in paraffin-embedded tissues. Surg Pathol 2:137, 1989.
79. Ordonez NG, Xiaolong J, Hickey RC: Comparison of HMB-45 monoclonal antibody and S-100 protein in the immunohistochemical diagnosis of melanoma. Am J Clin Pathol 90:385, 1988.
80. Smoller BR, McNutt NS, Hsu A: HMB-45 recognizes stimulated melanocytes. J Cutan Pathol 16:49, 1989.
81. Gown AM, Vogel AM, Hoak D, et al: Monoclonal antibodies specific for melanocytic tumors distinguish subpopulations of melanocytes. Am J Pathol 123:195, 1986.
82. Rode J, Dhillon AP: Neuron specific enolase and S100 protein as possible prognostic indicators in melanoma. Histopathology 8:1041, 1984.
83. Thomas P, Battifora H: Keratins versus epithelial membrane antigen in tumor diagnosis: An immunohistochemical comparison of five monoclonal antibodies. Hum Pathol 18:723, 1987.
84. Mazur MT, Shultz JJ, Myers JL: Granular cell tumor: immunohistochemical analysis of 21 benign tumors and one malignant tumor. Arch Pathol Lab Med 114:692, 1990.
85. Kliewer KE, Wen D-R, Cancilla PA, et al: Paragangliomas: assessment of prognosis by histologic, immunohistochemical, and ultrastructural techniques. Hum Pathol 20:29, 1989.
86. Miettinen M: Synaptophysin and neurofilament proteins as markers for neuroendocrine tumors. Arch Pathol Lab Med 111:813, 1987.
87. Miettinen M, Ekfors T: Alveolar soft part sarcoma: Immunohistochemical evidence for muscle cell differentiation. Am J Clin Pathol 93:32, 1990.
88. Coira BM, Sachdev R, Moscovic E: Skeletal muscle markers in alveolar soft part sarcoma. Am J Clin Pathol 94:799, 1990.
89. Ordonez NG, Ro JY, Mackay B: Alveolar soft part sarcoma: an ultrastructural and immunocytochemical investigation of its histogenesis. Cancer 63:1721, 1989.
90. Artlich A, Schmidt D: Immunohistochemical profile of meningiomas and their histological subtypes. Hum Pathol 21:843, 1990.
91. Hsu S-M: The use of monoclonal antibodies and immunohistochemical techniques in lymphomas: Review and outlook. Hematol Pathol 2:183, 1988.
92. Picker LJ, Weiss LM, Medeiros LJ, et al: Immunophenotypic criteria for the diagnosis of non-Hodgkin's lymphoma. Am J Pathol 128:181, 1987.
93. Knowles DM, Jakobiec FA, McNally L, et al: Lymphoid hyperplasia and malignant lymphoma occurring in the ocular adnexa (orbit, conjunctiva, and eyelids): A prospective multiparametric analysis of 108 cases during 1977 to 1987. Hum Pathol 21:959, 1990.
94. Medeiros LJ, Harris NL: Immunohistologic analysis of small lymphocytic infiltrates of the orbit and conjunctiva. Hum Pathol 21:1126, 1990.
95. Jakobiec FA, Neri A, Knowles DM: Genotypic monoclonality in immunophenotypically polyclonal orbital lymphoid tumors: A model of tumor progression in the lymphoid system. Ophthalmology 94:980, 1987.
96. Medeiros LJ, Andrade RE, Harris NL, et al: Lymphoid infiltrates of the orbit and conjunctiva: comparison of immunologic and gene rearrangement data. Lab Invest 60:61A, 1989.
97. Sklar J: What can DNA rearrangements tell us about solid hematolymphoid neoplasms? Am J Surg Pathol 14(Suppl 1):16, 1990.
98. Cossman J, Uppenkamp M, Sundeen J, et al: Molecular genetics and the diagnosis of lymphoma. Arch Pathol Lab Med 112:117, 1988.
99. Lindquist TD, Orcutt JC, Gown AM: Monoclonal antibodies to intermediate filament proteins: Diagnostic specificity in orbital pathology. Surv Ophthalmol 32:421, 1988.
100. Rodrigues MM: Monoclonal antibodies in ophthalmology. Am J Ophthalmol 99:720, 1985.
101. Rootman J, Quenville N, Owen D: Recent advances in pathology as applied to orbital biopsy. Ophthalmology 91:708, 1984.
102. Messmer EP, Font RL: Applications of immunohistochemistry to ophthalmic pathology. Ophthalmology 91:701, 1984.

103. Nadji M, Ganjei P: Immunocytochemistry in diagnostic cytology: A 12-year perspective. Am J Clin Pathol 94:470, 1990.
104. Reifler DM, Kini SR, Kennerdell JS, et al: Immunocytologic methods in the diagnosis of orbital tumors. Henry Ford Hosp Med J 33:180, 1985.
105. Rice BA, Foster CS: Immunopathology of cicatricial pemphigoid affecting the conjunctiva. Ophthalmology 97:1476, 1990.
106. Hoang-Xuan T, Rodriguez A, Zaltas MM, et al: Ocular rosacea: A histologic and immunopathologic study. Ophthalmology 97:1468, 1990.
107. Sacks EH, Jakobiec FA, Wieczorek R, et al: Immunophenotypic analysis of the inflammatory infiltrate in ocular cicatricial pemphigoid. Ophthalmology 96:236, 1989.
108. Sacks EH, Wieczorek R, Jakobiec FA, et al: Lymphocytic subpopulations in the normal human conjunctiva. Ophthalmology 93:1276, 1986.
109. Sacks E, Rutgers J, Jakobiec FA, et al: A comparison of conjunctival and nonocular dendritic cells utilizing new monoclonal antibodies. Ophthalmology 93:1089, 1986.

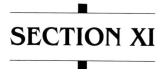

SECTION XI

Neuroophthalmology

Edited by

JOSEPH F. RIZZO III and SIMMONS LESSELL

Chapter 190

Overview

SIMMONS LESSELL

Neuroophthalmology is concerned with neurogenic disorders of vision, eye movements, pupils, and eyelids. Because there are no distinct boundaries between neuroophthalmology and the several related ophthalmic and neurologic subspecialties, this section contains information that overlaps with material presented elsewhere in these volumes but offers a neuroophthalmic perspective.

The ophthalmologist has a unique opportunity to diagnose and analyze certain neurologic disorders. A variety of neurologic symptoms can bring the patient initially to the ophthalmologist. Headache, for example, alleged to be the most prevalent of all symptoms, is commonly assumed to originate from the eye, which is a misconception reinforced by the frequent localization of pain to the eye or periorbital region. The ophthalmologist has the responsibility of deciding whether the headache reflects underlying structural disease and must determine how the patient should best be evaluated and managed. Double vision, transient visual loss, ptosis, and enlarged pupils are examples of other symptoms that are potentially indicative of serious neurologic disorders and that are likely to stimulate ophthalmic referral. Obviously, ophthalmologists must have a broad working knowledge of neurologic disorders and their eye manifestations. Finally, the ophthalmologist is probably the only physician equipped by training and experience to recognize the ocular origin of symptoms that might otherwise be erroneously attributed to lesions in the nervous system.

Chapter 191, which follows immediately, provides information on the clinical examination of patients with neuroophthalmic disorders. The neuroophthalmic history and physical examination remain the "gold standard," even in this era of sophisticated neuroimaging and electrophysiology, and are heavily emphasized.

The other sections are divided into neurogenic disorders of motility (Chapters 192 to 198), neurogenic disorders of vision (Chapters 199 to 209), and specific neurologic diseases of importance to the ophthalmologist (Chapters 210 to 215).

Ocular motility can be affected by lesions at several levels of the neuromuscular system, and this hierarchy is reflected in the organization of the various sections. Cannon discusses supranuclear aspects, and Halmagyi discusses the problems that arise from brain stem or cerebellar defects. Newman's section is devoted to disorders of the third, fourth, and sixth cranial nerves. Autonomic lesions, often manifested in the pupil and accommodation, are the subject of Bienfang's section. Disorders of the most peripheral portions of the motor apparatus—the eye muscles and their end-plates—are discussed in sections by Cogan and Borchert.

The section on sensory neuroophthalmology is also divided along anatomic lines, starting in the periphery. Rizzo describes neuroophthalmic retinal lesions. Sadun next discusses optic atrophy and papilledema, which are two of the most important eye signs of neurologic disease. The next six sections by Wray, Glaser, Katz, Feldon, Lessell, and Hepler review the optic neuropathies, including those of inflammatory, demyelinative, vascular, neoplastic, toxic, deficiency, and hereditary origin. Traumatic optic neuropathies are not included here but can be found in Chapter 280. Chiasmal disorders are the subject of Gittinger's section. Hedges discusses the retrochiasmal disorders of the visual pathway, and Mesulam discusses the so-called higher disorders of visual function that involve suprastriate processing.

Each of the last five sections is devoted to a neurologic disease that commonly presents with neuroophthalmic findings. Prominent among these are cerebrovascular diseases, which remain leading causes of death and disability. Caplan's section on stroke and transient ischemic attacks places these topics in perspective for the ophthalmologist. This is followed by Pruitt's section, which highlights pertinent aspects of neurooncology. Multiple sclerosis, discussed in the next section by Wall, is a prime example of a neurologic disorder that is likely to present initially to the ophthalmologist. The role of the ophthalmologist may be central in dealing with migraine and pseudotumor cerebri, which are discussed in the last two sections by Coppeto and Corbett.

Chapter 191

Clinical Examination

SIMMONS LESSELL

Nowhere in ophthalmology is the medical history as important as it is in the evaluation of patients with neuroophthalmic problems. The interview with the patient and any appropriate friends or relatives is best conducted by the physician and should not be delegated to nurses or technicians. History-taking is a dynamic transaction that requires an interrogator who has a broad knowledge of disease and does not lend itself to standardized questions or questionnaires. Guided by the patient's answers, each succeeding question aims to further define the location and nature of the patient's lesions. All available medical records should also be scrutinized. With inpatients, one is well advised to read the entire hospital chart. At minimum, a full past neurologic and ophthalmic history should be obtained in addition to the chief complaint and history of the present illness. A good history is one that permits the ophthalmologist to predict what, if anything, will be found when the patient is examined.

All elements of a full ophthalmic examination are incorporated in the neuroophthalmic examination and are not enumerated here. What follows is a discussion of elements that deserve special emphasis or modification in the neuroophthalmic context.

Regardless of the setting in which the patient is evaluated, an accurate, best-corrected Snellen visual acuity reading must be obtained at every examination. The patient should be pushed to the limits of his or her vision, using whatever lenses or other devices effect the best acuity. It is a rare patient who cannot see at least one line more than he or she alleges. If all the letters are read on a line, some letters will be legible on the next smaller line. Force the patient to guess. If a reduced Snellen chart is used to examine a patient in bed, carefully control the distance at which the chart is held. Snellen acuity fractions have little meaning if the numerator is inaccurate.

The neuroophthalmic visual-field test is tailored to the individual patient and situation. Confrontation testing is possible even in demented, agitated, or confused patients and also in infants, and this testing should be attempted. More formal testing is feasible in most other patients and is an integral part of the initial evaluation. A tangent screen examination offers some advantages over other techniques and is probably underutilized in the era of computerized perimetry. If symptoms and signs suggest the presence of small scotomas in the central portions of the field, a tangent screen examination at 1 or 2 m with small white and colored test objects is sometimes the only method of locating and characterizing the defects. Tubular constriction, such as one encounters in hysteria and malingering, is best demonstrated on the tangent screen. Perimetry offers several advantages, including the capacity to explore the entire extent of the field, excellent monitoring of fixation, and reproducibility. Computerized perimetry eliminates the potential biases introduced by the examiner in noncomputerized techniques. Noncomputerized perimetry, however, has the advantage of allowing flexibility. Thus, the examiner can make modifications during testing in order to concentrate on areas of particular interest and can alter the pace and duration of the procedure to accommodate the patient. We prefer noncomputerized projection perimetry for the screening of routine neuroophthalmic patients. If a defect is demonstrated and serial visual field tests are indicated, computerized perimetry is the method of choice.

Maculopathies and optic neuropathies share many symptoms, and both must be considered in the differential diagnosis of nonrefractive visual loss in patients with normal anterior segments. Dyschromatopsia is a common finding in optic neuropathies and can help to distinguish between neural and other forms of visual impairment. Color vision should be tested in each eye with pseudoisochromatic plates, and the results should be recorded as the number of plates correctly identified over the number presented. Useful information can also be obtained by having the patient make an inter-eye comparision of color intensity while viewing a red object.

Several other tests also help in differential diagnosis. Patients can be asked to make a brightness comparison between the two eyes, and there are even devices that permit measurement of inter-eye brightness disparity. Brightness sense is reduced in optic neuropathies. The delayed recovery from glare that characterizes some maculopathies can also be quantitated. The metamorphopsia of retinopathies may be identified by using Amsler's grids.

Pupils are best examined by careful inspection in dim light with the patient looking into the distance. Note the size and shape, and measure the pupils if there are any abnormalities. Reactions to light and near should also be recorded. Compare the extent of any anisocoria in dim and bright light. A relative afferent pupillary defect may be detected by swinging a flashlight from one eye to the other and showing that the pupils always dilate when the light is moved to one of the eyes. Relative afferent pupil defects can be quantitated with neutral density filters.

There are a host of lid signs of neuroophthalmic significance. Lid retraction is present if sclera shows above the corneal limbus. Lag may be evident when the patient follows a target moving slowly down. If there is ptosis, it is important to determine if it is increased with fatigue, accompanied by weakness of the orbicularis oculi, or associated with an elevated lower lid. Elevation of a ptotic lid on downgaze or attempted ocular adduction is a sign of aberrant regeneration of the third nerve. In the Marcus Gunn jaw-winking syndrome, a ptotic lid elevates with jaw movements. Palpation of the lids is an essential part of the examination of patients with ptosis.

The neuroophthalmic ocular motility examination goes beyond measuring phorias, tropias, ductions, and vergences. One should be alert to detect the abnormal head postures that result from disordered ocular motility. Inspection of the eyes during steady fixation in the primary position reveals nystagmus or other intrusions. The patient's capacity to execute rapid (saccadic) and slow (pursuit) movements in the vertical and horizontal planes and the range of these movements may provide useful localizing clues. Note if there is spontaneous nystagmus in any direction and characterize the nystagmus as completely as possible. Nystagmus and other adventitious eye movements missed on gross inspection may be detected during slit-lamp examination or direct ophthalmoscopy. Ocular dysmetria is manifested as inaccurate refixations with undershoots or overshoots. By eliciting nystagmus with an opticokinetic target, one can demonstrate asymmetries that help in cerebral localization. Down-rotating targets elicit the retractory movements in pretectal lesions.

Although the neuroophthalmic examination is not a complete neurologic examination, the physician will have learned a great deal about the neurologic status of the patient before the formal examination has begun. Gait, station, and coordination can be observed as the patient is greeted and accompanied to the office. Deficits in language, memory, speech, mood, behavior, hearing, and orientation will be evident while taking the history. Facial, orbital, and cranial asymmetries and anomalies, skin lesions, and adventitious movements of the face or limbs tend to be obvious. Auscultation for bruits over the carotids, the orbits, and head; testing of olfaction; cranial sensation; and motility can be added when appropriate.

The care of patients with neuroophthalmic problems is likely to be shared with nonophthalmologists, and therefore it is imperative that the ophthalmologist communicate clearly with the other physicians. Nothing less than prompt, legible, coherent narrative reports, free of special ophthalmic abbreviations, are required.

Chapter 192

Basic Mechanisms of Ocular Motor Control

STEPHEN C. CANNON

CLASSIFICATION OF EYE MOVEMENTS

Our understanding of ocular motor control has advanced rapidly during the last 30 yr, in part, because the *purpose* of eye movements can be defined so clearly: To maintain high acuity, images must be held steadily on the retina. Image motion of only a few degrees per second leads to significant blurring.[1] Two disturbances potentially cause image motion across the retina—movement of the observer or motion of the visual object of interest—and five distinct types of eye movements have evolved to counteract these disturbances or to bring new objects of interest onto the fovea (Table 192–1). Recognition of these five functionally, and to a large part anatomically, distinct subsystems of ocular motor control is a tremendous aid to critically observing and understanding both normal and pathologic eye movements.

Vestibuloocular and optokinetic eye movements stabilize images on the retina during head rotation by counterrolling the eyes through an angle equal to that of the head, but opposite in direction. Angular acceleration of the head deflects the cupula of the semicircular canal, which in turn changes the firing rate of the vestibular afferent nerve and leads to a compensatory eye rotation within 14 to 19 msec.[2] The latency of the vestibuloocular reflex (VOR) is shorter than any visual feedback system (approximately 100 msec), but owing to the mechanical properties of the canals this reflex decays during sustained rotations. The mechanism of compensatory eye movements during sustained head rotation gradually shifts from the VOR to optokinetic nystagmus (OKN), which is driven by visual cues.[3–5] Thus, the VOR and OKN keep images stationary on the retina and *maintain constant gaze* (eye position relative to the earth) by generating slow eye movements equal to and opposite head motion.

In contrast saccadic, smooth pursuit, and vergence eye movements *shift gaze* to bring new objects of interest onto the fovea. Saccades are rapid conjugate eye movements that redirect the fovea toward an object in the retinal periphery. They are optimized, in part, for speed, and there is a relatively consistent relationship between

Table 192–1. Functional Classification of Eye Movements

Type of Eye Movement	Purpose of Eye Movement
Vestibuloocular reflex (VOR)	Slow, conjugate eye movements to stabilize *gaze* (eye position in space) during head rotation by turning the eyes opposite to the direction of head motion. Large-amplitude head rotations generate nystagmus with a slow compensatory phase and a fast, resetting quick phase.
Optokinetic response	Slow, conjugate eye movements elicited by persistent rotation of the visual surround. Augments the VOR for sustained rotations.
Saccades	Rapid, conjugate eye movements to shift *gaze* and bring objects in the visual periphery onto the fovea. Saccades may be voluntary or triggered as quick phases of nystagmus.
Smooth pursuit	Slow, conjugate eye movements for tracking objects with the fovea.
Vergence	Slow, disconjugate eye movements to independently direct both foveae at a single target.

After Leigh RJ, Zee DS: The Neurology of Eye Movements. Philadelphia, FA Davis, 1983.

saccade amplitude and peak velocity.[6] The quick phases of nystagmus that rapidly turn the eyes toward the direction of self-rotation, between the compensatory slow phases of vestibular or optokinetic nystagmus, have the same dynamics and use the same neural machinery as saccades.[7] Smooth pursuit movements utilize visual feedback to track small objects and thus keep their image on the fovea. The smooth pursuit system may also have a role in the suppression of the VOR, while tracking an object with head movements[8] (see VOR cancellation later). Vergence movements are slow disconjugate changes in horizontal eye position that redirect each fovea independently toward an object in response to disparity between the images of one object on both retinas or as an accompaniment of accommodation in response to blurring.

OCULAR MOTOR CONTROL SIGNALS: A SYNTHESIS

To effectively interpret abnormal eye movements, one must first have a clear understanding of how the central nervous system (CNS) normally controls eye movement.[9, 10] Our understanding of the neuroanatomy and firing patterns of neurons that code for eye movements has advanced to the stage at which specific functions have been attributed to various anatomic components of the CNS. Furthermore, from a synthesis of the interconnections between these components, accurate predictions can be made on how the overall oculomotor system will behave when one element is impaired.[11]

Motoneuron: The Final Output

Motoneurons of the third, fourth, or sixth cranial nerve are, of course, the final output of the central nervous system for controlling eye movement. Knowing how a motoneuron's firing pattern must change in order to move or hold the eye is a prerequisite for understanding the necessity of and logic for all the signals* carried by premotor neurons.

*Signals and commands refer to the neuronal firing patterns, measured as the instantaneous discharge rate (reciprocal of interspike interval), that create subsequent eye movements.

Physically, the resistance to moving the eye arises from the inertia, viscosity, and elasticity of the globe and orbital connective tissue.[12] Inertia and viscosity are applicable only during motion of the eye. To hold the eye stationary at an eccentric orbital position, the extraocular muscles must generate enough force to overcome the elastic restoring forces of the orbital tissues that tend to pull the eye centripetally to the primary position. When a monkey fixates on a target, motoneurons discharge regularly at a constant rate (Fig. 192–1*A*).[13–15, 231] At fixation points further in the pulling direction for the muscle's motoneuron (the "on" direction), the discharge rate increases. In the primary or "straight ahead" position, the firing rate of most motoneurons is well above zero. The tonic firing rate in the primary position is approximately 100 spikes/sec. Consequently there is a resting tension in the muscles, for example about 12 g for horizontal recti.[16, 17] As the eye fixates further in the off direction the firing rate decreases until it reaches zero (ceases to discharge) at some threshold orbital position. The motoneuron firing rate is linearly proportional to eye position for fixation points above the threshold for firing. The sensitivity or slope (change in firing rate per degree of eye rotation) varies from one cell to another and has an average value of 4.0 (spikes/sec)/degree.

When the eyes are moving, there is an additional modulation in motoneuron firing rate that varies linearly with eye velocity.[13, 14] By measuring the instantaneous firing rate of a motoneuron as the eye passes by a fixed position at different speeds, the variation in motoneuron firing rate with eye velocity can be measured independently from any eye position effects. Figure 192–1*B* shows the discharge pattern of a motoneuron recorded during smooth pursuit eye movements in an awake monkey. At the times labeled 1 and 2 the eye position is the same, and yet the motoneuron firing rate is different. At point 1 the eye is moving in the "off" direction for this motoneuron, and therefore the firing rate is less than at point 2 where smooth pursuit is in the "on" direction. Over the range of about ±100 degrees/sec the change in primate motoneuron firing rate varies linearly with eye velocity, with an average sensitivity of 0.95 (spike/sec)/(degree/sec). The linear relationship implies that this additional component in neuronal discharge, above the eye-position dependence,

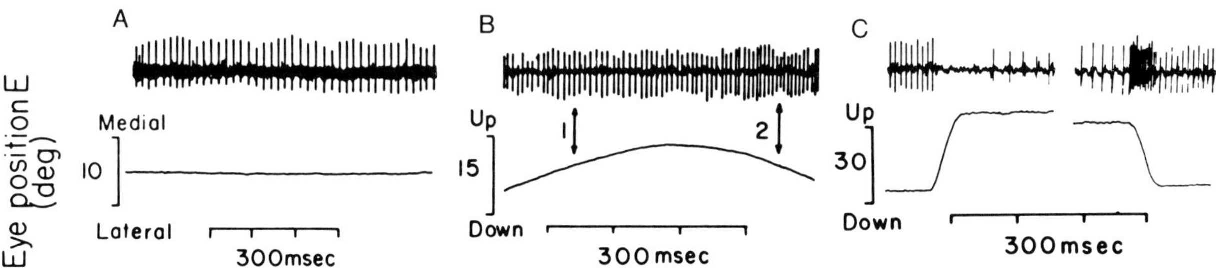

Figure 192–1. Firing patterns of motoneurons in the monkey during fixation *(A)*, smooth pursuit *(B)*, and saccades *(C)*. *A*, During fixation, both the eye position *(bottom trace)* and the firing rate *(top trace)* are steady. *B*, With smooth pursuit, the firing rate is much lower when the eye passes by a given position in the off direction (time 1) than when it passes the same position in the on direction (time 2). This demonstrates an eye-velocity dependence of the firing rate, in addition to the eye-position dependence. (*A* and *B*, From Robinson DA, Keller EL: The behavior of eye movement motoneurons in the alert monkey. Bibl Ophthal 82:7, 1972.) *C*, Before or after a saccade, the motoneuron discharge rate is steady. The cell exhibits bursts of firing (the *pulse*) for saccades in the on direction and then maintains a new, higher, steady discharge rate after the saccade (the *step*). In the off direction, premotor inhibition may silence the motoneuron during the saccade. (*C*, From Robinson DA: Oculomotor unit behavior in the monkey. J Neurophysiol 33:393, 1970.)

is required to overcome a retarding force on the globe proportional to eye velocity, that is a simple linear viscous drag. Because eye velocity may reach several hundred degrees per sec during saccades or quick phases of nystagmus, the eye velocity–dependent portion of motoneuron firing rate may be quite pronounced (see Figure 192–1*C*). Motoneuron firing rate is only weakly related to eye acceleration.[18] Thus, the viscoelastic properties of the globe and extraocular muscles dominate over the inertial load of the globe. The latter effect only becomes significant when examining fine details of motoneuron behavior during large, rapid saccades.

It is meaningless to consider which component of motoneuron discharge rate, eye position or eye velocity, is more "important." Both components are required to overcome the viscoelastic retarding force of the globe and bring the eyes on target. The eye-position signal is constant whenever the eyes are held stationary at the completion of an eye movement, and thus is called the *tonic* component. (See the portions of the record in Figure 192–1*C* before or after the saccade.) The eye velocity–encoded modulation is a transient change in motoneuron discharge rate during the eye movement and is referred to as the *phasic* component (see Fig. 192–1*C*, during the eye movement). The change in firing rate for a single motoneuron varies consistently with eye position and eye velocity, regardless of which oculomotor subsystem generated the movement. There are not separate "smooth pursuit" or "VOR" motoneurons,[19] nor are vergence movements encoded by a separate population of motoneurons.[20]

Neural Integrator: A Final Common Pathway

Motoneuron firing rate varies with both eye position and eye velocity. Recordings from premotor neurons in the brain stem, however, have shown that commands for all conjugate eye movements originate as eye velocity–encoded signals only, with no eye position component. For example, neurons in the paramedian pontine reticular formation (PPRF) discharge transiently in a direction-specific manner during saccades or quick phases of nystagmus and are otherwise silent.[21, 22] Their instantaneous firing rate (reciprocal of interspike interval) is a brief *pulse* that encodes the eye-velocity signal for rapid eye movements[18]; hence the name burst neurons. After a saccade, when the eye remains stationary, there is a *step* change in motoneuron firing rate—the eye-position signal (see Fig. 192–1*C*). Since there are no neuron collateral projections within a pool of motoneurons and proprioceptive feedback from extraocular muscles does not provide an eye position signal to motoneurons,[23] a premotor network of neurons must generate the eye-position command from the only available information, the eye-velocity signal. Position is the integral (in the mathematical sense) of velocity, and the neural network that performs this function has been called the *neural integrator.*[24]

Other conjugate eye movement signals are also generated as eye velocity commands. Primary vestibular afferent fibers discharge with a high resting rate that is modulated in proportion to head velocity, which equals the eye velocity command during the VOR.[25] Second-order neurons in the vestibular nucleus also carry the eye velocity signal for optokinetic movements,[26] and the firing rate of gaze-velocity Purkinje cells of the flocculus modulates in proportion to smooth pursuit velocity.[27]

Theoretical arguments[28] and experimental lesions[29–31] have demonstrated that there is one neural integrator shared by all of the oculomotor subsystems to generate the eye position signal for horizontal conjugate eye movements and have led to the concept of the *final common integrator* (Fig. 192–2). All eye movements are initially generated as eye-velocity signals on premotor neurons ($\dot{E}'$ in Fig. 192–2). Eye velocity signals from each oculomotor subsystem both project to motoneurons and converge upon the neural integrator that generates the eye-position signal sent to the motoneuron. Except for burst neurons, all premotor neurons have high resting discharge rates, similar to the primary vestibular afferents described earlier. The eye velocity signal is encoded as a change from this background rate, and homolateral premotor pathways are modulated in opposite directions—increased firing rate for pathways

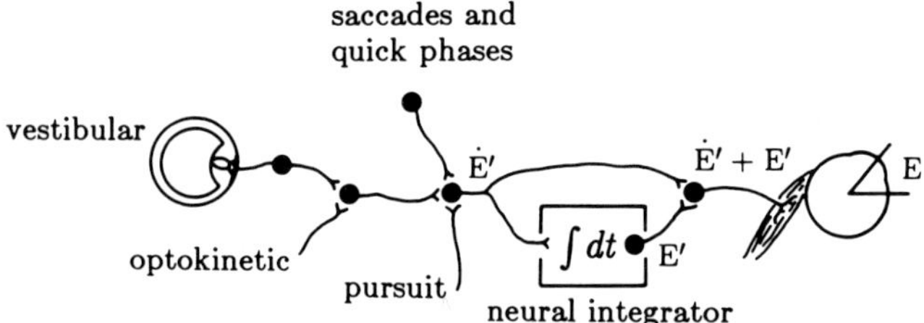

Figure 192–2. The final common integrator hypothesis. All conjugate eye movements (E) are initiated as eye-velocity commands (Ė′) that converge upon the neural integrator where eye-velocity signals are converted to eye-position commands (E′). Both the eye-velocity and the eye-position commands are then relayed to the motoneurons. This representation is schematic and is intended only to show the premotor signal processing of eye-movement commands; it does not represent actual anatomic pathways. Most likely, the "neural integrator" both converts the eye-velocity command to the eye-position signal and adds the former to the latter on the *same* population of neurons.[232] This possibility is supported by the fact that most premotor neurons that carry the eye-position signal also encode eye-velocity commands, whereas purely eye-position–encoding neurons are rare. (From Cannon SC, Robinson DA: Loss of the neural integrator of the oculomotor system from brain stem lesions in monkey. J Neurophysiol 57:1383, 1987.)

to agonist and decreased rate to antagonist muscle groups. Integration of this "push-pull" eye velocity signal, independent from the background firing rate, requires that the integrator be constructed from lateral inhibitory projections interconnecting homolateral structures in the brain stem.[32, 232] Because of this interdependence, there are not separate integrators for leftward and rightward movements, and a unilateral lesion of the integrator network affects eye movements in both the ipsilateral and contralateral directions.[29]

The integrity of the neural integrator is most readily evaluated clinically by examining saccades. Unlike ongoing slow eye movements (smooth pursuit, VOR, OKN), there is no eye velocity signal at the end of a saccade, and the eye position signal can be tested in isolation. The entire premotor command becomes the output from the neural integrator, and consequently, a major function of the neural integrator is to form a gaze-holding network. The inability to maintain eccentric eye position is the hallmark of neural integrator malfunction and is clinically manifest as gaze-evoked nystagmus:conjugate, centripetal drift of the eyes with an exponential time course, interrupted by quick phases that beat eccentrically to bring the eyes on target.

A qualitative evaluation of integrator function may be performed at the bedside. Instruct the patient to fixate on a target about 20 degrees from the center, either horizontally or vertically. Normally steady gaze is maintained, although at extreme positions beyond 20 degrees most patients show a few beats of nystagmus. Persistent nystagmus with quick phases beating eccentrically, in the direction of the fixation target, indicates integrator impairment. Gaze-evoked nystagmus becomes more pronounced (faster slow-phase drift) with targets placed further eccentrically. Any form of nystagmus with a slow-phase velocity that *varies* with *orbital position* is attributable in part to integrator malfunction.[29, 33] After maintaining eccentric gaze for tens of seconds, the nystagmus may diminish, then recur and beat in the opposite direction when the eyes are brought back to the primary position where there previously was no nystagmus. This *rebound nystagmus*[34] is particularly common with cerebellar lesions[35, 36] and may be the result of attempts by the nervous system to null the drift during gaze-evoked nystagmus.

Quantitatively, integrator performance is measured by the time constant of the exponential drift in eye position. The time constant is equal to the amplitude of the change in eye position (from a neutral orbital position where no nystagmus occurs) divided by the initial velocity of the drift. This number represents the time that would be required for the eye position to drift 63 percent back toward the rest position if no quick phases were made. Normally the eyes drift very little, even in the absence of vision, so that the drift velocity is small and the time constant is large (approximately $>$ 20 sec[37]). A time constant of 10 sec or less creates clinically appreciable nystagmus, and a lower limit of 0.2 sec is constrained by the mechanics of the orbit.[12]

The neural integrator for horizontal eye movements resides anatomically at the pontomedullary junction, in the rostral half of the medial vestibular nucleus (MVN) and the adjacent nucleus prepositus hypoglossi (NPH).[29–31] Lesions in this region simultaneously cause severe gaze-evoked nystagmus and highly abnormal slow eye movements (VOR, optokinetic, and smooth pursuit), all characterized by a step change in eye *position* whenever the stimulus would normally elicit a constant eye *velocity*—precisely the defect predicted from an absence of the neural integrator in Figure 192–2. *The superior vestibular nucleus (SVN) in the pons and the interstitial nucleus of Cajal in the mesencephalon form the analogous circuit for vertical eye movements.*[38] Although lesions in the MVN/NPH cause the most severe damage to the neural integrator for horizontal eye movements, other CNS structures, particularly the *flocculus* of the cerebellum,[39–41] strongly influence the performance of this network such that lesions outside the brain stem can degrade integrator performance. In addition to structural lesions of the vestibulocerebellum, cerebellopontine angle, or pontomedullary junction, drugs are another common cause of gaze-evoked nystagmus, particularly anticonvulsants[42] or sedatives.

Horizontal Gaze Pathways

The abducens nucleus in the pons is the final assembly site for horizontal eye movements.[43] Forty to sixty percent of the nucleus is composed of motoneurons[44, 45] whose axons exit the brain stem ventrally and innervate the ipsilateral lateral rectus. The remaining cells are either interneurons that project to flocculus[46] or internuclear neurons whose axons decussate to the contralateral medial longitudinal fasciculus (MLF) and project rostrally to synapse with motoneurons of the medial rectus subdivision of the contralateral oculomotor nucleus[47] (Fig. 192–3). Functionally the firing patterns of abducens motoneurons and internuclear neurons are

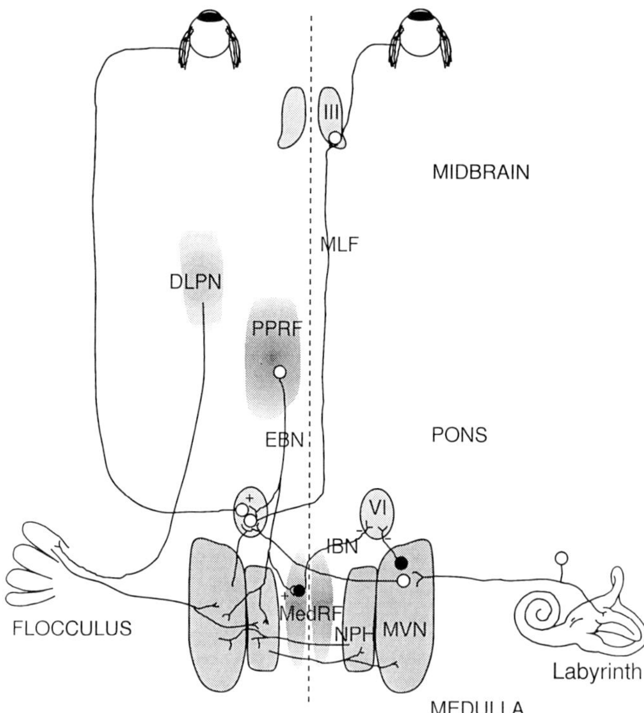

Figure 192–3. Pathways for the control of horizontal conjugate eye movements. The abducens nucleus (VI) contains motoneurons that innervate the ipsilateral lateral rectus and internuclear neurons to the contralateral medial rectus subdivision of the oculomotor nucleus (III) via the medial longitudinal fasciculus (MLF). Horizontal canal afferents project primarily to the medial vestibular nucleus (MVN) and the flocculus. Second-order vestibular neurons in the MVN excite neurons in the contralateral VI nucleus. Excitatory burst neurons (EBN) lie within the paramedian pontine reticular formation (PPRF) and project to the ipsilateral abducens nucleus and the vestibular nuclear complex. Inhibitory burst neurons (IBN) are caudal to the abducens nucleus in the paramedian medullary reticular formation (MedRF) and inhibit the contralateral abducens nucleus. Reciprocal commissural connections between the nucleus propositus hypoglossi (NPH) and the MVN probably form the anatomic substrate for the neural integrator. Smooth pursuit commands project from the dorsolateral pontine nuclei (DLPN) to the flocculus and then to the MVN-NPH complex. For simplicity, only pathways for leftward eye movement are illustrated; all projections have bilateral counterparts. Filled circles represent inhibitory neurons; open circles, excitatory neurons.

very similar, although the eye velocity and eye position sensitivity may be slightly greater for internuclear neurons.[48] Anatomically they are intermingled within the nucleus so that it is not possible to have a partial lesion of the abducens nucleus that selectively destroys motoneurons or interneurons. Consequently, lesions of the abducens *nucleus* cause a loss of *conjugate* ipsilateral horizontal eye movement.[49] Adduction of the contralateral eye during vergence is spared and demonstrates that this input to the medial rectus subdivision of the oculomotor complex is not conveyed by the internuclear neurons. A more ventral lesion in the basis pontis may interrupt the *fascicles* of the abducens and facial nerves while leaving the nucleus intact and thus cause a *monocular* paresis of abduction in the ipsilateral eye, ipsilateral facial weakness, and a contralateral hemiplegia (Millard-Gubler syndrome). Adduction of the contralateral eye is spared, and the patient experiences horizontal diplopia when looking away from the hemiplegia (toward the brain stem lesion).

The internuclear fibers of the MLF convey all the commands for adduction of the ipsilateral eye during versions (conjugate eye movements). Both the eye position and eye velocity components of the motor command for all types of horizontal eye movements are present in the MLF, which appears to simply relay these commands to the medial rectus motoneurons.[50] Thus a complete unilateral lesion of the MLF, rostral to the level of the abducens nucleus in the pons, causes a paresis of adduction in the ipsilateral eye during conjugate eye movements. Adduction is preserved for convergence, unless the lesion is in the most rostral portion of the MLF, where vergence input enters the oculomotor complex.[51] Abduction in this same eye may be slow or "fractionated,"[52] possibly because of impaired inhibition or disfacilitation of the medial rectus. Frequently, abduction nystagmus occurs in the contralateral eye. With lateral gaze, the eye drifts centripetally and is reset with saccades that may undershoot, overshoot, or bring the eye on target.[53] Owing to the paresis of adduction in the ipsilateral eye, the nystagmus is "dissociated" with larger amplitude and faster quick phases in the abducted eye. The constellation of adduction paresis with or without abduction nystagmus in the contralateral eye is called an *internuclear ophthalmoplegia* (INO). There is disagreement about the underlying mechanism of the abduction nystagmus.[52, 54–56] Recent evidence, however, has demonstrated that the nystagmus diminishes after patching one eye for days[54] and that it is not present in primates after acute experimental lesions of the MLF induced by lidocaine injections.[57] *Consequently, the nystagmus is thought to be due, at least in part, to an adaptive mechanism that attempts to chronically compensate for the adduction paresis.*[54] An INO is named for the side with weak adduction; that is, a left INO produces adduction paresis of the left eye and nystagmus in the right eye when the patient attempts to fixate a target on the right owing to a lesion of the left MLF. A less complete lesion of the MLF may cause only a subtle slowing of adducting saccades in the ipsilateral eye with normal abduction in the contralateral eye. Because medial rectus motoneurons are distributed to three disparate regions of the oculomotor complex,[58] a nuclear lesion cannot cause paresis of adduction in isolation. Many causes of internuclear ophthalmoplegia have been reported[9] (vascular, neoplastic, demyelinating, infectious, toxic, metabolic, and degenerative), and myasthenia gravis may mimic an INO by causing slow saccades.[59] Lesions of the MLF are particularly common in multiple sclerosis and may be bilateral. In addition to bilateral adduction paresis and abduction nystagmus, *a bilateral INO is associated with impaired vertical smooth pursuit and VOR as well as vertical gaze-evoked nystagmus.*[60, 61]

Large brain stem lesions may involve one entire abducens nucleus and the ipsilateral MLF. The nuclear lesion causes a complete conjugate palsy of ipsilateral gaze as outlined earlier. The MLF just rostral to the abducens nucleus contains axons of internuclear neurons originating from the contralateral abducens nucleus. Consequently, the commands to both medial rectus subdivisions of the oculomotor complex are interrupted—signals to the ipsilateral subdivision from the axonal lesion in the MLF and signals to the contralateral subdivision from the destruction of the soma of internuclear neurons. The overall result is a bilateral paralysis of adduction (INO) and an ipsilateral loss of abduction for all types of conjugate eye movements. Vergence may be preserved. Because the ipsilateral eye is paralyzed in the horizontal plane and half of the horizontal movements are lost in the contralateral eye, this constellation of signs has been labeled the "one-and-a-half" syndrome.[62, 63] It is important to recognize that this syndrome occurs with *unilateral* lesions of the brain stem and that this bilateral defect in horizontal gaze need not be due to bilateral or multiple lesions.

The supranuclear organization of horizontal eye movements converges on the pontomedullary junction of the brain stem. The eye position signal for all conjugate horizontal eye movements is formed by the neural integrator in the MVN/NPH, as described earlier. This complex is a supranuclear site of convergence for horizontal eye velocity commands generated by every type of conjugate eye movement (see Figs. 192–2 and 192–3). The eye velocity signals arise from separate subsystems that are described in later sections. Briefly, the eye velocity command during the VOR originates from afferents of the horizontal canals that enter the lateral medulla and project primarily to the ipsilateral MVN and vestibulocerebellum. The optokinetic signal follows an extrageniculate pathway from the retina via the accessory optic system to eventually reach the MVN.[64, 65] Excitatory burst neurons of the PPRF, rostral to the abducens nucleus, convey the eye velocity signal for saccades and quick phases.[18] These cells project to the ipsilateral abducens nucleus and the MVN/NPH[66] and receive input from the superior colliculus,[67] frontal eye field (FEF),[68] and vestibular nuclei.[69] The eye velocity command for smooth pursuit originates in the ipsilateral hemisphere,[70–72] projects to ipsilateral dorsolateral pontine nuclei (DLPN),[73, 74] and courses through the flocculus[41, 75] before impinging on the neural integrator.

Although lesions of the midbrain affect primarily vertical eye movements (see later), *mesencephalic lesions may cause deficits for movement in the horizontal plane because corticofugal projections that participate in the control of horizontal eye movement must traverse the midbrain.* Unilateral stimulation of the mesencephalic reticular formation in the monkey elicits horizontal gaze, the direction of which depends on the site of the electrode in the rostrocaudal direction. Stimulation in the rostral midbrain produces contralateral conjugate eye deviation; whereas at sites caudal to this region, near the level of the trochlear nucleus, passage of electric current elicits ipsilateral movements.[76] This decussation appears to be limited to pathways concerned with saccades, because patients with horizontal eye movement abnormalities due to a unilateral lesion in the mesencephalon have defective saccades in the contralateral direction (reduced peak velocity and hypometria) but impaired smooth pursuit ipsilaterally.[77]

Vertical Gaze Pathways

Unlike horizontal movements of the eyes or limbs that are dominantly controlled by one side of the nervous system (contralateral hemisphere—ipsilateral motor nuclei with a decussation of descending fibers), vertical eye movements arise from *bilateral* activation of homolateral structures in the brain.[78] *For example, focal seizures commonly elicit contraversive eye deviation, whereas vertical eye movements occur with generalized seizures.* For approximately 90 percent of the population, bilateral eyelid closure causes upward eye movement (Bell's phenomenon),[79] but no rotation occurs when one lid is closed. Electrical stimulation of structures within the brain elicits purely vertical eye movements only if paired regions or midline commissural tracts are involved.[76] Finally, conjugate paralysis of vertical gaze occurs only from bilateral,[76, 80] midline,[80] or rarely paramedian lesions adjacent to major commissural pathways.[81]

The control of vertical and torsional eye movements is organized in the mesencephalon[82] (Fig. 192–4). Analogous to the horizontal system, a neural integrator forms a supranuclear final common pathway for vertical eye velocity commands. *The interstitial nucleus of Cajal (INC) lies within the MLF, lateral to the rostral half of the oculomotor complex,*[83] *and most likely is the locus of the integrator for vertical eye movements,*[38] *perhaps in conjunction with reciprocal connections to the SVN since bilateral MLF lesions impair vertical gaze-holding.*[61] *The rostral interstitial nucleus of the medial longitudinal fasciculus (riMLF) contains short-lead burst neurons that activate 5 to 10 msec before vertical saccades.*[84, 85] (Cells that burst selectively for upward saccades are intermixed with neurons that have downward preferred directions.) No neurons in the riMLF burst for horizontal saccades. (Conversely the PPRF, where the premotor commands for horizontal saccades arise, contains some neurons with vertical direction selectivity[86] and that begin to discharge 20 to 150 msec before the onset of a saccade.[87]) Furthermore, anatomic tracer studies have demonstrated a projection from the PPRF to the riMLF, and *large bilateral lesions of the PPRF that abolish horizontal gaze can also eliminate vertical saccades.*[80] All of these results imply that the PPRF serves as a major input to the riMLF.[82] The eye velocity commands for vertical smooth pursuit and the VOR project to the mesencephalon via the MLF and *brachium conjunctivum.*[88] Chronic bilateral lesions of the MLF severely impair these eye movements.[61]

Although total paralysis of vertical eye movements is clinically more common than direction-specific palsies, upward,[80, 89] and in rare cases downward,[90, 91] eye movements may be selectively impaired, which suggests separate pathways for these movements. Stimulation and lesion studies in monkey[92] and clinicopathologic correlations in humans[81, 90] suggest that *pathways for upward eye movement are located more caudoventrally in the **medial** riMLF whereas projections carrying downward signals are rostrodorsally situated in the **lateral** riMLF. The medial fibers carrying upward saccadic motor commands decussate in the posterior commissure, where*

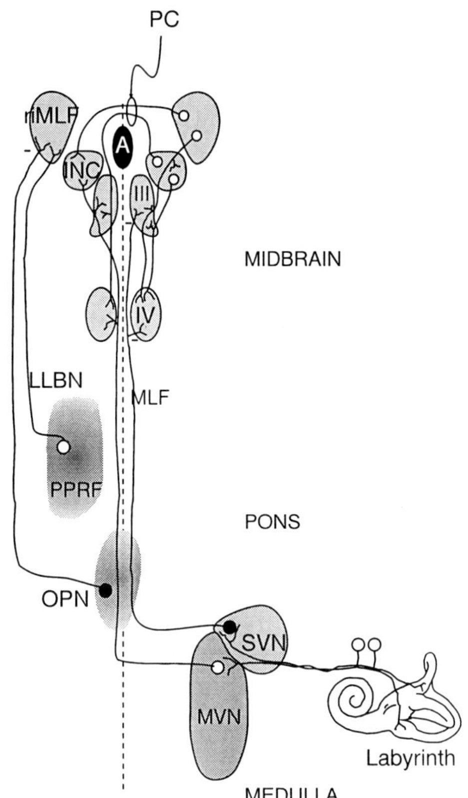

Figure 192–4. Pathways for the control of vertical conjugate eye movements. Vestibular afferents from the anterior and posterior canals project to the superior vestibular nucleus (SVN) and the medial vestibular nucleus (MVN). Projections from second-order vestibular neurons ascend in the medial longitudinal fasciculus (MLF) and the brachium conjunctivum (not shown) to motoneurons of the trochlear (IV) and oculomotor (III) nuclei and to the interstitial nucleus of Cajal (INC). Vestibular projections in the ipsilateral MLF are inhibitory and arise from the SVN. Long-lead burst neurons (LLBN) ascend from the paramedian pontine reticular formation (PPRF) to the rostral interstitial nucleus of the MLF (riMLF), in which medium-lead burst neurons encode vertical saccades and quick phases of nystagmus. Burst neuron axons for upward saccades decussate rostral to the Sylvian aqueduct (A) in the posterior commissure (PC), whereas those innervating depressor motoneurons pass laterally and course through the INC. The INC and its reciprocal connections with the vestibular nucleus may form the neural integrator for vertical eye movements. Smooth pursuit eye movement commands project from the flocculus to the vestibular nucleus and then traverse many of the same pathways used in the vertical vestibuloocular reflex. Filled circles represent inhibitory neurons; open circles, excitatory neurons. (OPN, omnipause neurons.)

upward smooth pursuit and VOR signals also cross the midline. This distinctive pathway for upward motor commands explains the selective palsy of upgaze in the pretectal syndrome[78] (also called Parinaud's syndrome: upgaze palsy, pupillary light-near dissociation, lid retraction, and convergence-retraction nystagmus).[93, 94] *Upward eye movements may also be conjugately impaired with a unilateral lesion confined to the oculomotor nucleus.*[77] This lesion is effectively "bilateral" for the superior rectus muscles, because the motoneurons of one nucleus innervate the contralateral superior rectus via a projection that passes through the contralateral oculomotor nucleus.[95] Paralysis of downgaze with intact upgaze occurs much less commonly. *Bilateral infarctions more laterally placed in the riMLF can cause a selective loss of downward eye movements in humans.*[90, 91] The unpaired posterior thalamosubthalamic paramedian artery arises from the posterior cerebral artery and supplies this territory. Interruption of blood flow in this vessel has been implicated as the cause of small bilateral infarctions with paralysis of downgaze.[82] Bilateral congenital lesions at the mesencephalic-diencephalic junction have been reported in a case of vertical oculomotor apraxia.[96] Downward saccades and vertical smooth pursuit were absent, but the vertical VOR was intact, and a combination of head movement and blink was used to change gaze in the vertical plane.

SACCADES AND QUICK PHASES OF NYSTAGMUS

Saccades and quick phases of nystagmus abruptly accelerate and decelerate the globe to shift the direction of gaze and bring the image of new objects onto the fovea. They are the fastest eye movements in the oculomotor repertoire. Under normal conditions these movements are very reproducible and machine-like, which has enabled quantitative performance criteria to be developed for the clinical evaluation of the saccadic system.

Latency. Of all the quantitative indices of saccadic performance, latency is the most variable because it depends on size of target displacement, illumination, target-shift schedule, difficulty of discrimination task, attention, and many other parameters of cognitive processing. The initial motion of a visually guided saccade begins about 180 to 250 msec after the presentation of a target in the periphery. If all visual stimuli are extinguished before presenting a new target, then the distribution of latencies becomes bimodal: one cluster of measurements at the usual latency and another with a mean of 100 to 130 msec. These "express" saccades are postulated to have a shorter latency, because in this paradigm the process of removing fixation on the previous target has been completed before the new target is presented.[97] Increased latency of saccades in all directions occurs frequently with diffuse degenerative disorders of the cerebrum or basal ganglia, such as Alzheimer's disease,[98] parkinsonism,[99] or Huntington's disease.[100] In patients with unilateral frontal lobe lesions, contralaterally directed saccades are delayed, especially for targets presented in a predictable pattern.[101]

Peak Velocity–Amplitude Relationship. Peak velocity increases monotonically with saccade amplitude and attains much higher values than the maximum speed for slow eye movements. For example, a large 40-degree saccade may reach a peak velocity of 500 to 600 degrees/sec. The relationship between saccade amplitude and peak velocity has been called the "main sequence."[6] Because this relationship is so reproducible, the main sequence can be used to determine whether pathologic, rapid-appearing eye movements of unknown type are attributable to disorders of the saccadic control system (on the main sequence) or independent from it (peak velocity lower than predicted by the main sequence). Part of the evidence that saccades and quick phases of nystagmus are both members of the same oculomotor subsystem is based on the finding that they both fall on the same main sequence.[7] Saccade peak velocity is not under voluntary control, although it may vary with ambient illumination or vigilance of the patient.

Accuracy. The initial movement in a visually guided saccade usually does not bring the eyes directly on target.[102] Thus, some degree of saccadic dysmetria is normal. The first saccade toward a target often falls short (undershoots) by approximately 10 percent of the target amplitude.[103, 104] The percentage of saccades that are hypometric increases with increasing target displacement; thus virtually all saccades over 30 degrees in amplitude undershoot the target. From a control systems standpoint, it is unclear why the saccadic system has evolved to incorporate this error, although many hypotheses have been proposed.[105–107] The primary saccade is hypometric, followed by a corrective saccade after a normal 192-msec latency. The same pattern of correction occurs with hypermetric saccades that normally occur much less frequently and are not as dependent on amplitude. Saccadic dysmetria is believed to originate from an error in the size of the *pulse* of innervation supplied by the burst neurons (see later and the section on the neural integrator). The ability to adaptively adjust the amplitude of the pulse, to correct persistent dysmetria, is dependent on midline cerebellar structures.[108]

A second form of error in saccadic accuracy occurs when the amplitude of the pulse of innervation from the burst neurons is not matched to that of the step change in discharge rate from the neural integrator (Fig. 192–5; see also Fig. 192–2). This *pulse-step mismatch* causes the eye to immediately drift exponentially toward its final position with a time constant of 192 msec, governed by the viscoelastic nature of the globe. This *conjugate* drift after a saccade is called a *glissade.*[109] Disconjugate drifts at the end of a saccade may be normal vergence movements. If the pulse is too small relative to the step, then the eye drifts further in the direction of movement. Conversely, a pulse that is too large causes the initial motion to overshoot the rest position and the eye drifts backward. Lesion studies in monkeys have demonstrated that the flocculus of the cerebellum is required to adaptively adjust the pulse-step match and thus eliminate postsaccadic drift.[41, 108]

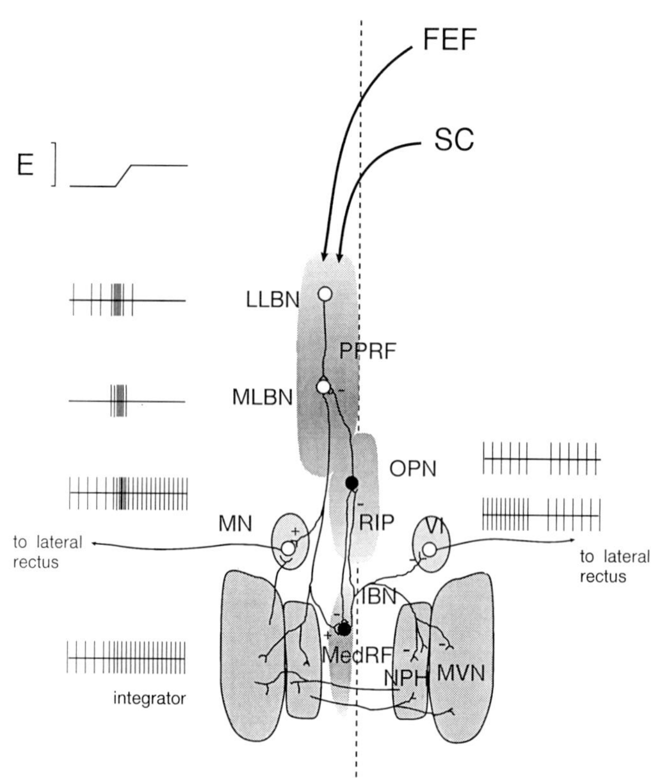

Figure 192–5. Simplified schematic of the brain stem saccade generator for horizontal eye movements. Change in eye position (E) and neuronal discharge patterns during a leftward saccade are shown for the various cells types as insets. Inputs to this brain stem circuit arise primarily from the superior colliculus (SC) and the frontal eye field (FEF). These signals decussate in the midbrain and excite burst neurons in the contralateral half of the paramedian pontine reticular formation (PPRF). Long-lead burst neurons (LLBN) discharge with a stuttering onset and excite medium-lead burst neurons (MLBN), which encode the eye velocity signal for the saccade. Omnipause neurons (OPN) are located in the ventrocaudal border of the PPRF in the nucleus raphe interpositus (RIP). These cells tonically inhibit burst neurons except for saccades. Inhibitory burst neurons (IBN) lie caudal to the abducens nucleus (VI) in the dorsomedial medullary reticular formation (MedRF) and inhibit the contralateral motoneurons. The discharge pattern of the IBN is similar to that of the excitatory MLBN and is not shown. The eye position signal is generated from the eye velocity command by the neural integrator in the medial vestibular nucleus (MVN) and the nucleus prepositus hypoglossi (NPH). The discharge pattern of motoneurons (MN) encodes both the eye-velocity (burst or pulse) and the eye-position (step from the neural integrator) commands. Filled circles represent inhibitory neurons; open circles, excitatory ones. Internuclear neurons from the abducens nucleus to the oculomotor complex are omitted for clarity.

Brain Stem Saccade Generator

The final stages of neuronal processing for the generation of saccades have been mapped out in the brain stem with a combination of anatomic and physiologic techniques (reviewed in reference 110). The primary components are the burst neurons, pause cells, neural integrator, and motoneurons as shown schematically in Figure 192–5.

Burst neurons are located in the PPRF, which lies ventral to the MLF and extends from the level of the abducens to the trochlear nuclei, and in the riMLF in the midbrain. The anatomy of these cell groups in the reticular formation has been reviewed extensively in a recent monograph.[111] Medium-lead burst neurons of the caudal PPRF begin to discharge between 5 and 15 msec before the onset of ipsilateral horizontal saccades and are otherwise inactive. The intensity of firing during the burst is proportional to the eye velocity during the saccade, and the duration of the burst is approximately equal to the transit time of the saccade.[5] Because burst neuron activity determines the speed of a saccade, the main sequence (peak eye velocity–amplitude relationship) is a direct measure of the integrity of these cells.

In the absence of mechanical restrictions, disorders of neuromuscular transmission, or myopathies, *slow saccades indicate dysfunction of burst neurons.* Unilateral excitotoxin lesions restricted to the PPRF in a monkey cause a selective loss of ipsilateral saccades and quick phases, while the VOR and gaze-holding remain normal.[112] In most clinical reports, lesions usually extend beyond the PPRF and also cause some degree of impairment for ipsilateral smooth pursuit and slow phases of vestibular nystagmus.[112, 113] Excitatory medium-lead burst neurons project to neurons of the ipsilateral abducens nucleus and the NPH and MVN. *Inhibitory burst neurons* are located in the dorsal medullary reticular formation, just caudal to the level of the abducens nucleus, and monosynaptically inhibit neurons in the contralateral abducens nucleus.[114] This projection provides the inhibitory signal to the antagonist motoneurons.

Burst neurons in the rostral PPRF are of the long-lead variety. They begin to discharge irregularly many tens of milliseconds before a saccade and have a more gradual rise time for the burst. *Unlike medium-lead burst neurons, the long-lead ones discharge for vertical as well as horizontal saccades.* Long-lead burst neurons may provide information to the medium-lead burst cells of the caudal PPRF for horizontal saccades and those of the riMLF for vertical saccades.

Pause cells have high spontaneous discharge rates and cease firing immediately before and during saccades in any direction. These cells are located close to the dorsal midline, just rostral to the abducens nuclei,[22] in a cell group that has been named the *nucleus raphe interpositus.*[115] Experimental lesions of the PPRF that extend caudally into the pause cell region disrupt vertical as well as horizontal saccades.[112] For every cell that was examined, excitatory and inhibitory burst neurons have been shown to receive monosynaptic inhibition from pause neurons.[116] *It has been proposed that pause cells tonically inhibit the activity of burst neurons so that the generation of extraneous saccades is suppressed.* Long-lead burst neurons may inhibit pause cells and thus release medium-lead burst cells from inhibition.[117]

The neural integrator and motoneurons have been described in previous sections. In accordance with Figures 192–2 and 192–5, the medium-lead burst neurons that convey the saccadic eye velocity signal have been shown to project to both of these regions.[66]

A wiring diagram can be constructed from the various brain stem cell types that encode saccadic eye movements. Figure 192–5 schematically depicts the anatomic connections for the generation of horizontal saccades. Not shown in Figure 192–5 are the feedback pathways in the brain stem saccade generator that cause the burst cells to fire until some internal representation of eye movement matches the desired trajectory for the saccade. The existence of this feedback has been demonstrated most clearly in two studies. First, electrical stimulation was applied to the primate PPRF[118] or superior colliculus[119] (a major source of input to the PPRF) after a visual target had been extinguished, but before a saccade could be initiated. The stimulation moved the eye to a new position in the dark, and yet the visually triggered saccade brought the eye to target location with a normal latency. Some internal feedback signal, independent of vision, corrected for the electrically induced perturbation. Second, in a patient with extremely slow saccades due to a degenerative disorder affecting the pons and cerebellum, saccades could be redirected midflight with visual feedback.[120] Although normal saccades are too fast for processing of visual information and in a practical sense are therefore ballistic, the existence of this feedback pathway has an important clinical consequence. The response of burst neurons is vigorous, even for small amplitude saccades. Thus the gain (intensity of burst neuron firing/change in eye position) is large, and a time delay in a feedback pathway may cause the system to become unstable and oscillate. This instability is avoided by turning off the burst cells with strong inhibition by pause cells during intersaccadic intervals. *Ocular flutter* is a *paroxysm of back-to-back horizontal saccades without a normal intersaccadic latency and has been attributed to a defect in the normal inhibition of burst neurons by pause cells.*[120] The precise pathway of this feedback system, and even which oculomotor signal is monitored (eye position[15] or eye velocity[121]), remains to be elucidated.

Higher-Level Control of Saccades

The superior colliculus (SC), FEF, striate and prestriate (posterior parietal) cortices, basal ganglia, thalamus, and cerebellum all participate in the supranuclear control of the brain stem saccade generator. A general scheme of the role that these separate regions play in the execution of saccades has recently emerged.[110, 122] The SC and FEF form parallel descending pathways to the brain stem saccade generator. In monkeys lesions of one or the other structure cause only mild and transient deficits in saccades, whereas combined lesions lead to a permanent inability to make visually guided saccades in the contralateral direction.[123] The collicular pathway is a phylogenetically older tectobulbar system that may have evolved to generate involuntary, reflexive, or searching movements that reorient gaze to visual or auditory stimuli. The pars reticulata division of the substantia nigra (SNPr) tonically inhibits the deep layers of the SC and may act as a gate to suppress extraneous triggering of saccades from the colliculus. The corticobulbar pathway from the FEF is more concerned with volitional saccades to visual or remembered targets. Cells in the intermedullary lamina of the posterior medial thalamus discharge in relation to saccades,[124] and lesions of the thalamus and adjacent SC in primates cause inaccuracies in the amplitude of saccades that are proportional to the position of the eye in the orbit.[125] This led to the hypothesis that the thalamus plays an important role in computing coordinate transformations (retinotopic to craniotopic) required to locate objects in space. The cerebellum forms reciprocal connections to brain stem nuclei and adaptively controls the metrics of saccades. *Midline structures (dorsal vermis and fastigial nuclei) modify the pulse intensity of burst neurons to prevent dysmetria. The lateral vestibulocerebellum (flocculus and paraflocculus) maintains the pulse-step match to reduce postsaccadic drifts (glissades)*[41, 108] *and optimizes the neural integrator performance that improves eccentric gaze-holding.*[39, 41]

The SNPr-SC and FEF pathways are the major inputs to the brain stem saccade generator, and the participation of these structures in the generation of saccades is described later.

Superior Colliculus

The superior colliculus is functionally and anatomically divided into deep and superficial layers.[126] The superficial layers are part of the afferent limb of the visuomotor system and are exclusively sensory. They receive inputs from the retina and visual cortex and project to the pulvinar.[127] Cells in these layers discharge in response to visual stimuli and are organized in a retinotopic fashion.[128] The deep layers provide an efferent motor command to the brain stem saccade generator. Electrical stimulation of the primate deep SC elicits conjugate, contralateral saccades with a latency of 20 to 30 msec: never smooth pursuit, nystagmus, or vergence.[129] The deep layers are organized into a motor map such that any suprathreshold stimulus elicits a saccade of fixed amplitude and direction. These parameters are determined by the *location* of the stimulation and not by the intensity. Single-unit recordings from the deep layers showed cells that burst 18 to 20 msec before saccades in the movement field defined by the location of the cell. The motor and sensory maps are aligned in register,[130] yet there is little anatomic evidence[131] and no physiologic evidence[131] of direct connections between the deep and superficial layers.

Lesions isolated to the superior colliculus have not been described in humans. In primates, small lesions placed at the site of a recording electrode cause an increase in the latency of contralateral saccades within the movement field defined previously by recording.[132] The defect is *transient,* and the animal recovers in 1 to 7 days. Subsequent studies reported decreased peak velocity or hypometria, but these results were more variable and may have been caused by extension of the lesion outside the confines of the SC. The most reproducible lesion effects were produced by microinjecting lidocaine[133] or an agonist of the inhibitory amino acid transmitter gamma-aminobutyric acid (GABA)[134] into the SC. Saccades to visual targets within the movement field of the injection site had dramatically increased latencies with normal accuracy, whereas saccades to "remembered" locations after extinguishing the target light were both delayed and hypometric. In contrast to these transient deficits, collicular lesions combined with ablation of either the FEF[123] or striate cortex[135] cause a permanent deficit in visually guided saccades to the contralateral hemifield.

Basal Ganglia

The substantia nigra exerts an inhibitory influence on the ipsilateral superior colliculus. The nonpigmented (nondopaminergic) cells of the pars reticulata (SNPr) project to the intermediate layer of the SC. These nigral cells discharge tonically at 80 spikes/sec and decrease their activity during contralateral saccades to visual or remembered targets, although this reduction is less tightly coupled to the movement than that of pause cells in the brain stem.[136] The axon terminals contain the inhibitory amino acid transmitter, GABA.[137, 138] Electrical stimulation of the SNPr inhibits cells in the SC, and this effect is blocked by iontophoretic application of GABA antagonists[139] into the SC. The pharmacologic basis of the nigrocollicular control of saccades has been elucidated by selectively microinjecting GABA agonists or antagonists.[134, 140] Local injection of muscimol, a GABA agonist, into the SC increases the latency, or at times even abolishes, saccades of the amplitude and direction that would have caused a maximal response in cells at this site. Saccades in other directions are normal. Conversely, injection of bicuculline, a GABA antagonist, into the SC induces repetitive, irrepressible saccades into the movement field. Muscimol injected into the SNPr (whose cells are GABAergic and contain postsynaptic GABA receptors) suppresses the nigrocollicular inhibition and also causes irrepressible saccades to the side contralateral to the injection. This suggests that tonic, GABA-induced inhibition of the SC may be exerted by the SNPr to maintain fixation and that the normal initiation of visually guided saccades arises from a combination of decreased nigrocollicular inhibition and increased corticocollicular excitation from the FEF. Inputs to the SNPr come primarily from the caudate that receives projections from the FEF, many other regions of the cortex, and the medial thalamus.

Although Parkinson's disease is caused primarily by the loss of dopaminergic neurons in the SNPc, the SNPr is also affected possibly through either SNPc → caudate → SNPr loops or direct dendrodendritic connections within the nigra. Saccades are mildly impaired in patients with parkinsonism, particularly for predictive tracking in which the latency is increased, the amplitude is persistently hypometric, and the peak velocity is mildly slowed.[99, 141, 142] These deficits are similar to those made by monkeys attempting saccades to remembered targets after muscimol injection into the SC and suggest that in parkinsonism there may be an impaired ability to turn off the nigrocollicular inhibition for predictive saccades. Conversely, patients with Huntington's disease have difficulty in suppressing saccades to targets in the periphery.[143] This may be a consequence of a decrease in tonic inhibition in the nigrocollicular pathway (similar to injecting muscimol in SNPr or bicuculline in SC of monkeys), perhaps due to a loss of cells in the striatum, which is the major source of input to the SNPr. The hypothesis of an increased inhibition for parkinsonism and a decreased inhibition for Huntington's disease is, however, overly simplistic because other features such as slow hypometric saccades in Huntington's disease[98] are not reconcilable with this scheme.

FEF

The FEF, Brodmann area 8, was defined more than a century ago as a region of frontal cortex where electrical stimulation elicited contraversive saccades. Modern studies using microstimulation[144, 145] have mapped its location to the posterior segment of the anterior bank of the arcuate sulcus. Some neurons in this region discharge before saccades, whereas others phasically discharge after the eye begins to move.[146, 147] This finding has raised questions about whether these cells are responsible for the initiation of saccades or carry an internal feedback copy of the motor command (corollary discharge or efferent copy). Afferents to the FEF originate in prestriate cortex, cingulate cortex, the contralateral FEF, and the thalamus. The FEF projects heavily to the SC, basal ganglia, and thalamus, with only a modest projection directly to the PPRF.[148] The extracollicular pathway does, however, form a functionally important input to the brain stem saccade generator, because visually guided saccades are relatively unimpaired with a single lesion confined to the collicular branch of this parallel efferent system. Acute, unilateral lesions in the frontal lobe cause a transient ipsilateral deviation of gaze, an inability to initiate contralateral saccades, and contralateral neglect.[101] After hours to days the eyes return to the midline, and visually guided saccades return to normal. The rate and extent of recovery depend on an intact contralateral frontal lobe.[149] Subtle saccadic deficits may persist chronically after unilateral frontal lobe lesions. The latency during predictive tracking with saccades is increased. Patients with subtotal frontal lobectomy for epilepsy surgery are unable to avoid making saccades to suddenly appearing targets ("visual grasp reflex"), particularly in the contralateral hemifield.[150] Thus the FEF participates in the decision of where to look and how to trigger the brain stem saccade generator, which in turn controls the trajectory of the movement.

VOR AND OPTOKINETIC RESPONSE

VOR

The VOR and optokinetic system counterrotate the eyes during head-turning to stabilize images on the retina. Patients with vestibular disorders may complain of dysequilibrium, dizziness, or vertigo—a false sense of self-rotation relative to the environment while at rest—due to an imbalance of vestibular tone. This is often manifested as spontaneous nystagmus when the head is motionless that may be apparent only with specific head positions, with fixation removed, or with ophthalmoscopy or electrooculography.[9, 151] Impairment of the dynamic response of the VOR leads to *oscillopsia,* an illusory movement of the environment while the head is moving. A simple bedside check of dynamic VOR function may be performed by testing acuity with a near-vision card. If rapid head-shaking at 2 cycles/sec decreases the acuity by several lines compared with that when the head is motionless, then the dynamic response of the VOR is abnormal.

The performance of the VOR is largely determined by the mechanical properties of the peripheral vestibular apparatus. Over the frequency range of most natural head rotations,[152] the change in discharge rate of the vestibular afferent nerve is proportional to head angular velocity.[25] This head-velocity signal generates a slow-phase eye velocity that is approximately equal to head velocity for rotations up to 350 degrees/sec.[153] The gain (eye velocity/ head velocity) for high-frequency rotation in the dark is about 0.95 but differs considerably between individuals and varies even for one person depending on the instructions to the subject.[154] The change in discharge rate of the vestibular afferent is produced by deflection of the cupula within the semicircular canal. The combination of endolymph and cupula acts as an overdamped pendulum, so that for sustained rotation of the head (zero or very low frequency change in speed) the head velocity signal encoded by the afferent fibers decays exponentially with a time constant of 5 to 10 sec.[9] This signal is augmented centrally by "velocity storage" that lengthens the time constant of the decay of slow-phase velocity for the VOR in the dark to 10 to 15 sec.[155] The latency of the VOR is 15 to 20 msec.[156] Thus the VOR is optimized to rapidly generate compensatory eye movements in response to transient rotations of the head. It responds more quickly than the optokinetic or smooth pursuit system that relies on visual feedback. The latter augment the VOR so that eye velocity matches head velocity more closely and so that during sustained rotations for which the vestibular signal diminishes, compensatory eye movements continue.

The mirror symmetry of the semicircular canals within the temporal bones causes canal pairs lying in the same plane to be driven in push-pull. For example, head rotation to the left increases the discharge rate of the afferent from the left horizontal canal, whereas the discharge rate from the right decreases. It is the difference between the firing rate of the left and right afferents that elicits slow-phase eye movements. With the head motionless, the signals from all push-pull canal pairs must balance. Otherwise the brain stem acts on false information and generates pathologic nystagmus with slow phases in the plane of the canal pair mismatch. Peripheral lesions often affect the entire labyrinth on one side, and the combination of horizontal, anterior, and posterior canal paresis causes a mixed horizontal-torsional nystagmus with slow phases toward the lesioned side. The upward and downward imbalance of the anterior and posterior canals cancels so that, in general, *purely vertical nystagmus does not arise from peripheral disorders and implies a pathologic change in central pathways*. Compensation for inherent inequalities between afferent pairs and rebalancing afferent signals after lesions of the peripheral vestibular apparatus are performed by the cerebellum, inferior olive, and vestibular nuclei.[157, 158] Interestingly, the reduction of spontaneous nystagmus after labyrinthectomy is not dependent on vision, although readjustment in the gain of the VOR is dependent on an intact geniculostriate system.[159] Smooth pursuit and the optokinetic system partially suppress the nystagmus originating from a lesion in the labyrinth. Nystagmus of central origin, however, often impairs smooth pursuit and optokinetic pathways. Therefore, a reduction in the slow-phase velocity when switching from darkness to light (or switching from blurred vision with Frenzel lenses to normal acuity) is a reliable sign of a peripheral lesion.[151]

The central connections of the VOR have been characterized classically as a three-neuron arc: vestibular afferent, vestibular nuclear neuron, and oculomotor neuron.[160] Although this basic projection has been demonstrated anatomically (see Fig. 192–3), the polysynaptic influence of parallel pathways is clearly important.[19, 161] Commissural inhibitory projections between the vestibular nuclei[162] augment the push-pull head-velocity signal from canal pairs, may form part of the neural integrator,[29, 32] and may contribute to the balance of the resting vestibular tone.[163] Vestibular afferents also project as mossy fiber inputs to the vestibulocerebellum (flocculus, paraflocculus, nodulus, and uvula). Cerebellar projections inhibit the vestibular nuclei, and this side loop is critical for adaptive adjustment of the VOR gain.[2, 164, 165] This also explains why cerebellar lesions are often accompanied by an inappropriately high VOR gain.[166, 167]

Normally, objects are tracked with a combination of eye and head movement. The latter stimulate the canals and would elicit an inappropriate VOR (hold *gaze stationary*) by rotating the eyes opposite to the head motion, away from the target. During head pursuit the VOR is *cancelled* so that the eyes remain stationary in the orbit. Clinically, VOR cancellation is easily tested by having a patient visually fixate the thumb of an outstretched arm while rotating to and fro on a swivel chair with the lights on. With adequate VOR cancellation, the eyes should remain stationary with no detectable nystagmus. The performance of VOR suppression is similar to that of the smooth pursuit system,[168] and most patients with a deficit in smooth pursuit also have impaired VOR cancellation.[8] There are, however, a few reported cases of a dissociation between impairment of smooth pursuit and VOR cancellation,[169] and vestibular neuron activity during VOR cancellation in the monkey is inconsistent with a simple linear addition of smooth pursuit and VOR signals to effect cancellation.[48, 170]

Optokinetic System

OKN is the visually induced pattern of nystagmus elicited by motion of images over the entire visual field. This occurs either during self-rotation or in the laboratory by rotation of the visual scene around a stationary subject. In humans, OKN is generated primarily by the smooth pursuit system and the phylogenetically older, subcortical optokinetic system (OKS) is largely vestigial.* The optokinetic system is best demonstrated in lower, afoveate mammals that have no smooth pursuit. In the rabbit, smooth movements of small visual targets elicit no smooth eye movements. If the rabbit is completely surrounded by a patterned optokinetic drum that is rotated in the dark at constant speed, then when the lights come on nystagmus occurs with a gradual build-up in slow-phase eye velocity that eventually matches drum velocity.[171] If the lights are then extinguished, the eyes continue to move and optokinetic afternystagmus (OKAN) persists for several seconds in complete darkness. In rabbit or humans, the braking deceleration required to stop self-rotation stimulates the canals and generates postrotatory nystagmus with slow phases in the opposite direction (compared with pre-rotatory nystagmus). The time course of postrotatory vestibular nystagmus in the dark matches that of OKAN, and it has been proposed that the function of OKAN is to cancel postrotatory vestibular nystagmus when the VOR and OKS have been stimulated simultaneously by prolonged rotation in the light.[4, 172] The optokinetic system is a subcortical visual pathway from the retina to the nucleus of the optical tract in the pretectum and the nuclei of the accessory optical system in the midbrain (the dorsal, lateral, and medial terminal nuclei),[65] and then via unknown polysynaptic pathways to the vestibular nucleus, and finally to ocular motoneurons (Fig. 192–6). It has been proposed that the OKS evolved in parallel with the VOR to sustain compensatory eye movements for prolonged self-rotation in which the canal signal decays.

In humans or monkeys, smooth pursuit movements elicited by following a small target stop abruptly when the lights are turned off. Consequently, the best method to examine the optokinetic system in humans is to electronically record OKAN, that is, the afternystagmus in the dark, following a prolonged period of constant-velocity, full-field image motion in the light. The clinical utility of this test is limited because OKAN in humans may be absent in approximately 10 percent of normal people,[173] has a highly variable time constant (2 to 85 sec), and achieves a velocity of only 10 to 30 percent of that during OKN with a maximum velocity of 15 to 20 degrees/sec.[3] Nevertheless, some aspects of the human OKS have clinical relevance. For example, cortical blindness from bilateral occipital lobe lesions does not obliterate ocular responses to sustained, full-field stimulation because of the intact subcortical OKS,[174] and the presence of these movements should not be interpreted as a sign of hysterical blindness. Because the vestibular nuclei are an obligate step in the OKS, lesions of the peripheral labyrinth that alter central vestibular tone abolish OKAN in humans[175] and monkeys[176] but leave smooth pursuit (and therefore OKN) unimpaired. The hand-held "optokinetic drum" used at the bedside is a useful test for qualitatively observing directional asymmetries in OKN, but it is a test of smooth pursuit and not the optokinetic system. With parietal lesions, slow-phase tracking is impaired when the stripes move toward the lesioned side and an obvious directional asymmetry occurs.[177–179] Abnormal quick phases with a directional preponderance may also cause an asymmetric OKN and must be distinguished from defective slow phases.[173]

*The two components of the optokinetic response have been assigned many synonymous terms. The contribution from the smooth pursuit system has also been called direct OKN, active OKN, or foveal pursuit. The component from the subcortical optokinetic system is also referred to as indirect OKN, passive OKN, or full-field pursuit.

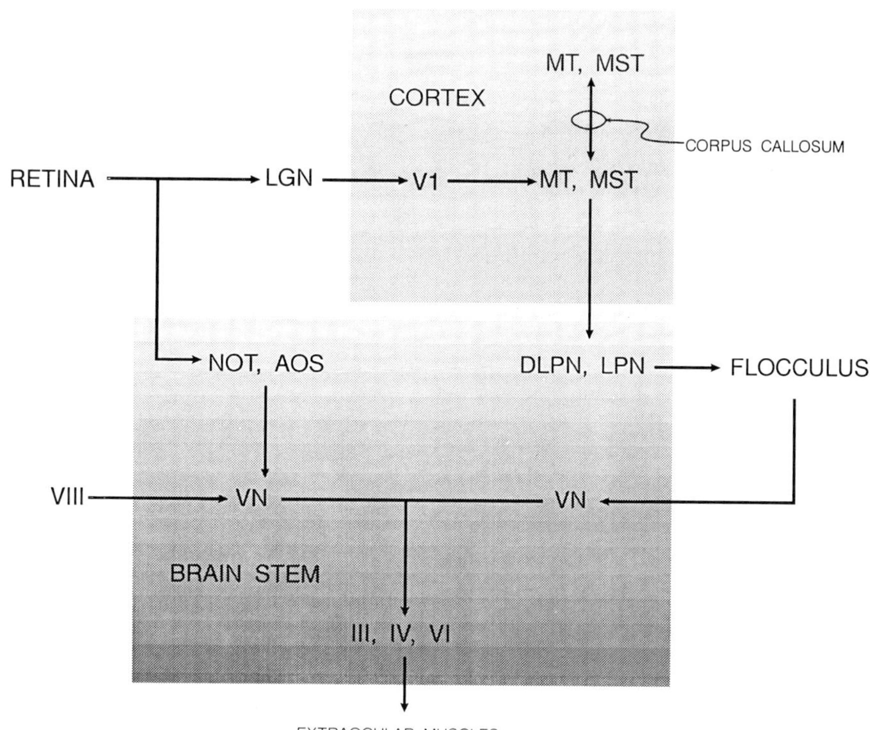

Figure 192–6. Supranuclear control of visual tracking. The afferent limb of the smooth pursuit pathway begins in the retina, synapses in the lateral geniculate nucleus (LGN), continues to the primary visual cortex (V1), and then projects to the middle temporal area (MT) in the occipitoparietal cortex. This sensory system encodes information about target motion in the contralateral hemifield. Corticocortical pathways project from the MT to both the ipsilateral and the contralateral medial superior temporal areas (MST). Thus the MST receives input from both hemifields. Neurons in the MST discharge during ipsilateral smooth pursuit even when vision is temporarily occluded. This motor signal descends ipsilaterally to the lateral and dorsolateral pontine nuclei (LPN, DLPN) and to the accessory optic system (not shown, for clarity). The smooth pursuit command then passes through the flocculus and finally via a polysynaptic pathway through the neural integrator in the vestibular nucleus (VN) to the motoneurons in the III, IV, and VI nuclei. The optokinetic system is an extrastriate pathway that in lower mammals is almost entirely crossed from one eye to the contralateral nucleus of the optic tract (NOT) and the accessory optic system (AOS). These midbrain nuclei also receive cortical inputs from the geniculostriate system. Efferents from the NOT and the AOS project widely to multiple levels of the brain stem and the diencephalon. The pathway to the vestibular nuclear complex is emphasized because second-order vestibular neurons encode optokinetic signals and interruption of the tonic discharge from primary vestibular afferents (VIII) disrupts optokinetic afternystagmus.

SMOOTH PURSUIT

The tracking of small targets against a patterned background is accomplished by the smooth pursuit system, which is present only in species with well-developed foveal vision and is more dependent on cortical input than any other type of eye movement. Smooth pursuit is elicited by target motion (velocity, not position displacement)[180] with a latency of 80 to 130 msec.[181] The performance of smooth pursuit is quantified as the gain (eye velocity/target velocity),[182] which is slightly less than 1 for randomly moving targets at low speeds (< 40 degrees/sec) and increases for predictable target motion.[183] Although humans are capable of generating smooth pursuit with a gain of 0.9 for target speeds up to 100 degrees/sec,[184] tracking at these velocities is inaccurate and requires many corrective saccades to recapture the target. The limiting factor for smooth pursuit performance may be a saturation of the neural representation of the peak eye acceleration required to compensate for retinal slip of images.[185] Lesions of the cortex, brain stem, or cerebellum that impair smooth pursuit decrease the *gain* and are accompanied by "saccadic" or "cogwheel" pursuit with an increased number of corrective "catch-up" saccades. A complete absence of smooth pursuit with no slow eye movements between these saccades is exceedingly rare.

The neural substrate for smooth pursuit has been elucidated from a combination of neural recordings and both clinical and experimental lesions. The sensorimotor transformation from the detection of image motion to movement of the eyes may be artificially divided into afferent and efferent limbs.[71] Sensory information about the speed and direction of target motion in the contralateral hemifield is encoded retinotopically on cells in striate cortex (area V_1[186] and the occipitoparietal cortex (in the monkey, the middle temporal area [MT] as shown in Fig. 192–6).[187, 188] Acute striate lesions cause a scotoma in the contralateral hemifield, and no eye movements are made toward visual targets in the blind hemifield.[189, 190] Recovery takes weeks to months, and saccades to *stationary* targets contralateral to the lesion are virtually normal. A persistent deficit, however, occurs in the ability to *perceive motion* of objects in the contralateral hemifield.[191] Thus saccades to moving targets are inaccurate, because the motor command fails to take into account the motion of the target that occurs between the observation of the target and the execution of the movement. This same persistent scotoma for motion perception severely impairs smooth pursuit in all directions for extrafoveal targets in the contralateral hemifield.[191] Small excitotoxin lesions in extrafoveal regions of MT cause a similar deficit with impaired initiation of smooth pursuit in all directions for targets moving within the lesioned field.[192] MT projects to the adjacent medial superior temporal area (MST) of parietal cortex as well as to the contralateral MST via the corpus callosum.[71] The efferent limb of the smooth pursuit signal appears to begin in MST. Neurons in dorsomedial MST continue to modulate their firing rates during smooth pursuit even when the target is momentarily blanked.[72] Thus, this nonvisual signal carried by these cells appears to be related to the generation of smooth pursuit rather than the perception of image motion. Excitotoxin lesions in lateral-anterior MST (or foveal MT) produce a deficit in the maintenance of pursuit in the ipsilateral direction regardless of which hemifield is stimulated by target motion.[193] This motor deficit in the efferent limb of smooth pursuit has no retinotopic (hemifield) lateralization because MST receives visual motion information from both hemifields via the input from ipsilateral and contralateral MT.[71] Electrical microstimulation of anterior-lateral MST accelerates ipsilateral smooth pursuit so that the eyes move faster than the target, and conversely decelerates contralateral smooth pursuit.[194] Other areas of prestriate and parietal cortex form parallel cortical pathways that participate in smooth pursuit by shifting visual attention and the perception of motion.[195]

An asymmetry in ocular tracking with a greater deficit when following objects toward the lesioned side has been recognized clinically for more than half a century.[178] Only recently has this been appreciated to be a defect in the smooth pursuit system.[177, 196, 197] Quantitative eye movement recording with testing paradigms designed to separate impaired motion perception and decreased motor performance has demonstrated two distinct deficits in human smooth pursuit.[198] These two forms of deficit correlate with the "afferent" and "efferent" functions of MT and MST in the simian brain. The most common clinical deficit was an asymmetry in visual tracking with decreased smooth pursuit gain for predictable or random targets moving toward the lesioned side, within either visual hemifield. Superposition of the computed tomography (CT)–defined lesions in these patients showed a common involvement in Brodmann areas 39 and 40 and varying amounts of underlying white matter. Some of these patients also had difficulty tracking objects moving in either direction within the contralateral hemifield. This form of smooth pursuit deficit is comparable with the impairment produced by lesions of MST in monkeys.[193] One patient with a temporoparietal hemorrhage in Brodmann areas 19 and 37 reported that objects moving in the contralateral hemifield appeared to jump from one position to the next without smooth continuous transitions. Saccades to moving targets in this hemifield were inaccurate, whereas saccades to static objects were on target. The initiation of smooth pursuit was impaired for targets moving in either direction within the impaired hemifield. This patient's oculomotor deficits were permanent but were otherwise similar to the effects of lesions in primate area MT.[192] Although these observations support the conceptual model of smooth pursuit derived from primate experiments, clinicopathologic studies in humans suggest the system is more complex and may involve other cortical areas. For example, frontal lobe lesions also impair smooth pursuit,[199, 200] and hemidecortication does not completely abolish ipsilateral smooth pursuit.[197] Furthermore, it has not been possible to identify the human analogs of areas MT and MST more precisely than the region of the temporooccipitoparietal junction (areas 19, 37, 39, and 40).[70, 71, 195]

The smooth pursuit signal projects subcortically from MST (and other regions of the inferior parietal lobule[201]) to the ipsilateral dorsolateral pontine nuclei (DLPN)[202] and to the accessory optic system. Smooth pursuit–related responses have been recorded from cells in DLPN,[203] and excitotoxin lesions placed there significantly decrease the gain of ipsilateral tracking.[73] The DLPN projects to the flocculus and dorsal vermis of the cerebellum, structures where pursuit-related signals have been recorded[27, 204, 205] and where lesions in monkeys[41] and humans[166] are known to impair smooth pursuit. This smooth pursuit velocity signal then projects to the MVN and NPH, where the final pursuit command (eye velocity and eye position) is assembled and relayed to ocular motoneurons.

VERGENCE

Binocular alignment of the visual axes requires disconjugate eye movements when objects at various distances are viewed in the midsagittal plane: convergence for near targets and divergence for far. Refixation, in general to a new arbitrary target, requires a combined conjugate and disconjugate eye movement.[206] The amplitudes of these two components are not necessarily divided equally between the two eyes. For example, one eye may make a large saccade with only a small vergence movement, whereas the fellow eye makes a relatively smaller saccade in combination with a larger vergence movement.[207] This inequality in the planning strategy of oculomotor control may be a consequence of ocular dominance.[208] These disconjugate movements to align images on corresponding retinal positions of both eyes are *fusional* vergence movements. The attempts by the fusional vergence system to align images are strong, even when each eye independently views different images simultaneously that cannot be overlapped.[209] Fusional vergence corrects the slight misalignment of the eyes that occurs in many normal individuals when one eye is covered (phoria). Blur, the loss of image sharpness, elicits accommodative vergence. With monocular viewing to remove fusional cues, refixating on a near target along the same line of sight produces a vergence movement (accommodative) in the occluded eye. In addition to lens accommodation and convergence, the pupil constricts thus completing the *near-triad* response. A step change in either retinal disparity or blur produces a slow exponential change in eye position with a dominant time constant of 200 msec that may require 1 sec or more to complete. The peak velocity of vergence eye movements increases from 50 degrees/sec for vergence changes of 5 degrees to up to 150 to 200 degrees/sec for vergence changes of 35 degrees.[210]

The supranuclear control of vergence movements is poorly understood. Neurons have been identified in the mesencephalic reticular formation, dorsal and dorsolateral to the oculomotor complex, that change their firing rate in proportion to vergence angle, but are unaffected by conjugate angle of gaze.[211] Other cells burst before vergence movements and appear to convey an eye-velocity signal.[212] The response of most cells is the same, whether artificial cues are presented to stimulate fusional or accommodative vergence independently or both together. This suggests that these neurons are near the motor output stage of the vergence system since the effects of separate sensory stimuli have been combined. A small subset of cells responded preferentially to fusional or accommodative cues.[205] The source of sensory input to these cells is unknown. A class of cortical neurons in the cat encodes retinal disparity,[213] which may be the neuronal signal for depth perception and a stimulus for vergence. Electrical stimulation of prestriate cortex produces a near triad in anesthetized monkeys.[214, 215] The parietal cortex[195, 216] and cerebellum[217] may also participate, but the functional role of these areas in the generation of vergence is unknown.

A separate group of motoneurons has never been identified that generates only vergence movements.[20] Every motoneuron that encodes vergence movements also carries signals for conjugate eye movements, although the sensitivity of motoneuron firing rate for the two types of movement may not be identical.[218] Medial and lateral rectus motoneurons must be reciprocally innervated so that the antagonist muscle relaxes when the agonist contracts. The pathway for coupling these motoneurons is unknown. It is independent from the MLF since lesions there do not abolish vergence,[61] and the firing pattern of physiologically identified internuclear neurons in the abducens nucleus is inappropriate to convey convergence signals.[219] A projection from the oculomotor nucleus to the abducens nucleus has been identified anatomically,[220] and this may effect the coordination between these motor nuclei during vergence.

Disorders of vergence may be organic or functional. Spasm of the near reflex with intermittent convergence, miosis, and accommodation is often a functional disturbance. Although this presentation has been mistaken for bilateral abducens nerve palsies and other neurologic disorders, several distinguishing features provide reliable clues to the correct diagnosis. Patients are often young, female, and complain vehemently about diplopia, blurred vision, and headache (from prolonged voluntary convergence). Pronounced miosis with limited abduction on attempted lateral gaze, and yet full range of eye movements with monocular viewing (ductions) or oculocephalic maneuvers are virtually pathognomonic.[220] Spasm of the near reflex has been observed with a wide variety of organic disorders of the nervous system, but this is rare and usually asymptomatic.[221] Paresis of convergence in association with abnormalities in vertical gaze occurs commonly with mesencephalic lesions (Parinaud's syndrome). There may also be light-near dissociation of pupillary reflexes and convergence-retraction nystagmus. The latter is elicited by moving an optokinetic tape downward. Slow-phase downward tracking is normal, but upward quick phases are replaced by rapid convergence movements with globe retraction owing to co-contraction of extraocular muscles. Convergence effort may also enhance or diminish many forms of nystagmus that arise from disorders in conjugate oculomotor systems.[9]

Clinical Methods for Measuring Eye Movements

Accurate measurement of eye movements has become essential for the description of both normal and abnormal ocular motility. With practice, the examiner can detect movements of 1 degree at the bedside[222] or even motions of 10 min of arc with ophthalmoscopy.[223] These qualitative observations are obviously noninvasive and inexpensive and are able to detect motion about all three rotational axes. However, no permanent record is produced for further analysis, different types of rapid eye movements and oscillations may be difficult to distinguish, and some eye movements are appreciated only in darkness. The ideal eye movement recording system does not exist, and one must weigh the cost and benefits of accuracy, sensitivity, expense, portability, and patient demands inherent with each technique. From a technical standpoint, the optimal system would: (1) measure eye rotation in all three directions; (2) be linear over a range exceeding 90 degrees, yet be sensitive enough to detect motion of only a few minutes of arc; (3) be insensitive to head motion; (4) have a broad dynamic range from zero to several hundred hertz; (5) require no physical contact with the eye; and (6) obscure no part of the visual field. Several reviews have described how each available class of measuring device attempts to achieve these goals,[208, 224–226] and only the three techniques in common clinical use are described herein.

The electrooculogram (EOG) is the most commonly used technique for measuring and recording eye movements. It is simple, inexpensive, and noninvasive yet is also the most artifact prone. The steady corneoretinal potential difference of approximately 1 mV acts as the dipole that generates the EOG signal. Differential recordings are made by placing surface electrodes on opposite sides of the orbit (medial and lateral canthi for horizontal eye movements, upper and lower lids for vertical). Torsional rotations cannot be measured. The amplitude of the EOG signal is approximately 20 μV/degree[227] and is contaminated by electrical signals from galvanic skin responses, EMG of facial muscles, and lid movement artifacts that make recording of vertical eye movements very limited. Furthermore, the amplitude of the corneoretinal potential varies with illumination.[228] For all these reasons the EOG must be recalibrated frequently, at least every 5 min, so that an accuracy of 0.5 degree can be achieved over a range of ±30 degrees horizontally. AC-coupled amplifiers are often used to cancel the slow drift that appears in the EOG signal, but this technique obscures the absolute eye-position information of the EOG so that position-dependent abnormalities might be missed. Despite these shortcomings, DC-coupled EOG remains the preferred method in most clinical laboratories. A particularly important advantage of the EOG is that it is independent of head motion and is thus suited for positional or rotational testing.

Many optical techniques for measuring eye movements have been developed: corneal reflection, double-image Purkinje image tracker, optical lever, and others,[208, 224] but for clinical testing most systems are based on differential reflection of light from the border of the iris and conjunctiva (limbus). Photodiodes are positioned on opposing sides of the eye so that rotation brings more of the dark iris, and therefore less reflected light, under one detector while the opposite one receives an increase in light reflected from the white conjunctiva. Infrared illumination and detectors are used to eliminate artifacts from ambient light sources. The photodiodes must be firmly attached to the head, because any motion of the detector relative to the head produces a signal that may be confused with actual eye rotation. For example, a 100-μm displacement of the detector causes the same signal that 0.5 degree of eye rotation would produce.[224] Usually the detectors are mounted on eyeglass frames, and considerable patient cooperation is required to achieve an accurate recording. As with EOG, lid movements severely limit the ability to record vertical eye movements. The operational range for horizontal eye movements is ±20 degrees with a resolution of 0.5 degree. The photodiode signal has less high-frequency noise than the EOG so that the former may be more desirable when eye velocity is to be measured from electronic differentiation of the eye-position signal.

The magnetic search coil technique has become widely accepted as the most accurate means of measuring eye movements. This method is based on the principle that voltage generated in a "search coil" of wire placed in an alternating magnetic field (spatially uniform and artificially generated) is proportional to the sine of the angle between the plane of the search coil and the axis of the magnetic field.[229] A pair of search coils can be imbedded into an annular scleral contact lens so that horizontal, vertical, and torsional eye movements can be measured.[230] A light contact lens in combination with fine flexible lead wires ensures that the lens remains fixed to the globe and that no appreciable external forces are imparted to the eye. The system measures rotation of the search coil relative to the magnetic field. Consequently, eye position can be measured relative to the orbit when the head is fixed relative to the externally applied magnetic field, or alternatively both head and eye position in space can be measured with an earth-fixed magnetic field and a second coil can be fixed to the head. The operational range is ±50 degrees, with a resolution of 0.25 degree and a band width of 0 to 1000 Hz. Unfortunately, many patients find the scleral contact lens uncomfortable, even with topical anesthetics, and the search coil–contact lens assembly is expensive and frequently needs to be replaced. Therefore, for routine screening, most clinicians use the EOG or infrared reflection techniques and reserve magnetic search coil measurements for situations that require either high accuracy, large vertical, or torsional eye movement recordings.

REFERENCES

1. Westheimer G, McKee SD: Visual acuity in the presence of retinal-image motion. J Opt Soc Am 65:1275, 1975.
2. Lisberger SG, Pavelko TA: Vestibular signals carried by pathways subserving plasticity of the vestibulo-ocular reflex. J Neurosci 6:346, 1986.
3. Cohen B, Henn V, Raphan T, Dennett D: Velocity storage, nystagmus, and visual-vestibular interactions in humans. Ann N Y Acad Sci 374:421, 1982.
4. Cohen B, Matsuo V, Raphan T: Quantitative analysis of the velocity characteristics of optokinetic nystagmus and optokinetic after-nystagmus. J Physiol (Lond) 270:321, 1977.
5. Robinson DA: Linear addition of optokinetic and vestibular signals in the vestibular nucleus. Exp Brain Res 30:447, 1977.
6. Bahill AT, Clark MR, Stark L: The main sequence: A tool for studying human eye movements. Math Biosci 24:191, 1975.
7. Sharpe JA, Troost BT, Dell'Osso LF, Daroff RB: Comparative velocities of different types of fast eye movements in man. Invest Ophthalmol 14:689, 1975.
8. Halmagyi GM, Gresty MA: Clinical signs of visual-vestibular interaction. J Neurol Neurosurg Psychiatry 42:934, 1979.
9. Leigh RJ, Zee DS: The neurology of eye movements, 2nd ed. Philadelphia, FA Davis, 1991.
10. Sharpe JA: Supranuclear disorders of horizontal eye motion. Semin Neurol 6(2):155, 1986.
11. Robinson DA: The use of control systems analysis in the neurophysiology of eye movements. Annu Rev Neurosci 4:463, 1981.
12. Robinson DA: The mechanics of human saccadic eye movement. J Physiol (Lond) 174:245, 1964.
13. Robinson DA: Oculomotor unit behavior in the monkey. J Neurophysiol 33:393, 1970.
14. Fuchs AF, Luschei ES: Firing patterns of abducens neurons of alert monkeys in relationship to horizontal eye movements. J Neurophysiol 33:382, 1970.
15. Schiller PH: The discharge characteristics of single units in the oculomotor and abducens nuclei of the unanesthetized monkey. Exp Brain Res 10:347, 1970.
16. Robinson DA, O'Meara DM, Scott AB, Collins CC: Mechanical components of human eye movements. J Appl Physiol 26:548, 1969.
17. Collins CC: The human oculomotor control system. *In* Lennerstrand G, Bach-y-Rita P (eds): Basic Mechanisms of Ocular Motility and Their Clinical Implications. Oxford, Pergamon, 1975, pp 145–180.
18. VanGisbergen JAM, Robinson DA, Gielen SA: A quantitative analysis of the generation of saccadic eye movements by burst neurons. J Neurophysiol 45:417, 1981.
19. Skavenski AA, Robinson DA: Role of abducens neurons in the vestibuloocular reflex. J Neurophysiol 36:724, 1973.
20. Keller EL, Robinson DA: Abducens unit behavior in the monkey during vergence movements. Vision Res 12:369, 1972.
21. Henn V, Cohen B: Coding of information about rapid eye movements in the pontine reticular formation of alert monkeys. Brain Res 108:307, 1990.
22. Keller EL: Participation of the medial pontine reticular formation in eye movement generation in monkey. J Neurophysiol 37:316, 1974.
23. Keller EL, Robinson DA: Absence of a stretch reflex in extraocular muscles of the monkey. J Neurophysiol 34:908, 1971.
24. Robinson DA: Eye movement control in primates. Science 161:1219, 1968.

25. Fernandez C, Goldberg JM: Physiology of peripheral neurons innervating semicircular canals of the squirrel monkey. II: Response to sinusoidal stimulation and dynamics of peripheral vestibular system. J Neurophysiol 35:661, 1971.
26. Waespe W, Henn V: Neuronal activity in the vestibular nuclei of the alert monkey during vestibular and optokinetic stimulation. Exp Brain Res 27:523, 1977.
27. Miles FA, Fuller JH: Visual tracking and the primate flocculus. Science 189:1000, 1975.
28. Robinson DA: Oculomotor control signals. *In* Lennerstrand G, Bach-y-Rita P (eds): Basic Mechanisms of Ocular Motility and Their Clinical Implications. Oxford, Pergamon Press, 1975, pp 337–374.
29. Cannon SC, Robinson DA: Loss of the neural integrator of the oculomotor system from brain stem lesions in monkeys. J Neurophysiol 57(5): 1383, 1987.
30. Cheron G, Gillis P, Godaux E: Lesions in the cat prepositus complex: Effects on the optokinetic system. J Physiol (Lond) 372:95, 1986.
31. Cheron G, Godaux E, Laune JM, VanDerkerlen B: Lesions in the cat prepositus complex: Effects on the vestibulo-ocular reflex and saccades. J Physiol (Lond) 372:75, 1986.
32. Cannon SC, Robinson DA, Shamma S: A proposed neural network for the integrator of the oculomotor system. Biol Cybern 49:127, 1983.
33. Cannon SC, Zee DS: The neural integrator of the oculomotor system. Curr Neuro Ophthalmol 1:123, 1988.
34. Hood JD, Kayan A, Leech J: Rebound nystagmus. Brain 96:507, 1973.
35. Yamazaki A, Zee DS: Rebound nystagmus: EOG analysis of a case with a floccular tumour. Br J Ophthalmol 63:782, 1979.
36. Sharpe JA: Rebound nystagmus—A cerebellar sign? JAMA 227:648, 1974.
37. Becker W, Klein HM: Accuracy of saccadic eye movements and maintenance of eccentric eye positions in the dark. Vision Res 13:1021, 1973.
38. Fukashima K: The interstitial nucleus of cajal and its role in the control of movements of the head and eyes. Progr Neurobiol 29:107, 1987.
39. Robinson DA: The effect of cerebellectomy on the cat's vestibuloocular integrator. Brain Res 71:195, 1974.
40. Westheimer G, Blair SM: Oculomotor defects in cerebellectomized monkeys. Invest Ophthalmol 12:618, 1973.
41. Zee DS, Yamazaki A, Butler PH, Gucer G: Effects of ablation of flocculus and paraflocculus on eye movements in primate. J Neurophysiol 46:878, 1981.
42. Remler BF, Leigh RJ, Osorio I, Tomsak RL: The characteristics and mechanisms of visual disturbance associated with anticonvulsant therapy. Neurology 40:791, 1990.
43. Henn V, Hepp K, Buttner-Ennever JA: The primate oculomotor system. II: Premotor system. Hum Neurobiol 1:87, 1982.
44. Porter JD, Guthrie BL, Sparks DL: Innervation of monkey extraocular muscles: localization of sensory and motoneurons by retrograde transport of horseradish peroxidase. J Comp Neurol 218:208, 1983.
45. Spencer RF, Porter JD: Innervation and structure of extraocular muscles in the monkey in comparison to those of the cat. J Comp Neurol 198:649, 1981.
46. Langer T, Fuchs AF, Scudder CA, Chubb MC: Afferents to the flocculus of the cerebellum in the rhesus macaque as revealed by retrograde transport of horseradish peroxidase. J Comp Neurol 235:1, 1985.
47. Graybiel AM, Hartweig EA: Some afferent connections of the oculomotor complex in the cat: An experimental study with tracer techniques. Brain Res 81:543, 1974.
48. Fuchs AF, Scudder CA, Kaneko CR: Discharge patterns and recruitment order of identified motoneurons and internuclear neurons in the monkey adbucens nucleus. J Neurophysiol 60:1874, 1988.
49. Carpenter MB, McMasters RE, Hanna GR: Disturbances of conjugate horizontal eye movements in the monkey. I: Physiological effects and anatomical degeneration resulting from lesions of the abducens nucleus and nerve. Arch Neurol 8:231, 1963.
50. Pola J, Robinson DA: Oculomotor signals in the medial longitudinal fasciculus of the monkey. J Neurophysiol 41:245, 1978.
51. Kupfer C, Cogan DG: Unilateral internuclear ophthalmoplegia: A clinicopathological case report. Arch Ophthalmol 75:485, 1966.
52. Feldon SE, Hoyt WF, Stark L: Disordered inhibition in internuclear ophthalmoplegia: Analysis of eye movement recordings with computer simulations. Brain 103:113, 1980.
53. Baloh RW, Yee RD, Honrubia V: Internuclear ophthalmoplegia. I: Saccades and dissociated nystagmus. Arch Neurol 35:484, 1978.
54. Zee DS, Hain TC, Carl JR: Abduction nystagmus in internuclear ophthalmoplegia. Ann Neurol 21:383, 1987.
55. Stroud MH, Newman NM, Keltner JL, Gay AJ: Abducting nystagmus in the medial longitudinal fasciculus (MLF) syndrome—Internuclear ophthalmoplegia. Arch Ophthalmol 92:2, 1974.
56. Pola J, Robinson DA: An explanation of eye movements seen in internuclear ophthalmoplegia. Arch Neurol 33:447, 1976.
57. Gamlin PDR, Gnadt JW, Mays LE: Lidocaine-induced unilateral internuclear ophthalmoplegia: Effects on convergence and conjugate eye movements. J Neurophysiol 62:82, 1989.
58. Buttner-Ennever JA, Akert K: Medial rectus subgroups of the oculomotor nucleus and their abducens input in the monkey. J Comp Neurol 197:17, 1981.
59. Glaser JS: Myasthenic pseudo-internuclear ophthalmoplegia. Arch Ophthalmol 75:363, 1966.
60. Baloh RW, Yee RD, Honrubia V: Internuclear ophthalmoplegia. II: Pursuit, optokinetic nystagmus, and vestibulo-ocular reflex. Arch Neurol 35:490, 1978.
61. Evinger C, Fuchs AF, Baker R: Bilateral lesions of the medial longitudinal fasciculus in monkeys: Effects on the horizontal and vertical components of voluntary and vestibular induced eye movements. Exp Brain Res 28:1, 1977.
62. Fisher CM: Some neuro-ophthalmological observations. J Neurol Neurosurg Psychiatry 30:383, 1967.
63. Pierrot-Deseilligny C, Chain F, Serdaru M, et al: The 'one-and-a-half' syndrome: Electro-oculographic analyses of five cases with deductions about the physiological mechanisms of lateral gaze. Brain 104:665, 1981.
64. Mustari MJ, Fuchs AF: Discharge patterns of neurons in the pretectal nucleus of the optic tract (NOT) in the behaving primate. J Neurophysiol 64:77, 1990.
65. Cooper HM, Magnin M: A common mammalian plan of accessory optic system organization revealed in all primates. Nature 324:457, 1986.
66. Strassman A, Highstein SM, McCrea RA: Anatomy and physiology of saccadic burst neurons in the alert squirrel monkey. J Comp Neurol 249:337, 1986.
67. Waespe W, Cohen B, Raphan T: Role of the flocculus and paraflocculus in optokinetic nystagmus and visual-vestibular interactions: Effects of lesions. Exp Brain Res 50:9, 1983.
68. Schnyder H, Reisine H, Hepp K, Henn V: Frontal eye field projection to the paramedian pontine reticular formation traced with wheat germ agglutinin in the monkey. Brain Res 329:151, 1985.
69. McCrea RA, Strassman A, May E, Highstein SM: Anatomical and physiological characteristics of vestibular neurons mediating the horizontal vestibulo-ocular reflex in squirrel monkey. J Comp Neurol 264:547, 1987.
70. Morrow MJ, Sharpe JA: Cerebral hemispheric localization of smooth pursuit asymmetry. Neurology 40:284, 1990.
71. Tusa RJ, Ungerleider LG: Fiber pathways of cortical areas mediating smooth pursuit eye movements in monkeys. Ann Neurol 23:174, 1988.
72. Newsome WT, Wurtz RH, Komatsu H: Relation of cortical areas MT and MST to pursuit eye movements. II: Differentiation of retinal from extraretinal inputs. J Neurophysiol 60:604, 1988.
73. May JG, Keller EL, Suzuki DA: Smooth-pursuit eye movement deficits with chemical lesions in the dorsolateral pontine nucleus of the monkey. J Neurophysiol 59:952, 1988.
74. Mustari MJ, Fuchs AF, Wallman J: Response properties of dorsolateral pontine units during smooth pursuit in rhesus macaque. J Neurophysiol 60:664, 1988.
75. Stone LS, Lisberger SG: Visual responses of Purkinje cells in the cerebellar flocculus during smooth-pursuit eye movements in monkeys. I: Simple spikes. J Neurophysiol 63:1241, 1990.

76. Bender MB, Shanzer S: Oculomotor pathways defined by electrical stimulation and lesions in the brain stem of monkey. *In* Bender MB (ed): The Oculomotor System. New York, Harper & Row, 1964, pp 81–140.
77. Zackon DH, Sharpe JA: Midbrain paresis of horizontal gaze. Ann Neurol 16:495, 1984.
78. Bender MB: Comments on the physiology and pathology of eye movements in the vertical plane. J Nerv Ment Dis 130:456, 1960.
79. Hall AJ: Some observations on the acts of closing and opening the eyes. Br J Ophthalmol 20:257, 1936.
80. Christoff N: A clinicopathologic study of vertical eye movements. Arch Neurol 31:1, 1974.
81. Ranalli PJ, Sharpe JA, Fletcher WA: Palsy of upward and downward saccadic, pursuit, and vestibular movements with a unilateral midbrain lesion. Neurology 38:114, 1988.
82. Buttner-Ennever JA, Buttner U, Cohen B, Baumgartner G: Vertical gaze paralysis and the rostral interstitial nucleus of the medial longitudinal fasciculus. Brain 105:125, 1982.
83. Pasik T, Pasik P: Experimental models of oculomotor dysfunction in the rhesus monkey. *In* Meldrum BS, Marsden CD (eds): Advances in Neurology. New York, Raven Press, 1975, pp 77–89.
84. King WM, Fuchs AF: Reticular control of vertical saccadic eye movements by mesencephalic burst neurons. J Neurophysiol 42:861, 1979.
85. Buttner-Ennever JA, Buttner U: A cell group associated with vertical eye movements in the rostral mesencephalic reticular formation of the monkey. Brain Res 151:31, 1978.
86. Henn V, Cohen B: Coding of information about rapid eye movements in the pontine reticular formation of alert monkey. Brain Res 108:307, 1976.
87. Luschei ES, Fuchs AF: Activity of brain stem neurons during eye movements of alert monkeys. J Neurophysiol 35:445, 1972.
88. Highstein SM, Reisine H: Synaptic and functional organization of vestibulo-ocular reflex pathways. Prog Brain Res 50:431, 1979.
89. Pasik P, Pasik T, Bender MB: The pretectal syndrome in monkeys. I: Disturbances of gaze and body posture. Brain 92:521, 1969.
90. Halmagyi GM, Evans WA, Hallinan JM: Failure of downward gaze. Arch Neurol 35:22, 1978.
91. Trojanowski JQ, Wray SH: Vertical gaze ophthalmoplegia: Selective paralysis of downgaze. Neurology 30:605, 1980.
92. Kompf D, Pasik T, Pasik P, Bender MB: Downward gaze in monkeys: Stimulation and lesion studies. Brain 102:527, 1979.
93. Keane JR, Davis RL: Pretectal syndrome with metastatic malignant melanoma to the posterior commissure. Am J Ophthalmol 82:910, 1976.
94. Keane JR: The pretectal syndrome: 206 patients. Neurology 40:684, 1990.
95. Bienfang DC: Crossing axons in the third nerve nucleus. Invest Ophthalmol 14:927, 1975.
96. Ebner R, Lopez L, Ochoa S, Crovetto L: Vertical ocular motor apraxia. Neurology 40:712, 1990.
97. Fischer B, Ramsperger E: Human express saccades: Extremely short reaction times of goal directed eye movements. Exp Brain Res 57:191, 1984.
98. Fletcher WA, Sharpe JA: Alzheimer's disease: Saccadic eye movement dysfunction. Ann Neurol 16:495, 1984.
99. White OB, Saint-Cyr JA, Tomlinson RD, Sharpe JA: Ocular motor deficits in Parkinson's disease. II: Control of the saccadic and smooth pursuit systems. Brain 106:571, 1983.
100. Lasker AG, Zee DS, Hain TC, et al: Saccades in Huntington's disease: Slowing and dysmetria. Neurology 38:427, 1988.
101. Sharpe JA: Adaptation to frontal lobe lesions. *In* Keller EL, Zee DS (eds): Adaptive Processes in Visual and Oculomotor Systems. Oxford, Pergamon Press, 1986, pp 239–246.
102. Becker W: Metrics. *In* Wurtz RH, Goldberg ME (eds): The Neurobiology of Saccadic Eye Movements. Amsterdam, Elsevier, 1989, pp 13–68.
103. Weber RB, Daroff RB: The metrics of horizontal saccadic eye movements in normal humans. Vision Res 11:921, 1971.
104. Henson DB: Investigation into corrective saccadic eye movements for refixation amplitudes of 10 degrees and below. Vision Res 19:57, 1979.
105. Becker W: The control of eye movements in the saccadic system. Bibl Ophthalmol 82:233, 1972.
106. Robinson DA: Models of the saccadic eye movement control system. Kybernetik 14:71, 1973.
107. Henson DB: Corrective saccades: Effects of altering visual feedback. Vision Res 18:63, 1978.
108. Optican LM, Robinson DA: Cerebellar-dependent adaptive control of the primate saccadic system. J Neurophysiol 44:1058, 1980.
109. Weber RB, Daroff RB: Corrective movements following refixation saccades: Type and control system analysis. Vision Res 12:467, 1972.
110. Wurtz RH, Goldberg ME: The Neurobiology of Saccadic Eye Movements. Amsterdam, Elsevier, 1989.
111. Buttner-Ennever JA: Neuroanatomy of the Oculomotor System. Amsterdam, Elsevier, 1988.
112. Henn V, Lang W, Hepp K, Reisine H: Experimental gaze palsies in monkeys and their relation to human pathology. Brain 107:619, 1984.
113. Pierrot-Deseilligny C, Goasguen J, Chain F, Lapresle J: Pontine metastasis with dissociated bilateral horizontal gaze paralysis. J Neurol Neurosurg Psychiatry 47:861, 1984.
114. Hikosaka O, Igusa Y, Nako S, Shimazu H: Direct inhibitory synaptic linkage of pontomedullary reticular burst neurons with abducens motoneurons in the cat. Exp Brain Res 33:337, 1978.
115. Buttner-Ennever JA, Cohen B, Pause M, Fries W: Raphe nucleus of the pons containing omnipause neurons of the oculomotor system in the monkey, and its homologue in man. J Comp Neurol 267:307, 1988.
116. Nako S, Curthoys IS, Markham CH: Direct inhibitory projection of pause neurons to nystagmus-related pontomedullary reticular burst neurons in the cat. Exp Brain Res 40:283, 1980.
117. Hepp K, Henn V, Vilis T, Cohen B: Brain stem regions related to saccade generation. *In* Wurtz RH, Goldberg ME (eds): The Neurobiology of Saccadic Eye Movements. Amsterdam, Elsevier, 1989, pp 105–212.
118. Sparks DL, Mays LE, Porter JD: Eye movement induced by pontine stimulation: Interaction with visually-triggered saccades. J Neurophysiol 58:300, 1987.
119. Sparks DL, Mays LE: Spatial localization of saccade targets. I: Compensation for stimulation-induced perturbations in eye position. J Neurophysiol 49:45, 1983.
120. Zee DS, Robinson DA: A hypothetical explanation of saccadic oscillations. Ann Neurol 5:405, 1979.
121. Scudder CA: A new local feedback model of the saccadic burst generator. J Neurophysiol 59:1455, 1988.
122. Zee DS: Ocular motor control: The cerebral control of saccadic eye movements. *In* Lessell S, VanDalen JTW (eds): Neuroophthalmology. Amsterdam, Elsevier, 1984, pp 141–156.
123. Schiller PH, True SD, Conway JL: Deficits in eye movements following frontal eye-field and superior colliculus ablations. J Neurophysiol 44:1175, 1980.
124. Schlag-Rey M, Schlag J: Visuomotor functions of central thalamus in monkey. I: Unit activity related to spontaneous eye movements. J Neurophysiol 51:1149, 1984.
125. Albano JE, Wurtz RH: Deficits in eye position following ablation of monkey superior colliculus, pretectum, and posterior-medial thalamus. J Neurophysiol 48:318, 1982.
126. Casagrande VA, Harting JK, Hall WC, Diamond IT: Superior colliculus of the tree shrew (Tupaia glis): Evidence for a structural and functional subdivision into superficial and deep layers. Science 177:444, 1972.
127. Robinson DL, McClurkin JW: The visual superior colliculus and pulvinar. *In* Wurtz RH, Goldberg ME (eds): The Neurobiology of Saccadic Eye Movements. Amsterdam, Elsevier, 1989, pp 337–360.
128. Cynader M, Berman N: Receptive-field organization of monkey superior colliculus. J Neurophysiol 35:187, 1972.
129. Robinson DA: Eye movements evoked by collicular stimulation in the alert monkey. Vision Res 12:1795, 1972.
130. Schiller PH, Stryker M: Single-unit recording and stimulation in superior colliculus of the alert rhesus monkey. J Neurophysiol 35:915, 1972.
131. Edwards SB: The deep cell layers of the superior colliculus: Their reticular characteristics and structural organization. *In*

Hobson JA, Brazier MAB (eds): The Reticular Formation Revisited. New York, Raven Press, 1980, pp 193–209.
132. Wurtz RH, Goldberg ME: Activity of superior colliculus in monkey. IV: Effects of lesions on eye movements. J Neurophysiol 35:575, 1972.
133. Hikosaka O, Wurtz RH: Saccadic eye movements following injection of lidocaine into the superior colliculus. Exp Brain Res 61:531, 1986.
134. Hikosaka O, Wurtz RH: Modification of saccadic eye movements by GABA-related substances. I: Effect of muscimol and bicuculline in monkey superior colliculus. J Neurophysiol 53:266, 1985.
135. Mohler CW, Wurtz RH: Role of striate cortex and superior colliculus in visual guidance of saccadic eye movements in monkeys. J Neurophysiol 40:74, 1977.
136. Hikosaka O, Wurtz RH: Visual and oculomotor functions of monkey substantia nigra pars reticulata. I: Relation of visual and auditory responses to saccades. J Neurophysiol 49:1230, 1983.
137. Dichiara G, Porceddu ML, Morelli ML, et al: Evidence for a GABAergic projection from the substantia nigra to the ventromedial thalamus and to the superior colliculus of the rat. Brain Res 176:273, 1979.
138. Araki M, McGeer PL, McGeer EG: Presumptive gamma-aminobutyric acid pathways from the midbrain to the superior colliculus studied by a combined horseradish peroxidase-gamma-aminobutyric acid transaminase pharmacohistochemical method. Neuroscience 13:433, 1984.
139. Chevalier G, Thierry AM, Shibazaki T, Feger J: Evidence for a GABAergic inhibitory nigrotectal pathway in the rat. Neurosci Lett 21:67, 1984.
140. Hikosaka O, Wurtz RH: Modification of saccadic eye movements by GABA-related substances. II: Effects of muscimol in monkey substantia nigra pars reticulata. J Neurophysiol 53:292, 1985.
141. DeJong JD, Melvill Jones G: Akinesia, hypokinesia, and bradykinesia in the oculomotor system of patients with Parkinson's disease. Exp Neurol 32:58, 1971.
142. Bronstein AM, Kennard C: Predictive ocular motor control in Parkinson's disease. Brain 108:925, 1985.
143. Leigh RJ, Newman SA, Folstein SE, et al: Abnormal ocular motor control in Huntington's disease. Neurology 33:1268, 1983.
144. Robinson DA, Fuchs AF: Eye movements evoked by stimulation of frontal eye fields. J Neurophysiol 32:637, 1969.
145. Bruce CJ, Goldberg ME, Stanton GB, Bushnell MC: Primate frontal eye fields. II: Physiological and anatomical correlates of electrically evoked eye movements. J Neurophysiol 54:714, 1985.
146. Bizzi E, Schiller PH: Single unit activity in the frontal eye fields of unanesthetized monkeys during head and eye movement. Exp Brain Res 10:151, 1970.
147. Bruce CJ, Goldberg ME: Primate frontal eye fields. I: Single neurons discharging before saccades. J Neurophysiol 53:603, 1985.
148. Leichnetz GR, Goldberg ME: Higher centers concerned with eye movement and visual attention: Cerebral cortex and thalamus. *In* Buttner-Ennever JA (ed): Neuroanatomy of the Oculomotor System. Amsterdam, Elsevier, 1988, pp 365–419.
149. Steiner I, Melamed E: Conjugate eye deviation after acute hemispheric stroke: Delayed recovery after previous contralateral frontal lobe damage. Ann Neurol 16:509, 1984.
150. Guitton D, Buchtel HA, Douglas RM: Disturbances of voluntary saccadic eye movement mechanisms following discrete unilateral frontal lobe removals. *In* Lennerstrand G, Zee DS, Keller EL (eds): Functional Basis of Ocular Motility Disorders. Oxford, Pergamon Press, 1982, pp 497–500.
151. Baloh RW, Honrubia V: Clinical Neurophysiology of the Vestibular System. Philadelphia, FA Davis, 1979.
152. Grossman GE, Leigh RJ, Abel LA, et al: Frequency and velocity of rotational head perturbations during locomotion. Exp Brain Res 70:470, 1988.
153. Pulaski PD, Zee DS, Robinson DA: The behavior of the vestibulo-ocular reflex at high velocities of head rotation. Brain Res 222:159, 1981.
154. Barr CC, Schulthesis LW, Robinson DA: Voluntary, non-visual control of the human vestibuloocular reflex. Acta Otolaryngol 81:365, 1976.
155. Raphan T, Matsuo V, Cohen B: Velocity storage in the vestibulo-ocular reflex arc (VOR). Exp Brain Res 35:229, 1979.
156. Lisberger SG: The latency of pathways containing the site of motor learning in the monkey vestibulo-ocular reflex. Science 225:74, 1984.
157. Ito M: Cerebellar control of the vestibulo-ocular reflex: Around the flocculus hypothesis. Annu Rev Neurosci 5:275, 1982.
158. Llinas R, Walton K: Vestibular compensation: A distributed property of the central nervous system. *In* Asanuma H, Wilson VJ (eds): Integration in the Nervous System. New York, Igaku-Shoin, 1979, pp 1140–1153.
159. Fetter M, Zee DS, Proctor LR: Effect of lack of vision and of occipital lobectomy upon recovery from unilateral labyrinthectomy in rhesus monkey. J Neurophysiol 59:394, 1988.
160. Lorente de No R: Vestibulo-ocular reflex arc. Arch Neurol Psychiatry 30:245, 1933.
161. Baker R, Evinger C, McCrea RA: Some thoughts about the three neurons in the vestibular ocular reflex. Ann N Y Acad Sci 374:171, 1981.
162. Shimazu H, Precht W: Inhibition of central vestibular neurons from the contralateral labyrinth and its mediating pathway. J Neurophysiol 29:467, 1966.
163. Galiana HL, Flohr H, Melvill Jones G: A Reevaluation of intervestibular nuclear coupling: Its role in vestibular compensation. J Neurophysiol 51:242, 1984.
164. Ito M, Shida T, Yagi N, Yamamoto M: The cerebellar modification of rabbit's horizontal vestibulo-ocular reflex induced by sustained head rotation combined with visual stimulation. Proc Jpn Acad 50:85, 1974.
165. Robinson DA: Adaptive gain control of vestibuloocular reflex by the cerebellum. J Neurophysiol 39:954, 1976.
166. Zee DS, Yee RD, Cogan DG, et al: Ocular motor abnormalities in hereditary cerebellar ataxia. Brain 99:207, 1976.
167. Baloh RW, Yee RD, Kimm J, Honrubia V: The vestibulo-ocular reflex in patients with lesions involving the vestibulo-cerebellum. Exp Neurol 72:141, 1981.
168. Lisberger SG, Evinger C, Johanson GW, Fuchs AF: Relationship between eye acceleration and retinal image velocity during foveal smooth pursuit in man and monkey. J Neurophysiol 46:229, 1981.
169. Chambers BR, Gresty MA: The relationship between disordered pursuit and vestibulo-ocular reflex suppression. J Neurol Neurosurg Psychiatry 46:61, 1983.
170. Giolli RA, Blanks RHI, Torigoe Y, Williams D: Projections of medial terminal accessory optic nucleus, ventral tegmental nuclei, and substantia nigra of rabbit and rat as studied by axonal transport of horseradish peroxidase. J Comp Neurol 232:99, 1985.
171. Collewijn H: Optokinetic eye movements in the rabbit: Input-output relations. Vision Res 9:117, 1969.
172. Ter Braak JWG: Untersuchungen uber optokinetischen Nystagmus. Arch Neerlandaises de Physiol 21:309, 1936.
173. Baloh RW, Yee RD, Honrubia V: Clinical abnormalities of optokinetic nystagmus. *In* Lennerstrand G, Zee DS, Keller BJ (eds): Functional Basis of Ocular Motility Disorders. New York, Pergamon Press, 1982, pp 311–320.
174. Ter Braak JWG, Schenk VWD, Van Vliet AGM: Visual reactions in a case of long-lasting cortical blindness. J Neurol Neurosurg Psychiatry 34:140, 1971.
175. Zee DS, Yee RD, Robinson DA: Optokinetic responses in labyrinthine-defective human beings. Brain Res 113:423, 1976.
176. Uemura T, Cohen B: Vestibulo-ocular reflexes: Effects of vestibular nuclear lesions. *In* Brodal A, Pompeiano O (eds): Progress in Brain Research: Basic Aspects of Central Vestibular Mechanisms. Amsterdam, Elsevier, 1972, pp 515–528.
177. Baloh RW, Yee RD, Honrubia V: Optokinetic nystagmus and parietal lobe lesions. Ann Neurol 7:269, 1980.
178. Fox JC, Holmes G: Optic nystagmus and its value in the localization of cerebral lesions. Brain 49:333, 1926.
179. Smith JL: Optokinetic Nystagmus. Springfield, IL, CC Thomas, 1963.
180. Rashbass C: The relationship between saccadic and smooth tracking eye movements. J Physiol (Lond) 159:326, 1961.
181. Robinson DA: The mechanics of human smooth pursuit eye movements. J Physiol (Lond) 180:569, 1965.

182. Baloh RW, Kumley WE, Sills AW, et al: Quantitative measurement of smooth pursuit eye movements. Ann Otol Rhinol Laryngol 85:111, 1976.
183. Michael JA, Melvill Jones G: Dependence of visual tracking capability upon stimulus predictability. Vision Res 6:707, 1966.
184. Meyer CH, Lasker AG, Robinson DA: The upper limit of human smooth pursuit velocity. Vision Res 25:561, 1985.
185. Lisberger SG, Morris EJ, Tychsen L: Visual motion processing and sensory-motor integration for smooth pursuit eye movements. Annu Rev Neurosci 10:97, 1987.
186. Hubel DH, Wiesel TN: Receptive fields and functional architecture of monkey striate cortex. J Physiol (Lond) 195:215, 1968.
187. Zeki SM: Representation of central visual fields in prestriate cortex in monkey. Brain Res 14:271, 1969.
188. Maunsell JR, VanEssen DC: Functional properties of neurons in middle temporal visual area of the macaque monkey. I: Selectivity for stimulus direction, speed, and orientation. J Neurophysiol 49:1127, 1983.
189. Mohler C, Wurtz RH: Role of striate cortex and superior colliculus in visual guidance of saccadic eye movements in monkeys. J Neurophysiol 40:74, 1977.
190. Newsome WT, Wurtz RH, Dursteler MR, Mikami A: Punctate chemical lesions of striate cortex in the macaque monkey: Effect on visually guided saccades. Exp Brain Res 58:392, 1985.
191. Segraves MA, Goldberg ME, Deng S, et al: The role of striate cortex in the guidance of eye movements in the monkey. J Neurosci 7:3040, 1987.
192. Newsome WT, Wurtz RH, Dursteler MR, Mikami A: Deficits in visual motion perception following ibotenic acid lesions of the middle temporal visual area of the macaque monkey. J Neurosci 5:825, 1985.
193. Dursteler MR, Wurtz RH, Newsome WT: Pursuit and optokinetic deficits following chemical lesions of cortical areas MT and MST. J Neurophysiol 60:940, 1988.
194. Komatsu H, Wurtz RH: Modulation of pursuit eye movements by stimulation of cortical areas MT and MST. J Neurophysiol 62:31, 1989.
195. Sakata H, Shibutani H, Kawano K: Functional properties of visual tracking neurons in posterior parietal association cortex of the monkey. J Neurophysiol 49:1364, 1983.
196. Troost BT, Daroff RB, Weber RB, Dell'Osso LF: Hemispheric control of eye movements. II: Quantitative analysis of smooth pursuit in a hemispherectomy patient. Arch Neurol 27:449, 1972.
197. Sharpe JA, Lo AW, Rabinovitch HE: Control of the saccadic and smooth pursuit systems after cerebral hemidecortication. Brain 102:387, 1979.
198. Thurston SE, Leigh RJ, Crawford T, et al: Two distinct deficits of visual tracking caused by unilateral lesions of cerebral cortex in humans. Ann Neurol 23:266, 1988.
199. Pyyko I, Dahlen AI, Schalen L, Hindfelt B: Eye movements in patients with speech dyspraxia. Acta Otolaryngol (Stockh) 98:481, 1984.
200. Sharpe JA, Bondar RL, Fletcher WA: Contralateral gaze deviation after frontal lobe haemorrhage. J Neurol Neurosurg Psychiatry 48:86, 1985.
201. Glickstein M, May J, Mercer BE: Corticopontine projection in the macaque: The distribution of labeled cortical cells after large injections of horseradish peroxidase in the pontine nuclei. J Comp Neurol 235:343, 1985.
202. Glickstein M, Cohen JL, Dixon B, et al: Corticopontine visual projections in macaque monkeys. J Comp Neurol 190:209, 1980.
203. Suzuki DA, Keller EL: Visual signals in the dorsolateral pontine nucleus of the alert monkey: Their relationship to smooth-pursuit eye movements. Exp Brain Res 53:473, 1984.
204. Noda H, Suzuki DA: The role of the flocculus of the monkey in fixation and smooth pursuit eye movements. J Physiol (Lond) 294:335, 1979.
205. Suzuki DA, Noda H, Kase M: Visual and pursuit eye movement-related activity in posterior vermis of monkey cerebellum. J Neurophysiol 46:1120, 1981.
206. Westheimer G, Mitchell AM: Eye movement responses to convergent stimuli. Arch Ophthalmol 55:848, 1956.
207. Kenyon RV, Ciuffreda KJ, Stark L: Unequal saccades during vergence. Am J Optom Physiol Opt 57:586, 1980.
208. Robinson DA: Control of eye movements. *In* Brooks VB (ed): Handbook of Physiology—The Nervous System. II: Bethesda, MD, American Physiological Society, 1981, pp 1275–1320.
209. Westheimer G, Mitchell DE: The sensory stimulus for disjunctive eye movements. Vision Res 9:749, 1969.
210. Erkelens CJ, Steinman RM, Collewijn H: Ocular vergence under natural conditions. II: Gaze shifts between real targets differing in distance and direction. J Physiol (Lond) 236:441, 1989.
211. Mays LE: Neural control of vergence eye movements: Convergence and divergence neurons in the midbrain. J Neurophysiol 51:1091, 1984.
212. Mays LE, Porter JD, Gamlin PDR, Tello CA: Neural control of vergence eye movements: Neurons encoding vergence velocity. J Neurophysiol 56:1007, 1986.
213. Barlow HB, Blakemore C, Pettigrew JD: The neural mechanism of binocular depth discrimination. J Physiol (Lond) 193:327, 1967.
214. Jampel RS: Representation of the near response on the cerebral cortex of the macaque. Am J Ophthalmol 48:573, 1959.
215. Jampel RS: Convergence, divergence, pupillary reactions, and accommodation of the eyes from faradic stimulation of macaque brain. J Comp Neurol 115:371, 1960.
216. Sakata H, Shibutani H, Kawano K: Spatial properties of visual fixation neurons in posterior parietal association cortex of the monkey. J Neurophysiol 43:1654, 1980.
217. Hosoba M, Bando T, Tsukahara N: The cerebellar control of accommodation of the eye in the cat. Brain Res 153:495, 1978.
218. Mays LE, Porter JD: Neural control of vergence eye movements: Activity of abducens and oculomotor neurons. J Neurophysiol 52:743, 1984.
219. Gamlin PDR, Gnadt JW, Mays LE: Abducens internuclear neurons carry an inappropriate signal for ocular convergence. J Neurophysiol 62:70, 1989.
220. Maciewicz RJ, Spencer RF: Oculomotor and abducens internuclear pathways in the cat. *In* Baker R, Berthoz A (eds): Control of Gaze by Brain Stem Neurons. Amsterdam, Elsevier, 1977, pp 99–108.
221. Rabinowitz L, Chrousos GA, Cogan DC: Spasm of the near reflex associated with organic disease. Am J Ophthalmol 103:582, 1987.
222. Yarbus AL: Eye Movements and Vision. New York, Plenum, 1967.
223. Zee DS: Ophthalmoscopy in examination of patients with vestibular disorders. Ann Neurol 3:373, 1978.
224. Carpenter RHS: Movements of the Eyes. London, Pion, 1988.
225. Young LR, Sheena D: Survey of eye movement recording methods. Behav Res Methods Instrum 7:397, 1975.
226. Collewijn H, Van Der Mark F, Jansen TC: Precise recording of human eye movements. Vision Res 15:447, 1975.
227. Shackel B: Eye movement recording by electro-oculography. *In* Venables PH, Martin I (eds): Manual of Psychophysical Methods. Amsterdam, North-Holland, 1967, pp 229–334.
228. Gonshor A, Malcolm R: Effect of changes of illumination level on electro-oculography. Aerospace Med 41:138, 1971.
229. Robinson DA: A method of measuring eye movement using a scleral search coil in a magnetic field. IEEE Trans Bio-Med Electron 10:1246, 1963.
230. Ferman L, Collewijn H, Jansen TC, Van den Berg AV: Human gaze stability in the horizontal, vertical and torsional direction during voluntary head movements, evaluated with a three-dimensional scleral induction coil technique. Vision Res 27:811, 1987.
231. Robinson DA, Keller EL: The behavior of eye movement motoneurons in the alert monkey. Bibl Ophthalmol 82:7, 1972.
232. Cannon SC, Robinson DA: An improved neural-network model for the neural integrator of the oculomotor system: More realistic neuron behavior. Biol Cybern 53:93, 1985.

Chapter 193

Central Eye Movement Disorders

G. MICHAEL HALMAGYI

The organization of the ocular motor system is one of the clearest examples of neural hierarchy. "Upper" motoneurons in the frontal eye fields and posterior parietal cortex activate pre–motoneurons in the pons and midbrain. These pre–motoneurons in turn activate interneurons in the abducens nucleus and "lower" motor neurons in the abducens, oculomotor nuclei, and trochlear nuclei. Interneurons and lower motoneurons are also directly activated by the disynaptic vestibuloocular reflex arc (Fig. 193–1). Although the physiologic validity of this scheme may be questioned, its clinical utility is not in doubt and it is used throughout this chapter.

Because eye movement disorders are caused by lesions and diseases of the nervous system, the diagnosis of eye movement disorders does require some familiarity with the principles and methods of neurologic diagnosis. (For more details of the clinical method in neurologic diagnosis see references 1 and 2.) The aim of this chapter is to review briefly but systematically eye movement disorders that are caused by lesions and diseases of the central nervous system and that can pose a problem for the practicing ophthalmologist. Many patients with serious, treatable neurologic diseases first present with isolated eye movement disorders. In such cases, the entire diagnosis and subsequent management depends on the correct evaluation of the eye movement disorder. Only clinically important eye movement disorders are discussed here, and many of these can be confidently diagnosed clinically. For further details of eye movement disorders, the reader is referred to comprehensive monographs by Leigh and Zee,[3] to a handbook of neuro-ophthalmology by Miller,[4] and to a regular review of neuroophthalmology by Lessell and van Dalen.[5] For a discussion of the special problems of eye movement disorders in children, the reader is referred to a textbook of pediatric ophthalmology edited by Taylor[6]; for a discussion of eye movements in coma, the reader is referred to Chapter 198.

PRINCIPLES OF NEUROLOGIC DIAGNOSIS

A diagnosis is an answer to a question. A neurologic diagnosis consists of five answers to five questions.

Question 1. "Where is the lesion?" The answer to this question is the topographic diagnosis reached by the process of neurologic localization. It states whether the lesion involves a single location or several locations in the nervous system, or alternatively whether it affects a particular system or class of neurons in the neural hierarchy. For example, whereas a left lateral medullary infarct is a unifocal lesion and multiple sclerosis causes multifocal lesions, amyotrophic lateral sclerosis affects a class of neurons.

Question 2. "What is the activity of the lesion?" The answer to this question is the physiologic diagnosis. It states whether the lesion is producing deficient excitatory neural activity leading to neurologic hypofunction or whether it is producing excessive excitatory neural activity (perhaps through deficient inhibitory neural activity or denervation hypersensitivity) leading to neurologic hyperfunction. For example, in a patient with a dorsal midbrain lesion, downgaze palsy represents deficient neural activity, whereas oculogyric crises represent excessive neural activity.

Question 3. "How old is the lesion?" The answer to this question is the chronologic diagnosis. The physiologic diagnosis must take into account lesion-induced neural plasticity and denervation hypersensitivity, because both of these mechanisms progressively alter the pattern of neurologic dysfunction that occurs after an acute lesion. An example of neural plasticity is the contraversive saccadic palsy that occurs with acute unilateral cerebral hemisphere lesions. In contrast to the saccadic palsy that occurs with pontine lesions, the saccadic palsy that occurs with cerebral hemisphere lesions resolves within 2 to 3 wk. The pendular nystagmus that follows weeks to months after acute lesions of the central tegmental tract is an example of denervation hypersensitivity.

Question 4. "What is the nature of the lesion?" This is the pathologic diagnosis. For example in a patient with a left one-and-a-half syndrome due to a left pontine lesion, it should be determined whether the lesion is due to demyelination, neoplasm, infarction, or some other recognized pathologic process.

Question 5. "What is the cause of the lesion?" This is the etiologic diagnosis. For example in a patient with a left cerebral hemisphere infarct, it should be determined whether this is due to thrombosis or to embolism, and if it is due to embolism, then what is the source of the embolus.

The answers to these five questions are found by considering two entirely different sources of information. The answers to "Where is the lesion?"; "What is the activity of the lesion?"; and "How old is the lesion?" are found by considering the precise pattern of neurologic dysfunction as revealed by the neurologic examination. "What is the nature of the lesion?" and "What is the cause of the lesion?" are answered first by considering the temporal profile of evolution and resolution of neurologic dysfunction as revealed in the history; second, by searching for evidence of systemic disease; and

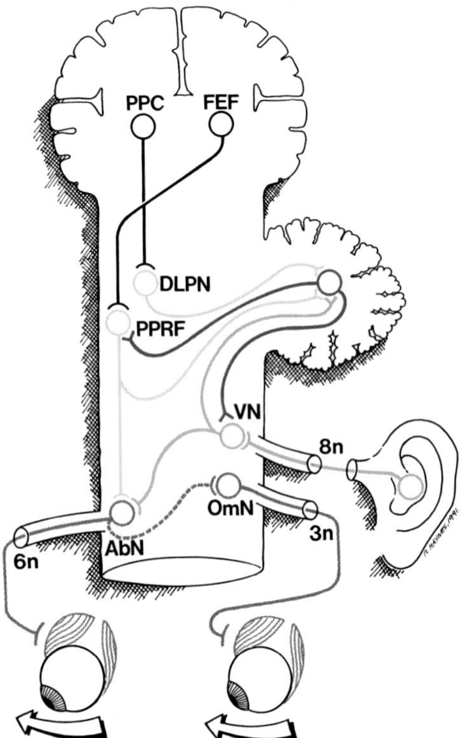

Figure 193–1. Schematic representation of the hierarchical organization of the ocular motor system. The example shown is the organization of rightward eye movements. *Level 1 (black)*: A supranuclear, or "upper," ocular motoneuron for rightward saccades projects from the frontal eye fields (FEF) of the left cerebral hemisphere to a premotor neuron (shown in blue) in the paramedian reticular formation of the right pons (PPRF). A supranuclear ocular motoneuron for rightward smooth pursuit projects from the right posterior parietal cortex (PPC) to a pre–motoneuron to the dorsolateral nucleus of the right pons (DLPN). *Level 2 (blue)*: A pre-motor neuron for rightward saccadic eye movements and a pre–motoneuron for rightward smooth pursuit project from the right PPRF and the right DLPN to "lower" ocular motoneurons (shown in brown) in the right abducens nucleus (AbN) (abducens motoneuron) and in the left oculomotor nucleus (OmN), (medial rectus motoneuron). *Level 3 (brown)*: The motoneurons project to the extraocular muscles *(level 6 [brown])* through the abducens (6n) and oculomotor (3n) nerves. An abducens interneuron is shown by the interrupted brown line. Brain stem pre–motoneurons also project to cerebellar neurons *(level 4 [purple])*, which project back to the pre–motoneurons. *Level 5 (yellow)*: A primary vestibular neuron from the left labyrinth projects to a secondary vestibular neuron in the left vestibular nucleus (VN) via the left vestibular nerve (8n). These neurons represent the afferent limb of the vestibuloocular reflex arc. The secondary vestibular neuron projects to the "lower" ocular motoneurons and interneurons in the right abducens nucleus to produce a rightward eye movement response to a leftward head rotation stimulus.

third, by evaluating the results of any special investigations.

It remains a cardinal rule of neurologic diagnosis that the pattern of neurologic dysfunction reflects only the site, age, and activity of the lesion and not its nature or cause. In other words only the site, age, and activity of a lesion—and not its nature or cause—are able to influence the pattern of neurologic dysfunction. The neurologic examination, which is the evaluation and analysis of the pattern of neurologic dysfunction, can therefore, only determine the site, age, and activity of a lesion and not its nature or cause. The nature and the cause of a lesion can only influence the temporal profile of the neurologic dysfunction, and this profile cannot be determined by a single neurologic examination.

Even so, accurate localization of a lesion can help to determine its nature. Different pathologic processes have a predilection for different sites in the nervous system. For example, a lesion in the lateral medulla is usually an infarct and not a tumor or a hemorrhage. Conversely, a correct pathologic diagnosis can suggest the likely site of a lesion. For example a patient known to have neurofibromatosis-2, will, by definition, eventually develop bilateral 8th cranial nerve lesions. In practice, however, it may only be possible to determine either the site of the lesion or nature of the lesion, but not both. Consider a patient with an internuclear ophthalmoplegia (INO) and ipsilateral lower motoneuron facial nerve palsy. Although there is no doubt that the lesion is in the ipsilateral pontine tegmentum, in the absence of historical details or positive investigations, the nature of the lesion cannot be determined. By contrast, in a patient with opsoclonus and a pelvic malignancy, although the paraneoplastic nature of the lesion is not in doubt, the site of the lesion causing the eye movement disorder can only be presumed.

NOMENCLATURE OF LESIONS OF THE OCULAR MOTOR SYSTEM

The aim of this section is to define certain descriptive terms used to categorize lesions that involve the nervous system in general and the ocular motor system in particular.

Focal Lesions Versus Diffuse Diseases. Focal lesions involve all adjacent neural structures within one or more circumscribed region of the nervous system. In contrast, diffuse disorders affect a class or category of neurons or excitable cells in the nervous system. Chronic progressive external ophthalmoplegia, myasthenia, Fisher's syndrome, Huntington's disease, and olivopontocerebellar degeneration are examples of diffuse diseases of the nervous system that produce eye movement disorders.

Intrinsic Versus Extrinsic Lesions. Lesions within the skull, which affect the brain, can be divided into those that arise within the substance of the brain itself and those that arise outside the substance of the brain, and only involve the brain secondarily, by compression or by invasion. This distinction is particularly relevant in the case of intracranial neoplasms. Intrinsic neoplasms are usually malignant and incurable, whereas extrinsic neoplasms are usually benign and potentially curable.

Central Versus Peripheral Lesions. Deciding whether the patient with an eye movement disorder has a central or a peripheral lesion is the basic minimum requirement of diagnosis. These two terms can be used in either a physiologic sense or in an anatomic sense. In the anatomic sense "central" is synonymous with "intrinsic" and "peripheral" is synonymous with "extrinsic." In the physiologic sense "central" is synonymous with "supranuclear" and "peripheral" is synonymous with "infranuclear." In this chapter "central" and "peripheral" are used in their anatomic sense.

Nuclear-Infranuclear Versus Supranuclear Lesions. Nuclear-infranuclear lesions comprise lesions of the ocular motor neurons—their cell bodies, their axons within the brain stem fascicles and within the cranial nerves themselves, the neuromuscular junction, and the extraocular muscles. Infranuclear lesions may be central or peripheral. An infranuclear lesion that involves the axons of the ocular motor neurons as they emerge from the motor nuclei in fascicles within the brain stem is clearly central. On the other hand a lesion that involves the same axons within a cranial nerve from its origin in the brain stem to the extraocular muscles is clearly peripheral. Nuclear-infranuclear lesions typically cause diplopia due to paralytic strabismus. Ocular motor neurons can be driven from above, in a hierarchical sense: (1) by saccadic inputs from the frontal cortex and superior colliculus, via reticular burst neurons; (2) by pursuit and optokinetic inputs from the parietal cortex; and (3) by vergence inputs (Fig. 193–1). Supranuclear lesions are lesions that affect any of these inputs, and they typically cause gaze palsies, nystagmus, and spontaneous or involuntary eye movements. All supranuclear and nuclear lesions are central, whereas infranuclear lesions may be either central or peripheral. The terms "upper motoneuron" and "lower motoneuron," traditionally used in clinical neurology, are essentially synonymous with the terms "supranuclear" and "nuclear-infranuclear," traditionally used in clinical neuro-ophthalmology.

Intracranial Versus Extracranial Lesions. Peripheral lesions of the ocular motor cranial nerves can arise outside the skull (e.g., in the postnasal space), as well as within the skull, or at the various exit foramina through the skull.

Restrictive Orbital Lesions. It is important to distinguish cases in which an ocular motor palsy is only apparent and is not due to a lesion of the ocular motor system itself but due to mechanical restriction of the motion of one or both eyes. Mechanical restriction occurs in orbit diseases when extraocular muscles are entrapped or infiltrated, and the resultant eye movement disorder can closely mimic those resulting from central or peripheral lesions.

Vestibuloocular Reflex Arc Lesions. The most potent segmental drive to brain stem ocular motor neurons is from the semicircular canals via the vestibular nuclei. This reflex arc consists of three neurons: the first is in Scarpa's ganglion; the second is in the vestibular nucleus; the third is the ocular motor neuron itself. Evaluation of the vestibuloocular reflex in the neuroophthalmologic examination is analogous to the evaluation of the tendon reflex in the general neurologic examination: Just as integrity of a tendon reflex demonstrates integrity of the spinal levels involved in the spinal reflex, integrity of the vestibuloocular reflex indicates integrity of the brain stem levels involved in the vestibuloocular reflex. In a conscious, alert patient, just as in a comatose patient, loss or impairment of the vestibuloocular reflexes indicates a lesion of the reflex arc.

CLINICAL EXAMINATION OF DISORDERED EYE MOVEMENTS

Magnetic Resonance Imaging (MRI) and the Diagnosis of Eye Movement Disorders

At this stage one may well ask "What is the point of such an elaborate process and such a detailed examination when it is so easy to show a lesion on MRI?" In some cases this is a perfectly valid point. MRI can provide a welcome short cut for the busy clinician confronted by a patient who has a difficult eye movement disorder. Consider a young man presenting with headache and an upgaze palsy. If the MRI shows a large mass lesion in the dorsal third ventricle, clearly any other midbrain eye movement disorders will only be of academic interest. But what if the MRI is normal? Does that really exclude a dorsal midbrain lesion? Or what if the MRI shows several areas of increased signal intensity in the subcortical white matter? Does that mean the patient has multiple sclerosis? Experienced clinicians know that in the absence of a considered clinical diagnosis, it can be dangerous to order, and misleading to interpret, radiologic images. It is dangerous practice to abbreviate the clinical examination and then attribute the clinical abnormalities to an abnormality demonstrated on MRI. Consider a middle-aged woman with poorly controlled hypertension presenting with episodic diplopia, definitely horizontal, possibly vertical, who is shown on MRI to have several small areas of increased signal intensity in the subcortical white matter and in the brain stem. In this case, it would be possible to make the diagnosis of cerebrovascular disease with multiple lacunar infarcts. However, it is only when careful examination reveals that in addition to a vertical heterotropia and a large controlled exophoria, she has bilateral asymmetric limitation of adduction amplitude in both eyes with normal saccadic velocities, that the possibility of myasthenia gravis will be seriously considered.

Oculography and the Diagnosis of Eye Movement Disorders

The role of oculography in the diagnosis of eye movement disorders is best explained by analogy with perimetry in the diagnosis of visual field disorders. Although we all examine the visual fields by confrontation, particularly in a patient suspected of having a visual field defect, we do not consider confrontation perimetry to be an adequate substitute for computerized perimetry. In the same way, in a patient suspected of having an eye movement disorder, clinical examination of the eye movements is not an adequate substitute for computerized oculography (Fig. 193–2). While the aim of this chapter is to help clinicians to recognize certain classic eye movement disorders, particularly when they occur in isolation, clinical recognition is not a substitute

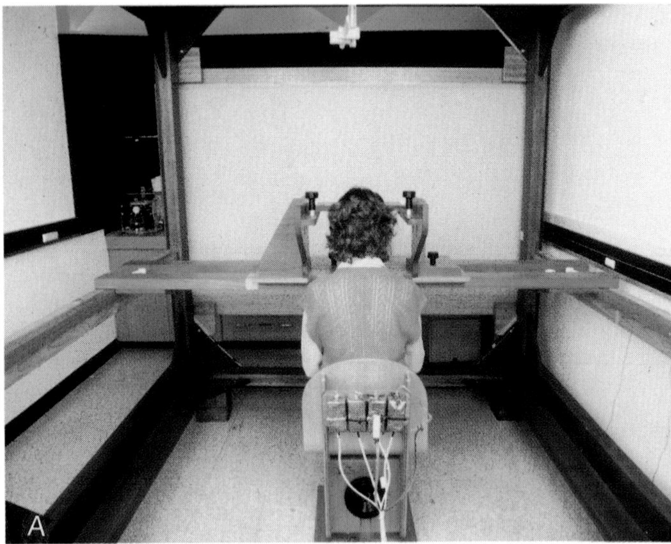

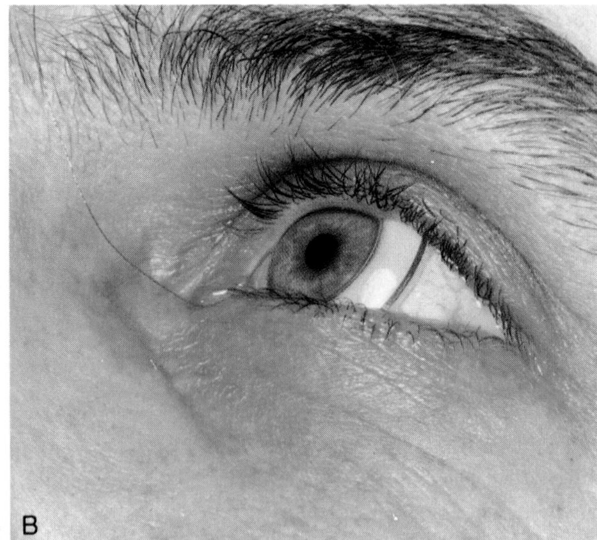

Figure 193–2. Magnetic search coil system for the diagnosis of eye movement disorders by computerized oculography. *A*, The patient sits at the center of a magnetic field generated by induction coils within the 2 × 2 × 2 m timber frame (CNC Engineering, Seattle) and views targets presented by rear projection onto the opaque Plexiglas screen. The patient's head is firmly restrained, and devices within the magnetic field, such as the head holder and the seat, are nonmetallic. *B*, Eye movements are detected by a fine copper wire search coil, embedded within silicon-rubber annular scleral contact lens that is worn on one eye or on both eyes (Skalar, Delft). The search coil detects changes in the orientation of the eye with regard to the magnetic field. Such systems can simultaneously measure horizontal, vertical, and torsional eye movements with an accuracy to 0.1 degree and 2 degrees/sec.

for quantitative analysis and evaluation, particularly in a patient with multiple, subtle, interrelated eye movement disorders.

Video Recordings of Eye Movement Disorders

In a patient with an eye movement disorder, a video recording of the eye movements is an essential part of the patient's permanent medical record. Although a videotape is no substitute for computerized oculography, it can serve as a baseline against which further developments can be checked and can also be used in order to obtain at least a preliminary neuroophthalmic opinion. Furthermore, videotapes[7] and computer simulation programs[8] are both excellent self-teaching aids for those who wish to learn how to recognize eye movement disorders clinically.

Aim of the Eye Movement Examination

The aim of the eye movement examination is to check the integrity of the six levels of the ocular motor system (see Fig. 193–1): (1) the "upper" motor neurons in the cerebral cortex that are responsible for the correct timing and targeting of voluntary saccades and of smooth pursuit eye movements; (2) the pre-motor neurons in the brain stem that are responsible for the speed and accuracy of smooth pursuit and for all saccadic eye movements; (3) the "lower" motor neurons that are responsible for the activation of the extraocular muscles; (4) the cerebellar neurons that are responsible for the correct synthesis and interaction of visual and vestibular eye movements; (5) the neurons of the vestibuloocular reflex arc that are responsible for the rapid involuntary activation of the "lower" motor neurons; and (6) the extraocular muscles themselves that are responsible for moving the eyes.

Method of the Eye Movement Examination

All clinicians have their individual style, and the method described here is only one of many. However, most clinicians experienced in dealing with eye movement disorders should try to answer the following 11 questions during the examination. Nevertheless, even if disordered eye movements appear to be the only sign of neurologic disease, it can be a mistake to try to make a neurologic diagnosis in a patient with disordered eye movements without a visual sensory, followed by a general neurologic examination. The eye movement examination itself seeks to determine: (1) if there is any abnormality of eye position; (2) if there is any abnormality of reflex eye movement; (3) if there is any abnormality of voluntary eye movement; (4) if there is any nystagmus or any other spontaneous, involuntary eye movement.

Question 1. Is there a manifest strabismus or are the eyes straight? The methods of the strabismus examination are not reviewed here. However, it should be noted that a comitant strabismus can be the legacy of a lower ocular motor lesion: A patient who has had a nuclear-infranuclear lesion causing an incomitant strabismus with limitation of the range and saccadic velocity of eye motion can still have a residual comitant strabismus after the range and velocity of eye motion have recovered.

Question 2. Is there limitation of the range of movement of either eye, or does each eye move to its full orbital range? It is important to determine whether each eye has a full range of motion within the orbit. If there is limitation of the range of motion of one eye, is it horizontal or vertical? It should be possible to nominate the extraocular muscle(s) that would have to be weak to produce the particular pattern of limited movement. Difficulties arise if there is limitation of movement of both eyes, particularly if the limitation is conjugate, because conjugate limitation of movement can occur in supranuclear as well as in nuclear-infranuclear ocular motor lesions and also with mechanical restriction of eye movement.

Question 3. Is there impairment of the latency, accuracy, or velocity of voluntary saccadic movements, or do the two eyes move together rapidly and accurately to the full orbital range? The integrity of the saccadic system is tested by asking the patient to make horizontal, vertical, and then oblique saccades between two targets 20 to 30 degrees to either side of the primary position. The examiner should note: (1) the latency, velocity, and accuracy of the saccades; (2) the trajectory of oblique saccades; (3) whether saccades are more easily initiated with the head free than with the head fixed; and (4) whether each saccade is accompanied by a blink. Particular note should be taken of the maximal saccadic velocity that can be generated by supposedly paretic muscles. Slowing of saccadic eye motion with preservation of the full range of eye motion can only be due to a supranuclear ocular motor lesion; a nuclear-infranuclear lesion that reduces saccadic velocity also reduces the range of ocular motion. As a corollary, a marked reduction in the range of eye motion with preservation of normal saccadic velocity within the remaining range of motion is characteristic of mechanical restriction and of myasthenic muscle weakness. Clinically, it is possible to recognize dissociated saccadic slowing of one eye with respect to the other in approximately 50 per cent of cases.[9]

Question 4. Is there impairment in the accuracy or velocity of smooth pursuit? Smooth pursuit is tested by asking the patient to follow a small target moving smoothly, horizontally, or vertically. Normal subjects can accurately pursue a target moving at up to 1 cycle every 2 sec, 20 degrees to each side, or up and down. Impairment of smooth pursuit is reflected in catch-up saccades. Pursuit deteriorates with age and is normally worse in the downward direction than in the upward direction.

Question 5. Is there impairment of optokinetic nystagmus? Genuine "full-field" optokinetic nystagmus is difficult to test clinically. It can sometimes be produced by moving a page from a full-sized newspaper before the patient's eyes. An assistant moves the page, while the examiner watches the patient's eyes. Tracking the moving stripes on a tape or small drum is more a test of pursuit than of optokinetic nystagmus.

Question 6. Is there any impairment of vestibuloocular reflexes or are they intact? Rapid "doll's head" or oculocephalic maneuvers elicit horizontal and vertical vestibuloocular reflexes in conscious as well as in unconscious patients and can detect severe unilateral as well as bilateral vestibular deficits. A corrective or compensatory saccade, during or immediately after a rapid passive head rotation, indicates a severe peripheral vestibular deficit on the side of the head rotation.[10] Horizontal nystagmus after rapid horizontal head shaking indicates a unilateral peripheral vestibular lesion on the side opposite the quick phases of the head-shaking nystagmus.[11] In patients with bilateral peripheral vestibular deficits, rapid horizontal or vertical head motion produces saccadic compensatory eye movements and oscillopsia.[12]

Question 7. Is there any abnormality of vestibuloocular reflex suppression or is it intact? The efficacy of vestibuloocular reflex suppression can be evaluated by observing the patient's ability to keep his or her gaze fixed on the thumb of his or her outstretched hand, while oscillating or being oscillated *en bloc*.[13] Horizontal vestibuloocular reflex suppression can be tested with the seated patient being passively oscillated on a regular office chair or with the patient standing and twisting at the waist (i.e., turning from side to side). Vertical vestibuloocular reflex suppression can be tested with the patient standing and actively bowing up and down by bending at the waist. Any quick phases seen to occur in the direction of head motion indicate failure of vestibuloocular reflex suppression in that direction.

Question 8. Is there any abnormality of vergence movements or are they intact? Vergence eye movements to a combined fusional and accommodative stimulus can be tested by asking the patient to fix on his or her own thumb as it is slowly moved toward the bridge of his or her nose. The ability to converge the eyes progressively and the associated pupillary constriction to near range are noted. By using a near card instead of a thumb, the near point of convergence can be measured as the closest distance at which the image is still single. Presbyopic patients must wear their reading correction for this test.

Question 9. Is there any abnormality of head posture or head movement, of lid posture or lid movement (closing, opening, and blinking), of pupil size or pupil reflexes, of facial sensation or corneal reflexes, or of hearing or balance? The posture and movement of associated structures, as well as functions mediated by adjacent cranial nerves, should also be examined. For example, abnormalities of head posture occur with vertical extraocular muscle palsies and with the ocular tilt reaction.[14] Abnormalities of head movement occur with congenital nystagmus and ocular motor apraxia. Abnormalities of lid posture occur with supranuclear lesions and with nuclear-infranuclear lesions. Abnormalities of lid movement occur with nuclear-infranuclear lesions and with extrapyramidal disorders. Abnormalities of the pupils occur with both central and peripheral lesions. Abnormalities of trigeminal nerve function occur with both supranuclear and nuclear-infranuclear lesions. Abnormalities of vestibular function, apart from vestibuloocular reflex abnormalities, occur with both supranuclear and nuclear-infranuclear lesions. Abnormalities of cochlear nerve function may occur with peripheral vestibular lesions.

Question 10. Could the eye movement disorder be caused by mechanical restriction of eye motion rather than by a disorder of the ocular motor system? Mechanical restriction of eye motion due to infiltration or entrapment of extraocular muscles can cause an apparent paresis of antagonist muscles and produce the clinical appearance of a nuclear-infranuclear lesion or even a supranuclear lesion. Typically, the restricted eye moves normally to the point of restriction and then moves no further. There may even be retraction of the eyeball. Consider, for example, a patient with Graves' disease affecting the right inferior rectus and right inferior oblique. Although the eyes are straight in the primary position, the patient develops increasing right hypotropia with increasing upward gaze. Upward saccades have normal velocity from downgaze to center, even though the eye does not move much above the horizontal meridian. Mechanical restriction can be confirmed with a forced duction test. The forced duction test is, however, not entirely specific for restriction, because it can also be positive in cases of long-standing paralytic strabismus with secondary contracture of the unopposed antagonist.

Question 11. Are there any spontaneous or inducible involuntary eye movements, ocular oscillations, or nystagmus? This section of the examination is fully considered below.

COMMON SYNDROMES OF DISORDERED EYE MOVEMENT

In considering the localization of some common eye movement disorders, it can be helpful to categorize certain syndromes. Although this is inherently an artificial process, particularly because several of these syndromes may be found at one time in one patient, considering eye movement disorders as syndromes reduces clinical data processing to manageable proportions. The syndromes discussed here are predominantly those that can be found in conscious, cooperative adults with virtually no other neurologic abnormalities. The reader is referred elsewhere for consideration of the special problems of children with eye movement disorders[6] and eye movement disorders in comatose patients (see Chap. 198). Patients with the syndromes discussed here can and do present to the ophthalmologist's office. In these cases, the entire neurologic diagnosis depends on the correct interpretation of the eye movement disorder. It is then up to the ophthalmologist to decide whether the patient has a benign, possibly long-standing disorder requiring only reassurance (e.g., congenital nystagmus, Duane's syndrome), a potentially serious but curable disorder (e.g., myasthenia, basal meningioma), or a serious and potentially lethal disorder (e.g., nasopharyngeal cancer, pontine glioma).

It is worth noting that whereas brain stem eye movement disorders are often symptomatic and are easily detectable at the bedside, cerebellar eye movement disorders are usually asymptomatic and are more difficult to detect, and cerebral eye movement disorders are almost always asymptomatic and difficult to demonstrate clinically even with special examination techniques. *One of the cardinal features of the brain stem control of eye movements is that it is plane specific: horizontal eye movements are controlled in the pons, whereas vertical eye movements are controlled in the midbrain. With some caveats, therefore, it can be generally assumed that an eye movement disorder that is limited either to the horizontal or to the vertical plane is due to a brain stem lesion.*

Horizontal Eye Movement Disorders

All the premotor structures required for horizontal gaze are located in the pons. Therefore, a horizontal gaze palsy indicates a lesion in the pons, and with a few rare exceptions involvement of horizontal gaze in a more complex eye movement disorder indicates involvement of the pontine tegmentum.

ABDUCTION PALSIES

The cardinal symptom of abduction palsy is an esotropia that causes an uncrossed, horizontal diplopia. The diplopia is worse for distance than for near and is worse in unilateral cases on gaze to the affected side than on gaze to the normal side.

Peripheral Lesions. The most common cause of an isolated unilateral abduction palsy is a lateral rectus palsy caused by an intracranial or extracranial peripheral lesion of the abducens nerve. Nonetheless, central lesions causing a real or apparent, unilateral, or bilateral abduction palsy should be excluded.

Pontine Lesions. Focal pontine lesions involving abducens fascicles emerging through the basis pontis can cause an isolated unilateral lateral rectus palsy.[15–17] Duane's syndrome is a special case of a pontine lesion with congenital absence of abducens motoneurons in one or in both abducens nuclei.[18] In addition to abduction palsy, there is ptosis and globe retraction on adduction.[19] This is caused by aberrant innervation of the lateral rectus muscle by branches from the oculomotor nerve.

Midbrain-Thalamic Lesions. Unilateral midbrain-thalamic lesions can cause an esotropia due to a contralateral abduction palsy, perhaps through disinhibition of vergence pathways. This disorder has been called "thalamic esotropia" and "pseudoabducens" palsy.[20–22] In some cases, the abduction palsy can be overcome by vestibular stimulation.

Bilateral Abduction Palsy. Bilateral isolated abduction palsy is rarely due to a single focal central lesion. The most common central causes of bilateral abduction palsy are divergence palsy, convergence spasm, and Wernicke-Korsakoff syndrome. Acute acquired esotropia or divergence palsy can be difficult to distinguish from bilateral mild lateral rectus palsies,[23] particularly because the two disorders are usually due to the same pathologic process, namely intracranial hypertension. Convergence spasm (or rather, "spasm of the near reflex") causes esotropia due to overaction of both medial recti. The bilateral miosis, which is less obvious with monocular occlusion,[24] helps to differentiate convergence spasm from bilateral abduction palsy. In most cases of convergence spasm, no organic lesion can be found.[25] In Wernicke-Korsakoff syndrome there are multiple petechial hemorrhages in several regions of the brain stem including the pontine tegmentum, which may explain the common finding of bilateral abduction palsy.[26]

ADDUCTION PALSIES

The cardinal symptom of adduction palsy is exotropia, which causes a crossed horizontal diplopia that is worse in unilateral cases on gaze to the normal side than on gaze to the affected side.

Peripheral Lesions. When adduction palsy is due to a peripheral oculomotor nerve lesion, it is not an isolated finding but is accompanied by vertical muscle palsies and often by lid and pupil changes as well. The diagnosis of a partial or a branch, peripheral oculomotor nerve lesion causing predominantly or exclusively an adduction palsy should be made with caution, only after other diagnoses have been excluded. The syndrome of "congenital adduction palsy with synergistic divergence" may be a variant of Duane's syndrome due to aplasia of medial rectus motoneurons with aberrant innervation of the medial rectus muscle by axons from the abducens nerve.[27]

Midbrain Lesions. Midbrain lesions that involve the oculomotor nucleus or fasciculus can produce an adduction palsy in association with equally evident ipsilateral vertical muscle palsies. The appearance may be that of an inferior oculomotor nerve branch palsy[28] or a total oculomotor nerve palsy.[29] In contrast, midbrain lesions that involve the medial longitudinal fasciculus (MLF) can produce an isolated adduction palsy due to INO.

Pontine Lesions. Pontine lesions that involve the MLF can cause an isolated adduction palsy due to INO. The eyes are usually orthotropic in INO, even if the adduction palsy is complete. If there is any exotropia at all, it is only in lateral gaze. This helps to distinguish adduction palsy due to an *inter*nuclear ophthalmoplegia from adduction palsy due to an *infra*nuclear ophthalmoplegia. Unilateral lesions of the pons, which extend from the MLF to the adjacent abducens nucleus, paralyze all conjugate horizontal movements of the ipsilesional eye as well as adduction of the contralesional eye. This is the "one-and-a-half syndrome": an ipsiversive gaze palsy plus a contraversive INO.[30–32] In some cases, a normal range of adduction can be produced in each eye by convergence. If the patient habitually fixates with the horizontally immobile ipsilesional eye, the contralesional eye that has intact lateral rectus innervation will be exotropic. This appearance is called "paralytic pontine exotropia" (Fig. 193–3).[33] Adductor palsies due to INO can be distinguished from adductor palsies due to

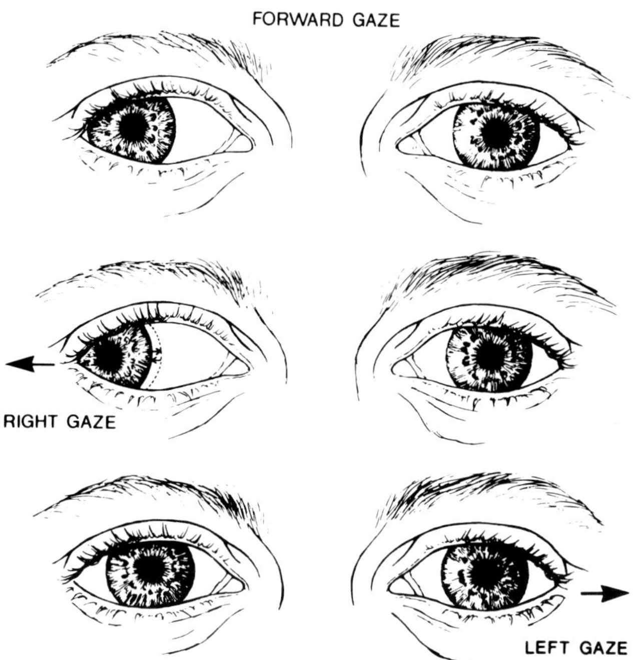

Figure 193–3. Paralytic pontine exotropia. In the primary position, the patient fixates with the horizontally immobile left eye; the right eye is moderately exotropic. On attempted rightward gaze, the right eye abducts normally, but the left eye fails to move. On attempted leftward gaze, the right eye moves to the midline, but the left eye again fails to move. Vertical saccadic movements and vergence movements can be normal. The lesion in this case involves the left pontine paramedian reticular formation and the adjacent left medial longitudinal fasciculus. (From Sharpe JA, Rosenberg MA, Hoyt WF, et al: Paralytic pontine exotropia. A sign of acute unilateral pontine gaze palsy and internuclear ophthalmoplegia. Neurology 24:1076, 1974.)

infranuclear ophthalmoplegia if it can be shown that medial rectus motoneurons can still be normally activated by vergence or that there is impairment of the vertical vestibuloocular reflex.[34] Whereas complete lesions of the MLF cause a loss of all inputs except vergence to medial rectus motoneurons, partial lesions may cause only a saccadic palsy of adduction of the ipsilesional eye. The maximal velocity of adducting saccades is reduced, but there is no reduction of the normal maximal amplitude of adduction (Fig. 193–4). However in these partial cases of INO, an abduction overshoot of the other eye will be evident with or without subsequent beats of abducting (dissociated) nystagmus. Some MLF lesions cause an adduction palsy due to INO that is bilateral and exotropic in the primary position ("wall-eyed" bilateral INO) (Fig. 193–5). The anatomic basis of the exotropia is unknown.[35] Although it is not possible to distinguish clinically between a pontine INO and a midbrain INO, MRI may help.[36–38] Since the MLF carries vestibular signals from the vestibular nuclei in the medulla to the vertical eye muscles in the midbrain, lesions of the MLF (especially bilateral lesions) produce a vertical vestibuloocular reflex palsy. The principal symptom of this is visual: head movement oscillopsia. In patients with adduction palsies, it is important to check if vertical head-shaking impairs visual acuity.

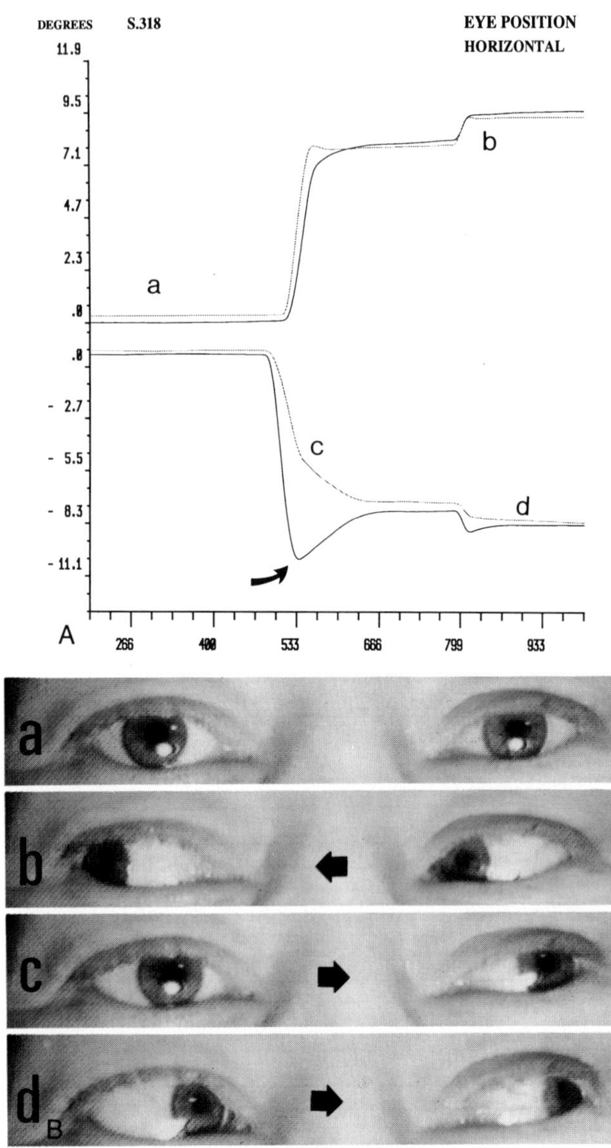

Figure 193–4. Left internuclear ophthalmoplegia. *A*, Binocular search coil recordings of horizontal eye movements with the system shown in Figure 193–2. Upward deflections indicate rightward eye movements; downward deflections indicate leftward eye movements. Movements of the right eye are shown in interrupted lines; movements of the left eye, in continuous lines. An attempted 10-degree leftward saccade reveals slow adduction of the right eye (peak velocity = 148 degrees/sec, in contrast to 400 degrees/sec for left eye abduction). There is also the characteristic abduction overshoot of the left eye *(arrow)*. The mild slowing of left eye adduction and the slight right eye abduction overshoot during the rightward saccade could be normal. (a, b, c, and d) refer to the video frames in *B*. *B*, Single frames from a video recording of the patient with the left internuclear ophthalmoplegia whose oculographic recordings are shown in *A*. There was no abnormality in the primary position (a). There was no limitation of the amplitude of adduction of the left eye and therefore no exotropia on holding gaze to the left *after* the leftward saccade (d); however, because of the delay in adduction of the right eye, there was in fact a marked exotropia *during* the leftward saccade (c). There was no delay in adduction of the left eye during a rightward saccade (b). The patient did experience momentary horizontal diplopia when looking to the left.

HORIZONTAL GAZE DEVIATION

A tonic gaze deviation can be due either to underactivity of a contraversive gaze mechanism or to overactivity of an ipsiversive gaze mechanism. Tonic horizontal gaze deviations can be due either to unilateral cerebral hemisphere lesions or to unilateral pontine lesions. There are several differences between pontine and cerebral gaze deviations.

Cerebral Hemisphere Lesions. The tonic head and eye deviation that occurs with large acute unilateral destructive cerebral hemisphere lesions has the following characteristics: (1) it is usually ipsilesional but can be contralesional; (2) it is always temporary; (3) saccadic and smooth pursuit eye movements opposite to the gaze deviation are impaired; (4) vestibular eye movements opposite to the gaze deviation are preserved; (5) the patient invariably has other neurologic signs of a large acute unilateral cerebral hemisphere lesion (e.g., hemiplegia, aphasia). (For a review see reference 39). A unilateral epileptogenic cerebral hemisphere lesion can also cause head and eye deviation during a partial or a generalized seizure. The gaze deviation is paroxysmal and is usually, but not always, contraversive. This deviation may be associated with epileptic nystagmus.[40, 41] Chronic unilateral cerebral hemisphere lesions can also cause "spasticity of conjugate gaze." This is a tonic, usually contraversive, deviation of the eyes, apparent under closed lids or during forced eye closure. In contrast to tonic gaze deviation, spasticity of gaze can occur in patients with no other neurologic deficits.[42]

Pontine Lesions. In contrast to the tonic gaze deviation produced by cerebral hemisphere lesions, the tonic gaze deviation produced by pontine lesions involving the abducens nucleus is always contralesional and is accompanied by a permanent loss of all ipsilesional eye movements.

HORIZONTAL GAZE PALSIES

Unilateral Horizontal Gaze Palsy. A unilateral horizontal gaze palsy is characteristic of a unilateral pontine

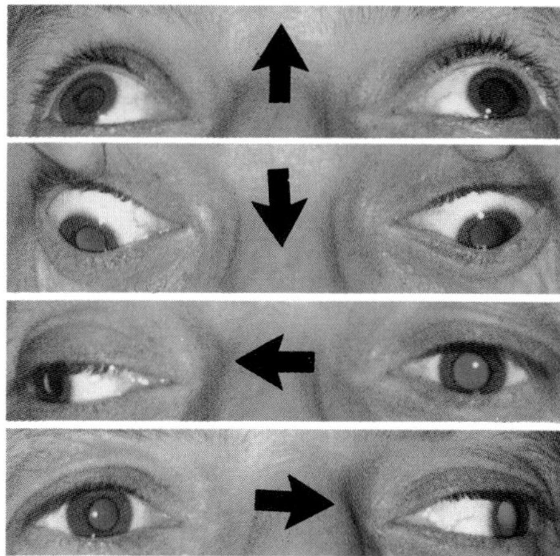

Figure 193–5. "Wall-eyed" bilateral internuclear ophthalmoplegia (WEBINO syndrome). The patient not only had an advanced bilateral internuclear ophthalmoplegia with inability to adduct either eye past the midline, but he also had a bilateral exotropia with alternating fixation. Although vertical saccades were normal, he had, as expected, a severe vertical vestibular palsy that produced vertical oscillopsia during head movement. Convergence was absent in this patient; however, it is preserved in some patients with the WEBINO syndrome.

lesion. The palsy can affect all types of eye movement in the one direction, or there can be a selective saccadic palsy. A unilateral horizontal saccadic palsy indicates a focal lesion involving the pontine paramedian reticular formation (PPRF). All ipsilesional saccadic eye movements, including the quick phases of vestibular and optokinetic nystagmus, are either slow or absent, whereas all contralesional saccadic eye movements and all eye movements produced by vestibular, pursuit, or optokinetic stimulation are normal.[43, 44] In contrast, unilateral abducens nucleus lesions destroy both abducens motoneurons and abducens interneurons and therefore cause a total loss of all conjugate ipsilesional eye movements.[45, 46] Occasionally a unilateral midbrain lesion produces, in addition to a vertical gaze palsy and a nuclear oculomotor nerve palsy, a contralesional saccadic palsy.[47, 48]

Bilateral Horizontal Gaze Palsy. A bilateral pontine lesion involving the PPRF can cause a bilateral selective saccadic palsy with preservation of vestibular and optokinetic horizontal eye movements.[49] In the acute stage of the lesion, vertical saccadic eye movements may be involved as well.[50, 51] More often, however, an isolated bilateral horizontal saccadic palsy with intact vertical saccades indicates a hereditary nervous system degeneration such as Huntington's disease[52] or Gaucher's disease.[53] An extensive bilateral pontine lesion involving the abducens nuclei causes a total loss of all horizontal eye movements, apart from vergence eye movements that may be substituted during attempted lateral gaze (see Fig. 193–19).[54, 55] In Möbius syndrome, there is a congenital bilateral horizontal conjugate gaze palsy due to aplasia of abducens motoneurons and interneurons, as well as bilateral facial and hypoglossal palsies due to aplasia of those nuclei. There may be characteristic abnormalities on CT and MRI.[56]

OCULAR MOTOR APRAXIA

The essential defect in ocular motor apraxia is an impairment of voluntary saccadic eye movements with a relative preservation of reflex saccadic eye movements (i.e., the quick phases of vestibular or optokinetic nystagmus). It usually affects only the horizontal eye movement system and can follow bilateral basal ganglia or cerebral hemisphere lesions.[57] In the congenital form the corpus callosum can be hypoplastic,[58] but whether this is the actual site of lesion is not known. Thrusting head movements and blink-saccade synkinesis can be prominent. The blinks break fixation, and the head thrusts can generate an anticompensatory vestibular quick phase. An oculomotor apraxia is found in some patients with ataxia-telangiectasia.[59] A purely vertical oculomotor apraxia can occur with midbrain-thalamic lesions.[60]

LATEROPULSION

The effects of lateropulsion on eye movements can be clearly seen as a unilateral bias in saccadic amplitude. Lateropulsion occurs with unilateral lesions of the cerebellum or lateral medulla. Unilateral lateral medullary lesions involving the vestibular nucleus cause ipsiversive lateropulsion, in which there is an ipsiversive tonic bias of resting eye position and of saccadic amplitude (Fig. 193–6).[61] During voluntary eye closure and sometimes even during blinks, the eyes deviate toward the side of the lesion and have to make a centering saccade to refixate as soon as the eyes are opened. All ipsiversive saccadic eye movements are hypermetric, whereas all contraversive saccadic eye movements are hypometric. Vertical saccades have a parabolic ipsiversive trajectory. In contrast, unilateral cerebellar hemisphere lesions can cause contraversive lateropulsion.[62, 63]

Vertical Eye Movement Disorders

ELEVATOR-DEPRESSOR PALSIES

There is a wide differential diagnosis of sites of lesions causing unilateral or bilateral asymmetric impairment of vertical eye movements, the chief symptom of which is vertical diplopia.

Peripheral Lesions. Isolated unilateral peripheral trochlear nerve lesions cause isolated weakness of the superior oblique muscle. This results in a vertical and torsional diplopia and a unilateral hypertropia and excyclotropia that is worse on adduction, depression, and ipsilateral head tilt.[64] Bilateral peripheral trochlear nerve lesions, if symmetric, may produce mainly esotropia and bilateral excyclotropia[65] with hypertropia of each adducting eye only in lateral gaze. Bilateral superior oblique paralysis should be differentiated from overaction of the inferior obliques[66] and from physiologic hyperdeviation in lateral gaze.[67] In a patient with a vertical paralytic strabismus but no pupil involvement, the diagnosis of a partial peripheral oculomotor nerve lesion should be made only after disorders have been excluded.

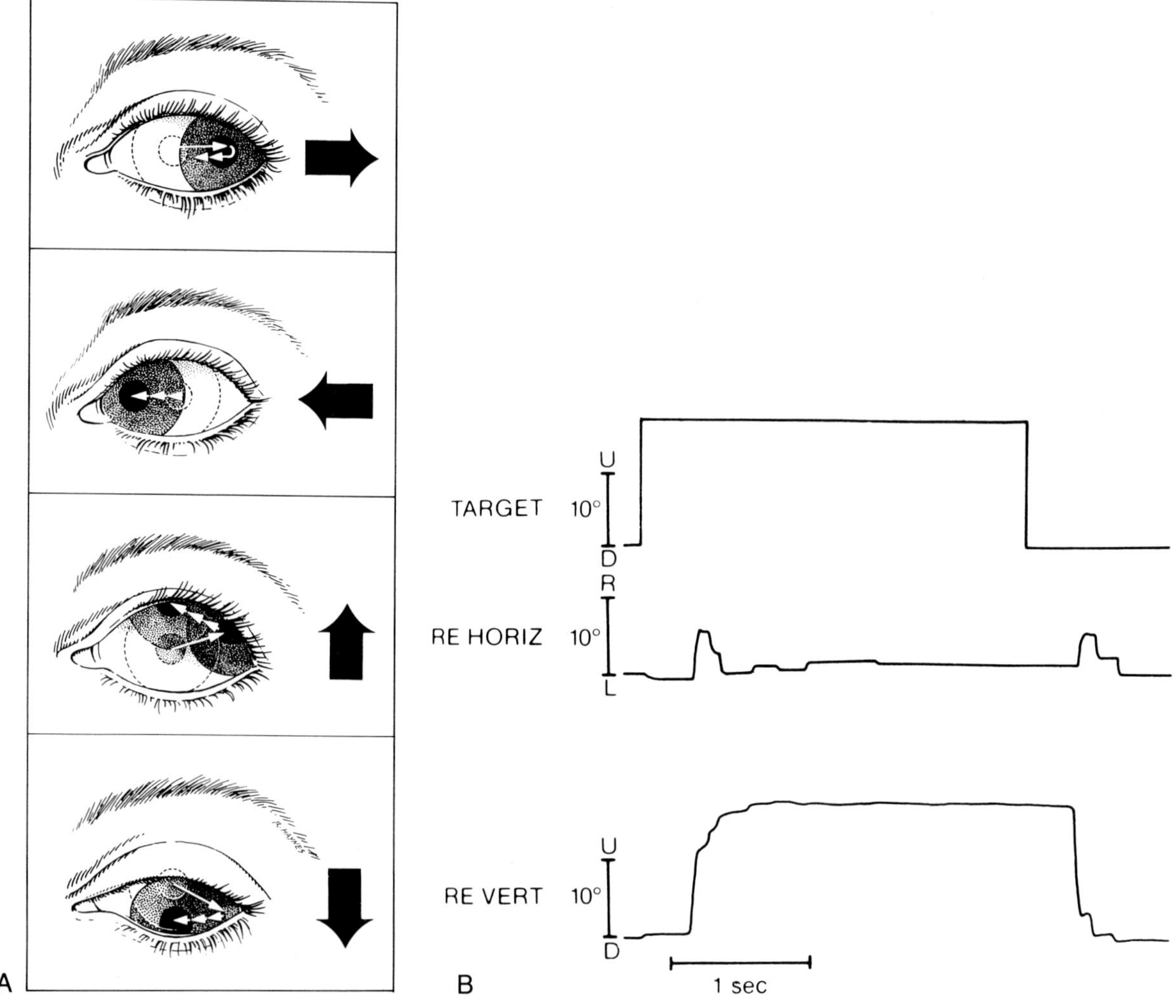

Figure 193–6. Lateropulsion. *A*, Leftward lateropulsion in a patient with a left lateral medullary infarct. (Only the left eye is shown.) The single leftward saccade in response to a 20-degree leftward target overshot the target, so that a single rightward corrective saccade was required in order to fixate the target. Saccades to a 20-degree rightward target undershot the target, so that three small rightward saccades were required in order to fixate the target. Vertical saccades to 20-degree upward and 20-degree downward targets also had an unintended leftward component, so that several small rightward saccadic components were required in order to fixate the target. (Adapted from Kommerell G, Hoyt WF: Lateropulsion of saccadic eye movements. Electro-oculographic studies in a patient with Wallenberg's syndrome. Arch Neurol 28:313, 1973. Copyright 1973, American Medical Association.) *B*, Rightward lateropulsion in a patient with a left cerebellar infarct: The upward saccade in response to the 20-degree upward target had an unintended 5 degree rightward component, which was then corrected by two leftward saccades. (U, up; D, down; R, right; L, left; RE HORIZ, right eye horizontal position; RE VERT, right eye vertical position.) (From Ranalli PJ, Sharpe JA: Contrapulsion of saccades and ipsilateral ataxia: A unilateral disorder of the rostral cerebellum. Ann Neurol 20:311, 1986.)

Skew Deviation and the Ocular Tilt Reaction. Skew deviation is defined as a vertical strabismus due to a supranuclear lesion. It has been reported with lesions throughout the brain stem and cerebellum. When skew deviation is bilateral and alternating (bilateral abducting hypertropia), it indicates a lesion either in the dorsal midbrain[68] or caudal medulla.[69] Bilateral skew deviation can be difficult to distinguish from bilateral superior oblique palsies[65] and from asymptomatic hyperdeviation in lateral gaze.[67] Skew deviation is of more localizing value when it is unilateral and associated with head and eye torsion as part of the "ocular tilt reaction." The ocular tilt reaction is a head-eye postural synkinesis that consists of torsion of the head, torsion of both eyes, and hypotropia all to one side. It appears to be an otolithic righting reflex and occurs in patients with lesions of both the peripheral and central vestibular system.[70]

Midbrain Lesions. A unilateral midbrain lesion that involves the trochlear nucleus or fasciculus may cause a typical unilateral superior oblique palsy on the side opposite the lesion.[71] A bilateral midbrain lesion that involves both trochlear fascicles can cause a bilateral superior oblique palsy.[72, 73] A unilateral midbrain lesion, which involves the interstitial nucleus of Cajal, produces an ocular tilt reaction that is either tonic and contralesional or paroxysmal and ipsilesional (Fig. 193–7). An ocular tilt reaction can be distinguished clinically from a unilateral superior oblique palsy: Although both show hypotropia and head tilt to one side, patients with unilateral superior oblique palsy have an excyclotropia of the hypertropic eye, whereas patients with an ocular tilt reaction have incyclotropia of the hypertropic eye and excyclotropia of the hypotropic eye. A midbrain lesion involving the oculomotor nucleus or fasciculus

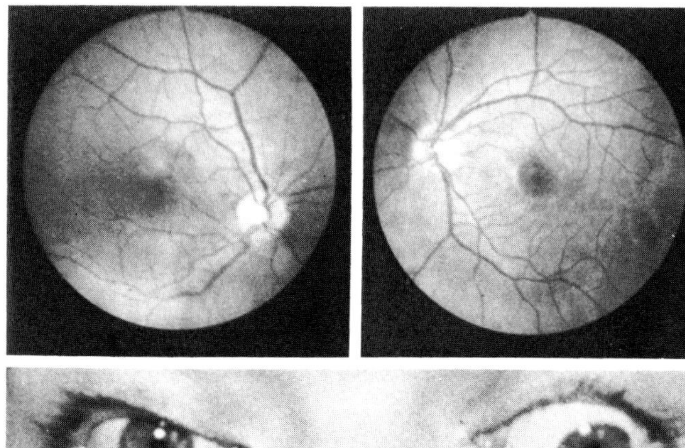

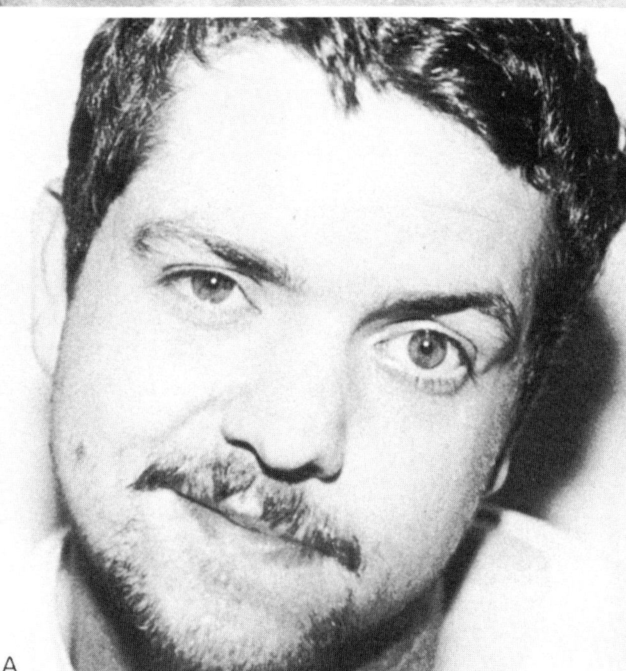

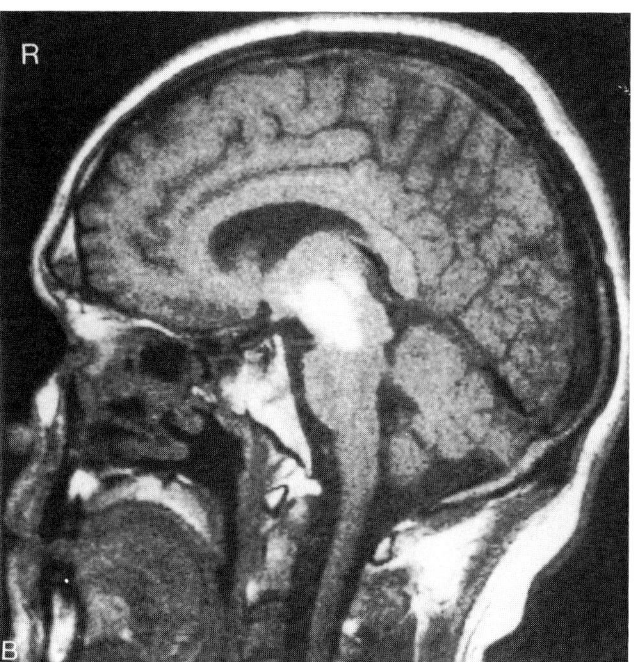

Figure 193–7. Tonic contraversive ocular tilt reaction caused by a unilateral midbrain-thalamic lesion. *A*, The patient had a leftward ocular tilt reaction consisting of a leftward head tilt, left hypotropia, and leftward torsion of each eye, as shown in the fundus photographs. *B*, The lesion, a hemorrhage caused by a right (R) midbrain-thalamic arteriovenous malformation, is shown on T_1-weighted parasagittal MRI. (From Halmagyi GM, Brandt T, Dieterich M, et al: Tonic contraversive ocular tilt reaction due to unilateral mesodiencephalic lesion. Neurology 40:1503, 1990.)

can also cause a paralytic vertical strabismus. There may be a total peripheral type of oculomotor nerve palsy,[29] an inferior branch palsy[28] or an isolated inferior oblique palsy,[74] or inferior rectus[75] palsy. With improvements in MRI, more cases of supposed peripheral oculomotor nerve palsy may be shown to be caused by focal midbrain lesions. Unilateral lesions of the oculomotor nucleus not only paralyze all the muscles innervated by the oculomotor nerve but also the contralateral superior rectus producing an apparent upgaze palsy. The ipsilesional superior rectus muscle, which is normally innervated by axons from contralesional superior rectus motoneurons passing through the lesioned oculomotor nucleus, is actually spared.[76] Paralysis of elevation of one eye with no primary position hypotropia can occur as an isolated congenital disorder[77] and in patients with presumed midbrain lesions.[78]

Medullary Lesions. Unilateral medullary lesions that involve the vestibular nucleus produce a tonic ipsilesional ocular tilt reaction. The patient has vertical diplopia due to the ipsilesional hypotropia. There can be a torsional element to the diplopia because the excyclotropia of the ipsilesional eye is usually greater than the incyclotropia of the contralesional eye (see Fig. 193–18).[14, 79]

Peripheral Vestibular Lesions. Acute unilateral lesions of the labyrinth or the vestibular nerve invariably produce asymptomatic ipsilesional conjugate ocular torsion.[80] In some cases, there is a complete ocular tilt reaction, with vertical diplopia due to the ipsilesional hypotropia.[81]

VERTICAL GAZE DEVIATION

A tonic vertical gaze deviation can be either due to underactivity of contraversive gaze mechanisms or due to overactivity of ipsiversive gaze mechanisms. For example, acute lesions at the midbrain-thalamic junction can produce a tonic upward gaze deviation due to a downward gaze palsy or a tonic downward gaze deviation due to an upward gaze palsy. The gaze palsy may be total or selectively saccadic. Tonic vertical deviation can also be due to overactivity of the ipsiversive gaze mechanism. For example, in patients with spasms of upward gaze due to oculogyric crises[82] or to epileptic seizures,[83] the upward gaze deviation may represent overactivity of the normal midbrain upward gaze mechanisms, caused by a temporary depression of normal tonic inhibitory activity from higher centers.

VERTICAL GAZE PALSIES

A vertical gaze palsy generally indicates a lesion of the dorsal midbrain: either a bilateral lesion involving the rostral interstitial nucleus of the medial longitudinal fasciculus (riMLF)[84] or a unilateral lesion of the riMLF, usually but not always extending to involve the posterior commissure.[85] There are three exceptions to this rule: (1) mechanical restriction of extraocular muscles in orbital disorders such as Graves' disease can produce an apparent vertical gaze palsy; (2) large acute pontine lesions involving the PPRF bilaterally can produce a temporary vertical saccadic palsy as well as a permanent horizontal saccadic palsy; (3) certain diffuse degenerative disorders of the nervous system can produce a selective unidirectional or bidirectional vertical saccadic palsy. The vertical gaze palsies that occur with midbrain lesions can assume several different patterns with respect to the direction and type of the eye movement affected. A vertical gaze palsy can selectively affect only upgaze, or only downgaze, or it can affect both; it can selectively affect only saccadic eye movements or only vestibulo-ocular reflex eye movements, or it can affect both. A vertical gaze palsy can occur in isolation, or in association with other eye movement disorders, and pupil or eyelid abnormalities, all of which constitute the various elements of Parinaud's dorsal midbrain syndrome.[86–88] A vertical gaze palsy due to a focal midbrain lesion can selectively affect only saccades, either only upward saccades, or only downward saccades,[89] or saccades in both directions.[85, 90] In such cases all horizontal eye movements as well as vertical eye movements produced by vestibular stimulation and by forced eye closure (Bell's phenomenon) are spared. Vertical saccadic palsies can also occur in certain degenerative disorders of the nervous system, such as Steele-Richardson-Olszewski disease,[91] or adult Niemann-Pick disease.[92] It is however more usual for a vertical gaze palsy due to a focal midbrain lesion to affect all types of eye vertical movements—either only downward eye movements[93, 94] or only upward eye movements[95, 96] or eye movements in both directions.[97] In a total upgaze palsy, the eyes do not move above the horizontal meridian, even with strong vestibular stimulation or with forced eye closure. The velocity of downward saccades may also be reduced. An isolated upward gaze palsy can be congenital[98] and can also occur as an incidental finding in the elderly. In a total downgaze palsy, the eyes do not move below the horizontal meridian, even with strong vestibular stimulation. In some cases, the velocity of upward saccades can also be reduced (Fig. 193–8).

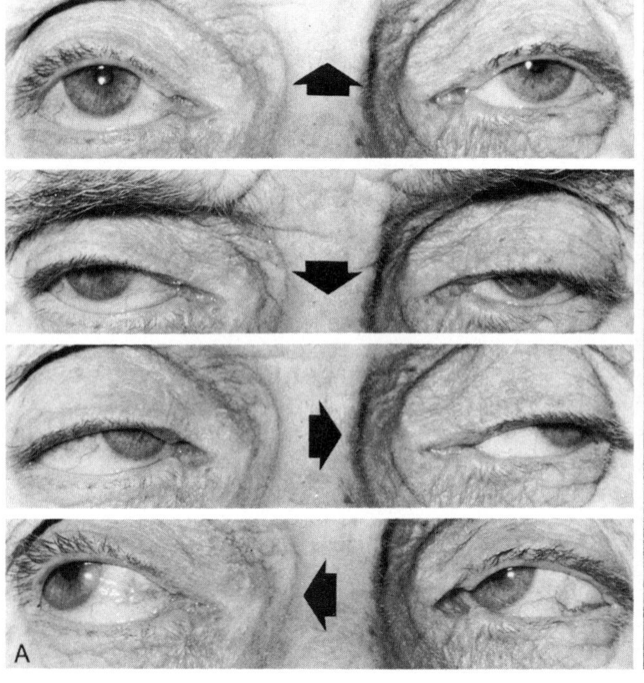

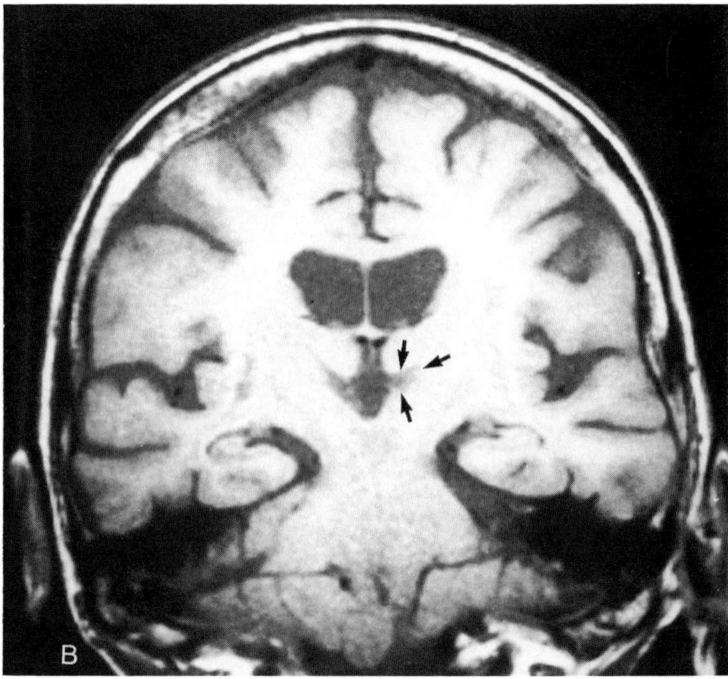

Figure 193–8. Total downgaze palsy. *A*, The patient could make no eye movements at all below the horizontal meridian. Downward saccades *to* the vertical meridian were slow. Upward eye movements were slightly restricted, but this is not necessarily abnormal at the age of 83 yr, since upward saccades were of normal velocity. There was also bilateral asymmetric ptosis. *B*, T_1-weighted MRI showed bilateral symmetric lesions at the midbrain-thalamic junction in the region of the rostral interstitial nucleus of the medial longitudinal fasciculus; three *arrows* show the lesion on the left. The patient had mitral stenosis with atrial fibrillation and had presented 15 yr previously with transient confusion and permanent downgaze palsy (Case 1[247]). She had presumably suffered a "top-of-the-basilar" syndrome[248] caused by embolic occlusion of the posterior thalamic-subthalamic artery.

MONOCULAR VERTICAL GAZE PALSIES AND THE VERTICAL ONE-AND-A-HALF SYNDROME

Some patients with presumed midbrain lesions develop a monocular upward ophthalmoplegia with no primary position hypotropia.[78] Vertical one-and-a-half syndrome describes the combination of a vertical gaze palsy in one direction and a monocular vertical ophthalmoplegia in the other direction with no primary position heterotropia.[99, 100] Patients with the vertical one-and-a-half syndrome have had unilateral dorsal midbrain lesions on the side of the monocular ophthalmoplegia.

VERTICAL VESTIBULOOCULAR REFLEX PALSY

Bilateral MLF lesions produce a selective deficit of vertical vestibuloocular reflexes. Horizontal vestibuloocular reflexes and vertical saccades are normal.[34] The only detectable evidence of an INO can be a reduction in the maximal velocity of adducting saccades and a subtle abduction overshoot (see Fig. 193–4). Patients with vertical vestibuloocular reflex palsies often present for ophthalmic opinion complaining of oscillopsia or blurred vision.

Global Gaze Disorders

TOTAL SACCADIC PALSY

Absence of all saccadic eye movements, reflex and voluntary, horizontal and vertical, with preservation of vestibuloocular reflex eye movements (and in some cases pursuit and optokinetic eye movements as well), can be produced acutely by bilateral PPRF lesions.[50] In practice, however, global saccadic palsies are found in patients with advanced degenerative diseases such as olivopontocerebellar degeneration, Huntington's disease,[52] or Steele-Richardson-Olszewski disease.[91]

TOTAL OPHTHALMOPLEGIA

Both supranuclear and nuclear-infranuclear lesions can cause total loss of all eye movements,[101] but seldom in isolation. In patients with total ophthalmoplegia, the diagnosis depends on the presence of other findings. For example in patients with total external ophthalmoplegia due to myopathy or myasthenia, there is the characteristic combination of ptosis and weakness of orbicularis oculi. In patients with multiple cranial neuropathies, there are generally also other abnormalities involving the eyelids, pupils, or trigeminal sensation. In patients with brain stem lesions such as in Wernicke's disease,[26] other deficits such as amnesia or ataxia are evident. Even in cases with total ophthalmoplegia in which it is not even certain if the lesion is central or peripheral or both (e.g., Fisher's syndrome),[102] there are other signs such as ataxia and areflexia to help with the diagnosis.

Pursuit Palsies

GLOBAL PURSUIT PALSY

Selective impairment of only smooth pursuit eye movements is common in practice but is rarely due to a focal lesion. When a clinically significant pursuit deficit does occur, it is usually in the context of, and in the direction of, a saccadic palsy or a gaze-evoked nystagmus. In patients with drug intoxication or with degenerative diseases involving the cerebral or cerebellar cortex or the basal ganglia, a global pursuit deficit may be the principal disorder of eye movements. Pursuit, especially downward pursuit, deteriorates with age.[103]

UNILATERAL PURSUIT PALSY

These comments notwithstanding, an isolated unilateral or asymmetric deficit of horizontal smooth pursuit occurs with unilateral cerebral[104, 105] and cerebellar hemisphere lesions (Fig. 193–9). Unilateral thalamic[106] and brain stem lesions[47, 107–110] can produce ipsiversive, contraversive, or bidirectional horizontal pursuit defects. Congenital nystagmus, even when it is only present in lateral gaze and not in the primary position, produces the appearance of reversed pursuit, a specific, usually bidirectional abnormality confined to the horizontal plane (Fig. 193–10). In some cases, unilateral reversed pursuit (i.e., unilateral, pursuit-induced nystagmus) can be the only manifestation of a *forme fruste* of congenital nystagmus.[111] Abnormalities of pursuit are generally accompanied by similar defects in vestibuloocular reflex suppression.[13, 112]

OPTOKINETIC REFLEX PALSIES

It is difficult to test optokinetic eye movements clinically, and most clinical tests of optokinetic nystagmus actually test the pursuit system and not the optokinetic system. Nevertheless, a so-called optokinetic tape or drum can be a convenient way to show pursuit defects in patients with unilateral cerebral or cerebellar lesions, to elicit pursuit-induced congenital nystagmus, or to elicit reflex saccadic eye movements (i.e., quick phases) in patients with disorders such as INO or Parinaud's syndrome.

VESTIBULOOCULAR REFLEX SUPPRESSION

Patients with clinically evident defects of vestibuloocular reflex suppression often have parallel defects of smooth pursuit. In the absence of a spontaneous or gaze-evoked nystagmus, ipsilateral vestibuloocular reflex suppression defects occur in patients with unilateral cerebral or cerebellar lesions (see Fig. 193–21). Bilateral horizontal vestibuloocular reflex suppression defects occur in congenital nystagmus. Global defects of vestibuloocular reflex suppression occur in diffuse cerebellar degeneration and in drug intoxication.[113, 114]

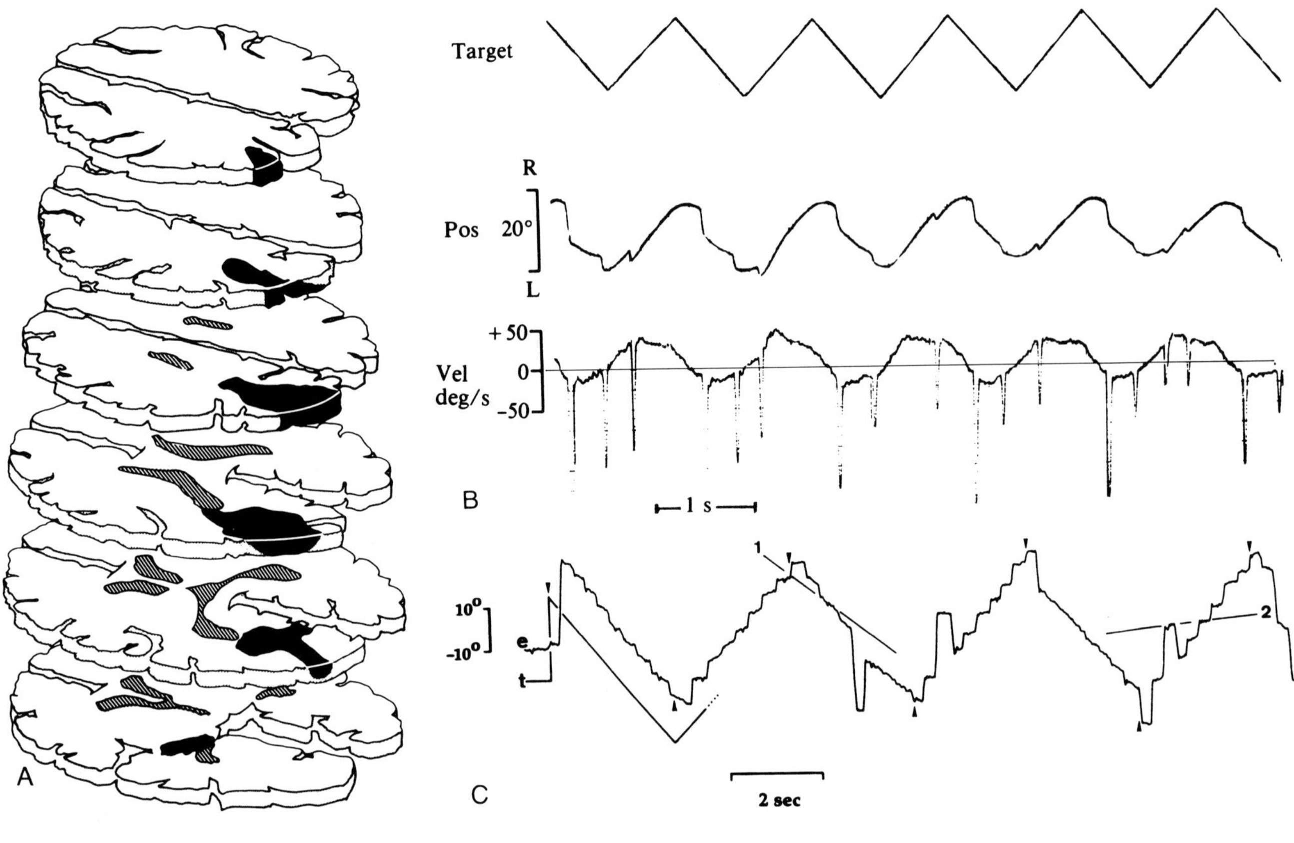

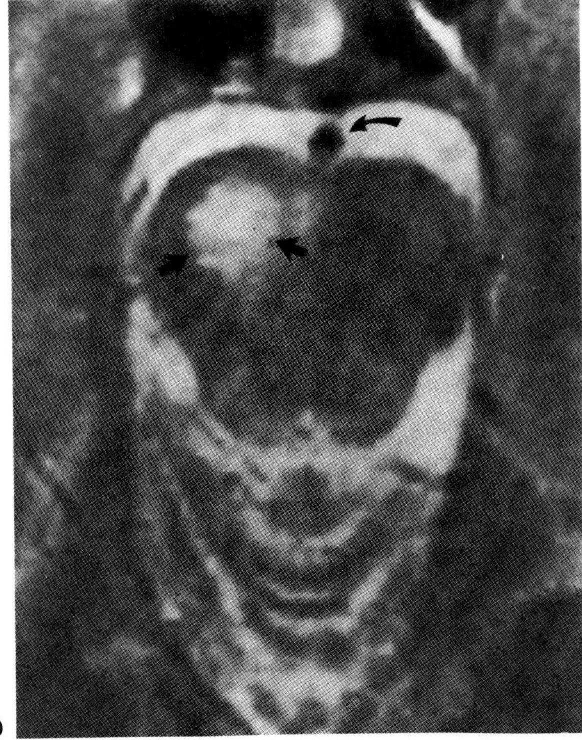

Figure 193–9. Unilateral smooth pursuit palsy. *A*, Oculographic recordings of horizontal pursuit in a patient with a left hemidecortication. The target moved to the left and then to the right at a constant velocity of 30 degrees/sec. Leftward (i.e., ipsilesional) smooth pursuit was defective (velocity [vel] 15 degrees/sec or less), and there were several leftward catch-up saccades, whereas rightward smooth pursuit velocity slightly exceeded target velocity. Horizontal saccades were normal. (R, right; Pos, position.) (From Sharpe JA, Lo AW, Rabinovitch HE: Control of saccadic and smooth pursuit systems after cerebral hemidecortication. Brain 102:387–403, 1979. By permission of Oxford University Press.) *B*, Three-dimensional reconstruction of the site of lesion in areas 19 and 39 of the posterior parietal cortex, in a group of patients with an ipsilesional smooth pursuit deficit. (From Morrow M, Sharpe JA: Cerebral hemispheric localization of smooth pursuit asymmetry. Neurology 40:284, 1990.) *C*, Oculographic recordings of horizontal smooth pursuit in a patient with a right pontine lesion *(D)*. The target (t) moved to the left and then to the right at a constant velocity of 25 degrees/sec. Rightward smooth pursuit was defective (eye velocity < 8 degrees/sec, shown as the slope of line 1), whereas leftward smooth pursuit was normal (>15 degrees/sec, slope of line 2). Horizontal saccades are normal. *D*, T_2-weighted MRI showing the right pontine lesion *(straight arrows)* in the patient whose oculographic recordings are shown in part C. *Curved arrow* indicates basilar artery. (From Thier P, Bachor A, Faiss J, et al: Selective impairment of smooth-pursuit eye movements due to an ischemic lesion of the basal pons. Ann Neurol 29:442, 1991.)

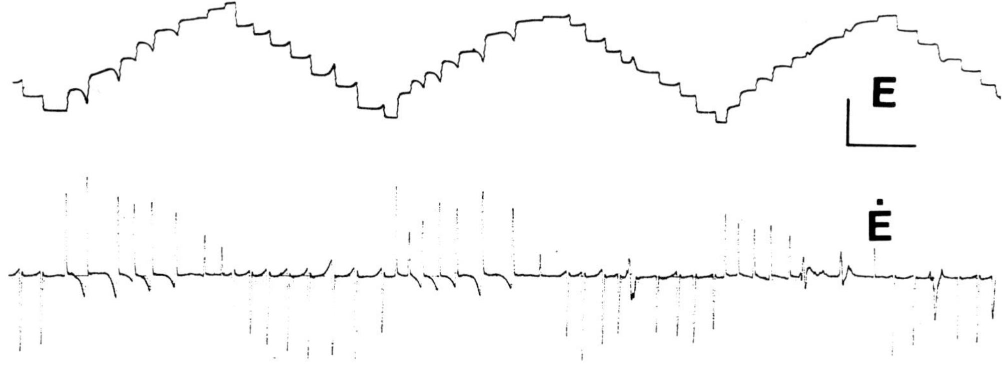

Figure 193–10. Bilateral pursuit-induced congenital nystagmus. Oculographic recordings of the left eye showing that attempted pursuit of a target (not shown) moving to the left and then to the right at a constant velocity of 10 degrees/sec induces a jerk nystagmus with the characteristic increasing-velocity, slow-phase waveform of congenital nystagmus. The nystagmus quick phases beat in the direction of the attempted smooth pursuit. The patient had presented at age 28 with headache and was found to have first-degree left-beating and first-degree right-beating nystagmus, but no primary position nystagmus. Other investigations (in retrospect, unnecessary) including MRI and lumbar puncture, all yielded normal results. Pursuit-induced nystagmus, also called "reversed" pursuit, is pathognomonic of congenital nystagmus.[249] Upward deflections indicate rightward eye movements; downward deflections indicate leftward eye movements. (Bars represent 10 degrees, 150 degrees/sec, and 1 sec. E, eye position; Ė, eye velocity.)

Vestibuloocular Reflex Palsies

Patients with vestibular diseases can present with visual symptoms.[115] In most cases the visual symptoms relate to, and can be reproduced by, head motion. A severe unilateral peripheral vestibular lesion causes a selective deficit of vestibuloocular reflex eye movement during rapid ipsilesional head rotation.[10] A selective defect of all vestibuloocular reflex eye movements indicates bilateral peripheral vestibular lesions.[116] A selective deficit of vertical vestibuloocular reflex eye movements, with intact horizontal vestibuloocular reflexes, occurs in bilateral MLF lesions.[34] In such cases, the only other clinically detectable evidence of INO may be a reduction in the maximal velocity of adducting saccades and a subtle abduction overshoot (see Fig. 193–4).

Vergence Disorders

Isolated vergence disorders are seldom attributable to neurologic disease. For example, convergence palsy or insufficiency seldom indicates neurologic disease unless it is accompanied by other signs of a dorsal midbrain lesion, such as vertical gaze palsy or dissociation of the near-triad (preservation of miosis and accommodation). Similarly, an excess of convergence due to convergence spasm is difficult to attribute to neurologic disease unless it occurs with other signs of a lesion at the midbrain-thalamic junction. Convergence spasm can easily be distinguished from bilateral abductor palsies by the accompanying miosis.[25] In contrast divergence palsy or insufficiency is difficult to distinguish from mild chronic bilateral abductor palsies. Although convergence-retraction nystagmus is pathognomonic of a dorsal midbrain lesion, and is often accompanied by convergence palsy, it is not actually a disorder of the vergence system—rather it is a disorder of reciprocal inhibition in the saccadic system[117, 118]; it should not be confused with the various types of convergence-evoked nystagmus,[119] particularly voluntary nystagmus.[120]

Nystagmus and Related Ocular Oscillations

Some types of nystagmus can be recognized and diagnosed clinically. To make a specific diagnosis in a patient with nystagmus, the examination should provide answers to the following questions:

1. Can the patient maintain steady binocular fixation on a near and on a distant target, or is there a saccadic instability, and if so is it voluntary or involuntary?
2. Is the nystagmus present in the primary position of gaze?
3. What is the direction and trajectory of the nystagmus: horizontal, vertical, torsional, or elliptical?
4. What is the waveform of the nystagmus: is it pendular or jerk, and what is its approximate frequency?
5. What is the effect of eccentric gaze position on the nystagmus: is it gaze-evoked or gaze-paretic?
6. Is the nystagmus conjugate or disconjugate? If it is disconjugate, is it dissociated (mainly or only in one eye) or is it disjunctive (equal and opposite in the two eyes)?
7. Is the nystagmus influenced by any maneuvers such as head-shaking, changes in head posture, convergence, monocular visual occlusion, binocular visual occlusion, eye closure, or hyperventilation?
8. Does the nystagmus have a periodicity?
9. Is the nystagmus associated with any ocular or gaze palsies?
10. Is the nystagmus associated with any other involuntary movements, for example of the eyelids, palate, or eardrum?
11. Is the nystagmus symptomatic, and in particular is it causing oscillopsia?

DOWNBEAT NYSTAGMUS

Downbeat nystagmus may or may not be present in the primary position; if it is, it beats directly downward.[121] It may be accentuated on either downward or upward gaze. It is, however, in lateral gaze that the identifying characteristics become evident: both the frequency and slow-phase velocity of the nystagmus increase, and the nystagmus beats obliquely downward (Fig. 193–11). In some patients the nystagmus is influenced both by vertical semicircular canal and by otolithic stimulation.[122] Downbeat nystagmus can be intermittent.[123] About a third of patients with downbeat nystagmus can be shown to have bilateral lesions involving the cerebellar flocculus, most commonly a type 1 Chiari malformation (see Fig. 193–11). In about half the patients with downbeat nystagmus, no cause for the nystagmus can be found.

PRIMARY POSITION UPBEAT NYSTAGMUS

The characteristic feature of primary position upbeat nystagmus is that by definition it is present in the primary position of gaze. Like downbeat nystagmus, it may be accentuated on either upward or downward gaze and in the supine posture. It beats obliquely upward on lateral gaze. Most patients with primary position upbeat nystagmus can be shown to have focal brain stem lesions in the tegmental gray matter, either at the pontomesencephalic junction or at the pontomedullary junction involving the prepositus hypoglossi nucleus[124, 125] or the ventral tegmental pathway of the upward vestibuloocular reflex.[126]

TORSIONAL NYSTAGMUS

A persistent torsional jerk nystagmus is usually caused by a lesion of the lateral medulla involving the vestibular nuclei.[127–129] It is occasionally due to a midbrain-thalamic lesion involving the interstitial nucleus of Cajal.[130] In patients with lateral medullary infarcts, the nystagmus is contralesional; that is, the quick phases beat away from the side of the lesion. Torsional nystagmus can be present in the primary position but is characteristically accentuated on lateral rather than on upward or downward gaze. Even if absent in the primary position, it can be direction-fixed and beats in the same direction on both leftward and rightward gaze. It can also be influenced by otolithic stimulation and can be accentuated in the lateral position when the intact side is dependent.

SEE-SAW NYSTAGMUS

Lesions at the midbrain-thalamic junction (usually bilateral, but sometimes unilateral)[130, 131] can cause a vertically symmetric but disjunctive, pendular nystagmus, characteristically composed of half cycles in which one eye elevates and intorts while the other eye depresses and extorts. Although the half-cycles resemble the ocular tilt reaction, the nystagmus is insensitive to otolithic stimulation. A jerk waveform see-saw nystagmus has also been reported.[130, 132]

PERIODIC ALTERNATING NYSTAGMUS

Periodic alternating nystagmus is a primary position horizontal nystagmus that changes direction in a crescendo-decrescendo fashion, characteristically every 90 sec (Fig. 193–12).[133] Some patients with periodic alternating nystagmus have bilateral lesions, malformations, or degenerations involving the vestibular nuclei and vestibulocerebellum. Some have congenital nystagmus or are blind, and others have a variety of diffuse or multifocal neurologic diseases such as drug intoxication or multiple sclerosis.

ACQUIRED PENDULAR NYSTAGMUS

The waveform of acquired pendular nystagmus, as the name indicates, is its most characteristic feature. When it is exclusively horizontal, there may be some difficulty in distinguishing acquired from congenital pendular nystagmus, but not when it is vertical or ellipsoidal or when it has a different trajectory in the two eyes.[134] It can affect one eye, or both eyes, equally or unequally, and it can be associated with similar, although not necessarily synchronous, oscillations of other regions such as the palate, face, eardrum, and diaphragm (Fig. 193–13).[135] In some cases, there is a lesion somewhere in the dentate nucleus of the cerebellum, the superior cerebellar peduncle, the red nucleus, the decussation of Wernekink,

---

Figure 193–11. Downbeat nystagmus and Chiari malformation. *A*, Oculographic recordings from a patient with idiopathic, isolated downbeat nystagmus. *Top rows*: Gaze-evoked nystagmus with the patient looking in sequence: center → 30 degrees right → center → 30 degrees left → center → 20 degrees up → center → 20 degrees down → center. Note that the downbeat nystagmus was absent in the primary position and appeared only in lateral gaze and (paradoxically) in upward gaze. *Middle rows*: Modulation of downbeat nystagmus by vertical vestibular stimulation. Downward head movement increased the downbeat nystagmus, whereas upward head movement abolished it. *Bottom rows*: Modulation of downbeat nystagmus by otolithic stimulation. The downbeat nystagmus was most marked when the patient was in the supine posture. (H, horizontal; V, vertical; R, right; U, up; L, left; D, down.) (From Halmagyi GM, Rudge P, Gresty MA, et al: Downbeating nystagmus: A review of 62 cases. Arch Neurol 40:777, 1983. Copyright 1983, American Medical Association.) *B*, A mild type 1 adult-form Chiari malformation, of the variety typically associated with downbeat nystagmus, shown on T_1-weighted MRI. The tip of one of the cerebellar tonsils *(open arrow)* extends well below the occipital rim of the foramen magnum *(straight arrows)*. The curved arrow indicates the site where upward and backward protrusion of the odontoid process of C2 can indent and angulate the pontomedullary junction in more advanced cases of Chiari malformation. *C*, Off-axis parasagittal reconstruction of a CT scan with intrathecal contrast provides more information than can MRI about the relationship between the skeletal abnormalities and the brain abnormalities in Chiari malformations. The upper border of the reconstructed CT image is indicated by the white line on the MRI. In the axial CT image the asymmetry of the tonsillar descent is evident *(short arrows)*. The exact relationship of the posterior lip of the foramen magnum *(long straight arrows)*, the first three vertebral bodies (1, 2, 3), and the tip of the odontoid (D) to the ectopic cerebellum *(open arrow)* is clearly shown. This type of anatomic information is important in the planning of surgery for patients with Chiari malformations.

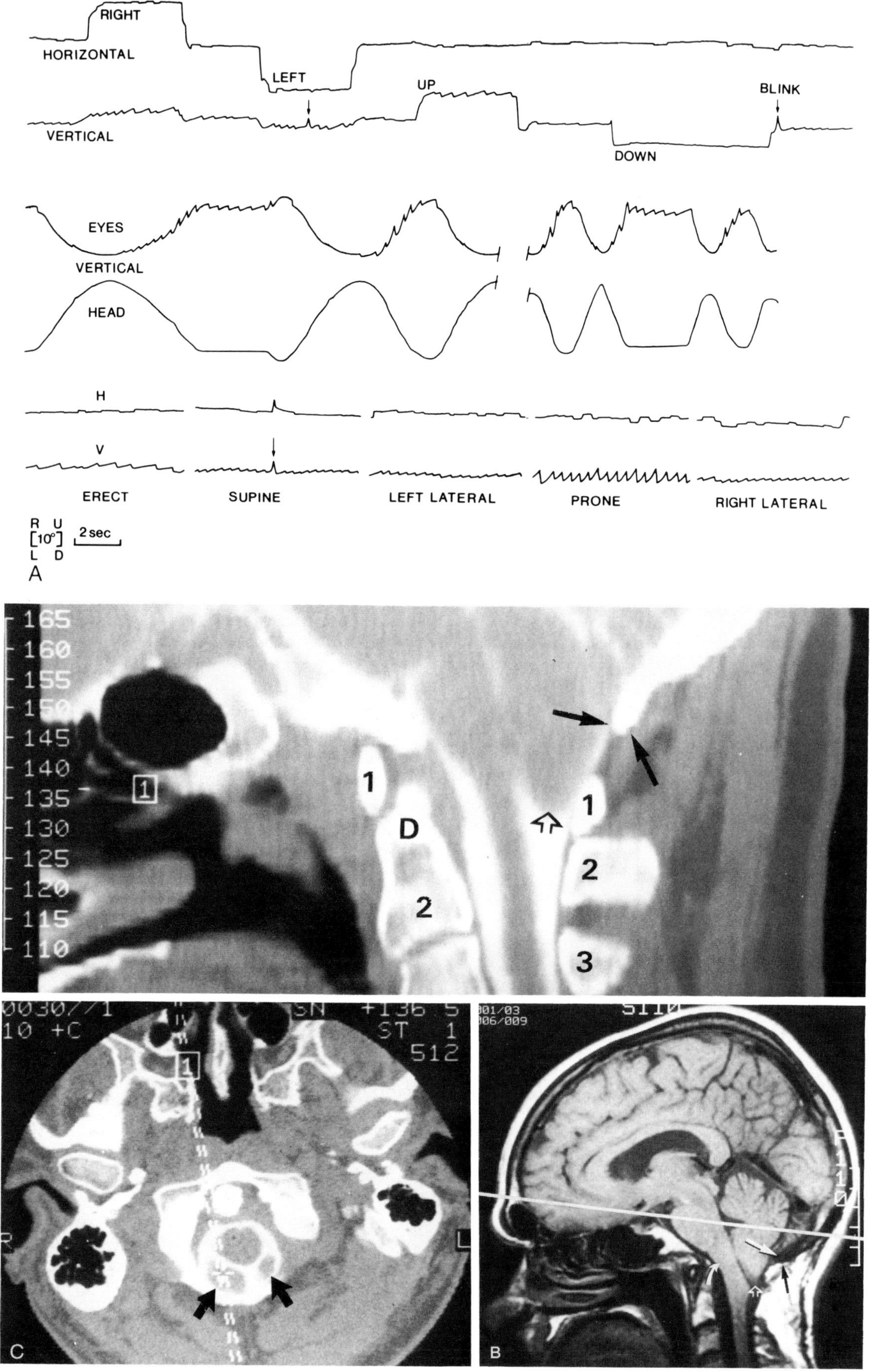

Figure 193–11 *See legend on opposite page*

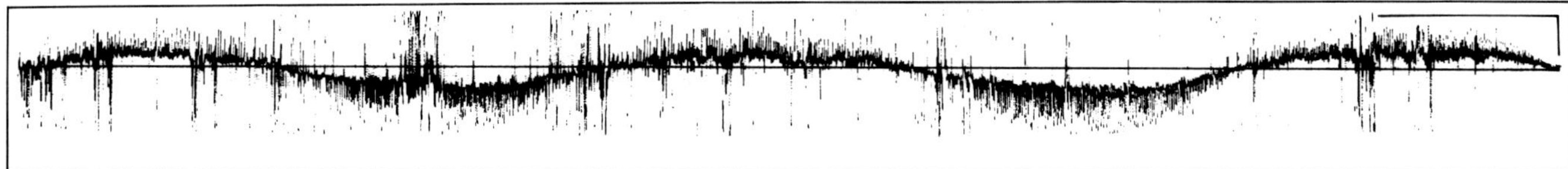

Figure 193–12. Periodic alternating nystagmus. Oculographic recording shows the characteristic 90-sec reversals in slow-phase direction and the sinusoidal changes in slow-phase velocity. The center line indicates zero eye velocity. The patient had advanced cerebellar degeneration. Upward deflections indicate rightward eye movements; downward deflections indicate leftward eye movements. (Bars represent 50 degrees/sec and 60 sec.)

the central tegmental tract, the inferior olive, the inferior cerebellar peduncle or the cerebellar cortex, a neural circuit known as the "myoclonic triangle."[136, 137] In these cases, the pendular nystagmus could be due to denervation hypersensitivity, because it begins weeks to months after an acute lesion occurs. The pseudohypertrophic degeneration of the inferior olivary nucleus that also occurs in these cases can be shown by MRI.[138, 139] Acquired pendular nystagmus can also occur with lesions around the optic chiasm[140] and in acquired blindness, in which case it may only affect the blind eye.[141] A pendular waveform convergence nystagmus occurs in spasmus nutans[140] and in some patients with Chiari malformations.[142]

CONVERGENCE-RETRACTION NYSTAGMUS

The characteristic feature of convergence-retraction nystagmus is the appearance of disjunctive convergent saccades causing retraction of the globes. The nystagmus can occur either spontaneously or when triggered by (attempted) upward saccades.[86, 117] The lesion responsible for convergence retraction nystagmus is in the dorsal midbrain, and the other components of the dorsal midbrain syndrome, such as abnormalities of the pupils, eyelids, and vertical gaze, can usually be found.[88]

PERIPHERAL VESTIBULAR NYSTAGMUS

The characteristics of peripheral vestibular nystagmus are so constant and so well known that it should be easy to recognize clinically. (For a review see reference 143). (1) Peripheral vestibular nystagmus does not occur in isolation: A patient who has nystagmus of peripheral vestibular origin experiences vertigo. (2) Pathologic peripheral vestibular nystagmus can be either persistent and horizontal, or paroxysmal and torsional, but is (almost) never exclusively vertical. (3) Peripheral vestibular nystagmus always indicates unilateral or at least asymmetric bilateral vestibular lesions; bilateral symmetric vestibular lesions do not cause peripheral vestibular nystagmus. (4) Peripheral vestibular nystagmus is always unidirectional, the quick phases beating away from the underactive labyrinth or toward the overactive labyrinth. (5) In the absence of brain stem or cerebellar dysfunction (including drug intoxication), horizontal vestibular nystagmus is markedly suppressed by visual fixation and therefore is only apparent if special examination techniques are used (e.g., ophthalmoscope[144] or Frenzel glasses). For all these reasons, peripheral vestibular nystagmus is rarely encountered in ophthalmic practice and should not be diagnosed if it occurs in the presence of visual fixation in an upright patient who has no vertigo.

Unilateral Vestibular Hypofunction. Immediately after acute complete deafferentation of one intact labyrinth, by either labyrinthectomy or vestibular neurectomy in an otherwise healthy subject with an intact contralateral labyrinth, there is in addition to intense vertigo, a brisk contraversive horizontal nystagmus. The nystagmus is apparent on examination in the primary position, but only in the absence of visual fixation (Fig.

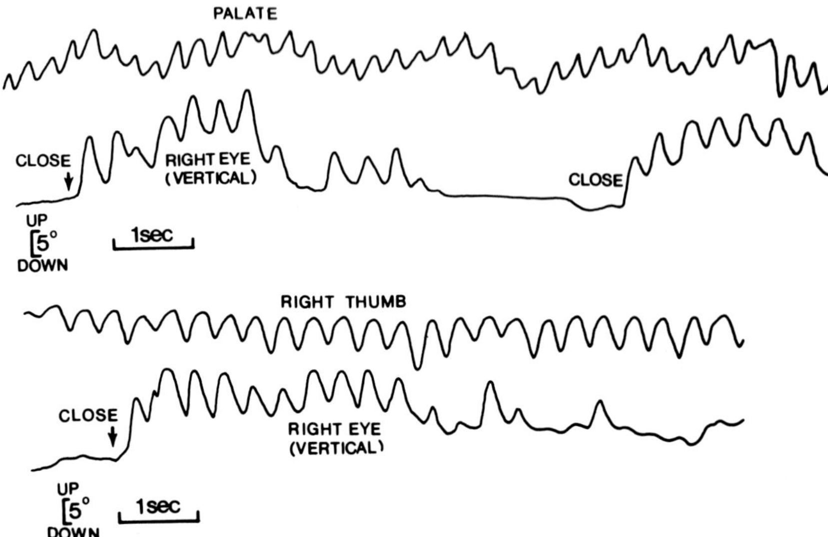

Figure 193–13. Pendular nystagmus. Oculographic recordings from the right eye show a regular 3- to 4-Hz vertical pendular oscillation of the eyes, which was present only when the eyes were closed. (It was absent even in the dark.) There was a synchronous pendular oscillation (i.e., tremor) of the palate and of the right thumb. Pendular nystagmus is caused by a lesion anywhere in the myoclonic triangle. This lesion was in the central tegmental tract in the midbrain. (Amplitude calibrations apply only to the eye movement.)

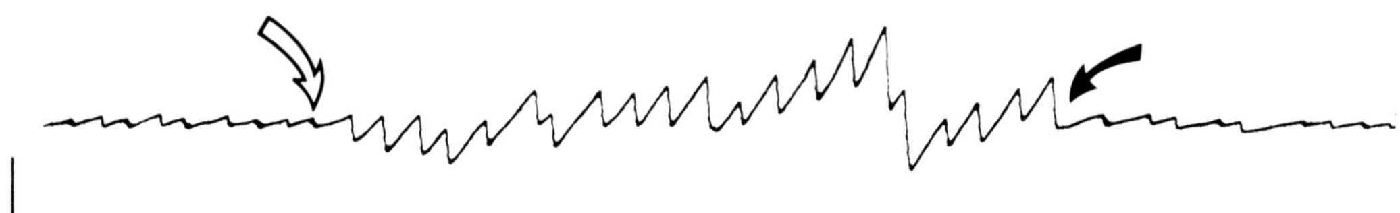

Figure 193–14. Peripheral vestibular nystagmus. Oculographic recording shows a left-beating primary-position nystagmus that was obvious only when visual fixation was removed *(open arrow)* and was quickly suppressed again when visual fixation was permitted *(filled arrow)*. Peripheral vestibular nystagmus can be detected clinically by viewing the fundus of one eye while occluding the other.[144] The patient had acute right vestibular neuritis. Upward deflections indicate rightward eye movements; downward deflections indicate leftward eye movements. (Bars represent 10 degrees and 1 sec.)

193–14). After about 1 wk, the vertigo and the nystagmus largely resolve. The nystagmus is then only apparent in the absence of visual fixation, especially after vigorous head-shaking.[11]

Unilateral Vestibular Hyperfunction. Attacks of endolymphatic hydrops, particularly when due to Menière's disease, may begin with vestibular *hyper*function rather than *hypo*function.[145] The mechanism may be temporary impairment of inhibitory vestibular efferent neurons. In these cases, unlike in cases of unilateral vestibular hypofunction, the nystagmus is ipsilesional—that is, the quick phases beat toward the side of the lesioned ear. The paretic contraversive nystagmus that follows this irritative ipsiversive nystagmus can then be followed by a second type of ipsiversive nystagmus called "recovery" nystagmus.[146]

Benign Paroxysmal Positioning Nystagmus. Sequestration of utricular otoconia onto the cupular surface of the posterior semicircular canal (cupulolithiasis) could be the cause of the syndrome of benign paroxysmal positioning vertigo. The condition is usually unilateral and is provoked by rapidly reclining or by turning the patient onto the affected side.[147] This provokes a brief attack of intense vertigo accompanied by brisk primary position torsional nystagmus beating toward the affected, lowermost labyrinth. Sometimes, another brief attack occurs on resuming the upright posture, but this time the nystagmus beats in the opposite direction. Benign paroxysmal positioning nystagmus is apparent in the presence of visual fixation. Any positional or positioning nystagmus that does not conform to these criteria, particularly if not accompanied by much vertigo, should in the first case be presumed to be a central positional nystagmus caused by a lesion of the vestibular nuclei or vestibulocerebellum.

CONGENITAL NYSTAGMUS

In patients with symptoms and signs of neurologic disease, it is important to recognize that a nystagmus could be of congenital rather than of acquired origin. A patient who does not have oscillopsia, despite a primary-position horizontal jerk nystagmus that has an eccentric null position but that is unaltered by vertical position, has congenital nystagmus. If, however, the nystagmus is only present on far lateral gaze or has largely a pendular waveform or a torsional component, then diagnostic difficulties may arise. In such cases it may be helpful to note whether optokinetic nystagmus is reversed and whether the nystagmus can be induced by smooth pursuit (see Fig. 193–10) or by attempted vestibuloocular reflex suppression. These features are all characteristic of congenital nystagmus. Oculographic recordings can be helpful in confirming the diagnosis.[148] The mechanism of congenital nystagmus is unknown.

LATENT NYSTAGMUS

True latent nystagmus is a type of congenital nystagmus that is only present with monocular viewing and then beats toward the viewing eye.[148] It is absent with binocular viewing. Manifest latent nystagmus is a type of congenital nystagmus associated with congenital esotropia, which is present when both eyes are open but beats in a different direction depending on which eye is viewing (i.e., always toward the viewing eye). Latent nystagmus is also associated with alternating hyperphoria (dissociated vertical deviation). When patients with latent nystagmus develop incidental neurologic symptoms such as headache or vertigo, there is always the danger that the nystagmus will be mistakenly attributed to neurologic disease.

GAZE-EVOKED NYSTAGMUS

Gaze-evoked nystagmus is a common, easily recognized clinical finding of limited localizing value. It is a jerk nystagmus that is by definition absent in the primary position and is only present in eccentric gaze. It may be sustained or unsustained. If it is unsustained, it may be followed on refixation to the primary position by rebound nystagmus. Unilateral gaze-evoked nystagmus, particularly if accompanied by a pursuit palsy, suggests a lesion in the ipsilateral cerebral or cerebellar hemisphere. Gaze-evoked nystagmus also occurs with brain stem lesions. Bilateral horizontal together with vertical gaze-evoked nystagmus commonly occurs with structural brain stem and cerebellar lesions, diffuse metabolic disorders, and drug intoxication (Fig. 193–15).

REBOUND NYSTAGMUS

Rebound nystagmus is a jerk nystagmus that beats away from the previous direction of eccentric gaze and that lasts for 3 to 25 sec after the eyes return to the primary position (see Fig. 193–15). It is found in association with a decaying gaze-evoked nystagmus in patients with cerebellar lesions and diseases and also in

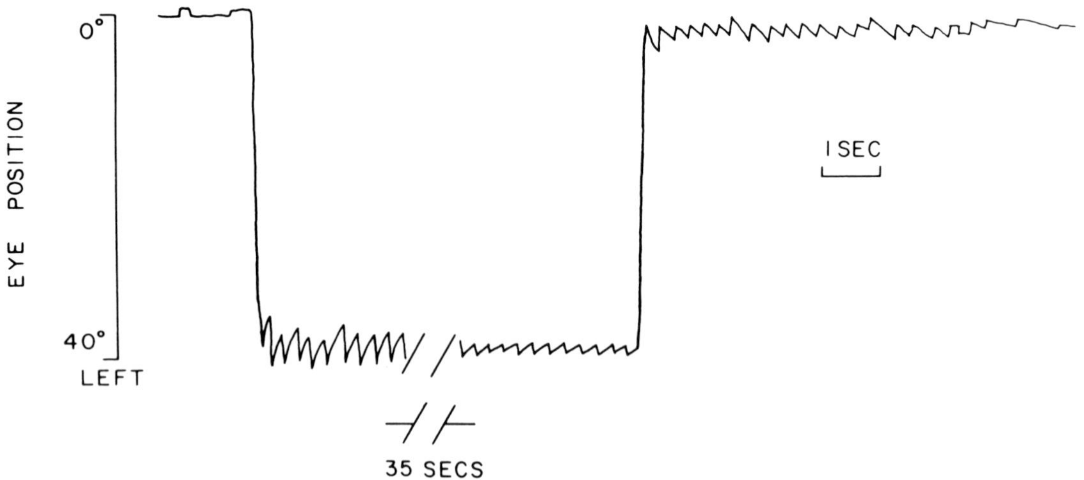

Figure 193–15. Gaze-evoked nystagmus and rebound nystagmus. Oculographic recordings show that at first there was no primary position nystagmus. When the patient looked 40 degrees to the left, there was a vigorous left-beating, gaze-evoked nystagmus that diminished during the 40 sec or so of eccentric fixation. When the patient made a saccade back to center, there was a transient primary-position, right-beating "rebound" nystagmus. The patient had hereditary cerebellar degeneration. (From Zee DS, Yee RD, Cogan DG, et al: Ocular motor abnormalities in hereditary cerebellar ataxia. Brain 99:207, 1976. By permission of Oxford University Press.)

patients with lesions of the perihypoglossal nucleus in the medulla.[149, 150]

EPILEPTIC NYSTAGMUS

Paroxysmal nystagmus can occur during many different types of epileptic seizures.[83, 151] The nystagmus does not occur in isolation but in association with other ictal phenomena, such as altered consciousness and tonic head-eye deviation. The nystagmus is usually conjugate horizontal and contraversive but may be monocular, ipsiversive, vertical, or even retractory.

NYSTAGMUS SECONDARY TO OPHTHALMOPLEGIA

Nystagmus, especially an unsustained dissociated nystagmus, occurs in patients with peripheral ocular motor palsies, particularly myasthenic palsies, and particularly if the patient habitually fixates with the paretic eye. The nystagmus represents the workings of a central adaptive mechanism that is attempting to compensate for the ophthalmoplegia. It is sometimes difficult to decide whether a patient with nystagmus and ophthalmoplegia has a lesion of the central oculomotor system causing both ophthalmoplegia and nystagmus or a lesion of the peripheral oculomotor system causing an ophthalmoplegia with a secondary nystagmus.

VOLUNTARY NYSTAGMUS

Many normal subjects can learn to make rapid to-and-fro horizontal saccades. A convergence effort is usually required to initiate and maintain these oscillations. This should not be confused with ocular flutter which is an involuntary saccadic oscillation that occurs in patients with cerebellar disease (Fig. 193–16).[120, 152]

SACCADIC INTRUSIONS AND OSCILLATIONS

Spontaneous saccadic oscillations form a continuum from square-wave jerks to opsoclonus. Four different types can be distinguished clinically.

1. *Square-wave jerks*. These jerks are pairs of small (1 to 2 degree) oppositely directed horizontal saccades intruding inappropriately on fixation. The first saccade of the pair takes the eyes away from fixation, while the second returns the eyes to fixation after a 200-msec or so intersaccadic interval. Square-wave jerks can occur in normal, particularly older subjects.[153] Patients with diseases of the cerebrum, cerebellum, or basal ganglia may have almost continuous square-wave jerks.[154, 155] Saccadic oscillations may be induced by blinking.[156]
2. *Macro square-wave jerks*. These jerks are larger (5 to 30 degree) involuntary saccades that occur singly or in bursts, during fixation or immediately after saccadic refixation.[157]
3. *Macrosaccadic oscillations*. These oscillations are crescendo-decrescendo bursts of saccades across fixation (Fig. 193–17). The intersaccadic intervals are normal.[157]
4. *Ocular flutter and opsoclonus*. These are bursts of inappropriate saccades without an intersaccadic interval. Flutter comprises bursts of inappropriate mainly horizontal saccades,[158] whereas opsoclonus comprises bursts of horizontal, vertical, and torsional saccades.[159] Voluntary nystagmus can sometimes be mistaken for ocular flutter. Macro square-wave jerks, macrosaccadic oscillations, and ocular flutter have all been found in patients with focal lesions of the cerebellum. Patients with these disorders also show dysmetric errors of their refixation saccades. Opsoclonus on the other hand has not been found in patients with focal cerebellar lesions but has by inference been attributed to cerebellar Purkinje cell dysfunction.[160]

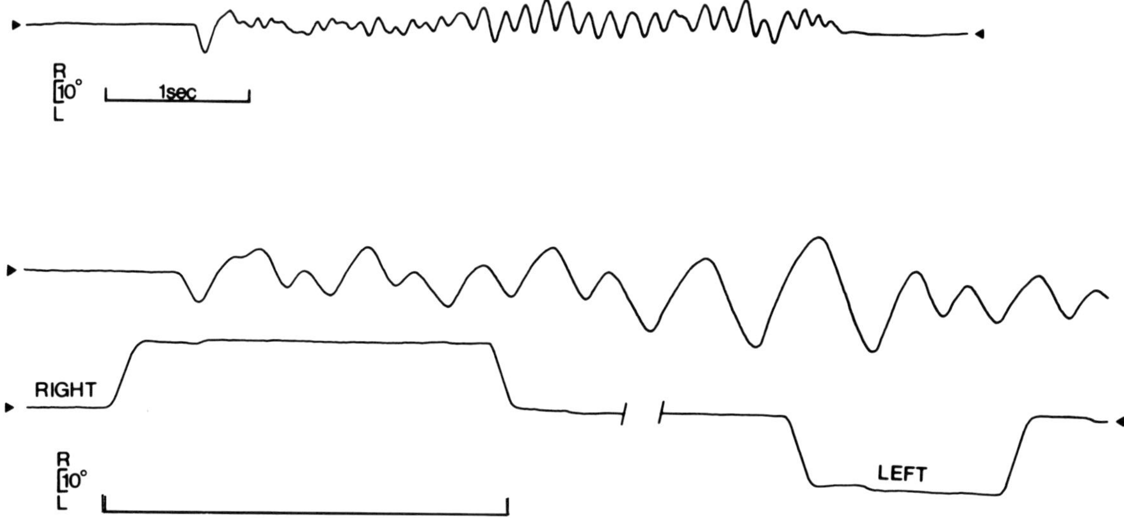

Figure 193–16. Voluntary nystagmus. Oculographic recordings show a low-amplitude rapid irregular 6- to 7-Hz horizontal pendular oscillation of the eyes. On a faster time scale *(bottom rows)*, the normal saccadic structure of voluntary nystagmus is evident. Arrowheads indicate the primary position of gaze. (R, right; L, left.)

Myasthenia Gravis

Ocular myasthenia, the great mimic, merits special mention. (For a recent review see reference 161 and Chapter 196.) There is often a delay in the correct diagnosis of myasthenia, either because it is not suspected or because it mimics another eye movement disorder. Although there is still dispute about the parameters worth observing,[162–166] there are several clinical situations in which a Tensilon test is worthwhile in a patient with disordered eye movements: (1) Ptosis, particularly if fatigable and if accompanied by a lid twitch with centering, upward saccades; (2) Weakness of orbicularis oculi, particularly in association with ptosis or ophthalmoplegia; (3) Decrease in the range of ocular motion in one direction without a commensurate decrease in saccadic eye velocity. In myasthenia, saccades may be of supernormal velocity.[167] In contrast, in patients with lesions of the ocular motoneuron, nerve, or muscle, any decrease in the range of ocular movement is accompanied by a similar decrease in the saccadic velocity of that movement.[168] Limitation of the range of ocular motion with normal saccadic velocity is found not only in ocular myasthenia but also in restrictive orbital lesions.

Disorders of Ocular Motoneuron Function

Some disorders of peripheral ocular motoneurons do not simply cause loss or deficiency of neural function, but rather excessive or inappropriate neural function.

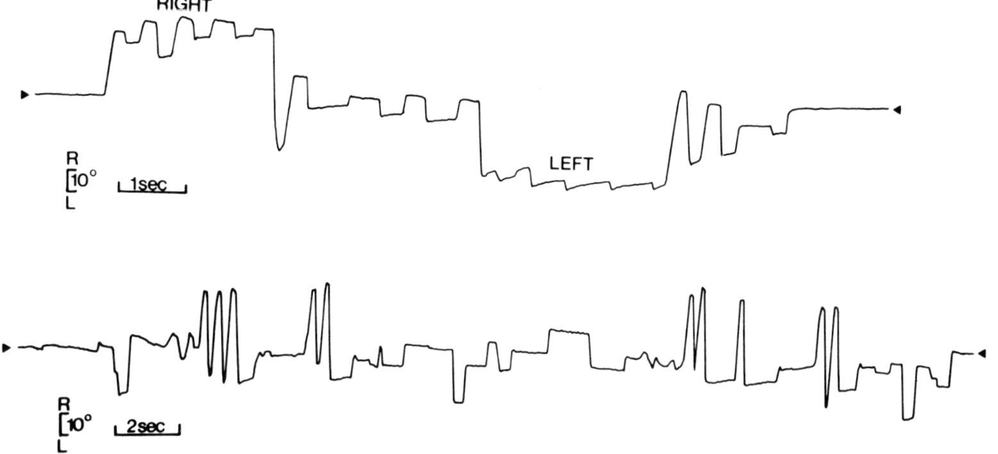

Figure 193–17. Saccadic oscillations. Oculographic recordings of macro square-wave jerks *(top row)* and ocular flutter *(bottom row)*. Macro square-wave jerks consist of 5- to 10-degree involuntary to-and-fro horizontal saccades, often across fixation and with a normal intersaccadic interval. Ocular flutter consists of a similar burst of saccades without an intersaccadic interval. (R, right; L, left.)

OCULAR NEUROMYOTONIA

Neuromyotonia is a syndrome of repetitive spontaneous activity of single motor units following maximal voluntary contraction. It is rarely accompanied by any appreciable muscle contraction. It can be differentiated on electrophysiologic criteria from other spontaneous motor unit discharges, such as fasciculation, myotonia, myokymia, and spasm. "Ocular neuromyotonia" is the name given to an ocular motor disorder that usually follows parasellar radiation therapy, in which there appears to be either a spontaneous contraction of extraocular muscles or a delayed relaxation of extraocular muscles after voluntary contraction.[169–171] This may result in a transient, intermittent incomitant strabismus sometimes appearing after sustained gaze deviation. The strabismus is due to sustained contraction of the agonist, giving the appearance of a palsy of the antagonist. There has not so far been electrophysiologic confirmation of the neuromyotonic nature of the motor unit discharges.

SUPERIOR OBLIQUE MYOKYMIA

Myokymia is a syndrome of repetitive spontaneous discharges of motor units firing rapidly, in doublets or triplets, in relative isolation. Superior oblique myokymia is a syndrome of intermittent, rapid, repetitive contraction of the superior oblique muscle, which causes paroxysmal monocular torsional oscillation and oscillopsia. The ocular oscillation can be seen with a slit lamp and can be heard with a stethoscope.[172] To date, there has not been electrophysiologic confirmation of the myokymic nature of the motor unit discharges.

OCULAR MOTOR NERVE SYNKINESIS

A normal synkinesis is the simultaneous activation of muscles supplied by different peripheral nerves or by different branches of the same nerve. A pathologic synkinesis is a syndrome that occurs when, following a lesion of one or more peripheral nerves, muscles are reinnervated by peripheral nerves apart from their own. The nerve palsy that precedes synkinesis may or may not be clinically evident. In Duane's syndrome there is, in the absence of the abducens nerve, annexation of the lateral rectus muscle by branches of the oculomotor nerve.[18] The functional result is a congenital oculomotor-abducens synkinesis. In congenital adduction palsy with synergistic divergence, there may be an abducens-oculomotor synkinesis due to annexation of the medial rectus by branches from the abducens nerve.[27] In the typical Marcus Gunn jaw-winking syndrome, there is a congenital trigeminooculomotor synkinesis. Some patients with Duane's syndrome also have a trigemino-oculomotor synkinesis.[173] A trigeminoabducens synkinesis may occur after trauma,[174, 175] and facial synkinesis is a common complication of facial nerve palsy. A synkinesis between various branches of the oculomotor nerve leads to a characteristic constellation of signs, including lid elevation on attempted adduction or depression, retraction or adduction on attempted elevation or depression, and miosis on adduction. Suggested mechanisms of synkinesis include misdirection of regenerating axons, ephaptic transmission across demyelinated axons, and synaptic reorganization at the level of the motor nuclei.[176]

DISORDERED EYE MOVEMENTS PRODUCED BY FOCAL BRAIN LESIONS

This section summarizes the various eye movement disorders seen in patients with focal brain lesions. For more detail and for more references on eye movement disorders in patients with focal brain stem and cerebellar lesions, in this case infarcts, the reader is referred to a review by Bogousslavsky and Meienberg.[177]

Lesions of the Medulla

Focal lesions of the medulla can produce several different eye movement disorders, sometimes in isolation. Since these disorders can produce visual symptoms, patients with medullary lesions can first present to the ophthalmologist. Three neural structures are involved in the genesis of medullary eye movement disorders: the vestibular nucleus, the olivary nucleus, and the perihypoglossal nucleus.

ANATOMY AND PHYSIOLOGY

The vestibular nucleus has four parts: medial, lateral, superior, and inferior. The medial and superior vestibular nuclei are concerned with eye movement control and contain the second neuron of the three-neuron vestibuloocular reflex. Vestibular nucleus neurons project directly to abducens motoneurons in the contralateral abducens nucleus. They also project indirectly via contralateral abducens interneurons and the ipsilateral MLF to medial rectus motoneurons in the ipsilateral oculomotor nucleus, and via the contralateral MLF to the vertical ocular motoneurons in the contralateral oculomotor nucleus. Unilateral lesions of the vestibular nucleus produce three main eye movement disorders: a predominantly torsional nystagmus, an ocular tilt reaction (Fig. 193–18), and lateropulsion (see Fig. 193–6). Some patients with acute unilateral vestibular nucleus lesion also have an irresistible illusion of visual tilt, even in the absence of any eye movement disorder. These illusions may be extreme and frightening—for example, the room can appear to be inverted.[178] They are probably due to involvement of otolithic elements in the vestibular nucleus. The medulla also contains the olivary nuclei. The inferior olivary nucleus receives input from the contralateral dentate nucleus in the cerebellum via the red nucleus in the midbrain and the central tegmental tract. Inferior olivary neurons then project to cerebellar Purkinje cells via the inferior cerebellar peduncle. Although the role of the olive in normal ocular motor control is not clear, lesions of the inferior olive or its

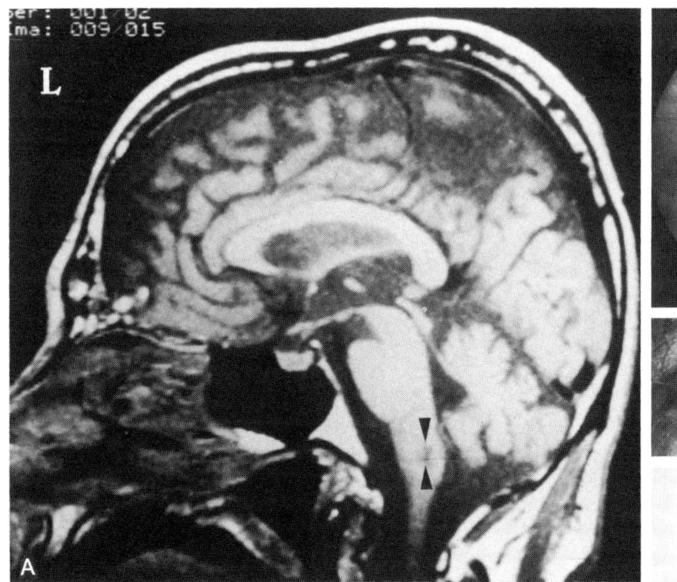

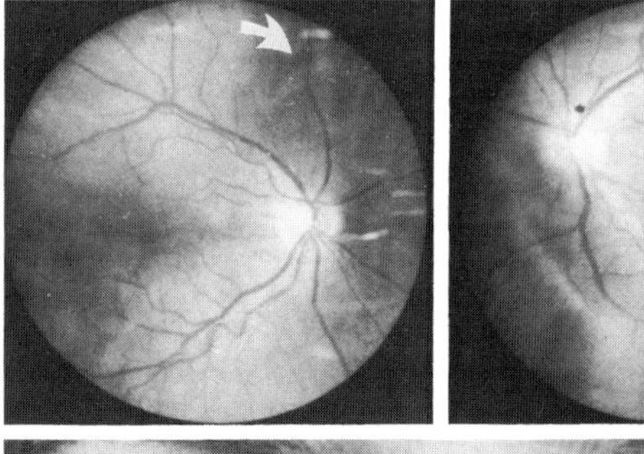

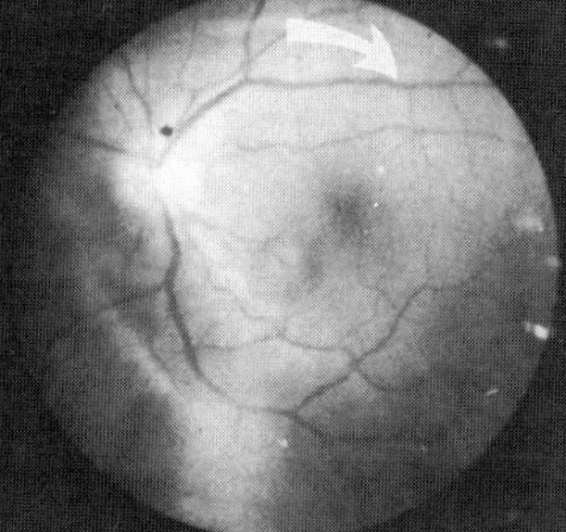

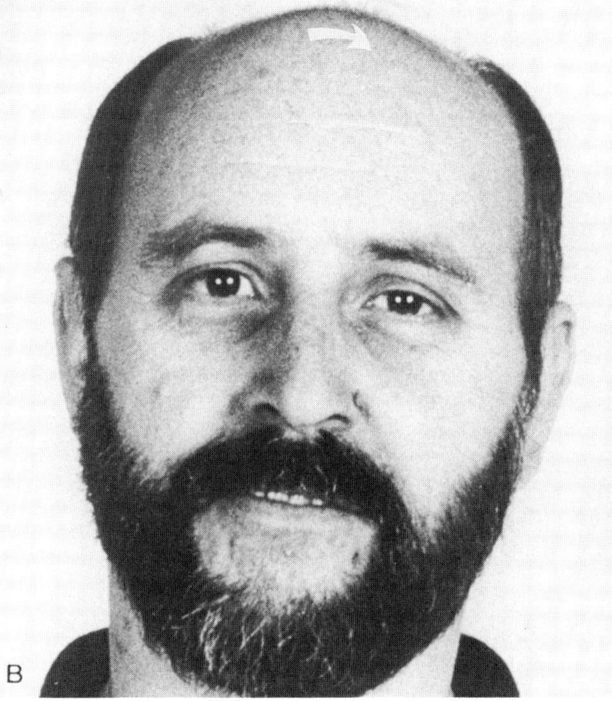

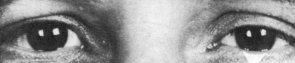

Figure 193–18. Medullary lesion with eye movement disorder. *A*, Left (L) lateral medullary infarct *(arrowheads)* involving the left vestibular nucleus, shown by parasagittal T_1-weighted MRI. *B*, The patient had left Horner's syndrome and a leftward ocular tilt reaction with left hypotropia, leftward head tilt, and dysconjugate leftward ocular torsion, about 20 degrees (excyclotropia) in the left eye but only about 5 degrees (incyclotropia) in the right eye. He also had loss of pain and temperature sensation on the left side of the face and on the right side of the body. (Courtesy of T Brandt, M.D.)

connections produce a distinctive eye movement disorder: pendular nystagmus (see Fig. 193–13). In contrast to the olivary nucleus, the role of the perihypoglossal nucleus (prepositus hypoglossi nucleus) in oculomotor control is well recognized. It is the site of integration of horizontal eye velocity signals into eye position signals. Lesions of perihypoglossal nucleus produce gaze-evoked nystagmus (Table 193–1).

Lesions of the Pons

The pons contains many structures necessary for eye movement control. These structures are closely packed in the dorsal pons, so that patients with small focal lesions of the pontine tegmentum commonly develop isolated disorders of eye movement (Fig. 193–19). Since the ocular motor structures in the pons are largely concerned with the control of conjugate horizontal eye movement, dorsal pontine lesions characteristically produce a selective disorder of horizontal eye movement. Except in the acute stage, vertical eye movements and vergence eye movements are entirely spared.

ANATOMY AND PHYSIOLOGY

The three key structures in the understanding of pontine eye movement disorders are the abducens nu-

Table 193–1. MEDULLARY EYE MOVEMENT DISORDERS

Eye Movement Disorder	Structure Involved
Torsional nystagmus	Vestibular nucleus[127]
Lateropulsion	Vestibular nucleus[61]
Ocular tilt reaction	Vestibular nucleus[14]
Pendular nystagmus	Olivary nucleus[134–139]
Horizontal gaze-evoked nystagmus	(?) Perihypoglossal nucleus[108, 150]
Primary-position upbeat nystagmus	(?) Perihypoglossal nucleus[124, 125]

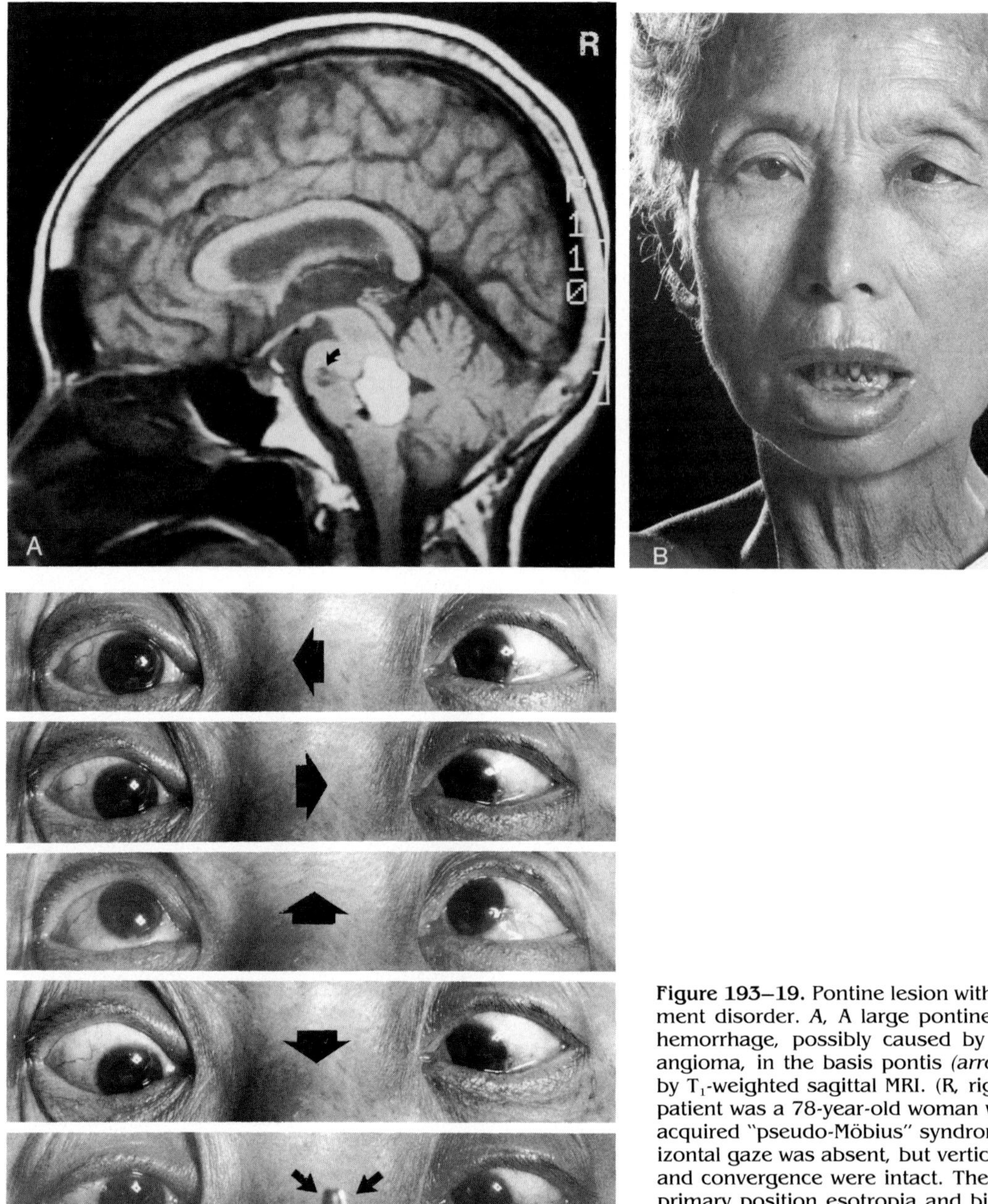

Figure 193–19. Pontine lesion with eye movement disorder. *A*, A large pontine tegmental hemorrhage, possibly caused by a capillary angioma, in the basis pontis *(arrow)*, shown by T_1-weighted sagittal MRI. (R, right.) *B*, The patient was a 78-year-old woman who had an acquired "pseudo-Möbius" syndrome. *C*, Horizontal gaze was absent, but vertical saccades and convergence were intact. There was also primary position esotropia and bilateral total facial palsy, but no disturbance of consciousness and no long-tract signs.

cleus, the PPRF, and the MLF (Table 193–2). Abducens nucleus contains not only the motoneurons that innervate the ipsilateral lateral rectus muscle but also contains the interneurons that project via the contralateral MLF to innervate medial rectus motoneurons in the contralateral oculomotor nucleus. Abducens interneurons in fact provide all input required for conjugate eye movement to the medial rectus motoneurons. The abducens nucleus receives input from the ipsilateral PPRF and from the contralateral vestibular nucleus. From burst neurons in the PPRF it receives the high-frequency neural discharges that are required to produce all ipsiversive horizontal saccadic eye movements. From the vestibular nucleus, it receives neural discharges required to produce smooth compensatory eye movements in response to vestibular or optokinetic stimulation. The MLF not only provides all input (except vergence) to medial rectus motoneurons but it also carries the vertical vestibular signal from the vestibular nuclei in the medulla to the vertical oculomotor neurons in the midbrain.

Lesions of the Midbrain

The dorsal midbrain, in a manner similar to the dorsal pons, contains many structures necessary for eye movement control. The major difference between the dorsal midbrain and the dorsal pons is that whereas the dorsal pons controls horizontal eye movement, the dorsal midbrain controls vertical and vergence eye movement.

Table 193–2. PONTINE EYE MOVEMENT DISORDERS

Eye Movement Disorder	Structure Involved
Abduction palsy	Abducens fascicle[15–17]
Horizontal saccadic palsy	PPRF*[43, 44]
Horizontal gaze palsy	Abducens nucleus[45, 46, 51]
Adduction palsy	MLF†[34–38]
Vertical vestibular palsy	Bilateral MLF[34]
One-and-a-half syndrome	Abducens nucleus + MLF[31, 32]
Horizontal gaze-paretic nystagmus	(?)
Primary position upbeat nystagmus	(?) Ventral tegmental VOR pathway[124, 125]
Pendular nystagmus	Central tegmental tract[134–139]

*PPRF, pontine paramedian-reticular formation.
†MLF, medial longitudinal fasciculus.

Lesions of the dorsal midbrain characteristically produce a selective disorder of vertical and vergence eye movements (Fig. 193–20). Horizontal conjugate eye movements may be entirely spared. The midbrain ocular motor structures are all closely packed, thus patients with small focal lesions of the dorsal midbrain commonly develop isolated disorders of eye movement. Dorsal midbrain lesions can produce many different vertical ophthalmoplegias, some of which can be difficult to distinguish from eye movement disorders that are of benign, congenital, nonorganic, or peripheral origin.

ANATOMY AND PHYSIOLOGY

The four key structures in the understanding of midbrain eye movement disorders are the oculomotor-trochlear nucleus, the riMLF, the interstitial nucleus (of Cajal), and the posterior commissure (Table 193–3). The oculomotor-trochlear nucleus receives input from the riMLF, interstitial nucleus, and vestibular nuclei. From burst neurons in the riMLF, it receives the high-frequency neural discharges that are required to produce all vertical and torsional saccadic eye movements. From the vestibular nuclei via the interstitial nucleus, it re-

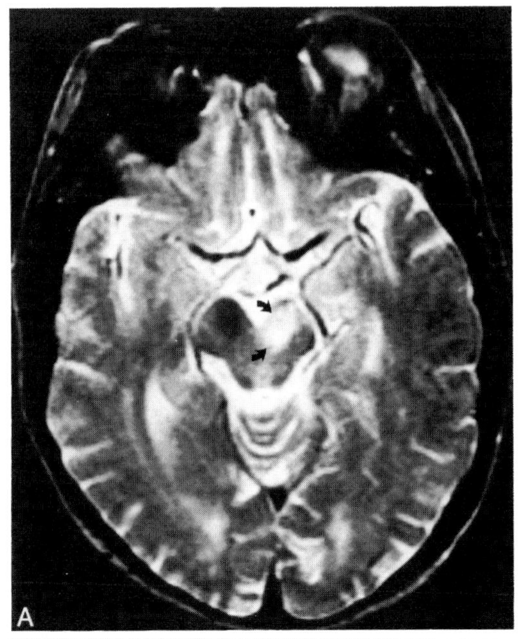

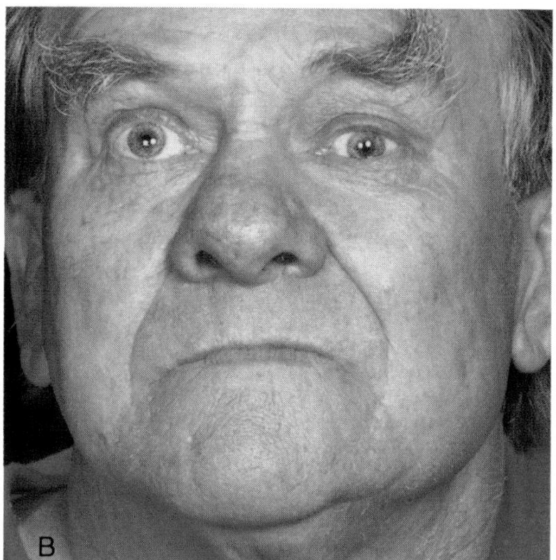

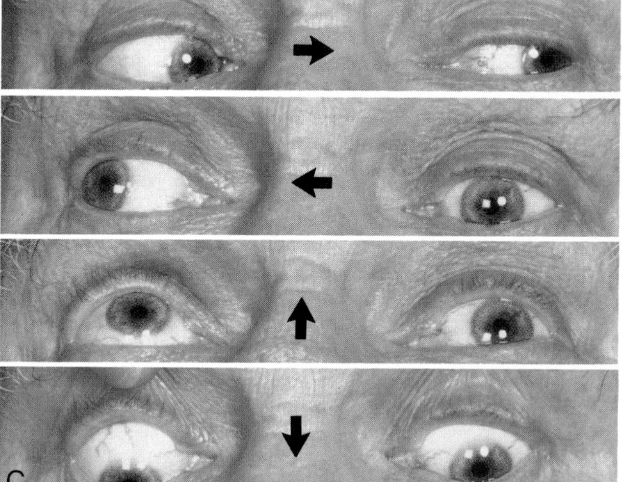

Figure 193–20. Midbrain lesion with eye movement disorder. *A*, An infarct in the ventral midbrain caused by a "top of the basilar" embolus is shown on T_2-weighted MRI. The lesion *(arrows)* involves the left pyramidal tract and the emergent fibers of the left oculomotor nerve. *B, C*, On presentation the patient had a pupil-sparing, but otherwise complete, left third-nerve palsy (shown here partly recovered) as well as right hemiparesis.

Table 193–3. MIDBRAIN EYE MOVEMENT DISORDERS

Eye Movement Disorder	Structure Involved
Third nerve palsy	Oculomotor nucleus or fasciculus[28, 29, 76]
Fourth nerve palsy	Trochlear nucleus or fasciculus[71–73]
Ocular tilt reaction	(?) Interstitial nucleus of Cajal[70]
Vertical gaze palsies:	
Selective saccadic	
Upward	(?) Bilateral riMLF,* lateral[84]
Downward	(?) Bilateral riMLF, medial[89]
Bidirectional	(?) Bilateral riMLF[85, 90]
Nonselective total	
Upward	Posterior commissure[86]
Downward	(?) Bilateral riMLF, medial[93, 94]
Bidirectional	(?) Bilateral riMLF[97]
Monocular upward palsy	(?)[78]
Vertical one-and-a half palsy	(?) Bilateral riMLF[99, 100]
Internuclear ophthalmoplegia	MLF[34]
Pendular nystagmus	Superior cerebellar peduncle[134–139]
Convergence-retraction nystagmus	Posterior commissure[117, 118]
Seesaw nystagmus	(?) Interstital nucleus of Cajal[130–132]
Gaze-evoked upbeat nystagmus	(?)[34]
Primary position upbeat nystagmus	(?) Ventral tegmental VOR pathway[124, 125]
Convergence palsy	(?)
Pseudoabducens palsy	(?) Posterior commissure[20]
Horizontal gaze paresis	(?) Crus cerebri[47, 48]

*riMLF, rostral interstitial nucleus of the medial longitudinal fasciculus.

ceives neural discharges that are required to produce smooth compensatory eye movements in response to vestibular or optokinetic stimulation. From the interstitial nucleus itself, it receives the tonic discharges necessary for eccentric gaze-holding. The internal organization of the oculomotor-trochlear nucleus also has clinical relevance. First, medial rectus motoneurons are not found in a single subnucleus but in three different locations. Second, the oculomotor-trochlear nucleus on one side innervates all the intortors of the contralateral eye (superior rectus and superior oblique) and all the extortors of the ipsilateral eye (inferior rectus and inferior oblique). Projections from one riMLF to the other, and from the interstitial nucleus to the contralateral oculomotor-trochlear nucleus all pass through the posterior commissure.

Lesions of the Cerebellum

There is ample evidence from single neuron and from lesion studies in animals that the cerebellum is intimately involved in eye movement control. Clinical observations are more difficult to interpret, because in many patients with diseases or focal lesions of the cerebellum the brain stem is also involved. Nevertheless, patients with cerebellar lesions do have a consistent pattern of eye movement disorders, and it is possible to ascribe some of these to the cerebellar lesion and in some cases to a lesion within certain parts of the cerebellum (Fig. 193–21).

ANATOMY AND PHYSIOLOGY

Three key structures in cerebellar eye movement disorders are the vestibulocerebellum (flocculus, paraflocculus, nodulus, and uvula), the dorsal vermis, and the dentate nucleus (Table 193–4). The vestibulocerebellum receives input from the vestibular nuclei, the

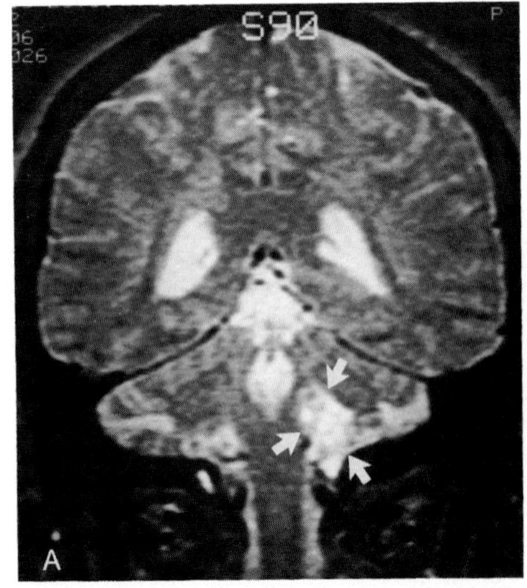

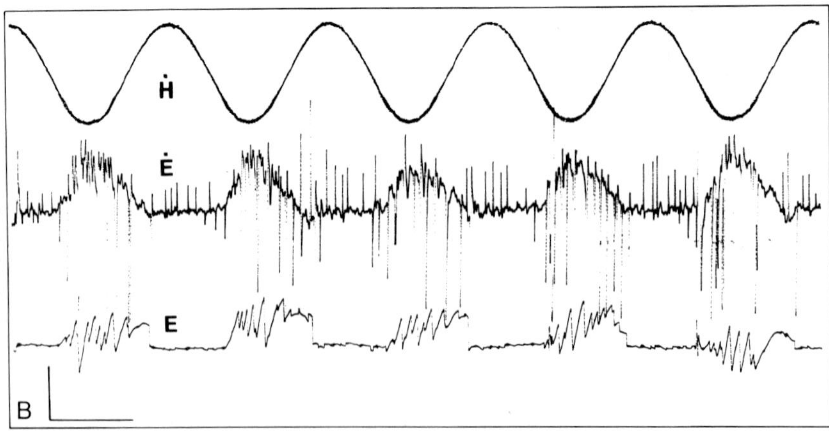

Figure 193–21. Cerebellar lesion with eye movement disorder. *A,* A low-grade glioma *(arrows)* arising in the left cerebellar flocculus is shown on T_2-weighted MRI. The patient presented with mild gait ataxia and was found to have no eye movement disorder apart from impairment of leftward smooth pursuit and leftward vestibuloocular reflex suppression. *B,* Oculographic recordings were made while the patient was being oscillated in a rotating chair at 0.1 Hz with a peak velocity of 50 degrees/sec and while the patient attempted to fixate the target light, which was moving with the chair. During rightward chair (i.e., head) motion, there was no eye movement; the rightward vestibuloocular reflex was totally suppressed. In contrast, during leftward chair motion, there was brisk left-beating nystagmus, indicating failure of leftward vestibuloocular reflex suppression. Upward deflections indicate rightward head and eye movement; downward deflections indicate leftward head and eye movement. (Ḣ, chair (head) velocity; Ė, eye velocity; E, eye position. Bars indicate 20 degrees, 50 degrees/sec, and 100 msec.)

Table 193–4. CEREBELLAR EYE MOVEMENT DISORDERS

Eye Movement Disorder	Structure Involved
Gaze-evoked horizontal nystagmus	Flocculus[179]
Downbeat nystagmus	Flocculus[121, 179]
Rebound nystagmus	Flocculus[149, 179]
Persistent positional nystagmus	(?) Nodulus[147]
Periodic alternating nystagmus	(?) Nodulus[133, 180]
Saccadic dysmetria	Fastigial nucleus[157–159]
Saccadic oscillations	(?)[157–160]
Ipsiversive pursuit paresis	Flocculus[179]
Ipsiversive VOR suppression paresis	Flocculus[179]
Pendular nystagmus	Dentate nucleus, superior peduncle[136, 139]
Skew deviation	(?)[69]
Contraversive lateropulsion	Lobulus simplex, crus I, vermal lobe V[62, 63]

perihypoglossal nuclei, and the inferior olivary nucleus. Its main output is back to the vestibular nuclei. Flocculus Purkinje cells are normally involved in the control of smooth pursuit eye movements and in the control of vestibuloocular reflex gain. Experimental lesions of the flocculus produce an eye movement syndrome resembling that found in humans with cerebellar ectopia due to Chiari malformation.[179] Experimental lesions of the nodulus can produce a form of periodic alternating nystagmus.[180] The dorsal vermis receives inputs from, and sends outputs via the fastigial nucleus to the PPRF. The dorsal vermis is normally involved in the control of saccadic eye movements, and experimental lesions of the vermis can produce saccadic dysmetria and macrosaccadic oscillations. The role of the dentate nucleus in eye movement control is not clear. However, lesions of the dentate or its output through the superior cerebellar peduncle can produce pendular nystagmus.

Lesions of the Thalamus-Subthalamus

Unilateral lesions originating in the thalamus produce disordered eye movements (Table 193–5). Whether or not these disorders are actually due to the lesion in the thalamus itself, or whether they are in fact due to involvement by extension or compression of the numerous oculomotor structures situated in the adjacent dorsal midbrain, is not clear. Normally the intralaminar nuclei of the thalamus are involved in saccade generation, and thalamic lesions do produce subtle, clinically inapparent disorders of saccadic control that are detectable only with computerized oculography.

Table 193–5. THALAMIC EYE MOVEMENT DISORDERS

Eye Movement Disorder	Structure Involved
Tonic contraversive gaze deviation ("wrong-way" eyes)	(?) Intralaminar nuclei[39]
Tonic downward gaze deviation	(?)[22, 30]
Esotropia	(?)[21, 22]

Lesions of the Basal Ganglia

Focal lesions of the basal ganglia do not produce clinically apparent eye movement disorders. In contrast, diffuse degenerative diseases of the basal ganglia, particularly Parkinson's disease and Huntington's disease in their advanced stages, do produce prominent disorders of eye movement.[181] Patients with advanced Parkinson's disease show several clinically detectable abnormalities that include small multistep hypometric saccades, square-wave jerks, poor smooth pursuit, limited head movements with refixation, and upgaze paresis. The preservation of saccadic velocity helps to differentiate advanced Parkinson's disease from Steele-Richardson-Olszewski disease, which is another, superficially similar disease that also involves the basal ganglia. The latter is characterized by a vertical saccadic palsy that occurs early in the disease and in fact gives it the descriptive name "Progressive Supranuclear Palsy." A saccadic palsy can also occur in Huntington's disease. In contrast to Steele-Richardson-Olszewski disease, in Huntington's disease the saccadic palsy occurs late in the course of the disease and tends to affect horizontal saccades before it affects vertical saccades.

Lesions of the Cerebral Hemispheres

The ability to fixate, refixate, and track moving visual targets is controlled by the cerebral hemispheres. Not surprisingly, therefore, cerebral hemisphere lesions frequently produce disordered eye movements, and many different disorders of saccadic and smooth pursuit eye movements can be found with computerized oculography in patients with focal cerebral lesions. However, with few exceptions, these disorders are either asymptomatic and too subtle to be clinically detectable or are only found in the presence of other obvious major neurologic abnormalities. Only clinically evident cerebral eye movement abnormalities are considered here.

ANATOMY AND PHYSIOLOGY

Several cortical areas are known to be involved in the preparation and initiation of saccadic movements, including the frontal lobe—particularly the frontal eye fields, and the parietal lobe—particularly the lateral intraparietal area (Table 193–6). These areas project to each other, and to the brain stem saccade generators in the pontine and midbrain reticular formations, the PPRF, and the riMLF, via the superior colliculi. Smooth pursuit and optokinetic eye movements are initiated in the posterior parietal cortex. From here smooth pursuit appears to follow a complicated pathway via the contralateral dorsolateral pontine nucleus, contralateral cere-

Table 193–6. CEREBRAL EYE MOVEMENT DISORDERS

Eye Movement Disorder	Structures Involved
Ipsiversive pursuit and optokinetic paresis	Parietal lobe[105]
Square wave jerks	(?)[154, 155]
Spasticity of conjugate gaze	(?)[42]
Tonic ipsiversive gaze deviation	(?)Frontal lobe[39]
Tonic contraversive gaze deviation ("wrong-way" eyes)	(?) Frontal lobe[39]
Epileptic gaze deviation and nystagmus	(?)[40, 41, 83, 151]
Oculomotor apraxia	Bilateral frontal and parietal lobes[57]
Loss of anti-saccades	Bilateral frontal lobe lesions[250]

bellar flocculus, and vestibular nucleus. The final pursuit pathway from the vestibular nucleus to the ocular motor nuclei may be the same as that taken by the vestibulo-ocular reflex.

Lesions of the Eye

Patients with severe bilateral visual loss have a jerk nystagmus with both horizontal and vertical components. The frequency, direction, and amplitude of the nystagmus varies in an aperiodic way.[182] The nystagmus is superimposed on an irregular wandering of gaze direction. Some patients with severe monocular visual loss develop drifting movements or even a regular pendular nystagmus of the blind eye.[141] The pendular nystagmus may have a vertical or elliptical waveform.

Lesions of the Ear

Lesions and diseases of the vestibular labyrinth may produce eye movement abnormalities and visual symptoms. Patients with bilateral vestibular loss frequently complain of vertical oscillopsia during head motion. Loss of all vestibular function can be verified clinically by the presence of compensatory saccades in response to rapid head turns during attempted fixation.[8] Aminoglycoside toxicity is the best recognized cause of a total vestibuloocular reflex palsy. These antibiotics can destroy all vestibular function with affecting cochlear function.[183] Occasionally, oscillopsia on head motion is caused by a total loss of vestibular function on only one side. The ocular tilt reaction that accompanies acute unilateral loss of vestibular function may produce vertical diplopia due to the skew deviation (ipsilesional hypotropia).

ANATOMIC DIAGNOSIS

Even if it is not possible after the clinical examination to make a precise anatomic diagnosis, it should be possible to decide the basic question of whether the eye movement disorder is of central or peripheral origin. The following rules may help to decide.

1. A monocular ophthalmoplegia is usually due to a peripheral lesion, but certain central lesions such as fascicular lesions of the oculomotor or abducens nerve and INO should be considered.
2. A conjugate binocular ophthalmoplegia that is direction or plane specific is usually due to a central lesion or disorder, but certain peripheral lesions such as myasthenia, Fisher's syndrome, and Graves' disease should be considered.
3. A conjugate binocular ophthalmoplegia selectively affecting a certain class of eye movements (e.g., saccades or pursuit) is of central origin. The exception to this rule is the loss of vestibuloocular reflexes due to bilateral peripheral vestibular disease.
4. A complex disconjugate binocular ophthalmoplegia could be due either to a central lesion (e.g., a horizontal or vertical "one-and-a-half" syndrome), or a peripheral lesion (e.g., myasthenia, multiple cranial nerve palsies).
5. A primary-position, or gaze-evoked involuntary eye movements in an upright patient without vertigo, severe visual loss, or ophthalmoplegia is always due to a central lesion or disorder, but the disorder may be entirely benign (e.g., square-wave jerks, voluntary nystagmus, congenital nystagmus).

ETIOLOGIC DIAGNOSIS

To make a pathologic-etiologic diagnosis it is necessary to consider: (1) the history—in particular the temporal profile of the neurologic deficit, its rate of evolution, progression, and regression; (2) the site of the lesion; (3) whether there are in fact multiple lesions; (4) the appearance of the lesion or lesions on neuroimaging. The following is a list of etiologic diagnoses worth considering in any patient with an eye movement disorder that is difficult to localize and proves to be "MR-negative."

Myasthenia. Myasthenia gravis should be considered in any patient with ophthalmoplegia, especially if there is also ptosis, weakness of orbicularis oculi or if there is nystagmus. Muscle fatigability can be a more reliable sign than a positive result on a Tensilon test. A negative Tensilon test, antibody test, or a negative result on peripheral muscle electromyography do not exclude the diagnosis of ocular myasthenia.[161]

Orbit Lesions. Orbit lesions, particularly blowout fractures and Graves' disease, should be considered in the differential diagnosis of ophthalmoplegia. Ocular movement is restricted by infiltration or entrapment of extraocular muscles or of other orbital tissues. Forced duction tests may help to make the diagnosis.

Fisher's Syndrome. A complex ophthalmoplegia may occur with any of the three variants of idiopathic demyelinating polyneuropathy: Fisher's syndrome,[101] chronic relapsing polyneuropathy,[184, 185] or Guillain-Barré syndrome.[186] In Fisher's syndrome, there is usually ataxia and areflexia and sometimes iridoplegia as well as ophthalmoplegia. It is still not certain whether the lesions responsible for Fisher's syndrome are supranuclear or infranuclear, or both.[186–188]

Drugs. Psychotropic and anticonvulsant drugs are the most common drugs that produce eye movement disorders and visual symptoms.[189] The eye movement disorders are usually a result of acute toxicity and are reversible, but the eye movement disorders produced by certain drugs such as lithium, phenothiazines, ethyl alcohol, and aminoglycosides can be permanent.

Gaze palsy: Baclofen,[190] barbiturates,[191] carbamazepine,[192] phenytoin,[193] tricyclics[194]
Internuclear ophthalmoplegia: Phenothiazines,[195] tricyclics[196]
Divergence palsy: Benzodiazepines[197]
Convergence spasm: Phenytoin[198]
Bilateral vestibular palsy: Aminoglycosides (permanent)[183]
Oculogyric crises: Carbamazepine,[199] lithium,[200] phenothiazines and butyrophenones,[201] metoclopramide[202]
Opsoclonus: Lithium,[203] L-tryptophan,[204] tricyclics,[205] phenytoin, benzodiazepine,[206] metyrosine[207]
Downbeat nystagmus: Carbamazepine,[208] ethyl alcohol (reversible[209] and irreversible[210]), lithium (permanent[211, 212]), phenytoin[213]
Primary position upbeat nystagmus: Tobacco[214]
Periodic alternating nystagmus: Phenytoin[215]
Pendular nystagmus: Toluene (irreversible[216])
Positional nystagmus: Ethyl alcohol[217]
Gaze-evoked nystagmus, impaired pursuit, and vestibuloocular reflex suppression: Marihuana,[218] ethyl alcohol,[219] sedatives, anticonvulsants[189]

Wernicke-Korsakoff Syndrome. Acute Wernicke's encephalopathy causes a complex symmetric or asymmetric horizontal and vertical ophthalmoplegia, with horizontal and vertical nystagmus.[26] If the ophthalmoplegia is obvious, then there will be obvious mental changes and ataxia and there may be characteristic changes on MRI.[219] Acute Wernicke's disease is a medical emergency requiring parenteral thiamine. Although the eye movement abnormalities resolve rapidly after the administration of thiamine, a delay in treatment may result in a severe permanent amnesic state (Korsakoff syndrome).

Paraneoplastic Syndrome. Patients with occult malignancies can present with a variety of nonmetastatic, paraneoplastic neurologic disorders. The primary tumor frequently arises in the lung, breast, or female reproductive tract. Paraneoplastic cerebellar degeneration can cause a variety of eye movement disorders such as saccadic oscillations including opsoclonus,[160] periodic alternating nystagmus,[220] and downbeat nystagmus.[221] Paraneoplastic encephalomyelitis can produce internuclear ophthalmoplegia[222] and gaze palsies.[223] Since the primary tumor is often undetectable radiologically, antibody tests may have an important role in diagnosis.[224, 225]

Chronic Meningitis. Chronic meningitis[226] due to tuberculosis[227] or cryptococcosis,[228] boriellosis,[229] cysticercosis,[230] sarcoidosis,[231] or cancer[232, 233] can cause bilateral ophthalmoplegia due to multiple cranial nerve palsies.

Whipple's Disease. Whipple's disease of the central nervous system can at first produce a vertical saccadic palsy and then later a global saccadic palsy,[234, 235] as well as a horizontal disjunctive pendular nystagmus that has been called "oculomasticatory myorhythmia."[236]

Steele-Richardson-Olszewski Disease. Patients with Steele-Richardson-Olszewski disease frequently present with visual symptoms due to a vertical saccadic palsy. Vertical vestibuloocular reflexes are typically preserved and lend the disease its alternative descriptive name "Progressive Supranuclear Palsy."[237] Eventually horizontal saccades and smooth pursuit are also disordered.[238] The ocular palsy combined with profound axial, particularly nuchal, rigidity produce a major visual disability as well as a characteristic appearance.[91]

Huntington's Disease. A horizontal saccadic palsy can be an early feature of Huntington's disease, before dementia and chorea become obvious. Later there may be a global saccadic palsy.[52, 239]

Hereditary Metabolic Diseases. Several groups of inherited metabolic diseases can present with eye movement disorders.

Mitochondrial encephalomyopathy: Involvement of the oculomotor system in mitochondrial disorders can produce chronic progressive external ophthalmoplegia due to extraocular myopathy, such as in the Kearns-Sayre syndrome[240] or see-saw nystagmus in adult Leigh's disease.[241]
Lipidoses: Niemann-Pick disease[92] and Tay-Sachs disease[242] produce a vertical saccadic palsy; Gaucher's disease[53] and DAF syndrome[243] produce a horizontal gaze palsy.
Bassen-Kornzweig disease: In abetalipoproteinemia, there may be a progressive ophthalmoplegia that may resemble bilateral wall-eyed internuclear ophthalmoplegia, bilateral ptosis, or signs of primary aberrant oculomotor nerve regeneration. It is not known whether the ophthalmoplegia is due to central or peripheral lesions.[244, 245]
Louis Bar disease: In ataxia-telangiectasia there is impairment of horizontal and vertical saccades, resulting in thrusting head movements of the type seen in congenital oculomotor apraxia. Some patients with ataxia-telangiectasia also have periodic alternating nystagmus or other cerebellar eye movement disorders. Patients with ataxia-telangiectasia have a widespread immunoparesis, and the serum levels of α fetoprotein are raised.[59] A similar syndrome with oculomotor apraxia but without immunologic changes, serologic changes, or telangiectasia has also been described.[246]

REFERENCES

1. Adams RD, Victor M: Principles of Neurology, 4th ed. New York, McGraw-Hill, 1989.
2. Caplan LR: The Effective Clinical Neurologist. Oxford, Blackwell 1990.
3. Leigh RJ, Zee DS: The Neurology of Eye Movements, 2nd ed. Philadelphia, FA Davis, 1991.

4. Miller NR: Walsh and Hoyt's Clinical Neuro-Ophthalmology, 4th ed, vol. 2. IV: The Ocular Motor System. Baltimore, Williams & Wilkins, 1985, pp 559–998.
5. Lessell S, van Dalen JTW (eds): Current Neuro-Ophthalmology, vol. 2. Chicago, Year Book, 1988.
6. Taylor D (ed): Pediatric Ophthalmology. Oxford, Blackwell, 1990, pp 595–616.
7. Daroff RB: Eye Movement Disorders. Dallas TX, Professional Information Library, 1988.
8. Huygen PLM: Computer simulation of eye movement disorders for teaching and training in ocular motor pathology. Adv Otorhinolaryngol 42:81–84, 1988. (Software available from Department of Otolaryngology, Academic Hospital, Nijmegen, POB 9101, 6500HB, Nijmegen, The Netherlands.)
9. Meienberg O, Muri R, Rabineau PA: Clinical and oculographic examinations of saccadic eye movements in the diagnosis of multiple sclerosis. Arch Neurol 43:438, 1986.
10. Halmagyi GM, Curthoys IS: A clinical sign of canal paresis. Arch Neurol 45:737, 1988.
11. Hain TC, Fetter M, Zee DS: Head-shaking nystagmus in patients with unilateral peripheral vestibular lesions. Am J Otolaryngol 8:36, 1987.
12. Baloh RW, Jacobson K, Honrubia V: Idiopathic bilateral vestibulopathy. Neurology 39:272, 1989.
13. Halmagyi GM, Gresty MA: Clinical sign of visual-vestibular interaction. J Neurol Neurosurg Psychiatry 42:934, 1979.
14. Brandt T, Dieterich M: Pathological eye-head coordination in roll: Tonic ocular tilt reaction in mesencephalic and medullary lesions. Brain 110:649, 1987.
15. Donaldson D, Rosenberg NL: Infarction of abducens nerve fascicles as a cause of isolated sixth nerve palsy related to hypertension. Neurology 38:954, 1988.
16. Johnson LN, Hepler RS: Isolated abducens nerve paresis from intrapontine fascicular abducens nerve injury. Am J Ophthalmol 108:459, 1989.
17. Bronstein A, Morris J, DuBoulay G, et al: Abnormalities of horizontal gaze: Clinical, oculographic and magnetic resonance imaging findings. I: Abducens palsy. J Neurol Neurosurg Psychiatry 53:194, 1990.
18. Miller NR, Kiel SM, Green WR, et al: Unilateral Duane's retraction syndrome (type 1). Arch Ophthalmol 100:1468, 1982.
19. Raab EL: Clinical features of Duane's syndrome. J Pediatr Ophthamol Strabismus 23:64, 1986.
20. Masdeu JC, Brannegan G, Rosenburg A, et al: Pseudoabducens palsy with midbrain lesions. Ann Neurol 8:103, 1980.
21. Gomez CR, Gomez SM, Selhorst JB: Acute thalamic esotropia. Neurology 38:1759, 1988.
22. Hertle RW, Bienfang DC: Oculographic analysis of acute esotropia secondary to thalamic hemorrhage. J Clin Neuro Ophthalmol 10:21, 1990.
23. Curran RE: True and simulated divergence palsy as a precursor of benign sixth nerve palsy. Binocular Vision Q 4:125, 1989.
24. Newman NJ, Lessell S: Pupillary dilatation with monocular occlusion as a sign of non-organic oculomotor dysfunction. Am J Ophthalmol 108:461, 1989.
25. Griffin JF, Wray SH, Anderson DP: Misdiagnosis of spasm of the near reflex. Neurology 26:1018, 1976.
26. Victor M, Adams RD, Collins GH: The Wernicke-Korsakoff Syndrome and Related Neurologic Disorders due to Alcoholism and Malnutrition, 2nd ed. Philadelphia, FA Davis, 1989.
27. Cruysberg JRM, Mtanda AT, Duinkerke-Eerola KU, Huygen PLM: Congenital adduction palsy with synergistic divergence: A clinical and electro-oculographic study. Br J Ophthalmol 73:68, 1989.
28. Ksiazek S, Repka MX, Maguie A, et al: Divisional oculomotor nerve paresis caused by intrinsic brain stem disease. Ann Neurol 26:714–718, 1989.
29. Breen LA, Hopf HC, Farris BK, et al: Pupil-sparing oculomotor nerve palsy due to midbrain infarction. Arch Neurol 48:105, 1991.
30. Fisher CM: Some neuro-ophthalmological observations. J Neurol Neurosurg Psychiatry 30:383, 1967.
31. Wall M, Wray SH: The one-and-a-half syndrome—A unilateral disorder of the pontine tegmentum: A study of 20 cases and a review of the literature. Neurology 33:971, 1983.
32. Deleu D, Solheid C, Michotte A, et al: Dissociated ipsilateral horizontal gaze palsy in one-and-a-half syndrome. Neurology 38:1278, 1988.
33. Sharpe JA, Rosenberg MA, Hoyt WF, et al: Paralytic pontine exotropia: A sign of acute unilateral pontine gaze palsy and internuclear ophthalmoplegia. Neurology 24:1076, 1974.
34. Ranalli PJ, Sharpe JA: Vertical vestibulo-ocular reflex, smooth pursuit and eye-head tracking dysfunction in internuclear ophthalmoplegia. Brain 111:1299, 1988.
35. McGettrick P, Eustace P: The w.e.b.i.n.o. syndrome. Neuro-ophthalmology 5:109, 1985.
36. Atlas SW, Grossman RI, Savino P, et al: Internuclear ophthalmoplegia: MR-anatomic correlation. AJNR 8:243, 1987.
37. Mutschler V, Eber AM, Rumbach L, et al: Internuclear ophthalmoplegia: Clinical and topographic correlation using magnetic resonance imaging. Neuro-ophthalmology 10:319, 1990.
38. Alexander JA, Castillo M, Hoffman JC: Magnetic resonance findings in a patient with unilateral internuclear ophthalmoplegia: Neuroradiological-clinical correlation. J Clin Neuro Ophthalmol 11:58, 1991.
39. Tijssen CC: Horizontal conjugate eye deviation: A clinical and electrophysiologic study. Bull Soc Belge Ophthalmol 237:1989.
40. McLachlan RS: The significance of head and eye turning in seizures. Neurology 37:1617, 1987.
41. Wyllie E, Luders H, Morris HM, et al: The lateralizing significance of versive head and eye movements during epileptic seizures. Neurology 36:606, 1986.
42. Sullivan HC, Kaminski HJ, Maas EF, et al: Lateral deviation of the eyes on forced lid closure in patients with cerebral lesions. Arch Neurol 48:310, 1991.
43. Nishida T, Tychsen L, Corbett J: Resolution of saccadic palsy after treatment of brainstem metastasis. Arch Neurol 43:1196, 1986.
44. Kommerell G, Henn V, Bach M, et al: Unilateral lesion of the paramedian pontine reticular formation: Loss of rapid eye movements with preservation of vestibulo-ocular reflex and pursuit. Neuro-ophthalmology 7:93, 1987.
45. Pierrot-Deseilligny CH, Goasguen J: Isolated abducens nucleus damage due to histiocytosis. X:Brain 107:1019, 1984.
46. Bronstein A, Rudge P, Gresty MA, et al: Abnormalities of horizontal gaze: Clinical, oculographic and magnetic resonance imaging findings. II: Gaze palsy and internuclear ophthalmoplegia. J Neurol Neurosurg Psychiatry 53:200, 1990.
47. Zackon DH, Sharpe JA: Midbrain paresis of horizontal gaze. Ann Neurol 16:495, 1984.
48. Masdeu JC, Rosenberg M: Midbrain-diencephalic horizontal gaze paresis. J Clin Neuro Ophthalmol 7:227, 1987.
49. Baloh RW, Furman J, Yee RD: Eye movements in patients with absent voluntary horizontal gaze. Ann Neurol 17:283, 1985.
50. Hanson MR, Hamid MA, Tomsak RL, et al: Selective saccadic palsy caused by pontine lesions: Clinical physiological and pathological correlations. Ann Neurol 20:209, 1986.
51. Dominguez RO, Bronstein AM: Complete gaze palsy in pontine haemorrhage. J Neurol Neurosurg Psychiatry 51:150, 1988.
52. Collewijn H, Went LN, Tamminga EP, et al: Oculomotor defects in patients with Huntington's disease and their offspring. J Neurol Sci 86:307, 1988.
53. Winkelman MD, Banker BQ, Victor M, et al: Non-infantile neuronopathic Gaucher's disease: A clinicopathologic study. Neurology 33:994, 1983.
54. Bogousslavsky J, Regli F: Convergence and divergence synkinesis: A recovery pattern with benign pontine hematoma. Neuro-ophthalmology 4:219, 1984.
55. Brusa G, Meneghini S, Piccardo A, et al: Regressive pattern of horizontal gaze palsy. Neuro-ophthalmology 7:301, 1987.
56. Kuhn MJ, Clark HB, Morales A, et al: Group III Mobius syndrome: CT and MR findings. AJNR 11:903, 1990.
57. Pierrot-Deseilligny CH, Gauthier J-C, Loron P: Acquired ocular motor apraxia due to bilateral frontoparietal infarcts. Ann Neurol 23:199, 1988.
58. Borchert MS, Sadun AA, Sommers JD, et al: Congenital oculomotor apraxia: Findings with magnetic resonance imaging. J Clin Neuro Ophthalmol 7:104, 1987.
59. Stell R, Bronstein AM, Plant GT, et al: Ataxia telangiectasia: A reappraisal of the ocular motor features and their value in the diagnosis of atypical cases. Mov Disord 4:320, 1989.

60. Ebner R, Lopez L, Ochoa S, et al: Vertical ocular motor apraxia. Neurology 40:712, 1990.
61. Kommerell G, Hoyt WF: Lateropulsion of saccadic eye movements: Electro-oculographic studies in a patient with Wallenberg's syndrome. Arch Neurol 28:313, 1973.
62. Ranalli PJ, Sharpe JA: Contrapulsion of saccades and ipsilateral ataxia: A unilateral disorder of the rostral cerebellum. Ann Neurol 20:311, 1986.
63. Uno A, Mukuno K, Sekiya H, et al: Lateropulsion in Wallenberg's syndrome and contrapulsion in the proximal type of superior cerebellar artery syndrome. Neuro-ophthalmology 9:75, 1989.
64. Scott WE, Kraft SE: Classification and surgical treatment of superior oblique palsies. I: Unilateral superior oblique palsies. Paediatric Ophthalmology and Strabismus. Transactions of the New Orleans Academy of Ophthalmology. New York, Raven Press, 1986, pp 15–38.
65. Scott WE, Kraft SE: Classification and surgical treatment of superior oblique palsies. II: Bilateral superior oblique palsies. Paediatric Ophthalmology and Strabismus. Transactions of the New Orleans Academy of Ophthalmology. New York, Raven Press, 1986, pp 265–291.
66. Simonsz HJ, Kolling GH, Kaufmann H, et al: The length-tension diagrams of human oblique muscles in trochlear palsy and nystagmus sursuadductorius. Doc Ophthalmol 70:227, 1988.
67. Slavin ML, Potash SD, Rubin SE: Asymptomatic hyperdeviation in peripheral gaze. Ophthalmology 95:778, 1988.
68. Moster ML, Schatz NJ, Savino PJ, et al: Alternating skew deviation on lateral gaze (bilateral abducting hypertropia). Ann Neurol 23:190, 1988.
69. Keane JR: Alternating skew deviation: 47 patients. Neurology 35:725, 1985.
70. Halmagyi GM, Brandt T, Dieterich M, et al: Tonic contraversive ocular tilt reaction due to unilateral meso-diencephalic lesion. Neurology 40:1503, 1990.
71. Keane JR: Trochlear nerve palsies with brainstem lesions. J Clin Neuro Ophthalmol 6:242, 1986.
72. Guy JR, Friedman WF, Mickle JP: Bilateral trochlear nerve paresis in hydrocephalus. J Clin Neuro Ophthalmol 9:105, 1989.
73. Tachibana H, Mimura O, Shiomi M, et al: Bilateral trochlear nerve palsies from a brainstem hematoma. J Clin Neuro Ophthalmol 10:35, 1990.
74. Castro O, Johnson LN, Mamourian AC: Isolated inferior oblique paresis from brain stem infarction. Arch Neurol 47:235, 1990.
75. Pusateri TJ, Sedwick LA, Margo CE: Isolated inferior rectus muscle palsy from a solitary metastasis to the oculomotor nucleus. Arch Ophthalmol 105:675, 1987.
76. Dehane I, Marchau M, Vanhooren G: Nuclear oculomotor nerve paralysis. Neuro-ophthalmology 7:219, 1987.
77. Bell JA, Fielder AR, Viney S: Congenital double elevator palsy in identical twins. J Clin Neuro Ophthalmol 10:32, 1990.
78. Ford CS, Schwartze GM, Weaver RG, et al: Monocular elevation paresis caused by an ipsilateral lesion. Arch Neurol 34:1264, 1984.
79. Dieterich M, Brandt TH, Fries W: Otolith function in man: Results from a case of otolith Tullio phenomenon. Brain 112:1377, 1989.
80. Curthoys IS, Dai MJ, Halmagyi GM: Human ocular torsional position before and after unilateral vestibular neurectomy. Exp Brain Res 85:218, 1991.
81. Halmagyi GM, Gresty MA, Gibson WPR: Ocular tilt reaction with peripheral vestibular lesion. Ann Neurol 6:80, 1979.
82. Leigh RJ, Foley JM, Remler BF, et al: Oculogyric crisis: A syndrome of thought disorder and ocular deviation. Ann Neurol 22:13, 1987.
83. Kaplan PW, Lesser RP: Vertical and horizontal epileptic gaze deviation and nystagmus. Neurology 39:1391, 1989.
84. Buttner-Ennever J, Buttner U, Cohen B, et al: Vertical gaze paralysis and the rostral interstitial nucleus of the medial longitudinal fasciculus. Brain 105:125, 1982.
85. Bogousslavsky J, Miklossy J, Regli F, et al: Vertical gaze palsy and selective unilateral infarction of the rostral interstitial nucleus of the medial longitudinal fasciculus. J Neurol Neurosurg Psychiatry 53:67, 1990.
86. Pierrot-Deseilligny P, Chain F, Gray F, et al: Parinaud's syndrome: Electro-oculographic and anatomical analyses of six vascular cases with deductions about vertical gaze organization in the premotor structures. Brain 105:667, 1982.
87. Baloh RW, Furman JM, Yee RD: Dorsal midbrain syndrome: Clinical and oculographic findings. Neurology 35:54, 1986.
88. Keane JR: The pretectal syndrome: 206 patients. Neurology 40:684, 1990.
89. Buttner-Ennever JA, Acheson JF, Buttner U, et al: Ptosis and supranuclear downgaze palsy. Neurology 39:385, 1989.
90. Heide W, Fahle M, Koenig E, et al: Impairment of vertical motion detection and downgaze palsy due to rostral midbrain infarction. J Neurol 237:432, 1990.
91. Kristensen MO: Progressive supranuclear palsy—20 years later. Acta Neurol Scand 71:177, 1985.
92. Fink JK, Filling-Katz MR, Sokol J, et al: Clinical spectrum of Niemann-Pick disease type C. Neurology 39:1040, 1989.
93. Trojanowski JQ, Wray SH: Vertical gaze ophthalmoplegia: Selective paralysis of downward gaze. Neurology 30:605, 1980.
94. Jacobs L, Heffner RR, Newman RP: Selective paralysis of downward gaze caused by bilateral lesions of the mesencephalic periaqueductal gray matter. Neurology 35:516, 1985.
95. Thames PB, Trobe JD, Ballinger WE: Upgaze paralysis caused by lesion of the periaqueductal gray matter. Arch Neurol 41:437, 1984.
96. Bogousslavsky J, Miklossy J, Deruaz JP, et al: Unilateral left paramedian infarction of the thalamus and midbrain: A clinicopathological study. J Neurol Neurosurg Psychiatry 49:686, 1986.
97. Ranalli PJ, Sharpe JA, Fletcher WA: Palsy of upward and downward saccadic, pursuit and vestibular movements with unilateral midbrain lesion: Pathophysiologic correlation. Neurology 38:114, 1988.
98. Tychsen L, Imes RK, Hoyt WF: Bilateral congenital restriction of upward eye movement. Arch Neurol 43:95, 1986.
99. Bogousslavsky J, Regli F: Upgaze palsy and monocular paresis of downward gaze from ipsilateral thalamo-mesencephalic infarction: A vertical one-and-a-half syndrome. J Neurol 231:43, 1984.
100. Deleu D, Buisseret T, Ebinger G: Vertical one-and-a-half syndrome: Supranuclear downgaze paralysis with monocular elevation palsy. Arch Neurol 46:1361, 1989.
101. Keane JR: Acute bilateral ophthalmoplegia: 60 cases. Neurology 36:279, 1986.
102. Zasorin NL, Yee RD, Baloh RW: Eye-movement abnormalities in ophthalmoplegia, ataxia, and areflexia (Fisher's syndrome). Arch Ophthalmol 103:55, 1985.
103. Zackon DH, Sharpe JA: Smooth pursuit in senescence. Acta Otolaryngol 1987;104:290–297.
104. Sharpe JA, Lo AW, Rabinovitch HE: Control of saccadic and smooth pursuit systems after cerebral hemidecortication. Brain 102:387–403, 1979.
105. Morrow M, Sharpe JA: Cerebral hemispheric localization of smooth pursuit asymmetry. Neurology 40:284, 1990.
106. Brigell M, Babikian V, Goodwin JA: Hypometric saccades and low-gain smooth pursuit from a thalamic hemorrhage. Ann Neurol 15:555, 1984.
107. Waespe W, Martin P: Pursuit eye movements in a patient with a lesion involving the vestibular nuclear complex. Neuro-ophthalmology 7:195, 1987.
108. Waespe W, Wichmann W: Oculomotor disturbances during visual-vestibular interaction in Wallenberg's lateral medullary syndrome verified by magnetic resonance imaging. Brain 113:821, 1990.
109. Johnston JL, Sharpe JA, Morrow MJ: Paresis of contralateral smooth pursuit and normal vestibular smooth eye movements after unilateral brain stem lesions. Ann Neurol 31:495, 1992.
110. Thier P, Bachor A, Faiss J, et al: Selective impairment of smooth-pursuit eye movements due to an ischemic lesion of the basal pons. Ann Neurol 29:442, 1991.
111. Kelly BJ, Rosenberg ML, Zee DS, et al: Unilateral pursuit-induced congenital nystagmus. Neurology 39:414, 1989.
112. Chambers BR, Gresty MA: The relationship between disordered pursuit and vestibulo-ocular reflex suppression. J Neurol Neurosurg Psychiatry 46:61, 1983.
113. Zee DS, Yee RD, Cogan DG, et al: Ocular motor abnormalities in hereditary cerebellar ataxia. Brain 99:207, 1976.
114. Baloh RW, Jenkins HA, Honrubia V, et al: Visual-vestibular interaction in cerebellar atrophy. Neurology 29:116, 1979.

115. Halmagyi GM, Henderson CJ: Visual symptoms of vestibular disease. Aust N Z J Ophthalmol 16:177, 1988.
116. Bronstein AM, Hood JD: Oscillopsia of peripheral vestibular origin: Central and cervical compensatory mechanisms. Acta Otolaryngol 104:307, 1987.
117. Ochs AL, Stark L, Hoyt WF, et al: Opposed adducting saccades in convergence-retraction nystagmus: A patient with the sylvian aqueduct syndrome. Brain 102:497, 1979.
118. Oohira A, Goto K, Ozawa T: Convergence nystagmus: An observation of horizontal and vertical components. Neuro-ophthalmology 6:313, 1986.
119. Oliva A, Rosenberg M: Convergence-evoked nystagmus. Neurology 40:161, 1990.
120. Shults WT, Stark L, Hoyt WF, et al: Normal saccadic structure of voluntary nystagmus. Arch Ophthalmol 95:1399, 1977.
121. Halmagyi GM, Rudge P, Gresty MA, et al: Downbeating nystagmus: A review of 62 cases. Arch Neurol 40:777, 1983.
122. Gresty M, Barratt H, Rudge P, Page N: Analysis of downbeat nystagmus: Otolithic vs semicircular canal influences. Arch Neurol 43:52, 1986.
123. Yee RD, Baloh RW, Honrubia V: Episodic vertical oscillopsia and downbeating nystagmus in a Chiari malformation. Arch Ophthalmol 102:723, 1984.
124. Keane JR, Itabashi HH: Upbeat nystagmus: Clinicopathogic study of two patients. Neurology 37:491, 1987.
125. Hirose G, Kawada J, Tsukada K, et al: Upbeat nystagmus: Clinicopathological and pathophysiological considerations. J Neurol Sci 105:159, 1991.
126. Ranalli PJ, Sharpe JA: Upbeat nystagmus and the ventral tegmental pathway of the upward vestibulo-ocular reflex. Neurology 38:1329, 1988.
127. Morrow M, Sharpe JA: Torsional nystagmus in the lateral medullary syndrome. Ann Neurol 24:390, 1988.
128. Thrush DC, Foster JB: An analysis of nystagmus in 100 consecutive patients with communicating syringomyelia. J Neurol Sci 20:381, 1973.
129. Lopez L, Bronstein AM, Gresty MA: Torsional nystagmus: A neuro-otological and MRI study of 35 cases. Brain (in press)
130. Halmagyi GM, Hoyt WF: See-saw nystagmus due to a unilateral meso-diencephalic lesion. J Clin Neuro Ophthalmol 11:79, 1991.
131. Kanter DS, Ruff RL, Leigh RJ, et al: Seesaw nystagmus and brain stem infarction. Neuro-ophthalmology 7:279, 1987.
132. Dehaene I, Zandijcke M: See-saw jerk nystagmus. Neuro-ophthalmology 4:261, 1984.
133. Furman JMR, Wall III C, Pang D: Vestibular function in periodic alternating nystagmus. Brain 113:1425, 1990.
134. Gresty MA, Ell JJ, Findley LJ: Acquired pendular nystagmus: Its characteristics, localizing value and pathophysiology. J Neurol Neurosurg Psychiatry 45:431, 1982.
135. Nakada T, Kwee IL: Oculopalatal myoclonus. Brain 109:431, 1086.
136. Cordonnier M, Goldman S, Zegers de Beyl D, et al: Reversible acquired pendular nystagmus after brain stem haemorrhage. Neuro-ophthalmology 5:47, 1985.
137. Keane JR: Acute vertical ocular myoclonus. Neurology 36:86, 1986.
138. Zarranz JJ, Fontan A, Forcadas I: MR imaging of presumed olivary hypertrophy in palatal myoclonus. AJNR 11:1164, 1990.
139. Revel MP, Mann M, Brugieres P, et al: MR appearance of hypertrophic olivary degeneration after contralateral cerebellar hemorrhage. AJNR 12:71, 1991.
140. Gottlob I, Zubcov A, Catalano RA, et al: Signs distinguishing spasmus nutans (with and without central nervous system lesions) from infantile nystagmus. Ophthalmology 97:1166, 1990.
141. Yee RD, Jelks GW, Baloh RW, et al: Uniocular nystagmus in monocular visual loss. Ophthalmology 86:511, 1979.
142. Mossman SS, Bronstein AM, Gresty MA, et al: Convergence nystagmus with Arnold-Chiari malformation. Arch Neurol 47:357, 1990.
143. Baloh RW, Honrubia V: Clinical Neurophysiology of the Vestibular System, 2nd ed. Philadelphia, FA Davis, 1990.
144. Zee DS: Ophthalmoscopy in examination of patients with vestibular disorders. Ann Neurol 3:373, 1978.
145. Dohlman GF: Further remarks on the mechanism producing symptoms in Menière's disease. J Otolaryngol 9:285, 1980.
146. Parnes LS, McClure JA: Rotatory recovery nystagmus: An important localizing sign in endolymphatic hydrops. J Otolaryngol 19:96, 1990.
147. Brandt TH: Positional and positioning vertigo and nystagmus. J Neurol Sci 95:3, 1990.
148. Dell'Osso LF: Nystagmus, saccadic intrusions/oscillations and oscillopsia. *In* Lessell S, van Dalen JTW (eds): Current Neuro-ophthalmology, vol. 2. Chicago, Year Book Medical Publishers, 1988, pp 147–182.
149. Bondar RL, Sharpe JA, Lewis AJ: Rebound nystagmus in olivocerebellar atrophy: A clinico-pathological correlation. Ann Neurol 15:474, 1984.
150. Cannon SC, Robinson DA: Loss of the neural integrator of the oculomotor system from brain stem lesions in the monkey. J Neurophysiol 57:1383, 1987.
151. Tusa R, Kaplan PW, Hain TC, et al: Ipsiversive eye deviation and epileptic nystagmus. Neurology 40:662, 1990.
152. Hotson JR: Convergence-initiated voluntary flutter: A normal intrinsic capability in man. Brain Res 294:299, 1984.
153. Shallo-Hoffman J, Sendler B, Muhlendyck H: Normal square wave jerks in differing age groups. Invest Ophthalmol Vis Sci 31:1649, 1990.
154. Sharpe JA, Herishanu YO, White OB: Cerebral square wave jerks. Neurology 32:57, 1982.
155. Fukazawa T, Tashiro K, Hamada T, Kase M: Multisystem degeneration: Drugs and square wave jerks. Neurology 36:1230, 1986.
156. Hain TC, Zee DS, Mordes M: Blink-induced saccadic oscillations. Ann Neurol 19:299, 1986.
157. Selhorst JB, Stark L, Ochs AL, Hoyt WF: Disorders in cerebellar ocular motor control. II: Macrosaccadic oscillation: An oculographic, control system and clinico-anatomical analysis. Brain 99:509, 1976.
158. Bergenius J: Saccade abnormalities in patients with ocular flutter. Acta Otolaryngol 102:228, 1986.
159. Zee DS, Robinson DA: A hypothetical explanation of saccadic oscillations. Ann Neurol 5:405, 1979.
160. Anderson NE, Budde-Steffen, Rosenblum MK, et al: Opsoclonus, myoclonus, ataxia and encephalopathy in adults with cancer: A distinct paraneoplastic syndrome. Medicine 67:100, 1988.
161. Schmidt D: Myasthenia gravis. *In* Lessell S, van Dalen JTW (eds): Current Neuro-ophthalmology, vol. 2. Chicago, Year Book Medical Publishers, 1988, pp 257–291.
162. Daroff RB: The office Tensilon test for myasthenia gravis. Arch Neurol 43:843, 1986.
163. Daroff RB: Lancaster test with Tensilon for myasthenia. Arch Neurol 44:47, 1987.
164. Seybold M: The office Tensilon test for ocular myasthenia gravis. Arch Neurol 43:842, 1986.
165. Younge BR, Bartley GB: Lancaster test with Tensilon for myasthenia. Arch Neurol 44:472, 1987.
166. Rosenberg ML: Spasm of the near reflex mimicking myasthenia gravis. J Clin Neuro-ophthalmol 6:106, 1986.
167. Oohira A, Goto K, Sato Y, et al: Saccades of supernormal velocity: Adaptive response to ophthalmoplegia in a patient with myasthenia gravis. Neuro-ophthalmology 7:203, 1987.
168. Yee RD, Whitcup SM, Williams IM, et al: Saccadic eye movements in myasthenia gravis. Ophthalmology 94:219, 1987.
169. Shults WT, Hoyt WF, Behrens M, et al: Ocular neuromyotonia: A clinical description of six patients. Arch Ophthalmol 104:1028, 1986.
170. Lessell S, Lessell I, Rizzo JF: Ocular neuromyotonia after radiation therapy. Am J Ophthalmol 102:766, 1986.
171. Salmon JF, Steven P, Abrahamson MJ: Ocular neuromyotonia. Neuro-ophthalmology 8:181, 1988.
172. Hoyt WF, Keane JR: Superior oblique myokymia. Report and discussion on five cases of benign intermittent uniocular microtremor. Arch Ophthalmol 84:461, 1970.
173. Erme M, Henn V: Familial Duane's syndrome with synkinetic jaw movements. Neuro-ophthalmology 7:211, 1987.
174. McGovern ST, Crompton JL, Ingham PN: Trigemino-abducens synkinesis: an unusual case of aberrant regeneration. Aust N Z J Ophthamol 14:275, 1986.
175. Nelson SK, Kline LB: Acquired trigemino-abducens synkinesis. J Clin Neuro Ophthalmol 10:111, 1990.

176. Sibony PA, Lessell S, Gittinger JW: Acquired oculomotor synkinesis. Surv Ophthalmol 28:382, 1984.
177. Bogousslavsky J, Meienberg O: Eye-movement disorders in brain stem and cerebellar stroke. Arch Neurol 44:141, 1987.
178. Ropper AH: Illusion of tilting of the visual environment: A report of five cases. J Clin Neuro Ophthalmol 3:147, 1983.
179. Zee DS, Yamazaki A, Butler PH, et al: Effects of ablation of flocculus and paraflocculus on eye movements in primate. J Neurophysiol 46:878, 1981.
180. Cohen B, Hedwig D, Raphan T: Baclofen and velocity storage: A model of the effects of the drug in the vestibulo-ocular reflex in the rhesus monkey. J Physiol (Lond) 393:703, 1987.
181. Kennard C, Lueck CJ: Oculomotor abnormalities in diseases of the basal ganglia. Rev Neurol (Paris) 145:587, 1989.
182. Leigh RJ, Zee DS: Eye movements of the blind. Invest Ophthalmol Vis Sci 19:328, 1980.
183. Proctor LR, Glackin RN, Smith CR: A test battery for detection of vestibular toxicity in man. *In* Lerner SA, Metz GJ, Hawkins JE (eds): Aminoglycoside Ototoxicity. Boston, Little Brown, 1981, pp 285–294.
184. Donaghy M, Earl CJ: Ocular palsy preceding chronic relapsing polyneuropathy by several weeks. Ann Neurol 17:49, 1985.
185. Chalmers AC, Miller RG: Chronic inflammatory polyradiculoneuropathy with ophthalmoplegia. J Clin Neuro Ophthalmol 6:166, 1986.
186. Dehaene I, Martin K, Geens K, et al: Guillain-Barré syndrome with ophthalmoplegia: Clinicopathologic study of the central and peripheral nervous systems including oculomotor nerves. Neurology 36:851, 1986.
187. Ropper A: Absence of CNS lesions in autopsied patients with Miller Fisher syndrome. Arch Neurol 42:15, 1985.
188. Panegyres PK, Mastaglia FL: Guillain-Barré syndrome with involvement of the central and autonomic nervous system. Med J Aust 150:655, 1989.
189. Remler BF, Leigh RJ, Osoria I, et al: The characteristics and mechanisms of visual disturbance associated with anticonvulsant therapy. Neurology 40:791, 1990.
190. Paulson GW: Overdose of lioresal. Neurology 26:1105, 1976.
191. Edis RH, Mastaglia FL: Vertical gaze palsy in barbiturate intoxication. Br Med J 1:144, 1977.
192. Mullaly WJ: Carbamazepine-induced ophthalmoplegia. Arch Neurol 39:64, 1982.
193. Fredericks CA, Gianotta SL, Sadun AA: Dilantin-induced long-term bilateral total external ophthalmoplegia. J Clin Neuro Ophthalmol 6:22, 1986.
194. Pulst S-M, Lombroso CT: External ophthalmoplegia and alpha spindle coma in imipramine overdose. Ann Neurol 14:587, 1983.
195. Cook FF, Davis RG, Russo LS: Internuclear ophthalmoplegia caused by phenothiazine intoxication. Arch Neurol 38:465, 1981.
196. Barret LG, Vincent FM, Arsac PL, et al: Internuclear ophthalmoplegia in patients with toxic coma: Frequency, prognostic value, diagnostic significance. J Toxicol Clin Toxicol 20:373, 1983.
197. Arai M, Fujii S: Divergence paralysis associated with ingestion of diazepam. J Neurol 237:45, 1990.
198. Guiloff RJ, Whiteley A, Kelly R: Organic convergence spasm. Acta Neurol Scand 61:252, 1980.
199. Berchou RC: Carbamazepine induced oculogyric crises. Arch Neurol 36:522, 1979.
200. Sandyk R: Oculogyric crisis induced by lithium carbonate. Eur Neurol 23:92, 1984.
201. FitzGerald PM, Jankovic J: Tardive oculogyric crises. Neurology 39:1434, 1989.
202. Edwards M, Koo MWL, Tse R-KK: Oculogyric crisis after metoclopramide. Optom Vis Sci 66:179, 1989.
203. Cohen WJ, Cohen NH: Lithium carbonate, haloperidol and irreversible brain damage. JAMA 230:1283, 1974.
204. Baloh RW, Dietz J, Spooner JW: Myoclonus and ocular oscillations induced by L-tryptophan. Ann Neurol 11:95, 1982.
205. Au WJ, Keltner JL: Opsoclonus with amitryptiline overdose. Ann Neurol 6:87, 1979.
206. Dehaene I, Van Vleymen B: Opsoclonus induced by phenytoin and diazepam. Ann Neurol 21:216, 1987.
207. Tychsen L, Sitaram N: Catecholamine depletion produces irrepressible saccadic eye movements in humans. Ann Neurol 25:444, 1989.
208. Chrousos GA, Cowdry R, Schuelein M, et al: Two cases of downbeat nystagmus and oscillopsia associated with carbamazapine. Am J Ophthalmol 103:221, 1987.
209. Rosenberg ML: Reversible downbeat nystagmus secondary to excessive alcohol intake. J Clin Neuro Ophthalmol 7:23, 1987.
210. Zasorin NI, Baloh RW: Downbeat nystagmus with alcoholic cerebellar degeneration. Arch Neurol 41:1301, 1984.
211. Corbett JJ, Jacobson DM, Thompson HS, et al: Downbeat nystagmus and other ocular motor defects caused by lithium toxicity. Neurology 39:481, 1989.
212. Halmagyi GM, Lessell I, Curthoys IS, et al: Lithium-induced downbeating nystagmus. Am J Ophthalmol 107:664, 1989.
213. Berger JR, Kovacs AG: Downbeat nystagmus with phenytoin. J Clin Neuro Ophthalmol 2:209, 1982.
214. Sibony PA, Evinger C, Manning KA: Tobacco-induced primary position upbeat nystagmus. Ann Neurol 21:53, 1987.
215. Campbell WW: Periodic alternating nystagmus in phenytoin intoxication. Arch Neurol 37:178, 1980.
216. Maas EF, Ashe J, Spiegel P, et al: Acquired pendular nystagmus in toluene addiction. Neurology 41:282, 1991.
217. Money KE, Myles WS: Heavy water nystagmus and the effects of alcohol. Nature 247:404, 1974.
218. Baloh RW, Sharma S, Moskowitz H, et al: Effect of alcohol and marijuana on eye movements. Aviat Space Environ Med 50:18, 1979.
219. Victor M: MR in the diagnosis of Wernicke-Korsakoff syndrome. AJNR 11:895, 1990.
220. Halperin JJ, Richardson EP, Ellis J, et al: Paraneoplastic encephalomyelitis and neuropathy. Arch Neurol 38:773, 1981.
221. Guy JR, Schatz NJ: Paraneoplastic downbeating nystagmus. J Clin Neuro Ophthalmol 8:269, 1988.
222. Boghen D, Sebag M, Michaud J: Paraneoplastic optic neuritis and encephalomyelitis. Arch Neurol 45:353, 1988.
223. Pillay N, Gilbert JJ, Ebers GC, et al: Internuclear ophthalmoplegia and optic neuritis: Paraneoplastic effects of bronchial carcinoma. Neurology 34:788, 1984.
224. Dalmau J, Furneaux HM, Gralla RJ, et al: Detection of anti-HU antibody in the serum of patients with small cell lung cancer—Quantitative Western blot analysis. Ann Neurol 27:544, 1990.
225. Luque FA, Furneaux HM, Ferzinger R, et al: Anti Ri: An antibody associated with paraneoplastic opsoclonus and breast cancer. Ann Neurol 29:241, 1991.
226. Swartz MN: Chronic meningitis—Many causes to consider. N Engl J Med 317:957, 1987.
227. Traub M, Colchester ACF, Kingsley DPE, et al: Tuberculosis of the central nervous system. Q J Med 53:81, 1984.
228. Tan CT: Intracranial hypertension causing visual failure in cryptococcal meningitis. J Neurol Neurosurg Psychiatry 51:911, 1988.
229. Finkel MF: Lyme disease and its neurologic complications. Arch Neurol 45:99, 1988.
230. Keane JR: Neuro-ophthalmic signs and symptoms of cysticercosis. Arch Ophthalmol 100:1445, 1982.
231. Stern BJ, Krumholz A, Johns C, et al: Sarcoidosis and its neurological manifestations. Arch Neurol 42:909, 1985.
232. Olson ME, Chrnik NL, Posner JB: Infiltration of the leptomeninges by systemic cancer. Arch Neurol 30:122, 1974.
233. Wasserstrom WR, Glass JP, Posner JB: Diagnosis and treatment of leptomeningeal metastases from solid tumors: Experience with 90 patients. Cancer 49:759, 1982.
234. Finelli PF, McEntee WJ, Lessell S: Whipple's disease with predominantly neuro-ophthalmic manifestations. Ann Neurol 1:247, 1977.
235. Adams M, Rhyner PA, Day J, et al: Whipple's disease confined to the central nervous system. Ann Neurol 21:104, 1987.
236. Schwartz MA, Selhorst JB, Ochs AL, et al: Oculomasticatory myorhythmia: A unique movement disorder occurring in Whipple's disease. Ann Neurol 20:677, 1986.
237. Troost BT, Daroff RB: The ocular motor defects in progressive supranuclear palsy. Ann Neurol 1:397, 1977.
238. Pierrot-Deseilligny CH, Rivaud S, Pillon B, et al: Lateral visually guided saccades in progressive supranuclear palsy. Brain 112:471, 1989.
239. Leigh RJ, Parhad IM, Clark AW, et al: Brain stem findings in Huntington's disease: Possible mechanism for slow vertical saccades. J Neurol Sci 71:247, 1985.

240. Moraes CT, Di Mauro S, Zeviani M, et al: Mitochondrial DNA deletions in progressive external ophthalmoplegia and Kearns-Sayre syndrome. N Engl J Med 320:1293, 1989.
241. Halmagyi GM, Pamphlett R, Curthoys IS: Seesaw nystagmus and ocular tilt reaction due to adult Leigh's disease. Neuro-ophthalmology 12:1, 1992.
242. Jampel RS, Quaglia ND: Eye movements in Tay-Sachs disease. Neurology 14:1013, 1964.
243. Cogan DG, Chu FC, Bachman DM, et al: The DAF syndrome. Neuro-ophthalmology 2:7, 1981.
244. Yee RD, Cogan DG, Zee DS: Ophthalmoplegia and dissociated nystagmus in abetalipoproteinemia. Arch Ophthalmol 94:571, 1976.
245. Cohen DA, Bosley TM, Savino PJ, et al: Primary aberrant oculomotor nerve regeneration with abetalipoproteinemia. Arch Neurol 42:821, 1985.
246. Aicardi J, Barbosa C, Andermann E, et al: Ataxia-ocular motor apraxia: A syndrome mimicking ataxia telangiectasia. Ann Neurol 24:497, 1988.
247. Halmagyi GM, Evans WA, Hallinan JM: Failure of downward gaze: The site and nature of the lesion. Arch Neurol 38:22, 1978.
248. Caplan L: "Top of the basilar syndrome." Neurology 30:72, 1980.
249. Halmagyi GM, Gresty MA, Leech J: Reversed optokinetic nystagmus (OKN): Mechanism and clinical significance. Ann Neurol 7:429, 1979.
250. Currie J, Ramsden B, McArthur C: Validation of a clinical anti-saccadic eye movement test in the assessment of dementia. Arch Neurol 48:644, 1991.

Chapter 194

Third-, Fourth-, and Sixth-Nerve Lesions and the Cavernous Sinus

NANCY J. NEWMAN

ANATOMY

The final common pathway for oculomotor control consists of the three pairs of ocular motor nerves and the muscles that they innervate. The nerves originate in paired nuclei within the midbrain and pons, and their axons course as fascicles through the brain stem parenchyma, run freely for variable distances within the subarachnoid space, pass through the cavernous sinus, and enter the orbit to supply the extraocular muscles.

The oculomotor nerve (third cranial nerve) supplies motor innervation for the superior rectus, medial rectus, inferior rectus, inferior oblique and levator palpebrae superioris muscles and also parasympathetic input to the pupillary constrictor and ciliary muscles. Cell bodies reside in the midbrain in a nuclear mass straddling the vertical midline (Fig. 194–1).[1–4] Each target muscle has a subnucleus devoted exclusively to its function. Most rostral and dorsal are the visceral nuclei (Edinger-Westphal nuclei and adjacent structures) that supply parasympathetic innervation to the pupillary sphincters and ciliary muscles via the ciliary ganglia.[5] Caudal and dorsal, the "caudal central nucleus" is a single midline structure that innervates the levator palpebrae superioris muscles, subserving upper lid elevation. The cell bodies in the superior rectus subnuclei send their axons directly across the midline to join the contralateral oculomotor fascicles.[6] The other subnuclei project ipsilaterally to their individual extraocular muscles.

The oculomotor fascicles refer to the portion of the nerve that travels through the brain stem parenchyma to exit ventrally. The fascicles pass through the substance of the red nuclei and the medial cerebral peduncles (Fig. 194–2). Upon leaving the brain stem, the nerve enters the subarachnoid space and courses forward and laterally between the posterior cerebral artery above and the superior cerebellar artery below (Fig. 194–3) to run briefly alongside the posterior communicating artery. At this level, the pupillary fibers are located dorsally and peripherally. The nerve then pierces the dura and enters the cavernous sinus (Fig. 194–4). Within the anterior aspect of the cavernous sinus, the third nerve divides so that two divisions of the oculomotor nerve pass through the superior orbital fissure and enter the orbit (Fig. 194–5). The superior division contains axons destined for the levator palpebrae superioris and superior rectus muscles. The inferior division carries the motor fibers to the medial rectus, inferior rectus, and inferior oblique muscles, as well as the preganglionic parasympathetic pupillomotor fibers to the ciliary ganglion.

The trochlear nerve (fourth cranial nerve) provides innervation to the superior oblique muscle only. Its nucleus is located in the midbrain, just beneath the cerebral aqueduct, caudal to the oculomotor nuclear complex (Fig. 194–6). The axons exit dorsally and cross within the anterior medullary velum that lies just caudal to the inferior colliculi. Thus, innervation to the superior oblique muscles is strictly contralateral. After decussation, the nerve runs forward in the subarachnoid space around the mesencephalon and cerebral peduncles, along the free edge of the tentorium, between the posterior cerebral and superior cerebellar arteries (Fig. 194–7; see also Fig. 194–3). It enters the cavernous

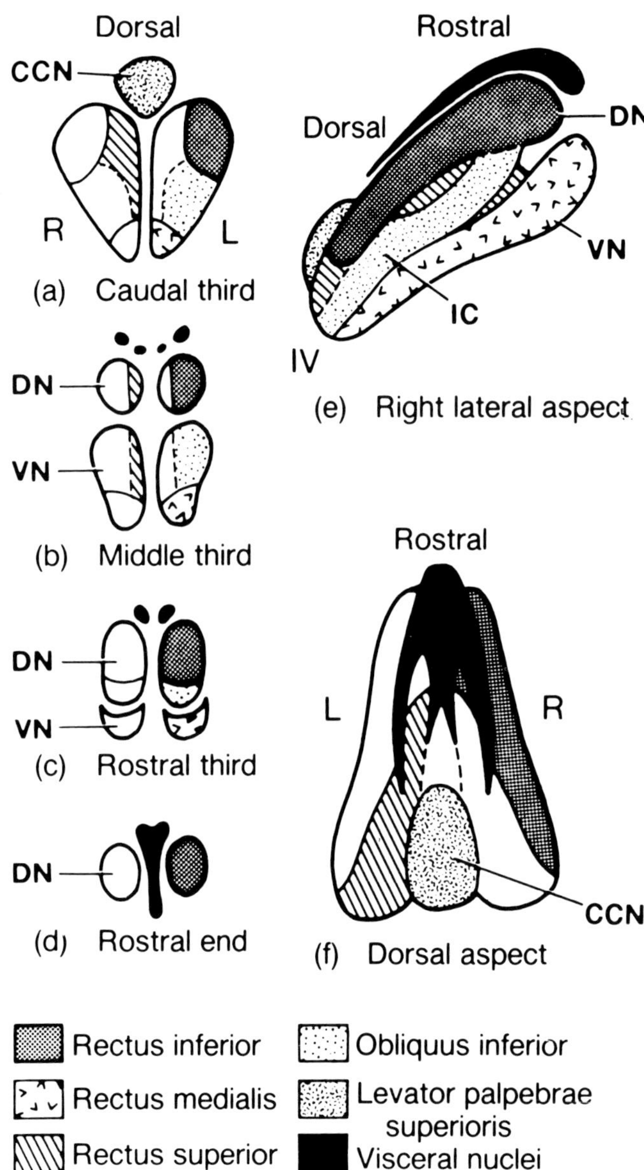

Figure 194–1. Warwick's schema of topographic organization within the oculomotor nucleus. Note the caudal dorsal midline position of the motor pool for the levator palpebrae superioris (CCN, caudal central nucleus). The motor pool of the superior rectus is contralateral to the extraocular muscle that it innervates. (R, right; L, left; DN, dorsal nucleus; IC, intermediate column; IV, region of the trochlear nucleus; VN, ventral nucleus.) (From Miller NR: Walsh and Hoyt's Clinical Neuro-ophthalmology, 4th ed, vol 2, p 569. Copyright 1985, the Williams & Wilkins Co., Baltimore. Redrawn from Warwick R: Representation of extra-ocular muscles in oculomotor nuclei of monkey. J Comp Neurol 98:449–503, 1953.)

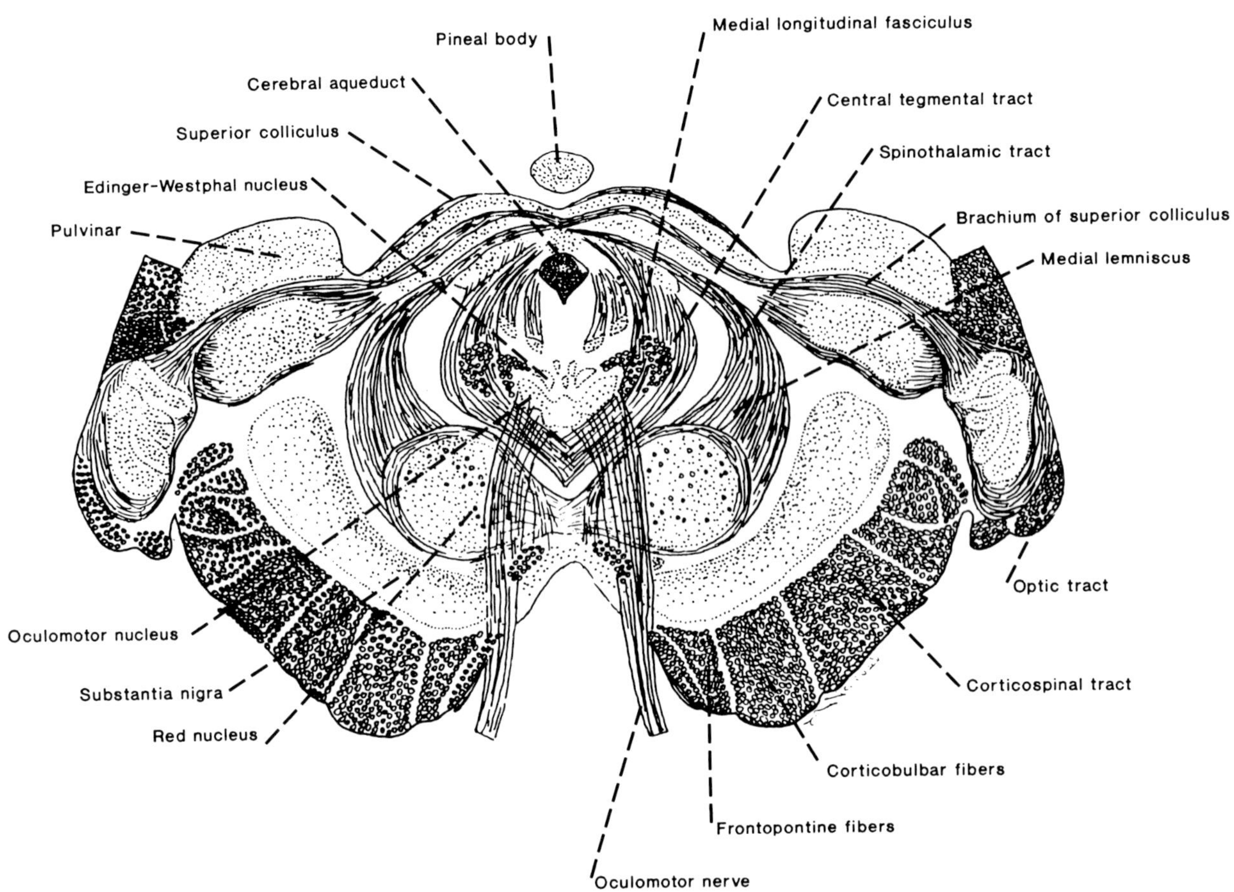

Figure 194–2. Cross section of the midbrain at the level of the superior colliculi and the oculomotor nerves. (Adapted from Ferner H [ed]: Pernkopf Atlas der topographischen und angewandten Anatomie des Menschen, 3rd ed, vols 1 and 2. Baltimore-Munich, Urban & Schwarzenberg, 1987, p 91.)

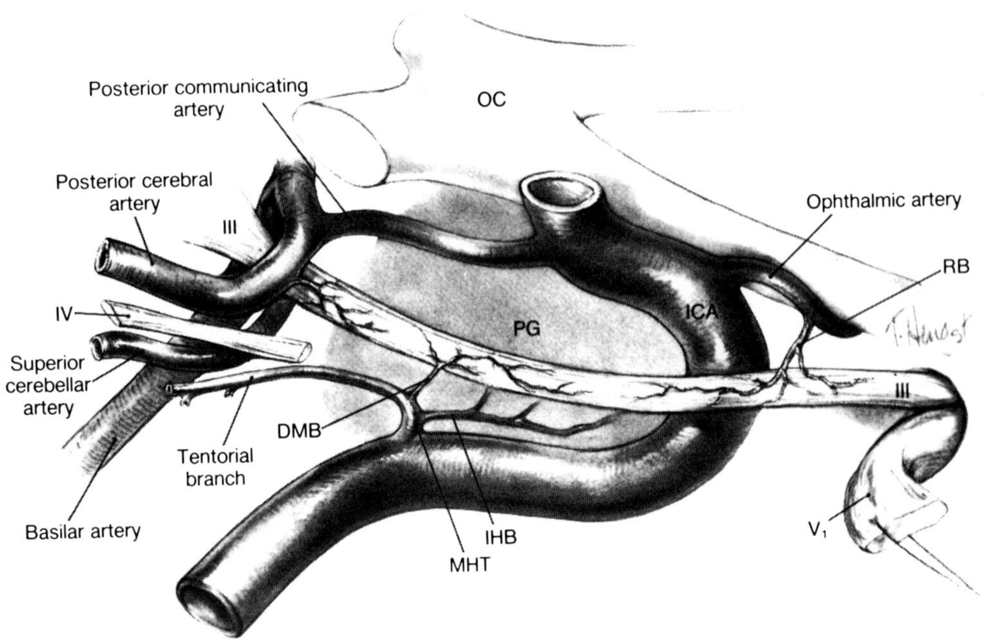

Figure 194–3. Lateral view of the subarachnoid and intracavernous portions of the oculomotor nerve (III) and its vascular supply. (DMB, dorsal meningeal branches; MHT, meningohypophyseal trunk; ICA, internal carotid artery; IHB, inferior hypophyseal branches; RB, recurrent collateral branches of the ophthalmic artery; IV, trochlear nerve; V_1, ophthalmic division of the trigeminal nerve; OC, optic chiasm; PG, pituitary gland.) (From Miller NR: Walsh and Hoyt's Clinical Neuro-ophthalmology, 4th ed, vol 2, p 577. Copyright 1985, the Williams & Wilkins Co., Baltimore. Redrawn from Nadeau SE, Trobe JD: Pupil sparing in oculomotor palsy: A brief review. Ann Neurol 13:143–148, 1983.)

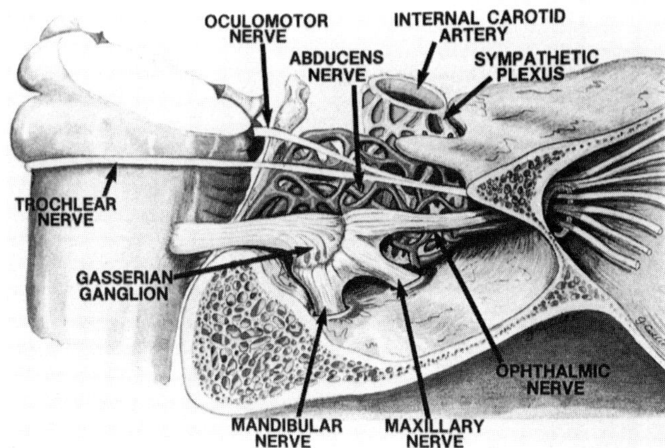

Figure 194–4. A coronal section of the right cavernous sinus viewed anteriorly. (From Kline LB, Acker JD, Post MJD: Computed tomographic evaluation of the cavernous sinus. Ophthalmology 89:374–385, 1982.)

sinus just below the oculomotor nerve (see Fig. 194–4). Although the trochlear nerve passes through the superior orbital fissure (see Fig. 194–5), it enters the orbit outside of the annulus of Zinn (a position unique for the ocular motor nerves) and crosses above the superior rectus muscle en route to innervate the superior oblique muscle.

The abducens nerve (sixth cranial nerve) supplies the lateral rectus muscle. Its nucleus is located in the pons in the floor of the fourth ventricle, at the level of the facial colliculi (Fig. 194–8). Loops of the fascicular portion of the facial nerve (seventh cranial nerve) course ipsilaterally around the abducens nucleus, creating the facial genu. The abducens nucleus contains both cell bodies destined to innervate the lateral rectus via the abducens nerve and interneurons whose axons run in the contralateral medial longitudinal fasciculus to the medial rectus subnucleus.[7] The abducens fascicles run ventrally through the substance of the pons, in close proximity to the facial nucleus and nerve, the trigeminal nuclei and tract, the superior olivary complex, the central tegmental tract, and the corticospinal fibers (see Fig. 194–8). The nerve enters the subarachnoid space at the junction of the pons and medulla, just lateral to the pyramids. It courses upward along the surface of the clivus to pierce the dura and run beneath the petroclinoid ligament into the cavernous sinus (see Fig. 194–4). Entrance into the orbit is through the superior orbital fissure (see Fig. 194–5) and the annulus of Zinn. Branches of the sixth nerve innervate the lateral rectus muscle.

The cavernous sinus is a trabeculated venous sinus located between folds of dura on either side of the sella turcica (see Fig. 194–4). Within the substance of the sinus runs the intracavernous portion of the internal carotid artery (as it bends into its siphon), surrounded by the sympathetic plexus. Also "free floating" within the sinus, just lateral to the carotid, is the abducens nerve.[8] In distinction, the third and fourth cranial nerves are located within the dural folds of the lateral wall of the cavernous sinus, along with the first division of the trigeminal nerve.[9] The second division of the trigeminal nerve travels in the dura of the middle fossa just lateral to the cavernous sinus.

This anatomic relationship is maintained as the ocular motor nerves and the first division of the trigeminal nerve travel forward through the superior orbital fissure. Most superior and lateral within this bone canal are the lacrimal and frontal branches of the trigeminal nerve, with the fourth nerve just below. More ventral and medial are the superior division of the third nerve, the nasociliary branch of the trigeminal nerve, the inferior division of the third nerve, the sixth nerve, and the superior ophthalmic vein.

SYMPTOMS AND HISTORY

The classic presenting symptoms of a patient with an abnormality in third, fourth, or sixth cranial nerve function are double vision, droopy lid, or, less fre-

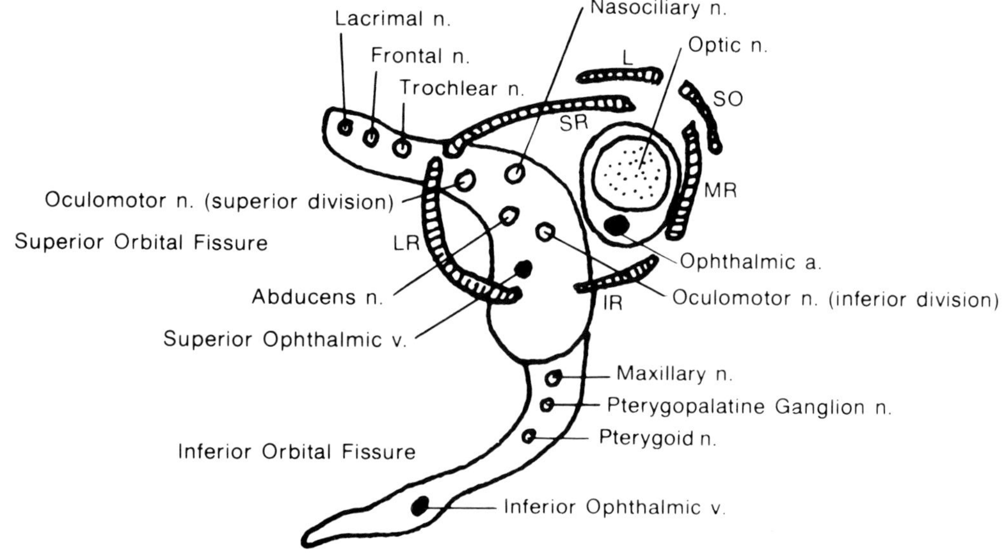

Figure 194–5. Orbital apex, superior and inferior orbital fissure. Note that the trochlear nerve lies outside the muscle cone. (n., nerve; a., artery; v., vein; MR, medial rectus; IR, inferior rectus; LR, lateral rectus; SR, superior rectus; L, levator; SO, superior oblique.) (Reprinted with permission from Basic and Clinical Science Course, Section 5: Neuro-Ophthalmology 1991–1992. San Francisco, American Academy of Ophthalmology, 1991, p 79.)

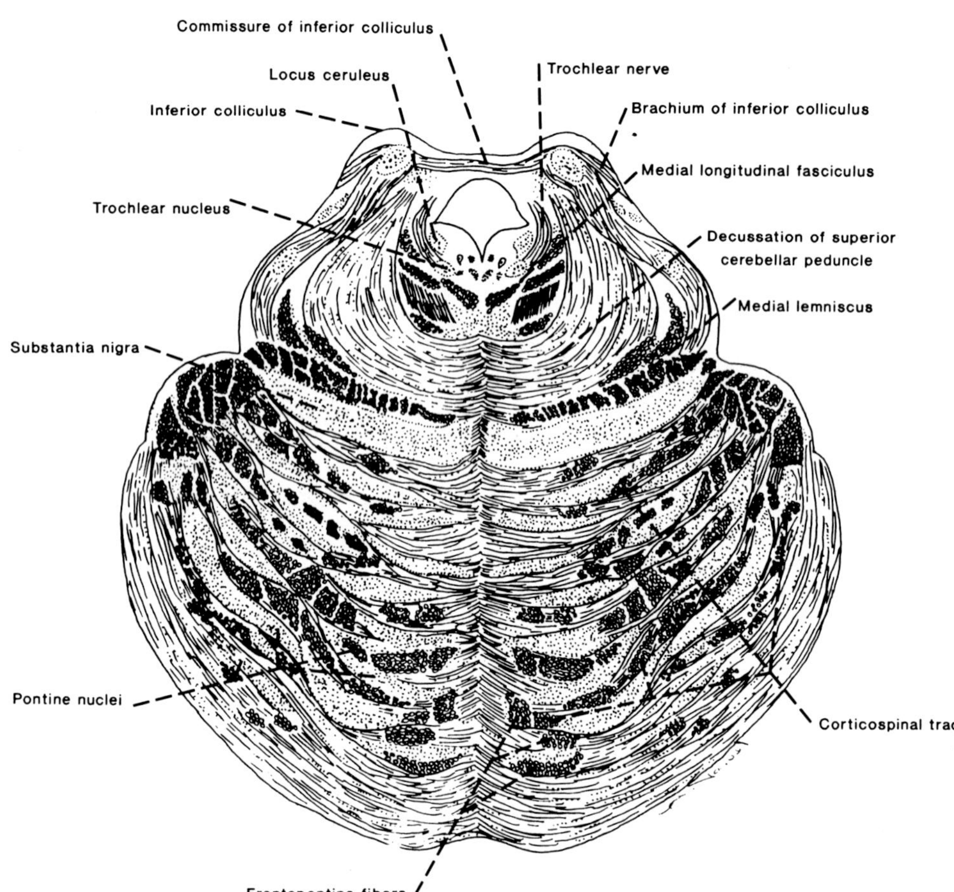

Figure 194–6. Cross section of the brain stem at the level of the inferior colliculi and the trochlear nerves. (Adapted from Ferner H [ed]: Pernkopf Atlas der topographischen und angewandten Anatomie des Menschen, 3rd ed, vol 1. Baltimore-Munich, Urban & Schwarzenberg, 1987, p 93.)

quently, awareness of an enlarged pupil or blurred monocular vision at near range.

The onset of diplopia is almost always characterized by a patient as "sudden." It may manifest initially in an intermittent fashion or may be perceived as a blurring of binocular vision that clears with monocular occlusion when there is only a modest separation of images. Historical features that help to predict the nature and localization of the problem include monocularity versus binocularity (i.e., does occlusion of one eye eliminate the diplopia?), direction of separation of images (horizontal, vertical, diagonal, torsional), direction of gaze in which there is greatest separation, change with near versus distant viewing, and diurnal variation. True monocular diplopia, especially that which clears with pinhole or refraction, is optical in origin, with extremely rare exception.[10–14] There are few reports of "neurogenic" (usually localized to lesions in the parietooccipital cortex) monocular diplopia.[11, 15–18]

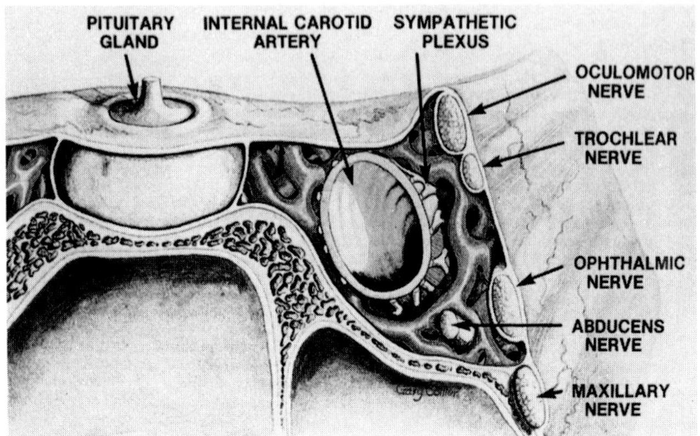

Figure 194–7. The right cavernous sinus viewed laterally. (From Kline LB: The Tolosa-Hunt syndrome. Surv Ophthalmol 27:82, 1982.)

An abnormality of the abducens nerve is the most likely cause of strictly horizontal double vision, especially if it is worse at a distance than nearby, and worse on lateral gaze. Fourth-nerve lesions typically manifest as vertical or diagonal diplopia that is worse with near viewing. The onset of a third cranial nerve lesion may be heralded by ptosis. If ptosis is complete, diplopia may not be recognized. Raising the lid may result in perception of vertical or horizontal diplopia. Infrequently, early oculomotor nerve compression may cause unilateral internal ophthalmoplegia (pupillary dilatation and accommodative paralysis) without the other characteristic features of third-nerve involvement, such as ptosis and ophthalmoplegia.[19, 20] Patients or those around them may note the anisocoria, and the observant patient may be aware of blurring of monocular near vision.

Associated symptoms are of extreme importance in the evaluation of the third, fourth, and sixth cranial nerves. The patient must be asked about headache or localized pain of the orbit, globe, or periorbital region, a red or protruding eye, visual involvement, facial or body numbness or weakness, hearing loss, tinnitus, self-

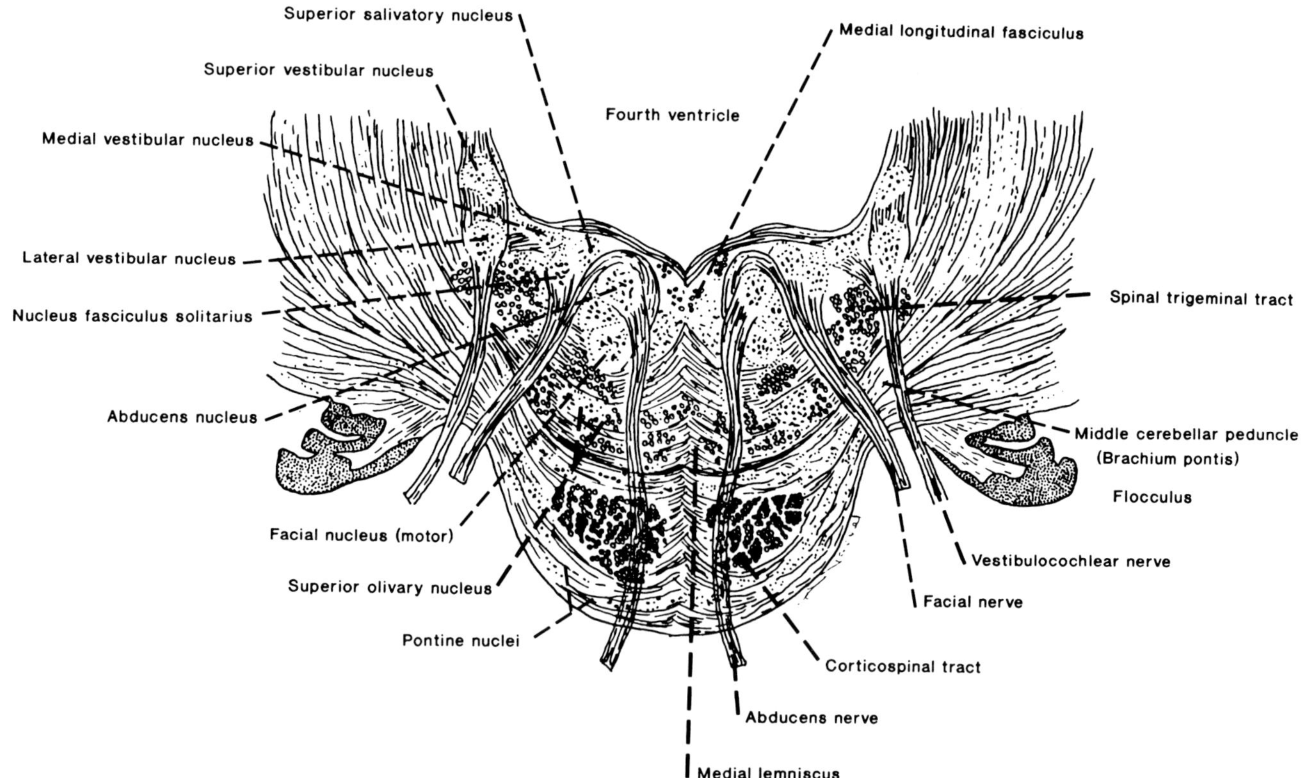

Figure 194–8. Cross section of the pons at the level of the abducens and the facial nerves. (Adapted from Ferner H [ed]: Pernkopf Atlas der topographischen und angewandten Anatomie des Menschen, 3rd ed, vol 1. Baltimore-Munich, Urban & Schwarzenberg, 1987, p 90.)

audible bruits, loss of smell or taste, or any previous episodes of neurologic or ophthalmic dysfunction.

TECHNIQUES OF EXAMINATION

The patient with a suspected ocular motor nerve palsy must be observed for obvious ocular deviation, ptosis, palpebral fissure asymmetry, lagophthalmos, facial asymmetry, head tilt, proptosis, conjunctival injection, or chemosis. During visual assessment, binocularity of the diplopia is verified by monocular occlusion. Associated abnormalities of visual acuity, color vision, or visual fields may be important localizing features. If there is ptosis, one must look for lid fatigue or lid-twitch, because these might indicate myasthenia gravis. The pupils should be assessed for relative size and reactivity. Special attention must be given to testing corneal sensation, although several situations, including chronic contact lens wear, aging, previous cataract surgery, and concurrent use of topical medications, may make interpretation problematic.[21] The sensory function of the three divisions of the trigeminal nerve should be tested with light touch and pinprick compared on either side of the face. Sometimes, subtle asymmetry in sensory function can be revealed by testing the perception of cold (the flat side of a piece of metal such as the handle of a reflex hammer or the end of a tuning fork is usually sufficient). First-, seventh-, and eighth-nerve function should always be tested. Olfactory pathways can be screened by using coffee or other substances that have easily identified odors. Facial nerve function is assessed by having the patient smile, puff out his or her cheeks, forcibly close his or her eyes, and wrinkle his or her forehead. Simple tests of hearing include the ticking of a watch, finger rubbing, and whispering common two-syllable words.

Ocular motility should be assessed monocularly (ductions) and binocularly (versions and vergence) with tests of saccadic and pursuit movements. The extent of movement is ascertained for each of the nine diagnostic positions of gaze as defined by the primary actions of the 12 extraocular muscles (Fig. 194–9). The nature and extent of the deviations of the eyes in relation to each other may be assessed subjectively with the red glass or Maddox rod and confirmed objectively by the alternate-cover test. The latter test can provide quantifiable measurements that help to localize the underacting muscles and allow for careful follow-up.

When confronted with a patient with a complaint referrable to cranial nerve dysfunction, the problem must be approached in an orderly, logical, and, above all, anatomic manner. Localization of the lesion helps to determine the differential diagnosis and subsequent management.

ABNORMALITIES IN THIRD-NERVE FUNCTION

Third-nerve palsies may be partial or complete, congenital or acquired, isolated, or accompanied by signs

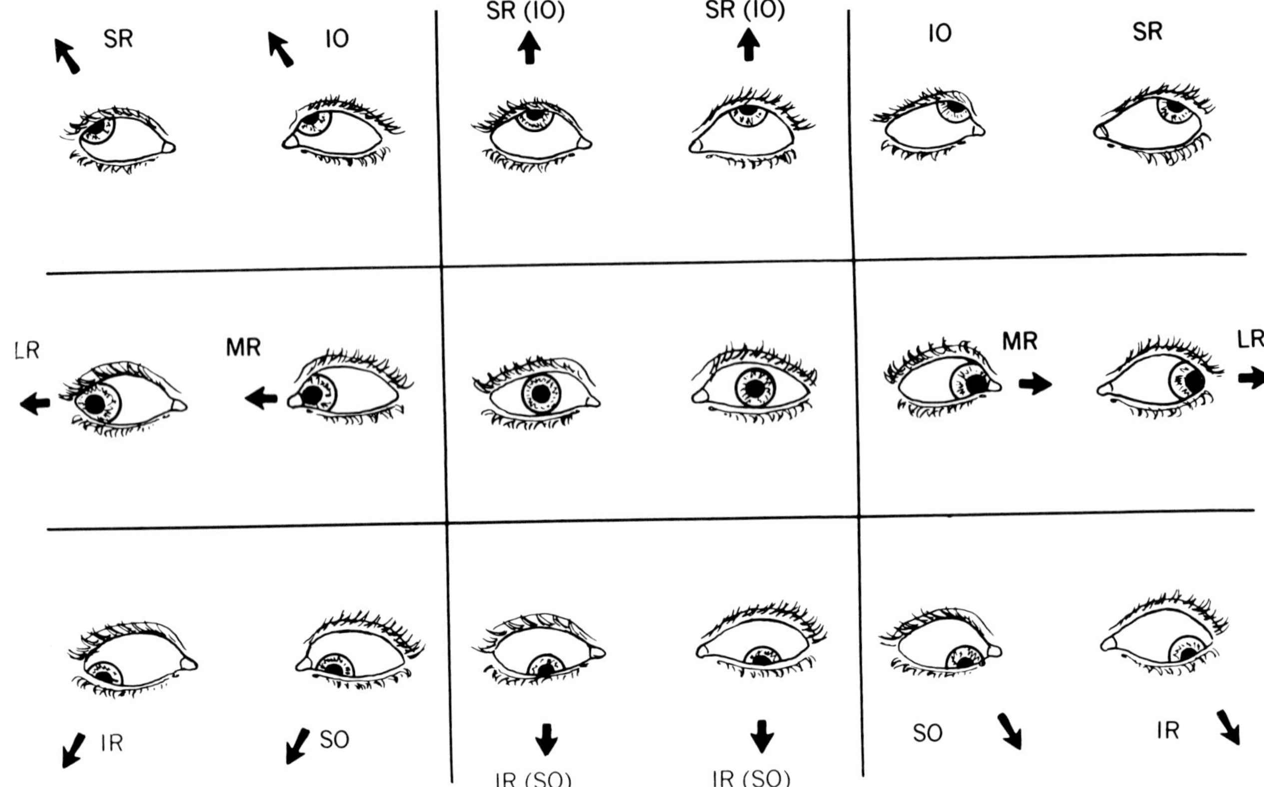

Figure 194–9. The principal actions of the extraocular muscles. (SR, superior rectus; IO, inferior oblique; LR, lateral rectus; MR, medial rectus; IR, inferior rectus; SO, superior oblique.) (From Von Noorden G: Atlas of Strabismus, 4th ed. St. Louis, CV Mosby, 1983, p 19.)

of more extensive neurologic involvement. They can result from lesions anywhere along the anatomic pathway from the nucleus to the muscle.

Congenital

Oculomotor nerve palsies present at birth are presumed secondary to maldevelopment, intrauterine injury, or birth trauma.[22–27] Although relatively rare compared with acquired lesions, they constitute nearly half of the third-nerve palsies documented in children.[23, 28, 29] Typically, they are unilateral and isolated, although bilaterality and accompanying neurologic signs are reported occasionally.[26, 27–30] Some degree of ptosis and ophthalmoplegia is the rule. The pupil is usually involved (either miotic because of presumed aberrant regeneration or dilated), but pupillary sparing has been noted in some cases.[26] The location of the lesion probably varies among cases. The significant occurrence of aberrant regeneration suggests that some of the lesions are along the peripheral course of the nerve,[23, 25, 28] but modern neuroimaging has demonstrated more central loci.[27] Except in cases of obvious birth trauma in which some recovery is expected, most congenital oculomotor nerve palsies are permanent.[23, 27]

Acquired

A listing of all the possible causes of acquired oculomotor nerve dysfunction would likely encompass all known pathologic processes and would be of little use to the clinician faced with diagnosis and management. However, when the lesion can be localized to a specific anatomic site along the course of the nerve (either by the accompanying signs or the particular nature of the palsy), a somewhat more limited and manageable differential diagnosis emerges (Table 194–1).

Lesions involving the oculomotor nucleus should have a particular constellation of clinical signs reflecting the unique anatomy as described earlier. Although a unilateral, stereotactically placed experimental lesion could conceivably result in bilateral ptosis, contralateral superior rectus dysfunction, and abnormalities of the remaining muscles ipsilaterally, the clinical picture is more likely that of a complete ipsilateral oculomotor nerve palsy with additional contralateral ptosis and superior rectus dysfunction.[6, 31–34] If the nuclear lesion is rostral, pupillary involvement is likely and lid function may be spared.[35, 36, 36a] Conversely, with caudal lesions, bilateral ptosis may be a prominent or even isolated finding.[34, 37–40] The most common cause of lesions of the oculomotor nucleus is vascular compromise, usually a result of thrombotic occlusion of small perforating vessels off the basilar artery or embolic or thrombotic occlusive disease of larger vessels ("top of the basilar syndrome").[34, 41–44] Other causes to consider include small intraparenchymal hemorrhage from presumed vascular malformations, metastatic neoplasms, and abscesses.[36, 37, 45, 46]

Classically, the differentiating feature of fascicular from peripheral nerve lesions has been the accompanying neurologic signs reflecting the fascicles' location

Table 194–1. ACQUIRED THIRD-NERVE LESIONS

Locations	Other Symptoms/ Signs	Common Causes
Nucleus	Complete 3rd plus contralateral ptosis and contralateral superior rectus weakness	Vascular occlusion Hemorrhage Metastasis
Fascicles	Contralateral hemiparesis (Weber's), contralateral tremor (Benedikt's), ipsilateral ataxia (Nothnagel's)	Vascular occlusion Hemorrhage Neoplasm Demyelination
Subarachnoid space	Typically isolated	Aneurysm Microvascular neoplasm Meningitis Herniation Trauma
Cavernous sinus	4th, 6th, V1, V2, oculosympathetic dysfunction; pain may be prominent	Neoplasm Inflammation Aneurysm Microvascular thrombosis Anteriovenous fistula
Orbit	Proptosis, visual loss	Trauma Neoplasm Inflammation

within the parenchyma of the brain stem. Several syndromes have been recognized (Fig. 194–10): Third-nerve palsy and ipsilateral cerebellar ataxia may result from involvement of the fascicles and the brachium conjunctivum (Nothnagel's syndrome),[47] oculomotor palsy and contralateral tremor may reflect a lesion in the region of the red nucleus (Benedikt's syndrome),[48] and third-nerve dysfunction plus contralateral hemiparesis implicates involvement of the ipsilateral cerebral peduncle (Weber's syndrome).[49]

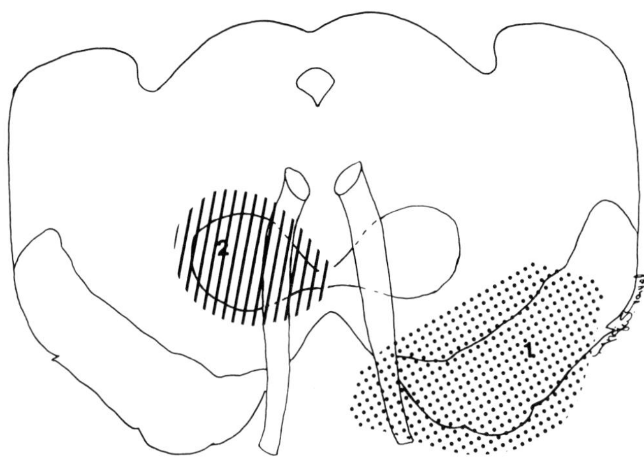

Figure 194–10. Cross section of the midbrain at the level of the oculomotor nerves depicting the location of lesions responsible for Weber's syndrome (1) and Benedikt's syndrome (2).

With the advent of more sensitive neuroimaging such as magnetic resonance imaging (MRI), isolated and even pupil-sparing oculomotor nerve dysfunction has been shown to occasionally result from fascicular lesions.[50–55] MRI has also demonstrated that a lesion of the fascicles can cause isolated dysfunction of either the superior or inferior division of the third nerve.[51, 52] This suggests that functional organization of the oculomotor nerve into divisions may occur within the fascicles prior to the anatomic separation seen grossly within the anterior cavernous sinus. The causes of fascicular oculomotor nerve lesions are nearly identical to those of lesions of the nuclear complex, with vascular causes heading the list, followed by infiltrative and inflammatory causes.[52, 54, 56–59] Because the fascicles are white matter tracts, the diagnosis of demyelinating disease must also be considered.[52, 60, 61]

Third-nerve involvement in the subarachnoid space is more often presumed clinically than demonstrated pathologically or with sophisticated neuroimaging. The subarachnoid space is the most likely site of injury in cases of isolated oculomotor palsies. Involvement may be partial or complete, although most commonly there is progression to total involvement over time.

Because of the dorsal and peripheral location of the pupillary fibers, a dilated pupil may be the first sign of a compressive lesion in the subarachnoid space.[19, 20, 62, 63] A common cause of an isolated oculomotor nerve palsy with significant pupillary involvement in adults is an intracranial aneurysm,[64–69] typically originating at the junction of the posterior communicating and the internal carotid arteries (Fig. 194–11). Almost without exception, there is pain (although sometimes modest) and eventually other evidence of oculomotor nerve involvement. Other locations of aneurysmal dilatation that have been shown to cause third-nerve palsies include the top of the basilar artery and the junction of the basilar and superior cerebellar arteries.[70–73] Diabetic "microvascular" oculomotor palsies are also commonly painful and can have some pupil involvement in 10 to 20 percent of

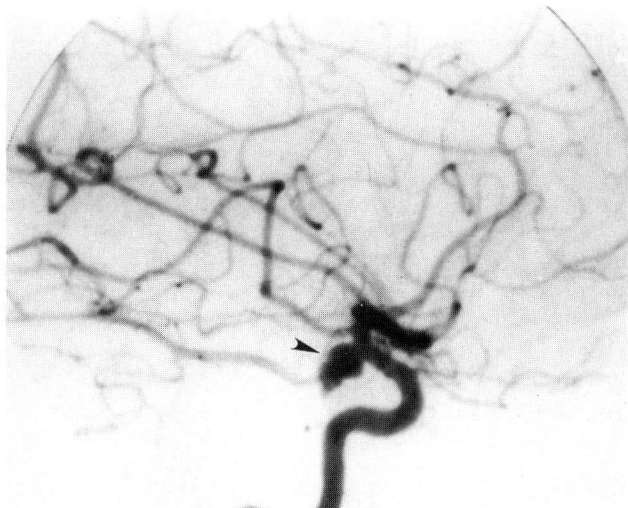

Figure 194–11. Cerebral angiogram in a patient with a painful third nerve palsy. An aneurysm is present at the junction of the posterior communicating and carotid arteries *(arrow)*.

cases.[64, 68b, 74] Other causes of oculomotor nerve dysfunction in the subarachnoid space include compressive or infiltrating neoplasms or inflammatory lesions, ischemia, meningitis (infectious, inflammatory, or neoplastic), compression by large dolichoectatic vessels or cerebral structures shifted by expanding supratentorial lesions or edema, and trauma.[65, 68a, 68b, 74–96] The trauma necessary for third-nerve damage is typically severe enough to have caused skull fractures and loss of consciousness.[77, 79, 86, 97] Beware the oculomotor palsy apparent after minor trauma, because it may reflect an underlying mass lesion.[80, 91] Third-nerve dysfunction may be a component of a generalized polyneuropathy or the Miller Fisher variant of the Guillain-Barré syndrome.[98–101, 101a]

There are no specific distinguishing features of third-nerve involvement in the cavernous sinus. Although bifurcation of the nerve into its two divisions typically occurs in the anterior cavernous sinus,[102, 103] there is evidence that a functional bifurcation occurs more proximally along the course of the oculomotor nerve, probably within the brain stem,[51, 52, 104] making localization of a divisional paresis problematic. To clinically distinguish a cavernous sinus location of an oculomotor nerve palsy, one must note the company it keeps. Dysfunction of the trochlear and abducens nerves, the first or second division of the trigeminal nerve, the oculosympathetics, and the venous drainage of the eye and orbit may be apparent. Pain may be a prominent feature. The pupil may be small or midsized and poorly reactive because of concurrent oculosympathetic involvement.[105] Causes include neoplastic (pituitary tumors, craniopharyngioma, meningioma, nasopharyngeal carcinoma, schwannoma, metastatic lesions), inflammatory (Tolosa-Hunt, sarcoid), aneurysmal compression, ischemia, cavernous sinus thrombosis, and arteriovenous fistulas.[103, 106–124]

Orbital lesions may cause third-nerve palsies that respect the anatomic bifurcation of the nerve or that reflect individual muscle involvement. Commonly associated clinical features include proptosis and visual loss. Causes include trauma, neoplasms, and inflammation.[125–128]

Most studies reviewing the causes of oculomotor nerve palsies do not distinguish isolated from nonisolated palsies, nor do they list causes by location.[64, 66, 68, 68a, 68b] A large number of cases are recorded as "undetermined" cause and a larger proportion still, those of vascular origin, remain of uncertain location. Newer, more sensitive neuroimaging modalities, such as MRI, are localizing more of these lesions and even providing clues about pathogenesis,[52–54] but most third-nerve palsies remain poorly characterized. Vascular lesions causing oculomotor nerve palsies were believed to occur most frequently along the nerve's subarachnoid or intracavernous course,[78, 112] although fascicular involvement was later demonstrated in some cases.[54, 58, 129] Conditions frequently associated with third-nerve dysfunction include diabetes mellitus, hypertension, giant cell arteritis, systemic lupus erythematosus, syphilis, and migraine.[54, 64, 65, 74, 130–143] The site of third-nerve involvement in "viral" syndromes remains unknown.[23, 144, 145]

The phenomenon of "pupillary sparing" bears special mention. True pupillary sparing implies that each of the extraocular muscles innervated by the oculomotor nerve is involved to some extent, but the pupil remains of normal size and reactivity.[74, 94, 146–148] Oculomotor nerve palsies without dysfunction of *all* of the muscles innervated by the third nerve that also do not involve the pupil are not "pupillary sparing." The distinction becomes very important in management (see later). The cause of most isolated pupil-sparing third-nerve palsies is believed to be vascular, frequently associated with diabetes mellitus or systemic hypertension.[54, 55, 64, 65, 68a, 68b, 74, 94, 140, 147] The explanation for this may be anatomic in that the peripherally located pupillary fibers may receive more collateral blood supply than the main nerve trunk.[112, 149] Vascular third-nerve palsies may be quite painful but usually resolve after 2 to 4 mo. Rarely, isolated pupillary-sparing oculomotor nerve palsies may be secondary to compressive lesions, although the majority of these cases have incomplete palsies.[73, 94, 129, 146, 148, 150–157]

Special Syndromes

CYCLIC OCULOMOTOR PARESIS

This is an uncommon but dramatic condition typically seen in patients with known congenital third-nerve palsies.[23, 25, 158–161] The classic scenario is that of alternating baseline paresis with episodes lasting seconds of pupillary miosis, increased accommodation, elevation of a previously ptotic upper lid, and adduction of the eye. In some cases, the spasms can be brought on by voluntary efforts in the direction of paretic muscles. The cause is unknown, but most authors speculate some element of aberrant regeneration after nerve or nuclear damage.

ABERRANT REGENERATION

Although this phenomenon has been demonstrated or suspected in virtually every peripheral nerve that has had partial damage, the oculomotor nerve is particularly interesting in this regard because of its many branches and target structures. Signs include elevation of the upper lid with attempted downgaze (pseudo-Graefe's sign) (Fig. 194–12), upgaze, or adduction, segmental constriction of the pupil with movement in the direction of action of muscles innervated by the third nerve, retraction of the globe with attempted vertical gaze (presumably secondary to co-contraction of the superior and inferior recti), or adduction of the eye with attempted up- or downgaze.[162–169] Oculomotor synkinesis is generally believed to reflect the misdirection of regenerating fibers after partial damage to the peripheral portion of the nerve.[163, 168] However, other theories involving more central mechanisms have been proposed.[165, 169]

Oculomotor nerve synkinesis is most commonly seen 2 to 3 mo after injury to the nerve by trauma or compression from aneurysms or tumors. Ischemic lesions (i.e., secondary to diabetes) rarely if ever result in aberrant regeneration,[165, 170] and the presence of syn-

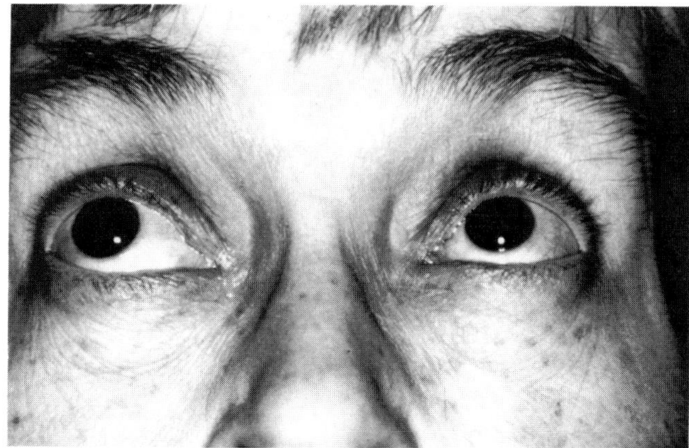

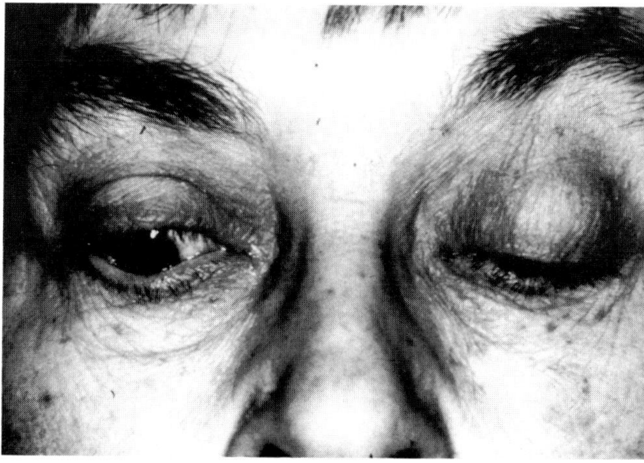

Figure 194–12. A pseudo-Graefe sign is shown in a patient with a right cavernous sinus aneurysm and aberrant regeneration of branches of the third nerve. On attempted downgaze *(bottom)*, the right lid elevates.

kinesis requires a careful search for a nonischemic cause. Slowly growing mass lesions are likely to be responsible for the phenomenon of "primary" oculomotor nerve synkinesis, in which a recognizable paretic phase does not precede development of the aberrant movements.[165, 171–173] A case of presumed contralateral oculomotor synkinesis following unilateral trauma prompted a critical review of the literature.[169]

NEUROMYOTONIA

Episodic involuntary contractions of the muscles innervated by the oculomotor nerve have been described in patients without baseline ocular motility abnormalities.[174, 175] The contractions are brief and myotonic and can sometimes be brought on by looking in the direction of action of the involved muscle. Most of these patients have a history of previous radiation therapy to either the parenchymal or peripheral course of the ocular motor nerves. Neuromyotonia of the fourth and sixth cranial nerves has also been reported. Neuromyotonia may respond to membrane-stabilizing agents, such as carbamazepine.[174–176]

Management

An evaluation of the patient with a third-nerve palsy depends on the associated symptoms and signs, the pattern of oculomotor nerve involvement, and the age of the patient (Table 194–2). If the patient has findings localizable to the nerve's nuclear or fascicular course within the brain stem, MRI or at least high-resolution computed tomography (CT) is indicated. Accompanying meningeal signs (e.g., global headache, stiff neck, and depressed level of consciousness) or other cranial nerve involvement, especially if bilateral, should prompt an evaluation of the cerebrospinal fluid by lumbar puncture. Localization to the cavernous sinus warrants neuroimaging, preferably MRI with gadolinium. High-resolution CT scanning with thin coronal and axial views, after the administration of a contrast agent, is in several respects still superior to MRI if an orbital locus is suspected.

The approach to the patient with an isolated third-nerve palsy differs among clinicians, and some of the issues remain controversial.[94, 147, 148, 177, 178] The sudden onset of a painful third-nerve palsy with associated meningeal signs demands an emergent neurologic evaluation, regardless of the patient's age or the extent of third-nerve involvement, including those that spare pupillary function. The work-up should include CT scanning without (looking for blood in the subarachnoid space) and with (looking for an intracranial aneurysm) intravenous contrast, and cerebral angiography. CT scanning alone will miss a significant proportion of cerebral aneurysms.[179] The sensitivity of MRI in the detection of aneurysms is likely better than CT but is as yet undetermined. Although most aneurysms are seen by angiography of the ipsilateral carotid circulation, the basilar circulation must also be studied to exclude a more posterior location. The contralateral carotid circulation should also be evaluated, because approximately 20 percent of patients have more than one aneurysm.[180–182]

All patients under the age of 40 who present with an isolated third-nerve palsy of any extent should also have complete neurologic evaluation, including a cerebral

Table 194–2. EVALUATION OF THIRD-NERVE DYSFUNCTION

Nonisolated		
Brain stem symptoms/signs	→	MRI
Meningeal symptoms/signs	→	MRI, LP
Orbital symptoms/signs	→	CT
Isolated		
< Age 40	→	CT/MRI, ± LP, cerebral angiography
> Age 40		
Pupil-sparing	→	glucose, ESR, close observation
Pupil-involved	→	glucose, ESR, CT/MRI, ± cerebral angiography

Key: CT, computed tomography; ESR, erythrocyte sedimentation rate; LP, lumbar puncture; MRI, magnetic resonance imaging.

angiogram. There is some controversy about the application of this rule to children under the age of 10, in whom aneurysms are extremely rare.[147, 148, 183, 184] Patients over the age of 40 who present with an isolated, pupil-sparing, but otherwise complete third-nerve palsy, even in the presence of pain, can usually be assumed to have a vasculopathic etiology. Minimal work-up in the known diabetic patient would consist of a measurement of systemic blood pressure, serum glucose, and sedimentation rate. If there is no history of diabetes, a glucose tolerance test or a serum hemoglobin Alc level should be obtained. These patients must be observed closely for the next week for evidence of pupillary involvement. The patient over age 40 with an isolated complete oculomotor nerve palsy with pupillary involvement or a partial third-nerve palsy presents the most difficult management issue. All these patients should have at least the minimal blood work-up as outlined earlier and a neuroimage performed, preferably the more sensitive MRI. The majority of these patients ultimately come to cerebral arteriogram. The use of new noninvasive techniques of MRI angiography in this setting awaits further experience.[185]

The majority of third-nerve palsies of ischemic etiology resolve within 3 mo. Compressive or traumatic oculomotor nerve palsies may take longer to improve, and incomplete recovery with or without synkinesis is more likely. Despite rare reports of continued improvement in third-nerve palsies years after onset,[186–188] once the deficit has stabilized (usually within 6 mo after injury) it is unlikely that there will be further recovery. The chronic oculomotor palsy, especially in younger age groups, requires subsequent serial neuroimaging over the years, especially as the sensitivities of our techniques improve.[189]

Various surgical procedures have been used to provide binocular fusion in at least primary position after third-nerve palsy and to correct vision-limiting or cosmetically annoying upper lid ptosis. However, complete oculomotor nerve palsies rarely allow for a completely satisfactory surgical result.[190, 191] The Scott procedure (transposition of the insertion of the superior oblique tendon to a point anterior and medial to the insertion of the superior rectus muscle without trochleotomy) combined with large recessions of the lateral rectus muscle of involved eyes and, occasionally, recess/resect procedures of horizontal recti muscles of noninvolved eyes can result in satisfactory cosmetic outcome and alignment in primary position in some cases.[192] In the correction of acquired strabismus, the use of adjustable sutures is encouraged.[193] The role of botulinum toxin injection in the management of acute or chronic third-nerve paresis has not been adequately investigated.[194]

Microvascular third-nerve palsies, especially in diabetics, may be exquisitely painful during the acute phase. Intense pain may require analgesics for 1 to 2 wk.

ABNORMALITIES IN FOURTH-NERVE FUNCTION

Trochlear nerve palsies are the most common cause of vertical malalignment of the eyes.[64, 66, 68, 68a, 195] Given the mechanical arrangement of the superior oblique muscle, this vertical deviation is worse with attempted downgaze and gaze to the side opposite the paretic muscle. This is the basis for the first two steps of the "Three-Step Test" (Fig. 194–13)[196–198] in which first the higher eye is identified (reflecting the relative decrease in tonic downward input from the superior oblique), then the direction of horizontal gaze in which this vertical deviation worsens is noted. In the third step, the patient's hyperdeviation is compared on head tilt left and right. The two intorters of each eye are the superior oblique and superior rectus muscles. If the superior oblique is paretic, the superior rectus, on attempted intortion, will further elevate the eye, because this is its primary function. Thus, the vertical deviation worsens when the head is tilted in such a way that intortion is necessary (i.e., toward the side of the paretic superior oblique). Other causes of vertical strabismus, such as paralysis of more than one vertical muscle, dissociated vertical divergence, previous muscle surgery, contracture of the vertical recti, myasthenia gravis, thyroid ophthalmopathy, and skew deviation, may have a positive three-step test and cause errors in diagnosis.[199, 199a] History and associated findings on examination, as well as careful observation of versions into all the diagnostic fields of gaze, help to distinguish isolated trochlear palsy from these other conditions. Patients typically compensate for a superior oblique palsy by tilting the head to the opposite side. Another clue to trochlear nerve paresis in the observant patient is a torsional component to the vertical diplopia: The two vertically separated images are not parallel, but rather approach each other as if to meet in the direction of the involved eye.[200] Detection of bilateral fourth-nerve palsies may be difficult, especially if the damage is asymmetric and the less involved nerve paresis is "masked."[201, 202] Clues to bilaterality include greater than 12 degrees of subjective excyclotorsion, a chin-down posture, lack of head tilt, a large "V" shift, observation of fundus torsion on ophthalmoscopy, and a reversal of hypertropia, however minimal, on cover testing in the oblique fields of gaze or on contralateral head tilt.

Congenital

Although the cause of congenital trochlear nerve palsies is unknown, they occur commonly.[28, 203] They may remain compensated and unrecognized during childhood, only to become manifest later either spontaneously or after minor trauma. Clues to their congenital nature include a head tilt seen on old photographs and the demonstration of large vertical fusional amplitudes (nonstrabismic patients usually only fuse 3- to 6-prism diopters vertically).[204]

Acquired

Involvement of the trochlear nerve at the nuclear or fascicular level may be recognized by associated brain stem findings (Table 194–3). If the process occurs before the decussation of the fascicles, the superior oblique

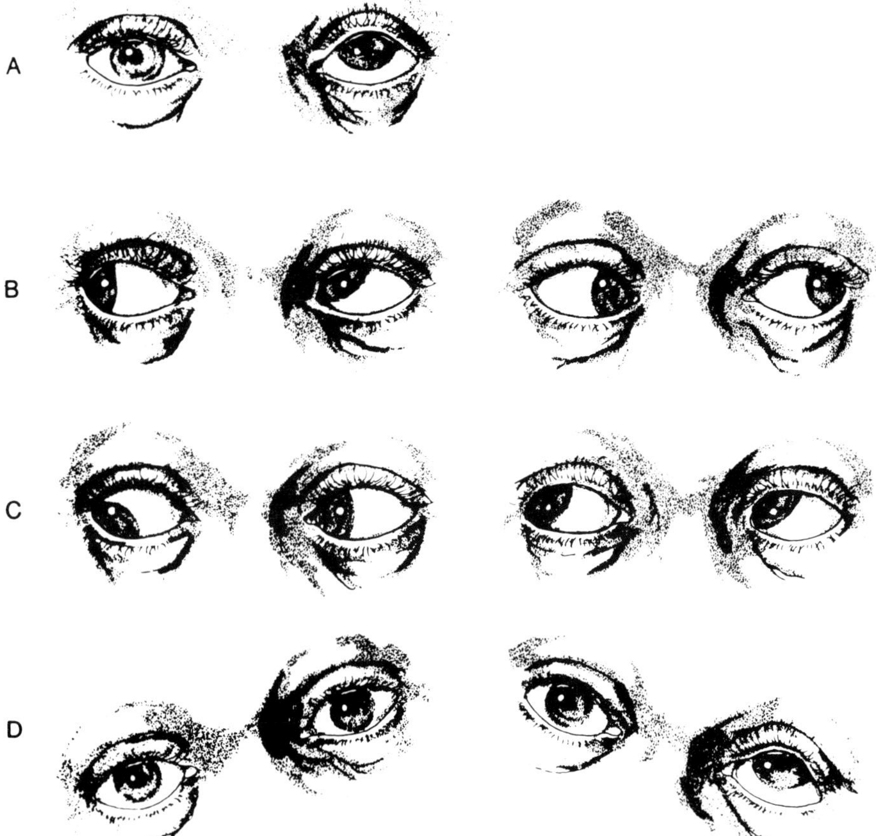

Figure 194–13. The diagnosis of vertical ocular deviation. The steps in diagnosis of a left superior oblique palsy are shown. *A,* In primary position, there is a left hypertropia. This could be caused by weakness of elevators of the right eye or depressors of the left eye. *B,* The deviation becomes worse on gaze to the right. This implies weakness of the right superior rectus or the left superior oblique. *C,* In right gaze, the deviation is more marked when the eyes look down. This implies weakness of the left superior oblique muscle. *D,* When the head is tilted to the right, no vertical deviation of the eyes is detectable. (This would be the patient's preferred head position.) When the head is tilted to the left, the left hypertropia is exaggerated. Steps *A, B,* and *D* constitute the "Three Step Test" (see text). (From Leigh RJ, Zee DS: The Neurology of Eye Movements, 2nd ed. Philadelphia, FA Davis, 1991, p 314.)

palsy is seen contralateral to the other parenchymal signs such as a "first-order neuron" Horner's syndrome.[205, 206] The causes of such lesions include small infarcts and hemorrhages, intrinsic mass lesions, and external compression or trauma.[42, 195, 206–213] Bilateral fascicular damage at the level of the superior medullary velum may be a primary site of trochlear nerve damage secondary to trauma or hydrocephalus.[212, 214–217] Trauma is the most common cause of bilateral fourth-nerve palsy.[202]

Table 194–3. ACQUIRED FOURTH-NERVE LESIONS

Location	Other Symptoms/ Signs	Common Causes
Nucleus	Contralateral Horner's syndrome	Vascular occlusion Hemorrhage Neoplasm Trauma
Fascicles	Frequently bilateral	Trauma Hydrocephalus
Subarachnoid space		Trauma Microvascular meningitis
Cavernous sinus	3rd, 6th, V1, V2, oculosympathetic dysfunction	Neoplasm Inflammation Microvascular thrombosis
Orbit	Brown's syndrome	Neoplasm Inflammation Trauma

The dorsal exit of the trochlear nerve and its long course around the brain stem and along the tentorial edge make it particularly susceptible to the effects of trauma and neurosurgical manipulation.[77, 96, 97, 218–220] It is here in the subarachnoid space that inflammatory and possibly ischemic processes may result in fourth-nerve dysfunction.[92, 212]

Lesions of the fourth nerve within the cavernous sinus are rarely if ever isolated. Associated oculomotor, abducens, or trigeminal nerve or oculosympathetic dysfunction helps to localize the problem. Neoplastic, inflammatory, and infiltrative causes are essentially the same as those discussed earlier in relation to oculomotor nerve abnormalities in the same location.

Neoplastic, inflammatory, ischemic, and traumatic processes within the orbit may affect the trochlear nerve, the superior oblique muscle, or the trochlear tendon or its sheath. In Brown's syndrome, congenital or acquired, there is restriction of elevation when the eye is adducted.[221] This is presumed secondary to restricted passive movement of the superior oblique tendon through the trochlea. A "click" is typically felt as this restriction is released. In the acquired forms, such as those seen with rheumatoid arthritis and other connective tissue abnormalities, pain and tenderness of the superomedial orbit may be prominent.

It is likely that the actual incidence of fourth-nerve palsy is higher than usually reported, reflecting the frequent difficulty in routine recognition and diagnosis.

When an etiology is known, the most common cause is trauma, although the exact locus of involvement remains unclear.[64, 66, 68, 68a, 68b, 195, 203, 212] About a third of the trochlear nerve palsies reported in large series are of undetermined etiology, with another 15 to 35 percent ascribed to presumed vascular disease. As with oculomotor nerve palsies of similar cause, it is unknown where an ischemic lesion occurs along the course of the fourth nerve.

Special Syndromes

SUPERIOR OBLIQUE MYOKYMIA

Superior oblique myokymia is a monocular nonrhythmic twitching of the superior oblique muscle that occurs in otherwise healthy young adults.[222, 223] Symptoms may be described as blurred vision, especially with reading, vertical or torsional diplopia, or true oscillopsia. Fine vertical or intorsional monocular movements are best viewed at the slit lamp and can sometimes be induced by directing the patient to look in the primary direction of action of the superior oblique muscle. The phenomenon is intermittent and may be self-limiting or persistent. For some patients, the symptoms are bothersome enough to require intervention. Successful medical therapy has been achieved with carbamazepine and possibly low-dose propranolol.[224, 225] A single case of superior oblique myokymia as the presenting sign of a cerebellar tumor with tectal compression and hydrocephalus suggests that neuroimaging is indicated in this usually benign condition.[226]

Management

The nonisolated fourth-nerve palsy requires an evaluation determined by the presumed location of the lesion (Table 194–4). Thus, if a mesencephalic or cavernous sinus locale is likely, MRI is indicated. If a meningeal process is suspected, cerebrospinal fluid analysis is necessary. Orbital lesions may be best evaluated with high-resolution CT scanning.

Table 194–4. EVALUATION OF FOURTH-NERVE DYSFUNCTION

Nonisolated		
Brain stem symptoms/signs	→	MRI
Meningeal symptoms/signs	→	MRI, LP
Orbital symptoms/signs	→	CT
Isolated		
Evidence of decompensated congenital palsy	→	No work-up
History of head trauma or neurosurgery	→	CT/MRI
< Age 40	→	CT/MRI, ± Tensilon test, observation
> Age 40	→	glucose, ESR, ± Tensilon test, observation

Key: CT, computed tomography; ESR, erythrocyte sedimentation rate; LP, lumbar puncture; MRI, magnetic resonance imaging.

The main differential diagnosis of isolated trochlear nerve paresis is skew deviation, ocular myopathies, and myasthenia gravis. A fourth-nerve palsy can usually be distinguished from skew deviation by the latter's frequent association with other brain stem signs or symptoms and the former's torsional diplopia with cyclodeviation.[200] However, this distinction can sometimes be quite difficult to make. Thyroid ophthalmopathy is rarely restricted to a single muscle, and orbital myositis affecting only the superior oblique is typically very painful. Disorders of the neuromuscular junction can mimic any single ocular muscle paralysis, and diagnosis depends on the presence of diurnal variation and ultimately the development of other associated signs.

In the patient with evidence of a decompensated congenital trochlear nerve palsy (i.e., previously documented head tilt and large fusional amplitudes), further work-up is usually not necessary. The patient with clearly documented precipitating head trauma or neurosurgical procedure probably deserves at least a noncontrast CT scan to rule out complicating hydrocephalus or hemorrhage. The diagnosis of a nontraumatic, noncongenital isolated fourth-nerve palsy should prompt a systemic evaluation for vascular risk factors, including hypertension, diabetes, and, when appropriate, giant cell arteritis. There should be a low threshold for performing a Tensilon test. Further evaluation can probably be avoided as long as careful observation documents nonprogression and the continued absence of associated signs.

The majority of acquired trochlear nerve palsies of traumatic, vascular, or "undetermined" etiology improve over time, usually within 6 mo. In the interim, monocular occlusion or vertical prisms[227] may help the patient symptomatically. In some cases, the nerve will have suffered permanent damage or transection. Various surgical procedures have been proposed involving the paretic muscle, its antagonist, or the contralateral yoke muscle.[228, 229, 229a] Especially with regard to surgical correction, a distinction between unilateral and bilateral fourth-nerve dysfunction preoperatively is crucial to avoid a second surgical procedure.[201, 202, 229a]

ABNORMALITIES IN SIXTH-NERVE FUNCTION

Although the abducens nerve may appear to be a simple arrangement of one nerve supplying a single ipsilateral extraocular muscle, the unique organization of its nucleus and the surrounding brain stem structures provides for a rich assortment of congenital and acquired clinical syndromes. An examination of the patient with suspected sixth-nerve palsy must include a close inspection of the function of the other cranial nerves of pontine origin and of the motility of the contralateral eye.

Congenital

A unilateral, isolated, congenital abduction deficit is an unusual finding, which is usually transient and most

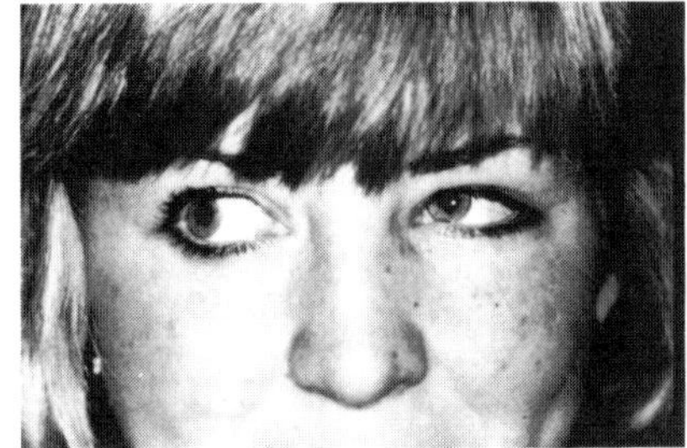
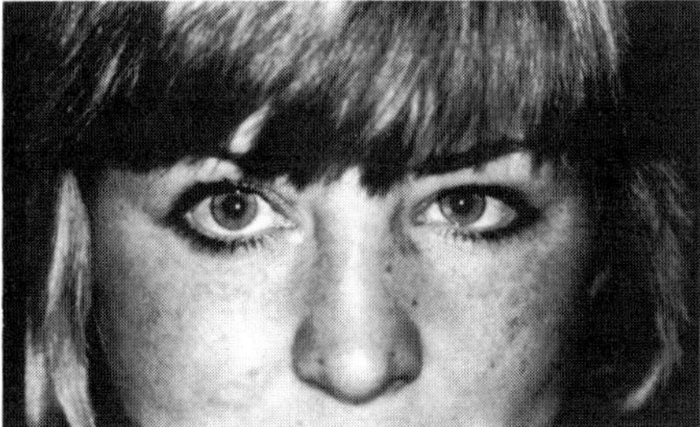
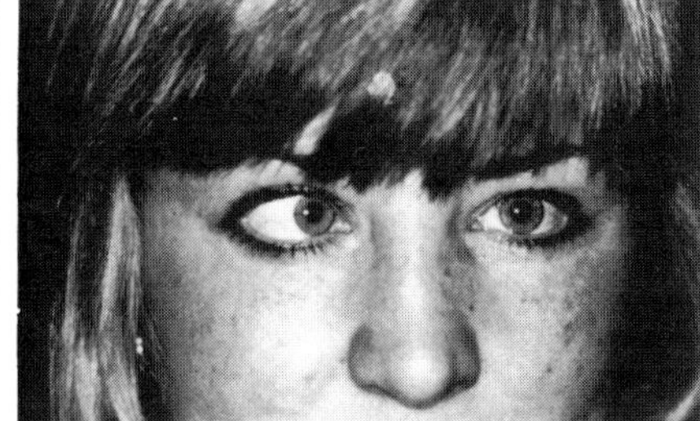

Figure 194–14. A patient with Duane's retraction syndrome of the left eye. There was no abduction of the left eye on attempted gaze to the left *(right panel)*. With gaze to the right *(left panel)*, the left globe retracts, and there is consequent palpebral fissure narrowing.

likely related to birth trauma.[230] Less rare, but also uncommon, are isolated congenital horizontal gaze palsies.[231–234] More frequently, these are associated with other neurologic or skeletal abnormalities.[235–237] The most common constellation of congenital findings involving sixth-nerve dysfunction fall under the headings of Möbius' syndrome and Duane's retraction syndrome.

In Möbius' syndrome, facial diplegia is associated with abnormalities of horizontal gaze, usually complete absence of horizontal motility.[238–243] Head movements and convergence (if preserved) are substituted. Other neurologic and musculoskeletal abnormalities are common. Etiologies are heterogeneous, including maldevelopment, intrauterine insults such as infections or hypoxia, or trauma.

Duane's retraction syndrome is characterized by unilateral or bilateral abduction deficits, variable abnormalities of adduction, and globe retraction with consequent palpebral fissure narrowing on attempted adduction (Fig. 194–14).[244–250] Clinical findings are bilateral in about one fifth of patients. Most patients are female and the left eye is involved more often than the right. Visual abnormalities such as diplopia or amblyopia are surprisingly infrequent. Three types of Duane's retraction syndrome have been described[250]: type I demonstrates abnormal abduction with preserved adduction; type II consists of relatively normal abduction but limited adduction; type III involves abnormalities of both abduction and adduction. The likely cause of this syndrome is an anomaly of innervation involving the third and sixth nerves. The most common reported pathology is a congenital absence of abducens neurons with innervation of the lateral rectus muscle by branches of the oculomotor nerve.[251, 252] Interneurons within the sixth-nerve nucleus destined for the contralateral medial rectus subnucleus are spared. Retraction of the globe with consequent narrowing of the palpebral fissure in some cases reflects co-contraction of the lateral and medial recti on attempted adduction. Other congenital neurologic and skeletal abnormalities may occur in up to 50 percent of patients with Duane's syndrome.[248, 253–255]

Acquired

Because of the diffuse intermixing within the sixth-nerve nucleus of neuronal cell bodies that project to the ipsilateral abducens nerve and those whose axons are destined for the contralateral medial longitudinal fasciculus, lesions of the nucleus result in abnormalities of ipsilateral horizontal gaze. Furthermore, the close proximity of the facial nerve fascicle as it loops around the abducens nucleus frequently results in a peripheral facial palsy as part of the clinical picture. The causes of lesions of the abducens nucleus are the same as those associated with other intraparenchymal brain stem lesions, namely infarction; infiltration; hemorrhage; trauma; and neoplastic, infectious, or inflammatory compression (Table 194–5).[256–264] In addition, the presumed metabolic lesions

Table 194–5. ACQUIRED SIXTH-NERVE LESIONS

Location	Other Symptoms/ Signs	Common Causes
Nucleus	Horizontal gaze palsy, peripheral seventh-nerve dysfunction	Vascular occlusion Hemorrhage Neoplasm Inflammation Metabolic
Fascicles	Contralateral hemiparesis (Raymond's), contralateral hemiparesis, and ipsilateral seventh-nerve palsy (Millard-Gubler)	Vascular occlusion Hemorrhage Neoplasm Inflammation Demyelination
Subarachnoid space		Meningitis Increased ICP* Neoplasm Microvascular Trauma Dolichoectasia Aneurysm
Petrous ridge	Gradenigo's syndrome	Inflammation Infection Thrombosis Neoplasm Trauma
Cavernous sinus	May be isolated or first involved; 3rd, 4th, V1, V2, oculosympathetic dysfunction	Neoplasm Inflammation Aneurysm Microvascular thrombosis Arteriovenous fistula
Orbit	Rarely isolated	Neoplasm Inflammation Dental anesthesia

*ICP, intracranial pressure.

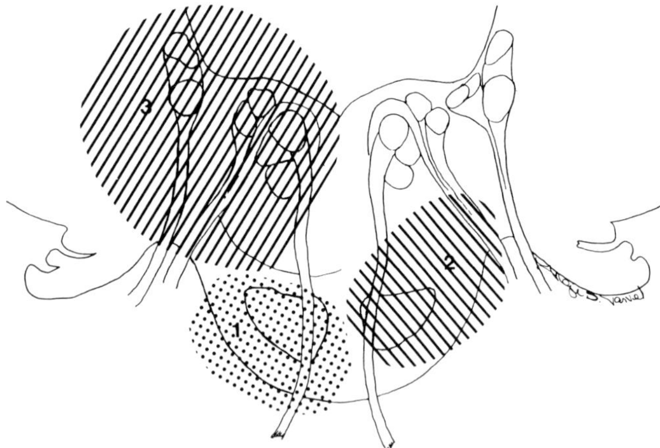

Figure 194–15. Cross section of the pons at the level of the abducens nerves depicting the location of lesions responsible for Raymond's syndrome (1), Millard-Gubler syndrome (2), and Foville's syndrome (3).

in Wernicke-Korsakoff syndrome are believed to involve the sixth-nerve nucleus.[265]

As with third-nerve palsies from fascicular injury, abducens nerve dysfunction secondary to involvement of the fascicle should be recognizable by the associated brain stem findings. Several specific syndromes reflecting particular localization have been described (Fig. 194–15). Foville's syndrome combines an abduction or horizontal gaze deficit with ipsilateral facial weakness, ipsilateral loss of taste, ipsilateral facial analgesia, ipsilateral Horner's syndrome, and ipsilateral deafness.[266] The structures affected are the abducens fascicle or nucleus, the facial nerve fascicle, the nucleus of the tractus solitarius, the spinal tract of the trigeminal nerve, the central tegmental tract, and the cochlear nuclei, respectively. If the lesion is located more ventrally in the pons, Raymond's syndrome or Millard-Gubler syndrome may be manifest. The former is a combination of sixth-nerve palsy and contralateral hemiplegia secondary to involvement of the abducens fascicle as it courses through the ipsilateral pyramidal tract.[267] Millard-Gubler syndrome combines an abduction deficit with contralateral hemiplegia and ipsilateral facial paralysis, implying involvement of the abducens fascicle, the pyramid, and the facial nerve fascicle.[268, 269] Modern imaging techniques have demonstrated that fascicular sixth-nerve damage may indeed be clinically isolated and indistinguishable from abducens nerve damage elsewhere along its course.[270, 271] The relative frequency of such an occurrence remains as yet undetermined. Causes of fascicular damage are the same as those listed for nuclear lesions, with the addition of demyelinating disease.[272, 273]

Abducens nerve lesions in the subarachnoid space may be isolated or associated with other peripheral cranial nerve involvement, unilateral or bilateral. Meningeal processes, including infectious, inflammatory, and neoplastic etiologies, may present with abduction deficits.[84, 92, 264, 274] Elevated intracranial pressure from any cause frequently results in unilateral or bilateral sixth-nerve palsies, presumably from nonspecific "stretching" of the nerves along their course between the pons and the petrous apex.[275–277] The same pathogenesis may be implicated in cases of abducens palsy following trauma, neurosurgical manipulation, cervical traction, and lumbar puncture.[96, 97, 214, 278–284] Tumors may involve the subarachnoid portion of the sixth nerve, either in isolation (e.g., with clivus chordomas, nasopharyngeal carcinomas, intrinsic neurinomas, and meningiomas) or with evidence of other neurologic abnormalities, as typically seen with exophytic intrinsic posterior fossa tumors or acoustic neuromas (Fig. 194–16).[285–287] Vascular compression of the nerve by dolichoectatic vessels is also possible.[288, 289] Although less common than third-nerve involvement, aneurysmal compression may result in a sixth-nerve palsy, almost always in association with a severe headache.[68a, 71, 290, 291]

Where the sixth nerve enters the dura above the clivus

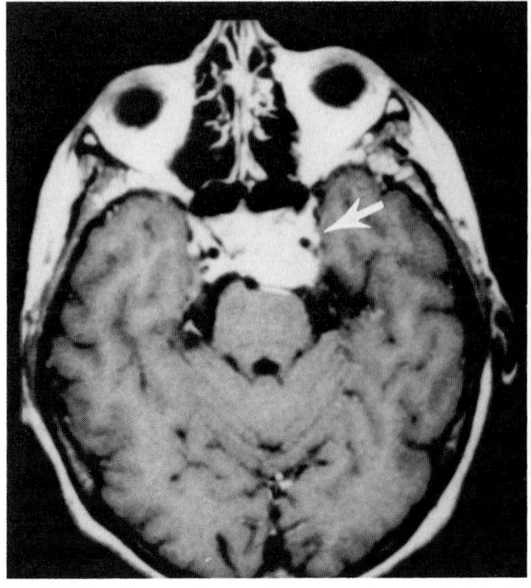
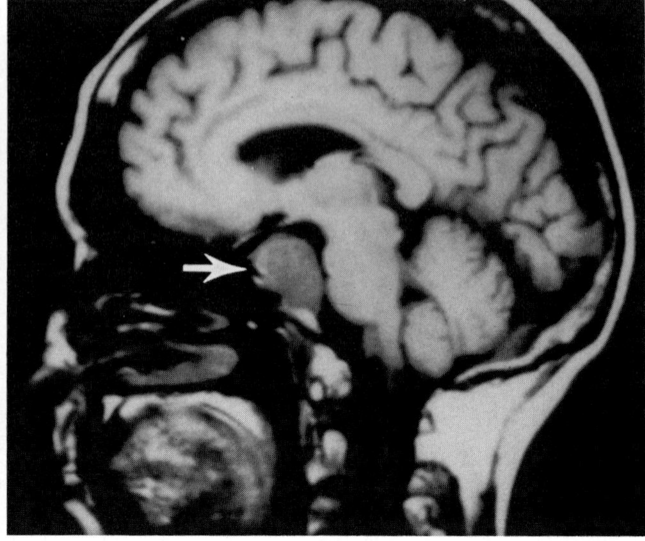

Figure 194–16. Axial *(left)* and sagittal *(right)* magnetic resonance images of the brain of a patient with bilateral sixth-nerve palsies. A clivus chordoma *(arrows)* is demonstrated.

and along the petrous ridge, it is susceptible to processes involving the adjacent mastoid air cells, such as mastoiditis. The resultant symptom complex, Gradenigo's syndrome, reflects inflammation in this region and consists of abducens palsy, severe facial and eye pain (from involvement of the adjacent gasserian ganglion), and sometimes facial paralysis.[292–295] Lateral sinus thrombosis with inferior petrosal sinus involvement or tumors along the petrous ridge may mimic this syndrome. This is presumably also the site of traumatic sixth-nerve palsies associated with basal skull fractures of the temporal bone.[126] The combination of abducens palsy and loss of tearing with or without involvement of the second division of the trigeminal nerve localizes the lesion to the sphenopalatine fossa. The cause is commonly metastatic tumor or nasopharyngeal carcinoma.[296]

In the cavernous sinus, the sixth nerve is susceptible to involvement by all the same processes mentioned earlier with regard to third- and fourth-nerve lesions in this location. The particular location of the abducens nerve floating relatively freely within the substance of the sinus rather than within a flap of dura, however, makes it frequently the first inhabitant of the cavernous sinus to be involved by any of these pathologic processes (see Fig. 194–4). This is particularly true when the cause of the lesion is vascular, such as carotid-cavernous fistulas, dural shunts, and intracavernous aneurysms.[297–300] Ischemia, inflammation, both infectious and noninfectious, and neoplasms may also involve the intracavernous sixth nerve, usually in association with other cranial nerve involvement.[117, 122, 301, 302] The combination of oculosympathetic dysfunction and ipsilateral abduction deficit is usually localized to the cavernous sinus, where the sympathetics anatomically run with the abducens nerve over a short course.[303–305]

Isolated orbital involvement of the abducens nerve is rare because of the relatively short course of the nerve prior to its innervation of the lateral rectus muscle. An orbital location of paralysis has been postulated for those sixth-nerve palsies occurring after dental anesthesia.[306, 307]

As with presumed ischemic lesions of the oculomotor and trochlear nerves, the exact location of isolated sixth-nerve palsies that occur in the setting of diabetes mellitus, hypertension, giant cell arteritis, or migraine remains unknown.[64, 66, 68, 308–311] It is probable that the majority of these lesions localize to the subarachnoid or intracavernous portion of the sixth nerve. As noted earlier, however, at least some of these ischemic lesions involve the fascicular, intraparenchymal nerve.[270, 271] The transient abducens palsy, which is seen especially in children, is presumed to be of viral or postinfectious origin and is also of indeterminant location.[293, 312–314]

Special Syndromes

Divergence weakness is characterized by acquired uncrossed horizontal diplopia at distance that resolves at a near range and is not worsened by horizontal gaze to either side.[315–318] It is frequently associated with entities that typically produce sixth-nerve palsies, such as elevated intracranial pressure, head trauma, meningeal processes, and intracranial mass lesions. Although it has been argued that this entity merely reflects early bilateral sixth-nerve palsies,[319, 320] the absence of worsening on horizontal gaze in either direction would suggest that this is not the case.[321] Evaluation and management should be the same as that for bilateral sixth-nerve palsies.

Management

Sixth-nerve palsies in conjunction with other cranial nerve or neurologic involvement require sophisticated neuroimaging, ideally MRI for a sensitive view of the brain stem and cavernous sinus (Table 194–6). Processes that localize to the subarachnoid space require cerebrospinal fluid analysis, including measurement of the opening pressure, and possibly cerebral angiography. If facial pain or numbness is an associated feature, immediate neuroimaging of the petrous ridge is appropriate.

An evaluation of the isolated, unilateral, nontraumatic abducens palsy depends on the age of the patient. In children with or without an antecedent viral illness or vaccination, observation alone is sufficient after careful neurologic assessment. Initially, an examination every 2 wk is necessary to determine if progression or additional neurologic involvement occurs. Similarly, in the elderly population, an isolated sixth-nerve paresis is likely to be ischemic in etiology and therefore ultimately transient and not indicative of underlying neurologic disease. A minimum work-up would include a glucose tolerance test (or serum glucose measurement in the already diagnosed diabetic), and an erythrocyte sedimentation rate, looking for evidence of giant cell arteritis. Even those isolated ischemic sixth-nerve palsies localized by MRI to the fascicular portion of the nerve usually recover, suggesting little prognostic importance in determining the exact location of these lesions. The initial evaluation of the young adult who presents with a truly isolated sixth-nerve palsy remains a controversial issue. Most clinicians obtain at least a neuroimage and

Table 194–6. EVALUATION OF SIXTH-NERVE DYSFUNCTION

Nonisolated		
Brain stem symptoms/signs	→	MRI
Meningeal symptoms/signs	→	MRI, LP
Orbital symptoms/signs	→	CT
Elevated ICP symptoms/signs	→	MRI, LP
Isolated		
< Age 15	→	close observation
< Age 40	→	CT/MRI, ± LP, ± Tensilon test, close observation
> Age 40	→	glucose, ESR, ± Tensilon test, close observation
Bilateral	→	MRI, LP

Key: CT, computed tomography; ESR, erythrocyte sedimentation rate; ICP, intracranial pressure; LP, lumbar puncture; MRI, magnetic resonance imaging.

possibly a lumbar puncture on these patients, although the majority of these work-ups prove to be negative. A thorough systemic and neurologic evaluation is mandatory. Bilateral sixth-nerve palsies suggest elevated intracranial pressure or a meningeal process and require neuroimaging. If the result is negative, lumbar puncture should be done.

Presumed ischemic abducens lesions generally resolve within 3 to 4 mo of onset. Similarly, the isolated sixth-nerve palsies in children usually completely recover within 4 mo.[312] These patients must be followed carefully to ensure nonprogression and continued clinical isolation. If at any time additional neurologic abnormalities develop, more extensive investigation should be pursued (see earlier). The chronic, isolated sixth-nerve palsy may reflect slow-growing basilar skull neoplasms, such as schwannomas or meningiomas.[301, 322–325] An abducens palsy that does not resolve by 6 mo requires a complete evaluation.

Simplest management for a sixth-nerve palsy is monocular occlusion, sometimes only over the portion of the temporal field in which horizontal diplopia occurs. Prisms are rarely helpful. After a sixth-nerve palsy has stabilized and underlying causes have been either ruled out or deemed nonprogressive, various surgical procedures can be performed to better align the eyes in primary position.[191, 326–328] Procedures usually involve resection of the lateral rectus muscle and recession of the poorly opposed medial rectus muscle. Transposition of the vertical recti may be necessary for the eye to be maintained in a straight position. Most surgeons prefer 6 to 12 mo of stable measurements before intervention.

The use of botulinum toxin in the treatment of abducens nerve palsies has added a new therapeutic option for transient symptomatic relief.[194, 329–332] The toxin is injected into the ipsilateral unopposed medial rectus muscle, thus reducing the tonic opposition to the weak lateral rectus and allowing for fusion. It is possible that the use of this treatment in acute lesions may reduce the tendency for fibrosis and contracture to develop, but at this time there is no randomized controlled study proving this. If used in acute lesions, one must be assured of the underlying diagnosis, because it is possible that botulinum toxin can mask progression and the involvement of other extraocular muscles. Botulinum toxin in chronic abducens palsy may provide an adjunct to muscle surgery.[331–333]

ABNORMALITIES OF MORE THAN ONE OCULAR MOTOR NERVE

A special situation exists when more than one ocular motor nerve is involved either unilaterally or bilaterally. Of primary importance is the exclusion of processes that may mimic neurogenic palsies, such as ocular myopathies and disorders of neuromuscular transmission. Once the problem has been diagnosed as multiple ocular motor nerve paralysis, localization is paramount. Common locations for multiple infranuclear nerve involvement are the subarachnoid space and the cavernous sinus/superior orbital fissure.

Although the brain stem contains all the ocular motor nerves and their nuclei, it would be difficult to have a pathologic process that involved the cranial nerves without also affecting the adjacent brain stem parenchyma with resultant disorders of supranuclear motility and neurologic motor and sensory dysfunction. There are rare reports of patients with severe amyotrophic lateral sclerosis who have abnormal ocular motility, possibly on the basis of lower ocular motor neuron degeneration, although supranuclear mechanisms may be primary.[334–336]

Meningeal disease, however, may affect multiple cranial nerves with minimal systemic or neurologic abnormality. Infectious and neoplastic seeding of the subarachnoid space can result in dysfunction of numerous cranial nerves, including the ocular motor nerves.[83, 84, 88, 92, 274, 337] Noninfectious inflammatory causes, such as neurosarcoidosis and Behçet's syndrome, have also been implicated.[338, 339] Head trauma with presumed shearing of multiple cranial nerves,[77, 96, 97, 126] base of the skull tumors, particularly along the clivus,[285, 340] and possibly dolichoectatic vasculature[289] may also result in a picture of multiple cranial neuropathies.

The anatomy of the cavernous sinus makes it a likely location of lesions resulting in multiple ocular motor nerve dysfunction. Traversing this paired trabeculated structure that flanks the sphenoid sinus and pituitary fossa are the third, fourth, and sixth cranial nerves, the first and, posteriorly, the second divisions of the trigeminal nerve, and the carotid artery with its surrounding sympathetic plexus (see Fig. 194–4). In close proximity is the pituitary gland medially within the sella turcica and the optic nerves and chiasm superiorly. Disease processes within or adjacent to the cavernous sinus can result in clinical syndromes reflecting dysfunction of various combinations of these structures, both unilateral and bilateral. To clinically distinguish cavernous sinus from superior orbital fissure syndromes is difficult and is of questionable value. The same structures continue forward into the fissure, and the disease processes usually do not respect any anatomic boundary.

Of the ocular motor nerves, the sixth nerve is probably affected most commonly by lesions intrinsic to the cavernous sinus because of its relatively free-floating position.[103, 117, 297–299] Because of its more superior position adjacent to the pituitary fossa, the third nerve may be the first to be involved with lateral expansion of tumors within the pituitary fossa.[106, 111, 113, 341–343] The combination of oculosympathetic and oculomotor nerve dysfunction may result in a small or midsized, poorly reactive pupil.[105, 344] Blockage of venous outflow can cause proptosis, ocular chemosis, and infection.[108, 121, 123, 345–347] There may be concurrent visual loss and visual field defects localizing to the optic chiasm or posterior optic nerves.[106, 113, 341–343] Pain is a common manifestation of cavernous sinus disease and likely reflects involvement of the trigeminal nerve.[122]

It is misleading, however, to think of "painful ophthalmoplegia" as a separate clinical entity with specific etiologic significance. At best, there is some localizing value of this symptom complex to the cavernous sinus/parasellar/superior orbital fissure region, although

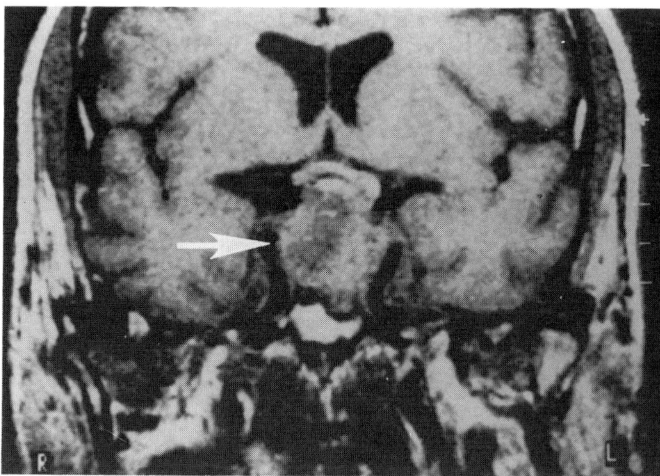

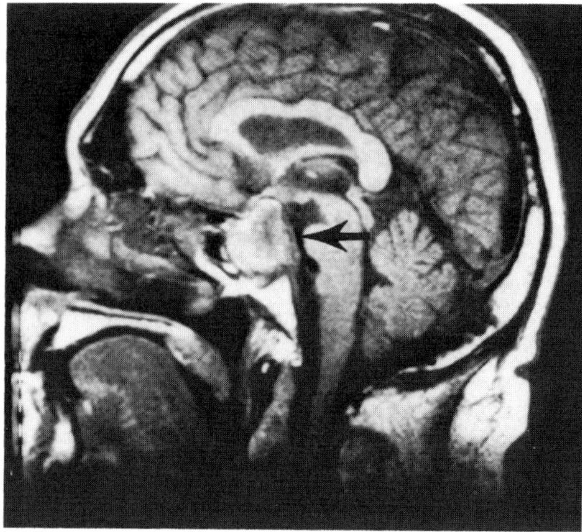

Figure 194–17. Coronal *(left)* and sagittal *(right)* magnetic resonance images of the brain of a patient with pituitary apoplexy. The patient presented with headache and with complete ptosis and ophthalmoplegia on the left. MRI revealed a large pituitary tumor with areas of inhomogeneous intensity that were suggestive of previous hemorrhage *(arrows)*.

orbital, meningeal, and even posterior fossa disease may present in a similar fashion. With regard to etiology, inflammatory, infiltrative, neoplastic, and vascular disease can all result in nonspecific painful ophthalmoplegia.

The disease processes that can involve the cavernous sinus are many and varied. They fall into three major categories: neoplasms, vascular lesions, and inflammation. In all three, the lesions may result from disease intrinsic to the sinus or from compression or extension from adjacent structures. Lateral extension of pituitary adenomas may result from either tumor growth or sudden expansion from pituitary apoplexy (Fig. 194–17).[106, 113, 341–343, 348, 349] Meningiomas, craniopharyngiomas, nasopharyngeal carcinomas, and metastatic tumors comprise the other common neoplasms in this region.[103, 106, 111, 350–357] Schwannomas within the sinus usually originate from branches of the trigeminal nerve, although the ocular motor nerves are rarely implicated.[358]

Vascular lesions within the cavernous sinus include aneurysms, arteriovenous fistulas, and venous thrombosis. The last two commonly result in bilateral clinical manifestations. Aneurysms within the sinus are frequently large upon presentation and cause much of their dysfunction by compression of adjacent structures.[103, 111, 359–363] The risk of catastrophic rupture is less than with cerebral aneurysms outside the cavernous sinus because of the enclosed nature of the sinus.[103, 364] Fistulas may be high-flow, as seen with direct communication of the carotid artery with venous blood within the sinus,[108, 121, 298, 299, 345–347] or low-flow, as seen with dural shunts in which small arteries feeding the dura communicate with the sinus directly.[297, 365–367] The former are usually secondary to trauma and can present quite a dramatic clinical picture of severe proptosis, chemosis, infection, ophthalmoplegia, visual loss, and bruit (Fig. 194–18). Superior ophthalmic veins are prominent on contrast-enhanced CT scanning (Fig. 194–19). The low-flow shunts occur spontaneously, usually in elderly women. Their clinical presentation depends on the particular direction of venous drainage: If anterior, they may have many findings similar to those seen with carotid-cavernous fistulas,

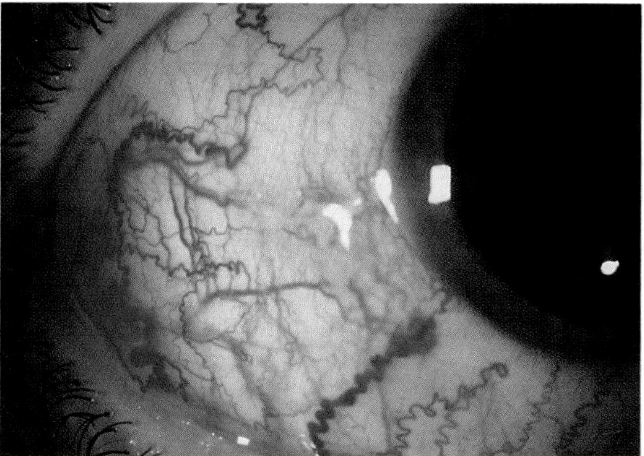

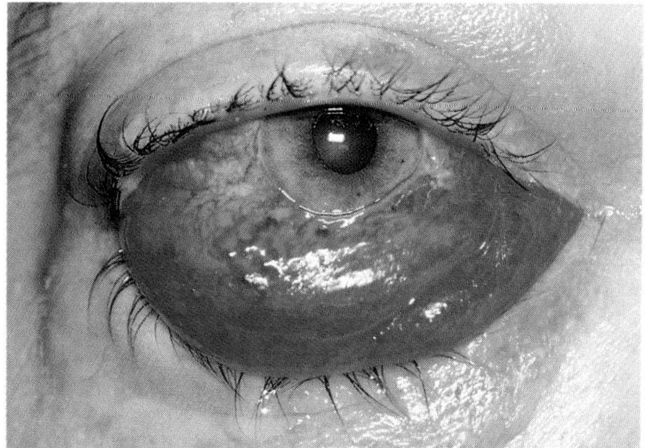

Figure 194–18. Conjunctival appearance in patients with carotid-cavernous fistulas. The eye on the left illustrates the arterialization of conjunctival vessels with the characteristic corkscrew appearance. The patient whose eye appears on the right had a traumatic fistula with resultant severe chemosis and proptosis.

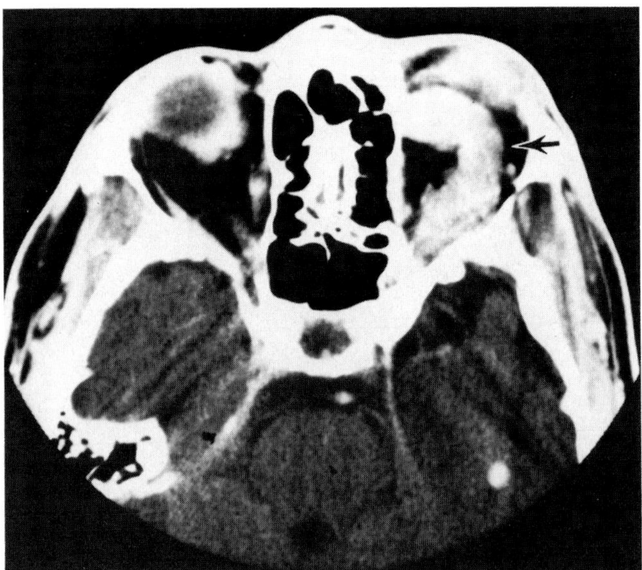

Figure 194–19. CT scan of a severely enlarged superior ophthalmic vein *(arrow)*.

although usually less severe; if posterior, isolated ocular motor nerve palsies without other ocular signs may result.[124] Cavernous sinus thrombosis presents with a clinical picture similar to carotid-cavernous fistulas, but the patients commonly have prominent systemic manifestations of sepsis.[123, 368–370] Paranasal sinus and local skin infections are the most frequent cause. Fungal infections, such as mucormycosis and aspergillus, may mimic cavernous sinus thrombosis, because their pathogenesis probably also involves some element of thrombophlebitis and obstruction of venous outflow.[371–374]

Inflammation within the cavernous sinus may result from infectious causes or be idiopathic. Ophthalmoplegia associated with herpes zoster infection may be localized to the cavernous sinus. The third, fourth, and sixth nerves may be involved, either isolated or in combination, and frequently to partial degree.[127, 375] In the Tolosa-Hunt syndrome, nonspecific, noninfectious granulomatous inflammation results in hemicranial or periorbital pain associated with ipsilateral ophthalmoplegia of any or all of the ocular motor nerves.[107, 109, 111, 116, 120, 122, 376] Sensory loss in the distribution of the ipsilateral ophthalmic or maxillary division of the trigeminal nerve and oculosympathetic paralysis may also be present. Typically, there is a dramatic response of symptoms and signs to corticosteroid therapy, enough to prompt some clinicians to suggest a trial of corticosteroids as a diagnostic test.[377] However, several authors have since emphasized the nonspecificity of steroid responsiveness in the painful parasellar syndrome and have reported cases of steroid-sensitive cavernous sinus syndromes secondary to neoplasms and aneurysms.[111, 114, 115, 118, 120, 122, 357]

The Guillain-Barré syndrome typically presents as an ascending motor paresis affecting limb, respiratory, and bulbar musculature, secondary to a peripheral polyneuropathy.[99, 101, 101a, 378–383] On occasion, the ocular motor nerves may be involved. A variant of this disorder, described by C. Miller Fisher, presents with multiple ocular motor nerve palsies, areflexia, and limb ataxia.[100, 101a, 384, 385] As with all cases of Guillain-Barré syndrome, there should be fewer than 5 to 10 white blood cells within the cerebrospinal fluid, and the protein is eventually elevated after 1 to 2 wk. The patient may report an antecedent viral illness. The actual location of the pathology in the Miller Fisher syndrome has been a matter of some debate, and both peripheral and central nervous system involvement have been proposed.[101a, 384, 386–392] In any of the variants of Guillain-Barré syndrome, there may be rapid deterioration to respirator dependency.

Acute botulism, typically secondary to the ingestion of food contaminated with *Clostridium botulinum*, results in a flaccid paresis, swallowing problems, pupillary dilatation and poor reactivity, and various degrees of ophthalmoparesis.[393–395] The toxin blocks transmission at cholinergic synapses. Cutaneous squamous cell carcinoma of the face may cause multiple cranial nerve involvement, with ophthalmoplegia as a result of perineural spread.[125, 396]

Management

The patient with multiple ocular motor nerve palsies should be carefully evaluated neurologically, ophthalmologically, and systemically for any associated findings that may help to localize and characterize the underlying pathology. If the brain stem, intracranial, or cavernous sinus regions are suspect, neuroimaging, specifically MRI, should be performed. CT scanning may be helpful in detecting orbital lesions, skull base tumors, and orbital venous outflow abnormalities. If the process has resulted in a painful parasellar syndrome and neuroimaging does not provide a definitive diagnosis, cerebral angiography should be performed of both the anterior and posterior circulations in search for an aneurysm. Cerebrospinal fluid analysis is indicated if signs and symptoms suggest a process in the subarachnoid space, or if the Miller Fisher syndrome is suspected.

Management of multiple ocular motor nerve palsies depends entirely on the underlying pathology. Treatment of neoplastic and infectious diseases is guided by the nature of the process and its location. In addition to antimicrobial therapy, anticoagulation may be used in the treatment of cavernous sinus thrombosis.[123, 369, 370] Arteriovenous communications can be treated with selective vessel occlusion by the angiographically guided placement of balloons or occluding substances or with ipsilateral carotid occlusion.[121, 397–401] Many dural shunts close off spontaneously, especially after angiography, and therapy may be best reserved for patients with medically unmanageable elevated intraocular pressure, visual loss, progressive ischemia to the retina or anterior segment of the eye, intractable diplopia, or an unacceptable level of discomfort.[365, 366, 400, 402] If other causes of the painful parasellar syndrome have been excluded, the Tolosa-Hunt syndrome may be treated with steroids.[122] This diagnosis must be periodically reconsidered, especially if new signs or symptoms appear in the patient. Treatment of the variants of the Guillain-Barré syndrome is typically supportive, although plasmapheresis has been shown to shorten the course and reduce the severity of the disease if performed early in its course.[403]

REFERENCES

1. Warwick RJ: Representation of the extraocular muscles in the oculomotor nuclei of the monkey. J Comp Neurol 98:449, 1953.
2. Büttner-Ennever JA, Akert K: Medial rectus subgroups of the oculomotor nucleus and their abducens internuclear input in the monkey. J Comp Neurol 197:17, 1981.
3. Büttner-Ennever JA, Grob P, Akert K: A transsynaptic autoradiographic study of the pathways controlling the extraocular eye muscles using [125I]B-IIb tetanus toxin fragment. Ann N Y Acad Sci 374:157, 1981.
4. Porter JD, Guthrie BL, Sparks DL: Innervation of monkey extraocular muscles: Localization of sensory and motor neurons by retrograde transport of horseradish peroxidase. J Comp Neurol 218:208, 1983.
5. Burde RM, Loewy AD: Central origin of oculomotor parasympathetic neurons in the monkey. Brain Res 193:434, 1980.
6. Bienfang DC: Crossing axons in the third nerve nucleus. Invest Ophthalmol 14:927, 1975.
7. Destombes J, Horcholle-Bossavit G, Rouviere A: Données récentes concernant le noyau oculomoteur externe: Centre du mouvement oculaire horizontal. J Fr Ophtalmol 6:605, 1983.
8. Harris FS, Rhoton AL Jr: Anatomy of the cavernous sinus: A microsurgical study. J Neurosurg 45:169, 1976.
9. Umansky F, Nathan H: The lateral wall of the cavernous sinus: With special reference to the nerves related to it. J Neurosurg 56:228, 1982.
10. Fincham EF: Monocular diplopia. Br J Ophthalmol 47:705, 1963.
11. Records RE: Perspectives in refraction: Monocular diplopia. Surv Ophthalmol 24:303, 1980.
12. Amos JF: Diagnosis and management of monocular diplopia. J Am Optom Assoc 53:101, 1982.
13. Hirst LW, Miller NR, Johnson RT: Monocular polyopia. Arch Neurol 40:756, 1983.
14. Coffeen P, Guyton DL: Monocular diplopia accompanying ordinary refractive errors. Am J Ophthalmol 105:451, 1988.
15. Bender MB: Polyopia and monocular diplopia of cerebral origin. Arch Neurol 54:323, 1945.
16. Kinsbourne M, Warrington EK: A study of visual perservation. J Neurol Neurosurg Psychiatr 26:468, 1963.
17. Meadows JC: Observations on a case of monocular diplopia of cerebral origin. J Neurol Sci 18:249, 1973.
18. Safran AB, Kline LB, Glaser JS, et al: Television-induced formed visual hallucinations and cerebral diplopia. Br J Ophthalmol 65:707, 1981.
19. Payne JW, Adamkiewicz J Jr: Unilateral ophthalmoplegia with intracrania aneurysm: Report of a case. Am J Ophthalmol 68:349, 1969.
20. Crompton JL, Moore CE: Painful third nerve palsy: How not to miss an intracranial aneurysm. Aust J Ophthalmol 9:113, 1981.
21. Martin XY, Safran AB: Corneal hypoesthesia. Surv Ophthalmol 33:28, 1988.
22. Norman MG: Unilateral encephalomalacia in cranial nerve nuclei in neonates: Report of two cases. Neurology 24:424, 1974.
23. Miller NR: Solitary oculomotor nerve palsy in childhood. Am J Ophthalmol 83:106, 1977.
24. Mellinger JF, Gomez MR: Agenesis of the cranial nerves. *In* Vinken PJ, Bruyn GW (eds): Handbook of Clinical Neurology, vol 30, part 1. New York, Elsevier, 1977, pp 395–414.
25. Victor DI: The diagnosis of congenital unilateral third-nerve palsy. Brain 99:711, 1976.
26. Balkan R, Hoyt CS: Associated neurologic abnormalities in congenital third nerve palsies. Am J Ophthalmol 97:315, 1984.
27. Hamed LM: Associated neurologic and ophthalmologic findings in congenital oculomotor nerve palsy. Ophthalmology 98:708, 1991.
28. Harley RD: Paralytic strabismus in children: Etiologic incidence and management of the third, fourth, and sixth nerve palsies. Ophthalmology 86:24, 1980.
29. Keith CG: Oculomotor nerve palsy in childhood. Aust N Z J Ophthalmol 15:181, 1987.
30. Flanders M, Watters G, Draper J, et al: Bilateral congenital third cranial nerve palsy. Can J Ophthalmol 24:28, 1989.
31. Pierrot-Deseilligny C, Schaison M, Bousser MG, Brunet P: Syndrome nucléaire du nerf moteur oculaire commun: à propos de deux observations cliniques. Rev Neurol 137:217, 1981.
32. Bogousslavsky J, Regli F, Ghika J, et al: Internuclear ophthalmoplegia, prenuclear paresis of contralateral superior rectus, and bilateral ptosis. J Neurol 230:197, 1984.
33. Bogousslavsky J, Regli F: Atteinte intra-axiale du nerf moteur oculaire commun dans les infarctus mésencéphaliques. Rev Neurol 140:263, 1984.
34. Biller J, Shapiro R, Evans LS, Haag JR, Fine M: Oculomotor nuclear complex infarction: Clinical and radiological correlation. Arch Neurol 41:985, 1984.
35. Elliot RL: Encephalitis with ophthalmoplegia. Confin Neurol 31:194, 1969.
36. Keane JR, Zaias B, Itabashi HH: Levator-sparing oculomotor nerve palsy caused by a solitary midbrain metastasis. Arch Neurol 14:210, 1984.
36a. Bryan JS, Mamed LM: Levator-sparing nuclear oculomotor palsy. Clinical and magnetic resonance imaging findings. J Clin Neuro Ophthalmol 12:26, 1992.
37. Stevenson GC, Hoyt WF: Metastasis to midbrain from mammary carcinoma: Cause of bilateral ptosis and ophthalmoplegia. JAMA 186:514, 1963.
38. Growdon JH, Winkler GF, Wray SH: Midbrain ptosis: A case with clinicopathologic correlation. Arch Neurol 30:179, 1974.
39. Meienberg O, Mumenthaler M, Karbowski K: Quadriparesis and nuclear oculomotor palsy with total bilateral ptosis mimicking coma: A mesencephalic "locked-in syndrome"? Arch Neurol 36:708, 1979.
40. Conway VH, Rozdilsky B, Schneider RJ, Sundaram M: Isolated bilateral complete ptosis. Can J Ophthalmol 18:37, 1983.
41. Kubik CS, Adams RD: Occlusion of the basilar artery: A clinical and pathological study. Brain 69:73, 1946.
42. Masucci EF: Bilateral ophthalmoplegia in basilar-vertebral artery disease. Brain 88:97, 1965.
43. Caplan LR: "Top of the basilar" syndrome. Neurology 30:72, 1980.
44. Mehler MF: The neuro-ophthalmologic spectrum of the rostral basilar artery syndrome. Arch Neurol 45:966, 1988.
45. Durward QJ, Barnett HJM, Barr HWK: Presentation and management of mesencephalic hematoma: Report of two cases. J Neurosurg 56:123, 1982.
46. Dierssen G, Trigueros F, Sanz F, et al: Surgical treatment of a mesencephalic tuberculoma: Case report. J Neurosurg 49:753, 1978.
47. Nothnagel H: Topische Diagnostik der Gehirnkrankheiten. Berlin. A. Hirschwald, 1879.
48. Benedikt M: Tremblement avec paralysie croisée du moteur oculaire commun. Bull Med 3:547, 1889.
49. Weber HD: A contribution to the pathology of the crura cerebri. Med Chirurg Trans 28:121, 1865.
50. Wilkins DE, Samhouri AM: Isolated bilateral oculomotor paresis due to lymphoma. Neurology 29:1425, 1979.
51. Guy J, Savino PJ, Schatz NJ, et al: Superior division paresis of the oculomotor nerve. Ophthalmology 92:777, 1985.
52. Ksiazek SM, Repka MX, Maguire A, et al: Divisional oculomotor nerve paresis caused by intrinsic brain stem disease. Ann Neurol 26:714, 1989.
53. Castro O, Johnson LN, Mamourian AC: Isolated inferior oblique paresis from brain stem infarction: Perspective on oculomotor fascicular organization in the ventral midbrain tegmentum. Arch Neurol 47:235, 1990.
54. Hopf HC, Gutmann L: Diabetic 3rd nerve palsy: Evidence for a mesencephalic lesion. Neurology 40:1041, 1990.
55. Breen LA, Hopf HC, Farris BK, et al: Pupil-sparing oculomotor

nerve palsy due to midbrain infarction. Arch Neurol 48:105, 1991.
56. Wilson WB, Sharpe JA, Deck JHN: Cerebral blindness and oculomotor nerve palsies in toxoplasmosis. Am J Ophthalmol 89:714, 1980.
57. Loseke N, Retif J, Noterman J, et al: Inferior red nucleus syndrome (Benedikt's syndrome) due to a single intramesencephalic metastasis from a prostatic carcinoma: Case report. Acta Neurochirurg 56:59, 1981.
58. Bogousslavsky J, Regli F: Nuclear and prenuclear syndromes of the oculomotor nerve. Neuro-ophthalmology 3:211, 1983.
59. Antworth MV, Beck RW: Third nerve palsy as a presenting sign of acquired immune deficiency syndrome. J Clin Neuro Ophthalmol 7(3):125, 1987.
60. Newman NJ, Lessell S: Isolated pupil-sparing third-nerve palsy as the presenting sign of multiple sclerosis. Arch Neurol 47:817, 1990.
61. Galer BS, Lipton RB, Weinstein S, et al: Apoplectic headache and oculomotor nerve palsy: An unusual presentation of multiple sclerosis. Neurology 40:1465, 1990.
62. Sunderland S, Hughes ESR: The pupillo-constrictor pathway and the nerves to the ocular muscles in man. Brain 69:301, 1946.
63. Kerr FWL, Hollowell OW: Location of pupillomotor and accommodation fibers in the oculomotor nerve: Experimental observations on paralytic mydriasis. J Neurol Neurosurg Psychiatry 27:473, 1964.
64. Rucker CW: Paralysis of the third, fourth, and sixth cranial nerves. Am J Ophthalmol 46:787, 1958.
65. Green WR, Hackett ER, Schlezinger NS: Neuro-ophthalmologic evaluation of oculomotor nerve paralysis. Arch Ophthalmol 72:154, 1964.
66. Rucker CW: The causes of paralysis of the third, fourth and sixth cranial nerves. Am J Ophthalmol 61:1293, 1966.
67. Soni SR: Aneurysms of the posterior communicating artery and oculomotor paresis. J Neurol Neurosurg Psychiatry 37:475, 1974.
68. Rush JA, Younge BR: Paralysis of cranial nerves III, IV, and VI: Cause and prognosis in 1000 cases. Arch Ophthalmol 99:76, 1981.
68a. Richards BW, Jones FR, Younge BR: Causes and prognosis in 4,278 cases of paralysis of the oculomotor, trochlear, and abducens cranial nerves. Am J Ophthalmol 113:489, 1992.
68b. Berlit P: Isolated and combined pareses of cranial nerves III, IV and VI. A retrospective study of 412 patients. J Neurol Sci 103:10, 1991.
69. Huige WM, van-Vliet AG, Bastiaensen LA: Early symptoms of subarachnoid haemorrhage due to aneurysms of the posterior communicating artery. Doc Ophthalmol 70:251, 1988.
70. Trobe JD, Glaser JS, Quencer RC: Isolated oculomotor paralysis: The product of saccular and fusiform aneurysms of the basilar artery. Arch Ophthalmol 96:1236, 1978.
71. McKinna AJ: Eye signs in 611 cases of posterior fossa aneurysms: Their diagnostic and prognostic value. Can J Ophthalmol 18:3, 1983.
72. Boccardo M, Ruelle A, Banchero MA: Isolated oculomotor palsy caused by aneurysm of the basilar artery bifurcation. J Neurol 233:61, 1986.
73. Lustbader JM, Miller NR: Painless, pupil-sparing but otherwise complete oculomotor nerve paresis caused by basilar artery aneurysm. Arch Ophthalmol 106:583, 1988.
74. Goldstein JE, Cogan DG: Diabetic ophthalmoplegia with special reference to the pupil. Arch Ophthalmol 64:592, 1960.
75. Johnson RT, Yates PO: Clinico-pathological aspects of pressure changes at the tentorium. Acta Radiol 46:242, 1956.
76. Keefe WP, Rucker CW, Kernohan JW: Pathogenesis of paralysis of the third cranial nerve. Arch Ophthalmol 63:585, 1960.
77. Heinze J: Cranial nerve avulsion and other neural injuries in road accidents. Med J Aust 2:1246, 1969.
78. Weber RB, Daroff RB, Mackey EA: Pathology of oculomotor nerve palsy in diabetics. Neurology 20:835, 1970.
79. Memon MY, Paine KWE: Direct injury of the oculomotor nerve in craniocerebral trauma. J Neurosurg 35:461, 1971.
80. Eyster EF, Hoyt WF, Wilson CB: Oculomotor palsy from minor head trauma: An initial sign of basal intracranial tumor. JAMA 220:1083, 1972.
81. Kass MA, Keltner JL, Gay AJ: Total third nerve paralysis: Recovery in a case of meningococcic meningitis. Arch Ophthalmol 87:107, 1972.
82. Hopkins EW, Poser CM: Posterior cerebral artery ectasia: An unusual cause of ophthalmoplegia. Arch Neurol 29:279, 1973.
83. Little JR, Dale AJD, Okazaki H: Meningeal carcinomatosis: Clinical manifestations. Arch Neurol 30:138, 1974.
84. Olson ME, Chernik NL, Posner JB: Infiltration of the leptomeninges by systemic cancer: A clinical and pathologic study. Arch Neurol 30:122, 1974.
85. Scotti G: Internal carotid origin of a tortuous posterior cerebral artery: A cause of ophthalmoplegia. Arch Neurol 31:273, 1974.
86. Caplan LR, Zervas NT: Survival with permanent midbrain dysfunction after surgical treatment of traumatic subdural hematoma: The clinical picture of a Duret hemorrhage? Ann Neurol 1:587, 1977.
87. Jordan K, Marino J, Damast M: Bilateral oculomotor paralysis due to neurosyphilis. Ann Neurol 3:90, 1978.
88. Carroll WM, Mastaglia FL: Optic neuropathy and ophthalmoplegia in herpes zoster oticus. Neurology 29:726, 1979.
89. Rush JA, Kramer LD: Biopsy-negative cranial arteritis with complete oculomotor nerve palsy. Ann Ophthalmol 11:209, 1979.
90. Lesser RL, Simon RM, Leon H, et al: Cryptococcal meningitis and internal ophthalmoplegia. Am J Ophthalmol 87:682, 1979.
91. Lesser RL, Geehr RB, Higgins DD, et al: Ocular motor paralysis and arachnoid cyst. Arch Ophthalmol 98:1993, 1980.
92. Swaminathan TR, Kalyanaraman S, Narendran P: Ocular manifestations of central nervous system tuberculosis correlated with CT scan findings. *In* Henkind P (ed): ACTA: XXIV International Congress of Ophthalmology. Philadelphia, JB Lippincott, 1982, pp 841–845.
93. Leunda G, Vasquero J, Cabezudo J, et al: Schwannoma of the oculomotor nerves: Report of four cases. J Neurosurg 57:563, 1982.
94. Nadeau SE, Trobe JD: Pupil sparing in oculomotor palsy: A brief review. Ann Neurol 13:143, 1983.
95. Durand JR, Samples JR: Dolichoectasia and cranial nerve palsies: A case report. J Clin Neuro Ophthalmol 9:249, 1989.
96. Keane JR: Neurologic eye signs following motorcycle accidents. Arch Neurol 46:761, 1989.
97. Adam T, Schumacher M: Traumatic lesions of the optic, oculomotor, trochlear, and abducens nerves—computer tomographic findings. Neurosurg Rev 11:231, 1988.
98. Baker AB: Guillain-Barré's disease (encephalomyelo-radiculitis): A review of 33 cases. Lancet 63:384, 1943.
99. Haymaker W, Kernohan JW: The Landry-Guillain-Barré syndrome: A clinicopathologic report of 50 fatal cases and a critique of the literature. Medicine 28:59, 1949.
100. Fisher CM: An unusual variant of acute idiopathic polyneuritis (syndrome of ophthalmoplegia, ataxia and areflexia). N Engl J Med 255:57, 1956.
101. Munsat TL, Barnes JE: Relation of multiple cranial nerve dysfunction to the Guillain-Barré syndrome. J Neurol Neurosurg Psychiatry 28:115, 1965.
101a. Berlit P, Rakicky J: The Miller Fisher syndrome. Review of the literature. J Clin Neuro Ophthalmol 12:57, 1992.
102. Susac JO, Hoyt WF: Inferior branch palsy of the oculomotor nerve. Ann Neurol 2:336, 1977.
103. Trobe JD, Glaser JS, Post JD: Meningiomas and aneurysms of the cavernous sinus: Neuro-ophthalmologic features. Arch Ophthalmol 96:457, 1978.
104. Guy JR, Day AL: Intracranial aneurysms with superior division paresis of the oculomotor nerve. Ophthalmology 96:1071, 1989.
105. Meadows SP: Intracavernous aneurysms of the internal carotid artery: Their clinical features and natural history. Arch Ophthalmol 62:566, 1959.
106. Jefferson G: The Bowman lecture: Concerning injuries, aneurysms, and tumors involving the cavernous sinus. Trans Ophthalmol Soc UK 73:117, 1953.
107. Tolosa E: Periarteritic lesions of the carotid siphon with the clinical features of a carotid infraclinoid aneurysm. J Neurol Neurosurg Psychiatry 17:300, 1954.
108. Henderson JW, Schneider RC: The ocular findings in carotid-cavernous fistula in a series of 17 cases. Am J Ophthalmol 48:585, 1959.
109. Hunt WE, Meager JN, LeFever HE, et al: Painful ophthalmo-

plegia: Its relation to indolent inflammation of the cavernous sinus. Neurology 11:56, 1961.
110. Thomas JE, Waltz AG: Neurological manifestations of nasopharyngeal malignant tumors. JAMA 192:95, 1965.
111. Thomas JE, Yoss RE: The parasellar syndrome: Problems in determining etiology. Mayo Clin Proc 45:617, 1970.
112. Asbury AK, Aldredge H, Hershberg R, Fisher CM: Oculomotor palsy in diabetes mellitus: A clinical-pathological study. Brain 93:555, 1970.
113. Hollenhorst RW, Younge BR: Ocular manifestations produced by adenomas of the pituitary gland: Analysis of 1000 cases. *In* Kohler PO, Ross GT (eds): Diagnosis and Treatment of Pituitary Tumors. New York, Elsevier, 1973, pp 53–64.
114. Fowler TJ, Earl CJ, McAllister VL, et al: Tolosa-Hunt syndrome: The dangers of an eponym. Br J Ophthalmol 59:149, 1975.
115. Hunt WE: Tolosa-Hunt syndrome: One cause of painful ophthalmoplegia. J Neurosurg 44:544, 1976.
116. Lenzi GL, Fieschi C: Superior orbital fissure syndrome: Review of 130 cases. Eur Neurol 16:23, 1977.
117. Neetens A, Selosse P: Oculomotor anomalies in sellar and parasellar pathology. Ophthalmologica 175:80, 1977.
118. Coppeto JR, Hoffman H: Tolosa-Hunt syndrome with proptosis mimicked by giant aneurysm of posterior cerebral artery. Arch Neurol 38:54, 1981.
119. Kline LB, Galbraith JG: Parasellar epidermoid tumor presenting as painful ophthalmoplegia. J Neurosurg 54:113, 1981.
120. Salomez JL, Rousseaux M, Petit H, et al: L'ophtalmoplégie douloureuse de Tolosa-Hunt: Limites du syndrome. Rev Otoneuroophtalmol 53:463, 1981.
121. Debrun G, Lacour P, Venuela F, et al: Treatment of 54 traumatic carotid-cavernous fistulas. J Neurosurg 55:678, 1981.
122. Kline LB: The Tolosa-Hunt syndrome. Surv Ophthalmol 27:79, 1982.
123. Clifford-Jones RE, Ellis CJK, Stevens JM, Turner A: Cavernous sinus thrombosis. J Neurol Neurosurg Psychiatry 45:1092, 1982.
124. Hawke SHB, Mullie MA, Hoyt WF, et al: Painful oculomotor nerve palsy due to dural-cavernous sinus shunt. Arch Neurol 46:1252, 1989.
125. Moore CE, Hoyt WF, North JB: Painful ophthalmoplegia following treated squamous cell carcinoma of the forehead: Orbital apex involvement from centripetal spread via the supraorbital nerve. Med J Aust 1:657, 1976.
126. Van Vliet AGM: Post-traumatic ocular imbalance. *In* Vinken PJ, Bruyn GW (eds): Handbook of Clinical Neurology. New York, Elsevier, 1976, pp 73–104.
127. Kattah JC, Kennerdell JS: Orbital apex syndrome secondary to herpes zoster ophthalmicus. Am J Ophthalmol 85:378, 1978.
128. Rootman J, Goldberg C, Robertson W: Primary orbital schwannomas. Br J Ophthalmol 66:194, 1982.
129. Fleet WS, Rapcsak SZ, Huntley WW, et al: Pupil-sparing oculomotor palsy from midbrain hemorrhage. Ann Ophthalmol 20:345, 1988.
130. Alpers BJ, Yaskin HE: Pathogenesis of ophthalmoplegic migraine. Arch Ophthalmol 45:555, 1951.
131. Ver Brugghen A: Pathogenesis of ophthalmoplegic migraine. Neurology 5:311, 1955.
132. Walsh JP, O'Doherty DS: Explanation of the mechanism of ophthalmoplegic migraine. Neurology 10:1079, 1960.
133. Hollenhorst RW, Brown JR, Wagner HV, et al: Neurologic aspects of temporal arteritis. Neurology (Minneap) 10:490, 1960.
134. Friedman AP, Harter DH, Merritt HH: Ophthalmoplegic migraine. Arch Neurol 7:320, 1962.
135. Johnson RT, Richardson EP: The neurological manifestations of systemic lupus erythematosus: A clinical-pathological study of 24 cases and review of the literature. Medicine 47:337, 1968.
136. Meadows SP: Temporal or giant cell arteritis: Ophthalmic aspects. *In* Smith JL (ed): Neuro-ophthalmology, vol 4. St. Louis, CV Mosby, 1968, pp 178–189.
137. Vijayan N: Ophthalmoplegic migraine: Ischemic or compressive neuropathy? Headache 20:300, 1980.
138. Graham E, Holland A, Avery A, et al: Prognosis in giant-cell arteritis. Br Med J 282:269, 1981.
139. Sergott RC, Glaser JS, Berger LJ: Simultaneous, bilateral diabetic ophthalmoplegia: Report of two cases and discussion of differential diagnosis. Ophthalmology 91:18, 1984.
140. Teuscher AU, Meienberg O: Ischaemic oculomotor nerve palsy: Clinical features and vascular risk factors in 23 patients. J Neurol 232:144, 1985.
141. Bregman DK, Harbour R: Diabetic superior division oculomotor nerve palsy. Arch Ophthalmol 106:1169, 1988.
142. Katz N, Rimmer S: Ophthalmoplegic migraine with superior ramus oculomotor paresis. J Clin Neuro Ophthalmol 9:181, 1989.
143. Rosenstein ED, Sobelman J, Kramer N: Isolated, pupil-sparing third nerve palsy as initial manifestation of systemic lupus erythematosus. J Clin Neuro Ophthalmol 9:285, 1989.
144. Hertenstein JR, Sarnat HB, O'Connor DM: Acute unilateral oculomotor palsy associates with ECHO 9 viral infection. J Pediatr 89:79, 1976.
145. Salazar A, Martinez H, Sotelo J: Ophthalmoplegic polyneuropathy associated with infectious mononucleosis. Ann Neurol 13:219, 1983.
146. Boghen D: Pupil sparing oculomotor palsy. Ann Neurol 14:698, 1983.
147. Trobe JD: Isolated pupil-sparing third nerve palsy. Ophthalmology 92:58, 1985.
148. Trobe JD: Third nerve palsy and the pupil: Footnotes to the rule. [Editorial] Arch Ophthalmol 106:601, 1988.
149. Dreyfus P, Hakim S, Adams R: Diabetic ophthalmoplegia. Arch Neurol 77:337, 1957.
150. Henderson JW: Intracranial arterial aneurysms. Trans Am Ophthalmol Soc 54:349, 1955.
151. Cogan DG, Mount HTJ: Intracranial aneurysms causing ophthamoplegia. Arch Ophthalmol 70:757, 1963.
152. Daily EJ, Holloway JA, Murto RE, et al: Evaluation of ocular signs and symptoms in cerebral aneurysms. Arch Ophthalmol 71:463, 1964.
153. Kasoff I, Kelly DL Jr: Pupillary sparing in oculomotor palsy from internal caroid aneurysm: Case report. J Neurosurg 42:713, 1975.
154. Roman-Campos G, Edwards KR: Painful ophthalmoplegia: Oculomotor nerve palsy without mydriasis due to compression by aneurysm. Headache 19:43, 1979.
155. Keane JR: Aneurysms and third nerve palsies. Ann Neurol 14:696, 1983.
156. O'Connor PS, Tredici TJ, Green RP: Pupil-sparing third nerve palsies caused by aneurysm. Am J Ophthalmol 95:395, 1983.
157. Kissel JT, Burde RM, Klingele TG, et al: Pupil-sparing oculomotor palsies with internal carotid-posterior communicating artery aneurysms. Ann Neurol 13:149, 1983.
158. Loewenfeld IE, Thompson HS: Oculomotor paresis with cyclic spasms: A critical review of the literature and a new case. Surv Ophthalmol 20:81, 1975.
159. Fells P, Collin JRO: Cyclic oculomotor palsy. Trans Ophthalmol Soc UK 99:192, 1979.
160. Bateman DE, Saunders M: Cyclic oculomotor palsy: Description of a case and hypothesis of the mechanism. J Neurol Neurosurg Psychiatry 46:451, 1983.
161. Friedman DI, Wright KW, Sadun AA: Oculomotor palsy with cyclic spasms. Neurology 39:1263, 1989.
162. Hepler RS, Cantu RC: Aneurysms, third nerve palsies: Ocular status of survivors. Arch Ophthalmol 77:604, 1967.
163. Forster RK, Schatz NJ, Smith JL: A subtle eyelid sign in aberrant regeneration of the third nerve. Am J Ophthalmol 67:696, 1969.
164. Czarnecki JSC, Thompson HS: The iris sphincter in aberrant regeneration of the third nerve. Arch Ophthalmol 96:1606, 1978.
165. Lepore FE, Glaser JS: Misdirection revisited: A critical appraisal of acquired oculomotor nerve synkinesis. Arch Ophthalmol 98:2206, 1980.
166. Spector RH, Faria MA: Aberrant regeneration of the inferior division of the oculomotor nerve. Arch Neurol 38:460, 1981.
167. Sebag J, Sadun AA: Aberrant regeneration of the third nerve following orbital trauma: Synkinesis of the iris sphincter. Arch Neurol 40:762, 1983.
168. Sibony PA, Lessell S, Gittinger JW: Acquired oculomotor synkinesis. Review. Surv Ophthalmol 28:382, 1984.
169. Guy J, Engel HM, Lessner AM: Acquired contralateral oculomotor synkinesis. Arch Neurol 46:1021, 1989.
170. O'Day J, Billson F, King J: Ophthalmoplegic migraine and aberrant regeneration of the oculomotor nerve. Br J Ophthalmol 64:534, 1980.
171. Schatz NJ, Savino PJ, Corbett JJ: Primary aberrant oculomotor

regeneration: A sign of intracavernous meningioma. Arch Neurol 34:29, 1977.
172. Boghen D, Chartrand JP, Laflamme P, et al: Primary aberrant third nerve regeneration. Ann Neurol 6:415, 1979.
173. Cox TA, Wurster JB, Godfrey WA: Primary aberrant oculomotor regeneration due to intracranial aneurysm. Arch Neurol 36:570, 1979.
174. Lessell S, Lessell IM, Rizzo JF: Ocular neuromyotonia after radiation therapy. Am J Ophthalmol 102:766, 1986.
175. Shults WT, Hyot WF, Behrens M, et al: Ocular neuromyotonia. A clinical description of six patients. Arch Ophthalmol 104:1028, 1986.
176. Ricker K, Mertens HG: Okuläre neuromyotonie. Klin Monatsbl Augenheilkd 156:837, 1970.
177. Burde RM, Savino PJ, Trobe JD: Clinical Decisions in Neuro-Ophthalmology. St. Louis, CV Mosby, 1985, pp 184–185.
178. Miller NR: Walsh and Hoyt's Clinical Neuro-Ophthalmology, 4th ed. Baltimore, Williams & Wilkins, 1985, p 680.
179. Binet FE, Angtuaco EJC: Radiology of intracranial aneurysms. *In* Wilkins RW, Rengachary SS (eds): Neurosurgery. New York, McGraw-Hill, 1985, pp 1341–1354.
180. Bigelow NH: Multiple intracranial arterial aneurysms. Arch Neurol Psychiatry 73:76, 1955.
181. Stehbens WE: Aneurysms and anatomical variation of cerebral arteries. Arch Pathol 75:45, 1963.
182. Wilson FMA, Jaspan T, Holland IM: Multiple cerebral aneurysms—A reappraisal. Neuroradiology 31:232, 1989.
183. Gabianelli EB, Klingele TG, Burde RM: Acute oculomotor nerve palsy in childhood. Is arteriography necessary? J Clin Neuro Ophthalmol 9:33, 1989.
184. Fox AJ: Angiography for third nerve palsy in children. J Clin Neuro Ophthalmol 9:37, 1989.
185. Ross JS, Masaryk TJ, Modic MT, et al: Intracranial aneurysms: Evaluation by MR angiography. AJNR 11:449, 1990.
186. Hamer J: Incidence and prognosis of oculomotor palsy after subarachnoid hemorrhage due to ruptured aneurysms of the posterior communicating artery. *In* Sammii M, Jannetta PJ (eds): The Cranial Nerves. Berlin, Springer-Verlag, 1981, pp 237–240.
187. Hamer J: Prognosis of oculomotor palsy in patients with aneurysms of the posterior communicating artery. Acta Neurochir (Wien) 66:173, 1982.
188. Golnik KC, Miller NR: Late recovery of function after oculomotor nerve palsy. Am J Ophthalmol 111:566, 1991.
189. Abdul-Rahim AS, Savino PJ, Zimmerman RA, et al: Cryptogenic oculomotor nerve palsy: The need for repeated neuroimaging studies. Arch Ophthalmol 107:387, 1989.
190. Saunders RA, Rogers GL: Superior oblique transposition for third nerve palsy. Ophthalmology 89:310, 1982.
191. Reinecke RD: Surgical management of third and sixth cranial nerve palsies. Int Ophthalmol Clin 25:139, 1985.
192. Gottlob I, Catalano RA, Reinecke RD: Surgical management of oculomotor nerve palsy. Am J Ophthalmol 111:71, 1991.
193. Nelson LB, Wagner RS, Calhoun JH: The adjustable suture technique in strabismus surgery. Int Ophthalmol Clin 25:89, 1985.
194. Metz HS, Mazow M: Botulinum toxin treatment of acute 6th and 3rd nerve palsy. Graefes Arch Clin Exp Ophthalmol 226:141, 1988.
195. Burger LJ, Kalvin NH, Smith JL: Acquired lesions of the fourth cranial nerve. Brain 93:567, 1970.
196. Haagedorn A: A new diagnostic motility scheme. Am J Ophthalmol 25:726, 1942.
197. Parks MM: Isolated cyclovertical muscle palsy. Arch Ophthalmol 60:1027, 1958.
198. Hardesty HH: Diagnosis of paretic vertical rotators. Am J Ophthalmol 56:811, 1963.
199. Kushner BJ: Errors in the three-step test in the diagnosis of vertical strabismus. Ophthalmology 96:127, 1989.
199a. Moster ML, Bosley TM, Slavin ML, Rubin SE: Thyroid ophthalmopathy presenting as superior oblique paresis. J Clin Neuro Ophthalmol 12:94, 1992.
200. Trobe JD: Cyclodeviation in acquired vertical strabismus. Arch Ophthalmol 102:117, 1984.
201. Kraft SP, Scott WE: Masked bilateral superior oblique palsy: Clinical features and diagnosis. J Pediatr Ophthalmol Strabismus 23:264, 1986.
202. Kushner BJ: The diagnosis and treatment of bilateral masked superior oblique palsy. Am J Ophthalmol 105:186, 1988.
203. Younge BR, Sutula F: Analysis of trochlear nerve palsies: Diagnosis, etiology, and treatment. Mayo Clin Proc 52:11, 1977.
204. Parks MM: Ocular Motility and Strabismus. Hagerstown, MD, Harper & Row, 1975.
205. Coppeto JR: Superior oblique paresis and contralateral Horner's syndrome. Ann Ophthalmol 15:681, 1983.
206. Guy J, Day AL, Mickle JP, et al: Contralateral trochlear nerve paresis and ipsilateral Horner's syndrome. Am J Ophthalmol 107:73, 1989.
207. Khawam E, Scott AB, Jampolsky A: Acquired superior oblique palsy: Diagnosis and management. Arch Ophthalmol 77:761, 1967.
208. Chapman LI, Urist MJ, Folk ER, et al: Acquired bilateral superior oblique muscle palsy. Arch Ophthalmol 84:137, 1970.
209. Coppeto JR, Lessel S: Cryptogenic unilateral paralysis of the superior oblique muscle. Arch Ophthalmol 96:275, 1978.
210. Krohel GB, Mansour AM, Petersen WL, et al: Isolated trochlear nerve palsy secondary to a juvenile pilocytic astrocytoma. J Clin Neuro Ophthalmol 1:119, 1982.
211. Wise J, Gomolin J, Goldberg LL: Bilateral superior oblique palsy: Diagnosis and treatment. Can J Ophthalmol 18:28, 1983.
212. Mansour AM, Reinecke RD: Central trochlear palsy. Surv Ophthalmol 30:279, 1986.
213. Keane JR: Trochlear nerve pareses with brainstem lesions. J Clin Neuro Ophthalmol 6:242, 1986.
214. Yoss RE, Rucker CW, Miller RH: Neurosurgical complications affecting the oculomotor, trochlear, and abducent nerves. Neurology 18:594, 1968.
215. Cobbs WH, Schatz NJ, Savino PJ: Midbrain eye signs in hydrocephalus. Ann Neurol 4:172, 1978.
216. Cobbs WH, Schatz NJ, Savino PJ: Nontraumatic bilateral fourth nerve palsies: A dorsal midbrain sign. Ann Neurol 8:107, 1980.
217. Guy JR, Friedman WF, Mickle JP: Bilateral trochlear nerve paresis in hydrocephalus. J Clin Neuro Ophthalmol 9:105, 1989.
218. Sydnor CF, Seaber JH, Buckley EG: Traumatic superior oblique palsies. Ophthalmology 89:134, 1982.
219. Lavin PJM, Troost BT: Traumatic fourth nerve palsy: Clinicoanatomic correlations with computed topographic scan. Arch Neurol 41:679, 1984.
220. Grimson BS, Ross MJ, Tyson G: Return of function after intracranial suture of the trochlear nerve. J Neurosurg 61:191, 1984.
221. Wilson ME, Eustis HS, Parks MM: Brown's syndrome. Surv Ophthalmol 34:153, 1989.
222. Hoyt WF, Keane JR: Superior oblique myokymia: Report and discussion on five cases of benign intermittent uniocular microtremor. Arch Ophthalmol 84:461, 1970.
223. Rosenberg ML, Glaser JS: Superior oblique myokymia. Ann Neurol 13:667, 1983.
224. Susac JO, Smith JL, Schatz NJ: Superior oblique myokymia. Arch Neurol 29:432, 1973.
225. Tyler TD, Ruiz RS: Propranolol in the treatment of superior oblique myokymia. Arch Ophthalmol 108:175, 1990.
226. Morrow MJ, Sharpe JA, Ranalli PJ: Superior oblique myokymia associated with a posterior fossa tumor: Oculographic correlation with an idiopathic case. Neurology 40:367, 1990.
227. Bixenman WW: Vertical prisms. Why avoid them? Surv Ophthalmol 29:70, 1984.
228. Von Noorden GK: Burian-Von Noorden's Binocular Vision and Ocular Motility: Theory and Management of Strabismus, 2nd ed. St. Louis, CV Mosby, 1980.
229. Knapp P: Treatment of unilateral fourth nerve paralysis. Trans Ophthalmol Soc UK 101:273, 1981.
229a. Maruo T, Iwashige H, Akatsu S, et al: Superior oblique palsy: Results of surgery in 443 cases. Binocular Vis Quart 6:143, 1991.
230. Reisner SH, Perlman M, Ben-Tovim N, Dubrawski C: Transient lateral rectus muscle paresis in the newborn infant. J Pediatr 78:461, 1971.
231. Phillips WH, Dirion JK, Graves GO: Congenital bilateral palsy of the abducens. Arch Ophthalmol 8:355, 1932.
232. Zweifach PH, Walton DS, Brown RH: Isolated congenital horizontal gaze paralysis: Occurrence of the near reflex and ocular retraction on attempted lateral gaze. Arch Ophthalmol 81:345, 1969.

233. Hoyt CS, Billson FA, Taylor H: Isolated unilateral gaze palsy. J Pediatr Ophthalmol 14:343, 1977.
234. Ehrenberg M, Jay WM, Sidrys LA, et al: Congenital bilateral horizontal gaze palsy in a brother and sister. J Pediatr Ophthalmol Strabismus 17:224, 1980.
235. Sharpe JA, Silversides JL, Blair RDG: Familial paralysis of horizontal gaze: Associated with pendular nystagmus, progressive scoliosis, and facial contraction with myokymia. Neurology 25:1035, 1975.
236. Riley E, Swift M: Congenital horizontal gaze palsy and kyphoscoliosis in two brothers. J Med Genet 16:314, 1979.
237. Yee RD, Duffin RM, Baloh RW, et al: Familial, congenital paralysis of horizontal gaze. Arch Ophthalmol 100:1449, 1982.
238. Harlan GC: Congenital paralysis of both abducens and both facial nerves. Trans Am Ophthalmol Soc 3:216, 1880.
239. Chisolm JJ: Congenital paralysis of the sixth and seventh pairs of cranial nerves in an adult. Arch Ophthalmol 11:323, 1882.
240. Möbius PJ: Über angeborene doppelseitige abducens-facialislähmung. Muench Med Wochenschr 35:91, 1888.
241. Henderson JL: The congenital facial diplegia syndrome: Clinical features, pathology and aetiology. Brain 62:381, 1939.
242. Baraitser M: Genetics of Möbius syndrome. J Med Genet 14:415, 1977.
243. Towfighi J, Marks K, Palmer E, et al: Möbius syndrome: Neuropathologic observations. Acta Neuropathol 48:11, 1979.
244. Duane A: Congenital deficiency of abduction, associated with impairment of adduction, retraction movements, contraction of the palpebral fissure and oblique movements of the eye. Arch Ophthalmol 34:133, 1905.
245. Gifford H: Congenital defects of abduction and other ocular movements and their relation to birth injuries. Am J Ophthalmol 9:3, 1926.
246. Gundersen T, Zeavin B: Observations on the retraction syndrome of Duane. Arch Ophthalmol 55:576, 1956.
247. Kirkham TH: Inheritance of Duane's syndrome. Br J Ophthalmol 54:323, 1970.
248. Pfaffenbach DD, Cross HE, Kearns TP: Congenital anomalies in Duane's retraction syndrome. Arch Ophthalmol 88:635, 1972.
249. Isenberg S, Urist MJ: Clinical observations in 101 consecutive patients with Duane's retraction syndrome. Am J Ophthalmol 84:419, 1977.
250. Huber A: Electrophysiology of the retraction syndromes. Br J Ophthalmol 58:293, 1974.
251. Hotchkiss MG, Miller NR, Clark AW, et al: Bilateral Duane's retraction syndrome: A clinical-pathologic case report. Arch Ophthalmol 98:870, 1980.
252. Miller NR, Kiel SM, Green WR, et al: Unilateral Duane's retraction syndrome (type 1). Arch Ophthalmol 100:1468, 1982.
253. Cross HE, Pfaffenbach DD: Duane's retraction syndrome and associated congenital malformations. Am J Ophthalmol 73:442, 1972.
254. Ramsay J, Taylor D: Congenital crocodile tears: A key to the aetiology of Duane's syndrome. Br J Ophthalmol 64:518, 1980.
255. Miller NR: Walsh and Hoyt's Clinical Neuro-Ophthalmology, 4th ed. Baltimore, Williams & Wilkins, 1985, p 695.
256. Bennet AH, Savill T: A case of permanent conjugate deviation of the eyes and head, the result of a lesion limited to the sixth nucleus: With remarks on associated lateral movement of the eyeballs, and rotation of the head and neck. Brain 12:102, 1889.
257. Minor RH, Kearns TP, Millikan CH, et al: Ocular manifestations of occlusive disease of the vertebral-basilar arterial system. Arch Ophthalmol 62:112, 1959.
258. Urist MJ: Lateral gaze palsy in diabetic lateral rectus paralysis. Ann Ophthalmol 6:583, 1974.
259. Bicknell JM, Carlow TJ, Kornfeld M, et al: Familial cavernous angiomas. Arch Neurol 35:746, 1978.
260. Goto N, Kaneko M, Hosaka Y, et al: Primary pontine hemorrhage: Clinicopathologic correlation. Stroke 11:84, 1980.
261. Klingele TG, Schultz R, Murphy MG: Pontine gaze paresis due to traumatic craniocervical hyperextension: Report of two cases. J Neurosurg 53:249, 1980.
262. Meienberg O, Büttner-Ennever JA, Kraus-Ruppert R: Unilateral paralysis of conjugate gaze due to lesion of the abducens nucleus. Neuro-ophthalmology 2:47, 1981.
263. Pierrot-Deseilligny C, Goasguen J, Chain F, et al: Pontine metastasis with dissociated bilateral horizontal gaze paralysis. J Neurol Neurosurg Psychiatry 47:159, 1984.
264. Hamed LM, Schatz NJ, Galetta SL: Brain stem ocular motility defects and AIDS. Am J Ophthalmol 106:437, 1988.
265. Cogan DG, Victor M: Ocular signs of Wernicke's disease. Arch Ophthalmol 51:204, 1954.
266. Foville A: Note sur une paralysie peu connue de certains muscle de l'oeil, et sa liaison avec quelques points de l'anatomie et la physiologie de la protuberance annulaire. Bull Soc Anat Paris 33:373, 1858.
267. Raymond A, Cestan B: Le syndrôme protuberantie supérient. Gaz Hôpit Civils et Militaires 76:829–834, 1903.
268. Millard B: Bull Soc Anat Paris 31:217–221, 1856.
269. Gubler A: Hemiplegie alternée d'une lesion du pont et la documentation de la preuve de la décussation. Gaz Hebd Med Chirurg 3:749–754, 789–792, 811–816, 1856.
270. Donaldson D, Rosenberg NL: Infarction of abducens nerve fascicle as cause of isolated sixth nerve palsy related to hypertension. Neurology 38:1654, 1988.
271. Johnson LN, Hepler RS: Isolated abducens nerve paresis from intrapontine, fascicular abducens nerve injury. Am J Ophthalmol 108:459, 1989.
272. Walsh FB, Hoyt WF: Clinical Neuro-Ophthalmology, 3rd ed. Baltimore, Williams & Wilkins, 1969, pp 985–986.
273. Bronstein AM, Morris J, du Boulay G, et al: Abnormalities of horizontal gaze: Clinical, oculographic and magnetic resonance imaging findings. I: Abducens palsy. J Neurol Neurosurg Psychiatry 53:194, 1990.
274. Swartz MN, Dodge PR: Bacterial meningitis: A review of selected aspects. II: Special neurologic problems, postmeningitis complications and clinicopathological correlations. N Engl J Med 272:954, 1965.
275. Lundberg N: Continuous recording and control of ventricular fluid pressure in neurosurgical practice. Acta Psychiatry Neurol Scand 36(Suppl 149):1, 1960.
276. Van Allen MW: Transient recurring paralysis of ocular abduction: A syndrome of intracranial hypertension. Arch Neurol 17:81, 1967.
277. Keane JR: Bilateral sixth nerve palsy: Analysis of 125 cases. Arch Neurol 33:681, 1976.
278. Bryce-Smith R, MacIntosh RR: Sixth nerve palsy after lumbar puncture and spinal analgesia. Br Med J 1:275, 1951.
279. Crouch ER Jr, Urist MJ: Lateral rectus muscle paralysis associated with closed head trauma. Am J Ophthalmol 79:990, 1975.
280. Rozario RA, Stein BM: Complications of halo-pelvic traction: Case report. J Neurosurg 45:716, 1976.
281. Thorsen G: Neurologic complications after spinal anesthesia. Acta Chir Scand Suppl 121:1, 1977.
282. Insel TR, Kalin NH, Risch SC, et al: Abducens palsy after lumbar puncture. N Engl J Med 303:703, 1980.
283. Black P McL, Chapman PH: Transient abducens paresis after shunting for hydrocephalus. J Neurosurg 55:467, 1981.
284. Rosa L, Carol M, Bellegarrique R, et al: Multiple cranial nerve palsies due to a hyperextension injury to the cervical spine. J Neurosurg 61:172, 1984.
285. Miller SJH: Ocular signs of chordoma. Proc R Soc Med 65:522, 1972.
286. Bing-huan C: Neurinoma of the abducens nerve. Neurosurgery 9:64, 1981.
287. Kline LB, Glaser JS: Bilateral abducens palsies from clivus chordoma. Ann Ophthalmol 13:705, 1981.
288. Liboni W, Baggiore P, De Mattei M, et al: An unusual case of focal symptomatology, monoparalysis of the abducent nerve and vertebrobasilar ectasia. Minerva Med 74:919, 1983.
289. Smoker WRK, Corbett JJ, Gentry LR, et al: High-resolution computed tomography of the basilar artery. 2:Vertebrobasilar dolichoectasia: Clinical-pathologic correlation and review. AJRN 7:61, 1986.
290. Dumas S, Shults WT: Abducens paresis: A rare presenting sign of posterior-inferior cerebellar artery aneurysm. J Clin Neuro Ophthalmol 2:55, 1982.
291. Coppeto Jr, Chan Y-S: Abducens nerve paresis caused by unruptured vertebral artery aneurysm. Surg Neurol 18:385, 1982.
292. Gradenigo G: A special syndrome of endocranial otitic compli-

cations (paralysis of the motor oculi externus of otitic origin). Ann Otol Rhinol Laryngol 13:637, 1904.
293. Robertson DM, Hines JD, Rucker CW: Acquired sixth-nerve paresis in children. Arch Ophthalmol 83:574, 1970.
294. Yamashita J, Asato R, Handa H, et al: Abducens nerve palsy as an initial symptom of trigeminal schwannoma. J Neurol Neurosurg Psychiatry 40:1190, 1977.
295. de Graaf J, Cats H, de Jager AE: Gradenigo's syndrome: A rare complication of otitis media. Clin Neurol Neurosurg 90:237, 1988.
296. Miller NR: Walsh and Hoyt's Clinical Neuro-Ophthalmology, 4th ed. Baltimore, Williams & Wilkins, 1985, p 703.
297. Newton TH, Hoyt WF: Dural arteriovenous shunts in the region of the cavernous sinus. Neuroradiology 1:71, 1970.
298. Brismar G, Brismar J: Spontaneous carotid-cavernous fistulas: Clinical symptomatology. Acta Ophthalmol 54:542, 1976.
299. De Keizer RJW: Spontaneous carotid-cavernous fistulas. Neuro-ophthalmology 2:35, 1981.
300. Rapport R, Murtagh FR: Ophthalmoplegia due to spontaneous thrombosis in a patient with bilateral cavernous carotid aneurysms. J Clin Neuro Ophthalmol 1:225, 1981.
301. Sakalas R, Harbison JW, Vines FS, et al: Chronic sixth nerve palsy: An initial sign of basisphenoid tumors. Arch Ophthalmol 93:186, 1975.
302. Lavin PJM, Younkin SG, Kori SH: The pathology of ophthalmoplegia in herpes zoster ophthalmicus. Neuro-ophthalmology 4:73, 1984.
303. Abad JM, Alvarez F, Blazquez MG: An unrecognized neurological syndrome: Sixth nerve palsy and Horner's syndrome due to traumatic intracavernous aneurysm. Surg Neurol 16:140, 1981.
304. Gutman I, Levartovski S, Goldhammer Y, et al: Sixth nerve palsy and unilateral Horner's syndrome. Ophthalmology 93:913, 1986.
305. Striph GG, Burde RM: Abducens nerve palsy and Horner's syndrome revisited. J Clin Neuro Ophthalmol 8:13, 1988.
306. Cooper JC: Deviation of eye and transient blurring of vision after mandibular nerve anesthesia: Report of a case. J Oral Surg 20:151, 1962.
307. O'Connor M, Eustace P: Tonic pupil and lateral rectus palsy following dental anaesthesia. Neuro-ophthalmology 3:205, 1983.
308. Lillie WI: Temporary abducens nerve paralysis not associated with other general or neurologic abnormalities. Arch Ophthalmol 28:548, 1942.
309. Shrader EC, Schlezinger NS: Neuro-ophthalmologic evaluation of abducens nerve paralysis. Arch Ophthalmol 63:84, 1960.
310. Johnston AC: Etiology and treatment of abducens paralysis. Trans Pac Coast Otolaryngol Ophthalmol Soc 49:259, 1968.
311. De Renzi E, Nichelli P: Ophthalmoplegic migraine with persistent abducens nerve palsy. Eur Neurol 15:227, 1977.
312. Knox DL, Clark DB, Schuster FF: Benign VI nerve palsies in children. Pediatrics 40:560, 1967.
313. Scharf J, Zonis S: Benign abducens nerve palsy in children. J Pediatr Ophthalmol 12:165, 1975.
314. Werner DB, Savino PJ, Schatz NJ: Benign recurrent sixth nerve palsies in childhood: Secondary to immunization or viral illness. Arch Ophthalmol 101:607, 1983.
315. Bruce GM: Ocular divergence: Its physiology and pathology. Arch Ophthalmol 13:639, 1935.
316. Chamlin N, Davidoff LM: Divergence paralysis with increased intracranial pressure: Further observations. Arch Ophthalmol 46:145, 1951.
317. Moller PM: Divergence paralysis. Acta Ophthalmol 48:325, 1970.
318. Rutkowski PC, Burian HM: Divergence paralysis following head trauma. Am J Ophthalmol 73:660, 1972.
319. Jampolsky A: Ocular divergence mechanisms. Trans Am Ophthalmol Soc 68:730, 1970.
320. Kirkham TH, Bird AC, Sanders MD: Divergence paralysis with raised intracranial pressure: An electro-oculographic study. Br J Ophthalmol 56:776, 1972.
321. Von Noorden GK: Burian-Von Noorden's Binocular Vision and Ocular Motility: Theory and Management of Strabismus, 2nd ed. St. Louis, CV Mosby, 1980.
322. Savino PJ, Hilliker JK, Casell GH, et al: Chronic sixth nerve palsies: Are they really harbingers of serious intracranial disease? Arch Ophthalmol 100:1442, 1982.
323. Currie J, Lubin JH, Lessell S: Chronic isolated abducens paresis from tumors at the base of the brain. Arch Neurol 40:226, 1983.
324. Del Priore LV, Miller NR: Trigeminal schwannoma as a cause of chronic, isolated sixth nerve palsy. Am J Ophthalmol 108:726, 1989.
325. Galetta SL, Smith JL: Chronic isolated sixth nerve palsies. Arch Neurol 46:79, 1989.
326. Von Noorden GK: Burian-Von Noorden's Binocular Vision and Ocular Motility: Theory and Management of Strabismus, 2nd ed. St. Louis, CV Mosby, 1980.
327. Wybar KC: Management of sixth nerve palsy and Duane's retraction syndrome. Trans Ophthalmol Soc UK 101:276, 1981.
328. Lee DA, Dyer JA, O'Brien PC, et al: Surgical treatment of lateral rectus muscle paralysis. Am J Ophthalmol 97:511, 1984.
329. Scott AB, Kraft SP: Botulinum toxin injection in the management of lateral rectus palsy. Ophthalmology 92:676, 1985.
330. Fitzsimmons R, Lee JP, Elston JS: Treatment of sixth nerve palsy in adults with combined botulinum toxin chemodenervation and surgery. Ophthalmology 95:1535, 1988.
331. Murray ADN: Early and late botulinum toxin treatment of acute sixth nerve palsy. Aust N Z J Ophthalmol 17:239, 1989.
332. Elston JS: Botulinum toxin. Aust N Z J Ophthalmol 17:209, 1989.
333. Armenia JV, Sigal MB: Abducens paralysis repaired with muscle transposition and intraoperative botulinum toxin. Ann Ophthalmol 19:416, 1987.
334. Walsh FB, Hoyt WF: Clinical Neuro-Ophthalmology, 3rd ed. Baltimore, Williams & Wilkins, 1969, pp 937–938.
335. Harvey DG, Torack RM, Rosenbaum HE: Amyotrophic lateral sclerosis with ophthalmoplegia: A clinicopathologic study. Arch Neurol 36:615, 1979.
336. Hayashi H, Kato S, Kawada T, et al: Amyotrophic lateral sclerosis: oculomotor function in patients on respirators. Neurology 37:1431, 1987.
337. Kay MC, McCrary JA: Multiple cranial nerve palsies in late metastatis of midline malignant reticulosis. Am J Ophthalmol 88:1087, 1979.
338. Wiederholt WC, Siekert RG: Neurological manifestations of sarcoidosis. Neurology 15:1147, 1965.
339. Wolf SM, Schotland DL, Phillips LL: Involvement of nervous system in Behçet's syndrome. Arch Neurol 12:315, 1965.
340. Givner I: Ophthalmologic features of intracranial chordoma and allied tumors of the clivus. Arch Ophthalmol 33:397, 1945.
341. Weinberger LM, Adler FH, Grant FC: Primary pituitary adenoma and the syndrome of the cavernous sinus: A clinical and anatomic study. Arch Ophthalmol 14:1197, 1940.
342. Chamlin M, Davidoff LM, Feiring EH: Ophthalmologic changes produced by pituitary tumors. Am J Ophthalmol 40:353, 1955.
343. Robert CM Jr, Feigenbaum JA, Stern WE: Ocular palsy occurring with pituitary tumors. J Neurosurg 38:17, 1973.
344. Dust G, Reinecke M, Behrens-Baumann W, et al: Schmerzhafte ophthalmoplegie ohne mydriasis: Oculomotoriusparese und läsion sympathischer fasern (Raeder syndrom) durch druck eines aneurysmas der A. carotis interna. Nervenarzt 52:85, 1981.
345. Elliot AJ: Ocular manifestations of carotid-cavernous fistulas. Postgrad Med 15:191, 1954.
346. Sanders MD, Hoyt WF: Hypoxic ocular sequelae of carotid-cavernous fistulae. Br J Ophthalmol 53:82, 1969.
347. Palestine AG, Younge BR, Piepgras DG: Visual prognosis in carotid-cavernous fistula. Arch Ophthalmol 99:1600, 1981.
348. Rovit RL, Fein FM: Pituitary apoplexy: A review and reappraisal. J Neurosurg 37:280, 1972.
349. Wakai S, Fukushima T, Teramoto A, et al: Pituitary apoplexy: Its incidence and clinical significance. J Neurosurg 55:187, 1981.
350. Smith JL, Wheliss JA: Ocular manifestations of nasopharyngeal tumors. Trans Am Acad Ophthalmol Otolaryngol 66:659, 1962.
351. Godtfredsen E, Lederman M: Diagnostic and prognostic roles of ophthalmoneurologic signs and symptoms in malignant nasopharyngeal tumors. Am J Ophthalmol 59:1063, 1965.
352. Barlett JR Jr: Craniopharyngiomas: A summary of 85 cases. J Neurol Neurosurg Psychiatry 34:37, 1971.
353. Finn JE, Mount LA: Meningiomas of the tuberculum sellae and planum sphenoidale: A review of 83 cases. Arch Ophthalmol 92:23, 1974.
354. Kennedy HB, Smith RJS: Eye signs in craniopharyngioma. Br J Ophthalmol 59:689, 1975.

355. Greenberg HS, Deck MDF, Vikram B, et al: Metastasis to the base of the skull: Clinical findings in 43 patients. Neurology 31:530, 1981.
356. Mills RP, Insalaco SJ, Joseph A: Bilateral cavernous sinus metastasis and ophthalmoplegia: Case report. J Neurosurg 55:463, 1981.
357. Spector RH, Fiandaca MS: The "sinister" Tolosa-Hunt syndrome. Neurology 36:198, 1986.
358. Schubiger O, Valavanis A, Hayek J, et al: Neuroma of the cavernous sinus. Surg Neurol 13:313, 1980.
359. Wilson CB, Myers FK: Bilateral saccular aneurysms of the internal carotid artery in the cavernous sinus. J Neurol Neurosurg Psychiatry 26:174, 1963.
360. Barr HWK, Blackwood W, Meadows SP: Intracavernous carotid aneurysms: A clinical-pathological report. Brain 94:607, 1971.
361. Huber A: Eye signs and symptoms of intracranial aneurysm. Neuro-ophthalmology 2:203, 1982.
362. Markwalder TM, Meienberg O: Acute painful cavernous sinus syndrome in unruptured intracavernous aneurysms of the internal carotid artery: Possible pathogenetic mechanisms. J Clin Neuro Ophthalmol 3:31, 1983.
363. Kupersmith MJ, Berenstein A, Choi IS: Percutaneous transvascular treatment of giant carotid aneurysms: Neuro-ophthalmologic findings. Neurology 34:328, 1984.
364. Pool JL, Potts DG: Aneurysms and Arteriovenous Anomalies of the Brain. New York, Harper & Row, 1965.
365. Phelps CD, Thompson HS, Ossonig KC: The diagnosis and prognosis of atypical carotid-cavernous fistula (red-eyed shunt syndrome). Am J Ophthalmol 93:423, 1982.
366. Grove AS Jr: The dural shunt syndrome: Pathophysiology and clinical course. Ophthalmology 90:31, 1983.
367. Keltner JL, Satterfield D, Dublin AB, et al: Dural and carotid cavernous sinus fistulas. Diagnosis, management, and complications. Ophthalmology 94:1585, 1987.
368. Tveteras K, Kristensen S, Dommerby H: Septic cavernous and lateral sinus thrombosis: Modern diagnostic and therapeutic principles. J Laryngol Otol 102:877, 1988.
369. DiNubile MJ: Septic thrombosis of the cavernous sinuses. Arch Neurol 45:567, 1988.
370. Levine SR, Twyman RE, Gilman S: The role of anticoagulation in cavernous sinus thrombosis. Neurology 38:517, 1988.
371. Gass JDM: Ocular manifestations of acute mucormycosis. Arch Ophthalmol 65:226, 1961.
372. Green WR, Font RL, Zimmerman LE: Aspergillosis of the orbit: Report of ten cases and review of the literature. Arch Ophthalmol 82:302, 1969.
373. Lehrer RI, Howard DH, Sypherd PS, et al: Mucomycosis. Ann Intern Med 93:93, 1980.
374. Forteza G, Burgeno M: Rhinocerebral mucormycosis. Presentation of two cases and review of the literature. J Craniomaxillofac Surg 16(2):80, 1988.
375. Archimbault P, Wise JS, Rosen J, et al: Herpes zoster ophthalmoplegia. Report of six cases. J Clin Neuro Ophthalmol 8:185, 1988.
376. Hunt WE, Brighton RP: The Tolosa-Hunt syndrome: A problem in differential diagnosis. Acta Neurochir Suppl (Wien) 42:248, 1988.
377. Smith JL, Taxdal DSR: Painful ophthalmoplegia: The Tolosa-Hunt syndrome. Am J Ophthalmol 61:1466, 1966.
378. Guillain G, Barré J-A, Strohl A: Sur un syndrome de radiculonévrite avec hyperalbuminase due liquide céphalo-rachidien sans réaction cellulaire: remarques sur les caractères cliniques et graphiques des réflexes tendineux. Bull Soc Med Hop Paris 40:1462, 1916.
379. Guillain G, Kreis B: Sur deux cas de polyradiculo-névrite avec hyperalbuminose du liquide céphalo-rachidien sans réaction cellulaire. Paris Med 2:224, 1937.
380. Guillain G: Les polyradiculonévrites avec dissociation albumi-nocytologique et à evolution favorable. (Syndrome de Guillain et Barré). J Belge Neurol Psychiatry 38:323, 1938.
381. Van Bogaert L, Maere M: Les polyradiculonevrites craniennes bilaterales avec dissociation albumino-cytologique: Formes craniennes de polyradiculonévrites du type Guillain et Barré. J Belge Neurol Psychiatry 38:275, 1938.
382. Kennedy RH, Danielson MA, Mulder DW, et al: Guillain-Barré syndrome: A 42-year epidemiologic and clinical study. Mayo Clin Proc 53:93, 1978.
383. McKhann GM: Guillain-Barré syndrome: Clinical and therapeutic observations. Ann Neurol 27(Suppl):S13, 1990.
384. Grunnet ML, Lubow M: Ascending polyneuritis and ophthalmoplegia. Am J Ophthalmol 74:1155, 1972.
385. Blau I, Casson I, Lieberman A, et al: The not-so-benign Miller Fisher syndrome: A variant of the Guillain-Barré syndrome. Arch Neurol 37:384, 1980.
386. Derakhshan I, Lotfi J, Kaufman B: Ophthalmoplegia, ataxia and hyporeflexia (Fisher's syndrome): With a midbrain lesion demonstrated by CT scanning. Eur Neurol 18:361, 1979.
387. Dennig D: Ophthalmoplegia in Fisher's syndrome: A combination of peripheral, internuclear, and supranuclear lesions. Psychiatr Neurol Med Psychol (Leipz) 34:731, 1982.
388. Keane JR, Finstead BA: Upward gaze paralysis as the initial sign of Fisher's syndrome. Arch Neurol 39:781, 1982.
389. Meienberg O, Ryffel E: Supranuclear eye movement disorders in Fisher's syndrome of ophthalmoplegia, ataxia, and areflexia. Arch Neurol 40:402, 1983.
390. Meienberg O: Lesion site in Fisher's syndrome. Arch Neurol 41:250, 1984.
391. Dehaene I, Martin JJ, Geens K, et al: Guillain-Barré syndrome with ophthalmoplegia: Clinicopathologic study of the central and peripheral nervous systems, including the oculomotor nerves. Neurology 36:851, 1986.
392. Ropper AH: Three patients with Fisher's syndrome and normal MRI. Neurology 38:1630, 1988.
393. Cherington M: Botulism. Ten-year experience. Arch Neurol 30:432, 1974.
394. Barker WH Jr, Weissman JB, Dowell VR, et al: Type B botulism outbreak caused by a commercial food product: West Virginia and Pennsylvania, 1973. JAMA 237:456, 1977.
395. Terranova W, Palumbo JN, Breman JG: Ocular findings in botulism type B. JAMA 241:475, 1979.
396. Clouston PD, Sharpe DM, Corbett AJ, et al: Perineural spread of cutaneous head and neck cancer: Its orbital and central neurologic complications. Arch Neurol 47:73, 1990.
397. Mullan S: Treatment of carotid-cavernous fistulas by cavernous sinus occlusion. J Neurosurg 50:131, 1979.
398. Viñuela FV, Debrun GM, Fox AJ, et al: Detachable calibrated leak balloon for superselective angiography and embolization of dural arteriovenous malformations. J Neurosurg 58:817, 1983.
399. Theron J, Olivier A, Melancon D, et al: Left carotid-cavernous fistula with right exophthalmos: Treatment by detachable balloon: Case report and literature review. Neuroradiology 27:349, 1985.
400. Kupersmith MJ, Berenstein A, Choi IS, et al: Management of nontraumatic vascular shunts involving the cavernous sinus. Ophthalmology 95:121, 1988.
401. Hanneken AM, Miller NR, Debrun GM, et al: Treatment of carotid-cavernous sinus fistulas using a detachable balloon catheter through the superior ophthalmic vein. Arch Ophthalmol 107:87, 1989.
402. Sergott RC, Grossman RI, Savino PJ, et al: The syndrome of paradoxical worsening of dural-cavernous sinus arteriovenous malformations. Ophthalmology 94:205, 1987.
403. McKhann GM, Griffin JW, Cornblath DR, et al: Plasmapheresis and Guillain-Barré syndrome: Analysis of prognostic factors and the effect of plasmapheresis. Ann Neurol 23:347, 1988.

Chapter 195

Neuroophthalmology of the Pupil and Accommodation

DON C. BIENFANG

This chapter is intended to be an introduction to neuroophthalmic problems of the pupil and accommodation. For each subject there are extensive references, but at the outset I would like to recommend major reviews on the subject by Thompson, Miller, Zinn, Alexandridis, Burde.[1–9]

Pupillary size is determined by an interplay between the sympathetic and the parasympathetic nervous systems. The clinical neuroophthalmic entities to be considered are most simply divided into afflictions of one or the other, and thus it is useful to consider them separately.

NEUROANATOMY OF PUPILLARY CONSTRICTION (Fig. 195–1)

The two major stimuli that constrict the pupil are light falling on the retinal photoreceptors[10] and the effort of the near reflex and accommodation.[11–14] The afferent pathway for the pupillary light reflex travels together with the pathway concerned with vision but bypasses the lateral geniculate nucleus to synapse on nuclei in the pretectum, mainly the olivary nucleus. It is likely that the fibers to the pretectal nuclei are collaterals of the axons that synapse on the lateral geniculate nucleus.[15, 16] Functionally, there are connections from these pretectal nuclei to their partners on the other side. Also, fibers from these nuclei pass ipsilaterally and ventrally on their way to the Edinger-Westphal nucleus or they decussate in the posterior commissure to reach the contralateral Edinger-Westphal nucleus of the third nerve nuclear complex. Thus, there is ample opportunity for both ipsilateral and contralateral input from the pretectal nuclei to the Edinger-Westphal nucleus accounting for the symmetry of pupillary light reactions when light is shined in only one eye. The small cell bodies of the Edinger-Westphal nucleus appear to fuse as a midline structure in some anatomic sections, but functionally it behaves as a paired nucleus with all the parasympathetic axons remaining ipsilateral and passing into the ipsilateral third cranial nerve to reach the ciliary ganglion in the orbit.[17, 18]

The connections between the occipital cortex and the pretectal nuclei that serve the miosis of the near reflex[17, 19–21] pass near the paths[22–28] that link the occipital cortex and the oculomotor nuclei. There is something about the way that these fibers serving the miosis of the near reflex are "wired" into the mesencephalon[29–32] that allows such entities as central nervous system syphilis and dorsal midline tumors to damage the pupillary light reflex paths and spare the near reaction pathways.

The convergence portion of the near reaction is accomplished by co-contraction of the medial recti through coordinated stimulation of both medial recti subnuclei or a special portion of this nucleus called Perlia's nucleus. How the axons that stimulate this motor portion of the third-nerve complex relate to those from the pretectum that cause pupillary miosis and contraction of the muscles of the ciliary body of the eye (which causes the change in focus of the lens) is not well understood.

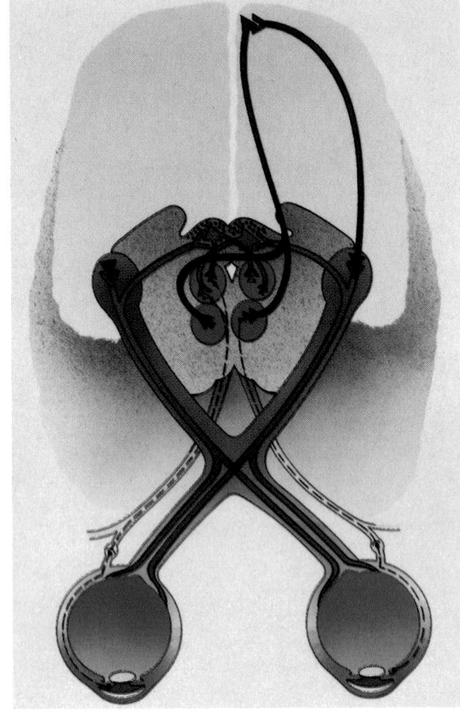

Figure 195–1. This is a diagram of the parasympathetic pathways serving the pupil and accommodation. The Edinger-Westphal nucleus is artificially divided into two parts to emphasize its separate, yet shared functions in the pupillary light reaction and accommodation. The drawing also emphasizes the extensive crossing within the mesencephalon that keeps the pupillary reactions normally symmetric. There are some asymmetries of input from the nasal versus temporal retina, but for clinical purposes these are seldom important. For simplicity the efferent pupillary light pathway is shown for the right eye, and the efferent accommodative and pupillary near-pathway is shown for the left eye.

The parasympathetic fibers destined for the pupil and the ciliary body travel on the surface of the third cranial nerve into its central root in the orbit and synapse on the ciliary ganglion.[33, 34] Most fibers emerging from the ciliary ganglion via the short ciliary nerves are destined for the ciliary muscle to stimulate change in the thickness of the lens (i.e., accommodation). Only a small percentage reach the sphincter muscle of the iris.[29]

NEUROANATOMY OF PUPILLARY DILATATION: THE SYMPATHETIC PATHWAYS (Fig. 195–2)

The first neuron, the central neuron, of the sympathetic chain originates in the posterior hypothalamus[35] and passes caudally and ipsilaterally around the red nucleus through the brain stem and into the upper spinal cord to synapse on the ciliospinal center of Budge, which is in the intermediate gray column at the level of C8–T2. The second or preganglionic neuron emerges from the spinal cord via the ventral roots of C8–T2 and enters the paravertebral sympathetic chain at the stellate ganglion. Most fibers pass out of the stellate ganglion and over the apex of the lung via the ansa subclavia and then go back into the ganglion chain to synapse in the superior cervical ganglion high in the neck. Some of the third-order or postganglionic neurons travel on the internal carotid artery to reach the cavernous sinus, where they leave the artery to join the first division of the fifth cranial nerve entering the orbit through the superior orbital fissure and the globe via the long ciliary nerve to reach the dilator muscle of the iris. For the purpose of later discussion it is important to know that sympathetic fibers of this group also innervate Müller's muscle of the upper and lower lids. Third-neuron fibers on the external carotid supply the piloerector muscles and sweat glands of the majority of the face.

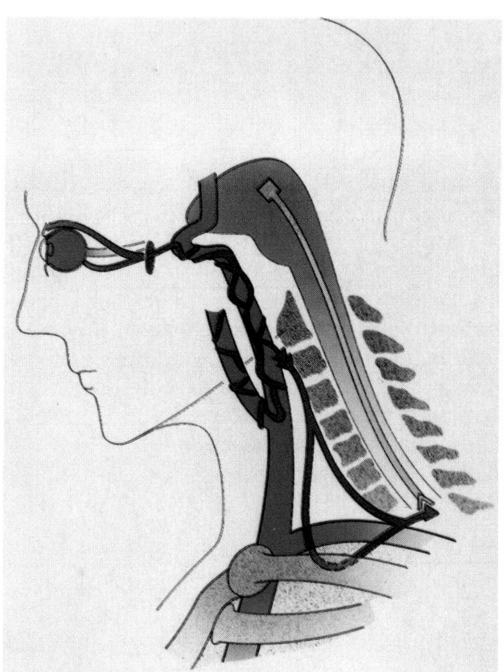

Figure 195–2. A diagram of the major landmarks of the three neuron sympathetic chains to the eye.

LIGHT REFLEX

Pupillary constriction reduces the light falling on the retina, decreases some lens aberrations, and increases the depth of field of vision. Miosis induced by light falling on the retinal receptors is sensitive to the rate of change of the illumination. Thus, going quickly from dark to bright light induces the maximum rate of pupillary change. With prolonged illumination there is a gradual adaptation of the retina, which allows the pupil to dilate slightly. The cones are most sensitive to light parallel to the cell, whereas the rods are also sensitive to oblique illumination. Since the pupillary response to cone illumination is greater than that to rod, direct light induces more pupillary response than indirect illumination of the same magnitude.[36]

Since both pretectal nuclei send axons to the ipsilateral and contralateral Edinger-Westphal nucleus, light falling on one retina normally causes both pupils to constrict—the direct and consensual response.

NEAR REFLEX AND ACCOMMODATION

Three events occur when someone looks at a near object: The medial recti both contract, the ciliary body contracts to change the shape of the lens moving the plane of focus closer to the eye, and the pupil becomes smaller.[37, 38] These three events can be separated from each another experimentally, and thus they involve adjacent but separate neuroanatomic pathways. The cortical organization of this system is poorly understood.[39] It is clear that target blur, which must be sensed in the occipital cortex, is the stimulus for accommodation.[40] Pathways from the cortex pass through the mesencephalon near, but separate from, the pretectal path for the light reflex and ultimately reach the Edinger-Westphal nucleus for miosis and accommodation and the medial rectus subnucleus for convergence.

PSYCHOSENSORY REFLEXES

Pain in or around the eye usually induces miosis on the affected side and also to some extent on the other side. In states of arousal, the increased sympathetic tone tends to cause the pupils to dilate. Thus, people with large pupils may appear to be more interesting and attractive. In depressed mental states such as sleepiness, the pupils tend to be small.[41]

PHARMACOLOGY OF THE PUPIL

Except for the synapse of the third-order or postganglionic neuron that uses norepinephrine as its transmitter, all the other synapses in the sympathetic nervous system and all of the synapses in the parasympathetic nervous system use acetylcholine. Acetylcholine is enzymatically degraded at the synapse by acetylcholinesterase. Norepinephrine is inactivated by catecholomethyl transferase or monoamine oxidase.

The literature on the effect of systemic and topical drugs on the eye is vast, and much of it has little practical application in ophthalmology. Two areas of interest worthy of discussion include topical drugs in regular use and systemic drugs, especially controlled substances, which affect pupil size.

Topical cocaine dilates the pupil by inhibiting reabsorption of norepinephrine released at the postganglionic axon terminal. Topical hydroxyamphetamine and tyramine dilate the pupil by artificially releasing norepinephrine from the postganglionic sympathetic neuron. Phenylephrine and epinephrine dilate the pupil through a direct effect on the dilator muscle. Hexamethonium blocks transmission of acetylcholine at the superior cervical ganglion; guanethidine blocks release of norepinephrine at the neuromuscular junction; and thymoxamine and dapiprazole block the receptors on the dilator muscle, as atropine blocks receptors of the constrictor muscle. Dapiprazole can be used to counteract mydriasis induced by sympathomimetics.

Pilocarpine and methacholine are parasympathetic agents that act directly on the sphincter of the pupil and on the ciliary muscle. Carbachol is the parasympathetic equivalent of hydroxyamphetamine and acts by releasing acetylcholine from nerve terminals. A number of drugs, including edrophonium, echothiophate, and physostigmine, potentiate the effect of acetylcholine on the pupillary sphincter by blocking the degradation by acetylcholinesterase—nerve gases used in chemical warfare act this way. Chronic use of miotic agents can result in a pupillary rigidity that persists after the drug is stopped. Atropine is an example of one drug that blocks the receptor site for acetylcholine on the pupillary sphincter and ciliary muscle.

Among the controlled substances, morphine and the other members of its class of central nervous system pain suppressants cause miosis by stimulating the Edinger-Westphal nucleus. When nalorphine is given to a person with miosis induced by morphine, the pupil will dilate. Nalorphine causes miosis in a normal pupil. Cocaine dilates the pupil when given topically and systemically.

When a postganglionic autonomic axon is damaged, the effector cell (the ciliary muscle and sphincter of the pupil for the parasympathetic system and the dilator of the pupil for the sympathetic system) becomes supersensitive to its transmitter and drugs similar to it. Supersensitivity occurs within days for the acetylcholine-type drugs and within weeks for the norepinephrine-related drugs.

CLINICAL EVALUATION OF THE PUPIL

Details of pupillary function in various disease states are considered in specific sections. In many cases the problem is anisocoria. The pathologic pupil is the one with deficient reactivity. Which pupil either does not dilate as well as its fellow in the dark or does not constrict as well in the light? Measurement of pupil size in a bright, evenly lit room[36] and in relative darkness gives this information and leads to more focused questioning and testing. Photography may help to quantitate these measurements.[42] Anisocoria with normal reactivity at one time or another is common in normal subjects.[43–45]

Since the pupil can be affected by local disease, a routine ophthalmologic examination with special emphasis on the slit-lamp examination is mandatory. The slit lamp is necessary to detect the small pupil of a corneal abrasion or the dilated pupil of angle-closure glaucoma. Abnormalities of the iris structure and segmental pupillary sphincter reactions are only visible with slit-lamp magnification. In some cases it is helpful to measure the amount of residual accommodation with an accommodative target. In persons over 40 yr of age, the influence of age is a complicating variable that influences accommodation. Testing of the pupillary near reaction must be done on a target that is more interesting than a flashlight.

The pupil is innervated both by parasympathetics (via the third cranial nerve) and by the sympathetic nervous system. The position of the upper lid is controlled by the third cranial nerve (the levator palpebrae superiorus) and by the smaller Müller's muscle, which is innervated by the sympathetic nervous system, and opposed by the orbicularis oculi that closes the lids. Damage to the function of the superior division of the third cranial nerve or the ocular sympathetics can cause ptosis of the upper lid. Ptosis due to levator palpebrae dysfunction is greater in almost all cases than that from Müller's muscle dysfunction, which usually leads to only 1 to 2 mm of ptosis.

Disorders that affect pupillary size and accommodation can affect other nerves in the vicinity of the pupillomotor pathways, especially those serving the eye. Special attention should be paid to an evaluation of the historical and clinical aspects of the second, third, fourth, fifth, and sixth cranial nerves. Since higher disorders of eye movement and visual function may be related to pupillary dysfunction, testing of gaze and visual fields may be helpful. The devious course of the sympathetics through the spine, chest, and neck require some attention to neck and lung in the history and physical examination. It is often useful to ask probing questions about possible exposure to topical pupillary dilators or constrictors. Patients often forget the exposure that causes the pupillary change. Old photographs examined under high magnification can be extremely helpful.

CLINICOPATHOLOGIC STATES

Categorization is according to the most obvious characteristic, the pupil size. The diagnostic groups become better defined as further tests are applied and the definitive characteristics emerge. An example is the syphilitic Argyll-Robertson pupil, which is always small;

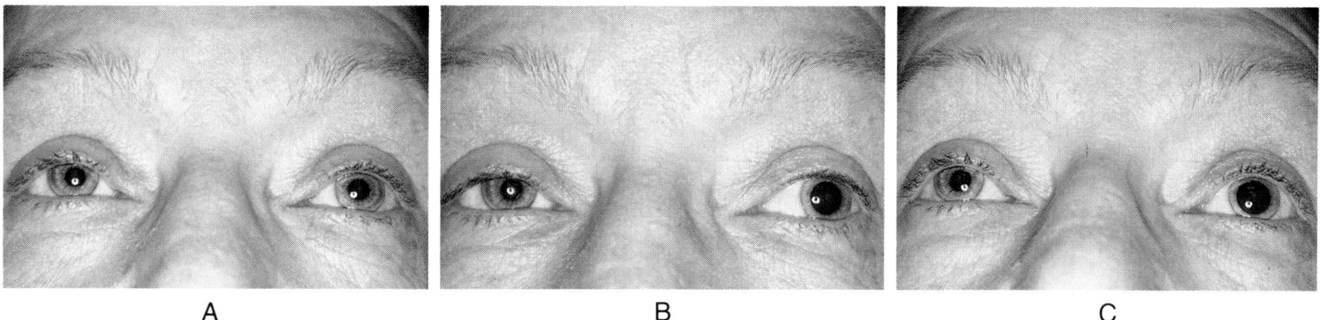

Figure 195–3. An example of postganglionic Horner's syndrome. *A*, Right-sided Horner's syndrome. *B*, Only the left pupil dilates after cocaine 4 percent is instilled into both eyes. *C*, The left pupil dilates much better than the right pupil after OH-amphetamine 1 percent is instilled in both eyes.

more importantly it is unreactive to light but reactive to a near stimulus.

PUPILS THAT DO NOT DILATE WELL IN THE DARK AND THE PUPIL THAT IS TOO SMALL

This pupil is small because the sympathetic nervous system is not functioning well or because the parasympathetic nervous system is overfunctioning.

HORNER'S SYNDROME

Sympathetic Failure (Figs. 195–3 and 195–4)

Horner's syndrome is almost always a unilateral condition with the following features. The pupil on the affected side is smaller than its fellow and dilates less well in the dark.[46] The upper lid on the affected side is slightly ptotic. The pupil on the affected side dilates less well to cocaine drops that does its fellow. Other features are less constant and less useful. These are ipsilateral ocular hypotony, loss of facial sweating,[47, 48] increased amplitude of accommodation, higher position of the lower lid, and the response of the pupil to epinephrine 1/1000.

Congenital Horner's syndrome has a lighter colored iris on the affected side.[49]

The relative miosis and the mild ptosis of Horner's pupil are due to the failure of the sympathetic nervous system to dilate the affected pupil and to stimulate Müller's muscle of the lid. Some patients with Horner's syndrome have a segmental spasm of the dilator muscle, which gives a tadpole-shaped pupil[50] that resembles the picture seen with the local application of epinephrine to the eye. Since the β_2-adrenergic receptors of the ciliary body are denervated, one might expect decreased aqueous secretion, hypotony, and increased accommodation, but apparently too many other factors supervene.

The sympathetic fibers to the face that cause sweating reach the skin via the external carotid artery. Horner's pupil due to a lesion distal to the carotid bifurcation does not affect sweating. Tests for sweating are cumbersome and are often difficult to interpret. Loss of sweating, when detectable, usually indicates a preganglionic lesion.

There is a muscle in the lower lid analogous to the Müller's muscle of the upper lid. Its influence on the lower lid position is not as constant as Müller's muscle and therefore dysfunction causes an unpredictable effect.

Cocaine dilates a normal pupil by enhancing the effect of norepinephrine by preventing its re-uptake into the nerve terminal.[51, 52] Pupillary testing with cocaine is an extremely reliable test. Any dysfunction of the sympathetic nerves (first-, second-, or third-order) decreases the amount of transmitter at the myoneural junction of the pupillary dilator muscle, and therefore cocaine has

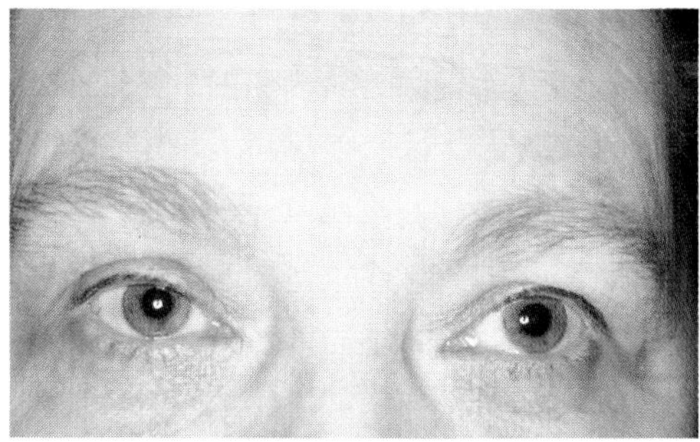

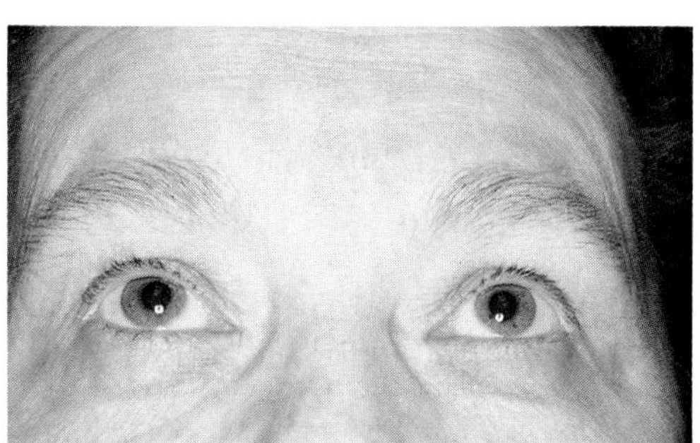

Figure 195–4. *A*, An example of a preganglionic Horner's pupil that appeared after chest surgery. *B*, Both pupils dilate after OH-amphetamine 1 percent is administered.

less effect. Cocaine is used in solution from 2 to 10 percent. The test is done by placing two drops separated by 5 min in each eye and re-measuring the pupil size in 30 min. As little as 0.5 mm less dilatation on one side is strongly suggestive of Horner's syndrome.[53–55] One need only measure the postcocaine asymmetry without paying any attention to the asymmetry before the cocaine was applied. A postcocaine anisocoria of 0.8 mm or more in a set of pupils that has not been altered by topical medications is overwhelmingly likely to indicate Horner's syndrome.[55, 56] It is very important that the cornea has not been tactilely or chemically manipulated before the drops are instilled. Such maneuvers can disrupt the corneal epithelium and enhance penetration of cocaine into the anterior chamber. Cocaine only identifies a Horner's pupil; it does not localize the damage to a particular neuron of the sympathetic chain.

Hydroxyamphetamine 1 percent acts by driving transmitter out of the third neuron terminal onto the pupillary dilator muscle.[57, 58] The pupil should dilate less if the third or postganglionic neuron is damaged, but the pupil should dilate normally if the third neuron is normal, no matter what the state of the preganglionic or central neurons. Thus in a postganglionic Horner's syndrome, hydroxyamphetamine dilates the miotic pupil less well than does the normal pupil.[59] Since topical cocaine alters the corneal epithelium, one cannot do the hydroxyamphetamine test the same day as the cocaine test.

A Horner's pupil due to a postganglionic neuron dysfunction should result in denervation hypersensitivity of the dilator of the iris.[52] However, use of 1/1000 epinephrine has not proved to be a reliable test.[60]

The hydroxyamphetamine test may be falsely localizing in children, perhaps due to transsynaptic degeneration.[61] Although an excellent test, one occasionally encounters patients with Horner's syndrome with preganglionic lesions that are well identified because they have been induced by surgery but that give confusing results when tested with hydroxyamphetamine.[62]

All the aforementioned chemical testing assumes that the pupil is free to move and has not been altered by local chemicals or disease.

Localization in Horner's Syndrome

The course of the sympathetic nerves to the eye dictates that each of the links of the three neuron chains is more exposed to certain pathologic entities than the others. Although there are exceptions, it has been a long-standing dictum that the third or postganglionic neuron is affected by conditions that are benign, whereas the preganglionic or central neurons are affected in more serious conditions. Thus the hydroxyamphetamine test should by itself separate "benign" from the more serious conditions.[63] One should avoid the temptation to depend entirely on the drug testing however. Other information is usually available.[64] The central neuron, running from the hypothalamus to the spinal cord, is almost never affected in isolation from other obvious and usually profound neurologic signs. It is usually the case that the other neurologic signs and symptoms are of chief concern and that Horner's syndrome is of ancillary interest.

The second member of the sympathetic chain, the preganglionic neuron, which passes from the spinal cord through the chest and into the neck, is vulnerable to spine pathology,[65] tumors,[66, 67] prior surgery, and injury. Arm pain is a symptom to be aware of in patients with chest tumors. Exquisite imaging of the chest and neck is available by computed tomography. Congenital Horner's syndrome is most commonly due to obstetric injury to the brachial plexus or the neck.

The third neuron or the postganglionic neuron has usually been associated with idiopathic "vascular" diseases. Head trauma is another common cause.[68] Infections of the intracavernous portion of the internal carotid by fungi in immunocompromised patients can cause Horner's syndrome before other structures within the cavernous sinus are affected. Children with acquired Horner's syndrome often have significant pathology.[49]

Horner's Syndrome with Pain

A special clinical combination frequently encountered is that of postganglionic Horner's syndrome with pain in a trigeminal distribution. If there is no evidence for any other neurologic dysfunction, these cases almost always fall into a "vascular" or idiopathic course. The head pain can be very severe, and with Horner's syndrome comes in attacks similar to those suffered by a migraneur, thus suggesting a common etiology. Raeder's syndrome is classically seen in middle-aged men and presents, like "cluster" headaches, with repeated attacks for several weeks and is then quiescent for several months only to return.[69, 70]

These distinctions may be artificial. It is important to separate two groups: Those without other neurologic signs in which case the condition is likely to be repetitive but benign, from those with other neurologic signs who deserve a more complete neuroradiologic work-up with the suspicion of more severe underlying pathology.[68, 71]

BILATERAL SMALL PUPILS

Pupils are small in infants because the dilator muscle is poorly developed, and they are also small in the elderly.[72, 73] They are relatively larger in teenagers. They become small during drowsiness.[74] There are numerous topical (e.g., parasympathomimetics) and systemic (e.g, morphine-related analgesics, pesticides, and related chemical weapons) drugs that cause intense miosis.[75–79] It should be remembered that intense local pain in or around the eye causes bilateral miosis worse on the affected side.[80] Patients with Argyll-Robertson pupils will have miotic pupils.[81] This condition is considered later with Adie's pupil. Finally, esotropia, myopia, and small pupils should suggest spasm of the near reflex, which is considered later.

FAILURE OF THE PUPIL TO CONSTRICT TO LIGHT (Fig. 195–5)

Failure of the pupil to constrict to light can mean an inadequate input on the afferent or visual side, the relative afferent pupillary defect, a dysfunction of the intermediate neurons of the protectum on which the afferent axons from the ganglion cells synapse, or a dysfunction of the neurons from the Edinger-Westphal nucleus to the ciliary ganglion or from the ciliary ganglion to the eye. It could also mean that the pupillary sphincter is unable to constrict due to local influences. These entities are separable on clinical grounds.

If the problem with the pupil light reflex is only due to the prechiasmal afferent or visual side, then the intactness of the motor side can be demonstrated by stimulating the healthy optic nerve with light on the retina and seeing that both pupils react. If the problem is in the afferent or visual system, there is also some evidence of dysfunction of vision: color appreciation and brightness sense may be depressed,[82, 83] there may be depressed visual acuity, there may be visual field defects,[84] or a depression of the amplitude of latency of the visual evoked potential.[85] In most cases, one optic nerve will be dysfunctional.[86] There is an asymmetric light reaction because the pupillary reaction in both eyes to direct light stimulation of the affected optic nerve is less than that in both eyes when the normal optic nerve is stimulated by light on the retina. What is remarkable about this test is that opacities of the ocular media, particularly cataracts, have so little effect on this light reaction.[87, 88] In fact, if enough light is excluded from one eye by patching or its equivalent, the increased retinal sensitivity of this eye creates a relative afferent defect in the fellow eye after the patch is removed and both eyes are tested by direct light.[89, 90] It is also true that only the most obvious retinal lesions depress the pupillary light reaction.[91–93] A problem arises if both optic nerves are dysfunctional or if there is chiasmal disease.[94] The eye with the larger visual field defect will have the less pupillary light reaction to direct input. With optic tract lesions, the pupillary light reaction to direct stimulation is slightly depressed in the eye contralateral to the affected tract, Behr's pupil.[95, 96] This is due to an excess of fibers from the nasal retina over the temporal retina.

An eye with strabismic or anisometropic amblyopia can have an afferent light defect.[97–99] It seems, however, that one would need histologic evidence that the optic nerve was indeed normal before one could be certain of this being possible. One must always be concerned in such cases about the possibility of an underlying optic neuropathy. Patients with congenital achromatopsia and congenital stationary night blindness show a transient pupillary constriction to darkness.[100]

The test for a relative afferent pupillary light defect can be done in a variety of ways.[101, 102] The Marcus-Gunn test involves covering one eye and then the other eye. Both pupils are larger, Kestenbaum's number, when the eye with the more normal nerve is covered.[103] This test is not as effective in rooms with uneven

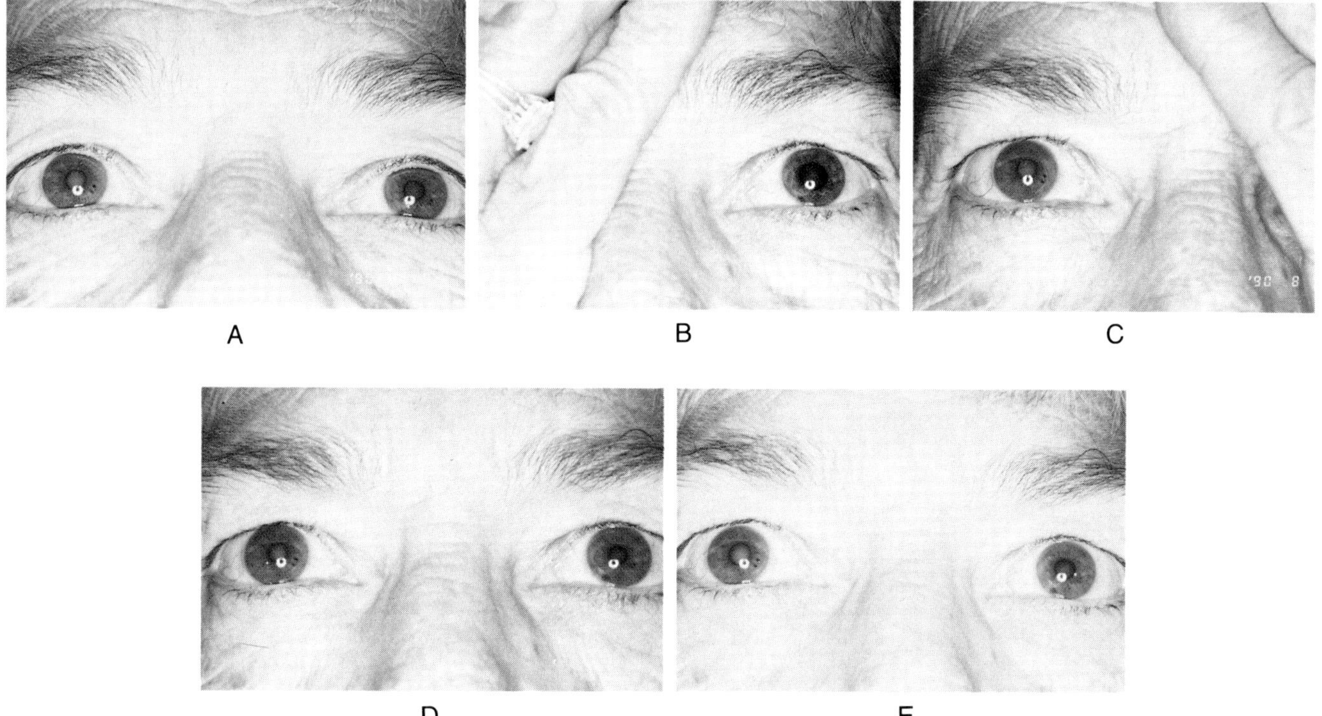

Figure 195–5. The afferent pupillary light reflex. *A,* A patient with a dense cataract in the right eye and an optic neuropathy in the left eye. *B,* When the right eye is covered, the left pupil dilates because the major afferent light input to the pretectal nuclei has been eliminated. *C,* When the left eye is covered, the pupil size remains unchanged. *D,* Both pupils constrict when light is shone in the right eye (notice the two light reflexes on the right cornea). *E,* Both pupils dilate when light is shone in the left eye.

illumination. The swinging flashlight test in which a light is rapidly shone into one eye and then the other eye has the additional advantage of contrasting a pupil that constricts when light hits it with one that dilates when illuminated.[104, 105] The afferent input when the eye with the healthy nerve is illuminated constricts both pupils. When light is passed over the bridge of the nose to the fellow eye, both pupils begin to dilate. When light strikes the eye with the dysfunctional nerve, both pupils continue to dilate because the afferent input is less.[106, 107] In cases in which one pupil is anatomically altered (e.g., after cataract surgery), the fellow eye can be observed instead, the "reverse pupillary light reaction."

A bright light works best, but because it rapidly bleaches the retina, it can only be used for a few cycles before the light reaction weakens to a point at which a distinction between the two eyes cannot be made.[108–110] It is then best to allow the patient to rest for a while before retesting. Furthermore, the pupils should be of the same size.[111] Anisocoria becomes significant for this test when it is 2 mm or greater. Finally, the light must go directly into the eye to be completely effective.[112] This can be a problem when the eyes are not aligned. When the narrow beam of the slit lamp is shone at the pupillary edge, the pupil constricts and eliminates the light from falling on the retina, thus causing the pupil to dilate. The number of times this cycle is repeated in 1 min is depressed with lesions of the afferent system giving a sense of quantitation to the analysis.[113–120] Another way of quantitating the pupillary light reaction is to place filters of graduated density in log units before the more normal afferent system until the swinging flashlight test is symmetric.[121]

FAILURE OF THE PUPILLARY LIGHT REFLEX—LESIONS INVOLVING THE PATHWAY FROM THE PRETECTAL NUCLEI TO THE EDINGER-WESTPHAL NUCLEUS (Fig. 195–6)[122]

Abnormalities result from brain stem lesions affecting supranuclear or nuclear pupil pathways. Pupils show a symmetric failure of the light reaction in both eyes with relative preservation of the near reflexes.[123, 124] Perfectly symmetric optic nerve disease could cause this but could be detected by the loss of vision. In the examples to be discussed, vision should be unaffected. To be discussed later are Adie's pupil and some third-nerve palsies with regeneration, but these are usually unilateral conditions and can easily be separated from pretectal cases by associated findings.

The two main conditions that are discussed are the syphilitic Argyll-Robertson pupil and the pupil that can be seen with compression of the pretectum by tumor or in pretectal stroke—Parinaud's pupil. Such pupils have also been reported in diabetes mellitus, myotonic dystrophy, familial amyloidosis, multiple sclerosis, and encephalitis.

The Argyll-Robertson pupil of central nervous system syphilis is bilateral; it has a small irregular shape; it is in an eye with vision; and it reacts to accommodative effort.[125, 126]

By contrast, in Parinaud's syndrome, the pupils are larger and there is impaired upward gaze. Larger lesions may cause convergence-retraction nystagmus. An extensive review of this situation can be found in Vogel's article.[127]

The anatomy that explains the aforementioned situation seems to be that the supranuclear accommodative fibers run below the hemidecussated supranuclear light reaction fibers in the pretectum and thus can be spared. It is well known that vertical gaze is represented in a compact manner in the pretectum. In Parinaud's syndrome, vertical gaze and the light reaction are affected. The miotic pupils of central nervous system syphilis are thought to be due to a disinhibition of the Edinger-Westphal nucleus, perhaps similar to that seen in sleep and that induced by morphine. However, more than one explanation for this may be possible.[128, 129] The irregularity of the pupil in the Argyll-Robertson pupil is due to iris atrophy.

UNILATERAL DILATED PUPIL

A lesion affecting the parasympathetic pathway from the Edinger-Westphal nucleus to the ciliary ganglion via

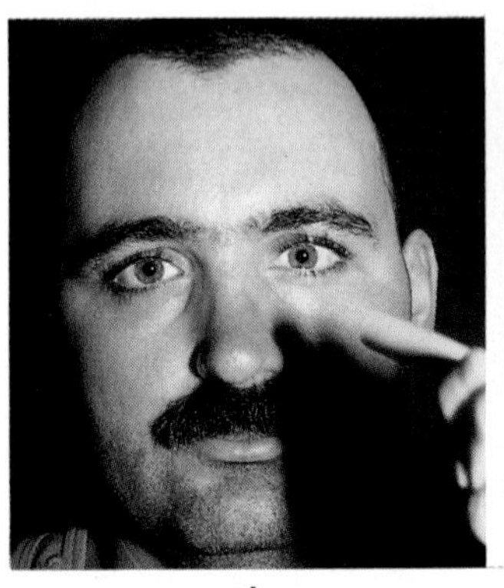
A

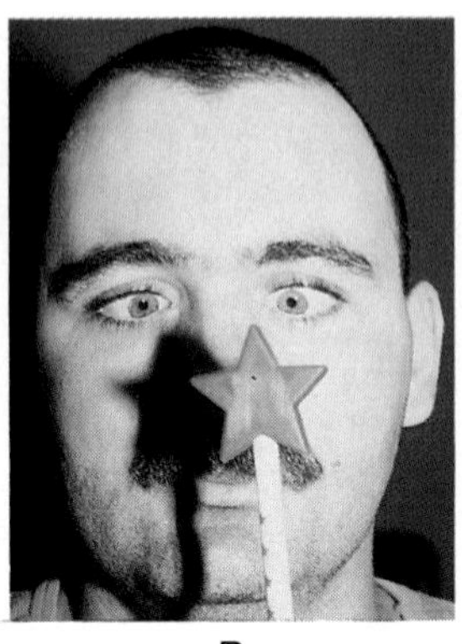
B

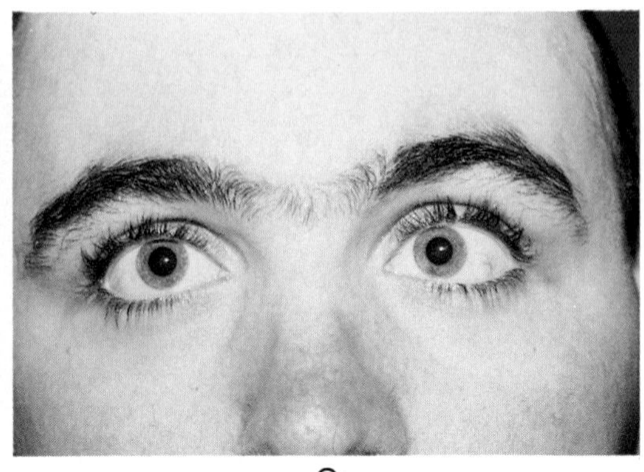
C

Figure 195–6. Parinaud's syndrome. *A,* A patient with a pineal cytoma pressing on the pretectum shows a poor pupillary light reaction. *B,* The near reaction of the pupils is good. *C,* Attempted upgaze is poorly done. (Photos courtesy of Joseph Rizzo, M.D.)

the third cranial nerve or a lesion of the ciliary ganglion or its axon to the ciliary body and the constrictor muscle of the pupil will dilate the pupil and paralyze accommodation. The issue of the importance of the dilated pupil in cases of third cranial nerve palsy is covered in Chapter 194. Some special issues deserve emphasis here. Aberrant regeneration of the third nerve is common when a third-nerve palsy includes a dilated pupil. With regeneration of the nerve the ciliary ganglion can be reinnervated by an aberrant axon, thus when the patient attempts to direct the affected eye into a particular direction, the pupil constricts.[130]

It is mentioned later that denervation hypersensitivity of the pupillary sphincter muscle is a characteristic of dysfunction of the ciliary ganglion and its axons. Adie's pupil is the most commonly recognized cause, and the denervation hypersensitivity can be detected by the use of topical methacholine (2.5 percent) or solutions of pilocarpine (0.1 percent). However, there is evidence to suggest that there can be transsynaptic degeneration at the ciliary ganglion, leading to denervation hypersensitivity in cases of a pupil involving preganglionic third cranial nerve palsies.[131, 132]

There are unusual cases of pupillary dilation that are seemingly due to involvement of the nucleus of the third cranial nerve.[133] During the paretic phase of cyclic congenital third-nerve palsies, the pupil is dilated; it constricts during the phase of third-nerve function.[134]

It has previously been mentioned that transient or permanent anisocoria with no apparent pathology is common—"simple, central anisocoria."[135] Patients who have asymmetric pupil size but no apparent failure to dilate in the dark or constrict in the light fall into this category. Anisocoria is always less in the light than in the dark because of the mechanical limits on pupillary constriction. Such patients have no other signs or symptoms.

It should be recognized that young adults with migraine suffer from intermittent dilatation of the pupil, often in an oval fashion with or without a headache. These patients should not have any other signs and in particular should not have double vision if they are to be placed in this category.[136, 137]

Damage to or disease of the ciliary ganglion or its axons paralyzes the pupillary sphincter muscle and causes the pupil to dilate and paralyze the ciliary muscle, which causes failure of accommodation. There are a number of disease states that can cause this to happen (Fig. 195–7), and Adie's pupil is the most common.[138–140] It is seen in young adults and in women more than men and starts with a unilaterally dilated pupil that is unreactive to light or near and poor accommodation. Within a few weeks, the accommodation may start to return but does not always return to normal. However, the pupil light reaction becomes unusual.[141] The pupil is almost always slightly dilated on the affected side.[142] Constriction of the pupil in light and dilatation in the dark and after prolonged near fixation are very sluggish, hence the term "tonic pupil." The degree of anisocoria varies depending on the amount of time that has passed since the level of illumination has changed. The pupillary near reaction is better than the light reaction. If one examines the pupil at high magnification, one can see that segments of the pupil constrict to light, whereas other segments are passively stretched, "vermiform" (worm-like) movements.[143] The pupil exhibits denervation hypersensitivity to weak solutions of pilocarpine or mecholyl and constricts more than the fellow, normal eye.[144] Although there is a certain degree of corneal anesthesia, there is not an increase in corneal permeability.[145, 146] Attempts to make the patient more comfortable over the long term with chronic use of pilocarpine drops are only occasionally successful.

Adie's pupil is idiopathic and annoying but is benign.[147] There is not much histopathology available[148]; a unifying hypothesis that could account for the clinical picture and its evolution is that described by Lowenfeld and Thompson, who suggest that the initial phase of complete pupillary and accommodative paralysis reflects damage to the ciliary ganglion or ciliary nerve.[149, 150] With time there is regeneration, but only partial reinnervation of the ciliary body and the pupil with the tonically acting neurons. The pupillary sphincter is only partially reinnervated, which accounts for the denervation hypersensitivity and the vermiform movements. The pupil moves sluggishly in light and dark because it is innervated by a tonic neuron rather than a phasic neuron.

It is thought that Adie's pupil represents a mild dysfunction of the autonomic nervous system. There are entities with more widely spread and troublesome autonomic dysfunction. The mildest of these is seen in Adie's syndrome when there is depression of the tendon jerks in addition to the ocular findings. This association is very common and reflects the additional disturbances of the dorsal root ganglia of the spinal cord.[151–153] Ross described tonic pupils, altered deep tendon reflexes, and segmental hypohidrosis.[154–158] Acute pandysautonomia and Fisher's syndrome may manifest tonic pupils.[159–161]

The aforementioned conditions seem to be part of a spectrum of neurologic dysfunction. Tonic pupils can rarely be seen in specific disease states other than the aforementioned idiopathic conditions: sarcoidosis,[162] neurosyphilis (supporting the need for serologic testing in patients with Adie's pupil),[163, 164] temporal arteritis,[165, 166] Charcot-Marie-Tooth disease,[168] and following preganglionic third-nerve palsies, epidemic nephropathy,[167] dental anesthesia,[169] and botulism.[168] The list is almost endless. Further details can be found in volume 2 of Miller's edition of Walsh and Hoyt's *Clinical Neuro-Ophthalmology*.[170]

IRIDOPLEGIA DUE TO DRUGS

The pharmacology of such agents has been mentioned earlier, but some special clinical situations deserve emphasis.

Bilateral dilated pupils from systemic drugs are rarely a clinical problem. The degree of dilatation is usually not striking, and the symmetry of the pupils is reassuring. Those medications that act as cycloplegics, espe-

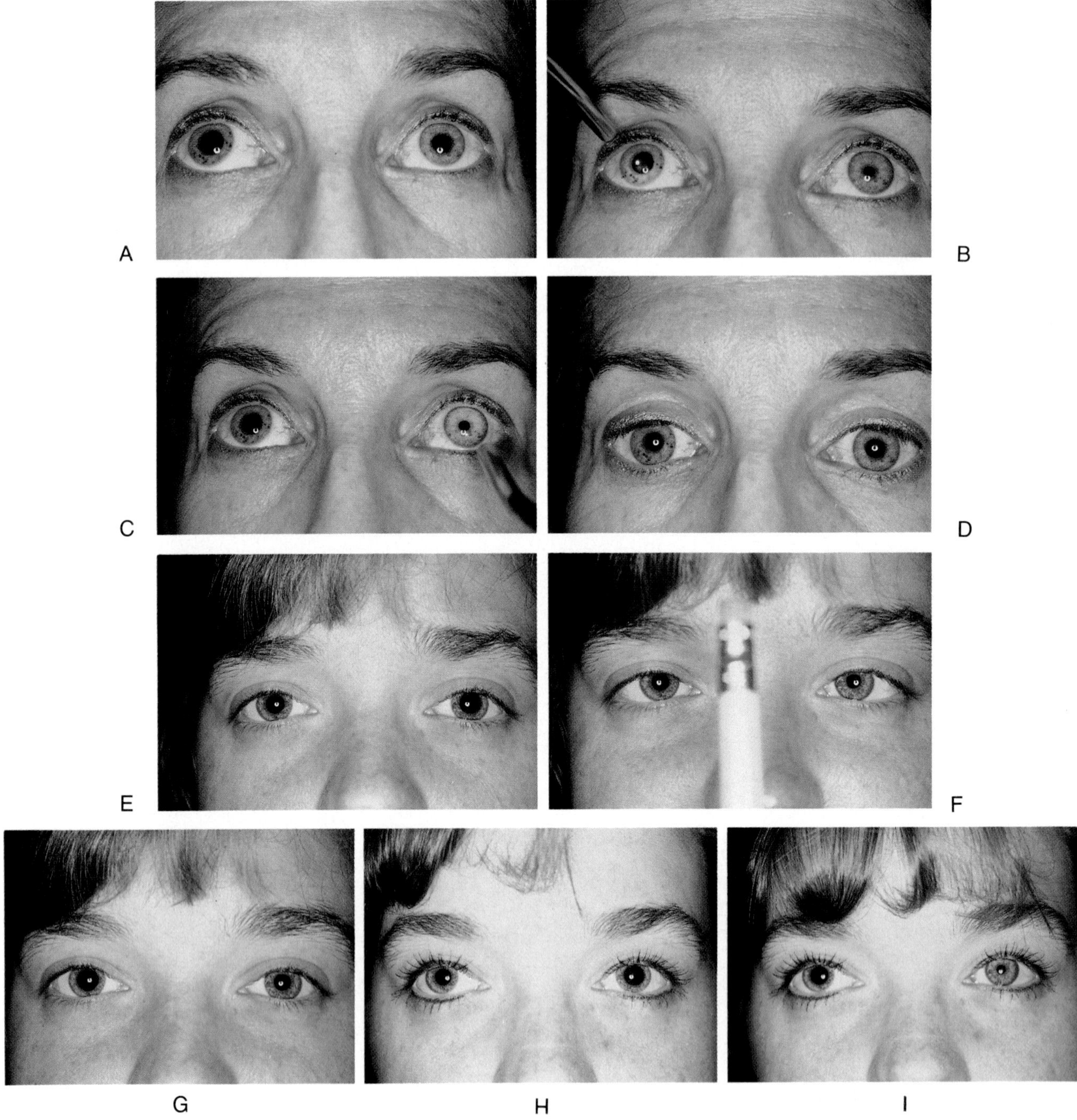

Figure 195–7. Adie's pupil. *A,* Right Adie's pupil in room light. *B* and *C,* To direct and consensual light, the right pupil constricts poorly. *D,* There is much better constriction of the right pupil to the near reflex. *E,* Left Adie's pupil. *F,* The left pupil constricts on near fixation. *G,* Immediately after prolonged near fixation, the left pupil dilates slowly—dilation lag. *H,* Left-sided Adie's pupil. *I,* Hypersensitive response of the left pupil after pilocarpine (0.1 percent) is instilled in both eyes.

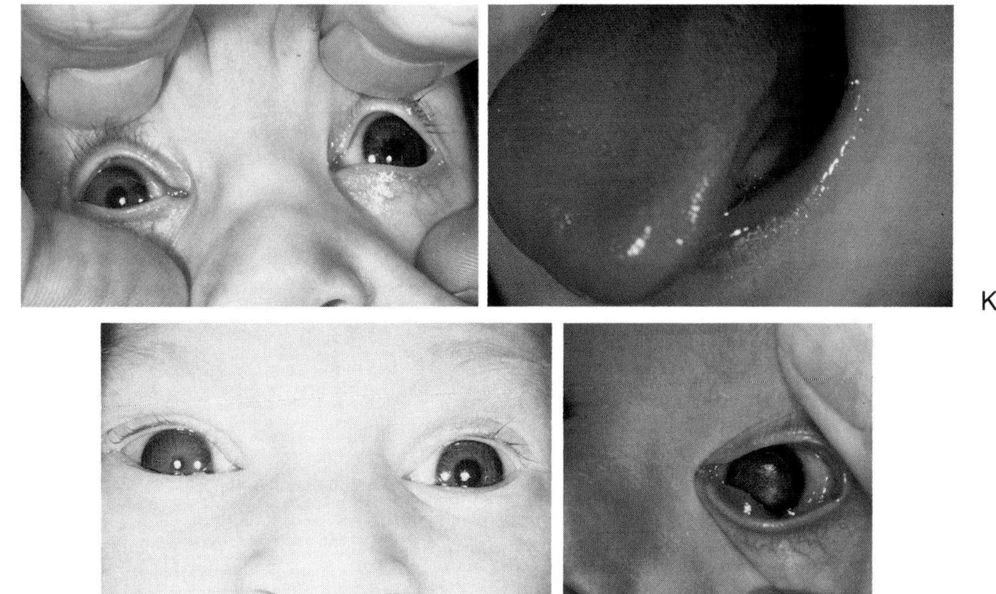

Figure 195–7 *Continued J,* Congenital hereditary dysautonomia. *K,* Characteristic smooth tongue. *L,* Hypersensitive response of the right pupil to methacholine (2.5 percent), which is instilled in the right eye. *M,* Corneal abrasions are common in this condition.

cially antidepressants in young people, are more annoying by virtue of their effect on accommodation.

Unilateral dilated pupils present more of a problem. The way in which the drug got into the eye may not be clear (e.g., with the use of scopolamine patches),[172, 173] or it may be deliberately concealed by malingerers.

The fear is that a fixed dilated pupil may be a sign of an impending neurologic catastrophe. In the healthy patient with no other neurologic findings and intact mentation, this is almost never the case. When a pupil is dilating because of third cranial nerve compression, it does not usually get as large as that induced by an atropine or adrenergic-like drop. One may apply 0.5 or 1 percent pilocarpine drops to both eyes.[174] If the pupil is dilated due to a lesion of the third nerve or ciliary ganglion, the dilated pupil constricts as well or better than the normal side. Pupils dilated by eye drops constrict less well. The test is dramatic in cases in which a long-acting atropine-like drug has been used. When the drops start to wear off and when weaker agents are used, the asymmetry of the response to pilocarpine is less dramatic.

COMA AND UNCAL HERNIATION

Assessment of pupil function may be helpful in patients in coma.[174] Depending on the site of the lesion, many of the pupillary abnormalities mentioned previously are present to help in localizing the lesion. A supratentorial lesion can cause an advancing caudal to rostral brain stem dysfunction, which when it involves chiefly the mesencephalon is characterized by bilateral dilated and fixed pupils. The prognosis for a full recovery after this stage is poor. An exception is that following lightning injury, when the pupil is an unreliable indicator of the severity of brain stem hypoxia.[175]

When there is uncal herniation, the only neurologic findings may be an altered level of consciousness and a unilateral dilated pupil.[176] Since the process deteriorates rapidly, it is important to intervene if possible to relieve the expanding supratentorial lesion as soon as possible.

SUMMARY

The pupil can be an important clue to diagnosis. It is tempting to be caught up in the rich variety of pharmacologic tests and to place the pupil in one category or another. One should avoid this temptation and treat it as one would any other neurologic sign. Pupils should be considered along with the company they keep and should not be judged in isolation.

REFERENCES

1. Thompson HS, Daroff R, Frisen L, Glaser JS: Topics in Neuro-Ophthalmology. Baltimore, Williams & Wilkins, 1979.
2. Miller NR: Walsh and Hoyt's Clinical Neuro-Ophthalmology, 4th ed. Baltimore, Williams & Wilkins, 1985.
3. Zinn K: The Pupil. Springfield, Charles C Thomas, 1972.
4. Alexandridis E: The Pupil. New York, Springer-Verlag, 1985.
5. Thompson HS, Pilley FJ: Unequal pupils: A flow chart for sorting out the anisocorias. Surv Ophthalmol 21:45–48, 1976.
6. Burde RM: Clinician's guide to the pupil. Int Ophthalmol Clin 17:134–156, 1977.
7. Thompson HS: The pupil and accommodation. Neuro-ophthalmology (Excerpta Medica) 1:226–240, 1980.
8. Thompson HS: The pupil. Curr Neuro-Ophthalmol 1:201–216, 1988.
9. Thompson HS: The pupil. Curr Neuro-Ophthalmol 2:213–220, 1989.
10. Alpern M, Campbell FW: The spectral sensitivity of the consensual light reflex. J Physiol 164:478–507, 1962.
11. Alexandridis E: Lichtsinn and pupillenreaktion. *In* Dodt E, Schrader KE: Die normale und die gestorte Pupillenbewegung. Munich, Bergmann, 1973.
12. Alexandridis E: Pupillographische Untersuchung der Netzhautempfindlichkeit des Taubenauges. Graefes Arch Clin Exp Ophthalmol 172:139–151, 1967.
13. Alexandridis E: Pupillographische Untersuchung der Netzhautempfindlichkeit eines Stabchenmonochromaten. Pflugers Arch 294:67, 1967.

14. Alexandridis E: Bestimmung der Dunkeladaptationskurve mit Hilfe der Pupillenlichtreflexe. Ber Dtsch Ophthalmol Ges 68:274–277, 1968.
15. Ranson SW, Magoun HW: The central path of the pupilloconstrictor reflex in response to light. Arch Neurol Psychiatry (Chicago) 30:1193–1204, 1933.
16. Crosby EC, Humphrey T, Laurel EW: Correlative Anatomy of the Nervous System. New York, Macmillan, 1962.
17. Clarke RJ, Coimbra CJP, Alessio ML: Oculomotor areas involved in the parasympathetic control of accommodation and pupil size in the marmose. Braz J Med Biol Res 18(3):373–379, 1985.
18. Christensen HD, Koss MC, Gherezghiher T: Synaptic organization in the oculomotor nucleus. Ann NY Acad Sci 473:382–399, 1986.
19. Jampel RS: Representation of the near response on the cerebral cortex of the macaque. Am J Ophthalmol 48:573–582, 1959.
20. Bando T: Pupillary constriction evoked from the posterior medial lateral suprasylvian (PMLS) area in cats. Neurosci Res (6):472–485, 1985.
21. Barris RW: A pupilloconstrictor area in the cerebral cortex of the cat and its relationship to the pretectal area. J Comp Neurol 63:353–368, 1936.
22. Hamann K-U, Hellner KA, Muller-Jensen A, et al: Videopupillographic and VER investigations in patients with congenital and acquired lesions of the optic radiation. Ophthalmologica 178:348–356, 1979.
23. Koerner F, Teuber H-L: Visual fields defects of the missile injuries to the geniculo-striate pathways in man. Exp Brain Res 18:88–113, 1973.
24. Alexandridis E, Krastel H, Reuther R: Pupillenreflex Storungen bei Läsionen der Oberen Sehbahn. Graefes Arch Clin Exp Ophthalmol 209:199–208, 1979.
25. Harms H: Grundlagen, Methodik und Bedeutung der Pupillenperimetrie. Graefes Arch Clin Exp Ophthalmol 149:1–68, 1949.
26. Harms H: Hemianopische Pupillenstarre. Klin Monatsbl Augenheilkd 118:133–147, 1951.
27. Harms H: Moglichkeiten und Grenzen der Pupillomotorischen Perimetrie. Klin Monatsbl Augenheilkd 129:518–534, 1956.
28. Harms H, Aulhorn E, Ksinsik R: Die Ergebnisse Pupillomotorischer Perimetrie bei Sehhirnverletzten und die Vorstellungen uber Verlauf der Lichtreflexbahn. *In* Dodt E, Schrader KE: Die normale und die gestorte Pupillenbewegung. Munich, Bergmann, 1973.
29. Warwick R: The ocular parasympathetic nerve supply and its mesencephalic sources. J Anat 88:71–93, 1954.
30. Sillito AM, Zbrozyna AW: The localization of the pupilloconstrictor function within the mid-brain of the cat. J Physiol 211:461–477, 1970.
31. Hultborn H, Mori K, Tsukahara N: The neuronal pathway subserving the pupillary light reflex. Brain Res 159:255–267, 1978.
32. Shoumura K, Imai H: Pupillary responses evoked by electrical stimulation of area pretectalis in cats. Jpn J Ophthalmol 30(4):436–452, 1986.
33. Kerr KW, Hollowell OW: Location of pupillomotor and accommodation fibers in the oculomotor nerve: Experimental observation on paralytic mydriasis. J Neurol Neurosurg Psychiatry 27:473–481, 1964.
34. Sunderland S, Hughes ESR: The pupilloconstrictor pathway and the nerves to the ocular muscles in man. Brain 69:301–309, 1946.
35. Parkinson D: Further observations on the sympathetic pathways to the pupil. Anat Rec 220(1):108–109, 1988.
36. Spring KH, Stiles WS: Variation of pupil size with change in the angles at which the light stimulus strikes the retina. Br J Ophthalmol 32:340–346, 1948.
37. Marg E, Morgan MW Jr: Further investigation of the pupillary near reflex. Am J Optom Physiol Opt 27:217–225, 1950.
38. Marg E, Morgan MW Jr: The pupillary near reflex: The relation of pupillary diameter to accommodation and various components of convergence. Am J Optom Physiol Opt 26:183–189, 1949.
39. Jampel RS: Representation of the near response on the cerebral cortex of the macaque. Am J Ophthalmol 48:573–582, 1959.
40. Phillips S, Stark L: Blur: A sufficient accommodative stimulus. Doc Ophthalmol 43:65–89, 1977.
41. Lowenstein O, Feinberg R, Loewenfeld IE: Pupillary movements during acute and chronic fatigue: A new test for the objective evaluation of tiredness. Invest Ophthalmol 2:138–157, 1963.
42. Czarnecki JSC, Pilley SFJ, Thompson HS: The analysis of anisocoria. Can J Ophthalmol 14:297–302, 1979.
43. Lam BL, Thompson HS, Corbett JJ: The prevalence of simple anisocoria. Am J Ophthalmol 104:69–73, 1987.
44. Roarty JD, Kelner JL: Normal pupil size and anisocoria in newborn infants. Arch Ophthalmol 108:94–95, 1990.
45. Meyer BC: Incidence of anisocoria and difference in size of palpebral fissures in 500 normal subjects. Arch Neurol Psychiatry 57:464–468, 1947.
46. Pilley SFJ, Thompson HS: Pupillary dilation lag in Horner's syndrome. Br J Ophthalmol 59:731–735, 1975.
47. Salvesen R, DeSouza CD, Sjaastad O: Horner's syndrome sweat gland and pupillary responsiveness in two cases with a probable third neuron dysfunction. Cephalgia 9:63–70, 1989.
48. Rosenberg ML: The friction sweat test as a new method for detecting facial anhidrosis in patients with Horner's syndrome. Am J Ophthalmol 108:443–447, 1989.
49. Sauer C, Levinsohn MW: Horner's syndrome in childhood. Neurology 26:216–220, 1976.
50. Thompson HS, Zackon DH, Czarnecki JSC: Tadpole shaped pupils caused by segmental spasm of the iris dilator. Am J Ophthalmol 96:467–477, 1983.
51. Lepore FE: Diagnostic pharmacology of the pupil. Clin Neuropharmacol 8(1)27–37, 1985.
52. Schafer WD, Leinwald B: Die Bedeutung des Cocain-Adrenaline-Testes beim Hornerschen Symptomenkomplex. *In* Dodt E, Schrader KE: Die normale und die gestorte Pupillenbewegung. Munich, Bergmann, 1973.
53. Van der Wiel HL, Van Gijn J: The diagnosis of Horner's syndrome: Use and limitations of the cocaine test. J Neurosurg Sci 73:311–316, 1986.
54. Friedman JR, Whiting DW, Kosmorsky GS, et al: The cocaine test in normal patients. Am J Ophthalmol 98:808–810, 1984.
55. Kardon RH, Denison CE, Brown CK, et al: Critical evaluation of the cocaine test in the diagnosis of Horner's syndrome. Arch Ophthalmol 108:384–387, 1990.
56. Moster ML: The cocaine test in Horner's syndrome. Arch Ophthalmol 108:1667, 1990.
57. Cremer SA, Thompson HS, Digre KB: Hydroxyamphetamine mydriasis in Horner's syndrome. Am J Ophthalmol 110:71–76, 1990.
58. Heitman K, Bode DD: The paradrine test in normal eyes. J Clin Neuro-Ophthalmol 6:228–231, 1986.
59. Thompson HS, Menscher JH: Adrenergic mydriasis in Horner's syndrome: Hydroxyamphetamine test for diagnosis of postganglionic defects. Am J Ophthalmol 72:472–480, 1971.
60. Newman NM, Levin PS: Testing the pupil in Horner's syndrome. [Letter] Arch Neurol 44(5):471, 1987.
61. Weinstein JM, Zwifel TJ, Thompson HS: Congenital Horner's syndrome. Arch Ophthalmol 98:1074–1078, 1980.
62. Maloney WF, Younge BR, Moyer NJ: Evaluation of the causes and accuracy of pharmacologic localization in Horner's syndrome. Am J Ophthalmol 90:394–402, 1980.
63. Thompson HS: Diagnosing Horner's syndrome. Trans Am Acad Ophthalmol Otolaryngol 83:840–842, 1977.
64. Thompson BM, Corbett JJ, Kline LB, et al: Pseudo-Horner's syndrome. Arch Neurol 39(2):108–111, 1982.
65. Safran MJ, Greenwald MJ, Rice HC, et al: Cervical spine dislocation presenting as an isolated Horner's syndrome. Arch Ophthalmol 108:327–328, 1990.
66. Giles CL, Henderson JW: Horner's syndrome: An analysis of 216 cases. Am J Ophthalmol 46:289–296, 1958.
67. Grimson BS, Thompson HS: Drug testing in Horner's syndrome. *In* Glaser JS, Smith JJ (eds): Neuro-Ophthalmology. St. Louis, CV Mosby, 1975.
68. Grimson BS, Thompson HS: Horner's syndrome: Overall view of 120 cases. *In* Thompson HS, Daroff R, Frisen L, Glaser JS: Topics in Neuro-Ophthalmology. Baltimore, Williams & Wilkins, 1979.
69. Grimson BS, Thompson HS: Reader's syndrome: A clinical review. Surv Ophthalmol 24:199–210, 1980.
70. Cohen DN, Zakov ZN, Salanga VD, et al: Reader's paratrigeminal syndrome. Am J Ophthalmol 79:1044–1049, 1975.

71. Jarett WH: Horner's syndrome with geniculate zoster. Am J Ophthalmol 63:326–330, 1967.
72. Loewenfeld IE: Pupillary changes related to age. *In* Thompson HS, Daroff R, Frisen L, Glaser JS: Topics in Neuro-Ophthalmology. Baltimore, Williams & Wilkins, 1979.
73. Birren JE, Casperson RC, Botwinick J: Age changes in pupil size. J Gerontol 5:216–225, 1950.
74. Pressman MR, DiPhillipo MA, Fry JM: Senile miosis: The possible contribution of disordered sleep and daytime sleepiness. J Gerontol 41:629–634, 1986.
75. Creighton FJ, Ghodse AH: Naloxone applied to conjunctiva as a test for physical opiate dependence. Lancet 1(8641):747–750, 1989.
76. Higgins ST, et al: Pupillary response to methadone challenge in heroin users. Clin Pharmacol Ther 37(4):460–463, 1985.
77. Pickworth WB, et al: Morphine-induced mydriasis and inhibition of pupillary light reflex and fluctuation in the cat. J Pharmacol Exp Ther 234(3):603–606, 1985.
78. Loimer N, Schmid R, Grunberger J, et al: Naloxone induces miosis in normal subjects. Psychopharmacology 101:282–283, 1990.
79. Fedder IL, Vlasses PH, Mojaverian P: Relationship of morphine-induced miosis to plasma concentration in normal subjects. J Pharm Sci 73(10):1496–1497, 1984.
80. Moses RA: Adler's Physiology of the Eye. St. Louis, CV Mosby, 1970.
81. Dalso CC, Bortz DL: Significance of the Argyll-Robertson pupil in clinical medicine. Am J Med 86:199–202, 1989.
82. Lam BL, Thompson HS: Brightness sense and optic nerve disease. Am J Ophthalmol 108(4):462–463, 1989.
83. Sadun AA, Lessell S: Brightness sense and optic nerve disease. Arch Ophthalmol 103(1):39–43, 1985.
84. Thompson HS, Montague P, Cox TA, et al: The relationship between visual acuity, pupillary defect and visual field loss. Am J Ophthalmol 93:681–688, 1982.
85. Cox TA, Thompson HS, Hayreh SS, et al: Visual evoked potential and pupillary signs: A comparison in optic nerve disease. Arch Ophthalmol 100:1603–1607, 1982.
86. Cox TA, Thompson HS, Corbett JJ: Relative afferent pupillary defects in optic neuritis. Am J Ophthalmol 92:685–690, 1981.
87. Thompson HS: Do cataracts influence pupillary responses? Int Ophthalmol Clin 18:109–111, 1978.
88. Sadun AA, Bassi CJ, Lessell S: Why cataracts do not produce afferent pupillary defects. Am J Ophthalmol 110(6):712–714, 1990.
89. Lam BL, Thompson HS: A unilateral cataract produces a relative afferent pupillary defect in the contralateral eye. Ophthalmology 97:334–338, 1990.
90. Dubois LG, Sadun AA: Occlusion induced afferent pupillary defect. Am J Ophthalmol 107:306–307, 1989.
91. Thompson HS, Watzke RC, Weinstein JM: Pupillary dysfunction in macular disease. Trans Am Ophthalmol Soc 78:311–317, 1980.
92. Jiang MQ, et al: Pupillary defects in retinitis pigmentosa. Am J Ophthalmol 99(5):607–608, 1985.
93. Servais GE, Thompson HS, Hayreh SS: Relative afferent pupillary defect in central retinal vein occlusion. Ophthalmology 93:301–303, 1986.
94. Lowenstein O: Clinical pupillary symptoms in lesion of the optic nerve, optic chiasm and optic tract. Arch Ophthalmol 52:385–403, 1954.
95. Bell RA, Thompson HS: Optic tract lesions and relative afferent pupillary defects. *In* Thompson HS, Daroff R, Frisen L, Glaser JS: Topics in Neuro-Ophthalmology. Baltimore, Williams & Wilkins, 1979.
96. Smith SA, Smith SE: Contraction anisocoria: Nasal versus temporal illumination. Br J Ophthalmol 64:933–934, 1980.
97. Portnoy JZ, Thompson HS, Lennarson L, et al: Pupillary defects in amblyopia. Am J Ophthalmol 96:690–614, 1983.
98. Kase M, Nagata R, Yoshida A, et al: Pupillary light reflex in amblyopia. Invest Ophthalmol Vis Sci 25:467–471, 1984.
99. Firth AY: Pupillary responses in amblyopia. Br J Ophthalmol 74:676–680, 1990.
100. Price MJ, Thompson HS, Judisch GF, et al: Pupillary constriction to darkness. Br J Ophthalmol 69:205–211, 1985.
101. Cox TA: Pupillary testing using the direct ophthalmoscope. Am J Ophthalmol 105(4):427–428, 1988.
102. Fison PN, Garlich DJ, Smith SE: Assessment of unilateral afferent pupillary defects by pupillography. Br J Ophthalmol 63:195–199, 1979.
103. Jiang MQ, Thompson HS, Lam BL: Kestenbaum's number as an indicator of pupillomotor input asymmetry. Am J Ophthalmol 107:528–530, 1989.
104. Levatin P: Pupillary escape in disease of the retina or optic nerve. Arch Ophthalmol 62:768–779, 1959.
105. Thompson HS, Corbett JJ, Cox TA: How to measure the relative afferent pupillary defect. Surv Ophthalmol 26:39–42, 1981.
106. Cox TA: Initial pupillary constriction in the alternating light test. Am J Ophthalmol 101(1):120–121, 1986.
107. Cox TA: Pupillographic characteristics of simulated relative afferent pupillary defects. Invest Ophthalmol Vis Sci 30:1127–1131, 1989.
108. Browning DJ, Tiedeman JS: The test light affects quantitation of the afferent pupillary defect. Ophthalmology 94:53, 1987.
109. Johnson LN: The effect of light intensity on measurement of the relative afferent pupillary defect. Am J Ophthalmol 109:481–482, 1990.
110. Thompson HS, Jiang MQ: Intensity of the stimulus light influences the measurement of the relative afferent pupillary defect. Ophthalmology 94:1360–1362, 1987.
111. Thompson HS: Putting a number on the relative afferent pupillary defect. *In* Thompson HS, Daroff R, Frisen L, Glaser JS: Topics in Neuro-Ophthalmology. Baltimore, Williams & Wilkins, 1979.
112. Spring KH, Stiles WS: Variation of pupil size with change in the angle at which the light stimulus strikes the retina. Br J Ophthalmol 32:340–346, 1948.
113. Martyn CN, Ewing DJ: Pupil cycle time: A simple way of measuring an autonomic reflex. J Neurol Neurosurg Psychiatry 49(7):771–774, 1986.
114. Milton JG, et al: Irregular pupil cycling as a characteristic abnormality in patients with demyelinative optic neuropathy. Am J Ophthalmol 105(4):402–407, 1988.
115. Hamilton W, Drewry RD: Edge-light, pupil cycle time and optic nerve disease. Ann Ophthalmol 15:714–721, 1983.
116. Weinstein JM, Gilder JCV, Thompson HS: Pupil cycle time in optic nerve compressions. Am J Ophthalmol 89:263–267, 1980.
117. Miller SD, Ewing EJ: The pupil cycle time. *In* Thompson HS, Daroff R, Frisen L, Glaser JS: Topics in Neuro-Ophthalmology. Baltimore, Williams & Wilkins, 1979.
118. Miller SD, Thompson HS: Edge-light pupil cycle time. Br J Ophthalmol 62:495–500, 1978.
119. Miller SD, Thompson HS: Pupil cycle time in optic neuritis. Am J Ophthalmol 85:635–642, 1978.
120. Thompson HS: The pupil cycle time. J Clin Neuro Ophthalmol 7(1):38–39, 1987.
121. Rosenberg ML, Oliva A: The use of crossed polarized filters in the measurement of the relative afferent pupillary defect. Am J Ophthalmol 110:62–65, 1990.
122. Behrens MM: Failure of the light reaction. Trans Am Acad Ophthalmol Otolaryngol 83:827–831, 1977.
123. Thompson HS: Pupillary light-near dissociation: A classification. Surv Ophthalmol 19:290–292, 1975.
124. Thompson HS: Light-near dissociation of the pupil. Ophthalmologica 189:21–23, 1984.
125. Loewenfeld IE: The Argyll-Robertson pupil, 1869–1969: A critical survey of the literature. Surv Ophthalmol 14:199–299, 1969.
126. Kerr FWL: The pupil-functional anatomy and clinical correlation. Smith JL (ed): Neuro-Ophthalmology Symposium, vol 4. St. Louis, CV Mosby, 1972.
127. Vogel R: Parinaud's syndrome and other related pretectal syndromes. Ophthalmic Semin 1(3):287–370, 1976.
128. Sears ML: The cause of the Argyll-Robertson pupil. Am J Ophthalmology 72:488–489, 1971.
129. McCrary JA: The pupil in syphilis. Smith JL (ed): Neuro-Ophthalmology Symposium, vol 4. St. Louis, CV Mosby, 1968.
130. Czarnecki JS, Thompson HS: The iris sphincter in aberrant regeneration of the third nerve. Arch Ophthalmol 96:1606–1610, 1978.
131. Coppeto JR, et al: Tonic pupils following oculomotor nerve palsies. Ann Ophthalmol 17(9):585–588, 1985.

132. Jacobson DM: Pupillary responses to dilute pilocarpine in preganglionic third nerve disorders. Neurology 40:804–808, 1990.
133. Shuaib A, Israelian G, Lee MA: Mesencephalic hemorrhage and unilateral pupillary deficit. J Clin Neuro Ophthalmol 9:47–49, 1989.
134. Loewenfeld IE, Thomas HS: Oculomotor paresis and cyclic spasms: A critical review of the literature and a new case. Surv Ophthalmol 20:81–124, 1975.
135. Loewenfeld IE: "Simple central" anisocoria: A common condition, seldom recognized. Trans Am Acad Ophthalmol Otolaryngol 83:832–839, 1977.
136. Miller NR: Intermittent pupillary dilatation in a young woman. Surv Ophthalmol 31:65–68, 1986.
137. Woods D, O'Connor PS, Fleming R: Episodic unilateral mydriasis and migraine. Am J Ophthalmol 98:229–234, 1984.
138. Hepler RS: Adie's tonic pupil. Trans Am Acad Ophthalmol Otolaryngol 83:843–846, 1977.
139. Thompson HS: Adie's syndrome: Some new observations. Trans Am Ophthalmol Soc 75:587–626, 1977.
140. Thompson HS, Daroff R, Frisen L, Glaser JS: Topics in Neuro-Ophthalmology. Baltimore, Williams & Wilkins, 1979.
141. Bell RA, Thompson HS: Ciliary muscle dysfunction in Adie's syndrome. Arch Ophthalmol 96:638–644, 1978.
142. Rosenberg ML: Miotic Adie's pupils. J Clin Neuro Ophthalmol 9:43–45, 1989.
143. Thompson, HS: Segmental palsy of the iris sphincter in Adie's syndrome. Arch Ophthalmol 96:1615–1620, 1978.
144. Bourgon P, Pilley FJ, Thompson HS: Cholinergic hypersensitivity of the iris sphincter in Adie's tonic pupil. Am J Ophthalmol 85:373–377, 1978.
145. Purcell JJ, Krachmer JH, Thompson HS: Corneal sensation in Adie's syndrome. Am J Ophthalmol 84:496–500, 1977.
146. Utsumi T: Corneal permeability in patients with tonic pupil. J Clin Neuro Ophthalmol 10:52–55, 1990.
147. Thompson HS, Burmeister LF, Meek ES: A search for serum antibodies in Adie's syndrome. Graefes Arch Clin Exp Ophthalmol 205:29–32, 1977.
148. Harriman DGF: Pathologic aspects of Adie's syndrome. Adv Ophthalmol 23:55–73, 1970.
149. Loewenfeld IE, Thompson HS: The tonic pupil: A reevaluation. Am Ophthalmol 63:46–87, 1967.
150. Loewenfeld IE, Thompson HS: Mechanism of tonic pupil. Ann Neurol 10:275–276, 1981.
151. Selhorst JB, Madge G, Ghatak NR: The neuropathology of the Holmes-Adie syndrome. [Abstract] Ann Neurol 16:138, 1984.
152. Ulrich J: Morphological basis of Adie's syndrome. Eur Neurol 19:390–395, 1980.
153. Miyasaki JM, Ashby P, Sharpe JA, et al: On the cause of the hyporeflexia in the Holmes-Adie syndrome. Neurology 38:262–265, 1988.
154. Ross AT: Progressive selective sudomotor denervation. Neurology 8:811, 1958.
155. Hedges TR, Gegner EW: Ross' syndrome (tonic pupil plus). Br J Ophthalmol 59:387–391, 1975.
156. Drummond PD, Edis RH: Loss of facial sweating and flushing in Holmes-Adie syndrome. Neurology 40:847–849, 1990.
157. Petajan JH, Danforth RC, D'Allesio DD, et al: Progressive sudomotor denervation and Adie's syndrome. Neurology 15:172–175, 1965.
158. Lucy DD, Allen MW van, Thompson HS: Holmes-Adie's syndrome with segmental hypohidrosis. Neurology 17:763–769, 1967.
159. Okada F, Shintomi Y, Noguchi K, et al: Two cases of Hashimoto's thyroiditis with pupillary disturbances. Eur Neurol 29:174–176, 1989.
160. Yee RD, Trese M, Zee DS, et al: Ocular manifestation of acute pandysautonomia. Am J Ophthalmol 81:740–744, 1976.
161. Okajima T, Imamura S, Kawasaki S, et al: Fisher's syndrome: A pharmacological study of the pupils. Ann Neurol 2:63–65, 1977.
162. Kupersmith MJ, Alekic SN: Bilateral pupillary cholinergic sensitivity in a case of sarcoidosis. Neuro Ophthalmology 4:15–20, 1984.
163. Englestein ES, Ruderman MI, Troiano RA: Dilated tonic pupils in neurosyphilis. [Letter] J Neurol Neurosurg Psychiatry 49(12):1455–1457, 1986.
164. Fletcher WA, Sharpe JA: Tonic pupils in neurosyphilis. Neurology 36(2):188–192, 1986.
165. Bronster DJ, Rudolph SH, Shanzer S: Pupillary light-near dissociation in cranial arteritis. Neuro Ophthalmology 3:65–70, 1983.
166. Currie J, Lessell S: Tonic pupil with giant cell arteritis. Br J Ophthalmol 68:135–138, 1984.
167. Parssinen O, Kuronen J: Tonic pupillary reaction after epidemic nephropathy and transient myopia. Am J Ophthalmol 108:201–202, 1989.
168. Keltner JL, Swisher CN, Gay AJ: Myotonic pupils in Charcot-Marie-Tooth disease. Arch Ophthalmol 93:1141–1148, 1975.
169. O'Connor M, Eustace P: Tonic pupil and lateral rectus palsy following dental anesthesia. Neuro Ophthalmology 3:205–208, 1983.
170. Miller NR: Walsh and Hoyt's Clinical Neuro-Ophthalmology, 4th ed, vol 2. Baltimore, Williams & Wilkins, 1985, pp 492–493.
171. Love DC: Anisocoria from scopolamine patches. [Letter] JAMA 254(13):1720–1721, 1985.
172. Price BH: Anisocoria from scopolamine patches. [Letter] JAMA 253(11):1561, 1985.
173. Thompson HS, Newsome DA, Loewenfeld IE: The fixed dilated pupil: Sudden iridoplegia or mydriatic drops? A simple diagnostic test. Arch Ophthalmol 86:21–27, 1971.
174. Plum F, Posner JB: The Diagnosis of Stupor and Coma, 3rd ed. Philadelphia, FA Davis, 1980.
175. Abt JL: The pupillary responses after being struck by lightning. [Letter] JAMA 254(23):3312, 1985.
176. Sunderland S: The tentorial notch and complications produced by herniations of the brain through that aperture. Br J Surg 45:422–438, 1958.

Chapter 196

Myasthenia Gravis

DAVID G. COGAN

Myasthenia gravis is a disease of striated muscles. More precisely, it is a disease of the myoneural junction in which the chemical transmitter, acetylcholine, is unable to bind to the receptors of the postsynaptic membrane and is thus unable to transmit the nerve impulse to the muscle fibers. This disease occurs at any age, involves either sex, and characteristically intensifies with fatigue (myasthenia). Myasthenia gravis begins insidiously by weakness of one or more muscles; ptosis and diplopia often comprise the initial manifestations. From a pathogenetic point of view, the block is caused by the development of an antibody to acetylcholine receptors on the myoneural junction; it is, in fact, an exceptionally well-documented example of the autoimmune category.

HISTORY AND DEVELOPMENT OF BACKGROUND KNOWLEDGE

Early Observations. Willis[1] is credited with providing the first clinical description of myasthenia gravis in 1672, but his contribution remained unrecognized until discovered by Guthrie in 1903.[2] Except for Willis' report, the medical literature is surprisingly devoid of any description of myasthenia gravis until the end of the 19th century when, almost simultaneously, a burst of case reports documented the fatigue-related ptosis, diplopia, dysphonia, dysphagia, respiratory paralysis, and general weakness. It was variously designated the Erb-Goldflam symptom complex or the Jolly syndrome.[3] Although the symptoms underwent spontaneous remission in some patients, the disease was fatal in most patients. This accounts for the addition of *gravis* to myasthenia gravis.

The first American case may have been that of the native American Chief, Opechankanough, who led the slaughter of the colonists at Jamestown and is said to have been carried into battle on a litter because of his alleged myasthenia.[4]

During the first half of the 20th century, progress crucial to the understanding of myasthenia gravis came about through advances in physiology rather than through medicine. Whereas the excitatory process at the neuromuscular junction was initially believed to be simply a matter of electrical transmission, Loewi[5] demonstrated a circulating humoral substance ("vagusstoff"). Dale[6] found that this substance was acetylcholine acting at the myoneural end-plates. Cholinesterase was shown to hydrolyse the residual acetylcholine and thus account for the transitoriness on repetitive stimulation. Physostigmine potentiated the response by inhibiting the action of the esterase at the junction between the nerve terminal and the muscle fiber.

This work, together with analogous effects of physostigmine on curare poisoning, prompted Walker, a London ophthalmologist, to try physostigmine on one of her patients who had myasthenic ptosis. The result was, of course, dramatic (Fig. 196–1). Walker submitted a modest, almost apologetic, letter to Lancet[7] describing this epochal event and concluding "I think this effect of physostigmine is important." This marked the first demonstration of a crucial method for the diagnosis and treatment of a heretofore fatal disease.

Pursuant to the above and concurrent with it has been a wealth of physiologic, cytochemical, and electron microscopic observations on the function and ultrastructure of the myoneural junction (see reviews by Lester,[8] Lennon,[9] and Drachman[10]). Suffice it to say that the myoneural junction of skeletal muscles consists of bulbous terminals of the nerve fibers that contain vacuoles surfeited with acetylcholine (Fig. 196–2). These vacuoles are strategically arranged to discharge their contents into the "space" between the nerve fiber membrane and the muscle cell. The ocular muscles have end-organs (Fig. 196–3) similar to those in other skeletal muscles, but they differ also in having multiple end-plates for each muscle fiber and in having other myoneural junctions that end within (hypolemmal), instead of on, the muscle fiber.[11, 12] The bulbous enlargement of the nerve terminal has a presynaptic portion that evidently induces fusion of the vacuoles with the postsynaptic portion overlying the muscle fiber. This postsynaptic membrane, in turn, has multiple folds that invaginate the muscle cell, providing a large surface area of contact. At the same time, acetylcholine esterase is present in the lamina between the postsynaptic membrane of the nerve and the sarcolemma of the muscle. The liberated acetylcholine opens the calcium channels of the muscle and allows influx of sodium and loss of potassium from the muscle fiber, a depolarization responsible for contraction of the muscle fiber. Nowhere else in the body has the infrastructure of neural transmission been so well documented as in the case of this myoneural junction, nor has it had such exquisite applicability to a diseased state as in the case of myasthenia gravis.

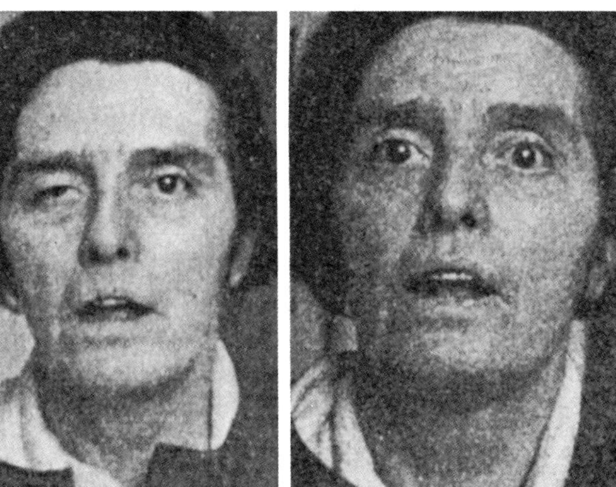

Figure 196–1. Photograph of Walker's patient before and 30 min after receiving an injection of physostigmine salicylate (1/60 g). (From Walker MB: Treatment of myasthenia gravis with physostigmine. Lancet 1:1200, 1934.)

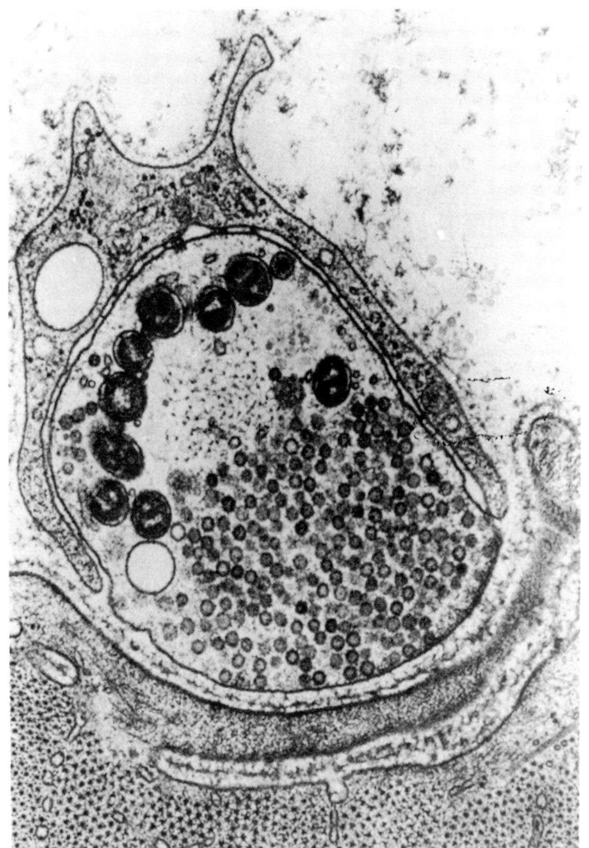

Figure 196–2. Electron micrograph of a myoneural junction. The circumscribed central area is the bulbous enlargement of a terminal nerve fiber containing acetylcholine vacuoles *(lower half)* and mitochondria *(upper half)*. The bulbous terminal is surrounded above by a Schwann cell and below by the postsynaptic space separating it from the muscle cell. ×71,400. (From Lester HA: The response to acetylcholine. Scientific American 236:106, 1977.)

RECENT TRENDS

In the second half of the 20th century the concept of autoimmunity applied to myasthenia gravis, first suggested by Simpson,[13] has been the dominant theme. The burgeoning literature is summarized in several reviews and is presented in detail in the quinquennium publications of the Myasthenia Symposium Foundation.[14–18]

Autoimmunity is a pathologic state in which the body fails to recognize some component or components of tissue as part of self. The tissue component assumes the role of an antigen, prompting the generation of specific antibodies with consequent cascade of immunologic reactions. In the case of myasthenia gravis, an antibody to acetylcholine receptors is present in 90 per cent of patients' sera. The binding of this antibody to the receptor blocks the neural transmission and eventually destroys the receptors. The concomitant anatomic change is an attenuation and ultimate loss of the folds of the postsynaptic membrane. The ocular muscles may represent a special case, because the antibody found in general myasthenia gravis is often minimal or absent in purely ocular myasthenia gravis.[14, 19–21] This difference presumably reflects the antigenic differences in the end-organs of the ocular muscles compared with other skeletal muscles.[22] The pathology of the ocular muscles in myasthenia gravis consists of lymphorrhagia compatible with an immunologic reaction (Fig. 196–4).

The reason why the body loses its recognition of self is unclear. Suggested causes are viral, inflammatory, drug-induced (D-penicillamine,[23, 24] chloroquine[25]), or neoplasms. In the latter case, a remote tumor generates an antigen shared with otherwise unrelated tissues. Thymomas present a prime illustration of autoimmunity. The tumor shares an antigen with the acetylcholine receptors and induces an antibody reaction that results in typical myasthenia gravis. Other examples of autoimmune states with which myasthenia is occasionally associated are hyperthyroidism, Hashimoto's thyroiditis, rheumatoid arthritis, lupus erythematosus, pemphigus, Guillain-Barré syndrome, and some forms of diabetes (Fig. 196–5). Present investigations are directed toward mitigating the immunologic reaction by manipulating the reactive lymphocytes or by washing out the antibody by plasmapheresis.

SIGNS AND SYMPTOMS WITH EMPHASIS ON OCULAR EFFECTS

The ocular signs often comprise the first, and sometimes the only, manifestation of myasthenia gravis. The disease can usually be recognized with reasonable certainty on the basis of the eye signs alone, if one is aware of the diverse modes of presentation and if one is familiar with the appropriate testing procedures. Yet myasthenia gravis is one of the most frequent cases of misdiagnosis. Drooping of the lids and diplopia are the prime ocular signs (Fig. 196–6). At first glance the appearance may suggest an abiotrophic form of progressive external ophthalmoplegia, peripheral nerve palsy, dysthyroid myopathy, or orbital disease. The reverse may also be the case wherein intracranial lesions masquerade as myasthenic symptoms[26]; nevertheless, various clues, some obvious and some bordering on the arcane, are usually sufficient to establish the diagnosis.

The history is often highly suggestive and may in itself be diagnostic. The onset is typically insidious, but occasionally abrupt, and is related to fatigue. The first ocular symptoms may be associated with prolonged ocular fixation, such as after an automobile trip that has necessitated hours of concentration on watching the road. Some patients attribute their difficulties to sunlight exposure or glare with attendant squinting. At times, a debilitating infection precipitates the initial symptoms. Rest, especially a night's sleep, restores the ocular functions for a few hours, but as the day continues, ptosis and diplopia increase. This diurnal variation is practically a pathognomonic symptom.

The periodicity is also characteristic. The symptoms may last for some days or weeks, then they disappear and recur at irregular intervals. The reason for this coming and going is obscure. The ocular signs may coincide with general muscular weakness or may remain

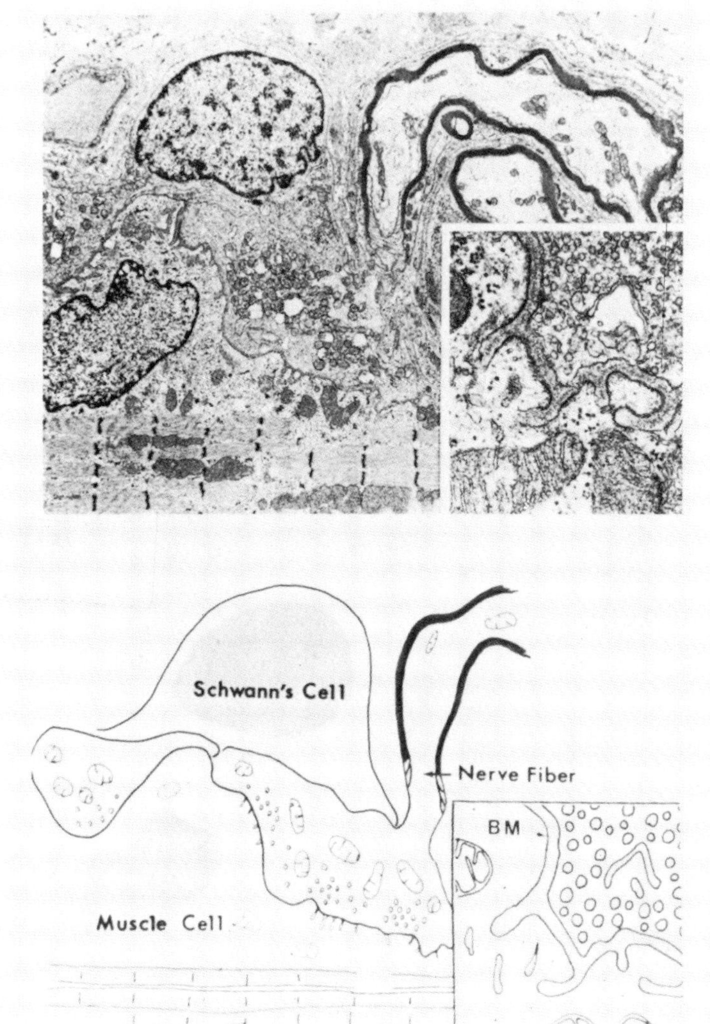

Figure 196–3. Electron micrograph *(top)* and diagram *(bottom)* of a myoneural junction from an ocular muscle. A convoluted nerve with lightly stained axoplasm, mitochondria, and darkly stained myelin sheath occupies the upper right of the photograph. As the nerve approaches the junction, it loses its myelin and enlarges into a bulbous tip containing abundant mitochondria and vacuoles. A Schwann cell is evident in the lower third by its nucleus, sarcoplasm, and striated fibers. ×5755. Insert shows details of the myoneural junction with a presynaptic membrane on the side of the nerve, a postsynaptic membrane on the side of the muscle, and a synaptic cleft in between. ×240,900. (Photograph by T. Kuwabara. From Cogan DG: Ocular myasthenia. *In* Rose FC [ed]: The Eye in General Medicine. London, Chapman and Hall, 1983, pp 151–171.)

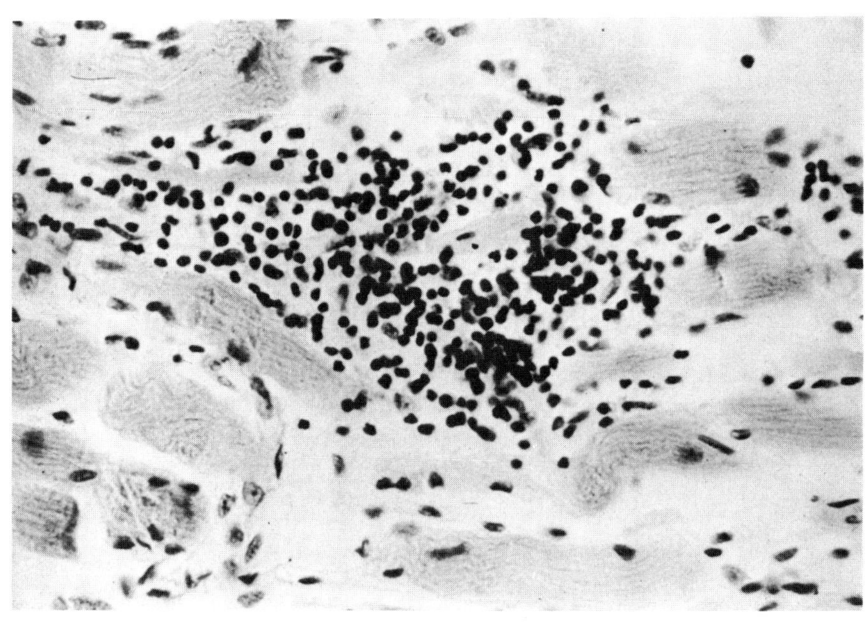

Figure 196–4. Lymphorrhagia in ocular muscle of patient who died in myasthenic crisis: Hematoxylin and eosin. ×255. (From Cogan DG: Ocular myasthenia. *In* Rose FC [ed]: The Eye in General Medicine. London, Chapman and Hall, 1983, pp 151–171.)

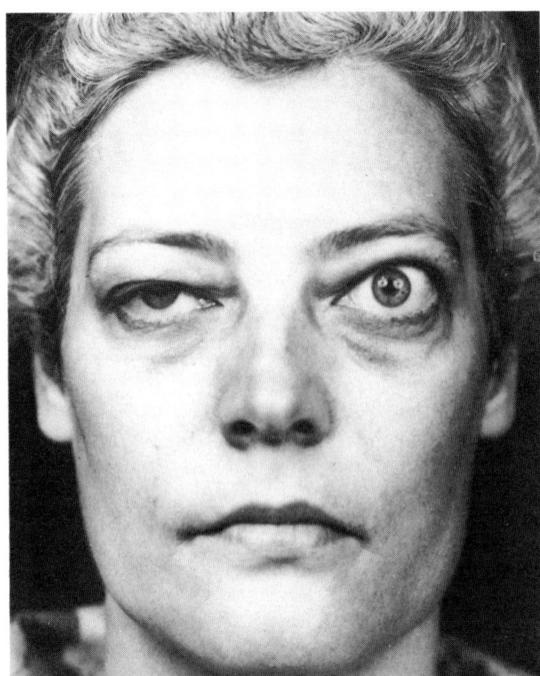

Figure 196–5. Multiple autoimmune diseases. The patient, a 40-year-old woman, had signs of current or previous hyperthyroidism/hypothyroidism, recurrent optic neuritis (presumably multiple sclerosis), lupus erythematosus, and myasthenia gravis.

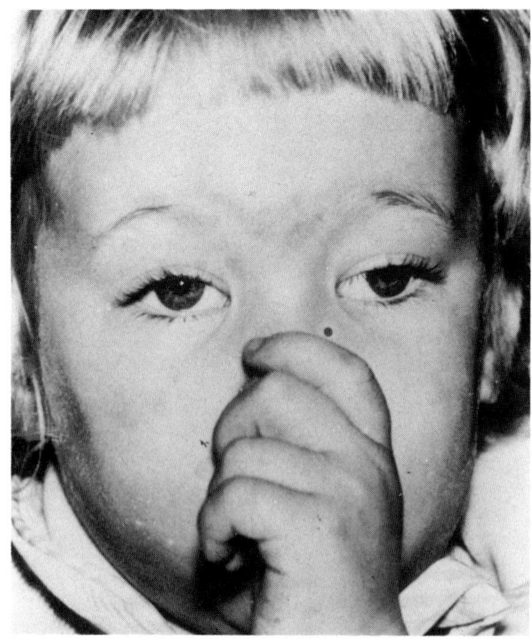

Figure 196–7. Infantile myasthenia gravis. The patient, a 2-year-old girl, had developed drooping of the eyelids and intermittent exotropia 5 weeks previously. The signs increased with fatigue and at the end of the day. They were relieved temporarily by intramuscular injection of 0.25 mg of prostigmine. There were no other neurologic signs. (From Cogan DG: Ocular myasthenia. *In* Rose FC [ed]: The Eye in General Medicine. London, Chapman and Hall, 1983, pp 151–171.)

as isolated signs for months, years, or indefinitely (ocular myasthenia).

No particular age or race is predisposed, but women are more susceptible to the disease before 40 yr of age and men are more susceptible after 40 yr of age.[27] When it occurs in infancy or early childhood, the eyes are likely to be solely affected (Fig. 196–7). Such cases are often the most refractory to treat.

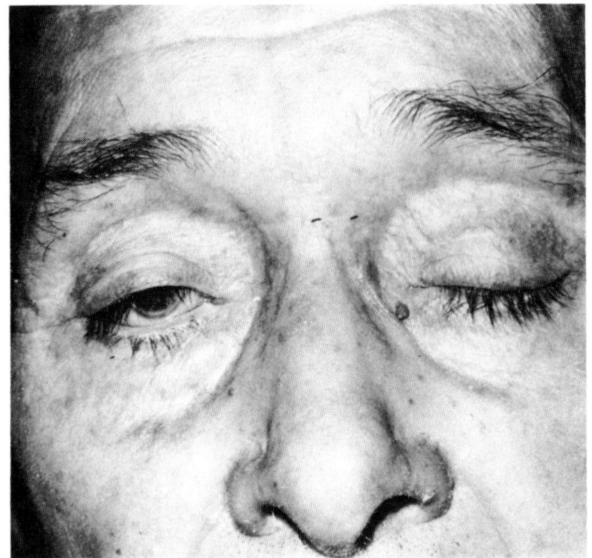

Figure 196–6. Typical appearance of myasthenia gravis, in a 76-year-old man. Eyelid drooping of 2 mo duration with compensatory furrowing of brow. (From Cogan DG: Ocular myasthenia. *In* Rose FC [ed]: The Eye in General Medicine. London, Chapman and Hall, 1983, pp 151–171.)

Ptosis is usually the most conspicuous sign and is then customarily asymmetric in the early stages. The increase of the ptosis on maintained upward gaze is especially characteristic (Fig. 196–8). This phenomenon may be best elicited by elevating one lid manually while observing the opposite lid. The patient is asked to avoid blinking during the test. This maneuver avoids the extra effort that would mask the effect. As the unassisted lid droops, it frequently makes oscillatory up-and-down movements that are highly characteristic. These oscillations have a frequency of 3 to 4 Hz but are irregular. The irregularity distinguishes them from the flutter seen occasionally in otherwise normal persons on closure of the eyes.

The lid twitch is also highly characteristic of myasthenic ptosis and occurs in one third to one half of all myasthenic patients with ptosis.[28] This twitch is elicited by having the patient look alternately from a downgaze to a forward gaze position. As the patient looks upward, the ptotic lid momentarily elevates above its eventual position, giving a twitch-like appearance. Occasionally, several oscillations accompany the twitch. This momentary overshoot of the lid appears to be caused by the rest period for the levator during the downgaze. It also occurs on first opening the eyes after closure or with a blink of the eyes.

Weakness of the orbicularis muscle also occurs in many ophthalmopareses, including myasthenia, but a special "peek sign" has been described with myasthenia.[29] On gentle closure of the eyes, the orbicularis is unable to maintain the eyes shut. In consequence, the

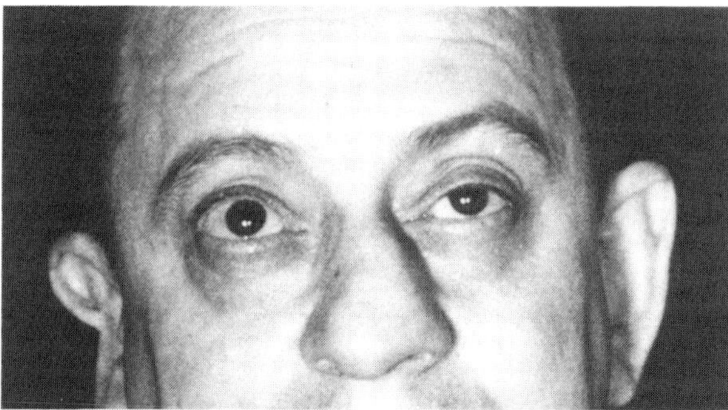

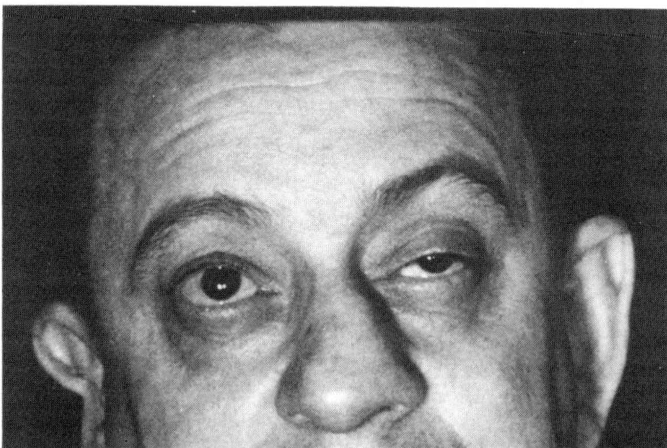

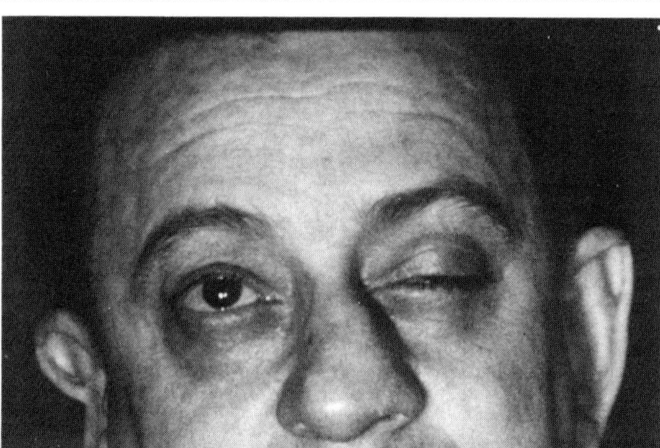

Figure 196–8. Increasing ptosis on maintained upward gaze. Three frames from a moving picture strip showing the progressive ptosis over a 3-min period as the patient maintained fixation above the horizontal meridian. (From Cogan DG: Myasthenia gravis: A review of the disease and a description of lid twitch as a characteristic sign. Arch Ophthalmol 74:218, 1965. Copyright 1965, American Medical Association.)

partial opening gives the appearance of peeking by the patient. This weakness of the orbicularis muscle may expose the patient to a risk of exposure keratitis.

A curious phenomenon may occur at times when the more ptotic lid is elevated manually. The opposite lid then droops (Fig. 196–9). Rapid repetition of this maneuver produces a curious effect that has been called "see-saw" ptosis. As with other myasthenic phenomena, it disappears after an injection with edrophonium.

A paradoxic retraction of one lid may occur with myasthenia[30] and is then usually associated with ptosis of the opposite side (Fig. 196–10). In such cases, the eye with the maximal ptosis also has a weakness of upward gaze. When the patient exerts effort to open the eye, the innervational spillover causes retraction of the opposite, less ptotic lid.[31] It disappears on downward

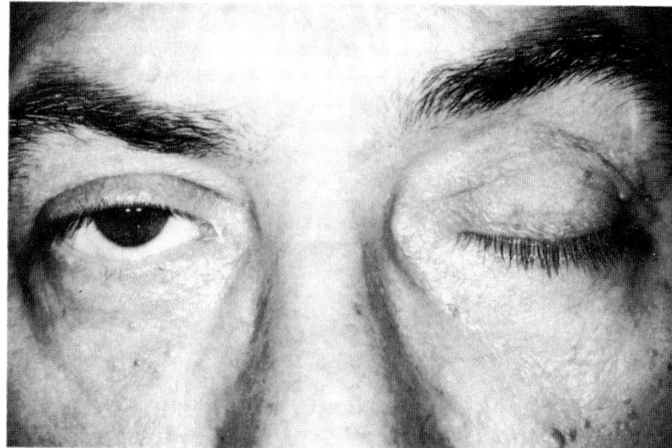

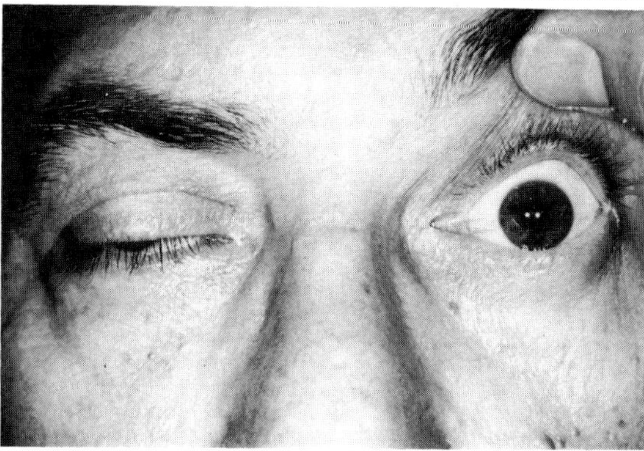

Figure 196–9. "See-saw" ptosis in a 60-year-old man with myasthenic ptosis of 2½ mo duration, which is more marked in the left eye. Manual elevation of the left lid results in an increased ptosis of the right eyelid, producing the "see-saw" effect.

gaze. Lid retraction in the presence of paresis of upward gaze is, of course, not limited to myasthenia, but the combination of lid retraction of one eye and ptosis of the other eye is unusual in any other condition, and its disappearance with the use of edrophonium is essentially pathognomonic.

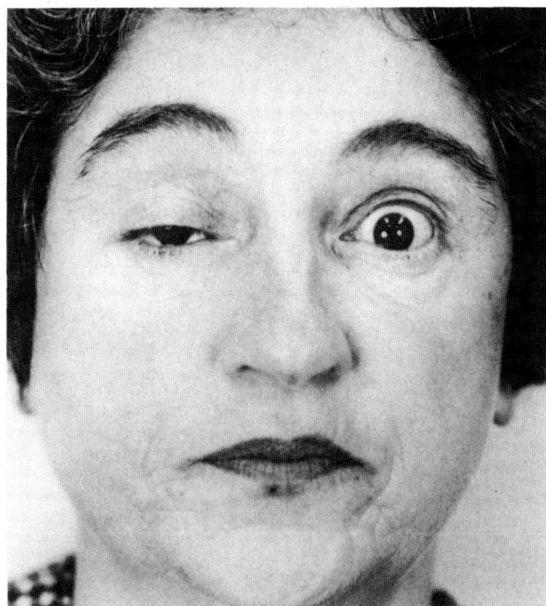

Figure 196–10. Ptosis of one eye and paradoxic lid retraction of opposite eye. (From Cogan DG, Chu FC: Ocular manifestations of myasthenia gravis. *In* Smith JL [ed]: Neuro-ophthalmology Focus, 1982. New York, Masson, 1982, pp 131–138.)

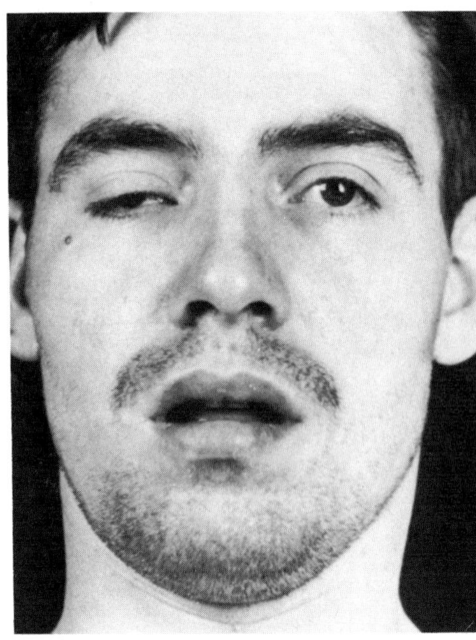
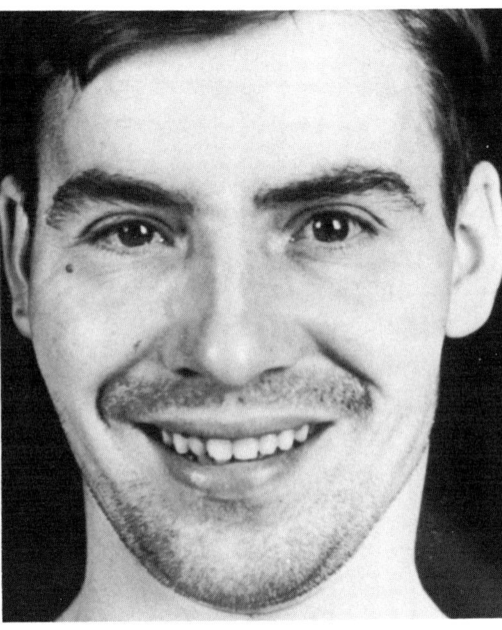

Figure 196–11. Myasthenia gravis before and after treatment with prostigmine. The 28-year-old patient had developed ptosis of the right eyelid as a first symptom 2 months previously; when the eyelid was passively raised, the patient complained of diplopia. The ptosis and diplopia were worse in the evening when the patient was fatigued. Dysphonia, dysphagia, and some weakness of the extremities developed a few weeks before the pictures were taken. The first picture was taken as the patient attempted to smile, revealing profound ptosis and weakness of the facial muscles. The second picture was taken 15 min after he received a diagnostic dose (1.5 mg) of prostigmine. (From Cogan DG: Neurology of the Ocular Muscles, 2nd ed. 1963. Courtesy of Charles C Thomas, Publisher, Springfield, Illinois.)

Above all else, the most characteristic aspect of myasthenic ptosis is an unequivocal responsiveness to anticholinesterase agents.[32] Edrophonium (Tensilon) administered intravenously to adults or prostigmine administered intramuscularly to children or adults results in a dramatic decrease of ptosis (Fig. 196–11). False-negative and false-positive results do occur, but they are infrequent, often raising doubt regarding the putative diagnosis or adequacy of the test procedure. Practically, they may be disregarded. Improvement by treatment with pyridostigmine (Mestinon) confirms the diagnosis but, surprisingly, the responsiveness to diagnostic tests with edrophonium does not reliably indicate the expected effectiveness of treatment with anticholinesterase agents.

Ophthalmoplegia of the ocular rotary muscles is, like that of the lids, usually insidious and variable in onset. Diplopia is not a presenting complaint if the ptosis occludes one eye. Although characteristically associated with ptosis, ophthalmoplegia occurs occasionally without involvement of the lids and may be curiously selective in the muscles affected. One or two muscles, commonly the medial recti, may alone be involved. In addition, fatigue may invoke an exaggerated endpoint nystagmus,[33] which, in combination with an adductive weakness, is a source of diagnostic confusion with internuclear ophthalmoplegia.

Myasthenic paresis of the ocular muscles usually produces a slow movement of the eyes similar to that occurring with other forms of paresis.[34] This finding is not surprising. What is surprising is that some patients with myasthenic paresis have abnormally rapid movements within their limited range of excursion. The result is a quiver-like or jelly-like movement that, when present, is highly characteristic of myasthenia.[35, 36] It is especially striking in persons whose range of movement is limited to 10 degrees in any direction. Then, as the patient looks about, the eyes show dart-like saccades that are diagnostically unmistakable. One speculation is that the pulse or phasic movements are less affected than are those of the step or tonic movements.

The same phenomena may be found with nonmyasthenic ophthalmoplegia but are less obvious. Although the movements of the eye may seem to be slow, careful observation and oculographic recording reveal a bimodal type of movement with a high velocity that is followed initially by a low-velocity glissade (intrasaccadic fatigue).[36] When present, this bimodal response is also characteristic of myasthenia.

Frequent, but not especially characteristic of myasthenia is some ocular instability, most evident on changes of fixation. This is usually asymmetric and is especially evident in the more paretic eye and is sometimes associated with oscillations of the lid. It suggests some defect in the effectiveness of signals to the muscles for stabilization of fixation. The instability that occurs with cerebellar lesions appears somewhat similar, but the eye movements are then, of course, conjugate.

Selective involvement of one or more ocular muscles may result in confusing syndromes. Rapid development of ophthalmoplegia in a child may suggest postinfectious encephalitis. Total external ophthalmoplegia in one eye may suggest a cavernous sinus syndrome or a lesion at the apex of the orbit. Concomitant involvement of the medial rectus of one eye and lateral rectus of the other eye may suggest a conjugate gaze defect of pontine origin. But probably the most frequent misdiagnosis is that of internuclear ophthalmoplegia as when the medial recti are preferentially involved (Fig. 196–12).[37–39] Unlike true internuclear ophthalmoplegia, however, nystagmus of the abducting eye is not regularly present, and vertical nystagmus is exceedingly rare. The correct diagnosis in all cases depends on such points as history of diurnal fluctuations, worsening on fatigue, ancillary

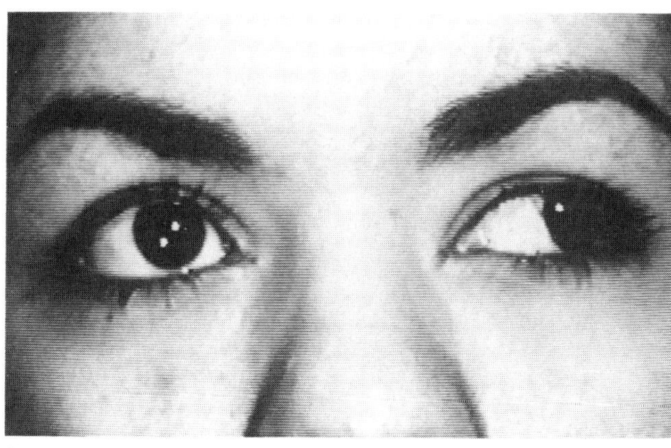

Figure 196–12. Pseudointernuclear ophthalmoplegia with myasthenia in a 25-year-old woman with weakness predominantly of adduction. (From Cogan DG, Chu FC: Ocular manifestations of myasthenia gravis. *In* Smith JL [ed]: Neuro-ophthalmology Focus, 1982. New York, Masson, 1982, pp 131–138.)

tests with anticholinesterase agents, and a characteristic decrement of action potentials in the skeletal, or rarely, in the ocular muscles.

The response of the ocular muscles to diagnostic anticholinesterase agents is often dramatic, but it is less regular and less complete than that of the lids. Similarly, treatment with anticholinesterase agents is less effective for the eye movements than it is for the lid movements; and both lids and eyes are generally less responsive than are the skeletal muscles. In general, ocular myasthenia is a difficult form of myasthenic disease to treat.

Similar to systemic myasthenia, ocular myasthenias may occasionally be associated with other diseases, notably hyperthyroidism, Hashimoto's disease, multiple sclerosis, lupus erythematosus, polymyositis, hemolytic anemia, and other autoimmune diseases (see Fig. 196–6).

Along with pseudointernuclear ophthalmoplegia and dysthyroid ophthalmoplegia, the chief cause of confusion for ocular myasthenia is abiotrophic progressive external ophthalmoplegia. This dystrophy has in common with myasthenia ptosis and ophthalmoplegia, either alone or with general weakness, and a progressive course beginning at any age. Distinctive features, however, that point to myasthenia are the relation to fatigue, the diurnal variation, the response to edrophonium, the asymmetry of the ptosis and of the ocular movements, and the absence of ragged red fibers in biopsy specimens of skeletal muscle.

A myasthenia-like condition, Eaton-Lambert syndrome, may simulate systemic myasthenia but is less likely to have ocular manifestations. It is associated with tumors elsewhere in the body, especially small cell carcinomas of the lung. It, too, is believed to have an underlying autoimmune basis with, in this case, immunologic sensitization to the presynaptic component of the myoneural junction. The entity differs from typical myasthenia in that muscle strength improves with use and its action potentials increase with repetitive stimulation of the nerve.

TREATMENT

Therapy is best supervised by neurologists according to a protocol tailored to each individual case.[32] It usually begins with empiric manipulation of the dose of anticholinesterase agents.[40] Pyridostigmine (Mestinon) is currently the most popular drug. A caveat, however: overdosage may provoke cholinergic symptoms with a myopathic weakness simulating myasthenia. Steroids, either alone or additive to other medication, are often used but are not advisable for long-term therapy. Thymomas should be looked for by roentgenography of the mediastinum and should be removed if present. Hyperplastic thymus tissue, common with myasthenia, may also indicate surgery or radiation for cases refractory to medication, but the benefits for ocular myasthenia are questionable.[41] Failing satisfactory control by the foregoing specific methods, an alternative is immunologic suppression by azathioprine, cyclophosphamide, cyclosporin,[42] or high-dose immunoglobulin.[43] None of these forms of treatment are, however, as effective for the eye signs as they are for other systemic manifestations of myasthenia. Rarely, surgery to the lids or eye muscles may be indicated, but surgical correction of ptosis engenders the risk of exposure keratitis due to orbicularis weakness. Finally, repeated plasmaphereses are indicated for acute crises in which paralysis of the respiratory muscles are threatened.

REFERENCES

1. Willis T: De Anima Brutorum. Oxford, England, Theatro Sheldoniano, 1672, p 404.
2. Guthrie LG: Myasthenia gravis in the seventeenth century. Lancet 1:330, 1903.
3. Viets HR: A historical review of myasthenia gravis from 1672 to 1900. JAMA 153:1273, 1953.
4. Marsteller HB: The first American case of myasthenia gravis. Arch Neurol 45:185, 1988.
5. Loewi O: Ueber humorale Uebertragbarkeit der Herznervenwirkung. Pflugers Arch 193:239, 1921.
6. Dale H: Chemical transmission of the effects of nerve impulses. Br Med J 1:835, 1934.
7. Walker MB: Treatment of myasthenia gravis with physostigmine. Lancet 1:1200, 1934.
8. Lester HA: The response to acetylcholine. Sci Am 326:107, 1977.
9. Lennon VA: Immunologic Mechanisms in Myasthenia Gravis—A Model Receptor Disease in Clinical Immunology Update Reviews for Physicians. New York, Elsevier, 1979, p 259.
10. Drachman DB: The biology of myasthenia gravis. *In* Cowan W (ed): Annual Review of Neurosciences, vol 4. Palo Alto, 1981, p 195.
11. Kupfer C: Motor innervation of extraocular muscles. J Physiol 153:522, 1960.
12. Dietert SE: The demonstration of different types of muscle fibers in human extraocular muscle by electron microscopy and cholinesterase staining. Invest Ophthalmol 4:51, 1965.
13. Simpson JA: Myasthenia gravis: A new hypothesis. Scott Med J 5:419, 1960.
14. Vincent A: Immunology of acetylcholine receptors in relation to myasthenia gravis. Physiol Rev 60:757, 1960.
15. Drachman DB, Adams RN, Josifek LF, Self SG: Functional activities of autoantibodies to acetylcholine receptors and the clinical severity of myasthenia gravis. N Engl J Med 307:769, 1982.
16. Lisak RB, Barchi RL: Myasthenia Gravis in Major Problems in Neurology, vol 11. Philadelphia, WB Saunders, 1982, p xi.

17. Myasthenia Gravis: Pathophysiology and Management. Sixth International Conference on Myasthenia Gravis Conference held December 2–4, 1980. Published in Annals of the New York Academy of Science; Grob D (ed), vol 377, 1981.
18. Myasthenia Gravis: Biology and Treatment. Seventh International Conference on Myasthenia Gravis held on March 4–7, 1986. Published in Annals of the New York Academy of Science; Drachman DB (ed), vol 505, 1987.
19. Lindstrom JM, Seybold ME, Lennon VA, et al: Antibody to acetylcholine receptor in myasthenia gravis: Prevalence, clinical correlates and diagnostic value. Neurology 26:1054, 1976.
20. Soliven BC: Sero-negative myasthenia gravis. Neurology 38:514, 1988.
21. Tsujihata M, Yoshimura T, Satoh A, et al: Diagnostic significance of IgG, C3, and C9 at the limb muscle motor end-plate in minimal myasthenia gravis. Neurology 39:1359, 1989.
22. Oda K, Shibasaki H: Antigenic difference of acetylcholine receptor between single and multiple forms of endplates of human extraocular muscle. Brain Res 449:337, 1988.
23. Katz LJ, Lesser RL, Merikangas JR, Silverman JP: Ocular myasthenia gravis after D-penicillamine administration. Br J Ophthalmol 73:1015, 1973.
24. Ferbert A: D-penicillamine-induced ocular myasthenia in psoriatic arthritis. Nervenarzt 60:576, 1989.
25. Sghirlanzi A, Mantegazza R, Mora M, et al: Chloroquine myopathy and myasthenia-like syndrome. Rinsho Shinkeigaku 29:1180, 1989.
26. Moorthy G: Ocular pseudomyasthenia or ocular myasthenia 'plus': A warning to clinicians. Neurology 39:1150, 1989.
27. Grob D, Brunner NG, Namba T: The natural course of myasthenia gravis and effect of therapeutic measures. Ann N Y Acad Sci 377:652, 1980.
28. Cogan DG: Myasthenia gravis: A review of the disease and a description of lid twitch as a characteristic sign. Arch Ophthalmol 74:217, 1965.
29. Osher RH, Griggs RC: Orbicularis fatigue: The "peek" sign of myasthenia gravis. Arch Ophthalmol 97:677, 1979.
30. Puklin JE, Sacks JG, Boshes B: Transient eyelid retraction in myasthenia gravis. J Neurol Neurosurg Psychiatry 39:44, 1976.
31. Gay AJ, Salmon JL, Windsor CE: Hering's law, the levators and their relationship in disease states. Arch Ophthalmol 77:157, 1967.
32. Drachman DB: Present and future treatment of myasthenia gravis. N Engl J Med 316:743, 1987.
33. Keane JR, Hoyt WF: Myasthenic (vertical) nystagmus: Verification by edrophonium tonography. JAMA 212:1209, 1970.
34. Metz HS, Scott AB, O'Meara DM: Saccadic eye movements in myasthenia gravis. Arch Ophthalmol 88:9, 1972.
35. Cogan DG, Yee RD, Gittinger J: Rapid eye movements in myasthenia gravis. I: Clinical observations. Arch Ophthalmol 94:1083, 1976.
36. Yee RD, Cogan DG, Zee DS, et al: Rapid eye movements in myasthenia gravis. II: Electro-oculographic analysis. Arch Ophthalmol 94:1465, 1976.
37. Glaser J: Myasthenic pseudo-internuclear ophthalmoplegia. Arch Ophthalmol 75:363, 1966.
38. Metz HS: Myasthenia gravis presenting as internuclear ophthalmoplegia. J Pediatr Ophthalmol 14:23, 1977.
39. Acers TE: Ocular myasthenia gravis mimicking pseudo-internuclear ophthalmoplegia and variable esotropia. Am J Ophthalmol 88:319, 1979.
40. Harvard CW, Fonseca V: New treatment approaches to myasthenia gravis. Drugs 39:66, 1990.
41. Evoli A, Batocchi AP, Provenzano C, et al: Thymectomy in the treatment of myasthenia gravis: Report of 247 patients. J Neurol 235:272, 1988.
42. Goulon M, Elkharrat D, Gajdos P: Treatment of severe myasthenia gravis with cyclosporin: A 12-month open trial. Presse Med 18:341, 1989.
43. Sakano T, Hamasaki T, Kinoshita Y, et al: Treatment for refractory myasthenia gravis. Arch Dis Child 64:1191, 1989.

Chapter 197

Diseases of the Ocular Muscles

MARK S. BORCHERT

EVALUATION OF OPHTHALMOPLEGIA AND SUSPECTED NEUROMUSCULAR DISEASES

Primary diseases of the extraocular muscles are quite unusual. Some of these diseases are so rare that no clinician could reasonably be expected to remember all of them or their characteristics. Nonetheless, the astute ophthalmologist should keep this general category of diseases in mind whenever evaluating a patient with ophthalmoplegia. The primary muscle diseases have several clinical characteristics in common that should cause the examining ophthalmologist to suspect their diagnosis.

In general, one should suspect muscle disease whenever ophthalmoplegia does not fit the pattern of a cranial nerve palsy (e.g., when only one of the muscles innervated by the third cranial nerve is involved). Isolated, acquired ptosis is one of the most common presentations of muscle disease.

Most primary muscle diseases are not confined to the extraocular muscles. Weakness of any other muscle group in the body should cause one to suspect neuromuscular disease. Weakness of the orbicularis oculi is particularly common and should be routinely checked in the ophthalmic examination. Ask the patient to forcefully squeeze his or her eyelids shut against the resistance of your thumb and index finger. Note how difficult it is to hold the eyelids open. Particularly note any asymmetry in the strength of orbicularis function in the two eyes. In children, orbicularis function should be assessed toward the end of the examination while administering dilating eyedrops. This will maximize the child's effort to close his eyelids and avoid loss of cooperation early in the examination.

Finally, if ophthalmoplegia is associated with retinal

Table 197–1. MYOPATHIC CAUSES OF OPHTHALMOPLEGIA

Static Ophthalmoplegia
Agenesis of extraocular muscles
Congenital fibrosis syndromes
Congenital myopathies
Central core
Centronuclear
Multicore
Progressive Ophthalmoplegia
Chronic progressive external ophthalmoplegia
Oculopharyngeal dystrophy
Myotonic dystrophy
Vitamin E deficiency
Inflammatory and infiltrative myopathies
Graves' disease
Idiopathic orbital myositis
Infectious myositis
Amyloidosis
Primary and metastatic muscle tumors
Episodic Ophthalmoplegia
Familial periodic paralysis
Muscular trauma and contusions
Ischemia and vasculitis
Disorders of neuromuscular junction
Myasthenia
Organophosphate poisoning
Eaton-Lambert syndrome
Botulism

degeneration, one should suspect a primary muscle disease.

Electromyography (EMG) is useful in distinguishing myopathic from neuropathic etiologies of weakness in affected muscles. Unfortunately, this technique is not routinely practical in diseases confined to the extraocular muscles. Furthermore, different types of myopathy often cannot be distinguished by EMG. Even the classic EMG findings of myasthenia gravis, a disease of the neuromuscular junction, can be mimicked by a myopathy such as chronic progressive external ophthalmoplegia.[1]

Diseases of the extraocular muscles can generally be divided according to whether their symptoms are static, progressive, or intermittent (Table 197–1). Secondary diseases of the extraocular muscles such as inflammatory and infiltrative disorders are not covered in this section. Diseases of the neuromuscular junction such as myasthenia gravis are also being covered elsewhere.

PROGRESSIVE OPHTHALMOPLEGIA

Mitochondrial Disorders

BACKGROUND AND BIOCHEMISTRY

Recently, muscle diseases associated with disruption in morphology and function of mitochondria have come to light. The most common mitochondrial cytopathy is chronic progressive external ophthalmoplegia (CPEO), or "ophthalmoplegia plus." This disorder was thought by many to represent a primary myopathy because of the typical histologic appearance of skeletal muscle biopsies from affected individuals. When stained with modified Gomori trichrome stain, small groups of irregular-appearing fibers stained dark red and were called ragged-red fibers (Fig. 197–1).[2] The belief that this disease was primarily a myopathy was difficult to reconcile with the frequent nonmuscular findings of peripheral neuropathy, ataxia, spasticity, deafness, retinopathy, optic atrophy, and dementia. When it was recognized that the ragged-red fibers were caused by accumulations of abnormal mitochondria within the myofibers, it became obvious that any cell dependent on aerobic metabolism could be affected. In fact, CPEO can occur with impairment of mitochondrial respiratory function even without the morphologic changes manifested by ragged-red fibers.[3] Many other diseases are now believed to be the result of mitochondrial dysfunction with or without morphologic changes in the mitochondria. Biochemical classification of the mitochondrial cytopathies is starting to develop. Defects in pyruvate utilization, oxidative phosphorylation, and respiratory chain function have been described.[4, 5] Lactic acidosis due to defective aerobic metabolism is a common finding. Presumably, many diseases remain to be identified and characterized, given the myriad of metabolic functions provided by the mitochondria.

By electron microscopy, the morphologic characteristics of the mitochondrial disorders are varied (Fig. 197–2). Some mitochondria appear empty or vacuolated, whereas others contain globular or crystalline inclusions. Abnormal size and shape or irregular cristae are common. Excessive accumulation of triglyceride droplets may histopathologically mimic lipid storage diseases. Similar morphologic changes may be seen in the various muscular dystrophies, polymyositis, and dermatomyositis. Consequently, deformities of the mitochondria cannot exclusively be relied on in making a diagnosis.

Mitochondrial DNA codes for 13 of the oxidative phosphorylation proteins. Among these are subunits of cytochromes b and c, and adenosine triphosphate (ATP)

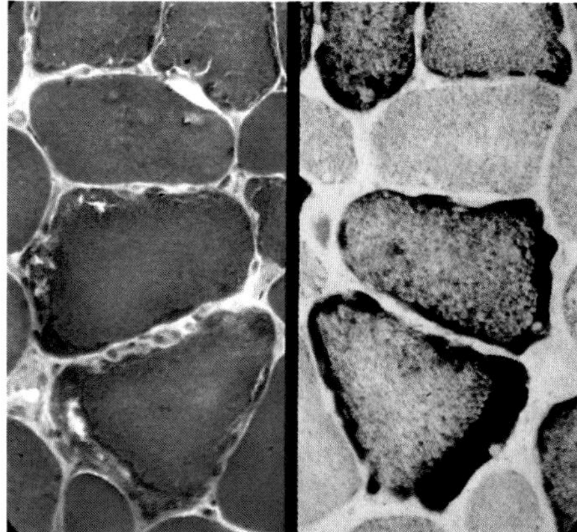

Figure 197–1. *Left,* modified trichrome stain of skeletal muscle demonstrating "ragged red" fibers. *Right,* mirror-mounted serial section stained for succinate dehydrogenase (specific for mitochondria). Note the subsarcolemmal accumulation of mitochondria corresponding to the red staining in modified trichrome. (Courtesy of W. K. Engel.)

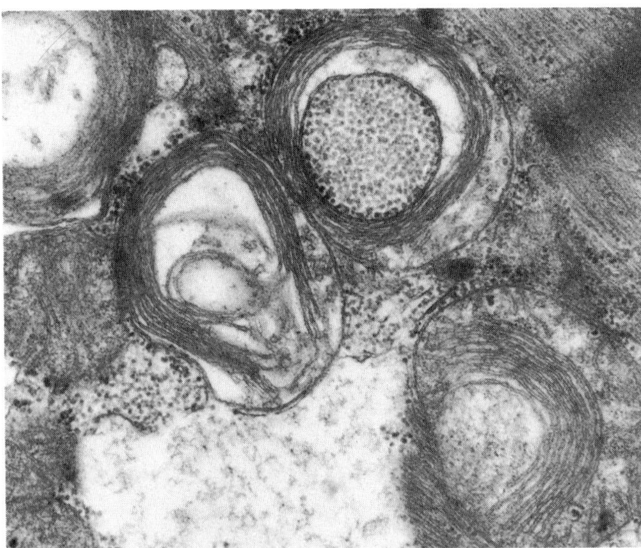

Figure 197–2. Abnormal mitochondria with cristae forming concentric membranous rings accumulated in the myocardium of a patient with Kearns-Sayre syndrome (× 42,000).

synthase.[7] Ninety percent of mitochondrial proteins are coded by nuclear DNA and are transmitted in a mendelian fashion. Mitochondrial DNA, on the other hand, is transmitted almost exclusively by the mother via the ovum. Since many copies of mitochondrial DNA may be transmitted to the offspring and since mitochondrial DNA replicates many times more frequently than nuclear DNA, the relative proportion of mutant and wild type of mitochondrial DNA may vary from one cell to another and from one individual to another, resulting in considerable phenotypic variability.

The clinical presentation of the mitochondrial cytopathies is varied, with considerable overlap among syndromes. Four distinct disorders transmitted by mitochondrial DNA are of ophthalmic importance. These are chronic progressive external ophthalmoplegia (CPEO) or Kearns-Sayre syndrome; myoclonus epilepsy with ragged-red fibers (MERRF), or Fukahara's disease; mitochondrial encephalopathy, lactic acidosis, and strokelike episodes (MELAS); and Leber's optic neuropathy (Table 197–2). Of these, only CPEO causes significant ophthalmoplegia.

CPEO AND KEARNS-SAYRE SYNDROME

Bilateral, often asymmetric, ptosis is usually the first sign of CPEO.[8] Patients use their brow muscles to elevate the eyelids. This usually begins before adolescence. Cases have been described with no ptosis at all.

Ptosis is usually followed within a few years by progressive external ophthalmoplegia. The ophthalmoplegia is usually symmetric, affecting both horizontal and upward gaze. Downward gaze is often spared. In those cases that develop strabismus, diplopia is unusual because of the slowly progressive nature of the ophthalmoplegia.

Often a patient's symptoms and signs are confined to ophthalmoplegia and ptosis. However, as with most diseases of the extraocular muscles, weakness of the orbicularis oculi is common. Eventually, most of the facial muscles may become involved. The ptosis may appear to worsen as the result of progressive weakness of the frontalis muscle. Weakness of the arms, legs, and muscles of mastication may mimic myasthenia gravis. Serum creatine kinase levels may be slightly elevated.

In 1958 Kearns and Sayre described two patients with chronic progressive ophthalmoplegia, atypical retinitis pigmentosa, and complete heart block.[9] Since then, many more cases have improved our understanding of the clinical spectrum of this disease. However, an argument continues as to whether Kearns-Sayre syndrome is a severe form of CPEO or a separate disease entity. Identical skeletal muscle mitochondrial DNA deletions have been found in cases of Kearns-Sayre syndrome and in cases of isolated CPEO, suggesting that they are the same disease.[10, 11] Phenotypic variability may be accounted for by the fact that patients with Kearns-Sayre syndrome have identical mitochondrial DNA deletions in other tissues, whereas patients with isolated CPEO who have had other tissue tested have the deletion only in muscle tissue. A higher concentration of mitochondria in extraocular muscles than in other skeletal muscles may account for the predominance of ocular motility problems in this disease.

The pigmentary retinopathy of Kearns-Sayre syndrome differs from retinitis pigmentosa in that it is typically confined to the posterior pole with a mottled appearance of the retinal pigment epithelium. Bone spicule formation is uncommon. Visual symptoms are usually mild if present at all. Electroretinography is usually normal or shows mildly attenuated a- and b-wave amplitudes.[12, 13]

Histopathologically, retinas in Kearns-Sayre syndrome suggest retinal pigment epithelial (RPE) dysfunction. They demonstrate RPE atrophy with overlying photoreceptor degeneration. The RPE cells show evidence of reduced phagocytosis of photoreceptor debris.[14–16] Macrophages containing photoreceptor outer segments have been noted within affected RPE.[17, 18] Peripheral photoreceptors are relatively spared, suggesting that this is not primarily a disease of the photoreceptors, in contradistinction to retinitis pigmentosa.[14]

Table 197–2. FEATURES OF THE MITOCHONDRIAL CYTOPATHIES

	CPEO+	MERRF	MELAS	Leber's
Ophthalmoplegia	+			
Retinal degeneration	+			
Optic atrophy		+		+
Cortical blindness			+	
Ataxia	+	+		
Seizures		+	+	
Cardiac dysrhythmia	+			+
Short stature	+	+	+	
Lactic acidosis	+	+	+	
Sensorineural deafness	+	+	+	
Ragged-red fibers	+	+	+	

Key: CPEO, Chronic progressive external ophthalmoplegia; MELAS, mitochondrial encephalopathy, lactic acidosis and strokelike episodes; MERRF, myoclonus epilepsy with ragged red fibers.

Other studies have shown predominantly peripheral retinal involvement although RPE degeneration was still out of proportion to photoreceptor degeneration.[18]

Cardiac dysfunction, particularly conduction disturbances and arrhythmia, may occur at any time during the course of the disease. Such disturbances can lead to sudden death. Electrocardiographic ST-depression without coronary artery disease may be seen.[19] Patients need to be warned of symptoms such as palpitations, lightheadedness, and shortness of breath. They should be followed by a cardiologist on a regular basis. Pacemaker insertion can be lifesaving. Unfortunately, heart failure due to congestive cardiomyopathy without conduction defects can also develop.[20]

Neurologic abnormalities include nystagmus, ataxia, hearing loss, and dementia.[18, 21] Spongiform degeneration of the cerebral cortex, basal ganglia, and brain stem is seen. Intracranial calcifications are common.[22]

Endocrine disturbances include growth retardation, hypogonadism, diabetes mellitus, thyroid abnormalities, hypoparathyroidism, and hyperaldosteronism.[23]

Genetics and Biochemistry

Mitochondrial DNA deletions varying from 1.3 to 8.0 kilobases (Kb) have been described in CPEO.[7, 10, 11, 24–26] These deletions affect subunits of oxidative phosphorylation enzymes as well as several transfer ribonucleic acid (tRNA) genes and therefore affect mitochondrial protein synthesis in general. This results in multiple problems in respiratory chain function. The size of the mitochondrial DNA deletions does not correlate with the severity of the disease.

Most cases appear to be due to spontaneous mitochondrial mutations within the oocyte or zygote, since few of the patients with mitochondrial DNA deletions have had a family history of the disease.[10, 11] Asymptomatic mothers of patients with known deletions have been tested and have shown no evidence of mitochondrial DNA deletions.[10] One patient had a 4.9-Kb deletion in muscle cells but not in lymphocytes or platelets, suggesting a somatic mutation or selective elimination of mutant mitochondria in certain cell lines.[25] Another patient with a similar 4.9-Kb deletion showed tremendous variability in the amount of mutant mitochondrial DNA from one tissue to another.[26]

Many patients with Kearns-Sayre syndrome show no detectable mitochondrial DNA deletions. This may be due to point mutations or deletions too small to detect with typical restriction fragment analysis techniques. Alternatively, the same defects in mitochondrial respiration could result from mutations in proteins encoded by nuclear DNA. The numerous reports of paternal and autosomal dominant transmission support this hypothesis.[13, 27]

There are many reports of reduced mitochondrial electron transport activity, particularly cytochrome *c* oxidase deficiency in patients with CPEO.[24, 28, 29] These deficiencies are not a consistent finding.[19] In some patients all ragged-red muscle fibers are histochemically deficient in cytochrome *c* oxidase.[24, 28] In other cases, cellular variability in cytochrome *c* oxidase activity has been described without correlation with ragged-red fibers.[30, 31] Cytochrome *c* oxidase deficiency may simply reflect muscle fiber degeneration, since it has been reported in several other neuromuscular diseases as well.[32] The heart may be particularly susceptible to the effects of decreased oxidative phosphorylation since, unlike skeletal muscle, it is dependent on fatty acid β-oxidation for its energy. The accumulation of nicotinamide-adenine dinucleotide phosphate (NADH) from cytochrome *c* oxidase deficiency results in inhibition of β-oxidation.

Treatment

Ubidecarenone, or coenzyme Q10 (CoQ), has been noted to be deficient in the serum and muscles of a few patients with Kearns-Sayre syndrome.[29, 33] This coenzyme is essential for normal mitochondrial respiration. Decreased CoQ levels have been found in other neuromuscular diseases, and are not present in all patients with Kearns-Sayre syndrome.[33, 34] Treatment of a few patients with mitochondrial cytopathies with CoQ has resulted in improved pyruvate metabolism, cardiac function, exercise tolerance, cerebrospinal fluid (CSF) protein levels, and ataxia, but it has had no effect on ophthalmoplegia, ptosis, or retinopathy.[19, 26, 29, 33, 35, 36]

Systemic steroids are contraindicated in CPEO since they can precipitate hyperglycemic, hyperosmolar coma in these patients.[18, 37]

OTHER MITOCHONDRIAL CYTOPATHIES

MELAS syndrome is characterized by seizures, vomiting, and lactic acidosis in the first few years of life. Episodes of hemiparesis, hemianopsia, and cortical visual loss are a prominent feature. Such episodes are believed to result from respiratory difficulties of cortical neurons, although problems with autoregulation of blood flow at the level of small pial arterioles has been suggested.[38] Patients usually recover from the strokelike episodes but are subject to multiple recurrences.

As in CPEO, patients with MELAS syndrome have ragged-red fibers with degeneration of skeletal and cardiac muscle fibers.[39] A genetic defect in MELAS syndrome has not yet been identified.[11] NADH-CoQ reductase deficiency has been reported in several patients with this syndrome.[39–41] Although there is considerable overlap with the other mitochondrial cytopathies, ocular myopathy consisting of ptosis, and abducens paresis has been reported only once.[40] Why clinical muscle weakness is not a prominent feature of this syndrome is unknown.

MERRF usually manifests with myoclonus in the second decade of life. This is followed by ataxia, weakness, and generalized seizures. Eventually, visual loss from progressive optic atrophy develops. Pure maternal transmission and defects of oxidative phosphorylation have been confirmed, but the mitochondrial DNA mutation has yet to be identified in this condition.[42]

Leber's optic neuropathy causes sudden, severe, central vision loss bilaterally. Both eyes are affected within a year of one another.[7] Vision loss usually strikes within the third decade, and there is a predilection for males.

This cytopathy is associated with cardiac dysrhythmias, but no other systemic manifestations are known. Some children with infantile bilateral striatal necrosis causing rigidity and mental retardation will develop Leber's optic neuropathy, indicating that this may represent a more severe form of the disease. A point mutation causing a conversion from argenine to histidine in the NADH dehydrogenase subunit 4 has been identified as a cause of Leber's optic neuropathy.[43]

Muscular Dystrophies

BACKGROUND AND OVERVIEW

The muscular dystrophies are characterized by progressive atrophy of skeletal muscles. Prototypical disease types are Duchenne's muscular dystrophy, facioscapulohumoral dystrophy, and limb-girdle muscular dystrophy. They are distinguished by clinical features and mode of inheritance. In general, they cannot be diagnosed histologically. Retinal telangiectasias similar to Coats' disease have been reported in many cases with facioscapulohumeral dystrophy.[44] Otherwise, only three forms of muscular dystrophy are of ophthalmic importance: oculopharyngeal dystrophy, Fukayama's syndrome, and myotonic dystrophy.

OCULOPHARYNGEAL DYSTROPHY

Oculopharyngeal dystrophy usually manifests in the third or fourth decade of life with dysphagia caused by weakness of the muscles of the hypopharynx.[45] This leads to lack of coordination between muscles of the pharynx and upper esophagus and regurgitation of food into the nasopharynx. Patients initially have difficulty with solid food, but eventually even liquids can be difficult to swallow without aspiration. They are at risk for aspiration pneumonia.

Dysphagia is followed within a few years by ptosis, which is usually bilateral but asymmetric. Eventually, varying degrees of external ophthalmoplegia develop. As with most myopathies, weakness of the orbicularis oculi is a common sign. Occasionally, other bulbar and limb-girdle muscle groups are involved.

Oculopharyngeal dystrophy occurs most commonly in French-Canadians as an autosomal dominant form that can be traced to a common ancestor who immigrated to Quebec from France in 1634.[46] Autosomal recessive and sporadic forms occur in other ethnic groups.

Tubulofilamentous intranuclear inclusions of characteristic size and location are seen in skeletal muscle biopsies by electron microscopy.[47] These inclusions are thought to be pathognomonic of this disease but are not present in all muscle fibers and must be specifically sought.[48] Rarely, ragged-red fibers are seen with modified Gomori trichrome stain.

FUKAYAMA'S SYNDROME

Fukayama's syndrome is a form of congenital muscular dystrophy predominantly affecting proximal muscle groups. It is an autosomal recessive condition reported in all ethnic groups, but concentrated in persons of Japanese descent.[49] Cerebral dysplasia thought related to abnormal migration of fetal cortical neurons leads to mental retardation, seizures, severe motor development delay, cortical blindness, and death in childhood.[50] Computerized tomographic scans of infants suggest delayed myelination of white matter in the brain.[51] Ocular findings include weakness of orbicularis oculi, strabismus, high myopia, anterior polar cataracts, nystagmus, optic nerve atrophy or hypoplasia, and chorioretinal degeneration with retinoschisis-like lesions or retinal detachment.[52] Ophthalmoplegia is not a feature of this disease. There is considerable overlap between this syndrome and the cerebroocular dysplasia–muscular dystrophy (Walker-Warburg) syndrome, which includes microphthalmia and dysmorphic facies.[53, 54]

MYOTONIC DYSTROPHY

Myotonic dystrophy is one of several myotonic conditions characterized by delayed relaxation of skeletal muscles after contraction. The electromyogram in all of the myotonias is diagnostic. It shows typical high-frequency, spontaneous, action potentials characterized as "dive bombers" by their sound. All types of myotonia may cause blepharospasm or difficulty opening the eyes after forced lid closure. Otherwise, only myotonic dystrophy has ocular findings. It is also the only myotonic condition with involvement of other organ systems, including cardiac and smooth muscles, brain, and bone. Such involvement can lead to congestive heart failure, dysphagia, constipation, incontinence, mental retardation, hyperostosis, and scoliosis. Testicular atrophy and baldness are common in men with this condition.

Myotonic dystrophy is an autosomal dominant condition with the onset of symptoms usually in second decade of life. Earlier onset often indicates a more severe course.

Myotonia is often the first symptom. This can be demonstrated clinically by shaking hands with the patient, who is then unable to release his or her grasp. It is aggravated by cold or anxiety and is often more severe in the morning. The myotonia is relieved by multiple repetitive movements. Eventually, muscle atrophy supervenes. This results in weakness of the limb muscles, particularly the leg extensors, and to a sunken appearance of the face with difficulty holding the head up.

Ptosis and weakness of the orbicularis oculi are the most frequent ocular manifestations of muscle involvement. Eighty-three percent of patients have abnormal eye movement recordings consisting of slow saccades with normal latencies and normal amplitudes.[55] Some investigators have found a selective impairment of pursuit.[56] EMG of the extraocular muscles shows myopathic changes similar to those in the limb muscles of these patients.[57] Varying degrees of ophthalmoplegia can be seen.[58]

Histologically, the extraocular muscles show degenerative changes similar to those of the other skeletal muscles.[59] These include rows of nuclei located centrally in the muscle fibers, disruption of myofilaments and sarcoplasmic reticulum, and focal accumulations of mitochondria. In late stages, atrophy and fibrosis are the typical findings.

Nearly all patients with myotonic dystrophy have cataracts. These usually appear as fine anterior and posterior, subcapsular, colored crystals. Spokelike cortical opacities along the suture lines are also common. Other ocular changes include pigmentary retinopathy with decreased vision similar to Kearns-Sayre syndrome and miotic, sluggishly reactive pupils.[60, 61]

Vitamin E Deficiency

Vitamin E deficiency results in diffuse damage to neurons and muscles, including disruption of myelin and sarcomeres, and inclusion body accumulations within muscle fibers.[62] Ocular motility problems include slow saccades, strabismus, and progressive external ophthalmoplegia.[63, 64] To what extent these problems are due to neuronopathy or myopathy is uncertain. Other problems include pigmentary retinopathy, acanthocytosis, areflexia, ataxia, and loss of vibratory sensation.[65, 66] Bassen-Kornzweig syndrome (abetalipoproteinemia with acanthocytosis and retinopathy) as a result of intestinal malabsorption of lipids now seems to be attributable entirely to vitamin E deficiency.

STATIC OPHTHALMOPLEGIA

Congenital Fibrosis Syndromes

Isolated agenesis of extraocular muscles is a rare occurrence but has been reported for nearly every muscle.[66] More commonly, one or more of the extraocular muscles may be involved with congenital fibrosis and may lead to limitation of ocular motility.[67] The full-blown syndrome manifests with bilateral ptosis, static external ophthalmoplegia, and downward deviation of the eyes. A few pedigrees with this constellation of findings have been reported with apparent autosomal dominant transmission.[68–71] We have observed one Cambodian family with three affected generations (Fig. 197–3). A sex-linked recessive form with bilateral ptosis, complete ophthalmoplegia, and high myopia has been described in one family in which the female carriers could be identified by absence of deep tendon reflexes.[72, 73] Pathologic evaluation has only revealed fibrosis of the extraocular muscles.[70, 71] One case of complete congenital fibrosis was associated with Marcus Gunn jaw-winking and synergistic divergence on attempted right gaze.[74] Such aberrant innervation is a common finding in the incomplete syndrome and suggests a neuropathic etiology with agenesis of cranial nerve nuclei similar to Duane's syndrome.[75] As with Duane's syndrome, such cases may be familial (Fig. 197–4).[76, 77] Cases of fibrosis of the extraocular muscles with additional orbital fibrotic bands adherent to the globe have been described and attributed to prenatal inflammation or trauma.[67, 78, 79]

Congenital Myopathies

The congenital myopathies are nonprogressive disorders of muscle cells, all of which have similar clinical findings of weakness, hypotonia, and delayed motor milestones. Entire groups of muscles may appear atrophic. These diseases are categorized by their histopathologic findings on muscle biopsy, although they all have the common characteristic of a size disproportion in the muscle fibers. Muscle biopsy should be considered in any child with ptosis or ophthalmoplegia combined with hypotonia or delayed motor development once myasthenia has been ruled out. Of these diseases, cen-

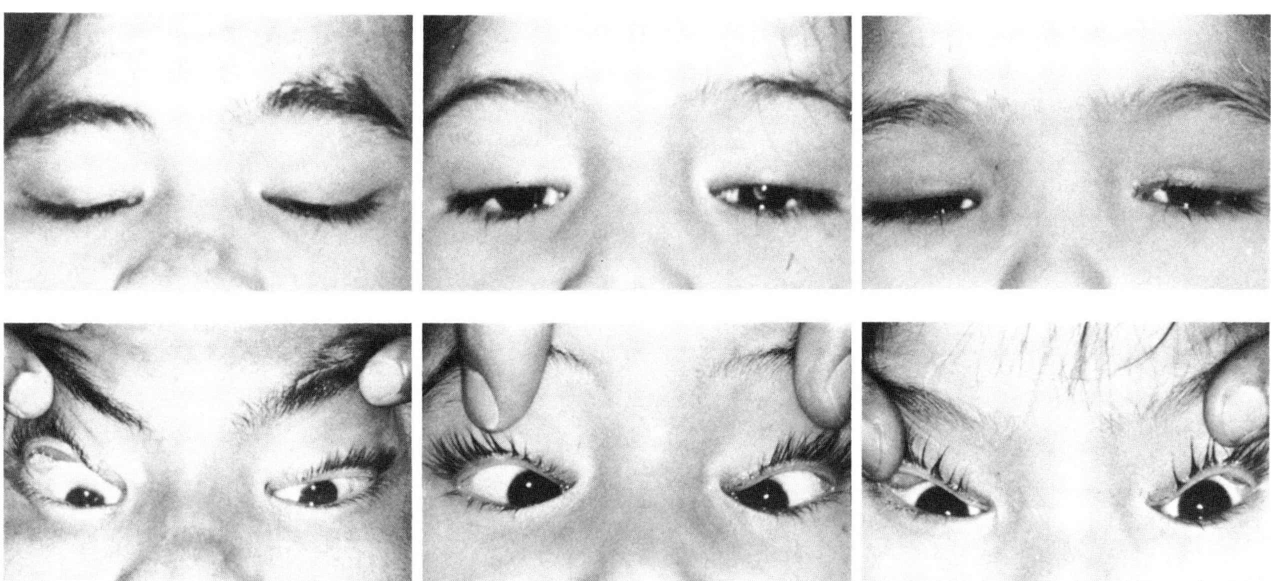

Figure 197–3. Patient (*left*) and his two children with complete congenital fibrosis syndrome. The eyes are fixed in convergent downgaze. There is bilateral ptosis with no levator function. The patient's father (not shown) had an identical condition.

tral core myopathy, centronuclear myopathy, and multicore disease affect the extraocular muscles, causing ptosis, ophthalmoplegia, or both.

CENTRAL CORE MYOPATHY

In this disease there is a characteristic blue staining of the central portion of nearly every muscle fiber with trichrome stain (Fig. 197–5*A*).[80] The disease appears to be autosomal dominant and predominantly affects the proximal muscle groups of the lower extremities.

CENTRONUCLEAR (MYOTUBULAR) MYOPATHY

This congenital myopathy is characterized by centrally located nuclei in many muscle fibers with the cytoplasm around the nuclei devoid of organelles or myofibrils (Fig. 197–5*B*).[81] On longitudinal sections, the nuclei appear lined up in rows like railroad cars. It was originally called myotubular myopathy because of histologic resemblance to myotubes of fetal muscle. Clinical manifestation includes atrophy of muscles of trunk and upper extremities, weakness of facial muscles, areflexia, ptosis, and external ophthalmoplegia. Most cases are sporadic. Those with identifiable modes of genetic transmission have characteristic clinical courses.

Patients with X-linked centronuclear myopathy have severe hypotonia at birth and often die early of respiratory problems.[82] Less severe cases with prolonged lifespan have been reported.[83] This form further resembles developing fetal muscle in that the muscles show a persistence of fetal cytoskeletal proteins vimentin and desmin.[84]

The autosomal recessive form of centronuclear myopathy usually manifests in the first year of life with delayed motor development.[48] This form may be very slowly progressive. These patients often develop a waddling gait with hypotrophy of the limb-girdle muscles and hypertrophy of the calves. They are usually confined to a wheelchair by the second decade of life. They have a typically myopathic, expressionless face with bilateral ptosis.

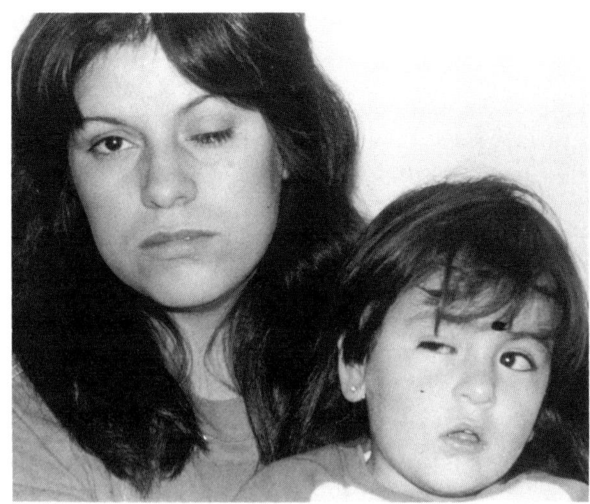

Figure 197–4. Mother and daughter with unilateral congenital fibrosis syndrome. Both patients had ptosis and double elevator palsy with levator synkinesis on adduction.

An autosomal dominant form of centronuclear myopathy with slowly progressive disability has been described.[85] Ocular motility disturbances are rare but may manifest as adult onset strabismus.[48] Patients with the autosomal dominant forms usually develop symptoms of proximal muscle group weakness in adolescence or adulthood, although infantile cases have been reported.[86] It is compatible with a normal life span.

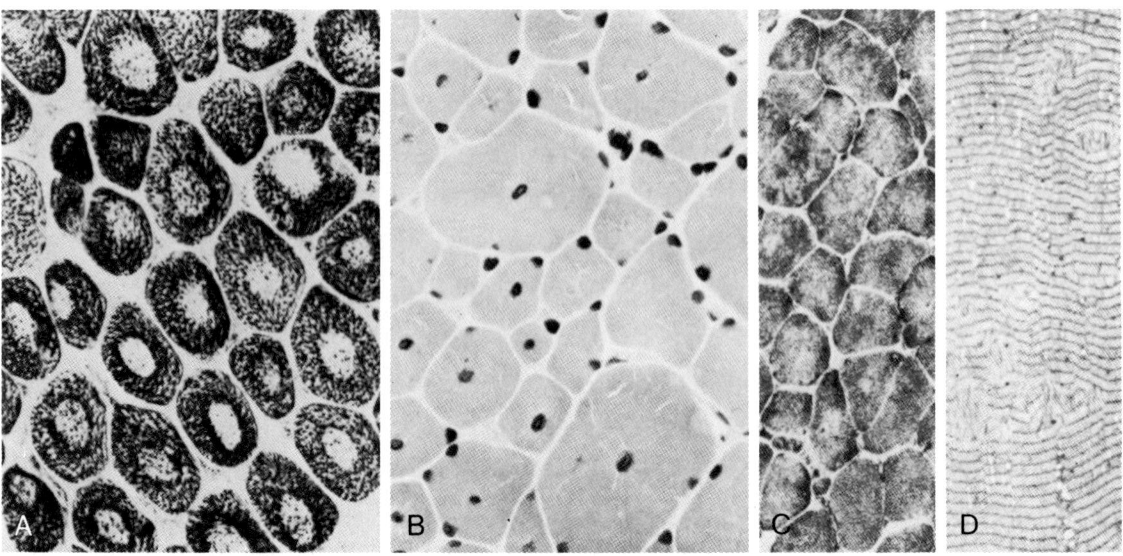

Figure 197–5. Skeletal muscle biopsies of congenital myopathies. *A*, Central core myopathy, cryostat cross section; NADH-tetrazolium reductase stain; × 135. *B*, Centronuclear myopathy, cryostat cross section; H & E stain; × 160. *C* Multicore disease, cryostat cross section; NADH-tetrazolium reductase stain; × 135. *D*, Multicore disease, epoxy-embedded longitudinal section; × 340. Foci of disrupted myofibrillar striations. (*A* to *D* from Fardeau M: Congenital myopathies. *In* Mastaglia FL, Walton J (eds): Skeletal Muscle Pathology. Edinburgh, Churchill Livingstone, 1982, pp 164, 171, 176, respectively.)

MULTICORE MYOPATHY

In this disease, foci of disrupted sarcomeres with loss of mitochondria cause irregularities in the cross-striations of muscle fibers with NADH-tetrazolium stain or electron microscopy (Fig. 197–5*C,D*).[87] The patients usually present with neonatal hypotonia. Many die in infancy of respiratory difficulties.[48] A few present in early childhood with difficulty walking, hypotrophic skeletal muscles, and facial weakness. Slowly progressive ocular involvement is common and runs the spectrum from ptosis to complete ophthalmoplegia.[88] Most cases appear sporadic, but autosomal recessive inheritance has been documented.[89]

Numerous other histologic types of congenital myopathies have been described, including fingerprint body myopathy, reducing body myopathy, zebra body myopathy, trilaminar muscle fiber disease, and nemaline myopathy. Clinical involvement of the extraocular muscles has rarely, if ever, been described in these diseases. A type of congenital myopathy with mild fiber-type variation and myofibrillar disorganization but no specific features (minimal change myopathy) has been described with complete ophthalmoplegia and ptosis in one case.[90] Undoubtedly, further congenital myopathies with extraocular muscle involvement will be described.

EPISODIC PARALYSIS AND OPHTHALMOPLEGIA

Familial periodic paralysis is a group of three distinct autosomal dominant disorders that have similar presentations but are distinguished by serum potassium levels at the time of an attack. In hypokalemic familial periodic paralysis, attacks begin with weakness of the extremities and progress to flaccid paralysis of most of the body. In the hyperkalemic and normokalemic varieties, attacks often begin with myotonia, followed by weakness and paralysis. Attacks last hours to days. Severe attacks can lead to death. Ophthalmoplegia is unusual, but ptosis or lid retraction is common. Treatment is directed at correcting the serum potassium levels.

All three varieties of familial periodic paralysis are characterized by central vacuolation of muscle fibers histologically. The underlying disorder is unknown but is believed to be related to alterations in muscle membrane permeability.[91]

REFERENCES

1. Krendel DA, Sanders DB, Massey JM: Single-fiber electromyography in chronic progressive external ophthalmoplegia. Muscle Nerve 10:299, 1987.
2. Olson W, Engel WK, Walsh GO, et al: Oculocraniosomatic neuromuscular disease with "ragged red" fibers. Arch Neurol 26:193, 1972.
3. Mitsumoto H, Aprille JR, Wray SH, et al: Chronic progressive external ophthalmoplegia (CPEO): Clinical, morphologic, and biochemical studies. Neurology 33:452, 1983.
4. Schapira AHV, Cooper JM, Morgan-Hughes JA, et al: Mitochondrial myopathy with a defect of mitochondrial-protein transport. N Engl J Med 323:37, 1990.
5. Schapira AHV, Cooper JM, Morgan-Hughes JA, et al: Molecular basis of mitochondrial myopathies: Polypeptide analysis in complex-I deficiency. Lancet 1:500, 1988.
6. DiMauro S, Bonilla E, Zeviani M, et al: Mitochondrial myopathies. Ann Neurol 17:521, 1985.
7. Wallace DC: Mitochondrial DNA mutations and neuromuscular disease. Trends Genet 5:9, 1989.
8. Walsh FB, Hoyt WF: Clinical Neuro-Ophthalmology, vol 2, 3rd ed. Baltimore, Williams & Wilkins, 1969.
9. Kearns TP, Sayre GP: Retinitis pigmentosa, external ophthalmoplegia, and complete heart block. Arch Ophthalmol 60:280, 1958.
10. Moraes CT, De Mauro S, Zeviani M, et al: Mitochondrial DNA deletions in progressive external ophthalmoplegia and Kearns-Sayre syndrome. N Engl J Med 320:1293, 1989.
11. Gerbitz KD, Obermaier-Kusser B, Zierz S, et al: Mitochondrial myopathies: Divergences of genetic deletions, biochemical defects and the clinical syndromes. J Neurol 237:5, 1990.
12. Beckerman BL, Henkind P: Progressive external ophthalmoplegia and benign retinal pigmentation. Am J Ophthalmol 81:89, 1976.
13. Leveille AS, Newell FW: Autosomal dominant Kearns-Sayre syndrome. Ophthalmology 87:99, 1980.
14. Eagle RC Jr., Hedges TR, Yanoff M: The atypical pigmentary retinopathy of Kearns-Sayre syndrome: A light and electron microscopic study. Ophthalmology 89:1433, 1982.
15. Eagle RC Jr., Hedges TR, Yanoff M: The Kearns-Sayre syndrome: A light and electron microscopic study. Trans Am Ophthalmol Soc 80:218, 1982.
16. McKechnie NM, King M, Lee WR: Retinal pathology in the Kearns-Sayre syndrome. Br J Ophthalmol 69:63, 1985.
17. Newell FW, Polascik MA: Mitochondrial disease and retinal pigmentary degeneration. *In* Shimizu K (ed): Ophthalmology. 23rd International Congress of Ophthalmology, Kyoto, 1978, Amsterdam, Excerpta Medica, 1979.
18. Flynn JT, Bachynski BN, Rodrigues MM, et al: Hyperglycemic acidotic coma and death in Kearns-Sayre syndrome. Trans Am Ophthalmol Soc 83:131, 1985.
19. Ogasahara S, Nishikawa Y, Yorifuji S, et al: Treatment of Kearns-Sayre syndrome with coenzyme Q_{10}. Neurology 36:45, 1986.
20. Kleber FX, Park JW, Hübner G, et al: Congestive heart failure due to mitochondrial cardiomyopathy in Kearns-Sayre syndrome. Klin Wochenschr 65:480, 1987.
21. Castaigne P, Laplane D, Escourolle R, et al: Ophthalmoplégie externe progressive avec spongiose des noyaux du tronc cérébral. Rev Neurol 124:454, 1971.
22. Seigel RS, Seeger JF, Gabrielsen TO, et al: Computed tomography in oculocraniosomatic disease (Kearns-Sayre syndrome). Radiology 130:159, 1979.
23. Doriguzzi C, Palmucci L, Mongini T, et al: Endocrine involvement in mitochondrial encephalomyopathy with partial cytochrome c oxidase deficiency. J Neurol Neurosurg Psychol 52:122, 1989.
24. Romero NB, Lestienne P, Marsac C, et al: Immunocytological and histochemical correlation in Kearns-Sayre syndrome with mtDNA deletion and partial cytochrome *c* oxidase deficiency in skeletal muscle. J Neurol Sci 93:297, 1989.
25. Shoffner JM, Lott MT, Voljavec AS, et al: Spontaneous Kearns-Sayre/chronic external ophthalmoplegia plus syndrome associated with a mitochondrial DNA deletion: A slip-replication model and metabolic therapy. Proc Natl Acad Sci 86:7952, 1989.
26. Shanske S, Moraes CT, Lombes A, et al: Widespread tissue distribution of mitochondrial DNA deletions in Kearns-Sayre syndrome. Neurology 40:24, 1990.
27. Bastiaensen LAK: On the heredity of mitochondrial cytopathies. Neuro-Ophthalmology 7:151, 1987.
28. Johnson MA, Turnbull DM, Dick DJ, et al: A partial deficiency of cytochrome *c* oxidase in chronic progressive external ophthalmoplegia. J Neurol Sci 60:31, 1983.
29. Bresolin N, Bet L, Binda A, et al: Clinical and biochemical correlations in mitochondrial myopathies treated with coenzyme Q_{10}. Neurology 38:892, 1988.
30. Turnbull DM, Johnson MA, Dick DJ, et al: Partial cytochrome oxidase deficiency without subsarcolemmal accumulation of mitochondria in chronic progressive external ophthalmoplegia. J Neurol Sci 70:93, 1985.
31. Müller-Hocker J, Johannes A, Droste M, et al: Fatal mitochon-

drial cardiomyopathy in Kearns-Sayre syndrome with deficiency of cytochrome-c-oxidase in cardiac and skeletal muscle. Virchows Arch [B] 52:353, 1986.
32. Yamamoto M, Koga Y, Ohtaki E, et al: Focal cytochrome c oxidase deficiency in various neuromuscular diseases. J Neurol Sci 91:207, 1989.
33. Zierz S, Jahns G, Jerusalem F: Coenzyme Q in serum and muscle of 5 patients with Kearns-Sayre syndrome and 12 patients with ophthalmoplegia plus. J Neurol 236:97, 1989.
34. Folkers K, Wolaniuk J, Simonsen R, et al: Biochemical rationale and the cardiac response of patients with muscle disease to therapy with coenzyme Q_{10} Proc Natl Acad Sci USA 82:4513, 1985.
35. Ogasahara S, Yorifuji S, Nishikawa Y, et al: Improvement of abnormal pyruvate metabolism and cardiac conduction defect with coenzyme Q_{10} in Kearns-Sayre syndrome. Neurology 35:372, 1985.
36. Goda S, Hamada T, Ishimoto S, et al: Clinical improvement after administration of coenzyme Q_{10} in a patient with mitochondrial encephalomyopathy. J Neurol 234:62, 1987.
37. Curless RG, Flynn J, Bachynski B, et al: Fatal metabolic acidosis, hyperglycemia, and coma after steroid therapy for Kearns-Sayre syndrome. Neurology 36:872, 1986.
38. Ohama E, Ohara S, Ikuta F, et al: Mitochondrial angiopathy in cerebral blood vessels of mitochondrial encephalomyopathy. Acta Neuropathol (Berl) 74:226, 1987.
39. Nishizawa M, Tanaka K, Shinozawa K, et al: A mitochondrial encephalomyopathy with cardiomyopathy: A case revealing a defect of complex I in the respiratory chain. J Neurol Sci 78:189, 1987.
40. Yamanaka R, Nomura Y, Segawa M, et al: MELAS, myoclonus, ataxia and deficiencies of complexes I and IV in muscle mitochondria. Acta Paediatr Jpn 29:761, 1987.
41. Kobayashi M, Morishita H, Sugiyama N, et al: Two cases of NADH-coenzyme Q reductase deficiency: Relationship to MELAS syndrome. J Pediatr 110:223, 1987.
42. Wallace DC, Zheng X, Lott MT, et al: Familial mitochondrial encephalomyopathy (MERRF): genetic, pathophysiological, and biochemical characterization of a mitochondrial DNA disease. Cell 55:601, 1988.
43. Wallace DC, Singh G, Lott MT, et al: Mitochondrial DNA mutation associated with Leber's hereditary optic neuropathy. Science 242:1427, 1988.
44. Gurwin EB, Fitzsimons RB, Sehmi KS, et al: Retinal telangiectasis in facioscapulohumeral muscular dystrophy with deafness. Arch Ophthalmol 103:1695, 1985.
45. Murphy SF, Drachman DB: The oculopharyngeal syndrome. JAMA 203:99, 1968.
46. Barbeau A: The syndrome of hereditary late onset ptosis and dysphagia in French-Canada. *In* Juhn (ed): Symposium uber progressive Muskeldystrophie, Myotonie, Myasthenie. Berlin, Springer-Verlag, 1966.
47. Bouchard JP, Gagné F, Tomé FMS, et al: Nuclear inclusions in oculopharyngeal muscular dystrophy in Quebec. Can J Neurol Sci 16:446, 1989.
48. Martin JJ: On some myopathies with oculomotor involvement. Acta Neurol Belg 87:207, 1987.
49. Fukuyama Y, Osawa M, Suzuki H: Congenital progressive muscular dystrophy of the Fukuyama type: Clinical, genetic and pathologic considerations. Brain Dev 3:1, 1981.
50. Takada K, Nakamura H, Takashima S: Cortical dysplasia in Fukuyama congenital muscular dystrophy (FCMD): A Golgi and angioarchitectonic analysis. Acta Neuropathol 76:170, 1988.
51. Yoshioka M, Saiwai S: Congenital muscular dystrophy (Fukuyama type)—Changes in the white matter low density on CT. Brain Dev 10:41, 1988.
52. Tsutsumi A, Uchida Y, Osawa M, et al: Ocular findings in Fukuyama-type congenital muscular dystrophy. Brain Dev 11:413, 1989.
53. Heggie P, Grossniklaus HE, Roessmann U, et al: Cerebro-ocular dysplasia–muscular dystrophy syndrome. Arch Ophthalmol 105:520, 1987.
54. Yoshioka M, Kuroki S, Kondo T: Ocular manifestations in Fukuyama-type congenital muscular dystrophy. Brain Dev 12:427, 1990.
55. Ter Bruggen JP, Bastiaensen LAK, Tyssen CC, et al: Disorders of eye movement in myotonic dystrophy. Brain 113:463, 1990.
56. von Noorden GK, Thompson HS, van Allen MW: Eye movements in myotonic dystrophy: An electrooculographic study. Invest Ophthalmol 3:314, 1964.
57. Davidson SI: The eye in dystrophia myotonica: With a report on electromyography of the extra-ocular muscles. Br J Ophthalmol 45:183, 1961.
58. Lessell S, Coppeto J, Samet S: Ophthalmoplegia in myotonic dystrophy. Am J Ophthalmol 71:1231, 1971.
59. Kuwabara T, Lessell S: Electron microscopic study of extraocular muscles in myotonic dystrophy. Am J Ophthalmol 82:303, 1976.
60. Mausolf FA, Burns CA, Burian HM: Morphologic and functional retinal changes in myotonic dystrophy unrelated to quinine therapy. Am J Ophthalmol 74:1141, 1972.
61. Thompson HS, Van Allen MW, von Noorden GK: The pupil in myotonic dystrophy. Invest Ophthalmol 3:325, 1964.
62. Werlin SL, Harb JM, Swick H, et al: Neuromuscular dysfunction and ultrastructural pathology in children with chronic cholestasis and vitamin E deficiency. Ann Neurol 13:291, 1983.
63. Yee RD, Cogan DG, Zee DS: Ophthalmoplegia and dissociated nystagmus in abetalipo-proteinemia. Arch Ophthalmol 94:571, 1976.
64. Brin MF, Fetall MR, Green PHA, et al: Blind loop syndrome, vitamin E metabsorption, and spinocerebellar degeneration. Neurology 35:338, 1985.
65. Brin MF, Emerson RG, Pedley TA, et al: The vitamin E deficiency syndrome: Occurrence, clinical characteristics, and electrophysiological features. Ann Neurol 14:109, 1983.
66. Miller NR: Walsh and Hoyt's Clinical Neuro-Ophthalmology, vol 2, 4th ed. Baltimore, Williams & Wilkins, 1985.
67. von Noorden GK: Congenital hereditary ptosis with inferior rectus fibrosis; Report of two cases. Arch Ophthalmol 83:378, 1970.
68. Hansen E: Congenital general fibrosis of the extraocular muscles. Acta Ophthalmol 46:469, 1968.
69. Lees F: Congenital, static familial ophthalmoplegia. J Neurol Neurosurg Psychiatry 23:46, 1960.
70. Holmes WJ: Hereditary congenital ophthalmoplegia. Trans Am Ophthalmol Soc 63:245, 1955.
71. Harley RD, Rodriguez MM, Crawford JS: Congenital fibrosis of the extraocular muscles. Trans Am Ophthalmol Soc 76:197, 1978.
72. Salleras A, Ortiz de Zarate JC: Recessive sex-linked inheritance of external ophthalmoplegia and myopia coincident with other dysplasias. Br J Ophthalmol 34:662, 1950.
73. Ortiz de Zarate JC: Recessive sex-linked inheritance of congenital external ophthalmoplegia and myopia coincident with other dysplasias: A reappraisal after 15 years. Br J Ophthalmol 50:606, 1966.
74. Brodsky MC, Pollock SC, Buckley EG: Neural misdirection in congenital ocular fibrosis syndrome: Implications and pathogenesis. J Pediatr Ophthalmol Strabismus 26:159, 1989.
75. Miller NR, Kiel SM, Green WR, et al: Unilateral Duane's retraction syndrome (type 1). Arch Ophthalmol 100:1468, 1982.
76. Sevel D, Kassar BS: Bilateral Duane syndrome: Occurrence in three successive generations. Arch Ophthalmol 91:492, 1974.
77. Kirkham TH: Inheritance of Duane's syndrome. Br J Ophthalmol 54:323, 1970.
78. Effron L, Price RL, Berlin AJ: Congenital unilateral orbital fibrosis with suspected prenatal orbital penetration. J Pediatr Ophthalmol Strabismus 22:133, 1985.
79. Prakash P, Menon V, Ghosh G: Congenital fibrosis of superior rectus and superior oblique: A case report. Br J Ophthalmol 69:57, 1985.
80. Shy GM, Magee KR: A new congenital nonprogressive myopathy. Brain 79:610, 1956.
81. Heckmatt JZ, Sewry CA, Hodes D, et al: Congenital centronuclear (myotubular) myopathy: A clinical, pathological and genetic study in eight children. Brain 108:941, 1985.
82. Barth PG, Van Wijngaarden GK, Bethlem J: X-linked myotubular myopathy with fatal neonatal asphyxia. Neurology 25:531, 1975.
83. Bruyland M, Liebaers I, Sacre L, et al: Neonatal myotubular myopathy with a probable X-linked inheritance: Observations on a new family with a review of the literature. J Neurol 231:220, 1984.
84. Sarnat HB: Myotubular myopathy: Arrest of morphogenesis of

myofibres associated with persistence of fetal vimentin and desmin. Can J Neurol Sci 17:109, 1990.
85. McLeod JG, Baker W, Lethlean AK, et al: Centronuclear myopathy with autosomal dominant inheritance. J Neurol Sci 15:375, 1985.
86. Torres CF, Griggs RC, Goetz JP: Severe neonatal centronuclear myopathy with autosomal dominant inheritance. Arch Neurol 42:1011, 1985.
87. Engel AG, Gomez MR, Groover RV: Multicore disease: A recently recognized congenital myopathy associated with multifocal degeneration of muscle fibers. Mayo Clin Proc 46:666, 1971.
88. Mukoyama M, Matsuoka Y, Kato H, Sobue I: Multicore disease. Clin Neurol 13:221, 1973.
89. Van Wijngaarden GK, Bethlem J, Dingemans KP, et al: Familial focal loss of striations. J Neurol 216:163, 1977.
90. Ohtaki E, Yamaguchi Y, Yamashita Y, et al: Complete external ophthalmoplegia in a patient with congenital myopathy without specific features (minimal change myopathy). Brain Dev 12:427, 1990.
91. Tomé FMS: Periodic paralysis and electrolyte disorders. *In* Mastaglia FL, Walton J (eds): Skeletal Muscle Pathology. Edinburgh, Churchill Livingstone, 1982.

Chapter 198

Eye Movements in Coma

JAMES R. KEANE

The ocular findings are the most important of the entire examination (of the comatose patient) and their interpretation at the bedside is often the mainstay of diagnosis.

C. MILLER FISHER[1]

EYE MOVEMENT LIMITATION

Diagnosis of Coma

Coma, like pornography, is difficult to define but easier to recognize when seen. There is an absence of purposeful responses to all stimuli in deep *coma*, whereas pain (but not speech) elicits voluntary responses and eye opening in *stupor* (moderate coma). In *drowsiness* (light coma), commands arouse the patient to speak.[1, 2] Such delightful terms as carus (deep sleep), typhomania (stupor and delirium), and cataphora (lethargy) are currently out of fashion.

The *Glasgow Coma Scale*[3] has gained deserved popularity as an attempt to quantitate the severity of coma in studies assessing outcome. Three factors, eye opening, motor response, and verbal response are given scores that depend on the level of reaction to various stimuli. Eye movements and pupillary responses are not included; the Glasgow score provides a limited description of the individual patient and no information about the cause of coma.

Several conditions should be distinguished from coma (Table 198–1): The *locked-in syndrome,*[4] in large part a tragic consequence of modern resuscitation capability, describes an awake but paralyzed patient who is unable to communicate. The usual cause is severe pontine infarction due to basilar artery occlusion,[5] but trauma[6, 7] and other conditions[2] may produce a deefferented state. Patients with locked-in syndrome respond by making eyelid and vertical eye movements that are mediated by the midbrain. Hearing is usually spared,[8] but every apparently comatose patient should be given a target to follow as well as being asked to open the eyes and look up and down.

The *chronic vegetative state,*[9] also mainly an iatrogenic problem, is an intractable social dilemma that is frequently highlighted in the news. Vegetative patients open their eyes and appear to be awake, but they exhibit no conscious awareness. In effect, the brain stem is awake and functioning, but bilateral cerebral damage (usually hypoxia) has put the cerebrum to sleep permanently.

Akinetic mutism refers to another variety of "vigilant coma," more ambiguous in definition and localization. Ophthalmic interest lies in the common association of akinetic mutism (usually hypokinetic hypophonia) with pretectal eye signs. The akinetic mute, dramatized by Sacks in *Awakenings,*[10] appears to be awake and has the capability of moving, but rarely demonstrates either.

Localization of Coma

Pupil and eye movement pathways lie adjacent to the brain stem ascending reticular formation that governs

Table 198–1. DIFFERENTIAL DIAGNOSIS OF COMA

Locked-in syndrome: awake but paralyzed
Chronic vegetative state: cerebrum asleep
Akinetic mutism: can respond but rarely does
Hysteria: feigned coma is rare

Table 198–2. COMA LOCALIZATION

Cerebral (bilateral): pupils and eye movements normal
Midbrain: pupils fixed, often total ophthalmoplegia
Pontine: tiny pupils; horizontal eye movement limitations

wakefulness. The neuroophthalmologic examination is key to diagnosing the location, and occasionally the origin, of coma (Table 198–2). When pupils and eye movements are intact, coma is caused by bilateral cerebral depression. Indeed, the presence of full horizontal eye movements, alone, indicates that the cause of coma is rostral to the midbrain.[1]

Vertical gaze paresis and bilateral third-nerve impairment indicate a *midbrain* origin of coma. Coma from *pontine* damage is associated with bilateral horizontal limitations: gaze palsy, internuclear ophthalmoplegia, and abducens nerve paresis. Eye movement limitation in deep coma can result from drug overdose, but the pupils are very rarely affected by *metabolic* conditions. (Neurologist Martin Samuels discusses the pupils in coma[11] and gives a cautionary hint to emergency room physicians concerning the fixed dilated pupil in a *conscious* patient: "Look on the chart—is there a big 'V' followed by gibberish? If the V is there, the phantom ophthalmologist has been around.")

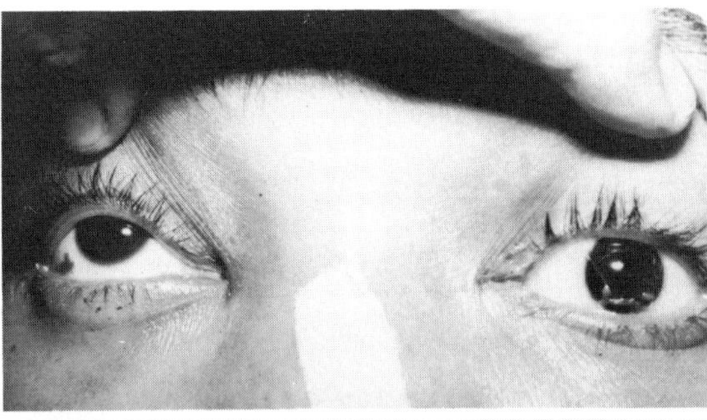

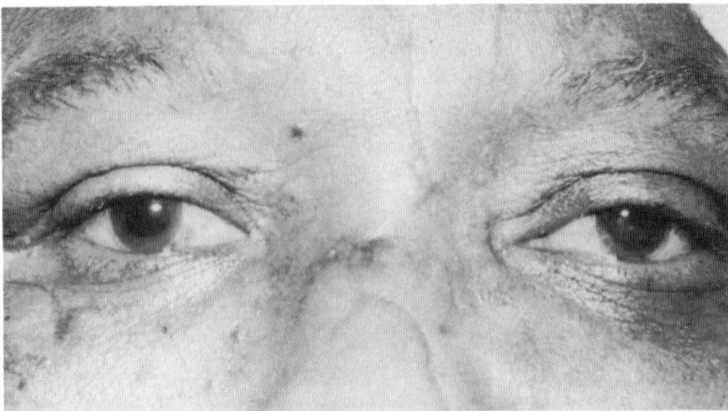

Figure 198–1. Comatose patients frequently show evidence of both old and new trauma. Left eye prosthesis inserted as a result of old trauma *(top)* and bilateral fixed and dilated pupils as a result of old trauma *(bottom;* note the scars) were interpreted as signs of acute tentorial herniation when patients were admitted in coma.

Examination of the Comatose Patient

History is the quintessence of neurologic diagnosis. Details concerning the patient in coma may be limited, and diagnostic confusion is often the result (Fig. 198–1). The neurologic examination of the comatose patient is less sure than that of the cooperative patient, but continued careful observation is mandatory.[1, 12] Many eye movement phenomena are intermittent and may be overlooked by a cursory examination. Stuporous patients, or those in light coma, may demonstrate their eye movement abilities spontaneously, but assistance from the vestibuloocular reflex (VOR) is required for most comatose patients.[13] The oculocephalic maneuver, using quick head movements to elicit opposite reflex eye movements, is helpful if successful. However, it provides a relatively weak vestibular stimulus and is further restricted by the numerous tubes that anchor the modern comatose patient's head, as well as concern for occult cervical spine fractures when trauma is a possibility. Serial cooling of each labyrinth, using prolonged ice water irrigation of the external auditory canals, is a powerful vestibular stimulus. If prior maneuvers do not evoke a full range of eye movements, caloric testing is required.[1, 2, 12]

In coma, saccades are absent and the unimpaired vestibular slow-phase response brings the eyes toward the irrigated ear. Vertical movements are much more difficult to elicit by oculovestibular maneuvers, but occasionally useful information can be obtained. In addition to help in localization, vestibular testing has considerable predictive value: 92 percent of comatose patients with absent VORs and 100 percent with absent VORs and pupillary responses will die.[14] (Granted, Hippocrates had concluded sometime before: "It is impossible to remove a strong attack of apoplexy and not easy to remove a weak attack."[15])

Other Ocular Clues

Eye signs other than eye movements are helpful in assessing coma[16] but can only be mentioned briefly here. *Papilledema* indicates intracranial mass effect and a probable neurosurgical emergency. *Retinal emboli* and occlusions suggest cerebral infarction as the cause of coma. Discrete retinal hemorrhages may suggest endocarditis, and mucormycosis should be considered when a cherry-red spot is seen in a comatose diabetic patient. Cerebral apoplexy accompanied by multiple retinal and *subhyaloid hemorrhages* indicates severe intracranial bleeding.[17]

Coma associated with an *afferent pupillary defect* may be the result of trauma, pituitary apoplexy, meningitis, or the effects of a large meningioma of the sphenoidal ridge. Thalamic hemorrhage with secondary ventricular bleeding may produce asymmetric, *small, fixed pupils*. Pretectal lesions produce equal, *midsized pupils* with impaired light reactions in patients who are more likely to be mute than comatose. Coma caused by midbrain lesions is accompanied by slightly larger, fixed pupils. When midbrain compression results from tentorial herniation, the contralateral pupil is initially fixed and small. *Very small (pontine) pupils* (Fig. 198–2) have long been recognized as an unusual and serious sign: In 1820,

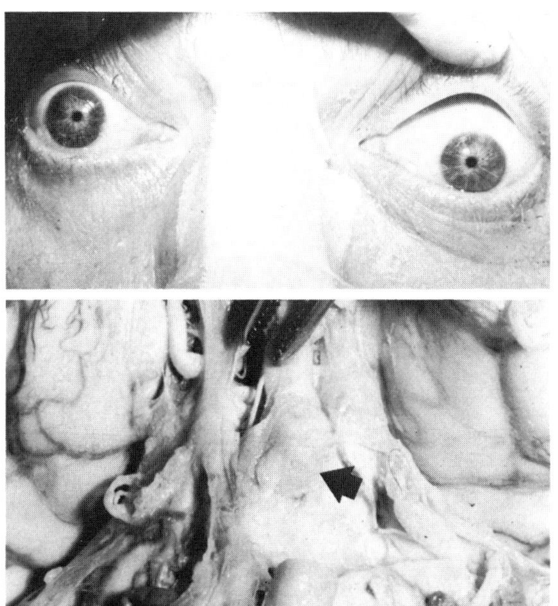

Figure 198–2. Small (reactive) pupils and skew deviation *(top)* were caused by large pontine infarct *(arrow)* associated with complete basilar artery occlusion *(bottom)*.

Cooke, who dated similar observations to Aretaeus, stated that "I never knew a person to recover from apoplexy when the pupil was greatly contracted."[18] By 1888, Gowers was more specific: "Great contraction occurs in and suggests opium poisoning, but it is also present in hemorrhage into the pons Varolii."[19]

Eyelid Abnormalities

Differences in eyelid position and tone should be noted before the eye movements are investigated. A slightly open lid suggests facial paresis (Fig. 198–3), as does a slower speed of lid closure upon releasing elevated lids. Symmetric slow lid closure is common in lighter stages of coma. This slow glide cannot be voluntarily imitated and is useful in eliminating the possibility of hysterical unconsciousness.[1] If the lids remain open when manually elevated, lid closure tone supplied by the facial nerve has been eliminated by bilateral pontine involvement, deepening coma, or death.

Bilateral lid retraction in a mute, unresponsive patient suggests pretectal dysfunction. Occasionally, upper pontine strokes result in persistent, strong levator tone.[20] The lids maintain their normal relationship with the globe during vertical eye movements but never close and predispose to early exposure keratopathy.

Myoclonic jerks are common following acute cerebral ischemia from cardiac arrest. Often, when the face is involved in such arrhythmic myoclonus, the eyelids simultaneously open and even retract for 1 or 2 sec with each myoclonic jerk. Occasionally, the lids participate in the periodic myoclonic jerks common in the late, unresponsive stages of subacute sclerosing panencephalitis (SSPE: slow rubella encephalitis) and Jakob-Creutzfeldt dementia.

Conjugate Eye Movement Limitation

The usual cause of a *cerebral gaze palsy* is a large hypertensive basal ganglia hemorrhage (Table 198–3).[21] Gaze toward the opposite side is paralyzed, and the eyes deviate strongly toward the lesion. As Hughlings Jackson noted in a more colorful era: "It has been likened to the conjugate deviation of the heads of two horses when an omnibus driver drops one of his reins, the other rein being 'in tone.' "[22] Paralysis of the opposite limbs is almost always present. Gaze deviation may be resistant to reversal by caloric testing initially, but after a few days, full horizontal eye movements can be evoked. Rarely, a supratentorial hemorrhage, usually located in the thalamus, produces unexplained contralateral gaze deviations.[23, 24] Saccadic eye movement pathways do not cross until they reach the caudal midbrain, and the reason for *"wrong-way" gaze deviation* remains unknown.

Pontine gaze palsies are less often accompanied by

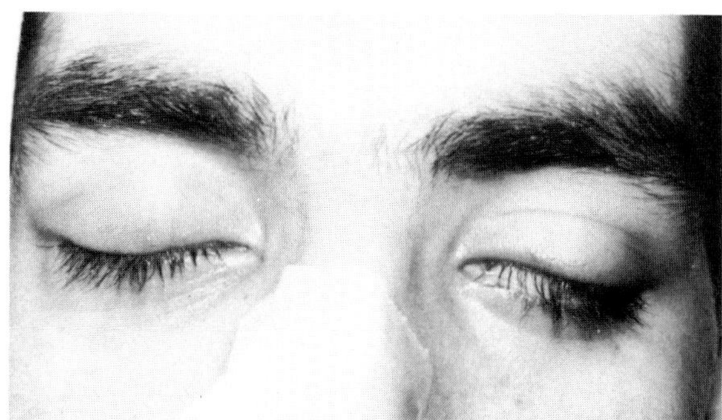

Figure 198–3. Incomplete closure of left eyelid indicates facial weakness.

Table 198–3. EYE MOVEMENT LIMITATION

Conjugate
Horizontal
Eyes forward: usually pontine damage
Eyes deviated to the side: usually cerebral
Vertical
Eyes forward: midbrain or pretectal dysfunction
Forced deviation
Upward: hypoxic encephalopathy likely
Downward: either pretectal or metabolic causes
Disconjugate
Oculomotor palsies
Internuclear ophthalmoplegia: upper stem damage
Skew deviation: posterior fossa dysfunction
Total ophthalmoplegia: midbrain stroke, pituitary apoplexy, meningitis

dramatic gaze deviations. When present, pontine gaze deviation is contralateral to the lesion, resistant to caloric reversal, and may be accompanied by extremity weakness opposite the lesion. (Gaze pathways cross above the pons, motor pathways below.) Pontine damage is usually bilateral in comatose patients with the result that the eyes are straight and do not respond to caloric stimulation.

Acute horizontal deviations without unilateral limb weakness are most often due to acute (contralateral) *cerebellar lesions* (Fig. 198–4)—usually hemorrhages. Hughlings Jackson had observed skew but not gaze deviation with cerebellar hemorrhage.[22] As the cerebellum is less differentiated than other regions of the central nervous system, removal of a damaged portion is much better tolerated. In carefully selected patients with large cerebellar strokes, acute neurosurgical intervention may be life-saving.[25]

Horizontal gaze deviations accompanying a *focal seizure* are usually opposite the seizure focus, but such transient gaze deviations are not good lateralizing signs.[26] Shifting horizontal eye deviations are common in patients in coma of cerebral origin, even in the absence of seizures. A unique "geotropic" horizontal gaze deviation has been noted in *hysteria*: the eyes deviate toward the ground regardless on which side the patient is lying.[27]

Upward eye deviation in coma is usually a sign of hypoxic encephalopathy,[28] but similar deviation occasionally follows lithium intoxication and heat stroke (Fig. 198–5). The common feature of these causes of coma is severe cerebellar damage. As coma lightens and upgaze deviation lessens, downbeat nystagmus often makes an appearance. The most likely explanation for forced upgaze in coma is that vestibulocerebellar damage acts to disinhibit upward gaze.[28, 29]

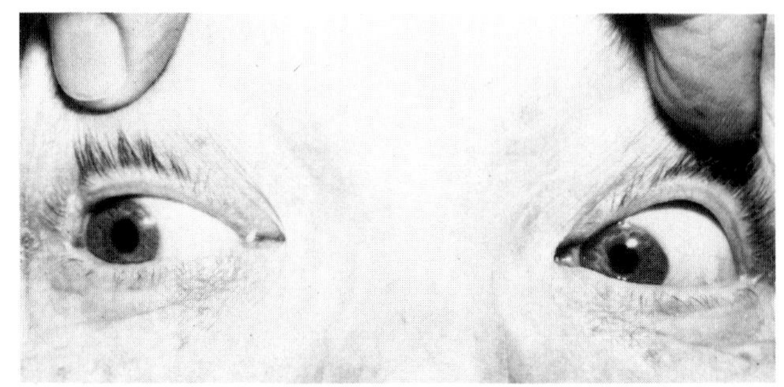

Figure 198–4. Right gaze deviation and mild skew deviation resulting from left cerebellar abscess.

An occasional case of forced upgaze represents an oculogyric crisis associated with a phenothiazine overdose. Upward eye deviation due to midbrain lesions is rare. Downward gaze impairment that could be expected to drive the eyes upward is usually balanced or overridden by upgaze limitation. The rare bilateral midbrain/subthalamic infarcts that do produce isolated downgaze paresis usually spare the reticular core controlling wakefulness. Even when midbrain lesions result from cardiorespiratory arrest,[30] additional cerebellar damage is usually present and may be causative. Brain tumors and other structural lesions do not appear to cause upward eye deviation in coma.

Forced downgaze in coma[31] is both more common and more ambiguous than upgaze deviation. It is seen with severe pretectal involvement in hydrocephalus (Fig. 198–6), thalamic hemorrhage, tentorial herniation,[32] and pineal region tumors.[33] Forced downgaze with esotropia "as if peering at the nose" was noted by Fisher to be a sign of medial thalamic hemorrhage.[23] Overall, however, exotropia is about as common as esotropia with pretectal

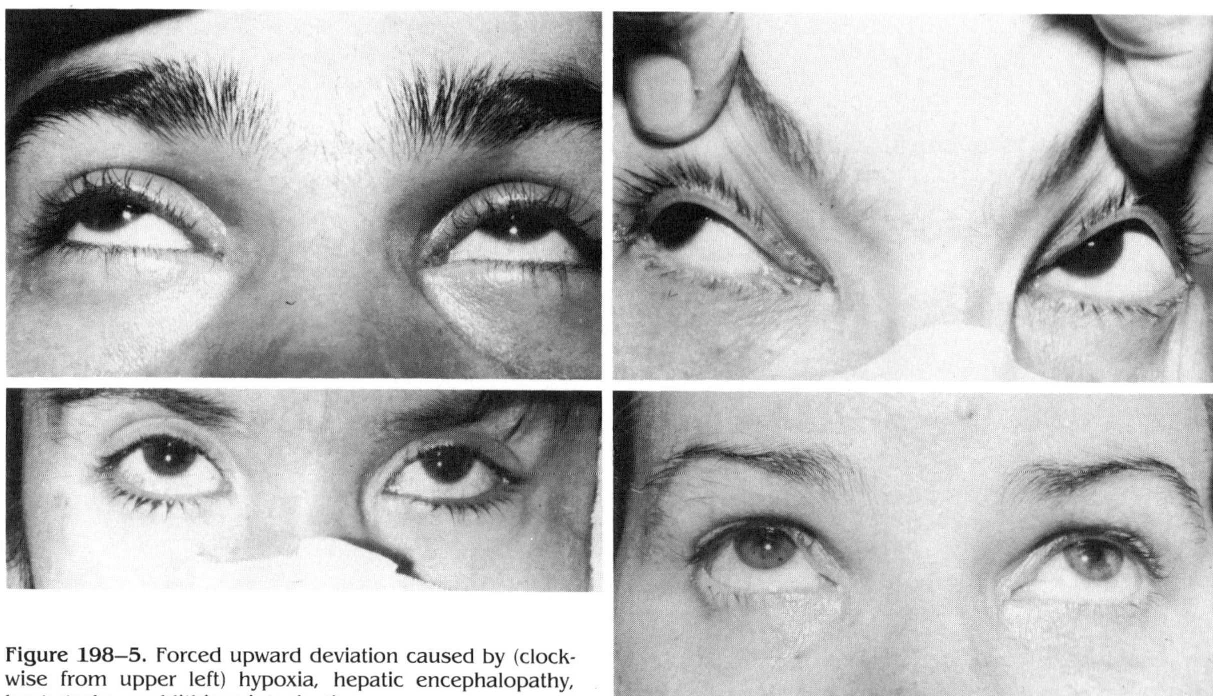

Figure 198–5. Forced upward deviation caused by (clockwise from upper left) hypoxia, hepatic encephalopathy, heat stroke, and lithium intoxication.

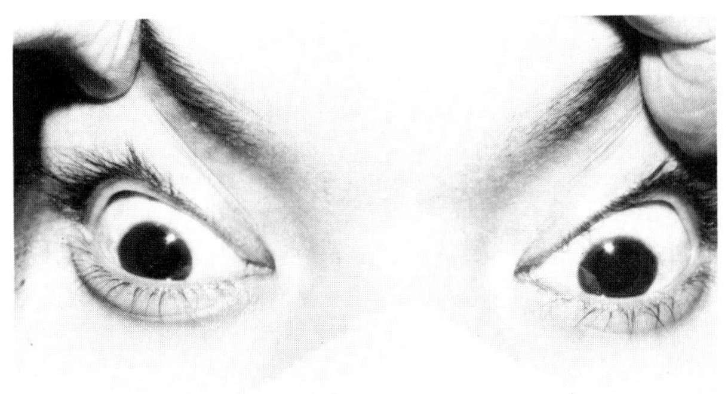

Figure 198–6. Forced downgaze with large, fixed pupils in akinetic, mute patient with cysticercal hydrocephalus.

dysfunction.[33] When normal pupils are associated with downward deviation of the eyes in a comatose patient, the cause is probably medical rather than surgical. Meningitis, subarachnoid hemorrhage, hepatic encephalopathy, and other metabolic abnormalities can cause downward eye deviation.[31] Patients who develop downward deviation during caloric testing may have sedative drug overdose as the cause of coma.[34]

Occasionally, one eyelid of a stuporous or comatose patient remains open and is even retracted to reveal a depressed globe (Fig. 198–7). The explanation for this curious appearance is that the patient has a fascicular third-nerve palsy superimposed on forced downgaze.[35] The combination of one ptotic lid and an opposite *elevated* eye (Fig. 198–8) is most unusual, because this situation requires forced upgaze in association with a third-nerve palsy.

Disconjugate Eye Movement Limitation

Coma blunts the neurologic examination and makes detection of minor ocular motor palsies impossible. Diagnosis of *third-nerve paresis* is aided by pupil and lid abnormalities and is relatively straightforward. Major *sixth-nerve palsies* can be confirmed by observation or caloric testing, but damage to the fourth nerve is rarely discernible in coma. *Internuclear ophthalmoplegia* is diagnosed by medial rectus limitation in the absence of pupillary or other evidence of a third-nerve palsy. However, caution is required concerning the diagnosis of bilateral internuclear ophthalmoplegia by caloric testing. The medial longitudinal fasciculus is sensitive to physiologic interruption by drug overdose[36] or even the deeper stages of coma, and bilateral medial rectus limitations on caloric testing do not necessarily indicate a structural pontine lesion. *Skew deviation*[37] is a supranuclear vertical divergence of the eyes that occurs with lesions throughout the posterior fossa. Vertical dissociation of the eyes must be obvious, persistent, and reasonably concomitant to justify the diagnosis of skew deviation in coma. The diagnosis of alternating skew deviation[38] is difficult in the drowsy, unlikely in the stuporous, and impossible in the comatose.

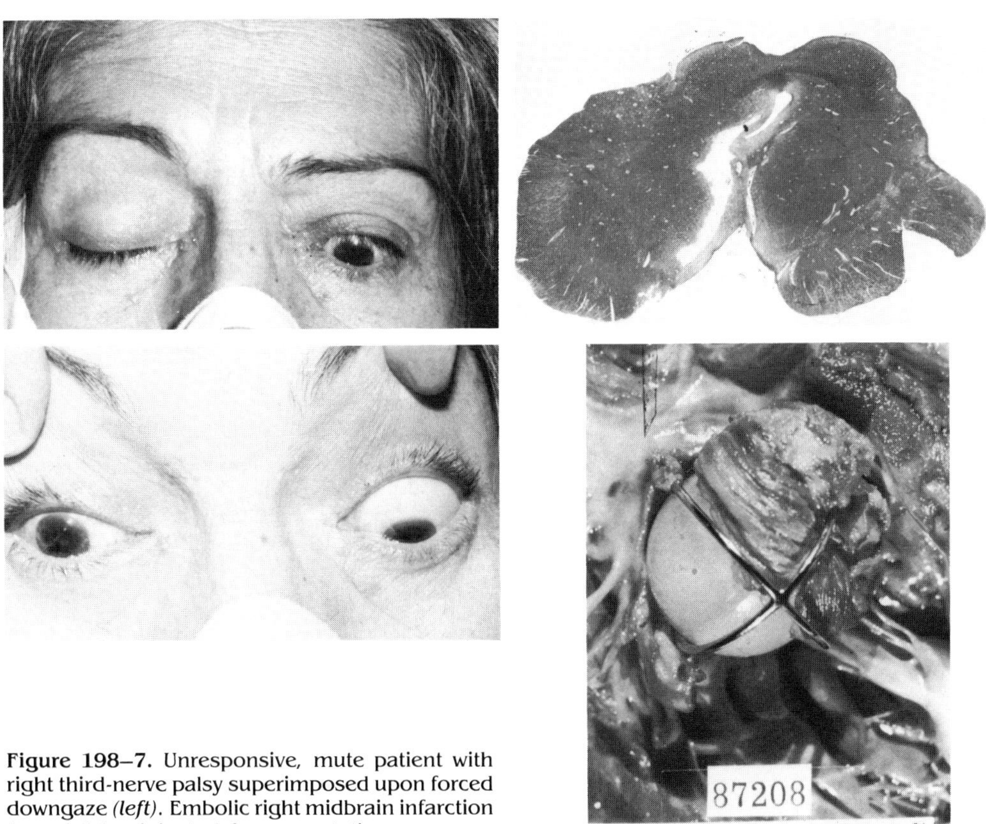

Figure 198–7. Unresponsive, mute patient with right third-nerve palsy superimposed upon forced downgaze *(left)*. Embolic right midbrain infarction *(top right)* originated from vegetations on prosthetic cardiac valve *(bottom right)*.

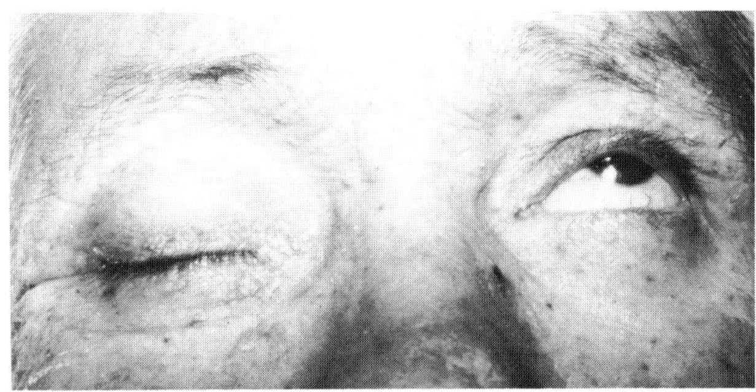

Figure 198–8. Another patient with a right third-nerve palsy caused by embolic (endocarditis) midbrain infarction has additional forced upgaze after cardiac arrest.

Complete Ophthalmoplegia

The usual cause of completely frozen eyes in coma is death. If a patient is stuporous, or at least shows some signs of life, and has fixed globes and pupils, midbrain infarction or hemorrhage is likely.[39] In such cases, bilateral third-nerve palsies combine with involvement of descending horizontal gaze pathways[40] to produce caloric-fast ophthalmoplegia. Within 1 wk, the horizontal gaze pareses remit to allow abduction. Less common but more treatable causes of bilateral ophthalmoplegia in coma include pituitary apoplexy, meningitis, and even sedative/antidepressant/anticonvulsant intoxication.[41]

SPONTANEOUS EYE MOVEMENTS

Horizontal Eye Movements

Roving eye movements are common in stupor and light coma (Table 198–4). Their slow, stately pace defies voluntary imitation and eliminates hysteria as a cause of unconsciousness. Roving movements are only roughly conjugate, and the eyes do not maintain a fixed relationship. Even so, they are often confused with skew deviation, internuclear ophthalmoparesis, or gaze palsies. The major diagnostic value of roving eye movements lies in the demonstration of a relatively full horizontal and vertical range of movements that eliminates a brain stem cause of coma.

Occasionally, roving eye movements are sufficiently regular to classify as *periodic alternating gaze* or *ping-pong gaze*.[42] When the lids are lifted, the eyes appear to be watching a very slow tennis match, moving from side to side in a 4- to 5-sec cycle, with brief pauses at each turnaround. Frequently the eyes move from corner to corner, but a unilateral bias is more common with movement from forward to far lateral gaze and back again. Fisher called these movements ocular agitation or restless eyes.[23] He correctly ascribed them to bilateral cerebral hemisphere damage, with asymmetric movements reflecting a recent insult superimposed on an older injury to the opposite hemisphere.

Nystagmus is rare in coma and tends to be overdiagnosed by inexperienced observers. The coarse, clonic jerks of *seizure nystagmus* are usually easy to identify, but, occasionally, continuous fine beats resembling vestibular nystagmus accompany documented seizure discharges. Most often, seizure nystagmus introduces a fit with accompanying ipsilateral head and eye deviation, followed by rhythmic jerking of the face and extremities on that side, and usually concluding with generalized clonus.[43] Rarely, nystagmus may be the only evidence of status epilepticus that is causing stupor.[44, 45]

Convergence-retraction "nystagmus" is a pretectal sign that may be seen in seemingly unresponsive patients with hydrocephalus or pretectal strokes and tumors.[33] Such patients are usually in a hypokinetic, hypophonic state rather than comatose and may respond if time is taken to allow for their extreme parkinsonian tempo. Saccades, especially upward attempted saccades, are often necessary to elicit convergence-retraction movements in awake individuals; however, stuporous or bradykinetic patients may exhibit continual spontaneous convergence movements.[46]

True repetitive *convergence movements* were seen in a young patient in coma following near-drowning.[47] Every 10 to 20 sec, 2 to 5 sec of marked esotropia and miosis would be superimposed on roving eye movements. Organic convergence spasm[48] is considerably less common than the hysterical variety,[49] but both occur almost exclusively in alert patients. Spasm of the near reflex occurring in a lethargic patient with metabolic encephalopathy showed convergence and miosis that lasted 5 to 20 sec and occurred 10 to 15 times/hr.[50]

Macrosaccadic oscillations typically appear in a patient recovering from the effects of a large hemorrhage in the dorsal cerebellar vermis. As stupor evolves into drowsiness, fixation attempts produce 10-sec crescendo-decrescendo bursts of alternating, wide-amplitude (up to 40 degrees) saccades.[51, 52]

Vertical Eye Movements

Patients with nystagmus are sometimes stuporous or mute but rarely comatose. Nystagmus occurs in patients recovering from sedative or anticonvulsant overdose. Vertical nystagmus is especially common following

Table 198–4. SPONTANEOUS EYE MOVEMENTS

Horizontal
Normal roving movements: stem working
Periodic alternating gaze: cerebral dysfunction
Nystagmus: rare, localizes to posterior fossa
Convergence-retraction "nystagmus": pretectal site
Macrosaccadic oscillations: acute cerebellar lesions
Vertical
Nystagmus
Upbeat: usually structural
Downbeat: often hypoxic
Ocular bobbing
Bobbing veritas: severe pontine damage
Bobbing varietals: less specific
"V"-pattern convergence nystagmus: acute hydrocephalus
Ocular myoclonus (myorhythmia): severe pontine stroke
Opsoclonus: no structural intracranial lesion
Ocular tilt reaction (paroxysmal): upper stem lesion

phencyclidine and lithium intoxications. *Downbeat nystagmus* is seen in stuporous patients recovering from coma associated with forced upgaze. Hypoxic encephalopathy following cardiac arrest is the usual cause.[28]

Upbeat nystagmus persisted as a young patient became stuporous with progressive respiratory failure.[53] An autopsy revealed a single midline area of medullary myelinolysis in the dorsal rostral medulla as the cause of nystagmus. Rarely, upward nystagmus is the only evidence of seizures in a comatose patient. An unresponsive man with a subdural hematoma showed two kinds of nystagmus associated with electroencephalogram documented seizure activity: right gaze deviation and nystagmus were followed by upgaze deviation and nystagmus.[45] A patient in coma from a pontine infarction had vertical/rotatory dissociated nystagmus.[54]

Ocular bobbing is a term coined by Miller Fisher to describe arrhythmic downward conjugate eye movements in three patients in coma from bilateral pontine tegmental strokes.[55] Downward movement, through one-fourth to one-third of the full range, was quicker than the slow return. The rate was highly variable and ranged from 2/min to 12/min. The patients were comatose with paralyzed horizontal eye movements but reactive pupils. A second, more diverse, group of five patients with atypical bobbing was included in the original article. These patients consisted of one with cerebellar hemorrhage, a case of monocular bobbing associated with a sixth-nerve palsy, several patients with preserved horizontal eye movement abilities, bobbing produced by caloric testing, simultaneous phasic pupillary movements, and a patient with locked-in syndrome with large, presumably voluntary, downward movements.

Ocular bobbing is not as common as the extensive literature would suggest, but the well-chosen name, the unexpected sight of these movements issuing from a deeply comatose patient, and curiosity about the mechanism have guaranteed interest. Unilateral bobbing is seen occasionally when the pontine lesion extends into the midbrain to involve one third nerve.[56] Much more common, however, is asymmetric bobbing, the eye with smaller downward excursions usually exhibiting a torsional component (Fig. 198–9).

A series of hyphenated bobbings have been described that threaten the term with homeopathic dilution. In brief, inverse bobbing (ocular dipping) has a slow downward movement and faster return[57]; reverse bobbing is fast upward with a slow return[58]; inverse/reverse bobbing (reverse dipping) is slow upward with a faster return[59]; obverse, converse, and perverse bobbing remain to be described. These adjectival attachments are seen in hypoxic/metabolic encephalopathy. None has proved to be of outstanding clinical utility, and the time has probably arrived for a bobbing moritorium. Clarification of the physiologic basis of spontaneous vertical movements in coma is obviously needed, and the knowledge that electrographic status epilepticus can be associated with a wide range of vertical eye movements in anoxic coma is a step in that direction.[60]

V-pattern convergence nystagmus resembles bobbing but functionally represents convergence nystagmus as-

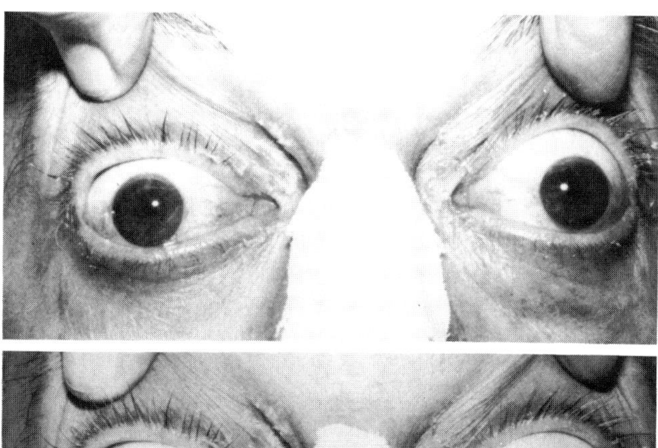

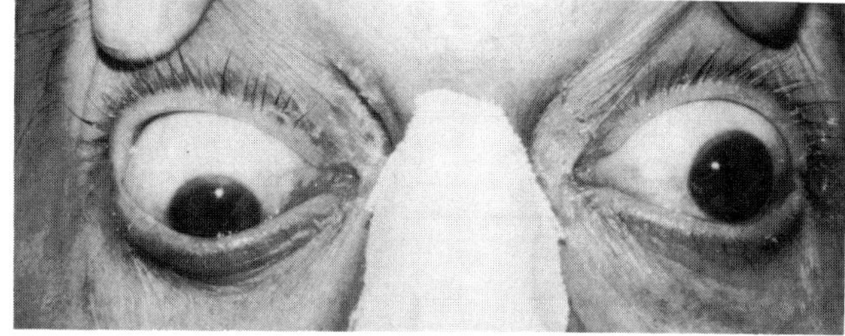

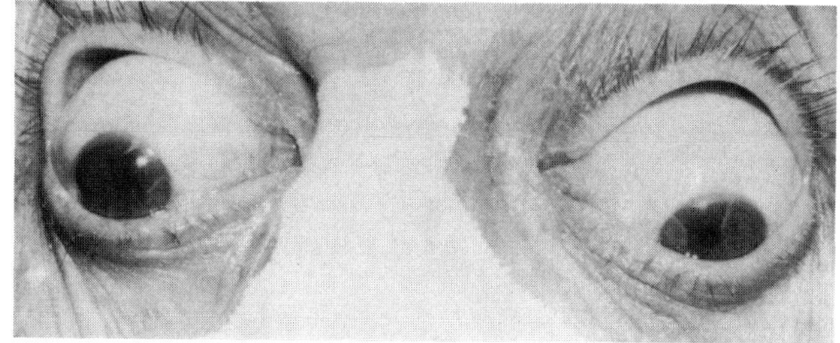

Figure 198–9. Patient with pontine infarction has unusual, asymmetric ocular bobbing. Sometimes one eye bobs lower *(middle)*, and sometimes the other eye does *(bottom)*.

sociated with downward eye deviations.[61] It is a pretectal sign, and the usual cause is obstructive hydrocephalus. In contrast to those with ocular bobbing, these patients usually have 4- to 6-mm fixed pupils and are in a hypokinetic mute state. The distinction is important, because patients with V-pattern convergence nystagmus are usually in need of prompt neurosurgical assistance.[33, 62]

Another vertical eye movement that is frequently confused with bobbing is *ocular myoclonus* (ocular myorhythmia).[63–65] This movement is a part of branchial (segmental) myoclonus, but unlike the usual palatal myoclonus, ocular myoclonus is often present immediately after an acute pontine stroke. The presentation is the same whether the patient is comatose or locked-in. Ocular myoclonus typically evolves in stages over several days. Initially resembling bobbing with irregular downward movements and slower return, the movements became more rhythmic, suggesting downbeat nystagmus, and finally become continuous rhythmic pendular movements oscillating at 2 to 3 cycles/sec.[63] Other elements of branchial myoclonus involving face, palate, tongue, chin, head, and extremities develop months after the stroke, survival permitting.

Opsoclonus is a rare, dramatic, chaotic, continuous discharge of saccades in all directions that may persist in stupor and coma.[66] Infectious or paraneoplastic encephalitis,[67] a hyperosmolar state,[68] and intoxications[69, 70] are the common causes in unconscious patients. Opsoclonus is very rarely associated with an intracranial mass and, in some of those cases, potentiating factors such as hyperosmolality are present.[71]

The intermittent *see-saw eye movements* that have been described in a comatose patient[72] probably represent a variety of the paroxysmal ocular tilt reaction. In this patient with diffuse brain stem trauma, both lids would open and retract, the eyes then vertically dissociated, and binocular cyclotorsion occurred toward the lower eye. These startling events initially occurred once or twice a minute but became nearly continuous midway through a 24-hr period of survival.

The *ocular tilt reaction*, described experimentally before World War I,[73] but not characterized until 1975,[74] consists of head tilt, skew deviation, and ocular cyclotorsion—all toward the same side. The causal lesion presumably interferes with otolith pathways regulating head and eye rolling. Both paroxysmal and fixed varieties of ocular tilt reactions occur, and the lesions producing tilts have been located in the midbrain/subthalamus, labyrinth, and lateral medulla.[75]

Some consider that Charcot's career marked the beginning and end of the "Golden Age" of observational neurology. As we approach the centenary (1993) of Charcot's death, it is striking to note that few of the observations mentioned in this chapter are more than 30 yr old. Miller Fisher, in particular, has contributed to almost every facet of the subject, in what is but one of his clinical enthusiasms. Future bedside observers will have to contend not only with the seductive distractions of modern brain scanning but also with progressive palisading of the bedside with tubes and monitors, as well as iatrogenic obscuration from curare and pentobarbital. Still, there is little doubt that the next edition of this book will forge further into the 19th century with additional important bedside observations concerning eye movements in coma.

REFERENCES

1. Fisher CM: The neurological examination of the comatose patient. Acta Neurol Scand 45 (Suppl 36), 1969.
2. Plum F, Posner JB: The Diagnosis of Stupor and Coma, 3rd ed. Philadelphia, FA Davis, 1980.
3. Teasdale G, Jennett B: Assessment and prognosis of coma after head injury. Acta Neurochir (Wien) 34:45, 1976.
4. Plum F, Posner JB: The Diagnosis of Stupor and Coma, 1st ed. Philadelphia, FA Davis, 1966.
5. Nordgren RE, Markesbery WR, Fukuda K, et al: Seven cases of cerebral medullary disconnexion: The "locked-in" syndrome. Neurology 21:1140, 1971.
6. Keane JR: Locked-in syndrome after head and neck trauma. Neurology 36:80, 1986.
7. Keane JR: Locked-in syndrome due to tentorial herniation. Neurology 35:1647, 1985.
8. Keane JR: Locked-in syndrome with deafness. [Letter] Neurology 35:1395, 1985.
9. Jennett WB, Plum F: The persistent vegetative state: A syndrome in search of a name. Lancet 1:734, 1972.
10. Sacks OW: Awakenings. Garden City, NY, Doubleday, 1974.
11. Samuels MA: A systematic approach to the comatose patient. Emerg Med 22:17, 1990.
12. Berger JR, Daroff RB: Intensive care evaluation of the comatose patient. *In* Green BA, Marshall LF, Gallagher RJ(eds): Intensive Care for Neurological Trauma and Disease. New York, Academic Press, 1982.
13. Leigh RJ, Hanley DF, Nunschauer FE 3rd, et al: Eye movements induced by head rotation in unresponsive patients. Ann Neurol 15:465, 1984.
14. Mueller-Jensen A, Neunzig HP, Emskotter T: Outcome prediction in comatose patients: Significance of reflex eye movement analysis. J Neurol Neurosurg Psychiatry 50:389, 1987.
15. Adams F: The Genuine Works of Hippocrates. New York, William Wood & Co, 1886, p 208.
16. Safran AB: Signes neuro-ophthalmologiques du coma. Schweiz Arch Neurol Neurochir Psychiatr 126:33, 1980.
17. Keane JR: Retinal hemorrhages: Significance in 100 patients with acute encephalopathy of unknown cause. Arch Neurol 36:691, 1979.
18. Cooke J: A Treatise on Nervous Diseases. London, Longman, Hurst, Tees, Orme, Brown, 1920, p 280.
19. Gowers WR: A Manual of Diseases of the Nervous System. Philadelphia, P Blakiston, Son & Co, 1888, p 535.
20. Keane JR: Spastic eyelids: Failure of levator inhibition in unconscious states. Arch Neurol 32:695, 1975.
21. Fisher CM: The pathology and pathogenesis of intracerebral hemorrhage. *In* Fields WS (ed): Pathogenesis and Treatment of Cerebrovascular Disease. Springfield, IL, Charles C Thomas, 1961.
22. Jackson JH: Cerebral hemorrhage and apoplexy. *In* Reynolds JR, Hartshorne H (eds): A System of Medicine, vol 1. Philadelphia, HC Lea's Son & Co, 1880.
23. Fisher CM: Some neuro-ophthalmological observations. J Neurol Neurosurg Psychiatry 30:383, 1967.
24. Keane JR: Contralateral gaze deviation with supratentorial hemorrhage. Arch Neurol 32:119, 1975.
25. Fisher CM, Picard EH, Polak A, et al: Acute hypertensive cerebellar hemorrhage: Diagnosis and surgical treatment. J Nerv Ment Dis 140:38, 1965.
26. Ochs R, Gloor P, Quesney F, et al: Does head-turning during a seizure have lateralizing or localizing significance? Neurology 34:884, 1984.
27. Henry JA, Woodruff GH: A diagnostic sign in states of apparent unconsciousness. Lancet 2:920, 1978.
28. Keane JR: Sustained upgaze in coma. Ann Neurol 9:409, 1981.
29. Nakada T, Kwee IL, Lee H: Sustained upgaze in coma. J Clin Neuro Ophthalmol 4:35, 1984.
30. Jacobs L, Heffner RR, Newman RP: Selective paralysis of downward gaze caused by bilateral lesions of the mesencephalic periaqueductal gray matter. Neurology 35:516, 1985.
31. Keane JR, Rawlinson DG, Lu AT: Sustained downgaze deviation: Two cases without structural pretectal lesions. Neurology 26:594, 1976.
32. Keane JR: Bilateral ocular motor signs after tentorial herniation in 25 patients. Arch Neurol 43:806, 1986.
33. Keane JR: The pretectal syndrome: 206 patients. Neurology 40:684, 1990.
34. Simon RP: Forced downward ocular deviation; occurrence during oculovestibular testing in sedative drug-induced coma. Arch Neurol 35:456, 1978.
35. Collier J: Nuclear ophthalmoplegia, with especial reference to retraction of the lids and ptosis and to lesions of the posterior commissure. Brain 50:488, 1927.
36. Hotson JR, Sachdev HS: Amitriptyline: another cause of internuclear ophthalmoplegia in coma. [Letter] Ann Neurol 12:62, 1982.
37. Keane JR: Ocular skew deviation. Arch Neurol 32:185, 1975.
38. Keane JR: Alternating skew deviation: 47 patients. Neurology 35:725, 1985.
39. Keane JR: Acute bilateral ophthalmoplegia: 60 cases. Neurology 36:279, 1986.
40. Zackon DH, Sharpe JA: Midbrain paresis of horizontal gaze. Ann Neurol 16:495, 1984.
41. Spector RH, Davidoff RA, Schwartzman RJ: Phenytoin-induced ophthalmoplegia. Neurology 26:1031, 1976.
42. Stewart JD, Kirkham TH, Matheison G: Periodic alternating gaze. Neurology 29:222, 1979.
43. Thurston SE, Leigh RJ, Osorio I: Epileptic gaze deviation and nystagmus. Neurology 35:1518, 1985.

44. Kanazawa O, Sengoku A, Kawai I: Oculoclonic status epilepticus. Epilepsia 30:121, 1989.
45. Kaplan PW, Lesser RP: Vertical and horizontal epileptic gaze deviation and nystagmus. Neurology 39:1391, 1989.
46. Segarra JM, Ojeman RJ: Convergence nystagmus. Neurology 11:883, 1961.
47. Keane JR: Convergence spasm. [Letter] Neurology 33:1637, 1983.
48. Keane JR: Neuro-ophthalmologic signs of hysteria. Neurology 32:757, 1982.
49. Dagi KR, Chrousos GA, Cogan DG: Spasm of the near reflex associated with organic disease. Am J Ophthalmol 103:582, 1987.
50. Moster ML, Hoenig EM: Spasm of the near reflex associated with metabolic encephalopathy. [Letter] Neurology 38:150, 1989.
51. Hoyt WF, Daroff RB: Supranuclear disorders of ocular control systems in man: Clinical, anatomical, and physiological correlations. *In* Bach-Y-Rita PB, Collins CC, Hyde JE(eds): The Control of Eye Movements. New York, Academic Press, 1971.
52. Selhorst JB, Stark L, Ochs AL, et al: Disorders in cerebellar ocular motor control. II: Macrosaccadic oscillation: An oculographic, control system and clinico-anatomical analysis. Brain 99:509, 1976.
53. Keane JR, Itabashi HH: Upbeat nystagmus: Clinicopathologic study of two patients. Neurology 37:491, 1987.
54. Nakanishi T, Tommonaga M, Ihar Y, et al: Dissociated nystagmus in a comatose patient. J Neurol 223:303, 1980.
55. Fisher CM: Ocular bobbing. Arch Neurol 11:543, 1964.
56. Susac JO, Hoyt WF, Daroff RB, et al: Clinical spectrum of ocular bobbing. J Neurol Neurosurg Psychiatry 33:771, 1970.
57. Ropper AH: Ocular dipping in anoxic coma. Arch Neurol 38:297, 1981.
58. Dell'Osso LF, Daroff RB, Troost BT: Nystagmus and saccadic intrusions and oscillations. *In* Glaser JS(ed): Neuro-ophthalmology, 2nd ed. Philadelphia, JB Lippincott, 1990.
59. Mehler MF: The clinical spectrum of ocular bobbing and ocular dipping. J Neurol Neurosurg Psychiatry 51:725, 1988.
60. Simon RP, Aminoff MJ: Electrographic status epilepticus in fatal anoxic coma. Ann Neurol 20:351, 1986.
61. Keane JR: Pretectal pseudobobbing. Arch Neurol 42:592, 1985.
62. Keane JR: Death from cysticercosis. West J Med 140:787, 1984.
63. Keane JR: Acute vertical ocular myoclonus. Neurology 36:86, 1986.
64. Stacy CB: Continuous vertical ocular flutter, asynchronous palatal myoclonus, and alpha coma. Neuro-ophthalmology 2:147, 1982.
65. Lawrence WH, Lightfoote WE: Continuous vertical pendular eye movements after brain stem hemorrhage. Neurology 25:896, 1975.
66. Digre KB: Opsoclonus in adults: Report of three cases and review of the literature. Arch Neurol 43:1165, 1986.
67. Anderson NE, Budde-Steffen C, Rosenblum MK, et al: Opsoclonus, myoclonus, ataxia, and encephalopathy in adults with cancer: A distinct paraneoplastic syndrome. Medicine 67:100, 1988.
68. Weissman B, Devereaux M, Chandar K: Opsoclonus and hyperosmolar stupor. [Letter] Neurology 39:1401, 1989.
69. Maccario M, Seelinger D, Snyder R: Thallotoxicosis with coma and abnormal eye movements (opsoclonus): Clinical and EEG correlations. [Abstract] Electroencephalogr Clin Neurophysiol 38:98, 1975.
70. Au WJ, Keltner JL: Opsoclonus with amitriptyline overdose. [Letter] Ann Neurol 6:87, 1979.
71. Keane JR, Devereaux MW: Opsoclonus associated with an intracranial tumor. Arch Ophthalmol 92:443, 1974.
72. Keane JR: Intermittent see-saw eye movements. Arch Neurol 35:173, 1978.
73. Muskens LJJ: An anatomico-physiological study of the posterior longitudinal bundle in its relation to forced movements. Brain 14:352, 1913–1914.
74. Westheimer B, Blair SM: The ocular tilt reaction—A brain stem oculomotor routine. Invest Ophthalmol 14:833, 1975.
75. Brandt T, Dieterich M: Pathological eye-head coordination in roll: Tonic ocular tilt reaction in mesencephalic and medullary lesions. Brain 110:153, 1987.

Chapter 199

Neuroophthalmologic Disease of the Retina

JOSEPH F. RIZZO III

The retina is a unique part of the brain partly because it can be visualized. This attribute permits observation of abnormalities that are associated with loss of vision. Ischemia is the most common mechanism of acute visual dysfunction, and this chapter primarily is devoted to this entity (see also Chap. 210).

CLINICAL MANIFESTATIONS OF RETINAL DISEASE

Optic nerve damage causes stereotypic patterns of visual loss. Vision is affected unilaterally, with a decline in central acuity, dyschromatopsia, and an afferent pupillary defect is present in most instances. Similarly, a lesion of the macula may present with these features. It can be difficult to ascertain the location of the lesion in some cases, but a few useful clinical guidelines make the task easier (Table 199–1). For instance, disease of the macula may result in substantial loss of central acuity but relatively well-preserved color vision. On the other hand, color vision is usually more affected by a lesion of the optic nerve. An afferent pupillary defect is usually present with disease of the optic nerve, and the likelihood of its presence with disease of the retina depends on the location and extent of damage. The distribution of visual field loss is another important parameter in identifying the location of the lesion (Fig. 199–1; see also Table 199–1). Optic nerve lesions often result in a nasal step defect or central, paracentral, or Bjerrum's scotoma. Retinal disease may cause diffuse visual loss if the central retinal artery is occluded, or visual loss may

Table 199–1. COMPARISON OF THE CLINICAL FEATURES OF CENTRAL RETINAL AND OPTIC NERVE DISEASE

	Central Retina	Optic Nerve
Central acuity	+ + + + +	+ + +
Color vision	+ +	+ + + + +
Afferent pupillary defect	+	+ + + + +
Visual fields defects	Central Midperipheral Ring scotomata Cross vertical meridian Constricted	Central/paracentral Arcuate ("Bjerrum") Altitudinal Nasal step Temporal wedge
Funduscopy	Pigmentary change Macular edema Narrowed arterioles Pale nerve (+/−) Normal	Swollen, pale, or normal nerve

This table is a summary of the most common features of disease of the central retina (macula) and optic nerve. These characteristics are not absolute and are useful only when considered as trends. The plus sign suggests the relative degree to which the clinical feature usually is present. Visual field defects resulting from disease limited to the macula would be present only in the central region.

be restricted to one sector if a branch artery is involved. Degenerative disease of the retina frequently causes midperipheral defects of the visual field that extend across the vertical meridian.

Ophthalmoscopy often discloses which of the neural structures are affected. Clinically observable abnormalities of either the retina or the retinal pigment epithelium are usually present with retinal diseases. Significant visual loss without funduscopic abnormalities occurs rarely. These cases can be vexing, and electrophysiologic tests can assist in establishing a diagnosis.

ISCHEMIA OF THE RETINA

Transient Retinal Ischemia

HISTORICAL PERSPECTIVE

A Conversation With C. Miller Fisher

"Isn't it funny that I went blind in the wrong eye!"

Dr. Miller Fisher, a compulsive note taker, recorded this comment by a patient who had experienced visual problems in the weeks before a stroke that rendered him paralyzed on the left side. "I'm paralyzed on the left side and it was my right eye that went blind," the bewildered patient remarked.

This comment did not have special meaning at the time that it was recorded. The then contemporary clinical wisdom recognized the association of internal carotid occlusion with hemiplegia and *permanent* blindness in the *opposite* eye (which, as was later learned, is an exceptionally rare coincidence). Nonetheless, the patient's message was logged.

One week later, another hemiplegic patient told me an almost identical story. This patient frequented a local tavern and had a tendency to drink more than was necessary. One night he told his friends that he had just lost vision in one eye. His friends reassured him that "it will be all right" as soon as he sobered up, and they were indeed correct. In a short time his vision returned to normal. The following week he suffered a stroke, and his hemiplegia, too, was on the "wrong side."

The first of these two patients died shortly thereafter from a carcinoma. I was away for the weekend and returned Sunday evening to learn of his death. I was told that the family of the patient requested an autopsy but they were told that an autopsy was not necessary, I suppose because it was Sunday. Although it was somewhat against my sensitivities, I called the widow to see if she would permit a postmortem examination at the funeral parlor, and she agreed. Remarkably, the right internal carotid artery was occluded by an atheroma.

These vignettes formed the basis for a revolutionary concept in neurology—transient visual loss could be a premonitory sign of impending stroke secondary to ipsilateral carotid atheromatous disease. Thus, a revised mind-set emerged, and new studies of stroke patients were undertaken.

I then surveyed old stroke patients at Queen Mary Veterans Hospital and St. Anne's Hospital in Montreal to determine the frequency of premonitory symptoms. I went to St. Anne's on Saturday and Sunday when families were visiting. It was amazing how often transient warning symptoms were reported.

In 1948, there was no treatment for stroke, and accurate diagnosis was not thought to be important. Patients with strokes were generally not admitted to the hospital but were nursed at home. Dr. Miller Fisher hoped that the prodromal symptoms that seemed to be so common might provide an opportunity to intervene before a permanent deficit occurred.

A greater appreciation of the incidence and severity of carotid artery disease was needed. The significant contributions of Moniz and colleagues, who introduced carotid angiography around 1937 and also described the first case of occlusion of the cervical portion of the internal carotid artery, added greatly to the understanding of the relationship of carotid artery disease and stroke.[1] Miller Fisher routinely began to remove carotid arteries from the neck at autopsy, as had been insightfully suggested four decades earlier by Chiari[2] and later by Hunt.[3] Within a period of months, Miller Fisher determined that carotid atheromatous disease was indeed common. Recognition that a diseased carotid artery could be a source for stroke resolved a then mysterious observation: Pathologic examinations of the middle cerebral arteries showed normal findings in patients who had suffered a stroke in the distribution of that artery, and normal vessels were also found in the other locations that were conventionally studied, such as the pulmonary veins, left auricle, left ventricle, and ascending aorta.

These observations, more fully expanded in Miller

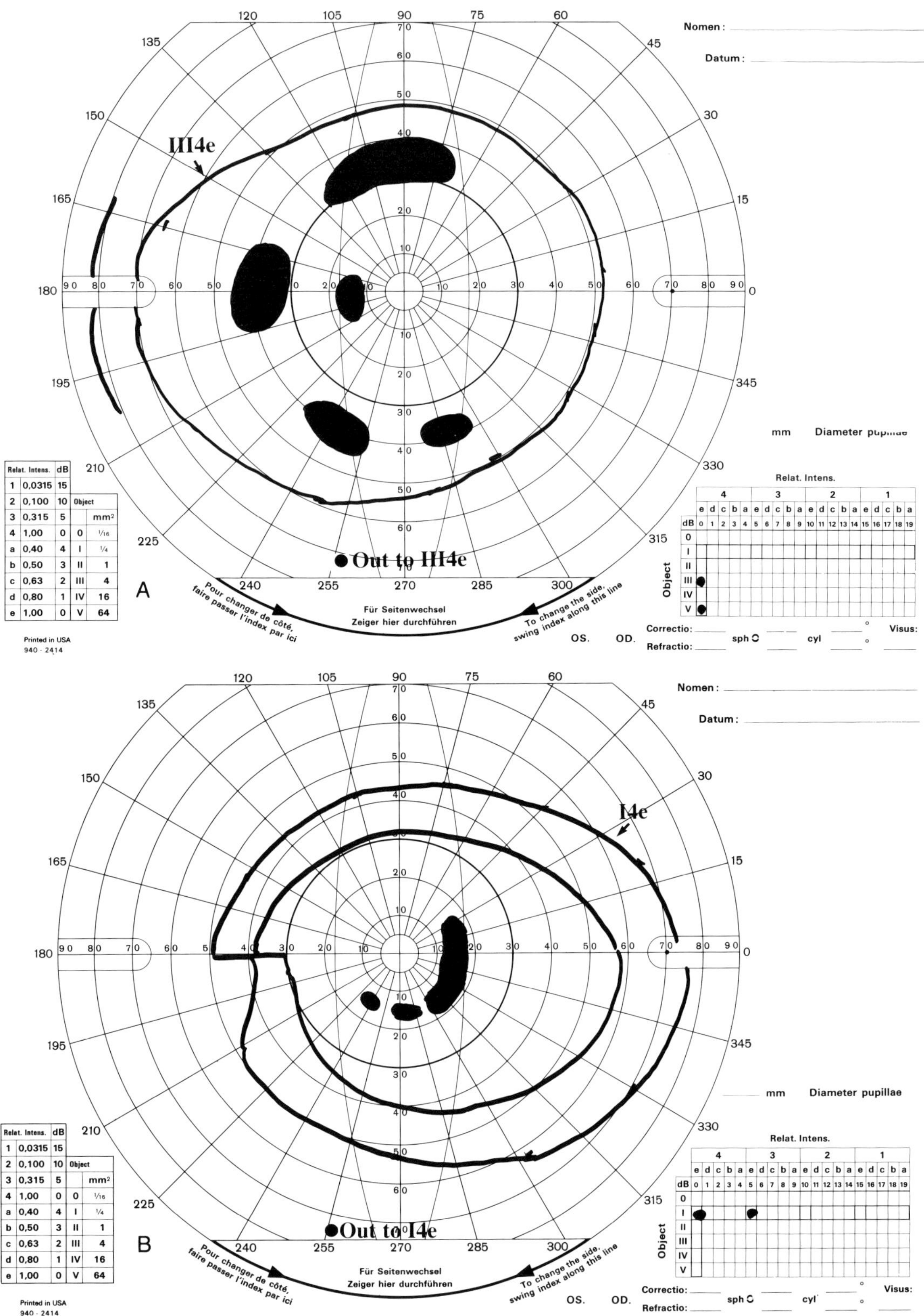

Figure 199–1. Common patterns of visual field defects associated with disease of the retina *(A)* and optic nerve *(B)*. *A,* Degenerative retinal disease often produces midperipheral scotomata that cross the vertical meridian. This field also shows generalized constriction. *B,* Visual field defects that respect the horizontal meridian are characteristic of optic nerve disease. The nasal step shown here has this characteristic. This field also shows nerve fiber bundle defects that are manifested by arcuate (Bjerrum's) scotomata and elongation of the blind spot (see also Table 199–1).

Fisher's landmark report in 1951,[4] led to the understanding that premonitory neurologic symptoms, most notably visual loss, were commonly associated with carotid atheromatous disease. Although transient unilateral blindness had been mentioned once previously in connection with carotid artery disease, the patient was "on the verge of fainting"[5] and the significance of the change in vision in that case is not ascertainable. Others had remarked on the phenomenon of transient visual loss, but it was the cogent work of Miller Fisher that has endured.

> *At lunch a vascular surgeon was recounting a new surgical approach to remove atheroma from iliac arteries. His discussion prompted suggestions that carotid plaque, being highly localized, would be well-suited for surgical removal.*

Therein the seed had been planted for a period of nearly unbridled optimism for surgical correction of carotid atherosclerotic disease. Despite decades of effort, the value of surgery or almost any other means of therapeutic intervention for patients with atherosclerotic cerebrovascular disease is unproved and highly controversial.

With "patience for patients," sagacious attention to detail and cunning, Miller Fisher achieved his legacy.[6–11] Working without a large budget or advanced technologies, he made profound contributions to the field of medicine. One lesson to be learned, among others, is the immense value of listening to patients and clinging to the transactions: "Experience is not experience unless it is retrievable," he is fond of commenting.

CLINICAL COMMENTS

Ischemia is the reduction in delivery of oxygen and other nutrients to tissues sufficient to cause metabolic compromise of cells. A decrease in either perfusion or oxygen-carrying capacity of the blood may be responsible for injury. The functional deficit may be temporary or permanent, depending on the degree of damage. Ischemia of the retina is one of the most common neuroophthalmologic disorders that prompts patients to seek the help of an ophthalmologist.

Fortunately, most instances of retinal ischemia are transient, and visual dysfunction is short-lived. The most common forms of transient visual loss are related either to migraine or to atherosclerotic carotid artery disease, and both have characteristic symptoms. Patients with migraine almost always report the presence of positive visual phenomena. The "subjective visual sensations" accompanying migraine were thoughtfully reviewed as long ago as 1895 by Gowers,[12] who explained that

> the migrainous sensation is deliberate, slow in evolution, occupying more minutes than seconds . . . yet the sensation, simple in character, is elaborate in form, the simple elements, developed in the most complex combinations, give rise to spectra that are extremely curious, and will one day, I doubt not, be most instructive.

Gowers's descriptions have withstood the test of time, but curiosity about the nature of the visual phenomena still exists. The physiologic and anatomic bases for even the routine symptoms have not been fully explained, but progress has been made in recent years.[13]

Positive phenomena, such as flashing lights or perception of movement, often occur with migraine. Headaches may or may not accompany the visual symptoms. The visual hallucinations often appear zigzag or angled. The term *fortification spectra* is commonly used to describe this feature, an analogy based on the architectural design historically used for fortresses. The images are usually arched and peripheral in location and tend to move slowly across the visual field. Flashing lights with or without color are commonly reported.

Visual symptoms associated with migraine commonly last longer than 25 min and as long as 1 hr or more.[14–16] Migraines may begin late in life or may recur after an absence of decades.[17] Rarely, classic visual symptoms of migraine may occur in patients with an arteriovenous malformation of the occipital lobe.[18–20]

In distinction, visual disturbances associated with atherosclerotic cerebrovascular disease usually appear as dark or gray. A descending shade or a veil may appear. Visual loss lasts for minutes (usually 10 to 15 min) and is not associated with pain. Vision usually returns to normal. It is often difficult, even for intelligent and aware patients, to distinguish unilateral from bilateral transient visual loss. *Transient monocular blindness* (TMB) and *amaurosis fugax* (fleeting blindness) are not synonymous; the former term more precisely defines the visual loss as being restricted to one eye.[21] Visual loss in migraine typically persists longer than that of atherosclerotic TMB. Temporal parameters, however, do not reliably distinguish the two conditions.[22]

Atherosclerotic stenosis may involve the internal and external circulations to the eye, resulting in a more pervasive circulatory disorder known as the ischemic ocular syndrome (see Ischemic Ocular Syndrome, later). Symptoms are often insidious, and visual loss may last only seconds. Visual loss may be precipitated by a change in posture or entry into an area of bright light.[38–44] The latter symptom may be analogous to a macular photostress test; delayed visual recovery may be caused by impaired regeneration of photopigment. Rarely the ischemic ocular syndrome may occur secondary to carotid artery dissection[45] or arteritis.

The causes of transient visual loss are numerous and varied (Table 199–2).[46] The arteritic form of ischemic optic neuropathy may occasionally present with premonitory episodes of transient visual loss.[47] Because arteritis can cause rapid and devastating visual loss, sedimentation rate should be determined in all cases of transient visual loss in patients over 55 yr of age.

CLINICAL FEATURES

Ophthalmoscopy during a period of transient visual loss was first reported around 1850, three decades after von Helmholtz (and, independently, Babbage) built the first ophthalmoscopes.[48] By 1959, 35 such observations had been reported.[49] The retina usually appears normal during spells of TMB. Several abnormalities have been described, however, including "boxcaring" (segmenta-

Table 199–2. CONDITIONS ASSOCIATED WITH TRANSIENT VISUAL LOSS

I. Cardiovascular
- Embolic
  - Arising from carotid artery, arch of aorta, cardiac valves or intracardiac (secondary to dyskinetic wall segments)
  - Paradoxical (passes through a cardial septal defect)
  - Carcinomatous
  - Disseminated atheroembolism[23]
- Stenotic vascular disease
  - Carotid or vertebral artery atherosclerotic disease
  - Ophthalmic artery disease (fibromuscular dysplasia)
  - Carotid artery dissection[24]
  - Carotid occlusive disease after irradiation[25]
- Cardiac
  - Mitral valve prolapse
  - Atrial myxoma
  - Marantic endocarditis
  - Arrhythmia
  - Dyskinetic wall segment
- Vasculitic
  - Temporal arteritis
  - Systemic lupus erythematosus

II. Hematologic
- Antiphospholipid antibody syndrome[26, 27]
- Polycythemia vera/thrombocytopenia
- Hypercoagulable states
  - Waldenstrom's macroglobulinemia
  - Antithrombin 3 deficiency
  - Protein S deficiency[28]
  - Protein C deficiency[29]
- Anemia

III. Local Orbital or Ocular Disease
- Angle-closure glaucoma
- Disc edema/papilledema[30]
- Optic nerve drusen and other disc anomalies
- Optic nerve sheath meningiomas[31–34]
- Orbital tumor adjacent to optic nerve
- Optic neuropathy associated with Graves' disease
- Photostress with maculopathy
- Pseudophakia
- Paraneoplastic photoreceptor retinopathy
- Ischemic ocular syndrome

IV. Miscellaneous
- Migraine: retinal, cortical
- Uthoff's symptom
- Hysteria/malingering
- Quinine, quinidine
- After cerebral angiography[35]
- Ornithine transcarbamoylase deficiency[36]
- Spontaneous anterior chamber microhyphema[37]
- Idiopathic

tion of the blood column that results from stasis) or engorgement of veins, reduced caliber of retinal arteries, white vessels, and swelling of the retina. A retinal embolus can be observed in some cases.[49] Some emboli lodge behind the optic nerve head and are not visible, and others enter the retinal circulation, fragment, and pass distally. Transient visual obscurations, which are more brief than spells of TMB and last only seconds, may be caused by anomalous optic nerves (e.g., optic nerve head drusen) or any situation marked by swelling of the optic nerve head.

TMB usually occurs in isolation. The simultaneous occurrence of TMB and a transient ischemic attack of the cerebral hemisphere is rare.[50]

MANAGEMENT

Patients typically present after one or more episodes of TMB, and the retina appears normal. Many disorders can cause TMB, and clinicians must have a strategy for approaching the diagnosis. Primary consideration must be given to those disorders with greatest potential for serious consequence. At the same time, clinicians should remember that common disorders occur most frequently. If a diagnosis is not evident after initial consideration, the less common causes should be reviewed, especially in patients younger than 40 yr.[51] Despite all efforts, a cause cannot be identified in many cases of TMB.[52, 53]

Most patients conform to one of two categories: (1) those who are young and otherwise healthy and (2) those who are either older than 55 yr or likely to have atherosclerosis (Fig. 199–2).[51, 54–57] Younger patients often have a history diagnostic of migraine or at least suggestive of it. Patients presumed to have migraine should not undergo invasive tests because migrainous visual loss is almost always benign.[55] *Migraine as a cause of permanent visual loss or neurologic dysfunction, the so-called complicated migraine, should be a diagnosis of exclusion.*[58–64]

Modification of dietary intake can ameliorate a patient's symptoms. Ingestion of red wine, tea, coffee, cheese, liver, and nuts, to name a few, can incite a migraine. Therapy is not necessary if transient disturbances of vision are the only symptoms or if headaches are relatively mild and infrequent. It is prudent to advise patients with frequent or severe headaches to stop smoking, especially female patients who are taking birth control pills, because these risk factors increase the risk of stroke. A comprehensive review of migraine is presented elsewhere (see Chap. 213).

Patients who have migraine and a history of seizures, cranial bruit, persistent visual field defect, or repetitive and stereotyped symptoms should be assessed more thoroughly. These patients occasionally harbor an arteriovenous malformation, and a magnetic resonance scan of the brain should be obtained.[18, 65–70] New-onset positive visual phenomena in an older patient may be a manifestation of ongoing ischemia of the occipital lobe(s).

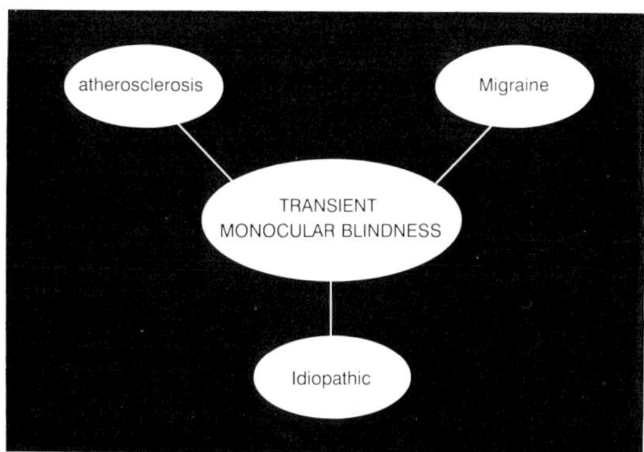

Figure 199–2. Representation of the most common causes of transient monocular blindness. (See Table 199–2 for a comprehensive list of causes of transient monocular blindness.)

Management of patients with TMB and atherosclerosis is more involved because of the higher risk of stroke.[51, 54, 71–83] Noninvasive evaluation of the carotid artery and the heart is useful in patients older than 40 yr. Noninvasive testing of the carotid arteries primarily provides information on the degree of stenosis. Ulceration of the carotid artery is much more difficult to detect noninvasively.[84, 85] The degree to which nonstenotic ulceration increases the risk of stroke is not settled.[86–89] Angiography remains the gold standard for detection of carotid atherosclerotic disease (Fig. 199–3).[51, 90]

Noninvasive study of the heart can detect abnormal valves, dyskinetic wall segments, and arrhythmias, all of which predispose to the formation of emboli. A Holter monitor is the preferred method to screen for intermittent cardiac arrhythmias. Anticoagulation may significantly reduce the risk of stroke in patients with atrial fibrillation.[86, 91–95]

Controversy exists about what degree of carotid artery stenosis is hemodynamically significant. Stenosis of 90 percent or greater, which corresponds to a 1-mm or less residual lumen, is accepted as being hemodynamically significant. Patients with such high-grade stenosis have an increased risk of hemispheric stroke, and the potential value of carotid endarterectomy is easier to appreciate in these cases. Surgery is not recommended for ulcerative disease of the carotid artery if hemodynamically significant stenosis is not also present.[87] Surgery is also not indicated for asymptomatic patients.

Patients who experience TMB and who have significant atherosclerotic disease of the carotid artery are at increased risk for

1. An episode of visual loss that is permanent
2. Cerebral stroke
3. Early mortality

The risk of permanent visual loss after an episode of transient visual loss is probably in the range of 1 percent/yr. The risk of cerebral stroke after an episode of transient cerebral ischemia is approximately 2 to 3 percent/yr. The risk of early mortality is three to five times greater than for age-matched controls, and coronary ischemia is the most common cause of early death of patients who have significant atherosclerosis.[51, 73–76, 78, 96–98] Furthermore, the presence of visible retinal emboli is a particularly unfavorable prognostic sign of early mortality.[99–101]

Carotid endarterectomy is known to reduce the risk of cerebral infarction after episodes of transient *cerebral* ischemia,[87, 96] but it has yet to be determined whether it reduces the risk of cerebral stroke after TMB. Furthermore, carotid endarterectomy does not influence the major cause of early death in older patients with TMB—myocardial infarction.[76, 98] Therefore, the value of carotid endarterectomy is to improve the quality of life by reducing the risk of stroke.[51, 71, 96, 102–109] Because restoration of carotid flow does not improve a persistent neurologic deficit, carotid endarterectomy is a prophylactic operation.[96]

Whatever the long-term benefits of carotid surgery, they must be compared with the combined risks of surgery and carotid angiography, which is a necessary prerequisite for surgery. The figures for morbidity and mortality associated with carotid endarterectomy vary greatly.[96, 102, 110, 111] Therefore, it is important to know the performance record of your hospital and surgical team.

Recommendations for carotid endarterectomy must be individualized. Guidelines have been proposed to help in the decision-making process. For instance, carotid endarterectomy should be considered for patients with TMB only if the surgical complication rate is 2 percent or less, assuming the patient does not have unusually high-risk factors.[102] For patients with cerebral transient ischemic attacks, a complication rate of 3 percent or less is acceptable, given the slightly higher risk of stroke in these patients.[102, 112]

It is prudent to have all patients with the atherosclerotic form of TMB evaluated by an internist.[51, 113] If hemodynamically significant disease of the carotid artery

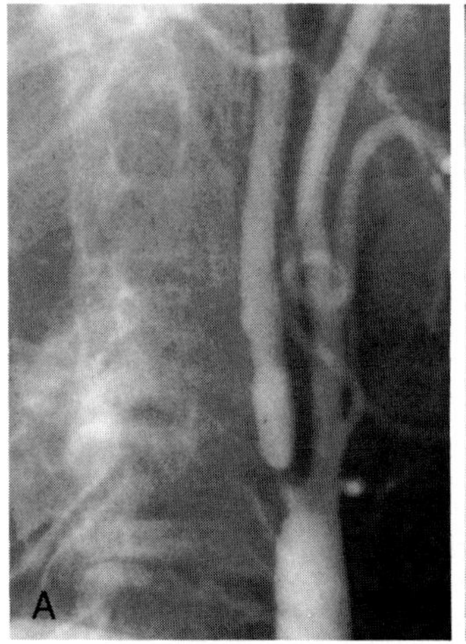

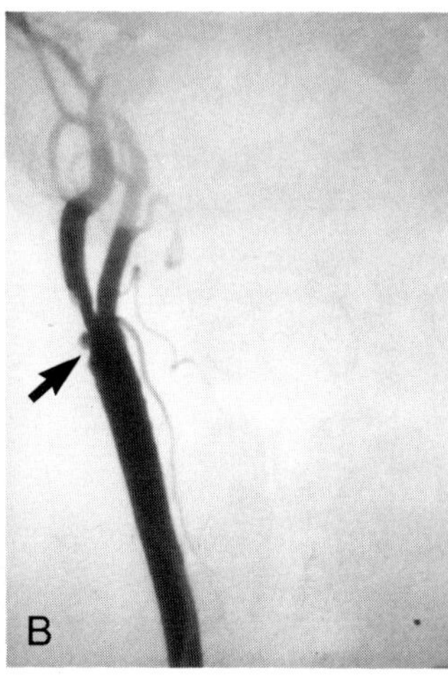

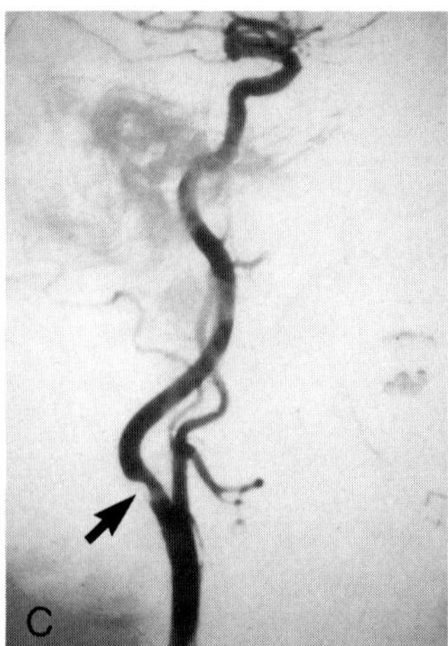

Figure 199–3. Carotid artery angiograms showing classic features of atherosclerotic disease. *A,* Lumen of the internal carotid artery is markedly narrowed. *B,* An area of ulceration *(large arrow)* can be identified by the concave pooling of the angiographic dye. *C,* An atherosclerotic plaque *(small arrow)* protrudes into the lumen of the artery.

is not demonstrated by noninvasive testing or if a patient is a poor surgical candidate or is unwilling to risk surgery, medical therapy with aspirin is thought to be beneficial.[114, 115] Generally, 65 mg/day of aspirin is recommended. Modification of risk factors (e.g., decreasing serum cholesterol level, controlling systemic hypertension) is a proven method of reducing the likelihood of myocardial infarction[116–119] and might also be effective in reducing the risk of stroke.

Infarction of the Retina

The central retinal artery arises from the ophthalmic artery and supplies blood to the inner two-thirds of the retina. Visual loss consequent to occlusion of the central retinal artery was first reported by von Graefe in 1859.[120] The duration of ischemia that can be tolerated depends on the severity of the insult. Retinal circulatory arrest of less than 96 min does not impair retinal function in monkeys.[121–123] A roughly similar time scale is considered applicable for humans even though some patients have demonstrated visual recovery after longer intervals, presumably because ischemia was less severe in those cases.[124, 125]

An embolus is probably the cause of most cases of occlusion of the central retinal artery. Emboli may not be visible if they lodge proximal to the lamina cribrosa or if they enter the retina proper, fragment, and then pass distally. Arteritis, secondary to temporal arteritis or other connective tissue diseases, is another important cause of central retinal artery occlusion (CRAO).

CRAO in children and young adults is rarely the result of embolization.[126] Important considerations in these patients include hemodynamic abnormalities (hemoglobulinopathies and hypercoagulable states, including the presence of antiphospholipid antibodies and use of birth control pills) and vasculitis (especially systemic lupus erythematosus).[127] A nonexhaustive list of infrequent causes includes Behçet's disease, syphilis, Takayasu's disease (usually in Japanese patients), homocystinuria,[128] Fabry's disease,[129] atrial myxoma,[130–133] fibromuscular dysplasia involving the ophthalmic artery, intravenous drug use, and cervical trauma with secondary carotid artery dissection.[24] Ultimately, migraine is often thought to be the culprit, although this diagnosis must be one of exclusion.

CLINICAL MANIFESTATIONS

Patients with CRAO usually experience a sudden profound loss of vision, although premonitory fluctuations in vision may occur. The retina becomes diffusely infarcted but swelling may be visible only within the posterior pole, where the nerve fiber layer is thickest. A cherry-red spot may be present in the macula (Fig. 199–4*A*). This spot develops because the fovea retains its blood supply via the choroidal circulation while the surrounding retina appears milky white when infarcted. Results of a funduscopic examination may be normal during the first 12 hr or so of ischemia.[124–126, 134–138] Less widespread infarction occurs if a branch artery is obstructed. Ischemia may be very localized and appear as a cotton-wool spot, which represents a microinfarction of the nerve fiber layer (Fig. 199–4*B*).

Occlusion may also occur more proximally at the level of the ophthalmic artery. In this situation, compromise of both retinal and choroidal circulations occurs, and the latter can disrupt the blood supply to the optic nerve. Temporal arteritis must be ruled out in patients older than 55 yr. It has been suggested that no light perception vision in cases of CRAO denotes coexistent impairment of the choroidal circulation.[135]

Emboli may be visible in the fundus. They are most commonly observed near the entrance of the retinal arteries into the fundus or at branch points along an artery. Emboli that are too large to pass into the retina may remain lodged in a retrolaminar location, invisible to the examiner. Emboli may remain visible at a particular location for years; others presumably break into smaller pieces and pass into a more peripheral location.

Many types of emboli have been identified (Table 199–3). The appearance of an embolus can sometimes provide a clue of its makeup and origin. For instance, a Hollenhorst's (cholesterol-laden) plaque is refractile and yellowish and usually arises from the carotid arteries

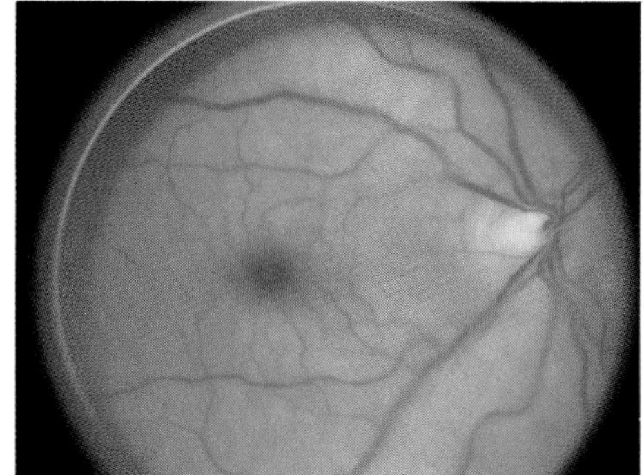

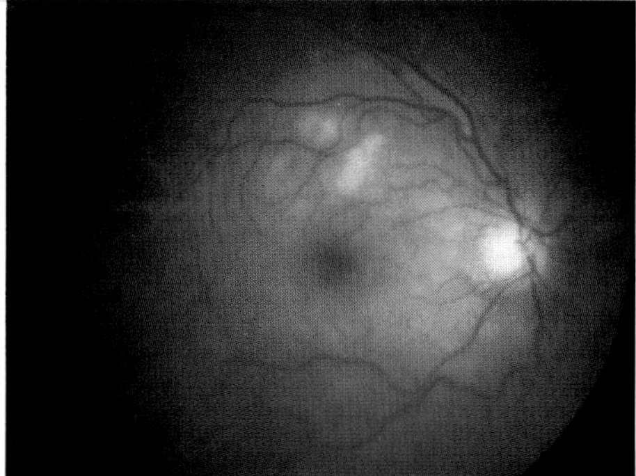

Figure 199–4. *A,* Cherry-red spot secondary to central retinal artery occlusion. The fovea remains red because its blood supply comes from the unaffected choroidal circulation. The retina surrounding the fovea swells in response to ischemia and appears white. Note that the caliber of the retinal arteries does not seem abnormal. *B,* Multiple cotton-wool spots. The retinal ischemia is less severe and has resulted in localized infarctions. Cotton-wool spots represent microinfarctions of the nerve fiber layer of the retina.

Table 199–3. TYPES OF RETINAL ARTERIAL EMBOLI

I. Endogenous	
Amniotic fluid	Bacteria
Cholesterol	Calcium
Fat	Parasites
Platelet-fibrin	Tumor
II. Exogenous	
Air	Cornstarch
Collagen	Oil
Talc	Particle embolization for cerebral vascular abnormalities

(Fig. 199–5). Emboli that appear dusky gray might represent a clump of platelets and fibrin. Emboli from the carotid arteries or cardiac valves may contain calcium and appear white. It is difficult, however, to ascertain the origin or composition of an embolus simply by visual inspection.

With severe compromise of the retinal circulation, groups of red blood cells can be observed to move to and fro within an artery. Swelling of the retina subsides after a period of days or weeks. At that time, the retinal arteries may appear normal or only slightly constricted and the diagnosis of prior CRAO may be less obvious. Rubeosis of the iris and neovascular glaucoma subsequently develop in less than 5 percent of patients. Rarely, artery to artery collaterals within the retina develop after CRAO, or simultaneous occlusion of the central retinal artery and vein may occur.[139] Optic atrophy usually becomes evident after CRAO. An electroretinogram (ERG), which is not necessary for the evaluation of CRAO, would demonstrate preservation of the a-wave and a loss of the b-wave, reflecting preservation of function of the outer retina which is supplied by the choroidal circulation.

MANAGEMENT

A recent CRAO is an emergency. Any patient who presents within 24 hr of onset should receive aggressive therapy designed to improve delivery of oxygen to the retina. The level of vision at presentation and the duration of visual loss generally correlate with visual prognosis. Few patients spontaneously recover much vision, with or without therapy.

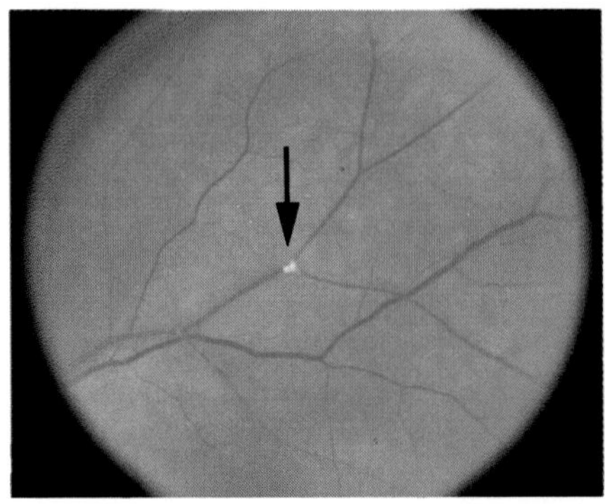

Figure 199–5. Cholesterol embolus *(arrow),* also known as a Hollenhorst's plaque. Cholesterol emboli are yellow and refractile and are usually found at bifurcations. They often give the illusion that they are larger than the blood vessel.

Treatment options, given in tandem, usually include intravenous acetazolamide and β-blocker eye drops to lower intraocular pressure, digital massage and paracentesis to dislodge the embolus, and carbogen inhalation (for 10 min, interrupted by a 5-min hiatus, times three) to increase retinal blood flow. Aspirin has also been used. None of these measures is known to be effective, but their combined use is accepted widely.[124, 140, 141]

Patients with CRAO should be evaluated in the same way as older patients who experience TMB (discussed earlier). Embolization is the most common mechanism underlying branch or central artery occlusion, and the diagnostic work-up should be designed to uncover potential sites of embolugenesis. Less common vascular disorders should be considered if the presentation is unusual or suggests one of the diagnoses listed in Table 199–2.

BRANCH AND CILIORETINAL ARTERY OCCLUSIONS

CLINICAL MANIFESTATIONS

Variations on the theme of CRAO occur. Cilioretinal arteries arise from the choroidal circulation, are present in up to 20 percent of normal people, and protect the macula during episodes of ischemia resulting from disrupted central retinal artery flow (Fig. 199–6).[142, 143] CRAO with sparing of the macula causes severe visual loss outside of the central 5 degrees but preserves central acuity. Isolated obstruction of the cilioretinal artery also may occur, in which case central vision is lost but peripheral vision is retained.[144–152] Patients with occlusion of the central retinal vein are susceptible to occlusion of the cilioretinal artery.[146, 153–155]

Like patients with CRAO, a significant number of patients with branch occlusions have systemic vascular disease, including carotid atherosclerotic disease and systemic hypertension. The incidence of such disease is lower, however, and the mortality rates are more favorable for patients with branch occlusions.[137, 156]

MANAGEMENT

The diagnostic evaluation is the same as for CRAO (described earlier). In short, an embolic source should be sought and an assessment of the patient's overall health should be made. Coincident involvement of both retinal and choroidal circulations should raise suspicion of temporal arteritis in patients older than 55 yr.

ISCHEMIC OCULAR SYNDROME

Marked impairment of both internal and external carotid artery perfusion can lead to slow and inexorable ischemia of the eye. The clinical presentation may be insidious. The earliest manifestations may be peripheral retinal hemorrhages, peripheral microaneurysms, tor-

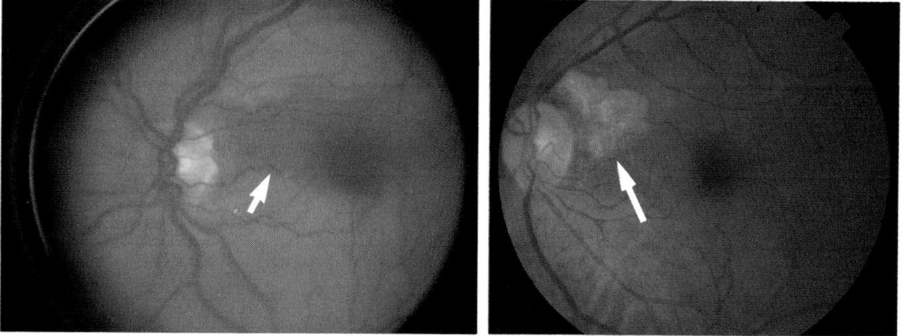

Figure 199–6. *A,* Retinal infarction with sparing within the distribution of the cilioretinal artery *(arrow). B,* Retinal infarction limited to the distribution of the cilioretinal artery *(arrow).*

tuous retinal vessels, and TMB (Fig. 199–7). Episodes of visual loss may be fleeting, lasting only seconds in some cases. Such brief spells are uncharacteristic of the more common form of TMB (discussed earlier). Visual loss may be precipitated by exposure to bright lights, presumably from impaired regeneration of photopigment within the nutritionally deprived photoreceptors. Fluorescein angiography is useful in that it may reveal choroidal hypoperfusion in cases in which only retinal compromise seemed present (Fig. 199–8). Although patients with ischemic ocular syndrome usually have significant atherosclerotic disease, this syndrome rarely may occur secondary to carotid artery dissection[45] or arteritis.

Progression of ischemia to the anterior segment occurs in many cases; the exact frequency of this complication is not known. It is clear, however, that the long-term potential for retaining vision is considerably diminished if the anterior segment becomes involved. Rubeosis of the iris, iritis, and folding of the cornea are the classic signs of anterior segment involvement. Neovascular glaucoma may develop and may be especially difficult to manage. The end result of anterior segment involvement can be a blind and painful eye.[38–45, 157–160] Acquired retinal arteriovenous communications may be observed.[161]

The speed of progression varies considerably from one patient to another. A stable course may persist for years despite the hypoperfusion, presumably because of added input from newly formed collateral channels. Cardiovascular disease is often the cause of mortality or significant morbidity in these patients.

The red eye and pain that are common manifestations of the advanced form of this syndrome may be misdiagnosed as ocular inflammation (i.e., iritis) or ocular infection (i.e., keratitis). The telltale findings of the posterior pole may be unobservable because of corneal clouding. Hence, ischemic ocular syndrome should be included in the differential diagnosis of ocular disorders associated with red eye that do not respond to treatment as anticipated.

MANAGEMENT

Noninvasive assessment of the carotid artery circulation should be obtained to verify the clinical suspicion of hemodynamically significant atheromatous disease. If the diagnosis is corroborated, panretinal photocoagulation (PRP) is the most commonly used treatment. This approach does not improve circulation to the needy eye, but it does reduce the metabolic demand of the most voracious element within the eye, the retina. PRP does seem to lessen the risk of progression from posterior to anterior segment ischemia,[44, 45] and involution of anterior segment neovascularization may occur after treatment. PRP does have the disadvantage of destroying discrete areas of the retina, resulting in constriction of peripheral vision.

If the suspicion of significant stenotic carotid vascular disease is confirmed by noninvasive carotid studies, carotid angiography can be considered for those patients who would agree to surgery and who do not have unacceptably great risk factors for surgery. Carotid endarterectomy would not be useful for a patient who already has advanced involvement of the anterior segment. The main indication for surgery would be to reduce the likelihood that the posterior form of the

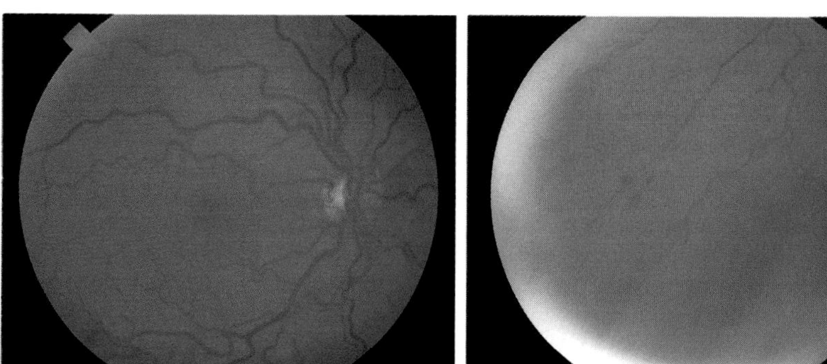

Figure 199–7. Clinical features of the ischemic ocular syndrome. *A,* Tortuous retinal arteries and veins. *B,* Dot hemorrhages in the peripheral retina.

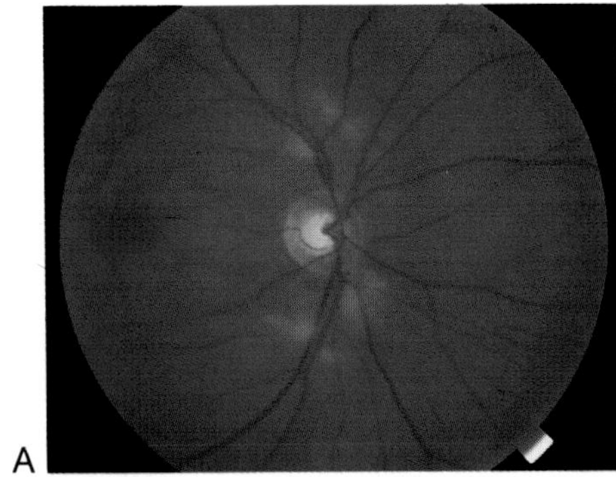

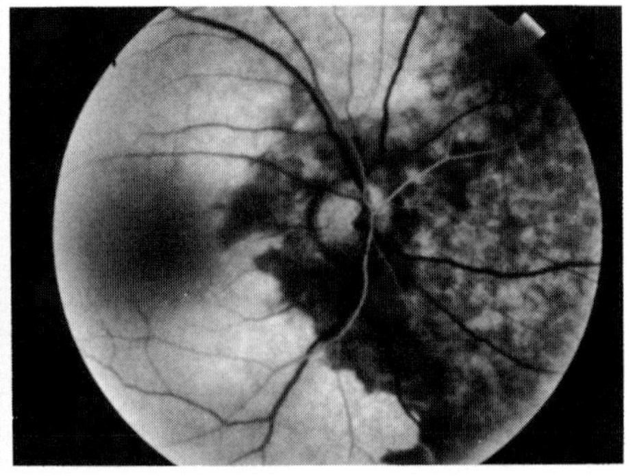

Figure 199–8. Impaired retinal and choroidal circulation. *A*, Multifocal retinal whitening denotes retinal ischemia. *B*, Fluorescein angiogram taken at 45 sec shows delayed filling of retinal circulation (retinal arteries are just beginning to fill, and the veins have yet to fill) and a large region of choroidal hypoperfusion that includes the optic nerve head. The funduscopic picture alone would not have illustrated the coexistent delay of the choroidal circulation. Decreased perfusion of both retinal and choroidal circulations can result from either severe stenosis of the internal and external carotid arteries (ischemic ocular syndrome), with compromise of the ophthalmic or proximal central retinal artery, or from a vasculitic process.

disease would progress anteriorly; surgery also might reduce the risk of stroke in patients who have experienced transient ischemic attacks of the brain. Superficial temporal artery–middle cerebral artery anastomosis has been advocated as therapy for this problem but has not been accepted widely.[43]

A paradoxical worsening may occur after carotid endarterectomy. The increased perfusion may cause further elevation of intraocular pressure and an increase in the size and the number of retinal hemorrhages, although the latter change is not clinically significant. Increased hemorrhaging may occur secondary to the sudden increase in pressure within vessels whose endothelium may have had diminished integrity after prolonged ischemia. The paradoxical response is usually short-lived.

The value of surgery in ischemic ocular syndrome is controversial. It is prudent to consider each case carefully with a team of specialists including an internist, neurologist, neuroradiologist, and neurovascular surgeon.

RETINAL VASCULAR OCCLUSIVE DISEASE ASSOCIATED WITH NEUROVASCULAR DISEASE

The coexistence of retinal and cerebral vascular events is usually a manifestation of carotid or cardiac atherosclerotic disease. Embolization is the most common mechanism leading to dysfunction. Vasculitis, especially in cases of temporal arteritis and systemic lupus erythematosus, is a relatively uncommon but important consideration in cases of combined retinal and cerebral vascular disease. Hypercoagulability should be considered in younger patients (discussed earlier).

Multiple recurrent retinovascular occlusions may occur in young and otherwise healthy persons. Some patients with this syndrome have had mitral valve prolapse, elevated levels of serum lipids, migraine headaches, or a history of intravenous injection of cocaine.[162] Antiphospholipid antibodies also may be associated with this presentation. Iritis may be present in some cases. Focal retinal arteritis is presumed to be the cause of the infarctions. Corticosteroids have not been beneficial. In one study, two of three patients who received anticoagulant therapy experienced a serious complication.[162]

Some patients with recurrent branch artery occlusions have had auditory symptoms. As such, this syndrome may overlap with another in which auditory symptoms occur together with arterial occlusive retinopathy and encephalopathy.[163–166] This latter condition may respond to steroids.[166]

Cerebroretinal vasculopathy is a syndrome that includes perifoveal and peripheral retinal capillary obliteration with formation of microaneurysms and central nervous system "pseudotumor" (see the caveat for the use of the term *pseudotumor*[51]). It seemingly is inherited in an autosomal dominant manner. Patients experience a reduction in central acuity, headache, loss of cognitive function, and seizures. The neuropathologic findings, which may be unique, are largely confined to the white matter of the frontoparietal regions of the brain.[86, 167]

PARANEOPLASTIC RETINOPATHY

In 1976, Sawyer and coworkers described three cases in which photoreceptor degeneration appeared to be the remote effect of cancer. The first of their cases serves as a paradigm for diagnosis and evaluation of this syndrome: A 65-year-old patient experienced progressive visual loss with ring scotomata and had markedly abnormal ERG findings; undifferentiated small cell carcinoma of the lung was eventually discovered. Postmortem examination of the eyes showed disintegration of the inner and outer segments of the rods and cones and widespread degeneration of the outer nuclear layer.[168]

Visual loss from paraneoplastic retinopathy may be acute or subacute and is often associated with positive visual phenomena. Diagnosis of this condition is usually predicated on abnormal ERG findings with normal fundi, absence of a family history of retinal disease, and a clinical course compatible with this disease. Visual field loss may be manifested by peripheral constriction, midperipheral ring scotomata that often cross the vertical meridian, and central defects (Fig. 199–9). Mild

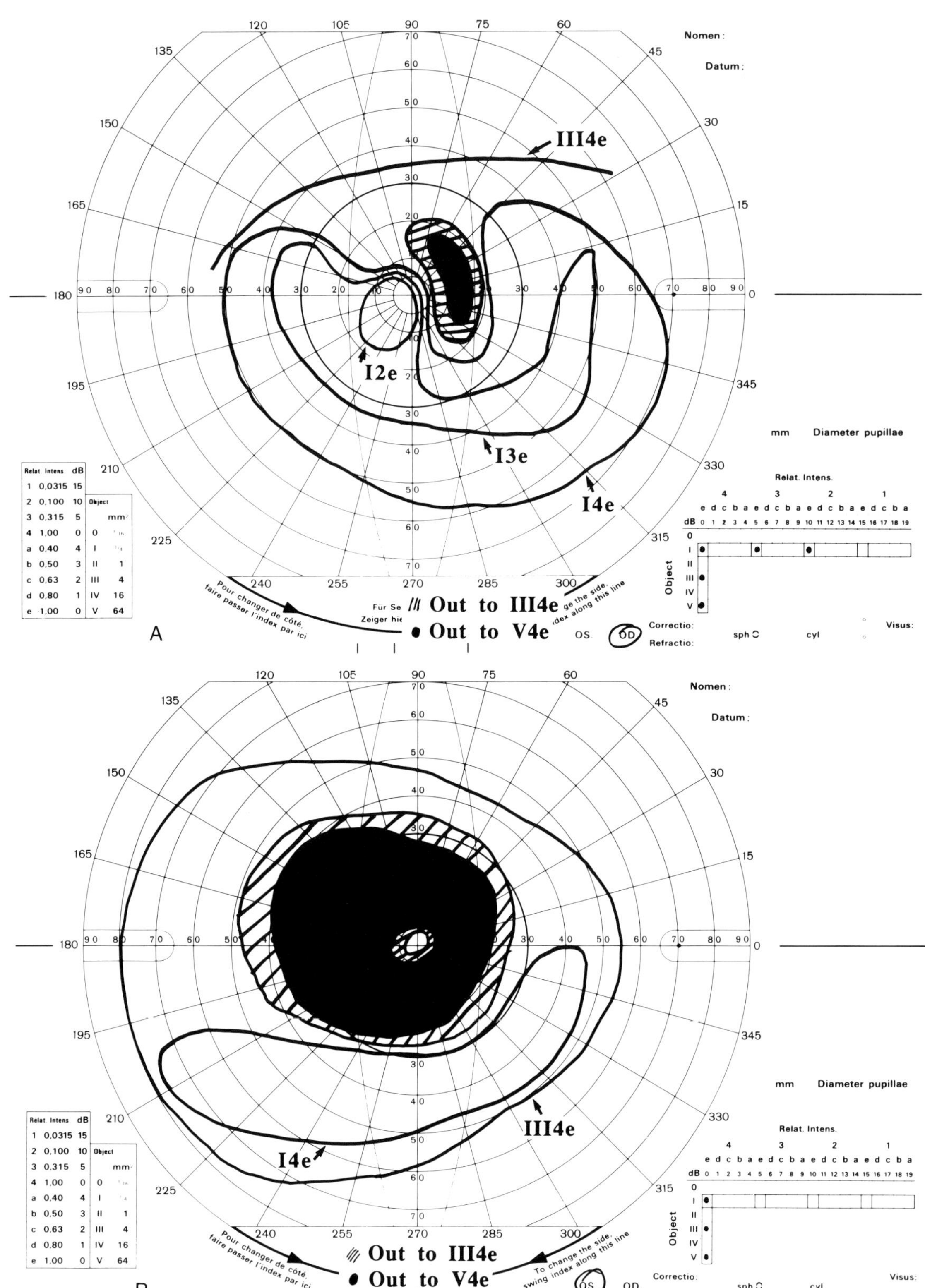

Figure 199–9. Goldmann's visual field test results. An arcuate scotoma was present O.D. *(B)*, and a ring scotoma was present O.S. *(A)*. Constriction of the peripheral isopters was present in both eyes.

pigmentary changes are occasionally visible in the fundi. Visual symptoms often antedate identification of the tumor. Older adults are usually affected, and small cell tumor of the lung is by far the most common tumor found in association with this syndrome. Adenocarcinoma of the breast, cervical carcinoma, endometrial carcinoma, and melanoma have also been associated with this syndrome.[168–183]

ERG may reveal reduced rod and cone amplitudes or absence of a detectable response. A distinctive ERG finding reported in association with melanoma was selective absence of the scotopic b-wave, a pattern typical of congenital stationary night blindness.[178]

Diagnosis may be aided by performing immunologic tests of a patient's serum. Enzyme-linked immunoassay (ELISA) and Western blot testing have proved to be useful in diagnosing the disease. These tests examine characteristics of antibodies present in the serum in different ways: ELISA provides quantification of any reaction between the patient's serum and retina, and the Western blot test determines the molecular weight of the antibody that reacts with the retina. These tests certainly have contributed to our understanding of this syndrome and have permitted identification of the cancer-associated retinopathy (CAR) antigen that is thought to contribute to the pathogenesis of this syndrome. These tests, however, may be neither highly specific nor sensitive. Nonetheless, such testing should be conducted for patients suspected or proved to have the visual paraneoplastic syndrome.

The pathogenesis of the syndrome is not known. There is substantial evidence that autoimmunity has a role—perhaps an immune response is mounted against the tumor, and one or more antibodies that are generated happen to cross-react with retinal proteins. Analogous situations are thought to occur in other types of paraneoplastic syndromes that involve the central nervous system. Antiretinal antibodies have been discovered in the serum of patients affected by the visual paraneoplastic syndrome,[169–171, 174, 175, 179, 183] but the mere presence of neuronal antibodies does not mean that a disease state exists (Fig. 199–10). Normal persons may have such antibodies without apparent ill effect. Presumably, the antibodies must have access to neurons to which they have an affinity in order for a disease to develop. The blood-retinal barrier would have to be transgressed for visual loss to occur as a consequence of a serum antibody.

Damage to the retina usually involves the photoreceptors, but variations on this theme have been reported. Selective involvement of ganglion cells has been reported.[169, 170, 174, 175] The paraneoplastic syndrome associated with melanoma (described earlier) produces an ERG pattern that suggests a block in signal transmission in the rod pathway distal to the photoreceptor.[178]

Visual fields may show dense midperipheral scotomata or central scotomata. Pathologic involvement of the retina may be patchy (see Fig. 199–10), thus accounting for the likewise patchy loss of visual field (see Fig. 199–9).[183] The funduscopic appearance of the retina is usually normal, although a mild increase in retinal pigmentation may be seen.

MANAGEMENT

Suspicion of this syndrome should prompt investigation for a tumor if one has not already become apparent. A chest film is the first test to order. Visual loss may be reversed at least temporarily with oral corticosteroids.

OTHER PARANEOPLASTIC SYNDROMES INVOLVING THE EYE

Paraneoplastic optic neuritis has been reported in a single patient who also had paraneoplastic encephalomyelitis. Postmortem examination demonstrated demyelination of the optic nerve.[184] Bilateral diffuse uveal melanocytic proliferation is another type of paraneoplastic syndrome. Exudative retinal detachment and rapid progression of cataract are additional features of this syndrome.[185]

PIGMENTARY AND OTHER DEGENERATIVE RETINOPATHIES ASSOCIATED WITH NEUROLOGIC DISEASE

Retinal dysfunction may occur together with more widespread neurologic degeneration. Retinal findings occasionally provide the first and most substantial clue to the diagnosis. For this reason, ophthalmologists should be familiar with this broad class of disease. I have summarized the effects on the retina by segregating the manifestations into one of three categories based on easy-to-recognize clinical features. Any simplification of this type has the disadvantage of not being absolute; some diseases show features of more than one group.

Retinal involvement associated with metabolic or neurodegenerative disease may take one of three forms:

1. Atrophy of particular cells, usually photoreceptors or ganglion cells
2. Deposition of storage materials within certain cells
3. Pigmentary reaction

A summary of diseases associated with each of these manifestations is provided below. Table 199–4 represents an amalgamation of several authoritative reviews,[186–190] with modifications and additions. In particular, the table is arranged to conform to the three general patterns of retinal involvement that may be observed with neurologic disease.

Atrophy of Particular Cells

One of the unique aspects of degenerative neurologic disease is the striking selectivity in the patterns of attrition of specific cells or systems. In one of the prototypic degenerative diseases, Friedreich's ataxia, the dorsal spinocerebellar tract degenerates (among other structures) but contiguous long tracts are relatively

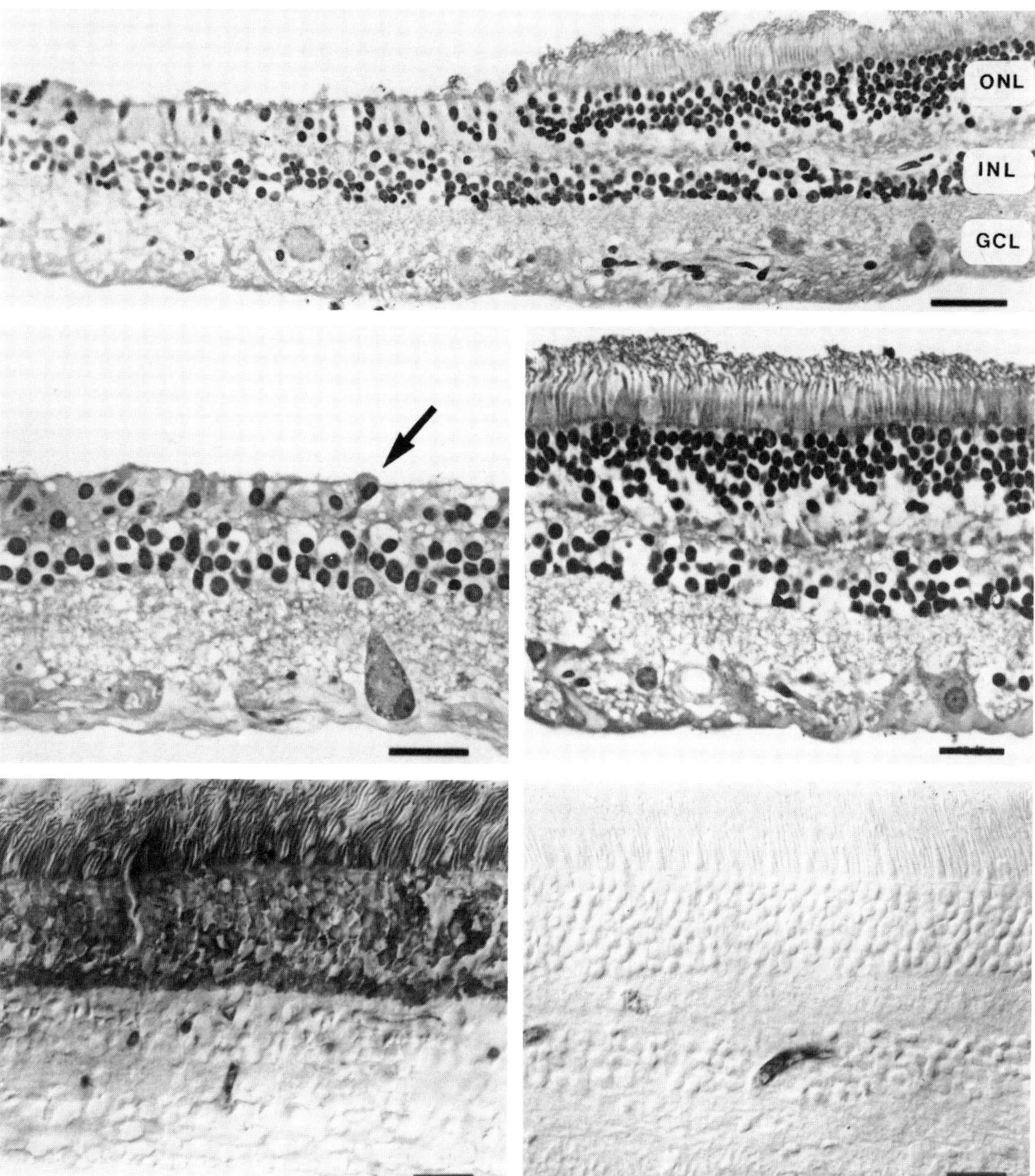

Figure 199–10. *Top and Center Rows,* Three micron sections of the postmortem human retina stained with cresyl violet. The top section was taken from the midperipheral retina and shows a transition from normal *(right side)* to grossly abnormal *(left side).* In the abnormal area, outer nuclear layer cells and the finger-like projections of the inner and outer segments are nearly absent. The outer plexiform layer is reduced in thickness. The inner retina appears similar across this section. In particular, the density of cells within the inner nuclear and ganglion cell layers appears normal for this region of retina. Horizontal bar = 60 μm. *Center Left,* This section was taken from the peripheral retina and shows degenerating profiles of outer nuclear layer cells *(arrow)* and an almost complete loss of inner and outer segments. Only a sparse outer nuclear cell layer that is a single cell in thickness remains. Compare it with the center right section, in which the outer nuclear layer is approximately seven cells thick. Horizontal bar = 30 μm. *Center Right,* This section was taken just beyond the peripheral edge of the macula and appears nearly normal. Horizontal bar = 30 μm. *Bottom,* Nomarski optics were used to visualize edges of cell bodies and other structures such as the inner and outer segments in normal postmortem human retinas. These structures can be imaged with this technique without the need for standard histochemical stains. Stain visible in the bottom sections is the insoluble reaction product of the immunohistochemical procedure. *Bottom Right,* This is a control for the immunohistochemistry in which normal serum was used; no staining of the retina is visible except in blood vessels, as expected. *Bottom Left,* The same procedure was performed using the serum of a patient with paraneoplastic photoreceptor retinopathy. Dark staining of the outer retina is visible and involves the outer segments. Compare the region of staining with the area of retina that had degenerated in the middle left section. Horizontal bars = 30 μm. (ONL, outer nuclear layer; INL, inner nuclear layer; GCL, ganglion cell layer.)

Table 199–4. RETINAL MANIFESTATIONS ASSOCIATED WITH PROGRESSIVE NEUROLOGIC DISEASE

Atrophy of Certain Retinal Cells

Cell type	*Associated Neurologic Disease*	*Other Features*
Photoreceptors	Spinocerebellar degenerations[191–194]	
	Neuronal ceroid lipofuscinosis[195, 196] (see also Associations with Pigmentary Retinopathy, later)	
Ganglion cells	Spinocerebellar degenerations[197]	
	Congenital deafness[198–200]	Progressive Autosomal dominant
	Deafness, ataxia limb weakness[201]	Autosomal dominant
	Deafness, spastic quadriplegia, mental deterioration[303, 203]	Autosomal recessive
	Juvenile diabetes mellitus, diabetes insipidus, hearing loss (DIDMOAD syndrome[204, 205])	Autosomal recessive
	Pyramidal tract signs, ataxia, mental retardation, urinary incontinence, pes cavus (Behr's syndrome[206, 209])	Autosomal recessive Often static after childhood
	Charcot-Marie-Tooth[210, 211]	Progressive weakness in intrinsic muscles of feet and anterior legs
	Hereditary motor and sensory neuropathy[212]	
	Extrapyramidal movement disorder, spastic paraplegia[213]	
	Riley-Day syndrome[214]	
	Inherited metabolic diseases	
	Lysosomal disorders:	
	Mucopolysaccharidoses[215]	
	Lipidoses	
	Pelizaeus-Merzbacher	
	Adrenoleukodystrophy, X-linked[216]	
	Infantile neuroaxonal dystrophy	
	Leigh's disease	
	Galactosialidosis[217]	
All retinal layers	Infantile amaurotic idiocy (Bielschowsky-Jansky)	Retinal pigmentation, progressive dementia, convulsions, early death

Deposition of Storage Material

Retinal Appearance	*Disease*
Cherry-red spot at macula[186, 187]	Tay-Sachs (90%) Sandhoff's[218] GM_1 gangliosidoses, type I Niemann-Pick Gaucher's (rare/questionable) Sialodoses Farber's lipogranulomatosis Metachromatic leukodystrophy
Grayish opacification around the fovea	Farber's lipogranulomatosis Metachromatic leukodystrophy
White annulus surrounding fovea ("macular halo")	Neimann-Pick[219, 220]
Vascular tortuosity	Fabry's[221]
Brownish discoloration of macula; progressive hypopigmentation of fundus	Neuronal ceroid lipofuscinosis[195, 196]
Scattered white spots	Gaucher's[222]
Bull's-eye maculopathy	Cerebellar ataxia[193]

Pigmentary Retinopathy

Lysosomal storage diseases	Gaucher's Infantile phytanic acid Juvenile GM_2 gangliosidosis with hexosaminidase A deficiency Mucolipodosis (type IV)[223] Neuronal ceroid lipofuscinosis Mucopolysaccharidoses
Other metabolic diseases	Abetalipoproteinemia Apoceruloplasmin deficiency Cystinuria Homocarnosinosis Hyperpipecolataemia McArdle's Refsum's

Table 199–4. RETINAL MANIFESTATIONS ASSOCIATED WITH PROGRESSIVE NEUROLOGIC DISEASE *Continued*

Retinal Appearance	*Disease*
Syndromes	Cockayne's
	Flynn-Aird
	Hooft's
	Joubert's
	Kearns-Sayre
	Laurence-Moon-Bardet-Biedl[224]
	Letterer-Siwe
	Marinesco-Sjögren
	Pelizaeus-Merzbacher
	Rud's
	Senior's
	Sjögren-Larsson
	Tuck-McLeod
	Usher/Hallgren
	Zellweger's
Specific diseases	Familial spastic paraparesis
	Friedreich's ataxia
	Hallervorden-Spatz
	Leber's congenital amaurosis (see text)
	Lytico-Bodig (amyotrophic lateral sclerosis-parkinsonism-dementia)[225]
	Spinocerebellar degeneration
Other	Congenital ophthalmoplegia
	Dystonia, blepharospasm
	Myoclonus epilepsy
	Myotonic dystrophy
	Osteogenesis imperfecta
	Progressive bulbar paralysis
Chorioretinal degeneration	Hyperornithinemia (gyrate atrophy), with muscle atrophy[226]
	Osteopetrosis[227, 228]

spared. Photoreceptors and ganglion cells appear to be most susceptible to degenerative processes that affect the retina (Fig. 199–11). Histopathologic examinations have been performed infrequently in these diseases, however, and it is possible that other cells also are affected. Little is known about the other cell types of the human retina, and it is possible that involvement simply has not been recognized.

Deposition of Storage Material

The cherry-red macular spot is the most common manifestation of the lysosomal storage diseases. The retinal appearance is the result of swelling of the perifoveal ganglion cells with metabolic storage products. The ring is only present in the perifoveal region, probably because of the high density of ganglion cells in this location. In contrast, the foveola does not contain ganglion cells, and the normal redness of the fundus background appears in the center of the white ring (see Fig. 199–11). The term *cherry-red spots* is also used for a similar appearance of the retina in some noninherited diseases, such as CRAO (see Fig. 199–4*A*), traumatic retinal edema, or quinine toxicity. A cherry-red spot may disappear as the retinal ganglion cells atrophy.

Pigmentary Reaction

Disease of photoreceptors is often accompanied by pigmentary reaction, which results from migration of the retinal pigment epithelium to the inner retina. The pigment often tracks along blood vessels ("bear tracks"), or it may clump. Great variability in the degree of pigmentation may be seen from one patient to another. Rarely, pigmentation may be unilateral. Attenuation of retinal arterioles is commonly observed, and a pale optic nerve head may be present (see Fig. 199–11).

MISCELLANEOUS

Big Blind Spot Syndrome

Fletcher and colleagues described a syndrome of enlargement of the blind spot in the absence of disc edema secondary to focal peripapillary retinopathy.[229] All of their patients exhibited absolute scotomata with steep margins and geographic features that centered on the blind spot, and four of the seven experienced positive visual phenomena in the region of the scotoma. Multifocal ERG demonstrated peripapillary retinal dysfunction. Central acuity and color vision were not affected; two patients had a mild afferent pupillary defect. Follow-up examinations of five patients showed resolution of the visual field defects. Interestingly, two of the patients had experienced prior episodes of blind spot enlargement that had resolved (Fig. 199–12).

One year later, two more patients with features similar to those described by Fletcher and colleagues were reported, but their funduscopic findings during the acute phase were characteristic of the multiple evanescent

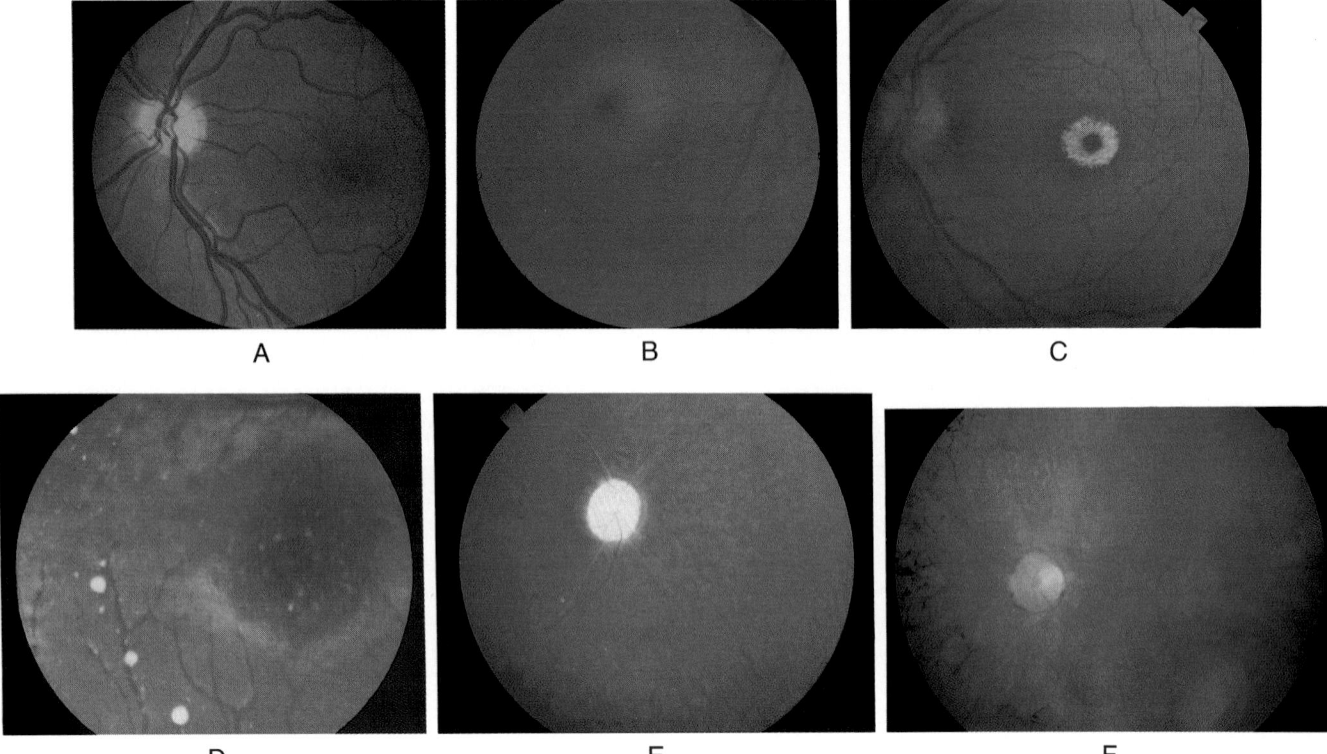

Figure 199–11. Funduscopic features of some neurodegenerative diseases that involve the retina. Examples of the three major categories of retinal pathology listed in Table 199–4 are shown. *A,* Marked atrophy of the optic nerve indicating the widespread loss of retinal ganglion cells in the Riley-Day syndrome. *B,* Cherry-red spot associated with Tay-Sachs disease, an example of deposition of storage material within the retina. The hexaminidase B enzyme defect results in abnormal accumulation of sphingolipids within neurons. Compare with Figure 199–4*A,* where the retinal pallor is much more diffuse. *C,* White annulus ("macular halo") surrounding the fovea in Nieman-Pick disease. *D,* White spots in the retina in a patient with Nieman-Pick disease. *E,* Marked optic atrophy and thinning of retinal arterioles with alteration in retinal pigment in a patient with neuronal ceroid lipofuscinosis. *F,* Pigmentary degeneration of the retina (best seen near the nasal border of the photograph) in a patient with Laurence-Moon-Bardet-Biedl syndrome. Thinning of retinal arterioles and optic atrophy are also present. (*B* and *D,* Courtesy of Dr. David Cogan.)

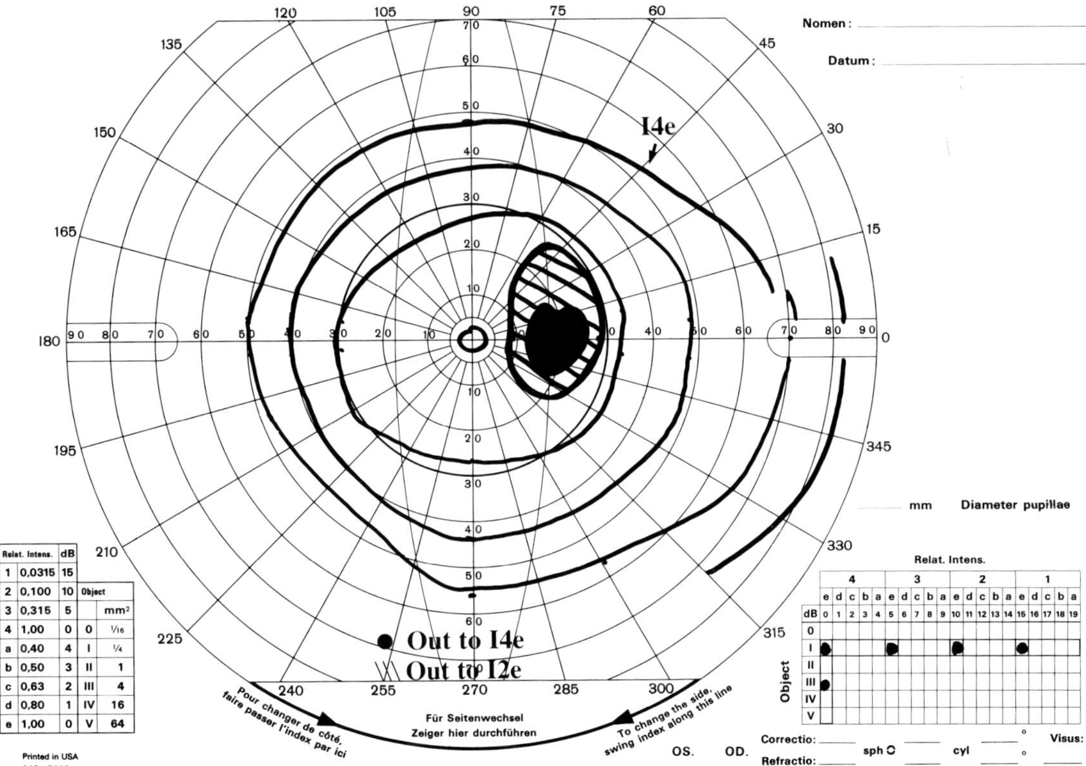

Figure 199–12. Visual field of a patient with the big blind spot syndrome. A large and dense scotoma is present around the blind spot.

white dot syndrome (MEWDS).[230] This syndrome, described in 1984, presents with characteristic small white spots deep to the retina or within it. Fletcher's group convincingly described similarities between MEWDS and the big blind spot syndrome. For instance, swelling of the optic nerve head, enlargement of the blind spot, and ERG abnormalities previously had been reported in some patients with MEWDS. The funduscopic findings of MEWDS are evanescent, partially explaining the source for diagnostic confusion between these disorders. The presence of optic neuropathy in MEWDS syndrome was emphasized by Dodwell and associates in a series of five patients who were initially misdiagnosed as having "optic neuritis, retrobulbar neuritis, and optic nerve edema and vitreitis."[232] There also appears to be a relationship between these syndromes and multifocal choroiditis.[233]

MEWDS syndrome has also occurred together with the acute macular neuroretinopathy syndrome.[234] This condition presents with an acute change in vision, sometimes progressive, with dense parafoveal scotomata and characteristic dark retinal lesions that correspond to the location of the field defect(s).[235]

The cause of these three syndromes is not known, but a virus has been suspected because of the occurrence of an antecedent viral illness, evidence of immune disturbance in some patients, and the suggestion that Epstein-Barr virus is related to multifocal choroiditis. Women are more often affected than men.

Antiphospholipid Antibodies

Antiphospholipid antibodies are a heterogeneous family of antibodies directed against phospholipids that include the lupus anticoagulant and antibodies to cardiolipin. These antibodies are more commonly discovered in women; persons who are younger than 50 yr and who have experienced stroke or cerebral transient ischemic attack; persons with a false-positive result on the rapid plasma reagin test; those with a history of thrombotic events, fetal loss, thrombocytopenia, or splinter hemorrhages under the nail beds; and those with a prolonged partial thromboplastin time in the absence of heparin therapy.[236–240] The presence of these antibodies should be suspected in patients with unexplained cerebral infarction, especially multiple small cortical infarcts, and in patients with atypical migraine-like headaches. The mechanism by which these antibodies cause neurologic disease, if indeed they do, has not been determined. The relationship between the presence of this antibody and progressive optic atrophy seems tenuous in one case report.[241]

Neurologic syndromes most frequently linked to the presence of antiphospholipid antibodies are thrombotic in character, including transient ischemic attacks, cerebral infarction, and acute ischemic encephalopathy.[237–241] Cardiogenic brain embolism and migrainous phenomena have also been reported.[238, 241, 243] Reported visual complications include amaurosis fugax, retinal arterial or

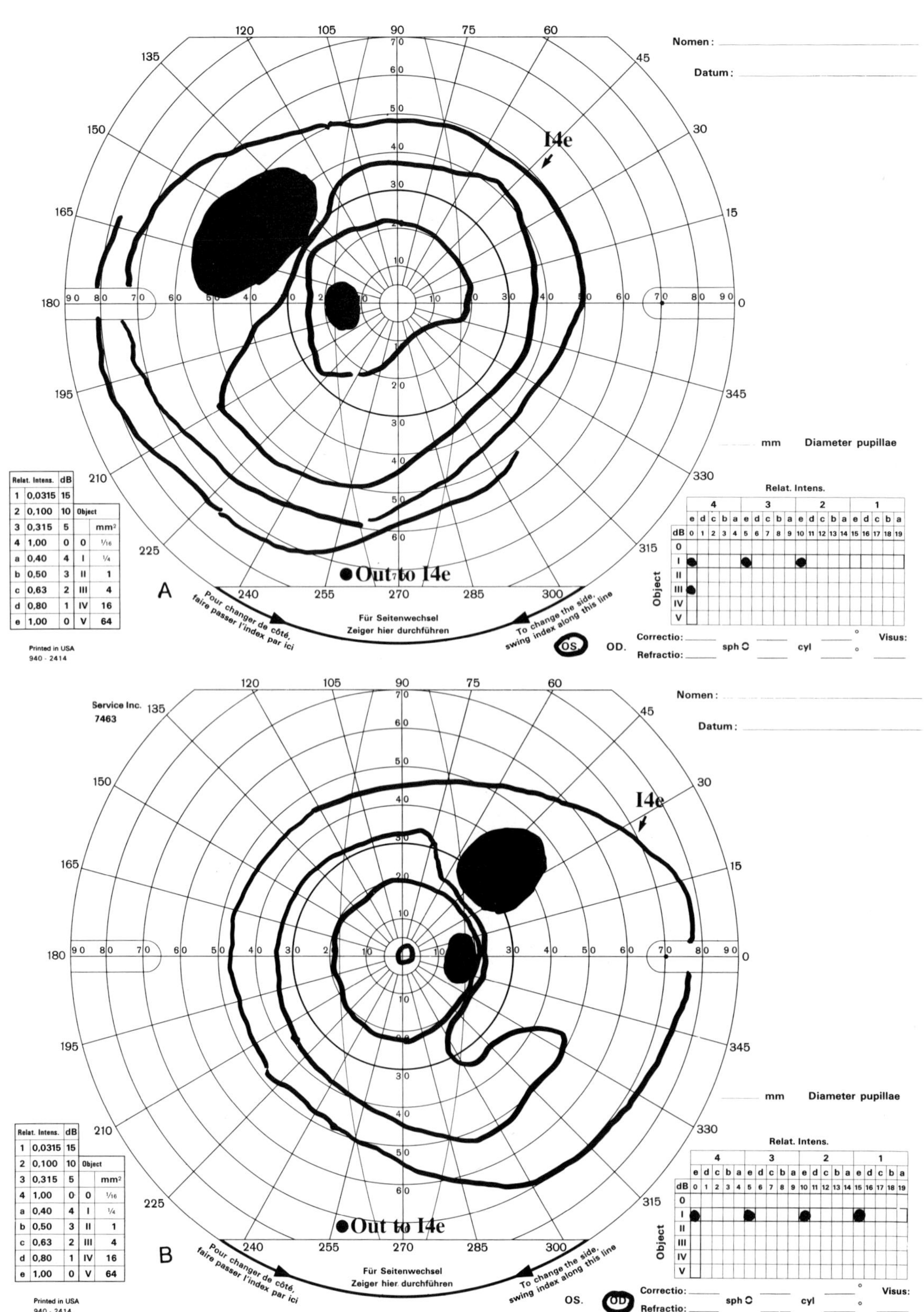

Figure 199–13. Visual fields of a 32-year-old woman with the antiphospholipid syndrome. Over the course of 10 years, she experienced two episodes of branch retinal artery occlusion. She has residual midperipheral scotomata in the temporal field of each eye.

venous occlusion, transient diplopia[238, 240, 241] (summarized in table form by Kleiner and colleagues[244]) and occipital ischemia.[238] Multiple episodes of branch retinal artery occlusion may occur (Fig. 199–13). A single case of recurrent ischemic optic neuropathy occurring over a 6-yr period was reported by Briley and associates, but the lack of clinical detail about what would be a highly unusual manifestation of ischemic optic neuropathy makes it difficult to interpret this presentation.[240]

The role of this family of antibodies as a cause of neurologic dysfunction has been controversial. Evidence for and against the role of antiphospholipid antibodies as a cause of ischemic brain disease was discussed by Levine and Welch in a review article.[236] The preponderance of evidence supports the notion that the coagulant-enhancing properties of these antibodies lead to an increased risk of neurovascular disease, especially among patients younger than 50 yr. A prospective study of 104 patients demonstrated that anticardiolipin antibodies were significantly more common in a group of patients suffering brain ischemia than in a group with nonischemic neurologic disorders.[244]

There is no consensus on therapy for patients who test positive for these antibodies. Some recommended treatments, including immunosuppression and anticoagulation, have a high risk of causing serious complications.[239, 241, 244] Strokes have occurred despite treatment with aspirin or a combination of warfarin and dipyridamole. Digre and colleagues speculated that treatment with antiplatelet medications, anticoagulants, or both reduced the frequency of amaurosis fugax.[239] Some diseases that involve the macula, however, also involve the extramacular retina and hence might present with the other types of field defects listed earlier.

REFERENCES

1. Moniz E, Lima A, de Lacerda R: Par thrombose de la carotide interne. Presse Med 45:977, 1937.
2. Chiari H: Über das Verhalten des Teilungswinkels der Carotis communis bie der Endarteriitis chronica deformans. Verh Dtsch Ges Pathol 9:326, 1905.
3. Hunt JR: The role of the carotid arteries, in the causation of vascular lesions of the brain, with remarks on certain special features of the symptomatology. Am J Med Sci 147:704, 1914.
4. Fisher CM: Occlusion of the internal carotid artery. Arch Neurol Psych 65:346, 1951.
5. Andrell PO: Thrombosis of the internal carotid artery: A clinical study of 9 cases diagnosed by arteriography. Acta Med Scand 114:336, 1943.
6. Adams RD, Richardson EP: Salute to C. Miller Fisher. Arch Neurol 38:137, 1981.
7. Fisher CM, Adams RD: Observations on brain embolism. J Neuropathol Exp Neurol 10:92, 1951.
8. Fisher CM: Transient monocular blindness associated with hemiplegia. Arch Ophthalmol 47:167, 1952.
9. Fisher CM, Cameron DG: Occlusion of the carotid arteries. Arch Neurol 3:468, 1953.
10. Fisher CM: Occlusion of the carotid arteries. Arch Neurol 72:187, 1954.
11. Fisher CM: Concerning recurrent transient cerebral ischemic attacks. Can Med Assoc J 86:1091, 1962.
12. Gowers WR: Subjective visual sensations. Trans Ophthalmol Soc UK 15:1, 1895.
13. Olesen J, Edvinsson L: Migraine: A research field matured for the basic neurosciences. Trends Neurosci 14:3, 1991.
14. Spector RH: Migraine. Surv Ophthalmol 29:193, 1984.
15. Hupp SL, Kline LB, Corbett JJ: Visual disturbances of migraine. Surv Ophthalmol 33:221, 1989.
16. O'Connor PS, Tredici TJ: Acephalgic migraine: Fifteen years experience. Ophthalmology 88:999, 1981.
17. Fisher CM: Late-life migraine accompaniments as a cause of unexplained transient ischemic attacks. J Can Sci Neurol 7:9, 1980.
18. Troost BT, Mark LE, Maroon JC: Resolution of classic migraine after removal of an occipital lobe AVM. Ann Neurol 5:199, 1979.
19. Troost BT, Newton TH: Occipital lobe arteriovenous malformations: Clinical and radiologic features in 26 cases with comments on the differentiation from migraine. Arch Ophthalmol 93:250, 1975.
20. Waltimo O, Hokkanen E, Pirskanen R: Intracranial arteriovenous malformations and headache. Headache 15:133, 1975.
21. Fisher CM: "Transient monocular blindness" versus "amaurosis fugax." Neurology 39:1622, 1989.
22. Goodwin JA, Gorelick PB, Helgason CM: Symptoms of amaurosis fugax in atherosclerotic carotid artery disease. Neurology 37:829, 1987.
23. Coppeto JR, Lessell S, Lessell IM, et al: Diffuse disseminated atheroembolism: Three cases with neuro-ophthalmic manifestations. Arch Ophthalmol 102:225, 1984.
24. Newman NJ, Kline LB, Leifer D, et al: Ocular stroke and carotid artery dissection. Neurology 39:1462, 1989.
25. Levinson SA, Close MB, Ehrinfeld, et al: Carotid artery occlusive disease following external cervical irradiation. Arch Surg 107:395, 1973.
26. Briley DP, Coull BM, Goodnight SH: Neurological disease associated with antiphospholipid antibodies. Ann Neurol 25:221, 1989.
27. Digre KB, Durcan FJ, Branch DW, et al: Amaurosis fugax associated with antiphospholipid antibodies. Ann Neurol 25:228, 1989.
28. Golub BM, Sibony PA, Coller BS: Protein S deficiency associated with central retinal artery occlusion. Arch Ophthalmol 108:918, 1990.
29. Coller BS, Owen J, Jesty J, et al: Deficiency of plasma protein S, protein C, or antithrombin III and arterial thrombosis. Arteriosclerosis 7:456, 1987.
30. Sadun AA, Currie JN, Lessell S: Transient visual obscurations with elevated optic discs. Ann Neurol 16:489, 1984.
31. Wright JE: Primary optic nerve meningiomas: Clinical presentation and management. Trans Am Acad Ophthalmol Otolaryngol 83:617, 1977.
32. Unsöld R, Hoyt WF: Blickinduzierte monokulare Obskurationen bei orbitalem Haemangiom. Klin Monatsbl Augenheilkd 174:715, 1979.
33. Orcutt JC, Tucker WM, Mills RP, et al: Gaze-evoked amaurosis. Ophthalmology 94:213, 1987.
34. Bradbury PG, Levy IS, McDonald WI: Transient uniocular visual loss on deviation of the eye in association with intraorbital tumours. J Neurol Neurosurg Psychiatr 50:615, 1987.
35. Silverman SM, Bergman PS, Bender MB: The dynamics of transient cerebral blindness: Report of nine episodes following vertebral angiography. Arch Neurol 4:333, 1961.
36. Snebold NG, Rizzo JF III, Lessell S, et al: Transient visual loss in ornithine transcarbamoylase deficiency. Am J Ophthalmol 104:407, 1987.
37. Kosmorsky GS, Rosenfeld SI, Burde RM: Transient monocular obscuration? Amaurosis fugax: A case report. Br J Ophthalmol 69:688, 1985.
38. Knox DL: Ischemic ocular inflammation. Am J Ophthalmol 60:995, 1965.
39. Ross-Russell RW, Ikeda H: Clinical and electrophysiological observations in patients with low pressure retinopathy. Br J Ophthalmol 70:651, 1986.
40. Jacobs NA, Ridgway AEA: Syndrome of ischaemic ocular inflammation: Six cases and a review. Br J Ophthalmol 69:681, 1985.
41. Ros MA, Magargal LE, Hedges TR, et al: Ocular ischemic syndrome: Long-term ocular complications. Ann Ophthalmol 19:270, 1987.

42. Michelson PE, Knox DL, Green WR: Ischemic ocular inflammation: A clinicopathologic case report. Arch Ophthalmol 86:274, 1971.
43. Young LHY, Appen RE: Ischemic oculopathy: A manifestation of carotid artery disease. Arch Neurol 38:358, 1981.
44. Carter JE: Chronic ocular ischemia and carotid vascular disease. Stroke 16:721, 1985.
45. Duker JS, Belmont JB: Ocular ischemic syndrome secondary to carotid artery dissection. Am J Ophthalmol 106:750, 1988.
46. Cogan DG: Blackouts not obviously due to carotid occlusion. Arch Ophthal 66:56, 1961.
47. Hayreh SS: Anterior ischaemic optic neuropathy: Differentiation of arteritic from non-arteritic type and its management. Eye 4:25, 1990.
48. Ramorino D: Due casi di ischemia dei vasi retinici. Ann Ottalmol Clin Ocul 6:25, 1877.
49. Fisher CM: Observations of the fundus oculi in transient monocular blindness. Neurology 9:333, 1959.
50. Pessin MS, Duncan GW, Mohr JP, et al: Clinical and angiographic features of carotid transient ischemic attacks. N Engl J Med 296:358, 1977.
51. Rizzo J: The retina. *In* Lessell S, van Dalen JTW (eds): Current Neuro-Ophthalmology, vol. 2. St. Louis, Mosby-Year Book, 1990, p 223.
52. Eadie MJ, Sutherland JM, Tyrer JH: Recurrent monocular blindness of uncertain cause. Lancet 1:319, 1968.
53. Fisher CM: Cerebral ischemia—Less familiar types. Clin Neurosurg 18:267, 1970.
54. Wray SH: Visual aspects of extracranial internal carotid artery disease. *In* Bernstein EF (ed): Amaurosis Fugax. New York, Springer-Verlag, 1988, p 81.
55. Poole CJM, Ross Russell RW, Harrison P, et al: Amaurosis fugax under the age of 40 years. J Neurol Neurosurg Psychiatry 50:81, 1987.
56. Tippin J, Corbett JJ, Kerber RE, et al: Amaurosis fugax and ocular infarction in adolescents and young adults. Ann Neurol 26:69, 1989.
57. Appleton R, Farrell K, Buncic JR, et al: Amaurosis fugax in teenagers: A migraine variant. Am J Dis Child 142:2331, 1988.
58. Fisher CM: Migraine accompaniments versus arteriosclerotic ischemia. Trans Am Neurol Assoc 93:211, 1968.
59. Lewis RA, Vijayan N, Watson C, et al: Visual field loss in migraine. Ophthalmology 96:321, 1989.
60. Coppeto JR, Lessell S, Sciarra R, et al: Vascular retinopathy in migraine. Neurology 36:267, 1986.
61. Raymond LA, Kranias G, Glueck H, et al: Significance of scintillating scotoma of late onset. Surv Ophthalmol 25:107, 1980.
62. Rothrock JF, Walicke P, Swenson MR, et al: Migrainous stroke. Arch Neurol 45:63, 1988.
63. Dorfman LJ, Marshall WH, Enzmann DR: Cerebral infarction and migraine: Clinical and radiologic correlations. Neurology 29:317, 1979.
64. Caplan LR: Migraine and vertebrobasilar ischemia. Neurology 41:55, 1991.
65. Walsh FB, Hoyt WF: Clinical Neuro-Ophthalmology, 3rd ed. Baltimore, Williams & Wilkins, 1969, p 1670.
66. Lees F: The migrainous symptoms of cerebral angiomata. J Neurol Neurosurg Psychiatry 25:45, 1962.
67. Pearee JMS, Foster JB: An investigation of complicated migraine. Neurology (Minneap) 15:333, 1965.
68. Featherstone HJ: Clinical features of stroke in migraine: A review. Headache 26:128, 1986.
69. Troost BT, Newton TH: Occipital lobe arteriovenous malformations: Clinical and radiologic features in 26 cases with comments on the differentiation from migraine. Arch Ophthalmol 93:250, 1975.
70. Selby G, Lance JW: Observations on 500 cases of migraine and allied vascular headache. J Neurol Neurosurg Psychiatry 23:23, 1960.
71. Glaser JS (ed) : Neuro-Ophthalmology, 2nd ed. Philadelphia, JB Lippincott, 1990.
72. Ellenberger C, Epstein AD: Ocular complications of atherosclerosis: What do they mean? Semin Neurol 6:185, 1986.
73. Hurwitz BJ, Heyman A, Wilkinson WE, et al: Comparison of amaurosis fugax and transient cerebral ischemia: A prospective clinical and arteriographic study. Ann Neurol 18:698, 1985.
74. Marshall J, Meadows S: The natural history of amaurosis fugax. Brain 91:419, 1968.
75. Parkin PJ, Kendall BE, Marshall J, et al: Amaurosis fugax: Some aspects of management. J Neurol Neurosurg Psychiatry 45:1, 1982.
76. Poole CJM, Ross Russell RW: Mortality and stroke after amaurosis fugax. J Neurol Neurosurg Psychiatry 48:902, 1985.
77. Harrison MJG, Marshall J: Arteriographic comparison of amaurosis fugax and hemispheric transient ischemic attacks. Stroke 16:795, 1985.
78. Ross Russell RW: Natural history of amaurosis fugax. *In* Bernstein EF (ed): Amaurosis Fugax. New York, Springer-Verlag, 1988, p 174.
79. Goodwin JA, Gorelick PB, Helgason CM: Symptoms of amaurosis fugax in atherosclerotic carotid artery disease. Neurology 37:829, 1987.
80. Harrison MJG, Marshall J: Prognostic significance of severity of carotid atheroma in early manifestations of cerebrovascular disease. Stroke 13:567, 1982.
81. Adams HP, Putman SF, Corbett JJ, et al: Amaurosis fugax: The results of arteriography in 59 patients. Stroke 14:742, 1983.
82. Bernstein EF, Dilley RB: Late results after carotid endarterectomy for amaurosis fugax. J Vasc Surg 6:333, 1987.
83. Harrison MJG: Angiography in amaurosis fugax. *In* Bernstein EF (ed): Amaurosis Fugax. New York, Springer-Verlag, 1988, p 227.
84. Eikelboom BC, Riles TR, Mintzer R, et al: Inaccuracy of angiography in the diagnosis of carotid ulceration. Stroke 14:882, 1983.
85. Otis SM: Noninvasive vascular examination in amaurosis fugax. *In* Bernstein EF (ed): Amaurosis Fugax. New York, Springer-Verlag, 1988, p 183.
86. Rizzo J: The retina. *In* Lessell S, van Dalen JTW (eds): Current Neuro-Ophthalmol, 3rd ed. St. Louis, Mosby-Year Book, 1991, p 237.
87. Caplan LR, Pessin MS: Symptomatic carotid artery disease and carotid endarterectomy. Annu Rev Med 39:273, 1988.
88. Moore WS, Boren C, Malone J, et al: Natural history of nonstenotic asymptomatic ulcerative lesions of the carotid artery. Arch Surg 113:1352, 1978.
89. Dixon S, Pais O, Raviola C, et al: Natural history of nonstenotic, asymptomatic ulcerative lesions of the carotid artery. Arch Surg 117:1493, 1982.
90. Chikos PM, Fisher LD, Hirsch JH, et al: Observer variability in evaluating extracranial carotid artery stenosis. Stroke 14:885, 1983.
91. Peterson P, Boysen G, Godtfredsen J, et al: Placebo controlled, randomized trial of warfarin and aspirin for prevention of thromboembolic complications in chronic atrial fibrillation: The Copenhagen AFASAK study. Lancet 1:175, 1989.
92. Peterson P, Boysen G: Prevention of stroke in atrial fibrillation. N Engl J Med 323:482, 1990.
93. Stroke Prevention in Atrial Fibrillation Study Group Investigators: Preliminary report of the stroke prevention in atrial fibrillation study. N Engl J Med 322:863, 1990.
94. The Boston Area Anticoagulation Trial for Atrial Fibrillation Investigators: The effect of low-dose warfarin on the risk of stroke in patients with non-rheumatic atrial fibrillation. N Engl J Med 323:1505, 1990.
95. Chesbro JH, Fuster V, Halperin JL: Atrial fibrillation—Risk marker for stroke. N Engl J Med 323:1556, 1990.
96. Easton JD, Hart RG, Sherman DG, et al: Diagnosis and management of ischemic stroke. I: Threatened stroke and its management. Curr Probl Cardiol 8:1, 1983.
97. Whisnant JP, Wiebers DO: Clinical epidemiology of transient cerebral ischemic attacks (TIA) in the anterior and posterior cerebral circulation. *In* Sundt TM (ed): Occlusive Cerebrovascular Disease: Diagnosis and Surgical Management. Philadelphia, WB Saunders, 1987, p 60.
98. Rokey R, Rolak LA, Harati Y, et al: Coronary artery disease in patients with cerebrovascular disease: A prospective study. Ann Neurol 16:50, 1984.
99. Savino PJ, Glaser JS, Cassady J: Retinal stroke: Is the patient at risk? Arch Ophthalmol 95:1185, 1977.

100. Howard RS, Ross Russell RW: Prognosis of patients with retinal embolism. J Neurol Neurosurg Psychiatry 50:1142, 1987.
101. Pfaffenbach DD, Hollenhorst RW: Morbidity and survivorship of patients with embolic cholesterol crystallization in the ocular fundus. Am J Ophthalmol 75:66, 1973.
102. Trobe JD: Carotid endarterectomy: Who needs it? Ophthalmology 94:725, 1987.
103. Jones S: Can carotid endarterectomy be justified? No. Arch Neurol 44:652, 1987.
104. American Neurological Association Committee on Health Care Issues: Does carotid endarterectomy decrease stroke and death in patients with transient ischemic attacks? Ann Neurol 22:72, 1987.
105. Winslow CM, Solomon DH, Chassin MR, et al: The appropriateness of carotid endarterectomy. N Engl J Med 318:721, 1988.
106. Scheinberg P: Controversies in the management of cerebral vascular disease. Neurology 38:1609, 1988.
107. Patterson RH: Can carotid endarterectomy be justified? Yes. Arch Neurol 44:651, 1987.
108. Hachinski V: Carotid endarterectomy. Arch Neurol 44:654, 1987.
109. Report of the American Academy of Neurology, Therapeutics and Technology Assessment Subcommittee: Interim assessment: Carotid endarterectomy. Neurology 40:682, 1990.
110. Stewart G, Ross-Russell RW, Browse NL: Long-term results of carotid endarterectomy for transient ischemic attacks. J Vasc Surg 4:600, 1986.
111. Browse NL, Ross-Russell R: Carotid endarterectomy and the Javid shunt: The early results of 215 consecutive operations for transient ischaemic attacks. Br J Surg 71:53, 1984.
112. Becker WL, Burde RM: Carotid artery disease: A therapeutic enigma. Arch Ophthalmol 106:34, 1988.
113. Adams HP, Kassell NF, Mazuz H: The patient with transient ischemic attacks: Is this the time for a new therapeutic approach? Stroke 15:371, 1984.
114. Antiplatelet Trialists' Collaboration: Secondary prevention of vascular disease by prolonged anti-platelet treatment. Br Med J 296:320, 1988.
115. Scheinberg P: Controversies in the management of cerebral vascular disease. Neurology 38:1609, 1988.
116. Rossouw JE, Lewis B, Rifkind BM, et al: The value of lowering cholesterol after myocardial infarction. N Engl J Med 323:1112, 1990.
117. Hypertension Detection and Follow-up Program Cooperative Group: Five year findings of the hypertensive detection and follow-up program. III: Reduction in stroke incidence among persons with high blood pressure. JAMA 247:663, 1982.
118. Whelton PK: Declining mortality from hypertension and stroke. South Med J 75:33, 1982.
119. Yatsu FM, Fisher CM: Atherosclerosis: Current concepts on pathogenesis and interventional therapies. Ann Neurol 26:3, 1989.
120. Von Graefe A: Ueber Embolie der arteria centralis retinae als Ursache plötzlicher Erblindung. Arch Ophthalmol 5:136, 1859.
121. Hayreh SS, Kolder HE, Weingeist TA: Central retinal artery occlusion and retinal tolerance time. Ophthalmology 87:75, 1980.
122. Hayreh SS, Weingeist TA: Experimental occlusion of the central artery of the retina. IV: Retinal tolerance time to acute ischaemia. Br J Ophthalmol 64:818, 1980.
123. Lessell S, Miller JR: Optic nerve and retina after experimental circulatory arrest. Invest Ophthalmol 14:146, 1975.
124. Perkins SA, Magargal LE, Augsburger JJ, et al: The idling retina: Reversible visual loss in central retinal artery obstruction. Ann Ophthalmol 19:3, 1987.
125. Duker JS, Brown GC: Recovery following acute obstruction of the retinal and choroidal circulations. Retina 8:257, 1988.
126. Brown GC, Magargal LE, Shields JA, et al: Retinal arterial obstruction in children and young adults. Ophthalmology 88:18, 1981.
127. Coppeto J, Lessell S: Retinopathy in systemic lupus erythematosus. Arch Ophthalmol 95:794, 1977.
128. Wilson RS, Ruiz RS: Bilateral central retinal artery occlusion in homocystinuria: A case report. Arch Ophthalmol 82:267, 1969.
129. Sher NA, Reiff W, Letson RD, et al: Central retinal artery occlusion complicating Fabry's disease. Arch Ophthalmol 96:815, 1978.
130. Jampol LM, Wong AS, Albert DM: Atrial myxoma and central retinal artery occlusion. Am J Ophthalmol 75:242, 1973.
131. Silverman J, Olwin JS, Graettinger JS: Cardiac myxomas with systemic embolization. Circulation 26:99, 1962.
132. Sybers HD, Boake WC: Coronary and retinal embolism from left atrial myxoma. Arch Pathol 91:178, 1971.
133. Manschot WA: Embolism of the central retinal artery originating from an endocardial myxoma. Am J Ophthalmol 48:381, 1959.
134. Brown GC, Magargal LE, Sergott R: Acute obstruction of the retinal and choroidal circulations. Ophthalmology 93:1373, 1986.
135. Brown GC, Magargal LE: Central retinal artery obstruction and visual acuity. Ophthalmology 89:14, 1982.
136. Appen RE, Wray SH, Cogan DG: Central retinal artery occlusion. Am J Ophthalmol 79:374, 1975.
137. Karjalainen K: Occlusion of the central retinal artery and retinal branch arterioles: A clinical, tonographic and fluorescein angiographic study of 175 patients. Acta Ophthalmol 109:12, 1971.
138. Gold D: Retinal arterial occlusion. Symposium: Retinal Vascular Disease. Trans Am Acad Ophthalmol Otol 83:392, 1977.
139. Richards RD: Simultaneous occlusion of the central retinal artery and vein. Trans Am Ophthalmol Soc 77:191, 1979.
140. Augsburger JJ, Magargal LE: Visual prognosis following treatment of acute central retinal obstruction. Br J Ophthalmol 64:913, 1980.
141. Ffytche TJ: A rationalization of treatment of central retinal artery occlusion. Trans Ophthalmol Soc UK 94:468, 1974.
142. Hayreh SS: The cilioretinal arteries. Br J Ophthalmol 47:71, 1963.
143. Justice J, Lehmann RP: Cilioretinal arteries. Arch Ophthalmol 94:1355, 1976.
144. Brown GC, Shields JA: Cilioretinal arteries and retinal arterial occlusion. Arch Ophthalmol 97:84, 1979.
145. Levy A: Obstruction of cilio-retinal artery. Trans Ophthalmol Soc UK 29:130, 1909.
146. Brown GC, Moffatt K, Cruess A, et al: Cilioretinal artery obstruction. Retina 3:182, 1983.
147. Zentmayer W: Embolism of a cilioretinal artery. Ophthalmol Rec 15:613, 1906.
148. Krauss F: Embolism of the cilioretinal artery. Ophthalmol Rec 16:196, 1907.
149. Levitt JM: Occlusion of the cilioretinal artery. Arch Ophthalmol 40:152, 1948.
150. Brosnan DW: Occlusion of a cilioretinal artery. Am J Ophthalmol 53:687, 1962.
151. Friedman MW: Occlusion of the cilioretinal artery. Am J Ophthalmol 49:684, 1959.
152. Perry HD, Mallen FJ: Cilioretinal artery occlusion associated with oral contraceptives. Am J Ophthalmol 84:56, 1977.
153. McLeod D, Ring CP: Cilio-retinal infarction after retinal vein occlusion. Br J Ophthalmol 60:419, 1976.
154. Schatz H, Fong ACO, McDonald HR: Cilioretinal artery occlusion in young adults with central retinal vein occlusion. Ophthalmology 98:594, 1991.
155. McLeod D: Cilio-retinal arterial circulation in central retinal vein occlusion. Br J Ophthalmol 59:486, 1975.
156. Liversedge LA, Smith VH: Neuromedical and ophthalmic aspects of central retinal artery occlusion. Trans Ophthalmol Soc UK 82:571, 1962.
157. Ross Russell RW, Page NGR: Critical perfusion of brain and retina. Brain 106:419, 1983.
158. Brown GC, Magargal LE, Simeone FA, et al: Arterial obstruction and ocular neovascularization. Ophthalmology 89:139, 1982.
159. Coppeto JR, Wand M, Bear L, et al: Neovascular glaucoma and carotid artery obstructive disease. Am J Ophthalmol 99:567, 1985.
160. Sturrock GD, Mueller HR: Chronic ocular ischaemia. Br J Ophthalmol 68:716, 1984.
161. Bolling JP, Buettner H: Acquired retinal arteriovenous communications in occlusive disease of the carotid artery. Ophthalmology 97:1148, 1990.
162. Gass JDM, Tiedeman J, Thomas MA: Idiopathic recurrent branch retinal arterial occlusion. Ophthalmology 93:1148, 1986.
163. Delaney WV, Torrisi PF: Occlusive retinal vascular disease and deafness. Am J Ophthalmol 82:232, 1976.
164. Monteiro MLR, Swanson RA, Coppeto JR, et al: A microangio-

pathic syndrome of encephalopathy, hearing loss, and retinal arteriolar occlusions. Neurology 35:1113, 1985.
165. von Sallmann L, Myers RE, Lerner EM II, et al: Vasculo-occlusive retinopathy in experimental allergic encephalomyelitis. Arch Ophthalmol 78:112, 1967.
166. Coppeto JR, Currie JN, Monteiro MLR, et al: A syndrome of arterial-occlusive retinopathy and encephalopathy. Am J Ophthalmol 98:189, 1984.
167. Grand MG, Kaine J, Fulling K, et al: Cerebroretinal vasculopathy: A new hereditary syndrome. Ophthalmology 95:649, 1988.
168. Sawyer RA, Selhorst JB, Zimmerman LE, et al: Blindness caused by photoreceptor degeneration as a remote effect of cancer. Am J Ophthalmol 81:606, 1976.
169. Kornguth SE, Klein R, Appen R, et al: Occurrence of anti-retinal ganglion cell antibodies in patients with small cell carcinoma of the lung. Cancer 50:1289, 1982.
170. Kornguth SE, Kalinke T, Grunwald GB, et al: Anti-neurofilament antibodies in the sera of patients with small cell carcinoma of the lung and with visual paraneoplastic syndrome. Cancer Res 46:2588, 1986.
171. Keltner JL, Roth AM, Chang RS: Photoreceptor degeneration: Possible autoimmune disorder. Arch Ophthalmol 101:564, 1983.
172. Buchanan TAS, Gardiner TA, Archer DB: An ultrastructural study of retinal photoreceptor degeneration associated with bronchial carcinoma. Am J Ophthalmol 97:277, 1984.
173. Klingele TG, Burde RM, Rappazzo JA, et al: Paraneoplastic retinopathy. J Clin Neuro Ophthalmol 4:239, 1984.
174. Grunwald GB, Klein R, Simmonds MA, et al: Autoimmune basis for visual paraneoplastic syndrome in patients with small-cell lung carcinoma. Lancet 1:658, 1985.
175. Grunwald GB, Kornguth SE, Towfighi J, et al: Autoimmune basis for visual paraneoplastic syndrome in patients with small cell lung carcinoma. Cancer 60:780, 1987.
176. Thirkill CE, Roth AM, Keltner JL: Cancer-associated retinopathy. Arch Ophthalmol 105:372, 1987.
177. Van Der Pol BAE, Planten JTH: A non-metastatic remote effect of lung carcinoma. Doc Ophthalmol 67:89, 1987.
178. Berson EL, Lessell S: Paraneoplastic night blindness with malignant melanoma. Am J Ophthalmol 106:307, 1988.
179. Thirkill CE, Fitzgerald P, Sergott RC, et al: Cancer-associated retinopathy (CAR syndrome) with antibodies reacting with retinal, optic-nerve, and cancer cells. N Engl J Med 321:1589, 1989.
180. Jacobson DM, Thirkill CE, Tipping SJ: A clinical triad to diagnose paraneoplastic retinopathy. Ann Neurol 28:162, 1990.
181. Nunez JAV, Velasco FB, Fernandez-Tejerina JC, et al: Degeneracion retiniana paraneoplasica. Med Clin (Barc) 88:431, 1987.
182. Crofts JW, Bachynski BN, Odel JG: Visual paraneoplastic syndrome associated with undifferentiated endometrial carcinoma. Can J Ophthalmol 23:128, 1988.
183. Rizzo JF III, Gittinger JW: Selective immunohistochemical staining in the paraneoplastic retinopathy syndrome. Ophthalmology 99:1286, 1992.
184. Boghen DR, Sebag M, Michaud J: Paraneoplastic optic neuritis and encephalomyelitis: Report of a case. Arch Neurol 45:353, 1988.
185. Gass JDM, Gieser RG, Wilkinson CP, et al: Bilateral diffuse uveal melanocytic proliferation in patients with occult carcinoma. Arch Ophthalmol 108:527, 1990.
186. Miller NR: Walsh and Hoyt's Clinical Neuro-Ophthalmology, vol 1. Baltimore, Williams & Wilkins, 1982, p 321.
187. Cogan DG: Heredodegenerations of the retina. *In* Smith JL (ed): Neuro-Ophthalmology. Symposium of the University of Miami and the Bascum Palmer Eye Institute, vol 2, St. Louis, CV Mosby 1965, p 44.
188. Kivlin JD, Sanborn GE, Myers GG: The cherry-red spot in Tay-Sachs and other storage diseases. Ann Neurol 17:356, 1985.
189. Kolodny EH, Cable WJL: Inborn errors of metabolism. Ann Neurol 11:221, 1982.
190. Coppeto JR, Lessell S: A familial syndrome of dystonia, blepharospasm, and pigmentary retinopathy. Neurology 40:1359, 1990.
191. Konigsmark BW, Weiner LP: The olivopontocerebellar atrophies: A review. Medicine 49:227, 1970.
192. Traboulsi EI, Maumenee IH, Green WR, et al: Olivopontocerebellar atrophy with retinal degeneration: A clinical and ocular histopathologic study. Arch Ophthalmol 106:801, 1988.
193. Hamilton SR, Chatrian G-E, Mills RP, et al: Cone dysfunction in a subgroup of patients with autosomal dominant cerebellar ataxia. Arch Ophthalmol 108:551, 1990.
194. Trauner DA: Olivopontocerebellar atrophy with dementia, blindness, and chorea: Response to baclofen. Arch Neurol 42:757, 1985.
195. Schochet SS Jr, Font RL, Morris HH: Jansky-Bielschowsky form of neuronal ceroid-lipofuscinosis: Ocular pathology of the Batten-Vogt syndrome. Arch Ophthalmol 98:1083, 1980.
196. Goebel HH, Zeman W, Damaske E: An ultrastructural study of the retina in the Jansky-Bielschowsky type of neuronal ceroid-lipofuscinosis. Am J Ophthalmol 83:70, 1977.
197. Carroll WM, Kriss A, Baraitser M, et al: The incidence and nature of visual pathway involvement in Friedreich's ataxia: A clinical and visual evoked potential study of 22 patients. Brain 103:413, 1980.
198. Hoyt CS: Autosomal dominant optic atrophy: A spectrum of disability. Ophthalmology 87:245, 1980.
199. Kollarits CR, Pinheiro ML, Swann ER, et al: The autosomal dominant syndrome of progressive optic atrophy and congenital deafness. Am J Ophthalmol 87:789, 1979.
200. Konigsmark BW, Knox DL, Hussels IE, et al: Dominant congenital deafness and progressive optic nerve atrophy. Arch Ophthalmol 91:99, 1974.
201. Sylvester PE: Some unusual findings in a family with Friedreich's ataxia. Arch Dis Child 33:217, 1958.
202. Nyssen R, van Bogaert L: La degenerescence systematisée optico-cochleo-dentelée. Rev Neurol 62:321, 1934.
203. Müller J, Zeman W: Degenerescence systematisée optico-cochleo-dentelée. Acta Neuropathol 5:26, 1965.
204. Lessell S, Rosman NP: Juvenile diabetes mellitus and optic atrophy. Arch Neurol 34:759, 1977.
205. Kocher GA, Spoor TC, Ferguson JG: Progressive visual loss, diabetes mellitus, and associated abnormalities (DIDMOAD syndrome). J Clin Neuro Ophthalmol 2:241, 1982.
206. Behr C: Die komplizierte, hereditar-familare optikusatrophie des kindesalters: Ein bisher nicht beschriebener symptomkomplex. Klin Monatsbl Augenheilkd 47:138, 1909.
207. Francois J: Les atrophies optiques héréditaires. J Genet Hum 24:183, 1976.
208. Francois J: Hereditary degeneration of the optic nerve (hereditary optic atrophy). Int Ophthalmol Clin 8:999, 1968.
209. Horoupian DS, Zucker DK, Moshe S, et al: Behr syndrome: A clinicopathologic report. Neurology 29:323, 1979.
210. Hoyt WF: Charcot-Marie-Tooth disease with primary optic atrophy. Arch Ophthalmol 64:925, 1960.
211. Burki E: Ophthalmologische befunde be der neuralen muckelatrophie: Charcot-Marie-Tooth, HMSN Typ 1. Klin Monatsbl Augenheilkd 179:94, 1981.
212. Sommer C, Schröder JM: Hereditary motor and sensory neuropathy with optic atrophy: Ultrastructural and morphometric observations on nerve fibers, mitochondria, and dense-cored vesicles. Arch Neurol 46:973, 1989.
213. Costeff H, Gadoth N, Apter N, et al: A familial syndrome of infantile optic atrophy, movement disorder, and spastic paraplegia. Neurology 39:595, 1989.
214. Rizzo J, Lessell S: Optic atrophy in familial dysautonomia. Am J Ophthalmol 102:463, 1986.
215. Collins MLZ, Traboulsi EI, Maumenee IH: Optic nerve head swelling and optic atrophy in the systemic mucopolysaccharidoses. Ophthalmology 97:1445, 1990.
216. Traboulsi EI, Maumenee IH: Ophthalmologic manifestations of X-linked childhood adrenoleukodystrophy. Ophthalmology 94:47, 1987.
217. Usui T, Sawaguchi S, Abe H, et al: Late-infantile type galactosialidosis: Histopathology of the retina and optic nerve. Arch Ophthalmol 109:542, 1991.
218. Brownstein S, Carpenter S, Polomeno RC, et al: Sandhoff's disease (G_{M2} gangliosidosis type 2): Histopathology and ultrastructure of the eye. Arch Ophthalmol 98:1089, 1980.
219. Matthews JD, Weiter JJ, Kolodny EH: Macular halos associated with Niemann-Pick type B disease. Ophthalmology 93:933, 1986.
220. Cogan DG, Chu FC, Barranger JA, et al: Macula halo syndrome: Variant of Niemann-Pick disease. Arch Ophthalmol 101:1698, 1983.

221. Bloomfield SE, David DS, Rubin AL: Eye findings in the diagnosis of Fabry's disease. JAMA 240:647, 1978.
222. Cogan DG, Chu FC, Gittinger J, et al: Fundal abnormalities of Gaucher's disease. Arch Ophthalmol 98:2202, 1980.
223. Riedel KG, Zwaan J, Kenyon KR, et al: Ocular abnormalities in mucolipidosis IV. Am J Ophthalmol 99:125, 1985.
224. Rizzo J, Berson E, Lessell S: Retinal and neurological findings in the Laurence-Moon-Bardet-Biedl phenotype. Ophthalmology 93:1452, 1986.
225. Cox TA, McDarby JV, Lavine L, et al: A retinopathy on Guam with high prevalence in Lytico-Bodig. Ophthalmology 96:1731, 1989.
226. Sipilä I, Simell O, Rapola J, et al: Gyrate atrophy of the choroid and retina with hyperornithinemia: Tubular aggregates and type 2 fiber atrophy in muscle. Neurology 29:996, 1979.
227. Keith CG: Retinal atrophy in osteopetrosis. Arch Ophthalmol 79:234, 1968.
228. Ruben JB, Morris RJ, Judisch GF: Chorioretinal degeneration in infantile malignant osteopetrosis. Am J Ophthalmol 110:1, 1990.
229. Fletcher WA, Imes RK, Goodman D, et al: Acute idiopathic blind spot enlargement: A big blind spot syndrome without optic disc edema. Arch Ophthalmol 106:44, 1988.
230. Hamed LM, Glaser JS, Gass JDM, et al: Protracted enlargement of the blind spot in multiple evanescent white dot syndrome. Arch Ophthalmol 107:194, 1989.
231. Singh K, de Frank MP, Shults WT, et al: Acute idiopathic blind spot enlargement: A spectrum of disease. Ophthalmology 98:497, 1991.
232. Dodwell DG, Jampol LM, Rosenberg M, et al: Optic nerve involvement associated with the multiple evanescent white-dot syndrome. Ophthalmology 97:862, 1990.
233. Khorram KD, Jampol LM, Rosenberg MA: Blind spot enlargement as a manifestation of multifocal choroiditis. Arch Ophthalmol 109:1403, 1991.
234. Gass JDM, Hameed LM: Acute macular neuroretinopathy and multiple evanescent white dot syndrome occurring in the same patients. Arch Ophthalmol 107:189, 1989.
235. Miller MH, Spalton DJ, Fitzke FW, et al: Acute macular neuroretinopathy. Ophthalmology 96:265, 1989.
236. Levine SR, Welch KMA: Antiphospholipid antibodies. Ann Neurol 26:386, 1989.
237. Levine SR, Deegan MJ, Futrell N, et al: Cerebrovascular and neurologic disease associated with antiphospholipid antibodies: 48 cases. Neurol 40:1181, 1990.
238. Brey RL, Hart RG, Sherman DG, et al: Antiphospholipid antibodies and cerebral ischemia in young people. Neurology 40:1190, 1990.
239. Digre KB, Durcan FJ, Branch DW, et al: Amaurosis fugax associated with antiphospholipid antibodies. Ann Neurol 25:228, 1989.
240. Briley DP, Coull BM, Goodnight SH: Neurological disease associated with antiphospholipid antibodies. Ann Neurol 25:221, 1989.
241. Gerber SL, Cantor LB: Progressive optic atrophy and the primary antiphospholipid antibody syndrome. Am J Ophthalmol 110:443, 1990.
242. Young SM, Fisher M, Sigsbee A, et al: Cardiogenic brain embolism and lupus anticoagulant. Ann Neurol 26:390, 1989.
243. Kleiner RC, Najarian LV, Schatten S, et al: Vaso-occlusive retinopathy associated with anti-phospholipid antibodies (lupus anticoagulant retinopathy). Ophthalmology 96:896, 1989.
244. Kushner MJ: Prospective study of anticardiolipin antibodies in stroke. Stroke 21:295, 1990.

Chapter 200

Optic Atrophy and Papilledema

ALFREDO A. SADUN

OPTIC ATROPHY

Optic atrophy is a misnomer. Although the term *atrophy* generally refers to physiologic involution or reduction, *optic atrophy* refers to cell death. In particular, optic atrophy represents the permanent loss of retinal ganglion cell axons always associated with retinal ganglion cell death in the retina. However, optic atrophy should not be considered a diagnosis; it is a pathologic end-point that is clinically discernible. Optic atrophy may be due to injury of the optic nerve head. However, because of anterograde and retrograde degeneration, it may reflect upstream injury of the retinal ganglion cells or downstream injury of the posterior optic nerve, optic chiasm, or optic tract. It is clinically very useful to try to differentiate optic atrophy into primary or secondary optic atrophy.

Primary Optic Atrophy

The term *primary optic atrophy* may be confusing because primary optic atrophy is, in fact, secondary to injury at any level of the retinal ganglion cell and its axon. A less confusing alternative term would be *simple optic atrophy*. The essence of primary or simple optic atrophy is a loss of optic nerve fibers with otherwise minimal disturbance of the optic nerve anatomy. In particular, primary optic atrophy is attended by only minimal gliosis.

Primary or simple optic atrophy can be a consequence of any injury of the retinal ganglion cell or its axon in the nerve fiber layer; the optic nerve head; the orbital, intracanalicular, or intracranial optic nerve; optic chiasm; optic tract; or lateral geniculate nucleus. However, the causes of primary or simple optic atrophy do not involve significant amounts of optic disc inflammation or optic disc edema.[1] Common causes of primary optic atrophy include anterior ischemic optic neuropathy, optic neuritis, and compressive lesions of the optic nerve, including orbital (e.g., optic nerve sheath meningioma), intracranial (e.g., olfactory groove meningioma), or optic chiasmic (e.g., pituitary adenoma) tumors.[2] Other ischemic, inflammatory, and compressive lesions can also produce primary or simple optic atrophy. Less common causes include posterior ischemic optic neuropathy, trauma, granulomatous inflammations of the optic nerve, or ophthalmic artery aneurysms that compress the optic nerve.[2, 3] Optic atrophy has been described in Alzheimer's disease[4, 5] and, to a lesser extent, occurs with age.[6, 7] In addition, long-standing disc edema can produce optic atrophy (Figs. 200–1 to 200–3). Glaucoma is a very common cause of optic atrophy.[8] All causes of primary or simple optic atrophy result in a loss of axons with some associated gliosis, a reduction in optic nerve diameter (Fig. 200–4), a diminution of number and size of blood vessels, and a slight thickening of the connective tissue septa.[1] Regional optic atrophy is histopathologically evident as zones of demyelination (Fig. 200–5).

Primary (simple) optic atrophy, in its severe form, is characterized funduscopically by an optic disc that appears white in appearance and has clearly delineated borders (Figs. 200–6 and 200–7). In some cases, the surface of the disc may appear waxy. Most important, no shaggy or gray, fuzzy gliotic reaction is seen overlying the disc or at its margins. It is this absence of a gliotic reaction that defines primary or simple optic atrophy and is the basis for its clinical distinction.

The pink or rose color of the disc is absent in primary or simple optic atrophy because of decreased blood perfusion. The loss of the normal pink color of the optic disc in optic atrophy may be a direct manifestation of capillary dropout. Others postulate that columns of optic nerve axons normally act as light pipes conducting the red color of capillaries to the surface; optic atrophy interferes with our fiberoptic view of disc capillaries.[9]

Optic atrophy may also be noted by a reduction in the number of small blood vessels crossing the disc margin (Kestenbaum's capillary number test), from a normal of about 10 down to 7 or even fewer (Figs. 200–6 and 200–7).[10, 11] In addition, constriction of the papillary or peripapillary blood vessels may occur, probably reflecting decreased inner retinal perfusion associated with the loss of retinal ganglion cells in optic atrophy. Quigley and colleagues have demonstrated histologically that optic disc capillaries drop out in proportion to axonal loss.[12] This is corroborated by measuring arteriolar diameters by fluorescein angiography[13] or by using noninvasive methods for measuring optic disc and retinal blood flow in patients with optic atrophy.[14, 15] Thinning of the nerve fiber layer associated with optic atrophy probably accounts for the alterations in light reflexes in the peripapillary retina and macula in patients with optic atrophy.[16] In certain forms of primary optic atrophy, such as in retinitis pigmentosa, the surface of the disc also takes on a shiny, waxy appearance. Optic disc atrophy may vary widely in appearance. The reduction of blood supply, disruption of axon columns, and formation of glial bridges may account for changes from slight temporal (disc) pallor to a chalk-white optic nerve head. However, the absence of optic disc color may be difficult to describe or quantitate.[10] Factors such as type of illumination, changes in the ocular media (e.g., cataract), and even weak ophthalmoscope batteries may influence the perception of optic disc coloration.[10]

The nature and extent of optic nerve injury also affect the disc appearance. The optic disc atrophy may be slight, moderate, or severe. The atrophy may be diffuse or confined to one sector. In anterior ischemic optic neuropathy, the atrophy is often limited to the upper or

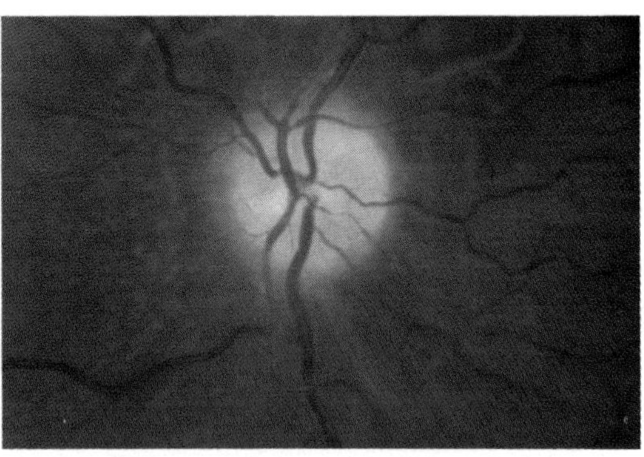

Figure 200–2. The same optic disc depicted in Figure 200–1, 2 mo after the intracranial pressure had been brought down to normal levels. The disc edema has resolved, leaving behind secondary optic atrophy. The changes associated with secondary optic atrophy can be fairly subtle. Despite the absence of severe disc pallor, visual restriction in this eye was extremely severe.

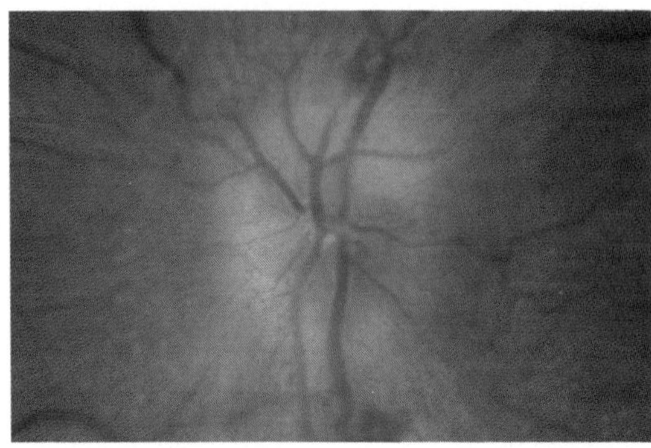

Figure 200–1. Chronic and resolving optic disc edema in an obese 15-year-old boy with pseudotumor cerebri. The intraocular pressure of 520 mm of water at diagnosis was brought down to under 200 mm for 10 days, leading to the partial resolution of this previously fulminate disc edema.

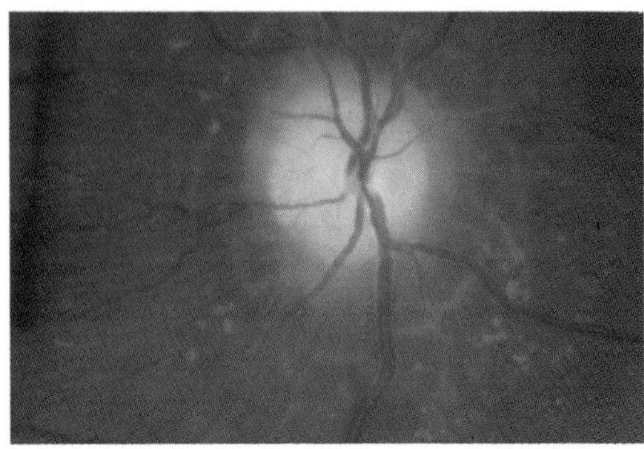

Figure 200–3. The other eye of the patient described in Figure 200–1. Secondary optic atrophy is seen in a slightly more severe form. Note the hazy, grayish margins. The patient's visual field was reduced to a central 5-degree island.

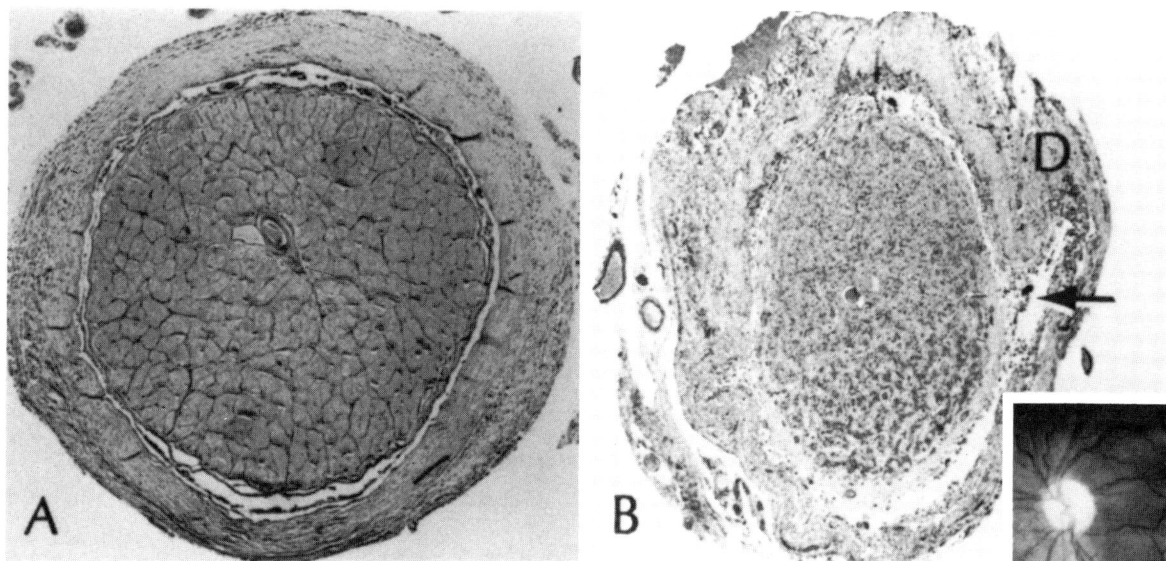

Figure 200–4. Optic atrophy. *A*, Normal optic nerve in cross section. H&E, ×8. *B*, Atrophic optic nerve at the same magnification shows shrinkage of the parenchyma, widening of the pial septa, gliosis, widening of the subarachnoid space (*arrow*), and redundant dura (D). H&E, ×8. *Inset*, Optic atrophy in a child. (From Duane TD, Jaeger EA [eds]: Biomedical Foundations of Ophthalmology, vol 3. New York, Harper & Row, 1985.

lower half of the disc. In chiasmal lesions, decussating fibers from the retina nasal to the fovea are primarily involved but the superior and inferior arcuate bundles are relatively spared, leading to atrophy in both temporal and nasal portions of the optic disc while the superior and inferior regions remain pink.[17] This so-called bow-tie or band optic atrophy is also seen in the eye contralateral to a unilateral optic tract lesion.[3, 18, 19] Such a lesion also causes temporal pallor of the ipsilateral optic disc because it involves the temporal retinal ganglion cells from that eye.

Over time, even sectoral involvement of the optic nerve appears to become more diffuse, probably reflecting at least a minor shift in position of the remaining intact axons. Optic atrophy from anterior ischemic optic neuropathy may, after 1 yr, look like diffuse optic atrophy or temporal pallor. Another important transformation in the appearance of optic atrophy can occur over time. Several months after the onset of atrophy, the optic disc may appear more excavated, giving the appearance of cupping similar to that in glaucoma.[20–22] It is unclear whether this reflects just a change in appearance or whether, in fact, optic atrophy proceeds to glaucomatous discs because of the inherent weakness of the optic disc brought on by the loss of the infrastructure of axons. Alternatively, the loss of optic nerve axons from aging may superimpose on the partly atrophied optic disc.[23, 24] It is possible that cases of low-tension glaucoma are in fact cases of optic atrophy secondary to other optic neuropathies, which in time transform into a cupped disc.[25] In at least some cases, the initially weakened optic disc becomes cupped and patients continue to show progressive visual field losses consistent with glaucoma.

The histopathologic findings of primary optic atrophy are unmistakable (Figs. 200–4 and 200–5).[1, 26, 27] The essence of primary optic atrophy is the absence of gliotic reaction on the surface of the optic disc. Nonetheless,

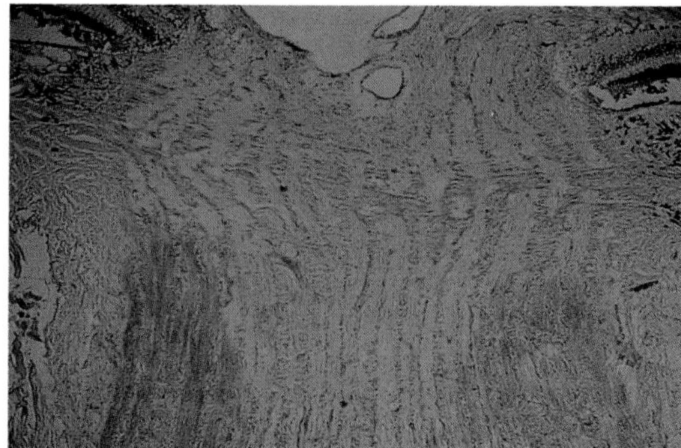

Figure 200–5. Sagittal view of atrophic optic nerve near the laminar cribrosa. Myelin stain demonstrates marked demyelination, reflecting optic atrophy particularly in the center and, to a lesser extent, the left side of the optic nerve. Wiegert, ×70.

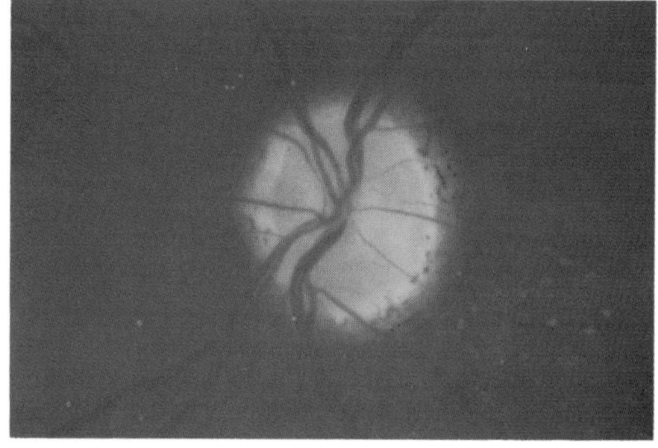

Figure 200–6. Primary optic atrophy. Extremely severe optic atrophy secondary to multiple episodes of optic neuritis. The patient's vision was reduced to no light perception.

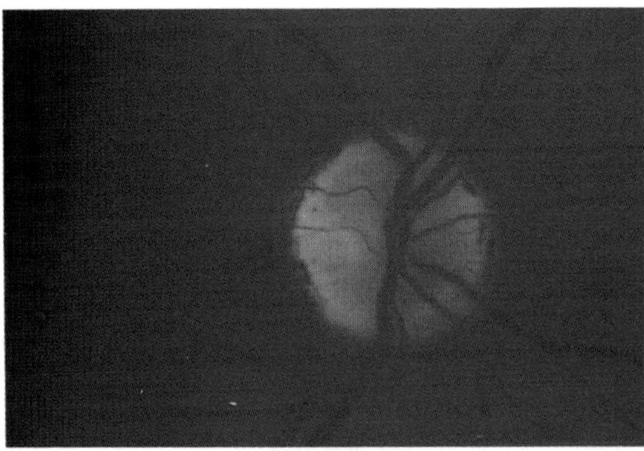

Figure 200–7. Other eye of the same patient depicted in Figure 200–6. Primary optic atrophy. This eye also had multiple episodes of optic neuritis; however, visual acuity was surprisingly good, 20/50. Note decreased number of blood vessels crossing disc margin (Kestenbaum's number).

some optic nerve axons are replaced by glia. Immediately after injury, microglia tend to accumulate. Proliferation of astrocytic glia follows shortly. Ultimately, as remyelination occurs, the number of oliogodendroglia may also be increased.[1]

Secondary Optic Atrophy

Secondary optic atrophy is sometimes referred to as *dirty optic atrophy*. Clinically, the distinction between primary and secondary optic atrophy is important because the latter is usually a consequence of severe papilledema (see Figs. 200–1 to 200–3). Secondary (dirty) optic atrophy reflects the disorganized appearance of the surface of the optic disc due to axonal injury in association with severe edema or inflammation at the optic nerve head.[1]

Although secondary optic atrophy most commonly occurs in cases of severe papilledema, it may also develop in cases of long-standing severe orbital inflammation. Patients with vitreous infections or severe uveitus, such as in unchecked Vogt-Koyanagi-Harada or Behçet's syndrome–associated uveitis, may be left with the appearance of a very fuzzy disc characteristic of secondary optic atrophy. More often, the observation of bilateral secondary optic atrophy provides an important clinical clue suggesting a past episode of prolonged severe papilledema. This finding is not uncommon in patients who have had undiagnosed or untreated pseudotumor cerebri (see Figs. 200–1 to 200–3).

The fundus has a characteristic appearance in secondary optic atrophy. The optic disc is grayish instead of pink or white. The margins appear fuzzy and blurred. The glial proliferation may be sufficient to give a raised appearance to the optic disc and its margins (see Fig. 200–3). The other funduscopic features of secondary optic atrophy are similar to those in primary optic atrophy. These include the absence of the pink color of perfusion, reduction in Kestenbaum's number, and constriction of the vasculature.[1, 25] However, because secondary optic atrophy is not characterized by a stark white optic disc, it may be misinterpreted as less severe than it really is (see Fig. 200–2).

Histopathologically, a great proliferation of glia is seen on the surface and edges of the optic disc. Astrocytes are seen throughout the optic disc and in heaps anterior to the disc. The other histologic features of optic atrophy remain the same, including loss of parenchyma due to loss of both myelin and axons with resultant shrinkage and widening of the septa. As in primary optic atrophy, the arachnoid and dural meninges thicken (see Fig. 200–4).[1]

Ascending Optic Atrophy

Ascending optic atrophy is characterized by degeneration of the axons at the level of the optic nerve head, secondary to retinal ganglion cell death in the retina. The degeneration begins at the cell body or at the site of disconnection between the axon and the cell body and then proceeds in an anterograde direction. Large axons may degenerate at a faster rate than small-caliber axons.[3] Degeneration that begins at the cell body and proceeds distally is termed *wallerian* or *ascending degeneration*. This degeneration follows the entire course of the axon from retinal cell body to nerve fiber layer, to optic nerve head, to optic nerve, to optic chiasm, to optic tract, and to axon terminals in the lateral geniculate nucleus. Degeneration at the optic disc (optic atrophy) can only occur in concert with retinal ganglion cell death.[28, 29] At the lateral geniculate nucleus, transsynaptic changes may be noted as well (Fig. 200–8).[30] Neurons in the layers of the lateral geniculate nucleus that correspond with the eye involved (layers 2, 3, and 5 receive ipsilateral ocular input) demonstrate shrinkage consisting of a reduction of cytoplasm and particularly of endoplasm reticulum (thus reducing their Nissl's staining). This does not represent transsynaptic degeneration because the lateral geniculate nucleus neurons are reduced in size rather than in number.[30] This transsynaptic anterograde atrophy of the lateral geniculate nucleus is seen in long-standing severe ocular disease, such as absolute glaucoma (see Fig. 200–8), or after trauma and enucleation of the eye.[31]

Descending Optic Atrophy

Descending optic atrophy occurs when the injury to the retinal ganglion cell axon is posterior to the optic nerve head (Figs. 200–9 to 200–11). The optic nerve degenerates in a retrograde (descending) direction, until the cell body in the retina eventually dies.[32] The time delay between the degeneration at the site of injury and the optic atrophy at the level of the disc probably varies only slightly with the distance between these two locations. At the maximum, it may take more than 1 mo for optic atrophy to occur after injury to the posterior portion of the optic tract.

Descending optic atrophy occurs with trauma to the orbital or intracranial optic nerve. Compressive lesions,

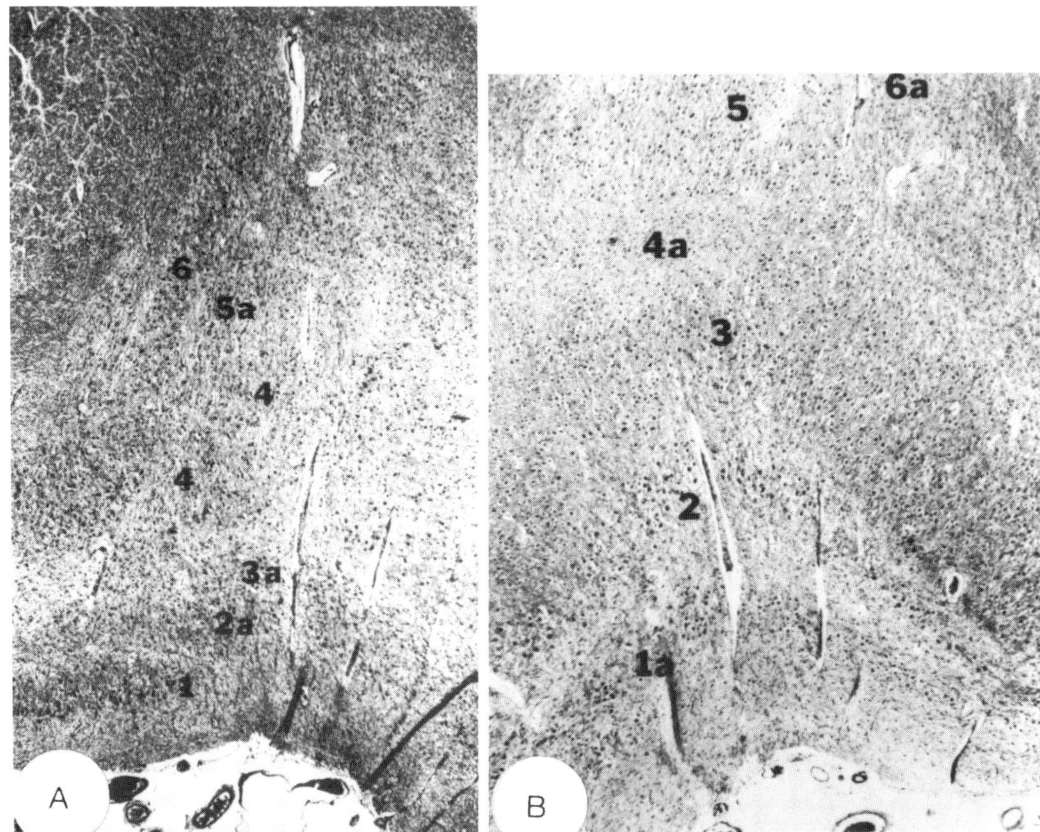

Figure 200–8. *A*, Lateral geniculate nucleus (LGN) demonstrating transsynaptic changes after long-term optic atrophy from absolute glaucoma. Cell bodies in layers 2, 3, and 5 receiving input from the ipsilateral glaucomatous eye have atrophied (a). *B*, High magnification of part *A*, demonstrating reduced Nissl's staining and cellular size of lateral geniculate neurons. Layers 1, 4, and 6 contain atrophic cell bodies (a). (From Sadun AA, Smythe BA, Schaechter JD: Optic neuritis or ophthalmic artery aneurysm? Case presentation with histopathologic documentation utilizing a new staining method. J Clin Neuro Ophthalmol 4:265–273, 1984.)

including tumors posterior to the optic nerve head, also produce descending optic atrophy. The most common tumors producing optic atrophy are sphenoid wing or optic nerve sheath meningiomas, optic nerve gliomas, pituitary adenomas, and chiasmal meningiomas. However, any form of compression, including that due to aneurysms or craniopharyngiomas, also produces descending optic atrophy. Inflammatory lesions such as optic neuritis are common causes of descending optic atrophy. Posterior ischemic optic neuropathy is an uncommon cause of descending optic atrophy. Toxic, metabolic, and nutritional lesions that affect the optic nerve posterior to the optic nerve head also produce descending optic atrophy.

Transsynaptic changes can also occur in a retrograde fashion. Thus, lesions affecting the optic radiations may lead to retrograde degeneration of lateral geniculate nucleus neurons.[31, 33] This can, usually over considerable time, lead to degeneration of the retinal ganglion cell and its axon, producing optic atrophy.[34] However, trans-

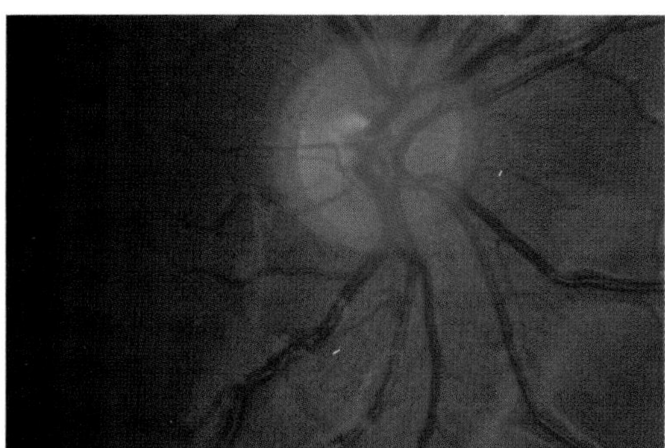

Figure 200–9. Normal right optic disc. Note pink coloration.

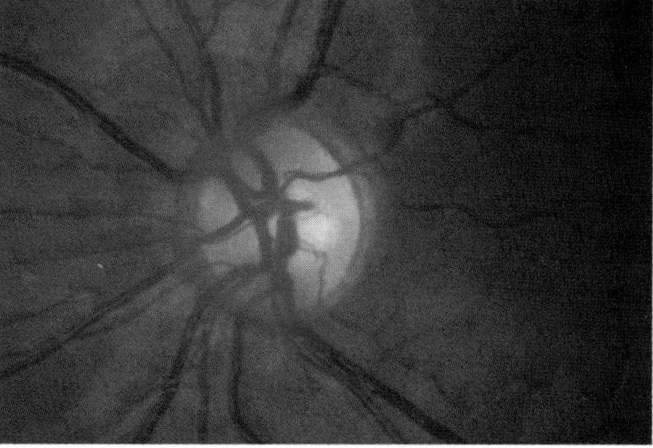

Figure 200–10. Left optic disc of patient in Figure 200–9. The patient had sustained complete transsection of the optic nerve at the level of the canal 22 days earlier. Note temporal pallor.

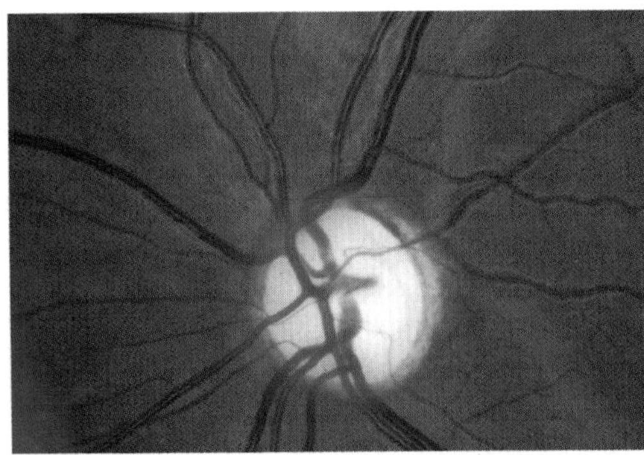

Figure 200–11. Same optic disc as in Figure 200–10. Note severe optic atrophy 2 mo after traumatic transsection of the optic nerve.

synaptic retrograde degeneration after injury to the visual cortex or optic radiations has been reported only infrequently in adults and only in cases with a very long-standing cortical lesion.[35, 36] More commonly, retrograde transsynaptic degeneration and optic atrophy have been reported in children and in animal studies.[31, 37]

Fundus Changes in Optic Atrophy

Severe optic atrophy always has a striking funduscopic appearance (see Figs. 200–6, 200–7, and 200–11). For the reasons described earlier, the normal pink color of the optic nerve head is lost. The temporal side of the disc usually appears paler than the nasal side (even in normal discs). In severe primary optic atrophy (see Figs. 200–6 and 200–7), the optic disc may appear chalk white with sharp margins. The blood vessels are likely to be constricted, and whether constricted or not, they appear to stand out in sharper relief in the peripapillary region. This is because of the drop-out of axons in the nerve fiber layer that normally surrounds the blood vessels.[38, 39] Other manifestations of nerve fiber layer losses can also be seen. The nerve fiber layer drop-out can be noted directly, especially by using a red-free filter, with a direct or indirect ophthalmoscope. Slitlike defects, wedge defects, and diffuse loss can be seen, as well as total atrophy.[39]

The pallor of the optic disc may be diffuse or confined to one sector, such as in anterior ischemic optic neuropathy. The appearance of secondary optic atrophy was described earlier. The margins of the disc are essentially hazy, and gliosis is seen overlying the disc. In mild cases of optic atrophy, greater reliance must be placed on looking for nerve fiber layer drop-out. Additionally, in young patients, it is often possible to see evidence of mild optic atrophy manifested by the loss of Gunn's dots. These are small bright reflectances in a hexagonal pattern seen best one to two disc diameters from the optic disc. The ophthalmoscope light catches the indentations in the internal limiting membrane produced by Müller's cell attachments. This parabolic reflection is lost with nerve fiber layer loss. Unfortunately, Gunn's dots are obliterated by various other retinal conditions as well as by age; this test is most useful in young patients in whom one eye can be used as a control for the other.

Histology

Microscopic examination of eyes and optic nerves from patients with optic atrophy demonstrates some ubiquitous findings. Shrinkage of the optic nerve is secondary to a loss of parenchyma (see Fig. 200–4).[1] This represents loss of retinal ganglion cell axons as well as the ensheathing myelin.[3] This loss also leads to a widening of the pial septa and other connective tissues. The subarachnoid space becomes larger, and the dura may become redundant (see Fig. 200–4). These changes may be limited to certain sectors of the optic nerve.[40] A small degree of gliosis is usually present, manifesting a proliferation of mainly astrocytes.[1] However, this gliosis is not as severe as it would be in an inflammatory condition of the optic nerve.

As the optic nerve axon degenerates, its myelin fragments and breaks down into spherules of lipid. Phagocytic macrophages attempt to engulf and remove this debris.[3] However, accumulations of lipid droplets often persist and may be remyelinated by oligodendrocytes in an apparent attempt to wall off this lipid material from adjacent intact axons.[41] Paraphenylene-diamine is a special stain that can identify remnants of axonal degeneration in the optic nerve even long after the injury (Figs. 200–12 and 200–13).[42, 43] After injury to the optic nerve and clinical optic atrophy, the paraphenylene-diamine technique reveals dark profiles that probably represent the reensheathment of myelin debris left behind after axonal death, as confirmed by electron microscopy (Fig. 200–14).[44]

Histopathologic study of the retina reveals depletion or complete loss of retinal ganglion cells and their axons that constitute the nerve fiber layer. The outer retinal layers may be completely normal. Histologic examination of the lateral geniculate nucleus may or may not show any changes, depending on the extent and duration of the optic atrophy. In cases of very severe monocular optic nerve loss of long duration, atrophy (true atrophy, not degeneration) may ensue in three of the six layers of the lateral geniculate nucleus that receive their afferents from the injured optic nerve.[31] Figures 200–8*A* and *B* depict a lateral geniculate nucleus from a patient who had absolute glaucoma on the ipsilateral side for 8 yr before death.

PAPILLEDEMA (DISC EDEMA)

Papilledema refers specifically to swelling of the optic disc that is believed to be secondary to increased intracranial pressure. Until this condition is ascertained, it is best to use the more generic term *optic disc edema*.[45, 46] Optic disc edema can be due to various causes reflecting pathology in the brain, eye, or optic nerve.

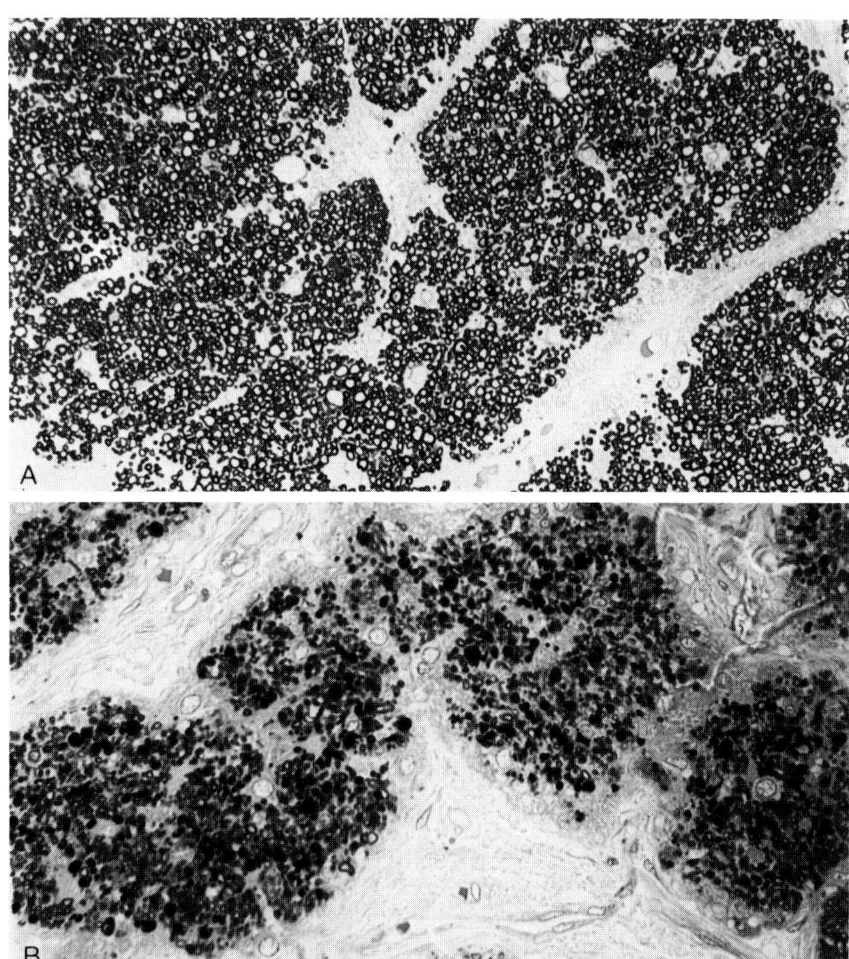

Figure 200–12. *A*, Cross section of a normal human optic nerve showing myelinated axon profiles. Paraphenylene-diamine, ×325. *B*, Cross section showing profiles indicative of axonal degeneration in human optic nerve. Paraphenylene-diamine, ×325.

A subarachnoid communication exists between the brain and the optic nerve; any increased intracranial pressure can be transmitted through the subarachnoid space to the optic nerve and nerve head.[45] Thus, increased intracranial pressure from tumor, from pseudotumor (benign intracranial hypertension), or from hydrocephalus may lead to anterior bulging of the optic nerve head. In order to rule out intracranial pathology as the cause of disc edema, it is usually wise to perform neuroimaging studies. Increased intracranial pressure in the absence of a space-occupying lesion or dilated ventricles usually leads to the diagnosis of pseudotumor cerebri.

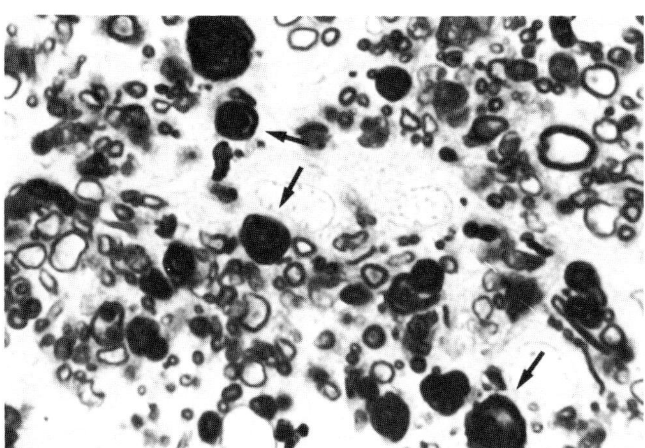

Figure 200–13. High magnification demonstrating optic nerve degeneration (*arrows*). Paraphenylene-diamine, ×1250.

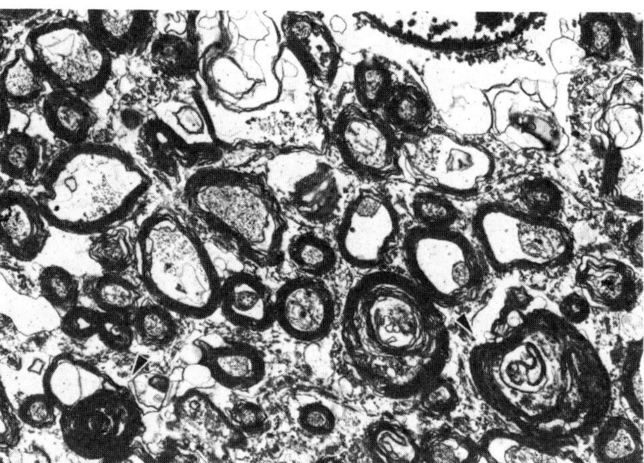

Figure 200–14. Electromicrograph showing ultrastructural characteristics of degenerating axons in the optic nerve (*arrows*). ×6400.

Local Factors of Disc Edema

Lesions of the optic nerve can produce optic disc edema. Intrinsic tumors such as optic nerve sheath meningioma or orbital gliomas, other orbital masses, infiltrative lesions such as leukemia, or inflammatory lesions all may lead to disc edema by producing blockage of axoplasmic flow and vascular congestion.[47] Anterior ischemic optic neuropathy often manifests as sectoral disc edema (Fig. 200–15).

Other factors that can increase the venous pressure at or near the lamina cribrosa include carotid cavernous sinus fistula, central retinal vein occlusion, increased orbital pressure due to trauma or surgery, or decreased intraocular pressure due to intraocular surgery, inflammation, or other causes.[47] Indeed, ocular hypotony due to any cause can result in optic disc edema.

Blockage of Axoplasmic Transport

The principal pathophysiologic finding of optic disc edema is blockage of axoplasmic transport. Orthograde axoplasmic transport has several components and occurs at various rates. The slow component generally progresses at 0.5 to 3.0 mm/day; the rapid flow occurs at a rate of 200 to 1000 mm/day.[48, 49] Retrograde axonal transport also occurs. Mechanical and vascular factors may produce a blockage of axoplasmic flow in the optic nerve.[49, 50] This blockage usually occurs at the level of the lamina choroidalis or lamina scleralis. This can be replicated experimentally by increasing intracranial pressure or by either reducing or increasing intraocular pressure.[51, 52] In a clinical setting, optic disc edema is probably produced by any event that increases venous pressure at or near the lamina cribrosa or that directly blocks axoplasmic flow.

Fundus Changes in Disc Edema

Ten clinical signs of optic disc edema can be seen by direct ophthalmoscopy.[45] Indirect ophthalmoscopy with a 20-D lens may reveal the most dramatic changes, although a 14-D lens is generally recommended. Alternatively, a 60-, 78-, or 90-D lens used in biomicroscopy provides an excellent stereoscopic view of the optic nerve head. We have found it useful to divide the ten funduscopic signs of disc edema into five mechanical and five vascular signs.[45] The five mechanical signs are as follows:

1. Anterior extension of optic nerve head (3 D = 1 mm of elevation)
2. Blurring of the optic disc margins
3. Filling in of the physiologic cup
4. Edema of the peripapillary nerve fiber layer
5. Retinal or choroidal folds

The five vascular signs are as follows:

1. Hyperemia of the optic disc (the Kestenbaum's number may be greater than 12)
2. Venous congestion (venous dilatation and tortuosity)
3. Peripapillary hemorrhages
4. Exudates in the disc or peripapillary area
5. Nerve fiber layer infarcts

Optic disc edema can be characterized as early, fully developed, chronic, or late (atrophic).[46, 53, 54] Early optic disc edema is marked by disc swelling, blurring of the optic disc margins, blurring of the nerve fiber layer, and optic disc hyperemia. The earliest changes may be flattening of the internal limiting membrane leading to loss of superficial light reflexes as seen by red-free direct ophthalmoscopy of the nerve fiber layer.[55] In fully developed optic disc edema, the optic nerve head is fully elevated and circumferential retinal folds (striae or Paton's lines) and choroidal folds are seen.[56] The vascular signs of fully developed disc edema consist of veins that are engorged and dusky, as well as peripapillary splinter hemorrhages. Hard exudates and hemorrhages may be noted around the disc or in the macula.[57, 58] Retinal hemorrhages may dissect anteriorly to the subhyaloid or vitreous spaces.[59] In chronic papilledema, the optic disc cup is completely obliterated; also noted are less disc hyperemia, fewer hemorrhages, but more prominent hard exudates (pseudodrusen) within the optic nerve head.[54] Chronic disc edema may persist for months or even years without change in appearance or severe visual impairment. Late optic disc edema is marked by secondary optic atrophy (see the preceding section) that is sometimes termed *postpapilledema atrophy* (see Figs. 200–1 to 200–3). There is less optic disc swelling, the retinal blood vessels have become narrowed and ensheathed, and the optic disc appears dirty gray and blurred secondary to the glial reaction. Optociliary shunt vessels sometimes develop.[60]

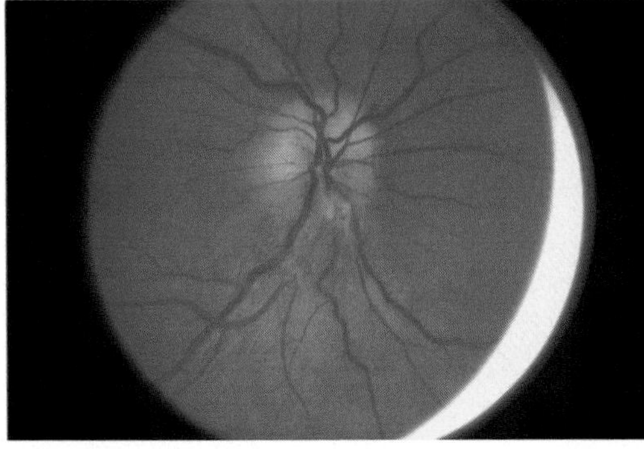

Figure 200–15. Sectoral optic disc edema. Hemidisc involvement in anterior ischemic optic neuropathy (AION). Partial resolution 10 days after acute event.

Histology of Optic Disc Edema

In acute optic disc edema, histopathologic examination reveals edema and vascular congestion. Peripapillary hemorrhages are seen primarily in the retinal nerve fiber layer, but they may overlie the optic disc or be noted in any layer of the retina or subretinal space.[46]

An increase in tissue mass causes the physiologic cup to be narrowed or completely obliterated. This increased tissue mass also causes the optic nerve head to protrude anteriorly to the vitreous. The small blood vessels are engorged and tortuous. Vacuoles of extracellular fluid accumulate in and anterior to the retinal lamina cribrosa posteriorly, and the subarachnoid space is enlarged with stretching of the subarachnoid strands.

Engorgement of axons in the retinal laminar portion of the optic nerve can be demonstrated by electron microscopy. The axons are swollen and filled with mitochondria, primarily anterior to the choroidal lamina cribrosa. The mitochondria themselves appear swollen and disrupted, and the fascicles of microtubules are also in disarray. It is important to note that the extracellular accumulation is minimal compared with the intracellular accumulation that results in the engorgement of axons.[61] Changes are seen also in the surrounding retina. The sensory retina is displaced away from the optic disc, and the outer layer of the retina may be buckled (retinal folds). The rods and cones are obliquely displaced away from their anchor near Bruch's membrane. Retinal detachment may occur in the peripapillary area.

In chronic disc edema, degeneration of retinal ganglion cell axons may occur.[1] This process proceeds in both an anterograde and retrograde fashion, thus degeneration and subsequent atrophy may occur anywhere from the retinal nerve fiber layer to the optic tract. Noted in conjunction with this secondary optic atrophy is gliosis, seen in both the optic nerve head and extending anteriorly in to the vitreous. The dirty gray appearance of the disc correlates with the histologic appearance of large glial nets on the surface and edges of the disc (see Secondary Optic Atrophy, discussed earlier).

Clinical Signs

Patients with papilledema (due to increased intracranial pressure) may demonstrate all of the signs and symptoms associated with the neurologic problem, including headache, nausea, and vomiting. However, disc edema per se may produce minimal or no visual symptoms. Unless the disc edema is chronic, there is generally little or no change in visual acuity. In early disc edema, the only visual field defect is that of an enlarged blind spot, generally secondary to the displacement of retina away from the optic nerve head. However, symptoms of transient obscurations of vision (TOVs) are characteristic of disc edema.[62, 63] TOVs are classically associated with papilledema. However, they may be seen in patients who have monocular or binocular disc edema and who do not have increased intracranial pressure. Disc edema, regardless of etiology, and even pseudopapilledema may produce TOVs.[62] Chronic disc edema may lead to severe and irreversible losses of visual field, contrast sensitivity, and eventually impairments in visual acuity and color vision.[58, 64]

Pseudopapilledema

Pseudopapilledema or, more correctly, pseudodisc edema, refers to abnormalities that produce elevation and irregularities of the optic nerve head that mimic disc edema. Hyaline bodies (optic disc drusen) may be embedded so deeply in the optic nerve head that they are not funduscopically obvious; however, they can usually be seen well on fluorescein angiography (by autofluorescence) and can be shown well by ultrasonography.[65, 66] These drusen may become larger and move anteriorly with time. Optic disc drusen are sometimes inherited as an autosomal trait with variable penetrance. The hyaline bodies are usually at the level of the lamina or just anterior to it and often become calcified. Congenital abnormalities of the optic nerve head may also mimic disc edema.[67] Tilted discs and Fuchs' coloboma may be confused with sectoral disc edema. The optic disc in hyperopic eyes often appears full; even with ultrasonography, the optic nerve head may be shown to extend anteriorly in a way that mimics optic disc edema.

REFERENCES

1. Sadun AA, Yanoff B, Fine BS: Pathology of the optic nerve. *In* Duane TD, Jaeger EA (eds): Biomedical Foundations of Ophthalmology. Philadelphia, JB Lippincott, 1985, pp 1–31.
2. Walsh FB, Hoyt WF: Clinical Neuro-ophthalmology, 3rd ed. Baltimore, Williams & Wilkins, 1969.
3. Miller NR: Optic atrophy. *In* Walsh FB, Hoyt WF: Clinical Neuro-ophthalmology, 4th ed. Baltimore, Williams & Wilkins, 1982, pp 329–342.
4. Sadun AA, Bassi C: Optic nerve damage in Alzheimer's disease. Ophthalmology 97:9, 1990.
5. Sadun AA, Bassi CJ: The visual system in Alzheimer's disease. *In* Cohen B, Bodis-Wallner I (eds): Vision and the Brain. New York, Raven Press, 1990, pp 331–347.
6. Johnson BM, Miao M, Sadun AA: Age-related decline of human optic nerve axon populations. Age 10:5, 1987.
7. Sadun AA, Johnson B, Miao M: Axon caliber populations in the human optic nerve: Changes with age and disease. Highlights in Neuro-Ophthalmology. Proceedings of the Sixth Meeting of the International Neuro-Ophthalmology Society. Amsterdam, Aeolus Press, 1987, pp 15–20.
8. Quigley HA, Dunkelberger GR, Green WR: Retinal ganglion cell atrophy correlated with automated perimetry in human eyes with glaucoma. Am J Ophthalmol 107:453, 1989.
9. Quigley HA, Anderson DR: The histological basis of optic disc pallor. Am J Ophthalmol 83:709, 1977.
10. Walsh FB, Hoyt WF: Clinical Neuro-ophthalmology, 3rd ed. Baltimore, Williams & Wilkins, 1969, pp 631–641.
11. Kant A: The ophthalmoscopic evaluation of optic atrophy. Am J Ophthalmol 32:1479, 1949.
12. Quigley HA, Hohman RM, Addicks EM: Quantitative study of optic nerve head capillaries in experimental optic disc pallor. Am J Ophthalmol 93:689, 1982.
13. Frisen L, Claesson M: Narrowing of the retinal arterioles in descending optic atrophy: A quantitative clinical study. Ophthalmology 91:1342, 1984.
14. Sebag J, Delori FC, Feke GT, et al: Anterior optic nerve blood flow decreases in clinical neurogenic optic atrophy. Ophthalmology 93:858, 1986.
15. Sebag J, Delori FC, Feke GT, Weiter JJ: Effects of optic atrophy on retinal blood flow and oxygen saturation in humans. Arch Ophthalmol 107:222, 1989.
16. Safran AB, Lupolover Y, Berney J: Macular reflexes in optic atrophy. Am J Ophthalmol 98:494, 1984.
17. Lundstrom M, Frisen L: Atrophy of optic nerve fibres in compression of the chiasm: Degree and distribution of ophthalmoscopic changes. Acta Ophthalmol 54:623, 1976.
18. Miller NR, Fine SL: The ocular fundus in neuro-ophthalmologic diagnosis. *In* Sights and Sounds in Ophthalmology, vol. 3. St. Louis, CV Mosby, 1977, pp 50–53.
19. Unsold R, Hoyt WF: Band atrophy of the optic nerve: The histology of temporal hemianopsia. Arch Ophthalmol 98:1637, 1980.

20. Blazar HA, Scheie HG: Pseudoglaucoma. Arch Ophthalmol 44:499, 1950.
21. Quigley H, Anderson DR: Cupping of the optic disc in ischemic optic neuropathy. Trans Am Acad Ophthalmol Otolaryngol 83:755, 1977.
22. Trobe JD, Glaser JS, Cassady JC: Optic atrophy: Differential diagnosis by fundus observation alone. Arch Ophthalmol 98:1040, 1980.
23. Behrens MM: Other optic nerve diseases. *In* Lessel S, Van Dalen JTW (eds): Current Neuro-Ophthalmology, vol 1. Chicago, 1988, pp 33–52.
24. Balazi AG, Rootman J, Drance SM, et al: The effect of age on the nerve fiber population of the human optic nerve. Am J Ophthalmol 97:760, 1984.
25. Trobe JD, Glaser JS, Cassady J, et al: Nonglaucomatous excavation of the optic disc. Arch Ophthalmol 98:1046, 1980.
26. Quigley H, Anderson D: The histologic basis of optic disc pallor in experimental optic atrophy. J Ophthalmol 83:709, 1977.
27. Henkind P, Charles NC, Pearson J: Histopathology of ischemic optic neuropathy. Am J Ophthalmol 69:78, 1970.
28. Anderson DR: Ascending and descending optic atrophy produced experimentally in squirrel monkeys. Am J Ophthalmol 76:693, 1973.
29. Radius RL, Anderson DR: Retinal ganglion cell degeneration in experimental optic atrophy. Am J Ophthalmol 86:673, 1978.
30. Smith LE, Sadun AA, Kenyon KR: Transsynaptic changes in the human visual system: Atrophy versus degeneration. Invest Ophthalmol Vis Sci 22(Suppl):76, 1982.
31. Beatty B, Sadun A, Smith L, Richardson E: Direct demonstration of transsynaptic degeneration in the human visual system: A comparison of retrograde and anterograde changes. J Neurol Neurosurg Psychiatry 45:143, 1982.
32. Quigley HA, Davis EB, Anderson DR: Descending optic nerve degeneration in primates. Invest Ophthalmol Vis Sci 16:841, 1977.
33. Van Buren JM: Transsynaptic retrograde degeneration in the visual system of primates. J Neurol Neurosurg Psychiatry 26:402, 1963.
34. Miller NR, Fine SL: The ocular fundus in neuro-ophthalmologic diagnosis. *In* Sights and Sounds in Ophthalmology, vol 3. St. Louis, CV Mosby, 1977, pp 50–53.
35. Weller RE, Kaas JH, Ward J: Preservation of retinal ganglion cells and normal patterns of retinogeniculate projections in prosimian primates with long-term ablations of striate cortex. Invest Ophthalmol Vis Sci 20:139, 1981.
36. Miller NR, Newman NM: Transsynaptic degeneration. Arch Ophthalmol 99:1654, 1981.
37. Weller RE, Kaas JH: Loss of retinal ganglion cells and altered retinogeniculate projections in monkeys with striate cortex lesions. Invest Ophthalmol Vis Sci 19 (ARVO Suppl):2, 1980.
38. Hoyt WF: Ophthalmoscopy of the retinal nerve fiber layer in neuroophthalmologic diagnosis. Aust J Ophthalmol 4:14, 1976.
39. Hoyt WF, Frisen L, Newman NM: Fundoscopy of nerve fiber layer defects in glaucoma. Invest Ophthalmol 12:814, 1973.
40. Quigley HA, Addicks EM, Green WR: Optic nerve damage in human glaucoma. III: Quantitative correlation of nerve fiber loss and visual field defect in glaucoma, ischemic neuropathy, papilledema and toxic neuropathy. Arch Ophthalmol 100:135, 1982.
41. Guillery RW: Light- and electron-microscopical studies of normal and degenerating axons. *In* Nauta WJH, Ebbesson SOE (eds): Contemporary Research Methods in Neuroanatomy. New York, Springer-Verlag, 1970, pp 77–105.
42. Sadun AA, Smith LEH, Kenyon KR: A new method for tracing visual pathways in man. J Neuropathol Exp Neurol 42:200, 1983.
43. Sadun AA: Neuroanatomy of the human visual system. I: Retinal projections to the LGN and pretectum as demonstrated with a new stain. Neuro-Ophthalmology 6:353, 1986.
44. Johnson BM, Sadun AA: Ultrastructural and paraphenylene studies of degeneration in the primate visual system: Degenerative remnants persist for much longer than expected. J Electron Microsc Tech 8:179, 1988.
45. Sadun AA, Rismondo V: Evaluation of the swollen disc. *In* Schachat AP (ed): Current Practice in Ophthalmology. Boston, Mosby Year Book, 1992, pp 177–186.
46. Miller NR: Papilledema: A sign of increased intracranial pressure. *In* Walsh FB, Hoyt WF (eds): Clinical Neuro-Ophthalmology, 4th ed. Baltimore, Williams & Wilkins, 1982, pp 175–211.
47. Glaser J: Neuro-Ophthalmology. Philadelphia, JB Lippincott, 1990, pp 64–68, 95, 107–8, 135–40.
48. Brady ST, Lasek RJ, Allen RD: Video microscopy for fast axonal transport of extruded axoplasm: A new model for study of molecular mechanisms. Cell Motil 5:81, 1985.
49. Minckler DS, Bunt AH: Axoplasmic transport in ocular hypotony and papilledema in the monkey. Arch Ophthalmol 95:1430, 1977.
50. Tso MOM, Hayreh SS: Optic disc edema in raised intracranial pressure. IV: Axoplasmic transport in experimental papilledema. Arch Ophthalmol 95:1458, 1977.
51. Hayreh MS, Hayreh SS: Optic disc edema in raised intracranial pressure. I: Evolution and resolution. Arch Ophthalmol 95:1237, 1977.
52. Tso MOM, Hayreh SS. Optic disc edema in raised intracranial pressure. III: A pathologic study of experimental papilledema. Arch Ophthalmol 95:1448, 1977.
53. Frisen L: Swelling of the optic nerve head: A staging scheme. J Neurol Neurosurg Psychiatry 45:13, 1982.
54. Hoyt WF, Beeston D: The Ocular Fundus in Neurologic Disease. St. Louis, CV Mosby, 1966.
55. Hoyt WF, Knight CL: Comparison of congenital disc blurring and incipient papilledema in red-free light—A photographic study. Invest Ophthalmol 12:241, 1973.
56. Keane JR: Papilledema with unusual ocular hemorrhages. Arch Ophthalmol 99:262, 1981.
57. Morris AT, Sanders MD: Macular changes resulting from papilloedema. Br J Ophthalmol 64:211, 1980.
58. Gittinger JW, Asdourian GK: Macular abnormalities in papilledema from pseudotumor cerebri. Ophthalmology 96:192, 1989.
59. Bird AC, Sanders MD: Choroidal folds in association with papilloedema. Br J Ophthalmol 57:89, 1973.
60. Eggers HM, Sanders MD: Acquired optociliary shunt vessels in papilloedema. Br J Ophthalmol 64:267, 1980.
61. Minckler DS, Tso MOM: A light microscopic, autoradiographic study of axoplasmic transport in the normal rhesus optic nerve head. Am J Ophthalmol 82:1, 1976.
62. Sadun AA, Currie JN, Lessell S: Transient visual obscurations with elevated optic discs. Ann Neurol 16:489, 1984.
63. Smith TJ, Baker RS: Perimetric findings in pseudotumor cerebri using automated techniques. Ophthalmology 93:887, 1986.
64. Wall M: Contrast sensitivity testing in pseudotumor cerebri. Ophthalmology 93:4, 1986.
65. Reifler DM, Kaufman DI: Optic disk drusen and pseudotumor cerebri. Am J Ophthalmol 106:95, 1988.
66. Beck RW, Corbett JJ, Thompson HS, Sergott RC: Decreased visual acuity from optic disc drusen. Arch Ophthalmol 103:1115, 1985.
67. Brown GC, Tasman WS: Congenital anomalies of the optic disc. New York, Grune & Stratton, 1983, pp 95–192.

Chapter 201

Optic Neuritis

SHIRLEY H. WRAY

Optic neuritis is the term used for inflammation of the optic nerve. It is a serious condition, which in young adults invariably leads to multiple sclerosis (MS). Overall 15 to 20 percent of cases with definite MS present with optic neuritis, and an additional 35 to 40 percent succumb to optic neuritis at some point during the course of the disease.[1–3] Because one study also indicates that approximately 75 percent of patients with optic neuritis seek medical attention early (usually within 2 wk of onset[4]), ophthalmologists are on the diagnostic front line: optic neuritis is one of the most important optic neuropathies in ophthalmic practice and its diagnosis is a diagnosis of potential gravity. This means that ophthalmologists must not only be alert to symptoms of optic neuritis, but they must also be prepared to assume responsibility for the much more serious condition to which these symptoms are linked.

Prevalence

Prevalence surveys for optic neuritis are reported in the United States (US),[5] England,[6] Finland,[7, 8] and Norway.[9] In the US study, done in Rochester, MN (1935 to 1964), the annual incidence of idiopathic optic neuritis was 6.4 new cases per 100,000 population.[5] In the English study, the reported annual incidence was 1.4 per 100,000 for optic neuritis and 3.0 for MS.[6] In Finland, the mean annual incidence of optic neuritis for the whole country was only 0.94 per 100,000[7]; however, optic neuritis incidence rates reported for medium- and high-risk MS areas were significantly higher. In an incidence study carried out (1970 to 1978) in Uusimaa, a medium-risk area, and Vaasa, a high-risk area for MS, the mean annual age-adjusted incidence of optic neuritis per 100,000 was 2.2 in Uusimaa and 2.5 in Vaasa.[8] It seems clear that prevalence rates for optic neuritis correlate with those for MS, and similar data from Norway support this.[9] Furthermore, because it is a factor in the observed geographic distribution of MS, race must also be considered in the optic neuritis-multiple sclerosis incidence configuration. Whites of northern European extraction are most susceptible to MS; whites of Mediterranean extraction are moderately susceptible; and African blacks and Asians are hardly susceptible at all.[10]

Age and Sex

Overall, the mean age of onset of optic neuritis is 29 to 30 yr.[1] The condition is rare in children,[11–20] in whom it is usually postinfectious or parainfectious[12–15]; often simultaneously bilateral[12, 13, 15, 19]; and generally characterized by a good visual prognosis.[15–17, 19] Children have a comparatively low risk (35 percent) of developing MS.[18–21]

Optic neuritis in patients 40 to 50 yr of age behaves similarly to the disorder in younger adults (18 to 39 yr of age).[22] In patients older than 50 yr of age, optic neuritis can be a misleading diagnosis, because other disorders, particularly ischemic optic neuropathy, commonly cause acute or subacute visual loss.[22]

In the New England region of the US, the incidence of optic neuritis in adult women exceeds that of men by a ratio of 1.8:1. The mean age of onset in women is 30.2 yr (range 9 to 55 yr, median of 29 yr). In men, the mean age of onset is 31.1 yr (range of 16 to 60 yr, median of 32 yr).[2]

CLINICAL SYMPTOMS OF THE CONDITION

Optic neuritis may be symptomatic or asymptomatic. Symptomatic cases present with a triad of symptoms: loss of vision, ipsilateral eye pain, and dyschromatopsia. The initial attack is unilateral in 70 percent of adult patients and bilateral in 30 percent.[4] The associated visual symptoms are movement phosphenes, sound-induced phosphenes, visual obscurations in bright light, and Uhthoff's symptom.

Subclinical asymptomatic cases of optic neuritis are detectable by a routine ophthalmic or neurologic examination since the presence of mild dyschromatopsia, temporal pallor of the optic disc, and slits in the nerve fiber layer are clear signs of the disease. Asymptomatic cases are also detectable electrophysiologically by visual evoked potential (VEP) tests[23] and are unmistakably detectable histologically by an examination of the optic nerves at autopsy. In one autopsy study of both optic nerves, in 18 cases of MS only 8 of 18 patients had been diagnosed with unilateral or bilateral optic neuritis while they were alive, yet 35 of the 36 optic nerves showed evidence of demyelination.[24]

Loss of Vision

A single plaque in a previously healthy optic nerve can cause a complete failure of vision. In a small number of patients it can be undetectable, and in such cases patients who retain 20/20 Snellen acuity may be undi-

Table 201–1. VISUAL ACUITY IN 108 EYES WITH ACUTE ISOLATED OPTIC NEURITIS AT THE ONSET, AT MAXIMUM ACUITY LOSS, AND AT 8 WK

	VA Initial (%)	VA Maximum (%)	VA At 8 wk (%)
20/15–20/60	52	34	74
20/70–NLP	48	66	25
20/200–NLP	38	54	20

From Wray SH, Scholl GB, Giffen C: Optic neuritis and gender. In preparation 1992.
NLP, no light perception.

agnosed despite visual symptoms such as blurred vision on exertion or movement phosphenes.

Decreased acuity as an isolated symptom occurs in 58 percent of cases of optic neuritis.[4] The rate at which vision fails varies. It may occur very rapidly, within hours (29 percent); fast, within 1 to 2 days (20 percent); slowly, within 3 to 7 days (23 percent); or chronically slowly, within 1 to 2 wk (7 percent). Initially acuity is unstable. Within 7 days of the onset, acuity may be less than 20/60 in 52 percent of eyes, 20/70 to 20/100 in 48 percent and worse than 20/200 in 38 percent (Table 209–1).[2] Data also show that a significant number of eyes continue to deteriorate initially and to suffer severe visual loss (an acuity of 20/200 or worse) before stabilizing and then improving (Table 201–1).[2]

Chronic progressive demyelinating optic neuropathy, characterized by slowly progressive visual loss without remission, is a rare variant of optic neuritis. It is due to a protracted production of micro plaques until the full cross section of the optic nerve is ultimately affected. Micro plaques in the chiasm or optic tracts may contribute to the impairment of vision, and chiasmal optic neuritis with bitemporal hemianopia is reported.[25] However, clinical signs of chiasmal or tract dysfunction are usually obscured by optic nerve plaques.

A further variant of chronic progressive demyelinating optic neuropathy is characterized by a slow, progressive loss of acuity punctuated by acute episodes of more profound visual loss and incomplete restoration of vision after each exacerbation.

Pain

The incidence of ipsilateral eye pain in unilateral optic neuritis ranges from 53 percent to 62 percent to 88 percent.[2, 4, 26] In one study, 115 patients with optic neuritis (62 percent) complained of pain during an attack in or behind the involved eye. In 39 patients (21 percent), it occurred only with eye movements. In 19 patients (16 percent), pain preceded a decrease in visual acuity. Headache in the involved eye region was reported by 40 patients (22 percent) and generalized headache by 24 patients (13 percent).[4]

In the typical case, pain is experienced as a dull ache or sinus pain, with or without tenderness of the globe. It reaches maximum severity within 24 to 36 hr and spontaneously abates within 48 to 72 hr. Pain persisting for 7 days is highly atypical in cases of optic neuritis, and other causes of optic neuropathy should first be ruled out.

The cause of the eye pain is unknown. It does not correlate with the severity of visual loss, or with the absence of optic disc swelling implying a retrobulbar optic neuropathy, or with enlargement of the optic nerves on computed tomography (CT). It may be that the pain occurs because of the tight fit of the swollen optic nerve within the bone of the optic canal, but a study of 42 adult patients with unilateral optic neuritis contradicts this hypothesis[27]: 37 of 42 eyes (88 percent) had orbital pain and the MR imaging data showed lesions in different sites along the course of the nerve yet identified only 15 of 44 eyes (34 percent) with plaques in the intracanalicular region of the nerve (Table 201–2).

Dyschromatopsia

Impaired color vision, dyschromatopsia, is always present in optic neuritis.[4, 19, 23, 28, 29] Typically the patient observes a reduced vividness of saturated colors. In color terminology saturation refers to the purity of color, and desaturation is the degree to which a color is mixed with white. Some patients who are shown a red target characterize the sensation as darker (i.e., red is shifted toward amber), whereas others say the color is bleached or lighter (i.e., red is shifted towards orange). In the absence of a macular lesion, color desaturation is a highly sensitive indicator of optic nerve disease.

Movement Phosphenes

Movement phosphenes can appear without a prior history of optic neuritis. They can occur before an attack of optic neuritis or may accompany visual loss during the attack. They may also occur 6 mo after full recovery when acuity is 20/20 and fundoscopy is normal.[30] In three patients with MS the phenomenon lasted for 3 wk, 7 mo, and 9 mo, respectively.[31] Their characteristics are as follows:

> They occur almost exclusively with horizontal eye movement and are best perceived in a dark room or in a dimly lit room with the eyes closed.

Table 201–2. FREQUENCY OF MR LESIONS AT EACH SITE IN 44 SYMPTOMATIC OPTIC NERVES

Site	Frequency of Involvement Number	%
Anterior	20/44	45
Midintraorbital	27/44	61
Intracanalicular	15/44	34
Intracranial	2/44	5
Optic chiasm	1/44	2

From Miller DH, Newton MR, van der Poel JC, et al: Magnetic resonance imaging of the optic nerve in optic neuritis. Neurology 38:175, 1988.

The eye sees a very brief flash of light that lasts for only 1 or 2 sec, even if lateral gaze is maintained.
Repeated eye movements cause temporary lulling of the phosphenes with reappearance after several minutes of rest. They occur unilaterally and ipsilateral to the affected eye.[31]

Movement phosphenes of retinal origin occur with vitreous traction as a prelude to retinal detachment. In optic neuritis, however, clinical evidence of optic nerve demyelination is associated with the phenomenon, and this suggests that the origin of the phosphenes is in the optic nerve rather than in the retina. Since no satisfactory explanation for the increased mechanical sensitivity of the demyelinated nerve axons exists, Lhermitte's symptom in MS of the spinal cord may be a useful analogy to consider.[30] This symptom is usually provoked by neck flexion and is described most often as an electric shock traveling down the spine. Here too, the precise mechanism is unknown, but experiment has shown that partially demyelinated spinal cord axons discharge spontaneously when subjected to minimal mechanical stress.[32] With this in mind, and as long as other causes are excluded, the acute development of movement phosphenes in young patients suggests the presence of a demyelinating optic neuropathy.

Sound-Induced Phosphenes

Phosphenes can also be precipitated by sudden noise when the patient is resting in the dark.[33–35] Sound-induced phosphenes are thought to be a pathologic variety of hypnagogic hallucinations. They can occur transiently in disease of the eye or of the optic nerve, including optic neuritis and compressive optic neuropathies.

Visual Obscurations in Bright Light

Obscuration of vision in bright light is a symptom of acute optic neuritis.[36] Patients with chronic optic neuritis in fact see better in dim light.[3, 36, 37] One patient with optic neuritis volunteered this symptom on finding that his vision in strong sunlight was much improved by tinted glasses,[38] and this effect is reported by approximately 50 percent of patients with optic neuritis who say that they see more clearly in a dimly lit environment than in bright sunlight.[37]

In patients with MS, the variability of seeing in different lighting conditions is related to the luminance of the background, with vision becoming more impaired as background lumination increases.[38] This luminance-dependent variability is due not to visual fatigue of the type reported in optic neuritis[39] but rather to a fluctuating interference in the transmission of visual signals. The likely site of the fluctuating interference is the demyelinated visual pathway, and there are two possible physiologic causes: intermittent conduction block and cross-excitation (ephaptic transmission) between affected nerve fibers at the demyelinating lesion.[40–43]

An increased variability in seeing may also explain the visual field phenomenon of flickering scotomata, revealed by use of the Tübingen perimeter with a patient with MS who reported that the test object appeared to flicker on and off in some areas.[44] This phenomenon, which I have personally confirmed in optic neuritis cases, occurs most commonly between 10 and 25 degrees of eccentricity. Since the test object is normally not greatly above threshold at this angle, any increase in threshold variability results in the object being seen intermittently (i.e., appearing to flicker on and off).

Uhthoff's Symptom

Uhthoff's symptom, episodic transient obscuration of vision with exertion, occurs in isolated optic neuritis[45, 46] and in MS.[47, 48] However, exertion is not the only provoking factor for Uhthoff's symptom (Table 201–3). Hot baths or showers account for 27.5 percent of cases, and hot weather accounts for another 27.5 percent of cases. Typically, the patient has blurring of vision in the affected eye after 5 to 20 min of exposure to the provoking factor. Color desaturation may also occur. After resting or moving away from heat, vision recovers to its previous level within 5 to 60 min; some patients experience a slow recovery that can take up to 24 hr. Uhthoff's symptom is also associated with toxic optic neuropathy due to chloramphenicol[49]; Friedreich's ataxia[50]; and Leber's optic neuropathy.[51] In MS cases an inverse Uhthoff's symptom may be present, characterized by improved vision in response to exercise,[52] beer drinking,[53] or 4-aminopyridine.[54]

Uhthoff's symptom occurs in 49.5 percent of patients with isolated optic neuritis.[46] In 16 percent of cases it develops within 2 wk of the onset of visual loss, and in 58 percent it occurs within 2 mo. Patients may experience a long period free of the symptom (3, 14, and 32 mo), followed by the return of the symptom without a recurrent attack of optic neuritis. Typically the transient visual episodes continue over several months to several years, and the frequency varies from sporadic to several episodes a day, with some cases noting an increase in frequency in the summer.

Table 201–3. FACTORS PROVOKING UHTHOFF'S SYMPTOM

Factor	No. of Patients	%
Physical exertion	21	52.5
Hot bath or shower	11	27.5
Hot weather	11	27.5
Stress, anxiety, anger	5	12.5
Tired, end of day	4	1.0
Hot food or drink	3	7.5
Cooking	2	5.0
Other specific activity*	3	7.5

From Scholl GB, Song H-S, Wray SH: Uhthoff's symptom in optic neuritis: Relationship to magnetic resonance imaging and development of multiple sclerosis. Ann Neurol 30:180, 1991.
*Working a cash register, playing the trumpet, and reading (1 patient each).

In optic neuritis, Uhthoff's symptom correlates significantly with multifocal white matter lesions on brain magnetic resonance imaging (MRI) ($P < .025$), and conversion to MS in patients followed for a mean of 3.5 yr is significantly greater in patient with Uhthoff's symptom ($P < .01$). Uhthoff's symptom also correlates with a higher incidence of recurrent optic neuritis.[46]

Uhthoff's symptom in MS can be detected by Farnsworth-Munsell 100-Hue testing and Octopus perimetry,[55] as well as by fluctuations of VEP amplitudes and contrast sensitivity.[56]

CLINICAL HISTORY OF THE CONDITION

The potential gravity of a diagnosis of optic neuritis requires a meticulous patient history. The physician must document:

1. The mode of onset and rate of progression of visual loss
2. The location, character, and severity of pain
3. Symptoms that indicate involvement of structures adjacent to the optic nerve; for example, the nasal sinuses,[57–59] the olfactory nerve, the chiasm, or the pituitary gland
4. A complete symptomatic inquiry for previous disease of the eye or central nervous system (CNS) for symptoms suggestive of demyelinating disease.

A complete medical history should include details of: pregnancy[60]; cancer[61]; mixed connective tissue syndrome combining the clinical features of autoimmune disease and systemic lupus erythematosus[62–68]; exposure to *Coxiella burnetii* (Q fever),[69] or to spirochetal diseases such as Lyme borreliosis[70, 71]; syphilis[72–75]; viral infection(s), such as Epstein-Barr virus (infectious mononucleosis)[76]; hepatitis B virus[77]; varicella-zoster[78]; human immunodeficiency virus (HIV), which is the etiologic agent of AIDS[73–75]; and cytomegalovirus.[79]

Details of all medications must be recorded, particularly those that can produce optic nerve or retinal toxicity (including ethambutol and isoniazid,[80] phenothiazines, and antineoplastic agents). Drug and alcohol use, recent head and eye trauma (and the medicolegal details), and stress and psychiatric disorder(s) must also be recorded.

CLINICAL SIGNS OF THE CONDITION

The clinical signs of optic neuritis are those of optic nerve disease. They include:

Visual acuity (distance and near)—reduced
Dyschromatopsia
Contrast sensitivity—impaired
Stereo-acuity—reduced
Visual field—generalized depression, particularly pronounced centrally
Afferent pupillary defect
Optic disc(s)—hyperemia and acute swelling

Acuity

The inability to see and to recognize foveated objects has traditionally been assessed in terms of visual acuity alone. In clinical practice the Snellen letter reading test for spatial vision, which assesses both the ability to detect a target and the ability to discriminate its shape, is the most familiar test. It represents recognition of a suprathreshold target at a high spatial frequency.

The fine degree of spatial resolution measured by Snellen acuity (better than 1 min of arc) is dependent on the functional properties of retinal neurons, the high cone density in the fovea, and the proportion of functional foveal cone outflow pathways.

The foveal cone pathway consists of a three-neuron chain. Each cone synapses with two bipolar cells, and then each bipolar cell synapses with a single P (parvo) ganglion cell. The parvosystem is all important for high-resolution vision and is characterized by color opponency, high spatial resolution, and low contrast sensitivity. In contrast, M (magno) ganglion cells, which are larger than P cells and which constitute the magnosystem are characterized by color ignorance, low spatial resolution, fast temporal resolution, stereopsis, and high contrast sensitivity (Table 201–4).[81]

A precise correlation between loss of optic nerve axons or P ganglion cells within the fovea and the level of acuity has not yet been determined, but it is estimated that an acuity of 0.5 (20/40) is supported by a reduction of 40 percent of the axons emanating from the papillomacular bundle.[82, 83] Data also indicate that a reduction of the number of macular ganglion cell layers from 6 to 3 can still support 20/25 acuity, suggesting that a substantial loss of macular outflow channels might have only a modest effect on acuity.[84]

In optic neuritis the severity of impairment of all visual functions tested, acuity, visual fields, color vision, and VEPs can be measured on a graded visual impairment scale (GVIS) that incorporates Snellen acuity (Tables 201–5 and 201–6).[85]

The GVIS classifies cases as monocular blindness (total, severe, moderate), monocular low vision (severe, moderate, mild), and normal vision (see Table 201–5).

Table 201–4. PROPERTIES OF PARVOCELLULAR (P) AND MAGNOCELLULAR (M) RETINAL GANGLION CELLS

Properties	P	M
Retinal distribution	Foveal	Extrafoveal
Receptive field size	Small	Large
Axonal velocity	Slow	Fast
Motion discharge rate	Low	High
Color opponency	Yes	Low
Responses to contrast	Sustained	10
Contrast gain	Low	
Spatial resolution	High	
% of total cells	90	

Modified from Livingstone MS, Hubel DH: Psychophysical evidence for separate channels for the perception of form, color movement, and depth. J Neurosci 7:3416, 1987.

Table 201–5. GRADED VISUAL IMPAIRMENT SCALE IN OPTIC NEURITIS

1. Monocular blindness
   a. Total
      No light perception
   b. Severe blindness
      Visual acuity <20/1,000, or light perception, hand motion only
   c. Moderate blindness
      (visual acuity or other visual deficits)
      Visual acuity 20/500 or 20/1,00
      Count finger at 1 m, central scotoma >10° at V_{4e}
2. Monocular low vision
   a. Severe visual impairment (visual acuity or other visual deficits)
      Visual acuity 20/200 to 20/400
      Central scotoma of <10° and V_{4e}
      Contrast sensitivity is severely impaired with abnormalities at all sensitivities tested
   b. Moderate visual impairment (visual acuity or other visual deficits)
      Visual acuity 20/70 to 20/160
      Relative central scotoma of <5°
      Arcuate scotoma within 20° of the central axis, or monocular peripheral depression of at least 10°
      Color vision impairment (8 to 15 misses with pseudoisochromatic color plates or error score of 720 with L'Anthony new color test)
      Contrast sensitivity impairment with 4 to 7 abnormalities
   c. Mild impaired vision or near-normal vision
      (visual acuity or other visual deficits)
      Visual acuity 20/30 to 20/60
      Impaired contrast sensitivity (<4 abnormalities)
      Impaired color vision (6 to 8 misses with pseudoisochromatic color plates or error score of 199 with L'Anthony new color test)
      No visual field defect
3. Normal vision
   Visual acuity 20/10 to 20/25
   All other visual parameters within normal limits

From Celesia GG, Kaufman DI, Brigell M, et al: Optic neuritis: A prospective study. Neurology 40:919, 1990.

Dyschromatopsia

Color vision, a P-ganglion cell function, is abnormal in patients with acute and recovered optic neuritis. Many clinicians consider the localized loss of red and green perception to be the most sensitive test of interference with optic nerve function[86, 87]; however, both red/green and blue/yellow color vision defects have been reported.[88, 89] Color vision defects are highly sensitive indicators of a previous attack of optic neuritis.[29, 90, 91]

Interestingly enough, the impairment in color perception does not occur at the cone receptor level but at a postreceptor, precortical level in the visual system, beyond which signals from more than one class of cone receptor are combined. At this precortical level there are thought to be three independent neural channels, two signaling chromatic changes in light and one indicating luminance changes.[92, 93]

Research in recent years has focused on the question of whether luminance (brightness) and color vision may be selectively affected in demyelinating optic nerve disease. The notion that chromatic mechanisms may be more severely affected than luminance mechanisms has until now been based on the remarkable ability of tests using colored stimuli to indicate disordered optic nerve function. The problem is that colors themselves contain both luminance and color differences. It is impossible to tell, for example, whether substituting a red target for a white one reveals a greater visual deficit due to its color difference from the background or whether this is due to its lower luminance contrast. Experiments to test independently luminance and chromatic mechanisms are not easy to design, and problems arise if stimuli used to test color vision differ in their spatial or temporal characteristics from those used to test luminance vision.

Investigators have used different experimental meth-

Table 201–6. VISUAL MEASURES OF THE AFFECTED EYE

	At Onset of ON*			Final Outcome		
		Abnormal			Abnormal	
Measure	*No. Tested*	*No.*	%	*No. Tested*	*No.*	%
Visual acuity	20	18	90	20	4	20
Color vision	20	20	100	20	4	20
Contrast sensitivity†	19	18	95	19	4	21
Visual field defect	20	20	100	20	4	20
GVIS‡	20	20	100	20	7	35
Marcus Gunn pupil	19	18	95	19	11	58
Disc edema (papillitis)	20	10	50	20	0	0
Disc pallor	20	1	5	19	9	47
VEPs§ at 60′	17	16	94	20	18	90
P-ERG‖ at 60′	16	3	19	19	0	0
MRI¶ brain	17	10	59	ND**	ND	ND
MRI optic nerve	11	1	9	ND	ND	ND

Modified from Celesia GG, Kaufman DI, Brigell M, et al: Optic neuritis: A prospective study. Neurology 40:919, 1990.
*ON, optic neuritis.
†Could not be tested in some patients due to severe visual loss.
‡GVIS, graded visual impairment scale.
§VEP, visual evoked potential.
‖P-ERG, pattern-electroretinogram.
¶MRI, magnetic resonance imaging.
**ND, not done.

ods and have drawn conflicting conclusions in comparisons of chromatic and achromatic sensitivity in optic neuritis. For example, a study that compared thresholds for the detection of a chromatic change from white with thresholds for a change in luminance,[94] and another experiment using a somewhat similar method,[95] have demonstrated selective chromatic losses. Sensitivities to red/green and blue/yellow stimuli have been shown to be equally impaired.[95]

On the other hand, experiments designed to exploit the difference in temporal or spatial characteristics of the luminance and chromatic mechanisms[96, 97] show reverse results; that is, a greater loss of luminance function (obtained at high frequencies) than chromatic function. Still others report that chromatic losses are nonselective and multiple hue in optic neuritis.[98, 99]

Attempts have been made to link chromatic and luminance changes identified psychophysically with anatomy (i.e., the parvo system or the magno system) and with physiologic data, but no simple relationship(s) have been identified (reviewed in references 100 to 102).[81, 100–104]

Physiologic evidence[105, 106] suggests that color and luminance are encoded by a single pathway and that many P ganglion cells are transmitting information both about the color and the luminance of a stimulus; that is, performing "double-duty." Some investigators regard contrast sensitivity as also linked to the parvocellular channel,[106] citing in evidence the selective destruction of P ganglion cells in the lateral geniculate nucleus of the macaque monkey when exposed to the neurotoxic chemical acrylamide, which reduces contrast sensitivity by almost a factor of 10 as well as depressing chromatic thresholds.[107]

If P ganglion cells perform "double-duty," then as red/green discrimination deteriorates so too should contrast vision. In fact, this is now clearly seen in MS, in which a red/green color deficit correlates strongly and positively with loss of contrast sensitivity.[108] This is a striking correlation, indicating damage to the same cells in the visual pathway.

Equally striking is the lack of any correlation between a blue/green color deficit and the loss of contrast sensitivity, and the evidence that the spatial distribution of damage to the foveal and perifoveal visual field helps determine deficits in hue discrimination. In one study,[89] an approximately equal number of eyes with optic neuritis had a blue/yellow (48 percent) versus red/green (52 percent) dyschromatopsia. The investigators found a strong association between the spatial distribution of damage to the visual field and the type of hue discrimination deficit. Eyes with greater field depression at the fovea, compared with the perifovea, showed a preponderance of red/green (68 percent) dyschromatopsia as opposed to blue/yellow (32 percent) dyschromatopsia. Eyes with greater perifoveal impairment showed a preponderance of blue/yellow (100 percent) dyschromatopsia. This relationship between the spatial distribution of visual field damage and the hue discrimination deficit is statistically significant in optic neuritis ($P = .002$) (Table 201–7).[89]

Table 201–7. THE SPATIAL DISTRIBUTION OF VISUAL FIELD DEFECT AND THE RELATIVE DYSCHROMATOPSIA AXIS IN OPTIC NEURITIS (29 EYES)

Spatial Distribution of Visual Field Defect	Relative Dyschromatopsia Axis	
	Blue/Yellow (n)	*Red/Green (n)*
Relative foveal sparing	7	0
Relative foveal impairment	7	15

From Silverman SE, Hart WM Jr, Gordon MO, et al: The dyschromatopsia of optic neuritis is determined in part by the foveal/perifoveal distribution of visual field damage. Invest Ophthalmol Vis Sci 31:1895–1902, 1990.
Fisher's exact test $P = .002$.

Color vision defects can be detected clinically using Hardy-Rand-Ritter or Ishihara pseudoisochromatic plates. More sensitive testing can be achieved with the Farnsworth-Munsell 100 Hue test. Using this test the author detected dyschromatopsia in all 23 cases (30 eyes) with optic neuritis, compared with 12/23 cases (13 eyes) tested with Ishihara plates. Dyschromatopsia was present when visual acuity had recovered to 20/40 or better.[29]

Contrast Sensitivity

Most patients with recovered optic neuritis and 20/20 Snellen acuity insist that vision in the affected eye(s) is imperfect.[109–113] Using psychophysical tests, such as contrast sensitivity measurements, investigators have been able to detect the hidden visual loss[114–119] (for reviews see references 120 and 121), and one important outcome of their findings is to protect patients with optic neuritis, who have difficulty seeing, from misdiagnosis as nonorganic cases of functional amblyopia. Another important outcome is the ability to determine the effect of spatial frequency of visual stimuli on visual loss.

Measurement of contrast sensitivity at individual spatial frequencies, typically ranging from 0.5 to 23 cycles/degree, can be performed using sinewave gratings displayed on a television monitor at variable contrast. Patients' responses are entered into a computer for tabulation. In humans, there is a sensitivity peak around 4 cycles/degree.

Plotting contrast sensitivity for various spatial frequencies (SF) has led to the detection of four basic patterns of selective loss in pathologic states: high SF, generalized SF, mid-frequency ("notch") SF, and low–mid-SF loss.

In optic neuritis[104, 115–120] and MS,[114, 121, 122] the pattern of loss in individual patients is variable; high, medium, or low SFs may be selectively affected or all spatial frequencies may be evenly affected. Although a low spatial frequency loss is the least common of these possibilities, all can occur.

Any of the four types of spatial loss may be accounted for by variations in the loss of contrast sensitivity within the area of visual field tested.[118] A central foveal field defect produces a contrast sensitivity deficit maximal at high spatial frequencies; a perifoveal field deficit predominantly affects medium-spatial frequencies; and peripheral field loss, sparing the fovea, causes a low-frequency loss.

Low-contrast letter wall charts provide the clinician with an easier method than sinewave gratings for measuring contrast sensitivity.[123, 124] Pelli-Robson low-contrast letter charts are used at a testing distance of 1m, at which distance the letters subtend a visual angle of 3 degrees. The test consists of 16 triplets of letters that range in contrast from approximately 96 percent to 1 percent. The letters are all the same size, and there are three letters on each line. Contrast sensitivity is defined as a reciprocal of the lowest contrast level at which the patient correctly identifies at least 60 percent of the letters (i.e., two-thirds).[124]

The Pelli-Robson charts discriminate normal from abnormal peak contrast function (a midrange spatial frequency) and give repeatable results.[125] The measurement of peak contrast sensitivity is an extremely effective indicator of subclinical optic neuritis, and for this reason it is unnecessary to measure individual spatial frequencies using different sinewave gratings.[126] However, the test is not useful in differentiating optic neuritis from maculopathies, and because it is a subjective test it is of no value in distinguishing organic from nonorganic factitious visual loss.[119]

Stereoacuity

There is a linear relationship between stereoacuity, a measurement of depth perception, and Snellen acuity. Individuals who have normal 20/20 vision in each eye and binocular fixation (no manifest strabismus) have an average stereopsis of 40 sec of arc. Stereoacuity is reduced as acuity decreases down to 20/200, at which level monocular and binocular responses become identical. The value of a normal stereoacuity in the presence of impaired Snellen acuity indicates either that the Snellen acuity for distance is incorrect or that the patient is claiming poor acuity and the visual loss is factitious.

Testing stereoacuity is straightforward. The Titmus polaroid 3-D vectograph stereoacuity test is recommended for both children and adults with optic neuritis.

Because optic nerve damage results in delayed transmission of impulses to the visual cortex, patients with unilateral or markedly asymmetric optic neuritis should experience the Pulfrich effect, a stereo illusion.[127] Pulfrich reported that when a small target oscillating in a frontal plane is viewed binocularly and one eye is covered with a filter that reduces light intensity, the target appears to move in a elliptic rather than a to-and-fro path. When the filter is placed over the right eye, the rotation appears counter clockwise; if it is placed over the left eye, the rotation appears clockwise. This stereo phenomenon is explained on the basis that the covered eye is more weakly stimulated than the uncovered eye, resulting in a delay in the transmission of visual signals to the visual cortex. This disparity in time, caused by the difference in latency between eyes, is interpreted as a disparity in space resulting in a stereo illusion. The magnitude of the effect is determined by the velocity of the target, the difference in retinal illumination between the two eyes, the basic level of retinal illumination, and the distance of the observer from the target. In practice the Pulfrich effect is rarely tested, yet it is thought to be a more sensitive indicator of optic nerve disease than the observation of an afferent pupil defect.[128–133] (For review and instructions for the construction of a Pulfrich apparatus see reference 132.)

Visual Field

Involvement of the visual field during an attack of optic neuritis, as well as following recovery, can be extremely variable.[4, 26, 134–136] Patchy demyelination of the optic nerve is the rule, and the sizes of the circumscribed plaques in the optic nerve differ.[24, 137] In addition areas of both complete and incomplete demyelination are present, and ultrastructural studies show a range of abnormalities on different fibers within the same plaque.[138]

In acute optic neuritis, the cardinal field defect is a widespread depression of sensitivity, particularly pronounced centrally as a cecocentral scotoma (Fig. 201–1*A–C*). An isolated central scotoma is atypical in demyelination; this pattern is more typical of Leber's hereditary optic atrophy or of a toxic nutritional optic neuropathy.

When acuity is severely impaired perimetric field charting is unreliable and confrontation testing is recommended.[139] As vision improves multiisopter kinetic Goldmann perimetry or computer-assisted automated static perimetry using a Humphrey Field Analyzer[140] or Octopus perimeter[141–143] are sensitive techniques for serial testing (Fig. 201–2*A* and *B*; see also Fig. 201–1*A–C*). Plotting the field of the contralateral eye is particularly important, because the detection of a subtle temporal depression may indicate the presence of a sella mass. A finding of generalized depression, paracentral scotomas,[141] or scattered nerve fiber bundle–related defect(s) between 5 and 20 degrees from fixation, may indicate sequelae of prior demyelinating optic neuropathy. Asymptomatic field loss may correlate with other defects of visual function in resolved optic neuritis.[104, 110]

Afferent Pupillary Defect

Unless there is an optic nerve lesion in the fellow eye from previously unrecognized optic neuritis, a unilateral relative afferent pupil defect (RAPD) will be present in the symptomatic neuritic eye. Normal pupillary responses consist of prompt, symmetric constriction (miosis) on exposure to light or on near convergence. Diminished response to a direct light stimulus, combined with a normal consensual pupillary response following stimulation of the contralateral eye, characterize RAPD. The best way to elicit RAPD is to perform a swinging flashlight test.[144] To perform this test, the examiner should maintain a rhythmic equal time alternation of the light from one eye to the other to avoid asymmetric retinal bleach.[145]

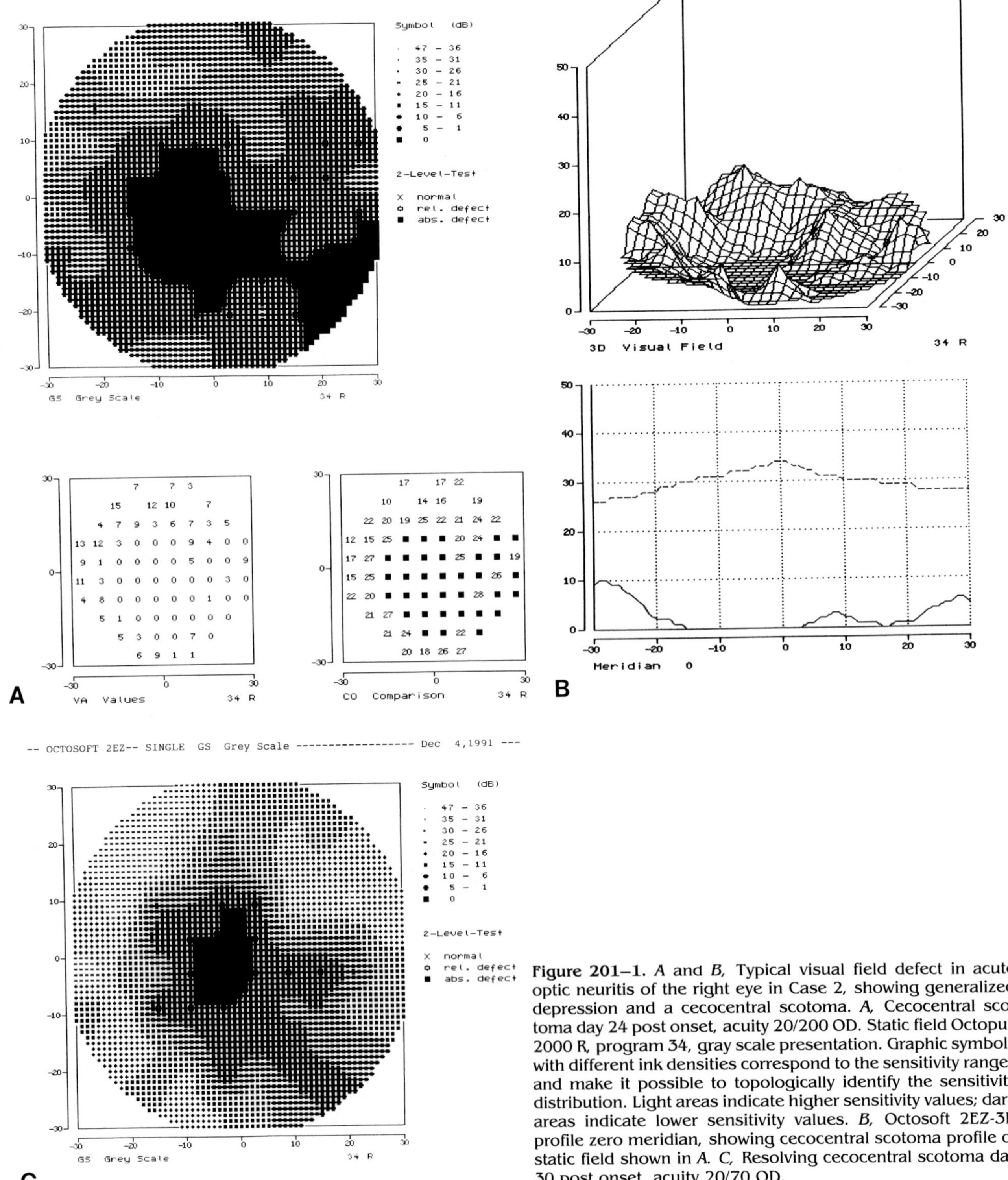

Figure 201–1. *A* and *B,* Typical visual field defect in acute optic neuritis of the right eye in Case 2, showing generalized depression and a cecocentral scotoma. *A,* Cecocentral scotoma day 24 post onset, acuity 20/200 OD. Static field Octopus 2000 R, program 34, gray scale presentation. Graphic symbols with different ink densities correspond to the sensitivity ranges and make it possible to topologically identify the sensitivity distribution. Light areas indicate higher sensitivity values; dark areas indicate lower sensitivity values. *B,* Octosoft 2EZ-3D profile zero meridian, showing cecocentral scotoma profile of static field shown in *A. C,* Resolving cecocentral scotoma day 30 post onset, acuity 20/70 OD.

An afferent pupil defect can be assessed even if one pupil is unreactive due to mydriatics, miotics, oculmotor palsy, or trauma. In such cases, when performing the swinging flashlight test, the direct and consensual responses of the single reactive pupil must be compared. The reactive pupil's direct light response reflects the afferent function of the ipsilateral eye; its consensual response reflects the afferent function of the contralateral eye.

A unilateral afferent pupillary defect can be roughly quantified by the use of graded neutral density filters. By placing a neutral filter in front of the normal eye, the examiner can effectively eliminate the relative afferent defect by "balancing" the visual loss in the two eyes. The filter density needed to balance the pupil defect is a measure of the loss of input to the affected eye and can be compared with earlier measurements for evidence of progression of a disease process.[146, 147]

In acute optic neuritis, the incidence of RAPD is 44 to 76 percent.[4, 26] In recovered optic neuritis, the incidence drops to 17 to 55 percent.[4, 26, 134] In the absence of a maculopathy, RAPD is a highly sensitive sign of an ipsilateral optic nerve lesion and can be seen in an eye with 20/20 vision.

Optic Disc

The appearance of the optic disc in 240 eyes affected acutely by optic neuritis was normal in 64 percent, swollen (papillitis [Fig. 201–3]) in 23 percent, blurred or hyperemic in 18 percent, and blurred with peripapillary hemorrhages around the disc in 2 percent. Temporal pallor was noted in 10 percent, suggesting a preceding attack of optic neuritis in the same eye.[4] In recovered optic neuritis, 6 mo after the first attack, a normal disc was present in 42 percent of eyes; temporal pallor was present in 28 percent; and total disc pallor was evident in 18 percent. Others have observed similar ophthalmoscopic findings in acute optic neuritis.[26, 148, 149] In MS in remission, optic pallor is present in 38 percent of cases.[150]

OCTOSOFT TREND

INTERZEAG AG Schlieren / Switzerland

	EX1	EX2	EX3	EX4	SUMMARY
date of exam.: m.d	10.05	10.17	10.28	12.21	
year	1988	1988	1988	1988	
program [examination]	34[02]	34[05]	34[06]	34[10]	
diameter of pupil	6.0	5.5	5.0	3.5	3.5 .. 6.0
TOTAL LOSS (whole f.)	2071	1277	248	85	920 +- 466
MEAN LOSS (per location)					
whole field	28.0	17.3	3.4	1.1	12.4 +- 6.3
upper nasal	27.4	14.4	2.0	.4	11.0 +- 6.3
lower nasal	28.2	18.3	3.4	.9	12.7 +- 6.4
upper temp.	27.4	13.8	3.5	2.1	11.7 +- 5.9
lower temp.	29.0	22.6	4.6	1.3	14.4 +- 6.8
ecc. 0 - 10	30.8	29.8	8.2	1.4	17.6 +- 7.5
10 - 20	28.9	21.4	4.2	2.1	14.2 +- 6.6
20 - 30	26.8	12.1	1.7	.7	10.3 +- 6.1
MEAN SENSITIVITY					
whole field(N:28.0)	*	*	*	*	* +- *
upper nasal(N:27.4)	*	*	*	*	* +- *
lower nasal(N:28.2)	*	*	*	*	* +- *
upper temp.(N:27.4)	*	*	*	*	* +- *
lower temp.(N:29.0)	*	*	*	*	* +- *
ecc. 0-10 (N:30.8)	*	*	*	*	* +- *
10-20 (N:28.9)	*	*	*	*	* +- *
20-30 (N:26.8)	*	*	*	*	* +- *
# of disturbed points	74	69	30	13	47 +- 15
RMS fluctuation	*	*	*	*	*
total fluctuation					8.7

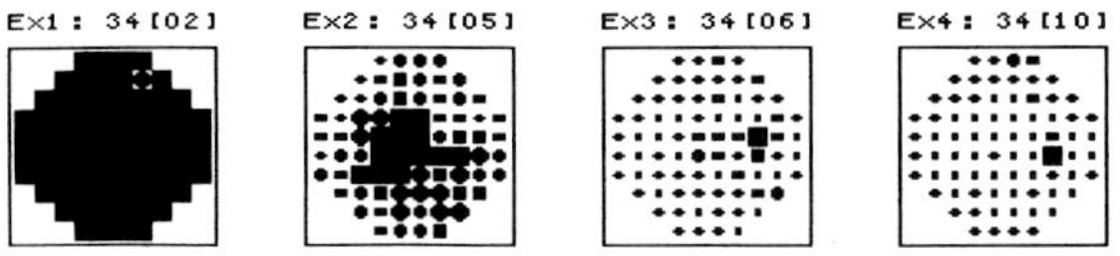

Ex1 : 34 [02] Ex2 : 34 [05] Ex3 : 34 [06] Ex4 : 34 [10]

A

Figure 201–2. *A,* Serial analysis, DELTA program SERIES mode, of a sequence of single visual field examinations in Case 2 with optic neuritis of the right eye. The columns designated EX1, EX2 refer to the examination sequence. The SUMMARY column shows the mean of all the examinations. *B,* The visual fields in both eyes of Case 2. Static field Octopus 2000R program 34 gray scale presentation (*top frame*). Octosoft 2EZ-3D profile at zero meridian (*bottom frame*). Optic neuritis OD recovered to 20/20 (*right frame*) compared to the unaffected left eye 20/15 (*left frame*). The fields are normal. The profile of the physiologic blind spot is shown at zero meridian.

Illustration continued on following page

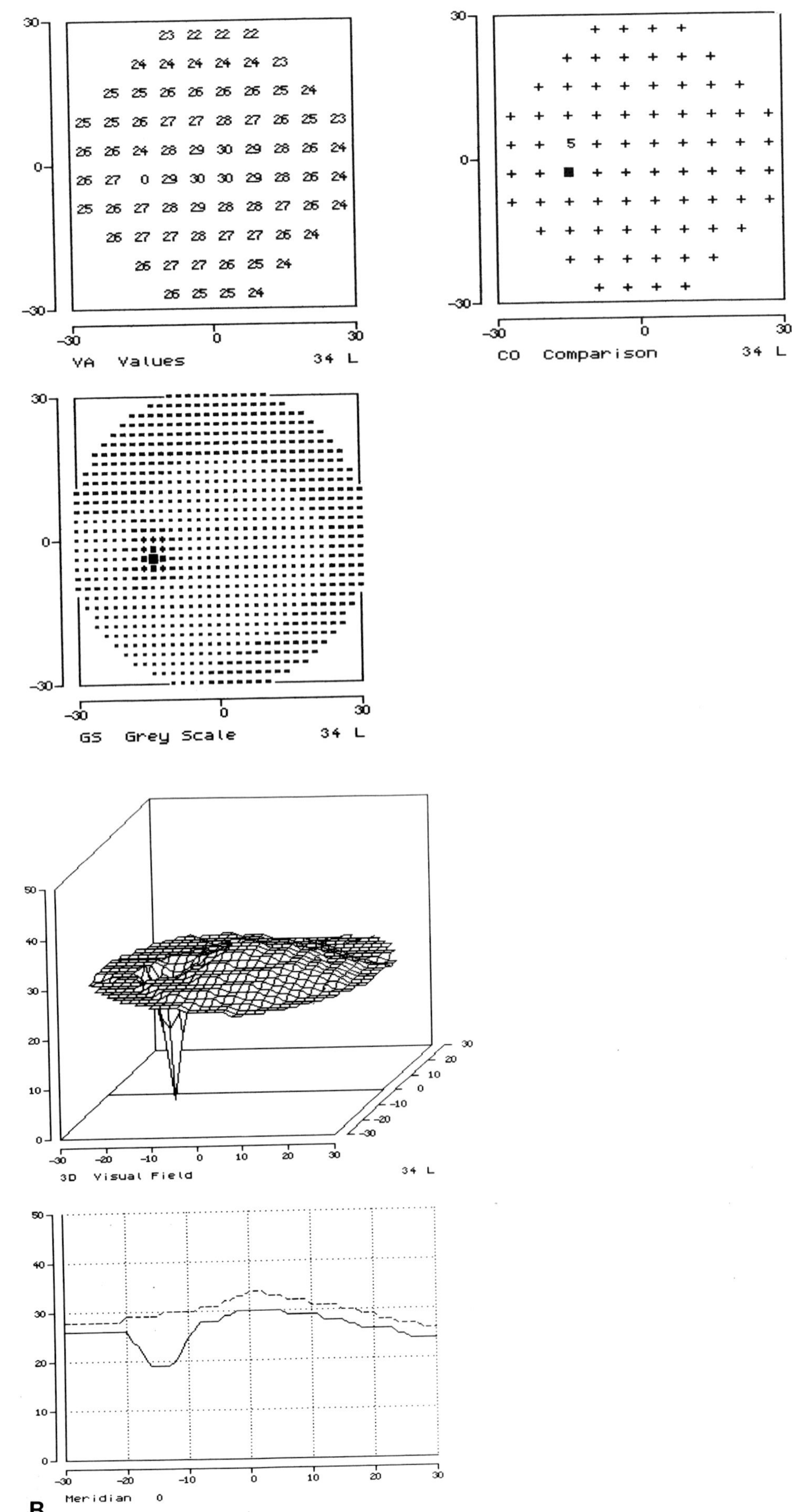

B

Figure 201–2 *Continued (B)*

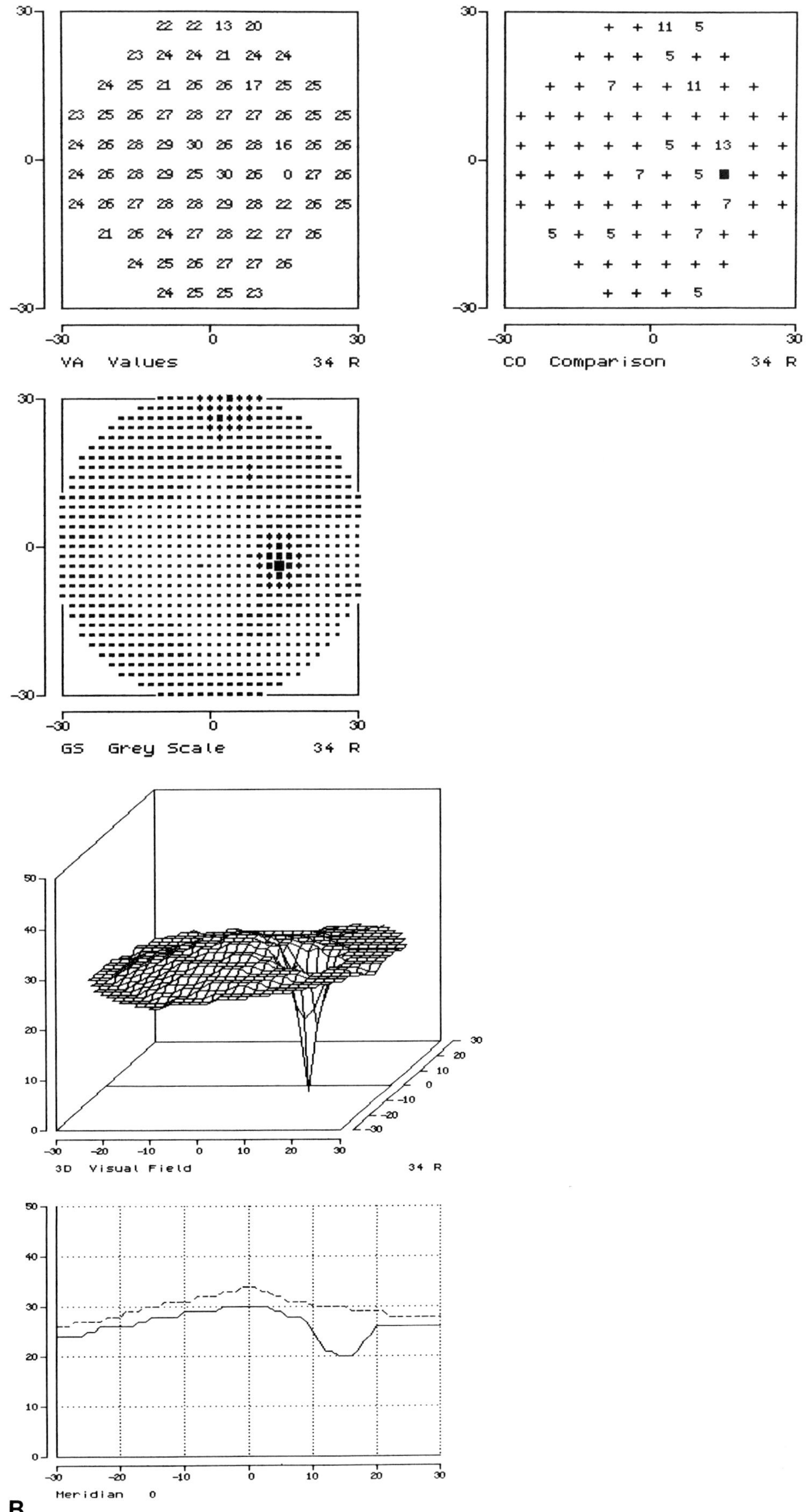

Figure 201–2 *Continued (B)*

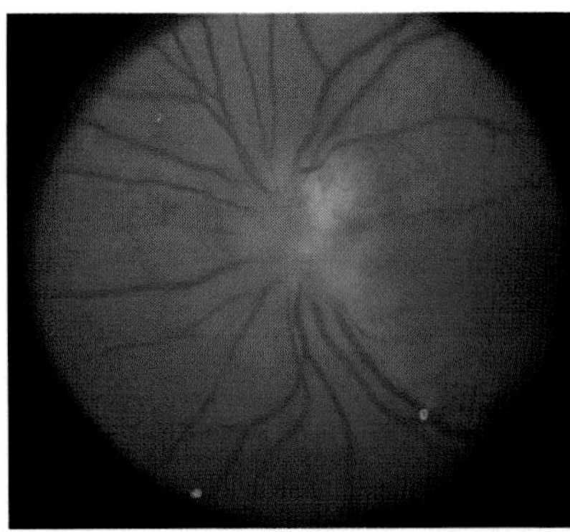

Figure 201–3. Fundus photograph of a swollen left optic disc in a patient with acute demyelinating optic neuritis and 20/100 acuity.

Retina

Two retinal signs are associated with optic neuritis and MS: retinal venous sheathing due to periphlebitis retinae and defects in the retinal nerve fiber layer.

Retinal venous sheathing, characterized by deposits of small, round or ill-defined confluent white exudate along a peripheral vein usually associated with vitreous cells, is present in 28 percent of patients with isolated optic neuritis. In a systematic study of 50 patients presenting with acute optic neuritis,[151] retinal vascular abnormalities or signs of inflammation were found in 14 patients; fluorescein leakage was evident in 10 patients; perivenous sheathing occurred in 6 patients; and cells in the vitreous were found in 6 patients and in the anterior chamber in 4 patients. In two patients, cells in the media were seen without retinal changes. After a mean follow-up of 3.5 yr, MS had developed in 8 of 14 patients with retinal vascular abnormalities or evidence of inflammation, and in 5 of 32 without. The difference is significant ($P > .02$).

Retinal venous sheathing in the eye with MS occurs as an apparently isolated asymptomatic condition, usually in both eyes.[152–154] The condition can resolve completely and can then recur. Some investigators[155] have concluded that virtually all patients with MS develop venous sheathing at some point in their lives. Others have reported an incidence of only 10 percent in the MS population that they studied and associate venous sheathing with progressive MS.[156] In this group of patients sheathing remained unchanged for periods varying from 5 to 11 mo, with an extreme of up to 2 yr.

The connection between venous sheathing and demyelination is important. The occurrence of perivenular abnormalities in a region free of myelin and oligodendrocytes shows that vascular changes in MS can occur independently of contiguous demyelination and in fact may be the primary event in the formation of a new lesion.

The finding of retinal venous sheathing in a patient in whom a diagnosis of optic neuritis or MS is suspected but not confirmed is of diagnostic significance.

Atrophy of the nerve fiber layer precedes the appearance of obvious optic atrophy and occurs in all types of optic neuropathy, regardless of the cause.[157, 158] In the eye with MS, insidious atrophy of retinal nerve fibers occurs without visual symptoms of optic nerve dysfunction.[44] Defects in the retinal nerve fiber layer due to axonal atrophy are seen in optic neuritis and MS as slits in the nerve fiber striations in the arcuate fiber bundles.[159] The incidence of retinal slits in MS is as high as 70 percent, and when slits are seen in the normal eye of a patient with contralateral optic neuritis, they constitute evidence for a second subclinical optic nerve lesion.[160]

Both focal and diffuse nerve fiber atrophy are detectable with the use of monochromatic red-free ophthalmoscopy through a dilated pupil. Red-free light magnifying fundus photography highlights the defects.[161, 162]

INVESTIGATIVE STUDIES

There is usually no need for investigative studies in a healthy adult presenting with typical acute, monosymptomatic, unilateral optic neuritis and an unremarkable medical history. Exceptions should be made for patients from areas where Lyme disease is endemic, and in such cases serology screening for antibody reactivity against *Borrelia burgdorferi* should be considered.[163]

When a deficit in optic nerve function is diagnosed by a thorough eye examination, the cause must be determined. Regular follow-up examination is essential until improvement in vision is recorded, since recovery of vision usually confirms the diagnosis of idiopathic optic neuritis. When there is no improvement, or if visual function declines, investigation is necessary to exclude a compressive optic neuropathy or some other type of optic neuropathy. In both cases the need for further investigation is self-evident, and the decision to investigate is growing less and less debatable.

It is no longer possible for ophthalmologists to ignore the potential for MS in a patient with optic neuritis, even though some ophthalmologists continue to dismiss the need for neuroimaging of the brain to uncover abnormal white matter signals, claiming that moving the patient into the category of MRI-supported MS is not beneficial because there is no specific treatment to reverse or halt the disease. These efforts to "do no harm" become efforts to protect the patient from a diagnosis of MS, and the problem becomes not just one of a patient's right to know. The ophthalmologist may be held responsible in the long term for not looking for lesion dissemination in space.

My own practice is to obtain an MRI within 6 wk of the onset of visual loss. I request T_1- and T_2-weighted images of the brain and orbits in the axial and sagittal planes with coronal views of the orbit back to the middle fossa to visualize the optic nerves and chiasm. The presence of white matter lesions on MRI tends to validate the clinical diagnosis of a demyelinating optic neuropathy and improves, beyond an educated guess, the prediction for MS.

Imaging Plaques

Before the use of brain CT and MRI, the presence of cerebrospinal fluid (CSF) pleocytosis and oligoclonal immunoglobulin provided paraclinical evidence of the dissemination of lesions and met the criteria for the diagnosis of laboratory-supported MS in isolated optic neuritis. They indicated an increased risk of progression to MS.[164]

Today, neuroimaging has supplanted the spinal tap. Brain and orbit CT is used to eliminate a compressive lesion or to evaluate the nasal sinuses. In optic neuritis, CT scanning can show enlargement and contrast enhancement of the affected nerve.[165, 166] Although these features are nonspecific and occur in association with raised intracranial pressure and papilledema, inflammatory pseudotumor, optic nerve sheath meningioma,[167] or glioma, the signs are transient in optic neuritis.[165]

Brain MRI, with and without gadolinium, is more sensitive than the CT for imaging multifocal plaques in the white matter (Fig. 201–4*A–E*). MRI abnormalities of this type occur in 56 to 72 percent of adult patients with isolated optic neuritis[46, 168–172] and in 90 to 98 percent of patients with clinically definite MS.[173–177] However, the lack of specificity of MRI findings for demyelination can lead to a false-positive diagnosis of MS, and as with other clinical signs such as nystagmus, the Babinski sign, or optic disc pallor, clinical judgment must be exercised.

Modification of the brain imaging technique using the STIR sequence (an inversion recovery sequence with a short inversion time) and a surface coil specially designed for orbit imaging increases the diagnostic potential of visualizing plaques in the optic nerve(s). Using this technique, investigators examined 37 adult patients (25 women and 12 men) with known optic neuritis.[27] Twenty-nine patients (78 percent) had isolated optic neuritis, and 8 patients (21 percent) had probable or definite MS.

Focal high-signal MRI lesions were detected in 84 percent of symptomatic optic nerves and in 20 percent of asymptomatic optic nerves. The mean longitudinal extent of the lesions measured 1 cm. Lesion sites were classified as: (1) anterior, when the lesion was in continuity with the nerve head and did not extend beyond

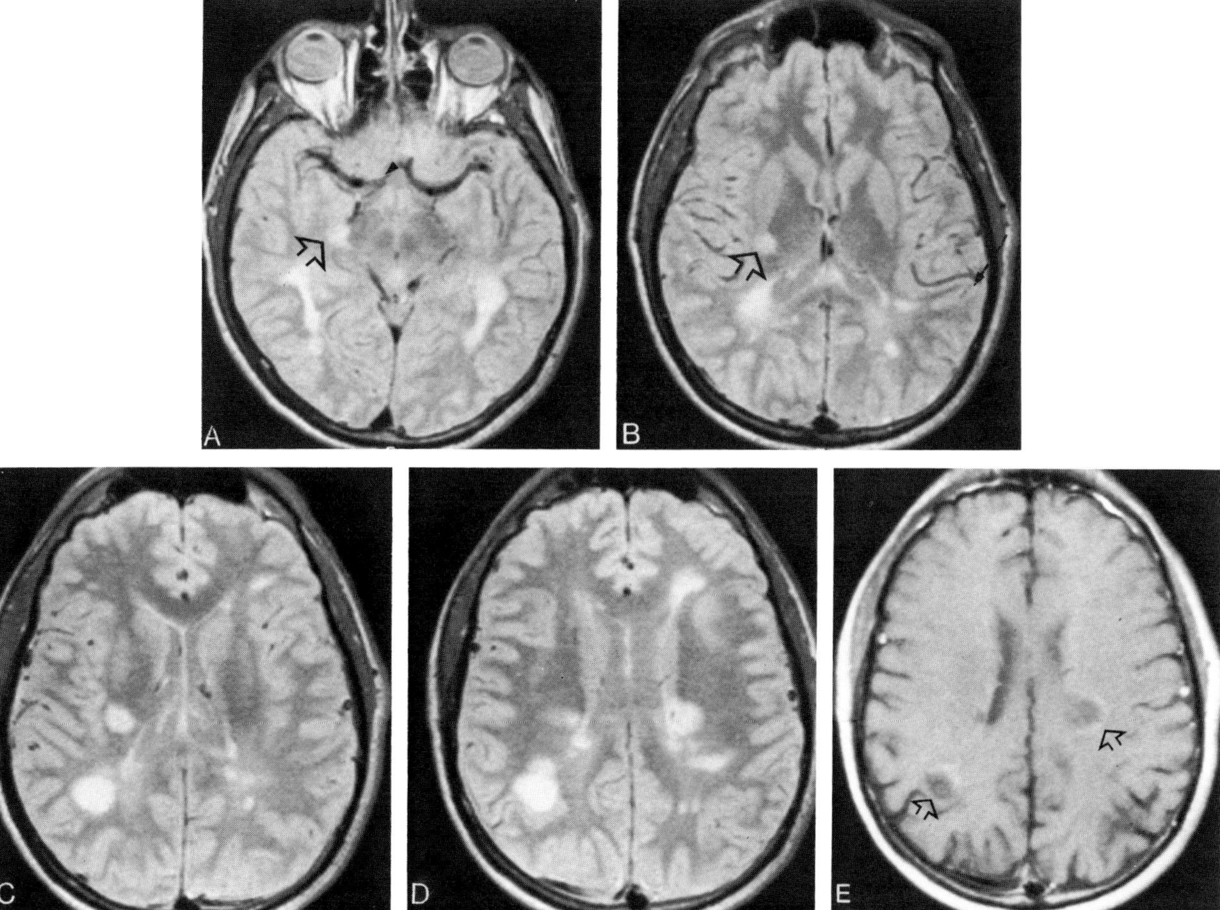

Figure 201–4. *A–E,* Axial views of the brain MRI of a man, 32 yr of age, with a left incongruous homonymous hemianopia. *A–D,* The T2 W1 proton image revealed multiple small hyperintense lesions in the cerebral white matter consistent with a diagnosis of multiple sclerosis. *A* and *B,* One plaque in the right lateral geniculate body (*arrow, top left frame*) extends superiorly into the putamen posteriorly (*arrow, top right frame*). *C* and *D,* Two of the largest plaques are seen in the right parietal lobe and in the corpus callosum. *E,* The T1 W1 proton image with gadolinium, axial view through the roof of the lateral ventricle, revealed ring enhancement of the right parietal (*arrow*) and corpus callosal (*arrow*) lesions consistent with active demyelination.

midorbit; (2) intraorbital, when it extended from midorbit to the optic canal; (3) intracanalicular, when it was within the optic canal; (4) intracranial, when that portion of the optic nerve was involved; and (5) chiasmal, when the chiasm was affected. Lesions frequently struck more than one site in continuity.

Table 201–2 shows the frequency of lesions at each site in the symptomatic optic nerves. The retrobulbar segment was most commonly involved with an incidence of 61 percent in the midintraorbital region. No additional lesions were seen with gadolinium-enhanced MRI, although in one patient gadolinium demonstrated intracranial nerve and chiasmal involvement that was not visible with the STIR sequence.

VEPs

VEPs in optic neuritis provide an objective extension of the ophthalmic examination. There are two tests: the pattern shift VEP and the pattern electroretinogram (PERG). In optic neuritis, the pattern VEP is the technique of choice: (1) to objectively confirm weak clinical evidence of visual dysfunction; (2) to detect subclinical abnormality; and (3) to demonstrate an organic cause for symptoms that might otherwise be suspected to be of psychogenic origin (e.g., blurred vision on exertion).

The pattern VEP tests the central and perifoveal visual field. While it is generated in cortical areas 17, 18, and 19, as is the flash VEP, it draws on different though overlapping pools of neurons. The waveform of the pattern VEP is triphasic. The major positive component, P100, is preceded and followed by smaller negative peaks (N75 and N145) (Fig. 201–5*A* and *B* top trace). The response is reproducible and is sensitive to conduction defects in the visual pathways.

The major change associated with optic nerve demyelination is prolongation of P100 latency (see Fig. 201–5*A* top trace).[178–182] P100 amplitude is not a reliable parameter because of relatively large normal variability in amplitude, and P100 amplitude is correlated with visual acuity. P100 latency, however, is not.[183, 184] When there is clinical evidence of optic neuritis, the incidence

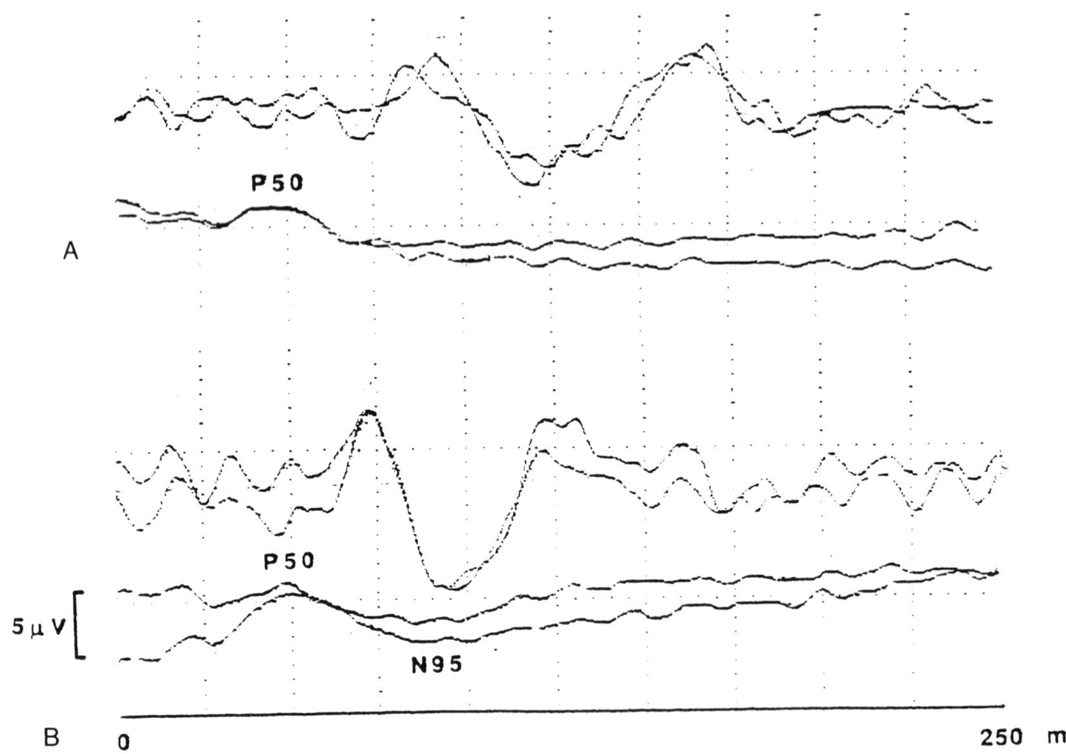

Figure 201–5. *A* and *B,* Simultaneous recording of the pattern VEP and PERG to 50′ checks in a patient with monocular optic neuritis in the right eye OD. *A,* Right eye Snellen acuity 20/20 −2. PVEP P100 latency 118.5 msec, amplitude 14uV (*top trace*) PERG P50 latency 45.5 msec, amplitude 2uV. The N95 wave is flat (*bottom trace*). *B,* Normal left eye, Snellen acuity 20/15; PVEP P100 latency 96.5 msec, amplitude 19.5 uV (*top trace);* PERG P50 latency 49 msec, amplitude 5 uV; N95 latency 99.5 msec, 1.6 uV (*bottom trace*).

Normal values for check size 50′ for PVEP and PERG

PVEP P100 latency mean 102 msec, upper limit 112.5 msec
P100 amplitude mean 11.4 uV, lower limit 4.7 uV

PERG P50 latency mean 48.5 msec, upper limit 53.5 msec
P50 amplitude mean 2.1 uV, lower limit 0.8 uV
N95 latency mean 93 msec, upper limit 100 msec
N95 amplitude mean 1.7 uV, lower limit 0.5 uV

Limits are based on 98 percent confidence intervals for the normal range. For PVEP n = 84, and for PERG n = 32. (Modified from Scholl GB, Song H-S, Winkler DE, et al: The pattern visual evoked potential and pattern electroretinogram in Drusen optic neuropathy. Arch Ophthalmol 110:75, 1992. Copyright 1992, American Medical Association.)

of P100 latency changes is very high, that is to say, 89 percent in 438 patients, with some studies above 95 percent. When there is no clinical evidence of optic nerve involvement, the incidence is much lower—51 percent in 715 patients.[185]

Delay in the P100 is usually present whatever the time interval following the attack of optic neuritis. One study found pattern VEP abnormalities 5 yr after the clinical episode,[181] and other investigators found P100 latency abnormalities as long as 15 yr later.[179] Only 5 percent of patients with abnormal pattern VEPs have the P100 latency return to normal following an episode of optic neuritis.

The difference in interocular P100 latency is also an indicator of optic nerve dysfunction in the pattern VEP, and this parameter has been used to provide evidence of optic nerve pathology in optic neuritis and MS.[181, 186–190] In MS, in the 20/20 eye with no history of optic neuritis, delayed latencies were found in the P100 in 38 percent of 23 patients and abnormal interocular latency differences in 67 percent.[190]

Several investigators have explored the correlation between pattern VEP abnormalities and the clinical eye examination in MS.[191–193] In a retrospective study, the striking finding was that when the pattern VEP was normal, no abnormalities were found in the neuroophthalmologic examination. When the pattern VEP was abnormal, the clinical examination was also normal to a surprising degree.[191] Other studies,[136, 192, 193] including those using automated Octopus perimetry,[142, 193] now indicate that a formal and careful visual field examination will reveal field defects even in asymptomatic eyes.

Despite the sensitivity of the pattern VEP in detecting optic nerve dysfunction, the prolongation of P100 latency produced by demyelinating plaques in optic neuritis and MS is indistinguishable from abnormalities secondary to compression,[194] glaucoma,[195] and CNS dopamine deficiency diseases.[196] Because of this lack of specificity, the ophthalmologist must decide if other procedures (e.g., neurology consultation or neuroimaging) are indicated to differentiate the possible causes of delayed conduction.

Pattern Electroretinogram

The PERG monitors the integrity of the central retinal ganglion cell layer. The PERG waveform consists of a prominent positive component at approximately 52 msec (P50), followed by a large negative component at approximately 93 msec (N95) (see Fig. 201–5*A* and *B* bottom trace). In some patients, a small early negative N35 component is also present.[197–199]

The PERG is of value in the improved interpretation of an abnormal pattern VEP, and, a PERG is required in order to make certain that a delay in the pattern VEP P100 in a patient with suspected optic nerve demyelination is not due to a more anterior visual dysfunction or to a maculopathy. To accomplish this, the PERG and pattern VEP must be recorded simultaneously (see Fig. 201–5*A* and *B*). In an optic neuropathy the results show a delayed pattern VEP P100 latency, a near-normal PERG P50 amplitude, and a small amplitude or absent PERG N95 component (see Fig. 201–5*A*). In an anterior visual pathway dysfunction or maculopathy, the major abnormality is a reduction in amplitude of the PERG P50 component with a normal N95 component and a delayed and small-amplitude pattern VEP P100.

Early investigators of the PERG in optic nerve demyelination limited their analysis of the changes in PERG to the P50 component.[200–207] Subsequently, they extended the analysis to include the later N95 component and demonstrated that the N95 can be selectively affected in optic nerve demyelination.[197, 208–210] This abnormality of PERG N95 is also present in drusen optic neuropathy.[211]

One study reports PERG changes in 141 patients with optic nerve demyelination in one or both eyes.[208] The overall incidence of PERG abnormality in 199 eyes with abnormally delayed pattern VEP P100 was 39.2 percent, with 84.6 percent of these PERG abnormalities being confined to the N95 component. The incidence of an abnormal PERG was greater (53.3 percent) in eyes with a history of optic neuritis than in those with subclinical demyelination (22.8 percent). The relatively low figure of 39.2 percent for abnormality of PERG in this series confirms previous suggestions that PERG is of little value in the diagnosis of optic nerve demyelination.[212, 213] The data do, however, support growing evidence that the P50 and N95 components of the PERG have different retinal origins.

DIFFERENTIAL DIAGNOSES OF THE CONDITION

Errors in the diagnosis of optic neuritis can be minimized if the ophthalmologist is alert to discrepancies in the clinical picture presented. These discrepancies include unusual features in the onset or course, for example, the absence of pain or onset over 50 yr of age, failure to remit, or the presence of neurologic abnormalities in the upper cranial nerves not attributable to MS.

Unilateral Optic Neuritis

The differential diagnosis of unilateral optic neuritis includes ischemic optic neuropathy, rhinogenous optic neuritis, Lyme borreliosis optic neuropathy, syphilis, HIV-associated optic neuropathies, and nonorganic factitious visual loss.

Ischemic optic neuropathy (anterior or posterior) cannot be distinguished from idiopathic optic neuritis by the age of the patient, even though most patients with ischemic optic neuropathy are in middle and late life and the condition is rare in persons younger than 40 yr of age. Acute anterior ischemic optic neuropathy is, however, characterized by a more abrupt onset, severe visual loss within minutes to hours, an altitudinal field defect (58 percent of cases), and pale swelling of the disc with flame-shaped peripapillary hemorrhages (for review see Chapter 202).

Rhinogenous optic neuritis can arise from sinus disease, and even though it is an infrequent cause of optic neuritis it can closely mimic unilateral idiopathic optic neuritis.[57–59, 214] The clinical history provides the clue, and rhinogenous optic neuritis should be suspected in any patient with recurrent attacks of visual loss that repeatedly occur with severe headache and a bad head cold. Nevertheless, the condition can be diagnostically difficult, and when missed, infection of the paranasal sinuses may be complicated by sphenoethmoiditis[215] or a sphenoid sinus mucocele.[58] Furthermore, a sinus mucocele may cause enlargement of the sella or calcification and simulate an intrasellar or suprasellar tumor,[216] or when vision improves with steroid therapy it can mimic steroid-sensitive optic neuritis. Thus, when sinus disease is suspected, a rhinologist should be consulted.

Lyme borreliosis optic neuritis is rare.[70, 71, 163, 217] The most common manifestation of optic nerve involvement in Lyme disease is optic disc edema, which occurs usually during the early stage of the illness and is associated with meningitis. In these patients, disc swelling is caused by papilledema or optic perineuritis. Treatment is not yet specific, however, in two patients with optic neuritis and CSF pleocytosis, treatment with intravenous ceftriaxone resulted in improved visual acuity. Two other patients who received oral antibiotics are also reported to have shown excellent recovery of visual acuity.[163] Serologic testing for Lyme disease is warranted for individuals with optic neuritis who reside in an endemic region, and patients with rising convalescent antibody levels or unexplained CSF pleocytosis should receive antibiotic treatment.[163] Unfortunately, currently available blood tests to detect antibodies are not very sensitive. The overall sensitivity of serology is 30 to 45 percent using indirect immunofluorescence antibody and 24 to 32 percent using enzyme-linked immunosorbent assay.[218]

Acute syphilitic optic neuritis is a manifestation of early infectious (secondary) neurosyphilis, and it is characterized by acute unilateral visual loss. In two reported cases, optic disc swelling preceded the development of the typical mucocutaneous lesions and was accompanied by mild signs of meningeal inflammation.[219] Other signs of ocular inflammation, such as uveitis or retinal vasculitis, were absent. In patients with syphilitic optic neuritis, involvement of the CNS must be confirmed and appropriate antibiotic therapy prescribed. Syphilitic optic perineuritis may also occur as a manifestation of meningeal inflammation in secondary syphilis.[220–222] This condition is characterized by inflammation of the optic nerve sheath and swelling of the optic disc. Normal acuity is usually preserved. The diagnosis of secondary syphilis is confirmed by serology. Serology tests for syphilis are of two classes: nontreponemal (reagin) tests such as the rapid plasma reagin (RPR) test and the Venereal Disease Research Laboratory (VDRL) slide test, and treponemal tests, such as the *Treponema pallidum* immobilization (TPI) and the fluorescent treponemal antibody absorption (FTA-ABS) test. The RPR and VDRL tests detect the presence of reagin antibodies in serum. They are equally sensitive and can be used for screening, in the assessment of treatment, and for follow-up. Both tests give positive results in the case of secondary syphilis. The VDRL test remains the standard test for use with spinal fluid and CSF serology need only be examined when the peripheral serology is positive or there is clinical evidence of CNS syphilis. In secondary syphilis, the VDRL titer usually reaches 1:32 or higher. The spinal fluid cell count and protein level can be normal. Treponemal tests detect antibodies directed against specific *T. pallidum* antigen(s). Their sensitivity and specificity far outweigh the nontreponemal tests, and therefore they are used to confirm the diagnosis. Once positive, they tend to remain so for life. They cannot however be used to monitor therapeutic responses. Therefore, TPI is the standard to which other tests are compared, and the FTA-ABS is the next most reliable test and is the one most widely available. False-negative FTA-ABS are reported in up to 15 percent of primary syphilitics, up to 5 percent each of latent and late syphilitics, and less than 1 percent of secondary syphilitics. For the ophthalmologist, the best practice is to obtain an FTA-ABS together with a VDRL test for syphilis.

HIV-associated optic neuropathies cover a spectrum of various types of infective optic neuritides: syphilitic optic neuritis[73–75]; papillitis or neuroretinitis of cytomegalovirus[79]; and hepatitis B optic neuropathy or acute retinal necrosis syndrome (herpes group) (for review see reference 223). The role of HIV itself as an agent in optic nerve disease is unknown, but a neurologic disease clinically and histologically indistinguishable from MS and associated with bilateral optic neuritis is reported in HIV type I infection.[224]

Nonorganic visual loss is often misdiagnosed as idiopathic optic neuritis. The disorder occurs at all ages and in both sexes and may be unilateral or bilateral. It often coexists with organic eye disorders or with MS (see Case 4). Nonorganic factitious visual loss must be suspected in any patient who claims impaired acuity and who has normal pupillary reflexes and no abnormality on fundus examination.

Simultaneous or Sequential Bilateral Optic Neuritis

When optic neuritis strikes both eyes, simultaneously or sequentially, the disorder must be distinguished from the following: Devic's disease, immune-mediated optic neuropathy, nutritional amblyopia, Jamaican optic neuropathy, Leber's hereditary optic neuropathy, and functional blindness.

Devic's disease, neuromyelitis optica,[225, 226] is an inflammatory CNS-demyelinating disease that is considered to be a variant of MS.[227, 228] Devic's disease affects both eyes simultaneously or sequentially in children,[229–231] in young adults,[225, 226, 229] and in the elderly[232–234] and is accompanied by transverse myelitis within days or weeks. The condition is rare in the US, and two investigators, in order to provide an updated clinical profile of neuromyelitis optica as well as to consider the prognostic implications of a single bout, have reported two cases of their own along with a review of 43 cases from the literature.[229] The data show that the presenting symptom was bilateral optic neuritis in 36 percent of patients, unilateral optic neuritis in 40 percent of patients, transverse myelitis in 13 percent of patients, and simultaneous optic neuritis and transverse myelitis in 11 percent of patients. The interval between the development of optic neuritis and transverse myelitis ranged from simultaneous onset to 7 wk; however, in 60 percent of patients, the interval was less than 1 wk. Furthermore, the severity of the optic neuritis and transverse myelitis tended to correlate, although the two conditions can be dissociated in their degree of severity. In most patients, the visual deficit was bilateral (91 percent) and usually severe, and unilateral or bilateral blindness occurred in 58 percent. Eighty-four percent of cases had an abnormal CSF during the acute stage of the illness: 62 percent had an elevated CSF protein and 61 percent had a CSF pleocytosis.

The neurologic outcome reported indicated that 79 percent of the patients improved neurologically, 14 percent had a poor outcome, and 16 percent died in the acute stages. Predictors of a poor outcome were older age, marked CSF pleocytosis, and severe myelitis. Forty-two percent of patients had a recurrence of demyelinating disease after initial recovery, suggesting a diagnosis of MS.

Neuromyelitis optica has also been reported in association with systemic lupus erythematosus (SLE)[235] and pulmonary tuberculosis.[236] Familial cases of acute optic neuropathy and myelopathy may be linked to an inherited mutation in mitochondrial DNA (mtDNA), possibly a cytochromic oxidase subunit 2 mutation at nucleotide (nt) position 7706.[237]

Immune mediated optic neuropathy may be associated with SLE. A review of optic neuropathy with SLE emphasizes that both disc swelling and a retrobulbar form occur attributable to small vessel ischemia.[238] Autoimmune optic neuritis is also reported in patients lacking the necessary immunologic criteria for a classification of SLE. In a small subset of female patients, it is characterized by progressive bilateral visual loss that is remarkably steroid responsive to high-dose corticosteroids and other immunosuppressive drugs.[239, 240]

Nutritional amblyopia due to vitamin deficiencies and tobacco-alcohol amblyopia should be readily distinguishable from the rare cases of bilateral progressive demyelinating optic neuropathy. Characteristically, both eyes are affected simultaneously and symmetric cecocentral scotoma are present. Clinically there are no distinguishing differences between tobacco amblyopia, tobacco-alcohol amblyopia, optic neuropathy of chronic alcoholism, or malnutrition optic neuropathy.[241–244] Dietary deficiency is the common denominator, and thiamine therapy improves vision in the early phase of the neuropathy despite continuing abuse of alcohol or tobacco. However, in young patients, even in the absence of a family history of optic neuropathy, Leber's hereditary optic neuropathy should be considered in the differential diagnosis, particularly because alcohol may act as a synergistic agent for the clinical expression of the mtDNA point mutations at nt position 11,778 and 3460 (see later). In elderly patients, the possibility of B_{12} or folate deficiency should not be overlooked.[245]

Jamaican optic neuropathy is characterized by bilateral visual loss (acuity < 20/200) and dense central scotoma.[246] The syndrome affects West African and Caribbean immigrants. These patients are well nourished, nonintoxicated, and nonreactive on serologic tests for syphilis. Yet no form of therapy affords relief, and there is no spontaneous recovery. The cause of this neuropathy is unknown.

Leber's hereditary optic neuropathy (LHON) is a maternally inherited disease that primarily affects young men.[247, 248] The male predominance ranges from 80 to 90 percent in most caucasians to approximately 60 percent in families from Japan. Approximately 50 to 60 percent of men at risk for LHON experience significant visual loss.[249–252] Among the women at risk, the occurrence rate is in the range of 8 to 32 percent. The neuropathy is characterized by painless subacute bilateral visual loss and central or cecocentral scotoma. The onset occurs typically between the ages of 12 and 30 yr, but otherwise classic LHON has been reported in younger and older individuals. Characteristically, impaired visual acuity occurs in one eye only, and sequential visual loss develops in the contralateral eye weeks or months later. Simultaneous visual loss is also reported,[252–255] but these cases may also include examples in which initial involvement of the first eye was not recognized. On rare occasions, loss of vision in the second eye may occur after a prolonged interval (up to 8 yr).[256, 257] Rarely, involvement may remain monocular.[258–260] Uhthoff's symptom may occur in patients with LHON as it does in patients with demyelinating optic neuritis. Maximimum visual acuity loss may range from no light perception to as good as 20/20, but most patients with LHON have acuities of worse than 20/200. And, in most patients, visual loss remains profound and permanent, although spontaneous improvement of some degree has been reported in 29 percent of patients in one study,[261] in 45 percent in another,[252] and in 11 of 13 patients in one Canadian pedigree.[254]

The fundoscopic abnormalities in LHON depend on the stage of the neuropathy. During the acute stage, circumpapillary telangiectatic microangiopathy is present with hyperemia of the disc, swelling of the peripapillary nerve fiber layer, vascular tortuosity, and absence of leakage from the disc or vessels on fluorescein angiography.[263, 264] When the typical funduscopic appearance of LHON is present in a patient or in his or her maternal relatives, it is a good corroborative sign.[260] However, some patients with LHON never exhibit the characteristic fundus findings,[255] thus their absence is not exclusionary. The telangiectatic microangiopathy resolves in time, and in the late stage of LHON optic atrophy develops with loss of the nerve fiber layer striations in the region of the papillomacular bundle. In most patients with LHON, visual dysfunction represents the only significant manifestation of the disease, although cardiac conduction abnormalities (notably the Wolff-Parkinson-White and Lown-Ganong-Levine syndromes) have been reported in Finnish families.[265]

Leber's hereditary optic neuritis is the first human

disease to be linked conclusively to an inherited mutation in mtDNA.[266] The diagnosis can be made by DNA sequencing of blood (two purple top tubes of blood per patient should be sent to the appropriate center for testing). A single nucleotide substitution occurs at position 11,778 in the ND-4 gene that codes for subunit 4 of complex I in the respiratory chain and accounts for about 40 to 60 percent of the cases of LHON worldwide. The mutation has also been reported in Asian patients with LHON.[267] A second mutation in complex I genes has been found in three independent Finnish LHON families at the nt 3460 mutation in ND-1 but in none of 60 maternally unrelated controls.[268] None of the families with the nt 3460 mutation had the previously reported nt 11,778 mutation. But the ophthalmologic findings in the affected individuals from the three families that had the ND-1 mutation were similar to those in families with the ND-4 mutation. Additional mutations at nt position 4,216 (ND-1), position 4,917 (ND-2), and position 13,708 (ND-5) have also been discovered, linked to the 11,778 mutation in Leber probands.[269] It thus appears that a mutation of distinct, functionally related complex I genes is the central pathogenetic feature of LHON, and a continued search for mutations is still needed in the small minority of LHON probands who do not harbor either the 11,778 or the 3460 point mutation to fortify the molecular genetic analysis. (For review see references 270 and 271.)

TREATMENT OF THE CONDITION

There is no specific treatment for optic neuritis, and the evidence is unconvincing that a retrobulbar injection of triamcinolone,[272] or prednisone by mouth, or daily intramuscular[273] or subcutaneous[274] injections of corticotrophin for 30 days, influence visual outcome.

In a 1977 controlled single-blind trial, 31 patients with optic neuritis were treated with a single retrobulbar injection of triamcinolone within the first 2 wk of visual loss. Thirty patients were untreated controls.[272] The results showed a trend toward more rapid recovery of vision in the treated group but no significant difference from the controls in visual acuity, color vision, or visual fields for the first 6 mo after treatment. The authors of this trial concluded that routine use of corticosteroids is not justified in unilateral optic neuritis when vision in the other eye is good. Shortening the period of visual disability in bilateral disease, or in unilateral disease when vision in the other eye is poor, was considered a justifiable indication for steroid therapy. (For review see references 275 and 276.)

In 1980 the effect of pulse intravenous 6-methylprednisolone (6-MP) therapy in MS was reported.[277] Intravenous 6-MP produced fast clinical improvement from acute relapse but failed to confer any lasting benefit on the course of the disease.[277–281]

In optic neuritis, a short course of high-dose intravenous 6-MP produced a similar rapid clinical improvement in 12 consecutive patients (9 women, 3 men).[282] Each received 6- MP (250 or 500 mg intravenously every 6 hr for 3 to 7 days) within 7 to 90 days of onset. The initial visual acuity ranged from no light perception to 20/30. Visual acuity was followed daily, and visual fields were charted on admission and every other day. After 3 to 7 days of 6-MP treatment the drug was abruptly discontinued, and either therapy was stopped or a rapidly tapered oral dose of corticosteroid was administered. After treatment, visual acuity and visual fields were followed weekly for 1 mo, monthly for 3 mo, and subsequently every 3 mo. There was no untreated control group in this study. The authors concluded that patients with optic neuritis may benefit from intravenous megadose corticosteroids.

Subsequent to this study, and in order to reevaluate the documented visual outcome, another investigator matched 26 untreated control cases of optic neuritis examined over 6 mo to the 12 6-MP treated cases and reported no significant difference in the final visual acuity between the treated patients and an untreated group regardless of whether the Snellen fraction ($t = -0.94$; degrees of freedom = 38; $P = 0.36$ [two-tailed]) or the log MAR ($t = -1.20$; degrees of freedom = 38; $P = 0.24$ [two-tailed]) acuity was used.[283]

This comparison, however, does not establish that treatment of optic neuritis with intravenous 6-MP does not work, only that the current data fails to show any long-term benefit if visual acuity is used as the final measurement. Nonetheless, caution is warranted because intravenous 6-MP treatment has potentially serious side effects, including psychologic disturbance, hypertension, hyperglycemia, and, more rarely, anaphylactic reactions, seizures, and sudden death.

A report of a possible harmful late effect of 6-MP therapy in optic neuritis supports this cautionary note.[284] Twenty-six patients with optic neuritis from southern Israel were treated in three ways. Six patients were treated with 6-MP, 1000 mg intravenously for 8 hr on 3 consecutive days with no oral steroid administered subsequently. Fourteen patients were treated with prednisone 1 mg/kg/day taken orally for 10 days and then tapered off during a period of 3 to 5 wk. Six patients were left untreated. Improved vision, measured as an improvement in visual acuity of at least one line on the Snellen chart, the number of recurrent attacks of optic neuritis, or conversion to MS were all recorded.

The results showed that 6-MP therapy improved vision faster (mean = 8 days) than did prednisone (mean of 32 days), or if cases were left untreated (mean of 40 days). All 6-MP treated cases improved and so did 12 of 14 patients taking prednisone. Only 3 of 6 untreated patients improved spontaneously.

Overall 30 percent (8 of 26) of patients had one or more recurrent attacks of optic neuritis. The 6-MP treated group suffered the highest number of recurrences. Patients were followed for 3 yr, and recurrent optic neuritis occurred in 4 of 6 patients in under 2 yr. One patient had five attacks, and two patients had three attacks in this period. In the prednisone group, recurrent optic neuritis occurred in 2 of 14 cases—in one case 10 mo and in the other case 5 yr after the first attack. Two of the six untreated patients, followed for up to 6 yr, suffered recurrent attacks—one patient 3 mo and the other 3 yr after the initial episode.

The conversion to MS was also significantly higher in the 6-MP treated group (5 of 6), compared with the prednisone group (1 of 4), and the untreated cases (0 of 6). In the 6-MP therapy patients, MS was diagnosed clinically within 7 to 18 mo of the first attack of optic neuritis.

The observation of a high rate of recurrent optic neuritis and an apparent increased conversion to MS in the 6-MP therapeutic group is both surprising and disturbing, even though the patient population was extremely small. Patient numbers were also small in the 1969 and 1974 corticotrophin trials. For example, patient numbers ranged from 44 to 54 cases with the individual group size (treated and untreated groups) varying from 21 to 28 cases per group. A letter to the editor of the *Archives of Ophthalmology* in 1981 critically addresses this issue.[285]

The need for a much larger and thus statistically more predictive sample has now been addressed by a multicenter randomized, controlled trial of corticosteroids in the treatment of acute optic neuritis.[286] Four hundred and fifty-seven patients were randomly assigned to receive oral prednisone therapy (Deltasone 1 mg/kg of body weight per day) for 14 days; intravenous methylprednisolone (Solumedrol, 250 mg every 6 hr) for 3 days, followed by oral prednisone (Deltasone 1 mg/kg/day [rounded to the nearest 10 mg]) for 11 days; or oral placebo for 14 days. Each treatment period was followed by a short course of oral prednisone, which was tapered and stopped. Visual function was assessed over a 6-mo follow-up.

The trial was designed to answer the following questions: Does treatment with either oral prednisone or intravenous methylprednisolone improve visual outcome in acute optic neuritis? Does either treatment speed the recovery of vision? What are the complications of treatment in relation to its efficacy?

The results showed that intravenous methylprednisolone followed by oral prednisone speeds the recovery of visual loss due to optic neuritis but results in only slightly better vision at 6 mo. Oral prednisone alone, as prescribed in this study, provided no benefit in terms of either the rate of recovery or the outcome at 6 mo, and the investigators concluded that this drug is ineffective treatment.

Surprisingly, prednisone was found to increase the risk of new episodes of optic neuritis. The data showed that 20 patients (13 percent) in the intravenous methylprednisolone group, 42 (27 percent) in the oral prednisone group, and 24 (15 percent) in the placebo group had at least one new episode of optic neuritis in either eye during the 6 to 24 mo of follow-up. Relative risk for oral prednisone compared with placebo was 1.79; 95 percent confidence interval, 1.08 to 2.95.

The results of this therapeutic trial are applicable to the care of most patients with an acute unilateral attack of optic neuritis. The message is clear. Do not prescribe prednisone.

The question still remains, however, with regard to whether intravenous methylprednisolone is the drug of choice to treat acute unilateral optic neuritis. In the trial, methylprednisolone compared with placebo was found to be beneficial during the first 15 days of visual loss to speed visual recovery. However, when the risk of serious side effects associated with high-dose intravenous methylprednisolone, and the inconvenience of hospitalization to the patient, and the expense are all considered, it is clear that this therapy is not justified, except perhaps in the case of the exceptional patient who requires the rapid return of stereoscopic vision essential to job skills (e.g., seamstress, dentistry).

PROGNOSIS

Visual Recovery

Although irreversible optic nerve damage occurs in 85 percent of patients with optic neuritis,[113] prognosis for the recovery of Snellen acuity is good. Sixty-five to 80 percent of cases regain 20/30 or better.[26, 85] Forty-five percent of these cases recover rapidly within the first 4 mo; 35 percent recover normal or near normal acuity at 1 yr; and 20 percent fail to make any significant improvement.

In a study to evaluate recovery, the GVIS was used to monitor prospectively the course of 20 cases of optic neuritis over 12 mo. No single visual impairment at the onset predicted final outcome, but the GVIS showed significant correlation between the initial classification and visual recovery. Of the six patients classified at the onset of optic neuritis as "low vision moderate," five patients recovered normal vision and one patient recovered to near-normal vision. Of the four patients initially classified as having "severe blindness," two were left with severe deficits—one patient with moderate blindness, the other with "low vision moderate." The remaining two patients recovered normal vision. Seven patients were left impaired as measured by the GVIS. The data were statistically evaluated by the Wilcoxon matched-pairs signed-rank test. The change between the initial visual scores (GVIS classification or score) and the scores at 12 mo is significant at a level of less than 0.01 for a two-tailed test.[85]

Other studies of recovered optic neuritis have evaluated single parameters of visual function other than Snellen acuity. Residual abnormalities in contrast sensitivity are reported in 63 to 100 percent of cases,[112, 114, 116, 117, 287, 288] color vision defects in 33 to 100 percent,[26, 29, 90, 110, 289] visual field loss in 62 to 100 percent,[26, 29, 134, 290] and light brightness sensitivity disturbance in 100 percent.[120]

Visual recovery in optic neuritis has also been correlated with MRI optic nerve lesions. The results show that in 37 patients, fast visual recovery occurred in 26 eyes (mean of 2 wk) and slow recovery in 10 (mean of 10.3 wk). Slow or poor recovery was associated either with extensive lesions in the optic nerve or with a lesion within the optic canal.[27]

The importance of this study lies in the correlation the imaging technique made possible between lesion length and location along the nerve and the time course for, and level of, visual recovery. Slow or poor visual recovery in long lesions is probably due to the demyelination of several internodes along the visual axon. In lesions within the optic canal, compression of the nerve may also play a role, and management of eyes with intracanalicular optic neuritis may warrant surgical decompression of the nerve.

Recurrent Optic Neuritis

Overall, in my own patient population in New England, optic neuritis recurred in 33 percent (33 of 101) of patients (36 percent of women, 25 percent of men) in one or the other eye during an 8-yr follow-up period. In 81 unselected patients with a first attack of acute idiopathic optic neuritis, the incidence of subsequent recurrent attacks of optic neuritis was significantly greater in patients with Uhthoff's symptom (18 of 40 or 47.5 percent) than in patients without Uhthoff's symptom (4 of 41 or 10 percent) ($P = .00017$).[46] In this particular study, we chose not to include a recurrent attack of optic neuritis as a second lesion in our statistical analysis for the overall incidence of MS in order to analyze other prognostic factors independently. However, the high incidence of recurrent optic neuritis in patients with Uhthoff's symptom has prognostic value and accords with other published data.[291, 292] Our analysis revealed a highly significant correlation between Uhthoff's symptom and the subsequent development of MS using other criteria.

In another prospective study of 86 patients with monosymptomatic optic neuritis who were followed for a median period of 12.9 yr, optic neuritis recurred in 14 of 86 patients (16.3 percent) during the observation period. Eight of these 14 patients (57 percent) were later diagnosed as having MS. Only 25 of 72 patients (32 percent) without recurrent optic neuritis progressed to MS. The risk for MS was significantly increased for patients with recurrent optic neuritis ($P = .0005$; Cox proportional hazard model with time-dependent covariates).[293] This result is at variance with data reported by others.[294–296]

Conversion to Multiple Sclerosis

Overall, the risk that an individual with optic neuritis will develop MS is high. The probability is that approximately one of two patients with optic neuritis will convert to MS in 15 yr.[295] At the lower end of probability, several studies suggest a conversion rate to MS of one third to one half[297–304] and at the higher end a rate of 60 percent,[305] 71 percent,[306] and even higher.[307, 308] For example, an updated study of 200 optic neuritis cases from Northern Ireland reveals an 88 percent rate of conversion to MS over a mean observation period of 18 yr.[307] Furthermore, using actuarial analysis, investigators in the United Kingdom predict that 75 percent of patients with optic neuritis will develop MS within 15 yr.[308]

What is evident is that the risk of MS does not decline with time (Fig. 201–6), and the search for a prognostic indicator that would identify the patient at risk at the onset of optic neuritis has been attempted in several studies.[293, 295, 296, 305, 306, 309, 310] Three risk factors have been identified: low age (Fig. 201–7),[295, 299] abnormal CSF at the onset,[306, 310] and early recurrence of optic neuritis.[309] Female gender,[295, 309] onset in the winter season,[293, 304] and the presence of HLA-DR2 antigen[308, 309] increase the risk of MS, but not significantly. Normal CSF at the onset of optic neuritis conferred a better prognosis but unfortunately did not preclude the development of MS.

PHYSICIAN-PATIENT RELATIONSHIP IN OPTIC NEURITIS

It is now inescapable that idiopathic optic neuritis is the vanguard symptom of MS, and the potential gravity of the diagnosis has been alluded to many times in the course of this chapter. As of this writing I have treated 689 patients with optic neuritis and MS, and I present a number of case histories here, first with the caveat that the course of a disease in any one individual can never be entirely typical; and second, in the hope that the cases present insight as well as information and give a sense of how one doctor deals with this disease. The cases range from a patient with painless monosymptomatic optic neuritis and MRI supported MS with conversion to clinical MS within 6 mo, to a patient with known MS, previous optic neuritis, and failure to respond to steroid therapy due to nonorganic visual loss.

CASE 1: *Painless Monosymptomatic Optic Neuritis, MRI Supported MS, and Conversion to Clinical MS Within 6 Mo*

A 40-year-old male probation officer presented with a 7-day history of progressive painless loss of vision in the left eye (OS), commencing with vision being

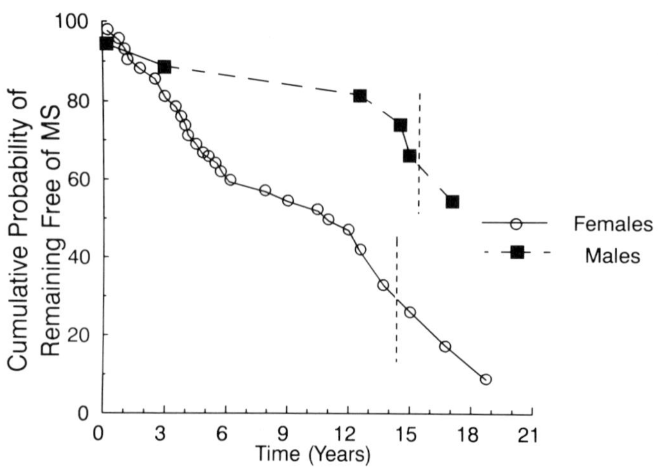

Figure 201–6. Kaplan-Meier life table analysis of the cumulative proportion remaining free of multiple sclerosis after an attack of uncomplicated optic neuritis as a function of time. A total of 42 women and 18 men are included. Curves are depicted separately for women and men. The vertical hatched lines reflect the mean follow-up for each group. (From Rizzo JF, Lessell S: Risk of developing multiple sclerosis after uncomplicated optic neuritis: A long-term prospective study. Neurology 38:185, 1988.)

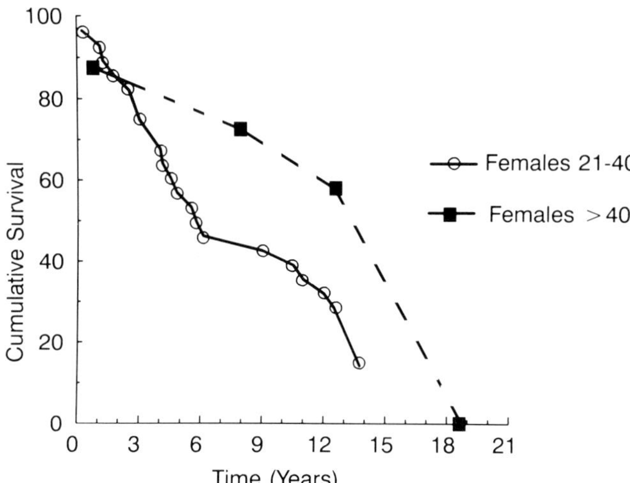

Figure 201–7. Kaplan-Meier life table analysis of the cumulative proportion remaining free of multiple sclerosis after an attack of uncomplicated optic neuritis as a function of time. This analysis is of women only. Curves are depicted for women who had their initial attack of optic neuritis between 21 and 40 yr of age (28 patients) and for those 41 yr or older (8 patients). The curve for the women over 40 yr is censored after 12.5 yr because of the effect caused by the conversion of the last remaining patient in this group. (From Rizzo JF, Lessell S: Risk of developing multiple sclerosis after uncomplicated optic neuritis: A long-term prospective study. Neurology 38:185, 1988.)

"blocked out like a screen in the midline." The night before the onset he had refereed an ice hockey game without noting blurring of vision, but he had felt unusually fatigued. During the next 7 days visual loss progressed so that he could no longer read newspaper print. Consultation with a retina specialist ruled out a retinal detachment, and he was referred for a neuroophthalmic opinion. His past history revealed no previous ophthalmic or CNS disease. A rhinoplasty was performed in 1974 for fracture of the nose, and surgery for a deviated nasal septum in 1977. His general health was excellent apart from borderline hypertension. Family history was negative for MS.

On examination he had no abnormality in the right eye (OD). Visual acuity (VA) OS: counting fingers at 3 inches, Ishihara plates 1/15 OS, stereopsis absent, and the visual field showed a dense cecocentral scotoma to II4e isopter. There was a 2+ afferent pupil defect OS, no exophthalmos, full eye movements, and a normal fundoscopic examination.

In order to rule out involvement of the contiguous nasal sinuses, a CT scan of the brain and orbits with contrast was obtained. The scan showed the optic nerves to be of normal size and no abnormality of the orbits, sinuses, or brain. On completion of the scan, which was performed on the day of presentation, the patient was told that he had an inflammation of the optic nerve (i.e., optic neuritis) and that his vision was likely to improve over the next 4 mo. Serial follow-up examinations were recommended, and the patient agreed to return. No mention was made of the association of optic neuritis with MS on the first visit, and the patient did not inquire further as to the cause at that time.

A follow-up examination 4 days later showed VA OS: 20/200 eccentrically. Static perimetry on the Octopus 2000 documented a cecocentral scotoma. Dyschromatopsia was evaluated by a Farnsworth-Munsell 100 Hue test, error score OD: 81, (normal), OS: 749 (abnormal). A simultaneous pattern VEP and PERG were normal OD. The pattern VEP was absent OS with a normal P50 component of the PERG and an absent N95 component. This study confirmed that there was no evidence of a subclinical optic neuropathy in the right eye. Absence of the pattern VEP in association with an absent PERG N95 OS was interpreted as being consistent with a demyelinating optic neuropathy.

Follow-up 1 wk later showed no change in the neuroophthalmic examination. On this occasion the patient asked whether he could have "inflammation elsewhere in the body." This question provided an opening for discussing the possibility of subclinical foci of inflammation elsewhere in the CNS and to recommend a brain MRI with and without gadolinium to determine whether other lesions were present. After discussion the patient decided to have an MRI. This showed a number of T_2 bright signal abnormalities within the centrum semiovale, corona radiata, and temporal lobes bilaterally, the largest of which measured approximately 1 cm in diameter. There were no lesions in the optic nerve(s), chiasm, or tract(s). Because of the age of the patient, the clinical history and the size and configuration of the lesions, the MRI appearance was read as being most consistent with MS, and I told the patient he had an abnormal MRI that supported a diagnosis of MS as the cause of the optic neuritis. I also told him that the abnormal T_2 signals represented focal defects in the blood-brain barrier and that foci that enhanced with gadolinium were acute and active but likely to resolve spontaneously. To confirm that the MRI abnormalities were subclinical, I performed a neurologic examination, which was normal. At this stage, the patient accepted the diagnosis of a demyelinating optic neuropathy, and an MRI supported diagnosis of possible MS. He asked no further questions but requested that the diagnosis should not be revealed to his wife.

Subsequently the patient contacted the national MS Society and researched the details of MS in medical textbooks. He returned 3 mo after the onset of visual loss, at which time VA OS was 20/20 and the field was normal. Dyschromatopsia, an afferent pupil defect, and optic atrophy OS were noted. He returned to his hobby of refereeing ice hockey games wearing a helmet and an eye shield. At this time he told his wife that he had recovered from an attack of MS.

Six months later he developed paresthesia in the right side of his face that was unaccompanied by any sensory loss. The symptom disappeared within 21 days. He diagnosed this episode as a second "bout of MS" but expressed optimism that his form of MS was mild because his symptom was so short-lived. He has remained asymptomatic for the past 28 mo.

Comment. The role of neuroimaging in evaluating a patient with monosymptomatic optic neuritis is controversial. In this case both the type of scan and when the scan was performed were directed by the immediate need to rule out sinus disease and by the patient's request to know the extent of the inflammatory CNS process. The patient then did what many male patients do in my experience, he started to do research in the literature on his own condition. However, prior to this time he had been introduced to the possibility of MS and he had been given a good prognosis for visual recovery. He told me that he was not depressed by what he read, and he was reasonably confident that he could deal with knowing that he probably had MS.

CASE 2. *Monosymptomatic Optic Neuritis Following Dental Work*

A 32-year-old woman photographer had a root canal procedure on her right upper molar tooth and 10 days later developed eyeball tenderness after rubbing the right eye (OD). The next day she developed pain on eye movement, blurred vision, and color desaturation. She consulted an ophthalmologist on the second day, and an examination showed VA OD: 20/40, OS: 20/20, Ishihara plates 4/15 OD, 15/15 OS. The next day pain abated, but visual acuity dropped further to 20/50 OD. The left eye remained normal throughout. By day 5, she was unable to see light OD.

Her past history was negative for ophthalmic and CNS disease, and her general health was excellent. The family history was positive for Alzheimer's disease, Parkinson's disease, and hypertension but negative for MS.

The ophthalmologist obtained a complete white blood count and sedimentation rate, which were normal; however, a brain and orbits contrast CT scan showed an enhancing lesion in the left frontal lobe. The patient was then referred to rule out a brain abscess.

On examination on day 7, she was extremely anxious, visual acuity OD was light perception, OS: 20/20, stereopsis absent, Ishihara plates 0/15 OD, 13/14 OS. There was a 3+ afferent pupil defect OD, no exophthalmos, full eye movements, and a normal fundus examination. A neurologic examination showed no abnormality. An emergency brain MRI showed multiple bilateral foci of prolonged T2 in the centrum semiovale. The left frontal lesion seen on the CT scan enhanced with gadolinium, but there was no mass effect. The MRI changes were interpreted as being consistent with chronic and active demyelinating disease.

On the same day, I told the patient that she did not have a brain abscess and that the CT and MRI abnormality in the frontal lobe represented an area of acute inflammation that was clinically inactive and likely to resolve but that could at this stage be associated with changes in the CSF. She agreed to a spinal tap on day 16, and the CSF contained 20 white blood cells per cu mm, 94 percent lymphocytes, a normal protein and sugar content, an elevated IgG index (normal range less than 0.66) and the presence of oligoclonal bands. The VDRL was nonreactive, and all cultures were negative.

At this point I told the patient that the CSF abnormalities together with the MRI findings represented an inflammatory demyelinating process consistent with acute MS and to her this was a diagnosis of lesser severity than an abscess in the brain. I reassured her that there was no evidence of infection of the CNS as a result of her diseased tooth, and I advised her that because visual acuity was likely to recover spontaneously no specific treatment was required.

On day 18 spontaneous improvement in vision commenced, and by day 24, VA was 20/200 OD with a dense cecocentral scotoma (see Fig. 201–1*A* and *B*). On day 30 VA was 20/70, and the cecocentral scotoma was resolving (see Fig. 201–1*C*). Serial static visual fields were recorded on the Octopus 2000 (see Fig. 201–2*A*). By day 45 VA was 20/25, J1 OD, and the visual field was normal (see Fig. 201–2*B*). There was persistent dyschromatopsia and optic atrophy.

To reevaluate the activity of her MS, I repeated the MRI 6 mo later. The scan showed persistent nonenhancing bilateral T2 foci in the centrum semiovale that were essentially unchanged in size, configuration, and number compared with the earlier study. The gadolinium-enhanced frontal lesion had resolved completely without a detectable scar. I informed the patient of these findings.

The patient has since remained asymptomatic for 3 yr. She has had a normal pregnancy and delivery and continues her career as a photographer but is aware of a reduced brightness sense in the right eye and desaturation of colors. She returns to see me once a year.

Comment. The main conclusion from this case, which supports previous studies,[177, 311] is that gadolinium is a sensitive marker of the blood-brain barrier impairment, which occurs consistently in new plaques. As such it should prove useful in monitoring therapeutic trials in MS, but because in this patient the active frontal CNS plaque was clinically inactive, no therapy was recommended.

The development of optic neuritis following a dental procedure is of additional interest in this case. While the MRI provided evidence of preexisting plaques as well as active demyelination, nothing in the MS literature indicates a time-linked relationship between a dental (or surgical) procedure and manifest symptoms of optic neuritis (see also the discussion following Case 3).

CASE 3. *A Patient With MS With Posttraumatic Optic Neuritis*

In 1988 a 27-year-old woman accountant developed transient numbness in the legs, gait ataxia, and difficulty initiating micturition. A neurologic examination showed only a right extensor plantar response. A brain and cervical spine MRI showed multiple T2 foci in the corona radiata and centrum semiovale bilaterally, and two well-defined circumscribed T2 lesions in the cervical spinal cord (one localized to the cervicomedullary junction and the second at the level of the second cervical vertebra). The first lesion enhanced following gadolinium; the second lesion did not enhance. A diagnosis of MS was made. The patient's symptoms resolved within 3 mo, and she remained asymptomatic until 1990.

In December 1990 she was a passenger in a commuter train crash. At the time of the collision she was seated, but the impact threw her forwards and she struck the right side of her head on the seat in front of her. She was then thrown backward and struck the back of her head on the headrest of her own seat. She was shaken but not knocked out and, despite the immediate onset of neck pain, she left the station and went to work. Within 2 hr after arriving at her office, she developed cloudy vision OD and went immediately to the emergency room of her local hospital. There she was told to see her neurologist. Six days later he documented VA 20/400 OD, a dense central field defect, normal funduscopy, and an otherwise normal neurologic examination. She complained on that occasion of an electric feeling down her spine on flexion of her neck (i.e., L'hermitte's sign). A diagnosis of whiplash was made, and treatment was started with a supportive neck collar. She was referred for a neuroophthalmic opinion 9 days after the accident.

A detailed history at the time of the neuroophthalmic examination revealed that in June, 1990, she had experienced a transient episode of painless visual blurring OD, uncorrected by glasses prescribed by both an optometrist and an ophthalmologist, but that within a few weeks her vision had returned to normal. The examination showed no abnormality OS, a VA 1/400 OD, a dense cecocentral field defect breaking out inferiorly to the I4e isopter, absent stereopsis, Ishihara plates 0/15, a 2+ afferent pupil defect, and a normal optic disc. A contrast CT scan of the brain and orbits with bone windows showed no abnormality, and in particular there was no orbit or optic canal fracture. A review of the 1988 brain and cervical spine MRI confirmed their original findings.

At this stage the differential diagnosis of the right optic nerve lesion rested between recurrent optic neuritis and posttraumatic optic neuropathy. Because I did not see her until 9 days after the accident, I elected not to treat her with high-dose steroids for acute posttraumatic optic neuropathy but rather to follow her conservatively, suspecting that she, being a known patient with MS, had recurrent optic neuritis.

Ten days later vision spontaneously improved, and 4 wk later VA was 20/70 OD. On this occasion she told me that she had brought suit against AMTRAK, claiming that the attack of optic neuritis was provoked by the physical and emotional trauma of the train crash. She considered that she was sensitive to stress and recalled that her initial MS attack occurred when she was nursing her mother who was terminally ill with cancer.

Comment. Several studies suggest a relationship between stress[312, 313] and trauma[307, 314] and exacerbation or worsening of symptoms in MS, including optic neuritis. The mechanism that these studies identify is either a posttraumatic alteration in the blood-brain barrier in patients who have had a head injury or a change in the patient's immune system. It is conceivable that one or both of these mechanisms played a role in this case; however, the issue to be considered is more complicated. The likelihood that a patient with MS will suffer recurrent attacks of optic neuritis is extremely high. Thus the crash trauma cannot be a cause in the sense of medical probability. On the other hand, the role of behavioral responses in immune regulation,[315] possibly through the modulation of immunologic activity by neural systems, is now clear.[316] Because there is evidence for ongoing abnormalities of immunoregulation in patients with MS, it is possible that behaviorally significant events can trigger the worsening of symptoms in MS via a change in immune regulation. In this patient's case, posttraumatic investigation of changes in her immune responsiveness might have provided evidence to support her claim.

CASE 4. *A Patient With Known MS, Previous Optic Neuritis, and Failure to Respond to Steroid Therapy due to Nonorganic Visual Loss*

A 42-year-old woman bookkeeper consulted a neurologist in May 1990 for a second opinion regarding a diagnosis of MS. She had been well until December 1989, when she noted right orbit pain and dimming of central vision OD. Her ophthalmologist diagnosed optic neuritis, and she was placed on 25 mg of prednisone every other day for 2 wk. Within 6 wk visual impairment had largely resolved, and by the end of 2 mo was "75 percent improved." A brain MRI showed multiple T2 images in the subcortical and periventricular white matter that were consistent with possible demyelination.

Her past history was negative for ophthalmic disease or symptoms to suggest disseminated demyelination of the nervous system. Her general health was good.

The neurologic examination documented VA OD: 20/30, OS: 20/20, decreased color saturation OD to red, and temporal pallor of the optic disc OD. The left optic nerve showed no abnormality, and the general neurologic examination was normal. The neurologist advised the patient that the history and findings of mild optic nerve damage OD, in the presence of a few bright spots on the brain MRI T_2-weighted images, was compatible with a diagnosis of early MS.

In November 1990 she returned to see her neurologist with a recurrence of right-sided eye pain and blurred vision and was uncertain whether her left eye was also involved. Two weeks previously she had consulted her ophthalmologist, who on examination found VA OD: 4/200, OS: 20/40. Automated visual fields showed no central scotoma in either eye, but there was a superior altitudinal defect and paracentral scotoma OD and a superior depression and tiny paracentral scotoma OS. His report failed to document the pupil reflexes and fundoscopic examination. The ophthalmologist started the patient on 10-mg tablets of prednisone—4 tablets as a single initial dose, followed by a tapering regimen over 18 days.

The neurologist found no abnormality on examination apart from the visual impairment. The patient declined a spinal tap. Because her vision was still impaired, the neurologist increased the prednisone to 60 mg/day for 1 wk, 40 mg/day for a second week, 20 mg/day for 4 days, 10 mg/day for 3 days, and 10 mg every other day for the fourth week. Reexamination at that time revealed a deterioration in her vision to OD: 20/200, OS: 20/800. She was then admitted to hospital as an emergency for intravenous 6-MP therapy and started on 1.5 g/day for 5 days. A neuroophthalmologist consulted on her case and found evidence of bilateral optic neuropathy with atypical features. The patient completed the 6-MP course and left hospital with no improvement in vision.

The patient came to see me for a second opinion and said that she would like to know the following: first, if the courses of prednisone and 6-MP were appropriate and given in a timely fashion; second, why her glasses were of no benefit to her; third, whether she should be on any treatment presently; and fourth, whether the diagnosis of MS was correct since she had no neurologic deficit in her arms or legs.

I found her initially to be both angry and hostile. This behavior was also documented by two physicians in the past. Visual acuity without her glasses was 20/400 OU, pinhole 20/200 − 1, with glasses 20/200 unimproved with a pinhole, with bifocals J4 OU. Color vision was absent, and she claimed that she could not see the Ishihara test plate 12, OU. She identified a red bottle top as red with either eye and a green bottle top as green. Stereopsis was present 60 sec of arc. Amsler grid showed no metamorphopsia and an intact grid pattern with each eye. The pupils were equal; OS reacted briskly to light and near; OD showed a 1+ afferent defect. The visual fields on Goldmann perimeter were full to 2 isopters, with marginal enlargement of the blind spots. Central static presentation of a I4e target showed no central scotoma OU. Ocular movements were full. There was no nystagmus, and a fundus examination showed temporal pallor of the right optic disc and a normal left optic disc. The macular and peripheral retina were normal OU.

Clear signs on this examination confirmed a right optic nerve lesion with an afferent pupil defect and optic atrophy. I could not confirm that the claimed acuity of 20/200 OU was organic. There was no central visual field defect; no significant loss of stereopsis; and 60 days after the onset of her visual symptoms OU, there was no afferent pupil defect or optic atrophy of the left eye. I diagnosed nonorganic visual loss OS and superimposed nonorganic acuity loss OD with a previous genuine attack of optic neuritis in the right eye.

I answered her questions as follows: first, I told her that the prednisone and 6-MP therapy had been initiated in an effort to reduce the period of visual loss but that steroids do not influence the ultimate level of visual recovery in MS/optic neuritis. The choice and course of drug treatment reflected the treating physician's preference and experience. Second, I told her that her glasses were of no benefit to her because her poor acuity was a reflection of stress. Third, I told her that I agreed with her neurologist's diagnosis of MS but that fortunately she had clinically inactive MS at this time and no inflammation of the optic nerve(s). I then went on to tell her that I had found a number of inconsistencies in her visual responses that alerted me to the possibility that she might be anxious or under stress. I inquired if there was anything in her job or personal life that might be stressful. She rapidly poured out her story. She worked in a hospital accounting department where an audit had been underway for 6 mo to find misplaced funds. During this time she was afraid that she might lose her job, and she had herself begun to suspect that anxiety was contributing to her fluctuating visual symptoms. I asked her to consider seeing a psychologist or psychiatrist for supportive therapy but she declined; however, she agreed to return in 1 mo for a follow-up visit. When she returned her acuity, 20/200 OU, was unimproved, and I documented identical signs to the initial examination. On this occasion I told her that an acuity of 20/200 could be labelled as legal blindness, but that such a label was not appropriate in her case since she was able to drive her car and use a calculator at work. At this point she interjected that she was "just stressed out" and she agreed to see a psychiatrist. She is now in therapy but has not yet returned for follow-up.

Comment. I found this patient to be an unwished-for challenge because of her hostile behavior. But I also found her to be a most instructive case because of the superimposition of nonorganic symptoms and indications on genuine signs of a monocular optic neuropathy in a patient with known MS who is under stress. Recognition of nonorganic illness is not easy, and in this patient the clinical clues were the presence of normal stereopsis despite a claimed acuity of 20/200, the absence of central scotoma in either eye, and the absence of optic atrophy in the left eye.

Every physician has a different technique for dealing with patients with nonorganic factitious visual loss. My own approach is as follows: when I diagnose nonorganic blindness, I tell the patient my diagnosis and I encourage him or her to seek psychiatric help. In my experience, this helps the patient to come to terms with the need for recovery. I continue to follow the patient to provide additional support during the course of his or her therapy.[313]

CONCLUSION

There is no question that essentially untreatable conditions place a special burden on the physician-patient relationship, and optic neuritis with its painful promise of multiple sclerosis is no exception. If the physician cannot treat the patient, the patient's needs and fears become part of the condition itself; and the patient's need to hope, the fear of being unable to cope, the physician's wish to reassure on the one hand and to tell it the way it is on the other, all contribute their own weight to the burden. The physician, facing each patient's different individual concerns, must try to tell the diagnostic truth in such a way that the patient is left to feel that it is possible for him or her to be in control of the changes that will occur in his or her life. Over the years, I have never ceased to be amazed by the resolve of so many of my patients to do just this and to resume, as far as they possibly can, the activities that were important to them before they became ill. I have been even more amazed at the gratitude that so many of them feel after being able to do so.

Acknowledgment

This manuscript was typed by Fran Christie. The author is indebted to her and conveys her thanks.

REFERENCES

1. Ebers GC: Multiple sclerosis and other demyelinating diseases. *In* Asbury AH, McKhann GM, McDonald WI (eds): Diseases of the Nervous System, vol 2. Philadelphia, WB Saunders, 1986, p 1268.
2. Wray SH, Scholl GB, Giffen C: Optic neuritis and gender. In preparation, 1992.
3. Lillie WI: The clinical significance of retrobulbar and optic neuritis. Am J Ophthalmol 17:110, 1934.
4. Nikoskelainen E: Symptoms, signs and early course of optic neuritis. Acta Ophthalmol 53:254, 1975.
5. Percy AK, Nobrega FT, Kurland LT: Optic neuritis and multiple sclerosis. Arch Ophthalmol 87:135, 1972.
6. Brewis M, Poskanzer DC, Rolland C, et al: Neurological disease in an English city. Acta Neurol Scand 42 (Suppl 24):1, 1965.
7. Wikstrom J: The epidemiology of optic neuritis in Finland. Acta Neurol Scand 52:196, 1975.
8. Kinnunen E: The incidence of optic neuritis and its prognosis for multiple sclerosis. Acta Neurol Scand 68:371, 1983.
9. Gronning M, Mellgren SI, Schive K: Optic neuritis in the two northernmost counties of Norway: A study of incidence and the prospect of later development of multiple sclerosis. Arctic Med Res 48:117, 1989.

10. Kurtzke JF: Epidemiology of multiple sclerosis. *In* Hallpike JF, Adams CWM, Tourtelotte WW (eds): Multiple Sclerosis, vol 3. Baltimore, Williams & Wilkins, 1983, p 47.
11. Kennedy C, Carroll FD: Optic neuritis in children. Arch Ophthalmol 63:747, 1960.
12. Selbst RG, Selhorst JB, Harbison JW, et al: Parainfectious optic neuritis: Report and review following varicella. Arch Neurol 40:347, 1983.
13. Purvin V, Hrisomalos N, Dunn D: Varicella optic neuritis. Neurology 38:501, 1988.
14. Riikonen R: The role of infection and vaccination in the genesis of optic neuritis and multiple sclerosis in children. Acta Neurol Scand 80:425, 1989.
15. Farris BK, Pickard DJ: Bilateral postinfectious optic neuritis and intravenous steroid therapy in children. Ophthalmology 97:339, 1990.
16. Earl CJ, Martin B: Prognosis in optic neuritis related to age. Lancet i:74, 1967.
17. Kriss A, Francis DA, Cuendet F: Recovery after optic neuritis in childhood. J Neurol Neurosurg Psychiatry 51:1253, 1988.
18. Kennedy C, Carter S: Relation of optic neuritis to multiple sclerosis in children. Pediatrics 28:377, 1961.
19. Parkin PJ, Heirons R, McDonald WI: Bilateral optic neuritis: A long-term follow-up. Brain 107:951, 1984.
20. Riikonen R, Donner M, Erkkila H: Optic neuritis in children and its relationship to multiple sclerosis: A clinical study of 21 children. Dev Med Child Neurol 30:349, 1988.
21. Riikonen R, Ketonen L, Sipponen J: Magnetic resonance imaging, evoked responses and cerebrospinal fluid findings in a follow-up study of children with optic neuritis. Acta Neurol Scand 77:44, 1988.
22. Jacobson DM, Thompson HS, Corbett JJ: Optic neuritis in the elderly: Prognosis for visual recovery and long-term follow-up. Neurology 38:1834, 1988.
23. Engell T, Trojaborg W, Raun NE: Subclinical optic neuropathy in multiple sclerosis: A neuro-ophthalmological investigation by means of visually evoked response, Farnsworth Munsell 100 Hue test and Ishihara test and their diagnostic value. Acta Ophthalmol 65:735, 1987.
24. Ulrich J, Groebke-Lorenz W: The optic nerve in multiple sclerosis: A morphological study with retrospective clinico-pathological correlations. Neuro-ophthalmology 3:149, 1983.
25. Reynolds WD, Smith JL, McCrary JA 3rd: Chiasmal optic neuritis. J Clin Neuro Ophthalmol 2:93, 1982.
26. Perkin GD, Rose CF: Optic Neuritis and its Differential Diagnosis. Oxford, Oxford University Press, 1979, p 206.
27. Miller DH, Newton MR, van der Poel JC, et al: Magnetic resonance imaging of the optic nerve in optic neuritis. Neurology 38:175, 1988.
28. Cox J: Colour vision defects acquired in diseases of the eyes. Br J Physiol Optics 18:3, 1961.
29. Griffin JF, Wray SH: Acquired color vision defects in retrobulbar neuritis. Am J Ophthalmol 86:193, 1978.
30. Earl CJ: Some aspects of optic atrophy. Trans Ophthalmol Soc 84:215, 1964.
31. Davis FA, Bergen D, Schauf C, et al: Movement phosphenes in optic neuritis: A new clinical sign. Neurology 26:1100, 1976.
32. Smith KJ, McDonald WI: Spontaneous and evoked electrical discharges from a central demyelinating lesion. J Neurol Sci 55:39, 1982.
33. Bender MD: Neuro-ophthalmology. *In* Baker AB, Baker LH (eds): Clinical Neurology, vol 1. Hagerstown, MD, Harper & Row, 1977, p 37.
34. Lessell S, Cohen MM: Phosphenes induced by sound. Neurology 29:1524, 1979.
35. Page NGR, Bolger JP, Sanders MD: Auditory evoked phosphenes in optic nerve disease. J Neurol Neurosurg Psychiatry 45:7, 1982.
36. Percival AS: Retrobulbar neuritis and associated conditions. Trans Ophthalmol Soc UK 46:392, 1926.
37. McDonald WI: Acute optic neuritis. Br J Hosp Med 18:42, 1977.
38. Patterson VH, Foster DH, Heron JR: Variability of visual threshold in multiple sclerosis: Effect of background luminance on frequency of seeing. Brain 103:139, 1980.
39. Sunga RN, Enoch JM: Further perimetric analysis of patients with lesions of the visual pathway. Am J Ophthalmol 70:403, 1970.
40. McDonald WI, Sears TA: The effects of experimental demyelination on conduction in the central nervous system. Brain 93:583, 1970.
41. Rasminsky M, Sears TA: Internodal conduction in undissected demyelinated nerve fibers. J Physiol 227:323, 1972.
42. Huizar P, Kuno M, Miyata Y: Electrophysiological properties of spinal motoneurons of normal and dystrophic mice. J Physiol 248:231, 1975.
43. Rasminsky M: Ectopic generation of impulses and cross-talk in spinal nerve roots of "dystrophic" mice. Ann Neurol 3:351, 1978.
44. Frisen L, Hoyt WF: Insidious atrophy of retinal nerve fibers in multiple sclerosis. Arch Ophthalmol 92:91, 1974.
45. Perkin GD, Rose FC: Uhthoff's syndrome. Br J Ophthalmol 60:60, 1976.
46. Scholl GB, Song H-S, Wray SH: Uhthoff's symptom in optic neuritis: Relationship to magnetic resonance imaging and development of multiple sclerosis. Ann Neurol 30:180, 1991.
47. Uhthoff W: Untersuchungen uber die bei der multiplen Herdsklerose vorkommenden Augenstorungen. Arch Psychiatry 21:303, 1889.
48. McAlpine D, Compston ND, Lumsden CE: Multiple Sclerosis. Edinburgh, Churchill Livingstone, 1955.
49. Godel V, Nemet P, Lazar M: Chloramphenicol optic neuropathy. Arch Ophthalmol 98:1417, 1980.
50. Nelson DA, Jeffreys WH, McDowell F: Effects of induced hyperthermia on some neurological diseases. Arch Neurol Psychiatry 79:31, 1958.
51. Smith JL, Hoyt WF, Susac JO: Ocular fundus in acute Leber optic neuropathy. Arch Ophthalmol 90:349, 1973.
52. Singh J, Menon V, Prakash P, et al: Inverse Uhthoff's symptom. Neuro-ophthalmology 4:95, 1984.
53. Alvarez SL, Jacobs NA, Murray IJ: Visual changes mediated by beer in retrobulbar neuritis—An investigative report. Br J Ophthalmol 70:141, 1986.
54. Jones RE, Heron JR, Foster DH, et al: Effects of 4-aminopyridine in patients with multiple sclerosis. J Neurol Sci 60:353, 1983.
55. Zrenner E: Detection of Uhthoff's symptom in disseminated sclerosis by the Farnsworth-Munsell 100 Hue test and the octopus perimetry. Dev Ophthalmol 9:182, 1984.
56. Wildberger H, Hofmann H, Siesfried J: Fluctuations of visual evoked potential amplitudes and of contrast sensitivity in Uhthoff's symptom. Doc Ophthalmol 65:357, 1987.
57. Sanborn GE, Kivlin JD, Stevens M: Optic neuritis secondary to sinus disease. Arch Otolaryngol 110:816, 1984.
58. Johnson LN, Hepler RS, Yee RD, et al: Sphenoid sinus mucocele (anterior clinoid variant) mimicking diabetic ophthalmoplegia and retrobulbar neuritis. Am J Ophthalmol 102:111, 1986.
59. Auerbuch G, Labadie EL, Van-Dalen JT: Reversible optic neuritis secondary to paranasal sinusitis. Eur Neurol 29:189, 1989.
60. Erkkila H, Raitta C, Iivanainen M, et al: Optic neuritis during lactation. Graefes Arch Clin Exp Ophthalmol 222:134, 1985.
61. Boshen D, Sebag M, Michaud J: Paraneoplastic optic neuritis and encephalomyelitis. Report of a case. Arch Neurol 45:353, 1988.
62. Hackett ER, Martinez RD, Larson PF, et al: Optic neuritis in systemic lupus erythematosus. Arch Neurol 31:9, 1974.
63. Cinefro RJ, Frenkel M: Systemic lupus erythematosus presenting as optic neuritis. Ann Ophthalmol 10:559, 1978.
64. Dutton JJ, Burde RM, Klingele TG: Autoimmune retrobulbar optic neuritis. Am J Ophthalmol 94:11, 1982.
65. Smith CA, Pinals RS: Optic neuritis in systemic lupus erythematosus. J Rheumatol 9:963, 1982.
66. Deutsch TA, Corwin HL: Lupus optic neuritis with negative serology. Ann Ophthalmol 20:383, 1988.
67. Gressel MG, Tomsak RL: Recurrent bilateral optic neuropathy in mixed connective tissue disease. J Clin Neuro Ophthalmol 3:101, 1983.
68. Fleet WS, Watson RT: Autoimmune optic neuritis: A potentially treatable form of visual loss. Ann Ophthalmol 18:144, 1986.
69. Schuil J, Richardus JH, Baarsma GS, et al: Q fever as a possible cause of bilateral optic neuritis. Br J Ophthalmol 69:580, 1985.

70. Gustafson R, Svenungsson B, Unosson-Hallnas K: Optic neuropathy in *Borrelia* infection. [Letter] J Infect 17:187, 1988.
71. Del-Sette M, Caponnetto C, Fumarola D, et al: Unusual neurological manifestations of Lyme disease: A case report. Ital J Neurol Sci 10:455, 1989.
72. Colombati S, Borri P, Tosti G, et al: Two cases of papillitis in patients with early syphilis. Bull Soc Belge Ophthalmol 220:69, 1986.
73. Zaidman GW: Neurosyphilis and retrobulbar neuritis in a patient with AIDS. Ann Ophthalmol 18:260, 1986.
74. Zambrano W, Perez GM, Smith JL: Acute syphilitic blindness in AIDS. J Clin Neuro Ophthalmol 7:1, 1987.
75. Carter JB, Hamill RJ, Matoba AY: Bilateral syphilitic optic neuritis in a patient with a positive test for HIV: Case report. Arch Ophthalmol 105:1485, 1987.
76. Jones J, Gardner W, Newman T: Severe optic neuritis in infectious mononucleosis. Ann Emerg Med 17:361, 1988.
77. Galli M, Morelli R, Casellato A, et al: Retrobulbar optic neuritis in a patient with acute type B hepatitis. J Neurol Sci 72:195, 1986.
78. Miller DH, Kay R, Schon F, et al: Optic neuritis following chickenpox in adults. J Neurol 233:182, 1986.
79. Grossniklaus HE, Frank KE, Tomsak RL: Cytomegalovirus retinitis and optic neuritis in acquired immune deficiency syndrome: Report of a case. Ophthalmology 94:1601, 1987.
80. Garrett CR: Optic neuritis in a patient on ethambutol and isoniazid evaluated by visual evoked potentials: Case report. Milit Med 150:43, 1985.
81. Livingstone MS, Hubel DH: Psychophysical evidence for separate channels for the perception of form, color movement, and depth. J Neurosci 7:3416, 1987.
82. Frisen L: Visual acuity and visual field tests: Psychophysical versus pathophysical objectives. *In* Kennard C, Rose FC (eds): Physiological aspects of clinical neuro-ophthalmology. Chicago, Year Book Med Pub, 1988.
83. Quigley HA, Sanchez RM, Dunkelberger GR, et al: Chronic glaucoma selectively damages large optic nerve fibers. Inv Ophthalmol Vis Sci 28:913, 1987.
84. Van Buren JM: The Retinal Ganglion Cell Layer. Springfield, IL, Charles C Thomas, 1963.
85. Celesia GG, Kaufman DI, Brigell M, et al: Optic neuritis: A prospective study. Neurology 40:919, 1990.
86. Gunn M, Buzzard T: Discussion on retro-ocular neuritis. Trans Ophthalmol Soc UK 17:107, 1897.
87. Kollner H: Die Storungen des Farbensinnes: Ihre Klinische Bedeutung und ihre Diagnose. Berlin, S Karger, 1912, p 114.
88. Ohta Y: Studies on acquired anomalous color vision: Color vision anomalies in patients with lesions of the retina, optic chiasma and post-occipital centre. *In* Colour '69: Proceedings of the First AIC Congress. (M. Richter [ed]) Gottingen, Musterschmidt, 1970, p 88.
89. Silverman SE, Hart WM Jr, Gordon MO, et al: The dyschromatopsia of optic neuritis is determined in part by the foveal/perifoveal distribution of visual field damage. Invest Ophthalmol Vis Sci 31(a):1895, 1990.
90. Lynn BH: Retrobulbar neuritis: A survey of the present condition of cases occurring over the last fifty-six years. Trans Ophthalmol Soc UK 79:701, 1959.
91. Rosen JA: Pseudoisochromatic visual testing in the diagnosis of disseminated sclerosis. Trans Neurolog Assoc 90:283, 1965.
92. Krauskopf J, Williams DR, Heeley DW: The cardinal directions of color space. Vision Res 22:1123, 1982.
93. Derrington AM, Lennie P, Krauskopf J: Chromatic response properties of parvocellular neurons in the macaque LGN. *In* Mollon JD, Sharpe LT (eds): Color Vision: Physiology and Psychophysics. London, Academic Press, 1983, p 245.
94. Fallowfield L, Krauskopf J: Selective loss of chromatic sensitivity in demyelinating disease. Invest Ophthalmol Vis Sci 25:771, 1984.
95. Mullen KT, Plant GT: Colour and luminance vision in human optic neuritis. Brain 109:1, 1986.
96. Alvarez SL, King-Smith PE: Dichotomy of psychophysical responses in retrobulbar neuritis. Ophthalmic Physiol Opt 4:101, 1984.
97. Foster DH, Snelgar RS: Test and field spectral sensitivities of color mechanisms obtained on small white backgrounds: Action of unitary opponent-color processes? Vis Res 23:787, 1983.
98. Foster DH, Snelgar RS, Heron JR: Nonselective losses in foveal chromatic and luminance sensitivity in multiple sclerosis. Invest Ophthalmol Vis Sci 26:1431, 1985.
99. Foster DH: Psychophysical loss in optic neuritis. *In* Hess RF, Plant GT (eds): Optic Neuritis. Cambridge, Cambridge University Press, 1986, p 152.
100. Schiller PH, Logothetis NK, Charles ER: Role of the color-opponent and broad-band channels in vision. Vis Neurosci 5:321, 1990.
101. Shapley R: Visual sensitivity and parallel retinocortical channels. Ann Rev Psychol 41:635, 1990.
102. Cavanagh P: Vision at equiluminance. *In* Kulikowski JJ, Murray IJ, Walsh V (eds): Vision and Visual Dysfunction. V: Limits of Vision. Boca Raton, FL, CRC Press, 1991, pp 234–250.
103. De Valois RL, De Valois KD: Neural coding of color. *In* Carterette EC, Friedman MP (eds): Handbook of Perception, vol 5. New York, Academic Press, 1975, p 117.
104. Wall M: Loss of P retinal ganglion cell function in resolved optic neuritis. Neurology 40:649, 1990.
105. Ingling CR, Martinez-Uriegas E: The spatiotemporal properties of the r-g X-cell channel. Vision Res 25:33, 1985.
106. Derrington AM, Lennie P: Spatial and temporal contrast sensitivities of neurones in lateral geniculate nucleus of macaque. J Physiol 357:219, 1984.
107. Merrigan WH, Eskin TA: Spatio-temporal vision of macaques with severe loss of P retinal ganglion cells. Vision Res 26:1751, 1986.
108. Travis D, Thompson P: Spatiotemporal contrast sensitivity and colour vision in multiple sclerosis. Brain 112:283, 1989.
109. Heron JR, Regan D, Milner BA: Delay in visual perception in unilateral optic atrophy after retrobulbar neuritis. Brain 97:69, 1974.
110. Burde RM, Gallin PF: Visual parameters associated with recovered retrobulbar optic neuritis. Am J Ophthalmol 79:1034, 1975.
111. Galvin RJ, Regan D, Heron JR: Impaired temporal resolution of vision after acute retrobulbar neuritis. Brain 99:255, 1976.
112. Sanders EACM, Volkers ACW, van der Poel JC, et al: Estimation of visual function after optic neuritis: A comparison of clinical tests. Br J Ophthalmol 70:918, 1986.
113. Fleishman JA, Beck RW, Linares OA, et al: Deficits in visual function after resolution of optic neuritis. Ophthalmology 94:1029, 1987.
114. Regan D, Silver R, Murray TJ: Visual acuity and contrast sensitivity in multiple sclerosis—Hidden visual loss; an auxiliary diagnostic test. Brain 100:563, 1977.
115. Frisen L, Sjostrand J: Contrast sensitivity in optic neuritis: A preliminary report. Doc Ophthalmol 17:165, 1978.
116. Zimmern RL, Campbell FW, Wilkinson IMS: Subtle disturbances of vision after optic neuritis elicted by studying contrast sensitivity. J Neurol Neurosurg Psychiatry 42:407, 1979.
117. Beck RW, Ruchman MC, Savino PJ, et al: Contrast sensitivity measurements in acute and resolved optic neuritis. Br J Ophthalmol 68:756, 1984.
118. Plant GT, Hess RF: Regional threshold contrast sensitivity within the central visual field in optic neuritis. Brain 110:489, 1987.
119. Lorance RW, Kaufman DO, Wray SH, et al: Contrast visual testing in neurovisual diagnosis. Neurology 37:923, 1987.
120. Hess RF, Plant GT: The psychophysical loss in optic neuritis: spatial and temporal aspects. *In* Hess RF, Plant GT (eds): Optic Neuritis. Cambridge, Cambridge University Press, 1986, p 109.
121. Regan D: Visual psychophysical tests in the diagnosis of multiple sclerosis. *In* Poser CM (ed): The Diagnosis of Multiple Sclerosis. New York, Thieme-Stratton, 1984, p 64.
122. Regan D, Maxner C: Orientation-dependent loss of contrast sensitivity for pattern and flicker in multiple sclerosis. Clin Vision Sci 1:1, 1986.
123. Regan D, Neima D: Low-contrast letter charts in early diabetic retinopathy, ocular hypertension, glaucoma, and Parkinson's disease. Br J Ophthalmol 68:885, 1984.
124. Pelli DG, Robson JG, Wilkins AJ: The design of a new letter chart for measuring contrast sensitivity. Clin Vision Sci 2:187, 1988.

125. Rubin GS: Reliability and sensitivity of clinical contrast sensitivity tests. Clin Vision Sci 2:169, 1988.
126. Glaser JS (ed): Neuro-ophthalmology, 2nd ed. Philadelphia, JB Lippincott, 1990, p 14.
127. Pulfrich C: Die stereoskopic im dienste der isochromen und heterochromen photometrie. Naturwissenschaften 10:553, 1922.
128. Grimsdale H: A note on Pulfrich's phenomenon with a suggestion on its possible clinical significance. Br J Ophthalmol 9:63, 1925.
129. Frisen L, Hoyt WF, Bird AC, et al: Diagnostic uses of the Pulfrich phenomenon. Lancet 2:385, 1973.
130. Rushton D: Use of the Pulfrich pendulum for detecting abnormal delay in the visual pathway in multiple sclerosis. Brain 98:283, 1975.
131. Lessell S: Neuro-ophthalmology. Arch Ophthalmol 93:434, 1975.
132. Sokol S: The Pulfrich stereo-illusion as an index of optic nerve dysfunction. Surv Ophthalmol 20:432, 1976.
133. Slagsvold JE: Pulfrich pendulum phenomenon in patients with a history of acute optic neuritis. Acta Ophthalmol 56:817, 1978.
134. Nikoskelainen E: Later course and prognosis of optic neuritis. Acta Ophthalmol (Copenh) 53:273, 1975.
135. Harms H: Role of perimetry in assessment of optic nerve dysfunction. Trans Ophthalmological Soc UK 96:363, 1976.
136. Patterson VH, Heron JR: Visual field abnormalities in multiple sclerosis. J Neurol Neurosurg Psychiatry 43:205, 1980.
137. McDonald WI: Pathophysiology of conduction in central nerve fibres. *In* Desmedt JE (ed): Visual Evoked Potentials in Man: New Developments. Oxford, Clarendon Press, 1977, p 427.
138. Prineas JW, Connell F: The fine structure of chronically active multiple sclerosis plaques. Neurology 28 (Suppl 68):684, 1978.
139. Burde RM: Confrontation testing. *In* Thompson HS, Daroff R, Frisen L, et al (eds): Topics in Neuro-Ophthalmology. Baltimore, Williams & Wilkins, 1979, pp 70, 71.
140. Beck RW, Bergstrom TJ, Lichter PR: A clinical comparison of visual field testing with a new automated perimeter, the Humphrey Field Analyzer, and the Goldmann perimeter. Ophthalmology 92:77, 1985.
141. Johnson LN, Hill RA: Correlation of afferent pupillary defect with visual field loss on automated perimetry. American Academy of Ophthalmology Annual Meeting Abstract 138, 1987.
142. Younge BR, Trautmann JC: Computer assisted perimetry in neuro-ophthalmic disease. Mayo Clin Proc 55:207, 1980.
143. Heijl A, Drance SM: A clinical comparison of three computerized automatic perimeters in the detection of glaucoma defects. Arch Ophthalmol 99:832, 1981.
144. Levatin P: Pupillary escape in disease of the retina or optic nerve. Arch Ophthalmol 62:768, 1959.
145. Thompson HS, Jiang MQ. Letter to the editor. Ophthalmology 94:1360, 1987.
146. Fineberg E, Thompson HS: Quantitation of the afferent pupillary defect. *In* Smith JL (ed): Neuro-ophthalmology Focus. New York, Masson, 1979, p 25.
147. Thompson JS, Corbett JJ, Cox TA: How to measure the relative afferent pupillary defect. Surv Ophthalmol 26:39, 1981.
148. Marshall D: Ocular manifestations of multiple sclerosis and relationship to retrobulbar neuritis. Trans Am Ophthalmol Soc 48:487, 1950.
149. Bradley WG, Whitty CWM: Acute optic neuritis: Its clinical features and their relation to prognosis for recovery of vision. J Neurol Neurosurg Psychiatry 30:531, 1967.
150. Zeller RW: Ocular findings in the remission phase of multiple sclerosis. Am J Ophthalmol 64:767, 1967.
151. Lightman S, McDonald WI, Bird AC, et al: Retinal venous sheathing in optic neuritis: Its significance for the pathogenesis of multiple sclerosis. Brain 110:405, 1987.
152. ter Braak JG, Herwaarden A: Ophthalmo-encephalomyelitis. Klin Monatsbl Augenheilk 91:316, 1933.
153. Rucker CW: Sheathing of the retinal veins in multiple sclerosis. Mayo Clin Proc 19:176, 1944.
154. Rucker CW: Retinopathy of multiple sclerosis. Trans Am Ophthalmol Soc 45:564, 1947.
155. Engell T, Andersen PK: The frequency of periphlebitis retinae in multiple sclerosis. Acta Neurol Scand 65:601, 1982.
156. Bamford CR, Ganley JP, Sibley WA, et al: Uveitis, perivenous sheathing and multiple sclerosis. Neurology 28:119, 1978.
157. Hoyt WF: Ophthalmoscopy of the retinal nerve fiber layer in neuro-ophthalmologic diagnosis. Aust J Ophthalmol 4:14, 1976.
158. Hoyt WF: Fundoscopic changes in the retinal nerve fiber layer in chronic and acute optic neuropathies. Trans Ophthalmol Soc UK 96:368, 1976.
159. Hoyt WF, Schlicke B, Eckelhoff RJ: Funduscopic appearance of a nerve fibre bundle defect. Br J Ophthalmol 56:577, 1972.
160. Feinsod M, Hoyt WF: Subclinical optic neuropathy in multiple sclerosis. J Neurol Neurosurg Psychiatry 38:1109, 1975.
161. Miller NR, George TW: Monochromatic (red-free) photography and ophthalmoscopy of the peripapillary retinal nerve fiber layer. *In* Smith JL (ed): Neuro-Ophthalmology Focus 1980. New York, Masson, 1979, p 43.
162. Ito H, Ozawa K, Suga S, et al: Red-free light magnifying photography in neuritis and some retinal vascular lesions. Folia Ophthalmol Jpn 79:1062, 1969.
163. Jacobson DM, Marx JJ, Dlesk A: Frequency and clinical signficance of Lyme seropositivity in patients with isolated optic neuritis. Neurology 41:706, 1991.
164. Sandberg-Wollheim M: Optic neuritis: Cerebrospinal fluid findings and clinical course. *In* Shimizu K, Oosterhuis JA (eds): XXIII Concilium Ophthalmologicum, Kyoto. International congress Series No 450. Amsterdam, Excerpta Medica 347, 1978.
165. Howard CW, Osher RH, Tomsak RL: Computed tomographic features in optic neuritis. Am J Ophthalmol 89:699, 1980.
166. Shiraki Y: Application of computerized tomography to a case of acute optic neuritis. J Univ Occupation Environ Health 3:173, 1981.
167. Schumacher M: Misinterpretation of unilateral swelling of the optic nerve. Klin Monatsbl Augenheilkd 181:202, 1982.
168. Ormerod IEC, McDonald WI, du Boulay EP, et al: Disseminated lesions at presentation in patients with optic neuritis. J Neurol Neurosurg Psychiatry 1986.
169. Jacobs L, Kinkel PR, Kindel WR: Silent brain lesions in patients with isolated optic neuritis: A clinical and nuclear magnetic resonance imaging study. Arch Neurol 43:452, 1986.
170. Johns K, Lavin P., Elliot JH, et al: Magnetic resonance imaging of the brain in isolated optic neuritis. Arch Ophthalmol 104:1486, 1986.
171. Miller DH, Ormerod IE, McDonald WI, et al: The early risk of multiple sclerosis after optic neuritis. J Neurol Neurosurg Psychiatry 51:1569, 1988.
172. Frederiksen JL, Larsson HB, Henriksen O, et al: Magnetic resonance imaging of the brain in patients with acute monosymptomatic optic neuritis. Acta Neurol Scand 80:512, 1989.
173. Young IR, Hall AS, Pallis CA, et al: Nuclear magnetic resonance imaging of the brain in multiple sclerosis. Lancet 2:1063, 1981.
174. Lukes SA, Crookes LE, Aminoff MJ, et al: Nuclear magnetic resonance imaging in multiple sclerosis. Ann Neurol 13:592, 1983.
175. Runge VM, Price AC, Kirshner HSA, et al: Magnetic resonance imaging of multiple sclerosis; study of pulse-technique efficiency. AJR 143:1015, 1984.
176. Ormerod IEC, Miller DH, McDonald WI, et al: The role of NMR imaging in the assessment of multiple sclerosis and isolated neurological lesions: A quantitative study. Brain 110:1579, 1987.
177. Paty DW, Oger JJF, Kastrukoff LF, et al: MRI in the diagnosis of MS: A prospective study with comparison of clinical evaluation, evoked potentials, oligoclonal banding and CT. Neurology 38:180, 1988.177.
178. Halliday AM, McDonald WI, Mushin J: Delayed visual evoked responses in optic neuritis. Lancet 1:982, 1972.
179. Halliday AM, McDonald WI, Mushin J: Visual evoked responses in the diagnosis of multiple sclerosis. Br Med J 4:661, 1973.
180. Halliday AM, Mushin J: The visual evoked potential in neuro-ophthalmology. Int Ophthalmol Clin 210:155, 1980.
181. Shahrokhi F, Chiappa KH, Young RR: Pattern shift visual evoked responses: Two hundred patients with optic neuritis and/or multiple sclerosis. Arch Neurol 35:65, 1978.
182. Halliday AM: The visual evoked potential in the investigation of diseases of the optic nerve. *In* Halliday AM (ed): Evoked Potentials in Clinical Testing. London, Churchill Livingstone, 1982, p 187.
183. Halliday AM, McDonald WI, Mushin J: Delayed pattern evoked

responses in optic neuritis in relation to visual acuity. Trans Ophthalmol Soc UK 93:315, 1973.
184. Halliday AM, MCDonald WI: Visual evoked potentials. *In* Stalberg E, Young RR (eds): Neurology I: Clinical Neurophysiology. London, Butterworths, 1981, p 228.
185. Chiappa KH (ed): Evoked Potentials in Clinical Medicine, 2nd ed. New York, Raven Press, 1990.
186. Asselman P, Chadwick DW, Marsden CD: Visual evoked responses in the diagnosis and management of patients suspected of multiple sclerosis. Brain 98:261, 1975.
187. Matthews WB, Small DG, Small M, et al: Pattern reversal evoked visual potential in the diagnosis of multiple sclerosis. J Neurol Neurosurg Psychiatry 40:1009, 1977.
188. Collins DWK, Black JL, Mastaglia FL: Pattern reversal visual evoked potential. J Neurol Sci 36:83, 1978.
189. Hoeppner T, Lolas R: Visual evoked responses and visual symptoms in multiple sclerosis. J Neurol Neurosurg Psychiatry 41:493, 1978.
190. Kupersmith MJ, Nelson JI, Seiple WH, et al: The 20/20 eye in multiple sclerosis. Neurology 33:1015, 1983.
191. Brooks EB, Chiappa KH: A comparison of clinical neuro-ophthalmological findings and pattern shift visual evoked potentials in multiple sclerosis. *In* Courjon J, Mauguiere F, Revol M (eds): Clinical Applications of Evoked Potentials in Neurology. New York, Raven Press, 1982, p 453.
192. van Buggenhout E, Ketelaer P, Carton H: Success and failure of evoked potentials in detecting clinical and subclinical lesions in multiple sclerosis patients. Clin Neurol Neurosurg 84:3, 1982.
193. Meienberg O, Flammer J, Ludin HP: Subclinical visual field defects in multiple sclerosis. J Neurol 227:125, 1982.
194. Halliday AM, Halliday E, Kriss A, et al: The pattern-evoked potential in compression of the anterior visual pathways. Brain 99:357, 1976.
195. Bobak P, Bodis-Wollner I, Harnois C, et al: Pattern electroretinograms and visual evoked potentials in glaucoma and multiple sclerosis. Am J Ophthalmol 96:72, 1983.
196. Bodis-Wollner I, Yahr MD, Mylin L, et al: Dopamine deficiency and delayed visual evoked potentials in humans. Ann Neurol 11:478, 1982.
197. Holder GE: Significance of abnormal pattern electroretinography in anterior visual pathway dysfunction. Br J Ophthalmol 71:166, 1987.
198. Berninger TA, Arden GB: The pattern electroretinogram. Eye 2 (Suppl): S257, 1988.
199. Tan CB, King PJL, Chiappa KH: Pattern ERG: Effects of reference electrode site, stimulus mode and check size. Electroencephalogr Clin Neurophysiol 74:11, 1989.
200. Arden GB, Vaegan, Hogg CR: Clinical and experimental evidence that the pattern electroretinogram (PERG) is generated in more proximal retinal layers than the focal electroretinogram (FERG). Ann NY Acad Sci 388:214, 1982.
201. Boschi MC, Frosini R, Scaioli V: Correlations among clinical data, pattern electroretinogram, visual evoked potential and retinal fibre layer findings in multiple sclerosis. Doc Ophthalmol 40:133, 1984.
202. Persson HE, Wanger P: Pattern reversal electroretinograms and visual evoked cortical potentials in multiple sclerosis. Br J Ophthalmol 68:760, 1984.
203. Porciatti V, Von Berger GP: Pattern electroretinogram and visual evoked potentials in optic nerve disease: early diagnosis and prognosis. Doc Ophthalmol 40:117, 1984.
204. Serra G, Carreras M, Tugnoli V, et al: Pattern electroretinogram in multiple sclerosis. J Neurol Neurosurg Psychiatry 47:879, 1984.
205. Celesia GG, Kaufman D: Pattern ERGs and visual evoked potentials in maculopathies and optic nerve disease. Invest Ophthalmol Vis Sci 26:726, 1985.
206. Celesia GG, Kaufman D, Cone SB: Simultaneous recording of pattern electroretinography and visual evoked potentials in multiple sclerosis. Arch Neurol 43:1247, 1986.
207. Kaufman DI, Lorance RW, Woods M, et al: The pattern electroretinogram: A long-term study in acute optic neuropathy. Neurology 38:1767, 1988.
208. Holder GE: Pattern ERG abnormalities in anterior visual pathway disease. Electroencephalogr Clin Neurophysiol 61:S135, 1985.
209. Holder GE: Abnormalities of the pattern ERG in optic nerve lesions; changes specific for proximal retinal dysfunction. *In* Barber C, Blum T (eds): Evoked Potentials. III: London, Butterworths, 1987, p 221.
210. Ryan S, Arden GB: Electrophysiological discrimination between retinal and optic nerve disorders. Doc Ophthalmol 68:247, 1988.
211. Scholl GB, Song H-S, Winkler DE, et al: The pattern visual evoked potential and pattern electroretinogram in Drusen optic neuropathy. Arch Ophthalmol 110:75, 1992.
212. Kirkham TH, Coupland SG: The pattern electroretinogram in patients with optic nerve disease. Can J Neurol Sci 10:256, 1983.
213. Ota E, Miyake Y: The pattern electroretinogram in optic nerve disease. Doc Ophthalmol 62:53, 1986.
214. Imachi J, Tajino M, Okamoto N, et al: Rhinogenous retrobulbar neuritis: Pathogenetic problems and case reports. Neuro-ophthalmology 1:273, 1981
215. Slavin M, Glaser JS: Acute severe irreversible visual loss with sphenoethmoiditis—"Posterior" orbital cellulitis. Arch Ophthalmol 105:345, 1987.
216. Goodwin JA, Glaser JS: Chiasmal syndrome in sphenoid sinus mucocele. Ann Neurol 4:440, 1978.
217. Schmutzhard E, Pohl P, Stanek G: Involvement of *Borrelia burgdorferi* in cranial nerve affection. Zentralbl Bakt Hyg A 263, 1986.
218. Lyme disease—Connecticut. JAMA 259:1147, 1988.
219. Weinstein JM, Lexow SS, Ho P, et al: Acute syphilitic optic neuritis. Arch Ophthalmol 99:1392, 1981.
220. Rush JA, Ryan EJ: Syphilitic optic perineuritis. Am J Ophthalmol 91:404, 1981.
221. McBurney J, Rosenberg ML: Unilateral syphilitic optic perineuritis presenting as the big blind spot syndrome. J. Clin Neuro Ophthalmol 7:167, 1987.
222. Lim SH, Hens LK, Puvanendran K: Secondary syphilis presenting with optic perineuritis and uveitis. Ann Acad Med Singapore 19:413, 1990.
223. Winward KE, Hamed LM, Glaser JS: The spectrum of optic nerve disease in human immunodeficiency virus infection. Am J Ophthalmol 107:373, 1989.
224. Berger JR, Sheremata WA, Resnick M, et al: Multiple sclerosis-like illness occurring with human immunodeficiency virus infection. Neurology 39:324, 1989.
225. Devic E: Myelite subaigue compliquée de névrite optique. Bull Med (Paris) 8:1033, 1894.
226. Gault F: De la neuromyelite optique aigue. Lyon, Thesis, 1894.
227. Kuroiwa Y, Igata A, Itahara K, et al: Nationwide survey of multiple sclerosis in Japan: Clinical analysis of 1084 cases. Neurology 25:845, 1975.
228. Shibasaki H, Kuroda Y, Kuroiwa Y: Clinical studies of multiple sclerosis in Japan: Classical multiple sclerosis and Devic's disease. J Neurol Sci 23:215, 1974.
229. Whitham RH, Brey RL: Neuromyelitis optica: Two new cases and review of the literature. J Clin Neuro Ophthalmol 5:263, 1985.
230. Arnold TW, Myers GJ: Neuromyelitis optica (Devic syndrome) in a 12 year old male with complete recovery following steroids. Pediatr Neurol 3:313, 1987.
231. Ko FJ, Chiang CH, Jons YJ, et al: Neuromyelitis optica (Devic's disease) report of one case. Acta Paediatr Sin 30:428, 1989.
232. Filley CM, Sternberg PE, Norenberg MD: Neuromyelitis optica in the elderly. Arch Neurol 41:670, 1984.
233. Ghezzi M, Giansanti M, Malentacchi GM, et al: Neuromyelitis optica in the old age: A clinico-pathological contribution. Ital J Neurol Sci 8:613, 1987.
234. Barbieri F, Buscaino GA: Neuromyelitis optica in the elderly. Acta Neurol 11:247, 1989.
235. Kenik JG, Krohn K, Kelly RB, et al: Transverse myelitis and optic neuritis in systemic lupus erythematosus: A case report with magnetic resonance imaging findings. Arthritis Rheum 30:947, 1987.
236. Silber MH, Willcox PA, Bowen RM, et al: Neuromyelitis optica (Devic's syndrome) and pulmonary tuberculosis. Neurology 40:934, 1990.
237. Johns DR, Hurke O, Griffin JW, et al: Molecular basis of a new mitochondrial disease: Acute optic neuropathy and myelopathy. Ann Neurol 30:234, 1991.

238. Jabs DA, Miller NR, Newman SA, et al: Optic neuropathy in systemic lupus erythematosus. Arch Ophthalmol 104:564, 1986.
239. Dutton JJ, Burde RM, Klingele TG: Autoimmune retrobulbar optic neuritis. Am J Ophthalmol 94:11, 1982.
240. Kupersmith MJ, Burde RM, Warren FA, et al: Autoimmune optic neuropathy: Evaluation and treatment. J Neurol Neurosurg Psychiatry 51:1381, 1988.
241. Samples JR, Younge BR: Tobacco-alcohol amblyopia. J Clin Neuro Ophthalmol 1:213, 1981.
242. Frisen L: Fundus changes in acute malnutritional optic neuropathy. Arch Ophthalmol 101:577, 1983.
243. Kupersmith MJ, Weiss PA, Carr RE: The visual-evoked potential in tobacco-alcohol and nutritional amblyopia. Am J Ophthalmol 95:307, 1983
244. van Noort BAA, Bos PJM, Klopping C, et al: Optic neuropathy from thiamin deficiency in a patient with ulcerative colitis. Doc Ophthalmologica 67:45, 1987.
245. Strambolian D, Behrens MM: Optic neuropathy associated with vitamin B_{12} deficiency. Am J Ophthalmol 83:465, 1977.
246. Fasler JJ, Rose FC: West Indian amblyopia. Postgrad Med J 56:494, 1980.
247. Leber T: Ueber hereditare und congenitalangelegte sehnervenleiden. Graefes Arch Exp Ophthalmol 17:249, 1871.
248. Von Graefe A: Ein ungewohnlicher fall von hereditare amaurose. Arch Fr Ophthalmol 4:266, 1858.
249. Nikoskelainen EK, Savontaus ML, Wanne OP, et al: Leber's hereditary optic neuroretinopathy, a maternally inherited disease: A genealogic study in four pedigrees. Arch Ophthalmol 105:665, 1987.
250. Seedorf T: Leber's disease. Acta Ophthalmol 46:4, 1968.
251. Seedorf T: The inheritance of Leber's disease: A genealogical follow-up study. Acta Ophthalmol 63:135, 1985.
252. van Senus AHC: Leber's disease in the Netherlands. Doc Ophthalmol 17:1, 1963.
253. Asseman R: La Maladie de Leber Étude Clinique et Génétique à Propos de 86 Cas Examinées. Lillie, Thèse, 1958.
254. Bird A, McEachern D: Leber's hereditary optic atrophy in a Canadian family. Can Med Assoc J 61:376, 1949.
255. Newman NJ, Lott MT, Wallace DC: The clinical characteristics of pedigrees of Leber's hereditary optic neuropathy with the 11778 mutation. Am J Ophthalmol 111:750, 1991.
256. Mathieu J: Contribution à l'Étude de la Neurité Optique Retro-Bulbaire Héreditaire. Paris, Thèse No. 117, 1901, p 51.
257. Taylor J, Holmes GM: Two families, with several members in each suffering from optic atrophy. Trans Ophthalmol Soc UK 33:95, 1913.
258. Carroll WM, Mastaglia FL: Leber's optic neuropathy: A clinical and visual evoked potential study of affected and asymptomatic members of a six generation family. Brain 102:559, 1979.
259. Nettleship E: Leber's disease: The Bowman Lecture. Trans Ophthalmol Soc UK 29 (Appendix VI): clix, 1909.
260. Nikoskelainen E, Hoyt WF, Numelin K: Ophthalmoscopic findings in Leber's hereditary optic neuropathy. II: The fundus findings in the affected family members. Arch Ophthalmol 101:1059, 1983.
261. Holloway TB: Leber's disease. Arch Ophthalmol 9:789, 1933.
262. Brunett JR, Bernier G: Study of a family of Leber's optic atrophy with recuperation. *In* Brunett JR, Barbeau A (eds): Progress in Neuro-ophthalmology. Amsterdam, Excerpta Medica, 1969, p 91.
263. Smith JL, Hoyt WF, Susac JO: Ocular fundus in acute Leber optic neuropathy. Arch Ophthalmol 90:349, 1973.
264. Nikoskelainen E, Sogg RL, Rosenthal AR, et al: Early phase in Leber hereditary optic atrophy. Arch Ophthalmol 95:969, 1977.
265. Nikoskelainen E, Wanne O, Dahl M: Pre-excitation syndrome and Leber's hereditary optic neuroretinopathy. Lancet 1:969, 1985.
266. Wallace DC, Singh G, Lott MT, et al: Mitochondrial DNA mutation associated with Leber's heredity optic neuropathy. Science 242:1427, 1988.
267. Yoneda M, Tsuji S, Yamauchi T, et al: Mitochondrial DNA mutation in a family with Leber's hereditary optic neuropathy. Lancet 1:1076, 1989.
268. Houponen K, Vilkki J, Aula P, et al: A new mtDNA mutation associated with Leber's hereditary optic neuroretinopathy. Am J Hum Genet 48:1147, 1991.
269. Johns DR, Berman J: Alternative, simultaneous complex I: mitochondrial DNA mutations in Leber's hereditary optic neuropathy. Biochem Biophys Res Comm 174:1324, 1991.
270. Morris MA: Mitochondrial mutations in neuro-ophthalmological diseases: A review. J Clin Neuro Ophthalmol 10:159, 1990.
271. Newman NJ: Leber's hereditary optic neuropathy. Ophthalmol Clin North Am 4:431, 1991.
272. Gould ES, Bird AC, Leaver PK, et al: Treatment of optic neuritis by retrobulbar injection of triamcinolone. Br Med J 1:1495, 1977.
273. Rawson MD, Liversedge LA: Treatment of retrobulbar neuritis with corticotrophin. Lancet 2:222, 1969.
274. Bowden AM, Bowden PMA, Friedmann AJ, et al: A trial of corticotrophin gelatin injection in acute optic neuritis. J Neurol Neurosurg Psychiatry 37:896, 1974.
275. Bird AC: Is there a place for corticosteroids in the treatment of optic neuritis? *In* Brockhurst RJ, Boruchoff SA, Hutchinson BT, Lessell S (eds): Controversy in Ophthalmology. Philadelphia, WB Saunders, 1977, p 822.
276. Wray SH: ACTH and oral corticosteroids in the treatment of acute optic neuritis. *In* Brockhurst RJ, Boruchoff SA, Hutchinson RT, Lessell S (eds): Controversy in Ophthalmology. Philadelphia, WB Saunders, 1977, p 830.
277. Dowling PC, Bosch VV, Cook SD: Possible beneficial effect of high dose intravenous steroid therapy in acute demyelinating disease and transverse myelitis. Neurology 30:33, 1980.
278. Buckley C, Kennard C, Swash M: Treatment of acute exacerbations of multiple sclerosis with intravenous methylprednisolone. J Neurol Neurosurg Psychiatry 45:179, 1982.
279. Newman PK, Saunders M, Tilley PJB: Methylprednisolone therapy in multiple sclerosis. J Neurol Neurosurg Psychiatry 45:941, 1982.
280. Goas JY, Marion JL, Missoum A: High dose intravenous methylprednisolone in acute exacerbations of multiple sclerosis. J Neurol Neurosurg Psychiatry 46:99, 1983.
281. Barnes MP, Bateman DE, Cleveland PG, et al: Intravenous methylprednisolone for multiple sclerosis in relapse. J Neurol Neurosurg Psychiatry 48:157, 1985.
282. Spoor TC, Rickwell DL: Treatment of optic neuritis with intravenous megadose corticosteroids: A consecutive series. Ophthalmology 95:131, 1988.
283. Wall M: Megadose corticosteroids for optic neuritis. Ophthalmology 95:1006, 1988.
284. Herishanu YO, Badarna S, Sarov B, et al: A possible harmful late effect of methylprednisolone therapy on a time cluster of optic neuritis. Acta Neurol Scand 80:569, 1989.
285. Cox TA, Woolson RF: Steroid treatment of optic neuritis. Arch Ophthalmol 99:336, 1981.
286. Beck RW, Cleary PA, Anderson MM, et al: A randomized controlled trial of corticosteroids in the treatment of acute optic neuritis. N Engl J Med 326:581, 1992.
287. Sjostrand J, Abrahamsson M: Suprathreshold vision in acute optic neuritis. J Neurol Neurosurg Psychiatry 45:227, 1982.
288. Arden GB, Guckoglu AG: Grating test of contrast sensitivity in patients with retrobulbar neuritis. Arch Ophthalmol 96:1626, 1978.
289. Wybar KC: The ocular manifestations of disseminated sclerosis. Proc R Soc Med 45:315, 1952.
290. VanDalen JTW, Greve EL: Visual field defects in multiple sclerosis. Neuro-ophthalmology 2:93, 1981.
291. Thomson DS: Blurring of vision on exercise. Trans Ophthalmol Soc UK 86:479, 1966.
292. Goldstein JE, Cogan DG: Exercise and the optic neuropathy of multiple sclerosis. Arch Ophthalmol 72:168, 1964.
293. Sandberg-Wollheim M, Bynke M: Cronqvist H, et al: A long-term prospective study of optic neuritis; evaluation of risk factors. Ann Neurol 27:386, 1990.
294. Cohen MM, Lessell S, Wolf PA: A prospective study of the risk of developing multiple sclerosis in uncomplicated optic neuritis. Neurology 29:208, 1979.
295. Rizzo JF, Lessell S: Risk of developing multiple sclerosis after uncomplicated optic neuritis: A long-term prospective study. Neurology 38:185, 1988.

296. Miller DH, Ormerod IEC, McDonald WI, et al: The early risk of multiple sclerosis after optic neuritis. Neurol Neurosurg Psychiatry 51:1569, 1988.
297. Taub RG, Rucker CW: The relationship of retrobulbar neuritis to multiple sclerosis. Am J Ophthalmol 37:494, 1954.
298. Collis WJ: Acute unilateral retrobulbar neuritis. Arch Neurol 13:409, 1965.
299. Bradley WG, Whitty CWM: Acute optic neuritis: Prognosis for development of multiple sclerosis. J Neurol Neurosurg Psychiatry 31:10, 1968.
300. Appen RE, Allen JC: Optic neuritis under 60 years of age. Ann Ophthalmol 6:143, 1974.
301. Lynn BH: Retrobulbar neuritis: A survey of the present condition of cases occurring over the last fifty-six years. Trans Ophthalmol Soc UK 79:701, 1959.
302. Hutchinson WM: Acute optic neuritis and the prognosis for multiple sclerosis. J Neurol Neurosurg Psychiatry 39:283, 1976.
303. Kahana E, Alter M, Feldman S: Optic neuritis in relation to multiple sclerosis. J Neurol 213:87, 1976.
304. Compston DAS, Batchelor JR, Earl CJ, et al: Factors influencing the risk of multiple sclerosis developing in patients with optic neuritis. Brain 101:495, 1978.
305. Corridori F, Salmaggi A, Bortolami C, et al: Prognostic value of cerebrospinal fluid electrophoresis in optic neuritis and suspected multiple sclerosis. Ital J Neurol Sci Suppl 6:77, 1987.
306. Nikoskelainen E, Frey H, Salmi A: Prognosis of optic neuritis with special reference to cerebrospinal fluid immunoglobulins and measles virus antibodies. Ann Neurol 9:545, 1981.
307. McAlpine D, Lumsden CE, Acheson ED: Multiple sclerosis: A reappraisal. Edinburgh, Churchill Livingstone, 1965, p 107.
308. Francis DA, Compston DAS, Batchelor JR, et al: A reassessment of the risk of multiple sclerosis developing in patients with optic neuritis after extended follow up. J Neurol Neurosurg Psychiatry 50:758, 1987.
309. Hely MA, McManis PG, Doran TJ, et al: Acute optic neuritis: A prospective study of risk factors for multiple sclerosis. J Neurol Neurosurg Psychiatry 49:1125, 1986.
310. Sandberg-Wollheim M: Optic neuritis: Cerebrospinal fluid findings and clinical course. *In* Shimizu K, Oosterhuis JA (eds): XXIII Concilium Ophthalmologicum Kyoto. International Congress Series No 450. Amsterdam, Excerpta Medica, 347, 1978.
311. Miller DH, Rudge P, Johnson G, et al: Serial gadolinium enhanced magnetic resonance imaging in multiple sclerosis. Brain 111:927, 1988.
312. Warren SG, Greenhill S, Warren KG: Emotional stress and the development of multiple sclerosis: Case-control evidence of a relationship. J Chron Dis 35:821, 1982.
313. Franklin GM, Nelson LM, Heaton RK, et al: Stress and its relationship to acute exacerbations in multiple sclerosis. J Neurol Rehab 2:7, 1988.
314. Poser C: Trauma and multiple sclerosis. J Neurol 234:155, 1987.
315. Ader R: Behaviorally conditioned modulation of immunity. *In* Ader R (ed): Neural Modulation of Immunity. New York, Raven Press, 1985.
316. Felten DI, Felten SY, Bellinger DL, et al: Noradrenergic sympathetic neural interactions with the immune system. Immunol Rev 100:225, 1987.

Chapter 202

The Ischemic Optic Neuropathies

JOEL S. GLASER

Infarction of the optic disc, and rarely of the retrobulbar portion of the optic nerve, unrelated to inflammation, demyelination, neural infiltration or metastasis, compression by mass lesion, or diffuse orbital congestion, is a poorly understood but well-recognized and unfortunately common cause of sudden loss of vision, especially in the presenescent and elderly population. Primary ischemic optic neuropathy (ION) is the most frequent basis of disc swelling in adulthood after 50 yr of age. By "ischemic," we also include other diverse subsets only infrequently associated with ION, including severe hypertensive episodes, juvenile diabetes, acute blood loss, collagen arteritis, radionecrosis, and paraneural inflammation. But when more specific mechanisms are evident, the clinical situation with regard to therapies and outcome differs substantially from the typical idiopathic, or perhaps "arteriosclerotic," form of ION. It is this *common* type that is first discussed.

COMMON ("ARTERIOSCLEROTIC," NONARTERITIC)

In contrast to inflammatory or demyelinative retrobulbar optic neuritis, ION characteristically involves the prelaminar portion of the optic nerve with a rather constant ophthalmoscopic appearance of disc swelling (thus, the alternate term "*anterior*" ION) (Fig. 202–1). In fact, the absence of disc swelling in the presence of acute monocular loss of vision makes a diagnosis of

Figure 202–1. *A,* Acute right disc swelling (*left*) and subsequent optic atrophy (*right*) in a 61-year-old hypertensive man. *B,* Acute left disc swelling (*left*) with nerve fiber layer and subretinal blood at the nasal disc margin. Fluorescein angiogram (*right*) shows normal arteriovenous flow with diffuse disc leakage. *C,* Right and left fundi showing acute disc swelling (R) coupled with previous optic atrophy (L), giving a picture of "Foster Kennedy syndrome." *D,* Left disc with superior hemipallor (*brackets*), corresponding to dense inferior altitudinal "hemianopic" field defect, attenuation of superior arterioles (*large arrows*), and pigment epithelium disturbance (*small arrows*) forming a "high-water line" as evidence of previous edema.

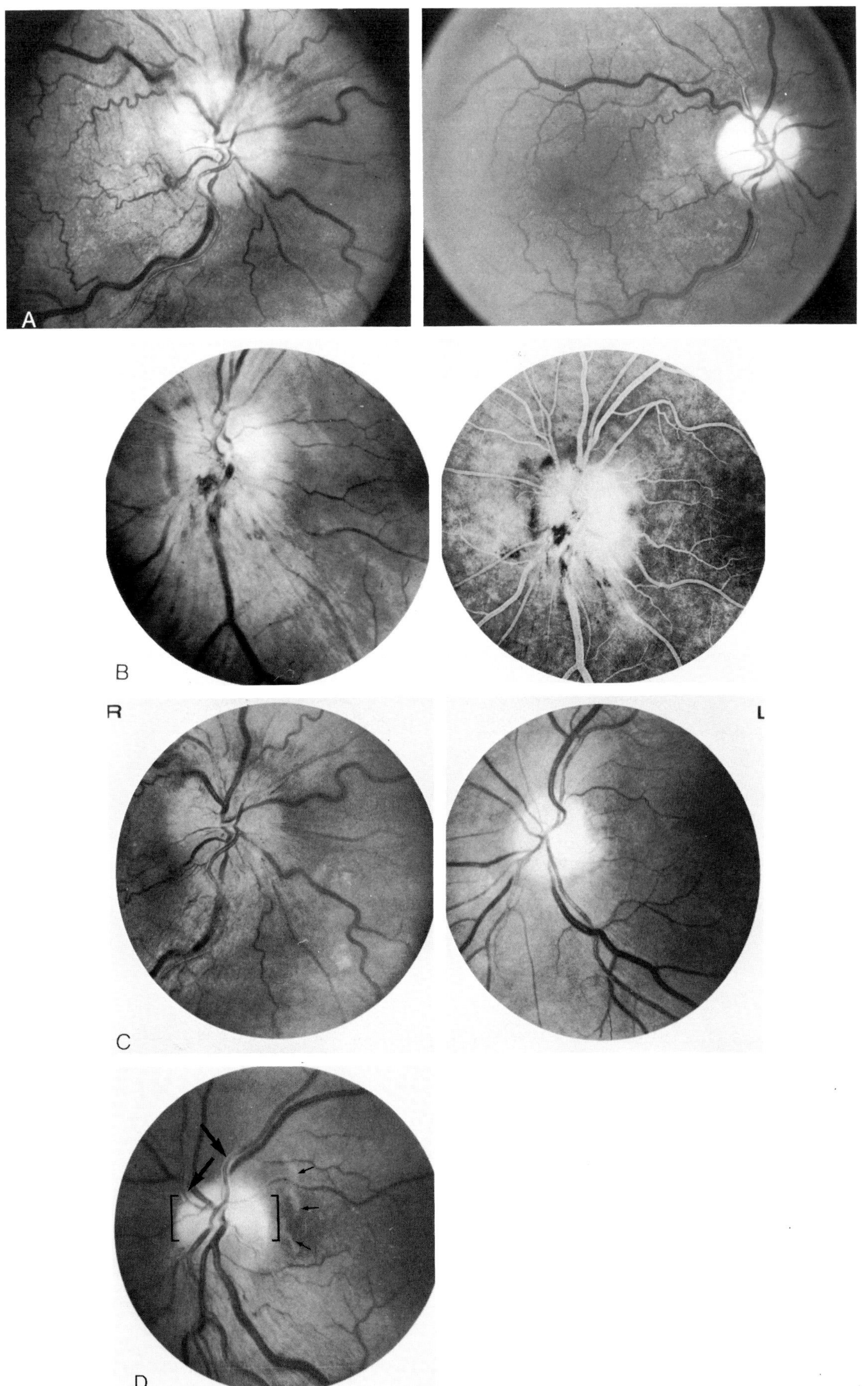

Figure 202–1 *See legend on opposite page*

See legend on opposite page

"simple" ischemic infarction untenable. The rare exception to this rule is retrobulbar ION associated with cranial arteritis (see later). Otherwise, abrupt visual loss in the elderly patient with a *normal* disc should bring to mind the possibility of a rapidly expanding basal tumor or carcinomatous infiltration of the optic nerve sheaths.

Common ION may be characterized as follows[1, 2]: Peak incidence is at age 60 to 70 yr, but on rare occasions ION may occur in the late 40s. The onset of altitudinal[1, 3] or other field defects (Fig. 202–2) is sudden and usually, but not invariably, involves the central fixational area and produces reduced acuity (Fig. 202–3); acuity may range from normal to nil, but tends to be more severely reduced in the arteritic form of ION (see later). The visual deficit is typically maximal at onset, but deterioration may progress for a few days to several weeks[2, 4]; recurrent disc infarcts in the same eye must be considered relatively rare.[5, 6] In a review of same eye recur-

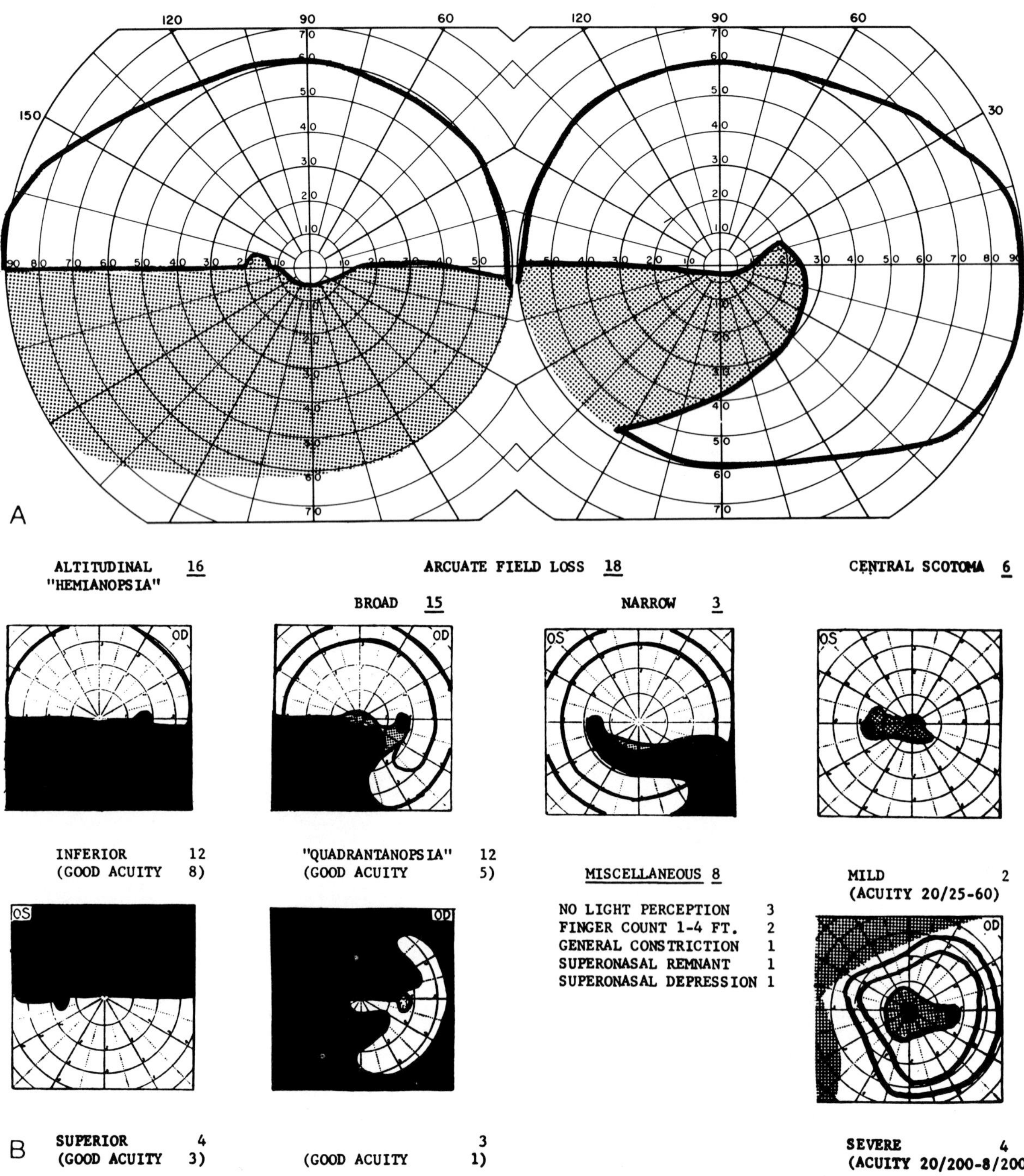

Figure 202–2. *A,* Visual field defects in common ischemic optic neuropathy. The right field shows a dense arcuate nerve fiber bundle defect extending from the blind spot into the inferonasal quadrant. The left field shows inferior altitudinal "hemianopic" depression. *B,* Visual field defects in nonarteritic ischemic optic neuropathy; 48 eyes in 34 patients (From Boghen DR, Glaser JS: Ischaemic optic neuropathy: The clinical profile and natural history. Brain 98:689, 1975. By permission of Oxford University Press.)

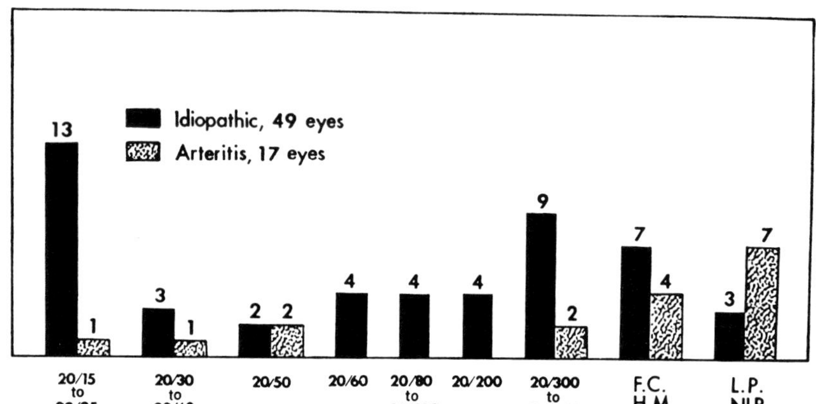

Figure 202–3. Visual acuity after stabilization, idiopathic versus arteritic ischemic neuropathy. FC, finger-counting; HM, hand movement; LP, light perception; NLP, no light perception. (From Boghen DR, Glaser JS: Ischaemic optic neuropathy: The clinical profile and natural history. Brain 98:689, 1975. By permission of Oxford University Press.)

rences, the period between episodes lasted from 10 days to 9 yr.[7] Unlike infarction with cranial arteritis, premonitory ocular symptoms do not occur, and significant eye or brow discomfort, or headache, is exceptional, unlike optic neuritis in which orbital ache or pain on eye movement is a prominent symptom.[8] Many patients indeed note the visual deficit upon awakening, but this is not a fixed rule.[9]

The optic disc is swollen to some degree (see Fig. 202–1), usually in a sector with small flame hemorrhages, and edema typically extends only a short distance beyond the border of the disc. A presymptomatic phase of disc swelling may be observed[10]; for example, a patient presents with characteristic ION with visual loss in one eye, and disc edema with good visual function surprisingly is found in the contralateral fundus; after a brief delay, disc edema progresses and vision declines. Perhaps this odd situation is related to chronic or subacute nerve ischemia with obstipation of axoplasm flow without significant nerve fiber infarction.

Clinical and experimental studies[11] indicate that ION is precipitated by insufficiency in posterior ciliary artery circulation and that branches of the peripapillary choroidal arterial system occlude, with consequent infarction of retinal nerve fiber bundles in the disc substance anterior to the lamina cribrosa. Olver and associates[12] have studied the morphology of the microvasculature of the retrolaminar area of the human optic nerve and describe an elliptical anastomosis ("circle of Zinn-Haller") of branches of the medial and lateral para-optic short posterior ciliary arteries. This ellipse is divided into superior and inferior portions by the entry points of these branches into the eye, providing a potential "altitudinal" blood supply to the retrolaminar optic nerve that may play a role in the pathogenesis of the altitudinal pattern of visual field defects frequently found in ION. The role of carotid embolic or occlusive disease is considered below.

Some small case studies[13] imply that chronic raised intraocular tension may play a role in ION, but in larger series[14] no evidence was found to support this hypothesis. Two cases are reported[15] of progressive ION immediately following transient pressure elevations induced by topical corticosteroid therapy for conjunctivitis, occurring in otherwise healthy adults with no known preceding ocular or systemic risk factors.

The visual field defects in ION vary but usually take the form of arcuate scotomas or "altitudinal hemianopias" of the superior or inferior half-fields (see Fig. 202–2). These altitudinal or nasal pseudoquadrantic defects are dense and easily discovered by hand or finger-counting confrontational field techniques. The localizing value of the position of the "vertex" of quadrantic and wedge-shaped defects has been emphasized by Kestenbaum: When the wedge originates at, or points toward, the blind spot, the defect is due to disease at the nerve head or just behind it. The differential diagnosis of such *arcuate* scotomas (i.e., with curvilinear or radial borders originating at the blind spot) includes: branch retinal artery occlusion, glaucoma, ischemic optic neuropathy, optic neuritis, hyaline bodies (drusen) of the optic disc, congenital optic pit, juxtapapillary inflammation and, very rarely, chiasmal interference. Central scotomas are the predominant field defects in about one sixth[1] to one fourth[9] of cases of common ION.

Optic atrophy ensues as disc edema resolves (see Fig. 202–1), and some small loss of disc tissue may be evident. Increased cup size may be observed, but rarely is glaucomatous excavation mimicked.[16] The ophthalmoscopic criteria that permit a retrospective diagnosis of optic atrophy of ischemic origin include arterial attenuation,[17] although Frisen[18] has quantitatively demonstrated a reduction in central retinal artery caliber of 17 to 24 percent in nonischemic, descending (retrobulbar nerve, chiasm lesions) optic atrophy.

Following ischemic infarction of one disc, there is great likelihood of second eye involvement, generally believed to sequentially occur in approximately 30 to 40 percent. Beri and associates[19] provide the following figures for 10-yr cumulative incidence rates: for patients 45 to 64 yr of age, 55.3 percent; for patients 65 yr or more, 34.4 percent; for patients under age 45, 75.9 percent; for patients with diabetes mellitus, 72.2 percent; for patients with arterial hypertension, 42.2 percent; for patients with diabetes and hypertension, 60.6 percent.

In common ION *simultaneous* bilateral disc infarction is practically unknown, and an underlying systemic disease such as cranial arteritis or severe renovascular hypertension must be suspected. The occurrence of *consecutive* disc infarction with fresh disc swelling in one eye, when combined with contralateral previous optic atrophy, mimics the ophthalmoscopic combination popularized as the "Foster Kennedy syndrome"[20] (see Fig. 202–1), but there are obvious functional differences that separate acute disc infarction from papilledema of raised pressure (Table 202–1). Ironically, then, the celebrated "diagnostic sign" of Foster Kennedy is most typical of alternating, consecutive ION and is exceedingly infrequent as a sign of intracranial frontal fossa masses.

Although the precise roles of diabetes and hypertension are not known, certainly the prevalence of these systemic disorders is significantly greater in patients with ION than in comparable age-matched groups[1, 2]; correlations with these diseases seem to be greater in patients under age 45 yr. Likewise, the association of cerebral and cardiac vascular disease[21] seems to be circumstantial, and that simple ION may be taken for a harbinger of future vascular events is moot. Indeed, in a study of magnetic resonance (MR) brain images in patients with ION,[22] there did not appear to be an increased incidence of subcortical white matter lesions (i.e., infarcts due to cerebral vascular disease). Giuffre[23] has reported that serum cholesterol, triglycerides and glucose are elevated in ION, and others have found a correlation of elevated concentrations of IgG anticardiolipin antibody in patients with arteritic ION but not in common ION.[24]

A series of funduscopic analyses have addressed the question of cup:disc ratio as a possible morphologic factor in the pathogenesis of common ION, culminating in the article by Beck and associates.[25] By observing the disc appearance of the normal fellow eyes of patients with ION, it is apparent that the optic cup is smaller or absent at a significant rate in common ION (but not different in arteritic ION); furthermore, one study[26] suggests that both the horizontal disc diameter and disc area are smaller in fellow eyes with ION than in controls ($P < .05$). Possibly, ischemic axons in the "crowded" setting of a small scleral canal are predisposed to infarction. However, as patients with common ION may have variably sized contralateral physiologic cups, and patients with arteritic ION may show contralateral cupless discs, no strong diagnostic distinction should be placed on the state of fellow eye cup:disc ratio.

No medical therapies have proved to be effective in restoring vision in acute ION, although systemic corticosteroid usage might theoretically reduce the focal impact of edema and, therefore, short-term trials are not unreasonable. The untoward effects of corticosteroids on diabetes, hypertension, and general well-being must be taken into account. Spontaneous significant recovery of vision is generally thought to be relatively rare, but Movsas and associates[2] documented that, of 116 eyes with acuity of 20/60 or worse, 21 percent improved by three or more lines, and of 126 eyes with acuity better than 20/60, 23 percent improved by three or more lines.

Optic nerve sheath fenestration with drainage of perineural subarachnoid cerebrospinal fluid has been investigated. Sergott and associates have performed this

Table 202–1. CLINICAL CHARACTERISTICS OF OPTIC NEURITIS, PAPILLEDEMA, AND ISCHEMIC OPTIC NEUROPATHY

	Optic Neuritis	Papilledema	Ischemic Neuropathy
Symptoms			
Visual	Rapidly progressive loss of central vision; acuity rarely spared	No visual loss; ± transient obscurations	Acute field defect, commonly altitudinal; acuity variable
Other	Tender globe, pain on motion; orbit or brow ache	Headache, nausea, vomiting; other focal neurologic signs	Usually none; cranial arteritis to be ruled out
Bilateral	Rarely in adults; may alternate in MS; frequent in children, especially papillitis	Always bilateral, with extremely rare exceptions; may be asymmetric	Typically unilateral in acute stage; second eye involved subsequently with picture of "Foster-Kennedy" syndrome
Signs			
Pupil	No anisocoria; diminished light reaction on side of neuritis	No anisocoria; normal reactions unless asymmetric atrophy	No anisocoria; diminished light reaction on side of disc infarct
Acuity	Usually diminished	Normal acuity	Acuity variable; severe loss (incl. NLP) common in arteritis
Fundus	Retrobulbar: normal; papillitis: variable degree of disc swelling, with few flame hemorrhages; cells in vitreous variable	Variable degrees of disc swelling, hemorrhages, cytoid infarcts	Usually pallid segmental disc edema with few flame hemorrhages
Visual prognosis	Vision usually returns to normal or functional levels	Good, with relief of cause of increased intracranial pressure	Poor prognosis for return; second eye ultimately involved in one third of idiopathic cases

From JS Glaser: Neuro-ophthalmology. Philadelphia, JB Lippincott, 1990, p 117.

type of surgery in a series of patients with the progressive form of nonarteritic ION.[27] Visual function (acuity or field) was improved in several cases, curiously including in two eyes (with long-standing visual loss) *contralateral* to the surgical decompression. Initial acuities as poor as hand motion to 20/400, improved to the 20/30 to 20/60 range. Likewise, Spoor and associates,[28] and Kelman and associates[29] have documented unqualified visual improvement. However, other nerve sheath decompression results are less sanguine,[30] and this therapy remains controversial.

CRANIAL (GIANT CELL) ARTERITIS

An arteritic form of ischemic optic neuropathy occurs with onset in a slightly older age-group (Fig. 202–4),[1, 25] usually with devastating visual loss (Table 202–2). As pointed out by Wagner and Hollenhorst, arteritis may result in a *retrobulbar* form of nerve infarction or may produce a picture similar to central retinal artery occlusion.[31] These authors also noted an appreciable incidence of fleeting premonitory visual symptoms similar to amaurosis fugax from carotid atheromatous emboli. Such episodes may be precipitated by changes from the supine to upright head position and suggest impending nerve infarction; bedrest with lowering of the head to flat or dependent levels is an important maneuver (of course, along with hospitalization for intensive corticosteroid therapy).

Very few cases of biopsy-proved cranial arteritis occur in patients younger than age 50 yr,[32] but in the population age 50 yr or over, annual *incidence* rates for cranial arteritis (CA) are estimated at 17.4[33] to 28.6[34] per 100,000; age-specific *prevalence* rate between ages 60 and 69 is 33/100,000, and over age 80, 844/100,000.[33] Most large series report a female:male preponderance of about 3:1.

Visual loss with arteritic ION tends to be more profound than with common ION (see Fig. 202–3)[1, 35]; levels of finger counting to no perception of light are not uncommon. At times, the optic disc is characterized by a milk-pale edema that may extend some considerable distance away from the optic nerve (Fig. 202–5), and central retinal artery occlusion with "cherry-red spot" also occurs. As mentioned, bilateral simultaneous ION is suggestive of CA and both therapy and laboratory investigations are bent toward that diagnosis. In 50 cases of arteritic ION,[19] 19 of the 20 bilateral patients had both eyes involved by the time of initial visits. When second eye infarction occurs in CA, it does so within days to weeks, longer intervals being exceptional. The prognostic value of this point bears emphasis: if the second eye is not yet involved, and patients are under adequate systemic corticosteroid therapy, the likelihood of bilateral visual loss becomes more remote with each passing week.

Other signs of orbital hypoxia include evidence of anterior segment ischemia: hyperemia of the conjunctival and episcleral vessels, mild-to-moderate corneal edema, lowered intraocular tension, anterior chamber cellular reaction, iris rubeosis, and rapidly progressive cataract. Irregular streaks and patches of chorioretinal pigmentary disturbances secondary to *choroidal ischemia* may appear weeks after visual loss, and considerable disc cupping may ensue, at times mimicking simple glaucoma.[36] Diplopia is infrequent, probably reflecting diffuse ischemia of extraocular muscles,[37] but symptomatic ophthalmoplegia of any degree may be obscured by the more dramatic complaint of severe visual loss.

Ocular pneumotonography, which measures the ocular pulsation induced by perfusion pressure in choroidal (posterior ciliary) and ophthalmic arteries, has been used[38] to distinguish common ION from arteritic ION. In patients with arteritic ION, ocular pulse amplitude was only 4 percent of pulse amplitude of patients with

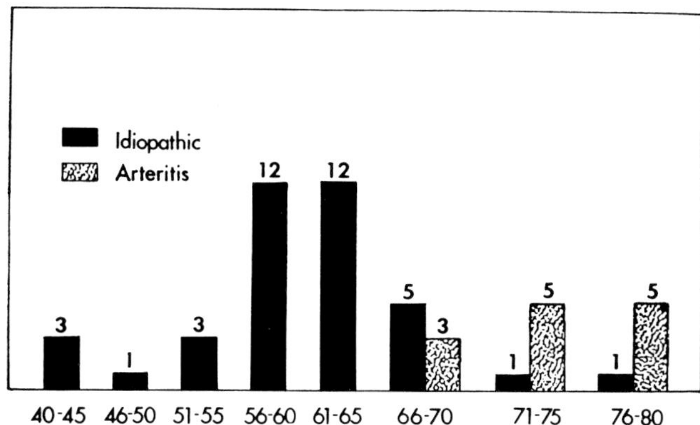

Figure 202–4. Relative age incidences (yr) of idiopathic and arteritic ischemic optic neuropathy. (From Boghen DR, Glaser JS: Ischaemic optic neuropathy: The clinical profile and natural history. Brain 98:689, 1975. By permission of Oxford University Press.)

Table 202–2. ISCHEMIC OPTIC NEUROPATHY

	Common ("Arteriosclerotic")	Cranial Arteritis
Age peak	60 to 65 yr	70 to 80 yr
Visual dysfunction	Minimal-severe	Usually severe
Second eye*	Approximately 40%	Approximately 75%
Fundus, acute	Swollen disc, often segmental	Swollen disc, normal disc, or central artery occlusion
Systemic	Hypertension approximately 50%	Malaise, weight loss, fever, polymyalgia, head pain
ESR (mm/hr)	Up to 40	Usually high (50 to 120)
Response to steroids	None	Systemic symptoms +; return of vision ±

From JS Glaser: Neuro-ophthalmology. Philadelphia, JB Lippincott, 1990, p 138.

*Simultaneous bilateral visual loss is highly suggestive of arteritis and practically excludes common type. Acute massive blood loss with hypotension may produce bilateral nerve infarction.

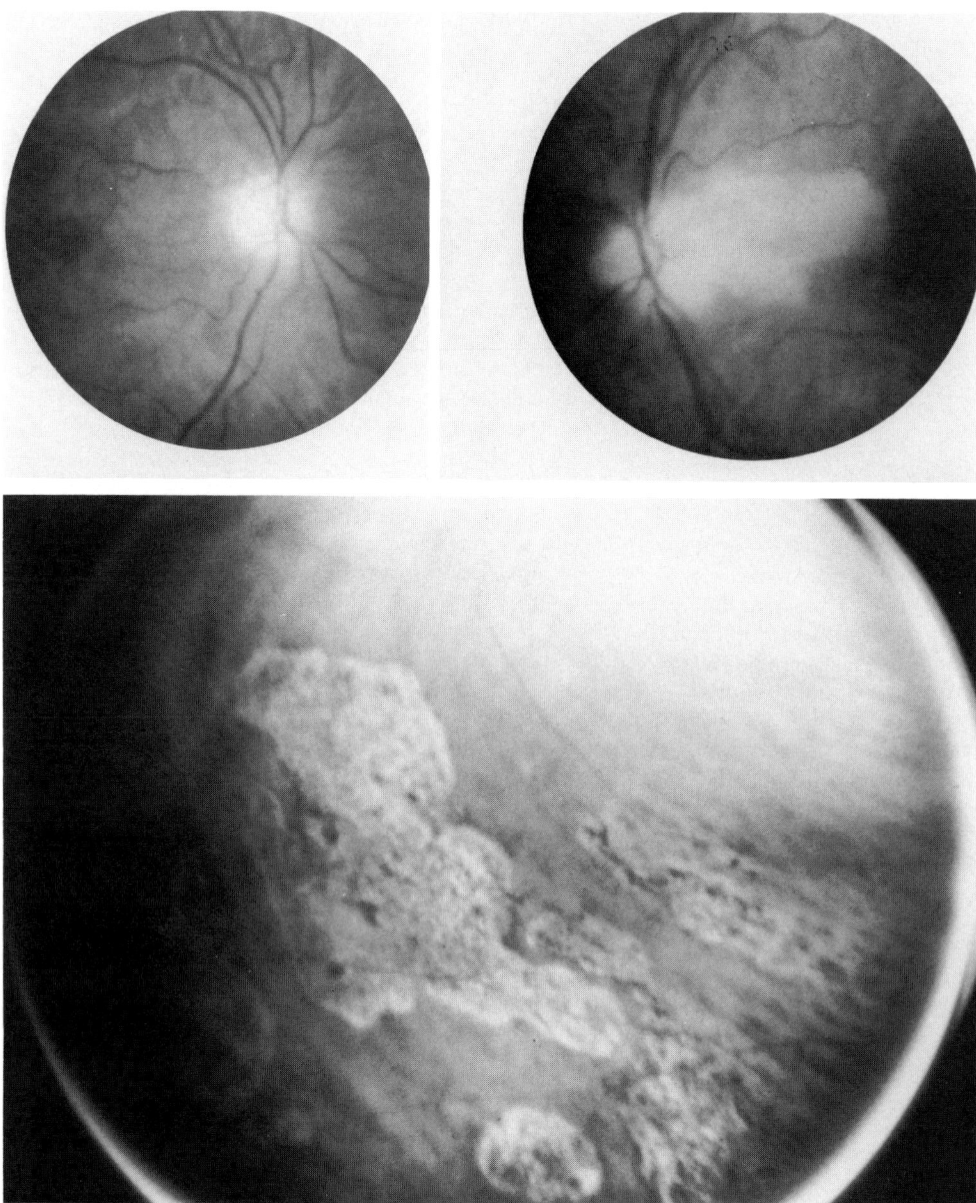

Figure 202–5. Arteritic ischemic neuropathy. *Top left,* Milky pale disc edema. *Top right,* Pale disc edema with infarction extending into the macular portion of the retina. *Bottom,* Choroidal infarcts.

arteritis but without ION, and only 6 percent of pulse amplitude of patients with nonarteritic ION. Moreover, half of patients with arteritic ION showed pulsation loss in the noninfarcted contralateral eye. Return of pulse amplitudes to a normal range can occur rapidly upon systemic corticosteroid therapy, although in some cases the pulse does not revert to normal levels. Bosley and associates[39] suggest that ocular pneumoplethysmography (OPG), measuring ocular pulse amplitude that reflects the volume changes in the globe with each cardiac cycle, provides a diagnostic accuracy of 94 percent for CA, rivaling the accuracy of erythrocyte sedimentation rate (ESR) determination or even temporal artery biopsy.

It is critical to discover, when possible, instances of ION due to cranial arteritis because prompt steroid therapy may be effective in restoring some degree of vision,[40–42] averting similar visual deficit in the other eye, and improving long-term systemic morbidity and mortality, although the Mayo series showed no statistically significant effect of arteritis on survivorship rates.[33] Patients with cranial arteritis may complain of weakness, weight loss, and fever. Myalgia of the large muscle masses of the shoulders, neck, thighs, and buttocks is common. These symptoms constitute *polymyalgia rheumatica,* which really cannot be clinically or histologically distinguished from cranial arteritis.[43] Other common complaints include pain in the jaw muscles precipitated by eating or talking (masseter "claudication"), chronic suboccipital headache (mistakenly attributed to cervical osteoarthritis, so common in this age group), and pain or tenderness of the scalp of the forehead or temples. A palpable, often nonpulsatile, temporal artery should be sought as a likely biopsy site.

The Westergren ESR is the most consistently helpful laboratory test in the confirmation of the diagnosis of arteritis. Cullen,[44] in comparing arteritic versus "arteriosclerotic" (common, idiopathic) ischemic optic neuropathy, found only 3 of 19 patients in the latter group with ESR greater than 30 mm/hr (mean of 26 mm), whereas only 3 of 25 patients with biopsy-positive arteritis had ESRs of 50 mm and below (mean of 84 mm; 70 mm or above in 80 percent). Cullen has also pointed out the rare occurrence of arteritis with normal ESR. In a series of 31 patients with temporal arteritis and severe visual impairment, Palm[45] reported the mean of the highest ESR values to be 96 mm, with a range of 50 to 145 mm. Hamrin[46] found mean ESR values of 106 mm (51 patients with positive biopsy) and 99 mm (42 patients with negative biopsy); for the entire series of 93 cases, the mean ESR was 103 ± 26.5 mm/hr (range 47 to 155 mm).

It is clear from the papers of Boyd and Hoffbrand[47] and Milne and Williamson[48] that ESR increases with age and is "elevated" (i.e., greater than 20 mm/hr) in apparently healthy elderly subjects. In at least 50 percent of persons with an ESR greater than 50 mm, no obvious reason was found.[48] Taking 20 mm/hr as upper limit of normal, bacteriuria, ischemic heart disease, and chronic respiratory symptoms show no association with a raised ESR. Miller and Green[49] provide the following rule for calculation of the maximum normal ESR at a given age: in men, (age in yr)/2; in women, (age in years +10)/2. We agree with the aforementioned authors and personally utilize 35 to 40 mm/hr (Westergren) as the upper limit of normal for the ESR in the elderly.

The affirmation provided by a positive artery biopsy is helpful when instituting long-term corticosteroid therapy in an elderly patient, but a negative biopsy in no way militates against a diagnosis of arteritis. Klein and associates have established the presence of "skip lesions" in temporal artery biopsies from patients with unequivocal cranial arteritis.[50] They also point out that a temporal artery that is normal to palpation may show histologic signs of inflammation and that patients with "skip lesions" do not have a more benign form of the disease. Therefore, it may be argued that arterial biopsy is superfluous since diagnosis or treatment is not altered by the results, especially in the full-blown case of cranial arteritis accompanied by significant ESR elevation, with or without symptoms of polymyalgia rheumatica. Others contend that multiple biopsies should be considered, especially in the "occult" form of CA, with no systemic signs or symptoms and normal or minimally elevated ESR.[51]

In the appropriately aged patient with systemic or cranial signs or symptoms, and normal or (usually) elevated sedimentation rate, *systemic* corticosteroid therapy (e.g., oral prednisone 80 to 100 mg/day, or intravenous methylprednisolone 250 mg every 6 hours) should be instituted immediately upon presumed diagnosis. In addition, retrobulbar depot steroid on the side of the acutely involved eye may be considered, although this latter strategy is not used widely. To reiterate: *In the patient with suspected arteritis, therapy should not be delayed for results of ESR or biopsy.* Symptomatic response to steroids, excluding vision, may be dramatic within 24 hr, with relief of headache and malaise. Recovery of vision is rare,[40–42, 52] in both the retrobulbar and ocular forms of arteritic ION.

Prolonged therapy should be dictated by symptomatic response to steroids and depression of the sedimentation rate. It is suggested that high dosage be maintained for approximately 4 wk, then tapered so long as the patient remains symptom free and the ESR is below 40 mm/hr (see earlier). Complications of prolonged steroid usage are well known and include gastric ulcers, myopathy and weakness, osteoporosis, and recrudescence of tuberculosis.

DIABETES MELLITUS

It is presently unclear whether a direct relationship exists between diabetes and acquired optic neuropathies, other than as an apparent risk factor for common ION (see earlier). A genetically determined progressive optic atrophy may be associated with juvenile diabetes, but the incidence in diabetes of retrobulbar neuritis or papillitis is probably no higher than in the nondiabetic population.

Skillern and Lockhart[53] collected 14 cases of "optic neuritis" in poorly controlled diabetics. Apparently, slowly progressive loss of vision was a common symptom (as opposed to the frequently apoplectic onset of ischemic optic neuropathy), and visual fields showed central scotomas or peripheral contraction. No mention was made of altitudinal defects, and only two patients demonstrated diabetic retinopathy. Of greater importance is the report by Lubow and Makley[54] of teenage patients with long-standing juvenile diabetes who presented with hemorrhagic swelling of one or both optic discs, mimicking papilledema of increased intracranial pressure (Fig. 202–6). Barr and associates[55] reported a series of 21 eyes in 12 juvenile diabetics and outlined a clinical profile consisting of symptoms of slightly blurred vision, minimal acuity and field deficits, general salutary outcome, and no consistent correlation with clinical control of hyperglycemia; diabetic retinopathy is usually of modest degree, and prognosis for proliferative retinopathy is uncertain. Neurodiagnostic studies are not indicated, and corticosteroid administration upsets diabetic control without providing any known therapeutic effect.

Although surely related to hypoxia of the prepapillary capillaries, "diabetic papillopathy" enjoys a much better visual prognosis than do most other forms of ischemic optic neuropathy.

INFREQUENTLY ASSOCIATED CONDITIONS

In 1973, Carroll originally called attention to a form of ischemic optic papillopathy occurring after uncomplicated *cataract extraction,* with sudden visual loss from 4 wk to 15 mo postoperatively.[56] About half of patients with initial eye affected may anticipate visual loss following operation on the second eye; three patients were in their 50s and the disc infarction occurred with both retrobulbar or general anesthesia. In Carroll's series, no

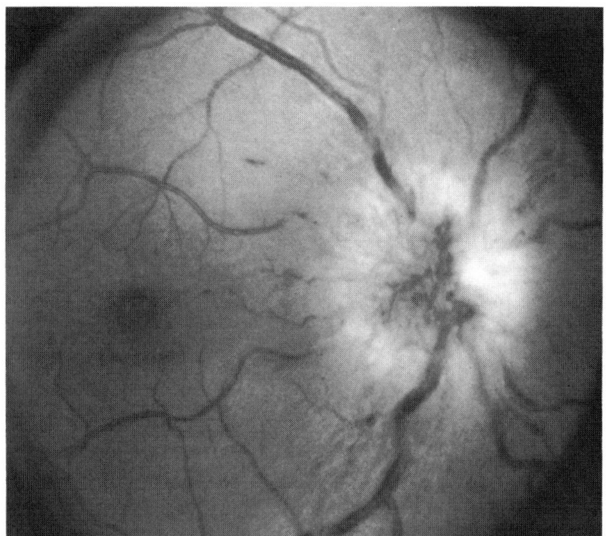

Figure 202–6. Papillopathy in juvenile diabetes. Note the florid capillary hyperemia on the disc surface and minimal background retinopathy. In this case, there is a small foveal edema cyst that reduced acuity.

patient experienced a loss of vision in a second eye unless subjected to cataract extraction and, therefore, Carroll speculated that "there is at least a localized occlusive vascular process involving the blood supply to the optic nerve" and that the operative procedure "tends to increase the occlusive disease over a period of weeks or months." Carroll also concluded that neither corticosteroids nor anticoagulants are effective therapies.

Perioperative data are incomplete to incriminate simple postoperative rise in ocular tension, although discs with marginal perfusion could be vulnerable. Hayreh's suggestion of lowering ocular tension when second eyes are at risk seems reasonable.[57]

Optic neuropathy following cataract extraction represents a distinct variant characterized by a circumscribed time course and high incidence of bilaterality, to the point of predictability, when the second eye is operated on (even in the fifth and sixth decades).[58]

Acute disc edema with visual loss, in patients not yet old enough to be included in what may comfortably be called the "vasculopathic" age group, falls into categories in which *collagen vascular* or *autoimmune arteritis* are suspected, or inflammatory neuritis may not be ruled out. This idiopathic ION of the "young" tends to be bilateral and recurrent.[59] The question of retinal arterial vasospasm is unanswered and, indeed, both unilateral and sequential bilateral disc infarctions have been reported in *migraine* [60, 61] and during cluster headache.[62]

Other varieties of ischemic disc swelling occur following marked or recurrent *blood loss*,[63] most frequently from the gastrointestinal tract, but peculiarly delayed by days to weeks. This seems an infrequent complication of pulmonary bypass surgery[64] or other general surgical procedures in which progressive postoperative red blood cell destruction drops hemoglobin levels[65]; visual loss has been reversed apparently by blood replacement. Bilateral *retrobulbar infarcts* with mild disc edema have been documented histologically.[66]

Knox and associates[67] have reported a variety of "*uremic*" optic neuropathy characterized by bilateral visual loss with disc swelling in patients with severe renal disease manifested by uremia, anemia, and hypertension. Improvement followed hemodialysis, except in one case of actual cryptococcal meningitis. However, Hamed and associates[68] contend that "uremic optic neuropathy" does not constitute a single pathophysiologic entity but includes complications of raised cerebrospinal fluid pressure, severe consecutive anterior ischemic optic neuropathy, and adverse reaction to hemodialysis itself. Bilateral ION is reported in a young woman with optic disc drusen and chronic hypotension, while undergoing renal dialysis.[69]

Carotid artery disease does not seem to play any regular role in ION; in fact, retinal arterial embolization and ION are mutually exclusive findings, except in the rarest of situations. Waybright and associates[70] documented three instances of typical ION with ipsilateral carotid occlusions, with retrograde filling of the ophthalmic artery by external carotid branches, perhaps indicating hypoperfusion of the nerve head, and Brown[71] reported a single case of abrupt visual loss at first with a normal disc, then with pale edema, in an eye suffering chronic hypoxia from complete carotid occlusion. From a series of 612 patients with acute ischemic hemispheric strokes due to internal carotid occlusions with "reversed flow in the ophthalmic artery," only three cases of simultaneous optic nerve infarction were uncovered.[72] Pulseless disease also has been complicated by ION.[73]

In a patient with atrial fibrillation,[74] emboli were found in the posterior ciliary arteries at autopsy, and Tomsak[75] recorded three patients with ION accompanied by retinal emboli, following coronary artery bypass surgery and cardiac catheterization.

Acute disc swelling attributed to ION has been reported in eclampsia,[76] porphyria,[77] and pseudoxanthoma elasticum with platelet hyperaggregability.[78]

Even as ION with disc swelling (i.e., *anterior*) does not constitute a single nosologic disorder, so retrobulbar (i.e., *posterior*) optic nerve ischemia does not connote distinctive etiology but represents a rare consequence of various diseases. This "posterior" ION variant consists of abrupt unilateral, rarely bilateral, visual loss without disc edema; other compressive, inflammatory, toxic, traumatic, or infiltrative causes should be rigorously excluded. Hayreh[79] has included cases of lupus and cranial arteritis, and Isayama and associates[80] reported 14 cases, 20 to 73 yr of age (6 less than 54 yr), with hypertension, diabetes, and infrequent carotid stenosis. Otherwise, polyarteritis nodosa,[81] acute internal artery occlusion,[82] blood loss,[52] and intraoperative hypotension[83] are all rare causes of posterior ION.

In those subsets of ischemic optic neuropathy in which a degree of inflammation plays some role, the use of systemic corticosteroid therapy seems reasonable.

REFERENCES

1. Boghen DR, Glaser JS: Ischaemic optic neuropathy: The clinical profile and natural history. Brain 98:689, 1975.
2. Movsas T, Kelman SE, Elman MJ, et al: The natural course of non-arteritic ischemic optic neuropathy. [Abstract] Invest Ophthalmol Vis Sci 42:951, 1991.

3. Traustason OI, Feldon SE, Leemaster JE, et al: Anterior ischemic optic neuropathy: Classification of field defects by Octopus (TM) automated static perimetry. Graefes Arch Clin Exp Ophthalmol 226:206, 1988.
4. Kline LB: Progression of visual field defects in ischemic optic neuropathy. Am J Ophthalmol 106:199, 1988.
5. Beck RW, Savino PJ, Schatz NJ, et al: Anterior ischemic neuropathy: Recurrent episodes in the same eye. Br J Ophthalmol 67:705, 1983.
6. Borchert M, Lessell S: Progressive and recurrent nonarteritic anterior ischemic optic neuropathy. Am J Ophthalmol 106:443, 1988.
7. Kao, LY, Huang L, Chen, TT: Anterior ischemic optic neuropathy—Recurrent attacks in one eye in a bilateral case. Ann Ophthalmol 21:71, 1989.
8. Beck RW: The clinical profile of optic neuritis: Experience of the Optic Neuritis Treatment Trial. Arch Ophthalmol 109:1673, 1991.
9. Rizzo JF, Lessell S: Optic neuritis and ischemic optic neuropathy: Overlapping clinical profiles. Arch Ophthalmol 109:1668, 1991.
10. Hayreh SS: Anterior ischemic optic neuropathy. V: Optic disc edema an early sign. Arch Ophthalmol 99:1030, 1981.
11. Hayreh SS: Anterior ischemic optic neuropathy. I: Terminology and pathogenesis. Br J Ophthalmol 58:955, 1974.
12. Olver JM, Spalton DJ, McCartney ACE: Microvascular study of the retrolaminar optic nerve in man: The possible significance in anterior ischemic optic neuropathy. Eye 4:7, 1990.
13. Katz B, Weinreb RN, Wheeler DT, et al: Anterior ischemic optic neuropathy and intraocular pressure. Br J Ophthalmol 74:99, 1990.
14. Kalenak JW, Kosmorsky GS, Rockwood EJ: Nonarteritic anterior ischemic optic neuropathy and intraocular pressure. Arch Ophthalmol 109:660, 1991.
15. Barrett DA, Schatz NJ, Glaser JS, et al: Progressive anterior ischemic optic neuropathy associated with transient increased intraocular pressure. J Clin Neuro Ophthalmol (in press).
16. Trobe JD, Glaser JS, Cassady J, et al: Nonglaucomatous excavation of the optic disc. Arch Ophthalmol 98:1046, 1980.
17. Trobe JD, Glaser JS, Cassady JC: Optic atrophy: Differential diagnosis by fundus observation alone. Arch Ophthalmol 98:1040, 1980.
18. Frisen L, Claesson M: Narrowing of the retinal arterioles in descending optic atrophy: A quantitative clinical study. Ophthalmology 91:1342, 1984.
19. Beri M, Klugman MR, Kohler JA, et al: Anterior ischemic optic neuropathy. VII: Incidence of bilaterality and various influencing factors. Ophthalmology 94:1020, 1987.
20. Lepore FE, Yarian DL: A mimic of the "exact diagnostic sign" of Foster Kennedy. Ann Ophthalmol 17:411, 1985.
21. Guyer DR, Miller NR, Auer CL, et al: The risk of cerebrovascular disease in patients with anterior ischemic optic neuropathy. Arch Ophthalmol 103:1136, 1985.
22. Jay WM, Williamson MR: Incidence of subcortical lesions not increased in nonarteritic ischemic optic neuropathy on magnetic resonance imaging. Am J Ophthalmol 104:398, 1987.
23. Giuffre G: Hematologic risk factors for anterior ischemic optic neuropathy. Neuro-ophthalmology 10:197, 1990.
24. Watts MT, Greaves M, Rennie IG, Clearkin LG: Antiphospholipid antibodies in the aetiology of ischaemic optic neuropathy. Eye 5:75, 1991.
25. Beck RW, Servais GE, Hayreh SS: Anterior ischemic optic neuropathy. IX: Cup-to-disc ratio and its role in pathogenesis. Ophthalmology 94:1503, 1987.
26. Mansour AM, Shoch D, Logani S: Optic disk size in ischemic optic neuropathy. Am J Ophthalmol 106:587, 1988.
27. Sergott RC, Cohen MS, Bosley TM, Savino PJ: Optic nerve decompression may improve the progressive form of nonarteritic ischemic optic neuropathy. Arch Ophthalmol 107:1743, 1989.
28. Spoor TC, Wilkinson MJ, Ramocki JM: Optic nerve sheath decompression for the treatment of progressive nonarteritic ischemic optic neuropathy. Am J Ophthalmol 111:724, 1991.
29. Kelman SE, Elman MJ: Optic nerve sheath decompression for nonarteritic ischemic optic neuropathy improves multiple visual function measurements. Arch Ophthalmol 109:667, 1991.
30. Jablons MM, Glaser JS, Schatz NJ, et al: Optic nerve sheath decompression for progressive ischemic optic neuropathy: Results in 26 patients. Arch Ophthalmol 110:(in press), 1992.
31. Wagner HP, Hollenhorst RW: The ocular lesions of temporal arteritis. Am J Ophthalmol 45:617, 1958.
32. Biller J, Asconape J, Weinblatt ME, et al: Temporal arteritis associated with a normal sedimentation rate. JAMA 247:486, 1982.
33. Hauser WA, Ferguson RH, Holley KE, et al: Temporal arteritis in Rochester, Minnesota, 1951 to 1967. Mayo Clin Proc 46:597, 1971.
34. Bengstsson BA, Malmvall BE: The epidemiology of giant cell arteritis including temporal arteritis and polymyalgia rheumatica: Incidences of different clinical presentations and eye complications. Arthritis Rheum 24:899, 1981.
35. Hayreh SS, Podhajsky P: Visual field defects in anterior ischemic optic neuropathy. Doc Ophthalmol Proc Ser 19:53, 1979.
36. Sebag J, Thomas JV, Epstein EL, et al: Optic disc cupping in arteritic anterior ischemic optic neuropathy resembles glaucomatous cupping. Ophthalmology 93:357, 1986.
37. Barricks ME, Traviesa DB, Glaser JS, Levy IS: Ophthalmoplegia in cranial arteritis. Brain 100:209, 1977.
38. Bienfang DC: Loss of the ocular pulse in the acute phase of temporal arteritis. Acta Ophthalmol (Copenh) 67 (Suppl 191):35, 1989.
39. Bosley TM, Savino PJ, Sergott RC, et al: Ocular pneumoplethysmography can help in the diagnosis of giant-cell arteritis. Arch Ophthalmol 107:379, 1989.
40. Model DG: Reversal of blindness in temporal arteritis with methylprednisolone. Lancet i:340, 1978.
41. Rosenfeld SI, Kosmorsky GS, Klingele TG, et al: Treatment of temporal arteritis with ocular involvement. Am J Med 80:143, 1986.
42. Diamond JP: Treatable blindness in temporal arteritis. Br J Ophthalmol 75:432, 1991.
43. Hamilton CR, Shelley WM, Tumulty PA: Giant cell arteritis: Including temporal arteritis and polymyalgia rheumatica. Medicine 50:1, 1971.
44. Cullen JF: Ischemic optic neuropathy. Trans Ophthalmol Soc UK 87:759, 1967.
45. Palm E: The ocular crisis of the temporal arteritis syndrome (Horton). Acta Ophthalmol 36:208, 1958.
46. Hamrin B: Polymyalgia arteritica. Acta Med Scand 533 (Suppl):1, 1972.
47. Boyd RV, Hoffbrand BI: Erythrocyte sedimentation rate in elderly hospital in-patients. Br Med J 1:901, 1966.
48. Milne JS, Williamson J: The ESR in older people. Gerontol Clin 14:36, 1972.
49. Miller A, Green M: Simple rule for calculating normal erythrocyte sedimentation rate. Br Med J 286:266, 1983.
50. Klein RG, Campbell RJ, Hunder GG, Carney JA: Skip lesions in temporal arteritis. Mayo Clin Proc 51:504, 1976.
51. Coppeto JR, Monteiro M: Diagnosis of highly occult giant cell arteritis by repeat temporal artery biopsies. Neuro-ophthalmology 10:217, 1990.
52. Lipton RB, Solomon S, Wertenbaker C: Gradual loss and recovery of vision in temporal arteritis. Arch Intern Med 145:2252, 1985.
53. Skillern PG, Lockhart G: Optic neuritis and uncontrolled diabetes mellitus in 14 patients. Ann Intern Med 51:468, 1959.
54. Lubow M, Makley TA: Pseudopapilledema of juvenile diabetes mellitus. Arch Ophthalmol 85:417, 1971.
55. Barr CC, Glaser JS, Blankenship G: Acute disc swelling in juvenile diabetes: Clinical profile and natural history of 12 cases. Arch Ophthalmol 98:2185, 1980.
56. Carroll FD: Optic nerve complications of cataract extraction. Trans Am Acad Ophthalmol Otolaryngol 77:623, 1973.
57. Hayreh SS: Anterior ischemic optic neuropathy. IV: Occurrence after cataract extraction. Arch Ophthalmol 98:1410, 1980.
58. Serrano LA, Behrens MM, Carroll FD: Postcataract extraction ischemic optic neuropathy. Arch Ophthalmol 100:1177, 1982.
59. Hamed LM, Purvin V, Rosenberg M: Recurrent anterior ischemic optic neuropathy in young adults. J Clin Neuro Ophthalmol 8:239, 1988.
60. O'Hara M, O'Connor PS: Migrainous optic neuropathy. J Clin Neuro Ophthalmol 4:85, 1984.
61. Katz B: Bilateral sequential migrainous ischemic optic neuropathy. Am J Ophthalmol 99:489, 1985.

62. Toshniwal P: Anterior ischemic optic neuropathy secondary to cluster headache. Acta Neurol Scand 73:213, 1986.
63. Hayreh SS: Anterior ischemic optic neuropathy. VIII: Clinical features and pathogenesis of post-hemorrhagic amaurosis. Ophthalmology 94:1488, 1987.
64. Sweeney PJ, Breuer AC, Selhorst JB, et al: Ischemic optic neuropathy: A complication of cardiopulmonary bypass surgery. Neurology 32:560, 1982.
65. Jaben SL, Glaser JS, Daily M: Ischemic optic neuropathy following general surgical procedures. J Clin Neuro Ophthalmol 3:239, 1983.
66. Johnson MW, Kincaid MC, Trobe JD: Bilateral retrobulbar optic nerve infarctions after blood loss and hypotension: A clinicopathologic case study. Ophthalmology 94:1577, 1987.
67. Knox DL, Hanneken AM, Hollows FC, et al: Uremic optic neuropathy. Arch Ophthalmol 106:50, 1988.
68. Hamed LM, Winward KE, Glaser JS, et al: Optic neuropathy in uremia. Am J Ophthalmol 108:30, 1989.
69. Michaelson C, Behrens M, Odel J: Bilateral anterior ischemic optic neuropathy associated with optic disc drusen and systemic hypotension. Br J Ophthalmol 73:767, 1989.
70. Waybright EA, Selhorst JB, Combs J: Anterior ischemic optic neuropathy with internal carotid artery occlusion. Am J Ophthalmol 93:42, 1982.
71. Brown GC: Anterior ischemic optic neuropathy occurring in association with carotid artery obstruction. J Clin Neuro Ophthalmol 6:39, 1986.
72. Bogousslavsky J, Regli F, Zografos L, et al: Optico-cerebral syndrome: Simultaneous hemodynamic infarction of optic nerve and brain. Neurology 37:263, 1987.
73. Leonard TJK, Sanders MD: Ischaemic optic neuropathy in pulseless disease. Br J Ophthalmol 67:389, 1983.
74. Liebermann MF, Shahi A, Grenn WR: Embolic ischemic optic neuropathy. Am J Ophthalmol 86:206, 1978.
75. Tomsak RL: Ischemic optic neuropathy associated with retinal embolism. Am J Ophthalmol 99:590, 1985.
76. Beck RW, Gamel JW, Willcourt RJ, et al: Acute ischemic optic neuropathy in severe preeclampsia. Am J Ophthalmol 90:342, 1980.
77. DeFrancisco M, Savino PJ, Schatz NJ: Optic atrophy in acute intermittent porphyria. Am J Ophthalmol 87:221, 1979.
78. Manor RS, Axer-Siegal R, Cohenn S, et al: Bilateral anterior ischemic optic neuropathy, pseudoxanthoma elasticum, and platelet hyperaggregability. Neuro-ophthalmology 6:173, 1986.
79. Hayreh SS: Posterior ischaemic optic neuropathy. Ophthalmologica 182:29, 1981.
80. Isayama Y, Takahashi T, Inoue M, et al: Posterior ischemic optic neuropathy. III: Clinical diagnosis. Ophthalmologica 187:141, 1983.
81. Hutchinson CH: Polyarteritis nodosa presenting as posterior ischemic optic neuropathy. J R Soc Med 77:1043, 1984.
82. Sawle GV, Sarkies NJC: Posterior ischaemic optic neuropathy due to internal artery occlusion. Neuro-ophthalmology 7:349, 1987.
83. Rizzo JF, Lessell S: Posterior ischemic optic neuropathy during general surgery. Am J Ophthalmol 103:808, 1987.

Chapter 203

Tumors of the Anterior Visual Pathways

STEVEN E. FELDON

Not infrequently, the ophthalmologist is called on to determine whether or not visual loss is caused by anterior visual pathway disease of infiltrative or compressive etiology. Although much of the diagnostic dilemma has been alleviated with the advent of advanced neuroimaging techniques, the clinical evaluation is still of paramount importance.

Tumors affecting the optic nerve should be suspected in any patient presenting with unilateral visual loss or proptosis that slowly progresses over months to years. "Corticosteroid-dependent" optic neuritis may be another presentation of optic nerve tumor. Occasionally, an asymptomatic tumor is discovered incidentally at the time of neuroimaging for evaluation of neurofibromatosis[1] or of a completely unrelated condition (e.g., headache).

Many lesions may compress or infiltrate the optic nerve secondarily (see Orbit), but this chapter is confined to the diagnosis and management of primary optic nerve tumors. Tumors of the optic nerve are divided primarily into those of glial origin and those of meningeal origin. Often, the clinical and radiologic presentations overlap sufficiently that, in the absence of histologic confirmation, no final diagnosis may be ascertained.

OPTIC NERVE GLIOMA OF CHILDHOOD (Table 203–1)

Presentation

The incidence of optic nerve glioma is estimated at 1.5 percent of children presenting with proptosis.[2] On the other hand, optic nerve glioma represents about 17 percent of the orbital tumors encountered in childhood.[3] In different series, the association with neurofibromatosis ranges from 10 to 70 percent.[4–13] Of patients with neurofibromatosis, optic nerve glioma is detected in about 15 percent.[1]

Diagnosis is usually made prior to 5 yr of age, but occasionally the presentation is in early adulthood.[14] About half of optic nerve gliomas are confined to the orbit, whereas half demonstrate intracranial extension.[15] Intracranial extension may be suspected clinically on the basis of precocious puberty, somnolence, or diabetes insipidus.

Table 203–1. SUMMARY

	Optic Nerve Glioma of Childhood	Optic Nerve Meningioma
Presentation	1.5% of children with proptosis Frequent association with neurofibromatosis Intracranial symptoms may include precocious puberty, somnolence, diabetes insipidus	3–5% of orbital tumors Rare bilateral involvement Frequently present in middle adulthood 3:1 female predominance Intracranial extension may cause anosmia, ophthalmoplegia, seizures, and pituitary dysfunction
Pathology	Fusiform swelling of optic nerve, if intraorbital Juvenile pilocystic astrocytoma; rarely other types Histologically benign appearance Frequent microcystoid changes Arachnoid proliferation may simulate meningioma Malignant degeneration is rare	Derived from arachnoidal cap cells Histologic features include whorls and psammoma bodies Histologic type may be fibroblastic, syncytial, angioblastic, or transitional Rare malignant degeneration occurs May arise within or adjacent to optic nerve Hyperostosis may occur adjacent to tumor Subfrontal lesions may compress prechiasmal nerve
Physical Findings	Typical of chronic optic nerve dysfunction Central scotomas common Bitemporal field defects if chiasm involved Sensory-induced strabismus may occur Optic disc may be edematous, infiltrated, or atrophic Rarely optociliary shunt vessels occur on disc Rarely neovascular glaucoma may be present	Proptosis common Optic disc may be swollen, pale, or normal (early) Triad: optociliary veins, disc pallor, and visual loss Visual fields may show central defects, peripheral constriction, or overall depression Bitemporal hemianopia present with chiasm involvement Ocular and motility disorders may occur depending on tumor location Subfrontal tumors may cause Foster Kennedy syndrome
Radiology	CT and MRI preferred to plain films or polytomography Intraorbital lesion appears as fusiform enlargement of optic nerve Intracanalicular extension causes enlargement and erosion of bone canal Intracranial mass may thicken chiasm or produce exophytic suprasellar/hypothalamic mass	CT or MRI are the preferred imaging techniques Coronal CT may demonstrate "railroad track" sign Apical and intracanalicular lesions may be difficult to image ("impossible meningioma") Rarely, pneumosinus dilatans may occur Hyperostosis may be present
Natural History	Slow or limited growth potential as a rule Occasional aggressive lesions encountered	Orbital lesions slowly progress to unilateral blindness Intracranial lesions may involve chiasm and adjacent structures
Treatment	*Isolated Orbital Lesions* Controversial—benefit is uncertain Radiation and chemotherapy may be used if progressive on imaging In patients younger than 5 yr of age, consider surgical removal if progression on imaging	*Orbital Lesions* Surgical removal is not advocated Stabilization and regression possible with radiation
	Intracranial Extension Hydrocephalus is a poor prognostic sign Exophytic growth is a poor prognostic sign Radiation and/or chemotherapy is controversial	*Orbital Lesions* Surgery for intracranial lesions is often beneficial Radiation benefit is controversial Hormone therapy may offer a treatment alternative in the future

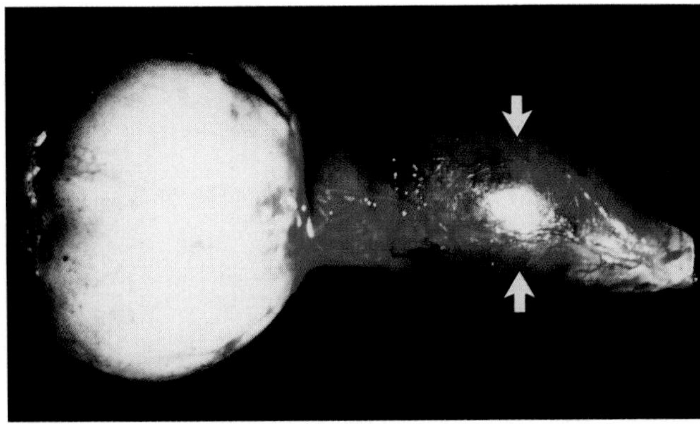

Figure 203–1. En bloc resection of intraorbital optic nerve glioma demonstrates fusiform enlargement of the optic nerve without disruption of the dural sheath.

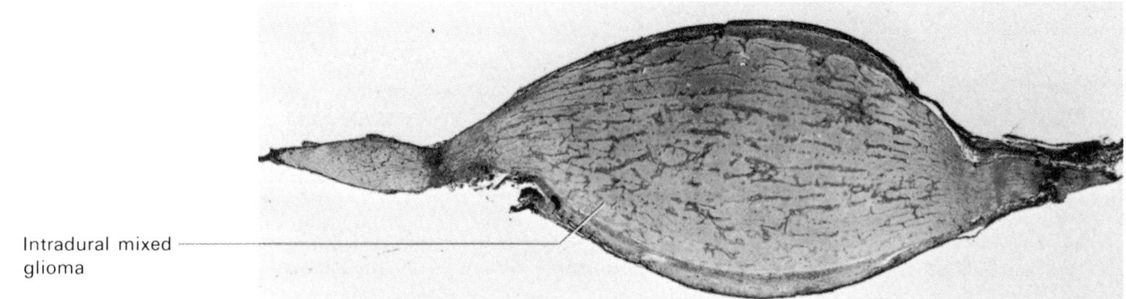

Figure 203–2. The glioma involves only the orbital segment of the nerve and is confined by the dura. There is no evidence of tumor in either stump. The subdural and subarachnoid spaces are obliterated by dense tissue. The septa between the enlarged fiber bundles are thicker than normal (Bodian stain). (From Lindenberg R, Walsh FB, Sacks JG: Neuropathology of Vision: An Atlas. Philadelphia, Lea & Febiger, 1973, p 127.)

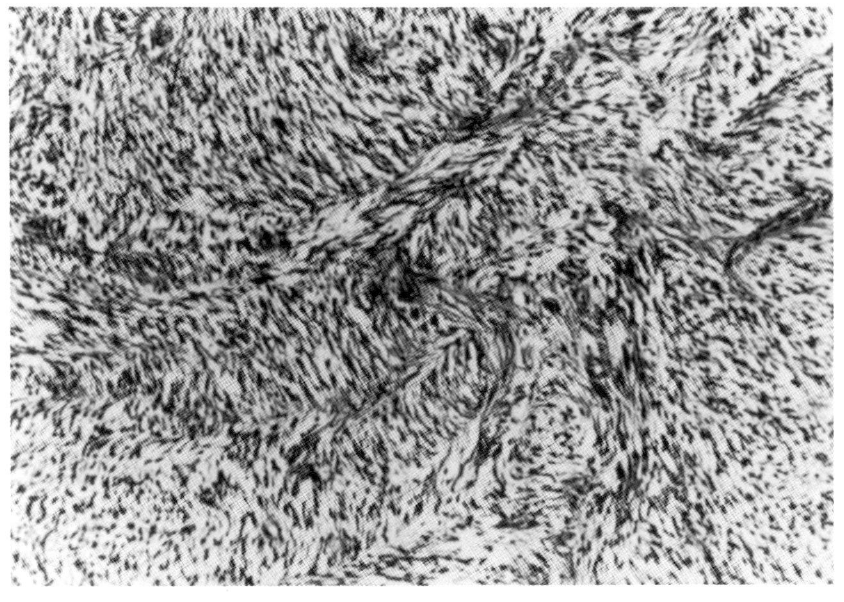

Figure 203–3. A typical compact pilocytic area in which the elongated tumor cells are arranged in interlacing fascicles. (From Yanoff M, Davis RL, Zimmerman LE: Juvenile pilocytic astrocytoma ("glioma") of optic nerve: Clinicopathologic study of sixty-three cases. *In* Jakobiec FA [ed]: Ocular and Adnexal Tumors. Birmingham, AL, Aesculapius Publishing, 1978, p 690.)

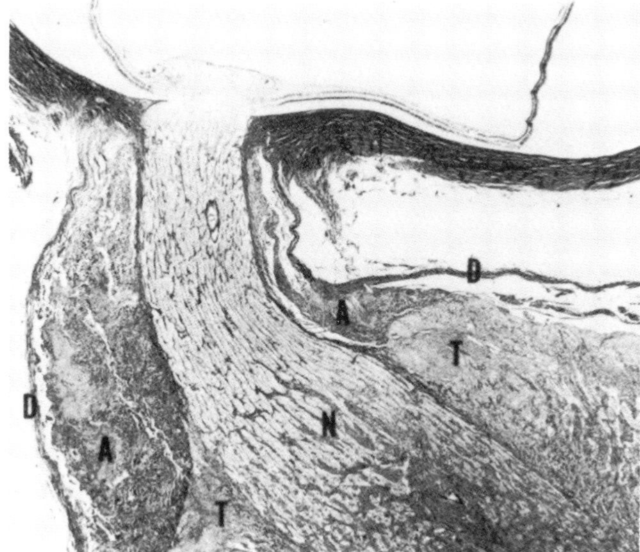

Figure 203–4. In this large orbital tumor, almost all of the mass close to the globe is located between the dura (D) and the nerve (N). Even at this low magnification, a distinction is easily made between areas of neoplastic invasion of the meninges by the tumor (T) and areas of reactive arachnoidal hyperplasia (A). The optic nerve head is markedly swollen. (From Yanoff M, Davis RL, Zimmerman LE: Juvenile pilocytic astrocytoma ("glioma") of optic nerve: Clinicopathologic study of sixty-three cases. *In* Jakobiec FA [ed]: Ocular and Adnexal Tumors. Birmingham, AL, Aesculapius Publishing, 1978, p 693.)

Pathology

When confined to the orbital portion of the optic nerve, a glioma often appears as a fusiform swelling (Figs. 203–1 and 203–2). Histologically, optic nerve glioma is generally characterized as a juvenile pilocytic astrocytoma, although mixed gliomas and oligodendrogliomas have been reported.[7, 12, 16, 17] The tumor may infiltrate the normal optic nerve substance (Fig. 203–3) or be confined primarily to the subarachnoid space (Fig. 203–4). Rarely, there is exophytic extension of the tumor outside the optic nerve sheath. The overall histologic appearance is benign, with a paucity of cellular atypia, mitosis, or tumor necrosis. Often, microcystoid extracellular spaces containing acid mucopolysaccharide produced by astrocytes are encountered (Fig. 203–5). Such spaces may constitute a major portion of the optic nerve mass.[18] Proliferation of arachnoid surrounding the optic nerve glioma (see Fig. 203–4) may simulate meningioma.[16] Malignant degeneration of optic nerve glioma is rare. In the glioma of one 4-year-old boy (Fig. 203–6), malignant degeneration of the distal portion of the tumor was encountered in an otherwise typical optic nerve glioma.

Physical Findings

Except in those circumstances when optic nerve gliomas are discovered incidentally and vision is normal, the eye findings are typical of chronic optic nerve dysfunction. An ipsilateral afferent pupillary defect is present, visual acuity is deficient, and there is acquired achromatopsia. Central scotomas are common, but temporal or bitemporal field loss may occur if the prechiasmal or chiasmal portion of the intracranial optic nerve is involved.[19] Sensory-induced strabismus may result from the visual loss. The optic nerve head may be edematous, infiltrated with tumor, or atrophic (Fig. 203–7). Rarely, optociliary shunt vessels may be present (see under meningioma). Also, neovascular glaucoma secondary to optic nerve glioma has been reported.[20, 21]

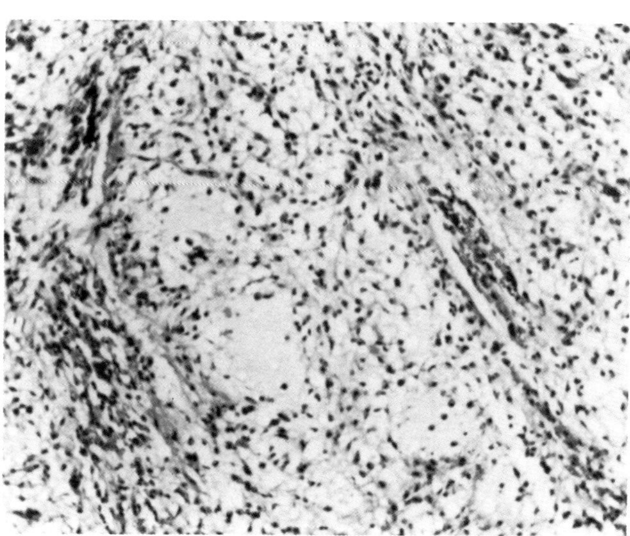

Figure 203–5. Mucoproteinaceous fluid is present in microcystic areas from a large glioma involving the intracranial optic nerve, chiasm, and hypothalamus. (From Yanoff M, Davis RL, Zimmerman LE: Juvenile pilocytic astrocytoma ("glioma") of optic nerve: Clinicopathologic study of sixty-three cases. *In* Jakobiec FA [ed]: Ocular and Adnexal Tumors. Birmingham, AL, Aesculapius Publishing, 1978, p 689.)

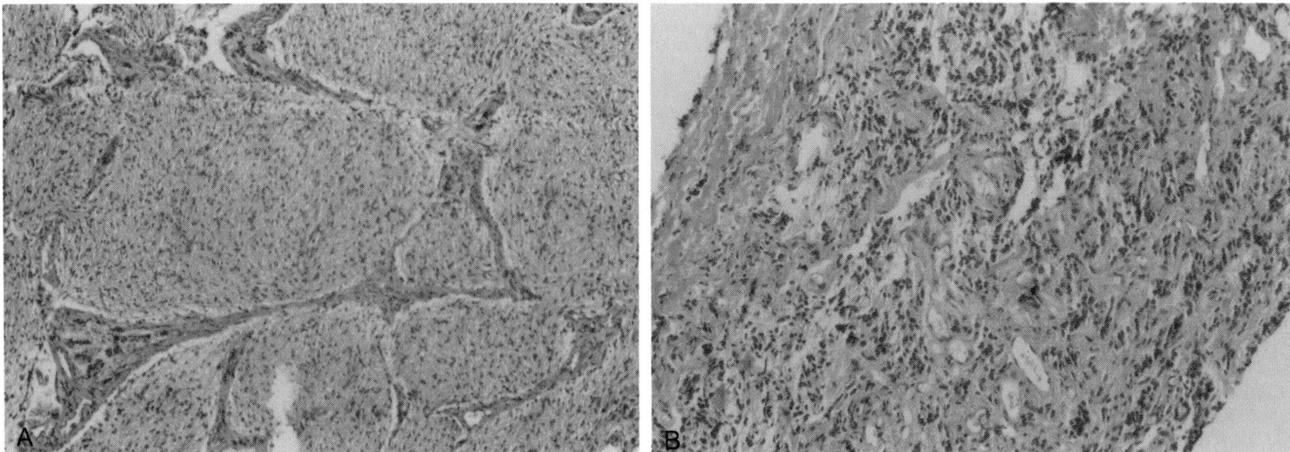

Figure 203–6. Histopathologic appearance of resected optic nerve glioma confined by radiologic criteria to the orbit; however, the proximal end of the specimen just anterior to the chiasm demonstrated microscopic invasion with tumor. *A*, Benign astrocytic infiltration spreading between septa of the intraorbital optic nerve. *B*, Distal section of same tumor at higher magnification demonstrates marked cellular atypia, which is consistent with malignant degeneration.

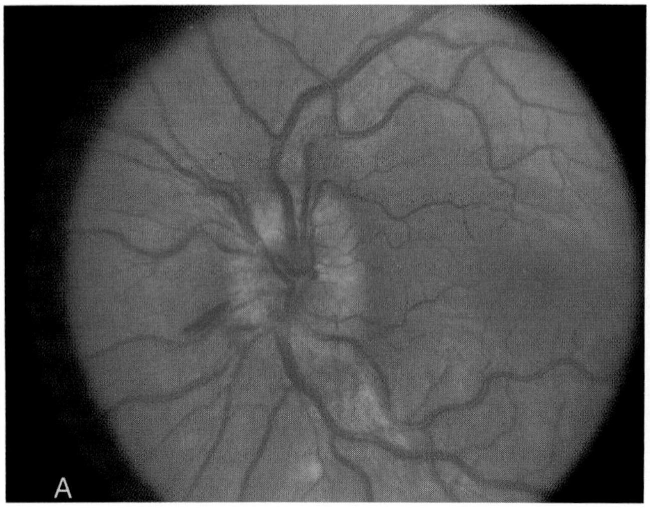

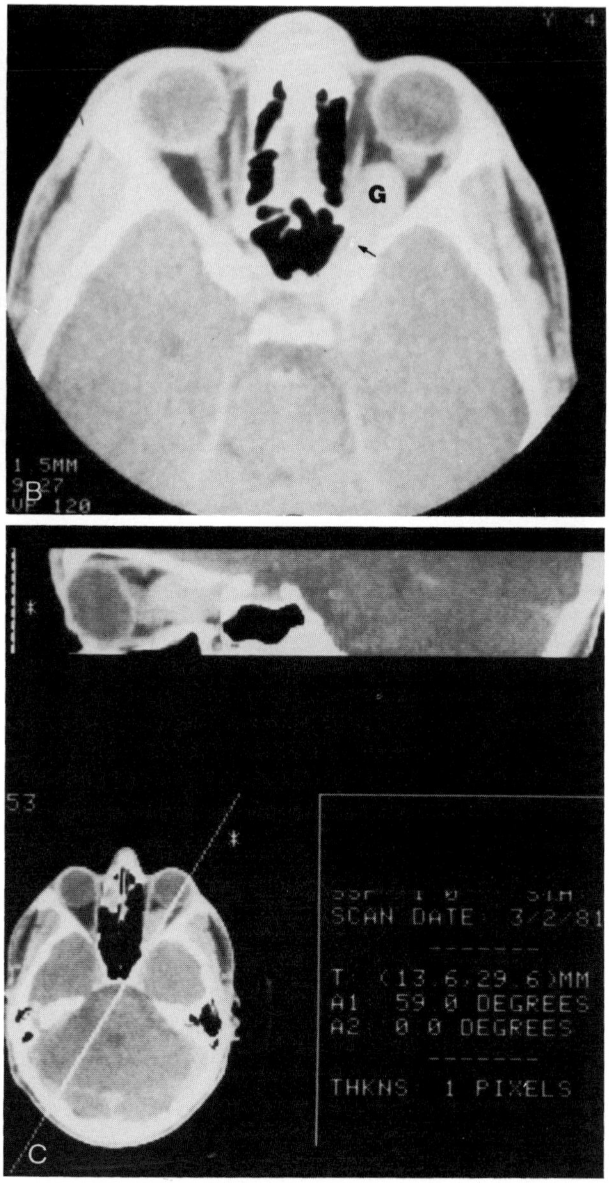

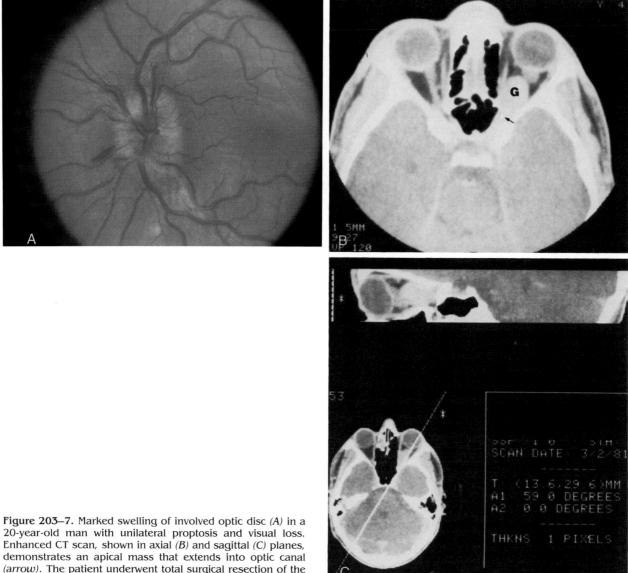

Figure 203–7. Marked swelling of involved optic disc *(A)* in a 20-year-old man with unilateral proptosis and visual loss. Enhanced CT scan, shown in axial *(B)* and sagittal *(C)* planes, demonstrates an apical mass that extends into optic canal *(arrow)*. The patient underwent total surgical resection of the lesion.

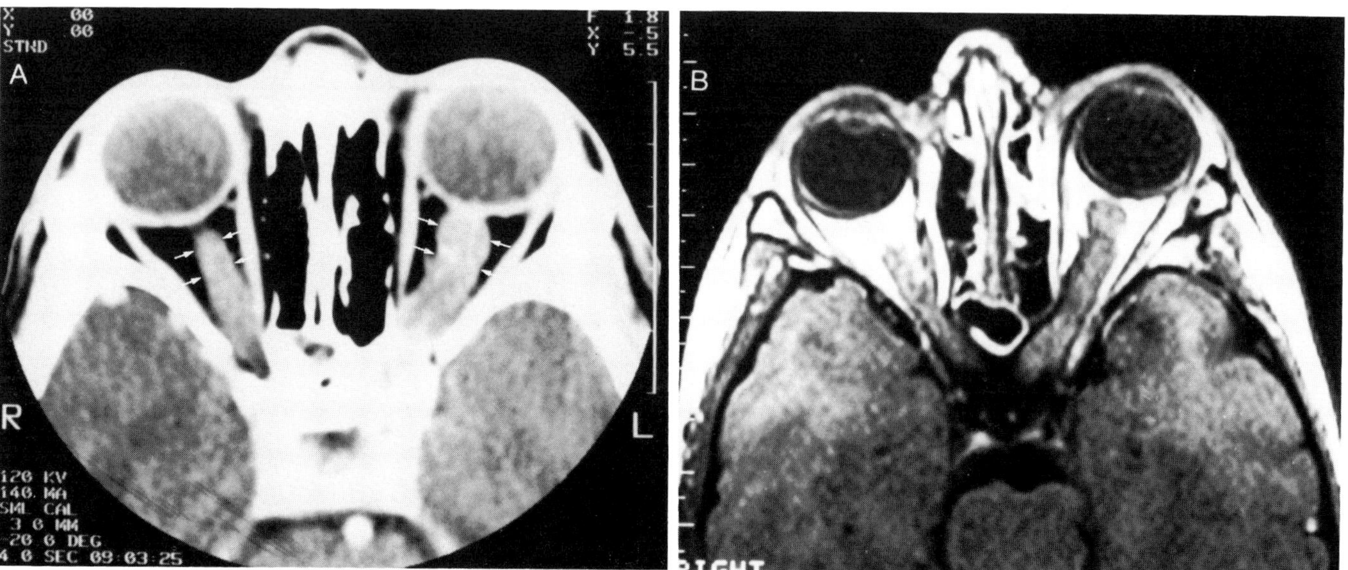

Figure 203–8. A 5-year-old boy with no stigmata or family history of neurofibromatosis presented with primarily left-sided proptosis and visual loss. Both CT scan *(A)* and T_1-weighted MRI scan *(B)* demonstrate bilateral asymmetric widening of the optic nerves *(arrows)* extending from the globe through the optic canals. Higher sections (not shown) document thickening of the optic chiasm as well. Optic disc, visual acuity, and visual fields in the right eye have remained normal over 3 years, without treatment.

Radiology

In the appropriate clinical setting, the diagnosis is readily confirmed radiologically. Plain roentgenograms or polytomography utilizing optic canal views may reveal bony enlargement,[22] but computed tomography (CT) and magnetic resonance imaging (MRI) are capable of imaging the fusiform enlargement of the optic nerve directly (Fig. 203–8).[1]

Natural History

The natural history of optic nerve glioma of childhood is highly controversial. Most tumors grow slowly or have self-limited growth, consistent with a benign hamartoma. However, some tumors are more aggressive, resulting in a rapid increase in ipsilateral proptosis and visual loss. Subsequent involvement of the chiasm and contralateral optic nerve have been described.[23] Rare cases of apparent remission of symptoms have also been reported.[24] Using a statistical review of the literature, with its obvious limitations in terms of accurate data collection, Alvord and Lofton[15] suggest that optic nerve gliomas are never benign hamartomas, with 100 percent projected progression of symptoms by 48 yr after presentation. Miller[25] asserts that "those patients who are most likely to have a relatively benign prognosis are those who present with mild proptosis, optic disc pallor, and neurofibromatosis, whereas those patients who are likely to experience symptomatic growth are those with moderate to severe proptosis, optic disc swelling, and no evidence of neurofibromatosis."

Treatment

Orbital Tumor. The variability in the natural history of optic nerve glioma has complicated the assessment of treatment. No treatment has been advocated by several experts.[7, 26] However, according to the survival analysis by Alvord and Lofton,[15] 70 percent of untreated patients will show progression within 3 yr and 7 percent will die of their disease. Thus, the decision to treat remains a controversial issue.

Radiation therapy of orbital gliomas has its advocates.[27, 28] Cases of clinical as well as radiologic improvement following treatment have been reported.[23] Some survival statistics accumulated by Alvord and Lofton[15] suggest that there is no associated progression or death with radiation of greater than 4500 rads.[15] On the other hand, radiation treatments for which the dose is not established have 25 percent progression at 5 yr and 50 percent progression at 10 yr. A 14 percent incidence of death is reported for this group.[15]

Progression of tumor, based on clinical and radiologic follow-up, may be considered, in the appropriate clinical setting, as an indication for complete surgical excision. The preferred technique is transcranial superior orbitotomy, preserving the globe.[29, 30] Although vision is lost due to surgery, further progression is only rarely encountered, and death secondary to the glioma almost never occurs.[15, 17, 31, 32] Incomplete excision may be associated with a worse prognosis.[11, 33, 34]

The author's opinion on treatment of optic nerve glioma isolated to the orbit is individualized and relies heavily on careful clinical and radiologic follow-up. Those lesions demonstrating little or no progression of visual loss should not receive treatment. Also those lesions demonstrating slow, progressive visual loss without radiologic evidence of intracanalicular or intracranial extension should not be treated. If the patient has evidence of rapid radiologic progression that threatens to extend intracranially and is greater than 5 yr of age, radiation therapy should be seriously considered. If the patient is under 5 yr of age, surgical excision may be preferable to preclude possible long-term side effects of radiation on immature brain tissue. Given the controversy regarding efficacy of therapy, the family should participate actively in the decision-making process. In the blind, proptotic eye, surgical excision may be advocated for improved cosmesis.

Intracranial Tumor. When the optic nerve glioma affects the chiasm, the natural history and the options for treatment are altered. In general, patients who do not develop hydrocephalus have a better chance of survival,[15] and several series suggest a relatively good prognosis,[26, 35] even without treatment. The study by Imes and Hoyt[35] documented that the chiasmal tumor was a cause of death in only 18 percent of patients followed for a mean of 20 yr. Fletcher and colleagues[36] suggest that patients demonstrating enlarged chiasm and optic nerves, without exophytic component, have a better prognosis than do those with large exophytic components. By 10 yr after presentation, 58 percent of untreated patients with hydrocephalus will have died, compared with 30 percent of treated patients.[15]

Although many studies suggest that all patients with chiasmal gliomas benefit significantly from radiation or chemotherapy,[6, 14, 15, 27, 28, 32, 33] some authors recommend treatment only for patients with hydrocephalus, progressive visual loss, or other complications.[7, 10, 37–42] A few studies have, in fact, failed to document significant benefit from radiation therapy, and these investigators do not recommend its use.[11, 13, 17, 26, 43–45]

MALIGNANT GLIOMA OF ADULTHOOD

Since the advent of CT scanning, the exceedingly rare malignant gliomas of the optic nerve and chiasm are more often being diagnosed premortem. In a review of the literature published in 1980, Spoor and associates reported only 26 cases,[46] and only a few cases have been reported since then.[47, 48] There is no apparent sexual predilection, and most patients are middle-aged.

Almost invariably, patients present with rapidly progressive unilateral or bilateral visual loss.[49] Eye pain or headache may accompany the visual loss. Bilateral blindness occurs within weeks of onset. Central scotomas, altitudinal field defects, and hemianopsias have all been reported. By ophthalmoscopy the optic disc may be normal in appearance; alternatively, edema or atrophy of the optic disc may be present. Often the initial presentation is suggestive of an anterior or posterior ischemic optic neuropathy.[46, 47, 50]

When the intraorbital portion of the optic nerve is affected, there may be proptosis, ophthalmoplegia, conjunctival chemosis, and venous stasis retinopathy, as well as evidence of both posterior and anterior segment ischemia.[46, 51] The ischemic changes may lead to the onset of neovascular glaucoma.[51]

Even with aggressive radiation therapy, there is invariably rapid spread of tumor intracranially, and death occurs within months. Histologically, the tumor may be characterized as either astrocytoma or glioblastoma multiforme.

OPTIC NERVE MENINGIOMA

Presentation

Optic nerve meningiomas account for less than 1 percent of all meningiomas and for only 3 to 5 percent of orbital tumors.[10, 52] Bilateral involvement is rare (Fig. 203–9). They most commonly present in patients 30 to 50 yr of age, but they may be found at any age. There is a 3:1 female predominance.[44] With intracranial extension, associated findings include anosmia, ophthalmoplegia, seizures, and pituitary dysfunction.

Pathology

Meningiomas probably arise from cap cells that line the outer arachnoidal surface. Meningiomas of the anterior visual pathway do not differ histopathologically from those found elsewhere in the central nervous system. Two characteristic features of most meningiomas are the presence of whorls and of psammoma bodies. Whorls are spindle-shaped cells that are concentrically packed, producing an onion-skin appearance in cross section. Psammoma bodies are concentric laminae of calcium deposits and are often seen in the degenerative centers of whorls. Some meningiomas, called fibroblastic, consist of elongated cells, suggestive of fibroblasts. Syncytial tumors have indistinct cell borders, and those with prominent vessels are called angioblastic. Transitional cell meningiomas have polygonal cells, which are often interspersed with prominent whorls. Malignancies are rare; however, when present, they demonstrate characteristic pleomorphism and mitotic figures.[53]

Optic nerve meningiomas may arise from within the optic nerve sheath as well as from meninges or rests of meningeal cell structures adjacent to the optic nerve (Fig. 203–10). Meningiomas arising within the optic nerve sheath may produce symptoms by localized extraneural expansion with resultant optic nerve compression; by circumferential extraneural growth, which produces ischemia of the optic nerve; or by actual invasion of the optic nerve tissue (Fig. 203–11). Meningiomas arising outside the optic nerve sheath may produce distal compression as they grow into the optic canal from the intracranial meatus. Occasionally, hyperostotic bone adjacent to the tumor or interosseous meningioma produces the optic nerve compression (Fig. 203–12). Subfrontal meningiomas may directly compress the prechiasmal portion of the optic nerve.

Physical Findings

Optic nerve meningiomas occurring within the nerve sheath or involving the sphenoid ridge are often associated with proptosis, in contrast to tumors that are intracanalicular or intracranial (Fig. 203–13). Swelling or pallor of the optic disc is a common sequela of optic nerve meningioma, although Knight and associates[54]

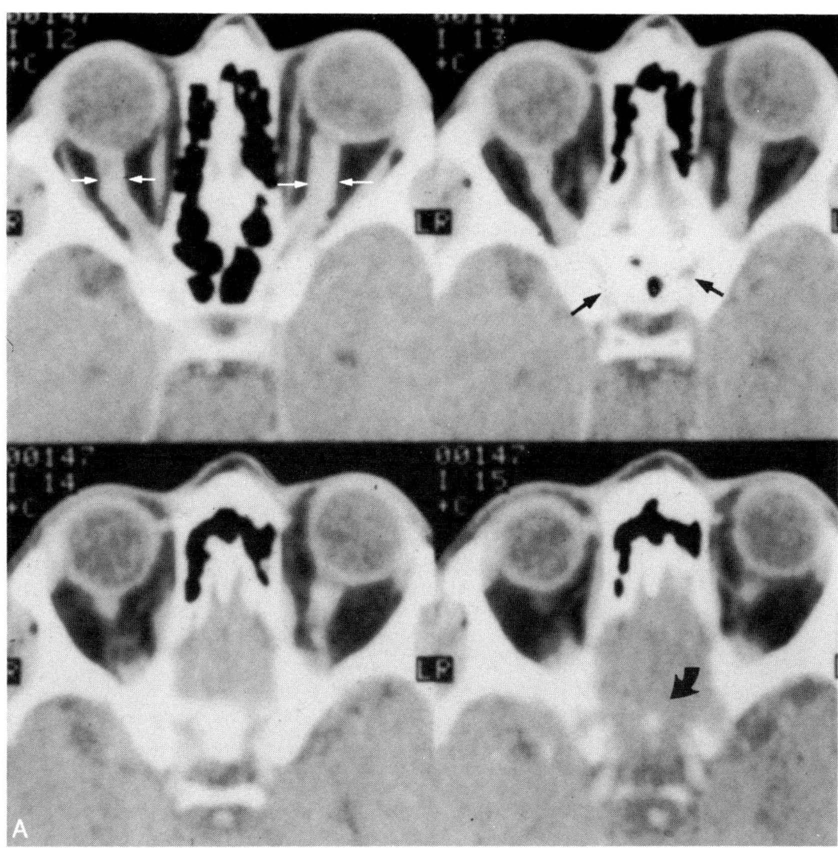

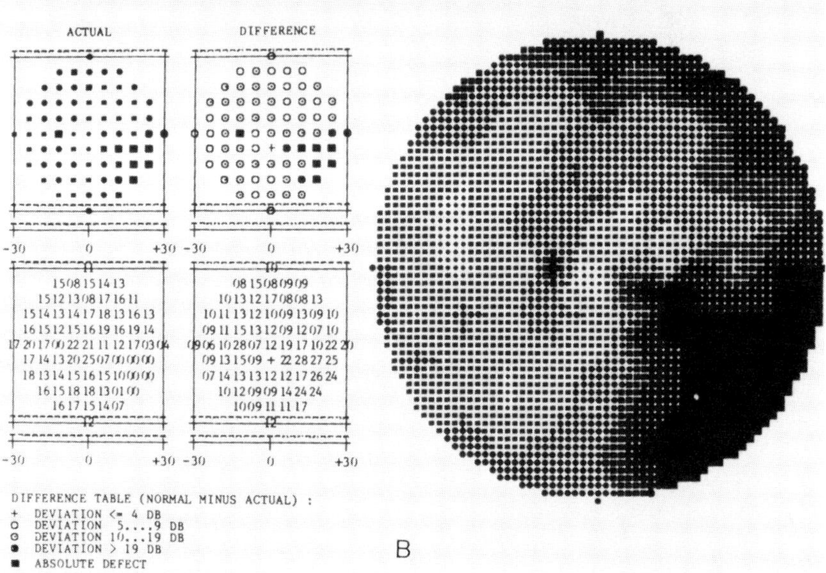

Figure 203–9. *A,* Four axial sections from the enhanced CT scan from a middle-aged woman with progressive visual loss in the left eye shows bilateral thickening of the optic nerve sheaths *(white arrows).* The low density of the optic nerve parenchyma results in the "railroad tracks" characteristic of meningiomas. The bony optic canals do not appear widened *(black arrows),* and there is no evidence of a common intracranial component *(curved black arrow). B,* The 30-degree central field of the patient's left eye, demonstrating an inferior nasal step superimposed on overall field depression. The visual field of the patient's right eye was normal.

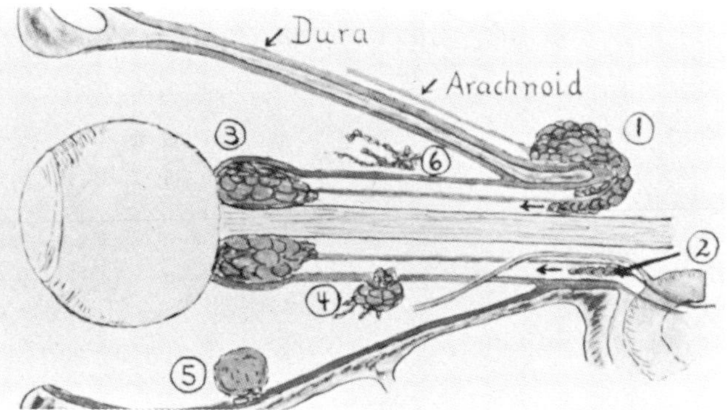

Figure 203–10. Diagram demonstrating possible locations of intraorbital meningiomas. Tumor cells may arise from the planum sphenoidale (1) or from the optic canal (2) and migrate into the subdural space of the intraorbital optic nerve. Tumors may also arise de novo from within the optic nerve sheaths and remain intradural (3) or become exophytic masses (4). Atopic nests of arachnoidal cells within the orbit (5 and 6) may also give rise to meningiomas. (From Lindenberg R, Walsh FB, Sacks JG: Neuropathology of Vision: An Atlas. Philadelphia, Lea & Febiger, 1973, p 143.)

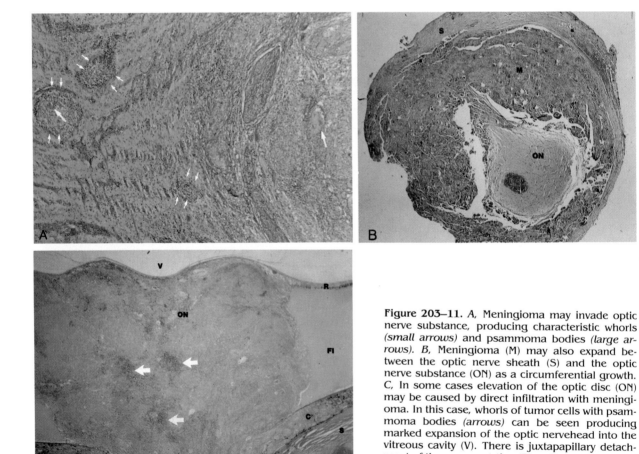

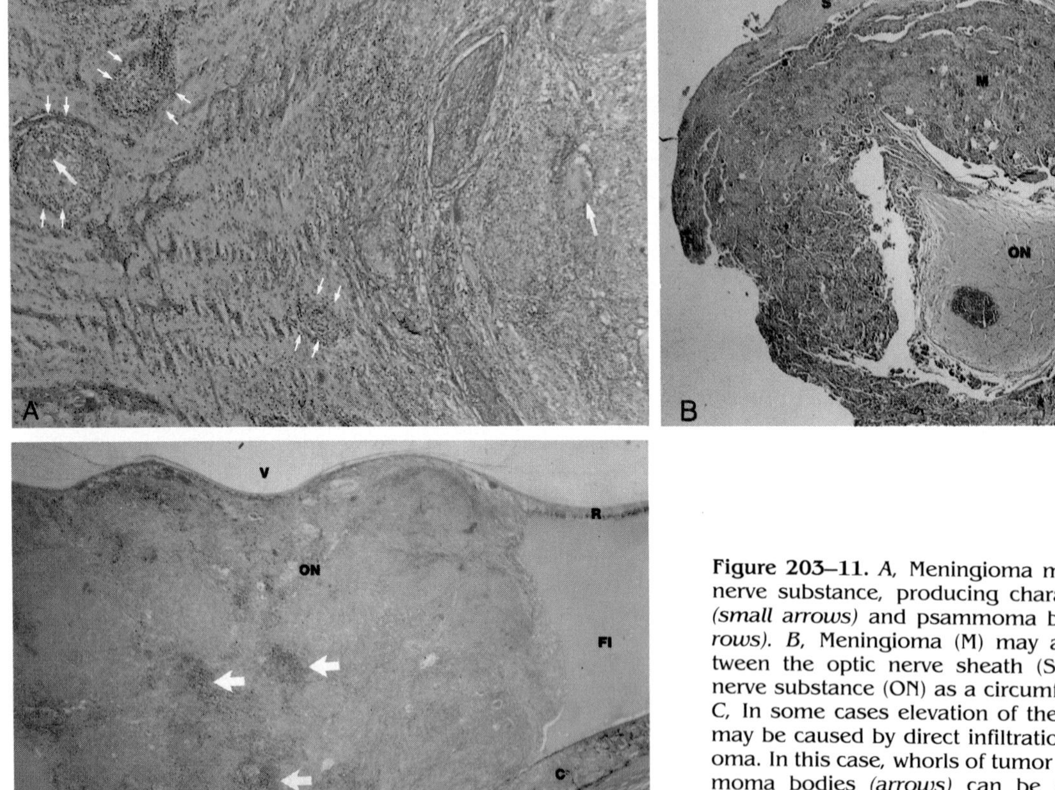

Figure 203–11. *A,* Meningioma may invade optic nerve substance, producing characteristic whorls *(small arrows)* and psammoma bodies *(large arrows). B,* Meningioma (M) may also expand between the optic nerve sheath (S) and the optic nerve substance (ON) as a circumferential growth. C, In some cases elevation of the optic disc (ON) may be caused by direct infiltration with meningioma. In this case, whorls of tumor cells with psammoma bodies *(arrows)* can be seen producing marked expansion of the optic nervehead into the vitreous cavity (V). There is juxtapapillary detachment of the sensory retina (R) and accumulation of subretinal fluid (F1). Even the juxtapapillary choroid (C) is slightly infiltrated by meningioma.

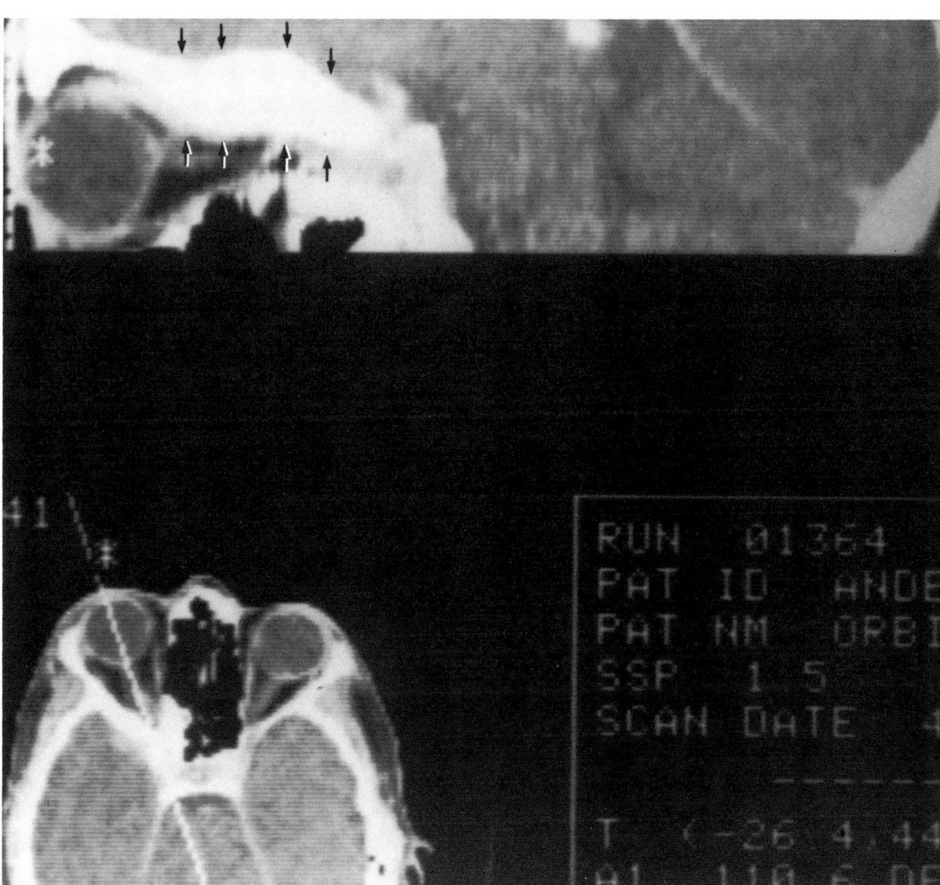

Figure 203–12. Enhanced CT scan in the sagittal plane demonstrates marked thickening of orbital roof *(arrows)*, causing compressive optic neuropathy within the orbital apex and optic canal. Primary intraosseous meningioma was diagnosed histopathologically at the time of transcranial resection. Postoperative vision was markedly improved.

have emphasized that the optic nerve may appear normal early in the course of the disease. The classic triad of optociliary veins (Fig. 203–14), disc pallor, and visual loss were described by Frisén and associates.[55] Most visual field defects caused by optic nerve tumors that spare the chiasm are centrocecal scotomas, followed by generalized constriction or overall depression.[52] Chiasmal involvement is associated with asymmetric, bitemporal hemianopia.[56] Other manifestations may include lid edema, chemosis, conjunctival injection, motility disorders, and choroidal folds, depending on the size and location of the tumor. A specific sign for subfrontal tumor is anosmia, which, in conjunction with ipsilateral visual loss and contralateral papilledema, is known as the Foster Kennedy syndrome (Fig. 203–15).

Radiology

Optic nerve sheath meningiomas are most easily visualized by CT or MRI scan as a fusiform enlargement of the optic nerve (Fig. 203–16). The optic canal may be enlarged. On CT scan there may be circumferential calcification or enhancement that looks like "railroad tracks" on axial CT section and a "double ring" on coronal sections.[57, 58] These characteristics may be less visible on MRI. The "impossible meningioma,"[59] confined to the optic canal, could not be detected prior to the availability of high-resolution imaging (Fig. 203–17). Occasionally, dilatation of adjacent air sinuses occurs—pneumosinus dilatans (Fig. 203–18). Hyperostosis may also occur adjacent to the tumor.[60, 61]

Natural History

Left alone, unilateral optic nerve meningiomas slowly but inexorably progress to produce blindness of the involved eye. Intraorbital and intracanalicular meningiomas extend intracranially only rarely. In contrast, tumors that begin intracranially often extend to involve the chiasm and other structures adjacent to the optic nerve.

Treatment

Treatment of intraorbital meningiomas of the optic nerve has proved to be controversial. Although the successful removal of exophytic meningiomas of the optic nerve has been described,[62] Kennerdell and colleagues[63] reviewed seven patients who underwent surgery and who had poor postoperative results, with blindness, central retinal artery occlusion, and recurrence. They concluded that "visual improvement (is) not worth the risk" of surgery. On the other hand, these same authors were more enthusiastic about the use of radiation therapy and reported six patients who had documented progressive visual loss and who received 5500 rads in divided doses. All patients improved with

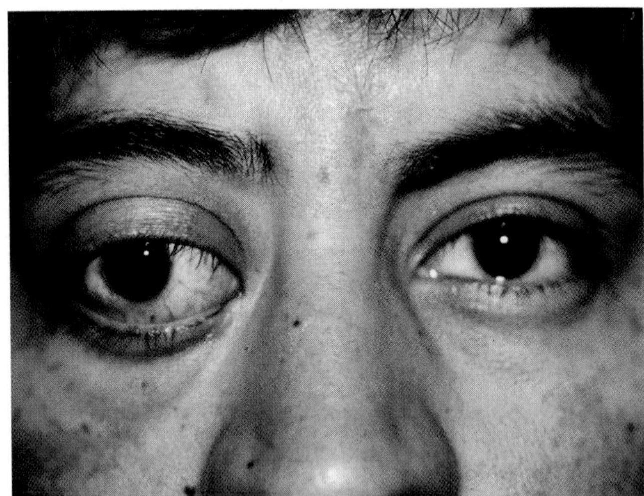

Figure 203–13. A patient with optic nerve meningioma and proptosis of the right eye.

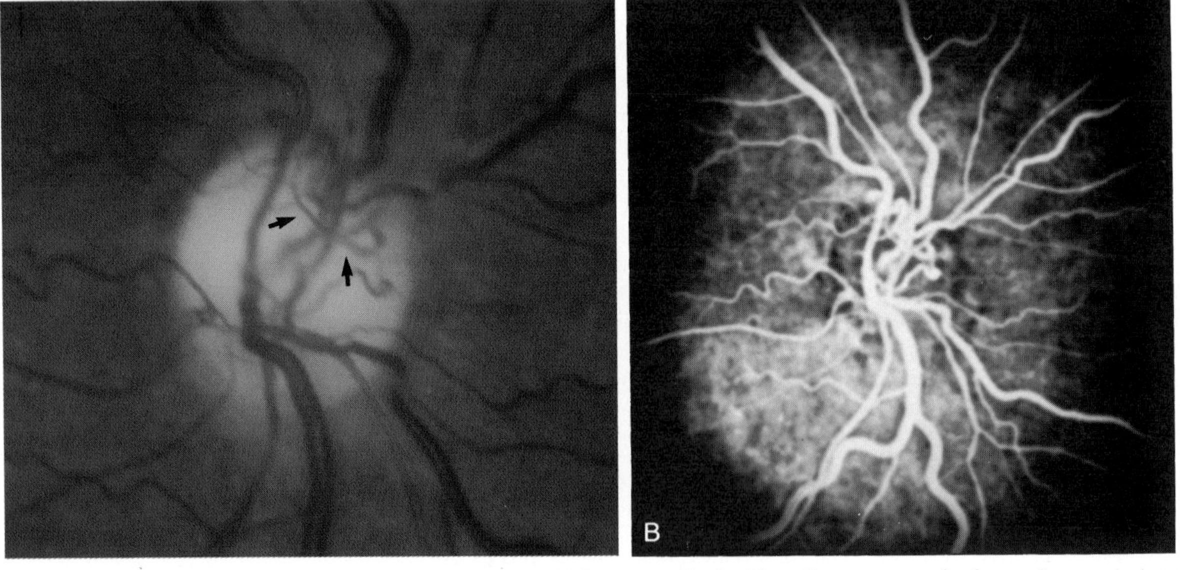

Figure 203–14. Disc photograph *(A)* and fluorescein angiogram *(B)* from a patient with optic nerve meningioma demonstrates pallor, blurred disc margins, and multiple optociliary shunt vessels *(arrows)*.

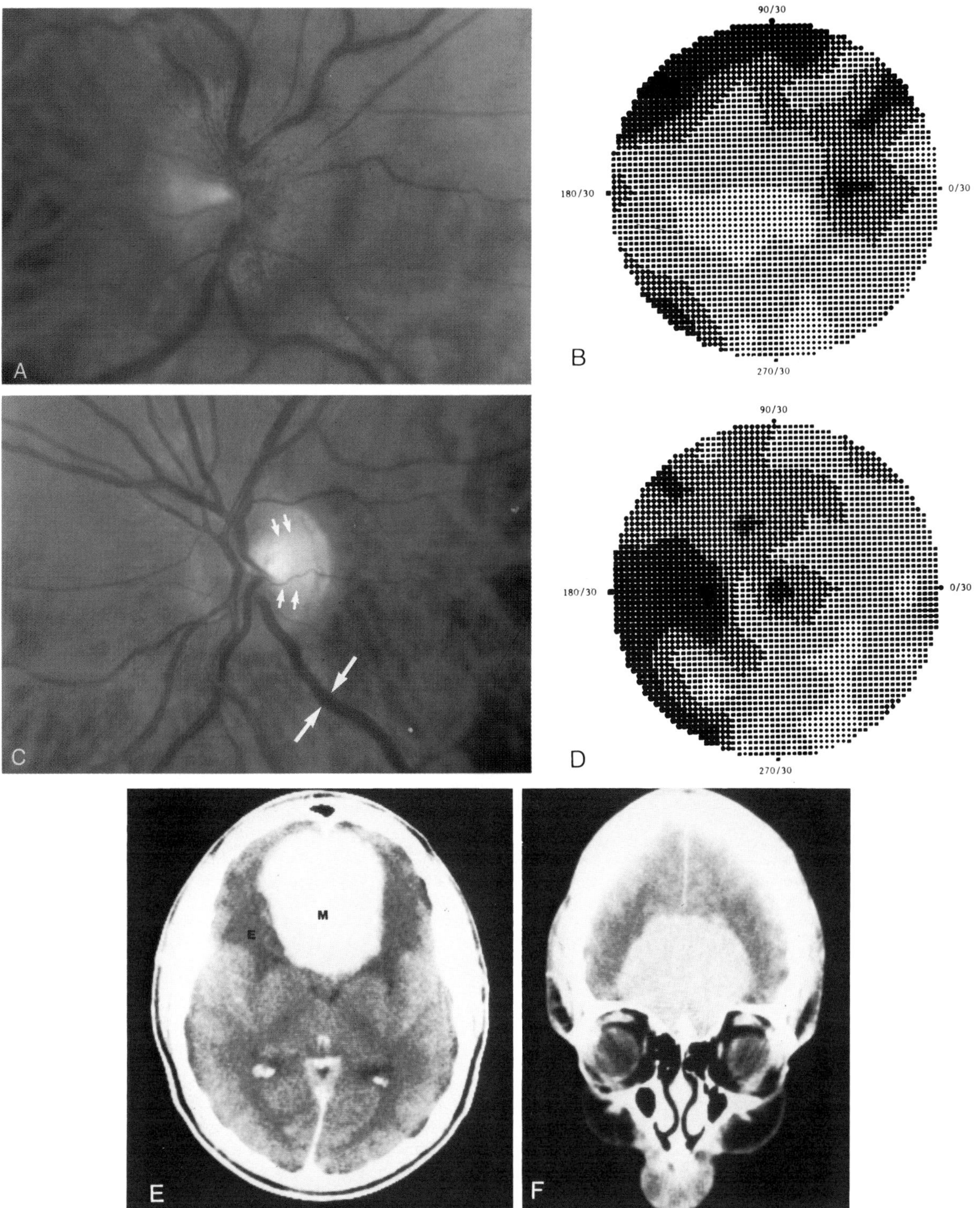

Figure 203–15. A middle-aged man with a 5-year history of anosmia and mild alteration of personality complained of decreased vision in the left eye. On ophthalmoscopy of the right eye *(A)*, the optic disc was edematous and there was dilatation of the retinal veins. Automated perimetry of the right eye *(B)* documented an enlarged blind spot and a possible early superior arcuate field defect. On ophthalmoscopy of the left eye *(C)*, the optic disc was mildly blurred nasally and showed marked temporal pallor *(small arrows)*. Dilated veins are apparent *(large arrows)* even in the absence of obvious disc edema. Automated perimetry of the left eye *(D)* documented an enlarged blind spot, a central scotoma, and superior field depression. A large subfrontal mass (M) with surrounding edema (E) was noted on an enhanced axial CT scan *(E)*. Coronal CT scan *(F)* shows the involvement extending to the olfactory groove. Sections obtained more posteriorly (not shown) suggested involvement of the prechiasmal portion of the optic nerves, especially on the left side. Histologic appearance of the tumor was typical of meningioma. Anosmia, unilateral optic nerve swelling, and contralateral optic atrophy caused by subfrontal masses are components of the Foster Kennedy syndrome. (From Jarus GD, Feldon SE: Clinical and computed tomographic findings in the Foster Kennedy syndrome. Am J Ophthalmol 93:317–322, 1982. Published with permission from The American Journal of Ophthalmology. Copyright by The Ophthalmic Publishing Company.)

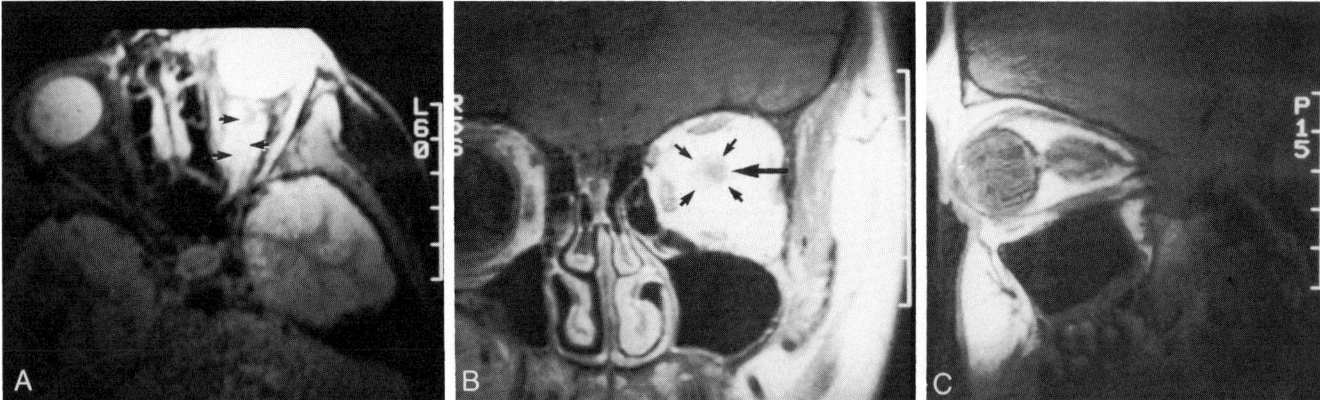

Figure 203–16. MRI scan from an 11-year-old girl with biopsy-proven unilateral optic nerve meningioma. Axial scan *(A)* using inversion recovery technique demonstrates the nerve *(arrows)* traversing through the tumor. T_1-weighted coronal scan *(B)* shows the tumor *(small arrows)* to be of different intensity from the optic nerve substance *(large arrow)*. T_1-weighted sagittal scan *(C)* documents typical fusiform thickening of the optic nerve.

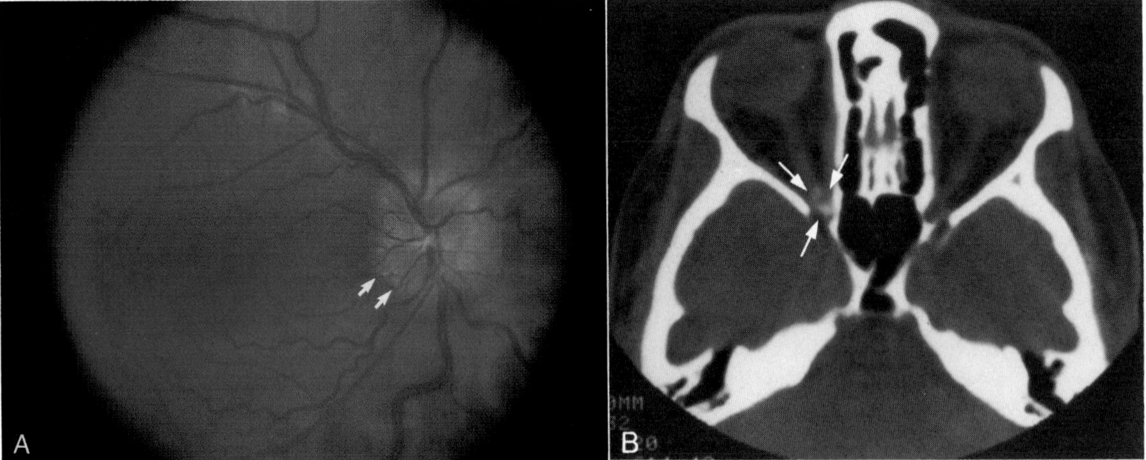

Figure 203–17. *A*, Chronic swelling of the right optic disc with presence of cytoid bodies *(arrows)* was associated with a 4-year history of progressive visual loss in a 41-year-old woman. Multiple work-ups failed to reveal evidence of a compressive lesion. A so-called "impossible" meningioma was suspected. Subsequently, high-resolution CT scan *(B)* demonstrated small calcific densities *(arrows)* consistent with a diagnosis of meningioma adjacent to the optic nerve at the level of the orbit apex and anterior optic canal.

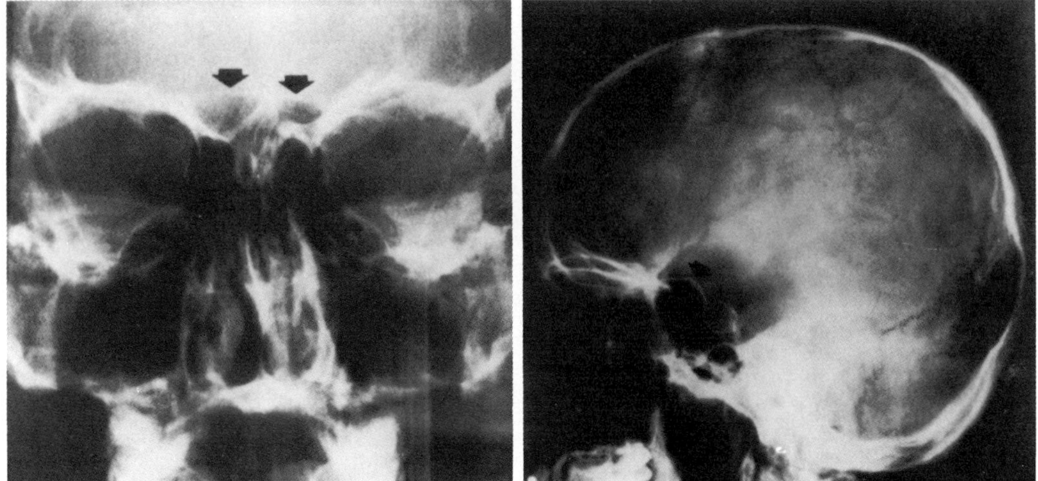

Figure 203–18. Plain skull films demonstrate pneumosinus dilatans in a case of bilateral optic nerve sheath meningiomas in anteroposterior *(left)* and lateral *(right)* views. Diffuse pneumatization of the sphenoid bone is present. The tuberculum sellae is distorted and displaced *(arrows)*. (From Hirst LW, Miller NR, Allan GS: Sphenoidal pneumosinus dilatans with bilateral optic nerve meningiomas: Case report. J Neurosurg 51:402–407, 1979.)

therapy, the improvement being retained for the 30 to 84 mo of follow-up.

Although invasion of the optic nerve parenchyma or sheath may occur with the optic nerve meningioma that has an intracranial component, localized compression is more frequently encountered. Therefore, it is not surprising that surgery may play a more important role in the management of this disease. In a series by Andrews and Wilson,[64] 15 of 38 (42 percent) patients had improved visual acuity, 11 (30 percent) were unchanged, and 10 (28 percent) worsened after surgery. Tuberculum meningiomas had the best prognosis for vision. In another report, Rosenstein and Symon[65] reported improvement of vision in 63 of 101 (62 percent) patients.

Radiation therapy has been considered as having little role in the treatment of intracranial meningiomas affecting the optic nerve.[66] However, Kupersmith and associates[67] reported a series of 20 patients, in which 12 (60 percent) improved and 4 (20 percent) stabilized.

Estrogen and progesterone receptors have been discovered on meningioma tumor cells. This finding has stimulated interest in hormonal treatment of patients with meningioma. In an in vitro study by Olson and colleagues,[68] meningioma cells were inhibited by RU486, β-estradiol, and progesterone. However, the latter two drugs also caused stimulation of tumor growth in some cultures. Tamoxifen stimulated growth of meningioma cells in vitro. The antiprogesterone mifepristone (RU486) produced 10 percent tumor shrinkage in 5 of 14 patients with unresectable meningiomas; ocular motility improved in two patients; automated visual fields improved in one patient during follow-up of only 3 to 31 mo.[69] The tumors in three patients progressed under treatment.

MISCELLANEOUS PRIMARY TUMORS OF THE OPTIC NERVE

Rarely, fusiform enlargement of the optic nerve occurs in association with unilateral, progressive visual loss which, on histologic examination, is neither glioma nor meningioma. Zimmerman and associates[70] described two cases of choristoma of the optic nerve extending into the chiasm in which coarse bundles of well-differentiated smooth muscle and mature adipose tissue were found. Primary arachnoid cysts may also occur within the optic nerve sheath and can cause optic disc edema or atrophy.[71, 72] Optociliary shunt vessels may be present on the disc.

SECONDARY INFILTRATIONS OF THE OPTIC NERVE

Inflammatory infiltration of the optic nerve is beyond the scope of this chapter. However, several neoplastic processes are worthy of mention. Leukemias, including acute myelogenous, monocytic, acute lymphatic, and chronic lymphatic types have been shown to infiltrate the optic nerve.[73] Lymphoreticular disease and multiple myeloma may also affect the optic nerve and chiasm.[74] Finally, carcinoma may infiltrate the optic nerve, producing symptoms either as an initial manifestation[75, 76] or as part of a more generalized meningeal involvement.[77]

REFERENCES

1. Lewis RA, Gerson LP, Axelson KA, et al: von Recklinghausen neurofibromatosis. II: Incidence of optic gliomata. Ophthalmology 91:929, 1984.
2. Crawford JS: The Eye in Childhood. Chicago, Year Book, 1967.
3. Porterfield JF: Orbital tumors in children: A report on 214 cases. Int Ophthalmol Clin 2:319, 1962.
4. Davis FA: Primary tumors of the optic nerve (a phenomenon of Recklinghausen's disease): A clinical and pathologic study with a report of five cases and a review of the literature. Arch Ophthalmol 23:735, 957, 1940.
5. Marshall D: Glioma of the optic nerve as a manifestation of von Recklinghausen's disease. Am J Ophthalmol 37:15, 1954.
6. Lloyd LA: Gliomas of the optic nerve and chiasm in childhood. Trans Am Ophthalmol Soc 71:488, 1973.
7. Miller NR, Iliff WJ, Green WR: Evaluation and management of gliomas of the anterior visual pathways. Brain 97:743, 1974.
8. Stern J, DiGiacinto GV, Housepian EM: Neurofibromatosis and optic glioma: Clinical and morphological correlations. Neurosurgery 4:524, 1979.
9. Stern J, Jakobiec FA, Housepian EM: The architecture of optic nerve gliomas with and without neurofibromatosis. Arch Ophthalmol 98:505, 1980.
10. Klug GL: Gliomas of the optic nerve and chiasm in children. Neuro-ophthalmology 2:217, 1982.
11. Rush JA, Younge BR, Campbell RJ, et al: Optic glioma: Long-term follow-up of 85 histopathologically verified cases. Ophthalmology 89:1213, 1982.
12. Yanoff M, Davis RL, Zimmerman LE. Juvenile pilocytic astrocytoma ("glioma") of optic nerve: Clinicopathologic study of sixty-three cases. *In* Jakobiec FA (ed): Ocular and Adnexal Tumors. Birmingham, AL, Aesculapius, 1978.
13. Wong IG, Lubow M: Management of optic glioma of childhood: A review of 42 cases. *In* Smith FJ (ed): Neuro-Ophthalmology: Symposium of the University of Miami and the Bascom Palmer Eye Institute, vol 6. St. Louis, CV Mosby, 1972.
14. Chutorian AM, Schwartz JF, Evans RA, et al: Optic gliomas in children. Neurology 14:83, 1964.
15. Alvord EC Jr, Lofton S: Gliomas of the optic nerve or chiasm: Outcome by patients' age, tumor site, and treatment. J Neurosurg 68:85, 1988.
16. Lindenberg R, Walsh FB, Sacks JG: Neuropathology of Vision: An Atlas. Philadelphia, Lea & Febiger, 1973.
17. Borit A, Richardson EP Jr: The biological and clinical behaviour of pilocytic astrocytomas of the optic pathways. Brain 105:161, 1982.
18. Anderson DR, Spencer WH: Ultrastructural and histochemical observations of optic nerve gliomas. Arch Ophthalmol 83:324, 1970.
19. Trobe JD, Glaser JS: Quantitative perimetry in compressive optic neuropathy and optic neuritis. Arch Ophthalmol 96:1210, 1978.
20. Buchanan TAS, Hoyt WF: Optic nerve glioma and neovascular glaucoma: Report of a case. Br J Ophthalmol 66:96, 1982.
21. Hovland KR, Ellis PP: Hemorrhagic glaucoma with optic nerve glioma. Arch Ophthalmol 75:806, 1966.
22. Holt JF: Neurofibromatosis in children. Am J Roentgenol 130:615, 1978.
23. McDonnell P, Miller NR: Chiasmatic and hypothalamic extension of optic nerve glioma. Arch Ophthalmol 101:1412, 1983.
24. Frohman LP, Epstein F, Kupersmith MJ: Atypical visual prognosis with an optic nerve glioma. J Clin Neuro Ophthalmol 5:90, 1985.
25. Miller NR: Tumors of neuroectodermal origin. *In* Walsh and Hoyt's Clinical Neuro-Ophthalmology, vol 3. Baltimore, Williams & Wilkins, 1988.
26. Hoyt WF, Baghdassarian SB: Optic glioma of childhood: Natural

history and rationale for conservative management. Br J Ophthalmol 53:793, 1969.
27. Taveras JM, Mount LA, Wood EH: The value of radiation therapy in the management of glioma of the optic nerves and chiasm. Radiology 66:518, 1956.
28. Throuvalas N, Bataini P, Ennuyer A: Les fiomes du chiasma et du nerf optique: L'apport de la radiothérapie transcutanée dans leur traitement. Bull Cancer 56:231, 1969.
29. Housepian EM: Surgical treatment of unilateral optic nerve gliomas. J Neurosurg 31:604, 1969.
30. Housepian EM: Transcranial orbital surgery. *In* Laws ER Jr (ed): The Diagnosis and Management of Orbital Tumors. Mount Kisco, NY, Futura, 1988.
31. Redfern RM, Scholtz CL: Long-term survival with optic nerve glioma. Surg Neurol 14:371, 1980.
32. Gaini SM, Tomei G, Arienta C, et al: Optic nerve and chiasm gliomas in children. J Neurosurg Sci 26:33, 1982.
33. Dosoretz DE, Blitzer PH, Wang CC, et al: Management of glioma of the optic nerve and/or chiasm: An analysis of 20 cases. Cancer 45:1467, 1980.
34. Iraci G, Peserico L, Galligioni F, et al: Anterior optic gliomas: Pros and cons of surgical and conservative treatment. Neuro-ophthalmology 3:179, 1983.
35. Imes RK, Hoyt WF: Childhood chiasmal gliomas: Update on the fate of patients in the 1969 San Francisco study. Br J Ophthalmol 70:179, 1986.
36. Fletcher WA, Imes RK, Hoyt, WF: Chiasmal gliomas: Appearance and long-term changes demonstrated by computerized tomography. J Neurosurg 65:154, 1986.
37. Heiskanen O, Raitta C, Torsti R: The management and prognosis of gliomas of the optic pathways in children. Acta Neurochirurg 43:193, 1978.
38. Lowes M, Bojsen-Møller M, Vorre P, et al: An evaluation of gliomas of the anterior visual pathways: A 10-year survey. Acta Neurochirurg 43:201, 1978.
39. Oxenhandler DC, Sayers MP: The dilemma of childhood optic gliomas. J Neurosurg 48:34, 1978.
40. DeSousa AL, Kalsbeck JE, Mealey J Jr, et al: Optic chiasmatic glioma in children. Am J Ophthalmol 87:376, 1979.
41. Guiffrè R, Bardelli AM, Taverniti L, et al: Anterior optic pathways gliomas: The dilemma of treatment. J Neurosurg Sci 26:61, 1982.
42. McFadzean RM, Brewin TB, Doyle D, et al: Glioma of the optic chiasm and its management. Trans Ophthalmol Soc UK 103:199, 1983.
43. Glaser JS, Hoyt WF, Corbett J: Visual morbidity with chiasmal glioma: Long-term studies of visual fields in untreated and irradiated cases. Arch Ophthalmol 85:3, 1971.
44. Bynke H, Kågström E, Tjernström K: Aspects of the treatment of gliomas of the anterior visual pathway. Acta Ophthalmol 55:269, 1977.
45. Packer RJ, Savino PJ, Bilaniuk LT, et al: Chiasmatic gliomas of childhood: A reappraisal of natural history and effectiveness of cranial irradiation. Childs Brain 10:393, 1983.
46. Spoor TC, Kennerdell JS, Martinez AJ, et al: Malignant gliomas of the optic nerve pathways. Am J Ophthalmol 89:284, 1980.
47. Rudd A, Rees JE, Kennedy P, et al: Malignant optic nerve gliomas in adults. J Clin Neuro Ophthalmol 5:238, 1985.
48. Barbaro NM, Rosenblum ML, Maitland, CG, et al: Malignant optic glioma presenting radiologically as a "cystic" suprasellar mass: Case report and review of the literature. Neurosurgery 11:787, 1982.
49. Hoyt WF, Meshel LG, Lessell S, et al: Malignant optic glioma of adulthood. Brain 96:121, 1973.
50. Manor RS, Israeli J, Sandbank U: Malignant optic glioma in a 70-year-old patient. Arch Ophthalmol 94:1142, 1976.
51. Hamilton AM, Garner A, Tripathi RC, et al: Malignant optic nerve glioma: Report of a case with electron microscope study. Br J Ophthalmol 57:253, 1973.
52. Wilson WB: Meningiomas of the anterior visual system. Surv Ophthalmol 26:109, 1981.
53. Rubinstein LJ: Tumors of the central nervous system. Second series, sixth fascicle. Washington, DC, Armed Forces Institute of Pathology, 1972.
54. Knight CL, Hoyt WF, Wilson CB: Syndrome of incipient prechiasmal optic nerve compression: Progress toward early diagnosis and surgical management. Arch Ophthalmol 87:1, 1972.
55. Frisén L, Hoyt WF, Tengroth BM: Optociliary veins, disc pallor and visual loss: A triad of signs indicating spheno-orbital meningioma. Acta Ophthalmol 51:241, 1973.
56. Grant FC, Hedges TR Jr: Ocular findings in meningiomas of the tuberculum sellae. Arch Ophthalmol 56:163, 1956.
57. Cohn EM: Optic nerve sheath meningioma: Neuroradiologic findings. J Clin Neuro-ophthalmol 3:85, 1983.
58. Jakobiec FA, Depot MJ, Kennerdell JS, et al: Combined clinical and computed tomographic diagnosis of orbital glioma and meningioma. Ophthalmology 91:137, 1984.
59. Susac JO, Smith JL, Walsh FB: The impossible meningioma. Arch Neurol 34:36, 1977.
60. Hirst LW, Miller NR, Allen GS: Sphenoidal pneumosinus dilatans with bilateral optic nerve meningiomas: Case report. J Neurosurg 51:402, 1979.
61. Wiggli U, Oberson R: Pneumosinus dilatans and hyperostosis: Early signs of meningiomas of the anterior chiasmatic angle. Neuroradiology 8:217, 1975.
62. Mark LE, Kennerdell JS, Maroon JC, et al: Microsurgical removal of a primary intraorbital meningioma. Am J Ophthalmol 86:704, 1978.
63. Kennerdell JS, Maroon JC, Malton M, et al: The management of optic nerve sheath meningiomas. Am J Ophthalmol 106:450, 1988.
64. Andrews BT, Wilson CB: Suprasellar meningiomas: The effect of tumor location on postoperative visual outcome. J Neurosurg 69:523, 1988.
65. Rosenstein J, Symon L: Surgical management of suprasellar meningioma. 2: Prognosis for visual function following craniotomy. J Neurosurg 61:642, 1984.
66. Wara WM, Sheline GE, Newman H, et al: Radiation therapy of meningiomas. Am J Roentgenol Rad Ther Nucl Med 123:453, 1975.
67. Kupersmith MJ, Warren FA, Newall J, et al: Irradiation of meningiomas of the intracranial anterior visual pathway. Ann Neurol 21:131, 1987.
68. Olson JJ, Beck DW, Schlechte J, et al: Hormonal manipulation of meningiomas in vitro. J Neurosurg 65:99, 1986.
69. Grunberg SM, Weiss MH, Spitz IM, et al: Treatment of unresectable meningiomas with the antiprogesterone agent mifepristone. J Neurosurg 74:861, 1991.
70. Zimmerman LE, Arkfeld DL, Schenken JB, et al: A rare choristoma of the optic nerve and chiasm. Arch Ophthalmol 101:766, 1983.
71. Harris GJ, Sacks JG, Weinberg PE, et al: Cyst of the intraorbital optic nerve sheaths. Am J Ophthalmol 81:656, 1976.
72. Miller NR, Green WR: Arachnoid cysts involving a portion of the intraorbital optic nerve. Arch Ophthalmol 93:1117, 1975.
73. Allen RA, Straatsma BR: Ocular involvement in leukemia and allied disorders. Arch Ophthalmol 66:490, 1961.
74. Kansu T, Orr LS, Savino PJ, et al: Optic neuropathy as initial manifestation of lymphoreticular diseases: A report of five cases. *In* Smith JL (ed): Neuro-ophthalmology Focus 1980. New York, Masson, 1979.
75. Susac JO, Smith JL, Powell JO: Carcinomatous optic neuropathy. Am J Ophthalmol 76:672, 1973.
76. Terry TL, Dunphy EB: Metastatic carcinoma in both optic nerves simulating retrobulbar neuritis. Arch Ophthalmol 10:611, 1933.
77. Katz JL, Valsamis MP, Jampel RS: Ocular signs in diffuse carcinomatosus meningitis. Am J Ophthalmol 52:681, 1961.

Chapter 204

Hereditary Optic Neuropathies

BARRETT KATZ

The hereditary optic neuropathies are a heterogeneous group of processes whose primary clinical signature is optic nerve dysfunction (Table 204–1). They share hereditary pronouncements, although specific causes remain unknown to us. The categorization of an optic neuropathy as hereditary does not preclude its being primarily metabolic, ischemic, or inflammatory in nature. Such processes may turn out to be primarily *retinal* or may rather be a unique declaration of an inborn error of metabolism that primarily affects the optic nerves. Our classification is one that is always changing and is only as current as our understanding of underlying pathophysiologic mechanisms (Table 204–2).

The *optic nerve* is a white matter *tract* of the central nervous system. It consists of myelinated nerve fibers, interstitial cells (including oligodendrocytes, astrocytes, and microglia), and fibrous vascular septae of pia matter. It has limited degrees of freedom in responding to injury or insult. The specific way in which the optic nerve responds to insult or biochemical dysfunction often constitutes enough of a recognizable gestalt to allow for the clinical differentiation of several entities linked by a common thread of heredity. It is in this context that we can speak of *hereditary optic neuropathies*.

An inherited optic neuropathy ought to be a bilateral process—one that is symmetric between eyes. It can be expected to culminate in a loss of central vision, dyschromatopsia, and changed anatomy of the optic nerve head that is recognizable clinically. Commonly, there are alterations of visual field and electrophysiologic function. Occasionally, there are associated neurologic findings. Our usual classification of the inherited optic neuropathies takes into account the *genetics of transmission* (whether mendelian or mitochondrial), the *age of presentation of the clinical illness*, and the *association* (or lack thereof) *of neurologic or systemic signs*.

OPTIC NEUROPATHIES INHERITED BY MENDELIAN PRINCIPLES

Dominant Optic Atrophy

Clinicians have long recognized an autosomally dominant optic atrophy (DOA) whose transmission seems to follow classic mendelian rules. It has been classified into two distinct entities, depending on the age of presentation. One group is an infantile variant, which is often accompanied by nystagmus; the second variant is one that presents later, during childhood years.[1–3] One has to be impressed, however, by the considerable interfamilial and intrafamilial variability of presentation and clinical parameters; the question regarding whether there are two distinct variants, or one with a spectrum of presentations, is still debated.

This abiotrophy of neural tissue generally presents in the first decade of life, although clinically one sees the first recognition and diagnosis of DOA at all ages. Not infrequently, an adult is first recognized as having a

Table 204–1. HEREDITARY OPTIC NEUROPATHIES

	Dominant Optic Atrophy	Recessive Optic Atrophy			Mitochondrial Optic Neuropathy
Variant	Juvenile	Simple/congenital	Complicated/Behr's	Associated with diabetes, deafness	Leber's hereditary optic neuropathy
Principles of inheritance	Mendelian dominant	Mendelian recessive	Mendelian recessive	Mendelian recessive	Mitochondrial
Age at onset (yr)	4–10	3–4	1–10	5–14	Teens–20s; up to 60s
Visual disability	Mild/moderate	Severe	Moderate	Severe	Moderate/severe
Expected acuity	20/20–20/200	20/200–HM	20/200	20/200–FC	20/200–FC
Color vision	Specific blue-yellow dyschromatopsia	Severe loss	Moderate loss	Severe loss	Severe loss
Nystagmus	Not expected	Expected	In 50%	Not expected	Not expected
Optic nerve head findings	Eventual temporal pallor Eventual temporal excavation	Diffuse pallor Vascular attenuation	Moderate temporal pallor	Severe temporal pallor	Disc edema (acute) Surface microangiopathy Eventual diffuse pallor
Course	Minimally progressive	Probably stable	Probably stable	Progressive	Stable (with rare improvement)
Genetic markers	None	None	None	None	Yes

*Adapted from Glaser JS (ed): Neuro-ophthalmology. Philadelphia, JB Lippincott, 1992.

Table 204–2. DIFFERENTIAL DIAGNOSIS OF BILATERAL SYMMETRIC LOSS OF CENTRAL VISION ASSOCIATED WITH DYSCHROMATOPSIA AND CHANGED OPTIC NERVE HEAD TOPOGRAPHY

Hereditary Optic Neuropathy
Dominant
Recessive
Leber's hereditary optic neuropathy
Associated with neurodegenerative syndromes
Toxic Optic Neuropathy and Deficiency States
Tobacco/alcohol amblyopia
Radiation optic neuropathy
Pernicious anemia
Vitamin deficiency
Demyelinating Optic Neuropathy
Ischemic Process
Anterior ischemic optic neuropathy
Retinal stroke
Pressure-Related Optic Neuropathy
Glaucoma
Carcinomatous Associated Optic Neuropathy
Infiltrative Optic Neuropathy
Sarcoid
Lymphoma
Leukemia
Congenital Anomaly of the Optic Nerve Head
Optic nerve dysplasia/hypoplasia
Structural Lesions Compressing Each Anterior Pathway
Post-papilledematous optic atrophy
Intracranial space occupying lesions
Chiasmal compression
Orbital Process
Dysthyroid orbitopathy with optic nerve compression
Retinal Process
Macular dystrophy
Rod/cone dystrophy

DOA when examined after another family member was diagnosed. It has not been recognized congenitally nor in infancy. Kline and Glaser,[4] Hoyt,[5] and Smith[6] have summarized the expected clinical profile of DOA. Affected individuals commonly cannot date a specific onset of visual symptomatology, although most patients report an onset of symptoms before 10 yr of age. Presentation may be earlier and may then be expected to be accompanied by nystagmus. Very few cases are observed to have optic atrophy before 10 yr of age, however.[6] The onset is insidious, almost imperceptible, with mild visual dysfunction occurring without nyctalopia or dramatic progression. As a rule, one sees symmetric involvement between eyes; on occasion, one sees asymmetric acuities. Vision ranges from 20/30 through 20/200. Both Kjer and Smith report that perhaps 40 percent of patients will have vision of 20/60, or better.[3, 6]

DOA declares itself in a recognizable and usually predictable matrix of optic atrophy characterized by pallor of the temporal aspect of each optic nerve head and associated temporal (sectoral) excavation of the optic disc; rarely, pallor may be diffuse (Fig. 204–1). The optic atrophy may be subtle or dramatic. There is an expected loss of both the nerve fiber layer within the papillomacular bundle and the superficial capillarity of the temporal aspect of the disc.

Plotting of the visual fields in this entity commonly reveals central, centrocecal, or paracentral scotomas, which are often associated with midzonal temporal depression. The moderate depression of temporal isopters can on occasion superficially resemble a bitemporal hemianopic defect. Peripheral fields are expected to be normal in DOA, however.

There is an associated acquired blue-yellow dyschromatopsia which, when present, may be helpful in supporting this clinical diagnosis.[7] A reflection of this dyschromatopsia can be demonstrated at tangent screen as an inversion of colored isopters. The isopter plotted with a blue test object is more constricted than the isopter plotted with a red test object (in contradistinction to normals or other optic neuropathies, in which the field plotted with a blue test object is larger than that mapped with a red test object). This color inversion of field would be predicted in patients with tritanopic deficits.[8]

Although the dominant pedigree of DOA is characteristic, it is not uncommon for patients to be ignorant of the familial nature of their disease. The diagnosis is often made in an asymptomatic affected patient as a direct consequence of recognition of a more severely affected family member, attesting to significant intrafamilial variation of its clinical declarations and often subtle disturbances of visual function.

Visual electrophysiologic profiles in affected individuals can be characterized by both diminished amplitudes and prolonged latencies of visually evoked response

A 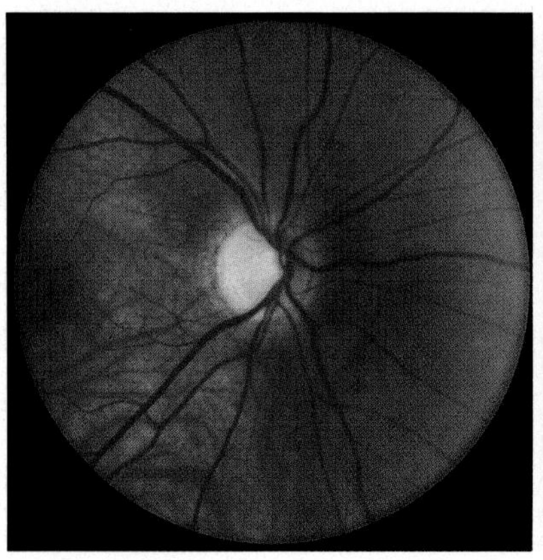

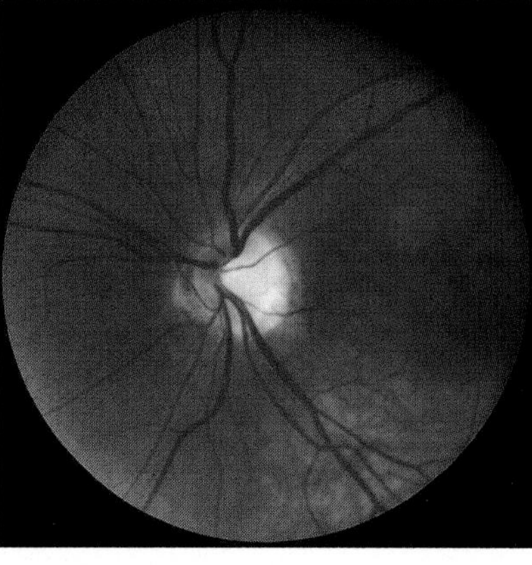 B

Figure 204–1. Typical appearance of optic nerve head in a dominant optic atrophy. Note pallor affecting temporal aspect of disc, with associated temporal excavation. *A*, O.D. *B*, O.S.

(VER). Whether the extent of VER anomaly corresponds to depressed acuity has yet to be determined. Patients with DOA are expected to be neurologically normal (although 10 percent of Kjer's early cases were said to show "mental abnormalities"). Concomitant hearing loss, mutism, and deuteronomalous color deficits have been recognized.[9] Whether such cases of "dominant optic atrophy plus" are separate nosologic entities or the extreme declaration of a single genetic disorder is not known.

Pathologic reflections of DOA include diffuse atrophy of the retinal ganglion cell layer, atrophy and loss of myelin within the optic nerves, thinning of the papillomacular bundle itself, and loss of temporal disc substance, which are all seen in the setting of normal inner and outer nuclear layers.[10, 11]

Clinical experience dictates that juvenile onset dominant optic atrophy is the most common of the heredofamilial optic abiotrophies. Most patients can be expected to partake of a "sighted education," with only mild progression of visual impairment, and lead productive and relatively normal lives. Some data suggest that the disease is not static, however. Kjer noted that none of his patients younger than 15 yr of age had acuities as severe as 20/200, whereas 20 percent of his patients 45 yr and older lost vision to these levels.[3] Spontaneous recovery has not been recognized. The diagnosis remains a clinical one, however, and necessitates examination of other family members for confirmation. When the clinical course shows dramatic progression, further neurologic investigation is imperative. The underlying pathophysiologic mechanisms and specific genetic markers remain to be discovered.

RECESSIVE OPTIC ATROPHY

Simple (Congenital) Optic Atrophy

A simple form of optic atrophy described as occurring with autosomal recessive transmission occurs, albeit rarely. As is true for most recessive disorders, signs and symptoms are more severe than those occurring in dominantly transmitted optic neuropathies. Visual disability is significant enough to allow it to be discovered before the child is 4 yr of age. There may be consanguinity between parents. A searching pendular "sensory" nystagmus can be present. Visual fields would be expected to be severely disturbed and optic discs more completely atrophic (possibly more deeply excavated) than in dominant optic atrophy. Peripapillary attenuation of the retinal arteriolar tree may suggest a tapetoretinal degeneration, although electroretinography would be expected to be normal. The disability is severe, stable, and predictably unassociated with other systemic or neurologic declarations.[12, 13]

Complicated (Infantile) Hereditary Optic Atrophy

Another variant of a recessively inherited optic atrophy has been described by Behr.[14] In this syndrome, optic atrophy can be recognized in early childhood in association with ataxia, mental retardation, pyramidal tract dysfunction, increased tonicity, urinary incontinence, and pes cavus. Though initially recognized only in males, subsequent reports seem to indicate no sexual predilection. The ensuing optic atrophy is severe, as is the associated visual disability. Nystagmus is expected to be present (reported in more than half of such patients). Optic nerve pallor may be predominantly temporal, and associated findings of dyschromatopsia are anticipated. Whether this nosologic entity ought truly to be separate and distinct remains controversial. The neurologic community often considers it to be a part of the continuum encompassing optic atrophy seen as a manifestation of the hereditary ataxias.[15, 16]

Autosomal Recessive Optic Atrophy Associated With Juvenile Diabetes

The association of juvenile onset diabetes mellitus and progressive visual loss with optic atrophy has been recognized since the late 1930s.[17] The clinical spectrum includes the development of neurosensory hearing loss, neurogenic bladder, and diabetes insipidus. Glucose intolerance usually presents before visual dysfunction. Visual acuity may remain normal early on, despite mild dyschromatopsia and recognized optic atrophy. As the optic neuropathy progresses, visual loss can become severe. Acuity can be dramatically affected, and patients can progress from mild through moderate to severe visual disability. Dyschromatopsia is an invariate feature, and visual fields are expected to show central scotomas with generalized constriction. Optic atrophy is often dramatic and may be associated with mild to moderate excavation of the disc itself. The optic neuropathy seems to be unrelated to the degree of underlying diabetic retinopathy, although this is controversial.

The association of neurosensory hearing loss and diabetes insipidus is variable. Both or either may begin in the first or second decade of life. Other anomalies have been recorded in these patients and include ptosis, ataxia, seizure diathesis, mental retardation, nystagmus, abnormal electroretinography, elevated cerebrospinal fluid protein, and short stature.[18] It is the slowly progressive nature of this inherited optic neuropathy and its association with underlying glucose intolerance that makes it distinctive. The specific metabolic defects precipitating such selective involvement of selected cranial nerves (and brain stem nuclei?) remain to be discovered.

OPTIC NEUROPATHIES NOT INHERITED BY MENDELIAN PRINCIPLES

Leber's Optic Neuropathy

Mitochondria are unique among cellular structures in that they contain their own genetic material; this is, generally, two to ten copies of a double-stranded circular

DNA molecule that differs from the DNA of the cell nucleus itself in several respects. It is transmitted exclusively by mothers; it contains very few noncoding sequences, and it has a slightly different genetic code. Mitochondrial DNA is thought to encode for a small group of specific proteins (all of which are components of the mitochondrial respiratory chain and oxidative phosphorylation system) in addition to two ribosomal RNAs and more than 20 transfer RNAs.[19] Defects within this small segment of the human genome are associated with specific disease entities of disparate clinical declarations: mitochondrial myopathies and encephalopathies (including infantile lactic acidosis), some cases of progressive external ophthalmoplegia, and some cases of both exercise-induced myopathy and Leigh's syndrome. The most recent addition to this list of alterations of mitochondrial DNA with clinical import is Leber's optic neuropathy.

In 1871 Leber described a disease of young males characterized by abrupt loss of central vision occurring in the second and third decades of life. Its genetics seemed to implicate an absence of transmission through men, with passage occurring through only the female line.[20] A clinical dictum had been that if a mother has clinical disease, one half of her sons and one third of her daughters would be affected. If the carrier mother is not recognized to have clinical disease, 50 percent of her sons and between 8 and 15 percent of her daughters will become clinically affected.[21]

Its age of onset is now recognized to vary widely. Although in the United States it occurs primarily in males (to a male: female ratio of 9 : 1) in differing locales, its sexual prevalence changes; thus in Japan, the ratio between male and female involvement is approximately 6 : 4, male to female. In Europe, the male incidence has been reported to be five times more frequent than involvement in women.

The initial symptom is usually blurred vision in one eye. This may be associated with subjective dyschromatopsia. Although one eye is affected first, the second eye can be expected to become involved within days or weeks. Intervals of involvement between eyes have extended to many years; nonetheless, it seems almost always to be a sequential bilateral optic neuropathy. All levels of visual loss have been recognized. Commonly, vision is lost to levels of 20/200; on occasion it is reduced to hand motions, light perception, or even no light perception. Accompanying visual field deficits are expected to be central or centrocecal in nature. While these scotomas are relative during the early stages of the disease, as visual loss progresses, scotomas become absolute.

Disc hyperemia and swelling are frequently mentioned in clinical descriptions of the entity. Rather specific signatures of altered anatomy comprise the classical ophthalmoscopic findings of acute Leber's optic neuropathy (Fig. 204–2*A*). There is a *circumpapillary telangiectatic microangiopathy*, a swelling of the nerve fiber layer around the disc (a pseudo-edema, yet without leakage from the disc or peripapillary region when studied by fluorescein angiography).[22] Prominent vascular tortuosity and fine arteriovenous shuntlike vessels can be demonstrated on fluorescein angiography (see Fig. 204–2*B*). Retinal striations may extend from the disc margin; there may be associated macular edema; and retinal hemorrhages can occur. This microangiopathy occurs not only in the presymptomatic phase of involved eyes but also in a high proportion of asymptomatic offspring of the female line. Increased shunting and disc hyperemia presage the acute phase of visual loss; the telangectatic microangiopathy can be thought of as an inherited marker of the disease, implying some risk of future optic nerve insult.

During the acute phase of visual loss, patients are otherwise well. Rarely, headaches and vertigo may be reported; some observers have interpreted these as signs

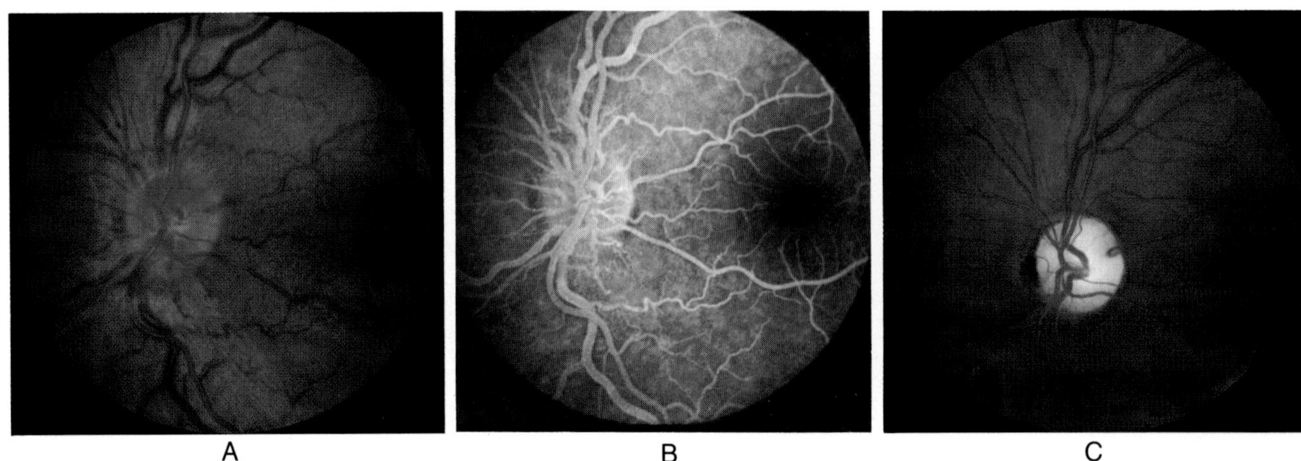

Figure 204–2. *A*, Typical appearance of optic nerve head during acute phase of Leber's optic neuropathy. Disc is edematous and hyperemic, with circumpapillary telangiectatic microangiopathy characterized by prominent vascular tortuosity of vessels on and just off the surface of the disc. *B*. Fluorescein angiogram in the same patient during acute phase, demonstrating fine arteriovenous shuntlike vessels within peripapillary retina and absence of leakage from the disc itself in spite of presence of disc edema. *C*, Late, atrophic phase of same nerve head, demonstrating loss of many of the previously visible telangiectatic vessels and diffuse pallor with nerve fiber layer loss. (Courtesy of Eeva Nikoskelainen, M.D.)

of meningeal inflammation and arachnoid involvement. After several weeks, the telangectatic vessels disappear, and the pseudo-edema of the disc resolves, with ensuing optic atrophy and loss of nerve fiber layer (see Fig. 204–2*C*). Whereas nerve fiber loss is most prominent in the papillomacular bundle, the entire nerve fiber layer commonly disappears, leaving the disc diffusely pale. There is a spectrum of presentations; some patients show relative preservation of the superior and inferior arcuate bundles, though some element of loss of extra macular nerve fiber layers is expected to occur in all cases.

Abnormalities of color perception have been documented, and changed visual evoked responses have been recorded after loss of central acuity. The Farnsworth-Munsell 100 Hue test may be abnormal before central acuity falls.[23] Relative stability of visual function after the acute episode is anticipated; a gradual decline or surprising improvement after many years of stationary vision has occasionally been observed.[24, 25] When this happens, visual acuity may recover in one eye only.[26] If such visual recovery occurs, further recurrence of visual failure is not expected.[27]

Observations of spontaneous recovery have made the assessment of possible treatment modalities problematic. Reports of improvement following hydroxycobalamine therapy have appeared.[28] Craniotomy with lysis of presumed optochiasmatic arachnoidal adhesions has been employed, although not commonly attempted outside of Japan.[29]

Visual loss is, most commonly, the only manifestation of Leber's disease. Disparate neurologic signs have been recognized—most commonly pyramidal, cerebellar, or peripheral in declaration. These include spastic paraparesis, hyperactive deep tendon reflexes, muscular wasting, changes in primary sensory modalities, ataxia, and pyramidal tract dysfunction.[30–32] As is true for many of the heredofamilial neurologic syndromes, associated defects in cardiac conduction are also recognized.[33] Neuroradiologic investigation and cerebrospinal fluid studies are expected to be normal in these patients during presymptomatic and acute stages.[34] Following the acute phase, imaging of the optic nerve with magnetic resonance imaging (MRI) or computed tomography (CT) may show increased optic nerve signal either unilaterally, or bilaterally, without associated white matter changes that are so common in patients with disseminated sclerosis.[35]

The analysis of mitochondrial DNA from patients with Leber's hereditary optic neuropathy and their relatives has shown a single mutation at one select base pair.[36] This mutation presumably leads to an amino acid alteration (arginine to histadine), altering the gene that encodes for a subunit of nicotinamide-adenine dinucleotide (NADH) dehydrogenase. This relatively conservative alteration (both amino acids are basic) culminates in some degradation of the enzyme complexes involved in complex I of the electron transport chain, resulting in dysfunction within the mitochondrial energy-producing pathways of oxidative phosphorylation. Although a specific abnormal protein has not yet been identified, reduced activity of an enzyme of this system (NADH-coenzyme Q oxidoreductase) has been demonstrated within platelets of four men with a Leber's-like hereditary optic neuropathy.[37]

It is difficult to explain how a widespread mitochondrial DNA defect interfering with respiratory chain function leads to the eventual development of subacute loss of vision in young adults. Such metabolic pathways are concerned with the generation of adenosine triphosphate (ATP); decreased catalytic activities of complex I, therefore, may result in insufficient energy availability for basic cellular metabolic requirements. Cellular pumps may be adequate for normal physiologic function for some finite time, yet they may not be able to withstand additional stress or further metabolic demands. The optic nerve may therefore function normally for many years, with ensuing visual loss as some additional factor or factors concur.

Some have suggested that not all families with clinical Leber's disease have this specific mutation; indeed, the disease has been recognized to occur in the absence of such a mutation.[38] Genetic analysis of some cases of Leber's disease (the minority) have demonstrated mixtures of both mutant and normal (wild) mitochondrial DNA molecules, speaking for a spectrum of genetic heteroplasmy. Such heteroplasmy has clinical relevance, because the normal (wild) DNA population of a patient's cells might reduce the impact of the mutant genotype.[39] The proportion of mutant mitochondrial DNA molecules has been shown to differ markedly across affected generations and even within tissues of an affected individual. This suggests that the *genotypic* analysis of the mitochondrial DNA from a single tissue (e.g., blood) would not necessarily indicate the *mitochondrial* DNA genotype of the optic nerve's environment, and therefore peripheral blood determinations (with their mitochondrial DNA signature) may not be a reliable predictor of the optic neuropathy. The presence of excessive amounts of wild-type mitochondrial DNA would be expected to reduce the extent of the respiratory complex deficiency; individuals whose optic nerve cells carried an abundance of the mutant mitochondrial DNA (with minimal heteroplasmy) might be expected to suffer the most severe insult to optic nerve metabolism. This mutation appears to be, then, neither a necessary nor sufficient criterion for the clinical disease. Presumably, additional factors are involved in the expression of the mutant phenotype. Indeed, environmental factors that might tend to reduce respiratory capacity or depression of the cellular respiratory metabolism might also be necessary for phenotypic expression. Additional modulating factors, such as anoxia from smoking and cyanide exposure, might explain the historic association of this entity with chronic cyanide intoxication[28] and still be consistent with most recent molecular genetic findings.[39, 40]

While a DNA marker has now been recognized for Leber's disease, we must know much more about the genetics of the mitochondrial DNA and its segregation before we can use molecular genotypes to make strict clinical correlations with the clinical disease as we know it.[39] Furthermore, we must await a final explanation of how this genetic defect of respiratory enzyme function causes such specific pathognomic change (the characteristic ophthalmoscopic findings) at a characteristic location (i.e., the intraocular segment of optic nerve) after some latency period measured in decades.

MISCELLANEOUS OPTIC NEUROPATHIES ASSOCIATED WITH SYSTEMIC AND NEUROLOGIC DISEASE

Simple and complex optic neuropathies, with varying patterns of inheritance and differing clinical symptomatology, have been described in many inherited systemic and metabolic syndromes. A large body of anecdotal and descriptive associations has evolved. Indeed, optic nerve dysfunction has become a part of the nosologic categorization in many neurodegenerative syndromes. There has been much confusion surrounding such optic nerve changes; suffice it to say that a continuum exists of genetic transmissibility and anatomic change culminating in the *final common pathway expression of optic atrophy* running through the spinocerebellar degenerations, inherited ataxias, heritable motor and sensory neuropathies, inherited deafness, and inborn errors of metabolism. The most important of the classic neurologic syndromes of which optic atrophy is a part are Charcot-Marie-Tooth disease, Friedreich's ataxia, and the association of juvenile diabetes with both hearing loss and progressive optic atrophy.[41–43]

The clinical experience with any one of these associations is not vast; nonetheless, some generalizations are possible. When optic atrophy is part of a larger systemic or neurologic syndrome, the optic atrophy usually is recognized concurrently with the more systemic signs of the disease, follows a progression that parallels the more generalized symptomatology of the larger process, and progresses to but moderate levels of visual disability. There appear to be no *specific* optic nerve head signs recognized in this heterologous group of entities. The nerve heads do appear atrophic; nerve fiber layer is lost; and other clinical signs of optic nerve dysfunction are apparent (e.g., loss of central vision, loss of color vision, and depressed field). Declarations are usually bilateral and symmetric.

REFERENCES

1. Jaeger W: Hereditary optic atrophies in childhood. J Genet Hum 15:312, 1966.
2. Lodberg CV, Lund A: Hereditary optic atrophy with dominant transmission: Three Danish families. Acta Ophthalmol 28:437, 1950.
3. Kjer P: Infantile optic atrophy with dominant mode of inheritance: A clinical and genetic study of nineteen Danish families. Acta Ophthalmol (Kbh) Suppl 54, 1959.
4. Kline LB, Glaser JS: Dominant optic atrophy: The clinical profile. Arch Ophthalmol 97:1680, 1979.
5. Hoyt CS: Autosomal dominant optic atrophy: A spectrum of disability. Ophthalmology 87:245, 1980.
6. Smith DP:Diagnostic criteria in dominantly inherited juvenile optic atrophy: A report of three new families. Am J Optom 49:183, 1972.
7. Krill AE, Smith VC, Pokorny J: Similarities between congenital tritan defects and dominant optic-nerve atrophy: Coincidence or identity? J Opt Soc Am 60:1132, 1970.
8. Miller NR: Discussion of paper by Hoyt. Ophthalmology 87:250, 1980.
9. Grehn F, Kommerell G, Ropers H-H, et al: Dominant optic atrophy with sensory neural hearing loss. Ophthalmic Pediatr Genet 1:77, 1972.
10. Johnston PB, Gaster RN, Smith VC, et al: A clinicopathologic study of autosomal dominant optic atrophy. Am J Ophthalmol 88:868, 1979.
11. Kjer P, Jensen OA, Klinken L: Histopathology of the eye: Optic nerve and brain in a case of dominant optic atrophy. Acta Ophthalmol 61:300, 1983.
12. Waardenburg PJ: Different types of hereditary optic atrophy. Acta Genet Statist Med 7:287, 1957.
13. Francois J: Mode d'héredité des heredo-dégénérescences du nerf optique. J Genet Hum 15:147, 1966.
14. Behr C: Die Komplizierte, Hereditar-familare optikusatrophie des kindesalters: Ein bisher nicht beschriebener symptomkomplex. Klin Monatsbl Augenheilkb 47:138, 1909.
15. Horoupian DS, Zucker DK, Moshe S, et al: Behr syndrome: A clinicopathologic report. Neurology 29:323, 1979.
16. Francois J: Hereditary degeneration of the optic nerve (hereditary optic atrophy). Int Ophthalmol Clin 8:99. 1968.
17. Wolfram DJ: Diabetes mellitus and simple optic atrophy among siblings. Mayo Clin Proc 13:715, 1938.
18. Lessell S, Rossman NP: Juvenile diabetes mellitus and optic atrophy. Arch Neurol 34:759, 1977.
19. Attardi G: The ellucidation of the human mitochondrial genome: A historical perspective. Bio Essays 5:34, 1987.
20. Leber T: Ueber hereditare und congenital angelegte schenervenleiden. Graefes Arch Clin Ophthalmol 17:249, 1871.
21. Seedorff T: Leber's disease. Acta Ophthalmol 48:187, 1970.
22. Smith JL, Hoyt WF, Susac JO: Ocular fundus in acute Leber's optic neuropathy. Arch Ophthalmol 90:349, 1973.
23. Nikoskelainen E, Sogg RL, Rosenthal AR, et al: The early phase in Leber's hereditary optic atrophy. Arch Ophthalmol 95:969, 1977.
24. Nikoskelainen E, Hoyt WF, Nummelin K: Ophthalmoscopic findings in Leber's hereditary optic neuropathy. II: The fundus findings in affected family members. Arch Ophthalmol 101:1059, 1983.
25. Lessell S, Gise RL, Krohel GB: Bilateral optic neuropathy with remission in young men: Variation on a theme by Leber? Arch Neurol 40:2, 1983.
26. Taylor J, Holmes GM: Two families, with several members in each suffering from optic atrophy. Trans Ophthalmol Soc UK 33:95, 1913.
27. Wallace DC: Leber's optic atrophy: A possible example of vertical transmission of a slow virus in man. Aust Ann Med 3:259, 1970.
28. Foulds WS, Cant JS, Chisholm IA, et al: Hydroxycobalamine in the treatment of Leber's hereditary optic atrophy. Lancet 1:896, 1968.
29. Imachi J, Nishizaki K: The patients of Leber's optic atrophy should be treated brain-surgically. Folia Ophthalmol Jpn 21:209, 1970.
30. Ford FR: Diseases of the nervous system in infancy, childhood and adolescence, 5th ed. Springfield, IL, Charles C Thomas, 1966, pp 291–293.
31. Lees F, MacDonald A-ME, Aldren Turner JW: Leber's disease with symptoms resembling disseminated sclerosis. J Neurol Neurosurg Psychiatry 27:415, 1964.
32. Bereday M, Cobb S: Relation of hereditary optic atrophy (Leber) to other familial diseases of the central nervous system. Arch Ophthalmol 48:669, 1952.
33. Rose FC, Bowden AN, Bowden PMA: The heart in Leber's optic atrophy. Br J Ophthalmol 54:388, 1970.
34. Nikoskelainen E: The clinical findings of Leber's hereditary optic neuropathy. Trans Ophthalmol Soc UK 104:845, 1985.
35. Kermode AG, Mosley IF, Kendall BE, et al: Magnetic resonance imaging in Leber's optic neuropathy. J Neurol Neurosurg Psychiatry 52:671, 1989.
36. Wallace DC, Singh G, Lott MT, et al: Mitochondrial DNA mutation associated with Leber's hereditary optic neuropathy. Science 242:1427, 1988.

37. Parker WC, Oley CA, Parks JK: A defect in mitochondrial electron-transport activity (NADH-coenzyme Q oxidoreductase) in Leber's hereditary optic neuropathy. N Engl J Med 320:1331, 1989.
38. Coppinger JN, Stone EM, Slavin ML, et al: Leber hereditary optic neuropathy in a sixth generation pedigree with a wild-type ND-4 gene. Invest Ophthalmol Vis Sci 31 (Suppl 4):1452, 1990.
39. Lott NT, Voljavec AS, Wallace DC: Variable genotype of Leber's hereditary optic neuropathy patients. Am J Ophthalmol 109:625, 1990.
40. Newman NJ, Wallace DC: Mitochondria and Leber's hereditary optic neuropathy. Am J Ophthalmol 109:726, 1990.
41. Hoyt WF: Charcot-Marie-Tooth disease with primary optic atrophy. Arch Ophthalmol 64:925, 1960.
42. Livingstone IR, Mastaglia FL, Edis R, Howe JW: Visual involvement in Friedreich's ataxia and hereditary spastic ataxia: A clinical and visual evoked response study. Arch Neurol 38:75, 1981.
43. Rosenberg RN, Chutorin A: Familial optico-acoustic nerve degeneration and polyneuropathy. Neurology 17:827, 1967.

Chapter 205

Toxic and Deficiency Optic Neuropathies

SIMMONS LESSELL

Neurogenic visual loss on a toxic or nutritional basis is by no means common but assumes significance out of all proportion to incidence for various reasons. In times and places of famine, these disorders may take on epidemic proportions. Even in societies that are generally spared the ravages of hunger, certain groups and individuals still suffer from undernutrition. Toxic visual disorders are a potential threat in the workplace and are a use-limiting side effect of some drugs. Toxic optic neuropathies are sometimes the focus of malpractice and product-liability litigation. Both toxic and nutritional optic neuropathies must also be considered by clinicians in the differential diagnosis of central or centrocecal scotomata, retrobulbar optic neuropathies, optic atrophy, and bilateral amblyopias.

Patients with toxic or nutritional visual disorders and normal fundi or optic atrophy are generally assumed to have primarily an optic neuropathy. However, the typical signs in these patients—visual impairment, dyschromatopsia, central visual field defect, and normal fundus or optic atrophy—are also compatible with lesions that primarily affect the inner retinal layers, the chiasm, or the optic tracts. Therefore, some of the disorders discussed in this section and assumed to be neuropathies might in the future be found to originate in the retina, chiasm, or tracts.

DEFICIENCY OPTIC NEUROPATHY

Symptoms and Signs.[1] A patient gradually becomes aware of a blur or cloud in the center of the visual field. Although only one eye may initially be involved, the symptom soon becomes binocular, and visual acuity gradually declines in both eyes. Deficiency optic neuropathy tends to be a symmetric disease. Strictly unilateral visual failure or a marked acuity difference between the two eyes is not a feature of this disorder. Some patients report that colors look faded. Pain is absent unless the deficiency state has also produced corneal lesions. There are no photisms, visual hallucinations, or metamorphopsia.

Visual acuity can be reduced to almost any level but rarely if ever extends to hand motions or total blindness. Dyschromatopsia is a constant feature. Central or centrocecal scotomata are the characteristic visual field defects of deficiency optic neuropathies. Careful perimetry can sometimes identify a dense "nucleus" within the centrocecal scotoma just temporal to fixation. Because of the symmetric nature of the visual loss, a relative afferent pupillary defect is not seen. In the early stages, the fundi look normal, but optic atrophy supervenes after a time (many weeks or months).

Laboratory Findings. Imaging studies yield normal results. Appropriate blood tests may show stigmata of generalized undernutrition or identify pertinent specific abnormalities, such as low vitamin B_{12} levels. The visual evoked response shows increased latency or low amplitude.

Differential Diagnosis. A distinction must first be made among retinal, neural, and psychogenic causes of bilateral visual loss. Retinopathies are more likely to cause metamorphopsia or photisms and may be associated with delayed glare recovery. Dyschromatopsia is less pronounced in retinopathies than it is in neuropathies and may be absent if the acuity is only slightly or moderately affected. Fluorescein angiography and electroretinography sometimes establish the basis of retinogenic visual impairment.

Psychogenic (hysterical or malingered) amblyopia is easily confused with deficiency optic neuropathies. In both disorders, objective clinical findings may be absent. Central and centrocecal visual field defects, however, are distinctly rare in psychogenic amblyopia. As discussed elsewhere (see Chapter 213), patients with psychogenic visual loss may have inconsistent results when acuities are tested at various distances. This does not occur in optic neuropathies. Nevertheless, the distinction between psychogenic and neurogenic visual loss can be exceedingly difficult to make, especially in the early stages of a symmetric disorder. Visual evoked responses offer an objective method of validating the organic basis of subnormal vision and may be required when there is an urgent need to establish the diagnosis. Of course, the issue is settled once optic atrophy develops.

Once having established the neural basis of visual loss, one must distinguish among the various bilateral retrobulbar optic neuropathies. Dominantly inherited (Kjer's) and mitochondrially inherited (Leber's) hereditary optic neuropathies cause progressive bilateral visual loss, occasionally with centrocecal scotomata. Without a family history, it might be impossible to recognize Kjer's disease in a malnourished individual, and one would have to treat the patient as if he or she had a nutritional disorder. A positive family history is also helpful in diagnosing Leber's hereditary optic neuropathy, but this information is not always available. A peripapillary telangiectatic microangiopathy and rarely pain are features of Leber's disease that help to make the correct diagnosis. Leber's disease, although ultimately bilateral, may cause profound visual loss in one eye months before the other eye is involved. This aspect is not found in deficiency optic neuropathies. The mitochondrial DNA deletion of patients with Leber's hereditary optic neuropathy can be detected in blood samples.

Bilateral inflammatory or demyelinative optic neuropathies cause more acute loss of vision and are usually accompanied by pain or tenderness. However, it may be difficult to distinguish bilateral optic neuritis from deficiency optic neuropathies. Clinical or magnetic resonance imaging signs of multiple sclerosis, present in more than half of the cases, would reveal the nature of the process. Syphilitic optic neuritis must always be considered in the differential diagnosis of retrobulbar optic neuropathies, and appropriate serologic tests should be performed if no firm alternative cause is identified.

Infiltration or compression of the anterior visual pathways by neoplasms or granulomas can cause slow symmetric visual loss and can occasionally even produce bilateral central or centrocecal scotomata.[2–4] Neuroimaging is the best method of ruling out such lesions and is indicated in all patients in whom the diagnosis of deficiency amblyopia is entertained.

The toxic optic neuropathies can present the most difficult problem in differential diagnosis, because they share most symptoms and signs. A history of exposure to a toxin that is known to affect the anterior visual pathways is usually the clue that leads to the diagnosis (discussed later).

Course and Prognosis. Untreated deficiency optic neuropathies can lead to profound bilateral visual loss but not to total blindness. Correction of the nutritional deficiency or appropriate vitamin therapy usually reverses the deficit if instituted within the first few months.

SPECIFIC DEFICIENCY DISORDERS

Alcohol-Tobacco Amblyopia

Sporadic cases of nutritional amblyopia are encountered, mainly among abusers of alcohol and tobacco, and there is continuing debate about the roles of toxins and dietary deficiency in the pathogenesis of the disorder in these individuals.[5] Perhaps it represents more than one disease. In any case, the opinion that visual loss could result from the combined or synergistic effects of tobacco and alcohol is in virtually complete disrepute. As discussed later, tobacco probably has an independent role in rare cases. Except in a few cases of acute intoxication, ethyl alcohol has not been shown to be toxic to the anterior visual pathway of humans or other primates. Instead, most experts agree that undernutrition is the central cause of amblyopia in habitual alcohol and tobacco abusers.

Clues to a nutritional cause can be elicited from the history. One needs to determine how much and what the patient eats. Verification of information by a friend or family member is helpful, because undernourished patients are likely to exaggerate their food intake and to underestimate their consumption of alcohol. The social history is pertinent. It may be necessary to calculate how much money patients have left to spend on food after they have met their fixed obligations and purchased alcohol and cigarettes. When reviewing a patient's general health, inquire about sensory symptoms in the limbs and about gait disturbances that might reflect a nutritional peripheral neuropathy.

Patients with nutritional amblyopia may appear thin and emaciated and have spindly limbs, and the stigmata of alcoholism are obvious even to a layman. Vision is impaired almost to the same degree in each eye, with dyschromatopsia and central or centrocecal scotomata. The optic discs are normal in the early stages; however, several clinicians have observed evanescent abnormalities in the peripapillary retina during the acute phase.[6, 7] They described hemorrhages and dilated, tortuous vessels in the nerve fiber layer. If left untreated, optic atrophy develops.

Imaging studies have not shown abnormalities in this disease, but these studies should be performed so that infiltrative or compressive lesions of the anterior visual pathway might be ruled out. The visual evoked response test has shown predominantly a reduction in amplitude and has not shown prolongation of latency.[8] A serologic test for syphilis, serum vitamin B_{12}, folate level, and transketolase level should be performed.[9] Referral to a neurologist is also indicated to look for neurologic manifestations of nutritional deficiency. The neurologist can decide if tests of peripheral nerve conduction or an examination of the cerebrospinal fluid is warranted.

Although there is little doubt that the bilateral amblyopia that occurs in alcoholic persons and malnourished individuals is a result of a dietary deficiency, the specific deficiency has yet to be identified. Recovery is associated with the institution of a nutritious diet that is usually supplemented with B vitamins. There are excellent medical and social reasons for convincing patients to stop or reduce drinking and smoking, but as generations of well-intentioned physicians have discovered, this is not easily accomplished. Fortunately, vision recovers anyway unless treatment has been inordinately delayed.

Vitamin B_{12} Deficiency

Although the hematologic and neurologic consequences of vitamin B_{12} deficiency are more familiar than the ophthalmic deficiency, an optic neuropathy can be an important and sometimes presenting feature. Dietary vitamin B_{12} deficiency may occur, especially in strict vegans. It is more commonly encountered with gastrointestinal disorders and after gastric or ileal resection. In some areas, fish tapeworm infestation leads to vitamin B_{12} deficiency. However, pernicious anemia is the context in which the disorder is most often encountered.

Pernicious anemia is an autoimmune disorder in which gastric atrophy indirectly results in malabsorption of vitamin B_{12} because of a lack of the intrinsic factor. It is mainly encountered in middle-aged or elderly Caucasians but occurs in all races. Megaloblastic anemia and its metabolic complications are the most prominent manifestations; however, most untreated patients also develop neurologic complications. These complications include numbness and tingling that spread proximally in the extremities from a peripheral neuropathy, as well as leg weakness, positive results on a Romberg's test, and extensor plantar responses from myelopathy (subacute combined degeneration of the spinal cord).

Bilateral demyelinative lesions have been produced in the anterior visual pathway of primates that were made experimentally deficient in vitamin B_{12}.[10–12] Similar lesions were found at autopsy in patients with subacute combined degeneration.[13] Abnormal visual evoked responses have been recorded in some visually asymptomatic patients with pernicious anemia.[14]

Several dozen reports have described cases of a retrobulbar optic neuropathy in patients with vitamin B_{12} deficiency.[15–19] Visual loss can be the initial symptom, before the development of anemia. The findings are typical of the deficiency optic neuropathies (discussed earlier). Serum vitamin B_{12} levels, which can be measured directly, are low in this disorder. Patients with abnormally low levels should be referred for evaluation by a hematologist. The capacity for visual recovery is considerable if therapy is instituted before marked optic atrophy supervenes. Hydroxocobalamin is the drug of choice.

Other Vitamin Deficiencies

Thiamine deficiency is sometimes blamed for the optic neuropathy that occurs in prisoners of war and in other extremely undernourished individuals. It has also been indicted in the few cases of amblyopia that have been associated with ketogenic and high-protein, low-carbohydrate diets.[20, 21]

A modest literature on experimental thiamine deficiency in animals has shown that (at least in rats) optic neuropathy may occur.[22] Thiamine deficiency is sometimes demonstrated (usually by documenting whole blood transketolase levels) in undernourished patients with presumed deficiency optic neuropathy,[9] and administration of the vitamin may reverse the visual loss.[23] However, when selective thiamine deficiency has been produced experimentally in human volunteers, visual symptoms and signs have not developed.[24, 25] The apparent therapeutic effect of thiamine in patients with deficiency amblyopia could actually result from the improvement in appetite rather than from correction of hypovitaminosis. In many cases, patients are treated with multiple vitamins, further clouding the issue of pathogenesis.

Although thiamine deficiency is central to the pathogenesis of such neurologic disorders as beriberi and Wernicke's encephalopathy, its role has not been established in deficiency optic neuropathies.

The role of other vitamin deficiencies is even less well established than that of thiamine. Deficiencies in folic acid, niacin, riboflavin, and pyridoxine all have been alleged to be factors, but the evidence is suggestive at best. Considering the prevalence of malnutrition, it is surprising that if hypovitaminosis causes deficiency optic neuropathy, so few cases have been reported.

TOXIC OPTIC NEUROPATHIES

General Considerations

Symptoms and Signs. The clinical findings in toxic optic neuropathies are similar to those found in deficiency optic neuropathies. Visual loss is typically painless, bilateral, and progressive, with central or centrocecal scotomata and late development of optic atrophy. However, in some intoxications, loss of vision is rapid; blindness may occur; and patients may recover incompletely, if at all. Disc edema, which is unknown in the deficiency optic neuropathies, is encountered in some intoxications.

The differential diagnosis is the same as it is for the deficiency optic neuropathies. In my experience, the disorders that are most often mistaken for a toxic optic neuropathy are idiopathic or demyelinative optic neuritis, Leber's hereditary optic neuropathy, factitious visual loss, and perichiasmatic tumors.

Laboratory tests are useful both for helping to establish the cause and for ruling out other diagnoses. An imaging study of the visual pathways is always justified and is almost always indicated. As mentioned earlier, infiltrative and compressive lesions of the anterior visual pathway can occasionally cause bilateral central or centrocecal scotomata, and bitemporal hemicentral scotomata are easily confused with these defects. If the history fails to identify exposure to a toxin in a patient with characteristic clinical findings of a toxic optic neuropathy, screening of the urine, blood, or even hair is indicated to establish exposure.

Table 205–1 lists the large number of substances blamed for toxic optic neuropathies. Some are undoubt-

Table 205–1. CAUSES OF TOXIC OPTIC NEUROPATHY

Amantidine	Iodopyracet (intravenous)
Amiodarone	Isoniazid
Amoproxan	Khat
Antipyrine	Lead
Arsenicals	Lysol (per cervix)
Aspidium	Methanol
Barbiturates	Methotrexate (intrathecal)
Caramiphen hydrochloride	Methyl acetate
Carbon disulfide	Methyl bromide
Carbon tetrachloride	Octamoxin
Carmustine (intracarotid)	Oil of chenopodium
Chloramphenicol	Oral contraceptives
Chlorodinitrobenzene	Penicillamine
Chlorpromazine	Pheniprazine
Chlorpropamide	Plasmocid
Cobalt chloride	Quinine
Deferoxamine	Sodium fluoride
Dinitrobenzene	Streptomycin
Dinitrotoluene	Sulfonamides
Disulfiram	Tamoxifen
Ergot	Thallium
Ethambutol	Thioglycolate
Ethchlorvynol	Tin
Ethyl alcohol	Tolbutamide
Favism	Toluene
5-Fluorouracil	Trichloroethylene
Halogenated hydroxyquinolines	Tricresyl phosphate
Hexachlorophene	Vincristine
Iodoform	Vinylbenzene

edly optic nerve toxins, whereas others are merely suspects. A few of these putative optic neurotoxins have been only rarely indicted in human optic neuropathies, despite considerable human exposure. That fact alone raises questions about their pathogenicity. The list is incomplete because one can expect that some drugs and other chemicals yet to be introduced will prove to be toxic, and some chemicals already in use are probably unrecognized neurotoxins.

There are pressing medical and legal reasons for establishing the toxic cause of an optic neuropathy. Stopping the toxic exposure is a keystone of therapy, and recognizing a toxin may prevent visual loss in others. In intoxications for which specific treatment is available, accurate diagnoses are essential.

The establishment of a toxic cause is also important in litigation concerning workers' compensation, product liability, and medical malpractice. Physicians should not invoke toxicity unless the evidence is compelling. First, there should be appropriate clinical findings. Eschew the diagnosis if pain is a manifestation or if the disorder is monocular or strikingly asymmetric. Second, a patient should have been unequivocally exposed to an optic neurotoxin. It is very helpful if one can identify similar illnesses in coworkers, or in others exposed to the same drug or chemical. Third, the visual symptoms should have first been noted during or very shortly after exposure. Fourth, other likely causes of an optic neuropathy should be ruled out by appropriate examinations and tests.

Methanol

Methanol is the most notorious optic nerve toxin. Methanol optic neuropathy is usually encountered sporadically in alcoholic individuals who have accidentally or intentionally consumed the toxin. Epidemics have occurred when methanol, which looks, smells, and tastes like ethanol, has been substituted for ethanol or added to it by bootleggers. Methanol can be toxic even in small quantities, and poisoning occurs with ingestion of less than half an ounce.

Experimental methanol intoxication has been studied extensively in monkeys.[26–28] These investigations documented the occurrence of disc edema and showed that the lesion is primarily a retrobulbar optic neuropathy. The investigators postulated that toxic metabolites of methanol penetrate the nerve and inhibit cytochrome oxidase. Postmortem investigations on human victims have shown a retrobulbar demyelinative optic neuropathy that Sharpe and associates ascribed to histotoxic anoxia in a vascular watershed.[29]

The clinical picture has been established from the plethora of reported cases.[30–34] Apart from nausea and nonspecific symptoms of inebriation, patients are well for 18 to 48 hr. Headache, dyspnea, vomiting, abdominal pain, and bilateral visual impairment then supervene. At this point, patients are in metabolic acidosis and may become comatose, suffer circulatory collapse, and die.

Visual loss is typically profound but may be reduced to any level. Pupillary dilatation accompanies near or total blindness. The discs are swollen and hyperemic, with edema extending into the peripapillary retina. Some patients may enjoy early or late improvement, but relapses are not unknown. Optic atrophy develops in 1 to 2 mo. Some cases are marked by cupping that is identical to that encountered in glaucoma.

Treatment includes correction of the acidosis, hemodialysis, and administration of ethanol to interfere with the metabolism of the methanol.

It is worth noting that methanol intoxication differs from most toxic and deficiency optic neuropathies in several respects. The visual loss is likely to be much more severe and acute than in other intoxications. Disc edema is an exceptional finding in this group of disorders. Methanol intoxication is also unusual in that systemic symptoms are prominent. Finally, the prognosis is generally worse in methanol optic neuropathy than it is in the other toxic optic neuropathies.

Ethambutol

Visual impairment was recognized as a serious side effect soon after ethambutol was introduced for the treatment of tuberculosis, and visual impairment remains a problem.[35] Ethambutol was originally distributed as the racemate, but after investigations showed that the toxicity was mainly from the levo isomer, only the dextro ethambutol has been used. This change and reduction of dosage probably account for reduced incidence and severity of toxic optic neuropathy. Nevertheless, the optic neuropathy occurs even in patients who are taking allegedly safe dosages.

Ethambutol's toxic effects on the anterior visual pathway have been well documented in rats and monkeys.[36, 37] It has been postulated that ethambutol neurotoxicity results indirectly from its chelating properties.

In patients taking 15 to 25 mg/kg/day for pulmonary tuberculosis, visual symptoms may appear in 4 mo to 1 yr. Onset may be earlier, and progression may be more rapid in the presence of renal disease. The picture is typical of the toxic and deficiency optic neuropathies, with slowly progressive, painless, symmetric loss of vision and central or centrocecal scotomata. Dyschromatopsia is a feature as it is in almost all optic neuropathies, but patients who are intoxicated with ethambutol may have special difficulty seeing the color green. Bitemporal visual field defects have been encountered, and it is notable that primary chiasmal lesions have been recognized in experimentally intoxicated animals.[38] The fundi remain normal until the late stage. The optic neuropathy of ethambutol is not accompanied by other ocular, neurologic, or systemic side effects.

Improvement follows cessation of ethambutol therapy. Rarely, vision continues to fail after the drug is discontinued or vision does not recover.

Halogenated Hydroxyquinolines

The halogenated hydroxyquinoline derivatives, which were commonly used as over-the-counter prophylactic agents for travelers' diarrhea in some parts of the world, were implicated in a large number of cases of myelopathy and optic neuropathy in Japan.[39, 40] The disorder, which came to be known as *subacute myelooptic neuropathy* (SMON), was reported in other countries as well. Ironically, halogenated hydroxyquinolines do not prevent travelers' diarrhea! Awareness of the cause and withdrawal of oral preparations of the drug from some markets have effected a dramatic reduction in incidence.

These agents are also used for the treatment of some chronic gastrointestinal diseases such as acrodermatitis enteropathica. Cases of toxic optic neuropathy have been reported in that setting, and there is evidence that in all situations the presence of colonic abnormalities predisposes patients to intoxication. In normal people, the neurotoxicity of these drugs is dose related. For example, in the case of iodochlorhydroxyquin, intoxication is infrequent at relatively low dose levels (750 to 1500 mg/day for up to 2 wk). The risk increases considerably after 2 wk, with more than one third of subjects manifesting neurologic abnormalities. Patients receiving higher doses show toxicity at an earlier stage.

Numerous autopsies have been conducted on patients with clioquinol intoxication. Degeneration of axons and myelin is found in the optic nerves, optic tracts, spinal cord, nerve roots, and peripheral nerves.[41] Drop-out of retinal ganglion cells has also been described.[42]

The following description is derived from the Japanese experience.[43] SMON from clioquinol afflicts all age groups but is most prevalent among older women. The early symptoms are abdominal, with pain and a sensation of fullness. The patient's urine, feces, and tongue may be green if iron has also been ingested. Numbness and sometimes pain develop in the legs, and most patients have an abnormal gait. Bladder disturbances also occur. An indistinct sensory level may be noted on the trunk. The legs can be weak, with hyperactive deep tendon reflexes and extensor plantar responses. Visual symptoms, which appear in 25 percent of cases, range from isolated dyschromatopsia to severe visual loss. As with methanol intoxication, total blindness can occur. In any case, the disturbance is bilateral and reasonably symmetric. After a time, optic atrophy develops.

It should be noted that there have been a few cases in which children treated with diiodohydroxyquin and dibrominated hydroxyquinoline have developed bilateral optic atrophy without other neurologic deficits.[44–47]

Cessation of the intoxicant is the only available therapy. Unfortunately, visual loss is not always reversible.

Tobacco

Although the very existence of the entity is controversial, heavy smoking can apparently cause visual loss. The disorder is apparently more prevalent in Great Britain than it is in the United States. Despite the increased use of tobacco, the incidence of the disease has declined. Some authorities believe that the rarity of the disease in relation to the prevalence of smokers implies a multifactorial etiology.[48] Low serum vitamin B_{12} levels have been suspected as one factor.[49, 50]

Tobacco amblyopia is overwhelmingly a disorder that occurs in men; women make up less than 1 percent of cases.[51] Most victims are undernourished elderly pipe smokers. Cigars, cigarettes, snuff, and chewing tobacco are less commonly implicated. Vision declines slowly, painlessly, and bilaterally, but perfect symmetry is not characteristic. Dyschromatopsia is invariable. Patients describe bilateral centrocecal scotomata, most marked for red or green targets, containing denser islands of reduced sensitivity. The fundi remain normal until a late stage.

Recovery occurs if patients stop smoking or are treated with injections of hydroxocobalamin. The recovery process is very slow, however, and may take many months. Color vision is regained later than acuity, and scotomata may be permanent.

REFERENCES

1. Lessell S: Toxic and deficiency optic neuropathies. *In* Smith JL, Glaser JS (eds): Neuro-Ophthalmology; Symposium of the University of Miami and the Bascom Palmer Eye Institute, vol 7. St. Louis, CV Mosby, 1973, pp 21–37.
2. Slavin ML: Acute, severe, symmetric visual loss with cecocentral scotomas due to olfactory groove meningioma. J Clin Neuro Ophthalmol 6:224, 1986.
3. Page NGR, Sanders MD: Bilateral central scotomata due to intracranial tumour. Br J Ophthalmol 68:449, 1984.
4. Gutman I, Behrens M, Odel J: Bilateral central and centrocaecal scotomata due to mass lesions. Br J Ophthalmol 68:336, 1984.
5. Brockhurst RJ, Boruchoff SA, Hutchinson BT, Lessell S (eds): Controversy in Ophthalmology. Philadelphia, WB Saunders, 1977, pp 841–874.
6. Frisén L: Fundus changes in acute malnutritional optic neuropathy. Arch Ophthalmol 101:577, 1983.
7. Carroll FD: Nutritional amblyopia. Arch Ophthalmol 76:406, 1966.
8. Kupersmith MJ, Weiss PA, Carr RE: The visual-evoked potential

in tobacco-alcohol and nutritional amblyopia. Am J Ophthalmol 95:307, 1983.
9. Dreyfus PM: Blood transketolase levels in tobacco-alcohol amblyopia. Arch Ophthalmol 74:617, 1965.
10. Agamanopolis DP, Victor M, Chester EM, et al: Neuropathology of experimental vitamin B_{12} deficiency in monkeys. Neurology 26:905, 1976.
11. Hind VMD: Degeneration in the peripheral visual pathway of vitamin B_{12}-deficient monkeys. Trans Ophthalmic Soc UK 90:839, 1970.
12. Chester EM, Agamanopolis DP, Harris JW, et al: Optic atrophy in experimental vitamin B_{12} deficiency in monkeys. Acta Neurol Scand 61:9, 1980.
13. Adams RD, Kubik CS: Subacute combined degeneration of the brain in pernicious anemia. N Engl J Med 231:1, 1944.
14. Troncoso J, Mancall EL, Schatz NJ: Visual evoked responses in pernicious anemia. Arch Neurol 36:168, 1979.
15. Hyland HH, Sharpe VJH: Optic nerve degeneration in pernicious anmenia. Can Med Assoc J 67:660, 1952.
16. Hamilton HE, Ellis PP, Sheets RF: Visual impairment due to optic neuropathy in pernicious anemia: Report of a case and review of the literature. Blood 14:378, 1959.
17. Lerman S, Feldmahn AL: Centrocecal scotomata as the presenting sign in pernicious anemia. Arch Ophthalmol 65:381, 1961.
18. Cohen H: Optic atrophy as the presenting sign in pernicious anemia. Lancet 2:1202, 1936.
19. Turner JAA: Optic atrophy associated with pernicious anemia. Brain 63:225, 1940.
20. Haag JR, Smith JL, Susac JO, et al: Optic atrophy following jejunoileal bypass. J Clin Neuro Ophthalmol 5:9, 1985.
21. Thompson RE, Felton JL: Nutritional amblyopia associated with jejunoileal bypass surgery. Ann Ophthalmol 14:848, 1982.
22. Rodger FC: Experimental thiamine deficiency as a cause of degeneration in the visual pathway of the rat. Br J Ophthalmol 37:11, 1953.
23. Carroll FD: Nutritional retrobulbar neuritis. Am J Ophthalmol 30:172, 1947.
24. Williams RD, Nason HL, Power MH, et al: Induced thiamine (vitamin B_1) deficiency in man. Arch Intern Med 71:38, 1943.
25. Williams RD, Nason HL, Wilder RM, et al: Observations on induced thiamine deficiency in man. Arch Intern Med 66:785, 1940.
26. Hayreh MS, Hayreh SS, Baumbach GL, et al: Methyl alcohol poisoning. III: Ocular toxicity. Arch Ophthalmol 95:1851, 1977.
27. Martin-Amat G, Tephly TR, McMartin KE, et al: Methyl alcohol poisoning. II: Development of a model for ocular toxicity in methyl alcohol poisoning using the rhesus monkey. Arch Ophthalmol 95:1847, 1977.
28. Baumbach GL, Cancilla PA, Martin-Amat G, et al: Methyl alcohol poisoning. IV: Alterations of the morphological findings of the retina and optic nerve. Arch Ophthalmol 95:1859, 1977.
29. Sharpe JA, Hostovsky M, Bilbao JM, et al: Methanol optic neuropathy: A histopathological study. Neurology 32:1093, 1982.
30. Benton CD, Calhoun FP: The ocular effects of methyl alcohol poisoning. Trans Am Acad Ophthalmol Otolaryngol 56:875, 1952.
31. Roe O: Clinical investigation of methyl alcohol poisoning with special reference to the pathogenesis and treatment of amblyopia. Acta Med Scand 113:558, 1943.
32. Kane RL: A methanol poisoning outbreak in Kentucky. Arch Environ Health 17:119, 1968.
33. Jacobson BM, Russell HK, Grimm JJ, et al: Acute methyl alcohol poisoning: Report of eighteen cases. US Naval Med Bull 44:1099, 1945.
34. Ziegler SL: The ocular menace of wood alcohol poisoning. Br J Ophthalmol 5:365, 411, 1921.
35. Carr RE, Henkind P: Ocular manifestations of ethambutol. Arch Ophthalmol 67:566, 1962.
36. Lessell S: Histopathology of experimental ethambutol intoxication. Invest Ophthalmol 15:765, 1976.
37. Schmidt IG, Schmidt LH: Studies on the neurotoxicity of ethambutol and its racemate for the rhesus monkey. J Neuropathol Exp Neurol 25:40, 1966.
38. Asayama T: Two cases of bitemporal hemianopsia due to ethambutol. Jpn J Clin Ophthalmol 23:1209, 1969.
39. Nakae K, Yamamoto K, Igata A: Subacute myelo-optico-neuropathy (S.M.O.N.) in Japan. Lancet 2:510, 1971.
40. Kono R: Subacute myelo-optic-neuropathy: A new neurological disease prevailing in Japan. Jpn J Med Sci Biol 24:195, 1971.
41. Sobue I, Mukoyama M, Takayanagi T, et al: Myeloneuropathy with abdominal disorders in Japan: Neuropathologic findings in seven autopsied cases. Neurology 22:1034, 1972.
42. Shiraki H: Neuropathology of subacute myelo-optic-neuropathy, SMON, in the human. Jpn J Med Sci Biol 28:101, 1975.
43. Sobue I: Clinical features of S.M.O.N. *In* Gent M, Shigematsu I (eds): Epidemiological Issues in Reported Drug-induced Illnesses—S.M.O.N. and Other Examples. Hamilton, Ontario, Canada, McMaster University Library Press, 1978.
44. Behrens M: Optic atrophy in children after diiodohydroxyquin therapy. JAMA 228:693, 1974.
45. Garcia-Perez A, Castro C, Franco A, et al: A case of optic atrophy possibly induced by quinoline in acrodermatitis enteropathica. Br J Dermatol 90:453, 1974.
46. Hache JC, Woillez M, Breuillard F, et al: La névrite optique des iodo-quinoleines. Bull Soc d'Ophthalmol Fr 73:501, 1973.
47. Berggren L, Hansson O: Treating acrodermatitis enteropathica. Lancet 1:52, 1966.
48. Foulds WS, Pettigrew AR: Tobacco-alcohol amblyopia. *In* Brockhurst RJ, Boruchoff SA, Hutchinson BT, Lessell S (eds): Controversy in Ophthalmology. Philadelphia, WB Saunders, 1977, pp 851–865.
49. Heaton JM, McCormick AJA, Freeman AG: Tobacco amblyopia—A clinical manifestation of vitamin B_{12} deficiency. Lancet 2:286, 1958.
50. Foulds WS, Chisholm IA, Bronte-Steward JM, et al: Vitamin B_{12} absorption in tobacco amblyopia. Br J Ophthalmol 53:393, 1969.
51. Traquair HM: Toxic amblyopia, including retrobulbar neuritis. Trans Ophthal Soc UK 50:351, 1930.

Chapter 206

Miscellaneous Optic Neuropathies

ROBERT S. HEPLER

The great majority of optic neuropathies in clinical practice fall into three major categories: compression by tumor, demyelination, and ischemia. These frequently encountered disorders are presented in detail in previous chapters. However, the clinician must be aware of the existence of other disease processes that can significantly affect optic nerve function. These relatively infrequent disorders should be considered when patterns of visual loss are atypical, when there are associated systemic diseases, or when there is disease in structures adjacent to the course of the optic nerves. Topic headings in this chapter include optic neuropathy associated with paranasal sinus disease, granulomatous inflammation of the optic nerves, and radiation-induced damage to the optic nerves. The subject of symptoms and signs generally associated with optic nerve disease has been presented in preceding chapters and applies to the topics in this chapter.

OPTIC NEUROPATHY ASSOCIATED WITH DISEASE OF ADJACENT SINUSES AND BONES

Anatomic Considerations

Reference to any neuroanatomic text illustrates the close proximity of the optic nerves to adjacent paranasal sinuses. In addition, the bone separation is normally thin in the lateral wall of the ethmoid sinus (lamina papyracea) and is easily breached by infectious agents, tumors, and surgical instruments. As if this weren't hazardous enough, local bone defects between the optic nerve and the adjacent ethmoid air cells are not infrequent. Computed tomography (CT) in 80 persons with ophthalmologic complaints, whose scans were considered to be normal, were reviewed to study the relationships between the optic nerves and the paranasal sinuses.[1] These authors found that 48 percent of posterior ethmoid air cells are separated from the optic nerve by the thin bony lamina of the optic canal and that 23 percent of all optic nerves project into the sphenoid sinus. It is not difficult to envision the spread of paranasal sinus disease toward the optic nerve via naturally occurring defects in the thin bone separations and via defects created by inflammation and local pressure on the thin bone, although the incidence of such occurrences is not known.

Acute and Chronic Sinusitis—Bacterial, Sterile, Fungal

CASE REPORT

Patient TG presented for an evaluation of reduced vision in the right eye, during her 17th week of pregnancy. Twelve days prior to ophthalmologic assessment, she developed aching pain in the right periorbital region, and 3 days later she awakened with loss of the bottom half of the field of vision in the right eye. Vision worsened 5 days later. Visual acuity measured OD finger counting superiorly, OS 20/20. Additional positive findings included mild erythema of the right lower lid, 2 mm of right proptosis, and tenderness of the right orbit on palpation. There was an afferent pupillary defect OD, and the right optic nerve was mildly elevated and hyperemic (Fig. 206–1). The left eye was normal. She had slight leukocytosis. With abdominal shielding a limited CT scan was performed, and it demonstrated right ethmoiditis. Transantral ethmoidectomy showed polypoid granulation tissue in the ethmoid and maxillary sinuses, and cultures grew only a few colonies of *Streptococcus viridans* species. Appropriate antibiotics were administered. Visual acuity OD returned to 20/30.

In the first half of this century, it was medically fashionable to attribute optic neuritis to adjacent sinus disease; this was probably not without some basis in the preantibiotic era, when bacterial sinusitis was more common and was a more serious infection than it is now. Tarkkanen and associates reviewed the records of 104 consecutive patients with optic neuritis in order to clarify the relationship of optic neuritis to otorhinolaryngological pathology.[2] Their study, performed before the advent of CT scanning, disclosed one patient in whom optic nerve involvement appeared attributable to paranasal sinus inflammation. Six of 12 patients with otolaryngologic pathology also had neurologic examination findings that suggested a diagnosis of probable multiple sclerosis. The conclusion of Tarkkanen and associates was that optic neuritis was caused by adjacent sinus inflammation with great infrequency.

This case, however, illustrates that *occasionally* sinus infection causes optic neuritis. Although such cases may be infrequently encountered, the importance of their recognition is great; identification of these cases and immediate, appropriate treatment may provide significant visual return. Unlike routine cases of demyelinative and nonarteritic anterior ischemic optic neuropathy, in which treatment probably does little good, these uncommon sinus infection–associated cases can be helped. This fact is one of the significant reasons for including CT or magnetic resonance imaging (MRI) in the assessment of patients with atypical optic neuritis.

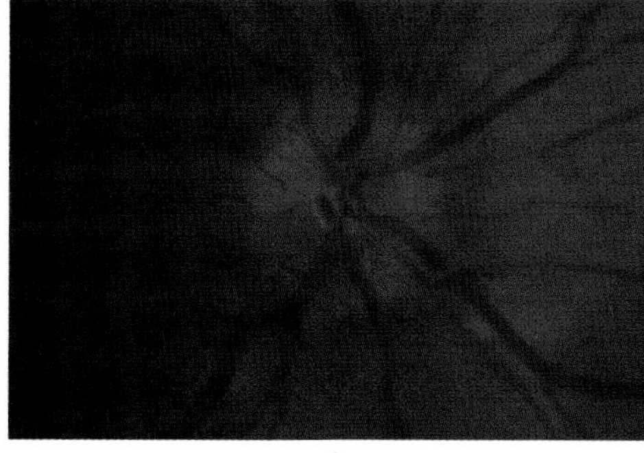
A

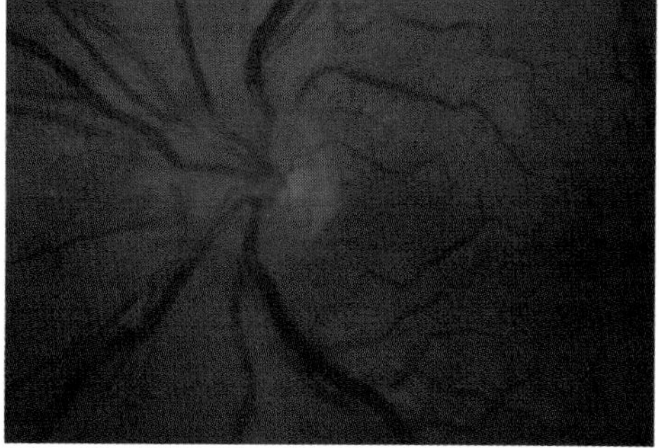
B

Figure 206–1. Swollen right disc and normal left disc (for comparison) in a patient with optic nerve inflammation due to adjacent paranasal sinus infection.

At least some cases of sphenoid and ethmoid sinusitis lead to orbital cellulitis and severe, permanent visual loss.[3] Three cases described by Slavin and Glaser had substantial signs of posterior orbital inflammation and probably involved pressure-related ischemia of the optic nerves as the mechanism of visual loss. Prompt paranasal sinus drainage and antibiotic administration may prevent blindness in such patients.

Goldberg and associates describe three cases in which cocaine abuse was the cause of optic neuropathy, associated with chronic sinusitis.[4] Their patients had scan findings of chronic sinusitis and diffuse bone destruction in the maxillary, sphenoidal, and ethmoidal sinuses; in one case, there was striking destruction of the nasal septum and turbinates. The underlying mechanism is chronic irritation of the upper respiratory mucosa leading to osteolytic sinusitis.

Fungal infections of the orbit may affect the posterior orbit and may cause cranial nerve impairment and blindness. Their origin is usually in one or more of the paranasal sinuses, and debility and immunocompromised state predispose their occurrence. Representative organisms are *Aspergillus fumigatus* and *Mucor* species. A case of *Aspergillus* infection in the ethmoid sinus and orbit occurred in a nondebilitated, nonketotic individual who had recently traveled to the Sudan—a hot, dry area in which infection with *Aspergillus* is much more common than in North America.[5] Fungal infections with agents such as *Aspergillus* can be remarkably indolent and should be considered in the differential diagnosis of atypical optic neuropathies, particularly in patients with chronic sinusitis. Another case of aspergillosis, this time in an immunocompromised woman, terminated in fatal hemorrhage from arteritic rupture of the internal carotid artery, having earlier caused blindness on the side with *Aspergillus* abscess of the ethmoid sinus.[6]

Aspergillosis may occur in the absence of an immunocompromised state, and the pain and reduced vision of posterior orbital involvement may be remarkably responsive to systemic steroids. Such a case was presented by Spoor and associates, who emphasize the danger in misinterpreting steroid responsiveness as indicating ordinary optic neuritis and the potential risks of treating patients with aspergillosis with steroids. Use of systemic steroids in such cases may contribute to a more rapidly progressive or even fatal outcome.[7]

Mucormycosis is well known in the context of poorly controlled, insulin-dependent diabetics who develop a rapid progression of cranial nerve palsies. This infection is believed to originate in the paranasal sinuses and to cause damage by a relatively selective arteritis accounted for by the organism's predilection to grow along and within arterial walls. The ophthalmic artery is not exempt: sudden blindness is one manifestation of this disorder. The spectrum of medical diseases predisposing to mucor becomes broader with time. Out-of-control diabetes has now been joined by a variety of other immunocompromised states showing susceptibility to mucor. The list now includes leukemia, lymphoma, multiple myeloma, carcinoma, anemia, septicemia, tuberculosis, thermal burns, extensive wounds, malnutrition, dehydration, severe diarrhea, gastroenteritis, hepatitis, cirrhosis, glomerulonephritis, acute tubular necrosis, uremia, pulmonary alveolar proteinosis, congenital heart disease, and treatment with antibiotics, folic acid antagonists, chemotherapeutic agents, corticosteroids, and ionizing radiation. Early diagnosis improves the likelihood of survival. Treatment of mucor involving the orbit traditionally has involved immediate exenteration combined with administration of amphotericin B, but selected cases may be managed successfully without exenteration.[8]

Paranasal Sinus Tumors

Most primary tumors of the paranasal sinuses, particularly those that affect the optic nerve, are malignant and present to the ophthalmologist with pain and cranial nerve palsies. Most such tumors are readily identified on CT or MRI scans. In a review of 36 patients with primary sphenoid sinus malignancy, headache was most often reported as the presenting symptom (in 16 patients), followed by diplopia (in 13 patients), and visual loss or visual obscurations (in 8 patients). Diagnosis by a CT or MRI scan followed by biopsy is usually not difficult, but unfortunately prognosis remains poor.[9]

Coppeto and associates reported a case of optic neuropathy associated with paranasal sinus lymphoma.[10] Their case emphasizes the need for histologic diagnosis in order to guide therapy.

Representative of the *benign* processes arising in the paranasal sinuses and affecting optic nerve function are polyps that invade the orbits and even the pituitary fossa, basal cisterns, and cavernous sinuses. Such a case, in which surgical management helped with regard to proptosis and paralytic strabismus aspects, but left the patient with visual field loss in one eye, was presented by Kaufman and associates.[11] This case, as is often true of patients with mucocele, had a past history of chronic inflammatory sinus disease. Such aggressive nasal/sinus polyps can erode bone of the lamina papyracea, sphenoid sinus, and orbital roof or floor.

Whatever the disease process, benign or malignant, there is risk of damage to the optic nerve in performance of ethmoid surgical procedures. Stankiemicz reviews the literature concerning this topic and discusses aspects of prevention.[12] He points out that direct injury to the optic nerve, which is one mechanism causing loss of vision in ethmoidectomy, has little in the way of promising treatment, and therefore must be avoided through knowledge of anatomic variations in the relationship between the optic nerves and ethmoid sinus. The second mechanism, orbital hematoma secondary to ethmoid surgery, can be managed with urgent orbital decompression to preserve vision.

Mucoceles

Mucoceles arise from the paranasal sinuses and usually follow long-standing symptoms of chronic sinusitis. They consist of cystic bone expansions of a sinus, containing mucoid debris trapped through obstruction of normal drainage through the sinus ostia. Frontal, sphenoid, or ethmoid sinuses can be involved, and the signs and symptoms vary accordingly. The most common manifestation arises from the frontal sinus and presents as a slowly progressive proptosis in which displacement of the involved eye is characteristically down and out. In this classic form, palpation confirms the presence of a mass in the upper nasal quadrant of the orbit. Unfortunately, however, diagnosis of mucoceles is often confused by the wide variety of their potential manifestations. Diagnosis is usually readily made via CT or MRI; therapy, by surgical resection and restoration of sinus drainage, produces excellent results.

Avery and associates present two cases that exemplify the ophthalmic effects of large frontal mucoceles; one patient had developed complete blindness in the involved eye.[13] Newton and associates present a rare case of bilateral posterior sphenoethmoidal mucocele with bilateral optic neuropathy.[14] As is not uncommon in the analysis of visual loss due to mucoceles, their case was initially considered to be optic neuritis; only after visual loss had declined to finger counting bilaterally was the proper diagnosis established by scanning.

Unusual variants of mucoceles test diagnostic acumen. Yue and associates present a case of unilateral blindness due to mucocele in the optic canal from mucocele originating in the posterior ethmoid.[15] Combined transcranial excision and transnasal drainage were followed by significant return of vision in the affected eye. Johnson and associates present two cases of anterior clinoid variant of sphenoid sinus mucocele.[16] In the first case, the mucocele initially mimicked diabetic ophthalmoplegia with pupil-sparing palsy of the oculomotor nerve.[16] Later, after resolution of the third-nerve problem, severe visual loss occurred, and reinvestigation disclosed that anterior clinoid mucocele was the cause. In their second case, a 59-year-old man reported having had episodic visual loss OS for 20 yr. As recently as 1975, visual acuity had declined to hand motions OS but then returned to 20/20 on administration of retrobulbar corticosteroid and oral steroid therapy. Reevaluation in 1985, during a time of reduction in vision to hand motions perception, demonstrated CT findings of opacification and expansion of the left anterior clinoid by a soft-tissue mass that was neuroradiologically consistent with mucocele (Fig. 206–2). A third case of optic canal involvement with visual loss due to mucocele, probably arising from the sphenoid sinus, was presented by Matsuoka and associates.[17]

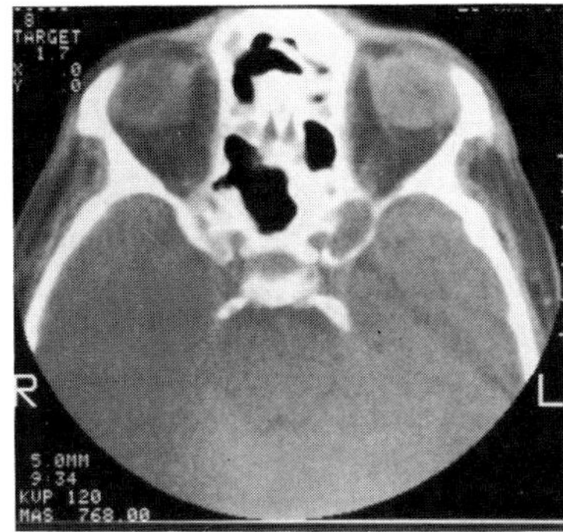

Figure 206–2. Left anterior clinoid mucocele.

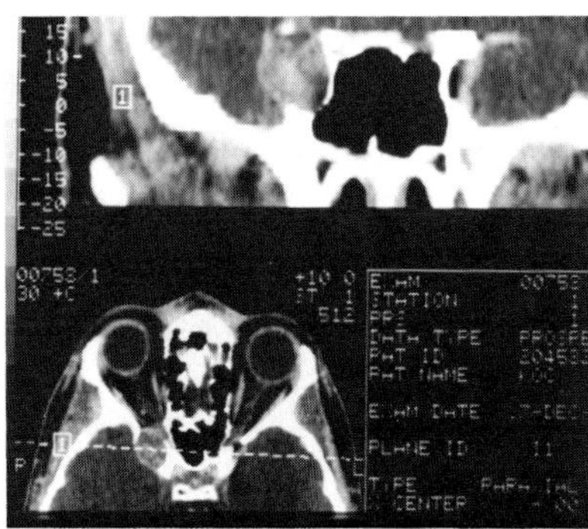

Figure 206–3. Right anterior clinoid hemangioma, simulating a mucocele.

Although mucoceles tend to present as indolent processes, they sometimes cause acute optic nerve dysfunction, with severe visual loss being present for only a few days or less.[18, 19] These acute cases, which are very likely to be initially misunderstood as optic neuritis cases, emphasize the importance of neuroimaging to detect treatable causes of acute optic neuropathy. Even with modern neuroimaging, there may be surprises in dealing with disorders in this area. The scan in Figure 206–3 is that of a patient who lost all vision in the right eye due to what was believed neuroradiologically to be an anterior clinoid mucocele. Unexpectedly, the neurosurgeon drew back blood when he attempted to aspirate it. This particular lesion turned out to be a hemangioma of the anterior clinoid, simulating a mucocele.

Pneumosinus Dilatans

Another abnormality arising in cranial bones with potential to affect vision is pneumosinus dilatans. Unfortunately, the term has been applied imprecisely to more than one clinical circumstance. Some have applied the term to the enlargement of a paranasal sinus adjacent to a tumor such as meningioma. A better definition is more general and refers to "all dilated, air-filled sinuses with outwardly bulging walls when the primary cause is uncertain."[20] The neuroradiologic criteria for diagnosis are further characterized as including enlargement of an air cell or an entire sinus, the presence of only air in the abnormal space, and the ballooning outward of the walls of the sinus. Figure 206–4 illustrates pneumosinus dilatans causing right eye blindness in a 17-year-old male.

The neuroophthalmic significance of pneumosinus dilatans is two-fold: first, reduced vision, optic atrophy, and/or bitemporal hemianopsia can result from anterior visual pathway compression of the enlarging sinus. Second, radiologic diagnosis of sphenoidal pneumosinus dilatans provides a warning to look for optic nerve sheath meningioma(s). Progressive visual loss was found, in one series of cases, to be due to intracanalicular meningiomas of the sheath of the optic nerve, which demonstrated sphenoid sinus pneumosinus dilatans.[21]

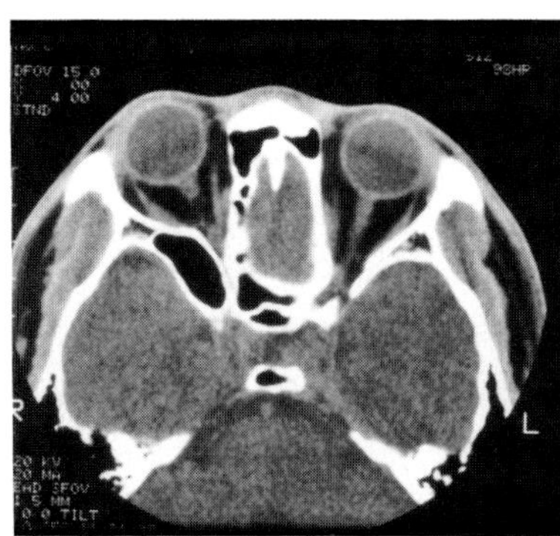

Figure 206–4. Pneumosinus dilatans compressing the right optic nerve.

Spoor and associates described a case of bilateral optic nerve sheath meningioma with pneumosinus dilatans in a patient with the Klippel-Trenaunay-Weber syndrome in whom the nerve sheath tumor was diagnosed by fine-needle aspiration biopsy.[22] Clearly, the presence of pneumosinus dilatans in a patient with unexplained visual loss calls for diligent search for optic nerve sheath meningioma.

Fibrous Dysplasia

Fibrous dysplasia is a developmental anomaly of bone, often affecting facial and orbital bones. The abnormality is apparent in childhood and stems from gradual replacement of normal bone by fibrous tissue. If the sphenoid bone is involved in the dysplastic process, optic nerve function can be impaired, even in adult years when most of the dysplastic growth has already occurred. Significant facial asymmetry is greater than that usually encountered with meningioma, aiding in the differential diagnosis. Neuroophthalmic involvement may include proptosis, exposure keratitis, and diplopia—but the main complication is visual loss either through gradual compromise of the optic canal or occasionally through abrupt optic nerve compromise.

CASE REPORT

A remarkable case combining both fibrous dysplasia *and* sphenoid sinus mucocele involved a young woman who experienced severe, acute loss of vision in the right eye in 1987, found to be due to pressure from a mucocele associated with her underlying fibrous dysplasia (Fig. 206–5). A craniotomy disclosed the mucocele, removal of which led to restoration of 20/25 acuity. In 1990 she again experienced abrupt loss of vision in the right eye, to the level of finger-counting acuity, and reexploration demonstrated a recurrence of mucocele, removal of which restored vision to her baseline 20/25 level.[23]

This case illustrates the potential for acute visual changes in this entity and the benefit of prompt, appropriate surgical therapy. Melen and associates[24] report a similar case, with striking improvement achieved by neurosurgical decompression.

INFLAMMATORY OPTIC NEUROPATHIES

The disease entities considered in this section include truly inflammatory disorders of the optic nerves—excluding ordinary optic neuritis of the sort frequently associated with multiple sclerosis and also inflammation secondary to adjacent primary inflammatory disease such as sinusitis, orbital cellulitis, and meningitis, all of which are dealt with elsewhere in this text.

Infectious Agents

The consideration of infectious agents as causes for optic neuritis is important because of the rising incidence of such occurrences and because of the potential for successful treatment of at least some infectious causes. The incidence is difficult to quantify with certainty, but it is rising in clinical experience because of the effects of the AIDS virus in lowering resistance to infection with agents previously seldom encountered in optic nerve infection; the frequency of such cases is also increasing because of the immunocompromising effects of drugs used in the treatment of a wide range of inflammatory diseases, as well as drugs used in the management of patients who have undergone renal, heart, and other transplant procedures.

SYPHILIS

The traditional circumstance in which syphilitic optic neuropathy is discovered involves a middle-aged or older individual, in whom serologic studies (performed because of otherwise unexplained optic atrophy) are markedly positive, leading to a diagnosis of tertiary syphilis. The discovery of serologic evidence of syphilis may come initially as a great surprise, particularly if the patient is a prominent figure in the social, religious, or political life of the community. History of exposure to syphilis may or may not be elicited when the patient is confronted by the serologic results.

The context in which to suspect syphilis must be broadened considerably in the modern world. Acute syphilitic optic neuritis may occur in primary (or secondary) syphilis—not just tertiary—as illustrated by two patients presented by Weinstein and associates.[25] Optic nerve dysfunction may be acute and severe, as exemplified by a case of acute syphilitic blindness associated with AIDS, in which a patient deteriorated from a documented level of 20/20 acuity OU to total blindness overnight.[26] Even in the case of severe visual loss reported by Zambrano and associates, acuity returned to 20/40 (with major field deficit) in at least one eye after the administration of high-dosage penicillin.

As befits its reputation as a mimic, syphilitic involvement of the optic nerve can take many forms. These include indolent optic atrophy, acute papillitis, gumma, passive disc edema associated with elevated cerebrospinal fluid (CSF) pressure in luetic meningitis and syphilitic perineuritis. The latter is defined by the presence

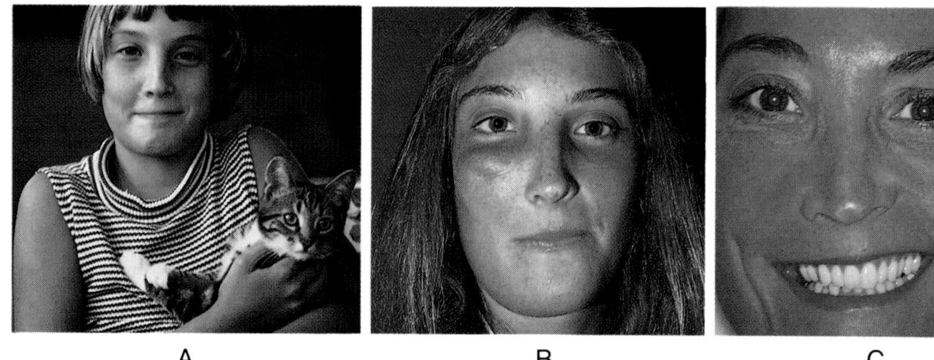

Figure 206–5. Progressive fibrous dysplasia at ages 12 (with cat "Mittens"), 19, and 29 yr. Facial asymmetry first noted at approximately 7 yr of age.

of swollen optic discs without visual loss and without raised CSF pressure. Syphilitic optic perineuritis is reported to occur in secondary syphilis and is distinguished from cases of syphilitic optic neuritis by preservation of good visual function.[27] Diagnosis requires neuroimaging and CSF analysis (pressure, cell count, and FTA-ABS). The presumed inflammation of the meningeal sheaths of the optic nerves is expected to respond quickly to penicillin treatment.[28]

Syphilitic neuroretinitis occurs most often in secondary syphilis and shows signs of inflammation in the optic nerves, as well as in the retina and sometimes in the vitreous. Four such cases presented by Folk and associates had similar features of papillitis, gray opaque retinal edema, retinal vasculitis, and vitreous inflammation, and all four patients developed neuroretinitis in either secondary or early tertiary phases of infection. All responded well to appropriate penicillin treatment.[29] Although almost complete visual recovery is the rule in suitably treated cases, cystoid macular edema and retinal ischemia may cause permanent visual loss.[30]

In summary, testing for syphilis is indicated in many clinical circumstances, including unexplained visual loss, optic atrophy, disc swelling, and retinal vasculitis cases—along with anterior and posterior uveitis, vitritis, cranial nerve paresis, and pupillary abnormality cases. The coexistence of syphilis and AIDS makes the laboratory testing for syphilis appropriate whenever testing for AIDS is done.[31] Regarding treatment of syphilis, the recommended dosage of penicillin has been increased in recent years, and the physician should consult current recommendations. Treatment dosage for patients with optic nerve-involved syphilis is appropriately based on treatment for neurosyphilis, which involves 2 to 4 million units of crystalline penicillin G given intravenously every 4 hr for 10 days. Lesser treatment, although considered adequate in the past, is now believed to be insufficient.

LYME DISEASE

Lyme disease relates to syphilis in that both are caused by spirochetal organisms that are fastidious and share at least some antigenic or serologic features: both cause systemic illness of variable manifestations; both are diagnosed on the basis of clinical and serologic evidence; and both are treated by penicillin or equivalent antibiotic therapy, the requisite dosage of which is uncertain. What is known in the United States as Lyme disease was first described after an outbreak was observed in Lyme, Connecticut in 1975. However, the disorder was well known in Europe before that time. The responsible organism, *Borrelia burgdorferi*, was reported in 1982.[32]

Clinical illness with Lyme disease involves three phases: following a tick bite (of which the patient may not be aware), there develops a skin lesion known as erythema chronicum migrans, in which a pruritic lesion commences near the site of the bite, gradually expands, and is followed by secondary annular lesions. This initial phase may be accompanied by systemic symptoms including malaise, fever, chills, headache, and neck stiffness. A physical examination during the initial phase may disclose organomegaly and painful lymphadenopathy, and conjunctivitis. In the second stage there are neurologic and cardiac disorders—including meningitis, cranial nerve palsies, Guillain-Barré–like syndrome, myocarditis, and occasionally optic neuritis or papilledema. In the third stage, which may occur months to years after the onset of the illness, there is chronic monoarticular or oligoarticular arthritis in approximately 60 percent of patients.[33]

An understanding of the ophthalmic significance of Lyme disease is still developing. However, it is apparent that most patients with this disorder do not seek ophthalmologic attention, although conjunctivitis is probably not infrequent in the first phase. Acute dysfunction of the seventh cranial nerve (Bell's palsy) is relatively common in the second stage, occurring in three of six cases of Lyme disease in the series reported by Winward and associates.[34] Uveitis has been reported, including a case that went on to enucleation (despite vigorous antibiotic and surgical therapy), and organisms were identified in the enucleated eye.[35] Optic neuritis occurring 6 mo after onset, despite treatment for Lyme disease, was attributed to this cause and appeared to respond to additional antibiotic treatment.[36] Although the incidence of conjunctivitis and Bell's palsy is relatively high in Lyme disease, uveitis and optic neuropathy are infrequent.

TUBERCULOSIS AND LEPROSY (HANSEN'S DISEASE)

Both of these diseases have a long history of being attributed as causes of ocular inflammatory disorder, primarily implicating keratitis and uveitis, caused by infestation or allergic reaction to *Mycobacterium tuberculosum* or *M. leprae*. Interest in cases of optic neuritis attributed to tuberculosis is expressed by Wilbrand and Saenger.[37] Publications giving evidence of tuberculous optic nerve disease in the modern era are scant. Despite a paucity of credible case reports in recent times, it does seem to be appropriate to include tuberculosis in the differential of potential causes of optic neuropathy, to be considered primarily when there is other evidence of systemic or central nervous system infection with *M. tuberculosum*.

Ocular findings in leprosy in the United States were presented by Spaide and associates.[38] Of 55 patients with biopsy-proven Hansen's disease, only eight patients had anterior segment inflammation. As in tuberculosis, it also appears reasonable to consider Hansen's disease as a cause of optic neuropathy but also to realize that such involvement must be very rare—at least in the United States.

TOXOCARA, TOXOPLASMA, CAT-SCRATCH FEVER, AND Q FEVER

These entities share the involvement of an animal vector. In terms of frequency of occurrence, toxoplasmosis and toxocara are much more frequent causes of disease than are Q fever and cat-scratch disease. *Toxocara canis* and *T. catis* are worms that complete their life cycle in dogs and cats, respectively. When eggs are ingested from feces-contaminated soil, a systemic infestation arises, with larvae passing through the intestinal wall of the human host and reaching all parts of the body. As the larvae travel through progressively smaller blood vessels, they are eventually trapped, and at that point the larvae burrow into adjacent tissue and remain there. The ophthalmologic manifestations most often involve a fundus granuloma in a child. In at least one case, acute neuroretinitis was observed in a child concurrently while he was experiencing the active disseminated stage of the infestation—visceral larval migrans.[39] Primary optic neuropathy due to *Toxocara* is seldom reported. Cox and associates report a case of bilateral toxocara optic neuropathy in a child exposed to puppies, who developed striking bilateral optic neuropathy in association with visceral larval migrans, with *Toxocara* ELISA titers supporting the diagnosis.[40]

Toxoplasma gondii is well recognized as a cause of necrotic retinitis. Cerebral involvement (encephalopathies, meningoencephalitis) has been considered rare, except in immunocompromised persons. However, acute acquired toxoplasmosis has been reported in an immunocompetent child.[41] Six cases of presumed toxoplasmic papillitis presented with ocular inflammation limited to the optic nerve head and adjacent vitreous.[42] Because of the absence of visible retinitis in these six patients, the diagnosis of toxoplasmosis was not considered initially in five of the six cases.

Cat-scratch disease is a systemic disorder (benign lymphoreticulosis) with regional lymphadenopathy preceded by a cat scratch. The causative organism is proposed to be a gram-negative pleomorphic bacillus, and the most common ophthalmologic manifestations are Parinaud's ocular glandular syndrome and neuroretinitis.[43] Optic neuritis followed typical cat-scratch disease in a young adult patient whose cat-scratch skin test was positive.[44]

Even cattle may harbor organisms capable of causing significant optic neuropathy. A farmer developed bilateral optic neuritis while suffering a febrile illness. Antibody titers to *Coxiella burnetii* increased as he was recovering from the systemic illness. Titers in his own animals were absent, but on the farm where he bought his calves, several cows were seropositive. The patient's wife had no antibodies against *C. burnetii*, and we are not informed concerning the antibody titers of the wife on the adjacent farm. The patient was treated with doxycycline with improved vision in one eye.[45]

CRYPTOCOCCOSIS AND ASPERGILLOSIS

Central nervous system and ocular involvement with cryptococcosis is one of the increasingly common accompaniments of the AIDS epidemic. The mechanisms that have been proposed for optic neuropathy in cryptococcosis have included effects of increased intracranial pressure, adhesive arachnoiditis around the optic nerves, and direct infiltration/inflammation of the optic nerves by cryptococcal organisms. Cryptococcal meningitis may be the initial clinical manifestation of AIDS, and thus it is appropriate to test for AIDS when evaluating cryptococcal meningitis.[46] Visual loss attributed to adhesive arachnoiditis was reported in two patients with AIDS who also had cytomegalovirus retinitis (one patient) and *Pneumocystis carinii* pneumonia (the other patient) but were treated without surgery.[47] In another patient with AIDS, whose CSF demonstrated *Cryptococcus neoformans* and opening pressure of 350 mm of water, nerve sheath fenestration surgery provided a specimen of optic nerve sheath that contained several yeast forms consistent with *C. neoformans*.[48] While their case had extensive adhesions between the dural sheath and the optic nerve observed at surgery, and organisms were found in the sheath biopsy, these authors believed that the mechanism of optic atrophy was direct invasion of the optic nerve by the organism. Vision was not improved by the nerve sheath fenestration in this particular case. The role of nerve sheath fenestration in cryptococcal meningitis is not yet clear.

Another fungal organism that occasionally has involved the optic nerve directly is *Aspergillus*. Visual loss due to infiltration with this organism is likely to occur in immunocompromised individuals, is likely to be indolent in clinical course, and is associated with pain and radiologic signs of sinus disease. "Painful ophthalmoplegia" (Tolosa-Hunt syndrome) is a promising (but incorrect) diagnosis early in the course of these *Aspergillus* cases, particularly when the patients respond well initially to systemic corticosteroid treatment—as they are likely to do. However, the steroids probably contribute to the ultimate bad outcome. One patient of this type, without associated proptosis or demonstrable sinus disease, had biopsy-proven diagnosis and treatment with amphotericin B, yet died despite treatment.[49]

One more mechanism of visual loss in cryptococcal and *Aspergillus* cases may be idiosyncratic reaction to amphotericin B. An intravenous test dose of 1 mg given to a patient with systemic lupus erythematosus, diffuse proliferative glomerulonephritis, and cryptococcal meningitis is blamed for sudden bilateral blindness 10 hr later, yet her fundi looked initially normal on clinical examination.[50]

VIRAL OPTIC NEUROPATHIES

Optic neuropathies associated with viral etiology can be divided into two major groups. The first class, parainfectious relationship, refers to optic neuropathy cases that characteristically *follow* acute viral infection elsewhere in the body, with the implication that the systemic viral infection stimulates an immune-mediated response in the optic nerve. The second, direct viral infestation, is exemplified by cases of herpes zoster or cytomegalovirus optic neuritis.

Typical parainfectious optic neuritis was presented in the case of a 10-year-old girl who, 1 mo after recovery from varicella, developed severe visual loss in both eyes. Visual recovery was excellent, but she was left with optic atrophy and acuity of OD 20/20, OS 20/25.[51] Selbst and associates point out that a good visual outcome is the rule but is not invariably the case; prognosis is more guarded in cases associated with herpes zoster than with the other viruses, probably because of the vasculitic component that is typical of zoster virus. Reported parainfectious cases have implicated all of the following: rubeola, rubella, mumps, varicella, herpes zoster, and infectious mononucleosis. Instructive reports on parainfectious optic neuritis include cases following chicken pox in adults[52]; chiasmal neuritis as part of Epstein-Barr virus infection[53]; and optic and auditory nerve involvement in Guillain-Barré syndrome after an influenza-like illness.[54] The fact that vision doesn't always return to good levels is exemplified in a case following varicella in a 14-year-old, in whom one eye did not improve above 20/400.[55]

A specific subgroup of parainfectious optic neuritis involves patients whose optic neuritis follows immunization. Associations have been made in a middle-aged patient immunized with bivalent 1973 to 1974 influenza formula[56] and in a surgical house officer immunized against swine and Victoria flu.[57] The patients in both reports recovered their sight. It seems reasonable to look for a common mechanism in these optic neuropathy cases, relating them to the more highly publicized Guillain-Barré cases that were noted in the media and in the courts and attributed to influenza immunization. As with the other parainfectious optic neuritis categories, the visual outcome is usually, but not always, excellent. A patient who received swine flu vaccination experienced severe loss of vision in one eye, with no return of vision and severe optic atrophy as sequelae.[58] Trivalent vaccination against measles, mumps, and rubella was followed by papillitis, which resolved with return of good vision in a 6-year-old boy.[59]

Neuroretinitis is a term applied to disc swelling and visual loss with peripapillary and macular exudates. While occasionally specifically connected with cat-scratch disease, more often it follows a seemingly pedestrian upper respiratory or other unremarkable viral illness. Typical features are illustrated by the following case.

CASE REPORT

A 23-year-old woman had what she considered to be an ordinary cold, so ordinary that she didn't even remember it until prompted during a review of her history. About 3 wk later, a decline in vision in the left eye was noted, and the referring physician noted acuity in the involved eye to be 20/200, with a swollen disc; the other eye was normal. Initially she presented no perimacular exudates, but when seen in consultation 3 wk after the onset of her visual loss, the fundus appearance was as shown in Figure 206–6. Three months later her vision had returned to 20/25, but she was bothered by differences in light and color sensitivity between the two eyes; furthermore, she had a minimal afferent pupillary defect and mild optic atrophy. The edema residues had almost completely gone.

A review of 12 patients with neuroretinitis disclosed that some were bilateral, and a time-relationship to antecedent viral disease was present in five of the 12 cases.[60] Neuroretinitis does not imply a risk of later development of multiple sclerosis; this leads to the useful recommendation of bringing back patients with papillitis, who don't initially have the typical macular exudates, for reexamination within 2 wk. Development of the macular star, as in this case report, is strong evidence against the development of multiple sclerosis.[61]

Direct viral infection of optic nerves may occur in otherwise normal individuals but is more likely to happen in immunocompromised persons and, in particular, patients with AIDS. Reference is made to a useful

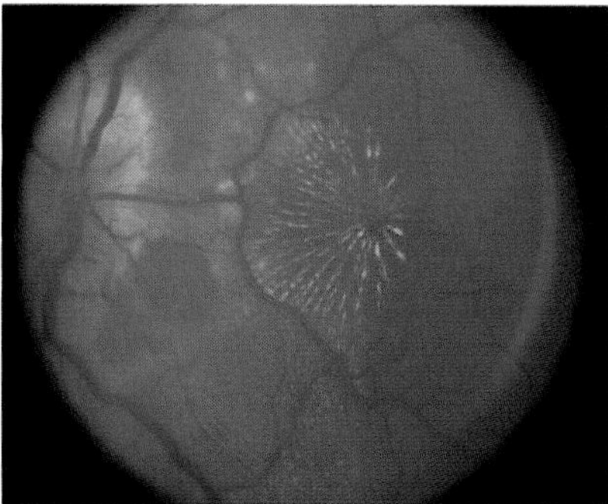

Figure 206–6. Characteristic fundus appearance in neuroretinitis.

review of the spectrum of optic nerve disease in patients with HIV infection.[62] These authors list the following as infectious disease entities to be considered in potentially HIV-infected patients with visual loss: cytomegalovirus (CMV), syphilis, toxoplasmosis, tuberculosis, cryptococcosis, herpes zoster, and herpes simplex. They present four patients, illustrating the first four in this list. The presence of ocular inflammatory disease in any of these categories calls for consideration of possible HIV positivity. More than one of the entities may coexist in the same patient; for instance, syphilis, which is treatable, may be present along with CMV. Although most of the entities are more likely to affect the retina in HIV-positive patients, all of the seven infections can also involve the optic nerves. HIV itself is not yet known to cause optic neuritis, but the virus is found throughout the body of affected individuals; because it is known to be neurotropic, it would not be surprising eventually to learn that it is capable of causing optic nerve injury. The nonviral entities (syphilis, toxoplasmosis, tuberculosis, and cryptococcosis) are discussed in greater depth earlier in this chapter.

CMV optic neuritis is described in a case that included pathologic confirmation.[63] Bilateral acute retrobulbar neuritis was attributed to epidemic keratoconjunctivitis in a patient who did not have AIDS but who was otherwise immunocompromised.[64] A case of optic neuritis, attributed to parainfectious mechanism related to infectious mononucleosis in a 61-year-old man, may have been caused instead by direct infection of the optic nerves, in view of the short time between systemic infection and the onset of visual loss.[65] A case of optic neuropathy associated with herpes simplex encephalitis was proved at autopsy to involve the optic nerves in the viral infection.[66]

Noninfectious Granulomatous Disease

The broad subject of systemic diseases that affect the eye, many of which can have optic nerve manifestations, is reviewed in Section 13: The Eye and Systemic Disease. A number of these are characterized by granulomatous inflammatory tissue responses (e.g., systemic lupus erythematosus, temporal arteritis, Wegener's granulomatosis, and sarcoidosis). The differential diagnosis of granulomatous inflammations includes those caused by specific infectious organisms (presented earlier in this chapter) and those that are believed to be noninfectious in etiology but are still manifested by granulomatous inflammation.[67]

Sarcoidosis is a chronic, idiopathic granulomatous disorder that is more common in blacks than in other racial groups in the American population. Frequent manifestations include pulmonary granulomas and the anterior and posterior uveitis that is well known to ophthalmologists (see Chapter 27). Sarcoidosis affects the nervous system in only an estimated 15 percent of patients, and direct involvement of the optic nerves with sarcoid granulomatous inflammation is estimated to be rare. However, 11 cases of sarcoidosis from the North Carolina area, demonstrating direct optic nerve involvement, were identified between 1952 and 1982 and were reported in one study.[68] Of these 11 patients, only two were previously known to have sarcoid when their visual symptoms appeared. These authors found neuroimaging of the optic nerves to be very important in suggesting the diagnosis, and they recommended consideration of sarcoid in the differential of cases that might be interpreted initially as optic nerve gliomas or optic nerve sheath meningiomas.

The presence of optociliary shunts, often interpreted as supporting the diagnosis of optic nerve sheath meningioma, can occur in cases of optic disc edema caused by sarcoidosis.[69] One of two patients, whose initial manifestation of sarcoidosis was optic nerve disease attributed to optic neuritis, also had an optociliary shunt vessel; biopsy of the optic nerve in both cases showed typical findings of sarcoidosis. The diagnosis of sarcoidosis is based on consistent clinical and radiologic findings, demonstration of noncaseating granulomas, and absence of potential causative organisms recoverable from body tissues or fluids. Frequent supporting features include hilar lymphadenopathy and elevated levels of serum angiotensin-converting enzyme (ACE). These and other aspects of the diagnosis of this systemic disorder are presented by Jordan and associates.[70]

Treatment of sarcoidosis depends mainly on the administration of systemic steroids, the benefit of which is likely to be impressive. Unfortunately, steroid treatment may need to be prolonged, with attendant side effects of treatment that may become difficult to manage. Immunosuppressive agents (azathioprine, chlorambucil) have been used with reported benefit in some cases. Such agents may potentiate corticosteroids or may replace them in patients who do not respond to steroids or who become jeopardized by long-term steroid administration yet still need treatment. Benefits of high-voltage radiation therapy, if any, were transient in four patients who did then appear to improve with immunosuppressive treatment.[71]

Although the following are not, strictly speaking, granulomatous optic neuropathies, it is appropriate nevertheless, in a section reviewing the broad subject of inflammatory diseases that can affect optic nerves, to mention them and to cite relevant reviews. Optic neuropathy can occur in patients with systemic lupus erythematosus (presumably due to small vessel obstruction) and corticosteroid treatment may help the optic neuropathy.[72] A presumed autoimmune optic neuropathy may occur primarily in young women whose laboratory studies point toward underlying collagen vascular disease but who do not have proven systemic lupus erythematosus. These patients need to be differentiated from the more common idiopathic optic neuritis or multiple sclerosis–associated optic neuritis patients, in terms of laboratory findings and treatment. Substantial corticosteroid treatment is indicated in cases of autoimmune optic neuropathy.[73] In a series of four biopsy-proven cases of idiopathic inflammatory perioptic disease, one patient showed chronic granulomatous inflammation (etiology unknown) without benefit from corticosteroids.[74] Another case of idiopathic, noninfectious optic nerve sheath inflammation developed bilateral loss of vision from optic nerve compression and infarction.[75] A case of Tolosa-Hunt syndrome (inflammatory cavernous sinus syndrome) involved the optic nerve and was found by frontotemporal craniotomy to be caused by infiltration with eosinophilic granuloma (histiocytosis X) in an HIV-positive patient.[76] The cases sampled here illustrate the wide range of infrequently encountered inflammatory optic neuropathies. The underlying cause is still a mystery in some cases.

RADIATION-INDUCED OPTIC NEUROPATHY

CASE REPORT

In February, 1971, a 57-year-old man experienced visual disturbance in both eyes. An initial diagnosis of giant cell arteritis led to corticosteroid treatment, with modest subjective improvement. An initial neuroophthalmologic examination in April, 1971, disclosed normal central acuity but substantial bitemporal field defects. A craniotomy was performed with what was believed to be total removal of a suprasellar chromophobe adenoma. He recovered from surgery well. His vision returned, except for a trace of residual bitemporal field defect. Despite the impression of total removal of the 1 × 1 cm tumor, it was elected to give postoperative radiation. Radiation therapy was planned to administer 5000 rads to the sella, by opposing lateral fields, over 1 mo. Treatment was concluded in November, 1971. In March, 1973, he reported recent decreased vision in the right eye, and acuity and fields worsened with appearance of optic atrophy OD. Follow-up examinations showed central acuity preservation at OD 20/200, OS 20/30 through 1977, although visual fields worsened in both eyes and the patient reported declining vision. Neuroimaging and CSF testing were repeated several times, but no cause was found for his deteriorating status. Throughout the 1980s the patient's optic atrophy increased, and when he was last seen in October, 1985, his acuity was OD light perception, OS 20/400. He had profound optic atrophy, constant somnolence, and dementia.

Re-review of the record of his irradiation treatment in 1971 indicates that he received 250 rads/day for 20 days.

Historical interest in damaging effects on the visual system focused primarily on cataractogenesis, it being perceived that the retina and optic nerve were resistant to adverse radiation effects. An early report in 1975 was based on three patients who developed delayed radiation damage to the optic nerves, pointing out that these adverse effects occurred after therapy utilizing currently acceptable radiation dosages.[77] These authors correctly suspected a microvascular mechanism and pointed to the probable importance of the *daily* dosage, in addition to the total dosage of radiation therapy.

Brown and associates studied the ophthalmoscopic findings in 14 patients who received radiation therapy from 1976 to 1981 for a variety of paranasal sinus and other tumors. They found acute disc swelling, peripapillary exudates, hemorrhages, and subretinal fluid. Fluoroscein angiography gave evidence of nerve head ischemia, which lasted for several weeks to several months, with subsequent optic atrophy. The average time for the acute radiation optic neuropathy in their series was 12.6 mo after conclusion of radiation, with a range from 3 to 22 mo. They found a patient who had received only 3500 rads, but who also had diabetes mellitus, which may have provided a contributing microvascular cause.[78]

Kline and associates studied four patients who received radiation therapy specifically for pituitary adenomas. Their patients had normal fundi at the onset of visual loss, but these patients subsequently developed optic atrophy. Kline and colleagues identified the peak incidence as occurring at 1 to 1½ yr. They observed that in this entity, it is not unusual for visual loss to be severe or even total; furthermore, the second eye may be involved a few weeks or months after the first. They also observed that dementia may accompany the visual deterioration.[79]

Usefulness of MRI scanning with gadolinium-DPTA enhancement was studied in 13 patients, two of whom had acute radiation-induced optic neuropathy. Gadolinium-enhanced MRI scanning showed enhancement of the radiation-damaged optic nerve in the acute phase, presumably because of increased permeability of the blood-brain barrier.[80] Zimmerman and associates also found MRI scans to be useful in diagnosis of three patients who had been irradiated for tumors in the parasellar region. They list as risk factors: more than 4800 rads of total dosage, more than 200 rads/day in fractional dosage, overlapping treatment fields, age younger than 12, and adjunctive chemotherapy.[81]

Nakissa and associates reported ocular complications after radiation therapy of paranasal sinus malignancies. They found that there is sometimes a long delay, as long as 12 yr in one case, between radiation therapy and radiation optic neuropathy. They believe that retinal and optic nerve vessels are probably similar in sensitivity to radiation, and they point out that all their patients who had more than 5000 rads to the posterior chamber had recognizable retinal vascular changes. Two patients who had more than 6800 rads in 6 to 7 wk lost sight 2 to 5 yr after treatment.[82]

Two patients, who received both cranial radiation (2400 rads) and prophylactic chemotherapy for acute lymphocytic leukemia, developed radiation optic neuropathy, proven by craniotomy and biopsy of the involved optic nerves, which showed characteristic microvascular occlusive changes.[83] Chemotherapy is presumed, therefore, to have a potentiating effect, allowing normally tolerated amounts of irradiation to cause optic neuropathy.

The differential diagnosis of radiation-induced optic neuropathy includes recurrent tumor, empty sella syndrome, secondary malignant tumors presumed to be caused by irradiation, adhesive arachnoiditis, and radiation-induced optic neuropathy. Reliance is placed on modern neuroimaging to rule out most of these, with occasional need for CSF analysis if arachnoiditis is a serious issue. A case of malignant glioma of the optic chiasm believed to be caused by radiation for a pituitary tumor 8 yr earlier provides a good example of radiation-induced tumors, although these are probably more often sarcomas.[84]

Treatment is ineffective. Systemic corticosteroids and hyperbaric oxygen therapy given to 13 patients provided no indication of benefit.[85] Prevention seems to be the only approach to management of this serious complication of radiation therapy. The risks of the complication rise with increasing total dosage and with increasing daily dosage. Although there must be individual variation in susceptibility, and patients with diabetes mellitus and those receiving chemotherapy may be even more sensitive, a current reasonable guideline seems to be to avoid exceeding 185 rads/day, for a total of no more than 5000 rads.[86] Treatment of pituitary adenomas with more than 5000 rads probably does not produce improved therapeutic results, while significantly increasing the risk of complications.[87]

REFERENCES

1. Bansberg SF, Harner SG, Forbes G: Relationship of the optic nerve to the paranasal sinuses as shown by computed tomography. Otolaryngol Head Neck Surg 96:331, 1987.
2. Tarkkanen J, Tarkkanen A: Otorhinolaryngological pathology in patients with optic neuritis. Acta Ophthalmologica 49:649, 1971.
3. Slavin ML, Glaser JS: Acute severe irreversible visual loss with sphenoethmoiditis-'posterior' orbital cellulitis. Arch Ophthalmol 105:345, 1987.
4. Goldberg RA, Weisman JS, McFarland JE, et al: Orbital inflammation and optic neuropathies associated with chronic sinusitis of intranasal cocaine abuse. Arch Ophthalmol 107:831, 1989.
5. Lowe J, Bradley J: Cerebral and orbital *Aspergillus* infection due to invasive aspergillosis of ethmoid sinus. J Clin Pathol 39:774, 1986.
6. Corvisier N, Gray F, Gherardi R, et al: Aspergillosis of ethmoid sinus and optic nerve, with arteritis and rupture of the internal carotid artery. Surg Neurol 28:311, 1987.
7. Spoor TC, Hartel WC, Harding S, et al: Aspergillosis presenting as a corticosteroid-responsive optic neuropathy. J Clin Neuro Ophthalmol 2:103, 1982.
8. Kohn R, Hepler RS: Management of limited rhino-orbital mucormycosis without exenteration. Ophthalmology 92:1440, 1985.
9. Harbison JW, Lessel S, Selhorst JB: Neuro-ophthalmology of sphenoid sinus carcinoma. Brain 107:855, 1984.
10. Coppeto JR, Monteiro MLR, Cannarozzi DB: Optic neuropathy associated with chronic lymphomatous meningitis. J Clin Neuro Ophthalmol 8:39, 1988.
11. Kaufman LM, Folk ER, Chow JM: Invasive sinonasal polyps causing ophthalmoplegia, exophthalmos, and visual field loss. Ophthalmology 96:1667, 1989.
12. Stankiewicz JA: Blindness and intranasal endoscopic ethmoidectomy: prevention and management. Otolaryngol Head Neck Surg 101:320, 1989.
13. Avery G, Tang RA, Close, LG: Ophthalmic manifestations of mucoceles. Ann Ophthalmol 15:734, 1983.
14. Newton N, Baratham G, Sinniah R, et al: Bilateral compressive optic neuropathy secondary to bilateral sphenoethmoidal mucoceles. Ophthalmologica 198:13, 1989.
15. Yue CP, Mann KS, Chan FLC: Optic canal syndrome due to posterior ethmoid sinus mucocele. J Neurosurg 65:871, 1986.
16. Johnson LN, Hepler RS, Yee RD, et al: Sphenoid sinus mucocele (anterior clinoid variant) mimicking diabetic ophthalmoplegia and retrobulbar neuritis. Am J Ophthalmol 102:111, 1986.
17. Matsuoka S, Nishimura H, Kitamura K, et al: Circular enlargement of the optic canal caused by paranasal sinus mucocele. Surg Neurol 19:544, 1983.
18. Fujitani T, Takahashi T, Asai T: Optic nerve disturbance caused by frontal and fronto-ethmoidal mucopyoceles. Arch Otolaryngol 110:267, 1984.
19. Wurster CF, Levine TM, Sisson CA: Mucocele of the sphenoid sinus causing sudden onset of blindness. Otolaryngol Head Neck Surg 94:257, 1986.
20. Reicher MA, Bentson JR, Halbach VV, et al: Pneumosinus dilatans of the sphenoid sinus. AJNR 7:865, 1986.
21. Hirst LW, Miller NR, Hodges FJ, et al: Sphenoid pneumosinus dilatans: A sign of meningioma originating in the optic canal. Neuroradiology 22:207, 1982.
22. Spoor TC, Kennerdell JS, Maroon JC, et al: Pneumosinus dilatans, Klippel-Trenaunay-Weber syndrome, and progressive visual loss. Ann Ophthalmol 13:105, 1981.
23. Weisman JS, Hepler RS, Vinters HV: Reversible visual loss caused by fibrous dysplasia. Am J Ophthalmol 110:244, 1990.
24. Melen O, Weinberg PE, Kim KS, et al: Fibrous dysplasia of bone with acute visual loss. Ann Ophthalmol 12:734, 1980.
25. Weinstein JM, Lexow SS, Ho P, et al: Acute syphilitic optic neuritis. Arch Ophthalmol 99:1392, 1981.
26. Zambrano W, Perez GM, Smith JL: Acute syphilitic blindness in AIDS. J Clin Neuro Ophthalmol 7:1, 1987.
27. Toshniwal P: Optic perineuritis with secondary syphilis. J Clin Neuro Ophthalmol 7:6, 1987.
28. Rush JA, Ryan EJ: Syphilitic optic perineuritis. Am J Ophthalmol 91:404, 1981.
29. Folk JC, Weingeist TA, Corbett JJ, et al: Syphilitic neuroretinitis. Am J Ophthalmol 95:480, 1983.
30. Arruga J, Valentines J, Mauri F, et al: Neuroretinitis in acquired syphilis. Ophthalmology 92:262, 1985.
31. Carter JB, Hamill RJ, Matoba AY: Bilateral syphilitic optic neuritis in a patient with a positive test for HIV. Arch Ophthalmol 105:1485, 1987.
32. Burgdorfer W, Barbour AG, Hayes SF, et al: Lyme disease: A tick-borne spirochetosis? Science 216:1317, 1982.
33. Winward KE, Smith JL, Culbertson WW, et al: Ocular Lyme borreliosis. Am J Ophthalmol 108:651, 1989.
34. Winward KE, Smith JL, Culbertson WW, et al: Ocular Lyme borreliosis. Am J Ophthalmol 108:651, 1989.
35. Steere AC, Duray PH, Kauffmann DJH, et al: Unilateral blindness caused by infection with the Lyme disease spirochete, *Borrelia burgdorferi*. Ann Intern Med 103:382, 1985.
36. Farris BK, Webb RM: Lyme disease and optic neuritis. J Clin Neuro Ophthalmol 8:73, 1988.
37. Wilbrand H, Saenger A: Die Erkrankungen des Opticusstammes. *In* Die Neurologie des Auges, vol 5. Wiesbaden, Verlag von JF Bergmann, 1913.
38. Spaide R, Nattis R, Lipka A, et al: Ocular findings in leprosy in the United States. Am J Ophthalmol 100:411, 1985.
39. Margo CE, Sedwick LA, Rubin ML: Neuroretinitis in presumed visceral larva migrans. Retina 6:95, 1986.
40. Cox TA, Haskins GE, Gangitano JL, et al: Bilateral toxocara optic neuropathy. J Clin Neuro Ophthalmol 3:267, 1983.
41. Confavreux C, Girard-Madoux P, Moulin T, et al: Acute acquired toxoplasmosis causing neuroptico-meningoencephalitis in an immunocompetent boy. J Neurol Neurosurg Psychiatry 48:715, 1985.
42. Folk JC, Lobes LA: Presumed toxoplasmic papillitis. Ophthalmology 91:64, 1984.
43. Dreyer RF, Hopen G, Gass DM, et al: Leber's idiopathic stellate neuroretinitis. Arch Ophthalmol 102:1140, 1984.
44. Brazis PW, Stokes HR, Ervin FR: Optic neuritis in cat-scratch disease. J Clin Neuro Ophthalmol 6:172, 1986.
45. Schuil J, Richardus JH, Baarsma GS, et al: Q fever as a possible cause of bilateral optic neuritis. Br J Ophthalmol 69:580, 1984.
46. Giberson TP, Kalyan-Raman K: Cryptococcal meningitis: Initial presentation of acquired immunodeficiency syndrome. Ann Emerg Med 16:802, 1987.
47. Lipson BK, Freeman WR, Beniz J, et al: Optic neuropathy associated with cryptococcal arachnoiditis in AIDS patients. Am J Ophthalmol 107:523, 1989.
48. Ofner S, Baker RS: Visual loss in cryptococcal meningitis. J Clin Neuro Ophthalmol 7:45, 1987.
49. Hedges TR, Leung LE: Parasellar and orbital apex syndrome caused by aspergillosis. Neurology 26:117, 1976.
50. Li PKT, Lai KN: Amphotericin B induced ocular toxicity in cryptococcal meningitis. Br J Ophthalmol 73:397, 1989.

51. Selbst RG, Selhorst JB, Harbison JW, et al: Parainfectious optic neuritis. Arch Neurol 40:347, 1983.
52. Miller DH, Kay R, Schon F, et al: Optic neuritis following chicken pox in adults. J Neurol 233:182, 1986.
53. Purvin V, Herr GJ, De Myer W: Chiasmal neuritis as a complication of Epstein-Barr virus infection. Arch Neurol 45:485, 1988.
54. Pall HS, Williams AC: Subacute polyradiculopathy with optic and auditory nerve involvement. Arch Neurol 44:885, 1987.
55. Purvin V, Hrisomalos N, Dunn D: Varicella optic neuritis. Neurology 38:501, 1988.
56. Perry HD, Mallen FJ, Grodin RW, et al: Reversible blindness in optic neuritis associated with influenza vaccination. Ann Ophthalmol 11:545, 1979.
57. Bienfang DC, Kantrowitz FG, Noble JL, et al: Ocular abnormalities after influenza immunization. Arch Ophthalmol 95:1649, 1977.
58. Cangemi FE, Bergen RL: Optic atrophy following swine flu vaccination. Ann Ophthalmol 12:857, 1980.
59. Kazarian EL, Gager WE: Optic neuritis complicating measles, mumps, and rubella vaccination. Am J Ophthalmol 86:544, 1978.
60. Maitland CG, Miller NR: Neuroretinitis. Arch Ophthalmol 102:1146, 1984.
61. Parmley VC, Schiffman JS, Maitland CG, et al: Does neuroretinitis rule out multiple sclerosis? Arch Neurol 44:1045, 1987.
62. Winward KE, Hamed LM, Glaser JS: The spectrum of optic nerve disease in human immunodeficiency virus infection. Am J Ophthalmol 107:373, 1989.
63. Grossniklaus HE, Frank KE, Tomsak RL: Cytomegalovirus retinitis and optic neuritis in acquired immune deficiency syndrome. Ophthalmology 94:1601, 1987.
64. Manor RS, Cohen S, Ben-Sira T: Bilateral acute retrobulbar optic neuropathy associated with epidemic keratoconjunctivitis in a compromised host. Arch Ophthalmol 104:1271, 1986.
65. Jones J, Gardner W, Newman T: Severe optic neuritis in infectious mononucleosis. Ann Emerg Med 17:361, 1988.
66. Johnson BL, Wisotzkey HM: Neuroretinitis associated with herpes simplex encephalitis in an adult. Am J Ophthalmol 83:481, 1977.
67. Krohel GB, Charles H, Smith RS: Granulomatous optic neuropathy. Arch Ophthalmol 99:1053, 1981.
68. Beardsley TL, Brown SVL, Sydnor CF, et al: Eleven cases of sarcoidosis of the optic nerve. Am J Ophthalmol 97:62, 1984.
69. Mansour AM: Sarcoid optic disc edema and optociliary shunts. J Clin Neuro Ophthalmol 6:47, 1986.
70. Jordan DR, Anderson RL, Nerad JA, et al: Optic nerve involvement as the initial manifestation of sarcoidosis. Can J Ophthalmol 23:232, 1988.
71. Gelwan MJ, Kellen RI, Burde RM, et al: Sarcoidosis of the anterior visual pathway: Successes and failures. J Neurol Neurosurg Psychiatry 51:1473, 1988.
72. Jabs DA, Miller NR, Newman SA, et al: Optic neuropathy in systemic lupus erythematosus. Arch Ophthalmol 104:564, 1986.
73. Kupersmith MJ, Burde RM, Warren FA, et al: Autoimmune optic neuropathy: evaluation and treatment. J Neurol Neurosurg Psychiatry 51:1381, 1988.
74. Dutton JJ, Anderson RL: Idiopathic inflammatory perioptic neuritis simulating optic nerve sheath meningioma. Am J Ophthalmol 100:424, 1985.
75. Margo CE, Levy MH, Beck RW: Bilateral idiopathic inflammation of the optic nerve sheaths. Ophthalmology 96:200, 1989.
76. Gross FJ, Waxman JS, Rosenblatt MA, et al: Eosinophilic granuloma of the cavernous sinus and orbital apex in an HIV-positive patient. Ophthalmology 96:462, 1989.
77. Schatz NJ, Lichtenstein S, Corbett JJ: Delayed radiation necrosis of the optic nerves and chiasm. *In* Smith JL, Glaser JS (eds): Symposium of the University of Miami and Bascom Palmer Eye Institute, vol VIII. St Louis, CV Mosby, 1975.
78. Brown GC, Shields JA, Sanborn G, et al: Radiation optic neuropathy. Ophthalmology 89:1489, 1982.
79. Kline LB, Kim JY, Ceballos R: Radiation optic neuropathy. Ophthalmology 92:1118, 1985.
80. Guy J, Mancuso A, Quisling RG, et al: Gadolinium-DPTA-enhanced magnetic resonance imaging in optic neuropathies. Ophthalmology 97:592, 1990.
81. Zimmerman CF, Schatz NJ, Glaser JS: Magnetic resonance imaging of radiation optic neuropathy. Am J Ophthalmol 110:389, 1990.
82. Nakissa N, Rubin P, Strohl R, et al: Ocular and orbital complications following radiation therapy of paranasal sinus malignancies and review of literature. Cancer 51:980, 1983.
83. Fishman ML, Bean SC, Cogan DG: Optic atrophy following prophylactic chemotherapy and cranial radiation for acute lymphocytic leukemia. Am J Ophthalmol 82:571, 1976.
84. Hufnagel TJ, Kim JH, Lesser R, et al: Malignant glioma of the optic chiasm eight years after radiotherapy for prolactinoma. Arch Ophthalmol 106:1701, 1988.
85. Roden D, Bosley TM, Fowble B, et al: Delayed radiation injury to the retrobulbar optic nerves and chiasm. Ophthalmology 97:346, 1990.
86. Parker R: Personal communication with the author, July 1991.
87. Aristizabal S, Caldwell WL, Avila J: The relationship of time-dose factors to complications in the treatment of pituitary tumors by irradiation. Int J Radiat Oncol Biol Phys 2:667, 1977.

Chapter 207

Chiasmal Disorders

JOHN W. GITTINGER JR.

THE CHIASM

The terms *chiasm, chiasma*, and *optic chiasm* derive from the Greek letter *chi* (χ) and refer to the gross anatomic appearance of the plate of neural tissue that extends from the optic nerves anteriorly to the optic tracts posteriorly and contains the axons and supporting tissues of the afferent visual system. Hoyt describes the chiasm as a flattened oblong structure approximately 4 mm thick, 12 mm wide, and 8 mm long, formed by the union of the intracranial optic nerves.[1] Bergland and associates measured the average width of the chiasm at autopsy as 10 mm.[2]

The chiasm is located at the junction of the floor and anterior wall of the third ventricle at the base of the brain. Obstructive hydrocephalus may produce an enlarged third ventricle, which, acting as a mass, compresses the chiasm.[3]

A semidecussation as the explanation for the existence of the chiasm was first postulated in writing by Sir Isaac

Newton in 1704 but did not achieve scientific recognition and clinical relevance until William Hyde Wollaston independently developed the concept and presented his own case of recurrent hemianopia to the Royal Society in 1824.[4, 5] Wollaston died 5 yr later of a right thalamic tumor.

Axonal Arrangement in the Anterior Visual Pathways

The chiasmal bar contains decussating axons from both optic nerves. Axons arising from retinal ganglion cells nasal to the fovea, which carry information from the temporal visual fields, cross the midline to join the axons from the temporal retinal ganglion cells and form the optic tracts. Each optic tract thus carries visual information from the contralateral visual fields of both eyes to the lateral geniculate bodies, fulfilling the physiologic rule that sensory input from one side of the body must be processed in the thalamus of the contralateral hemisphere.

Because the watershed for this decussation passes through the fovea, not the optic nerve, the blind spot lies entirely within the temporal visual field. Even with the blind spot, the temporal visual field has a larger area than the nasal visual field, and the majority (about 53 percent[6]) of axons in each optic nerve decussate. An exception is the visual system of albinos, in which additional nasal fibers, representing 20 degrees of temporal field, also decussate.[7] The basis for the anomalous distribution of ganglion cell axons in albinism is not understood.

Studies published in the early 1960s by Hoyt and coworkers clarify the distribution of chiasmal axons in primates.[8–10] After the retinal ganglion cells of macaque monkeys were destroyed focally by photocoagulation, their axons were traced through the chiasm and into the optic tract using Nauta's degeneration technique. This technique revealed that macular ganglion cell axons are widely distributed throughout the chiasm; only thin areas of anterior and posterior inferior chiasm are free of macular fibers. A group of crossed inferior quadrant extramacular ganglion cell axons extends forward into the posterior optic nerve. This "knee of von Willebrand" is the anatomic substrate for the superior quadrantic visual field defects in the contralateral eye found in some posterior optic nerve lesions.

Relationships of the Chiasm

VASCULAR RELATIONSHIPS

The visual pathways pass through the circle of Willis, and the chiasm is flanked by the supraclinoid segments of the carotid arteries. The anterior cerebral and anterior communicating arteries lie above the plane of the visual pathways, and the posterior communicating, posterior cerebral, and basilar arteries below. The arterial supply of the chiasm derives from all of these vessels, even in some cases the small anterior communicating artery.[11, 12]

Bergland and Ray divided the chiasmal arteries into a superior and an inferior group.[13] Because the inferior group supplies the chiasmal bar, they postulated that this arterial distribution makes the decussating axons more vulnerable to compression from below by pituitary adenomas and suggested that this would explain the evolution of chiasmal visual field defects observed in pituitary adenomas. The superotemporal fields are affected early, but the superonasal fields, whose undecussated axons lie laterally in the chiasm and are thus supplied by the superior group of arteries, are spared until late in the course. Hoyt, however, argues that the compressive force from a tumor could never exceed arterial perfusion pressure; thus, the pattern of arterial supply would not account for the selective vulnerability of decussating fibers.[1]

PITUITARY BODY

The most important relationship of the chiasm clinically is with the pituitary body or hypophysis. The infundibulum arises from the ventral diencephalon behind the chiasm and extends downward into the pituitary fossa to connect with the posterior lobe of the pituitary or neurohypophysis. The anterior lobe of the pituitary body, or adenohypophysis, forms from an embryologic structure connected to the pharynx known as *Rathke's pouch*.

The chiasm does not cap the pituitary fossa but rather lies about 1 cm above it, inclining forward as much as 45 degrees from the horizontal.[1] Tumors arising in the sella must be large before they impact on the visual pathways. As a consequence, radiologic enlargement of the bony sella is present in most patients in whom visual loss is secondary to pituitary tumor,[14] with only a few exceptions.[15] The converse is also true: A patient who has bitemporal visual field loss and a normal sella on plain films is unlikely to have a pituitary adenoma.

Cushing called attention to a chiasmal syndrome of optic atrophy, bitemporal hemianopia, and a normal sella as being characteristic of suprasellar meningiomas[16] but also described these same findings in rare pituitary adenomas and in craniopharyngiomas, optic gliomas, aneurysms, and chordomas.[17] Because of the emphasis on computed tomography (CT) and magnetic resonance imaging (MRI) in current practice, plain views of the sella are often not taken, although they may still have diagnostic value.

The chiasm usually lies directly above the pituitary fossa of the sella turcica, but because of normal variations in the length of the optic nerves, about 9 percent overlie the tuberculum sella anteriorly and about 11 percent overlie the dorsum sella posteriorly.[2] The former are termed *prefixed*, and the latter *postfixed*. A tumor growing out of the pituitary fossa impinges first on the posterior aspect of a prefixed chiasm, and a neurosurgeon may have difficulty reaching the tumor through a subfrontal approach.[12, 18]

VISUAL FIELD TESTING

The major role of ophthalmologists in the diagnosis and management of chiasmal disorders is to assess visual function accurately and to interpret the results. Failure to perform or to interpret visual fields properly is a common cause of delay in the diagnosis of chiasmal disorders.[19, 20] In the United States at least, this has become a significant medicolegal issue.

A comprehensive review of visual field testing techniques is beyond the scope of this discussion. All of the methods of plotting the visual field in current use—the tangent screen,[21] quantitative kinetic perimetry on Goldmann's perimeter,[22] suprathreshold static perimetry,[23, 24] and threshold static perimetry[25]—are capable of detecting visual field loss from chiasmal compression when properly applied. The use of colored stimuli in special modifications of kinetic perimetry[26] and confrontation techniques[27] has advocates but should probably be considered only supplementary to conventional perimetry.

The most important factor in ensuring detection of chiasmal visual field loss is testing on either side of the vertical meridian through fixation within the central 20 to 30 degrees from fixation.[28] The clinical principle is consistent with the earlier cited anatomic observations that the chiasm contains large macular projections. A useful rule is that any patient with unexplained reduction in visual acuity should have a visual field test to assess the possibility of chiasmal compression.

CLINICAL FINDINGS

Patterns of Visual Field Loss

(Table 207–1)

The classic chiasmal visual field defect is a bitemporal depression greater near fixation. When the chiasm is compressed from below by a pituitary adenoma, the pattern most often observed is a bitemporal superior hemianopia. Conversely, compression of the chiasm from above—as occurs with a craniopharyngioma or dysgerminoma (discussed later)—typically produces an inferior bitemporal hemianopia. In occasional patients, chiasmal compression does not produce a recognizable pattern of visual field loss.[29]

At surgery, large tumor masses are seen to distort and compress the chiasm, making specific localization from visual field defects alone moot. When the following discussion is compared with Adler and coworkers' review of this subject in 1948,[30] it will be apparent that little has been added in the past 50 yr to our knowledge of those visual field patterns with localizing value.

Table 207–1. PATTERNS OF VISUAL FIELD LOSS IN CHIASMAL DISORDERS

Bitemporal depressions
Bitemporal hemianopic scotomata
Monocular
Superior temporal defect
Central scotoma
Nerve fiber bundle defects
Hemianopic arcuate scotoma
Inferior altitudinal hemianopia
Binasal field defects
Homonymous hemianopias

BITEMPORAL HEMIANOPIC SCOTOMATA

Bitemporal hemianopic scotomata have been thought to suggest that the chiasm is being compressed from behind; however, Frisén found prefixed chiasms at surgery in only two of his eight patients with scotomatous bitemporal field defects; two others had postfixed chiasms.[31] Traquair suggested that this pattern of field loss denotes a more rapidly growing tumor,[32] an opinion supported by Sugita and coworkers' finding at surgery of hemorrhagic cysts in the pituitary adenomas of four of eight patients with such scotomatous defects.[33] Care must be taken to distinguish enlargement of the blind spots or bilateral centrocecal scotomata from true bitemporal scotomata.

MONOCULAR VISUAL FIELD DEFECTS

Monocular visual field defects were detected in 9 percent of the 1000 patients in the Mayo Clinic series. The most common monocular visual field defect (33 of 61 eyes) was a superior temporal defect.[34] Monocular temporal hemianopia in the absence of optic atrophy and a relative afferent pupillary defect is, however, a surprisingly common variant of psychogenic visual loss.[35] Testing of the visual fields binocularly usually confirms the nonphysiologic basis of this pattern of visual loss.[36]

A central or hemicentral scotoma accompanied by superior temporal visual field loss in the opposite eye points to compression at the junction of the optic nerve and chiasm.[37] This pattern of field loss is less often encountered with pituitary adenomas than it is with meningiomas and craniopharyngiomas,[31] although unilateral central[38] and centrocecal scotomata[39] are reported as the presentation of pituitary tumors. The hemianopic character of compressive visual loss should be apparent if attention is paid to differences in sensitivity across the vertical meridian through fixation during perimetric testing.[40]

NERVE FIBER BUNDLE DEFECTS

The nerve fiber bundle arrangement of the retina continues at least as far as the anterior chiasm.[41] A hemianopic arcuate scotoma suggests early chiasmal compression[42] and also points to the anterior chiasm. An inferior altitudinal hemianopia in one or both eyes may denote compression of the optic nerve against the roof of the inner opening of the optic canal.[43] Bilateral nerve fiber defects, with or without associated central scotomata, are occasionally reported in chiasmal compression.[44] The mechanism of such field loss is not known; impairment of circulation in the anastomotic prechiasmal arterial plexus has been postulated.[45]

BINASAL FIELD DEFECTS

At no place in the visual system do the axons arising in the two retinas temporal to fixation intermingle, and bilateral nasal field loss thus requires two anatomically distinct lesions. True binasal hemianopias respecting the vertical meridian through fixation are rarely encountered.[46] Their detection should raise the possibility of psychogenic visual loss.[47, 48] The most common cause of bilateral nasal field loss is optic nerve damage—glaucoma, optic disc drusen, and papilledema—but such field loss does not respect the vertical meridian through fixation and may point toward the blind spot (nerve fiber bundle defect).

Bilateral nasal field loss in the context of chiasmal compression suggests lateral compression of the chiasm, with the lesion lying on the side of the greater defect pressing the chiasm against the contralateral carotid artery.[49] Nasal field loss may also be encountered with optochiasmic arachnoiditis (discussed later) and as a postoperative defect.[50]

HOMONYMOUS HEMIANOPIA

Frisén distinguishes a median chiasmal syndrome, with bitemporal visual field defects, from a lateral chiasmal syndrome, with hemianopic patterns of visual field loss.[31] In median chiasmal syndromes, the visual acuities in both eyes reflect the severity of visual field loss. In lateral chiasmal syndromes, acuity in the contralateral eye is usually preserved.

Just as central scotomata and arcuate visual field defects point to the anterior chiasm/posterior optic nerve, homonymous hemianopias denote involvement at the posterior chiasm/anterior optic tract. Isolated optic tract lesions are uncommon, both because of the intimate relationship of the tract to the brain stem and because the nature of its vascular supply makes infarction rare. Characteristics of optic tract hemianopias include reduction in ipsilateral visual acuity, defects with both bitemporal and hemianopic character, incongruity, associated bow-tie optic atrophy (from selective involvement of decussated axons), and a contralateral relative afferent pupillary defect.[51–53]

Optic Disc

Axonal loss due to compression of the pregeniculate visual pathways eventually leads to disc pallor, and optic atrophy is encountered in patients presenting with pituitary adenomas and visual field defects. In the Mayo Clinic series studied between 1935 and 1972, disc pallor was recognized in 34 percent of eyes and field defects in 67 percent.[34] Unequivocal pallor of one or both discs was present in 28 of 50 patients with pituitary tumors encountered at the Guy's-Maudsley Neurosurgical Unit in London between 1953 and 1964.[54] With improved endocrinologic diagnosis, the percentage of patients with optic atrophy (and field defects) appears to be declining. Only 4 of 200 consecutive patients admitted to the neuroendocrine service at the Montreal General Hospital between 1976 and 1981 had optic atrophy.[55]

Optic atrophy is a late sign of chiasmal compression. Trobe and coworkers found that disc pallor was significantly but weakly correlated with the duration of visual symptoms and strongly correlated with persistent decreased postoperative acuity.[56]

Even before optic atrophy is recognizable, drop-out of axons in the peripapillary nerve fiber layers may be visible, especially photographically and ophthalmoscopically with red-free light.[57] Exclusive loss of decussating axons may produce bow-tie or butterfly optic atrophy, with pallor limited to the nasal and temporal disc.[58] This appearance is not usually encountered with compressive lesions because the nondecussating axons are simultaneously damaged.

Ocular Motility

Lateral to the sella turcica lie the cavernous sinuses, with the ocular motor cranial nerves. Processes such as pituitary adenomas may spread laterally and compress these nerves, producing ophthalmoplegia.[59, 60] Sudden enlargement of pituitary adenomas may present as painful ophthalmoplegia, with or without visual loss (see Pituitary Apoplexy, later). Patients in whom ptosis was the initial manifestation of a pituitary adenoma usually have other associated findings on neuroophthalmic examination.[61]

SEE-SAW NYSTAGMUS

Rhythmic intorsion and elevation of one eye accompanied by extorsion and depression of the other is appropriately called *see-saw nystagmus*, because the eyes appear to be riding a see-saw whose fulcrum is the nose. This unusual ocular motility disturbance is usually associated with bitemporal hemianopias caused by tumor or trauma,[62] but see-saw nystagmus has been a transient finding after isolated brain stem stroke.[63, 64] When trauma is the precipitating factor, a delay of weeks to months follows the severe head injury before see-saw nystagmus appears. Oscillopsia may signal the development of see-saw nystagmus.[65]

Vision appears to have a role in its pathogenesis, because see-saw nystagmus ceases when the eyes are closed and does not develop in blind patients. A lesion involving the Cajal's interstitial nucleus and its connections or dysfunction of the ocular counterrolling system mediated by the inferior olivary nucleus has been postulated. Although other causes must be considered—and see-saw nystagmus is encountered as a variant of congenital nystagmus[66]—the presence of see-saw nystagmus should prompt evaluation for a perichiasmal tumor.

Other Sensory Disturbances

Peripheral field and central visual loss in one eye are often asymptomatic. Photopsias and photophobia may be the presentation of various disorders of the anterior visual pathways including chiasmal compression.[67] Formed visual hallucinations are occasionally associated with the visual loss of chiasmal compression,[68, 69] but such hallucinations develop in other cases of visual loss involving the anterior visual system and are therefore nonspecific.[70]

NONPARETIC DIPLOPIA

A sensory phenomenon relatively specific to chiasmal visual field loss is nonparetic diplopia.[71] The two nasal hemifields do not overlap, and patients with a complete bitemporal hemianopia lose binocular fusional stabilization. In some cases, an underlying phoria may then produce doubling of images,[72] a phenomenon called *hemifield slide*.[73]

CHIASMAL SYNDROMES
(Table 207–2)

Pituitary Adenomas (Table 207–3)

By far the most common perichiasmal tumor, pituitary adenomas manifest in many ways. In general, tumors that secrete hormones such as prolactin, growth hormone, or adrenocorticotropic hormone are detected when they are small (i.e., less than 10 mm in diameter). Such microadenomas do not compress the visual pathways. Nonsecretory tumors are detected when they reach a size that produces visual symptoms. Some secretory adenomas, however, become macroadenomas before discovery or during follow-up.

Enlarging nonsecretory adenomas eventually cause hypopituitarism. A rule of thumb useful in the evaluation of visual loss is that an adenoma large enough to compress the chiasm is attended by altered pituitary function. Potent males or menstruating females are thus unlikely to have pituitary adenomas as the cause of their decreased vision. Another common symptom of pituitary adenomas is headache.[74]

Table 207–2. CAUSES OF CHIASMAL COMPRESSION/INFILTRATION

Tumors
Pituitary adenomas
Craniopharygiomas
Meningiomas
Germinomas
Optic gliomas
Malignant optic gliomas
Gangliogliomas
Choristomas
Chordomas
Cavernous hemangiomas
Leukemias and lymphomas
Metastatic tumors

Vascular Structures
Vessels
Aneurysms
Arteriovenous malformations

Other Processes
Sarcoidosis
Lymphoid hypophysitis
Pituitary abscess
Sphenoidal sinus mucocele
Empty sella syndrome
Arachnoid and other cysts

Table 207–3. MANIFESTATIONS OF PITUITARY TUMORS

- Nonvisual (endocrine):
  - Hypopituitarism
  - Acromegaly
  - Amenorrhea/galactorrhea
  - Cushing's syndrome
  - Headache
- Visual:
  - Visual loss
    - Decreased acuity
    - Visual field defects
    - Optic atrophy
  - Visual disturbances
    - Diplopia
    - Photophobia
    - Oscillopsia
    - Photopsias
    - Formed hallucinations
  - Ocular motility disturbances
    - Ptosis
    - Ophthalmoplegia
    - See-saw nystagmus

PITUITARY APOPLEXY

Sudden enlargement of a pituitary adenoma because of hemorrhage or infarction produces headache, visual loss, and ophthalmoplegia. This syndrome is usually called *pituitary apoplexy*. Some prefer to limit this designation to its original application—spontaneous infarction of nontumorous pituitary glands with subsequent hypopituitarism[75]—but the definition has in practice been expanded to any manifestation of a rapidly enlarging pituitary tumor, including sudden visual loss or ophthalmoplegia.[76] Various predisposing factors have been postulated, including head trauma, radiation therapy, anticoagulation, estrogen therapy, angiography,[77] atheromatous emboli,[78] and coughing.[79] Persons with diabetes, sickle cell trait, acromegaly, Cushing's disease, or pregnancy are sometimes considered to be at increased risk.[80] In many cases, no obvious precipitating factor is recognizable, and the tumor was previously asymptomatic.

Pituitary apoplexy presents both diagnostic and therapeutic problems.[81] Massive enlargement of a pituitary tumor mimics meningitis, encephalitis, or other causes of intracranial bleeding. Physicians evaluating patients with a severe headache and alteration of consciousness may not initially detect visual loss or ophthalmoplegia, and interpretation of noncontrast CT obtained to look for subarachnoid hemorrhage is difficult in the region of the chiasm. MRI, which is more sensitive to the presence of hemorrhage, improves diagnostic sensitivity[82] in this and other lesions near the chiasm.

Surgical intervention with corticosteroid coverage is indicated to decompress the visual pathways in patients with acute severe visual loss or alteration in consciousness. Conservative management may be warranted for ophthalmoplegia only, for minor degrees of visual loss, or when patients present some time after the onset of symptoms and are stable and conscious, because the swollen tumor mass may shrink spontaneously with time. The endocrinologic status of all patients with pituitary apoplexy must be monitored.

CHIASMAL APOPLEXY

Pituitary apoplexy should be distinguished from the less common chiasmal apoplexy, in which visual loss is the result of hemorrhage from an intrachiasmal vascular malformation or tumor or into an optic glioma.[83, 84] Cavernous hemangiomas (cavernous angiomas, cavernomas) of the chiasm, which appear on CT as circumscribed hyperdense lesions with moderate enhancement and on MRI as a heterogenous pattern of hypointensity and hyperintensity on T_1- and T_2-weighted images, characteristically present as chiasmal apoplexy and may be familial.[85, 86] Chiasmal apoplexy may be recurrent, and surgical evacuation of the bleed is sometimes warranted.[87, 88] Both cavernous hemangiomas and intrachiasmal vascular malformations may also cause gradual visual loss.[89] The presence of cutaneous or orbital malformations may provide a clue to the presence of intracranial vascular malformations.[90]

MANAGEMENT OF PITUITARY ADENOMAS

A primary goal of the treatment of pituitary adenomas is preservation of vision. Visual dysfunction is caused by compression of the visual pathways or ocular motor nerves or their vascular supplies. Relief of this compression may be accomplished surgically or medically.

Surgical treatment consists of transsphenoidal, transethmoidal, or transfrontal removal of the tumor. Since the 1950s there has been a movement toward transsphenoidal surgery, with numerous centers documenting a good visual response.[91–94] Among 714 patients who had pituitary adenomas and underwent transsphenoidal surgery at the Mayo Clinic between 1971 and 1982, 115 had decreased acuity preoperatively.[95] Fifty-three improved postoperatively, and two worsened. Similarly, of 230 patients with preoperative visual field abnormalities, 168 improved postoperatively and 10 worsened. Five patients with normal acuity and fields preoperatively had deficits postoperatively. Improvement in vision may be incomplete or delayed, and at least 10 wk should pass before the final effect of the surgery on vision is assessed.[96]

Transsphenoidal surgery is not without complications, including death, stroke, hemorrhage, visual loss, meningitis, cerebrospinal fluid rhinorrhea, ophthalmoplegia, permanent diabetes insipidus, hypopituitarism, and nasal septal perforation.[97] In eight series before 1983, the average complication rate was 2.3 percent, a rate Laws and coworkers considered acceptable.[97]

A measure that is an alternative or adjunct to surgery is bromocriptine for prolactin-secreting adenomas.[98] Administration of this dopamine agonist usually reduces the size of the tumor, improving visual and endocrine function and making surgical removal easier in some instances.[99, 100] Rapid improvement of visual loss may be accomplished with bromocriptine treatment alone.[101] Unfortunately, bromocriptine appears only to suppress, not cure, the tumor, which often regrows when the drug is discontinued.[102]

Bromocriptine may be especially useful when a prolactin-secreting adenoma invades the cavernous sinus or the middle or posterior cranial fossa—a situation in which complete surgical removal is difficult. In one case that I evaluated, administration of bromocriptine led to resolution of bitemporal hemianopia and fifth- and sixth-nerve palsy.[103]

Both the normal pituitary and pituitary adenomas tend to enlarge during pregnancy, with involution after delivery. The management of women who become pregnant during bromocriptine therapy or who are found to have a pituitary adenoma while pregnant is controversial.[104] Gemzell and Wang recommend monthly visual field testing during pregnancy.[105] Newman gives patients an Amsler's grid with red dots set across the vertical midline to allow them to monitor their own fields.[106]

The role of irradiation in the management of pituitary adenomas is also unclear. Radiotherapy has been used as an adjunct to surgery, when other treatment has failed, and as a primary therapy. Visual improvement after radiotherapy is documented, but some patients become blind after an interval of months to years.[107] The likelihood of radiation damage to the chiasm or optic nerves increases with fraction sizes greater than 250 rad.[108]

Causes of delayed visual loss after treatment include recurrence of the tumor, an empty sella syndrome, optochiasmatic arachnoiditis, and radionecrosis (discussed later). Differentiation among these mechanisms has become less difficult with improved neuroimaging techniques.

Meningiomas

Meningiomas arising from the dura of the tuberculum sellae and adjacent structures (including the sphenoid plane) compress the optic nerves and chiasm as they grow. Meningiomas developing in the parasellar, frontal, and subfrontal regions may also impinge on the chiasm.[109] In a monumental report, Cushing and Eisenhardt first called attention to a chiasmal syndrome of primary optic atrophy, bitemporal hemianopia, and a normal sella (at least when the tumor is small) in middle-aged patients as signaling the presence of a tuberculum sellae meningioma.[110] Symmetric bitemporal hemianopia was uncommon in Cushing and Eisenhardt's cases, and Huber points out that asymmetry of visual loss—many of his patients were blind in one eye and had a temporal hemianopia in the other—and slow progression are characteristic of meningiomas.[111] Visual loss may occasionally be rapidly progressive.[112]

In the pre-CT era, the detection and differential diagnosis of tuberculum sellae meningiomas were especially difficult, and the visual loss they caused was often attributed to chronic retrobulbar neuritis[113] or low-tension glaucoma. Abnormalities detectable on skull radiographs—including hyperostosis, calcification, blistering of the planum sphenoidale or tuberculum sellae, enlarged sella turcica, and erosion of the sella turcica, dorsum sellae, or anterior clinoids—are not always present. Expansion of the sinuses because of entrapment of air, known as pneumosinus dilatans, is also sometimes associated with meningiomas or may develop idiopathically and compress the chiasm and optic nerves.[114]

Even in the modern era, a small meningioma may escape detection. In a case reported on two occasions by Coppeto and Gahm,[115] bitemporal hemianopic scotomata were attributed to chiasmal compression by an intraventricular catheter, but CT 7 yr later demonstrated a meningioma of the planum sphenoidale.[116] (The significance of another possible case of compression of the chiasm by an intraventricular catheter reported in the interim is unclear.[117])

Earlier diagnosis of meningiomas of the tuberculum sellae with CT and MRI may improve visual prognosis.[118] In the series reported from the Neurological Institute of New York, 90 percent of patients with tumors 3 cm or smaller had improved visual acuity at hospital discharge, compared with 52 percent with larger tumors.[119] Despite the evolution of imaging techniques, preoperative angiography is considered essential in planning the surgical approach.[120]

Craniopharyngiomas

Hoffman[121] defines craniopharyngiomas as benign tumors that arise from squamous cell rests in the incompletely involuted hypophyseal-pharyngeal duct[122] or Rathke's pouch. Craniopharyngiomas are related to Rathke's pouch cysts, intrasellar cysts with linings of cuboidal or columnar and sometimes goblet cells, and to the epidermoid and dermoid cysts of this region.[123]

Craniopharyngiomas are presumed to be congenital tumors and have both a solid component that grows slowly and a cystic component that can expand rapidly. The tumor may be supra- or intrasellar, and rare instances of intrachiasmatic craniopharyngiomas mimic optic gliomas.[124] Extension into the third ventricle is common, and a few craniopharyngiomas are wholly intraventricular.[125] Craniopharyngiomas thus may present with signs of hydrocephalus or of brain stem and cerebellar compression.

DIAGNOSIS OF CRANIOPHARYNGIOMAS

Although craniopharyngiomas are more frequently encountered in childhood, they may present at any age.[126] Children with craniopharyngiomas present with visual loss, signs of increased intracranial pressure (headaches and vomiting), and growth disturbances. In pituitary adenomas, diabetes insipidus occurs almost exclusively postoperatively; however, this endocrinologic disorder may precede surgical intervention in craniopharyngiomas. In adults, visual loss and headaches are the common reasons to seek medical attention. Psychiatric symptoms including dementia are more common in adults than children. Unusual manifestations of craniopharyngiomas include recurrent meningitis due to leakage of cyst fluid[127, 128] and see-saw nystagmus (discussed earlier).

The varied manifestations of craniopharyngiomas result in frequent delay or misdiagnosis. Miller states that craniopharyngiomas are more likely than any other lesion of the anterior visual system to be mistaken for functional visual loss.[129] Like pituitary adenomas and meningiomas, craniopharyngiomas may cause monocular visual loss that is mistaken for optic neuritis.[130]

The pattern of visual field loss encountered in patients with a craniopharyngioma depends on the location and size of the tumor. The expected inferior bitemporal hemianopia, representing compression of the chiasm from above, is less common than an asymmetric bitemporal or homonymous hemianopia. At Wills Eye Hospital in Philadelphia, craniopharyngiomas were the most common tumor causing visual field defects localizable to the optic tract.[51]

Craniopharyngiomas in children usually calcify, thus simplifying their recognition and diagnosis on plain skull radiographs. In adults, in whom calcification is less common, the tumor may have a density similar to cerebrospinal fluid and brain, leading to difficulties in interpreting CT findings. MRI is more sensitive than CT in the diagnosis of such noncalcified craniopharyngiomas.[131]

MANAGEMENT OF CRANIOPHARYNGIOMAS

Complete surgical removal of craniopharyngiomas is more difficult than that of pituitary adenomas, and the parameters for optimal surgical management remain controversial.[132, 133] The major indication for surgery is to decompress the visual pathways, but the visual prognosis for patients with craniopharyngiomas after decompression is not as favorable as with pituitary adenomas.[134, 135] An approach used in some centers is subtotal resection followed by external beam irradiation,[136] but about one quarter recur symptomatically in 10 yr.[137] An alternative therapy used at the University of Michigan Medical Center is cyst aspiration with instillation of ^{32}P.[138]

Both surgery and radiation have significant side effects, especially on the developing brain of children with craniopharyngiomas. Frontal lobe abnormalities on MRI in survivors of craniopharyngioma led Stelling and coworkers to suggest gentle intraoperative retraction.[139] Secondary malignant gliomas follow irradiation.[140] The outcome in patients with craniopharyngioma is uncertain even when the tumor is promptly diagnosed and treated.

Other Chiasmal Tumors

GERMINOMAS

Suprasellar germinomas, also known as *ectopic pinealomas* or *atypical teratomas*, are germ cell tumors that characteristically manifest as the triad of visual loss, diabetes insipidus, and hypopituitarism in young persons.[141, 142] Diabetes insipidus usually precedes the visual loss. Although an inferior bitemporal defect might be expected as the result of compression of the chiasm from above, various chiasmal visual field defects that are encountered may be the result of tumor infiltration into the visual pathways.[143] Familial occurrence of suprasellar yolk sac tumors, another germ cell tumor, has been reported from Japan.[144] Germinomas are radiosensitive, and vision may improve after treatment.

OPTIC GLIOMAS

Although occasional reports describe gangliogliomas[145] or choristomas,[146] the vast majority of tumors of the anterior visual pathways are histologically benign pilocytic astrocytomas, called *optic gliomas*. Most optic gliomas are discovered in children. The much less common malignant optic glioma of adulthood is a glioblastoma involving the visual pathways, usually leading to death within 1 yr.[147] Rare instances of malignant evolution of childhood optic glioma may be related to radiation therapy.[148]

The prognosis for childhood optic gliomas depends on their location.[149] In general, the more anterior the tumor, the better the prognosis for life and vision. Optic gliomas are commonly associated with neurofibromatosis, and screening imaging studies performed on asymptomatic children with neurofibromatosis uncovers many incidental gliomas.[150]

Although gliomas of the optic nerve characteristically cause unilateral visual loss or proptosis, chiasmal gliomas produce bilateral visual loss and optic atrophy. Diagnosis is often delayed.[151] A presentation that causes much diagnostic difficulty is nystagmus in infancy.[152] Children with optic gliomas may have nystagmus indistinguishable from that of spasmus nutans, a benign developmental problem,[153] or of Leber's congenital amaurosis (and other congenital sensory disorders).[154] Optic atrophy may not be apparent initially. Other manifestations of chiasmal (opticohypothalamic) gliomas are diencephalic wasting, hypopituitarism, precocious puberty, and hydrocephalus.

The diagnosis of optic glioma is now usually made by imaging study; biopsy is seldom necessary.[155] Except for shunting of hydrocephalus and rare cases in which an extrinsic component compresses adjacent visual pathways, there is no established role for surgery beyond biopsy in those few instances in which the diagnosis is uncertain (i.e., when the tumor has a globular appearance and there is no associated diencephalic syndrome or neurofibromatosis).[156]

Despite and because of the poor prognosis, treatment of malignant optic glioma of adulthood with radiation therapy and chemotherapy is probably warranted.[157] Management of childhood optic gliomas remains controversial. The indolent nature of many childhood optic gliomas militates against radiotherapy or chemotherapy, with their attendant complications and uncertain clinical responses.[158] Pierce and coworkers at Children's Hospital in Boston advocate radiotherapy only when there is evidence of progressive disease in older children.[159] Two infants irradiated in their series developed carotid artery occlusion with collateral telangiectasia, the so-called moyamoya syndrome (see Small Vessels, later),[160] and chemotherapy has been suggested as an alternative or to allow postponement of radiation therapy in young children.[161]

CHORDOMAS

Chordomas arise from notochordal remnants in the base of the skull, especially the clivus but also the dorsum sellae and paranasal sinuses. Unilateral sixth-nerve palsy is the most common neurologic sign of chordoma; bilateral sixth-nerve palsy is the most characteristic.[162] Chordomas may extend forward and compress the chiasm or optic nerve, causing junctional defects or bitemporal hemianopia in a small percentage of cases.[163] Neetens and coworkers describe a woman who developed a chordoma 11 yr after removal of a pituitary adenoma.[164] Management of chordomas consists of subtotal resection and radiotherapy.

LEUKEMIAS AND LYMPHOMAS

Tumors that infiltrate the brain occasionally involve the chiasm. These include lymphomas—both Hodgkin's[165] and nonHodgkin's type[166]—chronic lymphocytic leukemia,[167] and multiple myeloma.[168] Plasmacytomas in multiple myeloma are especially difficult to distinguish pathologically from pituitary adenomas. Drug-induced pseudolymphoma may also involve the chiasm.[169] Results of treatment of true lymphomas in this region have been disappointing.

METASTATIC TUMOR

Carcinomas arising elsewhere in the body may metastasize to the pituitary body[170] or into preexisting pituitary adenomas.[171] Differentiation of metastatic disease from primary pituitary adenoma or other perichiasmal tumor is difficult preoperatively, but the possibility should be suggested by a history of cancer (especially of the breast) or the presence of diabetes insipidus or ophthalmoplegia.[172] An intrasellar metastasis may be the initial presentation of remote carcinomas.[173] Incidental pituitary metastases are encountered in autopsy series, and the primary tumor may not be identified.[174]

Vascular Disorders

LARGE VESSELS

The significance of compression of the chiasm by the larger arteries of the circle of Willis is controversial. Indentation of the chiasm and optic nerves by the carotid artery is encountered as an incidental finding at autopsy.[13] Instances of bitemporal visual field loss in which evaluation reveals only enlargement and elongation of arteries of the circle of Willis must therefore be interpreted with caution.[175–177] Although manipulation of an ectatic vessel seen to indent the chiasm may be followed by postoperative visual improvement, the role of such surgical intervention remains uncertain.[178]

Of more practical significance is the recognition of saccular aneurysms of the carotid artery that compress the chiasm and may be mistaken neuroradiologically for a tumor, with potentially disastrous consequences if surgical removal is attempted transsphenoidally. Although prolactin levels greater than 150 ng/ml or the presence of acromegaly or Cushing's disease is presumptive evidence that a tumor is present,[98] endocrinologic abnormalities including moderate hyperprolactinemia may confound a clinician.[179] Until recently, carotid angiography was recommended preoperatively to rule out aneurysm,[180] but the sensitivity of MRI of vascular structures may obviate this step.[181]

SMALL VESSELS (Table 207–4)

As a consequence of the richly anastomotic vascular supply of the chiasm, infarctions selectively involving this area are rare except in diseases in which multiple arteries are simultaneously involved—for example, giant cell arteritis, periarteritis nodosa, or systemic lupus erythematosus.[182, 183] Bilateral carotid occlusive disease producing collateral vascular networks, called *moyamoya disease* because of the angiographic resemblance of these vascular networks to puffs of smoke (*moyamoya* in Japanese), has been implicated in ischemic chiasmal syndromes.[184] Instances of apparent hemorrhagic infarction of the posterior optic nerve encountered on surgical exploration suggest that the vascular supply at the junction of the optic nerve and chiasm is tenuous[185] and may account for the central scotomata occasionally encountered as the presentation of pituitary adenomas.[186, 187]

RADIATION NECROSIS

Radiation necrosis of the visual pathways occasionally follows irradiation for pituitary adenomas[188, 189] but may also develop after radiation treatment of sinus carcinomas, a cavernous sinus meningiomas,[190] and other tumors in this region. In a case reported from Belgium in the pre-CT era, blindness and death followed treatment for a presumed basophilic adenoma, but no tumor was found at autopsy.[191] The probable pathogenesis is damage to capillary beds, a mechanism similar to that observed in radiation retinopathy.[192] The clinical diagnosis of radiation necrosis has largely been one of exclusion, but Zimmerman and coworkers demonstrate that areas of radionecrosis enhance with gadolinium on MRI, which should improve the recognition of this entity.[193] The risk of radiation necrosis appears to increase with concomitant chemotherapy.[194]

Table 207–4. NONCOMPRESSIVE CHIASMAL LESIONS

Ischemia
Demyelination
Radionecrosis
Drug toxicity
Optochiasmatic arachnoiditis
Head trauma

Trauma and Toxins

The midline location of the chiasm makes it vulnerable to the acceleration-deceleration forces of head trauma. Complete bitemporal hemianopias are observed after head trauma.[195, 196] Lindenberg and associates provide pathologic correlation in one case in which fatal head trauma split the chiasm in half. They suggest three possible mechanisms for the visual loss found clinically in theirs and other cases: a tear in the chiasm, contusion necrosis, and compression of the chiasm by swollen brain.[197] Delayed posttraumatic hemorrhage may also result in blindness (see Chiasmal Apoplexy, earlier).[198]

Grant considers the chiasm a favored site for the toxicity of chloramphenicol, ethambutol, hexachlorophene, and vincristine.[199] Pathologic confirmation of specific chiasmal toxicity is difficult to obtain, and chiasmal involvement may be suspected in many cases of toxic optic neuropathy because of centrocecal scotomata mimicking bitemporal hemianopia.[200] Reynolds and coworkers report centrocecal scotomata and more peripheral bitemporal field defects in a 37-year-old man with suspected ethchlorvynol toxicity.[201]

Inflammation and Infection

DEMYELINATION

Chiasmal neuritis has a course and significance similar to that of retrobulbar optic neuritis.[202] Purvin and coworkers describe a 13-year-old boy in whom chiasmal neuritis appears to have been caused by Epstein-Barr virus infection.[203] Because inflammation may enlarge the chiasm, the appearance on CT may be similar to optic glioma and lead to unnecessary surgical exploration.[204]

OPTOCHIASMATIC ARACHNOIDITIS

The designation *optochiasmatic arachnoiditis* usually refers to cases in which surgical exploration or autopsy has demonstrated localized inflammatory changes in the leptomeninges around the chiasm. The incidence of this disorder is directly related to the willingness of neurosurgeons to explore the region and perhaps to their interpretation of operative findings.[205] This definition includes some cases of demyelinating chiasmal neuritis,[206] but optochiasmatic arachnoiditis also has been reported after head trauma, with subarachnoid hemorrhage, in nasopharyngeal and sinus infections, and with various types of meningitis.[201] Specific causes include syphilis, tuberculosis,[207] cryptococcosis,[208] and rheumatoid pachymeningitis.[209]

When diagnosis is difficult, management is seldom straightforward. Surgical lysis of adhesions—an approach with a long history—is still performed in some noninfectious cases, but the justification for this therapy is unclear. Corticosteroids and cytotoxic agents are reportedly effective in some instances.[210]

SARCOIDOSIS

Neurosarcoidosis involving the chiasmal region should be considered especially in young blacks. The diagnosis is made by identifying noncaseating granulomas elsewhere in the body or in surgical specimens obtained at craniotomy.[211, 212] Treatment is with corticosteroids, radiotherapy, and cytotoxic agents,[213] but the visual prognosis must be considered guarded.

LYMPHOID HYPOPHYSITIS

Lymphoid hypophysitis is an inflammation that presents in young women as sometimes fatal hypopituitarism, usually in association with pregnancy, and appears to be an autoimmune reaction to the adenohypophysis.[214] The inflammatory process may produce an intrasellar mass that compresses the chiasm and mimics a pituitary adenoma[215] or that lies suprasellarly and mimics a meningioma.[216] The visual loss may respond to corticosteroids alone, although in most cases surgical biopsy has been required for diagnosis.

PITUITARY ABSCESS

Bacterial abscesses in the pituitary develop in patients with pituitary tumors, both preoperatively and postoperatively,[217] and occasionally in nontumorous pituitaries, both spontaneously and in association with sinus infections.[218] Preoperative diagnosis is difficult, but pituitary abscess should be considered in a patient with a known pituitary tumor and meningitis, in a patient with meningitis with visual field loss or an enlarged sella,[219] and in the differential diagnosis of pituitary apoplexy (discussed earlier).[220]

Fungal abscesses that arise in the sphenoidal sinus as a result of aspergillosis may mimic pituitary adenomas.[221, 222] The fungal mass, called an *aspergilloma*, is treated by surgical removal and systemic antifungal chemotherapy.[223]

Miscellaneous Nonneoplastic Lesions

SPHENOIDAL SINUS MUCOCELE

Mucoceles of the posterior ethmoidal and sphenoidal sinuses occasionally compress the chiasm.[224] The expanding mucocele may enlarge the sella turcica, mimicking a pituitary adenoma.[225] Differentiation on preoperative imaging studies may be difficult,[226] but when the diagnosis is made at surgery, drainage and removal of the lining membranes are usually curative.

ARACHNOID CYSTS

Intrasellar arachnoid cysts may present with headache, visual loss, galactorrhea, or hypopituitarism.[227] Suprasellar cysts cause obstructive hydrocephalus.[228] At surgery, by their appearance and pathology, arachnoid cysts are distinguished from pars intermedia cysts (which lie between the anterior and posterior lobe of the pituitary body), Rathke's pouch cysts (see Craniopharyngioma), cysticercosis, and epidermoid cysts.[229]

EMPTY SELLA SYNDROME

Overlapping in some cases with intrasellar arachnoid cysts is the so-called empty sella syndrome. Randall defines an empty sella as an extension of the normal subarachnoid space into the sella turcica and the empty sella syndrome as the effects of this extension, including flattening of the pituitary and enlargement of the sella.[230] The syndrome is usually subdivided into primary and secondary types. Primary empty sella is the result of an anatomic defect in the diaphragma sellae. Expansion of the subarachnoid space into the sella may be encouraged by increased intracranial pressure, such as occurs in pseudotumor cerebri, and primary empty sella is much more prevalent in women. Secondary empty sella follows treatment or spontaneous shrinkage of pituitary tumors. The distinction between primary and secondary forms is blurred, because an empty sella in a patient with pseudotumor may be considered secondary and that following spontaneous infarction of the pituitary, primary. An empty sella and a microadenoma may coexist.

Abnormalities in visual acuity or field are more commonly encountered in secondary than primary empty sella syndrome. Visual loss in empty sella syndrome is attributed to herniation of the chiasm into the sella, but such herniation may be demonstrated by MRI in cases without visual disturbance.[231] Progressive visual loss may be an indication for chiasmapexy, surgery to support the chiasm with muscle and bone, but unrelated ocular causes of decreased vision should of course be ruled out before such intervention is undertaken.[232]

CHIASMAL COMPRESSION BY A NON-NEOPLASTIC PITUITARY

A few reports suggest that pituitary enlargement in primary hypothyroidism[233] and pregnancy[104] causes field defects. Because even a normal-sized pituitary has been reported to impinge on the chiasm in a patient with a hypoplastic sella,[234] this possibility cannot be completely discounted, but Walsh and Hoyt suggest that most such defects are functional.[235]

Bitemporal Field Loss Not Caused by Chiasmal Disorders
(Table 207–5)

Just as binasal hemianopic defects may be the result of bilateral optic nerve or retinal disease, so can bitemporal hemianopia. Glaucoma in eyes with disc anomalies may result in progressive temporal—rather than the

Table 207–5. MIMICS OF CHIASMAL LESIONS

Bilateral optic nerve lesions
Glaucoma and other optic neuropathies
Disc anomalies
Testing artifacts
Psychogenic visual loss

characteristic nasal—field loss.[236] The presence of disc anomalies does not protect from chiasmal disorders, and cases in which two problems coexist are likely to cause diagnostic confusion.[237]

Bitemporal hemianopia as a false localizing sign has been reported with nasal fundus ectasia,[238] tilted discs and other disc anomalies,[239] sectorial retinal degeneration, papilledema (especially when choroidal folds are present[240]), and optic neuropathies.[241] Bitemporal field loss may be an artifact of either contact lenses or the corrective lenses used for testing on bowl perimeters.[242] Even psychogenic visual loss occasionally manifests as bitemporal hemianopia.[243]

SUMMARY

In both a literal and figurative sense, the chiasm is a crossroads of the the visual system. The anatomy, relations, and function of the chiasm make it an important structure clinically. Testing of the visual fields and imaging of this region should be considered in patients with unexplained visual loss, optic atrophy, various endocrinologic disorders, and some types of oculomotor dysfunction.

REFERENCES

1. Hoyt WF: Correlative functional anatomy of the optic chiasm—1969. Clin Neurosurg 17:179, 1970.
2. Bergland RM, Ray BS, Torack RM: Anatomical variations in the pituitary gland and adjacent structures in 225 autopsy cases. J Neurosurg 28:93, 1968.
3. Osler RH, Corbett JJ, Schatz NJ, et al: Neuroophthalmological complications of enlargement of the third ventricle. Br J Ophthalmol 62:536, 1978.
4. Rucker CW: The concept of a semidecussation of the optic nerves. AMA Arch Ophthalmol 59:159, 1958.
5. Reynolds TM: A nineteenth century view of the optic commissure. Surv Ophthalmol 32:214, 1987.
6. Kupfer C, Chumbley L, Downer J deC: Quantitative histology of optic nerve, optic tract and lateral geniculate nucleus of man. J Anat 101:393, 1967.
7. Russell-Eggitt I, Kriss A, Taylor DSI: Albinism in childhood: A flash VEP and ERG study. Br J Ophthalmol 74:136, 1990.
8. Hoyt WF, Luis O: Visual fiber anatomy in the infrageniculate pathway of the primate: Uncrossed and crossed retinal quadrant fiber projections studied with Nauta silver stain. Arch Ophthalmol 68:94, 1962.
9. Hoyt WF, Luis O: The primate chiasm: Details of visual fiber organization studied by silver impregnation techniques. Arch Ophthalmol 70:69, 1963.
10. Hoyt WF, Tudor RC: The course of parapapillary temporal retinal axons through the anterior optic nerve: A Nauta degeneration study in the primate. Arch Ophthalmol 69:503, 1963.
11. Dawson BH: The blood vessels of the human optic chiasma and their relation to those of the hypophysis and hypothalamus. Brain 81:207, 1958.
12. Rhoton AL, Harris FS, Renn WH: Microsurgical anatomy of the sellar region and cavernous sinus. *In* Glaser JS (ed): Neuro-Ophthalmology: Symposium of the University of Miami and the Bascom Palmer Eye Institute, vol 9. St. Louis, CV Mosby, 1977, p 75.
13. Bergland R, Ray BS: The arterial supply of the human optic chiasm. J Neurosurg 31:327, 1969.
14. Huber A: Roentgen diagnosis vs visual field. Arch Ophthalmol 90:1, 1973.
15. Johnson JC, Lubow M, Banerjee T, et al: Chromophobe adenoma and chiasmal syndrome without enlargement of the bony sella. Ann Ophthalmol 8:1043, 1976.
16. Cushing H: The chiasmal syndrome. Arch Ophthalmol 3:505, 1936.
17. Cushing H: The chiasmal syndrome of primary optic atrophy and bitemporal field defects in adults with a normal sella turcica. Arch Ophthalmol 3:505, 704, 1936.
18. Wilson P, Falconer MA: Patterns of visual failure with pituitary tumors: Clinical and radiological correlations. Br J Ophthalmol 52:94, 1968.
19. Moore KP, Wass JAH, Besser GM: Late diagnosis of pituitary and parapituitary lesions causing visual failure. Br Med J 293:609, 1986.
20. Foulds WS, Bronte-Stewart J, McClure E: Delayed diagnosis of optic nerve or chiasmal compression as a result of negative CT scanning. Trans Ophthalmol Soc UK 103:543, 1983.
21. Chamlin M, Davidoff LM: The 1/2000 field in chiasmal interference. Arch Ophthalmol 44:53, 1950.
22. Trobe JD, Acosta PC, Kirscher JP: A screening method for chiasmal visual-field defects. Arch Ophthalmol 99:264, 1981.
23. Schindler S, McCrary JA III: Automated perimetry in a neuro-ophthalmologic practice. Ann Ophthalmol 6:691, 1981.
24. Wirtschafter JD, Coffman SM: Comparison of manual Goldmann and automated static visual field using the Dicon 200 perimeter in the detection of chiasmal tumors. Ann Ophthalmol 16:733, 1984.
25. Younge BR, Trautmann JC: Computer-assisted perimetry in neuroophthalmic disease. Mayo Clin Proc 55:207, 1980.
26. Safran AB, Glaser JS: Statokinetic dissociation in lesions of the anterior visual pathways: A reappraisal of the Riddoch phenomenon. Arch Ophthalmol 98:291, 1980.
27. Frisén L: A versatile color confrontation test for the central visual field: A comparison with quantitative perimetry. Arch Ophthalmol 89:3, 1973.
28. Trobe JD, Acosta PC, Kirscher JP: A screening method for chiasmal visual-field defects. Arch Ophthalmol 99:264, 1981.
29. Kline LB: Chiasmal compression without bitemporal hemianopia. *In* Smith JL (ed): Neuro-Ophthalmology 1982. New York, Masson, 1981, p 223.
30. Adler FH, Austin G, Grant FC: Localizing value of visual fields in patients with early chiasmal lesions. Arch Ophthalmol 40:579, 1948.
31. Frisén L: The neurology of visual acuity. Brain 103:639, 1980.
32. Traquair HM: An Introduction to Clinical Perimetry, 4th ed. St. Louis, CV Mosby, 1944.
33. Sugita K, Sato O, Hirota R, et al: Scotomatous defects in the central visual fields in pituitary adenomas. Neurochirurgica 18:155, 1975.
34. Hollenhorst RW, Younge BR: Ocular manifestations produced by adenomas of the pituitary gland: Analysis of 1000 cases. *In* Kohler PO, Ross GT (eds): Diagnosis and Treatment of Pituitary Tumors. Amsterdam, Excerpta Medica, 1973, p 53.
35. Gittinger JW Jr: Functional monocular temporal hemianopsia. Am J Ophthalmol 101:226, 1986.
36. Keane JR: Hysterical hemianopia: The "missing half" field defect. Arch Ophthalmol 97:865, 1979.
37. Bird A: Field loss due to lesions at the anterior angle of the chiasm. Proc R Soc Med 65:519, 1972.
38. Walsh FB: The ocular signs of tumors involving the anterior visual pathways. Am J Ophthalmol 42:347, 1956.
39. Asbury T: Unilateral scotoma: As the presenting sign of pituitary tumor. Am J Ophthalmol 59:510, 1965.
40. Trobe JD, Glaser JS: Quantitative perimetry in compressive optic neuropathy and optic neuritis. Arch Ophthalmol 96:1210, 1978.
41. Hoyt WF: Anatomic considerations of arcuate scotomas associated with lesions of the optic nerve and chiasm: A Nauta axon degeneration study in the monkey. Bull Johns Hopkins Hosp 111:58, 1962.
42. Trobe JD: Chromophobe adenoma presenting with a hemianopic temporal arcuate scotoma. Am J Ophthalmol 77:388, 1974.
43. Schmidt D, Buhrmann K: Inferior hemianopia in parasellar and pituitary tumors. *In* Glaser JS (ed): Neuro-Ophthalmology: Symposium of the University of Miami and the Bascom Palmer Eye Institute, vol 9. St. Louis, CV Mosby, 1977, p 236.

44. Hupp SL, Savino PJ, Schatz NJ, et al: Nerve fibre bundle visual field defects and intracranial mass lesions. Can J Ophthalmol 21:231, 1986.
45. Manor RS, Ouaknine GE, Matz, et al: Nasal visual field loss with intracranial lesions of the optic nerve pathways. Am J Ophthalmol 90:1, 1980.
46. Cogan DG: Neurology of the Visual System. Springfield, IL, Charles C Thomas, 1966.
47. Pilley SFJ, Thompson HS: Binasal field loss and prefixation blindness. *In* Glaser JS, Smith JL (eds): Neuro-Ophthalmology: Symposium of the University of Miami and the Bascom Palmer Eye Institute, vol 8. St. Louis, CV Mosby, 1975, p 277.
48. Gittinger JW Jr: Functional hemianopsia: A historical perspective. Surv Ophthalmol 32:427, 1988.
49. O'Connell JEA: The anatomy of the optic chiasma and heteronymous hemianopia. Mayo Clin Proc 51:563, 1976.
50. Manor RS, Ouaknine GE, Matz S, et al: Nasal visual field loss with intracranial lesions of the optic nerve pathways. Am J Ophthalmol 90:1, 1980.
51. Savino PJ, Paris M, Schatz NJ, et al: Optic tract syndrome: A review of 21 patients. Arch Ophthalmol 96:656, 1978.
52. Savino PJ, Schatz NJ, Corbett JJ, et al: Visual field defects in optic tract disease. *In* Thompson HS (ed): Topics in Neuro-Ophthalmology. Baltimore, Williams & Wilkins, 1979, p 86.
53. Bender MB, Bodis-Wollner I: Visual dysfunction in optic tract lesions. Ann Neurol 3:187, 1978.
54. Wilson P, Falconer MA: Patterns of visual failure with pituitary tumours: Clinical and radiological correlations. Br J Ophthalmol 52:94, 1968.
55. Anderson D, Faber P, Marcovitz S, et al: Pituitary tumors and the ophthalmologist. Ophthalmology 90:1265, 1983.
56. Trobe JD, Tao AH, Schuster JJ: Perichiasmal tumors: Diagnostic and prognostic features. Neurosurgery 15:391, 1984.
57. Lundstrom M, Frisén L: Atrophy of optic nerve fibres in compression of the chiasm: Degree and distribution of ophthalmoscopic changes. Acta Ophthalmol 54:623, 1976.
58. Hoyt WF, Rios-Montenegro MM, Behrens MM, et al: Homonymous hemioptic hypoplasia. Br J Ophthalmol 56:537, 1972.
59. Symonds C: Ocular palsy as the presenting symptom of pituitary adenoma. Bull Johns Hopkins Hosp 11:72, 1962.
60. Robert CM Jr, Feigenbaum JA, Stern WE: Ocular palsy occurring with pituitary tumors. J Neurosurg 38:17, 1973.
61. Yen MY, Liu JH, Jaw SJ: Ptosis as the early manifestation of pituitary tumour. Br J Ophthalmol 74:188, 1990.
62. Walsh TJ: See-saw nystagmus revisited. *In* Smith JL, Katz RS (eds): Neuro-Ophthalmology Enters the Nineties. Hialeah, FL, Dutton Press, 1988, p 195.
63. Kanter DS, Ruff RL, Leigh RJ, et al: See-saw nystagmus and brainstem infarction; MRI findings. Neuro-Ophthalmology 7:279, 1987.
64. Nakada T, Kwee IL: Seesaw nystagmus: Role of visuovestibular interaction in its pathogenesis. J Clin Neuro Ophthalmol 8:171, 1988.
65. Frisén L, Wikklelsø C: Posttraumatic seesaw nystagmus abolished by ethanol ingestion. Neurology 36:841, 1986.
66. Zelt RP, Biglan AW: Congenital seesaw nystagmus. J Pediatr Ophthalmol Strabismus 22:13, 1985.
67. Safran AB, Kline LB, Glaser JS: Positive visual phenomena in optic nerve and chiasm disease: Photopsias and photophobia. *In* Glaser JS (ed): Neuro-Ophthalmology: In Memory of Dr. Frank B. Walsh, vol 10. St. Louis, CV Mosby, 1980, p 225.
68. Dawson DJ, Enoch BA, Shepherd DI: Formed visual hallucinations with pituitary adenomas. Br Med J 289:414, 1984.
69. Ram Z, Findler G, Gutman I, et al: Visual hallucinations associated with pituitary adenoma. Neurosurgery 20:292, 1987.
70. Lepore FE: Spontaneous visual phenomena with visual loss: 104 patients with lesions of retinal and neural afferent pathways. Neurology 40:444, 1990.
71. Nachtigaller H, Hoyt WF: Störingen des Scheindruckes bei bitemporaler Hemianopsie und Verschiebung der Sehachsen. Klin Monatsbl Augenheilkd 186:821, 1970.
72. Wybar K: Chiasmal compression: Presenting ocular features. Proc R Soc Med 70:307, 1977.
73. Lyle TK, Clover P: Ocular symptoms and signs in pituitary tumours. Proc R Soc Med 54:611, 1961.
74. Bynke O: Incidence of neuro-ophthalmic manifestations of pituitary adenomas in the referral area of Linkoping, Sweden, 1965–1984. Neuro-Ophthalmology 7:165, 1987.
75. Conomy JP, Ferguson JH, Brodkey JS, et al: Spontaneous infarction in pituitary tumors: Neurologic and therapeutic aspects. Neurology 25:580, 1975.
76. Senelick RC, van Dyk HL: Chromophobe adenoma masquerading as corticosteroid-responsive optic neuritis. Am J Ophthalmol 78:485, 1974.
77. Wakai S, Fukushima T, Teramoto A, et al: Pituitary apoplexy: Its incidence and clinical significance. J Neurosurg 55:187, 1981.
78. Sussman EB, Porro RS: Pituitary apoplexy: The role of atheromatous emboli. Stroke 5:318, 1974.
79. Rovit PL, Fein JM: Pituitary apoplexy: A review and reappraisal. J Neurosurg 37:280, 1972.
80. Reid RL, Quigley ME, Yen SSC: Pituitary apoplexy: A review. Arch Neurol 42:712, 1985.
81. Cardoso ER, Peterson EW: Pituitary apoplexy: A review. Neurosurgery 14:363, 1984.
82. Laconis D, Johnson LN, Mamourian AC: Magnetic resonance imaging in pituitary apoplexy. Arch Ophthalmol 106:207, 1988.
83. Maitland CG, Abiko S, Hoyt WF, et al: Chiasmal apoplexy: Report of four cases. J Neurosurg 56:118, 1982.
84. Lavin PJM, McCrary JA III, Roessmann U, et al: Chiasmal apoplexy: Hemorrhage from a cryptic vascular malformation in the optic chiasm. Neurology 34:1007, 1984.
85. Honegger J, Fahlbusch R, Lieb W, et al: Cavernous hemangioma of the optic chiasm. Neuro-Ophthalmology 10:81, 1990.
86. Corboy JR, Galetta SL: Familial cavernous hemangiomas manifesting with an acute chiasmal syndrome. Am J Ophthalmol 108:245, 1989.
87. Carter JE, Wymore J, Ansbacher L, et al: Sudden visual loss and a chiasmal syndrome due to an intrachiasmatic vascular malformation. J Clin Neuro Ophthalmol 2:163, 1982.
88. Moffit B, Duffy K, Lufkin R, et al: MR imaging of intrachiasmatic hemorrhage. J Comput Assist Tomogr 12:535, 1988.
89. Hassler W, Zentner J, Wilhelm H: Cavernous angiomas of the anterior visual pathways. J Clin Neuro Ophthalmol 9:160, 1989.
90. Sibony PA, Lessell S, Wray S: Chiasmal syndrome caused by arteriovenous malformations. Arch Ophthalmol 100:438, 1982.
91. Blaauw G, Braakman R, Cuhadar M, et al: Influence of transsphenoidal hypophysectomy on visual deficit due to a pituitary tumour. Acta Neurochir (Wien) 83:79, 1986.
92. Dagi TF, Kattah JC: Ocular and endocrine function in patients with pituitary tumors: Operative results following transnasal, transsphenoidal approach with marsupialization of the sella turcica. Am Surg 52:165, 1986.
93. Findlay G, McFadzean RM, Teasdale G: Recovery of vision following treatment of pituitary tumours: Application of a new system of visual assessment. Trans Ophthalmol Soc UK 103:212, 1983.
94. Harris PE, Afshar F, Coates P, et al: The effects of transsphenoidal surgery on endocrine function and visual fields in patients with functionless pituitary tumours. Q J Med 71:417, 1989.
95. Trautmann JC, Laws ER Jr: Visual status after transsphenoidal surgery at the Mayo Clinic, 1971–1982. Am J Ophthalmol 96:200, 1983.
96. Goldman JA, Hedges TR III, Shucart W, et al: Delayed chiasmal compression after transsphenoidal operation for a pituitary adenoma. Neurosurgery 17:962, 1985.
97. Laws ER Jr, Fode NC, Redmond MJ: Transsphenoidal surgery following unsuccessful prior therapy: An assessment of benefits and risks in 158 patients. J Neurosurg 63:823, 1985.
98. Barrow DL, Tindall GT: Pituitary adenomas: An update on their management with an emphasis on the role of bromocriptine. J Clin Neuro Ophthalmol 2:169, 1983.
99. Moster ML, Savino PJ, Schatz NJ, et al: Visual function in prolactinoma patients treated with bromocriptine. Ophthalmology 92:1332, 1985.
100. Lesser RL, Zheutlin JD, Boghen D, et al: Visual function improvement in patients with macroprolactinomas treated with bromocriptine. Am J Ophthalmol 109:535, 1990.
101. Grimson BS, Bowman ZL: Rapid decompression of anterior intracranial visual pathways with bromocriptine. Arch Ophthalmol 101:604, 1983.

102. Thorner MO, Perryman RL, Rogol AD, et al: Rapid changes of prolactinoma volume after withdrawal and reinstitution of bromocriptine. J Clin Endocrinol Metab 153:480, 1981.
103. King LW, Molitch ME, Gittinger JW Jr, et al: Cavernous sinus syndrome due to prolactinoma: Resolution with bromocriptine. Surg Neurol 19:280, 1983.
104. Sunness JS: The pregnant woman's eye. Surv Ophthalmol 32:219, 1988.
105. Gemzell C, Wang CF: Outcome of pregnancy in women with pituitary adenoma. Fertil Steril 31:363, 1979.
106. Newman SA: Advances in diagnosis and treatment of pituitary tumors. Int Ophthalmol Clin 26:285, 1986.
107. Rush SC, Newall J: Pituitary adenoma: The efficacy of radiotherapy as the sole treatment. Int J Radiat Oncol Biol Phys 17:165, 1989.
108. Harris JR, Levene MB: Visual complications following irradiation for pituitary adenomas and craniopharyngiomas. Radiology 120:167, 1978.
109. Wybar K: Chiasmal compression: Presenting ocular features. Proc R Soc Med 70:307, 1977.
110. Cushing H, Eisenhardt L: Meningiomas arising from the tuberculum sellae. Arch Ophthalmol 1:1, 1929.
111. Huber A: Eye Signs and Symptoms in Brain Tumors. St. Louis, CV Mosby, 1976, p 235.
112. Finn JE, Mount LA: Meningiomas of the tuberculum sellae and planum sphenoidale: A review of 83 cases. Arch Ophthalmol 92:23, 1974.
113. Udvarhelyi GB: Neurosurgical diagnosis and treatment of lesions involving the anterior visual pathways: Symposium on Neuro-Ophthalmology. Transactions of the New Orleans Academy of Ophthalmology. St. Louis, CV Mosby, 1976, p 98.
114. Reicher MA, Bentson JR, Halbach VV, et al: Pneumosinus dilatans of the sphenoid sinus. Am J Neuroradiol 7:865, 1986.
115. Coppeto JR, Gahm NH: Bitemporal hemianopic scotoma: A complication of intraventricular catheter. Surg Neurol 8:361, 1977.
116. Coppeto JR, Monteiro MLR: Bitemporal hemianopic scotomas from intraventricular catheter: The 'pinched-chiasm' syndrome? Neuro-Ophthalmology 9:343, 1989.
117. Slavin ML, Rosenthal AD: Chiasmal compression caused by a catheter in the suprasellar cistern. Am J Ophthalmol 105:560, 1988.
118. Trobe JD, Tao AH, Schuster JJ: Perichiasmal tumors: Diagnostic and prognostic features. Neurosurgery 15:391, 1984.
119. Kadis GN, Mount LA, Ganti SR: The importance of early diagnosis and treatment of the meningiomas of the planum sphenoidale and tuberculum sellae. Surg Neurol 12:367, 1979.
120. Yeakely JW, Kulkarni MV, McArdle CB, et al: High-resolution MR imaging of juxtasellar meningiomas with CT and angiographic correlation. AJNR 9:279, 1988.
121. Hoffman HJ: Craniopharyngiomas. Prog Exp Tumor Res 30:325, 1987.
122. Cobb CA, Youmans JR: Brain tumors of disordered embryogenesis in adults. *In* Youmans JR (ed): Neurological Surgery, 2nd ed, vol 5. Philadelphia, WB Saunders, 1982, p 2899.
123. Zulch KJ: Brain Tumors: Their Biology and Pathology. Berlin, Springer-Verlag, 1986.
124. Brodsky MC, Hoyt WF, Barnwell SL, et al: Intrachiasmatic craniopharyngioma: A rare cause of chiasmal thickening: Case report. J Neurosurg 68:300, 1988.
125. Cohen ME, Duffner PK: Craniopharyngiomas: Brain Tumors in Children: Principles of Diagnosis and Treatment. New York, Raven Press, 1984, p 193.
126. Crane TB, Yee RD, Hepler RS, et al: Clinical manifestations and radiologic findings in craniopharyngiomas in adults. Am J Ophthalmol 94:220, 1982.
127. Case 17–1980. Case records of the Massachusetts General Hospital. N Engl J Med 302:1015, 1980.
128. Krueger DW, Larson EB: Recurrent fever of unknown origin, coma, and meningismus due to a leaking craniopharyngioma. Am J Ophthalmol 84:543, 1988.
129. Miller NR: Walsh and Hoyt's Clinical Neuro-Ophthalmology, 4th ed. Baltimore, Williams & Wilkins, 1988, p 1393.
130. Cappaert WE, Kiprov RV: Craniopharyngioma presenting as unilateral central visual loss. Ann Ophthalmol 13:703, 1981.
131. Johnson LN, Hepler RS, Yee RD, et al: Magnetic resonance imaging of craniopharyngioma. Am J Ophthalmol 102:242, 1986.
132. Hoffman HJ: Craniopharyngiomas. Prog Exp Tumor Res 30:325, 1987.
133. Shillito J Jr: Treatment of craniopharyngiomas. Clin Neurosurg 33:533, 1986.
134. Repka MX, Miller NR, Miller M: Visual outcome after surgical removal of craniopharyngiomas. Ophthalmology 96:195, 1989.
135. McFadzean RM: Visual prognosis in craniopharyngioma. Neuro-Ophthalmology 9:337, 1989.
136. Cabezudo JM, Vaquero J, Areitio E, et al: Craniopharyngiomas: A critical approach to treatment. J Neurosurg 55:371, 1981.
137. Hoogenhout J, Otten BJ, Kazem I, et al: Surgery and radiation therapy in the management of craniopharyngiomas. Int J Radiat Oncol Biol Phys 10:2293, 1984.
138. Anderson DR, Trobe JD, Taren JA, et al: Visual outcome in cystic craniopharyngiomas treated with intracavitary phosphorus-32. Ophthalmology 96:1788, 1989.
139. Stelling MW, McKay SE, Carr WA, et al: Frontal lobe lesions and cognitive function in craniopharyngioma survivors. Am J Dis Child 140:710, 1986.
140. Liwnicz BH, Berger TS, Liwicz RG, et al: Radiation-associated gliomas: A report of four cases and analysis of postradiation tumors of the central nervous system. Neurosurgery 17:436, 1985.
141. Kageyama N, Belsky R: Ectopic pinealoma in the chiasma region. Neurology 11:318, 1961.
142. Bowman CB, Farris BK: Primary chiasmal germinoma: A case report and review of the literature. J Clin Neuro Ophthalmol 10:9, 1990.
143. Isayama Y, Takahashi T, Inoue M: Ocular findings of suprasellar germinoma: Long-term follow-up after radiotherapy. Neuro-Ophthalmology 1:53, 1980.
144. Nakasu S, Handa J, Hazama F, et al: Suprasellar yolk-sac tumor in two sisters. Surg Neurol 20:147, 1983.
145. Chilton J, Caughron MR, Kepes JJ: Ganglioglioma of the optic chiasm: Case report and review of the literature. Neurosurgery 26:1042, 1990.
146. Zimmerman LE, Arkfeld DL, Schenken JB, et al: A rare choristoma of the optic nerve and chiasm. Arch Ophthalmol 101:766, 1983.
147. Taphoorn MJB, de Vries-Knoppert WAEJ, Ponssen H, et al: Malignant optic gliomas in adults: Case report. J Neurosurg 70:277, 1989.
148. Wilson WB, Feinsod M, Hoyt WF, et al: Malignant evolution of childhood pilocytic astrocytoma. Neurology 26:322, 1976.
149. Alvord EC Jr, Lofton S: Gliomas of the optic nerve or chiasm: Outcome by patients' age, tumor site, and treatment. J Neurosurg 68:85, 1988.
150. Lewis RA, Gerson LP, Axelson KA, et al: Von Recklinghuasen neurofibromatosis. II: Incidence of optic gliomata. Ophthalmology 91:929, 1984.
151. Appleton RE, Jan JE: Delayed diagnosis of optic nerve glioma: A preventable cause of visual loss. Pediatr Neurol 5:226, 1989.
152. Lavery MA, O'Neill JF, Chu FC, et al: Acquired nystagmus in early childhood: A presenting sign of intracranial tumor. Ophthalmology 91:425, 1984.
153. Farmer J, Hoyt CJ: Monocular nystagmus in infancy and early childhood. Am J Ophthalmol 98:504, 1984.
154. Weiss AH, Biersdorf WR: Visual sensory disorders in congenital nystagmus. Ophthalmology 96:517, 1989.
155. Fletcher WA, Imes RK, Hoyt WF: Chiasmal gliomas: Appearance and long-term changes demonstrated by computerized tomography. J Neurosurg 65:154, 1986.
156. Fletcher WA, Imes RK, Hoyt WF: Chiasmal gliomas: Appearance and long-term changes demonstrated by computerized tomography. J Neurosurg 65:154, 1986.
157. Albers GW, Hoyt WF, Forno LS, et al: Treatment response in malignant optic glioma of adulthood. Neurology 38:1071, 1988.
158. Imes RK, Hoyt WF: Childhood chiasmal gliomas: Update on the fate of patients in the 1969 San Francisco study. Br J Ophthalmol 53:793, 1969.
159. Pierce SM, Barnes PD, Loeffler JS, et al: Definitive radiation therapy in the management of symptomatic patients with optic glioma: Survival and long-term effects. Cancer 65:45, 1990.

160. Okuno T, Prensky AL, Gado M: The moyamoya syndrome associated with irradiation of an optic glioma in children: Report of two cases and review of the literature. Pediatr Neurol 1:311, 1985.
161. Packer RJ, Sutton LN, Bilaniuk LT, et al: Treatment of chiasmatic/hypothalamic gliomas of childhood with chemotherapy: An update. Ann Neurol 23:79, 1988.
162. Bagan SM, Hollenhorst RW: Ocular manifestations of intracranial chordomas. Trans Am Ophthalmol Soc 78:148, 1980.
163. Takahashi T, Asai T, Isayama Y, et al: Chordoma. J Clin Neuro Ophthalmol 3:251, 1983.
164. Neetens A, Bultinck J, Martin JJ, et al: Intrasellar adenoma and chordoma. Neuro-Ophthalmology 2:123, 1980.
165. McFadzean RM, McIlwaine GG, McLellan D: Hodgkin's disease at the optic chiasm. J Clin Neuro Ophthalmol 10:248, 1990.
166. Cantore GP, Raco A, Artico M, et al: Primary chiasmatic lymphoma. Clin Neurol Neurosurg 91:71, 1989.
167. Howard RS, Duncombe AS, Owens C, et al: Compression of the optic chiasm due to a lymphoreticular malignancy. Postgrad Med J 63:1091, 1987.
168. Poon M-C, Prchal JT, Murad TM, et al: Multiple myeloma masquerading as chromophobe adenoma. Cancer 43:1513, 1979.
169. Galetta SL, Stadmauer EA, Hicks DG, et al: Reactive lymphohistiocytosis with recurrence in the optic chiasm. J Clin Neuro Ophthalmol 11:25, 1991.
170. Nelson PB, Robinson AG, Martinez AJ: Metastatic tumor of the pituitary gland. Neurosurgery 21:941, 1987.
171. van Seters AP, Bots GTAM, van Dulken H, et al: Metastasis of an occult gastric carcinoma suggesting growth of a prolactinoma during bromocriptine therapy: A case report with a review of the literature. Neurosurgery 16:813, 1985.
172. Max MB, Deck MDF, Rottenber DA: Pituitary metastasis: Incidence in cancer patients and clinical differentiation from pituitary adenoma. Neurology 31:998, 1981.
173. Buonaguidi R, Ferdeghini M, Faggionato F, et al: Intrasellar metastasis mimicking a pituitary adenoma. Surg Neurol 20:373, 1983.
174. Duvall J, Cullen JF: Metastatic disease in the pituitary: Clinical features. Trans Ophthalmol Soc UK 102:481, 1982.
175. Hilton GF, Hoyt WF: An arteriosclerotic chiasmal syndrome: Bitemporal hemianopia associated with fusiform dilation of the anterior cerebral arteries. JAMA 196:1018, 1966.
176. Matsuo K, Kobayashi S, Sugita K: Bitemporal hemianopia associated with sclerosis of the intracranial carotid arteries: Case report. J Neurosurg 53:566, 1980.
177. Slavin ML: Bitemporal hemianopia associated with dolichoectasia of the intracranial carotid arteries. J Clin Neuro Ophthalmol 10:80, 1990.
178. Post KD, Gittinger JW Jr, Stein BM: Visual improvement after surgical manipulation of dolichoectatic anterior cerebral arteries. Surg Neurol 14:321, 1981.
179. Krauss HR, Slamovits TL, Sibony PA, et al: Carotid artery aneurysm simulating pituitary adenoma. J Clin Neuro Ophthalmol 2:169, 1982.
180. Wolpert SM: The radiology of pituitary adenomas—An update. *In* Post KD, Jackson IMD, Reichlin S (eds): The Pituitary Adenoma. New York, Plenum, 1980, p 287.
181. Naheedy MH, Haag JR, Axar-Kia B, et al: MRI and CT of sellar and parasellar disorders. Radiol Clin North Am 25:819, 1987.
182. Walsh FB, Hoyt WF: Clinical Neuro-Ophthalmology. Baltimore, Williams & Wilkins, 1969, p 1883.
183. Lee KF: Ischemic chiasma syndrome. Am J Neuroradiol 4:777, 1983.
184. Ahmadi J, Keane JR, McCormick GS, et al: Ischemic chiasmal syndrome and hypopituitarism associated with progressive cerebrovascular occlusive disease. Am J Neuroradiol 5:367, 1984.
185. Schneideer RC, Kriss FC, Falls HF: Prechiasmal infarction with intrasellar and suprasellar tumors. J Neurosurg 32:197, 1970.
186. Schlezinger NS, Thompson RA: Pituitary tumors with central scotomas simulating retrobulbar optic neuritis. Neurology 17:782, 1967.
187. Sugita K, Sato O, Hirota T, et al: Scotomatous defects in the central visual field in pituitary adenomas. Neurochirurgica 18:155, 1973.
188. Hammer HM: Optic chiasmal radionecrosis. Trans Ophthalmol Soc UK 103:208, 1983.
189. Kline LB, Kim JY, Ceballos R: Radiation optic neuropathy. Ophthalmology 92:1118, 1985.
190. Pasquier F, Leys D, Dubois F, et al: Chiasm and optic nerve necrosis following radiation therapy: Report of two cases. Neuro-Ophthalmology 9:331, 1989.
191. Neetens A, Martin J, Rubbens MC: Iatrogenic roentgen encephalopathy. Neuro-Ophthalmology 1:203, 1981.
192. Brown GC, Shields JA, Sanborn G, et al: Radiation optic neuropathy. Ophthalmology 89:1489, 1982.
193. Zimmerman CF, Schatz NJ, Glaser JS: Magnetic resonance imaging of radiation optic neuropathy. Am J Ophthalmol 110:389, 1990.
194. Wilson WB, Perez GM, Kleinschmidt-Demasters BK: Sudden onset of blindness in patients treated with oral CCNA and low-dose cranial irradiation. Cancer 59:901, 1987.
195. Savino PJ, Glaser JS, Schatz NJ: Traumatic chiasmal syndrome. Neurology 30:963, 1980.
196. Elisevich KV, Ford RM, Anderson DP, et al: Visual abnormalities with multiple trauma. Surg Neurol 22:565, 1984.
197. Lindenberg R, Walsh FB, Sacks JG: Neuropathology of Vision: An Atlas. Philadelphia, Lea & Febiger, 1973, p 222.
198. Crowe NW, Nickles TP, Troost BT, et al: Intrachiasmal hemorrhage: A cause of delayed post-traumatic blindness. Neurology 39:863, 1989.
199. Grant WM: Toxicology of the Eye, 3rd ed. Springfield, IL, Charles C Thomas, 1986, p 23.
200. DeVita EG, Miao M, Sadun AA: Optic neuropathy in ethambutol-treated renal tuberculosis. J Clin Neuro Ophthalmol 7:77, 1987.
201. Reynolds WD, Smith JL, McCrary JA III: Chiasmal optic neuritis. J Clin Neuro Ophthalmol 2:93, 1982.
202. Spector RH, Glaser JS, Schatz NJ: Demyelinative chiasmal lesions. Arch Neurol 37:757, 1980.
203. Purvin V, Herr GJ, De Myer W: Chiasmal neuritis as a complication of Epstein-Barr infection. Arch Neurol 45:458, 1988.
204. Edwards MK, Gilmor RL, Franco JM: Computed tomography of chiasmal optic neuritis. Am J Neuroradiol 4:816, 1983.
205. Iraci G, Giordano R, Gerosa M, et al: Cystic suprasellar and retrosellar arachnoiditis: A clinical and pathologic follow-up case report. Ann Ophthalmol 11:1175, 1979.
206. Bell RA, Robertson DM, Rosen DA, et al: Optochiasmatic arachnoiditis in multiple sclerosis. Arch Ophthalmol 93:191, 1975.
207. Navarro IM, Peralta VHR, Leon JAM, et al: Tuberculous optochiasmatic arachnoiditis. Neurosurgery 9:654, 1981.
208. Takahashi T, Isayama Y: Chiasmal meningitis. Neuro-Ophthalmology 1:19, 1980.
209. Weinstein GW, Powell SR, Thrush WP: Chiasmal neuropathy secondary to rheumatoid pachymeningitis. Am J Ophthalmol 104:439, 1987.
210. Marus AO, Demakas JJ, Ross A, et al: Optochiasmatic arachnoiditis with treatment by surgical lysis of adhesions, corticosteroids, and cyclophosphamide: Report of a case. Neurosurgery 19:101, 1986.
211. Tang RA, Grotta JC, Lee KF, et al: Chiasmal syndrome in sarcoidosis. Arch Ophthalmol 101:1069, 1983.
212. Case records of the Massachusetts General Hospital (Case 10–1991). N Engl J Med 324:677, 1991.
213. Gelwan MJ, Kellen RI, Burde RM, et al: Sarcoidosis of the anterior visual pathway: Successes and failures. J Neurol Neurosurg Psychiatry 51:1473, 1988.
214. Gal R, Schwartz A, Gukovsky-Oren S, et al: Lymphoid hypophysitis associated with sudden maternal death: Report of a case and review of the literature. Obstet Gynecol Surv 41:619, 1986.
215. Hungerford GD, Biggs PJ, Levine JH, et al: Lymphoid adenohypophysitis with radiologic and clinical findings resembling a pituitary tumor. Am J Neuroradiol 3:444, 1982.
216. Stelmach M, O'Day J: Rapid change in visual fields associated with suprasellar lymphocytic hypophysitis. J Clin Neuro Ophthalmol 11:19, 1991.
217. Nelson PB, Haverkos H, Martinez AJ, et al: Abscess formation within pituitary tumors. Neurosurgery 12:331, 1983.

218. Marks PV, Furneaux CE: Pituitary abscesses following asymptomatic sphenoid sinusitis. J Laryngol Otol 98:1151, 1984.
219. Ford J, Torres LF, Cox T, et al: Recurrent sterile meningitis caused by a pituitary abscess. Postgrad Med J 62:929, 1986.
220. Domingue JN, Wilson CB: Pituitary abscesses: Report of seven cases and review of the literature. J Neurosurg 46:601, 1977.
221. Fuchs HA, Evans RM, Gregg CR: Invasive aspergillosis of the sphenoid sinus manifested as a pituitary tumor. South Med J 78:1365, 1985.
222. Larranaga J, Fandino J, Gomez-Bueno J, et al: Aspergillosis of the sphenoid sinus simulating a pituitary tumor. Neuroradiology 31:362, 1989.
223. Robb PJ: Aspergillosis of the paranasal sinuses (a case report and historical perspective). J Laryngol Otol 100:1071, 1986.
224. Goodwin JA, Glaser JS: Chiasmal syndrome in sphenoid sinus mucocele. Ann Neurol 4:440, 1978.
225. Abla AA, Maroon JC, Wilberger JE Jr, et al: Intrasellar mucocele simulating pituitary adenoma: Case report. Neurosurgery 18:197, 1986.
226. Schwaighofer BW, Sobel DF, Klein MV, et al: Mucocele of the anterior clinoid process: CT and MR findings. J Comput Assist Tomogr 13:501, 1989.
227. Meyer FB, Carpenter SM, Laws ER Jr: Intrasellar arachnoid cysts. Surg Neurol 28:105, 1987.
228. Muraji R, Epstein F: Diagnosis and treatment of suprasellar arachnoid cyst: Report of three cases. J Neurosurg 50:515, 1979.
229. Baskin DS, Wilson CB: Transsphenoidal treatment of nonneoplastic intrasellar cysts. J Neurosurg 60:8, 1984.
230. Randall RV: Empty sella syndrome. Compr Ther 10:57, 1984.
231. Kaufman B, Tomsak RL, Kaufman BA, et al: Herniation of the suprasellar visual system and third ventricle into empty sellae: Morphologic and clinical considerations. Am J Neuroradiol 152:597, 1989.
232. McFadzean RM: The empty sella syndrome: A review of 14 cases. Trans Ophthalmol Soc UK 103:537, 1983.
233. Yamamoto K, Saito K, Takai T, et al: Visual field defects and pituitary enlargement in primary hypothyroidism. J Clin Endocrinol Metab 57:283, 1983.
234. Elias Z, Powers SK, Grimson BS: Chiasmal syndrome caused by pituitary-sellar disproportion. Surg Neurol 28:395, 1987.
235. Walsh FB, Hoyt WF: Clinical Neuro-ophthalmology, 3rd ed. Baltimore, Williams & Wilkins, 1969, p 2124.
236. Chadwick AJ: Inversion of the disc and temporal field loss in chronic simple glaucoma. Br J Ophthalmol 52:932, 1968.
237. Keane JR: Suprasellar tumors and incidental optic disc anomalies. Arch Ophthalmol 95:2180, 1977.
238. Riise D: The nasal fundus ectasia. Acta Ophthalmol 126 Suppl:5, 1975.
239. Young SE, Walsh FB, Knox DL: The tilted disc syndrome. Am J Ophthalmol 82:16, 1976.
240. Frisén L, Holm M: Visual field defects associated with choroidal folds. *In* Glaser JS (ed): Neuro-Ophthalmology: Symposium of the University of Miami and the Bascom Palmer Eye Institute. St. Louis, CV Mosby, 1977, p 248.
241. Riise D: Neuro-ophthalmological patients with bitemporal hemianopsia (follow-up study on etiology). Acta Ophthalmol 48:685, 1970.
242. Gittinger JW Jr: Ophthalmological evaluation of pituitary adenomas. *In* Post KD, Jackson IMD, Reichlin S: The Pituitary Adenoma. New York, Plenum, 1980, p 259.
243. Mills RP, Glaser JS: Hysterical bitemporal hemianopia. Arch Ophthalmol 99:2053, 1981.

Chapter 208

Retrochiasmal Disorders

THOMAS R. HEDGES III

The role of the ophthalmologist in the clinical management of retrochiasmal disease is primarily diagnostic. Most of the therapeutic issues remain in the domain of the neurologist and neurosurgeon. The main ophthalmic tool for the diagnosis of retrochiasmal disorders is visual field testing, the performance and interpretation of which depends on a firm understanding of visual pathway anatomy. Associated neurologic findings and ancillary clinical tests supplement topographical diagnosis and assist neurologists and neurosurgeons in the workup that is primarily neuroradiologic. This chapter is primarily devoted to the discussion of topographic relationships of visual field abnormalities to anatomic structures using clinical neuroradiologic correlations as illustrations. Differential diagnosis of conditions that affect certain locations along the visual pathways are provided, but the reader is directed to other chapters for more detailed discussion of more common disorders.

OPTIC TRACT

Mastering the neuroophthalmic findings of optic tract disease requires an understanding of many neuroophthalmic principles. Pupillary abnormalities, eye movement disorders, and optic atrophy may accompany characteristic visual field defects.

When there is complete disruption of the optic tract on one side, a complete, macular splitting, hemianopia occurs; however, partial optic tract involvement is more common.[1–4] Even in complete optic tract lesions, macular-splitting hemianopia does not usually cause a reduction in visual acuity unless there is an extension of a lesion into the chiasm.[1] However, because of macular splitting, a false impression of reduced acuity may result from the inability of affected patients to read an entire line of letters on the acuity chart or individual letters that appear split.[5] Partial involvement of the optic tracts results in incongruous field defects that may be fairly small and central. Occasionally, one may even have the false impression that the visual field defect is unilateral (Fig. 208–1).

A variety of pupillary abnormalities occur with optic tract disease. When there is significant incongruity of visual field loss or complete hemianopia, there may be a relative afferent defect in the eye with greater visual field loss, most often contralateral to the lesion.[4, 6]

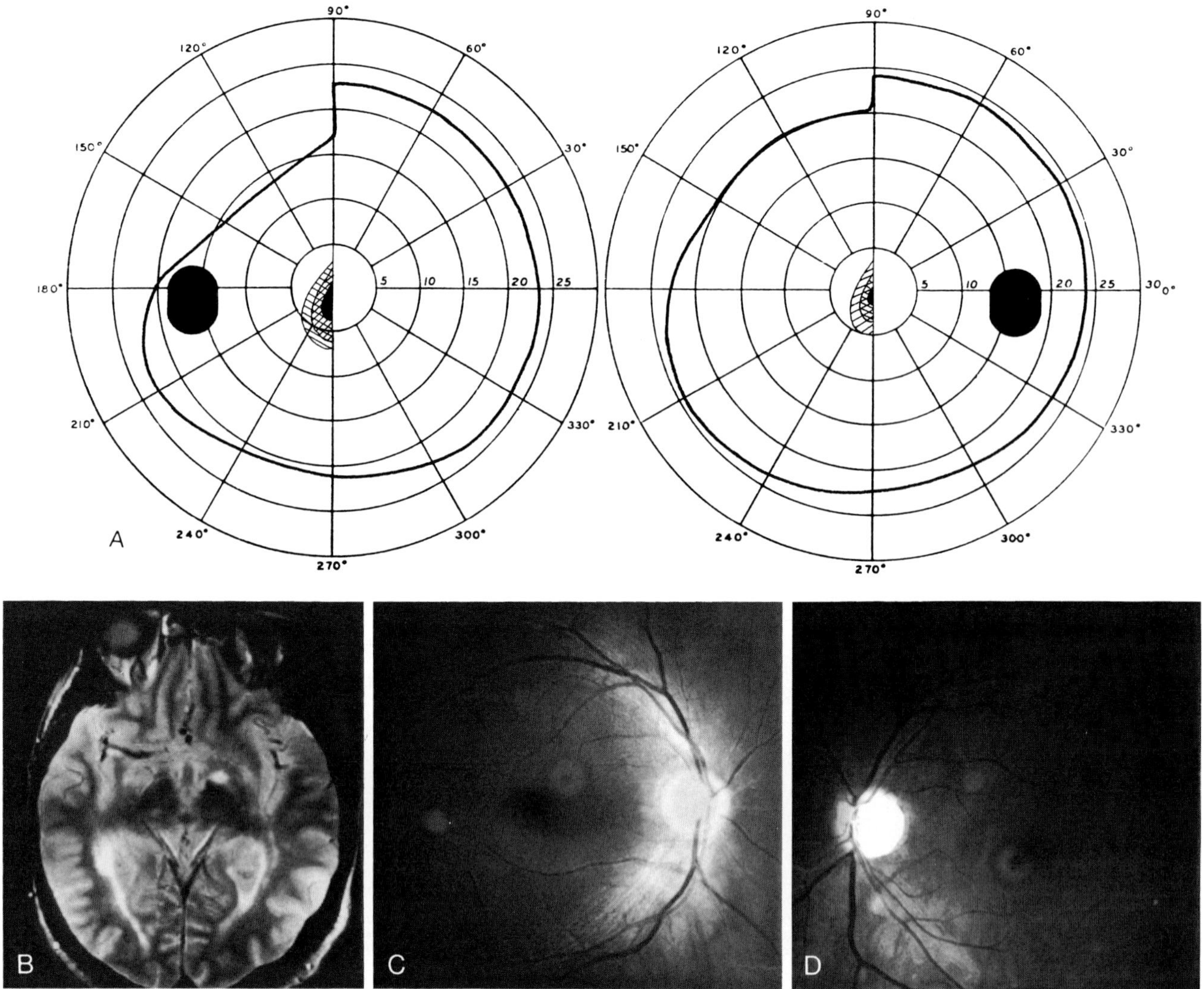

Figure 208–1. *A,* Incongruous, left, hemianopic scotomas that split fixation, due to demyelinating lesion of the contralateral optic tract shown on magnetic resonance imaging (*B*). *C* and *D,* Red-free nerve fiber–layer photographs of a patient with a complete left hemianopia due to an optic tract lesion. The contralateral eye (C) shows drop-out of nerve fibers temporal and nasal to the optic disc, with preservation of the superior and inferior nerve fibers. The nerve fiber layer in the left eye (*D*) is diffusely affected.

Pupillary defects in the absence of visual field loss have been reported.[4, 7] In these cases it is presumed that afferent pupillary fibers in the brachium of the superior colliculus of the midbrain have been damaged, whereas the remaining visual fibers within the optic tract are preserved. Hemianopic afferent pupillary dysfunction, referred to as Wernicke's hemianopic defect or pupillary hemiakinesia, has been demonstrated using a specially designed illuminating system.[8] However, pupillary hemiakinesia usually cannot be detected clinically because of diffusion of light normally used to test the pupil. Another interesting pupillary phenomenon that remains to be explained is Behr's pupil. In some patients with optic tract disease, the pupil contralateral to the lesion and ipsilateral to the visual field defect is larger than the fellow pupil. Although it was not observed in two reported series of patients[2, 3] and has not been produced experimentally,[6] it was identified in 3 of 21 patients described by Savino and associates.[1] One explanation for Behr's pupil might be that involvement of sympathetic input to the ipsilateral pupil may be damaged because of nearby hypothalamic injury.[9] Another pupillary abnormality that may occur in patients with optic tract lesions is due to third-nerve damage, which causes an enlarged and poorly reactive pupil ipsilateral to the lesion.

Other findings associated with optic tract damage may be due to involvement of the nearby hypothalamus. Various endocrine disturbances as well as memory deficits have been reported in a series of patients with optic tract lesions.[3] Involvement of the nearby pyramidal tract may lead to contralateral weakness. Headache, although nonspecific, is also a common finding.[1]

In patients who have chronic optic tract or lateral geniculate damage, so-called hemianopic optic atrophy occurs (see Fig. 208–1). This was emphasized by Hoyt as an indication of postchiasmal, previsual radiation involvement.[10] Although this phenomenon is characteristic of optic tract and lateral geniculate lesions, it rarely occurs in retrogeniculate lesions that are congenital. In the contralateral eye there is a loss of nerve fibers nasal to the fovea, which collects information from the temporal field. This also results in optic disc pallor, which has a bow-tie configuration. A more diffuse type of optic atrophy occurs in the eye ipsilateral to the lesion as nerve fibers temporal to the fovea subserving the nasal visual field degenerate. This sign is most useful in localizing complete homonymous hemianopia as pregeniculate. Hemianopic optic atrophy accompanied by an afferent pupillary defect confirms that the lesion is in the optic tract.

The differential diagnosis of optic tract lesions includes tumors of the basal region of the brain, such as craniopharyngioma, glioma, meningioma, pituitary adenoma, and ectopic pinealoma.[10] See-saw nystagmus may accompany gliomas as well as other conditions affecting the optic tract and nearby subthalamus and midbrain, where the control mechanism for the ocular tilt reaction is located.[11] Demyelinating disease probably affects the optic tracts more often than is recognized clinically, because many patients have preexisting optic neuritis that may reduce vision to the point at which retrochiasmal visual field defect cannot be detected.[12] A variety of vascular disorders including aneurysms and arteriovenous malformations,[1–3] as well as surgery for such lesions, can lead to optic tract damage. Optic tract injury may occur after temporal lobectomy from vasospasm[13] and occasionally from trauma,[1] including subdural hematoma. An abscess rarely affects the optic tract.[11]

The diagnosis of optic tract lesions usually can be made by using magnetic resonance imaging (MRI) scanning. It is important to clinically localize the lesion to the optic tract so that the radiologic study can be properly directed to that location. Lesions involving the optic tract are often so small that only careful attention to the region of the optic tract can identify them (see Fig. 208–1).

LATERAL GENICULATE BODY

Lateral geniculate body lesions are encountered pathologically more frequently than they are recognized clinically.[14] Perhaps this occurs because lateral geniculate lesions may be confused with other retrochiasmal disorders on physical examination.

As in optic tract disease, lateral geniculate involvement may cause complete, macular-splitting, homonymous hemianopia. When the lesion is partial, the resultant hemianopia is incongruous because of unequal involvement of the alternating layers of neurons subserving the two visual fields.[15] Macular vision may be spared in one or both visual fields depending on which layers of the lateral geniculate body are affected.[16] The visual field defects may also extend from the vertical meridian out into the periphery forming a sector type of hemianopia.[17, 18] The reverse may occur, resulting in a sector of preserved visual field along the horizontal meridian extending out into the periphery bordered by homonymous upper and lower quadrantic sectors of the visual loss (Fig. 208–2).[19]

Lateral geniculate lesions can be distinguished from optic tract lesions by preservation of pupillary responses, whereas most, but not all, optic tract lesions affect the pupils to some degree. On the other hand, the optic atrophy seen in lateral geniculate lesions is the same as that which occurs in optic tract lesions with a bow-tie or band type of atrophy occurring in the contralateral eye and diffuse optic atrophy occurring in the eye ipsilateral to the lesion.[16]

Neurologic signs and symptoms associated with lateral geniculate lesions may be caused by involvement of areas of the adjacent thalamic nuclei. This includes hemisensory defects such as contralateral loss of pain and temperature sensation. A possible thalamic syndrome related directly to the eyes has been referred to as central dazzle. This form of photophobia can be distinguished from ocular photophobia in that central dazzle is described as an exaggeration of brightness without discomfort in the eyes.[20, 21] Involvement of the nearby pyramidal tract may result in a contralateral hemiplegia.

Many reported lateral geniculate lesions have been due to infarcts, primarily involving the anterior and lateral choroidal arteries.[18, 19, 22] However, tumors also affect the lateral geniculate body along with arteriovenous malformations, trauma, and inflammatory disorders.[23]

As with optic tract lesions, carefully performed MRI is required to adequately identify small tumors or infarcts affecting the lateral geniculate.[24] Precise clinical localization of the findings to the lateral geniculate is helpful in identifying small lesions, by computed tomography (CT) scanning, or by MRI.

VISUAL RADIATIONS

Temporal Lobe

Anterior and inferior fibers of the optic radiations form Meyer's loop within the temporal lobe. Superior quadrantic visual field defects occur in patients with temporal lobe disease, because fibers within the temporal lobe carry information from the inferior retina. The visual field defects are characteristically incongruous, because fibers carrying information from identical points in the two visual fields are spatially separated. Incongruous, homonymous, wedge-shaped defects in the upper visual fields almost always indicate involvement of the temporal lobe.[25] The ipsilateral nasal visual field defect is usually denser, comes closer to fixation, involves more of the periphery, and extends more toward the inferior quadrant (Fig. 208–3).[26] Involvement of the more proximal portions of visual radiations results in a complete homonymous hemianopia with macular splitting.[26, 27]

Left-sided temporal lobe lesions affecting speech areas may result in expressive aphasia. Involvement of either temporal lobe may cause uncinate fits characterized by an aura of unusual taste or smell along with involuntary movements of the mouth and auditory or formed visual hallucinations.[28] A common cause of temporal lobe

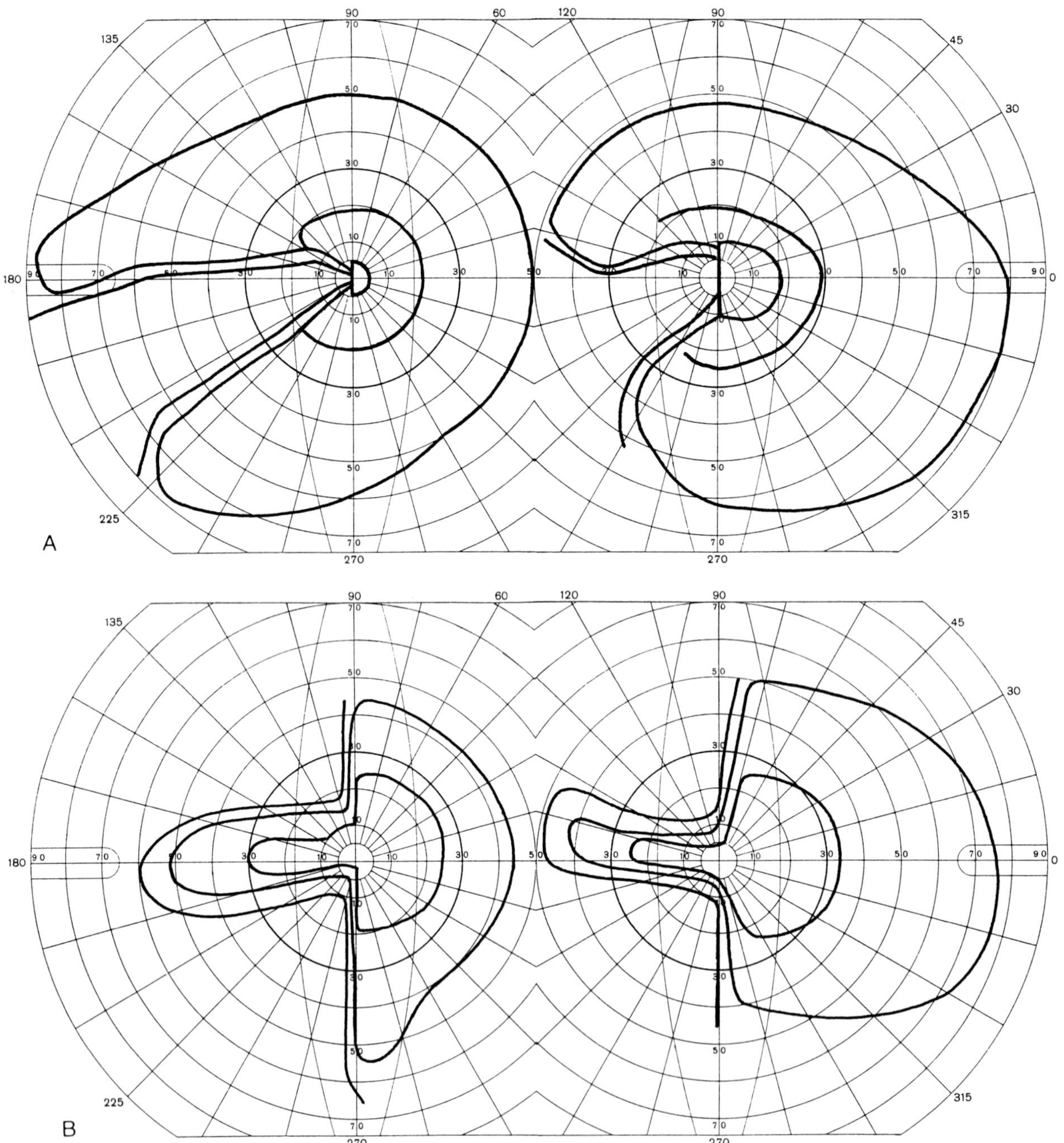

Figure 208–2. *A*, Hemianopic, sector defect splitting fixation due to lateral geniculate infarction. *B*, Superior and inferior homonymous defects with preservation of the horizontal sector visual field, and another patient with lateral geniculate damage. (Modified from Frisen L, Holmegaard L, Rosencrantz M: Sectorial optic atrophy and homonymous, horizontal sectoranopia: A lateral choroidal artery syndrome? J Neurol Neurosurg Psychiatry 41:374, 1978 and Frisen L: Quadruple sectoranopia and sectorial optic atrophy: A syndrome of the distal anterior choroidal artery. J Neurol Neurosurg Psychiatry 42:590, 1979.)

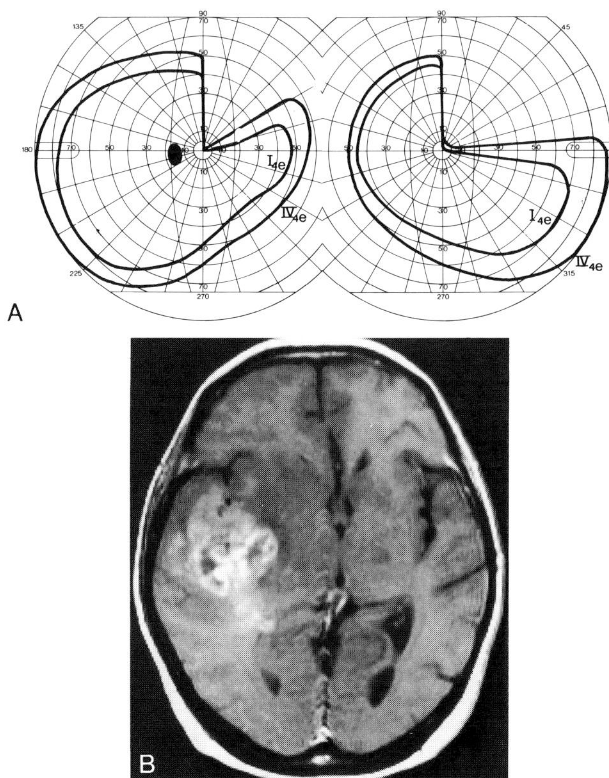

Figure 208–3. *A*, Incongruous, superior quadrantanopia due to a tumor involving the contralateral temporal lobe seen on magnetic resonance imaging (*B*).

epilepsy is a tumor, the surgical treatment of which may result in visual field loss. Usually, a significant amount of temporal lobe must be removed before vision is affected. Although Meyer's loop fibers may reach a position within 4 mm from the tip of the temporal horn, resections of the temporal lobe up to 8 cm may not cause visual field defects.[26, 27, 29, 30] Furthermore, the visual field defects following temporal lobectomy may be fairly congruous.[27]

Tumors that affect the temporal lobe include gliomas and metastases. Among vascular lesions, stroke is most common. Anterior choroidal artery infarction may affect the visual radiations of the temporal lobe as well as the lateral geniculate body. In this situation, contralateral hemiplegia with hemianesthesia tends to occur.[31] Rare conditions that may affect the visual radiations in the temporal lobe include demyelinating lesions,[12] abscess, congenital malformations, and trauma.[32]

Patients with incongruous superior quadrantic visual field defects that are associated with optic atrophy or afferent pupillary defects should be suspected of having temporal lobe disease. Most lesions in this area can be identified by either CT scanning or by MRI.

Parietal Lobe

Parietal lobe diseases may affect the upper fibers of the visual radiations and cause inferior visual field loss. Partial defects tend to be incongruous. More often than not, homonymous hemianopia of parietal origin is complete (Fig. 208–4). Wedge-shaped, quadrantic, inferior hemianopsias, analogous to those found with temporal lobe lesions, are rarely recorded.[33] In the posterior parietal lobe, fibers carrying information from corresponding retinal points tend to be fairly close in proximity, and disorders in this region tend to cause more congruous field defects than do more anterior lesions. Macular splitting almost always occurs when parietal lobe disease causes complete, homonymous hemianopia.

One of the problems encountered in testing visual fields in patients with right parietal lobe disease is due to an associated deficit in spatial orientation that may lead to neglect or inability to perform visual tasks in the left side of visual space.[34] Conversely, neglect of the left half of space may be difficult to demonstrate in patients with complete homonymous hemianopia. However, in patients with incomplete field defects, inattention can be distinguished from visual field loss using double simultaneous stimulation.[35] One can also use tasks of varying difficulty, requiring awareness of the two visual fields such as selecting specific letters out of a group of randomly placed letters.[36] Right-sided parietal lesions also cause difficulty in copying simple figures, drawing clocks, or constructing two-dimensional designs (constructional apraxia).[37]

Left parietal lobe lesions may be associated with finger agnosia, right-left disorientation, agraphia, and acalculia (Gerstmann syndrome).[38] Visual perceptual problems caused by left-sided parietal disease include word blindness and visual agnosia. These topics are dealt with in more detail in Chapter 209.

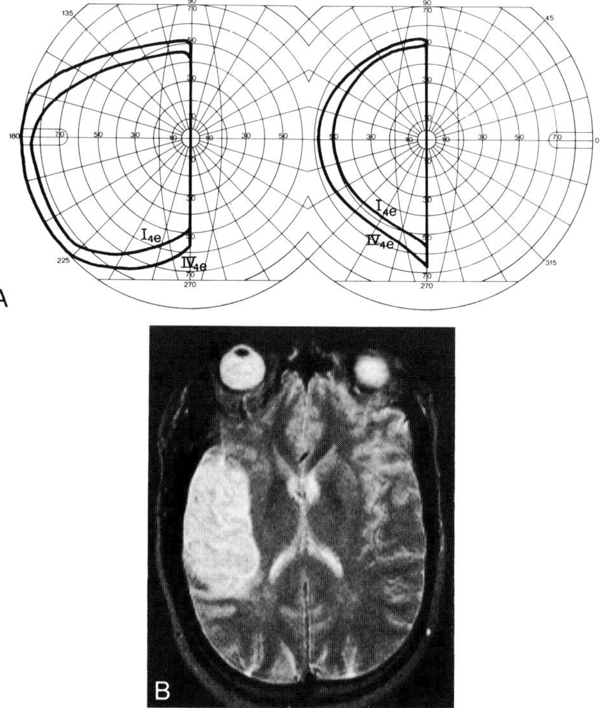

Figure 208–4. *A*, Complete homonymous hemianopia due to infarction of the contralateral parietal lobe seen on magnetic resonance imaging (*B*).

A useful ocular motor sign of parietal lobe dysfunction is loss of normal optokinetic responses.[39] Although optokinetic responses may be decreased in patients with occipital disease, deep parietal lobe lesions disrupt ipsilateral pursuit and responses to optokinetic targets directed toward the side of the lesion. Loss of optokinetic responses is not due to visual field loss. On occasion, patients with parietal lobe disease have normal visual fields but asymmetric optokinetic responses. Another ocular motor sign seen in patients with parietal disease is conjugate deviation of the eyes. Two phenomena have been described. The first is sustained, involuntary gaze deviation occurring *spontaneously toward* the side of frontoparietal lesions.[40] The second phenomenon, conjugate deviation of the eyes *away* from the side of parietal lesions *during forced eyelid closure*, was described by Cogan, who noted that this also occurred in some cases of temporal and occipital disease.[41]

Parietal lobe lesions do not cause pupillary abnormalities unless they are associated with damage to the adjacent optic tract. Optic atrophy is not observed unless the damage is congenital.[10]

The differential diagnosis of lesions involving the parietal lobe includes stroke due to middle cerebral artery occlusion, hypertensive cerebral hemorrhage, and hemorrhage within arteriovenous malformations and tumors.[33] Visual radiations may be affected by subdural hematoma[42] from blunt trauma or from penetrating injury. Primary and metastatic tumors affect the parietal lobe fairly commonly. Demyelinating disease is rarely recognized as a cause of parietal visual loss.[43] CT scanning and MRI show most of the aforementioned lesions.

OCCIPITAL LOBE

Unilateral disease of the occipital cortex is characterized by isolated, congruous, hemianopic, paracentral scotomas. Most occipital lesions, including those affecting the most posterior portions of the occipital lobe, tend to spare the central 5 degrees of the visual field (macular sparing).[44] The macular area is split only when the lesions extend anteriorly into the visual radiations.[45, 46] Some central visual field defects are so small that they may be perceived by the patient as being unilateral and may be misinterpreted by physicians as being due to macular disease. Frequently, Goldmann and automated perimetry are not sensitive enough to detect the field defect in one or both homonymous visual fields. In this situation, tangent screen visual field testing is necessary to identify a small, dense, congruous, hemianopic, paracentral scotoma that, with proper neuroradiologic studies, can be readily demonstrated to be due to a lesion in the occipital pole (Fig. 208–5).[47] An Amsler

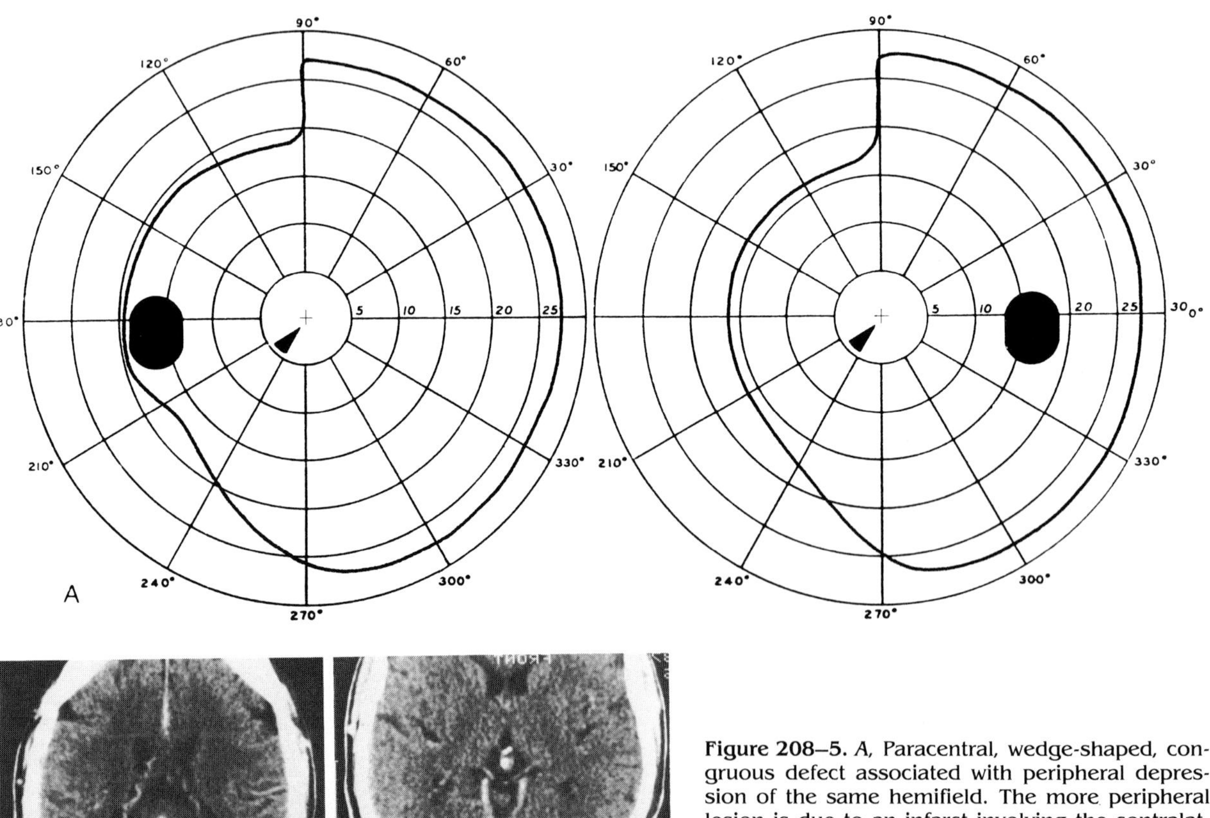

Figure 208–5. *A,* Paracentral, wedge-shaped, congruous defect associated with peripheral depression of the same hemifield. The more peripheral lesion is due to an infarct involving the contralateral, anterior calcarine cortex, demonstrated by the low-density area shown on the CT scan in *B.* The central visual field defect is due to a more recent infarct of the posterior, contralateral, occipital lobe shown as a higher-density, contrast-enhancing lesion on the CT scan (C).

grid may help to locate the area where a small defect is likely to be found. With larger occipital lesions, a quadrantic defect may be detected, sometimes respecting the horizontal meridian as well as the vertical meridian. A superior quadrantic defect indicates inferior calcarine disease and vice versa.[47] When both upper and lower calcarine cortices are affected, a complete hemianopia may result, most commonly with macular sparing. Furthermore, disease involving most of the calcarine cortex, except for the anterior tip, may be great enough to obliterate the smaller, ipsilateral nasal visual field but may not be large enough to obliterate the larger contralateral temporal visual field, causing sparing of the temporal crescent (Fig. 208–6).[48] Anterior calcarine lesions affecting only the temporal crescent of the contralateral visual field occur, but they are difficult to identify with certainty using perimetry.[49] Perception of motion in a visual field otherwise blind to static targets is a phenomenon described by Riddoch and is thought to be indicative of occipital lobe disease. However, the phenomenon of statokinetic dissociation has subsequently been found to occur in visual pathway lesions outside the occipital lobe.[50]

Signs and symptoms other than visual field loss occur in patients with occipital disease, but isolated loss of visual field is one of the hallmarks of occipital damage. Although most affected patients are aware of a problem with their vision, some patients may be unaware of their visual loss until they start bumping into objects or having automobile accidents. Others may become aware of preexisting visual loss when they lose vision in the contralateral visual field. Visual acuity may appear to be reduced in some patients with occipital disease in which splitting of fixation occurs or in whom a quadrantic defect encroaches upon fixation. Some patients also have difficulty with reading, even though their visual acuity and their ability to write are preserved. This syndrome of alexia without agraphia occurs in patients who have left posterior cerebral artery occlusions that result in damage to the left calcarine cortex along with

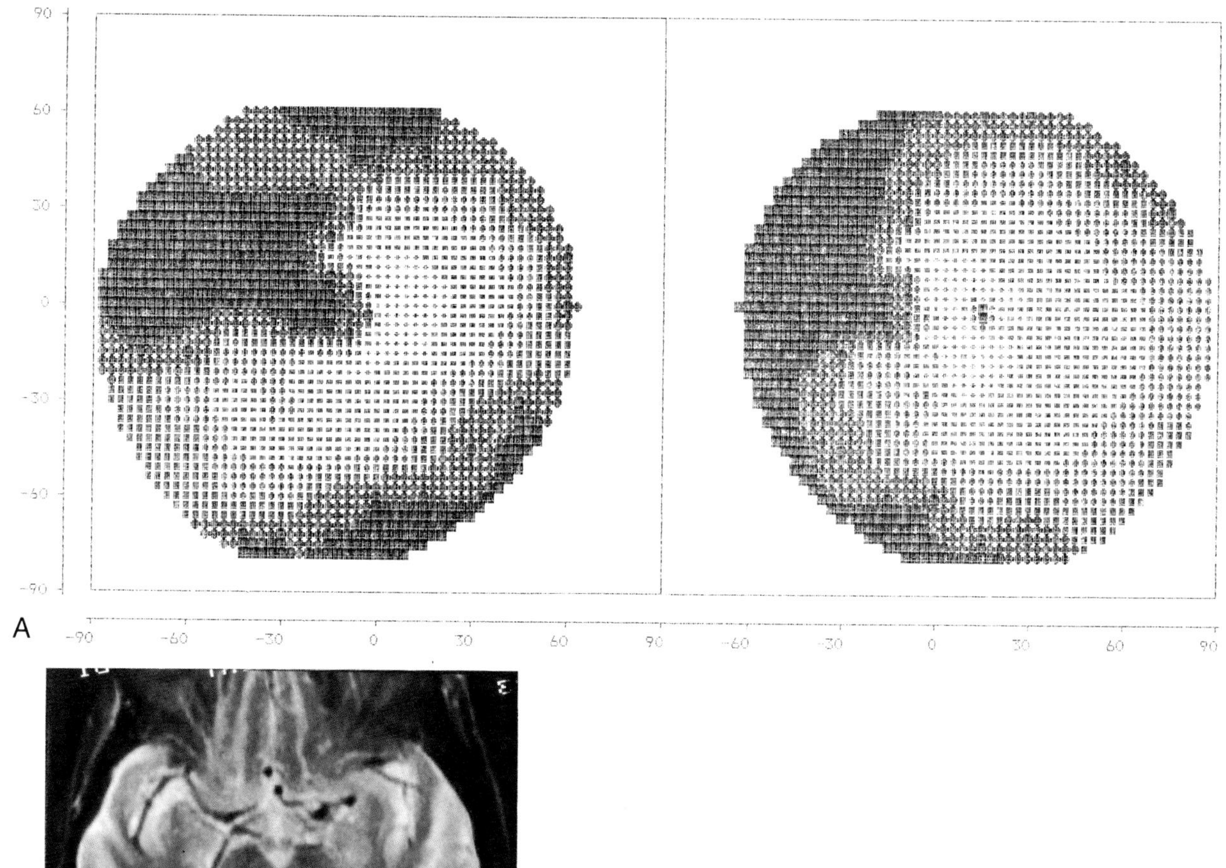

Figure 208–6. *A*, Automated visual field showing a left, homonymous defect that is congruous, except for sparing of the temporal crescent in the left visual field due to corresponding occipital infarct involving the posterior calcarine cortex with sparing of the anterior calcarine cortex seen on magnetic resonance imaging (*B*).

the splenium of the corpus collosum.[51] Information cannot be seen in the damaged left occipital cortex, and information that is seen by the intact right visual cortex cannot be transmitted across the corpus callosum to the language center on the left side of the brain.[52]

Headache occurs in patients with a variety of lesions affecting the occipital lobe, including a stroke. Occasionally, the pain may be referred to the eye.[53] Visual hallucinations occur in patients with a variety of occipital disorders, including stroke.[54] Visual agnosia, pure alexia, palinopsia, and dyschromatopsia are other important phenomena associated with occipital disease and are discussed in detail in Chapter 209.

The most common cause of unilateral occipital disease is stroke (Table 208–1).[46] In one review of 104 patients with isolated homonymous hemianopia from retrochiasmal disorders, 86 percent had posterior cerebral artery occlusions.[32] This finding has been confirmed more recently.[55] Commonly, patients with occipital stroke become acutely aware of their visual problem; however, occasionally the history may suggest a more insidious process that may be difficult to distinguish from the chronic onset of visual loss from a tumor, for example. In patients with vascular occlusion of the posterior cerebral artery or its branches, the visual loss may improve slightly and then remain stable without evidence of progression. This may also help to differentiate stroke from other types of lesions. In patients with occipital infarcts, it is important to rule out an embolic source.[46] This should include cardiac valvular disease and atrial fibrillation. Although localized disease within the posterior cerebral artery can occur,[56] this is unusual. A rare patient with complicated migraine may develop posterior cerebral artery occlusion, but in these cases an associated abnormality, particularly something that may result in hyperviscosity (e.g., polycythemia, leukemia, or dysproteinemia) must be investigated.[57, 58] These conditions should also be considered in other patients with posterior cerebral artery occlusion. Giant cell arteritis may affect the vertebrobasilar artery system and rarely may cause occipital infarction. Other vascular disorders including systemic lupus erythematosus may result in visual loss from occipital lobe involvement. It is of interest that patients with lupus frequently have positive visual experiences.[59] It is extremely unlikely, but possible, that the posterior cerebral artery circulation can be affected by disease in the carotid arteries.[60]

The posterior cerebral arteries may also become occluded after diffuse swelling of the brain, such as following hypoxia or injury in which one or both blood vessels may be occluded when they are compressed by the brain against the tentorial edge.[61, 62] Trauma to the neck, including chiropractic manipulation, may result in posterior cerebral artery occlusion.[63, 64] Venous occlusive disease may also lead to occipital injury, and this is something that has been reported to occur postpartum.[65, 66] Visual field defects may result from arteriovenous malformations,[67] especially when complicated by hemorrhage or treated by surgery or embolization. Occipital hemorrhage occurs from hypertension or coagulopathy, or within a tumor, particularly melanoma.

Occipital field defects may occur in isolation when they are secondary to occipital lobe tumors,[68] but often headache as well as other neurologic signs, including papilledema, occurs. Positive visual phenomena, such as brief flashes of colored shapes or formed images, may occur in such individuals, and the symptom of palinopsia (recurring images) is highly suggestive of a tumor, although this may follow an infarct.[69, 70] Tumors affecting the occipital lobe include gliomas, meningiomas, and metastatic tumors.

Bilateral occipital disease occurs on occasion, usually due to vascular disease (see Table 208–1).[71] Such a patient may be unaware of a preexisting hemianopic field defect until the contralateral visual field is involved.[72] In extreme situations, this may result in a keyhole of preserved visual field, which is sometimes complicated by encroachment close to fixation by quadrantic defects.[47] Patients with this type of field defect usually retain central vision but have difficulty due to visual field constriction. On a rare occasion, bilateral infarcts of either both superior or both inferior calcarine cortices result in bilateral altitudinal visual field defects that may be misinterpreted as being due to bilateral optic nerve head disease.[73]

The term cerebral blindness refers to a complete loss of vision due to bilateral lesions affecting the posterior visual pathways. The term cortical blindness is used if the disorder can be more discretely localized to the occipital cortex. However, the two syndromes are difficult to distinguish from a clinical point of view.[74] Both are defined as complete loss of all visual sensation, retention of normal pupillary reflexes, full extraocular movements, and absence of other cerebral abnormalities such as hemiplegia, sensory dysfunction, aphasia, or dementia.[75] However, some people make the distinction based on the lack of any associated symptoms in cortical blindness and the presence of other neurologic symptoms in patients with cerebral blindness. Purely cortical blindness is generally due to hypoxia or anoxia, whereas cerebral blindness may be due to vascular disease as well as a variety of toxic, degenerative, neoplastic, infectious, and traumatic conditions (see Table 208–1). Therefore, the distinction between cerebral and cortical blindness may be assumed on the basis of etiology.

It is sometimes difficult to distinguish acute bilateral optic nerve lesions from cortical blindness. Optic nerve lesions should be accompanied by sluggish pupillary responses to light and, with time, optic atrophy. Patients may occasionally develop anterior as well as posterior visual pathway dysfunction. Examples of diseases that do this are adrenal leukodystrophy (Shilder's disease)[76, 77] and severe hypotension, especially after cardiac bypass surgery.[78, 79]

Yet another problem in the diagnosis of cortical or cerebral blindness is the denial of visual loss, referred to as anosagnosia or Anton's syndrome. This phenomenon, which is usually temporary, can make it difficult to determine the date of onset of visual loss. It rarely occurs in patients with lesions involving other areas of the visual pathways.[80]

Visual evoked potentials may be of some use in the

Table 208–1. CAUSES OF OCCIPITAL LOBE DYSFUNCTION

Arterial Occlusive Disorders
Atherosclerosis of posterior cerebral artery
Arteritis
Systemic lupus erythematosus
Migraine
Fibromuscular dysplasia
Hypoplasia of posterior artery
Moya-moya disease
Transtentorial herniation with compression of posterior cerebral arteries
Vasospasm following subarachnoid hemorrhage
Severe hypotension

Venous Occlusion
Venous sinus thrombosis
Behçet's disease
Puerperal

Embolic Phenomena
Valvular heart disease
Subacute bacterial/marantic endocarditis
Atrial fibrillation
Myocardial infarction
Atrial myxoma
Fat emboli

Hematologic Disorders
Hypercoagulable states
Hyperviscosity syndromes
Severe hypotension
Sickle cell disease

Hemorrhage
Arteriovenous malformation
Hypertension
Tumor (melanoma)
Coagulopathy

Tumors
Metastatic
Lymphoma
Meningioma
Glioma
Arteriovenous malformation

Inflammation/Infection
Multiple sclerosis
Creutzfeldt-Jakob disease
Progressive multifocal leukoencephalopathy
Syphilis
Abscess
Meningitis
Encephalitis
Subacute sclerosing panencephalitis

Trauma
Contusion
Electrical injury
Penetrating injury
Drowning
Surgery

Congenital Defects

Toxins
Mercury
Lead
Ethanol

Metabolic Disorders
Adrenal leukodystrophy/other leukodystrophies
Hypoglycemia
Intermittent porphyria
Mitochondrial disease (MELAS)

Other
Postangiography
Postcardiopulmonary bypass
Ictal and postictal
Postventriculography

diagnosis and management of cortical blindness. In children who develop cortical blindness following head injury, preserved pattern visual evoked potentials may indicate a good prognosis for recovery of vision,[81, 82] although patients with relatively normal visual evoked potentials have been reported with radiologic evidence of occipital damage that did not recover.[83, 84]

Overall, the prognosis for recovery of at least central vision is good in patients with cerebral or cortical blindness.[85] However, a significant amount of time (possibly years) must be allowed to elapse before considering the chances for further recovery of vision to be unlikely following stroke or injury, especially in children who appear cortically blind.

Cortical injury following hypoxia, trauma, or drowning is associated with laminar necrosis.[86] In these situations recovery may not occur. In situations of hypoxia as well as after significant head injury, especially if there has been subdural intracranial hemorrhage, herniation of the brain over the tentorium compressing the posterior cerebral arteries may lead to bilateral cortical blindness that may not recover.[62, 63] Cortical blindness as well as homonymous hemianopia appears in some women in the postpartum period. This may be transient and has been thought to be due to cerebral venous thrombosis in many cases.[65, 66]

Transient cortical blindness may follow injury. This has been divided into three clinical syndromes: (1) juvenile (up to 8 yr of age) with blindness lasting for hours and excellent prognosis for recovery; (2) adolescent (8 yr of age through the teens) with delay of onset of blindness lasting minutes to hours and an excellent prognosis for recovery; and (3) adult, from severe head injury with blindness that may be protracted and with a variable visual outcome.[87] The association of migraine or seizure disorders increases susceptibility to posttraumatic transient cerebral blindness. Transient cerebral blindness and transient hemifield loss can follow seizures.[88, 89] Transient cortical blindness may also follow cerebral angiography, especially when the vertebrobasilar system is injected with a contrast agent.[90, 91] The prognosis for visual recovery is very good in almost all of these cases.

A CT scan demonstrates most occipital lesions. Contrast agents are helpful, especially in the acute phase of an infarct, during which the lesion may appear isointense with a normal brain. MRI, with gadolinium, is more sensitive in identifying occipital abnormalities, including small lesions and arteriovenous malformations. However, an occipital lesion may be overlooked on MRI or CT scanning, unless the neuroradiologist is specifically directed to the appropriate occipital lobe and the area within the occipital lobe that appears to be affected based on visual field findings (see Fig. 208–5). In any patient with cortical blindness, MRI with gadolinium enhancement reveals the most detail, especially with regard to subcortical involvement.

REFERENCES

1. Savino PJ, Paris M, Schatz NJ, et al: Optic tract syndrome. Arch Ophthalmol 96:656, 1978.
2. Newman SA, Miller NR: Optic tract syndrome: Neuro-ophthalmologic considerations. Arch Ophthalmol 101:1241, 1983.
3. Bender MB, Bodis-Wollner I: Visual dysfunctions in optic tract lesions. Ann Neurol 3:187, 1978.
4. Bell RA, Thompson HS: Relative afferent pupillary defect in optic tract hemianopias. AJO 85:538, 1978.
5. Lessell S, Lessell IM, Glaser JS: Topical diagnosis: Retrochiasmal visual pathways and higher cortical function. *In* Glaser JS (ed): Neuro-ophthalmology, 2nd ed., Philadelphia, JB Lippincott, 1990.
6. O'Connor PS, Kasdon D, Tredici TJ, Ivan DJ: The Marcus Gunn pupil in experimental tract lesions. Ophthalmology 89:160, 1982.
7. Forman S, Behrens MM, Odel JG, et al: Relative afferent pupillary defect with normal visual function. Arch Ophthalmol 108:1074, 1990.
8. Cox TA, Drewes CP: Contraction anisocoria resulting from half-field illumination. AJO 97:577, 1984.
9. Carmel PW: Sympathetic deficits following thalamotomy. Arch Neurol 18:378, 1968.
10. Hoyt WF, Rios-Montenegro EN, Behrens MM, Eckelhoff RJ: Homonymous hemioptic hypoplasia: Fundoscopic features in standard and red-free illumination in three patients with congenital hemiplegia. Br J Ophthalmol 56:537, 1972.
11. Hedges TR III, Hoyt WF: Ocular tilt reaction due to an upper brain stem lesion: Paroxysmal skew deviation, torsion, and oscillation of the eyes with head tilt. Ann Neurol 11:537, 1982.
12. Slavin ML: Acute homonymous field loss: Really a diagnostic dilemma. Surv Ophthalmol 34:399, 1989.
13. Anderson DR, Trobe JD, Hood TW, Gebarski SS: Optic tract injury after anterior temporal lobectomy. Ophthalmology 96:1065, 1989.
14. Lindenberg R, Walsh FB, Sacks, JG: Neuropathology of Vision: An Atlas. Philadelphia, Lea & Febiger, 1973.
15. Gunderson CH, Hoyt WF: Geniculate hemianopia: Incongruous homonymous field defects in two patients with partial lesions of the lateral geniculate nucleus. J Neurol Neurosurg Psychiatry 34:1, 1971.
16. Hoyt WF: Geniculate hemianopias: Incongruous visual defects from partial involvement of the lateral geniculate nucleus. Proc Austr Assoc Neurologists 12:8, 1975.
17. Smith RJS: Horizontal sector hemianopia of non-traumatic origin. Br J Ophthalmol 54:208, 1970.
18. Frisen L, Holmegaard L, Rosencrantz M: Sectorial optic atrophy and homonymous, horizontal sectoranopia: A lateral choroidal artery syndrome? J Neurol Neurosurg Psychiatry 41:374, 1978.
19. Frisen L: Quadruple sectoranopia and sectorial optic atrophy: A syndrome of the distal anterior choroidal artery. J Neurol Neurosurg Psychiatry 42:590, 1979.
20. Fisher CM: Some neuro-ophthalmological observations. J Neurol Neurosurg Psychiatry 30:383, 1967.
21. Cummings JL, Gittinger JW Jr: Central dazzle. A thalamic syndrome? Arch Neurol 38:372, 1981.
22. Helgason C, Caplan LR, Goodwin J, Hedges T III: Anterior choroidal artery-territory infarction. Arch Neurol 43:681, 1986.
23. Goldman JE, Horoupian DS: Demyelination of the lateral geniculate nucleus in central pontine myelinolysis. Ann Neurol 9:185, 1981.
24. Horton JC, Landau K, Maeder P, Hoyt WF: Magnetic resonance imaging of the human lateral geniculate body. Arch Neurol 47:1201, 1990.
25. Miller, NR: Walsh and Hoyt's Clinical Neuro-ophthalmology, 4th ed, vol. 1. Baltimore, Williams & Wilkins, 1982.
26. Van Buren JM, Baldwin M: The architecture of the optic radiation in the temporal lobe of man. Brain 81:15, 1958.
27. Falconer MA, Wilson JL: Visual field changes following anterior temporal lobectomy: Their significance in relation to "Meyer's loop" of the optic radiation. Brain 81:1, 1858.
28. Fite JD: Temporal lobe epilepsy: Association with homonymous hemianopsia. Arch Ophthalmol 77:71, 1967.
29. Bjork A, Kugelberg E: Visual field defects after temporal lobectomy. Acta Ophthalmol 35:210, 1957.
30. Marino R, Rasmussen T: Visual field changes after temporal lobectomy in man. Neurology 18:825, 1968.
31. Morello A, Cooper IS: Visual field studies following occlusion of the anterior choroidal artery. AJO 40:796, 1955.
32. Trobe JD, Lorber ML, Schlezinger NS: Isolated homonymous hemianopia. Arch Ophthalmol 89:377, 1973.

33. Lessell S, Lessell IM, Glaser JS: Typical diagnosis: Retrochiasmal visual pathways and higher cortical function. *In* Glaser JS: Neuro-ophthalmology. Philadelphia, JB Lippincott, 1990.
34. Heilman KM, Watson RT: The neglect syndrome—A unilateral defect in the orienting response. *In* Harnard S, Doyt RW, Goldstein L, et al (eds): Lateralization in the Nervous System. New York, Academic Press, 1977.
35. Albert MC: A simple test of visual neglect. Neurology 23:658, 1973.
36. Ladavas E: Is the hemispatial deficit produced by right parietal lobe damage associated with retinal or gravitational coordinates? Brain 110:167, 1987.
37. DeRenzi E: Visuo-spatial disorders. *In* Kennard C, Rose FC (eds): Physiological Aspects of Clinical Neuro-ophthalmology. Chicago, Year Book Medical Publishers, 1988.
38. Gerstmann J: Some notes on the Gerstmann syndrome. Neurology 7:866, 1957.
39. Baloh RW, Yee RD, Honrubia V: Optokinetic nystagmus and parietal lobe lesions. Ann Neurol 7:269, 1980.
40. Tijssen CC, van Gisbergen JAM, Schulte BPM: Conjugate eye deviation: Side, site, and size of the hemispheric lesion. Neurology 41:846, 1991.
41. Cogan DG: Neurologic significance of lateral conjugate deviation of the eyes on forced closure of the lids. Arch Ophthalmol 62:694, 1948.
42. Pevehouse BC, Bloom WH, McKissock W: Ophthalmologic aspects of diagnosis and localization of subdural hematoma: An analysis of 389 cases and review of the literature. Neurology 10:1037, 1960.
43. Beck RW, Savino PJ, Schatz NJ, et al: Plaque causing homonymous hemianopsia in multiple sclerosis identified by computed tomography. Am J Ophthalmol 94:229, 1982.
44. Bunt AH, Minckler DS: Foveal sparing: New anatomical evidence for bilateral representation of the central retina. Arch Ophthalmol 95:1445, 1977.
45. McAuley DL, Russell RW: Correlation of CAT scan and visual field defects in vascular lesions of the posterior visual pathways. J Neurol Neurosurg Psychiatry 42:298, 1979.
46. Pessin MS, Lathi ES, Cohen MB, et al: Clinical features and mechanism of occipital infarction. Ann Neurol 21:290, 1987.
47. Horton JC, Hoyt WF: The representation of the visual field in human striate cortex: A revision of the classic Holmes map. Arch Ophthalmol 109:816, 1991.
48. Benton S, Levy I, Swash M: Vision in the temporal crescent in occipital infarction. Brain 103:83, 1980.
49. Walsh TJ: Temporal crescent or half-moon syndrome. Ann Ophthalmol 6:501, 1974.
50. Safran AB, Glaser JS: Statokinetic dissociation in lesions of the anterior visual pathways. Arch Ophthalmol 98:291, 1980.
51. Benson DF, Tomlinson EB: Hemiplegic syndrome of the posterior cerebral artery. Stroke 2:559, 1971.
52. Caplan LR, Hedley-Whyte T: Cuing and memory dysfunction in alexia without agraphia. Brain 98:251, 1974.
53. Knox DL, Cogan DG: Eye pain and homonymous hemianopia. Am J Ophthalmol 54:1091, 1962.
54. Cogan DG: Visual hallucinations as release phenomena. Graefes Arch Clin Exp Ophthalmol 188:139, 1973.
55. Fujino T, Kigazawa K, Yamada R: Homonymous hemianopia: A retrospective study of 140 cases. Neuro-ophthalmology 6:17, 1986.
56. Pessin MS, Kwan ES, DeWitt LD, et al: Posterior cerebral artery stenosis. Ann Neurol 21:85, 1987.
57. Dorfman LJ, Marshall WH, Enzmann DR: Cerebral infarction and migraine: Clinical and radiologic correlations. Neurology 29:317, 1979.
58. Bogousslavsky J, Regli F, Van Melle G, et al: Migraine stroke. Neurology 38:223, 1988.
59. Brandt KD, Lessell S, Cohen AS: Cerebral disorders of vision in systemic lupus erythematosus. Ann Intern Med 83:163, 1975.
60. Pessin MS, Kwan ES, Scott RM, Hedges TR III: Occipital infarction with hemianopsia from carotid occlusive disease. Stroke 20:409, 1989.
61. Sato M, Tanaka S, Kohama A, Fujii C: Occipital lobe infarction caused by tentorial herniation. Neurosurgery 18:300, 1986.
62. Hoyt WF: Vascular lesions of the visual cortex with brain herniation through the tentorial incisura: Neuro-ophthalmologic considerations. Arch Ophthalmol 64:74, 1960.
63. Sherman DG, Hart RG, Easton JD: Abrupt change in head position and cerebral infarction. Stroke 12:2, 1981.
64. Gittinger JW: Occipital infarction following chiropractic cervical manipulation. J Clin Neuro Ophthalmol 6:11, 1986.
65. Beal MF, Chapman PH: Cortical blindness and homonymous hemianopia in the postpartum period. JAMA 244:2085, 1980.
66. Monteiro MLR, Hoyt WF, Imes RK: Puerperal cerebral blindness: Transient bilateral occipital involvement from presumed cerebral venous thrombosis. Arch Neurol 41:1300, 1984.
67. Troost BT, Newton TH: Occipital lobe arteriovenous malformations. Clinical and radiologic features in 26 cases with comments on differentiation from migraine. Arch Ophthalmol 93:250, 1975.
68. Parkinson D, Craig WM: Tumours of the brain, occipital lobe: Their signs and symptoms. Can Med Assoc J 64:111, 1951.
69. Lessell S: Visual hallucinations and related phenomena. Weekly Update: Neurology and Neurosurgery 2:48, 1979.
70. Young WB, Heros DO, Ehrenberg BL, Hedges TR III: Metamorphopsia and palinopsia: Association with periodic lateralized epileptiform discharges in a patient with malignant astrocytoma. Arch Neurol 46:820, 1989.
71. Symonds C, MacKenzie I: Bilateral loss of vision from cerebral infarction. Brain 80:415, 1957.
72. Bogousslavsky J, Van Melle G: Unilateral occipital infarction: Evaluation of the risk of developing bilateral loss of vision. J Neurol Neurosurg Psychiatry 46:78, 1983.
73. Newman RP, Kinkel WR, Jacobs L: Altitudinal hemianopia caused by occipital infarcts: Clinical and computerized tomographic correlations. Arch Neurol 41:413, 1984.
74. Aldrich MS, Alessi AG, Beck RW, Gilman S: Cortical blindness: Etiology, diagnosis, and prognosis. Ann Neurol 21:149, 1987.
75. Bergman PS: Cerebral blindness. Arch Neurol Psychiatry 78:568, 1957.
76. Traboulsi EI, Maumenee IH: Ophthalmologic manifestations of X-linked childhood adrenoleukodystrophy. Ophthalmology 94:47, 1987.
77. Sedwick LA, Klingele TG, Burde RM, et al: Schilder's (1912) disease: Total cerebral blindness due to acute demyelination. Arch Neurol 43:85, 1986.
78. Sabah AH: Blindness after cardiac arrest. Postgrad Med J 44:513, 1968.
79. Rizzo JF, Lessell S: Posterior ischemic optic neuropathy during general surgery. Am J Ophthalmol 103:808, 1987.
80. Lessell S: Higher disorders of visual function: Negative phenomena. *In* Glaser JS, Smith JL (eds): Neuro-ophthalmology. St. Louis, CV Mosby, 1975.
81. Kupersmith MJ, Nelson JI: Preserved visual evoked potential in infancy cortical blindness: Relationship to blindsight. Neuro-ophthalmology 6:85, 1986.
82. Sokol S, Hedges TR, Moskowitz A: Research report: Pattern VEPs and preferential looking acuity in infantile traumatic blindness. Clin Vis Sci 2:59, 1987.
83. Bodis-Woliner I, Atkin A, Raab E, Wolkstein M: Visual association cortex and vision in man: Pattern-evoked occipital potentials in a blind boy. Science 198:629, 1977.
84. Spehlmann R, Gross RA, Ho SU, et al: Visual evoked potentials and postmortem findings in a case of cortical blindness. Ann Neurol 2:531, 1977.
85. Zihl J, Von Cramon D: Restitution of visual function in patients with cerebral blindness. J Neurol Neurosurg Psychiatry 42:312, 1979.
86. Lindenberg R: Compression of brain arteries as the pathogenic factor for tissue necrosis and their areas of predilection. J Neuropathol Exp Neurol 14:223, 1955.
87. Greenblatt SH: Posttraumatic transient cerebral blindness: Association with migraine and seizure diatheses. JAMA 225:1073, 1973.
88. Walsh FB, Hoyt WF: Clinical Neuro-ophthalmology. Baltimore, Williams & Wilkins, 1969.
89. Salmon JH: Transient postictal hemianopsia. Arch Ophthalmol 79:523, 1968.
90. Horwitz NH, Wener L: Temporary cortical blindness following angiography. J Neurosurg 40:583, 1974.
91. Studdard WE, Davis DO, Young SW: Cortical blindness after cerebral angiography: Case report. J Neurosurg 54:240, 1981.

Chapter 209

Higher Visual Functions of the Cerebral Cortex and Their Disruption in Clinical Practice

MARSEL MESULAM

Advanced primates display a great diversity of visually guided behaviors. A correspondingly large number of cortical areas in these species become involved in the processing of visual information. Experimental observations during the last 20 yr have revolutionized our understanding of how these parts of the cerebral cortex are organized. This chapter introduces some of the current observations in this field and then focuses on relevant syndromes that can be encountered in clinical practice (Table 209–1).

ORGANIZATION OF CORTICAL VISUAL AREAS

The eye acts as an obligatory transducer for transforming light wave information into temporospatial patterns of neural activity. This information is relayed centrally along two parallel pathways: one directed to the lateral geniculate nucleus and the other to the superior colliculus. The first of these two pathways is by far the more dominant in controlling visually guided behaviors in primates.

The input from the eyes is subjected to initial sorting and reorganization within the four parvocellular and two magnocellular layers of the lateral geniculate nucleus. This information is then relayed through the geniculostriate pathway (optic radiations) to area V1 (also known as area 17, OC, calcarine cortex, primary visual cortex, striate area) in the occipital lobe of the ipsilateral hemisphere (Fig. 209–1).

Area V1 occupies the ventral and dorsal banks of the calcarine sulcus and contains a complete and orderly spatial mapping of the contralateral visual hemifield. There is a vertical inversion so that the superior quadrant is represented ventrally in calcarine cortex and the inferior quadrant dorsally. The neurons that receive input from the macular part of the visual fields are located most peripherally in area V1 (over the occipital pole of the human brain) and have the smallest receptive fields, yielding a relatively large cortical magnification factor per degree of visual field.[1]

In the primate brain, area V1 is the obligatory relay for the direct entry of visual information into neocortical circuitry. Its neurons are sensitive to orientation, direction, binocular disparity, speed, length, spatial frequency, wavelength and luminance. Thus area V1 encodes the basic information necessary for determining movement, stereopsis, color, form, and texture.[2, 3] Individual area V1 neurons that are preferentially sensitive to different aspects of visual information (e.g., color, steropsis, orientation, movement) are not distributed homogeneously but display a relative spatial segregation into an exquisitely organized multidimensional mosaic of columns, layers, and cytochemically (e.g., cyto-

Table 209–1. HIGHER VISUAL FUNCTIONS OF THE CEREBRAL CORTEX AND THEIR DISRUPTION IN CLINICAL PRACTICE

Organization of Cortical Visual Areas
Lateral geniculate nucleus and superior colliculus
Primary visual area (V1, striate area, calcarine cortex, area 17)
Parastriate area (V2, area 18, area OB)
Peristriate areas (area 19 [OA], V3, V4 [color coded], VP, MT-V5 [movement coded])
Downstream visual association pathways
Ventral: To mid- and inferotemporal cortex (the WHAT pathway)
Dorsal: To parietal and frontal cortex (the WHERE pathway)

Striate-Peristriate Syndromes
1. Blind sight: Accurate reaching or detection within the blind field
2. Anton's syndrome: Denial of cortical blindness
3. Akinetopsia: Inability to perceive visual motion
4. Achromatopsia: Inability to perceive, name, or match colors

Syndromes of Ventral Visual Association Pathways
Visual-Verbal Dissociations
1. Color anomia: Can match colors but cannot name them
2. Pure alexia (word blindness): Can write and match words but cannot read them
3. Object anomia (optic aphasia): Can recognize and match objects but cannot name them by visual inspection

Visual-Visual Dissociations
1. Prosopagnosia: Can match but cannot recognize new or familiar faces; can recognize other visually presented generic objects
2. Associative visual object agnosia: can match but cannot recognize objects or faces

Visual-Limbic Dissociations
1. Visual amnesia and hypoemotionality

Dysfunction of Temporal Lobe Visual Association Cortex
1. Visual distractibility
2. Visual integration deficits
3. Visual hallucinations

Syndromes of Dorsal Visual Association Pathways
1. Balint's syndrome: Simultanagnosia, oculomotor apraxia, and optic ataxia
2. Hemispatial neglect

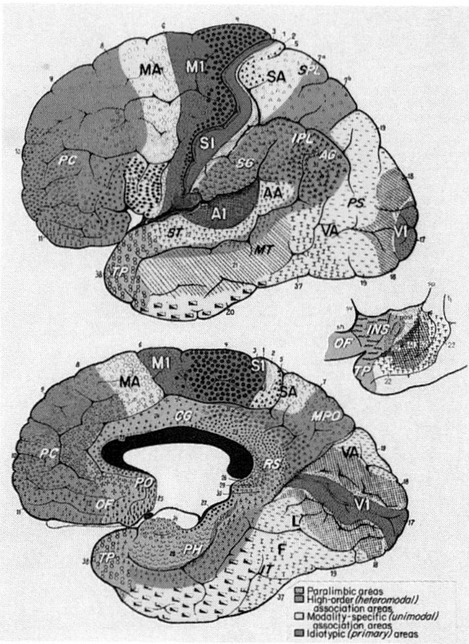

Figure 209–1. Distribution of functional zones in relationship to Brodmann's map of the human brain. The boundaries are not intended to be precise. Much of this information is based on experimental evidence obtained from laboratory animals and needs to be confirmed in the human brain. (AA, auditory association cortex; AG, angular gyrus; A1, primary auditory cortex; CG, cingulate cortex; F, fusiform gyrus; INS, insula; IPL, inferior parietal lobule; IT, inferior temporal gyrus; L, lingual gyrus; MA, motor association cortex; MPO, medial parietooccipital area; MT, middle temporal gyrus; M1, primary motor area; OF, orbitofrontal region; PC, prefrontal cortex; PH, parahippocampal region; PO, parolfactory area; PS, peristriate cortex; RS, retrosplenial area; SA, somatosensory association cortex; SG, supramarginal gyrus; SPL, superior parietal lobule; ST, superior temporal gyrus; S1, primary somatosensory area; TP, temporopolar cortex; VA, visual association cortex; V1, primary visual cortex.)

Note the very extensive areas of cortex denoted to visual processing. In the Brodmann nomenclature, these regions include areas 17 (V1), 18 (V2), 19, 20, 21, 37, and probably parts of 36.

chrome oxidase) differentiated modules. As shown in Figure 209–2, this spatial segregation can be traced back to the division of the lateral geniculate nucleus into four parvocellular layers in which color selectivity and spatial resolution are particularly high and two magnocellular layers in which the neurons are relatively color blind but highly sensitive to contrast.[4]

Area V1 projects to area V2, which is also known as the parastriate area, area 18, or area OB. Area V2 depends on neural input from area V1 for its visual information. It contains a representation of the entire contralateral visual hemifield. The response characteristics of its neurons are similar to those in area V1, but the receptive fields are larger, indicating that some integration of incoming information has taken place. According to classic concepts, the subsequent stage of visual processing was thought to occur in a homogeneous peristriate belt corresponding to area 19 or area OA. This view of a unitary and serial hierarchy is no longer accepted (Figs. 209–3 and 209–4). Anatomic and physiologic experiments in monkeys have shown that areas V1 and V2 give rise to multiple parallel pathways directed to several peristriate visual areas (e.g., V3, VP, V4, MT [V5]) that are partially coextensive with area 19.[2, 3] Receptive fields become larger with increasing synaptic distance from area V1, and the representation of the visual fields in peristriate areas is less complete and relatively disorganized.

At least two of the multiple peristriate areas, MT and V4, display a relative specialization for analyzing specific attributes of visual information. Area MT, located on the ventral bank of the caudal superior temporal sulcus in the monkey, contains many neurons sensitive to direction, velocity, and binocular disparity (stereopsis), whereas only a few of its neurons display color selectivity. In comparison to area V1 neurons whose preferred velocities range from 1 to 32 degrees/sec, for example, the range in MT extends from 2 to 256 degrees/sec.[2] Monkeys with MT lesions have more difficulty responding to moving stimuli than to stationary stimuli.[5] Observations based on positron emission tomography (PET) have revealed an area of increased activity over what appears to be the junction of areas 19, 37, and 39 when human subjects are instructed to attend to moving stimuli.[6, 7] This lateral occipitotemporal region of the human brain may constitute the homologue of area MT (V5) in the monkey.

The second peristriate area with a definable specialization is V4.[8] In the monkey brain, this area occupies the anterior bank of the lunate sulcus and probably the adjacent prelunate cortex. Area V4 contains color-coded neurons that can compensate for changes in the source of illumination, in a way that could provide a neural substrate for the perception of color constancy under variable illumination, such as in the Land effect.[8, 9] This area is thought to play a crucial role for color and perhaps also for form perception. Area V4 is the first point along occipitofugal visual pathways in which neurons display clear-cut attentional and task-related effects. Responses are of greater magnitude and more sharply tuned when the animal is engaged in more challenging tasks and there is a marked inhibition of neural reactivity to unattended stimuli.[10]

Studies based on PET show a relatively selective increase of activity in caudal parts of the lingual and fusiform gyri (areas 18, 19, and 37) when human subjects attended to color patterns, but not when they attended to gray patterns.[6, 7] In the human brain, the homologue to the color-coded part of area V4 may thus be located, at least in part, in the posterior aspects of the lingual and fusiform gyri (Fig. 209–5). An adjacent area in medial occipitotemporal cortex was also activated when subjects attended to stimulus shape,[7] supporting the suggestion that V4 or a closely related area may participate in form perception. An additional zone of activation by color was obtained laterally over what probably corresponds to the junction of areas 19 and 37.[7] Although this lateral occipitotemporal part of the human brain may also respond to color, the clinical evidence from patients with achromatopsia indicates that it may not be as critical for color perception as the more medially located lingual and fusiform region.

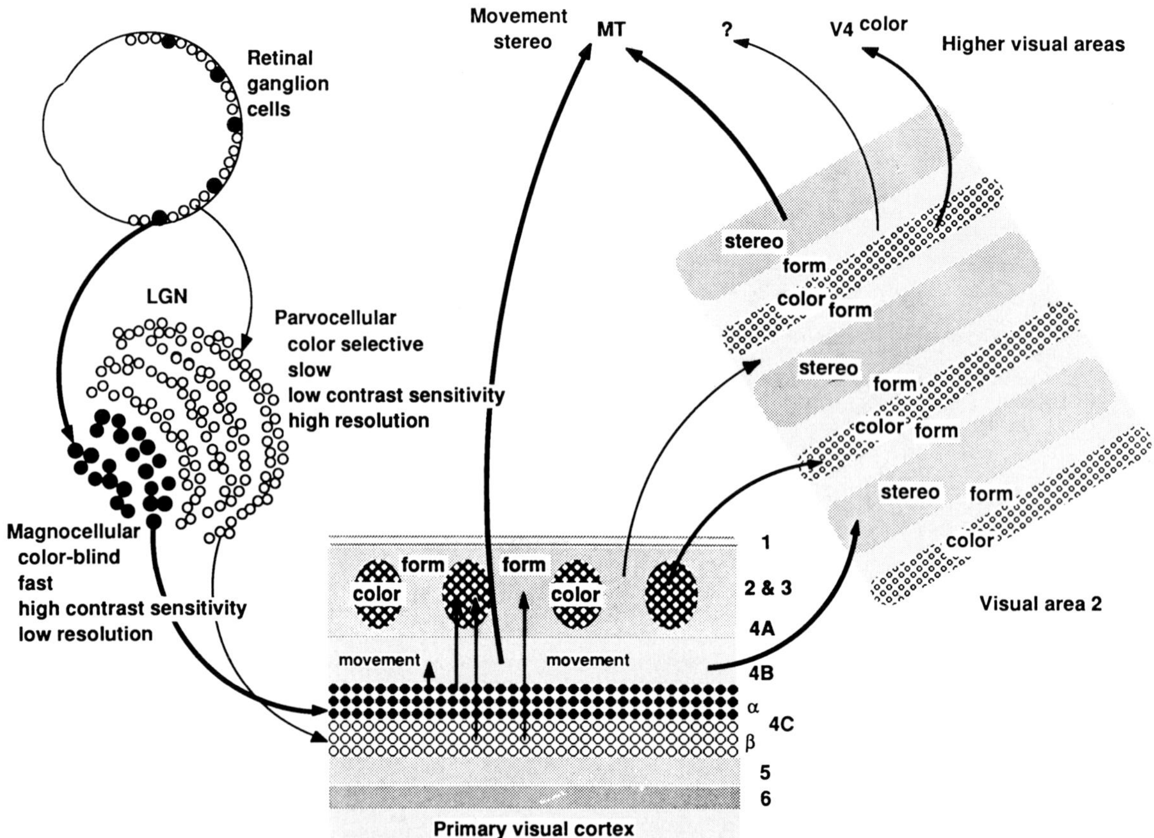

Figure 209–2. The functional segregation of the primate visual system. The cross-hatched areas in layers 2 and 3 of the primary visual cortex (V1) represent the color-sensitive cytochrome oxidase-positive blobs. Cytochrome oxidase staining of visual area 2 (V2) shows alternating sequences of thick (stereo), thin (color), and pale (form) stripes. The fate of projections from the pale stripes is not fully known, although there is some evidence that V4 may play a major role also in form discrimination. (From Livingstone M, Hubel D: Segregation of form, color, movement, and depth: Anatomy, physiology and perception. Science 240:740–749, 1988. Copyright 1988 by the American Association for the Advancement of Science.)

The further occipitofugal flow of visual information occurs along two divergent and parallel paths, one directed ventrally and the other dorsally.[11] The ventral pathway carries visual information originating mostly from V4 into midtemporal and inferotemporal visual association cortex (areas 20, 21, 37, and probably parts of 36 in the human brain and TEO-TE, TF, and TH in the monkey) and also into temporoparietal heteromodal regions (probably corresponding with ventral parts of area 39 in the human brain and the posterior banks of the superior temporal gyrus in humans and monkeys). This pathway sustains the type of information processing that is necessary for establishing visual object identity and has been designated the "what" pathway (Fig. 209–6). The dorsally directed occipitofugal pathway, on the other hand, takes a multisynaptic course to convey visual information, originating from MT as well as from V4, to dorsal heteromodal parietal cortex and to the frontal eye fields (area 8) of premotor association cortex. This pathway deals with the spatial attributes of visual information and has been designated the "where" pathway.[11] The connections along each of these pathways are reciprocal, providing the neural basis for interactive feedforward and feedback circuits.

Behavioral, physiologic, and anatomic experiments in monkeys provide considerable support for this dichotomous organization of visual processing. Along the ventral occipitofugal pathway, inferotemporal cortex neurons have large receptive fields that may cross the vertical meridian, display task-related response properties, show response inhibition to unattended stimuli in their receptive fields, and give selective group responses to complex stimuli such as faces.[10, 12] Lesions in posterior inferotemporal cortex (area TEO) of the monkey brain disrupt pattern discrimination, whereas lesions in anterior inferotemporal cortex (area TE) disrupt visual associative learning.[11] Anatomic experiments show that the inferotemporal cortex acts as a bottleneck for sustaining reciprocal interactions between the visual association cortex and the limbic system.[13, 14] Several independent lines of observation suggest that the resultant visuolimbic interactions are crucial for storing and activating distributed templates corresponding to visual experience and also for associating visual experience with the appropriate emotional-motivational states.[11, 15, 16] In keeping with these animal experiments, regional blood flow determinations in human subjects show increased midtemporal and inferotemporal activation (areas 37,

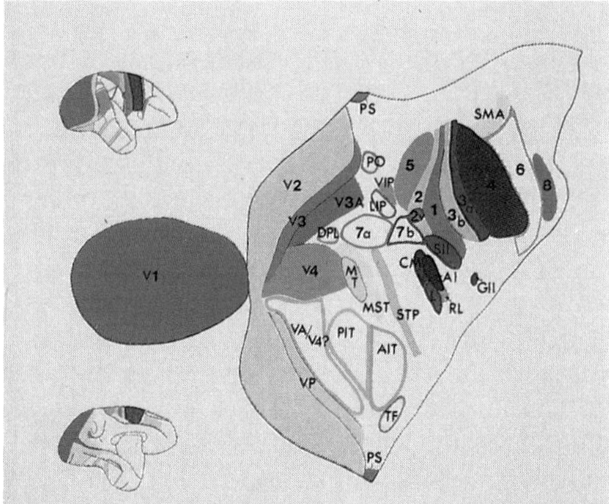

Figure 209–3. Cortical areas in the macaque monkey as represented on the lateral *(top)* and medial *(bottom)* surfaces of the hemispheres and an unfolded, two-dimensional map of the entire hemisphere (middle). (From Van Essen DC: Functional organization of primate visual cortex. *In* Peters A, Jones EG [eds]: Cerebral Cortex, Vol 3. New York, Plenum Publishing Corp, 1985.)

20, and 21) during the mental imagery of previously learned visual patterns, supporting the possibility that this part of visual association cortex (probably corresponding to area TE in the monkey) may provide a storage site for visual templates.[17, 18] Silent word reading and face matching tasks are associated with relatively selective posterior midtemporal (lateral parts of area 37) activation, suggesting that this region (probably corre-

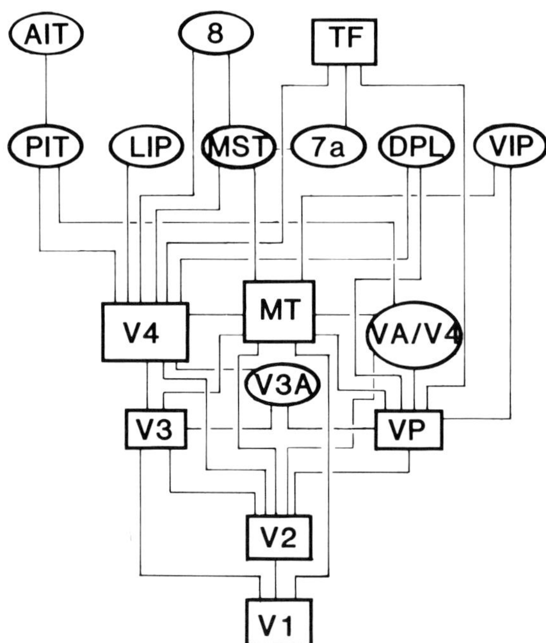

Figure 209–4. Corticocortical connections of visually related areas in the macaque brain. Wherever they have been studied specifically, these connections have been shown to be reciprocal. (From Van Essen DC: Functional organization of primate visual cortex. *In* Peters A, Jones EG [eds]: Cerebral Cortex, Vol 3. New York, Plenum Publishing Corp, 1985.)

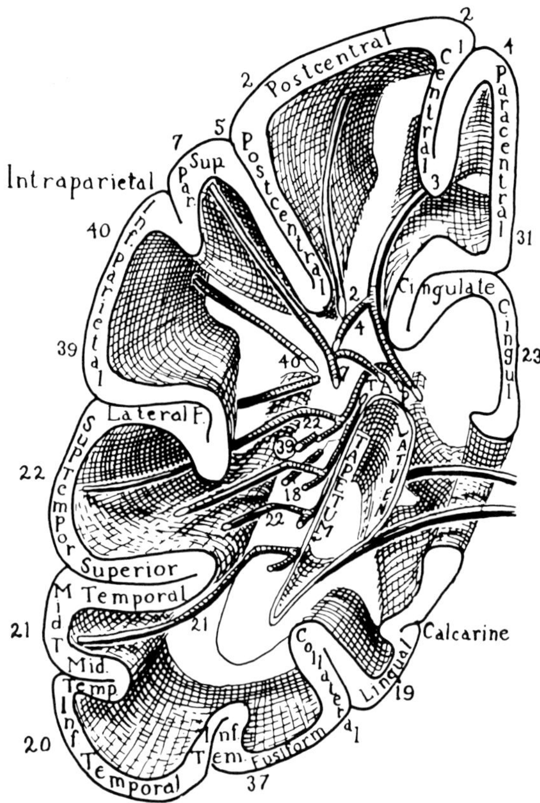

Figure 209–5. A coronal cross section of the human brain showing the location of the lingual and fusiform gyri. Numbers correspond to the Brodmann cytoarchitectonic designations shown in Figure 209–1. (From Krieg WJS: Architectonics of the Human Cerebral Fiber Systems. Evanston, IL, Brain Books, 1973. By permission of Oxford University Press.)

sponding to area TEO in the monkey) may be linked to the perception of complex visual patterns.[19, 20] These observations are consistent with the notion that the ventral occipitofugal pathways are specialized for encoding information related to the perceptual identity of visual objects and their relevance to past experience. In the human brain, this ventral pathway also plays the dominant role in conveying visual information into the language network of the left hemisphere, probably through the angular gyrus component of Wernicke's area (area 39).

Posterior parietal cortex constitutes one of the two major targets along the dorsal occipitofugal pathway. Visually responsive neurons of posterior parietal cortex (area 7a in the monkey) are not particularly sensitive to color, orientation, texture, or shape—properties that are important in determining the firing contingencies of neurons in midtemporal and inferotemporal visual association areas. Instead, the posterior parietal neurons are sensitive to large moving targets and to their spatial positions.[21, 22] Response enhancement occurs to stimuli that are to become the target of grasp, fixation, or other types of attentional focusing.[17] Analogous response contingencies are also detectable in the frontal eyefields (area 8), the second major target of the dorsal occipi-

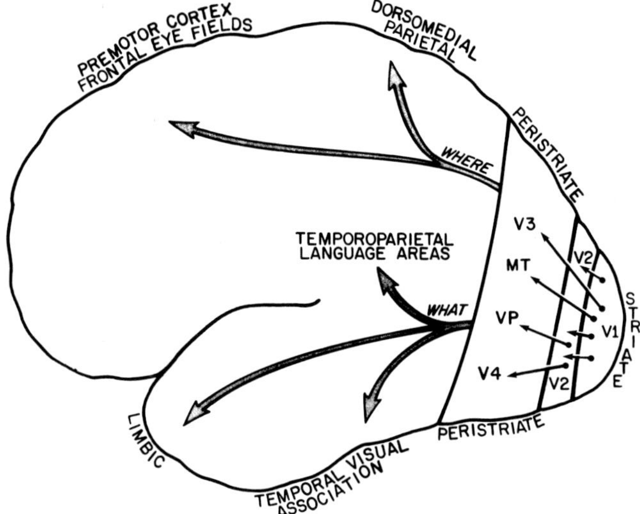

Figure 209–6. A schematic representation of visually related information streams in the human brain. The arrows point in the occipitofugal direction. However, all connections are also reciprocal, providing rich opportunities for feedforward-feedback interactions.

tofugal pathway. The frontal eyefields give rise to one of the two major parallel descending pathways (the other originates in the superior colliculus) that control saccadic eye movements. This part of the brain is related very closely to visual function. Almost half of all distal cortical neurons projecting to the frontal eye fields originate in the peristriate visual areas.[23] A neuron in the frontal eyefields may emit a burst of firing just before a saccadic eye movement towards a behaviorally relevant visual stimulus within its receptive (or motor) field or to its remembered site.[17] In monkeys, damage along the dorsal occipitofugal pathway results in visual neglect for the contralateral hemispace, abnormalities of visually guided hand movements, impaired performance in visuomotor mazes, and an inability to determine the relative position of stimuli in allocentric space.[24–27] These observations are in keeping with the notion that the dorsally directed occipitofugal pathway is concerned primarily with the location of visual stimuli, the visual guidance of movement, and the visuospatial distribution of attention. Studies with PET in human subjects have demonstrated selective increases of metabolic activity in the frontal eye fields and dorsal parietal cortex in tasks that include voluntary eye movements, active manual search, visuospatial localization, visuospatial imagery, and visuospatial attention.[20, 28–30]

This brief synopsis shows that the classic account of a hierarchical and unitary stream of cortical visual processing has been replaced by a new blueprint characterized by parallel routes, multiple hierarchies, reciprocal feedback-feedforward circuitry, and distributed nodes of convergence and divergence. The process starts in the occipital lobe but extends into the temporal lobe, parietal lobe, frontal cortex, and limbic system. The more precise details of this organization can only be investigated in experimental animals with the help of axonally transported tracers, single unit recordings, and focal cortical ablations. The few relevant anatomic observations and the emerging information from functional imaging studies, however, suggest that a similar, and perhaps even more intricate, organization is likely to exist in the human brain. Although the multiplicity of relevant cortical areas endows visually guided behaviors with exquisite flexibility, it also increases their vulnerability to a great variety of lesions, some of which involve the pertinent cortical areas directly and some of which interrupt their axonal interconnections. The resultant syndromes, which may initially appear quite confusing to the clinician, lend themselves to a relatively rational classification based on the experimentally established details of neural organization.

STRIATE-PERISTRIATE SYNDROMES

Blindsight. Damage to area V1 is associated with dense homonymous scotomas (field cuts) in the corresponding parts of the contralateral visual field. In clinical practice, the existence of a scotoma is determined by the patient's failure to report the existence of visual stimuli in the course of perimetry or similar testing procedures. Occasionally, however, if the patient is forced to reach towards a source of light or to distinguish a large X from an O within an otherwise hemianopic field, performance can be quite accurate. This phenomenon, designated "blindsight," may represent the residual visual function sustained by parallel inputs from the eye to the superior colliculus.[31] The role of the oculocollicular pathway in visual function is more substantial in lower animals than in humans. In monkeys, for example, nearly complete area V1 lesions abolish the ability to recognize complex objects but seem to leave intact the ability to locate visual events and avoid obstacles.[31]

Anton's Syndrome. This is a generic term used to designate the denial of blindness. The most usual setting involves bilateral infarctions in the territory of the posterior cerebral arteries. The anatomic correlates that distinguish Anton's syndrome from blindness without denial are not understood. Possible contributing factors include anosognosia associated with right hemisphere involvement or the agitated confusional state associated with damage to the medial occipitotemporal territory of the posterior cerebral arteries.

Akinetopsia. Zihl and associates described a patient with relatively intact visual fields, acuity, color perception, and object identification who reported a sudden loss in her ability to detect visual motion.[32] She had difficulty pouring tea because the fluid coming out of the spout appeared frozen like a glacier, and she could not tell when to stop because she could not perceive the fluid in the cup rising. The loss of movement perception was documented by psychophysical testing. A sagittal sinus thrombosis had caused bilateral lesions in lateral occipitotemporal cortex, including the junction of areas 19, 37, and 39.

In neurologically intact individuals, there is a selective increase of metabolic activity at the confluence of areas 19, 37, and 39 when subjects are attending to moving visual patterns.[6, 7] This area, a potential homologue of the motion-sensitive area MT (V5) in the human brain, was almost certainly damaged in this patient. Bilateral lesions are apparently necessary for the emergence of this rare syndrome. Unilateral lesions could conceivably disrupt movement perception in the contralateral hemifield, but the patient may not report the deficit and specific testing of motion perception may become necessary for its detection.

Central Achromatopsia. Central achromatopsia refers to an acquired loss of color perception resulting from central nervous system injury. The patient may report that colors are dull or drained, or that they seem to have been replaced by shades of gray. Especially in cases in which achromatopsia extends to only one hemifield (hemiachromatopsia) or to one quadrant, the patient may not report the symptom, and the deficit can only be revealed by specific questioning and testing of color perception. Within the achromatopic parts of the visual fields, the patient cannot match or name colors despite nearly normal acuity, stereopsis, movement perception, and the ability to identify objects.

The associated lesion is usually an embolic occlusion of the posterior cerebral artery. Contralateral hemiachromatopsia can occur with lesions of either hemisphere. The minimal lesion that can cause achromatopsia appears to be located in the ventromedial part of the occipital lobe, within the posterior aspects of the lingual and fusiform gyri,[33] a part of the human brain that may correspond, at least in part, to the color-coded area V4 as identified in the monkey brain.[6, 7]

Achromatopsia is relatively rare, because vascular lesions that destroy the critical region in the medial occipitotemporal area usually also extend into the adjacent area V1 cortex or to the optic radiations, leading to a hemianopic field within which color vision cannot be tested. Achromatopsia can be detected only if the lesion in the posterior linguofusiform area is also small enough to spare at least parts of area V1. Frequently, extension of the damage to ventral calcarine cortex (V1) causes an upper quadrantanopia, and there will be selective achromatopsia confined to the lower quadrant. More, rarely, strategically placed bilateral lesions that spare area V1 and the optic radiations may lead to full-field panachromatopsia.

The presence of akinetopsia and achromatopsia confirm the existence of multiple peristriate visual areas in the human brain, each displaying a relative specialization for processing specific attributes of visual information. The independent occurrence of these two syndromes also shows that the inputs from V1 to V2 to peristriate areas are organized in parallel rather than in series.

VENTRAL OCCIPITOFUGAL SYNDROMES: VISUOVERBAL, VISUOVISUAL, AND VISUOLIMBIC DISSOCIATIONS

The ventrally directed striatofugal pathways, organized at least in part along the inferior longitudinal fasciculus, have three major functions: (1) to convey visual information, probably via the angular gyrus, into the language network of the left hemisphere and into the corresponding parts of the right hemisphere; (2) to convey visual information into synaptically downstream components of visual association cortex in the middle and inferior temporal gyri (areas 20, 21, and 37) for perceptual processing, pattern identification, and the storage of distributed visual templates; (3) to convey neural information into limbic system structures such as the amygdala and hippocampal complex. Damage along these pathways, usually associated with stroke in the territory of the posterior cerebral arteries, causes complex deficits of visually guided function. The resultant deficits reflect combinations of visuoverbal, visuovisual, and visuolimbic dissociations. In clinical practice, visuoverbal dissociations lead to the syndromes of color anomia, pure alexia, and object anomia; visuovisual dissociations lead to prosopagnosia, object agnosia, and visual distractibility; visuolimbic dissociations lead to visual learning deficits and visual hypoemotionality.

Color Anomia. This diagnosis is made in nonaphasic patients who can match colors (and therefore have no achromatopsia) but who are unable to name colors. Usually, these patients also fail to point to colors named by the examiner. Thus, color anomia frequently represents a two-way deficit in the verbal labeling of color information. Queries about the color of blood or grass, however, are answered accurately. Color words thus retain their semantic associations (i.e., meaning) but cannot be matched to the appropriate visual stimulus, reflecting a visuoverbal dissociation confined to the domain of color. This diagnosis should be made only if naming in other categories is intact.

The responsible lesion is usually in the left occipital lobe and is almost always associated with a right homonymous hemianopia, so that color anomia is only seen within an otherwise intact left visual field. In addition to the involvement of area V1 or optic radiations, the critical lesion also involves the splenium of the corpus callosum or its radiations within the parasplenial white matter of the left occipital lobe.[33, 34] Since the callosal pathways are interrupted, color information from the intact left visual hemifield cannot be relayed to the language network in the left hemisphere, where the process of verbal labeling occurs. Color perception in the left hemifield remains preserved, because area V4 in the right hemisphere is intact. In such patients, color anomia represents a domain-specific callosal disconnection syndrome superimposed on a right hemianopia. Rarely, damage to splenial fibers in the right occipital lobe may lead to color anomia confined to the left visual field in a patient with otherwise intact visual fields.[35] Such clinical cases show that the naming of colors in the left hemifield requires the transcallosal transfer of visual information (from V4 or a closely related region of the right hemisphere) into the language network of the left hemisphere, probably via the angular gyrus. Pure alexia is a very frequent but not invariant correlate of color anomia.[34] The transcallosal visual pathways carrying information about color and about word forms are therefore not identical, although they seem to run in close anatomic proximity to each other. Visual object naming is spared, indicating that the transcallosal course of object-related visual information takes a different trajectory.

Pure Alexia. This condition, also known as word blindness, is one of the most dramatic examples of visuoverbal disconnection.[36] The patient with pure alexia can write, speak, and understand speech normally; has no difficulty with visual acuity, color perception, and object naming in the intact portion of the visual fields; but experiences a profound inability to read, even words that he or she may have written moments ago. Graphesthesia and the identification of anagram letters by palpation are intact, and the patient has no difficulty copying words that he or she cannot read. The term pure alexia is thus used to designate a domain-specific visual recognition (decoding) deficit for verbal material that is not secondary to underlying perceptual, graphomotor, or more general aphasic deficits.

The pathophysiologic considerations are similar to those of color anomia. The minimal lesion is located in the periventricular white matter of the left occipital lobe.[37] Such a lesion interferes with the transcallosal course of splenial fibers originating from the right occipitotemporal visual association areas and also with the rostral course of left hemisphere ventral occipitofugal association fibers directed toward the angular gyrus. This combination of lesions isolates the language network from information related to visual word forms. In such cases, pure alexia may be seen without hemianopia, color anomia, or object anomia, showing the existence of a distinct trajectory for the intrahemispheric and transcallosal course of visual information related to words.[37] In the most common clinical setting, however, right hemianopia (or achromatopsia) and color anomia (for the left hemifield) are frequent accompaniments because of the proximity of the critical lesion in the left occipital lobe to area V1, the optic radiations, area V4, and transcallosal fibers that carry color information. The preservation of object naming provides further indication that the fibers that carry object-related visual information into the language network have an anatomic arrangement that is considerably different from those that carry information related to color and words.

Transient amnesia is seen occasionally because of additional involvement of the left hippocampal complex, a region that is also in the territory of the posterior cerebral artery. As an alternative to the disconnection mechanism described earlier, it is also conceivable that a "cortical" form of pure alexia would arise from the selective involvement of a more downstream visual association area that could act as a repository of visual word-form templates and as a neural bottleneck for their relay into the language network. Studies with PET did, in fact, show an area of selective activation in the lateral occipitotemporal cortex at the lateral junction of areas 19 and 37 when subjects were visually exposed to words in a task that did not require semantic processing.[19] Assuming that an infarction of this area could constitute another cause of pure alexia, its proximity to Wernicke's area suggests that its destruction would almost always include additional damage to the language network. The resultant multimodal aphasia would make the diagnosis of pure alexia no longer appropriate.

Object Anomia (Optic Aphasia). This diagnosis is made in patients who fail to name objects by sight. Tactile palpation or hearing a characteristic sound made by the object leads to accurate naming. The distinction from visual agnosia is made by showing that the patient can indicate (by gesture or circumlocution) that he or she recognizes the nature or use of the object. The patient with this syndrome can draw the object, which he or she cannot name, and can tell if two objects are visually the same or different, ruling out the possibility that anomia is due to a failure of adequate percept formation. Object anomia thus represents a modality-specific deficit in the verbal tagging of visual information related to objects.

The associated lesion is almost always in the left occipitotemporal region, and there is almost always an associated right homonymous hemianopia. Color anomia and pure alexia are almost invariably present. The anatomic mechanism is similar to that of color anomia and alexia but probably involves a substantially more extensive disconnection of interhemispheric and intrahemispheric visual information from the language network of the left hemisphere.

Prosopagnosia. This diagnosis is made in patients who have lost the ability to recognize familiar faces (even their own) and to learn to recognize new ones. This is not a perceptual deficit, because the patient can describe facial features in detail and can match faces quite well in the Benton-Van Allen Test.[38] Correct recognition can be achieved through auditory cues (e.g., a familiar voice or chuckle) or a particularly salient visual marker (e.g., a characteristic piece of clothing or even posture). The deficit is therefore modality-specific and is most pronounced for the internal proprietary detail of complex visual patterns. Although the syndrome derives its name from the most salient feature, prosopagnosic patients invariably have a more widespread deficit for recognizing proprietary visual details of many generic patterns. They can easily identify the general class to which an object belongs but not the unique visual details that differentiate one member of this class from another.[33] For example, a prosopagnosic patient who cannot recognize his wife or son may have no difficulty in identifying a face as a face or even to determine its approximate age and gender. A patient may identify a car as a car or a house as a house but may not be able to determine the make of the car and may not be able to recognize the house as the specific one that belongs to him. The specific features of the syndrome may vary from one patient to another in a way that reflects the prior visual knowledge base. A birdwatcher, for example, may no longer identify the different species, and a farmer may no longer individually recognize his own cows even though the generic identification of birds and cows remains intact (see reference 33 for review).

The most commonly associated lesion is bilateral infarction in the medial occipitotemporal region, usually involving the lingual and fusiform gyri and the adjacent white matter.[33, 39] The damaged area is in the same general region as in cases of achromatopsia but extends more anteriorly. In the monkey brain, anterior inferotemporal cortex contains neuronal ensembles that encode visual information corresponding to individual faces.[12] The area damaged in human prosopagnosia may be enriched in this type of neuron. Because of the location of the critical lesion, prosopagnosic patients usually also display visual field deficits (especially upper quadrantanopia), achromatopsia, color anomia, and alexia. In some patients, however, prosopagnosia can occur without alexia, indicating that the anatomic substrates of object and word recognition are not identical.[40] The cause is usually an embolic occlusion of the posterior cerebral artery, but prosopagnosia can also emerge as an ictal (or immediately postictal) phenomenon.[33]

The syndrome of prosopagnosia introduces considerable insight into the anatomic basis of visual information processing in the human brain. Studies with PET have shown that a sector of lateral occipitotemporal cortex (areas 19 to 37) becomes selectively activated when human subjects are asked to perform a face-matching task.[20] This area (probably corresponding with area TEO in the monkey) is intact in prosopagnosia and allows the formation of visual "percepts," such as those that would be needed for successful performance in face-matching tasks. Recognition, however, requires the further occipitofugal relay of this information into high-order (downstream) unimodal, heteromodal, and paralimbic areas. These areas almost certainly contain widely distributed representational templates of faces and objects. Through such downstream connections and a subsequent computational architecture that is almost certainly based on parallel distributed processing, individual visual features (or percepts) can lead to recognition by activating the full sensorial attributes (visual and otherwise) of an object and its experiential relationship to the perceiver.

Visuolimbic interactions play a critical role in this process, especially in the binding and storage of new templates and in the activation of those formed in the relatively recent past.[16] The location of the critical lesions and some of the clinical features suggest that prosopagnosia is frequently associated with a considerable component of visuolimbic disconnection. Patients with this syndrome, for example, cannot learn new visual associations, even those that are unrelated to faces.[40] A visuolimbic disconnection, however, does not provide a sufficient anatomic substrate, since patients who are severely amnestic as a consequence of bilateral limbic lesions do not experience prosopagnosia. Such patients may not remember new faces and those that were first seen a short time before the onset of the amnesia, but they have no difficulty in recognizing familiar faces. Templates belonging to such familiar faces are presumably consolidated so extensively that they no longer depend on limbic structures for their activation. The key feature of prosopagnosia, the failure to recognize familiar faces, suggests that there is dysfunction at the level of areas that contain consolidated representations of familiar faces and that are critical for evoking the pertinent sensorial and experiential associations in response to visual information related to individual faces. Other components of the relevant templates seem to remain intact, because accurate recognition can be reached through alternative (e.g., auditory) channels.

Prosopagnosia, therefore, reflects a dysfunction at the level of an inferotemporal visual association area, which encodes visual components of object representations (templates) and which is essential for accessing the additional multimodal components of such templates through visual cues. From an anatomic point of view, it appears that this syndrome arises when parts of the linguofusiform gyri fail to receive input from upstream visual association areas or when they can no longer convey this information to downstream heteromodal areas. Such an outcome could result from interrupting the connections of this area or from directly damaging it. The central feature in the pathophysiology of prosopagnosia is, therefore, a disruption in the flow of visuovisual connections along the ventral occipital pathways.

Familiar faces elicit specific autonomic discharges from prosopagnosic patients who give no evidence of conscious recognition.[41, 42] This remarkable phenomenon suggests that the visual pathways necessary for evoking conscious identification of faces may differ from those that lead to their visceral and perhaps emotional recognition. The almost invariable existence of bilateral lesions in prosopagnosia emphasizes the unique contribution of each hemisphere to facial recognition. In fact, tachistoscopic experiments in split-brain patients show that each hemisphere can achieve facial recognition, but with distinct differences of information-processing strategies.[43]

Associative Visual Object Agnosia. The diagnosis of associative visual object agnosia is made when visually inspected objects cannot be named or recognized (through verbal description or pantomime) by a patient whose language and perceptual functions are otherwise adequate for the task. The adequacy of perceptual function is demonstrated by showing that the patient can draw the object and match those that are identical in appearance. The modality-specificity is demonstrated by showing that correct identification is achieved when the patient is allowed to palpate the object or to hear a characteristic sound associated with it. Performance is at its worst when the patient is shown an object and asked for a verbal response but improves if the patient is asked to point to objects named by the examiner. For the diagnosis to be made appropriately, it is necessary to show that there is no additional aphasia or dementia. The term apperceptive visual agnosia has been used to describe a different type of recognition deficit, one that is based on disorders of scanning, perceptual integration, and attention. The deficit in apperceptive agnosia is in the formation of percepts rather than in the subsequent stage of associative recognition.

In comparison to object anomia, in which visually presented objects can be recognized but not named because of a visuoverbal disconnection, associative object agnosia arises when visual information cannot activate either verbal or nonverbal associations related to that object. An otherwise adequate percept is therefore unable to elicit the associative linkages that lead to recognition.[44] In contrast to the visuoverbal disconnection of object anomia that can be caused by a unilateral left hemisphere lesion, the recognition deficits of associative object agnosia usually require the existence of bilateral lesions. The most commonly associated lesions are in the medial occipitotemporal region, which almost invariably involves the lingual and fusiform gyri of both hemispheres and the adjacent gray and white matter.[39] Frequently associated deficits include achromatopsia, color anomia, and alexia. Visual field deficits are common and are usually confined to upper quadrants, resulting from an extension of the ventral occipitotemporal lesion to the adjacent ventral calcarine cortex.

Associative object agnosia constitutes a more generalized form of prosopagnosia. In prosopagnosia, there is a recognition deficit confined to proprietary visual features that distinguish one member of a class from all the others. Generic identification of visual patterns, however, remains intact. In object agnosia, generic identification is also impaired. The critical feature in each syndrome is an interruption of ventral occipitofugal pathways so that the relevant representational templates cannot be accessed by visual information. There are at least two ways of conceptualizing the specific anatomic relationship of the lesions associated with prosopagnosia and object agnosia. One possibility is that the two share a common anatomic substrate. For example, if it takes X bits of information to specify a generic template of a face or a bird, it would take X + N bits to encode the additional proprietary features of an individual face or bird species. Accordingly, lesser damage to a common site could lead to prosopagnosia, whereas more extensive damage could cause object agnosia. This formulation is consistent with the fact that both syndromes are caused by lesions in the lingual and fusiform gyri and with the observation that every patient with object agnosia also has prosopagnosia, whereas the converse is not true.

As an alternative possibility, there could be two separate areas—a downstream area for identifying the proprietary features unique to individual faces and other objects (e.g., cars) and a synaptically upstream area where the level of encoding does not go beyond that of the general features shared by all members of the relevant object category. In such an arrangement, damage to the downstream area would cause prosopagnosia but not object agnosia since the afferent input to the upstream area would remain intact. Damage to the upstream area, on the other hand, would cause object agnosia as well as prosopagnosia. There is currently insufficient information to differentiate between these two alternative models, relating the anatomic substrates of face recognition to those of object recognition.

Visual Amnesia and Visual Hypoemotionality. Sensory information in each modality is conveyed to limbic structures (e.g., the amygdala and hippocampus) along a precisely organized downstream cascade of neural connectivity. One putative role of sensorilimbic interactions is to increase the durability of motivationally relevant memory traces; another role is to establish a code for binding the different fragments of experience into coherent events.[16] Limbic lesions lead to an impairment of new learning and an inability to retrieve information acquired within the recent past. The resultant amnesias are almost always multimodal. Lesions that interrupt sensorilimbic interconnections in only one modality but that leave limbic structures intact, however, can result in modality-specific amnesias. Object agnosia and prosopagnosia, for example, are modality-specific visual "memory" disturbances but with very special features. In addition to a visuolimbic disconnection, they also involve the destruction (or disconnection) of visual association areas that participate in the formation of relevant consolidated templates. The resultant deficit leaves basic visual perception intact but impairs the recognition of new and familiar visual patterns, even those that have been consolidated for many years. A lesion that causes only a visuolimbic disconnection but that spares the critical sectors of visual association cortex, however, would be expected to impair the learning of new visual associations and the recall of recently acquired ones but should leave consolidated visual knowledge such as the recognition of familiar faces and objects intact.

In at least one patient, a bilateral lesion in the occipital white matter (in the territory of the posterior cerebral artery) was associated with such a modality-specific recent memory loss.[40] The lesions were in a position to interfere with the relay of visual information into the limbic structures of the ventromedial temporal lobe. The patient had no prosopagnosia, object agnosia, or alexia but failed to acquire new visual associations despite adequate visuoperceptual function. The learning of verbal, tactile, and auditory material remained relatively intact. This patient was unable to learn to recognize new faces or to acquire spatial orientation in novel surroundings. This type of modality-specific disorder may not be rare but requires specialized testing for detection. The location of the critical lesions suggests that many of the patients are also likely to have prosopagnosia or object agnosia, in which case the specificity of the syndrome will be lost.

Another potential outcome of a visuolimbic disconnection is to interfere with the emotional impact of visual stimuli. At least two patients have been described in whom bilateral occipitotemporal infarctions were associated with a syndrome of visual hypoemotionality. One patient reported that flowers and landscapes had ceased to elicit the expected feeling of charm and beauty.[45] Another cancelled a subscription to *Playboy* because he no longer found the pictures stimulating even though music and tactile contact continued to provide pleasure.[46] Because of the location of the associated lesions, patients with visual hypoemotionality are frequently also prosopagnosic. However, prosopagnosic patients do not usually complain of visual hypoemotionality, and they continue to give the appropriate visceral (autonomic) responses to familiar faces, even those that they do not consciously recognize. The existence of hypoemotionality may therefore indicate that the medial occipitotemporal damage has resulted in a greater disruption of visuolimbic connections than is customarily found in prosopagnosia.

Visual Distractibility. An important aspect of visual function is the ability to focus awareness on the behaviorally important visual objects and to inhibit distraction by other sources of visual information. One patient with a lesion that involved lateral temporal visual association areas (areas 20 to 21) in the right hemisphere reported that he could no longer focus on the relevant aspects of the visual scene. When fishing, for example, he could not concentrate on the bobber and found his attention easily distracted by a bubble or dead leaf in the stream.[47] Persistent visual distractibility interfered with many of his professional and recreational activities. He had a partial left upper quadrantanopia (from a minor involvement of visual radiations) but no other difficulty in acuity, movement detection, color perception, or object identification. Experiments in monkeys show that neurons in area V4 and in the inferotemporal cortex inhibit responses to unattended stimuli in their receptive fields.[10] The clinical symptom of visual distractibility may reflect damage to this type of neuron. The symptoms may be most salient when the lesion is in the right hemisphere. Equivalent lesions in the left hemisphere may contribute to the emergence of alexia by increasing visual distractibility in the course of reading.

Visual Integration Deficits. The visuoverbal disconnection syndromes (i.e., pure alexia, color anomia, optic aphasia) have attracted a great deal of interest. They are caused by a disconnection of visual information from the language network in the left hemisphere. The syndromes associated with a disconnection of visual information from analogous parts of the right hemisphere remain poorly understood. A number of complex visuoperceptual tasks become severely disrupted after right hemisphere lesions, but not after left hemisphere lesions. These tasks include face-matching (Benton-Van Allen Test), the determination of line orientation (Judgment of Line Orientation Test), the mental rotation of visual patterns, the ability to recognize objects presented from unusual visual perspectives, and the ability to copy complex drawings. The exact anatomic correlate of each deficit remains obscure, even though "inferior parietal lobule" lesions are frequently invoked (see reference 47 for review). These disorders of complex visual processing may reflect, at least in part, an interference with the occipitofugal transfer of visual information into the parts of the right hemisphere that are homologous to components of the left hemisphere language network.

Visual Hallucinations. Hallucinations may occur in a large variety of clinical settings, including toxic metabolic encephalopathies (especially those associated with fever, infection, drug overdose, and withdrawal states), narcolepsy, Parkinson's disease, migraine, and idiopathic psychoses. Hallucinations associated with specific central nervous system lesions can be divided into two classes: ictal hallucinations and release hallucinations.

Ictal hallucinations, especially those arising in peristriate and temporal visual association areas, are associated with partial epilepsy. If the site of the epileptic discharge is in striate and peristriate areas, the hallucinations tend to take the form of flashes, simple geometric shapes, and colors. If the site is in the temporal lobe, especially in the right hemisphere, complex images and scenes are hallucinated. This anatomic correlation is consistent with the close association of temporal visual areas with stored templates of complex visual experiences. Ictal hallucinations tend to be brief, stereotyped, and sometimes restricted to a certain sector of the visual field.

Release hallucinations occur either when there is a major problem with the peripheral sensory apparatus (leading to sensory deprivation) or when there is central pathology in the brain, or both.[48] Loss of peripheral acuity, such as in macular degeneration and cataracts, may lead to vivid visual hallucinations in elderly individuals, even when no other evidence of psychiatric disturbance exists. The visual hallucinations may range from small animals to complex colorful scenes. In contrast to the ictal hallucinations, these hallucinations are continuous and repetitive. Initially, these release hallucinations are associated with fear, but eventually they result in annoyance and then resignation. The combination of pathologic alterations in the peripheral sensory apparatus with damage to the central nervous system is associated with the most florid hallucinations. The related central nervous system lesions can be anywhere along striate, peristriate, and temporovisual association areas. On rare occasions, central lesions alone (especially in the distribution of the basilar artery) may result in pure central release hallucinations. This condition is also known as peduncular hallucinosis. It has been suggested that the associated lesions permanently release hypothetical mechanisms that inhibit the daytime occurrence of dreaming.

DAMAGE ALONG DORSAL OCCIPITOFUGAL PATHWAYS: BALINT'S SYNDROME AND HEMISPATIAL NEGLECT

Dorsally directed occipitofugal pathways follow the general course of the dorsal longitudinal fasciculus and carry visual information into dorsal parietal cortex and the frontal eye fields (see Fig. 209–6). The associated clinical deficits are heteromodal and visuomotor rather than visuoassociative. Anatomic experiments in the monkey brain indicate that the dorsally directed occipitofugal pathway derives its visual information from area V4 as well as from area MT, whereas the information conveyed along the ventral occipitofugal pathways is principally derived from area V4.[2] Nonetheless, the influence of MT seems to predominate the neural activity of dorsal occipitofugal pathways, since visually responsive cells in posterior parietal cortex and the frontal eye fields display preferential response contingencies related to movement, spatial location, and visuomotor search rather than shape, orientation, or color. In keeping with these properties, behavioral observations indicate that the dorsal occipitofugal pathway is specialized for determining the location of visual stimuli, for coordinating their exploration in extrapersonal space, and for enabling their visuospatial synthesis into coherent scenes. In neurologically intact human subjects, studies with PET have shown a dorsal occipitoparietal area of selective activation at the confluence of areas 7 to 19 when subjects were engaged in a spatial localization task.[20] Furthermore, imagery tasks with a high visuospatial load (i.e., route finding) led to metabolic activation of the dorsal, parietal, and inferotemporal cortex, whereas imagery tasks with a lesser spatial load (i.e., comparing relative size of two objects) resulted in activation of only inferotemporal areas, suggesting that the activation of the dorsal parietal cortex was linked to the spatial load of the task.[29, 49] Damage to dorsal occipitofugal pathways does not cause agnosia or visual anomia but a different set of deficits that includes hemispatial neglect, optic ataxia, oculomotor apraxia, and simultanagnosia.

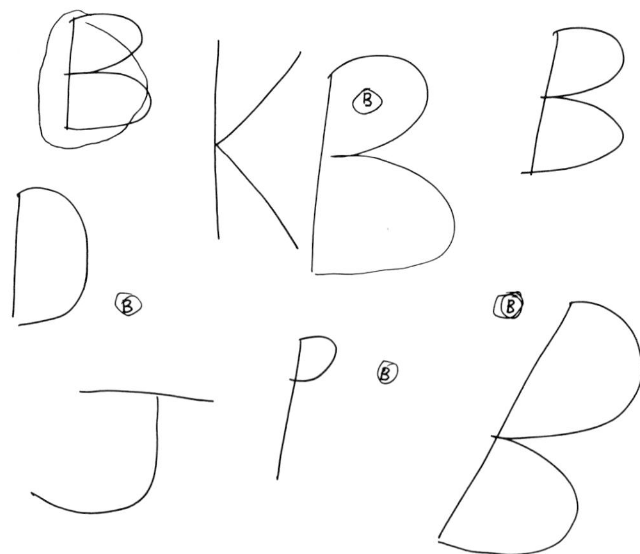

Figure 209–7. Test performance of a 68-year-old patient with simultanagnosia due to a degenerative disease of unknown etiology. The patient presented with a chief complaint of impaired reading abilities. In this search task, he was asked to circle all the B's. He does much better with the smaller letters that can be detected by single visual fixations. He misses the larger letters that require the integration of information across multiple fixations. No time limit was set. At the end of approximately 3 min, he stopped and stated that he had marked all the targets.

Balint's Syndrome. This diagnosis requires the existence of three components, the relative severity of which may vary from one patient to another. First, there is a tendency to misreach towards visual stimuli, whereas manual reaching to tactile and auditory stimuli remains intact. This component is known as *optic ataxia*. Second, there is an erratic pattern of oculomotor scanning and unpredictable spasms of fixation during visual search. Elementary eye movement abnormalities cannot account for this deficit, which is known as *oculomotor apraxia*. The third and usually most dramatic component of Balint's syndrome is known as *simultanagnosia* and refers to a severe disruption in the visuospatial synthesis of complex scenes.

The visuospatial synthesis of complex scenes is normally based on systematic scanning, during which multiple high-resolution "snapshots" from the center of gaze are integrated across multiple foveations. The scanning process is guided in reference to a continuously updated internal representation and requires a dynamic interaction between foveal and more peripheral visual information. Patients with simultanagnosia seem to get stuck on the information that falls within the center of gaze during a haphazardly directed fixation and cannot integrate this input with information coming from other segments of the same scene. When viewing the photograph of a person, for example, the patient may report seeing only a hat or a single feature such as an eye. When asked to read, the patient may fixate on single letters or single words and cannot synthesize the input into coherent words and sentences (Fig. 209–7).

These examples show that patients with Balint's syndrome may also experience severe impairments of face recognition and reading. However, the underlying mechanism is simultanagnosia rather than the visuoverbal and visuovisual disconnections underlying pure alexia and prosopagnosia. The recognition deficits caused by simultanagnosia are usually described as "apperceptive" in contrast to the "associative" agnosias that arise from lesions along ventral occipitofugal pathways. Determining the mechanisms associated with specific recognition deficits may have implications for rehabilitation strategies. Patients with pure disconnection alexias, for example, may show some improvement when the size of the letters is increased, whereas patients with the alexia of simultanagnosia improve when letters and words are made smaller so that meaningful chunks of information can be captured by single fixations (see Fig. 209–7). Patients with associative agnosia show some improvement if an object that they cannot recognize is moved about, whereas the recognition deficit of simultanagnosia is made worse by a similar maneuver. An inability to tell depth, reports of the erratic disappearance of objects in the line of gaze, and a difficulty in locating objects by visual search are common complaints of patients with simultanagnosia. A professional gardener, for example, experienced great difficulty in planting a bed of tulips because he could not locate the last bulb he had planted when he looked back after having picked up the next bulb from his basket.

Balint's syndrome is seen with bilateral lesions that involve the cortex and white matter of dorsal occipitoparietal areas. The etiology is usually based on an ischemic event in the posterior watershed zone, usually associated with a hypotensive event or saggital sinus thrombosis. This syndrome can also be seen in the course of degenerative diseases (e.g., Alzheimer's disease), when the underlying lesions are particularly intense in posterior parietal areas.[50] The optic ataxia and oculomotor apraxia of Balint's syndrome probably represent a dissociation of visual information from the frontal eye fields, whereas simultanagnosia probably represents a dissociation of visual information from dorsal parietal regions that participate in constructing and updating internal representations of extrapersonal space. Visual field deficits are almost always present, especially in the lower quadrants. Color perception, object identification (when the visual information can be incorporated by a single fixation), and acuity in the intact parts of the visual fields are relatively normal. The diagnosis of Balint's syndrome is almost impossible to make if the patient is severely aphasic, if there is also a dementia, or if visual fields are too compromised. For example, a patient who has scotomas in all quadrants on the basis of area V1 lesions and who is left with "tunnel" vision may experience many of the difficulties seen in simultanagnosia.

Hemispatial Neglect. Ventral occipitofugal pathways are important for modulating object-addressed attention and for inhibiting visual distractibility. Spatially addressed attention, however, is coordinated predominantly by the dorsal occipitofugal pathways. The most frequently encountered clinical disturbance of this process emerges in the form of hemispatial neglect.

The right hemisphere of the human brain contains the neural apparatus for distributing attention within the entire extrapersonal space, whereas the left hemisphere contains the neural apparatus for directing attention only to the contralateral right hemispace.[51–54] As a consequence of this right hemisphere dominance, left hemineglect caused by right hemisphere injury is more frequent, severe, and lasting than right hemineglect caused by left hemisphere injury. In fact, most clinicians see hemispatial neglect as a persistent phenomenon only in the left hemispace.

Hemispatial neglect is frequently multimodal, but its visual aspects are particularly salient. Patients with this syndrome ignore visual stimuli on the left, fail to explore and orient towards the left, and act as if the left side of space had been motivationally devalued. Some patients may fail to eat food on the left side of the tray or read the left half of each sentence. The copying of simple drawings reveals a tendency to omit detail on the left and an unusually large margin appears on the left side of the page when the patient is asked to write. Bilateral simultaneous stimulation reveals extinction on the left. There is increased resistance to leftward shifts of covert attention, and there is a failure to detect left-sided targets in tasks that require systematic visual scanning.[16, 52] Some patients may have a left hemianopia or left lower quadrantanopia. In other patients, the visual fields may be full, and there is usually no elementary loss of head or eye movement (except during the acute phase). Neglect behavior, therefore, reflects a disturbance of directed spatial attention rather than a complex combination of more elementary sensory motor deficits. Visual neglect is a deficit of looking, not of seeing (Fig. 209–8). Occasionally, however, the visual neglect may be so severe that it may lead to the mistaken diagnosis of hemianopia. In such patients, the demonstration of intact visual fields may require careful examination with special maneuvers.[51]

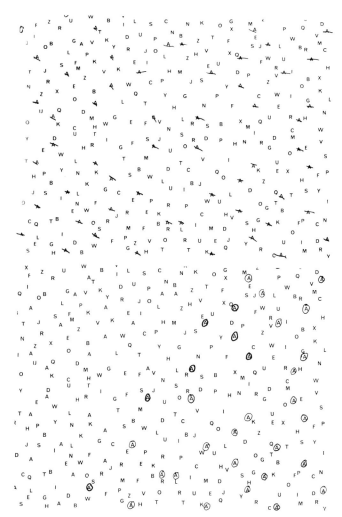

Figure 209–8. The performance of two different patients on a random letter cancellation task is shown. An 8 × 10 sheet of paper containing 15 As in each quadrant is placed directly in front of the patient, who is then asked to check or encircle all the As without moving the sheet of paper. No restriction is placed on head movement. *Top*, A 59-year-old right-handed woman had a left-sided stroke that left her with a dense right homonymous hemianopia. Despite the blind right hemifield, she does not miss any targets on the right. *Bottom*, A right-handed woman in her 70s had an infarct in the right frontal region. She developed a hemiparesis. Visual field testing did not reveal any hemianopia. These two patients demonstrate the independence of hemianopia from unilateral neglect. Visual neglect is an attentional, not a sensory deficit. (From Mesulam M-M [ed]: Principles of Behavioral Neurology. Philadelphia, FA Davis, 1985.)

The syndrome of visual neglect represents a disruption in the handling of visual information by a multifocal network that regulates the distribution of directed attention within the extrapersonal space. The three cortical foci of this network are located in the frontal eye fields, posterior parietal cortex, and the cingulate gyrus.[16, 51, 52] Damage to any one of these three components or to their interconnections in the right hemisphere can lead to hemispatial neglect for the left hemispace. Although this is not widely appreciated in clinical practice, the neglect that results from a lesion of the frontal eye fields can be at least as severe as the neglect that results from parietal lesions. There is a regional specialization within this network so that the frontal eye fields are more closely related to the coordination of exploratory and orienting movements, whereas the posterior parietal component is more closely related to the sensorial representation of extrapersonal space. In keeping with this organization, left hemispatial neglect caused by frontal lesions may be associated with a particularly severe disruption of exploratory scanning (as tested by the procedure shown in Fig. 209–8), whereas the neglect associated with parietal lesions may be more closely associated with visual extinction and with a resistance to internal (covert) attentional shifts.[55] In most patients with hemispatial neglect, extinction and exploratory motor impairments emerge in combination but with differences in relative severity in a way that reflects the site of the primary lesion.

CONCLUSIONS

Considerable advances have occurred in understanding the neurobiology of cortical visual processing. Clinical syndromes that were once considered baffling or even implausible can now be shown to be in keeping with the experimentally determined anatomy and physiology of visual pathways. Current concepts indicate that area V1 acts as a triage center for the multidimensional visual information coming from the eye. From area V1, visual information is conveyed along several parallel pathways into multiple peristriate areas, at least two of which, areas MT and V4, have identifiable specializations for movement detection and color perception, respectively. The further course of visual information occurs along two divergent occipitofugal pathways, one directed dorsally to parietal and premotor areas and the other ventrally to temporoparietal and limbic areas. Damage to the dorsal pathway interferes with visual reaching, oculomotor scanning, visuospatial integration, and spatial attention, whereas damage to the ventral pathway leads to alexia, optic aphasia, color anomia, visual amnesia, visual hypoemotionality, object agnosia, and prosopagnosia. Correct diagnosis of these syndromes may initially appear forbidding but should pose no problem if attention is paid to clinical definitions and testing strategies. This group of syndromes also provides particularly rich opportunities for probing the neurobiologic basis of human perception and cognition.

Acknowledgments

Supported in part by a Javits Neuroscience Investigator Award of the NINDS and an Alzheimer Research Center grant from the NIA. I am grateful to Dr. S. Weintraub for comments and to L. Christie for expert secretarial assistance.

REFERENCES

1. Fox P, Mintun MA, Raichle ME, et al: Mapping human visual cortex with positron emission tomography. Nature 232:806–809, 1986.
2. Van Essen DC: Functional organization of primate visual cortex. *In* Peters A, Jones EG (eds): Cerebral Cortex, vol. 3. New York, Plenum Publishing Company, 1985.
3. Felleman DJ, Van Essen DC: Distributed hierarchical processing in primate cerebral cortex. Cerebral Cortex 1:1–47, 1991.
4. Livingstone M, Hubel D: Segregation of form, color, movement, and depth: Anatomy, physiology and perception. Science 240:740–749, 1988.
5. Newsome WT, Wurtz RH, Dursteller MR, Mikami A: Deficits in visual motion processing following ibotenic acid lesions of the middle temporal visual area of the macaque monkey. J Neurosci 5:825–840, 1985.
6. Lueck CJ, Zeki S, Friston KJ, et al: The colour centre in the cerebral cortex of man. Nature 340:386–389, 1989.
7. Corbetta M, Miezin FM, Dobmeyer S, et al: Attentional modulation of neural processing of shape, color, and velocity in humans. Science 248:1556–1559, 1990.
8. Zeki S: Color coding in the cerebral cortex: The reaction of cells in monkey visual cortex to wavelengths and colors. Neurosci 9:741–765, 1983.
9. Land EH: The retinex theory of color vision. Sci Am 237:108–128, 1977.
10. Wise SP, Desimone R: Behavioral neurophysiology: Insights into seeing and grasping. Science 242:736–741, 1988.
11. Mishkin M, Ungerleider LG, Macko KA: Object vision and spatial vision: Two cortical pathways. Trends Neurosci 6:414–417, 1983.
12. Rolls ET, Baylis GC, Hasselmo ME, Nalwa V: The effect of learning on the face selective responses of neurons in the cortex of the superior temporal sulcus in the monkey. Exp Brain Res 76:153–164, 1989.
13. Van Hoesen GW: The differential distribution, diversity and sprouting of cortical projections to the amygdala in the rhesus monkey. *In* Ben Ari Y (ed): The Amygdaloid Complex. New York, Elsevier/North Holland, 1981.
14. Van Hoesen GW: The parahippocampal gyrus. Trends Neurosci 5:345–350, 1982.
15. Downer De C JL: Interhemispheric integration in the visual system. *In* Mountcastle VB (ed): Interhemispheric Relations and Cerebral Dominance. Baltimore, Johns Hopkins Press, 1962.
16. Mesulam M-M: Large-scale neurocognitive networks and distributed processing for attention, language and memory. Ann Neurol 28:597–613, 1990.
17. Goldberg ME, Segraves MA: Visuospatial and motor attention in the monkey. Neuropsychology 25:107–118, 1987.
18. Roland PE, Gulyas B, Seitz RJ, et al: Functional anatomy of storage, recall and recognition of a visual pattern in man. Neuro Rep. 1:53–56, 1990.
19. Petersen SE, Fox PT, Posner MI, et al: Positron emission tomographic studies of the cortical anatomy of single word processing. Nature 331:585–589, 1988.
20. Haxby JV, Grady CL, Horwitz B, et al: Dissociation of object and visual processing pathways in human extrastriate cortex. Proc Natl Acad Sci 88:1621–1625, 1991.
21. Lynch JC, Mountcastle VB, Talbot WH, Yin TCT: Parietal lobe mechanisms for directed visual attention. J Neurophysiol 40:362–389, 1977.
22. Zipser D, Andersen RA: A back-propagation programmed network that simulates response properties of a subset of posterior parietal neurons. Nature 331:679–684, 1988.
23. Barbas H, Mesulam M-M: Organization of afferent input to subdivisions of area 8 in the rhesus monkey. J Comp Neurol 200:407–431, 1981.
24. Heilman KM, Pandya DN, Geschwind N: Trimodal inattention following parietal lobe ablations. Trans Am Neurol Assoc 95:259–261, 1970.
25. Haaxma R, Kuypers HGJM: Intrahemispheric cortical connections and visual guidance of hand and finger movements in the rhesus monkey. Brain 98:239–260, 1975.
26. Petrides M, Iversen SD: Restricted posterior parietal lesions in the rhesus monkey and performance on visuospatial tasks. Brain Res 161:63–77, 1979.
27. Ungerleider LG, Brody BA: Extrapersonal spatial orientation: The role of posterior parietal, anterior frontal and inferotemporal cortex. Exp Neurol 56:265–280, 1977.
28. Fox PT, Fox JM, Raichle M, Burde RM: The role of cerebral cortex in the generation of voluntary saccades: a positron emission tomographic study. J Neurophysiol 54:348–370, 1985.

29. Roland PE, Friberg L: Localization of cortical areas activated by thinking. J Neurophysiol 53:1219–1243, 1985.
30. Roland PE, Larsen B: Focal increase of cerebral blood flow during stereognosis testing in man. Arch Neurol 33:551–558, 1976.
31. Weiskrantz L, Warrington EK, Sanders MD, Marshall J: Visual capacity in the hemianopic field following a restricted cortical ablation. Brain 97:709–728, 1974.
32. Zihl J, Von Cramon D, Mai N: Selective disturbance of movement vision after bilateral brain damage. Brain 106:313–340, 1983.
33. Damasio AR: Disorders of complex visual processing: Agnosias, achromatopsia, Balint's syndrome, and related difficulties of orientation and construction. *In* Mesulam M-M (ed): Principles of Behavioral Neurology. Philadelphia, FA Davis, 1985.
34. Mohr JP, Leicester J, Stoddard LT, Sidman M: Right hemianopia with memory and color deficits in circumscribed left posterior cerebral artery territory infarction. Neurology 21:1104–1113, 1971.
35. Zihl J, Von Cramon D: Colour anomia restricted to the left visual hemifield after splenial disconnexion. J Neurol Neurosurg Psychiatry 43:719–724, 1980.
36. Geschwind N: Disconnection syndromes in animals and man. Brain 88:237–294, 1965.
37. Greenblatt SH: Alexia without agraphia or hemianopsia. Brain 96:307–316, 1973.
38. Benton AL, Hamsher K de S, Varney W, Spreen D: Contributions to Neuropsychological Assessment. New York, Oxford University Press, 1983.
39. Alexander MP, Albert ML: The anatomical basis of visual agnosia. *In* Kertesz A (ed): Localization in Neuropsychology. New York, Academic Press, 1983.
40. Ross ED: Sensory-specific and fractional disorders of recent memory in man. I: Isolated loss of visual recent memory. Arch Neurol 37:193–200, 1980.
41. Bauer RM: Autonomic recognition of names and faces in prosopagnosia: A neuropsychological application of the guilty knowledge test. Neuropsychologia 22:457–469, 1984.
42. Tranel D, Damasio AR: Autonomic recognition of familiar faces by prosopagnosiacs: evidence for knowledge without awareness. Neurology 35:119–120, 1985.
43. Levy J, Trevarthen C, Sperry RW: Perception of bilateral chimeric figures following hemispheric deconnexion. Brain 95:61–78, 1972.
44. Teuber HL: Alteration of perception and memory in man. *In* Weiskranz L (ed): Analysis of Behavioral Change. New York, Harper & Row, 1968.
45. Habib M: Visual hypoemotionality and prosopagnosia associated with right temporal lobe isolation. Neuropsychologia 24:577–582, 1986.
46. Bauer RM: Visual hypoemotionality as a symptom of visual-limbic disconnection in man. Arch Neurol 39:702–708, 1982.
47. Mesulam M-M: Patterns in behavioral neuroanatomy: Association areas, the limbic system and hemispheric specialization. *In* Mesulam M (ed): Principles of Behavioral Neurology. Philadelphia, FA Davis, 1985.
48. McNamara ME, Heros RC, Boller F: Visual hallucinations in blindness: The Charles Bonnet syndrome. Int J Neurosci 17:13–15, 1982.
49. Goldenberg G, Podreka I, Steiner M, et al: Regional cerebral blood flow patterns in visual imagery. Neuropsychologia 27:641–664, 1989.
50. Hof, PR, Bouras C, Constantinidis J, Morrison JH: Balint's syndrome in Alzheimer's disease: Specific disruption of the occipito-parietal visual pathway. Brain Res 493:368–375, 1989.
51. Mesulam M-M: A cortical network for directed attention and unilateral neglect. Ann Neurol 10:309–325, 1981.
52. Mesulam M-M: Attention, confusional states and neglect. *In* Mesulam, M-M (ed): Principles of Behavioral Neurology. Philadelphia, FA Davis, 1985.
53. Weintraub SW, Mesulam M-M: Right cerebral dominance in spatial attention: Further evidence based on ipsilateral neglect. Arch Neurol 44:621–625, 1987.
54. Spiers P, Schomer D, Blume H, et al: Visual neglect during intracarotid Amytal testing. Neurology 40:1600–1601, 1990.
55. Daffner K, Ahern G, Weintraub S, Mesulam M-M: Dissociated neglect behavior following sequential strokes to the right hemisphere. Ann Neurol 28:97–101, 1990.
56. Krieg WJS: Architectonics of the Human Cerebral Fiber Systems. Evanston, IL, Brain Books, 1973.

Chapter 210

Transient Ischemia and Brain and Ocular Infarction

LOUIS R. CAPLAN

Much of the brain's function involves looking, seeing, and interpreting visual information. It follows that transient or persistent ischemia of the eye and brain often causes visual symptoms of one variety or another. Because ischemia of different regions causes quite different symptoms and signs, this chapter separately considers five anatomic regions that share relatively similar clinical characteristics and have their own unique blood supplies: the eye; the portion of the cerebral hemispheres supplied by the anterior circulation (the internal carotid arteries [ICAs] and their intracranial branches); the remainder of the cerebral hemispheres, which are supplied by the posterior cerebral arteries (PCAs), usually terminal branches of the basilar artery; and the brain stem and cerebellum, regions supplied by the vertebrobasilar arteries. The territories of the deep penetrating arteries within the anterior and posterior circulations are considered separately because the cause and treatment of lesions within their supply are different. This chapter relates symptoms and signs with the causative vascular lesions and suggests appropriate evaluations.

OCULAR ISCHEMIA

The nomenclature of eye ischemia is quite confusing. Hedges[1] and others suggest the following: *transient visual obscuration* (TVO) for very fleeting episodes lasting seconds, associated with papilledema or increased intracranial pressure[2]; *amaurosis fugax,* a brief fleeting attack of monocular partial or total blindness lasting seconds to a very few minutes; *transient monocular visual loss* (TMVL) or *transient monocular blindness* (TMB), a more persistent loss of vision lasting minutes or longer (although TMVL is more accurate, TMB has been a more customary designation); *transient bilateral visual loss* (TBVL), episodes affecting both eyes or one or both cerebral hemispheres and causing visual loss discernible with each eye; and *ocular infarction,* persistent ischemic damage to the eye with resulting persisting loss of vision.

Transient Monocular Visual Loss

SYMPTOMS AND SIGNS

Visual loss is most often described as graying, darkening, blurring, fogging, or dimming of vision. The entire field of vision may be affected, or altitudinal or lateralized sectors may be involved at the onset or for the duration of an attack. Some patients speak of a gray-black curtain that gradually descends or less often ascends or moves across the eye. At times patients see so-called positive visual phenomena such as scintillations, colored or bright displays, and streaks and shimmers.[3] Fisher's patient, examined during an attack of TMB, "likened the failure of vision to the snowing up of a television screen . . . colorless snowflakes were bright, shining, and jumping. As the cloud took form he could still see past or through it, but as the cloud became more dense, a total blackout occurred."[4] Attacks usually last a few minutes but can persist for hours; the frequency of attacks varies from many a day to single or widely spaced episodes. Attacks may continue in some patients for years but more often occur during a period of weeks to months. Strokes involving the eye or brain may develop at any time, but in most patients they do not.

Accompanying pain in the head or eye is said to be rare.[5] In one series of 37 patients with TMB, during the attack, only one had headache, consisting of a throbbing pain in the orbit and temporal and frontal regions.[3] However, in another series of 83 patients, all younger than 45 yr, headache was a prominent symptom accompanying visual loss in 41 percent of patients.[6] Orbital pain can be sharp and stabbing or aching in quality.[6] Ropper called attention to facial sensations accompanying TMB; he called these *transient ipsilateral paresthesias.*[7] Symptoms of tingling, warmthlike flushing, and feeling as if an area was twitching affected the eye, eyelid, periorbital region, or cheek and either preceded the visual loss by a minute or two or began simultaneously with TMB.[7] Some patients with attacks of TMVL also have attacks of brain dysfunction on the same side as the ocular symptoms. In one series of 95 patients with transient ischemic attacks (TIAs), ten had such episodes (referred to as *transient hemispheral attacks* [THAs]), but no patient had simultaneous hemispheral and eye ischemia.[8] In my experience, concurrent TMVL and ipsilateral hemispheral ischemia only occur in acute lesions affecting the ICA within the carotid siphon near the ophthalmic artery origin. Dissection of the ICA and embolus to the region are the most common such lesions, and in my opinion, the ocular ischemia involves the posterior choroidal arterial supply to the optic nerve rather than the central retinal artery and often causes persistent visual loss.[9–11]

In some patients, TMVL is precipitated by exposure to bright light. Presumably, in some patients with tenuous ocular perfusion, exposure of the retina to certain intensities of light increases retinal metabolic activity beyond the limits of the perfusion.[12] The attacks can be bilateral.[13] In such patients, attenuation of a previously normal visual evoked response in the affected eye can be demonstrated after bright light exposure.[14] TMVL can also be precipitated by assuming a sitting or upright posture or in some situations by reduced blood pressure (e.g., overzealous antihypertensive treatment or hypovolemia).[2, 12, 15] Patients with orthostatic or bright light–induced TMVL also often report dazzle, excessive contrast vision, flickering lights, photopsias, and dyschromatopsias.[2]

The most important and common ophthalmoscopic abnormality in patients with TMVL is embolic particles in the retinal arteries.[4, 16] The most frequently observed particles are cholesterol crystals, which although white, appear bright, often glinting, and orange-yellow, probably because the red blood cell column is seen beyond the crystals that reflect light.[5] These crystals are often small (10 to 250 μm in diameter), and they lodge at bifurcations, often not impeding flow. They disappear rather rapidly but may damage the vessel wall, producing a sheathing reaction. The blood column in adjacent veins often is segmented and flows slowly.[17] Fluorescein angiography, even after crystals are no longer visible by ophthalmoscopy, may show hyperfluorescent crystals or areas of fluorescein leakage caused by crystal-related endothelial damage.[18] Pressing on the eye may cause the cholesterol crystals to move, flip over, or "flash" so that they become more visible through the ophthalmoscope.[5, 18] In contrast, platelet or fibrin-platelet emboli are longer gray-white bodies that progress through the small retinal arteries, often with distal fragments breaking off.[5] Fisher, in his original observation of a patient's ocular fundus during an attack of TMVL, described and diagnosed a typical fibrin-platelet embolus.[4] Calcific emboli are chalky white and often remain in one location, blocking flow.[4, 6] Talc and other foreign body retinal emboli have been observed in the arteries of patients who inject drugs intended for oral use.[19] Myxoma and other tumor material and Roth's spots from infected embolic material can also be seen, as can petechiae related to fat emboli.

Some patients with TMVL, especially those with precipitation of visual blurring by bright light or orthostatic changes, have evidence of chronic ischemic ocular disease.[3, 20–23] The best-known findings are those of so-called venous stasis retinopathy: small dot and blot microaneurysms, especially at the midperiphery of the retina; hemorrhages; dilatation and darkening of retinal veins; disc swelling; and retinal clouding.[2, 20, 22] Also seen are dilated episcleral arteries, corneal edema, hyperemia of the conjunctiva, anterior chamber cells and flare, ischemia and rubeosis of the iris, and a dilated and poorly reactive pupil.[2, 21, 23, 24] Neovascularization can lead to increased intraocular pressure and glaucoma.[23]

CAUSES

Wray has classified TMVL into three different groups based mostly on probable pathogenesis.[2, 25] Type 1 TMVL is characterized by loss of all or a portion of vision in one eye, lasting seconds to minutes, with full recovery. Many of these attacks are probably due to embolism of one variety or another. Cholesterol crystals probably arise mostly from plaques in the ICA in the neck or carotid siphon or the aorta. Type 1 attacks have been correlated with "open" ICAs—that is, vessels without critical narrowing but with ulcerations.[8] Embolisms of carotid artery origin have been correlated with focal altitudinal, lateralized, or sector visual symptoms[26] and lengthier attacks.[3] Calcific emboli come mostly from calcified heart valves. Fibrin-platelet emboli arise mostly from the tail of clots formed in the ICAs and heart chambers. These thrombi can form because of cardiac or vascular disease or because of a hypercoagulable state. Less often, myxoma, other tumors, talc, and fat can serve as emboli that are visible in the fundus.

Type 2 TMVL includes visual loss thought to be due to hemodynamically significant occlusive low-flow lesions in the ICAs or ophthalmic arteries.[2, 25] The spells are either frequent and brief[3] or less rapid in onset and longer in duration. Recovery is often gradual. Attacks are also often precipitated by orthostatic changes, reduction in blood pressure, or exposure to bright light. Signs of chronic ocular ischemia may be present on examination. The most common pathology in this group is occlusion or "tight" stenosis of the ICA.[2, 3, 25] Takayasu's or giant cell temporal arteritis may involve aortic arch arteries and cause this type of TMVL.

Type 3 TMVL is thought to be due to vasoconstriction, so-called vasospasm. Some patients have a personal or family history of migraine. Vasospasm probably accounts for most attacks in women who are younger than 45 yr and who have TMVL.[6] Although the phenomenology of hemianopic migraine arising from the occipital cortex has been well characterized, the features of ocular migraine are less well defined. Retinal arteriolar and venous narrowing, retinal edema, dilated veins, and delayed filling of retinal arteries on fluorescein angiography have been described.[25, 27] Headache and eye pain are more frequent in this group.[3] Other, often young, patients seem to have a benign process with multiple attacks but lack features of the other two groups. They are also young, often under 30 yr, and possibly also have a migraine-like disorder.[2, 28]

Contrary to common opinion, ultrasonographic or angiographic evaluation of groups of patients with TMVL shows a rather low frequency of significant ICA narrowing, which has been found in less than a third of patients.[6, 29, 30] However, most patients who have both TMVL and ipsilateral attacks of hemisphere ischemia have severe occlusive disease of the ipsilateral ICA.[8] In nearly all series of patients in whom cholesterol crystals have been found in the fundus oculi, with or without symptomatic TMVL, the incidence of ICA disease is higher. The risk of stroke, coronary artery disease, and mortality is also increased in patients with visible cholesterol crystals in the retina.[16, 31, 32] TMVL in persons younger than 45 yr is usually benign, and many attacks in such individuals are probably vasospastic. TMVL can at times be caused by occlusive disease of the ophthalmic artery itself[33] or by occlusion of arteries supplying ophthalmic arteries with anomalous origins. In one patient, occlusive disease in an external carotid artery led to TMVL because the ophthalmic artery was fed by the middle meningeal artery, a branch of the external carotid artery.[34] When the ICA is occluded, emboli can pass from the external carotid artery through ophthalmic collaterals to the eye and also cause TMVL. Rarely, the ophthalmic artery arises from the middle cerebral artery (MCA), the posterior communicating artery, or the maxillary artery.[35] Ocular disorders such as hyphema, glaucoma, drusen of the optic nerve, vitreous floaters and hemorrhage, posterior staphylomas, and intraorbital masses can cause visual symptoms that mimic TMVL due to ischemia.[36] TBVL, when due to eye disease, is almost always associated with very severe occlusive disease of the ICAs or the vessels of the aortic arch.[13]

An evaluation of a patient with TMVL should be tailored to that individual and depends on age, sex, the presence of stroke, atherosclerotic risk factors, the presence of migraine, the nature of visual symptoms (Wray's types I to III), and results of ophthalmoscopy. Echocardiography, carotid ultrasonography, blood counts and coagulation studies, neuroimaging with computed tomography (CT) or magnetic resonance imaging (MRI), MR angiography and standard angiography, and ophthalmologic evaluation may be very helpful in some patients in determining the cause. A group of experienced physicians from different specialties have formulated a consensus statement about TMVL, sharing their advice and recommendations for evaluation and treatment.[36]

Ocular Infarction

Persistent eye ischemia has often been characterized as due to central retinal artery occlusion (CRAO), occlusion of a branch of the central retinal artery (BRAO), or ischemia of the optic nerve caused by disease of the posterior choroid artery supply of the nerve. The latter has usually been called *anterior ischemic optic neuropathy* (AION).

CENTRAL RETINAL ARTERY OCCLUSION

The central retinal artery (CRA) origin from the ophthalmic artery is quite variable. The vessel has intraorbital, intravaginal, and intraneural segments before piercing the dural sheath behind the eyeball to supply the retina.[35] To reach the fundus, the CRA penetrates the lamina cribrosa, a relatively inelastic, firm lattice composed of glia-lined collagen fibers at the level of the sclera.[37] At this point, the CRA narrows, and the tissue around the vessel is a mechanical barrier to dilatation. This area, not visible with an ophthalmoscope, is probably the region most often the site of embolic or inflammatory disease causing CRAO.[37] The most common causes of CRAO are embolic occlusion, thrombosis in situ, arteritis (especially due to temporal arteritis), vasospasm, and hypoperfusion due to glaucoma or severe proximal arterial occlusive disease.[37]

The major symptom is sudden painless blindness with persistent visual loss. Perception of hand movement or light can be preserved in parts of the visual field. The diagnosis is made by ophthalmoscopy, which shows partial or complete arrest of the retinal circulation. In 1859, von Graefe described the cardinal signs of a pale disc, attenuated arteries and veins, a cloudy retina, and a cherry-red spot in the macula in a patient who lost sight in an eye a week previously.[38, 39] He later saw segmental flow that gradually improved but without return of sight. Shortly after the occlusion, segmentation of the blood column with slow streaming of the veins is seen.[37] In the arteries, the blood is dark and clear areas may alternate with clumped cells, giving the appearance of segmentation, a process more prominent in adjacent veins. Retinal artery pressure as measured by an ophthalmodynamometer is very low. If occlusion of the CRA lasts more than 1 hr, the retina becomes infarcted. Swelling of the retinal ganglion cells causes loss of transparency and gives the retina a milky-white appearance. The central cherry-red macular appearance is due to accentuation of the normal fovea, through which the choroid appears red.[37] Retinal opacification disappearance and optic atrophy and loss of the retinal nerve fiber layer are found later.

Emergency treatment, advocated by some, includes anticoagulation with heparin, digital massage of the globe, paracentesis of the anterior chamber, and carbon dioxide inhalation.[37] The differential diagnosis is broad and varies with the age and sex of the patient and the existence of known medical conditions. Temporal arteritis is especially critical to diagnose. Advanced age, a history of prominent headache, malaise, anorexia, polymyalgia, tender temporal arteries, and a high sedimentation rate suggest the diagnosis. Suspected cases should be treated with corticosteroids until results of temporal artery biopsy are available. Occlusion of the CRA by thrombotic states is common, as is embolism to the vessel.

The incidence of various causes has varied among different series. Hypertension, smoking, and coronary artery disease are common.[32, 40, 41] Cardiac valve and other sources of cardiac origin embolism are often found[39] and accounted for 29 of 103 (28 percent) cases in one series.[40] The presence of ICA disease has varied. Wilson and colleagues found that 12 of 18 patients had carotid irregularities or stenosis on angiography.[40] In the series of Merchut and associates (which grouped CRAO and BRAO together), 29 of 34 (85 percent) patients had abnormal ICA on arteriography, of which 12 had occlusion or severe stenosis and 17 had plaques, ulcers, or stenosis of less than 60 percent.[41] The presence of cholesterol crystals in the fundus increased the likelihood of significant ICA disease. In the series of Chawluk and coworkers, patients with CRAO were studied with B-mode ultrasonography and integrated pulsed Doppler sonography; among 17 patients with CRAO, 24 percent had ICA occlusion and 36 percent had occlusive or ulcerated lesions indicating more ICA disease than in the patients with TMVL.[29] The results of investigations depend heavily on the age of subjects in a series. Among older subjects, ICA disease and temporal arteritis are more common; cardiac valvular disease is more often found in younger patients.

BRANCH RETINAL ARTERY OCCLUSION

BRAO shares with CRAO the fact that the occlusive process in the retina is visible with an ophthalmoscope. Branches of retinal arteries are occluded, and the visual defect and retinal ischemia are more focal and have an altitudinal, lateral, or scotomatous quality. In most series, the incidence of carotid artery and valvular disease is not very different from that in CRAO, but temporal arteritis is less often the cause.[29, 40, 41] In some patients with BRAO, cholesterol crystals are visible within the occluded artery; this feature makes the diagnosis of significant ICA disease more likely.

ANTERIOR ISCHEMIC OPTIC NEUROPATHY

The arterial supply of the optic nerve is quite different from that of the retina. The anterior portion of the optic nerve has a dual supply from branches of the CRA and from the posterior choroidal arterial system.[42, 43] Most of the nerve is usually supplied by the posterior choroidal system. The very far posterior portion of the nerve is fed by direct penetrators from the ophthalmic artery. Considerable individual variability is noted in the supply of the posterior choroidal arteries and their branches.[43] The choroidal artery branches are predominantly end arteries with little collateral capabilities.

Patients with AION usually develop painless visual loss in one eye, noted on awakening in the morning and not worsening thereafter. The degree of loss of acuity is variable but most often is not complete. Visual field defects depend on the region of the optic disc involved. Funduscopy, soon after the onset of symptoms, usually shows edema of the optic disc and splinter hemorrhages at the disc margins.[43] Optic atrophy develops later. When the ischemia is posterior to the disc, the optic disc may look normal. Subsequent involvement of the other eye is common.

AION is caused by ischemia of the optic nerve. The prevailing theory of its pathogenesis is that the ischemia is due to hypoperfusion of the nerve. Mean blood pressure in the various posterior choroidal arteries may be variable in both health and disease.[43] The vessels supplying the nerve may be similar to penetrating small cerebral vessels such as the lenticulostriates and may be susceptible to hypertension and diabetes as well as arteritis. The perfusion pressure and blood flow in the choroidal arterial system depend on many factors: intraocular pressure, mean blood pressure, vascular resistance, and autoregulation. Hayreh has written that the choroidal circulation has no autoregulatory capability, making its territory vulnerable to changes in perfusion pressure.[43]

The etiology of AION is customarily divided into arteritic and nonarteritic forms. Temporal (giant cell) arteritis is a very important cause of AION because involvement of the contralateral eye is very likely if the disorder is not treated with corticosteroids. In patients with bilateral arteritic AION, 95 percent have involvement of the second eye before the start of adequate corticosteroid systemic therapy and the rest develop it within 48 hr of treatment.[44] Weight loss, anorexia, jaw claudication, and high sedimentation rate suggest the diagnosis of temporal arteritis. Among nonarteritic cases, the incidence of severe hypertension and diabetes in young patients is high. Young diabetic patients also have a high incidence of involvement of the second eye.[44] In older patients without arteritis, there seem to be no major differences in risk factors from age-matched controls. Some observers have commented on the anatomy of the optic cup, which is very small or absent in AION. Overcrowding of nerve fibers in a small scleral canal may be an important factor in the development of AION in older persons.[43, 45, 46] Embolism and carotid artery occlusive disease are not common in patients with AION. They rarely have visible emboli or cholesterol crystals in the fundus, and their risk of stroke, myocardial infarction, and other vascular diseases is not substantially different from others of the same age.[47] Evaluation should be mostly directed at determining the presence or absence of temporal arteritis, and hypertension and diabetes mellitus, when present, should be controlled.

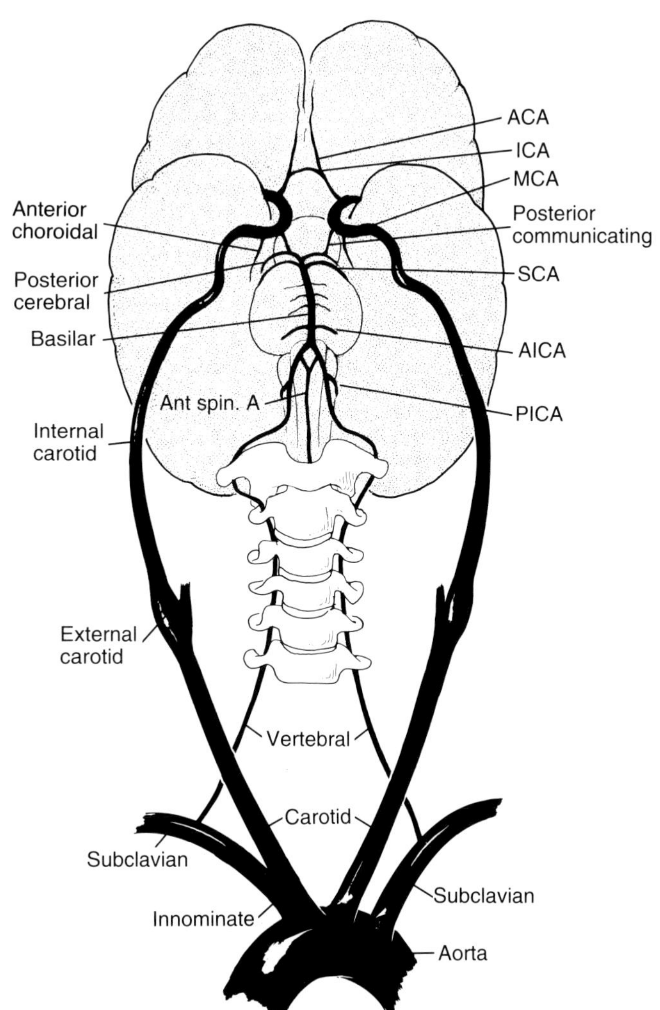

Figure 210–1. The major neck arteries and the intracranial circle of Willis. The relationship to the vertebral column and brain is illustrated.

HEMISPHERAL ISCHEMIA IN THE ANTERIOR CIRCULATION TERRITORY

Although the anterior portion of the cerebral hemispheres does not for the most part directly involve the visual radiations, dysfunction does affect looking and attention toward the contralateral visual field. The anterior choroidal artery does supply a portion of the optic radiations. The internal carotid artery courses cranially from its origin in the neck from the common carotid artery. Figure 210–1 depicts the vascular anatomy of the carotid artery and the vertebral artery in the neck, as well as the intracanial branches of these vessels. The first branch is the ophthalmic artery, which arises from the carotid siphon region. It usually originates after the ICA has emerged from the cavernous sinus, but in about 7.5 percent of patients the ophthalmic artery arises from the intracavernous portion.[35] After the anterior choroidal (AChA) and posterior communicating arteries emerge from the posterior portion of the supraclinoid ICA, the artery divides into its anterior cerebral artery (ACA) and MCA branches. Figure 210–2 reviews the distribution of these branches. The MCA has further important subdivisions into a superior trunk, whose branches supply the suprasylvian frontal and parietal lobes, and an inferior trunk, whose supply is the infrasylvian temporal lobe and inferior parietal lobule. The ACA, after giving off its deep Heubner's artery branches, travels around the corpus callosum to supply the paramedian frontal and parietal lobes. After its origin from the ICA, the AChA courses posterolaterally as it lies inferior and lateral to the optic tract, which it supplies through penetrating branches (Fig. 210–3). The AChA then courses to the medial side of the optic tract, passing between the medial temporal lobe laterally and the midbrain and thalamus medially. The AChA ends in the lateral geniculate body and the choroid plexus of the lateral ventricle. It also supplies a small portion of the geniculocalcarine tract near its origin from the lateral geniculate body.

ICA, MCA, ACA Territory Disease

The ICA, MCA, and ACA do not directly supply the optic radiations except the AChA supply described

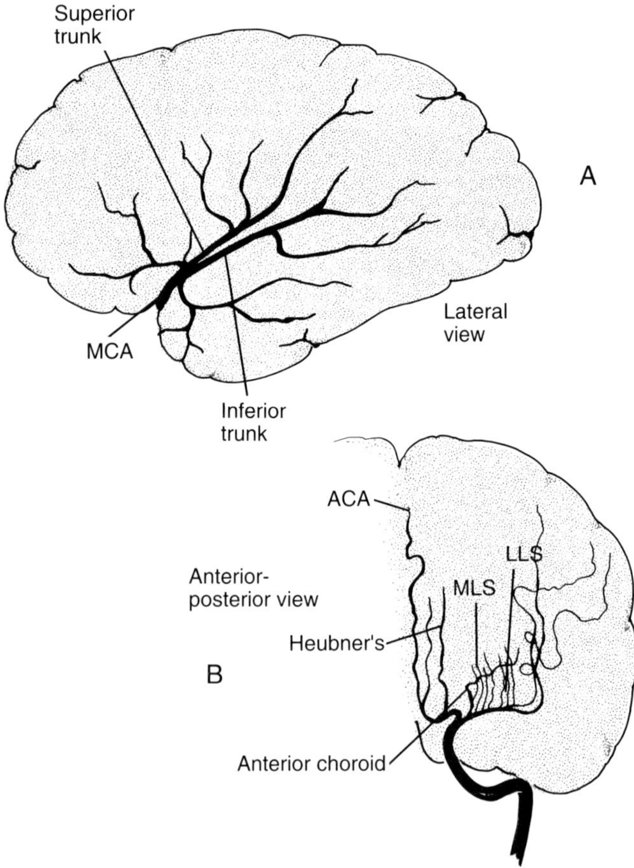

Figure 210–2. *A,* Lateral view of cerebral hemisphere showing middle cerebral artery branches. *B,* Coronal view of the blood supply of one cerebral hemisphere.

earlier and the MCA supply of the geniculocalcarine tract, especially the inferior fibers as they course adjacent to the temporal horn and atrium of the lateral ventricles. Patients with infarcts in the anterior portion of the cerebral hemispheres rarely complain of hemianopia, and a physician generally cannot map out a reliable, consistent visual field defect. We have already discussed ocular ischemia, which can of course result from ICA disease proximal to the ophthalmic artery origin.

ACA infarcts cause weakness of the contralateral lower extremity, as well as a weak shoulder shrug. A cortical type of sensory loss may also be found in the involved leg. Abulia is also often present, characterized by lack of spontaneity, prolonged latency in replying to queries or commands, and short, terse laconic replies with an inability to persevere at tasks. Infarction of the white matter near the corpus callosum and the anterior part of the callosum often causes a so-called anterior disconnection syndrome, in which language functions are performed poorly with the left hand.[48] Patients with this syndrome cannot correctly execute verbal commands with the left hand despite doing them normally with the right hand. They write aphasically with the left hand but produce normal written language (but poor penmanship) with their right hand. They also cannot correctly name objects in their left hand. The white matter pathways connecting the left hemisphere language region with the right frontal region controlling the left hand are affected. The medial frontal infarcts may cause inattention to visual, tactile, and auditory stimuli presented in the opposite side of space.[49, 50] When presented with an object to the left, patients with an ACA territory infarct may fail to look at or heed the object but when asked can usually say what it was. The eyes usually are not conjugately deviated.

MCA infarcts involving the entire territory usually cause severe contralateral hemiparesis and hemisensory loss with neglect of the contralateral visual, auditory, and somatosensory environment. Patients with a left MCA infarct are aphasic, whereas those with a right MCA infarct draw and copy poorly, have abnormal visual-spatial capabilities, and lack awareness or concern about their deficits.[51, 52] MCA territory infarcts can be clinically divided into superior and inferior division infarcts, which cause characteristic clinical manifestations on each side (Table 210–1).

Ischemia in the brain has traditionally been classified into arbitrarily defined categories depending on the time course and tempo of the symptoms. TIAs, reversible but more prolonged deficits, stroke in progress, and so-called completed strokes are examples of these time-based designations. Unfortunately, these designations do not determine the prognosis, the cause, or even whether or not the brain is damaged on neuroimaging tests.[56] These designations have long outlived their utility and never should be the sole basis for treatment. Physicians faced with patients with ischemia should base the treatment on the anatomy, pathology, and pathophysiology of the vascular process and not depend on current remedies for TIAs or other such deficits.[57] In the anterior circulation, patients with ischemia need evaluation irrespective of whether the symptoms are transient or fixed.[57]

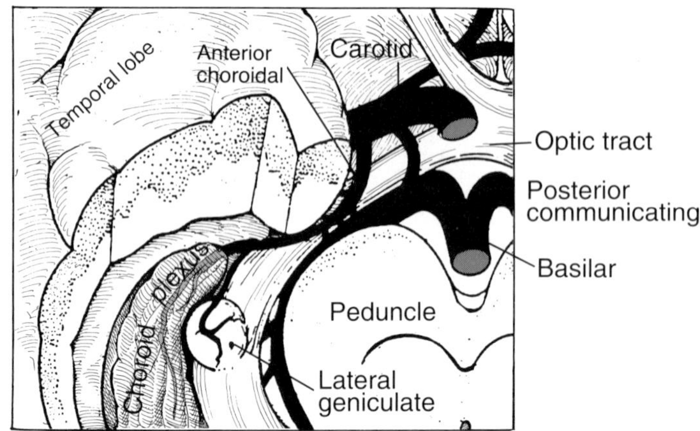

Figure 210–3. The course of the anterior choroidal artery. The artery arises from the internal carotid artery and courses along the optic tract between the cerebral peduncle and thalamus medially and the temporal lobe laterally. Its terminal branches to the choroid plexus of the lateral ventricle and to the lateral geniculate body are shown.

Table 210–1. SYMPTOMS AND SIGNS IN THE VARIOUS MCA TERRITORIES

Left MCA:	*Superior division*
	Right hemiplegia and hemisensory loss, sometimes partially sparing leg
	Neglect of right visual field
	Aphasia—Broca's or global types
	Inferior division
	Right hemianopia, especially involving upper quadrant (or superior quadrantanopia)
	Wernicke's aphasia
	Sometimes agitation, restlessness, and irascibility
Right MCA:	*Superior division*
	Left hemiplegia and hemisensory loss, sometimes partially sparing leg
	Severe neglect of left visual field
	Motor impersistence[53]
	Speech dysprosody (abnormal intonation and emphasis and its recognition)[54]
	Inferior division[55]
	Left hemianopia or upper quadrantanopia
	Poor drawing and copying ability
	Agitation and hyperactivity; sometimes delirium

CAUSE AND EVALUATION

The proximal ICA is very often the seat of atherosclerosis. Plaques usually develop on the posterior wall of the common carotid artery opposite the flow divider between the ICA and external carotid artery. The plaques then spread to the ICA. With time, plaques enlarge and, at a critical size, become complicated by fissures, ulcers, and deposition of fibrin-platelet clumps or red thrombin-dependent thrombi.[58] ICA lesions cause cerebral ischemia mostly by embolization of fibrin-platelet materials, plaque constituents, and thrombi. These materials block the ACA or the MCA or their branches. During the period after complete occlusion, low perfusion pressure supplied to the cerebral hemisphere, especially in border zone regions, can also lead to damage. Patients with ICA disease often have other systemic evidence of atherosclerosis such as coronary artery disease, as well as peripheral vascular occlusive disease with claudication. Smoking, hypercholesterolemia, and hypertension are also common risk factors in patients with ICA disease. There is a strong male predominance (2:1) among patients with severe ICA disease.[59] Whites, especially men, have a high incidence of ICA-origin atherosclerosis, whereas blacks and persons of Chinese and Japanese ancestry have more intracranial occlusive disease.[59] Dissection of the ICA is more often being recognized. Dissection usually involves the pharyngeal ICA and can be precipitated by trauma or can begin spontaneously. Pain in the neck, jaw, face, or head and ipsilateral Horner's syndrome, ipsilateral spells of TMVL, and THAs are frequent features.[60, 61] Infarcts occur if a clot embolizes from the region of dissection and travels intracranially. The ICA siphon is also a frequent site of atheroma formation.[62]

MCA and ACA occlusions are most often embolic, the source arising from the heart or atheromatous lesions in the ICA or the aortic arch. Intrinsic in situ narrowing of the MCA, MCA upper division, and ACA is more common in women, blacks, and Japanese and Chinese individuals.[59] Hypercoagulable states and migraine with vasoconstriction can also lead to occlusion of these intracranial arteries.

An evaluation of patients with anterior cerebral hemisphere ischemia must be individualized. Duplex scanning of the ICAs; transcranial Doppler ultrasound insonation of the ICA siphon,[63] ophthalmic artery, ACAs, and MCAs; neuroimaging in the form of MRI or CT; cardiac evaluation, especially echocardiography, electrocardiography, and rhythm monitoring; and hematologic evaluation are often helpful noninvasive tests that usually clarify the etiology of the ischemia. MRI angiography and angiography using arterial catheterization and opacification are needed in selected patients in whom noninvasive tests do not clarify the mechanism of ischemia. Treatment heavily depends on the cause.[64, 65]

Anterior Choroidal Artery Territory Ischemia

SYMPTOMS AND SIGNS

Infarction of the optic tract should cause an incongruent hemianopia with reduced pupillary reaction when light is shone from the hemianopia side (Wernicke's hemianopic pupillary reaction), but I am unaware of documentation of this syndrome. Ischemia of the geniculocalcarine tract usually causes a congruent homonymous hemianopia, often sparing the macula, with normal pupillary responses, but this finding is usually transient in patients with AChA occlusion because of the rich PCA collaterals.[66] The AChA supplies predominantly the hilum and anterolateral half of the lateral geniculate body.[67] Ischemia can lead to an upper quadrantanopia.[68] In other patients, hemianopia is found with sparing of a horizontal sector of the visual field.[68] Frisén has called this defect a *quadruple sector anopia* because of homonymous congruent defects in both upper and lower quadrants of each eye (Fig. 210–4).[69] The spared sector in the horizontal meridian is supplied by the lateral choroidal branch of the PCA.[70]

AChA territory infarcts are most often due to small artery occlusive disease, as found in hypertensive and diabetic patients.[68, 71] Embolism to the ICA siphon, aneurysms in this region with vasospasm, and mechanical injury during temporal lobectomy for epilepsy are occasional causes.[68] When infarcts are limited to AChA territory,[72] CT or MRI and noninvasive ultrasonography and echocardiographic testing suffice, and contrast angiography is seldom warranted. Treatment consists of risk factor reduction.

HEMISPHERAL ISCHEMIA IN THE TERRITORY SUPPLIED BY THE POSTERIOR CEREBRAL ARTERIES

Because the PCAs are ordinarily branches of the basilar artery, vascular lesions in these arteries often arise from disease of the vertebrobasilar (posterior)

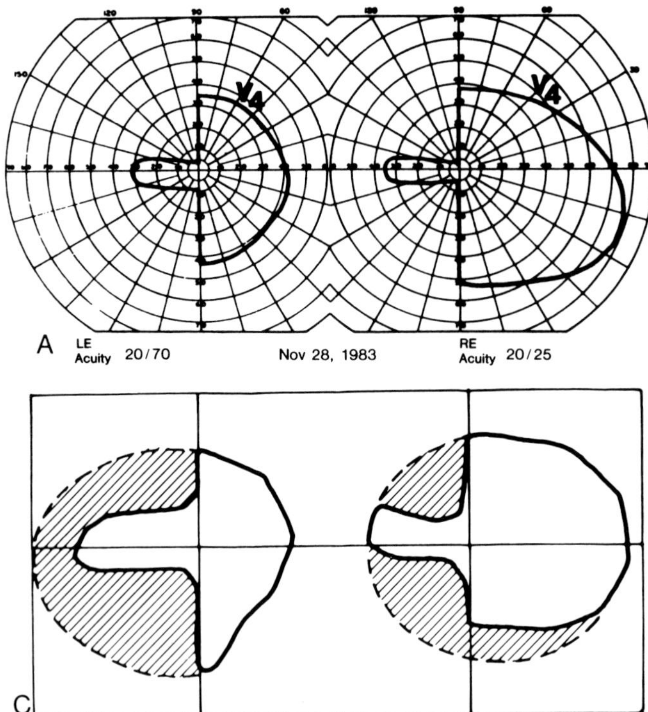

Figure 210–4. Visual field defects in patients with anterior choroidal artery territory infarcts. *A,* Initial visual field defect. *B,* Subsequent later visual field in the same patient. *C,* Frisen's diagram of visual field defect in a patient with anterior choroidal artery territory infarction. (From Helgason C, Caplan LR, Goodwin J, et al: Anterior choroidal artery-territory infarction. Report of cases and review. Arch Neurol 43:681, 1986. Copyright 1986, American Medical Association.)

circulation. As such, they are important to differentiate from lesions of ICA branches because the evaluation and treatments differ considerably. The basilar artery divides at the pontomesencephalic junction into the left and right PCAs. The proximal portion of the PCA is called the *basilar communicating artery,* and after its anastomosis with the posterior communicating artery branch of the ICA, the vessel is called the *PCA.* In about one third of patients, a fetal pattern persists in which the PCA predominantly originates from the ICA-posterior communicating artery and the basilar communicating artery is very hypoplastic.[73, 74] After giving off penetrating vessels to the thalamus and midbrain, the posterior choroidal arteries, which supply a portion of the lateral geniculate body, are given off. The PCA then divides after crossing the tentorial edge to extend branches to the inferior and medial temporal lobes and the occipital lobe. The PCA supplies the striate cortex along the calcarine fissure, usually with separate terminal branches of the calcarine artery supplying the upper trunk (cuneus) and the lower bank (fusiform and lingual gyri). Figure 210–5 depicts the PCA and its branches. Occipital infarcts sometimes selectively affect either the lower or upper bank of the calcarine fissure. Infarction of the entire unilateral PCA territory is much less common than ischemia limited to one or more branch territories.[74, 75] Bilateral simultaneous PCA hemispheral territory infarction occurs as a result of occlusion or embolism to the rostral basilar artery.[76, 77]

SYMPTOMS AND SIGNS—UNILATERAL

The most common symptom is a contralateral hemianopic visual defect. The PCA supplies the lateral geniculate body, the geniculocalcarine tract, and the striate visual cortex, and ischemia of any of these regions causes a contralateral visual field defect. Patients most often report a void, absence, or darkness in the opposite side, and in contrast to patients with MCA territory infarction, they are very aware of the visual defect. Neglect of objects within the blind field is often not present unless the lesion involves the bulk of the temporal lobe. Neglect is more common in large infarcts of the right PCA territory. Patients with striate infarcts can read entire newspaper headlines, although they may cant the paper to the side. They also usually retain reaction to visual threat, and optokinetic responses are preserved.[76] Ischemia limited to the upper calcarine bank causes a contralateral inferior quadrantanopia, and lower bank lesions cause an upper quadrantic defect. The macular region usually is partially spared. Some patients, although they see movement in the contralateral visual field, may be unable to distinguish the color, shape, or nature of objects. Hemiachromatopsia is also common. Visual perseverations and palinopsia may occur on the edge of the visual field defect, especially as the ischemia develops or clears.[78–80] Metamorphopsias, especially micropsia and macropsia, may involve parts of the abnormal visual field, and objects may seem very distorted or grotesque, like looking in a funhouse mirror.

Somatosensory abnormalities result from involvement of the somatosensory nuclei in the thalamus or the thalamoparietal radiations in the white matter destined for the parietal somatosensory cortices.[81] Paresthesias and subjective numb feelings affect the face, hand, arm, leg, and trunk. Objective sensory loss may be minimal or slight, even when the somatosensory nuclei are infarcted.

Left PCA territory infarcts may also cause disturbances of reading and naming, as well as visual agnosia.[74] Infarction of the left medial occipital lobe, often involv-

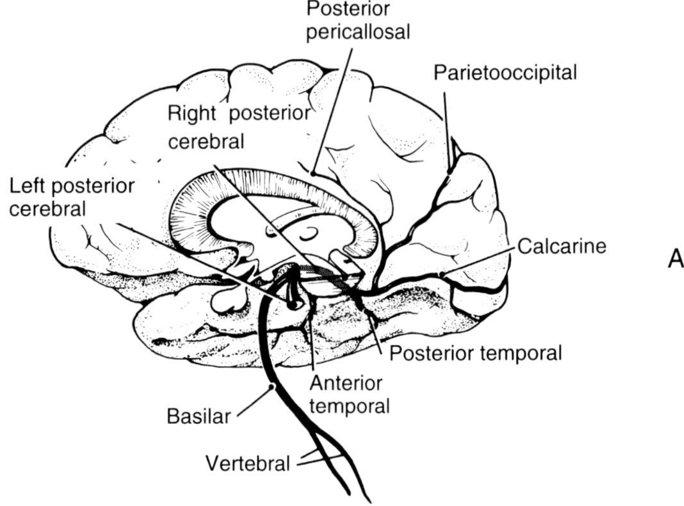

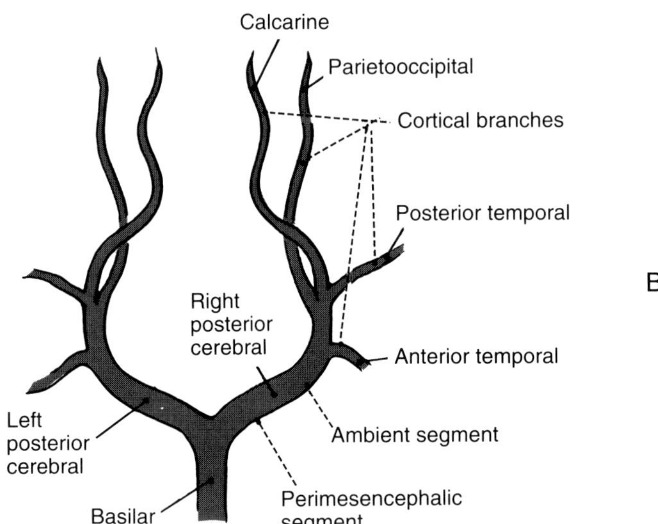

Figure 210–5. *A,* Sagittal drawing of cerebral hemispheres and vertebrobasilar arteries. The distribution of the posterior cerebral arteries to supply the temporal and occipital lobes is shown. *B,* The posterior cerebral arteries and their branches.

ing the corpus callosum, is the cause of a syndrome called *pure word blindness* or *alexia without agraphia.*[82] Although patients cannot read letters or words, they write and spell normally and are not aphasic in spoken language. They invariably cannot name colors but can match colors, can color objects appropriately, and tell what colors objects should be.[83] The syndrome has been explained by Geschwind and colleagues as a posterior disconnection syndrome.[83, 84] Anomic aphasia accompanies left temporal infarction; speech comprehension and repetition, reading, and writing are normal, but patients have difficulty recalling the names of objects or people. Some patients with left PCA infarct have a transcortical sensory aphasia syndrome in which they repeat spoken language correctly but have very poor comprehension.[85] Patients with left PCA infarction may show a syndrome of visual agnosia in which they have difficulty recognizing, naming, and characterizing objects shown to them; however, they can copy the objects, trace them, and recognize the same objects presented tactilely or verbally.[82] When the PCA lesion undercuts the inferior parietal lobule, elements of Gerstmann's syndrome may be present, including jargon aphasia, dyscalculia, agraphia, right-left confusion, and constructional dyspraxia.[82] Patients with infarction in the left hippocampus and medial temporal lobe may have an amnestic syndrome that can last as long as 6 mo.[74, 82] During this time, they cannot form new memories and learning is quite defective but other intellectual functions are preserved. Most reported patients have also had left thalamic infarcts. Bilateral medial temporal lesions are usually needed to cause a persistent amnestic disorder.[74, 82]

Right PCA infarction has been less well studied. Left visual neglect may be prominent, and patients often have abnormal drawing and copying functions. Patients may have difficulty reading words in their left visual field. Defective revisualization of objects and people and a lack of visual content in dreams have been characterized as the Charcot-Wilbrand syndrome.[74] Some patients with lesions in the right lingual and fusiform gyri, limbic cortical structures, show restless, agitated behavior. Abnormal recognition of faces may also accompany right occipital infarction, but most reported patients have had bilateral occipital infarcts.

Disorientation to place also occurs in patients with right occipitoparietal infarcts.[86]

Bilateral PCA territory infarction is relatively common. Symonds and Mackenzie pointed out that such patients were often cortically blind.[87] Amnesia and agitated delirium are also prominent findings in patients with large occipital, temporal bilateral PCA territory infarction.[76] When infarcts are bilateral but predominantly located below the calcarine fissure, patients often have aprosopagnosia and central achromatopsia. They cannot recognize names or match faces[88] but sometimes show psychophysiologic nonconscious signs of some recognition.[89] The color of things in the environment may appear distorted or lost. Some patients described a technicolor environment changing to black and white.[90] Patients with inferior occipital lesions can often find their way around well despite their upper quadrantanopia and visual deficits.[91] When the lesions are bilateral and involve the cuneus and structures superior to the calcarine sulcus, patients show features of Balint's syndrome and have difficulty finding their way about.[91, 92] In Balint's syndrome, the major features are *asimultagnosia* (piecemeal perception of visual space), *optical apraxia* (poor hand-eye coordination), and *apraxia of gaze* (difficulty directing the eyes on command or at will).[74, 76, 94–96] Bilateral medial temporal lobe lesions are attended by prominent amnesia.[76, 82, 97]

CAUSE AND EVALUATION

When the occipital and temporal lobes are simultaneously affected in their full PCA supply, the cause is nearly always embolism.[76, 77] Emboli arise most often from the heart but also may travel from occlusions in the more proximal vertebrobasilar arterial system, especially the vertebral artery at its origin in the neck and the intracranial vertebral artery. Cardiac arrest or severe hypotension can lead to bilateral patchy infarction in the border zone territories between the PCAs and MCAs and cause some of the same symptoms and signs, but the distribution on CT and MRI is different. Border zone ischemia spares the calcarine cortex. Hypotension and global hypoperfusion may also cause an amnestic syndrome due to hippocampal ischemia.

Unilateral PCA territory infarcts are also most often embolic. In a successive series of 35 patients with unilateral PCA occipital infarcts and both hemianopia and CT evidence of infarction, Pessin and colleagues found that the majority of patients had embolism to the PCA.[98] Cardiogenic embolism and embolism without a defined source were the largest etiologic groups, but some had embolism arising in thrombi in the intracranial vertebral arteries. Others have also noticed that artery-to-artery embolism from the vertebral artery to the PCA is common.[99] With an embryonic pattern of supply, the PCA can be fed primarily by the ICA. In that circumstance, a thrombus in the ICA can be the source of embolism to the PCA.[100] PCA stenosis does occur but not often.[101] PCA stenosis like other intrinsic intracranial arterial disease is more common in blacks, women, persons of Chinese or Japanese ancestry, and individuals with severe atherosclerosis and multiple vessel disease. TIAs consisting of temporary visual or sensory symptoms on the opposite side of the body have usually preceded a stroke.[101]

Patients with transient or persistent hemianopia or other symptoms or signs suggestive of PCA territory ischemia (e.g., hemisensory loss or amnesia) should have a CT or MRI scan. Noninvasive cardiac testing is important (echocardiography and rhythm monitoring), especially in patients with a history of coronary artery disease or arrhythmia and when findings on examination of the heart or on the electrocardiogram are abnormal. Duplex and Doppler scans of the extracranial ICA and vertebral artery (VA) are also an important part of the evaluation, as is transcranial Doppler insonation of the intracranial VA, basilar artery, and PCAs. When abnormalities are found, MR angiography or standard angiography of the posterior circulation may be needed to establish the vascular cause. Aspirin, warfarin, or other treatment then is prescribed, depending on the cause.[64, 65]

BRAIN STEM AND CEREBELLAR ISCHEMIA

The details of posterior circulation ischemia are vast and beyond the scope of this chapter. Comprehensive discussions are available.[102, 103] This section emphasizes mainly visual and oculomotor and vestibular phenomena that may present as "visual" symptoms. Brain stem and cerebellar ischemia patterns can be conveniently divided into four subgroups depending on the location of the occlusive or embolic vascular lesion: (1) the proximal arterial system in the neck (i.e., the subclavian and innominate arteries and their VA branches in the neck), (2) the intracranial VAs, (3) the basilar artery, and (4) penetrating artery branches to the pons, midbrain, and thalami. The common symptom complexes and brain stem and cerebellar areas of infarction are listed in Table 210–2. Categorizing patients with posterior circulation TIAs or strokes into one of these groups helps select evaluation and treatment.

Vascular Lesions of the Proximal Arterial System

The anatomy of the aortic arch is quite different on the two sides. On the left, the subclavian artery, usually arising as a direct branch from the aortic arch, ascends in the superior mediastinum before giving rise to the VA medial to the anterior scalene muscle. On the right, the subclavian originates from the innominate artery behind the sternoclavicular joint and arches above the clavicle before giving off the VA branch (see Fig. 210–1). The left subclavian artery is usually deeper and does not reach as high in the neck as the right. The relation of the VAs to their subclavian parents is different from the ICA–common carotid artery (CCA) relation. The VA is much smaller than the subclavian and is nearly perpendicular to it, whereas the ICA and CCA

Table 210–2. COMMON SYMPTOM COMPLEXES AND BRAIN STEM AND CEREBELLAR AREAS OF INFARCTION

Innominate, subclavian, and nuchal vertebral artery (V1 and V2 positions)
Subclavian steal
Transient medullary ischemia
Embolism to intracranial arteries, especially cerebellar and PCAs
Distal nuchal vertebral artery (V3) and intracranial vertebral artery (V4)
Lateral medullary syndrome
Cerebellar infarction (PICA territory)
Embolism to distal system, especially rostral basilar artery and PCA
Basilar artery
Proximal and midbasilar syndromes with pontine infarction
Rostral "top of the basilar" embolic occlusion—midbrain and thalamic infarction
Penetrating branch disease
Paramedian unilateral pontine infarcts
Paramedian unilateral thalamic infarcts—polar and hypothalamic-thalamic artery types
Lateral thalamic infarcts

PCA, posterior cerebral artery; PICA, posterior inferior cerebellar artery.

are almost equal in size and the ICA is nearly a 180 degree continuation. As a result, ulceration in the proximal VA occurs less often than in the proximal ICA but does occasionally occur at the VA-subclavian origin.[104] Also, many possibilities for formation of collateral circulation arise in the proximal VA through muscular branches of the vessel and from the adjacent thyrocervical trunk and branches of the external carotid artery in the neck. Atherosclerosis affects mostly the proximal subclavian or innominate arteries or the VA origin. Figure 210–6 reviews the most common sites for atherosclerosis in both the posterior and anterior circulations. After passing in the neck rostrally (V1), the artery enters the intravertebral foramen to course from C6 to C2 (called the *V2 segment*). In this latter position, the artery is interosseous and is seldom affected by atherosclerosis but is vulnerable to injury to the cervical vertebrae. Figure 210–1 shows the extracranial VA and its relation to the vertebral column.

SYMPTOMS AND SIGNS

The so-called subclavian steal syndrome is due to occlusion of the subclavian artery before the VA branch. Blood usually courses from the contralateral VA to the VA on the side of the subclavian artery occlusion and then flows into the subclavian artery beyond the block to supply the potentially ischemic arm.[102, 105, 106] The subclavian occlusion most often is asymptomatic and is detected during a noninvasive evaluation for carotid artery disease.[107] The most frequent symptoms relate to the ischemic arm and include fatigue, cramps, and coolness. Brain symptoms are the least frequent and usually consist of dizziness, momentary visual "blurring," and staggering. Although these symptoms can be precipitated by arm motion and exercise, they most often are not. Studies using Doppler techniques show that steal is usually from the opposite VA and is seldom accompanied by important brain stem ischemia.[108] With time, the symptoms of left subclavian steal disappear even without repair of the occlusive lesion. On the right side, the problem is less common but more severe: Clot formed in the subclavian artery can propagate proximally and embolize to the ICA and intracranial anterior circulation because the innominate artery gives off both VA and ICA branches.[102] Baseball pitchers, golfers, and cricket bowlers are especially susceptible to subclavian artery disease because of trauma to the artery by the rib cage during some arm motions.[109] Atherosclerotic disease of the proximal VA is most often encountered in patients with ICA, coronary, and peripheral vascular disease.[59] VA disease roughly parallels ICA disease and is most common in white men.[59]

Stenosis or occlusion of the proximal VA produces transient brain symptoms identical to those in the subclavian steal syndrome. Adequate collateral circulation invariably develops so that hemodynamically significant hindbrain ischemia does not persist. However, proximal VA occlusion, if and when it occurs, can serve as a source of embolism to the posterior circulation.[110]

EVALUATION AND TREATMENT

The subclavian artery and its supply to the arm can be readily studied by noninvasive ultrasonography and

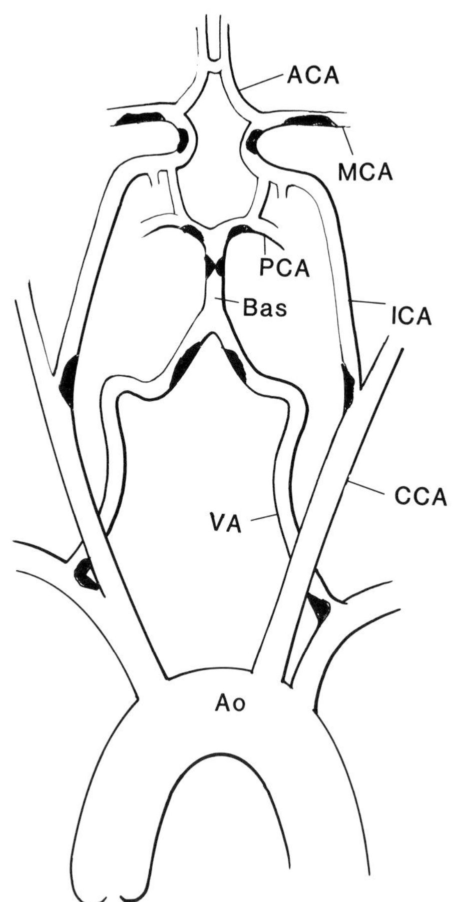

Figure 210–6. The major cerebrovascular branches of the aortic arch. The predilection sites for atherosclerosis are shown in black.

oscillographic and plethysmographic techniques.[102, 103] Duplex scan of the subclavian and VA origin are also helpful, and continuous-wave Doppler gives accurate information about the proximal VA. In uncertain cases, angiography serves to clarify the anatomy and pathology of this region. Brain MRI helps detect the unlikely possibility of brain stem or cerebellar infarction. Left subclavian occlusion usually requires no treatment unless the sufferer is an athlete dependent on arm function. On the right, surgery is usually indicated. For patients with occlusion of the VA in the neck, I give warfarin for a period of 4 to 6 wk during the time of most frequent embolization. After that, the clot has usually organized and become adherent and further occlusion is rare; collateral circulation has by that time become established. Aspirin might be given to patients who have irregularity and ulceration in the proximal vascular system and who do not have occlusion or severe stenosis of the vessels.

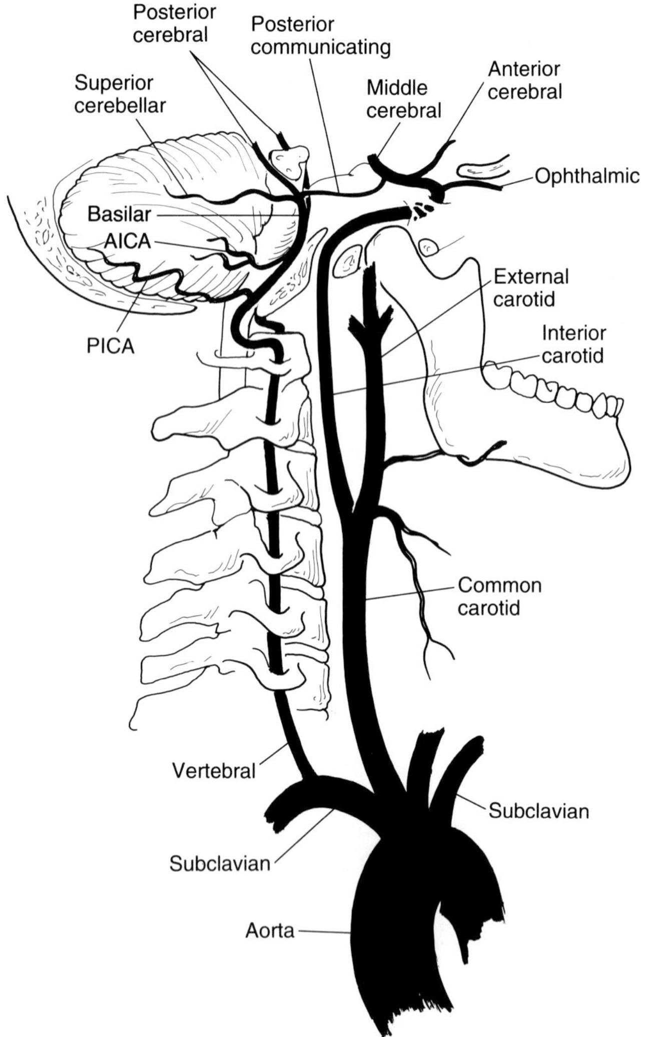

Figure 210–7. Lateral view of the aorta, neck, and inferior cranium showing the major extracranial arteries (internal carotid and vertebral arteries) and their major branches.

Occlusive Disease of the Distal Extracranial (V3) and Intracranial VA (V4)

The distal extracranial segment of the VA (V3) emerges from C2, then bends around the atlas before piercing the dura mater to enter the cranium through the foramen magnum. The artery has a tortuous course throughout this segment. It is anchored proximally in the bone and intracranially, but the third portion of the VA is movable and very vulnerable to trauma and to sudden movements or manipulations. Dissection, either traumatic or spontaneous, is common in this segment,[111] but atherosclerosis is rare. Temporal arteritis tends to involve the VA just before it pierces the dura.[112, 113]

The intracranial VA supplies predominantly the medulla and the posterior inferior surface of the cerebellum on each side. The major branches are the posterior inferior cerebellar arteries (PICAs) and the branches to the anterior spinal arteries that feed the medial medulla before coursing toward the spinal cord. Figure 210–7 reviews diagramatically the intracranial major posterior circulation branches. Atherosclerosis of the intracranial segment of the VA (V4) is common. Occlusive thrombi formed in the intracranial VA can propagate into the basilar artery or embolize distally into the rostral basilar artery or PCAs.[99, 110]

SYMPTOMS AND SIGNS

The two major regions of ischemia are the lateral medullary tegmentum and the cerebellum. These occur whether the vascular disease is in the distal extracranial VA or the intracranial VA segment. The cardinal symptoms of the lateral medullary syndrome are sharp pain in the ipsilateral eye or burning of the face, dizziness or vertigo, ataxia, hoarseness, clumsiness of the ipsilateral arm and leg, and difficulty standing or walking.[102, 114] The dizziness usually is a feeling of wavering or teetering, but spinning vertigo, nausea, and vomiting are possible. Oscillopsia and diplopia are sometimes mentioned.[102, 103, 114] The major ocular and oculomotor signs are an ipsilateral Horner's syndrome, nystagmus, and occasionally ocular pulsion toward the side of the lesion.[102, 103, 115, 116] The nystagmus is usually rotatory and horizontal and may be more coarse when looking to the side opposite the lesion. Hypometric saccades and poor smooth pursuit to the contralateral side are also often found.[116] Skewing and slight dysconjugacy of gaze with a lag of the abducting eye on gaze to the side of the lesion may be observed, and patients may tilt their head to compensate for the diplopia.[117] The lateral medullary syndrome is most often caused by occlusion of the intracranial VA before its PICA branch.[118] TIAs in patients with intracranial VA stenosis usually involve fragments of the lateral medullary syndrome.

Cerebellar ischemia causes gait ataxia and often clumsiness and dysmetria of the ipsilateral arm and leg. Dizziness, dysarthria, and vomiting are also common. Large cerebellar infarcts can produce increased pressure in the posterior fossa and hydrocephalus. Somnolence can be a symptom and can evolve to stupor, coma, and death if untreated.[102, 103] Oculomotor signs are seen in patients with large infarcts and include hypometric saccades to the lesion side, an ipsilateral conjugate gaze or seventh-nerve palsy, and head tilt.[103] Papilledema is occasionally present.[118] The underlying occlusive lesion is severe stenosis or occlusion of the intracranial VA before its PICA branch, either by atherostenosis or embolism.[110, 119, 120]

Transcranial Doppler ultrasonography using a foramen magnum window is an excellent means of studying the intracranial VA.[121] MR angiography and standard angiography can give reliable images of the vasculature. MRI is superior to CT in imaging medullary or cerebellar infarcts. I generally treat patients with recent thrombosis of the intracranial VA with warfarin for 4 to 6 wk. I use long-term warfarin for severe preocclusive stenosis of the intracranial VA. Bilateral severe occlusive disease of the intracranial VA can be a particularly malignant vascular lesion.[122] Persistent hypoperfusion of the medulla and cerebellum and rostral basilar artery territories causes motor and cerebellar symptoms, often with visual blurring due to occipital lobe ischemia. Treatment includes efforts to increase blood pressure and perfusion and sometimes surgery to unblock or bypass the occluded arteries.[102, 103, 122]

Basilar Artery Occlusive Disease

The basilar artery is formed at the medullopontine junction by the merging of the right and left intracranial VAs. The basilar artery then bifurcates at the pontomesencephalic junction into its terminal PCA branches. The major basilar artery branches are penetrating arteries to the pontine base and the short and long circumferential cerebellar arteries, the anterior inferior cerebellar artery (AICA), and the superior cerebellar arteries (SCA). The basilar artery irrigates primarily the pons. The basis pontis is supplied by penetrating branches at all levels; the tegmentum pontis is supplied more by the SCAs and branches that loop caudally from the rostral basilar artery.

SYMPTOMS AND SIGNS

The major symptoms and signs are motor and oculomotor. Occlusion of the basilar artery compromises primarily the penetrating arteries leading to the paramedian base and tegmentum.[102, 103, 123] The lateral regions that include mainly sensory and some cerebellar connections are usually spared. Motor symptoms are usually bilateral but may be asymmetric. At times, hemiplegia is obvious at onset.[124] Weakness, hyperreflexia, and extensor plantar responses are usually present. The basis pontis also contains the crossing pontocerebellar fibers on their way to and from the brachium pontis so that ataxia of the limbs or gait may be noted if the limbs are not paralyzed or too weak to determine coordination.

The oculomotor regions are the paramedian pontine reticular formation (PPRF), the medial longitudinal fasciculus (MLF), and the abducens nucleus. Unilateral lesions of the PPRF cause loss of voluntary lateral gaze to the lesion side and hypometric saccades from the contralateral field of motion directed ipsilaterally.[125] Reflex eye movements are preserved in lesions of the PPRF.[125] Involvement of the abducens nucleus causes an ipsilateral lateral gaze palsy for all eye movements, both voluntary and reflex.[125] MLF lesions lead to an inability to adduct the ipsilateral eye on gaze to the opposite side. PPRF lesions combined with lesions of the MLF on one side may produce a so-called one-and-a-half syndrome, in which the only preserved horizontal eye movement is abduction of the contralateral eye.[125, 126] Some data from MRI studies suggest that it is possible for a unilateral lesion of the tegmentum to cause a bilateral horizontal gaze palsy by involving the central raphe of the pons.[127] Ocular bobbing may be seen and probably represents preservation of vertical eye movements directed more rostrally at a time when horizontal eye movements are defective.[128] This condition is characterized by a brisk downward excursion of the eye, either unilaterally or bilaterally. Involvement of the pontine tegmentum can also cause ptosis and small reactive pupils.[126] Both horizontal and vertical nystagmus are also common.

When the rostral basilar artery is involved, the symptoms and signs are quite different. The findings in patients with a rostral basilar artery syndrome have been extensively reviewed elsewhere.[76, 77, 129] The neuroophthalmologic signs closely mimic those in patients with thalamic hematomas; they include abnormalities of upgaze and downgaze. Either upgaze or downgaze can be lost selectively. Unilateral or bilateral lesions in the pretectum in the region near the posterior commissure and the rostral interstitial nucleus of the MLF can cause selective upgaze palsies.[76, 129, 130] Hyperconvergence of one or both eyes is also common. The pupils on one or both sides may be small, oval, or poorly reactive.[102, 103] In addition, important abnormalities of alertness and behavior occur. Somnolence is due to lesions of the reticular activating system on both sides of the third ventricle or midbrain tegmentum. Amnesia, hallucinations, and apathetic behavior are also common.[76, 77, 102, 103, 129] When the lesion is limited to the rostral basilar artery, motor or sensory signs are often absent. Because the temporal and occipital lobe supply of the PCAs is also often ischemic, patients may also have prominent visual and sensory abnormalities and an agitated delirium.[76, 77]

Etiology, Evaluation, and Treatment

Occlusion of the basilar artery is most often thrombotic, occlusive thrombus being superimposed on gradually developing atherostenosis. Occlusions often occur at the origin of the basilar artery, where clot may have propagated from one VA. The middle and distal basilar arteries are often the site of the occlusive process.[131] Embolic occlusion of the basilar artery is also relatively common but until recently has not been well appreciated.[110] Occlusion of the rostral basilar artery is nearly always embolic, the donor site being the heart or proximal subclavian-vertebral artery system.

Transcranial Doppler is not particularly accurate at detecting basilar artery disease, which is often beyond the reach of the probe.[121] The distribution of the infarct on MRI can often be suggestive, and absence of the flow void in the basilar artery can suggest occlusion. MRI angiography or standard angiography is usually needed to corroborate the diagnosis and to image the proximal vascular system. Cardiac evaluation is also important in cases of suspected embolism, especially when a patient has no risk factors for cerebrovascular atherostenosis.

For acute basilar artery occlusions, it is critical to maintain optimal circulatory function in order to promote brain stem perfusion through collateral channels. I use short-term heparin, then warfarin anticoagulation to prevent propagation and embolization of a fresh clot. In patients with tight stenosis with some residual lumen, I use longer-term warfarin treatment. In the future, emergent use of thrombolytic and fibrinolytic agents such as recombinant tissue plasminogen activator may become the treatment of choice.[132–135]

PENETRATING ARTERY DISEASE IN THE ANTERIOR AND POSTERIOR CIRCULATIONS

Occlusion of penetrating arteries causes small deep infarcts or transient ischemia. The clinical findings, causes, and treatment in patients with penetrating artery disease are quite distinct from disease of large arteries.[136–139] The most important penetrating arteries are the medial and lateral lenticulostriate artery branches of the MCA, which supply the putamen and internal capsule region; Heubner's arteries, which are branches of the ACA supplying the caudate nucleus and subfrontal white matter; the thalamoperforating and thalamogeniculate branches of the rostral basilar artery and PCA; and the paramedian arteries to the pons, which originate from the basilar artery. Infarcts tend to be located mostly in the basal ganglia and internal capsules, the medial and lateral thalamus, and the paramedian pontine base.

SYMPTOMS AND SIGNS

Penetrating artery disease usually occurs in persons who are or have been hypertensive or who are diabetic. TIAs occur but less frequently than in patients with occlusion of larger extracranial or surface arteries. When TIAs do occur, they are often spaced over a short period of hours to days and do not continue for weeks or months. The TIAs are usually stereotyped and repetitive. The symptoms and signs of TIAs or strokes due to penetrating artery disease depend heavily on the location of the lesion. In the internal capsule or paramedian pons, the most frequent clinical symptom is motor paralysis on one side of the body, usually without sensory, visual, or cognitive abnormalities. The face, arm, and leg are most often involved, the reflexes on the hemiparetic side are exaggerated, and a Babinski sign is present. This syndrome has been called *pure motor hemiplegia* after Fisher.[140]

Ischemia in the lateral thalamus in the region of the somatosensory nuclei causes sensory symptoms and signs on one half of the body. The most common symptoms are paresthesias, but numbness also occurs. Examination usually does not show any major objective sensory loss.[141, 142] When the ischemia is due to occlusion of larger thalamogeniculate branches, the sensory loss is combined on the same side with hemiataxia and at times hemichorea.[81] Infarction in the medial thalamus can produce a behavioral syndrome with abulia or a syndrome of memory loss and upgaze palsy.[103] Infarction in the pons in the base or tegmentobasal junction can cause a combination of ataxia and weakness on one side of the body[143] or dysarthria and clumsiness of one hand.[144]

Because the lesions are small and deep, prominent headache, decreased alertness, vomiting, and loss of consciousness are not usual. Seizures are rare.

CAUSE AND EVALUATION

Two major pathologic conditions underlie lacunas and penetrating branch infarcts: lipohyalinosis and microatheroma. Hypertension causes an arteriopathy that involves mostly the media of penetrating arteries. Subintimal foam cells and fibrinoid material infiltrate the vessel walls. In places, whorls, tangles, and wisps of connective tissue obliterate the usual vessel layers.[145] Fisher referred to these changes as *segmental arterial disorganization, fibrinoid degeneration,* and *lipohyalinosis,* attempting to capture the pathologic nature of lipid and fibrinoid degeneration and disorganization of the arteries.[145] Ischemia is due to compromise of the lumen by the process involving the arterial wall. The same pathology can also lead to cerebral hemorrhage[146]; hypertensive intracerebral hemorrhage affects the same vascular distribution as lacunar infarction.

The other important pathologic condition that causes occlusion of penetrating branches is atherosclerosis. Miniature atheromas (called *microatheroma* by Fisher[145]) may block the orifice of penetrating branches. Alternatively, the atherosclerotic lesion in the parent artery can block the branch, or atheroma beginning in the parent vessel can spread into the orifice of the branch.[147–149] The two pathologies—atheromatous branch occlusion and lipohyalinosis—differ in two aspects, epidemiology and locus of occlusion in the artery. Lipohyalinosis is predominantly due to hypertension, whereas atheromatous occlusion often affects older patients with risk factors for atherosclerosis, but hypertension is not necessarily a cause. Atheromatous branch occlusion affects the origin of the artery, whereas lipohyalinosis usually involves the proximal and middle portions of the branch. This latter difference is academic but may be definable by MRI if the infarction involves the brain adjacent to the pial surface containing the origin of the branch.[149]

The diagnosis of penetrating branch disease is based on a combination of risk factors, time course, nature of clinical signs, lack of accompanying signs, and neuroimaging results. I agree with Miller that the diagnosis of lacunar infarction should not be made without a compatible CT or MRI scan.[150] Risk factors such as hypertension and diabetes should be present. The deficit should develop quickly or gradually during hours or a few days. The clinical deficit should reflect a deep lesion; pure motor hemiparesis, pure sensory stroke, and combinations of dysarthria, weakness, and ataxia are the most common clinical findings. Headache, seizures, vomiting, and loss of alertness or consciousness should not be present. Most important, neuroimaging studies should not show a superficial cortical infarct. A lacuna should be visible on CT or MRI, or no lesion may be apparent. In the brain stem, the infarct should conform to the territory of a single penetrating branch artery. Because infarcts can also be caused by occlusion of parent arteries such as the MCA and PCA, transcranial Doppler ultrasonography or MRI angiography may be needed in some cases to rule out occlusion of these arteries.[149] Occlusion of these intracranial arteries is especially common in blacks and persons of Chinese and Japanese ancestry.[59]

In some patients, the diagnosis of lacunar infarction is uncertain. Risk factors, clinical course, or the neurologic findings may be atypical. In that circumstance, investigation for occlusive disease of a larger artery should be pursued. If a lacuna can be confidently diagnosed, treatment consists of risk factor modification. Neither agents that modify platelet function, such as aspirin and ticlopidine, nor anticoagulants have been shown to be beneficial.

REFERENCES

1. Hedges TR: The terminology of transient visual loss due to vascular insufficiency. Stroke 15:907, 1984.
2. Burde RM: Amaurosis fugax, an overview. J Clin Neuroophthal 9:185, 1989.
3. Goodwin JA, Gorelick PB, Helgason C: Symptoms of amaurosis fugax in atherosclerotic carotid artery disease. Neurology 37:829, 1987.
4. Fisher CM: Observations of the fundus oculi in transient monocular blindness. Neurology 9:333, 1959.
5. Gautier JC: Clinical presentation and differential diagnosis of amaurosis fugax. *In* Bernstein EF (ed): Amaurosis Fugax. New York, Springer-Verlag, 1988.
6. Tippin J, Corbett JJ, Kerber RE, et al: Amaurosis fugax and ocular infarction in adolescents and young adults. Ann Neurol 26:69, 1989.
7. Ropper AH: Transient ipsilateral paresthesias (TIPs) with transient monocular blindness. Arch Neurol 42:295, 1985.
8. Pessin MS, Duncan GW, Mohr JP, et al: Clinical and angiographic features of carotid transient ischemic attacks. N Engl J Med 296:358, 1977.
9. Rivkin MJ, Hedges TR, Logigian E: Carotid dissection presenting as posterior ischemic optic neuropathy. Neurology 40:1467, 1990.
10. Bogousslavksy J, Regli F, Zografos L, et al: Opticocerebral syndrome: Simultaneous hemodynamic infarction of optic nerve and brain. Neurology 37:263, 1987.
11. Newman NJ, Kline LB, Leifer D, et al: Ocular stroke and carotid artery dissection. Neurology 39:1462, 1989.
12. Furlan AJ, Whisnant JP, Kearns TP: Unilateral visual loss in bright light. Arch Neurol 36:675, 1979.
13. Wiebers DO, Swanson JW, Cascino TL, et al: Bilateral loss of vision in bright light. Stroke 20:554, 1989.
14. Donnan GA, Sharbrough FW, Whisnant JP: Carotid occlusive disease: Effect of bright light on visual evoked response. Arch Neurol 39:687, 1982.
15. Russell RWR, Ikeda H: Clinical and electrophysiological observations in patients with low pressure retinopathy. Br J Ophthalmol 70:651, 1968.
16. Hollenhorst RW: Embolic retinal phenomena. Symposium on Neuro-Ophthalmology. Transaction of the New Orleans Academy of Ophthalmology. St. Louis, CV Mosby, 1976.
17. Muci-Mendoza R, Arruga J, Edward WO, et al: Retinal fluorescein angiographic evidence for atheromatous microembolism. Stroke 11:154, 1980.
18. Michelson JB, Friedlander MH: Angiography of retinal and choroidal vascular disease. *In* Bernstein EF (ed): Amaurosis Fugax. New York, Springer-Verlag, 1988.
19. Atlee W: Talc and cornstarch emboli in eyes of drug users. JAMA 219:49, 1972.
20. Kearns TP, Hollenhorst RW: Venous stasis retinopathy of occlusive disease of the carotid artery. Mayo Clin Proc 38:304, 1963.
21. Mills RP: Anterior segment ischemia secondary to carotid occlusive disease. J Clin Neuro Ophthalmol 9:200, 1989.
22. Carter JE: Chronic ocular ischemia and carotid vascular disease. *In* Bernstein EF (ed): Amaurosis Fugax. New York, Springer-Verlag, 1988.
23. Young LH, Appen RE: Ischemic oculopathy. Arch Neurol 38:358, 1981.
24. Fisher CM: Dilated pupil in carotid occlusion. Trans Am Neurol Assoc 91:230, 1966.
25. Wray SH: Visual aspects of extracranial internal carotid artery disease. *In* Bernstein EF (ed): Amaurosis Fugax. New York, Springer-Verlag, 1988.
26. Bruno A, Corbett JJ, Biller J, et al: Transient monocular visual loss patterns and associated vascular abnormalities. Stroke 21:34, 1990.
27. Kline LB, Kelly CL: Ocular migraine in a patient with cluster headaches. Headache 20:253, 1980.
28. Eadie MJ, Sutherland JM, Tyrer JH: Recurrent monocular blindness of uncertain cause. Lancet 1:319, 1968.
29. Chawluk JB, Kushner MJ, Bank WJ, et al: Atherosclerotic carotid artery disease in patients with retinal ischemic syndromes. Neurology 38:858, 1988.
30. Adams HP, Putnam S, Corbett JJ, et al: Amaurosis fugax: The results of arteriography in 59 patients. Stroke 14:742, 1983.
31. Pfaffenbach DD, Hollenhorst RW: Morbidity and survivorship of patients with embolic cholesterol crystallization in the ocular fundus. Am J Ophthalmol 75:66, 1973.
32. Savino PJ, Glaser JS, Cassady J: Retinal stroke: Is the patient at risk? Arch Ophthalmol 95:1185, 1977.
33. Weinberger J, Bender AN, Yang WC: Amaurosis fugax associated with ophthalmic artery stenosis: Clinical simulation of carotid artery disease. Stroke 19:290, 1980.
34. Weinberg PE, Patronas NJ, Kim K, et al: Anomalous origin of the ophthalmic artery in a patient with amaurosis fugax. Arch Neurol 38:315, 1981.
35. Hayreh SS: Arterial blood supply of the eye. *In* Bernstein EF (ed): Amaurosis Fugax. New York, Springer-Verlag, 1988.
36. Barnett JH, Bernstein EF, Callow AD, et al, the Amaurosis Fugax Study Group: Amaurosis fugax (transient monocular blindness): A consensus statement. *In* Bernstein EF (ed): Amaurosis Fugax. New York, Springer-Verlag, 1988.
37. Wray SH: Occlusion of the cerebral retinal artery. *In* Bernstein EF (ed): Amaurosis Fugax. New York, Springer-Verlag, 1988.
38. Von Graefe A: Ueber Embolie der Arteria centralis retinae als ursache plotzlicher erblindung. Graefes Arch Clin Exp Ophthalmol 5:136, 1859.
39. Appen RE, Wray SH, Cogan DG: Central retinal artery occlusion. Am J Ophthalmol 79:374, 1975.
40. Wilson LA, Warlow CP, Ross-Russell RW: Cerebrovascular disease in patients with retinal arterial occlusion. Lancet I:292, 1979.
41. Merchut MF, Gupta SR, Naheedy MH: The relation of retinal artery occlusion and carotid artery stenosis. Stroke 19:1239, 1988.
42. Hayreh SS: Blood supply of the optic nerve head and its role in optic atrophy, glaucoma, and edema of the optic disc. Br J Ophthalmol 53:721, 1969.
43. Hayreh SS: Acute ischemia of the optic nerve. *In* Bernstein EF (ed): Amaurosis Fugax. New York, Springer-Verlag, 1988.
44. Beri M, Klugman MR, Kohler JA, et al: Anterior ischemic optic

neuropathy. VIII: Incidence of bilaterality and various influencing factors. Ophthalmology 94:1020, 1987.
45. Beck RW, Servais GE, Hayreh SS: Anterior ischemic optic neuropathy. IX: Cup-disc ratio and its role in the pathogenesis. Ophthalmology 94:1503, 1987.
46. Doro S, Lessell S: Cup-disc ratio and ischemic optic neuropathy. Arch Ophthalmol 103:1143, 1985.
47. Savino PJ: Risk of cerebrovascular disease in patients with anterior ischemic optic neuropathy. *In* Bernstein EF (ed): Amaurosis Fugax. New York, Springer-Verlag, 1988.
48. Geschwind N, Kaplan E: A human cerebral deconnection syndrome. Neurology 12:675, 1962.
49. Heilman KM, Valenstein E: Frontal lobe neglect in man. Neurology 22:660, 1972.
50. Mesulam MM: A cortical network for directed attention and unilateral neglect. Ann Neurol 10:309, 1981.
51. Hier D, Mondlock J, Caplan LR: Behavioral defects after right hemisphere stroke. Neurology 33:337, 1983.
52. Hier D, Stein R, Caplan LR: Cognitive and behavioral deficits after right hemisphere stroke. Curr Concepts Cerebrovasc Dis (Stroke) 20:1, 1985.
53. Fisher CM: Left hemiplegia and motor impersistence. J Nerv Ment Dis 123:201, 1956.
54. Ross E: The aprosodias: Functional-anatomic organization of the affective components of language in the right hemisphere. Arch Neurol 38:561, 1981.
55. Caplan LR, Kelly M, Kase CS, et al: Infarcts of the inferior division of the right middle cerebral artery: Mirror image of Wernicke's aphasia. Neurology 36:1015, 1986.
56. Caplan LR: Are terms such as completed stroke or RIND of continued usefulness. Stroke 14:431, 1983.
57. Caplan LR: TIAs—We need to return to the question, what is wrong with Mr. Jones. Neurology 38:791, 1988.
58. Fisher CM, Ojemann RG: A clinico-pathologic study of carotid endarterectomy plaques. Rev Neurol 142:573, 1986.
59. Caplan LR, Hier DB, Gorelick PB: Race, sex and occlusive cerebrovascular disease. Stroke 17:648, 1986.
60. Fisher CM, Ojemann R, Roberson GS: Spontaneous dissection of cervico-cerebral arteries. Can J Neurol Sci 5:9, 1978.
61. Mokri B, Sundt TM, Houser OW, et al: Spontaneous dissection of the cervical internal carotid artery. Ann Neurol 19:126, 1986.
62. Caplan LR: Cerebrovascular disease: Large artery occlusive disease. *In* Appel S (ed): Current Neurology, vol. 8. Chicago, Year Book, 1988.
63. Caplan LR, Brass LM, DeWitt LD, et al: Transcranial Doppler ultrasound: Present status. Neurology 40:696, 1990.
64. Caplan LR, Stein R: Stroke: A clinical approach. Boston, Butterworth, 1986.
65. Caplan LR: Transient ischemic attacks. *In* Johnson R (ed): Current Therapy in Neurologic Disease. Philadelphia, BC Decker, 1985.
66. Pertuiset B, Aron D, Dilenge D, et al: Les syndromes de l'artere choroidienne anterieure: Étude clinique et radiologique. Rev Neurol 106:286, 1962.
67. Rhoton A, Kiyotaka F, Fradd B: Microsurgical anatomy of the anterior choroidal artery. Surg Neurol 12:171, 1979.
68. Helgason C, Caplan LR, Goodwin J, et al: Anterior choroidal artery-territory infarction: Report of cases and review. Arch Neurol 43:681, 1986.
69. Frisen L: Quadruple sectoranopia and sectorial optic atrophy: A syndrome of the distal anterior choroidal artery. J Neurol Neurosurg Psychiatry 42:590, 1979.
70. Frisen L, Holmegaard L, Rosencrantz M: Sectorial optic atrophy and homonymous, horizontal sectoranopia: A lateral choroidal artery syndrome. J Neurol Neurosurg Psychiatry 41:374, 1978.
71. Bruno A, Graff-Radford NR, Biller J, et al: Anterior choroidal artery territory infarction: A small vessel disease. Stroke 20:616, 1989.
72. Damasio H: A computed tomographic guide to the identification of cerebral vascular territories. Arch Neurol 40:138, 1983.
73. Szdzuy D, Lehman R: Hypoplastic distal part of the basilar artery. Neuroradiology 4:118, 1972.
74. Caplan LR: Posterior cerebral artery syndromes. *In* Vinken PJ, Bruyn GW, Klawans HL (eds): Handbook of Clinical Neurology, Vascular Diseases, Part I, vol. 53. Amsterdam, Elsevier Science, 1988.
75. Kinkel WR, Newman RP, Jacobs L: Posterior cerebral artery branch occlusion: CT and anastomotic considerations. *In* Berguer R, Bauer R (eds): Vertebrobasilar Arterial Occlusive Disease. New York, Raven Press, 1984.
76. Caplan LR: "Top of the basilar" syndrome. Neurology 30:72, 1980.
77. Mehler MF: The rostral basilar artery syndrome: Diagnosis, etiology, prognosis. Neurology 39:9, 1989.
78. Brust JC, Behrens M: "Release hallucinations" as the major symptom of posterior cerebral artery occlusion: A report of 2 cases. Ann Neurol 2:432, 1977.
79. Lance JW: Simple hallucinations confined to the area of a specific visual field defect. Brain 99:719, 1976.
80. Critchley M: Types of visual perseveration, palinopsia and illusory visual spread. Brain 74:267, 1951.
81. Caplan LR, DeWitt LD, Pessin MS, et al: Lateral thalamic infarcts. Arch Neurol 45:959, 1988.
82. Caplan LR, Hedley-White T: Cuing and memory dysfunction in alexia without agraphia—A case report. Brain 97:251, 1974.
83. Geschwind N, Fusillo M: Color naming defects in association with alexia. Arch Neurol 15:137, 1966.
84. Geschwind N: Disconnection syndromes in animals and man. Brain 88:237, 1965.
85. Kertesz A, Sheppard A, Mackenzie R: Localization in transcortical sensory aphasia. Arch Neurol 39:475, 1982.
86. Fisher CM: Disorientation to place. Arch Neurol 39:33, 1982.
87. Symonds C, Mackenzie I: Bilateral loss of vision from cerebral infarction. Brain 80:415, 1957.
88. Damasio AR, Damasio H, van Horsen GW: Prosopagnosia: Anatomic basis and behavior mechanisms. Neurology 32:331, 1982.
89. Tranel D, Damasio AR: Knowledge without awareness: An autonomic index of facial recognition by prosopagnosics. Science 228:1453, 1985.
90. Damasio AR, Yamada T, Damasio H, et al: Cerebral achromatopsia: Behavioral, anatomic and physiological aspects. Neurology 30:1064, 1980.
91. Levine D, Warach J, Farrah M: Two visual systems in mental imagery. Neurology 35:1010, 1986.
92. Holmes G: Disturbances of visual orientation. Br J Ophthalmol 2:449, 1918.
93. Riddoch G: Dissociation of visual perceptions due to occipital injuries with especial reference to appreciation of movement. Brain 40:15, 1917.
94. Balint R: Seeleneahmung des Schauens, optische ataxie und raumlicher storung der Aufmerksamkeit. Monatsschr Psychiatr Neurol 25:51, 1909.
95. Husain M, Stein J: Rezso Balint and his most celebrated case. Arch Neurol 45:89, 1988.
96. Hecaen H, Deajuriaguerra J: Balint's syndrome (psychic paralysis of visual function) and its minor forms. Brain 77:373, 1954.
97. Mohr JP: Posterior cerebral artery. *In* Barnett HJ, Mohr JP, Stein B, Yatsu F (eds): Stroke: Pathophysiology, Diagnosis and Management. New York, Churchill Livingstone, 1985.
98. Pessin MS, Lathi E, Cohen M, et al: Clinical features and mechanism of occipital infarction. Ann Neurol 21:290, 1987.
99. Koroshetz WJ, Ropper AH: Artery to artery embolism causing stroke in the posterior circulation. Neurology 37:292, 1987.
100. Pessin MS, Kwan E, Scott M, et al: Occipital infarction with hemianopsia from carotid occlusive disease. Stroke 20:409, 1989.
101. Pessin M, Kwan E, DeWitt LD, et al: Posterior cerebral artery stenosis. Ann Neurol 21:85, 1987.
102. Caplan LR: Vertebro-basilar occlusive disease. *In* Barnett HJM, Mohr JP, Stein B, Yatsu F (eds): Stroke Pathophysiology, Diagnosis, and Management. New York, Churchill Livingstone, 1986.
103. Caplan LR: Vertebrobasilar system syndromes. *In* Vinken PJ, Bruyn GW, Klawans HL (eds): Handbook of Clinical Neurology, Vascular Diseases, Part I, vol. 53. Amsterdam, Elsevier Science, 1988.
104. Pelouze GA: Plaque ulcerie de l'ostium de l'artère vertebrale. Rev Neurol 145:478, 1989.
105. Reivich M, Holling E, Roberts B, et al: Reversal of blood flow through the vertebral artery and the effect on the cerebral circulation. N Engl J Med 265:878, 1961.

106. Baker R, Rosenbaum A, Caplan LR: Subclavian steal syndrome. Contemp Surg 4:96, 1974.
107. Hennerici M, Aulich A, Sandmann W, et al: Incidence of asymptomatic extracranial arterial disease. Stroke 12:750, 1981.
108. Hennerici M, Kleman C, Rautenberg W: The subclavian steal phenomenon: A common vascular disorder with rare neurologic deficits. Neurology 38:669, 1988.
109. Fields WS, Lemak N, Ben-Menachem Y: Thoracic outlet syndrome: Review and reference to stroke in a major league pitcher. Am J Neuroradiol 7:73, 1986.
110. Caplan LR, Tettenborn B: Embolism in the posterior circulation. *In* Berguer R, Caplan LR (eds): Vertebrobasilar Arterial Disease. St. Louis, Quality Medical Publishers, 1992, pp 52–65.
111. Caplan LR, Zarins CK, Hemmatti M: Spontaneous dissection of the extracranial vertebral artery. Stroke 16:1030, 1985.
112. Wilkinson I, Russell R: Arteries of the head and neck in giant cell arteritis. Arch Neurol 27:378, 1972.
113. Goodwin J: Temporal arteritis. *In* Vinken PJ, Bruyn GW (eds): Handbook of Clinical Neurology, vol. 39. Neurological Manifestations of Systemic Diseases, Part II. Amsterdam, North-Holland, 1980.
114. Currier R, Giles C, Dejong R: Some comments on Wallenberg's lateral medullary syndrome. Neurology 12:778, 1961.
115. Kommerell G, Hoyt W: Lateropulsion of saccadic eye movements. Arch Neurol 28:313, 1973.
116. Meyer K, Baloh R, Krohel G, et al: Ocular lateropulsion: A sign of lateral medullary disease. Arch Ophthalmol 98:1614, 1980.
117. Estanol B, Lopez-Rios G: Neuro-otology of the lateral medullary infarct syndrome. Arch Neurol 39:176, 1982.
118. Fisher CM, Karnes W, Kubik C: Lateral medullary infarction: The pattern of vascular occlusion. J Neuropathol Exp Neurol 24:455, 1965.
119. Sypert GW, Alvord EC: Cerebellar infarction: A clinical pathology study. Arch Neurol 32:357, 1975.
120. Amerenco P, Hauw JJ, Henin D, et al: Les infarctus der territorie de l'artère cerebelleuse postero-inférieure. Etude clinico-pathologique de 28 cas. Rev Neurol 145:277, 1989.
121. Tetterborn B, Estol C, DeWitt LD, et al: Accuracy of transcranial doppler in the vertebrobasilar circulation. J Neurology 237:159, 1990.
122. Caplan LR: Bilateral distal vertebral artery occlusion. Neurology 33:552, 1983.
123. Kubik C, Adams RD: Occlusion of the basilar artery: A clinical and pathologic study. Brain 69:73, 1946.
124. Fisher CM: The "herald hemiparesis" of basilar artery occlusion. Arch Neurol 45:1301, 1988.
125. Pierrot-Deseilligny C, Chain P, Serraru M, et al: The one and a half syndrome: Electrophysiologic analysis of four cases with deductions about the physiological mechanism of lateral gaze. Brain 104:665, 1981.
126. Fisher CM: Some neuro-ophthalmological observations. J Neurol Neurosurg Psychiatry 30:383, 1967.
127. Bronstein AM, Rudge P, Gresty M, et al: Abnormalities of horizontal gaze. Clinical, oculographic and magnetic resonance imaging findings. II: Gaze palsy and internuclear ophthalmoplegia. J Neurol Neurosurg Psychiatry 43:200, 1990.
128. Fisher CM: Ocular bobbing. Arch Neurol 11:543, 1964.
129. Mehler MF: The neuro-ophthalmologic spectrum of the rostral basilar artery syndrome. Arch Neurol 45:966, 1988.
130. Zachon D, Sharpe JA: Midbrain paresis of horizontal gaze. Ann Neurol 16:495, 1984.
131. Pessin MS, Gorelick PB, Kwan E, et al: Basilar artery stenosis—Middle and distal segments. Neurology 37:1742, 1987.
132. Ferbert A, Bruchmann H, Brumen R: Clinical features of proven basilar artery occlusion. Stroke 21:1135, 1990.
133. Del Zoppo GJ, Zeumer H, Harker LA: Thrombolytic therapy in stroke: Possibilities and hazards. Stroke 17:595, 1986.
134. Sloan MA: Thrombolysis and stroke. Arch Neurol 44:748, 1987.
135. Pessin MS, Del Zoppo G, Estol CJ: Thrombolytic agents in the treatment of stroke. Clin Neuropharmacology 13:271, 1990.
136. Fisher CM: Lacunes, small deep cerebral infarcts. Neurology 15:774, 1965.
137. Fisher CM: Lacunar strokes and infarcts: A review. Neurology 32:871, 1982.
138. Mohr JP: Lacunes. Stroke 13:3, 1982.
139. Caplan LR: Lacunar infarction: A neglected concept. Geriatrics 31:71, 1976.
140. Fisher CM: Pure motor hemiplegia of vascular origin. Arch Neurol 13:30, 1965.
141. Fisher CM: Pure sensory stroke involving face, arm, and leg. Neurology 15:76, 1965.
142. Fisher CM: Pure sensory stroke and allied conditions. Stroke 13:434, 1982.
143. Fisher CM: Ataxic hemiparesis: A pathologic study. Arch Neurol 35:126, 1978.
144. Fisher CM: A lacunar stroke: The dysarthria—Clumsy hand syndrome. Neurology 17:614, 1967.
145. Fisher CM: The arterial lesions underlying lacunes. Acta Neuropathol 12:1, 1969.
146. Fisher CM: Pathological observations in hypertensive cerebral hemorrhage. J Neuropathol Exp Neurol 30:530, 1971.
147. Fisher CM, Caplan LR: Basilar branch occlusion: A cause of pontine infarction. Neurology 21:900, 1971.
148. Fisher CM: Bilateral occlusion of basilar artery branches. J Neurol Neurosurg Psychiatry 40:1182, 1977.
149. Caplan LR: Intracranial branch atheromatous disease. Neurology 39:1246, 1989.
150. Miller V: Lacunar stroke: A reassessment. Arch Neurol 40:129, 1983.
151. Feldmann E, Daneault N, Kwan E, et al: Chinese-white differences in the distribution of occlusive cerebrovascular disease. Neurology 40:1541, 1990.

Chapter 211

Brain Tumors

AMY PRUITT

Tumors of the brain, its meningeal coverings, and the spinal cord rank second only to stroke as the most common neurologic cause of death. Recent advances in diagnostic techniques and in perioperative management of cerebral edema have resulted in valuable palliative therapy for primary brain tumors. Improved treatment of systemic malignancies has led both to an increased incidence of neurologic complications of cancer and to more frequent involvement of specialists other than neurologists in the care of patients with metastatic brain tumors.

The role of the ophthalmologist in the clinical management of neurologic cancer may involve (1) recognition of signs and symptoms suggesting intracranial neoplasm, (2) use of appropriate diagnostic tests such as computed tomography (CT) or magnetic resonance imaging (MRI) to distinguish tumor from other causes of progressive neuroophthalmologic dysfunction, (3) urgent referral of patients to a neurologist for institution of emergency medication to control cerebral edema, and (4) appreciation of the prognosis and of the medical and ophthalmologic complications of the tumor and its therapy.

INCIDENCE AND CLASSIFICATION OF BRAIN TUMORS

Brain tumors can arise from the supporting tissue of the brain (gliomas), neurons, blood vessels, meninges, pituitary or pineal gland, cranial nerves, congenital rests, and lymphoreticular tissue, or they can spread to the intracranial contents from outside the central nervous system (CNS) (metastases). Table 211–1 provides a classification of brain tumors.

In persons younger than 20 yr, CNS tumors represent nearly 20 percent of malignancies, second to leukemia. Two thirds of the tumors in this age group are in the posterior fossa. The common tumors of childhood and adolescence are gliomas of the cerebellum, brain stem, and optic nerve; pinealomas; primitive neuroectodermal tumors; and craniopharyngiomas. Common tumors of midlife (20 to 60 yr) include meningiomas, gliomas of the cerebral hemispheres, and pituitary tumors. Malignant astrocytomas and metastases represent the bulk of tumors in late life. In all adult age groups, malignant astrocytomas are the most common primary brain tumor. With the exception of meningiomas and acoustic neuromas, intracranial tumors are slightly more common in men.

Table 211–1. CLASSIFICATION OF BRAIN TUMORS

Primary Tumors
- Tumors of glial origin (gliomas)
  - Astrocytoma (grades I, II)
  - Malignant astrocytoma (grades III, IV) (glioblastoma)
  - Oligodendroglioma
  - Ependymoma*
  - Choroid plexus papilloma
- Tumors of neuronal origin†
  - Medulloblastoma*
  - Neuroblastoma*
- Tumors of neural crest origin
  - Meningioma
  - Primary CNS melanoma
- Tumors of connective tissue origin
  - Sarcoma
- Tumors of lymphoreticular origin
  - Primary (non-Hodgkin's) CNS lymphoma
- Tumors of glands
  - Pituitary
    - Chromophobe adenoma
    - Acidophilic adenoma
    - Basophilic adenoma
    - Microadenoma
  - Pineal
    - Pineocytoma
    - Pineoblastoma
    - Germ cell tumors‡
      - Germinoma
      - Teratoma
      - Dermoid
      - Embryonal carcinoma
      - Choriocarcinoma
- Tumors of congenital rest origin
  - Notochord—chordoma*
  - Adipose cells—lipoma
  - Ectodermal derivatives—craniopharyngioma, teratoma, dermoid, colloid cysts
- Tumors of blood vessels
  - Hemangioblastoma
  - Angioma
- Tumors of the skull
  - Osteoma
  - Hemangioma
  - Granuloma (other tumors, including meningiomas, dermoids, chordomas, and metastases, may invade the skull)

Metastastic Tumors (in order of frequency found at autopsy)

Tumor	Frequency
Melanoma	50–80%
Lung	20–30%
Breast	20%
Renal	8–20%
Colorectal	1–5%
Ovarian	1%

- Tumors of the cranial nerves
  - Glioma of optic nerve
  - Neurofibroma
  - Schwannoma*

Modified from Escourolle R, Poirier J: Manual of Basic Neuropathology, 2d ed. Philadelphia, WB Saunders, 1978.

*More common in posterior fossa than supratentorially.

†Collectively known as *primitive neuroectodermal tumors.*

‡Although not glandular tumors exclusively, these cell types tend to occur near the pineal gland.

CNS, central nervous system.

CLINICAL MANIFESTATIONS OF BRAIN TUMOR

The symptoms and signs caused by brain tumors are determined by their size, location, invasiveness, and rate of growth. Although the brain can accommodate slowly growing tumors, both histologically benign and histologically malignant masses larger than 3 cm in diameter increase intracranial pressure. Vessels associated with a growing neoplasm contain fenestrations through which a plasma filtrate escapes, producing "vasogenic" cerebral edema and increasing the effective tumor volume. *Cerebral edema* is not synonymous with *raised intracranial pressure,* because considerable vasogenic edema may be present before the pressure begins to increase. Thus, clinically, a patient may have significant brain edema before evidence of papilledema develops, and the absence of this important neuroophthalmologic finding does not rule out brain tumor. Conversely, patients may have absent venous pulsations (in some patients a normal finding) and no cerebral edema or raised intracranial pressure.

Based on the mechanisms just described, brain tumors can produce both focal deficits and more generalized or "nonlocalizing" disturbances. With uncommon exceptions, primary brain tumors do not metastasize outside the CNS, although all glial tumors are capable of diffuse meningeal seeding. Patients with brain tumors usually have one or more of the following groups of symptoms: (1) headache with or without evidence of increased intracranial pressure; (2) progressive generalized decline in cognitive abilities or in specific neurologic functions such as speech, gait, or vision; (3) adult-onset seizures; and (4) focal neurologic symptoms and signs reflecting the anatomic site of the tumor. Headache is the initial symptom in half of patients with brain tumors. Traction on the dura, blood vessels, or cranial nerves results in pain. In most patients with supratentorial tumor, pain radiates to the side of the tumor mass, whereas patients with posterior fossa masses describe retroorbital, retroauricular, or occipital pain. Patients with tumors of the

Table 211–2. CLINICAL MANIFESTATIONS OF BRAIN TUMORS

Location	Ophthalmologic Signs and Symptoms	Associated Neurologic Signs and Symptoms	Common Tumor Types
Frontal lobe	Contralateral gaze paresis	*Subtle mentation disturbances, apathy, decreased spontaneity, urinary incontinence, gait disorder	Glioma Metastases Meningioma
Temporal lobe	Contralateral superior quadrantanopia	Personality change, memory deficit, auditory/gustatory/ olfactory hallucinations	Glioma Metastases Pituitary adenoma (large)
Parietal lobe	Contralateral hemianopia Asymmetric optokinetic nystagmus toward side of lesion	Dominant: dysphasia, contralateral hemiparesis Nondominant: spatial disorientation, inattention to contralateral side, constructional difficulties, contralateral hemiparesis	Glioma Metastases Meningioma
Occipital lobe	Contralateral hemianopia (possibly macula sparing) Dominant: difficulty naming colors, alexia without agraphia	Dominant: memory loss, dysnomia	Meningioma Metastases
Diencephalon	Disturbance of upward gaze, convergence, pupillary constriction (Parinaud's) Papilledema (due to obstructive hydrocephalus)	Neuroendocrine abnormalities (diabetes insipidus) Headache, emesis	Pineocytoma Pineoblastoma Germ cell tumors Glioma
Sella/parasellar region	Bitemporal hemianopia Cranial nerve III, IV, VI paresis	Neuroendocrine disturbances Facial hypesthesia Frontal headache	Pituitary adenomas Craniopharyngioma
Brain stem	Anesthetic cornea Diplopia (due to isolated cranial neuropathy, gaze paresis, or internuclear ophthalmoplegia)	Dysphagia, dysphonia Incoordination of limbs, crossed hemiparesis (ipsilateral cranial nerve signs with contralateral weakness)	Glioma Metastases
Cerebellum/cerebellopontine angle	Papilledema (due to obstructive hydrocephalus) Unilateral abducens palsy Brun's nystagmus	Unilateral limb ataxia, gait ataxia, nuchal headache, emesis Facial pain, numbness, or paresis Progressive unilateral hearing loss	Medulloblastoma (and other PNETs) Meningioma Acoustic neuroma Glioma
Leptomeninges (carcinomatous meningitis)	Papilledema (due to communicating hydrocephalus); painless or painful monocular visual loss; single or multiple, often painful cranial neuropathies; uveitis (lymphoma); disc edema (due to infiltrative optic neuropathy)	Headache, back pain, lumbosacral radiculopathy, urinary retention	Lymphoma Leukemia Metastases (breast, lung, melanoma, gastric) Glioma

*Tumors may be quite large and still produce very subtle signs.
PNETs, primitive neuroectodermal tumors.

pineal region, sella, parasellar and suprasellar regions, sphenoid wing, cerebellopontine angle, and orbit may first consult an ophthalmologist for diagnosis. Symptoms of localizing value, with special emphasis on ophthalmologic findings, are described in Table 211–2.

LABORATORY INVESTIGATIONS OF PATIENTS WITH BRAIN TUMOR

Advances in neuroradiology have contributed significantly to the diagnosis and management of CNS tumors.[1] Special diagnostic imaging techniques are described in Chapters 286 to 288. In general, suspected brain tumors are imaged with CT, MRI, or both. *Unenhanced CT* reveals calcium, cerebral edema, and blood. Tumors with a density that exceeds that of normal brain parenchyma and that are thus likely to be visible on unenhanced scans include meningioma, melanoma, primary CNS lymphoma, and some of the gliomas. *Iodinated contrast-enhanced CT* delineates intracranial tumors as small as 0.5 cm. Tumors commonly appear as ring-enhancing masses surrounded by variable amounts of edema. Ringlike enhancement can occur also in abscesses, toxoplasmosis lesions, recent cerebral infarctions or hemorrhages, and plaques of multiple sclerosis. Multiple lesions suggest metastatic disease, whereas primary brain tumors are more often solitary (Fig. 211–1). Initial CT may show no abnormality in small metastases, primary brain lymphoma, some glial tumors, or carcinomatous meningitis, and follow-up scans in 6 to 8 wk or MRI (discussed later) is indicated when clinical suspicion is high. CT is an excellent method for

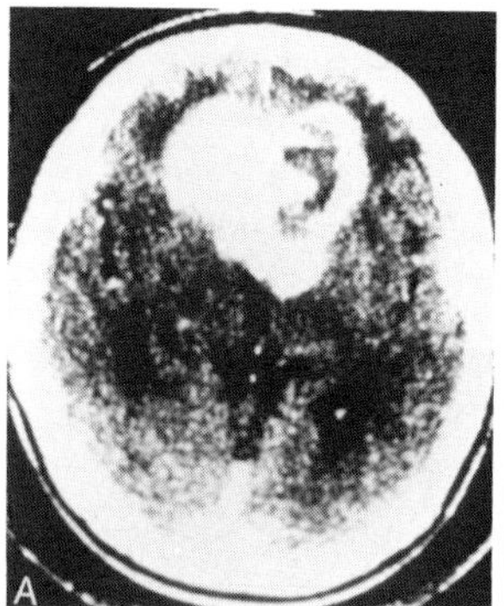

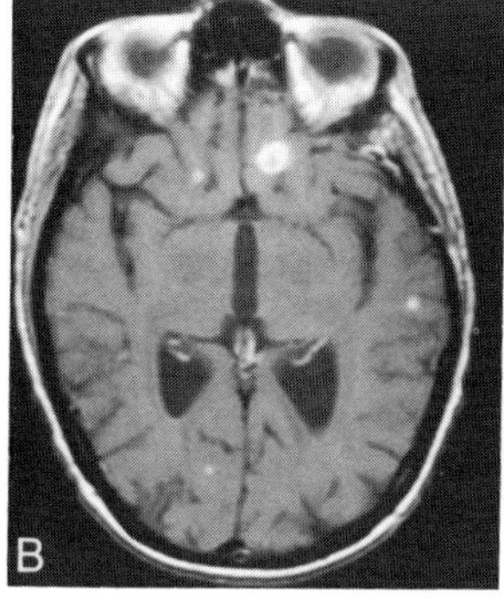

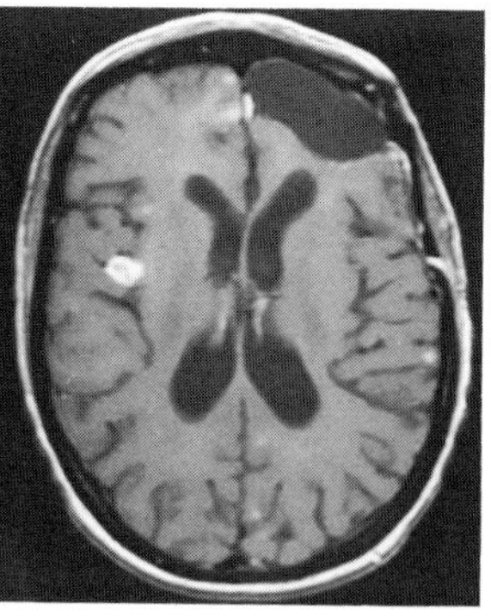

Figure 211–1. *A,* Large, heterogeneously enhancing lesion crossing the corpus callosum, consistent with malignant astrocytoma (glioblastoma). *B,* Multiple enhancing nodules in brain parenchyma and along the ependymal surface in a patient with metastatic melanoma. A large left frontal lesion that had hemorrhaged has been excised.

evaluating bony destruction in the orbit, sella, and clivus and thus is ideal for imaging orbital tumors, chordomas, and chondrosarcomas. Considerably less expensive than MRI, CT is also faster, which is a possible consideration in confused or uncooperative patients with cerebral neoplasm. CT is also preferable to MRI for imaging calcium and acute hemorrhage.

MRI is the procedure of choice for evaluating most cerebral infarctions, brain tumors, demyelination, and inflammatory processes. MRI is more sensitive than CT for detecting early gliomas (Fig. 211–2). When performed with intravenous gadolinium diethylenetriamine pentaacetic acid (GTPA), MRI can detect multiple metastases when CT would show only a solitary lesion. GTPA gives the same information as does iodinated contrast material in CT about integrity of the blood-brain barrier. MRI cannot distinguish radiation necrosis due to recurrent tumor or edema secondary to therapy from edema due to tumor growth. MRI is superior to CT for visualization of lesions in the brain, sella, and suprasellar and parasellar areas, as well as those close to the skull base and in the spinal cord.

Transfemoral angiography provides selective visualization of internal carotid and vertebral arteries and their branches. Malignant tumors are characterized by an angiographic "blush" with early draining veins. Although MRI is excellent for detecting vascular anomalies such as arteriovenous malformations and large aneurysms, angiography can provide definitive information about vascular anatomy that is also essential in preoperative neurosurgical planning. A particularly useful feature of angiography is its ability to demonstrate blood vessel supply to a tumor by branches of the external carotid artery, a finding supporting a diagnosis of meningioma.

Surgery is indicated for definitive diagnosis and for possible debulking in most primary brain tumors, as well as for some patients who have single metastatic tumors with systemic disease that is well controlled and with CNS disease that represents a life-limiting or quality-limiting factor.[2] It is always preferable to obtain tissue for confirmation of histologic diagnosis before initiating therapy for brain tumors, and such confirmation is mandatory for investigational protocols. Radiation doses are tailored to the type of cerebral malignancy, and specific chemotherapy is now available for several primary and secondary CNS malignancies. Because neither CT nor MRI can reliably distinguish abscess from tumor or recurrent tumor from radiation necrosis, repeat biopsy is encouraged after treatment if doubt exists about the pathologic condition and if the lesion is accessible.

Tumor biopsy can be performed through an open craniotomy or with CT- or MRI-guided stereotaxic techniques. Resection is attempted and may be curative for some primary tumors such as meningioma, pituitary adenomas, oligodendroglioma, and some low-grade astrocytomas. Partial resection improves symptoms and often allows better seizure control and reduced dependence on corticosteroids.

ACUTE TREATMENT OF BRAIN TUMORS

Acute management of brain tumor is directed at reducing cerebral edema, lowering intracranial pressure, and reducing seizure risk. Treatment with daily doses of corticosteroids such as dexamethasone (16 mg/day in four divided doses) or methylprednisolone (64 mg/day in four divided doses) is usually instituted immediately. Corticosteroids may not control symptoms caused by obstructive hydrocephalus, and emergency ventricular

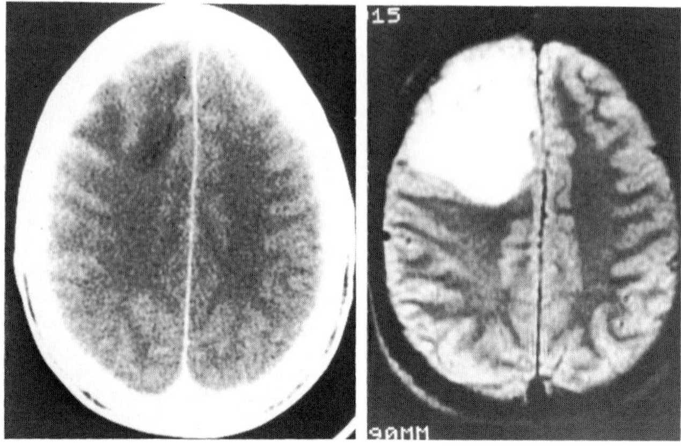

Figure 211–2. Comparable axial sections from contrast-enhanced computed tomography (CT) scan (*left*) and T_2-weighted magnetic resonance imaging (MRI) images. The patient had a right frontal oligodendroglioma, which is more vividly demonstrated on MRI than on CT.

drainage or shunting may be required. Anticonvulsant medications are usually prescribed for patients who have had seizures, although many physicians administer them prophylactically when a supratentorial tumor has been demonstrated.

PRIMARY BRAIN TUMORS

Malignant astrocytoma or glioblastoma, also referred to as grade III or IV astrocytoma, represents three fourths of the glial tumors diagnosed yearly in the United States.[3] This rapidly growing invasive tumor commonly occurs in the corpus callosum; in the frontal, parietal, and temporal lobes; and in the thalamus. Peak age of onset is between 40 and 70 yr. The tumor may be vascular, and CT and MRI demonstrate a usually solitary, heterogeneously enhancing lesion.

Treatment usually involves as much resection as feasible, followed by radiation therapy with or without chemotherapy.[3] Untreated, patients survive on average only about 17 wk, but with aggressive radiation therapy to 6000 cGy and chemotherapy with nitrosoureas or procarbazine, median survival is 62 wk.[4, 5] Other chemotherapy regimens being studied include combinations of procarbazine, vincristine, and cisplatin or carboplatinum.[6] Only 19 percent of patients are alive 18 mo after the diagnosis. Interstitial implantation of tumor with radioactive iodine or iridium seeds (bradytherapy)[7] is being investigated in attempts to improve both the dismal prognosis of this tumor and the serious sequelae such as dementia[8] and radiation necrosis[9] present in a high percentage of longer-term survivors.[10, 11]

Astrocytomas grades I and II occur throughout the brain and spinal cord, slowly infiltrating the white matter of these areas. Subcortical white matter in the cerebral hemispheres is the most common location in adults, whereas the optic nerve, cerebellum, and brain stem are the more typical locations in children. The tumors are avascular, with little or no contrast enhancement on CT or MRI. The natural history of these tumors reflects considerable variability in biologic aggressiveness. Patients may remain stable clinically for several years, with stable or minimally evolving areas of low density on CT or of T_2 signal abnormality on MRI. This variability in behavior has led to some uncertainty about proper treatment.

Treatment of low-grade astrocytomas generally involves resection of as much tumor as possible. For completely resected tumors, radiation therapy is generally not recommended, but postoperative radiation probably confers some benefit in incompletely resected lesions.[12] Because the benefit of treatment must be weighed against the consequences of high-dose cranial irradiation in a patient with life expectancy between 5 and 10 yr, a prospective controlled trial is under way to resolve the issue of efficacy of radiation for this class of tumor. In the meantime, clinical practice still can dictate deferring radiation if a patient is stable and the neuroradiologic studies show no growth. Attempts have been made to use positron emission tomography to determine metabolic changes in a tumor that might suggest that it is becoming more aggressive.[13, 14] Chemotherapy has no established role for low-grade astrocytomas. Life expectancy depends in part on the grade of the tumor, the patient's age, and the tumor location. Excision without further therapy may be curative for some astrocytomas, particularly those of the cerebellum or optic nerve, whereas even with aggressive chemotherapy and radiation median survival for brain stem astrocytomas averages 15 mo. Similar treatment considerations apply to the less common oligodendrogliomas.[15, 16]

Meningiomas usually are histologically benign, although they can invade adjacent skull, can recur after incomplete excision, and rarely metastasize extracranially. Common locations of meningiomas are the parasagittal falx, convexity near the coronal suture, sphenoid wing, olfactory groove, suprasellar region, and posterior fossa. Sphenoid wing meningiomas may become apparent to an ophthalmologist early in the course of the illness. For these tumors, a clinically useful classification involves distinction based on distance from the midline.[17] Outer sphenoid wing tumors may produce hyperostosis, exophthalmos, compression of the optic nerve, and seizures. Such meningiomas may appear in the en plaque configuration. Inner sphenoid wing tumors close to the optic nerve and chiasm generally produce diminished central vision in the ipsilateral eye and a temporal defect in the contralateral eye. Involvement of the superior orbital fissure may produce various patterns of ocular motor palsies (Fig. 211–3). Large tumors of this region can cause ipsilateral optic atrophy and contralateral papilledema (Foster Kennedy syndrome). Large olfactory groove meningiomas can present to an ophthalmologist as a combination of bilateral optic nerve and chiasmatic involvement. In general, meningiomas of the anterior visual pathways are smaller and have a shorter antecedent history than those involving the convexities or olfactory nerve, although meningiomas in any location can present during pregnancy with rapid increase in volume.[18]

Another situation in which ophthalmologists can become involved early in the diagnosis of meningiomas is in identifying patients with neurofibromatosis type 2. Patients from kindreds with this dominantly inherited disorder may be identified first by the presence of posterior lens opacities.[19] Such patients are at risk for bilateral acoustic neuromas[20] as well as for other tumors such as meningiomas, gliomas, and schwannomas of the cranial and spinal nerves.[21]

CT is an excellent tool for diagnosing meningiomas and reveals both bony erosion and calcification. MRI may be useful in imaging the parasellar or suprasellar extension of tumors. Angiography can be effective in the differential diagnosis of parasellar masses, because a tumor blush can be seen most frequently with meningiomas, and blood supply from meningohypophyseal branches of the internal carotid or middle meningeal branches of the external carotid artery can be confirmed.

Meningiomas are treated with surgical excision, if possible. Microsurgical techniques for tumors of the anterior visual pathways have improved visual outcome

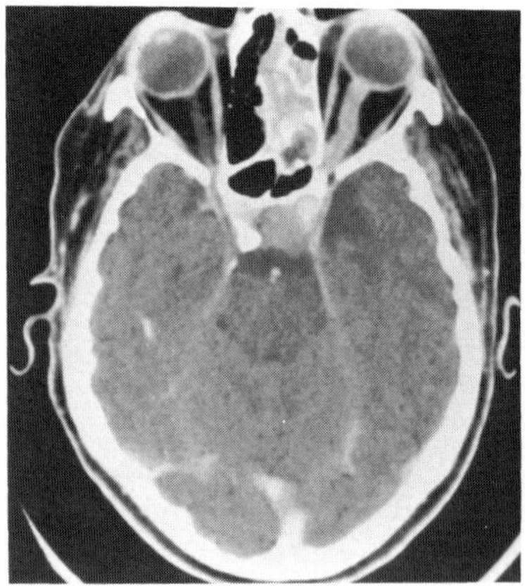

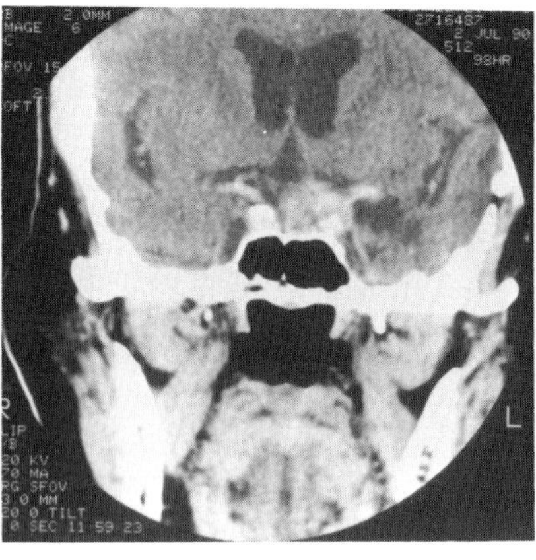

Figure 211–3. Axial *(left)* and coronal *(right)* images of parasellar region in a patient who had partial resection of a left sphenoid meningioma. A homogeneously enhancing mass arises at the level of the left anterior clinoid and extends anteriorly into the apex of the left orbit, medially into the sella turcica, and laterally along the edge of the tentorium. The left optic nerve is enlarged owing to entrapment at the level of the orbital apex. The patient had no vision O.S. and a partial left third-nerve palsy.

for these patients.[22] Incompletely excised tumors and tumors with invasive histologic characteristics are sometimes irradiated.[23, 24]

Because the population of immunosuppressed patients is growing as a result of AIDS, congenital immunodeficiency disease, or medical therapies for organ transplantation or autoimmune disease, *primary non-Hodgkin's CNS lymphoma* is being recognized with increasing frequency.[25] The tumor may be solitary or multicentric, is frequently in a periventricular location, and may seed the subarachnoid space. Ten percent of patients with this type of lymphoma may present with vitreal infiltration, often antedating the development of clinically evident lymphoma in the brain parenchyma or subarachnoid space.[26, 27] Ocular involvement may be due to direct extension of tumor through the meninges or optic nerve, or the eye may be another site of this multicentric neoplasm. Patients may report cloudy or blurred vision, and slit-lamp examination may reveal cells in the vitreous in an otherwise uninflamed-appearing eye. In one series, 40 percent of patients with ocular lymphoma had no symptoms at the time of positive findings on slit-lamp examination. Thus, all patients with CNS lymphoma should have slit-lamp examination as part of their initial evaluation. Results of a slit-lamp examination may be falsely negative, however, as may vitrectomy. A cellular infiltrate in the vitreous, choroid, or retina of a patient with primary non-Hodgkin's CNS lymphoma, should be equated with ocular extension and treated primarily with ocular radiation. However, because most patients in these series presented at a median interval of 9 mo before the diagnosis of CNS lymphoma, orbital irradiation may complicate subsequent CNS treatment. Ocular lymphoma sometimes responds to corticosteroids. Ocular relapse in a patient treated with cranial irradiation is difficult to treat because penetration of most chemotherapeutic agents into the vitreous is poor. All patients with primary non-Hodgkin's CNS lymphoma should have regular slit-lamp examination as part of their follow-up care.

CNS lymphoma is treated with corticosteroids and radiation after confirmation of diagnosis by biopsy or by cerebrospinal fluid (CSF) cytology. Several preirradiation chemotherapy regimens have been studied and appear promising. High-dose methotrexate administered intravenously has been used most extensively and has been demonstrated to achieve therapeutic levels in CSF and brain parenchyma.[25] Intravenous methotrexate is coupled with intrathecal instillation of methotrexate to treat meningeal lymphoma. With radiation treatment alone, median survival is 17 mo. Cases of temporary spontaneous remission have been reported, and the tumor's exquisite clinical and radiographic response to corticosteroids has been well documented.[25]

Tumors of the pineal region include pineocytomas, germ cell tumors, and glial tumors. These tumors may come to the attention of an ophthalmologist early in their course because of a characteristic presentation of limitation of conjugate upgaze, convergence and retraction of the eyes on attempted upgaze, light-near dissociation of the pupillary responses, and retraction of the eyelids (Parinaud's syndrome) with or without papilledema due to obstructive hydrocephalus. Hypothalamic invasion can lead to diabetes insipidus and to variable anterior pituitary insufficiency. Diplopia, headache, lethargy, and hydrocephalus are noted with larger lesions. The diencephalic syndrome of childhood characterized by emaciation, hyperkinesis, and a cheerful affect can be caused by invasive tumors of this region. Because germinomas are quite radiosensitive and some pineal tumors are chemotherapy responsive, early diagnosis is important. Some germ cell tumors may produce human chorionic gonadatropin or α-fetoprotein as serum markers.[28] Efforts to minimize radiation dose in the usually young patients afflicted by these neoplasms have led to trials of various preirradiation chemotherapy regimens for hypothalamic, parasellar, chiasmatic, and third ventricular glial tumors.[29]

Germ cell tumors are sometimes diagnosed by an ophthalmologist because of seeding of the subarachnoid space around the optic nerve, which may cause disc edema and visual loss. This may cause a CT or MRI picture of an enlarged optic nerve and may initially raise the diagnostic considerations of optic nerve glioma or meningioma, but cranial CT or MRI reveals the primary lesion. Conversely, marked monocular visual loss in the setting of a germ cell tumor, medulloblastoma, or other primitive neuroectodermal tumor is an indication for CT or MRI, with special attention to the orbits. Enlarged optic nerves should be investigated with lumbar puncture for CSF cytologic study in this setting. Indeed, virtually any primary or secondary brain neoplasm can seed the spinal subarachnoid space, and this complication is likely to be encountered more frequently by ophthalmologists as patients survive longer with CNS tumors.

Tumors of the posterior fossa are more common in children and adolescents. Low-grade astrocytomas of the brain stem are occasionally encountered by ophthalmologists because of the initial symptoms of diplopia or because of eye pain resulting from corneal dysfunction due to involvement of the ophthalmic division of the trigeminal nerve. Other symptoms and signs of brain stem astrocytomas include dysphagia, limb ataxia, dysphonia, and corticospinal signs of motor weakness or sensory disturbance. Hydrocephalus is rare with these astrocytomas.

Another common posterior fossa tumor arises from primitive multipotential precursor cells, which can give rise to either glial or neuronal mature cells. Several histologic varieties have been distinguished, the most common of which is the medulloblastoma. This tumor is usually located in the cerebellar vermis. Resection of the tumor is the first treatment step and is followed by radiation to the brain and entire neuraxis. Staging of disease involves MRI of the brain and spinal cord and CSF sampling for cytologic study. Recurrent tumors have been successfully treated with nitrosoureas, procarbazine, and vincristine, or with nitrogen mustard, vincristine, procarbazine, and prednisone (MOPP), and sometimes with methotrexate.[30] Extracranial metastases to the lung, liver, and bone have been reported. Five-year survival is reported to be nearly 75 percent. Because of the serious consequences of cranial irradiation in children, current efforts are directed at using pre-irradiation chemotherapy to try to reduce the dose of radiation administered.[31]

PITUITARY TUMORS

Pituitary adenomas represent 10 to 15 percent of intracranial neoplasms. Symptoms depend on the presence of pituitary hormone hypersecretion, the absence or diminution of hormones due to destruction of normal pituitary gland, and the direction of local expansion and invasion of adjacent structures. Pituitary tumors were previously classified by H&E staining into basophilic, acidophilic, or chromophobic types (see Table 211–1). Tumors are now classified both by size and by physiologic characteristics. Stage I tumors are microadenomas less than 10 mm in diameter. They may cause hormonal excess but do not cause hypopituitarism or mechanical problems. Stage II tumors are macroadenomas (greater than 10 mm) with or without suprasellar extension. Stage III tumors are distinguished from stage IV tumors by more significant destruction of the sella in the latter, although both may have sellar enlargement and suprasellar extension.[32] Physiologic classification by immunohistochemical staining or by serum hormone measurements divides tumors into nonsecreting and secreting types. From late adolescence through adulthood, the frequency of adenoma subtypes in decreasing order of occurrence is prolactinoma, nonsecreting adenoma, growth hormone–secreting adenoma, corticotroph cell adenoma, or glycoprotein-secreting adenoma. Prolactinomas produce amenorrhea-galactorrhea in women and testicular atrophy, gynecomastia, diminished body hair, and impotence in men. In men, in particular, the sometimes subtle effect of hyperprolactinemia or growth hormone hypersecretion may be overlooked, leading to an increased proportion of these types among the larger, more long-standing adenomas. Forty percent of nonfunctioning tumors are prolactinomas according to immunohistochemical study, and it is likely that increased sensitivity of assays and stimulation tests will increase the proportion of secreting tumors among microadenomas.[33]

Growth hormone–secreting tumors are the next most common type and cause acromegaly (Fig. 211–4). Next in frequency are adrenocorticotropic hormone (ACTH)–secreting adenomas, which cause the symptom complex of Cushing's disease: truncal obesity, abdominal striae, moon facies, and psychologic disturbances. Glycoprotein-secreting tumors (follicle-stimulating hormone [FSH], luteinizing hormone [LH], thyroid-stimulating hormone [TSH]) are the least common pituitary adenomas. However, gonadotroph-secreting adenomas are being recognized with increasing frequency.[34] In men, such tumors may come to light because of testicular enlargement or hypogonadism, but in postmenopausal women, whose basal levels of FSH and LH may be elevated, many apparently nonsecreting pituitary macroadenomas may now be demonstrated by thyrotropin-releasing hormone stimulation to be gonadotroph-secreting. About 15 percent of pituitary adenomas secrete more than one hormone, the most common combination being prolactin and growth hormone.

Prolactinomas in women and corticotroph-secreting adenomas in men are generally detected while still microadenomas. In general, tumors without endocrine symptoms are large at the time of diagnosis and present with structural problems. These tumors, therefore, may be disproportionately represented among the adenomas that come to the attention of an ophthalmologist. Severe frontal headaches occur in one half of patients with macroadenomas and result from pressure on the diaphragma sellae. Clinical signs referable to local expan-

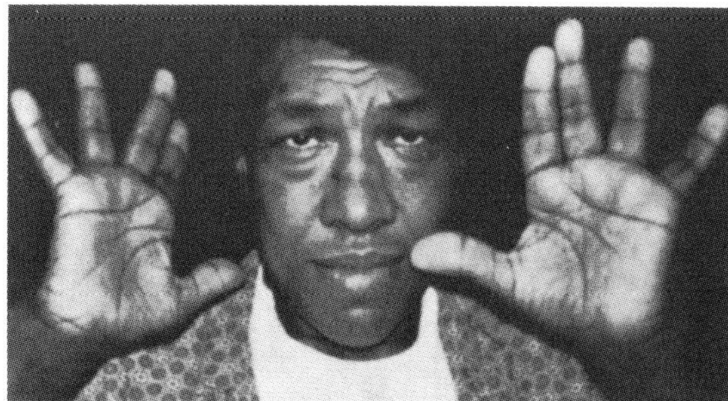

Figure 211–4. Patient with characteristic features of acromegaly. She reported a history of gradual enlargement and coarsening of her facial features, hands, and feet. An upper bitemporal defect was found on visual field examination. (From Laties AM: Neuro-ophthalmology. *In* Scheie HG, Albert DM [eds]: Textbook of Ophthalmology, 9th ed. Philadelphia, WB Saunders, 1977, p 507.)

sion assume two general patterns. Although the incidence of field defects from pituitary tumors is declining as a result of earlier diagnosis by sensitive hormonal assays and imaging techniques, tumors that extend predominantly upward involve the optic chiasm or optic nerves. The optic chiasm in 80 percent of normal persons is anterior and superior to the pituitary gland, overlying the pituitary fossa. In about 15 percent, the chiasm is anterior to the tuberculum sellae (prefixed), and in 5 percent it is postfixed over the dorsum sellae. Also, the chiasm is found at a variable distance from the sella (usually about 10 mm superior), and these anatomic variations account for different patterns of visual field loss. The typical field defect from pituitary adenoma is a bitemporal hemianopia, often superior greater than inferior. Depending on the position of the chiasm and the pattern of tumor growth, some patients may suffer complete loss of vision, with optic atrophy in one eye and a temporal defect in the opposite eye or occasionally a monocular defect that mimics nonpituitary lesions. Papilledema due to pituitary tumors is extremely rare and should lead to consideration of a different diagnosis. With marked suprasellar extension of an adenoma, symptoms may reflect hydrocephalus, hypothalamic compression, or subfrontal extension of the mass. Extension of the tumor up to or through the diaphragma sellae often causes pain that radiates to the frontal region.

The second pattern of clinical signs reflects lateral tumor extension with cavernous sinus invasion. The third cranial nerve is usually involved first, and pupillary reactivity may be preserved. Dysfunction of sixth and then fourth cranial nerves occurs later, and headache is often referred to the territories of the ophthalmic or mandibular divisions of the trigeminal nerve.

About 5 percent of patients suffer rapid progression of symptoms due to hemorrhage or partial necrosis or both of a pituitary adenoma. This syndrome, called *pituitary apoplexy,* usually develops rapidly over a few hours or a day but may have a longer evolution.[35] Upward expansion of tumor leads to rapid visual loss, impairment of consciousness, and hypothalamic involvement, whereas lateral expansion results in ophthalmoplegia and trigeminal nerve dysfunction with or without internal carotid artery compression. Downward expansion through the floor of the sella can result in epistaxis. Regardless of the direction of tumor expansion, patients experience sudden headache, usually retroorbital or frontal, often with vomiting. Extravasation of blood into the CSF may cause meningeal signs.

Factors predisposing to pituitary apoplexy include head trauma, sudden elevation of arterial pressure, pregnancy, childbirth, and anticoagulation, although in the majority of cases apoplexy occurs without clearly identifiable precipitants.[36] CT may show hemorrhagic adenomas with focal high signal intensity collections of blood or fluid levels (Fig. 211–5). Examination usually reveals a normal-appearing optic nerve and retina, unless optic atrophy was an antecedent. A major differential diagnostic consideration when a patient has a painful pupil-involving third-nerve palsy is expanding aneurysm, and emergent angiography may be necessary

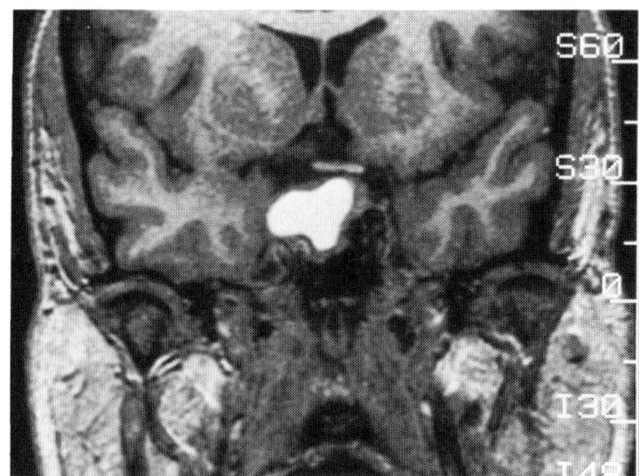

Figure 211–5. Patient sustained head trauma in a motor vehicle accident and developed hemorrhagic pituitary adenoma, presenting with headache and third-nerve palsy.

to distinguish these two conditions. Medical therapy includes administration of high-dose corticosteroids to reduce edema, hormonal replacement, and management of diabetes insipidus or inappropriate antidiuretic hormone secretion. Surgical decompression is mandatory if visual loss or decreased level of consciousness develops rapidly. Cases of laterally expanding apoplexy can be managed conservatively at times, and complete recovery from ophthalmoplegia has been reported.[35] Most patients subsequently have pituitary insufficiency requiring hormone replacement.

Diagnosis and treatment planning have been greatly facilitated by CT and MRI.[37, 38] The majority of microadenomas are isodense or slightly hyperdense compared with adjacent brain and demonstrate homogeneous enhancement with intravenous contrast. A minority have cystic formation or calcification. Calcification and continuity of the sella floor are better visualized with CT than with MRI, but MRI provides the most effective imaging of the sellar contents and allows for evaluation of the degree of suprasellar extension and involvement of the chiasm and cavernous sinus. MRI of pituitary macroadenomas features a relatively isointense signal of prolonged T_1 and T_2 compared with normal brain tissue (Fig. 211–6).[39] Cerebral angiography may be necessary to rule out cerebral aneurysms. The combination of clinical setting, CT, and MRI along with hormonal evaluation allows for discrimination among the disparate causes of parasellar lesions, including pituitary adenomas, craniopharyngiomas, meningiomas, aneurysms, infections such as mucormycosis, sarcoidosis,[40] and systemic neoplasms such as nasopharyngeal tumors or carcinoma of the sinus.

Laboratory investigation of anterior pituitary dysfunction includes determination of baseline growth hormone, prolactin, thyroid functions, FSH, LH, and testosterone. Sensitive thyrotropin-releasing hormone stimulation tests or dexamethasone suppression tests may be required to refine the diagnosis. Elevated prolactin levels are not necessarily diagnostic of a pituitary adenoma, and a number of other systemic causes including the postpartum state and use of oral contraceptives need to be ruled out.[41]

Physicians caring for patients with pituitary tumors have an extensive array of therapeutic options.[42] The

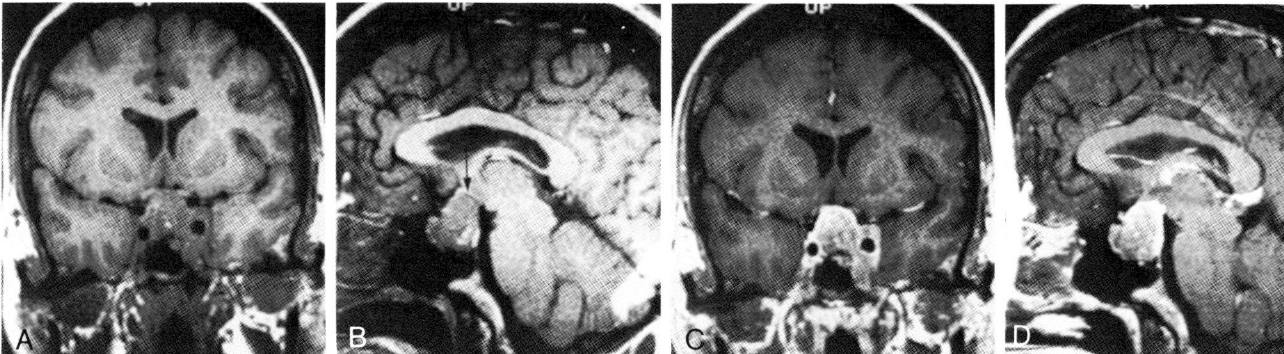

Figure 211–6. Growth hormone–secreting pituitary macroadenoma on coronal images with and without contrast *(A* and *C)* and on sagittal magnetic resonance image with and without contrast *(B* and *D)*. The intrasellar and suprasellar mass extends into the cavernous sinuses, particularly on the left side, with partial encasement of the cavernous segment of the internal carotid artery. Superiorly, the mass compresses the optic chiasm and the tuber cinereum *(B, arrow)*. (From Hasso AN, Shakudo M, Chadrycki E [eds]: MRI of the Brain. III: Neoplastic Disease. New York, Raven Press, 1991, p 178.)

goals of therapy must be individualized and range from restoration of fertility by reducing prolactin secretion to emergency decompression of an expanding tumor that is compromising vision. Some patients with small prolactinomas may not be treated at all, if adverse effects of hyperprolactinemia such as hypogonadism and decreased bone density can be eliminated. Patients' age and health are important considerations.

Traditional forms of therapy for pituitary tumors have included surgery or irradiation or both. Introduction of transsphenoidal surgery and microsurgical variations of this technique offer a favorable chance for cure in some patients with small tumors and for excellent visual recovery in larger tumors,[43] but recurrence rates are variable,[44, 45] and the effectiveness of surgical therapy alone is inversely related to the size of the tumor. Pituitary microsurgery with a cure rate of approximately 50 percent is the treatment of choice for Cushing's disease. Prognostic factors that can be evaluated by an ophthalmologist include the pattern of visual loss and involvement of the oculomotor nerves.[46] Relative contraindications to transsphenoidal surgery are extension of the tumor into the anterior or middle fossa and exclusively suprasellar tumors. Open craniotomy or radiation alone is then indicated.

Irradiation has cured many patients of acromegaly but is associated with numerous long-term sequelae, including pituitary insufficiency, seizures, atherosclerotic changes in cranial vessels,[47, 48] ocular neuromyotonia,[49, 50] the development of secondary benign[51] or malignant tumors,[52, 53] and the unusual complication of herniation of the visual system into the residual empty sella.[54] Different forms of radiation, such as heavy particles and proton beam therapy, available in some centers can deliver a more localized dose of radiation but are associated with a high incidence of postoperative hypopituitarism.

The newest, most specific form of therapy for hypersecreting pituitary adenomas is medical. The first successful drug was bromocriptine. By acting as a direct dopamine agonist, bromocriptine mimics dopamine's role as an inhibitor of prolactin secretion. It not only effectively reduces high prolactin levels in many patients but may also result in shrinkage of the tumor and relief of mechanical symptoms.[55] Withdrawal may lead to reexpansion of the tumor.[56] In as many as 80 percent of patients with prolactin-secreting microadenomas, medical therapy suffices to control symptoms and reduces prolactin to normal levels. For the remaining 20 percent with inadequate control, it provides a useful adjunct to subsequent surgery or radiation therapy. Bromocriptine has also been effective in patients with acromegaly, but the failure rate is higher than with prolactinomas. Somatostatin analogs have proved valuable in patients with acromegaly refractory to surgery, bromocriptine, and other therapies.[57, 58] This same analog (SMS-201-995) has now been reported to be successful therapy for the uncommon thyrotropin-producing pituitary adenomas.[59] Medical therapies may increasingly become primary therapy for hypersecreting microadenomas and macroadenomas and can be used before surgery to shrink tumors or as postoperative therapy for patients with incomplete tumor removal and persistently abnormal hormone levels.[60, 61] Management of pituitary adenomas often requires the combined or sequential use of multiple forms of therapy. Follow-up includes hormonal assay, neuroimaging studies, and neuroophthalmic evaluations at 6-mo intervals.[46]

Craniopharyngiomas are the second most common sellar-parasellar tumor. They occur primarily in children and young adults, arising from remnants of Rathke's pouch,[62] but approximately one quarter occur in adults older than 40 yr.[63] Endocrine dysfunction and visual signs similar to those of pituitary adenomas occur; however, in keeping with their usual location above the chiasm, the tumors first produce inferotemporal field defects that are usually more asymmetric than those with pituitary adenomas. Approximately 80 percent of patients present with visual complaints, and parasellar structures are involved in one third of adults. Papilledema is more common than with adenoma, because the tumor tends to invade the third ventricle and to produce hydrocephalus. A small number of tumors remain intrasellar. Cyst contents may occasionally spill, producing an acute aseptic meningitis.

Diagnosis is usually suggested by a patient's age and

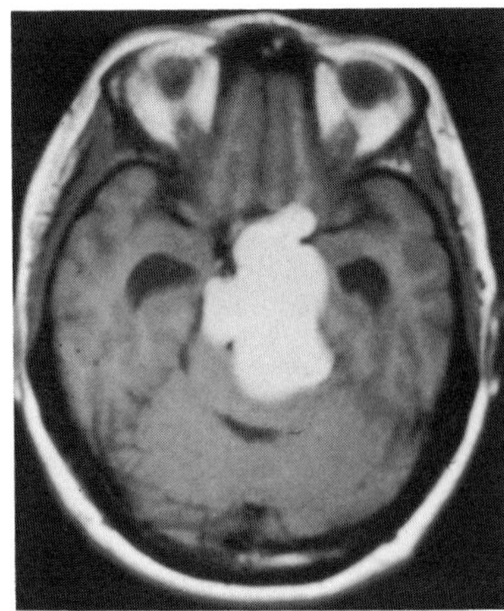

Figure 211–7. Large cystic component of a craniopharyngioma is vividly demonstrated on this axial T_1-weighted magnetic resonance image.

ocular manifestations. CT often reveals a calcified tumor, somewhat more common in children than in adults, and the lesion is often cystic. MRI may be a better diagnostic tool for this tumor, because the CT appearance may be deceptively normal if the tumor contains a large isodense cyst.[64] In these cases, MRI reveals a large area of T_2 signal abnormality reflecting the proteinaceous content of the cyst (Fig. 211–7).

Complete surgical excision of craniopharyngiomas is difficult and may result in significant deficits. Therefore, incomplete excision with postoperative radiation therapy of 4000 to 6000 cGy is usually recommended. The benefits of radiation must be balanced against the risks of this treatment, particularly in children.[65, 66] Proton beam therapy has also been used for this tumor, as has intracavitary stereotaxic radiation with ^{32}P or ^{198}Au colloid for tumors with large cysts.[67] Posttherapy hormone replacement is usually necessary.

SYSTEMIC CANCER AND THE NERVOUS SYSTEM

All systemic tumors have the potential to metastasize to the CNS, and one consequence of improved treatments for systemic neoplasms has been an increasing incidence of neurologic involvement by all types of metastatic cancer. Direct metastatic spread can take the form of parenchymal, epidural, or leptomeningeal involvement, whereas nonmetastatic complications of systemic cancer include vascular problems, paraneoplastic syndromes, metabolic abnormalities, and complications of treatment.

Sixty percent of cerebral metastases occur in the setting of previously diagnosed systemic cancer. In general, the clinical signs of metastases develop more quickly than do those of primary tumor, often with seizures or with a sudden strokelike onset. Tumors spread via hematogenous dissemination or may invade the brain parenchyma from adjacent bone (Fig. 211–8). Cancers of the lung in men and the breast in women account for the greatest absolute numbers of metastases, although melanoma is the tumor with the highest likelihood of spread to the CNS. For most patients, CNS metastasis occurs in the setting of advanced systemic malignancy. Major exceptions are melanoma and lung cancers. Twenty percent of patients with lung cancer present with cerebral metastasis antedating the discovery of the primary malignancy. Multiple metastases are present in one half of all types of metastatic brain tumors, with MRI revealing a slightly greater number of multiple metastases than CT.

The therapeutic plan for a patient with cerebral metastasis is dictated by the clinical status. Patients with solitary accessible lesions and little active systemic disease may be considered for surgery and postoperative radiation.[2] Patients with advanced systemic disease or multiple metastases are referred for radiation therapy. Three fourths of patients treated with radiation improve clinically, and one half are able to discontinue steroid medication. The cause of death of two thirds of patients with cerebral metastases is recurrent systemic tumor at a time of stable neurologic disease. Therefore, aggressive therapy of CNS metastases, particularly for patients with lung or melanoma primaries, may be indicated to preserve quality of life even when the tumor is known to have spread systemically. Chemotherapy has been of limited value for cerebral metastases, although consistent responses have been reported for testicular carcinoma, choriocarcinoma, and nasopharyngeal cancers, whereas isolated reports describe favorable responses to systemic chemotherapy of the breast, lung, and melanoma metastases.

Metastases to the skull base produce a number of syndromes depending on the area involved. The orbital syndrome presents as a painful ophthalmoplegia, diplopia, or visual loss. The parasellar syndrome results from metastasis to the petrous apex and sellar region with compression of cavernous sinus structures: Ipsilateral frontal or temporal headache and diplopia are noted. The middle fossa or gasserian ganglion syndrome is characterized by progressive facial numbness with oc-

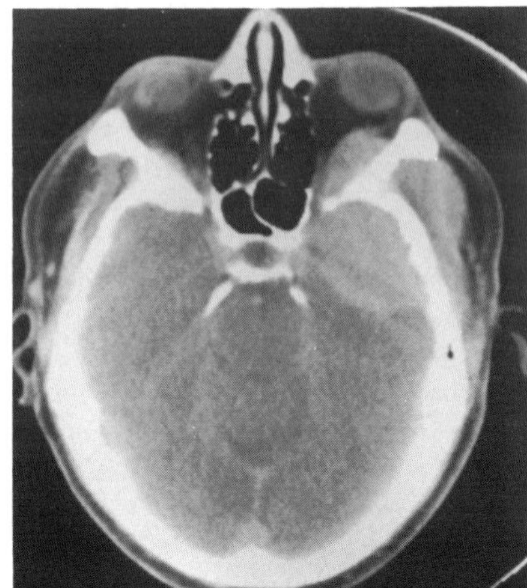

Figure 211–8. Metastatic testicular carcinoma invaded the orbit from a bony metastasis, producing exophthalmos and diplopia, and extended posteriorly to compress the left temporal lobe, producing partial complex seizures.

casional involvement of either the abducens or facial nerve. The jugular foramen syndrome includes retroauricular pain, hoarseness, and dysphagia. The occipital condyle syndrome is characterized by severe ipsilateral occipital headache, dysphagia, and dysarthria due to hypoglossal paresis. Although CT or MRI usually can detect the bone lesions, the clinical syndrome alone in the setting of known metastatic cancer at times suffices to establish the diagnosis and to dictate institution of radiation therapy.

Direct bone invasion of sinus and orbital structures may bring patients with nasopharyngeal or squamous cell cancers to an ophthalmologist. Sinus tumors can extend back directly to involve the orbital apex,[68] and tumors of various head and neck origins can disseminate via the cranial nerves (Fig. 211–9).[69] Isolated difficulty with lid eversion succeeded by facial numbness reflected early involvement of facial and trigeminal nerves in a patient with previously unrecognized squamous cell cancer that could be imaged by MRI.[70, 71]

A different form of CNS involvement by cancer reflects diffuse infiltration of the leptomeninges. Meningeal carcinomatosis is often manifested by painful cranial nerve and spinal root dysfunction. Painless or painful monocular visual loss can be an early symptom. The cranial nerve palsies are sometimes unilateral, reflecting contiguous spread of tumor down the brain stem, but the various cranial nerve palsies may be scattered. The presence of bilateral cranial neuropathies, particularly of the sixth nerve, could raise the question of direct brain stem invasion or of communicating hydrocephalus from impaired CSF flow and resorption. Contrast-enhanced CT or MRI is of some value in the diagnosis of leptomeningeal carcinomatosis. Suggestive findings include ventricular enlargement, enhancement of the leptomeninges, and nodular deposits near the ventricular surface (Fig. 211–10). Lumbar puncture for cytologic study is confirmatory, and the CSF formula usually

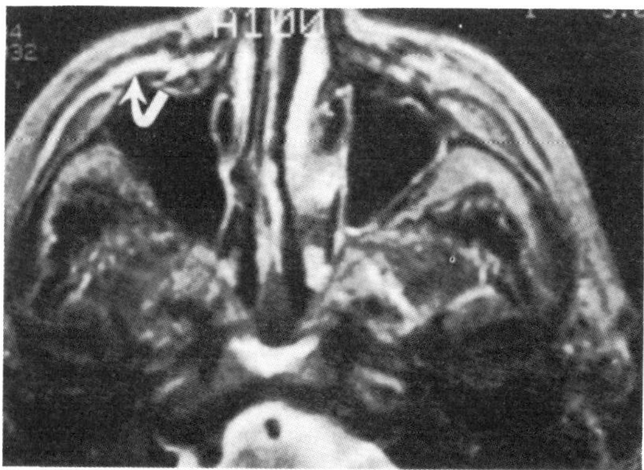

Figure 211–9. Axial T_2-weighted spin-echo image just inferior to the orbital rims shows a linear area of increased signal intensity (*arrow*) superficial to the right maxillary sinus. The patient presented with an isolated numb cheek initially in the infraorbital nerve distribution, with weakness of lower eyelid closure (numb cheek–limp lower lid syndrome) due to infiltration of the infraorbital nerve and distal branches of the facial nerve by squamous cell carcinoma. (From Brazis PW, Vogler JB, Shaw KE: The "numb cheek–limp lower lid" syndrome. Neurology 41:327, 1991.)

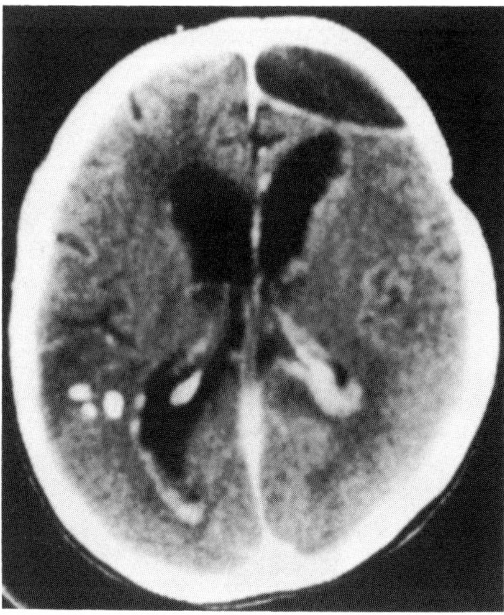

Figure 211–10. Multiple leptomeningeal deposits and parenchymal nodular deposits due to metastatic breast carcinoma. A primary tumor (astrocytoma) has been resected in the left frontal region.

includes hypoglycorrhachia, moderate pleocytosis, and elevated protein. Several lumbar punctures may be necessary to identify malignant cells. Carcinomatosis of the meninges is managed with combined cranial radiation and intrathecal chemotherapy with methotrexate or cytosine arabinoside instilled through an indwelling ventricular reservoir. Meningeal tumor due to leukemia, lymphoma, or breast carcinoma is more likely to respond to treatment, although for responding patients with solid tumors of other sites, median survival is on the order of 6 mo. Meningeal metastases from the lung or melanoma rarely respond, and survival is usually no more than 2 mo.

Unfortunately, successful treatment of many tumors is accomplished at the cost of some injury to normal tissue. Therapy-related complications can mimic recurrent tumor, infection, vascular disease, metabolic derangements, or paraneoplastic processes. Corticosteroids are the most commonly prescribed drugs for brain tumor management. Anticonvulsants, the second most commonly prescribed type of medication for these patients, can produce diplopia, confusion, and ataxia when present in excess.

Attempts to overcome the problem of chemotherapeutic drug delivery posed by the blood-brain barrier have led to intraarterial use of several agents.[11] Because the drugs are usually infused below the origin of the ophthalmic artery, a number of cases of retinopathy and optic neuropathy have been reported after the use of the nitrosoureas, cisplatin, and teniposide (Fig. 211–11). Carmustine (BCNU), the most commonly used nitrosourea, has produced ischemic optic neuropathy, retinal vasculitis, and a cavernous sinus syndrome when infused intraarterially. Teniposide has been reported to have a dose-related retinal toxicity, and intravenous cisplatin has been associated with pigmentary retinopathy. There is some suggestion that radiation and chemotherapy may

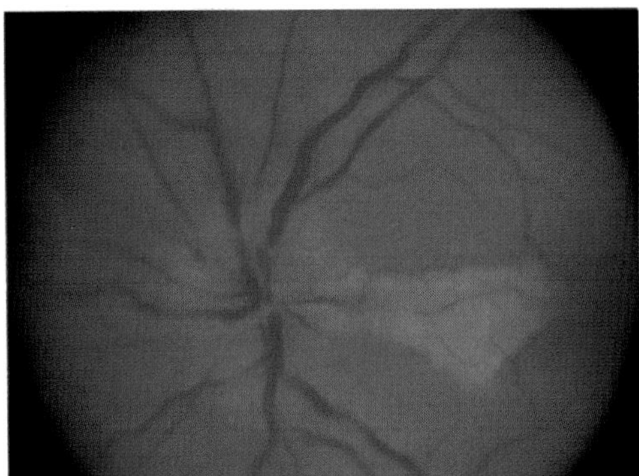

Figure 211–11. Ischemic optic neuropathy after infraophthalmic intraarterial BCNU infusion. The patient has a cilioretinal artery.

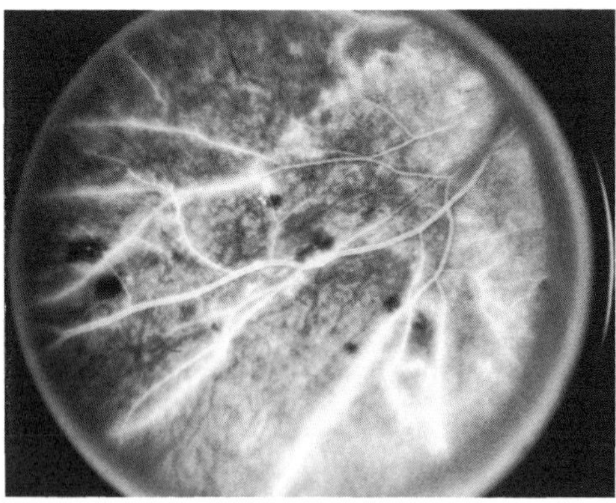

Figure 211–12. This patient with glioblastoma received 6000 cGy external beam irradiation to a left frontal tumor. The left eye developed neovascularization and hemorrhages near the disc; these were treated by laser photocoagulation, with some improvement in vision.

potentiate each other's neurotoxicity. Table 211–3 summarizes neurologic complications of chemotherapy likely to be encountered by an ophthalmologist.

Radiation therapy of the nervous system has been associated with acute, subacute, and chronic injury. Visual loss due to damage to the retina, optic nerve, and chiasm is a possible complication of radiation therapy directed at intracranial tumors that do not directly involve the visual system.[72–74] Macdonald and colleagues described 13 cases of radiation-induced optic neuropathy (RION) that developed between 7 and 26 mo (median 11 mo) after total doses of radiation that varied from 3000 to 6000 cGy and for indications that varied from prophylaxis of small cell lung carcinoma to definitive treatment for astrocytomas.[75] No clear correlation was noted between the dose and the interval after radiation until development of the ocular impairment. Eleven of the 13 patients had received systemic chemotherapy as well. Painless monocular visual loss developed initially and evolved in all patients. Reduced visual acuity, abnormal visual fields (often with an altitudinal defect), and abnormal funduscopic findings were the typical clinical findings. Seven patients had disc edema, one had optic atrophy, and four had normal fundi. Those with disc edema had swelling of the nerve head, hyperemia of the disc, telangiectasia of disc vessels, peripapillary and perimacular hemorrhages, cotton-wool spots, hard and soft exudates, and retinal arteriolar narrowing. Histologic changes paralleled those observed in chronic radiation injury of other parts of the brain and included axonal loss, demyelination, gliosis, and thickening and hyalinization of vessel walls.

Table 211–3. NEUROOPHTHALMIC COMPLICATIONS OF CANCER CHEMOTHERAPY

Problem	Drug	Route of Administration
Optic neuropathy or retinal damage	Nitrosoureas	Intraarterial, high-dose, intravenous
	Cisplatin	Intraarterial, high-dose, intravenous
	Carboplatin	Intraarterial
	Teniposide	Intraarterial
Cranial neuropathy	Vincristine	Intravenous
	Vinblastine	Intravenous
	Cisplatin	Intravenous, intraarterial

The diagnosis of RION is based on the clinical setting and on the funduscopic examination. Fluorescein angiography is of diagnostic value and reveals leakage of fluorescein and areas of capillary nonperfusion (Fig. 211–12). The differential diagnosis of RION and retinopathy is extensive when a patient with known CNS tumor and previous radiation therapy presents with the previously mentioned findings. Intracranial tumor recurrence with raised intracranial pressure must be ruled out, as must carcinomatous meningitis, chemotherapy-related complications,[76] cerebral venous sinus thrombosis with papilledema, the paraneoplastic syndrome of retinopathy with antiretinal antibodies,[77, 78] and idiopathic ischemic optic neuropathy. Radiation damage of the retina has been described at doses lower than those used in RION (1500 rad) in patients undergoing treatment for pituitary adenoma.[52]

In Macdonald's series, six patients showed some spontaneous improvement and one patient had full recovery of normal vision. Steroids were ineffective in the ten patients so treated in this series as well as in previously reported series.[75, 79] Other investigators have suggested the use of hyperbaric oxygen when RION has been present for less than 2 wk.[80] Laser photocoagulation can be of some benefit in patients with retinal exudates, microaneurysms, and hemorrhages due to radiation-induced retinopathy.[81]

Careful treatment planning and optic nerve shielding may reduce the incidence of this complication, but the need to include the visual system within some treatment portals, the variable threshold for optic nerve and retinal injury, and the requirement for potentially neurotoxic chemotherapy make it likely that this complication will persist.

REFERENCES

1. Stamovits TL, Gardner TA: Neuroimaging in neuroophthalmology. Ophthalmology 96:555, 1989.
2. Patchell R: A randomized trial of surgery in the treatment of single metastases to the brain. N Engl J Med 322:494, 1990.

3. Dropcho EJ: Glioma. *In* Johnson RT (ed): Current Therapy in Neurologic Disease, 3rd ed. Philadelphia, BC Decker, 1990.
4. Leibel S: Radiation therapy for neoplasms of the brain. J Neurosurg 66:1, 1987.
5. Walker MD, Green SB, Byar DP, et al: Randomized comparison of radiation therapy and nitrosoureas for the treatment of malignant glioma of the brain. N Engl J Med 303:1323, 1980.
6. Kornblith PL, Walker M: Chemotherapy for malignant gliomas. J Neurosurg 68:1, 1988.
7. Gutin PH: Recurrent malignant gliomas: Survival following interstitial bradytherapy with high activity iodine 125 sources. J Neurosurg 67:864, 1987.
8. DeAngelis LM, Delatter J-Y, Posner JB: Radiation-induced dementia in patients cured of brain metastases. Neurology 39:789, 1989.
9. DiChiro G, Oldfield E, Wright DC, et al: Cerebral necrosis after radiotherapy and/or intraarterial chemotherapy for brain tumors: PET and neuropathologic studies. AJR Am J Roentgenol 150:189, 1988.
10. Imperato JP, Paleologos NA, Vick NA: Effects of treatment on long-term survivors with malignant astrocytoma. Ann Neurol 28:818, 1990.
11. Stewart DJ: Intraarterial chemotherapy of primary and metastatic brain tumors. *In* Rottenberg DA (ed): Neurological Complications of Cancer Treatment. Boston, Butterworth-Heinemann, 1991.
12. Laws ER, Taylor WF, Clifton MS, et al: Neurosurgical management of low grade astrocytomas of the cerebral hemispheres. J Neurosurg 61:665, 1984.
13. Alavi JB, Alavi A, Chawluk J, et al: Positron emission tomography in patients with glioma: A predictor of prognosis. Cancer 62:1074, 1988.
14. Francavilla TL, Miletich RS, DiChiro G, et al: Positron emission tomography in the detection of malignant degeneration of low grade gliomas. Neurosurgery 24:1, 1989.
15. Bullard DE, Rawlings CE, Phillips B, et al: Oligodendroglioma: An analysis of the value of radiation therapy. Cancer 60:2179, 1987.
16. Ludwig CL, Smith MT, Godfrey AD, et al: A clinicopathological study of 323 patients with oligodendrogliomas. Ann Neurol 19:15, 1986.
17. Finn JE, Mount LA: Meningiomas of the tuberculum sellae and platum sphenoidale. Arch Ophthalmol 92:23, 1974.
18. Wan WL, Geller JL, Feldon SE, et al: Visual loss caused by rapidly progressive meningiomas during pregnancy. Ophthalmology 97:18, 1990.
19. Kaiser-Kupfer MI, Freidlin V, Datiles MB, et al: The association of posterior lens opacities with bilateral acoustic neuromas in patients with neurofibromatosis type 2. Arch Ophthalmol 107:541, 1989.
20. Martuza RL, Eldridge R: Neurofibromatosis type 2. N Engl J Med 318:684, 1988.
21. Mulvihill J, Parry D, Sherman J, et al: Neurofibromatosis 1 (von Recklinghausen's disease) and neurofibromatosis 2 (bilateral acoustic neuromas): An update. Ann Intern Med 113:39, 1990.
22. Rosenberg LF, Miller NR: Visual results after microsurgical removal of meningiomas involving the anterior visual system. Arch Ophthalmol 102:1019, 1984.
23. Kupersmith MJ, Warren FA, Newall J, et al: Irradiation of meningiomas of the intracranial anterior visual pathway. Ann Neurol 21:131, 1987.
24. Smith JL, McCrary J, Ray BS, et al: Managing menacing meningiomas. J Clin Neuro Ophthalmol 3:169, 1983.
25. Hochberg FH, Miller DS: Primary central nervous system lymphoma. J Neurosurg 68:835, 1988.
26. DeAngelis LM, Yaholom J, Heinemann M-H: Primary CNS lymphoma: Combined treatment with chemotherapy and radiotherapy. Neurology 40:80, 1990.
27. Qualman SS, Mendelsohn G, Mann RB, et al: Intraocular lymphomas: Natural history based on a clinicopathologic study of eight cases and a review of the literature. Cancer 52:878, 1983.
28. Jennings MT, Gelman R, Hochberg F: Intracranial germ cell tumors: Natural history and pathogenesis. J Neurosurg 63:155, 1985.
29. Packer RJ, Sutton LN, Bilaniuk LT, et al: Treatment of chiasmatic/hypothalamic gliomas of childhood with chemotherapy: An update. Ann Neurol 23:79, 1988.
30. Packer RJ: Chemotherapy for medulloblastoma/primitive neuroectodermal tumors of the posterior fossa. Ann Neurol 28:823, 1990.
31. Packer RJ, Sutton LN, Atkins TA, et al: A prospective study of cognitive deficits in children receiving whole brain radiotherapy. J Neurosurg 70:707, 1989.
32. Kovacs K, Horvath E: Pathology of pituitary tumors. Endocrinol Metab Clin North Am 16:529, 1987.
33. Black PM, Hsu DW, Klibanski A, et al: Hormone production in clinically nonfunctioning pituitary adenomas. J Neurosurg 66:244, 1987.
34. Daneshdoost L, Gennarelli TA, Bashey HM, et al: Recognition of gonadrotroph adenomas in women. N Engl J Med 324:589, 1991.
35. Riskind PN, Richardson EP: Clinicopathologic Conference 3–1986. N Engl J Med 314:229, 1986.
36. Cardoso ER, Peterson EW: Pituitary apoplexy: A review. Neurosurgery 14:363, 1984.
37. Abboud CF, Laws ER: Diagnosis of pituitary tumors. Endocrinol Metab Clin North Am 17:241, 1988.
38. Zimmerman RA: Imaging of intrasellar, suprasellar, and parasellar tumors. Semin Roentgenol 25:174, 1990.
39. Stadnik T, Stenenaert A, Beckers A, et al: Pituitary microadenomas: Diagnosis with two- and three-dimensional MR imaging at 1.5T before and after injection of gadolinium. Radiology 176:419, 1990.
40. Reichlin S, Vonsattel J-P: A 30-year-old man with polydipsia, hypopituitarism, and a mediastinal mass. N Engl J Med 324:677, 1991.
41. Koppelman MCS, Jaffe MJ, Reith KG, et al: Hyperprolactinemia, amenorrhea, and galactorrhea: A retrospective assessment of twenty-five cases. Ann Intern Med 100:115, 1984.
42. Klibanski A, Zervas N: Diagnosis and management of hormone-secreting pituitary adenomas. N Engl J Med 324:822, 1991.
43. Cohen DL, Cooper PR, Kupersmith MJ, et al: Visual recovery after transsphenoidal removal of pituitary adenomas. Neurosurgery 17:446, 1985.
44. Ciric I, Mikhael M, Stafford T, et al: Transsphenoidal microsurgery of pituitary macroadenomas with longterm follow-up results. J Neurosurg 59:395, 1984.
45. Guidetti B, Fraioli B, Cantore GP: Results of surgical management of 319 pituitary adenomas. Acta Neurochir 85:117, 1987.
46. Rush S, Kupersmith MJ, Lerch I, et al: Neuroophthalmic assessment of radiotherapy alone for pituitary microadenomas: Identification of prognostic factors. J Neurosurg 72:594, 1990.
47. Murros KE, Toole JF: The effect of radiation on carotid arteries: A review article. Arch Neurol 46:449, 1989.
48. Werner MH, Buser PC, Heinz ER, et al: Intracranial atherosclerosis following radiotherapy. Neurology 38:1158, 1988.
49. Lessell S, Lessell IM, Rizzo JF: Ocular neuromyotonia after radiation therapy. Am J Ophthalmol 102:766, 1986.
50. Shults WT, Hoyt WF, Behrens M, et al: Ocular neuromyotonia: A clinical description of six patients. Arch Ophthalmol 104:1028, 1986.
51. Iacono RP, Apuzzo ML, Davis RL, et al: Multiple meningiomas following radiation therapy for medulloblastoma. J Neurosurg 55:282, 1981.
52. Capo H, Kupersmith MJ: Efficacy and complication of radiotherapy of anterior visual pathway tumors. Neurol Clin 9:179, 1991.
53. Hufnagel TJ, Kim JH, Lesser R, et al: Malignant glioma of the optic chiasm eight years after radiotherapy for prolactinoma. Arch Ophthalmol 106:1701, 1988.
54. Kaufman B, Tomsak RL, Kaufman BA, et al: Herniation of the suprasellar visual system and third ventricle into empty sella: Morphologic and clinical considerations. AJNR 10:65, 1989.
55. Molitch ME, Elton RL, Blackwell RE, et al: Bromocriptine as primary therapy for prolactin-secreting macroadenomas: Results of a prospective multicenter study. J Clin Endocrinol Metab 60:698, 1985.
56. Thorner MO, Perryman RL, Rogol AD, et al: Rapid changes in prolactinoma volume after withdrawal and reinstitution of bromocriptine. J Clin Endocrinol Metab 53:480, 1981.
57. Barakat S, Melmed S: Reversible shrinkage of a growth hormone-secreting pituitary adenoma by a long-acting somatostatin analogue octreotide. Arch Intern Med 149:1443, 1989.
58. Comi RJ, Gesundheit L, Murray P, et al: Response of thyrotropin-

secreting pituitary adenomas to a long-acting somatostatin analogue. N Engl J Med 317:12, 1987.
59. Guillausseau PJ, Chanso P, Timsit J, et al: Visual improvement with SMS 201–995 in a patient with a thyrotropin-secreting pituitary adenoma. N Engl J Med 317:53, 1987.
60. Jordan RM, Kohler PO: Recent advances in diagnosis and treatment of pituitary tumors. Adv Intern Med 32:299, 1987.
61. Kohler PO: Treatment of pituitary adenomas. N Engl J Med 317:45, 1987.
62. Petito CK, DeGirolami U, Earle KM: Craniopharyngiomas: A clinical and pathological review. Cancer 37:1944, 1976.
63. Carmel PW, Antunes JL, Chang CH: Craniopharyngiomas in children. Neurosurgery 11:382, 1982.
64. Volpe BT, Foley KM, Howiesen J: Normal CAT scans in craniopharyngioma. Ann Neurol 3:87, 1978.
65. Fischer EG, Welch K, Belli JA, et al: Treatment of craniopharyngiomas in children: 1972–1981. J Neurosurg 62:496, 1985.
66. Ron E, Modam B, Boice JD, et al: Tumors of the brain and nervous system after radiotherapy in childhood. N Engl J Med 319:1033, 1988.
67. Pollack IF, Lunsford LD, Stamovits TL, et al: Stereotaxic intracavitary irradiation for cystic craniopharyngiomas. J Neurosurg 68:227, 1988.
68. Moore CE, Hoyt WF, North JB: Painful ophthalmoplegia following treated squamous cell carcinoma of the forehead: Orbital apex involvement from centripetal spread via the supraorbital nerve. Med J Aust 1:657, 1976.
69. Dodd GD, Dolan PA, Ballantyne AJ, et al: The dissemination of tumors of the head and neck via the cranial nerves. Radiol Clin North Am 8:445, 1970.
70. Brazis PW, Vogler JB, Shaw KE: The "numb cheek–limp lower lid" syndrome. Neurology 41:327, 1991.
71. Cohen MM, Lessell S: Retraction of the lower eyelid. Neurology 29:386, 1979.
72. Bagan SM, Hollenhorst RW: Radiation retinopathy after irradiation of intracranial lesions. Am J Ophthalmol 88:694, 1979.
73. Brown GC, Shields JA, Sanborn G, et al: Radiation optic neuropathy. Ophthalmology 89:1489, 1982.
74. Brown GC, Shields JA, Sanborn G, et al: Radiation retinopathy. Ophthalmology 90:1494, 1982.
75. Macdonald DR, Rottenberg DA, Schutz JS, et al: Radiation induced optic neuropathy. *In* Rottenberg DA (ed): Neurological Complications of Cancer Treatment. Boston, Butterworth-Heinemann, 1991.
76. Ashford AR, Donev I, Tiwari RP, et al: Reversible ocular toxicity related to tamoxifen therapy. Cancer 61:33, 1988.
77. Grunwald GR, Kornguth SE, Towfighi J, et al: Autoimmune basis for visual paraneoplastic syndrome in patients with small cell lung cancer: Retinal immune deposits and ablation of retinal ganglion cells. Cancer 60:780, 1987.
78. Thirkill CE, Fitzgerald P, Sergott RC, et al: Cancer-associated retinopathy (CAR syndrome) with antibodies reacting with retinal optic nerve and cancer cells. N Engl J Med 321:1589, 1989.
79. Chauduri PR, Austin DJ, Rosenthal R: Treatment of radiation retinopathy. Br J Ophthalmol 65:623, 1981.
80. Guy J, Schatz NJ: Hyperbaric oxygen in the treatment of radiation-induced optic neuropathy. Ophthalmology 93:1083, 1986.
81. Chee PHY: Radiation retinopathy. Am J Ophthalmol 66:860, 1968.

Chapter 212

Multiple Sclerosis

MICHAEL WALL

Multiple sclerosis is an inflammatory demyelinating disorder of central nervous system (CNS) white matter. It is characterized by multiple lesions confined to the CNS separated in both time and space. In addition the patient's symptoms and signs cannot be more accurately attributed to another disease process.

Few disorders lead to as much diagnostic confusion, uncertainty, and patients' anxiety as multiple sclerosis. The reasons for this are that the disorder (1) has protean manifestations because any white matter tract of the nervous system can be affected and (2) no laboratory test can diagnose the disease unequivocally. The diagnosis is therefore based on a combination of the clinical presentation and the laboratory evaluation.

The common presenting symptoms seen by ophthalmologists are monocular visual loss often accompanied by pain on eye movements (optic neuritis), visual blurring or horizontal diplopia (internuclear ophthalmoplegia), and various ocular oscillations. Uncommon presentations are visual loss attributable to chiasmal or retrochiasmal field defects, gaze palsies and third, fourth, and sixth cranial nerve palsies.

EPIDEMIOLOGY

The prevalence of multiple sclerosis varies with ethnic origin and latitude.[1] The prevalence is significantly greater in northern latitudes. This observation holds worldwide and is illustrated for the continental United States in Figure 212–1. Studies of migration patterns show that patients carry the risk imposed by the geographic location of the first 15 yr of life. A slightly increased risk is also noted among first-degree relatives. Also, the concordance of about 25 percent in monozygotic twins is higher than in dizygotic twins. Further support for a genetic basis comes from studies showing an association of specific HLA haplotypes in patients with multiple sclerosis.

Well-documented studies of changing prevalence in different regions suggest a causative environmental factor. For example, the incidence in the Faroe Islands increased dramatically coincident with the World War II arrival of British troops. Other regional clusters have been reported. Although many innovative models of

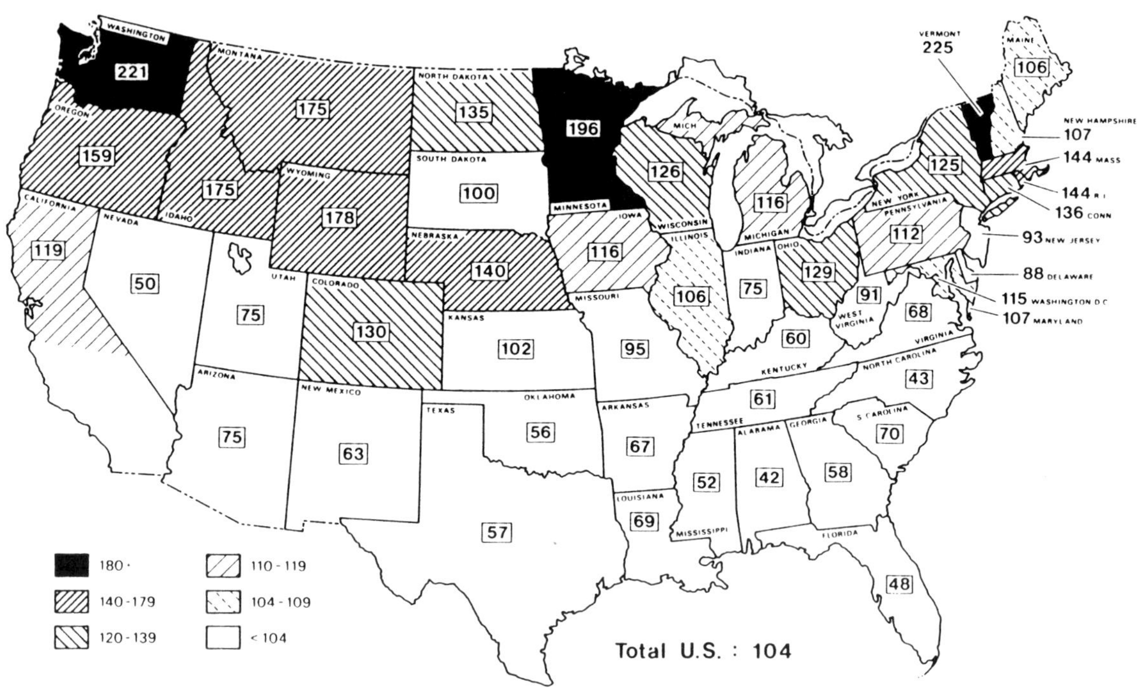

Figure 212–1. Geographic distribution of multiple sclerosis in United States veterans (case: control ratios × 100). (From Acheson ED: The pattern of the disease. *In* Matthews WB [ed]: McAlpine's Multiple Sclerosis, 4th ed. New York, Churchill Livingstone, 1985.)

viral transmission have been proposed, none have been proved.

PATHOLOGY

The characteristic plaque of multiple sclerosis is a sharply demarcated grayish-yellow lesion. About 90 percent of the plaques are located in the periventricular white matter. They are asymmetrically distributed in optic nerves and also appear in the optic chiasm and optic tract. Cerebellar and spinal cord white matter are other common locations.

Light microscopic study of acute lesions shows perivascular inflammation of venules (Fig. 212–2); the inflammatory response consists predominantly of activated T lymphocytes and macrophages. The resulting loss of myelin sheaths is assumed to be central to the pathophysiology of the disease. Interestingly, apparent demyelinating activity, whether it is found on neuroimaging procedures or at autopsy, may be asymptomatic. Remyelination follows demyelination, with subtotal recovery of function; the recovery occasionally appears complete to patients.

IMMUNOPATHOGENESIS

It is currently thought that multiple sclerosis is a type of autoimmune disorder. Accompanying the T-lymphocytic and macrophage destruction of CNS white matter are secretions of interleukins, resulting in production of oligoclonal IgG by plasma cells. In addition, alterations in T-cell populations including loss of suppressor T-cell function have been found in the blood of patients with multiple sclerosis.[2] Biopsy of an active lesion shows phenotypic heterogeneity of T lymphocytes, suggesting in situ exposure to many differentiating stimuli.[3] A review of the proposed immune mechanism can be found in Weiner and Hafler's comprehensive article.[4]

SYMPTOMS AND SIGNS

To ophthalmologists, the most common presentation of multiple sclerosis is optic neuritis.[5] This inflammatory disorder of the optic nerve causes progressive monocular visual loss occurring over 1 to 3 wk.[6] A central scotoma is usually found on kinetic perimetry, and various nerve fiber bundle defects or generalized depression of the visual field with automated static perimetry is noted. Snellen's acuity loss accompanies the clinical presentation, but acuity is seldom worse than 20/200. Pain is associated with movement of the involved eye in more than 90 percent of cases. Untreated, patients stabilize for 1 to 2 wk and then gradually recover over months, often with a return to normal or nearly normal Snellen's acuity. However, dyschromatopsia and contrast sensitivity loss with accompanying deficits on automated static perimetry better delineate a patient's incomplete recovery.[7] The optic disc may initially be edematous (about one fourth of the time) or normal. Optic disc pallor is

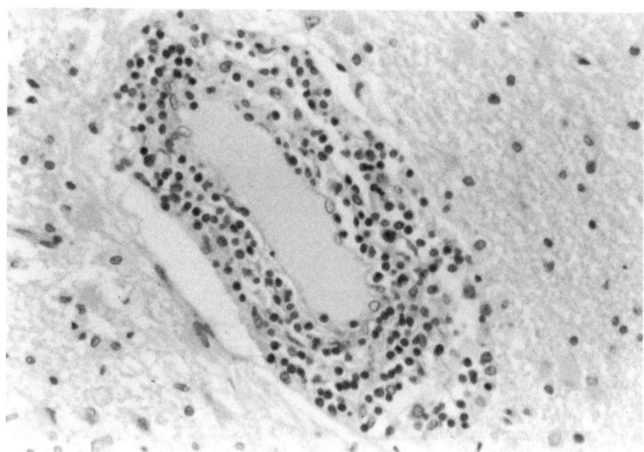

Figure 212–2. A characteristic multiple sclerosis lesion shown by light microscopy. Note the perivenular location of the inflammatory infiltrate.

a common sequel, as is the presence of a relative afferent pupillary defect even when visual acuity is normal. (See Chapter 201 for a more detailed discussion of optic neuritis.)

Because the pathologic lesion of multiple sclerosis is often a periventricular white matter plaque and the medial longitudinal fasciculus is a long white matter bundle located next to the ventricular system, internuclear ophthalmoplegia is a common presentation of the disorder. Internuclear ophthalmoplegia in a person younger than 50 yr is usually due to multiple sclerosis. The characteristic adduction deficit with nystagmus in the abducting eye is a dramatic clinical presentation. Convergence movements are characteristically normal. Skew deviation or gaze-evoked upbeating nystagmus may accompany the internuclear ophthalmoplegia. A "subclinical" form can be detected by having patients make large-amplitude horizontal saccades and observing lag of adduction on the involved side. This sign is especially useful to search for evidence of a second lesion in patients with optic neuritis.

A related disorder, the one-and-a-half syndrome, is characterized by a gaze palsy when looking toward the side of the lesion, with internuclear ophthalmoplegia on looking away from the lesion.[8] Associated findings are skew deviation and gaze-evoked nystagmus on upgaze or lateral gaze and less commonly on downgaze. Acutely, in the primary position, exotropia may be noted. Patients may also show limitation of upgaze, saccadic vertical pursuit, and loss of convergence. The location of the responsible lesion is the paramedian pontine reticular formation or sixth-nerve nucleus. The lesion extends to involve the internuclear fibers destined for the medial longitudinal fasciculus crossing from the contralateral sixth-nerve nucleus. In patients younger than 50 yr, this disorder, like internuclear ophthalmoplegia, is usually due to multiple sclerosis.

Many other types of ocular oscillations occur in multiple sclerosis. Primary position and gaze-evoked horizontal and vertical nystagmus signify posterior fossa demyelination. Various oscillations of cerebellar origin occur, including ocular dysmetria, rebound nystagmus, ocular flutter, ocular myoclonus, and opsoclonus. Failure to suppress the vestibuloocular reflex, tested by having patients fix on their thumb while the examining chair is rotated back and forth, is manifested by slippage of fixation in the direction opposite to the rotation; it occurs in 75 percent of tested patients with definite multiple sclerosis.[9] Patients with failure to suppress the vestibuloocular reflex report difficulty resolving images when their head is moving (e.g., reading road signs while in a moving car).

Evidence of bitemporal hemianopia and homonymous hemianopia[10, 11] is notably uncommon, even though plaques are common in the related sensory visual system structures. Cortical blindness or homonymous hemianopia due to the rare Schilder's disease probably represents a form of multiple sclerosis.[10] Third, fourth, and sixth cranial nerve palsies are also uncommon manifestations of demyelination. Retinal perivenous sheathing is sometimes present in multiple sclerosis; its pathogenesis is uncertain.[13]

The nonvisual symptoms and signs are best remembered by the predilection of multiple sclerosis for the major white matter bundles of the nervous system. Consequently, weakness from corticospinal tract disease, incoordination with cerebellar pathway lesions, and sensory disturbances with spinothalamic and posterior column system involvement are hallmarks of the disease. A clue to the diagnosis can be elicited by asking patients if they experience shocklike sensations down the spine, radiating into the extremities with neck flexion (Lhermitte's symptom). Unfortunately, this dramatic symptom may occur with any lesion of the posterior columns.

A common feature of symptoms of multiple sclerosis is that they may only become present or may worsen with elevated body temperature (Uhthoff's symptom). This may occur with the normal diurnal variation (Fig. 212–3),[14] exercise, a hot bath, or a febrile illness. Although multiple sclerosis is the disease in which patients most commonly report heat sensitivity, it occurs in other neurologic disorders.[15]

DIAGNOSTIC CRITERIA

Various diagnostic criteria have been proposed. These are most useful in research protocols because they rely heavily on abnormal laboratory findings. The most helpful clinical criteria are those developed by Schumacher (Table 212–1). In short, the diagnosis is established only when patients have two or more lesions of the nervous system in separate locations, when the lesions have occurred at different times and no other cause can be found. Therefore, a diagnosis of multiple sclerosis cannot be made after an episode of isolated optic neuritis regardless of the laboratory findings.

Erroneous diagnosis of multiple sclerosis is a major problem. Frequency of misdiagnosis, even in multiple sclerosis specialty clinics, has been estimated to be as high as 10 percent. Therefore, when a patient is first evaluated for multiple sclerosis, the diagnosis should be

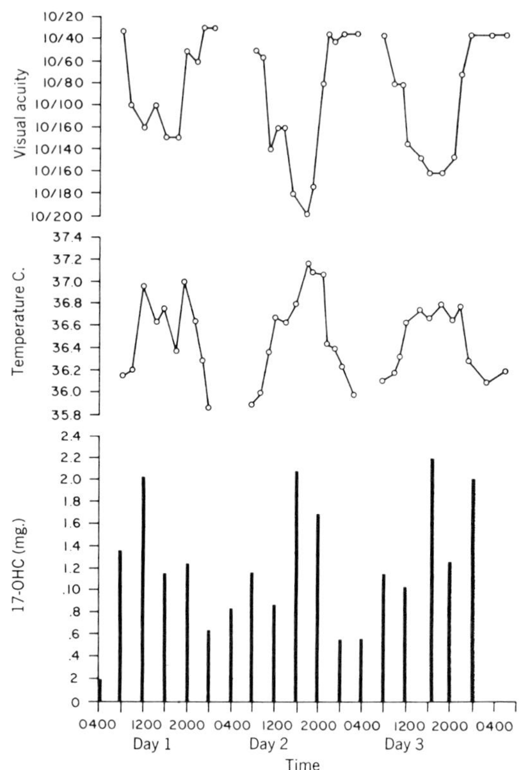

Figure 212–3. Visual acuity and oral temperature on consecutive days. Note the inverse relationship between acuity and temperature. (From Namerow NS: Circadian temperature rhythm and vision in multiple sclerosis. Neurology 18:417, 1968.)

questioned and care taken to ensure that Schumacher's criteria are fulfilled. Rudick and colleagues reviewed cases of misdiagnosis and identified five factors that are clues to misdiagnosis (Table 212–2).[16] Of note is the first feature listed—it is rare to have definite multiple sclerosis without visual system symptoms and signs.

DIFFERENTIAL DIAGNOSIS

The differential diagnosis consists mainly of disorders that subacutely affect multiple areas of the nervous system and can exacerbate and remit. Lupus erythematosus, sarcoidosis, polyarteritis, Behçet's disease, and

Table 212–1. SCHUMACHER'S CRITERIA FOR CLINICALLY DEFINITE MULTIPLE SCLEROSIS

Neurologic examination reveals objective abnormalities of central nervous system (CNS) function.
Analysis of history suggests involvement of two or more parts of the CNS.
CNS disease predominantly reflects white matter involvement.
Involvement of the CNS follows one of two patterns:
Two or more episodes, each lasting at least 24 hr and greater than 1 mo apart.
Slow or stepwise progression of signs and symptoms over at least 6 mo.
Age 10–50 yr at onset.
Signs and symptoms cannot be more accurately attributed to other disease processes.

Table 212–2. FEATURES CASTING DOUBT ON THE DIAGNOSIS OF MULTIPLE SCLEROSIS

Absence of eye findings
Optic nerve involvement
Oculomotor abnormalities
Absence of a clinical remission
Clinical presentation explained by a lesion in one location
Atypical clinical features
Absence of sensory findings
Absence of bladder involvement
Absence of cerebrospinal fluid abnormalities

syphilis are notable for this type of behavior.[1] Localization of the lesion to one site in the nervous system helps delineate disorders such as arteriovenous malformations and low-grade gliomas that can mimic a presentation of multiple sclerosis, especially the spinal progressive form. Another impersonator is Arnold-Chiari malformation accompanied by syringomyelia.

CLINICAL COURSE

Multiple sclerosis has an interesting natural history. Cases identified post mortem without apparent symptoms and signs during life have been documented, the so-called subclinical form.[17] About one third of patients have a benign form of the disease. Their disability throughout life is usually mild, except during exacerbations. A more severe form, characterized by moderate disability, allows most patients to continue a productive life. About one third of patients have a severe form and may become wheelchair bound or bedridden. The estimated 25-yr survival is 80 percent.[18]

Although patients characteristically have exacerbations and remissions, a chronic progressive form usually affects the spinal cord. Some researchers hypothesize an analog in the optic nerve (chronic progressive optic neuritis). Investigations, however, usually reveal another cause of this clinical presentation. Chronic progressive optic neuritis should only be diagnosed in the clinical setting of definite multiple sclerosis.

Isolated demyelination of the nervous system can occur—for example, idiopathic optic neuritis. However, optic neuritis is most commonly a harbinger of multiple sclerosis. Based on a life table analysis, Rizzo and Lessell in a New England population calculated that 74 percent of women and 34 percent of men with optic neuritis will develop multiple sclerosis within 15 yr.[19]

With the development of magnetic resonance imaging (MRI), serial studies of patients with definite multiple sclerosis show areas of apparent demyelinating activity that develop and resolve.[20] These transient abnormalities may or may not be accompanied by clinical symptoms or signs.

LABORATORY FINDINGS

Because no specific test is diagnostic for multiple sclerosis alone or in combination, many laboratory parameters are integrated with the clinical presentation to establish the diagnosis. Besides giving clues to the pathogenesis of the disease, the cerebrospinal fluid offers important diagnostic data and may suggest alternative diagnoses.

Cerebrospinal Fluid

Most patients with multiple sclerosis have normal spinal fluid cell counts (five or fewer lymphocytes). Less than 1 percent of patients have a white blood cell count greater than 25 per cubic millimeter, and all these are usually mononuclear cells.[1]

It has been known for many years that cerebrospinal fluid protein is usually elevated in multiple sclerosis. If the level is greater than 100 mg/dl, other diagnoses should be considered.

When the protein is fractionated, gamma globulin level is often elevated; more useful is the immunoglobulin electrophoretic pattern. The presence of oligoclonal bands in the gamma globulin region is more specific than either the total protein or the IgG level. This banding pattern is found in more than 90 percent of patients with clinically definite multiple sclerosis; however, it is also found in other CNS inflammatory and infectious disorders such as neurosyphilis and meningitis.[21]

Other protein indices that are commonly abnormal in multiple sclerosis are the IgG index (the ratio of IgG to albumin), the ratio of CSF IgG to serum IgG, and the IgG synthesis rate. The presence of myelin basic protein was initially thought to be a specific marker of multiple sclerosis; although it may be an antigenic stimulus in multiple sclerosis, it is found in other disorders that destroy myelin.

Evoked Potentials

An evoked potential (evoked response) is an electrical event in response to a nervous system stimulus. For example, strobe flash stimulation during an electroencephalogram (EEG) elicits a large potential. To improve definition of this potential, voltage averaging by a computer is used. The computer begins collecting data when a patient is stimulated (e.g., one shift of the checkerboard pattern) and records the voltages for 250 to 500 msec. Most stimuli produce small voltages that are hidden in the rhythms and noise of the EEG. Consequently, averaging of many potentials is necessary.

Although the strobe flash visual evoked response requires no cooperation by patients other than limited movement, it has little diagnostic utility because of its high variability—even between eyes of the same patient. Unfortunately, the pattern shift visual evoked response requires that patients focus and attend to the stimulus. The usual target is a checkerboard that remains isoluminant, with black squares alternating with white ones. In cooperative patients, it is a sensitive test of optic nerve demyelination, past or present. Because patients can focus in front of the stimulus monitor, causing a flat-line response, they should be required to count the pattern reversals accurately. Other evoked responses that show delay owing to demyelination are the clicks used for auditory brain stem evoked responses and the mild shocks used for somatosensory evoked responses. In clinically definite multiple sclerosis, at least one of the three evoked responses is abnormal more than 90 percent of the time.

Neuroimaging

Computed tomography (CT) has been used for many years in the assessment of multiple sclerosis; however, it is relatively insensitive. A more sensitive technique is MRI. The abnormalities due to multiple sclerosis are best seen on the T_2-weighted images. The lesions are irregular confluent areas of high signal intensity, usually in the periventricular white matter (Fig. 212–4).

The pathogenesis of the high signal intensity lesions is yet undetermined and reflects changes in water content that may or may not denote demyelination. Longitudinal studies have shown frequent occurrence of high signal intensity lesions developing and resolving without producing symptoms or signs.[20] The lesions of

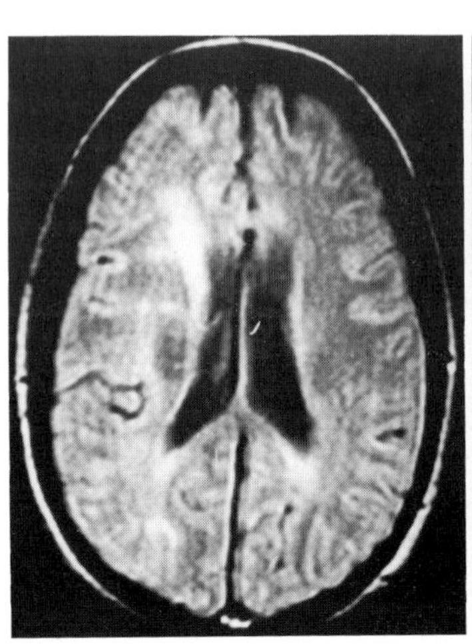

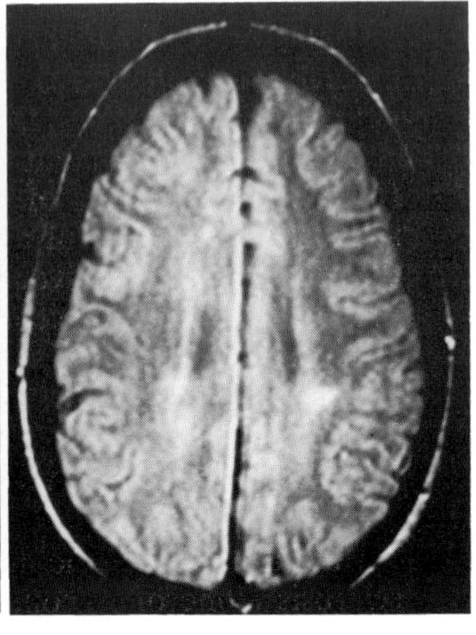

Figure 212–4. Characteristic example of T_2-weighted magnetic resonance images in a patient with definite multiple sclerosis. Note the numerous high-intensity signal white matter lesions in a periventricular location.

multiple sclerosis on MRI reach maximal size at about 4 wk and then gradually shrink, leaving a residual abnormality thought to be plaque. A biopsy specimen of one of these high signal intensity lesions showed histologic demyelination.[3]

Plaques in optic nerve can be demonstrated, but special techniques, such as those using fat suppression, are usually necessary, along with special surface coils. Patients with definite multiple sclerosis have abnormal MRI scans more than 90 percent of the time. The major disadvantage of MRI is that it is not specific. High-intensity signals in white matter are commonly seen in asymptomatic patients, especially those that have multiple risk factors for stroke. They are more likely to be due to multiple sclerosis if they (1) are greater than 6 mm in diameter, (2) are next to the ventricular system, (3) are infratentorial in location,[22] and enhance with gadolinium.

TREATMENT

Volumes of reports proclaim treatment efficacy in multiple sclerosis. Nearly all claiming effectiveness are flawed by their study design—usually lack of an adequate control group. A control group is especially important in treatment trials of multiple sclerosis, because with remyelination, patients improve without any therapy. Several controlled studies show promise for effective medical intervention. Treatment can be divided into symptomatic and immunologic types.

Symptomatic Treatment

Symptomatic treatment begins with education of patients. Patients should understand the natural history of multiple sclerosis. Anxiety may be alleviated when patients realize they may have a "benign form" of the disease. The National Multiple Sclerosis Society is an excellent source for current information. Patients should be warned that symptoms are usually temporarily worsened by heat. For example, taking a hot bath or shower, exercising, or even smoking a cigarette can induce enough elevation in temperature in the region of the optic nerve to cause blurring of vision. Visual function may improve if the patient keeps body temperature low by staying in a cool or cold environment. The reason for this is neural transmission is more efficient with cold temperatures.

Patients with optic neuritis may be helped by two other strategies. Patients may complain of visual distortions as objects approach them, such as misperceived veering of oncoming tennis balls, owing to delayed conduction through one optic nerve. These patients can be fitted with a neutral-density contact lens over the unaffected eye to alleviate this type of distortion. Some patients with the optic neuropathy of multiple sclerosis see better in dim light than bright light. This may be because of cross talk between neurons that have damaged myelin. Tinting of patient's spectacles may improve vision.

Patients with nystagmus may complain of blurring or oscillopsia. Pharmacotherapy, most notably clonazepam (Clonopin), can improve visual acuity in selected cases.[23, 24]

Potassium channel blockers to improve conduction in damaged nerve are under investigation. Both 4-aminopyridine[25] and digoxin[26] reportedly improve symptoms and conduction (lessen the delay on a visual evoked response). They appear to work best in patients with temperature-sensitive symptoms.

Immunologic Treatment

Immunologic therapy for multiple sclerosis has been the subject of intensive study.[4] Nonspecific types of immunosuppression therapy such as cyclophosphamide, azothiaprine, antilymphocyte globulin, plasma exchange lymphocytopheresis, thoracic duct drainage, and total lymphoid irradiation have been reported to be effective in altering the course of multiple sclerosis. The effects, however, have not been dramatic.

Specific types of immunotherapy are being developed.[4] Because evidence suggests loss of suppressor T-cell function,[2] methods to increase suppression are currently being investigated. Total lymphoid irradiation, besides its nonspecific effects, may decrease the number and function of helper T cells and stimulate suppressor cells. Both the cells triggering the immune response (the inducer T cells) and activated T cells are being attacked by creating monoclonal antibodies to destroy them. In fact, treatment of experimental allergic encephalomyelitis (the laboratory model for multiple sclerosis) with monoclonal antibodies directed toward activated T cells has been successful.[28]

Cyclosporine may prevent the production of interleukin-2, necessary for T-cell proliferation. Results of studies of this use for cyclosporine have not been impressive. Interferon has been used in clinical trials because it is immunoregulatory and antiviral (an unproven hypothesis for the cause of multiple sclerosis is a persistent viral infection). Preliminary studies are inconclusive. Interestingly, use of gamma interferon resulted in an increase in exacerbations in some patients.

Enthusiasm has been expressed for copolymer I, a peptide effective in treatment of experimental allergic encephalomyelitis. It was developed as an analog of myelin basic protein, and a double-blind study showed that patients with early-relapsing remitting disease had fewer exacerbations.[29] Confirmation awaits a large multicenter trial.

Many studies have used corticosteroids and adrenocorticotropic hormone to treat multiple sclerosis. No conclusive evidence shows that they change outcome, but they do shorten the course of an exacerbation.[30] Their utility is therefore in selected patients. For example, a patient who is blind in one eye from optic neuritis and who develops optic neuritis in the contralateral eye could be treated with corticosteroids to shorten the course of the disability. There is evidence that IV methylprednisolone is superior to oral corticosteroids (see Chap. 201).

When ophthalmologists diagnose optic neuritis, they usually face a dilemma in the approach to the patient. Because telling patients that they may have multiple sclerosis is so anxiety provoking, it is best to set aside some time (15 to 30 min) to discuss the disease. Most ophthalmologists do not have the background, knowledge, or experience to educate their patients fully about this disease. In this instance, it is advisable to tell patients they have "inflammation of the optic nerve." Referral to a neurologist for a complete discussion of multiple sclerosis is usually wise.

With improvements in technology, we are learning more about multiple sclerosis each year. Diagnostic techniques have improved, and many promising treatment strategies are currently under investigation. It is hoped that an effective treatment for this disease will be discovered in the near future.

REFERENCES

1. Acheson ED: The pattern of the disease. *In* Matthews WB (ed): McAlpine's Multiple Sclerosis, 4th ed. New York, Churchill Livingstone, 1985.
2. Reinherz EL, Weiner HL, Hauser SL, et al: Loss of suppressor T cells in active multiple sclerosis: Analysis with monoclonal antibodies. N Engl J Med 303:125, 1980.
3. Estes ML, Rudick RA, Barnett GH, et al: Stereotactic biopsy of an active multiple sclerosis lesion. Arch Neurol 47:1299, 1990.
4. Weiner HL, Hafler DA: Immunotherapy of multiple sclerosis. Ann Neurol 23:211, 1988.
5. Hess RF, Plant GT: Optic Neuritis. Cambridge, Cambridge University Press, 1986.
6. Bradley WG, Whitty CMW: Acute optic neuritis: Its clinical features and their relation to prognosis for recovery of vision. J Neurol Neurosurg Psychiatry 30:531, 1967.
7. Wall M: Loss of P retinal ganglion cell function in resolved optic neuritis. Neurology 40:649, 1990.
8. Wall M, Wray SH: The one and one-half syndrome—A unilateral disorder of the pontine tegmentum: A study of 20 cases and review of the literature. Neurology 33:971, 1983.
9. Sharpe JA, Goldberg HJ, Lo AW, et al: Visual-vestibular interaction in multiple sclerosis. Neurology 31:427, 1981.
10. Rosenblatt MA, Behrens MM, Zweifach PH, et al: Magnetic resonance imaging of optic tract involvement in multiple sclerosis. Am J Ophthalmol 104:74, 1987.
11. Beck RW, Savino PJ, Schatz NJ, et al: Plaque causing homonymous hemianopsia in multiple sclerosis identified by computed tomography. Am J Ophthalmol 94:229, 1982.
12. Sedwick LA, Klingele TG, Burde RM, et al: Schilder's (1912) disease: Total cerebral blindness due to acute demyelination. Arch Neurol 43:85, 1986.
13. Lightman S, McDonald WI, Bird AC, et al: Retinal venous sheathing in optic neuritis: Its significance for the pathogenesis of multiple sclerosis. Brain 110:405, 1987.
14. Namerow NS: Circadian temperature rhythm and vision in multiple sclerosis. Neurology 18:417, 1968.
15. Nelson DA, Jeffreys WH, McDowell F: Effects of induced hypothermia on some neurological diseases. Arch Neurol Psychiatry 79:31, 1958.
16. Rudick RA, Schiffer RB, Schwetz KM, et al: Multiple sclerosis: The problem of incorrect diagnosis. Arch Neurol 43:578, 1986.
17. Phadke JG, Best PV: Atypical and clinically silent multiple sclerosis: A report of 12 cases discovered unexpectedly at necropsy. J Neurol Neurosurg Psychiatry 46:414, 1983.
18. Wynn DR, Rodriguez M, O'Fallon WM, et al: A reappraisal of the epidemiology of multiple sclerosis in Olmsted County, Minnesota. Neurology 40:780, 1990.
19. Rizzo JF, Lessell S: Risk of developing multiple sclerosis after uncomplicated optic neuritis: A long-term prospective study. Neurology 38:185, 1988.
20. Willoughby EW, Grochowski E, Li DKB, et al: Serial magnetic resonance scanning in multiple sclerosis: A second prospective study in relapsing patients. Ann Neurol 25:43, 1989.
21. McLean BN, Luxton RW, Thompson EJ: A study of immunoglobulin G in the cerebrospinal fluid of 1007 patients with suspected neurological disease using isoelectric focusing and the log IgG-index: A comparison and diagnostic applications. Brain 113:1269, 1990.
22. Fazekas F, Offenbacher H, Fuchs S, et al: Criteria for an increased specificity of MRI interpretation in elderly subjects with suspected multiple sclerosis. Neurology 38:1822, 1988.
23. Currie JN, Matsuo V: The use of clonazepam in the treatment of nystagmus-induced oscillopsia. Ophthalmology 93:924, 1986.
24. Carlow TJ: Medical treatment of nystagmus and ocular motor disorders. Int Ophthalmol Clin 26:251, 1986.
25. Davis FA, Stefoski D, Rush J: Orally administered 4-aminopyridine improves clinical signs in multiple sclerosis. Ann Neurol 27:186, 1990.
26. Kaji R, Happel L, Sumner AJ: Effect of digitalis on clinical symptoms and conduction variables in patients with multiple sclerosis. Ann Neurol 28:582, 1990.
27. Hauser SL, Dawson DM, Lehrich JR, et al: Intensive immunosuppression in progressive multiple sclerosis: A randomized, three-arm study of high-dose intravenous cyclophosphamide, plasma exchange, and ACTH. N Engl J Med 308:173, 1983.
28. Schluesener HJ: Inhibition of rat autoimmune T cell activation by monoclonal antibodies. J Neuroimmunol 11:261, 1986.
29. Bornstein MB, Miller A, Slagle S, et al: A pilot trial of COP I in exacerbating-remitting multiple sclerosis. N Engl J Med 317:408, 1987.
30. Rose AS, Kuzma JW, Kurtzke JF, et al: Cooperative study in the evaluation of therapy in multiple sclerosis: ACTH vs. placebo. Neurology 20:1, 1970.

Chapter 213

Migraine and Other Head Pains

JAMES R. COPPETO

Migraine is to medicine what the proverbial elephant was to the seven blind men. The neurologist, ophthalmologist, general practitioner, physiologist, psychiatrist, pediatrician, and radiologist all notice a different aspect of the beast. The beast is easily recognized by all these observers only when it breaks the silence with its unmistakable and unique "roar": a small semicircle of jagged shimmering lines of light appearing near fixation and then expanding slowly and moving peripherally. In the absence of that roar there is often doubt and confusion; hence, operational definitions are required.

This discussion of migraine and other headaches relies heavily on the "Classification and diagnostic criteria for headache disorders, cranial neuralgias and facial pains" formulated by the Headache Classification Committee of the International Headache Society.[1] Although the classification is tentative, it fills the need for sound operational definitions for this group of disorders of obscure pathophysiology.[2] This classification, importantly, also recognizes the occasional association of supposedly primary types of headache with structural brain lesions: A structural brain lesion may trigger various types of headaches from which a patient has previously suffered, and it can occasionally trigger the first occurrence of a headache that has typical characteristics of migraine or cluster headache.[3–5]

MIGRAINE

Although most chronic recurring headaches are benign, every headache should be viewed with concern and its etiology sought.[6, 7]

Ophthalmologists require a broad understanding of the many aspects of migraine in order to evaluate whether a patient's symptoms may be related to migraine.[7] Moreover, ophthalmologists have an ethical and social responsibility when referring a patient to a neurologist or internist for therapy, to suggest what further investigations, if any, the patient or the patient's insurance company should be expected to undertake.

The terms *common migraine* and *classic migraine* are discarded as useless because, aside from the aura in so-called classic migraine, the differences between these two entities are small.[8–17] The terms *migraine without aura* and *migraine with aura* are preferable.

A fully developed migraine attack can be divided into four (sometimes overlapping) phases, each of which may have ophthalmologic manifestations: (1) premonitory symptoms (hours to days before a migraine attack), which may include heightened perceptions of taste and smell, arousal, exhilaration, sleep disorders, hypoactivity, abdominal discomfort, depression, craving for special foods, dulled mentation, yawning, and syncope; (2) aura (may be absent), a complex of focal neurologic symptoms immediately preceding and sometimes also accompanying the headache; (3) headache; and (4) postheadache alteration of mood or mentation, including drowsiness, lethargy, diuresis, or epiphora.[11, 18, 19]

Migraine Without Aura

Migraine without aura is diagnosed when at least five attacks of an idiopathic headache lasting 4 to 72 hr (not treated or unsuccessfully treated) have occurred. At least two of the four following characteristics must be present: unilaterality (at least at the onset), pulsation, moderate to severe intensity, and aggravation by routine physical activity. It must also be associated with nausea or photophobia and phonophobia.[1] In addition, at least one of the following is true: (1) History, physical examination, and neurologic examination do not suggest an underlying structural or toxic cause, or (2) if a cause is suggested, appropriate investigations exclude it, or (3) if such a disorder is present, it postdates the onset of the headache disorder. The headache attacks often alternate sides. Headache invariably on one side argues against migraine but does not rule it out.[11, 20] After the headaches starts, it may become nonpulsatile and diffuse. Migraine can begin at any age, and there is no specific migraine personality.[11]

Menstrual migraine is diagnosed when 90 percent of such attacks occur between 2 days before and the last day of the menses.

Migraine With Aura

Migraine with aura is defined in the same manner as migraine without aura, except in addition, a patient has had at least two attacks, each of which has at least three of the four following characteristics:

1. One or more fully reversible neurologic symptoms denoting focal cerebral cortical or brain stem dysfunction
2. At least one neurologic symptom that evolves gradually over more than 4 min or two or more different symptoms that occur in succession
3. No single neurologic symptom that lasts more than 60 min
4. Headache within 60 min of the onset of the aura or preceding the aura. Headache may be completely absent.

Most auras have a binocular visual component but often are also attended by coexisting symptoms in the extremities. The few patients who have suffered prominent extremity pareses or paresthesias with their auras virtually always have had visual auras as well. Therefore, a distinction between so-called ophthalmic and hemiparesthetic/hemiparetic migraine is useless, and these terms should be discarded.

Migraine probably can induce unpredictible vasospasm of the coronary arteries (Prinzmetal's variant angina), and an ophthalmologist's diagnosis of migraine may aid a cardiologist in his or her evaluation.[16, 21, 22]

Five general categories of auras have been described.[11] The first category includes primary visual, tactile (often beginning bilaterally), or other sensory disturbances (music, deafness, nausea, smell, taste, abdominal pain, vertigo, illusion of limb movement). Even though these are considered more or less specific sensory disturbances, patients often find these very difficult to describe because they are sometimes distorted beyond any familiar perceptions. Visual distortions may be misinterpreted as hallucinations of animals; elementary figures may transform into large patterns; emotional components may be unpredictably added to these perceptions—patients may develop a horror of annihilation in which they lose their sense of reality and identity and feel as if they are being swallowed by their scotoma.

The second type of aura is an alteration in the sensory threshold and excitability, such as the illusion of echos or heightened tactile sensations during the aura. The third type of aura includes alterations in level of consciousness and postural tone, which may begin with a heightened sense of awareness and arousal but may terminate in specific motor disturbances such as paralysis, twitch, or chorea. The fourth type of aura may be an alteration in mood, such as mortal fear, rapture, or time disorientation. The fifth type of aura consists of specific disturbances of higher cognitive functioning (described later).[11, 23, 24]

As discussed later, about 15 percent of attacks in patients with migraine with aura lack the headache. Probably less than 1 percent of the population experiences migraine aura without ever having headache.[11]

Visual auras usually occur before the headache but may occur during or after it. They may be as brief as 10 sec, although this is unusual.[25]

If a migraine aura persists during or after a headache, it is generally associated with basilar migraine stupor, periodic confusional states of childhood, or familial hemiplegic migraine (discussed later). The neurologic symptoms occasionally develop or intensify as the headache intensifies (interposed migraine).

The most common visual symptom of migraine is the fortification spectrum (teichopsia). Some alteration of perception (smudginess or focal dimness) typically heralds the teichopsia. A patient then sees a star-shaped figure paracentrally; it gradually spreads peripherally and assumes a concave, jagged scintillating edge that leaves a variable scotoma in its wake.[26] Scintillating scotomata can vary in location, shape, motion (rotation, oscillation, boiling), flicker, color, clarity (blurry, foggy), brightness, expansion, and migration.[27] In some cases, the scotoma crosses the vertical meridian, raising the possibility that it is originating in the retina. In this case, displacement of an eyeball with a finger may induce movement of the visual disturbance.

Other visual auras include simple or complex (visual associative) disturbances (Table 213–1). Facial and perioral edema or ecchymoses, analogous to migrainous nasal stuffiness due to engorged turbinates, may be a manifestation of an aura.[11, 40]

A subgroup, migraine with typical aura, is defined as fulfilling not just three but all four criteria listed earlier for migraine with aura. Visual auras are the most common. The auras next in frequency are unilateral paresthesias and numbness starting at any point on the body or face and spreading. Less common auras manifest as dysphasia and hemiparesis. When multiple sensory modalities are affected, the involvement occurs successively, not concurrently.

In migraine with prolonged aura, at least one aural symptom lasts more than 60 min and less than 8 days and neuroimaging studies are negative.

Migraine Aura Without Headache

Migraine aura without headache (acephalgic migraine) is identical to a migraine with an aura but without a headache. Patients with migraine with aura occasionally have the aura alone, especially as they age.[41] It is uncommon for patients, especially younger individuals, to experience typical aura without headache, but it is of no special significance because cases from migrainous families have the same prognosis for health as family members who do have headache after the aura.[41] When the first occurrence of a migraine aura is after 40 yr of age, a distinction from transient ischemic attacks may be difficult.[1] Although acephalgic auras are generally visual, they may also include cyclic vomiting and bilious attacks, abdominal pain (as an aura or instead of the headache), periodic diarrhea, periodic fever, periodic narcoleptic symptoms (including postprandial narcolepsy and hypnogogic hallucinations), and almost weekly mood changes.[11]

Characteristics that help to differentiate a migrainous scotoma without aura from scotomata or photopsias arising from other causes are the exclusive tendency of some migrainous scintillating scotomata to build up in size and migrate across the visual field, a march of paresthesias along the extremities, progression of sen-

Table 213–1. VISUAL SYMPTOMS ASSOCIATED WITH MIGRAINE[11, 27–39]

Teichopsia (scintillating scotoma)	Alternating dark and light rings around objects in one field, with hemianopia in the opposite field
Micropsia	Rippling
Photopsia	Disturbances of body image
Teopsia	Balint's syndrome (including misjudgment of distances)
Monocular diplopia	Illusion of movement
Monocular polyopia	Bitemporal hemianopia (occasionally with polyuria and suggesting chiasmal hypothalamic dysfunction)
Corona around objects	Temporal crescent defects
Palinopsia	Change in perception of color
Dimness	Achromatopsia
Asthenopic scotoma (disappearance of objects in the visual field after a latent time)	Diplopia within a scintillating scotoma
Change in the rate of movement, including jerky movement (such as the movement in a strobe light)	Spinning of vision with vertigo
Illusion of movement or tilting	Prosopagnosia
Visual alloesthesia (displacement of an object in space)	Bilateral visual blurring
Cyclic visual changes (illusions that come and go regularly)	Alexia without agraphia
Scotomata of almost any kind, with or without scintillations	Vivid afterimages
Hallucinations, often of distorted images	Turbulent visual imagery

sory disturbance from one modality to another in succession, duration of 15 to 30 min, occurrence of similar episodes in the past, a history of similar spells associated with a subsequent headache, a benign course, and possibly a strong family history of migraine.[42] Taking a careful history, preferably at a time when the ophthalmologist is not deluged by a flood of postoperative follow-up cases, is extremely important. Ask patients to compose a letter telling their story and to mail it to you before the next appointment.

Although the previously listed clues suggest migraine, the presence of atypical or complex neurologic and neuroophthalmologic symptoms does not necessarily signify transient ischemia due to vertebral or basilar artery disease.[43] The neuroophthalmologic symptoms may still be due to migraine.[42, 43] For example, Fisher has described eight syndromes (with or without headache) that he considers migrainous when neurologic investigations are negative and follow-up demonstrates a benign course: (1) atypical luminous phenomena alone; (2) complex visual phenomena lasting 30 sec to 30 min and including transient bilateral blindness (which he believes is rarely a sign of basilar atherosclerotic transient ischemia); (3) visual phenomena with paresthesias lasting 5 to 30 min and sometimes with an interval of more than 24 hr between the visual symptoms and the paresthesias; (4) visual symptoms and speech disturbances; (5) visual symptoms and brain stem disturbances; (6) visual symptoms, paresthesias, and speech disturbances; (7) visual symptoms, paresthesias, speech disturbances, and pareses; and (8) recurrence of an old stroke deficit.[29, 42] Fisher believes—and most investigators concur—that a past personal and family history of migraine is uncommon and irrelevant in diagnosing such cases. What common pathophysiology, if any, these complex benign neurologic syndromes share with usual migraine with aura is unknown. Perhaps an interaction of migrainous and microembolic or rheologic factors (mismatch of cerebral blood flow and neuronal function) triggering retinal or cortical electrical disturbances is the common denominator.[17, 44, 45] Fisher would agree with Schatz that before considering diagnosing migraine, one should perform an intensive neurologic investigation.[43] In summary, acephalgic migraine occurring between ages 50 and 80 yr often lacks a past personal and family history of migraine and generally runs a benign course, even though monocular cases are associated with a higher incidence of clinically occult cardiovascular disease than are binocular cases.[46–48] A diagnosis of migraine without headache should be made only after an unfruitful neurologic investigation, although when migraine occurs in younger individuals, neurologic findings are almost always negative.[43] Transient monocular scotomata are discussed in greater detail later.

Migraine With Acute-Onset Aura

Migraine with acute-onset aura is distinctive because the aura fully develops in less than 4 min, thereby somewhat resembling thromboembolic disease. Thromboembolic disease and other intracranial lesions should be ruled out by appropriate investigations. The diagnosis of migraine is nonetheless supported by a past personal or family history of migraine with a typical aura. Many cases simply represent an inaccurately reported history in which a patient does not recall that the aura took longer than 4 min to develop.[1]

Ophthalmoparesis With Migraine, Including Ophthalmoplegic Migraine

Ophthalmoplegic migraine is exceedingly rare and consists of repeated attacks of headache associated with pareses of one or more ocular motor cranial nerves in the absence of a demonstrable intracranial (especially parasellar) lesion.[1, 49] It should be considered last in the differential diagnosis of painful or painless ophthalmoplegia. Whether ophthalmoplegic migraine has any important relationship to any other form of migraine is uncertain, because the headache often lasts 1 wk or more and usually precedes the ophthalmoplegia (which itself is often protracted, lasting weeks).[1] Some authors require that it be diagnosed only if it evolves out of the background of typical migraine headaches and occurs during the evolution of a typical migraine headache.[50] It may be related to Tolosa-Hunt syndrome (cavernous sinusitis with painful cranial polyneuropathy), and both may respond to steroids.[51, 52]

Structural lesions must always be ruled out by appropriate diagnostic tests. Failure to adhere to these criteria accounts for the wide discrepancy in reported incidence and manifestations of ophthalmoplegic migraine in the literature. Repeated attacks may cause progressive oculomotor dysfunction that becomes permanent. The third nerve is most frequently involved, and the pupil is generally not spared, leading many to speculate that some form of compression by dilated blood vessels is implicated in the cause of the disorder.[28, 50, 53–55] However, in some reported cases, the pupil was spared during recurrent attacks.[56, 57] Aberrant regeneration is distinctly uncommon.[27, 50, 55]

Anterior Visual System Migraine

Like some other researchers, I believe that anterior visual system migraine (ocular or retinal migraine) is so uncommon that ocular or structural vascular disease must be ruled out by appropriate investigations in every supposed case.[46] Other investigators find it to be less than rare.[58] For diagnosis, one must document at least two attacks, each consisting of (1) fully reversible monocular scotoma or blindness lasting less than 60 min and confirmed by examination during the attack or (after proper instruction) by the patient's drawing of a monocular field defect during an attack and (2) headache following visual symptoms with a free interval of less than 60 min but possibly preceding the visual symptoms.[1] Such strict criteria are important, because recurrent spontaneous hyphemas, psychiatric disease, and many other disorders may convincingly masquerade as anterior visual system migraine, especially in patients with a past history of typical migraine.[59] A past history of migraine is not required for the diagnosis of anterior visual system migraine. Response to antimigraine medications may be misleading in the diagnosis of anterior visual system migraine because such medications actually have multiple mechanisms and sites of action.[43, 60–64]

Patients with anterior visual system migraine may not have evidence of other forms of migraine.[58] Symptoms may be invariably transient or may result in ocular stroke.[64] The somewhat long duration of the transient visual loss contrasts with the brevity of typical atherothrombotic transient ocular phenomena. However, atherothrombotic disease may occasionally produce spells of transient visual loss lasting longer than the usual 30 to 90 sec and even as long as an hour, and it may also produce photisms.[46] Moreover, facial paresthesias and even pain may precede or accompany transient visual loss due to retinal or optic nerve ischemia of any cause, making the mere presence of pain around the eye of dubious diagnostic value.[46, 65, 66] Anterior visual system migraine is a diagnosis of exclusion and depends on a carefully taken history and a search for other causes.

Conclusions about the mechanism of ocular migraine depend disproportionately and perhaps unreasonably on cases that eventuate in an ocular stroke. Ischemic ocular stroke in young adults is associated with identifiable risk factors, whereas transient attacks of ocular migraine generally are not. When ocular migraine results in stroke, powerful risk factors are often present. One or more of the following can be noted: ischemic optic neuropathy, branch retinal artery occlusion, central retinal artery occlusion, cilioretinal artery occlusion, and retinal vein occlusion.[67–70] That such cases terminating in stroke indeed may not be representative of migraine's mechanism of ocular dysfunction (which may be neurochemical rather than ischemic) is suggested by the fact that cases concluding in stroke tend to be associated with diseases or anomalies that could strongly predispose to ischemia. In this regard, bilateral sequential anterior ischemic optic neuropathies have been described in a migraine sufferer with small optic discs.[71] In such cases, migraine may have been coincidental or even a secondary reaction. Ocular stroke in other patients with migraine may have been related to the ingestion of Migril tablets, concurrent ocular trauma, retinal vascular anomalies, coexisting systemic vasculopathy, postprandial hyperlipidemia, antiphospholipid antibodies, or blood dyscrasias.[72–74] Whether mitral valve prolapse is a contributing or aggravating factor in ocular migraine stroke is debated. In some cases, particularly severe retching at the time of the headache may have been related to the precipitation of permanent ocular stroke.[75]

Ocular strokes occurring in patients with a past history of some form of migraine yet unassociated with a previous history compatible with recurrent ocular migraine often have another explanation.[59, 76] Isolated transient monocular scotomata with or without scintillations or similar photopsias but without headache and without a past history of typical ocular migraine should be particularly suspected as a manifestation of atherosclerotic carotid artery disease, especially in older patients, even if the patient has a past history of another form of migraine.[46, 47, 77]

Recurrent episodes of monocular visual loss without serious systemic symptoms, with or without headache and with an apparently benign outcome, cannot be viewed as diagnostic of ocular migraine even in patients with past history of migraine.

Pediatric Periodic Syndrome That May Be Precursors to or Associated With Migraine

Although some headaches in children may be similar to migraine in adults, many are not.[78–80] Nonetheless, migraine probably represents one of the most common types of headache in children.[81, 82] Children may have headaches with unusual auras. Not only are migraine attacks in children often less full blown than in adults, but headaches may not be reported at all, especially by younger children, making diagnosis difficult.[78, 83] A carefully taken personal and family history is important.[79] Children may also exhibit a heterogeneous variety of headache-free periodic syndromes, marked by personality change, abdominal pain, cyclic vomiting, paroxysmal vertigo, and alternating hemiplegia. The relationship of these symptoms to migraine may not be suspected by a physician. Psychologic stress may be a trigger, producing confusion with tension headache. Migraine, inordinately in children, may produce (and occasionally present as) acute confusional states. These may be prolonged and are frequently associated with disturbed vision.[84]

Visual symptoms occur in 4 to 40 percent of children with migraine and may lead to visual stroke.[79, 85, 86] The visual symptoms may occur before, during, or after the headache. Children should be encouraged to draw what they see during their attacks. These pleomorphic visual symptoms have been divided into three types: (1) visual impairment and binocular scotomata, including total bilateral blindness, partial hemianopias with halos around figures, altitudinal field defects, quadrantic field defects, peripheral field defects that travel centrally, (2) brightly colored flashing spots that enlarge into rings, and (3) small white stars. These visual apparitions or deficits may be stationary but usually are motile. Visual distortions or hallucinations are particularly common in children and in some forms have been termed the *Alice in Wonderland* syndrome. These include metamorphopsia, micropsia, macropsia, diplopia, inversion, undulation, and complex formed silent visual hallucinations.[28, 79, 87] The visual symptoms are occasionally monocular and in such cases have been said to be similar to the episodes of binocular visual impairment and scotoma. Children may occasionally have the typical visual auras occurring in adults.

Attacks of basilar migraine appear to be particularly common in migrainous children and young adults and may account for various eye movement disorders, including transient esotropia, ptosis, nystagmus, gaze palsy, and brain stem ocular palsies.[88] Paresthesias, sensory deficits, dysphasia, or hemipareses (including alternating hemiplegia) in children may have a similar cause.[53, 88–93] Seizure and coma may also occur.[87] Stroke or psychomotor deterioration may be sequelae.[87, 92, 93] Progression to more typical migraine in adulthood is not the rule.[79, 88, 92]

Children and young adults with migraine seem to be particularly prone to prominent and even permanent neurologic symptoms after relatively mild head trauma.[87, 94–99] The neurologic symptoms often develop after a latent period of 30 min or more.[100] Electroencephalographic findings may be abnormal at that time.[100] Under such circumstances, reported cases have been marked by acute confusional migraine, bilateral third-nerve palsies and total blindness, transient global amnesia, coma, transient anisocoria and unilateral numbness, and ophthalmoplegia. On follow-up, some of these patients are found to have developed the same symptoms without head trauma. The mechanism may be vasospasm.[100–102]

Complications of Migraine

The complications of migraine include status migrainosus and migrainous infarction. Status migrainosus is a migraine attack with a headache lasting longer than 72 waking hours despite treatment. It is usually associated with chronic overmedication.[1, 32]

In migrainous infarction, one or more symptoms persist more than 7 days or are associated with neuroimaging confirmation of ischemic infarction in the relevant area. Other causes of infarction must be ruled out by appropriate investigations.[1, 17]

Ischemic stroke in a migraine sufferer is logically divided into three types: (1) stroke due to another cause in a patient with a past history of migraine, (2) stroke due to another cause with migraine-like symptoms, and (3) stroke during the course of a typical migraine attack. Only the last variety of stroke qualifies as migrainous infarction. This does not mean that migraine is a contributor to stroke only in such cases. Moreover, because a stroke may trigger a migraine, not all cases of migrainous infarction are truly caused by migraine.[103]

What is the significance of stroke in a migraine sufferer? Although a population of patients with migraine would be expected to show an increased incidence of stroke, the evidence is conflicting.[104] Population studies show no significantly increased incidence of stroke in migraine sufferers or of migraine in patients with stroke, suggesting that stroke must be a rare complication of migraine.[105] However, small series suggest that migraine may predispose a patient to stroke due to a second cause. No direct relationship has been proved between migraine without aura and cerebral infarction. In one study, however, young patients with occipital strokes almost exclusively suffered migraine without aura and without other risk factors.[106] In order to prove an increased risk of stroke in migraine, it would be important to document that in a group of occipital strokes in young adults, migraine is many times more common than in the general population. What studies are available suggest that occipital strokes in young adults are, indeed, excessively associated with migraine, angiographically appear to be embolic, and, inexplicably, often occur in migraine without aura.[4, 5, 106–108] Migraine rarely causes stroke in the absence of other risk factors; all patients with apparent migraine-related stroke need thorough but tailored investigations, usually including cerebral angiography and very careful and complete echocardiography (including Valsalva's maneuver).[5, 73, 90, 104, 105, 109–119]

TENSION-TYPE HEADACHE

Tension-type headache is defined as recurrent or chronic bilateral headache of mild to moderate intensity and having a pressing or tightening quality. It does not worsen with physical activity and is not attended by nausea. Phonophobia or photophobia may be present. It is a very prevalent form of headache but has no ophthalmic manifestations.[120–124]

CLUSTER HEADACHE AND CHRONIC PAROXYSMAL HEMICRANIA

Cluster headache is diagnosed if a patient has experienced at least five attacks of severe pain (at times excruciating) that is strictly unilateral; maximal orbitally, supraorbitally, or temporally; lasts 15 to 180 min; and is associated with any of the following: conjunctival injection, lacrimation, nasal congestion, rhinorrhea, forehead and facial sweating, miosis, ptosis due to postganglionic oculosympathetic paresis, or eyelid edema.[1] During a cluster, the attack frequency is from once every other day to eight times a day. These cases are not known to be associated with a toxic cause or structural intracranial lesion. Cluster headache may be episodic (clusters last 7 to 360 days and are separated by pain-free periods of 14 days or longer) or chronic (clusters last more than 1 yr without remission or with remissions lasting less than 2 wk). Chronic cluster headache may arise de novo (primary) or from episodic cluster headache (secondary). During cluster periods, the pain may be spontaneous or induced by alcohol, histamine, or nitroglycerin and related vasodilators. The pain may alternate sides but usually not within the same cluster period. The pain is not relieved by sleep as readily as in migraine. It afflicts men 5 to 6 times more often than women and begins between the ages of 20 and 40 yr.

Chronic paroxysmal hemicrania is a variety of primary or secondary chronic cluster headache that occurs predominately in women, but the attacks are more brief (2 to 45 min) and more frequent (5 to 30 attacks a day on more than half of the days that they occur). By definition, indomethacin (150 mg/day or less) produces complete prophylaxis.[1]

Recurrent brief visual loss and ischemic papillitis have been reported to accompany chronic cluster headache.[63, 125] These associations may have been coincidental.[126]

Nitroglycerin (or other nitrates) may aggravate or precipitate cluster headache, and methysergide (Sansert), lithium, or ergots may intensify chronic paroxysmal hemicrania.

Differential Diagnosis of Cluster Headache

Lesions of the oculosympathetic fibers at the cervical carotid artery or distal to it can produce a complete or partial Horner's syndrome, head pain (by involvement of adjacent pain-sensitive structures), and occasionally other neurologic symptoms due to damage to adjacent structures. When the lesion is distal to the bifurcation of the common carotid artery, the ipsilateral side of the face sweats almost normally because the fibers depart with the external carotid artery. Such syndromes may bear a superficial resemblance to cluster headache but tend to be single episodes of variably protracted periocular pain unassociated with temporal clustering and often accompanied by other symptoms. For example, spontaneous or traumatic dissecting aneurysms of the carotid artery may produce pain in the forehead and orbit (sometimes increased with exercise) and neck pain or tenderness.[127] Throat or ear pain may occur and may be steroid responsive.[127] Coexisting features may include partial Horner's syndrome, scalp tenderness, dysgeusia, bruit, monocular scintillations (due to embolization), or transient monocular blindness. These symptoms only rarely occur together when atherosclerosis of the carotid artery is the cause. Dissecting aneurysm of the carotid can occasionally lead to internal carotid dilatation at the base of the skull.

After the carotid bifurcation, postganglionic oculosympathetic fibers travel to the carotid siphon and then leave the carotid plexus, travel briefly with the abducens nerve, and eventually enter the orbit with the ophthalmic division of the trigeminal nerve. Lesions along this route may produce postganglionic painless or painful Horner's syndrome, with the preservation of most facial sweating, but often with symptoms due to dysfunction of adjacent structures.[128–130] Decreased facial sensation or tic douloureux–like facial pains may be a clue to a lesion in this area. Patients with cluster headache may also have ticlike or ice pick–like facial pains. Some lesions that can produce this syndrome include carotid aneurysms, congenital carotid anomalies, atherosclerosis, fibromuscular dysplasia, trauma, tumors of the gasserian ganglion, metastatic tumor to the middle cranial fossa, infectious spread from dental abscesses, chronic sinusitis, osteitis of the petrous bone, basal arachnoiditis, basilar skull fractures, injection or transection of the gasserian ganglion, and gunshot wounds.[131–133] The pain may last for weeks and usually is not episodic or steroid responsive. Some investigators believe that if the only findings are a painful Horner's syndrome and, possibly, dysfunction of the fifth cranial nerve (with decreased sensation or tic douloureux limited to the ophthalmic division), the lesion is benign. These patients may be considered to have "true" Raeder's syndrome. The supposed pathogenesis of symptoms related to the trigeminal nerve in these cases of idiopathic benign Raeder's syndrome is an ischemic injury of the gasserian ganglion.[133] I believe such patients need careful follow-up.[134] Moreover, if symptoms last more than several weeks, an aneurysm at the base of the skull should be ruled out.

Treatment

The treatment of migraine and cluster headache is controversial but can be exceedingly simple.[135] Physicians should have their patients consider risk factors that may be operational and should be familiar with several lay publications on migraine to recommend to patients.[11] They should insist that their patient study their own premonitory signals and experiment with ways to abort the aura or headache.[136, 137] Attention to these two measures can appreciably reduce the frequency and severity of migraine attacks. Even if physicians do nothing more than listen to their migraine sufferers as they discuss their "tricks" for aborting their attacks, they will learn more to help their patients than might be learned from lectures by pharmacologists. Successful techniques to abort the aura and headache include sleep, exercise, caffeine, cold showers, digital superficial temporal artery massage (during the aura), and even vomiting.[11, 138, 139] Many patients can thwart migraine attacks by "figuring out just what to do" when premonitory signs appear. Yawning when not tired may be a signal for a patient to immediately douse his or her head in cold water!

The treatment of migraine can be satisfying yet fraught with potential complications.[28, 114, 115, 136, 140–142]

An acute attack of migraine may be completely relieved by acetylsalicylic acid or acetaminophen with or without codeine or barbiturates.[137, 143] Codeine and barbiturates may produce physical dependence and tolerance. Attempts to discontinue them may induce a headache misinterpreted as migraine and thus provoke patients to take more medications, thus creating a vicious cycle of daily headaches. Therefore, such medications containing codeine or barbiturates should not be taken for more than 2 days a week.

Ergotamine can be inhaled or used orally, sublingually, or as a suppository for an acute migraine attack. Use more than twice a week should be avoided because of rebound ergotamine headaches that are even more severe and more insidious than the rebound headaches associated with physical dependence on codeine and barbiturates.

Oral narcotics are rarely indicated for acute migraine attacks. Intractable acute attacks may require parenteral narcotics, parenteral dihydroergotamine, or systemic corticosteroids. In dehydrated patients, precautions should be taken against the complications of orthostatic hypotension. Antiemetics can be used if indicated.[137, 144]

The prophylaxis of migraine can be achieved with β-blockers, pizotyline, tricyclic antidepressants, calcium channel blockers, or methysergide.[27, 135, 137, 145, 146] Some β-blockers are ineffective, particularly β-blockers with intrinsic sympathomimetic activity.[137, 143, 147] Pizotyline circumvents many of the systemic complications of β-blockers but may stimulate appetite and produce weight gain. Tricyclic antidepressants seem to be effective regardless of any effect on mood. The reason is unknown. Calcium channel blockers may not be as effective as other prophylactic medications.[148] Methysergide provides excellent prophylaxis against migraine but can rarely cause coronary vasospasm or retroperitoneal fibrosis. Therefore, patients should be evaluated for cardiovascular disease and monitored closely during the initiation of therapy, and therapy should never be continued more than 3 to 5 mo in a row.[137] Beta-blockers probably should not be discontinued abruptly.

Cluster headache, like migraine, may be aborted with ergotamine. Prophylaxis can be achieved with methysergide with or without prednisone and sometimes with ergotamine in tapering doses. Lithium may be most effective in chronic, especially noncycling, cluster headache.[136, 149] Breathing 7 to 10 L/min of oxygen or vigorous exercise may abort an attack of cluster headache.[136]

Psychotherapy, traditional Chinese acupuncture, and biofeedback have also been used for migraine treatment and prophylaxis.[150] Children with uncontrolled migraine may respond to flunarizine or to anticonvulsant medications.[146, 151, 152]

Chronic intractable migraine is uncommon and generally secondary to overmedication and depression.[152] It usually requires hospitalization for careful detoxification.[153]

NONOCULAR EYE PAINS

A number of facial pain syndromes may on occasion produce one or more attacks of pain strictly localized to or near an eye, mimicking local ocular disease.[154] Although some of these attacks may qualify as cluster-like headache syndrome, some represent manifestations of less common validated syndromes or are defined entities, such as post–neck trauma dysautonomic cephalalgia.[155] Most head pains encountered defy diagnosis.

Idiopathic stabbing headache ("ice pick pains") are irregularly occurring momentary stabbing pains in the first division of the trigeminal nerve (orbit, temple, or parietal area). Local tissue damage and compression of the trigeminal nerve intracranially should be ruled out as causes. They are most common in migraine sufferers, especially around the time of a migraine attack. They may occur as a cluster headache is fading or in giant cell arteritis. They may be triggered by sudden postural change, physical exertion, dark-to-lighted environment transition, or head motion during a headache.[155] They often improve on indomethacin therapy (25 mg PO t.i.d.).

Headache associated with sexual activity (occasionally familial[156]) can be precipitated by masturbation or coitus. This headache usually starts as a dull bilateral ache while sexual excitement increases and suddenly becomes intense at orgasm. It may produce a partial Horner's syndrome.[132] It rarely produces stroke.[157, 158] Patients almost never volunteer coitus as the precipitant of the headache, and they must be specifically asked. Like migraine, it may be a sign of underlying pathophysiologic change.

Optic neuritis and diabetic oculomotor palsy may present as isolated eye pain for several days before visual loss or diplopia appears.

Headache associated with vascular disorders may produce predominantly periocular pain, such as occurs in posterior cerebral artery territory stroke, giant cell arteritis, dissecting aneurysms of the head, and paresthesias associated with ocular ischemia.[159] None of these pains are chronic, and most of these headaches remit within 1 mo of appropriate therapy for the underlying disorder. Thunderclap headache is a sudden severe and unusual headache that may herald subarachnoid hemorrhage but more often is a sign of impending migraine or tension headache.[160–162]

Headache with ischemic stroke (including Wallenberg's syndrome) usually begins at the onset of acute ischemic stroke but occasionally precedes a stroke by as much as 2 wk and rarely begins as late as 2 wk after the stroke. It may be strictly periocular and therefore mimic eye disease. Unruptured vascular malformations rarely produce eye pain. Arteriovenous malformations have not been proved to cause headaches or to mimic migraine closely. Saccular aneurysms may produce headache as a prelude to rupture and the attendant severe headache. Giant aneurysms may produce headache and even periocular pain without rupture, probably because they act as space-occupying lesions.

Arteritides, including giant cell arteritis, may produce headache, even with prominent periocular components.

Carotid or vertebral artery disease may cause pain primarily in the face. For example, carotid dissection produces ipsilateral pain combined with either (1) transient ischemic attack or ischemic stroke in the appropriate territory or (2) Horner's syndrome, arterial bruit, or tinnitus.

Carotodynia may be idiopathic or secondary to diseases of the carotid artery such as giant cell arteritis, atherosclerotic thrombosis, intraluminal hemorrhage, fibromuscular dysplasia, aneurysm, or aneurysmal dissection. The idiopathic form is a self-limited disorder of neck and face pain including tenderness, swelling, or increased pulsations over the carotid artery. The secondary form may be chronic and mimic cluster headache and cluster-like headache. Surgical denervation of the carotid bulb has been recommended for recalcitrant cases.[163]

Acknowledgments

I wish to thank my office staff and the staff of St. Mary's Hospital Library, Waterbury, CT.

REFERENCES

1. Sjaastad O: Classification and diagnostic criteria for headache disorders, cranial neuralgias and facial pain. Cephalalgia 8:9, 1988.
2. Capildeo R, Clifford Rose F: Towards a new classification of migraine. *In* Rose FC (ed): Advances in Migraine Research and Therapy. New York, Raven Press, 1982.

3. Behrman S: Migraine as a sequela of blunt head injury. Injury 9:74, 1977.
4. Broderich JP, Swanson JW: Migraine-related strokes: Clinical profile and prognosis in 20 patients. Arch Neurol 44:868, 1987.
5. Logan WR, Tegeler CH, Keniston WD, et al: Migraine and stroke in young adults. Neurology 34:206, 1984.
6. Silberstein SD: Treatment of headache in primary care practice. Am J Med 77(Suppl 3A):65, 1984.
7. Drexler ED: Severe headaches: When to worry, what to do. Postgrad Med 87:164, 1990.
8. Welch KMA: Migraine: A biobehavioral disorder. Arch Neurol 44:323, 1987.
9. Levine SR, Welch KMA, Ewing JR, et al: Cerebral blood flow asymmetries in headache-free migraineurs. Stroke 18:1164, 1987.
10. Welch KM, Levine SR, D'Andrea G, et al: Preliminary observations on brain energy metabolism in migraine studied by in vivo phosphorus 31 NMR spectroscopy. Neurology 39:538, 1989.
11. Sacks O: Migraine: Understanding a Common Disorder. Berkeley and Los Angeles, University of California Press, 1985.
12. Thie A, Fuhlendorf A, Spitzer K, et al: Transcranial Doppler evaluation of common and classic migraine. II: Ultrasonic features during attacks. Headache 30:209, 1990.
13. Dalessio DJ: Is there a difference between classic and common migraine? What is migraine, after all? Arch Neurol 42:275, 1985.
14. Kobari M, Meyer JS, Ichijo M, et al: Cortical and subcortical hyperfusion during migraine and cluster headache measured by Xe CT-CBF. Neuroradiology 32:4, 1990.
15. Skyhoj-Olsen T: Migraine with and without aura: The same disease due to cerebral vasospasm of different intensity. A hypothesis based on CBF studies during migraine. Headache 30:269, 1990.
16. Graham JR: The migraine connection. Headache 21:243, 1981.
17. Welch KM, Levine SR: Migraine-related stroke in the context of the international headache society classification of head pain. Arch Neurol 47:458, 1990.
18. Sahota PK, Dexter JD: Sleep and headache syndromes: A clinical review. Headache 30:80, 1990.
19. Blau JN: Resolution of migraine attacks: Sleep and the recovery phase. J Neurol Neurosurg Psychiatry 45:223, 1984.
20. Sjaastad O, Fredriksen TA, Sand T, et al: Unilaterality of headache in classic migraine. Cephalalgia 9:71, 1989.
21. Miller D, Waters DD, Warnica W, et al: Is variant angina the coronary manifestation of a generalized vasospastic disorder? N Engl J Med 304:763, 1981.
22. Leon-Sotomayor LA: Cardiac migraine: A report of twelve cases. Angiology 25:161, 1974.
23. Ardila A, Sanchez E: Neuropsychologic symptoms in the migraine syndrome. Cephalalgia 8:67, 1988.
24. Fuller GN, Guiloff RJ: Migrainous olfactory hallucinations. J Neurol Neurosurg Psychiatry 50:1688, 1987.
25. Klee A, Willanger R: Disturbances of visual perception in migraine. Acta Neurol Scand 42:400, 1966.
26. Gowers WR, Lond MD: Subjective visual sensations. Trans Ophthalmol Soc UK 15:1, 1895.
27. Hupp SL, Kline LB, Corbett JJ: Visual disturbances of migraine. Surv Ophthalmol 33:221, 1989.
28. Corbett JJ: Neuro-ophthalmic complications of migraine and cluster headaches. Neurol Clin 1:973, 1983.
29. Hoyt WF: Transient bilateral blurring of vision. Arch Ophthalmol 70:746, 1963.
30. Shiogal T, Takeuchi K, Akiyama R: Bitemporal hemianopsia as a prodromal symptom of ophthalmic migraine: A report of three cases. Jpn J Neuroophthalmol 1:96, 1984.
31. Kosmorsky G: Unusual visual phenomenon during acephalgic migraine. Arch Ophthalmol 105:613, 1987.
32. Haas DC: Prolonged migraine aura status. Ann Neurol 11:197, 1982.
33. Bigley GK, Sharp FR: Reversible alexia without agraphia due to migraine. Arch Neurol 40:114, 1983.
34. Jenkyn LR, Reeves AG: Aphemia with hemiplegic migraine. Neurology 29:1317, 1979.
35. Symonds C: Migrainous variants. Trans Med Soc Lond 67:237, 1951.
36. Fleishman JA, Segall JD, Judge FP: Isolated transient alexia: A migrainous accompaniment. Arch Neurol 40:115, 1983.
37. Abe K, Oda N, Araki R, et al: Macropsia, micropsia, and episodic illusion in Japanese adolescents. J Am Acad Child Adolesc Psychiatry 28:493, 1989.
38. Tychsen L, Hoyt WF: Hydrocephalus and transient cortical blindness. Am J Ophthalmol 98:819, 1984.
39. Sinoff SE, Rosenberg M: Permanent cerebral diplopia in a migraineur. Neurology 40:1138, 1990.
40. DeBroff BM, Spierings EL: Migraine associated with periorbital ecchymosis. Headache 30:260, 1990.
41. Whitty CWM, Oxon DM: Migraine without headache. Lancet 1:283, 1967.
42. Fisher CM: Late-life migraine accompaniments as a cause of unexplained transient ischemic attacks. Can J Neurol Sci 7:9, 1980.
43. O'Connor PS, Tredici TJ: Acephalgic migraine: Fifteen years experience. Am Acad Ophthalmol 86:414, 1978.
44. Coppeto JR: Migraine like accompaniments of vitreous detachment. Neuro-Ophthalmology 8:197, 1988.
45. Caplan LR, Weiner H, Weintraub RM, et al: "Migrainous" neurologic dysfunction in patients with prosthetic cardiac valves. Headache 16:218, 1976.
46. Goodwin JA, Gorelick PB, Helgason CM: Symptoms of amaurosis fugax in atherosclerotic carotid artery disease. Neurology 37:829, 1987.
47. Hedges TR, Lackman RD: Isolated ophthalmic migraine in the differential diagnosis of cerebro-ocular ischemia. Stroke 7:379, 1976.
48. Hedges TR: Isolated ophthalmic migraine: Its frequency, mechanisms, and differential diagnosis. *In* Smith JL (ed): Neuro-Ophthalmology, vol. 6. St. Louis, CV Mosby, 1972.
49. Miller NR: Solitary oculomotor nerve palsy in childhood. Am J Ophthalmol 83:106, 1977.
50. Bailey TD, O'Connor PS, Tredici TJ, et al: Ophthalmoplegic migraine. J Clin Neuro-Ophthalmol 4:225, 1984.
51. Erkulvrawatr S: Tolosa-Hunt syndrome or ophthalmoplegic migraine? Neurology 26:598, 1976.
52. Ruff T, Lenis A, Daiz JA: Atypical facial pain and orbital cancer. Arch Otolaryngol 111:338, 1985.
53. Friedman AP, Harter DH, Merritt HH: Ophthalmoplegic migraine. Arch Neurol 7:82, 1962.
54. Harrington DO, Flocks M: Ophthalmoplegic migraine. Arch Ophthalmol 49:643, 1953.
55. O'Day J, Billson F, King J: Ophthalmoplegic migraine and aberrant regeneration of the oculomotor nerve. Br J Ophthalmol 64:534, 1980.
56. Cruciger MP, Mazow ML: An unusual case of ophthalmoplegic migraine. Am J Ophthalmol 86:414, 1978.
57. Vijayan N: Ophthalmoplegic migraine: Ischemic or compressive neuropathy? Headache 20:300, 1980.
58. Tippin J, Corbett JJ, Kerber RE, et al: Amaurosis fugax and ocular infarction in adolescents and young adults. Ann Neurol 26:69, 1989.
59. Coppeto JR, Kawalick M: Ocular pseudomigraine after posterior chamber intraocular lens implantation. Am J Ophthalmol 102:393, 1986.
60. Kupersmith MJ, Warren FA, Hass WK: The non-benign aspects of migraine. Neuro-Ophthalmology 7:1, 1987.
61. Moskowitz MA: The neurobiology of vascular head pain. Ann Neurol 16:157, 1984.
62. Edmeads J: Migraine-resuscitation of the vascular theory. Headache 29:55, 1989.
63. Kline LB, Kelly CL: Ocular migraine in a patient with cluster headaches. Headache 20:253, 1980.
64. Kupersmith MJ, Hass WK, Chase NE: Isoproterenol treatment of visual symptoms in migraine. Stroke 10:299, 1979.
65. Ropper AH: Transient ipsilateral paresthesias (TIPs) with transient monocular blindness. Arch Neurol 42:295, 1985.
66. Protenoy RK, Abissi CJ, Lipton RB, et al: Headache in cerebrovascular disease. Stroke 15:1009, 1984.
67. Carroll D: Retinal migraine. Headache 10:9, 1970.
68. Connor RCR, Lond MB: Complicated migraine: A study of permanent neurological and visual defects caused by migraine. Lancet 2:1073, 1962.
69. Coppeto JR, Lessell S, Sciarra R, et al: Vascular retinopathy in migraine. J Clin Neuro Ophthalmology 6:196, 1986.

70. Brown GC, Magargal LF, Shields JA, et al: Retinal arterial obstruction in children and young adults. Ophthalmology 88:18, 1981.
71. Katz B: Bilateral sequential migrainous ischemic optic neuropathy. Am J Ophthalmol 99:489, 1985.
72. Eagling EM, Sanders MD, Miller SJH: Ischaemic papillopathy. Br J Ophthalmol 58:990, 1974.
73. Brown GC, Magargal LE, Shields JA, et al: Retinal arterial obstruction in children and young adults. Am Acad Ophthalmol 88:18, 1981.
74. Katz B, Bamford CR: Migrainous ischemic optic neuropathy. Neurology 35:112, 1985.
75. Victor DI, Welch RB: Bilateral retinal hemorrhages and disc edema in migraine. Am J Ophthalmol 84:555, 1977.
76. Kosmorsky GS, Rosenfeld SI, Burde RM: Transient monocular obscuration— Amaurosis fugax? A case report. Br J Ophthalmol 69:688, 1985.
77. Coppeto JR, Lessell S, Lessell I, et al: Diffuse disseminated atheroembolism: Three cases with neuro-ophthalmic manifestation. Arch Ophthalmol 102:225, 1984.
78. Jacobides GM: Migraine in children and adolescents. *In* Rose FC (ed): Advances in Migraine Research and Therapy. New York, Raven Press, 1982.
79. Brown JK: Migraine and migraine equivalents in children. Dev Med Child Neurol 19:683, 1977.
80. DuBois LG, Sadun AA, Lawton TB: Inner retinal layer loss in complicated migraine. Arch Ophthalmol 106:1035, 1988.
81. Prensky AL, Sommer D: Diagnosis and treatment of migraine in children. Neurology 29:506, 1979.
82. Jay GW, Tomasi LG: Pediatric headache: A one year retrospective analysis. Headache 21:5, 1981.
83. Hedges TR: Pediatric migraine. Am J Ophthalmol 95:844, 1983.
84. Ehyai A, Fenichel GM: The natural history of acute confusional migraine. Arch Neurol 35:368, 1978.
85. Rossi LN: Headache in childhood. Childs Nerv Syst 5:129, 1989.
86. Hachinski VC, Porchawka J, Steele JC: Visual symptoms in the migraine syndrome. Neurology 23:570, 1973.
87. Ferguson KS, Robinson SS: Life-threatening migraine. Arch Neurol 37:374, 1982.
88. Golden GS, French JH: Basilar artery migraine in young children. Pediatrics 56:722, 1975.
89. Durkan G, Troost BT, Slamovitis TL, et al: Recurrent painless oculomotor palsy in children: A variant of ophthalmoplegic migraine? Headache 21:58, 1981.
90. Dodge PR, Griffith JF: Some transient ocular manifestations of neurologic disease in children. *In* Smith JL (ed): Neuro-Ophthalmology vol. 3. St. Louis, CV Mosby, 1967.
91. Slavin ML: Transient concomitant esotropia in a child with migraine. Am J Ophthalmol 107:190, 1989.
92. Hockaday JM: Basilar migraine in childhood. Dev Med Child Neurol 21:455, 1979.
93. Siemes H, Casaer P: Alternating hemiplegia in childhood: Clinical report and single photon emission computed tomography study. Monatsschr Kinderheilkd 136:467, 1988.
94. Crosley CJ, Dhamoon S: Migrainous olfactory aura in a family. Arch Neurol 40:459, 1983.
95. Haan J, Ferrari MD, Brouwer OF: Acute confusional migraine: Case report and review of literature. Clin Neurol Neurosurg 90:275, 1988.
96. Venable HP, Wilson S, Allan WC, et al: Total blindness after trivial frontal head trauma: Bilateral indirect optic nerve injury. Neurology 28:1066, 1978.
97. Vohanka S, Zouhar A: Transient global amnesia after mild head injury in childhood. Activitas Nervosa Superior 30:68, 1988.
98. Bodian M: Transient loss of vision following head trauma. N Y State Med J 64:916, 1964.
99. Haas DC, Pineda GS, Lourie H: Juvenile head trauma syndromes and their relationship to migraine. Arch Neurol 32:727, 1978.
100. Haas DC, Lourie H: Trauma-triggered migraine: An explanation for common neurological attacks after mild head injury. J Neurosurg 68:181, 1988.
101. Call GK, Fleming MC, Sealfon S, et al: Reversible cerebral segmental vasoconstriction. Stroke 19:1159, 1988.
102. Ram Z, Hadani M, Spiegelman R, et al: Delayed nonhemorrhagic encephalopathy following mild head trauma. J Neurosurg 71:608, 1989.
103. Alsop RH, Brickner RM, Soltz SE: Unusual types of migraine. Bull Neurol Inst NY 4:403, 1935.
104. Hart RG, Miller VT: Cerebral infarction in young adults: A practical approach. Stroke 14:110, 1983.
105. Adams HP, Butler MJ, Biller J, et al: Nonhemorrhagic cerebral infarction in young adults. Arch Neurol 43:793, 1986.
106. Pessin MS, Lathi ES, Cohen MB, et al: Clinical features and mechanism of occipital infarction. Ann Neurol 21:290, 1987.
107. Sacquegna T, Andreoli A, Baldrati A, et al: Ischemic stroke in young adults: The relevance of migrainous infarction. Cephalalgia 9:255, 1989.
108. McAuley DL, Russell WR: Correlation of CAT scan and visual field defects in vascular lesions of the posterior visual pathways. J Neurol Neurosurg Psychiatry 42:298, 1979.
109. Weintraub MI: Migraine related to ocular stroke. Neurology 36:1410, 1986.
110. Webster MW, Chancellor AM, Smith HJ, et al: Patent foramen ovale in young stroke patients. Lancet 2:11, 1988.
111. Rothrock JF, Walicke P, Swenson MR, et al: Migrainous stroke. Arch Neurol 45:63, 1988.
112. Moen M, Levine SR, Newman DS, et al: Bilateral posterior cerebral artery strokes in a young migraine sufferer. Stroke 19:525, 1988.
113. Bevan H, Sharma K, Bradley W: Stroke in young adults. Stroke 21:382, 1990.
114. Smith JL: Permanent infarctions complicating migraine. J Clin Neuro-Ophthalmol 6:74, 1986.
115. Gilbert GJ: An occurrence of complicated migraine during propranolol therapy. Headache 22:81, 1982.
116. Leviton A, Malvea B, Graham JR: Vascular diseases, mortality, and migraine in the parents of migraine patients. Neurology 24:669, 1974.
117. Prendes JL: Cerebral infarction and migraine. Neurology 30:348, 1980.
118. Dorfman LJ, Marshall WH, Enzmann DR: Cerebral infarction and migraine: Clinical and radiologic correlations. Neurology 29:317, 1979.
119. Briley DP, Coull BM, Goodnight SH: Neurological disease associated with antiphospholipid antibodies. Ann Neurol 25:221, 1989.
120. Anderson CD, Franks RD: Migraine and tension headache: Is there a physiological difference? Headache 21:63, 1981.
121. Ziegler DK, Stephenson-Hassanein R: Migraine muscle-contraction headache dichotomy studied by statistical analysis of headache symptoms. *In* Rose FC (ed): Advances in Migraine Research and Therapy. New York, Raven Press, 1982.
122. Mikamo K, Takeshima T, Takahsasi K: Cardiovascular sympathetic hypofunction in muscle contraction headache and migraine. Headache 29:86, 1989.
123. Allen RA, Weinmann RL: The McGill-Melzack pain questionnaire in the diagnosis of headache. Headache 22:20, 1982.
124. Solomon S, Cappa KG, Smith CR: Common migraine: Criteria for diagnosis. Headache 28:124, 1988.
125. Toshniwal P: Anterior ischemic optic neuropathy secondary to cluster headache. Acta Neurol Scand 73:213, 1986.
126. Levy DE: Transient CNS deficits: A common, benign syndrome in young adults. Neurology 38:831, 1988.
127. Fisher CM: The headache and pain of spontaneous carotid dissection. Headache 22:60, 1982.
128. Raeder JG: "Paratrigeminal" paralysis of oculopupillary sympathetic. Brain 47:149, 1924.
129. Lance JW: Headache. Ann Neurol 10:1, 1981.
130. Appen RE, Sturm RJ: Raeder's paratrigeminal syndrome. Ann Ophthalmol 10:1181, 1978.
131. Cohen RJ, Taylor JR: Persistent neurologic sequalae of migraine: A case report. Neurology 29:1175, 1979.
132. Healy JF, Zyroff J, Rosenkrantz H: Raeder syndrome associated with lesions of the internal carotid artery. Radiology 141:101, 1981.
133. Lederman RJ, Salanga V: Fibromuscular dysplasia of the internal carotid artery—A cause of Raeder's paratrigeminal syndrome. Neurology 26:353, 1976.

134. Grimson BS, Thompson S: Raeder's syndrome: A clinical review. Surv Ophthalmol 24:199, 1980.
135. Gaudet RJ: Migraine prevention with β-blockers: A placebo effect? JAMA 254:3183, 1985.
136. Atkinson R, Appenzeller O: Headache. Postgrad Med J 60:841, 1984.
137. Edmeads JG: Migraine. Can Med Assoc J 138:107, 1988.
138. Van Gign J: Relief of common migraine by exercise. J Neurol Neurosurg Psychiatry 50:1700, 1987.
139. Lipton SA: Prevention of classic migraine headache of digital massage of the superficial temporal arteries during visual aura. Ann Neurol 19:515, 1986.
140. Whitney CM, Daroff RB: An approach to migraine. J Neurosci Nurs 20:284, 1988.
141. Mathew NT, Stubits E, Nigam MP: Transformation of episodic migraine into daily headache: Analysis of factors. Headache 22:66, 1982.
142. Katz B: Migrainous central retinal artery occlusion. J Clin Neuro Ophthalmol 6:69, 1986.
143. Edmeads J: Four steps in managing migraine. Postgrad Med J 85:121, 1989.
144. Dvorkin G, Andermann F, Melancon D, et al: Malignant migraine syndrome: Classical migraine, occipital seizures, and alternating strokes. Neurology 34:245, 1984.
145. Amery WK: Onset of action of various migraine prophylactics. Cephalalgia 8:11, 1988.
146. Sorge F, DeSimone R, Morano E, et al: Flunarizine in prophylaxis of childhood migraine: A double-blind, placebo-controlled, crossover study. Cephalalgia 8:1, 1988.
147. Joseph R, Steiner TJ, Schultz LU, et al: Platelet activity and selective beta-blockers in migraine prophylaxis. Stroke 19:704, 1988.
148. McArthur JC, Marek K, Pestronk A, et al: Nifedipine in the prophylaxis of classic migraine: A crossover, double-masked, placebo-controlled study of headache frequency and side effects. Neurology 39:284, 1989.
149. Damasio H, Lyon L: Lithium carbonate in the treatment of cluster headaches. J Neurol 224:1, 1980.
150. Sovak M, Kunzel M, Sternbach RA, et al: Mechanism of the biofeedback therapy of migraine volitional manipulation of the psychophysiological background. Headache 21:89, 1981.
151. Buda FB, Joyce RP: Pediatric migraine: Criteria for treatment and results of treatment with anti-convulsants. Ann Neurol 4:190, 1978.
152. Hansruedi I: Migraine treatment as a cause of chronic migraine. *In* Rose FC (ed): Advances in Migraine Research and Therapy. New York, Raven Press, 1982.
153. Bode DD: Ocular pain secondary to occipital neuritis. Ann Ophthalmol 11:589, 1979.
154. Vijayan N, Dreyfus PM: Posttraumatic dysautonomic cephalalgia. Arch Neurol 32:649, 1975.
155. Raskin NH, Schwartz RK: Icepick-like pain. Neurology 30:203, 1980.
156. Johns DR: Benign sexual headache within a family. Arch Neurol 43:1158, 1986.
157. Price RW, Posner JB: Chronic paroxysmal hemicrania: A disabling headache syndrome responding to indomethacin. Ann Neurol 3:183, 1978.
158. Massey EW: Effort headache in runners. Headache 22:99, 1982.
159. Monteiro MLR, Coppeto JR: Horner's syndrome associated with carotid artery atherosclerosis. Am J Ophthalmol 105:93, 1988.
160. Wijdicks EFM, Kerkhoff H, Van-Gijn J: Long-term follow-up of 71 patients with thunderclap headache mimicking subarachnoid hemorrhage. Lancet 2:68, 1988.
161. Day JW, Raskin NH: Thunderclap headache symptom of unruptured cerebral aneurysm. Lancet 1:1247, 1986.
162. Harling DW, Peatfield RC, Van Hille PT, et al: Thunderclap headache: Is it migraine? Cephalalgia 9:87, 1989.
163. De-Vries AC, Geuder J, Riles TS: Carotodynia managed by surgical denervation of the carotid bulb. Eur J Vasc Surg 4:325, 1990.

Chapter 214

Idiopathic Intracranial Hypertension (Pseudotumor Cerebri)

JAMES J. CORBETT

Idiopathic intracranial hypertension (IIH), commonly known as *pseudotumor cerebri* or *benign intracranial hypertension*, is a condition of unknown cause characterized by elevated cerebrospinal fluid (CSF) pressure and papilledema.[1] IIH is not an uncommon disorder; its incidence is at least 1 per 100,000 in the general population and increases to 19 per 100,000 in obese women of child-bearing age, the most commonly affected population.[2] In children, IIH has equal sex incidence.[1] The major symptoms are headache, transient visual obscurations in one or both eyes, blurred vision and horizontal diplopia,[3–5] pulsatile tinnitus, and pain in the neck, shoulders, back, and arms. Consciousness is not altered. Papilledema is the cardinal physical finding. Usually bilateral, papilledema may be grossly asymmetric or occasionally unilateral.[6] For practical purposes, visual loss caused by disc swelling is the major permanent sequel of IIH, because 10 to 25 percent of patients, including children, suffer serious visual loss.[3, 4, 7] IIH with a clearly identified cause is uncommon in adults but more common in children.

IIH DUE TO UNKNOWN CAUSE

The first and largest group of patients who fulfill Dandy's modified criteria[8] for IIH have no identifiable cause of high CSF pressure. A negative history, especially for medications, as well as a normal contrast-enhanced computed tomographic (CT) or magnetic resonance (MRI) scan and a lumbar puncture showing normal CSF contents and high pressure are required to call the condition idiopathic.

Symptomatic IIH (Table 214–1)

The second group, designated as having symptomatic intracranial hypertension, is of therapeutic importance because it presumes that the cause is known and that removing or altering the cause will cure the condition. Unfortunately, in many cases, this presumption is not borne out in practice.

Patients suffering from viral, bacterial, and fungal infections; tumors; and inflammatory and metabolic conditions that raise CSF pressure cannot be said to have IIH, even though they may have papilledema, headache, and no focal neurologic signs. Because all of these conditions can mimic IIH, lumbar puncture, after a CT or MRI scan, is absolutely mandatory to establish that the constituents of CSF are normal in every patient in whom IIH is a consideration.

NON-IIH

A third group of patients has "non-IIH."[9] The patient's body habitus, optic disc appearance, and symptoms (usually headache) suggest a diagnosis of IIH. The most common cause of this misdiagnosis of IIH in the era of modern imaging studies is the combination of migraine headache, anomalously elevated optic discs, obesity, normal findings on MRI or CT scan, and a physician's failure to perform a lumbar puncture to identify increased CSF pressure.

Table 214–1. SYMPTOMATIC FORMS OF INTRACRANIAL HYPERTENSION

This list of diseases and conditions associated with both papilledema and increased intracranial pressure *has been amended and updated. Note that computed tomography and magnetic resonance imaging studies, lumbar puncture results,* patient's history, and other abnormalities associated with many of these conditions would immediately exclude them as "idiopathic." However, many of the alleged causes of papilledema and increased cerebrospinal fluid pressure are unproved in any rigorous way. The long list of medications (under toxins) is largely anecdotal.

Renal Diseases
Chronic uremia

Developmental Diseases
Hydrocephalus
Syringomyelia
Craniostenosis
Aqueductal stenosis (adult type)

Toxic Conditions
Kepone (chlordecone)
Lead
Arsenic
Perhexiline maleate
Hypervitaminosis A
Nalidixic acid
Steroid withdrawal
Androgen therapy
Danazol
Dilantin
Lithium
Indomethacin and ketoprofen in Bartter's syndrome
Amiodarone
Tetracycline
Sulfamethoxazole
Nitrofurantoin
Penicillin

Allergic Diseases
Serum sickness
Allergies

Infectious Diseases
Bacterial
  Subacute bacterial endocarditis
Meningitis
Brucellosis
Lyme disease

Viral Diseases
Poliomyelitis
Acute lymphocytic meningitis
Coxsackie B virus encephalitis
Inclusion body encephalitis
Recurrent polyneuritis
Guillain-Barré syndrome

Parasitic Diseases
Sandfly fever
Trypanosomiasis
Torulosis
Neurocysticercosis

Metabolic/Endocrine
Treatment of hypothyroidism in children
Hyperalimentation of deprivation dwarfs
Hypoparathyroidism
Pseudohypoparathyroidism
Addison's disease
Scurvy
Diabetic ketoacidosis
Obesity
Eclampsia
Oral progestational agents
Menarche
Menstrual abnormalities
Pregnancy

Miscellaneous Diseases
Gastrointestinal hemorrhage
Lupus erythematosus
Sarcoidosis
Syphilis
Cerebrovascular malformation
Subarachnoid malformation
Paget's disease
Opticochiasmatic arachnoiditis
Cowden's syndrome
Ulcerative colitis
Turner's syndrome
Head trauma

Neoplastic Diseases
Leukemia
Spinal cord tumors
Any brain tumor, but especially gliomatosis cerebri

Hematologic Diseases
Infectious mononucleosis
Idiopathic thrombocytopenic purpura
Pernicious anemia
Polycythemia
Iron deficiency anemia
Hemophilia
Cryoglobulinemia
Cryofibrinogenemia
Monoclonal gammopathy
Abnormal fibrinogen
Hypocomplementemic urticarial vasculitis

Circulatory Diseases
Congestive heart failure
Mediastinal neoplasm
Dural sinus thrombosis
  Spontaneous
  Otogenic
  Behçet's disease
  Leukemia
  Traumatic
  Tumor (cholesteatoma, sarcoid, mestastasis, eosinophilic granuloma of temporal bone, glomus tumors)
Chronic pulmonary hypoventilation
Congenital cardiac lesion
  Atrial septal defect repair
  Ligation of patent ductus arteriosus
Superior vena cava obstruction

From Buchheit WA, Barton C: Nomenclature in intracranial pressure. N Engl J Med 280:938, 1969. Reprinted, by permission, from the New England Journal of Medicine.

IDIOPATHIC INTRACRANIAL PRESSURE WITHOUT PAPILLEDEMA

Some patients have headaches, normal findings on imaging, and increased CSF pressure but no papilledema and are reported as having "IIH without papilledema."[10] The major problem posed by IIH is visual loss, and the patients in this subgroup do not have papilledema. Headache control, not visual loss, is the issue. Symptomatic and prophylactic headache therapy for these patients is sufficient. Repeated lumbar puncture occasionally is helpful.

CLINICAL EVALUATION

History

One should especially ask about the use of vitamin A or multivitamins in large quantities, the recent use of nalidixic acid, and the use and discontinuation of corticosteroids — even topical steroids. Headache is a common symptom, although patients may rarely be discovered incidentally and have no symptoms or only nonspecific visual complaints with no headache. The headaches of IIH vary in intensity from mild to very severe; however, they are commonly characterized as the "worst of their life." Preexistent migraine may worsen with IIH.[11] There is no clear correlation between the height of the CSF pressure and the severity of the headache (Fig. 214–1).[12]

Monocular or binocular transient visual obscurations (TVOs) are very common.[5] Blurring or total loss of vision lasts seconds, rarely longer, and is frequently precipitated by some change in posture or the Valsalva maneuver. Regarded by some as a harbinger of visual failure,[4] TVOs may be alarming but have not definitely been proved to be predictive of serious visual loss.[3, 8]

Blurring of vision is a symptom that is possibly related to encroachment of the blind spot on fixation, but it remains poorly explained. Blurred vision may be a complaint despite no demonstrable visual acuity loss.[3, 4]

Diplopia, a much less common symptom,[5] is transient, almost always horizontal, and caused by sixth nerve paresis. In patients with vertical diplopia, other diagnoses should be considered, although studies have shown that most sixth nerve palsies commonly have a vertical component.

When persistent loss of vision is the presenting complaint, permanent severe visual loss is common. The causes of permanent visual acuity loss in IIH include optic disc infarction,[13, 14] macular changes,[15] subretinal hemorrhage,[16] and a combination of ischemic and compression damage to the optic nerves.[17]

Vision Assessment

Because visual loss is the most common and serious complication of IIH, visual function should be assessed using kinetic Goldmann's or static Humphrey's (24–2 or 30–2) perimetry and Snellen's visual acuity testing, as well as fundus photography in both the initial evaluation and the follow-up of these patients.[18] The importance of repeated ophthalmic observations of best corrected visual acuity, visual fields, and intraocular pressure, as well as careful examination for afferent pupil defects, cannot be overemphasized. The rare patients who have elevated intracranial pressure combined with increased intraocular pressure warrant special attention, because the risk of visual loss in these persons appears to be increased.[3]

PERIMETRY

In general, the field defects associated with IIH are disc related and analogous to glaucoma fields. In addition to the enlarged blind spot, they include nasal inferior constriction, arcuate defects, inferior altitudinal loss, and generalized constriction (Fig. 214–2). Kinetic Goldmann's perimetry using an Armaly-Drance testing strategy can detect field defects when about 30 percent of the optic nerve fibers are lost.[19] Static perimetry using the Humphrey's 24–2 is a more sensitive detector of visual field loss than the Goldmann's perimeter.[18] Repeated measurement of blind spot size alone is not

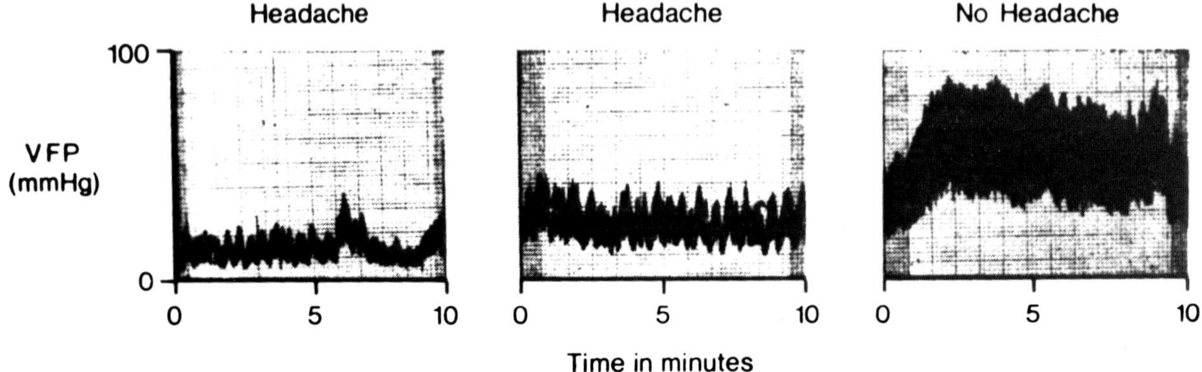

Figure 214–1. It is widely assumed that the severity of intracranial pressure elevation is the cause of headaches in idiopathic intracranial hypertension. This illustration of intraventricular pressure measurements shows that this is certainly not always the case. (From Johnston I, Paterson A: Benign intracranial hypertension II. CSF pressure and circulation. Brain 97:301, 1974. By permission of Oxford University Press.)

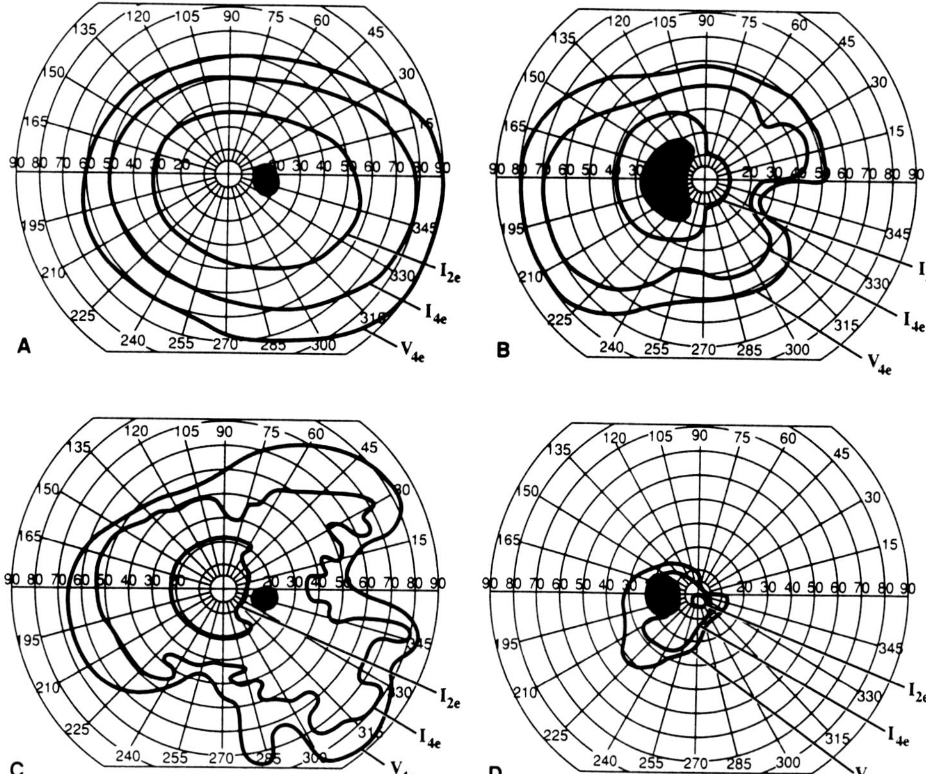

Figure 214–2. Typical visual field disturbances include (*A*) enlargement of the blind spot (a refractive scotoma); (*B*) nasal inferior (and less commonly, superior) quadrantic defects; (*C*) occasional temporal wedge defects; and (*D*) generalized constriction with preserved visual acuity.

adequate, because blind spot enlargement is largely refractive and can be seen in conditions unrelated to increased CSF pressure.[20]

RELATIVE AFFERENT PUPILLARY DEFECT (RAPD)

Asymmetries in afferent pupil function can alert a clinician to visual field loss that may not be recognized otherwise. The depth of the relative afferent pupillary defect (measured in log units with neutral density filters) is roughly proportional to the area of visual field lost.[21] Measurement of the RAPD provides objective evidence (but not an absolute measure) of asymmetric loss of visual field.

VISUAL ACUITY

Visual acuity is the least sensitive clinical measure of visual function in IIH. By the time serious changes in visual acuity occur, the disease is likely to have caused damage to the papillomacular bundle or collapse of the entire visual field. Disc swelling due to axoplasmic stasis causes loss of visual acuity by segmental anterior ischemic optic neuropathy,[13, 14] subretinal hemorrhage,[16] and macular changes secondary to hard exudates.[15] Occasionally, as if all of these were not bad enough, functional visual loss confounds the assessment of visual dysfunction in patients with IIH.[3] These patients make visual acuity and visual field testing unreliable indices of visual function. Such patients should probably have optic nerve sheath fenestration to be sure that visual loss does not occur.

FUNDUS PHOTOGRAPHY

Fundus photographs are widely available, and they provide graphic evidence of the clinical course of papilledema. They provide objective evidence of the efficacy of any treatment regimen. Photos are more accurate than memory (which serves everyone badly), verbal description, or even clinical drawings, which are usually too crude to be truly useful. Signs that may herald new visual deterioration, such as the appearance of multiple infarcts in the optic nerve fiber layer, subretinal or dot and blot hemorrhages, or new optociliary collateral veins, can be easily detected photographically. The fundus appearance from case to case is quite varied. Even in the same individual, papilledema may persist with gradual change over many years (Fig. 214–3). There is no pathognomonic ophthalmoscopic hallmark of papilledema caused by IIH that firmly sets it apart in appearance from other causes of optic disc swelling.

LABORATORY STUDIES

Lumbar puncture is mandatory for all patients suspected of having IIH. The diagnosis depends on demonstration of elevated CSF pressure (>250 mm H_2O) (Figs. 214–4 and 214–5).[22] Given the significance of this finding, a normal pressure measurement on the first spinal tap demands a second spinal tap before IIH can be ruled out. Rarely, continuous intracranial bolt monitoring is needed to establish the diagnosis firmly (Fig. 214–6).[1, 22] Although lumbar puncture is occasionally helpful in relieving headache, repeated lumbar puncture

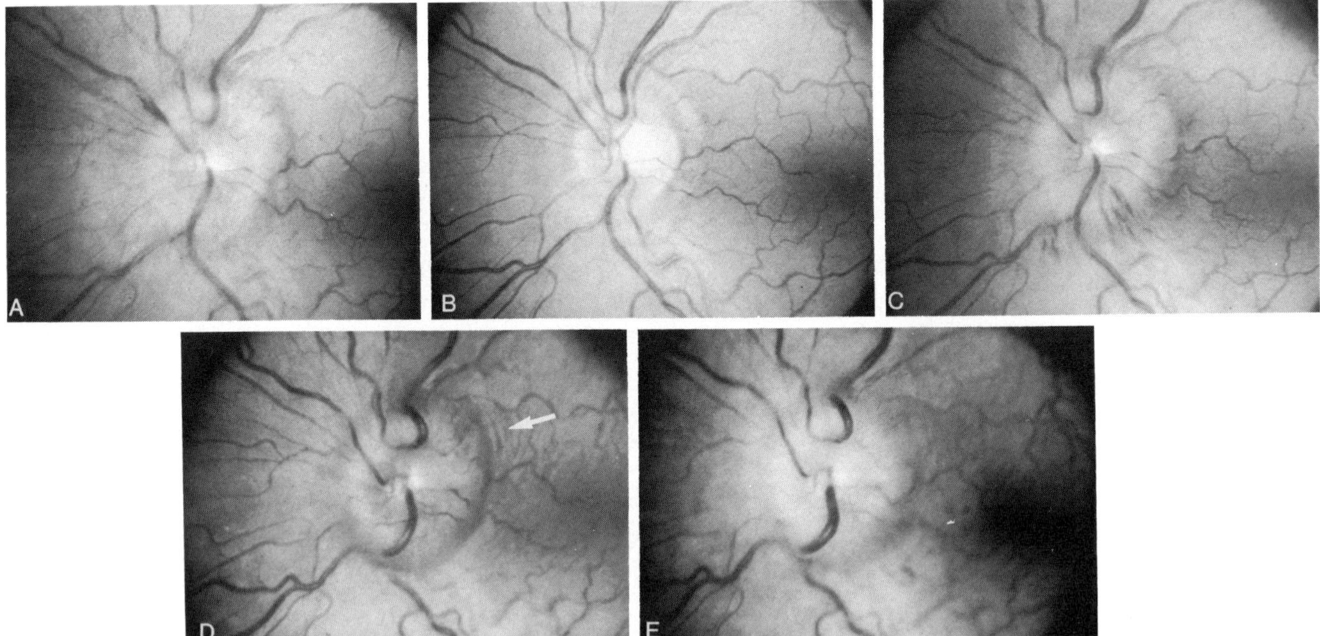

Figure 214–3. *A,* Obese 25-year-old woman with headaches and transient visual obscurations. Intracranial pressure never measured less than 550 mm H_2O. Treated with dexamethasone and acetazolamide with rapid resolution of headache and papilledema. *B,* Enlarged cup, preserved neuroretinal rim, and slight residual peripapillary swelling. *C,* Off the steroids and acetazolamide a month, papilledema returns. Steroids restarted but not acetazolamide because of gastrointestinal upset. *D,* Intraocular pressure rises to 26 to 28 mmHg; on repeated examination, visual field begins to constrict inferiorly and superiorly. The visual field was previously full. Peripapillary folds, which may be observed in instances of chronic swelling of the optic nerve head, are subtly visible. *E,* Within 2 months of restarting treatment, disc pallor denotes ischemic and compressive changes. Visual field strikingly and permanently constricted.

pressure measurements vary too much from hour to hour to help a physician make rational treatment decisions in IIH.[23] CSF must also be studied to rule out inflammation, tumor cells, and infection. In general, the CSF from patients with IIH contains normal or low protein (less than 20 mg/dl), normal glucose levels, and a normal cell count.

An extensive laboratory work-up is not indicated for most IIH patients, but some tests should always be performed. These include antinuclear antibody, Venereal Disease Research Laboratory testing, fluorescent treponemal antibody absorption, and serum calcium determinations to rule out hypoparathyroidism. Other endocrine studies are useful only if adrenal disease or hypoparathyroidism is seriously suspected.

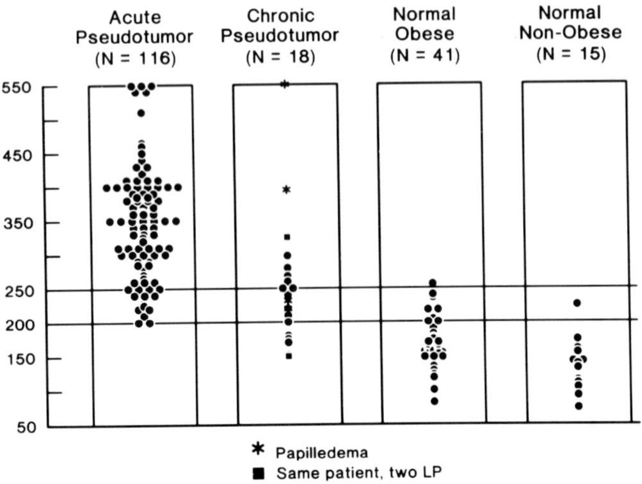

Figure 214–4. The pressures of patients with acute and chronic pseudotumor were statistically indistinguishable from one another. The pressures of normal obese and nonobese patients were statistically indistinguishable from each other but were significantly lower than those in the chronic or acute pseudotumor groups.

IMAGING TECHNIQUES

CT and MRI have largely replaced arteriography as the diagnostic tools in IIH. The ventricles are not

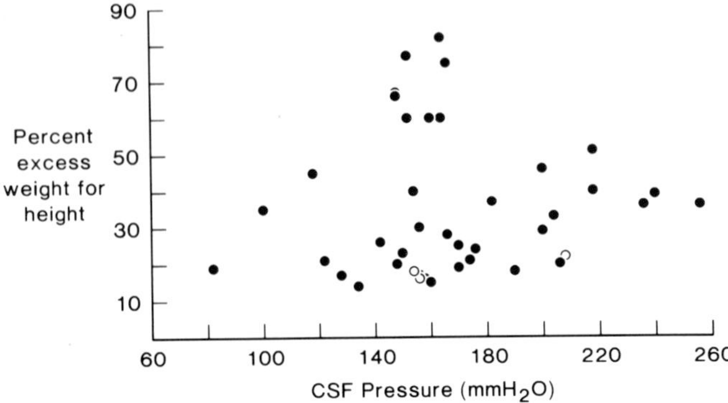

Figure 214–5. Scatter dot diagram showing the relationship of obesity to cerebrospinal fluid pressure. The most obese patients had pressures clustered clearly in the 140 to 160 mm H_2O (normal) range, whereas the highest pressures occurred in patients who were half as heavy as the most obese.

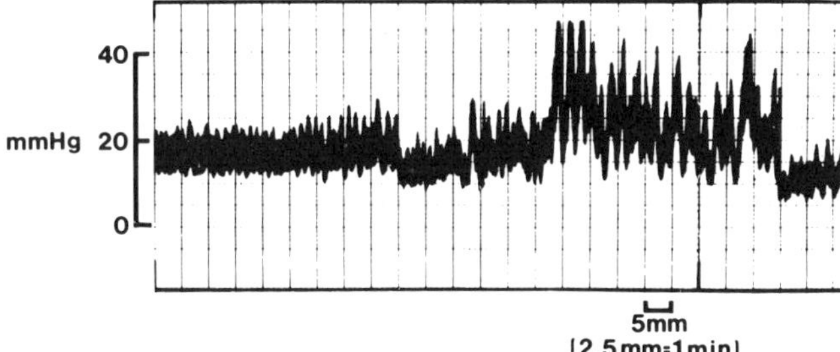

Figure 214–6. Continuous intracranial (subarachnoid bolt) cerebrospinal (CSF) pressure monitoring showing borderline elevation of CSF pressure with burst of high pressure waves. This patient had monocular papilledema, visual field loss, and normal CSF pressure on two spinal taps.

enlarged. Slitlike ventricles are not a useful sign to discriminate between normal persons and those with IIH.[24] Many patients have an empty sella turcica, which serves as indirect evidence that CSF pressure has been chronically elevated at least 6 months. Both MRI and CT are effective ways to screen for other possible causes of symptomatic intracranial hypertension such as tumor and hydrocephalus, and both can detect a sagittal or lateral sinus thrombosis (Figs. 214–7 and 214–8).

MRI provides the safest and least invasive tool for detecting venous sinus occlusions and underlying masses. However, if a patient is very obese, MRI may be limited by claustrophobia, space, or weight restrictions. Angiography is definitive for demonstrating a venous sinus obstruction, and MRI occasionally fails. Magnetic resonance angiography is a promising noninvasive vascular technique.

VISUAL EVOKED POTENTIAL

Flash and pattern visual evoked potentials (VEP) provide disappointingly little information about impending visual loss in IIH. Prolongation of VEP latency and central vision loss are among the last manifestations of visual loss due to papilledema. By the time the VEP is clearly abnormal, visual acuity is defective and permanent serious visual loss has usually occurred.[25]

SPECIFIC TREATMENT MODALITIES

Diet

Weight reduction should be suggested to all obese patients with IIH. Lowering caloric and sodium intake may be all that is therapeutically required for some asymptomatic patients. Because dieting is difficult for many people, weight programs should be prescribed with kindness and support, not "encouraged" by threats of blindness. Patients should be sent for professional dietary instruction, and some may benefit from commercial diet companies that support gradual weight loss. Vertical-banded gastroplasty and other bariatric operative procedures have been used with mixed success. Any

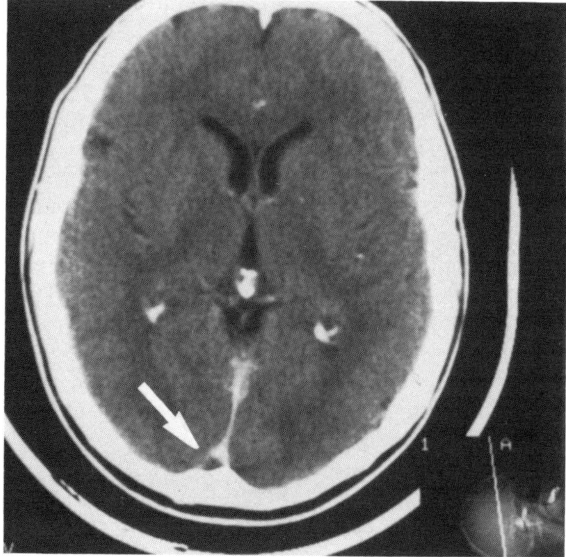

Figure 214–7. "Empty delta" sign in the superior sagittal sinus on computed tomography with contrast (*arrow*). The triangular dark spot denotes clot in the otherwise contrast-enhanced venous sinus.

surgical procedure poses the risk of intraoperative hypotension and ischemic damage to the swollen optic nerve heads.

Medication

When headache is the only symptom of IIH, treatment should be directed at its relief, preferably with standard headache remedies such as β-adrenergic blockers, calcium channel blockers, and nonsteroidal antiinflammatory drugs such as naproxen. Tricyclic antidepressants, although helpful for chronic headache, also stimulate

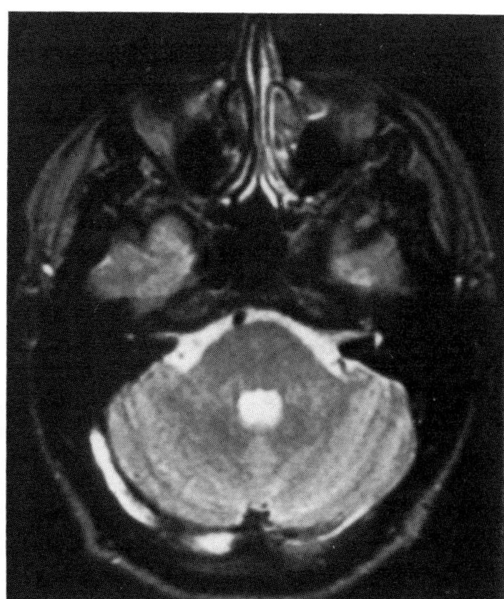

Figure 214–8. Transverse sinus occlusion in the same patient as Figure 214–7, seen well with magnetic resonance imaging (*arrow*).

appetite, and there is clearly a relationship between obesity and IIH.

Although carbonic anhydrase inhibitors such as acetazolamide have been used to treat IIH for years, their efficacy has never been studied prospectively in a randomized controlled clinical trial. Until such a trial is undertaken, the drugs of choice remain acetazolamide and furosemide. Acetazolamide, a strong carbonic anhydrase inhibitor, is prescribed at 1000 to 2000 mg daily (500 mg b.i.d. to q.i.d.). Furosemide is a weak carbonic anhydrase inhibitor and is prescribed at 40 to 160 mg/day (20 to 80 mg b.i.d.). Both acetazolamide and furosemide can decrease the frequency and severity of headaches and reduce the incidence of transient visual obscurations. Papilledema occasionally disappears completely with their use. Acetazolamide causes several side effects, including fatigue, nausea, anorexia, and tingling in the hands and feet and around the mouth. It also causes a mild metabolic acidosis (demonstrated by a serum bicarbonate level of 14 to 18 mEq/L) that does not require treatment and serves as an objective marker of patients' compliance. In rare instances, acetazolamide treatment may lead to renal stones, fatal hepatic dysfunction, and aplastic anemia. Potassium wasting occurs with both drugs, although it is more severe with furosemide, and patients may require substantial potassium replacement. Both drugs may be used for months to years.

Oral corticosteroids are often used and almost always are effective initially.[26, 27] When they are used in short courses of 2 to 6 weeks and tapered (a commonly advocated regimen), papilledema recurrence is the rule.[3] Prolonging corticosteroid treatment has obvious disadvantages. Weight gain, hair loss, acne, stretch marks, and a host of other more serious complications may occur. I personally do not use steroids for IIH; their efficacy is not clearly superior to acetazolamide or furosemide, and the side effects frequently add to patients' already low self-esteem.

Repeated Lumbar Punctures

Frequent lumbar punctures can be used for relief of headache, and some patients who respond favorably to the procedure return and request it. Unfortunately, spinal taps repeatedly performed have several drawbacks. They are painful and can be difficult to perform, especially in obese patients.

Anticipation of a painful procedure can lead to poor compliance by patients. Patients occasionally develop post–lumbar puncture headache and may need a blood patch. It is likely that individuals who benefit from repeated taps do so because CSF continues to leak from multiple needle holes in the lumbar theca. These holes may simulate a lumbar peritoneal shunt. Spinal epidermoid tumors may be the end result of repeated lumbar punctures, but this conclusion is not intuitive because the tumors may appear many years later.[28]

Surgery

Surgery is the treatment of choice for patients who are losing vision or, less commonly, for those who have severe headaches that do not respond to medication. Ordinarily, when a patient complains of visual field loss or diminished visual acuity or when a new visual field defect is discovered or a preexisting visual field abnormality enlarges, surgery should be performed without delay. Early intervention is the most effective way of arresting or reversing visual decline. Macular edema may cause decreased visual acuity, but it is risky to make that call and simply wait for improvement.

The indications for surgery in patients with IIH are as follows:

1. Development of a new visual field defect
2. Enlargement of a previously existing field defect
3. Presence of severe visual loss in one or both eyes at the time of first examination
4. Anticipated hypotension induced by treatment of high blood pressure or renal dialysis
5. Psychosocial reasons such as a patient's inability to perform visual field studies, noncompliance with medical treatment, an itinerant lifestyle, or a functional component to the presentation.
6. Headache unresponsive to standard headache nostrums.

SURGERY FOR VISUAL LOSS

The preferred surgical procedure is optic nerve sheath fenestration.[29–31] Done before vision is badly affected, this procedure effectively preserves or restores vision in 80 to 90 percent of patients. In this procedure, the surgeon makes a window or multiple incisions in the normally bulbous anterior dural covering of the optic nerve sheath using either a medial or lateral approach (Fig. 214–9). Although the mechanism of improvement has not been demonstrated conclusively, it appears that an outlet for continuous CSF drainage is created. As a result, the high CSF pressure no longer distends the sheath, and axoplasmic flow in the optic nerve is restored. Optic disc swelling cannot be sustained in the absence of a pressure differential.

SURGERY FOR HEADACHE

Before any surgery is recommended as a treatment for IIH-induced headache, heroic efforts should be made to relieve headache with usual antimigraine medications. Lumbar peritoneal shunt is an effective surgical method for relieving headaches due to IIH.[32] It has many complications and cannot be recommended for any patient who may require subsequent abdominal surgery (e.g., renal transplantation). Unfortunately, reoperation after lumbar peritoneal shunt is almost the rule, and the propensity for delayed and unrecognized shunt failure makes it particularly treacherous.[33] Shunts require careful long-term neurosurgical follow-up because shunt failure can occur 5 or more years after placement. Because IIH is most often a chronic condition, shunt failure can lead to abrupt return of papilledema and rapid visual failure. Optic nerve sheath fenestration is also effective in relieving headache in some patients; however, it is less reliable (60 to 65 percent) for this purpose than for preserving vision.[29–31]

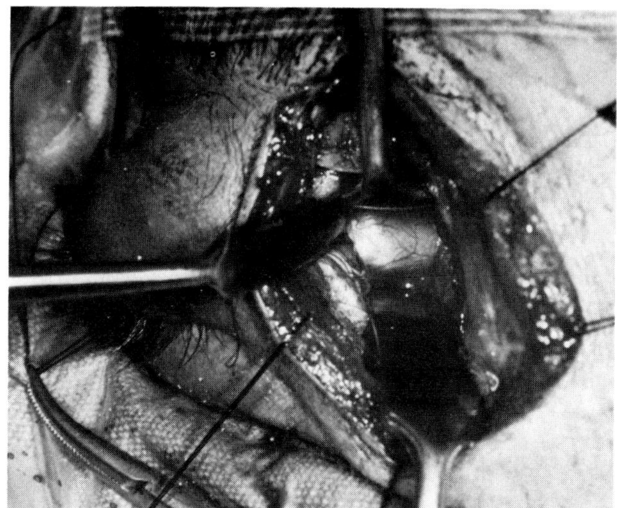

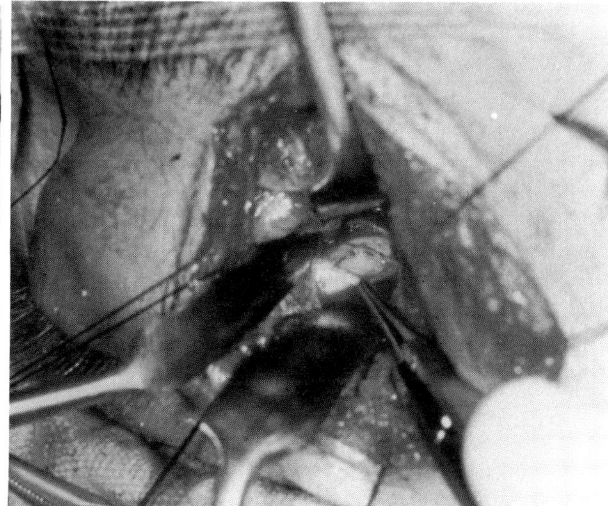

Figure 214–9. *A*, Optic nerve sheath visualized through a lateral orbitotomy. Before fenestration. *B*, Optic nerve sheath after 5 × 5-mm excision of dura and arachnoid (*arrow*). (Courtesy of Jeff Nerad, M.D.)

SPECIFIC TREATMENT PROBLEMS

Asymptomatic Patients

Asymptomatic patients who have no visual symptoms or visual loss and who were discovered incidentally to have IIH do not need to be treated. Patients like this should be monitored by an ophthalmologist in conjunction with a neurologist for at least 3 to 6 months. If visual problems appear, drug therapy should be initiated, preferably with acetazolamide or furosemide. Consider surgery if visual loss appears or progresses after medical treatment.

Headache

Patients whose primary clinical complaint is headache and whose vision loss is slight should be treated with standard medications for migraine headache. Patients with severe or persistent headaches may respond to lumbar puncture. The subgroup of patients with headache and high CSF pressure but no disc swelling are not at risk for visual loss.[10]

Serious Visual Loss

In patients who have serious loss of vision (such as diminished acuity or a progressive visual field defect), optic nerve sheath fenestration surgery should be performed before there is further visual decline, especially if a patient complains that visual loss was an early symptom. No single drug or combination of drugs has been proved effective in randomized prospective trials to prevent progressive visual loss, and no single or combination drug regimen has been proved more effective than any other. Therefore, patients with progressive visual loss should not be subjected to a long series of pharmacologic combinations and permutations before surgery is undertaken.

Surgical intervention is not a panacea, however. For patients with long-standing visual loss, atrophic discs, or rapid visual loss, even surgery cannot always recoup vision or prevent blindness. Careful documentation of a patient's visual acuity and visual fields, as well as fundus photographs of the optic disc during the course of treatment, is especially helpful in patients with serious vision defects and permanent visual defects, because patients may believe or allege that their treatment actually caused the visual loss.

Rapidly Progressive Visual Loss

Patients with rapidly progressive visual loss due to IIH are rare. Such patients are most commonly black men with systemic hypertension. Although their presenting symptoms may superficially resemble hypertensive encephalopathy, these patients do not have the rapid evolution of focal and generalized neurologic findings (e.g., altered consciousness and seizures) characteristic of this condition. Patients with this "hyperacute" or "malignant" form of IIH continue to pose a serious treatment challenge.

Occasional patients with the constellation of IIH, severe systemic hypertension, and rapid visual loss have lost vision to total blindness within a few days; others lose their vision despite rapid and aggressive treatment. Prompt treatment should be undertaken, preferably with optic nerve sheath fenestration or lumbar peritoneal shunt and the vigorous use of medications to reduce CSF production. Of special importance, however, is the management of elevated blood pressure; it should not be too vigorous until papilledema has subsided. Drastically lowering the mean arterial blood pressure may cause optic disc infarction.

Pregnancy and Headaches

Pregnant patients with severe headaches can be managed with relatively safe treatments during pregnancy, such as repeated lumbar puncture and β-adrenergic blockers. If headache is incapacitating, bedrest, narcotics, and lumbar peritoneal shunt as a last resort may be considered. If visual loss occurs during pregnancy, optic nerve fenestration is the safest way to preserve vision. IIH during pregnancy is not an indication for therapeutic abortion, and therapeutic abortion will not preserve vision.[34]

Renal Disease

Patients who have IIH and renal disease and who require hemodialysis may experience recurrent reductions in blood pressure and transient periods of severely elevated intracranial pressure due to shifts in fluid volume. Optic nerve sheath fenestration is the safest way to preserve vision if a patient with IIH must undergo hemodialysis.

PROGNOSIS

Once diagnosed, IIH runs a highly variable course; most cases last a year or longer. Occasional patients have short-lived episodes that resolve within months, but for many the condition lingers for years. Even in the absence of disc swelling, 75 to 80 percent of patients with IIH continue to demonstrate abnormal CSF pressure for a prolonged period.[3] The condition recurs in about 10 percent of patients and may reappear from weeks to many years after the initial symptoms.

REFERENCES

1. Corbett JJ: Problems in the diagnosis and treatment of pseudotumor cerebri. Can J Neurol 10:221, 1983.
2. Durcan J, Corbett JJ, Wall M: The incidence of pseudotumor cerebri: Population studies in Iowa and Louisiana. Arch Neurol 45:875, 1988.
3. Corbett JJ, Savino PJ, Thompson HS, et al: Visual loss in pseudotumor cerebri: Follow-up of 57 patients from five to 41 years and a profile of 14 patients with permanent severe visual loss. Arch Neurol 39:461, 1982.
4. Orcutt JC, Page NG, Sanders MD: Factors affecting visual loss in benign intracranial hypertension. Ophthalmology 91:1303, 1984.
5. Giuseffi V, Wall M, Siegal PZ, Rojas PB: Symptoms and disease associations in idiopathic intracranial hypertension (pseudotumor cerebri): A case-control study. Neurology 41:239, 1991.
6. Maxner CE, Freedman MI, Corbett JJ: Asymmetric papilledema and visual loss in pseudotumor cerebri. Can J Neurol Sci 14:593, 1987.
7. Lessell S, Rosman NP: Permanent visual impairment in childhood pseudotumor cerebri. Arch Neurol 43:801, 1986.
8. Wall M, George D: Visual loss in pseudotumor cerebri: Incidence and defects related to visual field strategy. Arch Neurol 44:170, 1987.
9. Meador CK: The art and science of nondisease. N Engl J Med 272:92, 1965.
10. Marcelis J, Siberstein SD: Idiopathic intracranial hypertension without papilledema. Arch Neurol 48:392, 1991.
11. Solomon SK, Wisoff H, Thorpy M: Symptoms of vascular headache triggered by intracranial hypertension. Headache 23:307, 1983.
12. Johnston I, Paterson A: Benign intracranial hypertension. II: CSF pressure and circulation. Brain 97:301, 1974.
13. Troost BT, Sufit RL, Grand MG: Sudden monocular visual loss in pseudotumor cerebri. Arch Neurol 36:440, 1979.
14. Green GJ, Lessell S, Loewenstein J: Ischemic optic neuropathy in chronic papilledema. Arch Ophthalmol 98:502, 1980.
15. Morris AT, Sanders MD: Macular changes resulting from papilledema. Br J Ophthalmol 64:211, 1980.
16. Morse PH, Leveille AS, Antel JP, et al: Bilateral juxtapapillary subretinal neovascularization associated with pseudotumor cerebri. Am J Ophthalmol 91:312, 1981.
17. Hayreh SS: Optic disc edema in raised intracranial pressure. VI: Associated visual disturbances and their pathogenesis. Arch Ophthalmol 95:1566, 1977.
18. Wall M, George D: Idiopathic intracranial hypertension: A prospective study of 50 patients. Brain 114:155, 1991.
19. Quigley HA, Addicks EM, Green WR: Optic nerve damage in human glaucoma. III: Quantitative correlation of nerve fiber layer loss and visual field defect in glaucoma, ischemic neuropathy, papilledema, and toxic neuropathy. Arch Ophthalmol 100:135, 1982.
20. Corbett JJ, Jacobson DM, Mauer RC, Thompson HS: Enlargement of blind spot caused by papilledema. Am J Ophthalmol 105:261, 1988.
21. Thompson HS, Montague P, Cox TA, Corbett JJ: The relationship between visual acuity, pupillary defect, and visual field loss. Am J Ophthalmol 93:681, 1982.
22. Corbett JJ, Mehta MP: Cerebrospinal fluid pressure in normal obese subjects and patients with pseudotumor cerebri. Neurology 33:1386, 1983.
23. Corbett JJ, Thompson HS: The rational management of idiopathic intracranial hypertension. Arch Neurol 46:1049, 1989.
24. Jacobson DM, Karanjia PN, Olson KA, Warner JJ: Computed tomography ventricular size has no predictive value in diagnosing pseudotumor cerebri. Neurology 40:1454, 1990.
25. Verplanck M, Kaufman DI, Parsons T, et al: Electrophysiology versus psychophysics in the detection of visual loss in pseudotumor cerebri. Neurology 38:1789, 1988.
26. Weisberg LA: Benign intracranial hypertension. Medicine 54:197, 1975.
27. Ahlskog JE, O'Neill BP: Pseudotumor cerebri. Ann Intern Med 97:249, 1982.
28. Batnitzky S, Keucher TR, Mealey J Jr, Campbell RL: Iatrogenic intraspinal epidermoid tumors. JAMA 237:148, 1977.
29. Corbett JJ, Nerad JA, Tse DT, et al: Results of optic nerve sheath fenestration for pseudotumor cerebri: The lateral orbitotomy approach. Arch Ophthalmol 106:1391, 1988.
30. Brourman ND, Spoor TC, Ramocki JM: Optic nerve sheath decompression for pseudotumor cerebri. Arch Ophthalmol 106:1378, 1988.
31. Sergott RC, Savino PJ, Bosley TM: Modified optic nerve sheath decompression provides long-term visual improvement for pseudotumor cerebri. Arch Ophthalmol 106:1384, 1988.
32. Johnston I, Besser M, Morgan MK: Cerebrospinal fluid diversion in the treatment of benign intracranial hypertension. J Neurosurg 69:195, 1988.
33. Repka MX, Miller NR, Savino PJ: Pseudotumor cerebri. Am J Ophthalmol 98:741, 1984.
34. Digre KB, Varner MW, Corbett JJ: Pseudotumor cerebri and pregnancy. Neurology 34:731, 1984.

Chapter 215

Nonorganic Visual Disorders

ROBERT S. HEPLER

A major problem in the practice of ophthalmology is the diagnosis and management of nonorganic visual disorders. This term describes visual symptoms (and sometimes signs) for which no organic disease can be identified as or reasonably theorized to be the cause. Less desirable terms commonly used in association with these disorders include hysteria, malingering, and psychosomatic and functional visual loss.

This subject is important in terms of frequency of occurrence, diagnostic difficulty for the physician, and cost to the patient and to society.[1] With regard to frequency, good data are not readily available; clinical experience would suggest that any reported frequency is probably understated when one includes not only impressive cases that used to be termed hysterical blindness and flagrant malingering but also the numerous patients with lesser manifestations of visual system complaints that would perhaps disappear if they could reduce stress in their lives. Societal trends toward increased litiginousness can be expected to increase the number of patients who report imaginary or magnified injuries to all physicians, including ophthalmologists. While some subspecialties (e.g., neuroophthalmology) will see more nonorganic patients than other subspecialties, even physicians dealing primarily with organic disease must be alert to nonorganic elaboration of physical symptoms and work out strategies for detecting and managing such patients.

This chapter emphasizes the complaint of nonorganic visual loss—most often noted in terms of central acuity, but sometimes involving peripheral field loss—but also reviews two ocular movement entities categorized as voluntary nystagmus and spasm of the near reflex. Also worthy of mention is Munchausen's syndrome, which occurs infrequently but tends to involve serious disturbance of function that is likely to be misinterpreted.

MANIFESTATIONS OF NONORGANIC VISUAL DISORDERS

As is the case with many medical disturbances, nonorganic visual disorders can present themselves in any number of ways. A partial list of some of the most common manifestations seen by this author follows.

Visual Loss

Case Report. A 7-year-old boy was evaluated urgently because of severe visual loss in the left eye, which occurred as he was playing ball with his older brother 24 hr earlier. The precise moment of visual loss occurred as he was trying (unsuccessfully) to catch a particularly fast ball. His pediatrician diagnosed migraine, as did the family ophthalmologist, who recorded visual acuity at finger counting in the involved eye. When vision did not return by morning, the patient was referred to a retina specialist who immediately performed fluorescein angiography. With loss of vision still unexplained, a magnetic resonance imaging (MRI) scan was performed, and arrangements were made for the patient to have a neurologic examination the following day. The extremely anxious parents took the patient for a neuroophthalmologic examination.

Visual acuity was recorded at 20/30 OD; light perception was OS. Light was equally bright in both eyes, and there was no afferent pupillary defect. Using the vertical prism test (described later in this chapter), the acuity was recordable at 20/60 OU. He correctly identified 3/9 stereo targets. On four-dot testing he indicated initially that he could not count any lights (with either eye!), then he reported seeing varying numbers of red, green, and yellow lights.

All other aspects of ophthalmic examination were normal. The patient and his parents were informed that his was a common type of visual disturbance in children and that it was very likely to resolve, without need for further testing. One month later, reexamination was entirely normal.

Comment. There was no indication that nonorganic visual loss entered into the differential diagnosis of the pediatrician, general ophthalmologist, or retina consultant—despite the clear discrepancies between symptoms and physical findings.

Patients who report reduced vision in one eye that cannot be correlated with relative afferent pupillary defect or fundus abnormalities are relatively easily detected—provided that the physician entertains the possibility of nonorganic visual loss. The problem most often lies primarily in not considering this diagnosis or in suspecting the diagnosis but not having readily at hand the skill and experience necessary to perform a few simple testing maneuvers that would conclusively identify the nature of the disorder. This is particularly unfortunate if the ophthalmologist handles this kind of case by initiating neuroimaging and neurologic consultation, because these steps will start a futile, expensive assessment that only serves to confuse the issue. It is not reasonable to hope that a neurologist will be better able than an ophthalmologist to make the correct diagnosis of nonorganic visual loss. Testing maneuvers (discussed at length below) rely heavily on observations of pupillary reactions, visual field testing, and techniques that, unknown to the patient, cause him to see with one eye when he thinks (perhaps subconsciously) that he is using the other.

It is fortunate for the physician that most patients complaining of nonorganic visual loss do so in only one eye, because our testing procedures are simple and effective in this case. Some patients, however, report mild-to-moderate visual loss in both eyes equally. The experienced clinician recognizes the patient complaining of reduction in vision to the range of 20/50 to 20/100 in both eyes as a tougher subject, because tricks to dissociate the two eyes clearly are not effective here and because overall visual function is still good enough to make the results of other tests unimpressive or nonapplicable (e.g., opticokinetic nystagmus, avoidance of objects, and face-in-the-mirror responses).

Apparent visual field abnormalities are frequently asymptomatic in patients who have other visual symptoms, such as central visual loss, particularly after mild trauma. This makes it important to deliberately test the person who claims to have reduced central vision, not just for best-refracted Snellen acuity but also for visual field function. Even though the patient may not report symptoms of peripheral visual field loss, his or her abnormal responses to peripheral field testing often gives valuable clues. Diffuse peripheral constriction, or patchy depression of sensitivity throughout the field when tested by automated perimetry, may be misinterpreted as reflecting disease when testing results have reasonably high false-negative and false-positive scores.

Some patients present complaining of impaired peripheral vision, most often "to the side" of an eye exposed to trauma. Even intelligent patients in this case are likely to be confused between monocular and homonymous field disturbance, and they may well give peculiar responses when testing first one eye, then the other, then both eyes together—creating a pattern unexplainable on an organic basis.[2]

The value of a *physician-performed* tangent screen examination cannot be overemphasized. It allows observation and encouragement of the patient, which help in the process of the assessment by yielding much more definitive contradictions in results than do those given by computerized printouts, which are difficult to interpret in patients with nonorganic problems.

Altered Motility

Voluntary nystagmus is the most frequently encountered nonorganic eye movement disorder. In fact, it isn't even necessarily a disorder, because many people are well aware of their own ability to perform this maneuver and may do it for no more sinister reason than to amuse (or bother) their friends. The same young person who knows how to do this may, however, in time of war deliberately confuse a physician in order to avoid the draft. Voluntary nystagmus usually requires convergence effort to initiate and sustain the movement. It is characterized by fast, low-amplitude pendular motions that are horizontal and conjugate. It takes effort to maintain these movements, and thus they are usually sustainable for only a few seconds at a time. Although they are almost always bilateral, Blair and associates reported two unilateral cases.[3] Since convergence mechanisms are involved, one should anticipate seeing significant pupillary miosis and accommodative changes while the process is occurring.

Spasm of the near reflex, elegantly described by Cogan and Freese in 1955,[4] is another perversion of the near synkineses but is less likely to be exhibited consciously compared with voluntary nystagmus. Spasm of the near reflex presents as an impressive acquired esotropia and is often said by the patient to have started after minor head trauma. It mimics bilateral VI paresis, which has fooled many clinicians into ordering neuroimaging and other studies. I recall a young woman who bumped her head in a minor car accident in the pre–computed tomography (CT) scanning era who presented with headache, blurred vision, and esotropia. These symptoms were misinterpreted in an emergency room as reflecting acute bilateral VI paresis. She promptly received bilateral burr hole taps by neurosurgeons who were looking for subdural hematomas. Fortunately, this is unlikely in the era of modern neuroimaging, but initial misdiagnosis of spasm of the near reflex is still more common than correct diagnosis.

Diagnosis of spasm of the near reflex begins with suspicion when presented with an otherwise healthy individual who has sudden bilateral onset of esotropia, pupillary miosis, and complaint of blurred vision. Confirmation of the diagnosis is established by examining visual acuity, eye movement, and pupillary size *under monocular conditions*. The previously apparent esotropia, miosis, and accommodative myopia disappear as if by magic when one eye at a time is tested. Treatment consists of reassurance, sometimes aided by temporary use of cycloplegic ophthalmic drops to impede the near synkineses.

Munchausen's Syndrome

Although infrequently encountered, the elaborate deceptions characteristic of Munchausen's syndrome are often very confusing to physicians, whose training and daily experience foster the belief that patients wish to get well and to minimize their own suffering. Such presumptions are false in the case of patients with Munchausen's syndrome. These patients present with contrived histories and even self-induced physical abnormalities. Patients' awareness of what they are doing varies from those who know full well what is going on, whose maneuvers are clearly related to secondary gain (e.g., patients seeking controlled substances) to those whose Munchausen's syndrome behavior reflects psychiatric disease. When evaluation of a patient discloses symptoms or signs that are difficult to explain by any known pathogenetic mechanism, it is wise to remember the existence of Munchausen's syndrome and to think about the patient's alleged medical problems from that perspective. If possible to identify other hospitals or physicians who have been involved in the patient's care, confirmation of Munchausen's syndrome may be supported.[5]

A relatively simple form of physician deception involves the patient who presents with a fixed, dilated pupil. This may occur innocently or may reflect deliberate manipulation. When deliberate, the patient is particularly likely to be someone who works in a medical environment with access to dilating drops. Presuming that there are no other objective signs of neurologic dysfunction—only the fixed, dilated pupils—it is good to test with miotic drops (which constrict the pupil involved in a true cranial nerve III palsy while leaving the pharmacologically blocked pupil dilated) before proceeding with expensive neuroimaging. Thompson and associates recommend using 0.5 percent pilocarpine solution to avoid getting a false-positive response in cases of incomplete atropinic mydriasis.[5]

GENERAL APPROACH TO EVALUATION

Physicians sometimes feel frustrated or even angry when trying to cope with patients who are either elaborating on true organic illness or who have no organic illness at all. However, by following certain recommendations successful evaluation and management can be achieved. It is important to remember that it is rare for the patient to have as much knowledge as the physician, who should therefore be able to keep control of the situation and emerge with the correct diagnosis. Some general suggestions include:

1. Approach such patients with, if anything, *extra* thoroughness. One is not entitled to take any shortcuts in the evaluation of this type of patient. Remember that coexistence of organic dysfunction with nonorganic elaboration is frequent, and the physician must attempt to separate the two. This cannot be done without a thorough review of the history and a complete ophthalmologic examination.
2. Approach the patient in a friendly, confident frame of mind. The patient is more likely to cooperate in giving the historical details and responses to testing that disclose nonorganic components if he or she perceives that the physician is supportive, interested in his or her welfare, and nonhostile.
3. Place special emphasis on skillful refraction, pupillary testing, and visual field testing in all cases, even when the presenting symptoms do not implicate visual field complaints. If given an opportunity, nonorganic patients frequently show nonorganic responses to field testing, which is most effectively performed by the physician at the tangent screen.

Useful Confirmatory Tests

Every neuroophthalmologist has his or her favorite maneuvers to demonstrate nonorganic visual loss—the list of potential clinical tests is extensive.[7–9] In practical application, what is important is for each clinician to have at least a few techniques that he or she has practiced sufficiently to allow skillfull and confident clinical application. I have found the following to be particularly useful.

Pupil Testing. The most common nonorganic visual symptom is monocular impairment of acuity. Particularly in this circumstance, the examiner must be skillful in looking for minimal afferent pupillary defects (e.g., swinging flashlight test, Marcus Gunn pupil). The light source must be bright, but not too bright. Advice at one time to use an indirect ophthalmoscopy light turned to a maximal setting is not good because of the photophobic response that it will generate and the severe retinal bleaching that also occurs. Remember that spurious afferent pupillary defects can seem to be present if asymmetry of stimulation is provided either by holding the light on one eye longer than the other or by examining a patient in whom unilateral dilatation with drops has allowed greater fundus illumination. If prior dilatation with drops or some other complicating factor seems to interfere with doing the swinging flashlight test, the patient can be asked to compare the brightness of light shown in the two eyes. The nonorganic patient often gives an inappropriate response, such as indicating that the light is much brighter in the eye with symptomatic visual reduction.[10]

The absence of correlation between claimed monocular visual loss and the occurrence of an afferent pupillary defect is one of the most important initial indications of nonorganicity.

Visual Fields. The goal is to demonstrate discrepancies that cannot be explained on an organic basis, and this is usually not difficult to achieve. Often, for example, the patient has had quantitative perimetry that showed diffuse reduction in sensitivity or peripheral constriction—obviously without objective signs of glaucoma or retinitis pigmentosa. Quickly counting fingers in the periphery in all four quadrants of both eyes requires less than 1 min to accomplish and gives valuable information that is likely not to match the automated perimetry printout.

At the tangent screen use a large object, such as a standard 8 ½ × 11-in piece of office paper to determine the isopter at the conventional 1-m distance (Fig. 215–1). Then move the patient several meters away—neither the size of the object (so long as it is large) nor the precise distance is critical—and note the nonexpansion of the field (Fig. 215–2). Since nonorganic patients are likely to demonstrate field defects, and because they subconsciously seem to want to demonstrate consistency, one can "help" them to do this by marking the tangent screen with a few black pins to assist them in remembering the isopter at 1 m while they are being tested at 3 m. More often than not, the isopters are the same regardless of distance from the screen.

Vertical Prism Test. With the patient's distance correction in place (if needed for best Snellen acuity), the examiner directs the patient to view the Snellen screen while the "bad" eye is occluded. An 8-diopter prism is placed base up over the "good" eye, with the prism

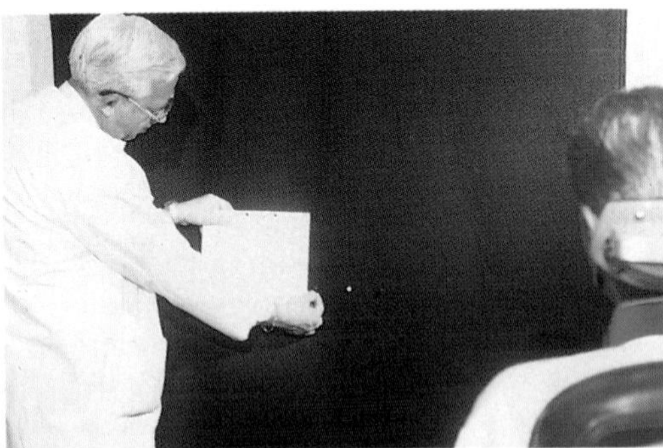

Figure 215–1. Tangent screen examination at 1 m, showing the constricted field.

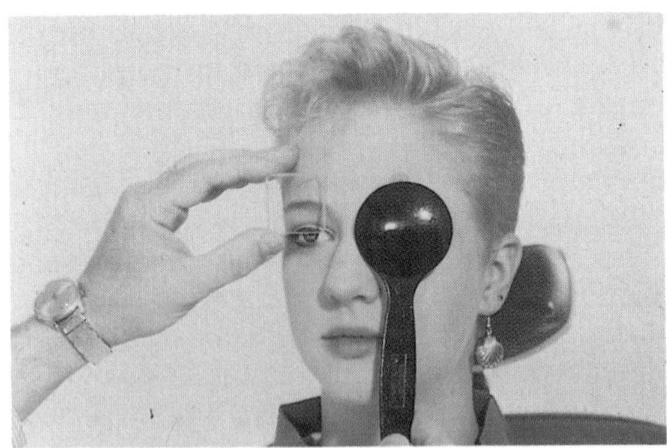

Figure 215–3. Prism-splitting fixation of the "better" eye.

edge transiently splitting the pupil (Fig. 215–3). One does not linger at this stage, but simply asks the patient whether he or she occasionally sees two charts, one above the other. The patient confirms that he or she does indeed see two charts, one above the other. The examiner than quietly moves the occluder away from the "bad" eye while simultaneously lowering the prism so that the "good" eye is now looking through the prism (Fig. 215–4). The patient now sees two charts, as he or she did a moment before, except that instead of seeing them monocularly as before, the patient is now seeing them binocularly. The examiner directs the patient to read the smallest print that he or she can see on the *bottom* chart, and then the smallest print that he or she can see on the *top* chart. Amazingly, an eye that was previously limited to 20/200 or worse acuity can now be demonstrated to see 20/20 (Figs. 215–5 and 215–6).

Magic Drop Test. After establishing a good rapport with the patient and an image of competence, the examiner indicates that he or she is going to do a test that involves some special eye drops and that these special eye drops dramatically, but temporarily, improve the vision "in cases like yours." With this setting of the stage the examiner excuses himself or herself long enough to go to an adjacent room, then the examiner returns with the special drops. The drops are actually something quite pedestrian, such as a topical anesthetic, but their nature is withheld by enclosing them in the examiner's hand—in case the patient might recognize the label as something that he or she has encountered in past examinations. The special drop is placed in the involved eye, and the patient is asked to read the Snellen chart with the distance correction and pinhole in a trial frame. Remarkably, thc previously impaired eye may see normally or near-normally.

In performing the magic drop test the patient is told that the improvement in vision is temporary, lasting only for the few minutes of the examination maneuver; this reassures patients who consciously or otherwise are not ready to give up their crutch permanently.

A surprising feature of both the vertical prism test and the magic drop test is that even intelligent, observant patients almost never detect the ruse that is being executed. I have never been accosted by someone who detected what was being done. Patients whose visual symptoms are consciously related to secondary gain are likely to be seen blinking and squinting, trying to figure out what they should be seeing in the vertical prism test, but even they often fall prey to the examiner's treachery. It should be acknowledged that neither the vertical prism test nor the magic drop test is infallible—there are patients who simply won't play the game! Even then, their responses may be revealing: with both eyes open during the vertical prism test, they may claim that they cannot see the chart at all, even though their "good" eye is open.

One of the most important benefits of these two tests is that they go beyond demonstrating nonorganic responses. They actually provide a measurement of the patient's true visual function when nonorganic elaboration has been removed. For instance, a patient with

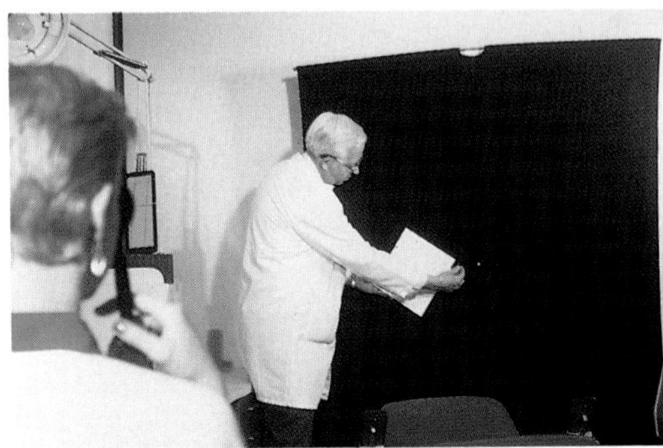

Figure 215–2. Tangent screen examination at 3 m, showing constriction identical to that seen in Figure 215–1.

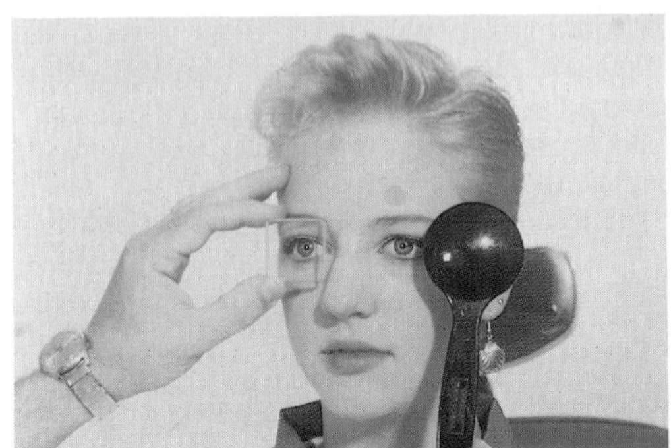

Figure 215–4. Both eyes uncovered and the prism lowered over the "better" eye.

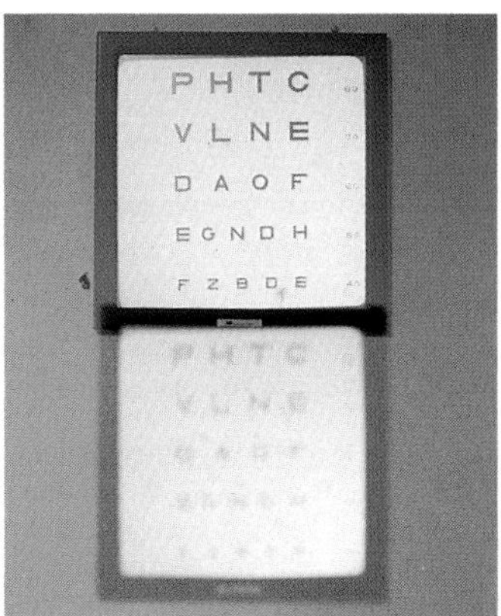

Figure 215–5. Photographic simulation of Snellen charts seen in the vertical prism test—one eye is pathologically blurred.

preexisting amblyopia ex anopsia reducing vision to 20/50, who is then injured in a traffic accident and claims to have no better than 20/200 as a result, can be demonstrated to retain his or her underlying 20/50.

This section deserves comment concerning the role of fluorescein angiography and visual evoked response (VER) testing. In the presence of normal fundus examination, it is *extremely* unlikely that fluorescein angiography will disclose an occult organic macular process that accounts for the patient's symptoms, particularly when the symptoms are monocular, and thus fluorescein angiography is very seldom helpful or indicated in the assessment of such cases.

VER testing, although seemingly logical in testing nonorganic patients, has proved in practice to be very disappointing and is actually used only occasionally by neuroophthalmologists. Reasons for the lack of success of VER in these cases include variability (and sometimes unreliability) in standardization of different VER laboratories, overinterpretation of minor variations, and voluntary alteration.[11] VER might be considered as one additional, *possibly* useful source of input in cases in which other testing has given ambiguous results, but only when the physician has reason to place confidence in the specific VER laboratory, and when the VER technician is appropriately alerted to watch for such maneuvers as deliberate closing of the eye being tested. Misinterpretation of VER has, unfortunately, befuddled the understanding of many a case of nonorganic visual loss.

MANAGEMENT AFTER NONORGANIC DYSFUNCTION HAS BEEN IDENTIFIED

Many issues of management have to do with what the patient (or referring physicians, attorneys, or claim examiners) are to be told. Clearly what is reported, and how it is presented, varies with the circumstances.

Having completed the thorough (and hopefully conclusive) clinical assessment, the physician must decide whether additional testing is still required. Fluorescein angiography and VER have been discussed earlier and are seldom useful adjuncts. Neuroimaging (CT or MRI scanning) often either have already been obtained by previous examiners or are not necessary when the nonorganic nature of the problem has been confirmed clinically. However, the physician must remember that patients who have nonorganic complaints or who elaborate their dysfunction do *occasionally* have a disease process, which may be detectable by CT or MR, that needs attention. If at all in doubt in this regard, it is better to order a scan than not to do so.

The next issue concerns the medical record. This should be completed with a detailed recording of the history and of the tests performed and their results. Having a meticulous record of the evaluation, the diagnostic impression is given next in terms of "nonorganic visual loss" (or spasm of the near reflex or some other impression). It is recommended that the following terms be avoided in verbal discussion and in written reports: hysteria; malingering; faking; crock; compensationitis; functional, conversion reaction. These terms tend either to be pejorative (which can lead to an angry patient acting out against the physician) or to imply a psychiatric evaluation. Most ophthalmologists would have difficulty establishing their credentials for the use of psychiatric terms, particularly in a court of law, and thus are better off to avoid them.

In writing reports in such cases, one useful approach is to record both the testing maneuvers performed and the results to provide an impression of "nonorganic visual loss" and then to conclude with the following statement under the heading "Comment": "It is not possible to account for the above findings on an organic basis." This concluding statement tells all who read it (e.g., attorneys, insurance carriers, other physicians) what is going on and avoids potentially embarrassing terminology.

What the patient is told at the conclusion of the evaluation varies with the circumstances. The patient seen under legal arrangements for an independent med-

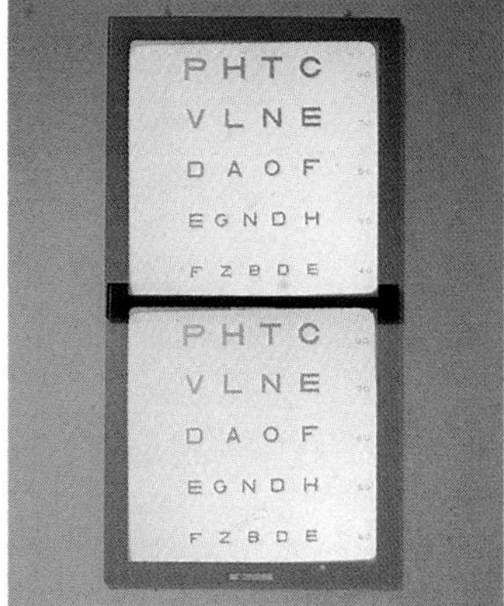

Figure 215–6. Photographic simulation in the vertical prism test—as seen in nonorganic visual loss.

ical examination need not (and in fact should not) be told anything about the evaluation. A friendly goodbye suffices. The physician does not get off the hook so easily when the patient is a child accompanied by understandably worried parents who may be particularly sensitive after having already spent thousands of dollars on scans and consultations. In the case of the patient who is a child—and this is very frequently the case—it is good to tell the patient that he or she has a common kind of visual problem, that it will get better on its own, and that it does not require more testing or painful examinations. This explanation to the child provides reassurance and has the additional benefit of being truthful. It is good to take the parents aside, by one means or another, to discuss the situation out of the child's earshot. Parents should leave the consultation realizing that children frequently react to stress (the origin may or may not be readily apparent) by having such symptoms, that they should think about situations at home or school to see whether there are problem areas that could be improved, that the child should not be punished for faking (because the child is really not aware of the mechanism of the visual disturbance), and that prompt recovery should be expected. The parents should also be informed that such visual disturbance does not generally indicate a need for psychiatric evaluation or care.[12–15] A follow-up examination by the referring physician in 6 to 8 wk is recommended to document the return of vision. Placebos (glasses, drops) are probably undesirable, because they tend to perpetuate the idea that there is something wrong that requires treatment.

REFERENCES

1. Keltner JL, May WN, Johnson CA, Post RB: The California syndrome: Functional visual complaints with potential economic impact. Ophthalmology 92:427, 1985.
2. Gittinger JW Jr: Functional monocular temporal hemianopsia. Am J Ophthalmol 101:226, 1986.
3. Blair CH, Goldberg MF, von Noorden GK: Voluntary nystagmus: Electro-oculographic findings in four cases. Arch Ophthalmol 77:349, 1967.
4. Cogan DG, Freese CG: Spasm of the near reflex. Arch Ophthalmol 73:752, 1955.
5. Rosenberg PN, Krohel GB, Webb RM, Hepler RS: Ocular Munchausen's syndrome. Ophthalmology 93:1120, 1986.
6. Thompson HS, Newsome DA, Loewenfeld IE: The fixed dilated pupil: Sudden iridoplegia or mydriatic drops? A simple diagnostic test. Arch Ophthalmol 86:21, 1971.
7. Smith CH, Beck RW, Mills RP: Functional disease in neuroophthalmology. Neurol Clin 1:955, 1983.
8. Kramer KK, La Piana FG, Appleton B: Ocular malingering and hysteria: Diagnosis and management. Surv Ophthalmol 24:89, 1979.
9. Keane JR: Neuro-ophthalmic signs and symptoms of hysteria. Neurology 32:757, 1982.
10. Thompson HS, Montague P, Cox TA, Corbett JJ: The relationship between visual acuity, pupillary defect, and visual field loss. Am J Ophthalmol 93:681, 1982.
11. Bumgartner J, Epstein CM: Voluntary alteration of visual evoked potentials. Ann Neurol 12:475, 1982.
12. Kathol RG, Cox TA, Corbett JJ, et al: Functional visual loss. I: A true psychiatric disorder? Psychol Med 13:307, 1983.
13. Kathol RG, Cox TA, Corbett JJ, et al: Functional visual loss. II: Psychiatric aspects in 42 patients followed for 4 years. Psychol Med 13:315, 1983.
14. Thompson HS: Functional visual loss. Am J Ophthalmol 100:209, 1985.
15. Kathol RG, Cox TA, Corbett JJ, Thompson HS: Functional visual loss: Follow-up of 42 cases. Arch Ophthalmol 101:729, 1983.

SECTION XII

Pediatric Ophthalmology

Edited by

RICHARD M. ROBB and DAVID S. WALTON

Chapter 216

Overview

RICHARD M. ROBB

Since the 1960s, pediatric ophthalmology has become an established subspecialty of ophthalmology in the United States. A young ophthalmologist wishing to specialize in pediatric ophthalmology can now choose among more than 30 postresidency fellowships available in the field. There are a number of recent textbooks devoted exclusively to the subject,[1–3] one in multiple volumes.[4] Therefore, in any comprehensive textbook of ophthalmology, pediatric ophthalmology must be represented. There are, however, conflicts between an anatomic or disease-oriented presentation of material and the segregation of subject matter according to age. In this section, there are discussions of the major eye problems that occur in childhood, even though their ramifications may extend into the adult years. Other eye diseases that may be present in childhood but have their major manifestations later or require treatment by other ophthalmic subspecialists are dealt with elsewhere. Some conditions are included in this section because they so clearly relate to the early development of the eye. Congenital nasolacrimal duct obstruction, optic nerve hypoplasia, and infantile glaucoma are among them. Ocular involvement in certain pediatric diseases is also considered, such as the iritis associated with juvenile rheumatoid arthritis, retinal involvement in the inherited cerebral lipidoses, and corneal opacification in the mucopolysaccharidoses. The ocular manifestations of childhood diabetes are discussed elsewhere because they mostly become apparent after the pediatric years.

The reader will quickly become aware of several themes that run through the following discussions of pediatric eye diseases. One is that *functional amblyopia* often compounds the visual loss of organic eye disease in pediatric patients. The threat of amblyopia often affects the nature and timing of treatment. This point is well illustrated by the current management of infantile cataracts. Amblyopia is also specifically considered in *Principles and Practice of Ophthalmology: Basic Sciences* (hereafter called *Basic Sciences*), Chapter 49. Another theme is the need to sort out *normal developmental changes* in eye structure and function from *pathologic changes* associated with disease. This need is especially apparent, for instance, when one is faced with the challenge of identifying possible retinal dysfunction in an infant whose visual development seems to be lagging. There is also a theme of the *difficulty of eye examinations* in preverbal and sometimes uncooperative children, whether one is attempting to test visual acuity, estimate an angle of strabismus, or measure the ocular pressure. Pediatric ophthalmologists often become quite skillful in obtaining diagnostic information under relatively unfavorable circumstances. A separate section on the examination of the pediatric patient has been included, and the reader is again referred to *Basic Sciences,* Chapter 42, for a discussion of methods of assessing early visual development.

A final theme is the tendency for pediatric ophthalmologists to be concerned with *early recognition and treatment* of children's eye problems. The advantages of early reversal of functional amblyopia associated with strabismus and of early rehabilitation of eyes with congenital monocular cataracts are obvious to all. It might be noted that there are also instances recounted on the following pages in which "earlier" is not necessarily better: Congenital nasolacrimal duct obstruction may resolve spontaneously without probing if given time, and the results of surgery for congenital blepharoptosis are often better if time is taken to assess the full development of levator function. The optimal timing for surgery to correct infantile esotropia may depend on specific features of the deviation. Still, in pediatric ophthalmology, one often has the opportunity for early restoration and long-term preservation of sight, and there is no gainsaying the satisfaction afforded by that kind of therapeutic intervention.

REFERENCES

1. Isenberg SJ: The Eye in Infancy. Chicago, Year Book Medical Publishers, 1989.
2. Taylor D: Pediatric Ophthalmology. London, Blackwell Scientific, 1990.
3. Nelson LB, Calhoun JH, Harley RD: Pediatric Ophthalmology, 3rd ed. Philadelphia, WB Saunders, 1991.
4. Harley RD: Pediatric Ophthalmology, 2nd ed. Philadelphia, WB Saunders, 1983.

Chapter 217

The Pediatric Eye Examination

CRAIG A. McKEOWN

Pediatric medical examinations present a number of unique challenges to the ophthalmologist, as well as to the pediatrician and family practitioner. There are significant and necessary differences between the design and function of adult and pediatric ophthalmology offices. Numerous pitfalls and problems exist with respect to eliciting and interpreting an accurate history from the child; therefore historical information is often obtained indirectly from adults. Children at various levels of development possess markedly different abilities to respond to clinical tests and display variable levels of cooperation, resulting in difficulties with subjective as well as objective examination techniques. A team approach to the pediatric patient is often helpful with respect to the systemic aspects of ophthalmic disorders and the potential effect of such abnormalities on the child's overall health and development.

With the exception of trauma, refractive error, and a few other disorders, ophthalmic disease tends to affect very young or elderly individuals. In many ophthalmology offices, the majority of patients represent a mature population, and waiting rooms tend to be places in which patients can read, converse quietly, or watch informative videotapes. This should be contrasted to a waiting room filled with young children, with the associated noise level and activity. Crying during and after eye drop administration, the need for diaper changes, and the occasional upset stomach add to the distinction. Such activities are often quite disconcerting to elderly patients.

The adult patient generally comes voluntarily to the ophthalmologist's office, anticipating the examination and the relatively mild discomfort associated with it. Adults usually attempt to perform at their highest level on subjective tests and provide full cooperation during the objective portions of the examination. Several aspects of the adult examination can be delegated to well-trained technicians while maintaining a consistent level of cooperation by the patient. In contrast, the child is often brought to the office without full comprehension of the impending examination. If the child has previously had an adverse experience in a physician's office, the level of anxiety may be exceptionally high.

THE OFFICE

Ideally, the eye examination should be a pleasant experience for the child, the parents, and the physician. Children often remember the office, the ophthalmologist, and details of the eye examination many years after the visit. Every effort should be made to provide the child with as favorable an encounter as possible. This improves the quality of information obtained from the examination and greatly enhances the child's level of cooperation on subsequent visits.

The child should be placed in an environment that is comfortable for the patient as well as the parents and other family members accompanying the child. In many pediatric ophthalmology offices, a separate play area is located adjacent to, but visible from, the family seating area. Children can either sit with their parents or move to the play area where they can be continually observed. This scheme greatly reduces the noise level in the seating area while providing the children with an enjoyable wait (Fig. 217–1). It may be helpful to have a separate, small eye drop room, which geographically separates the unpleasant experience of drop administration from the

A

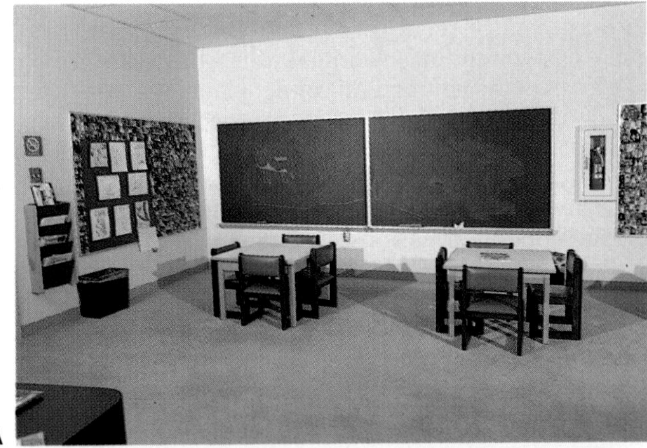

B

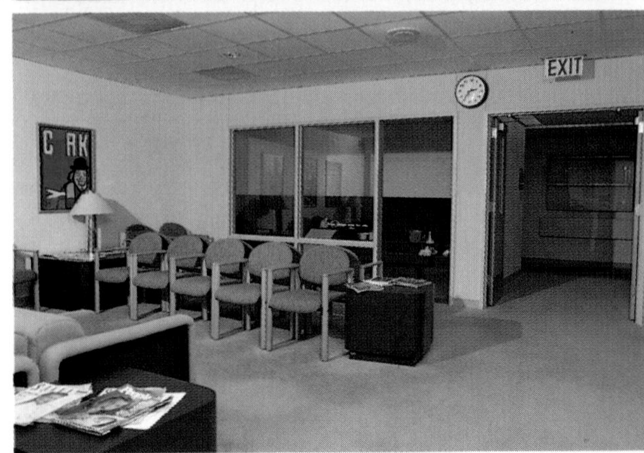

Figure 217–1. *A,* A well-designed waiting room with blackboards, children's tables, and chairs. *B,* Seating is available for parents and other family members with a separate but easily observed play area.

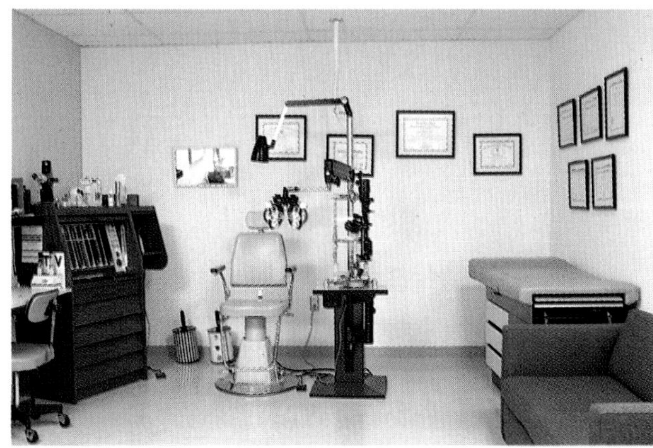
A

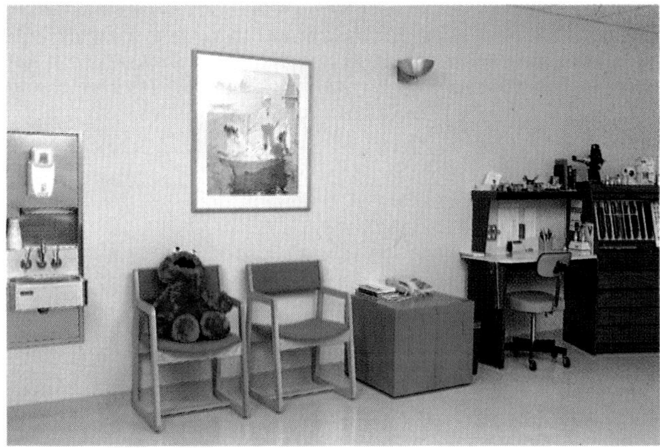
B

Figure 217–2. *A* and *B*, Spacious, parlor-like examining room with couch and chairs for extra family members that may accompany the pediatric patient.

examination room itself. In some offices, personnel other than the ophthalmologist administer the drops, which may avoid inducing an association between the physician and the drops.

The design of the examining room is important in establishing an environment that places the child immediately at ease. Ideally, the examining room should be large and comfortable, imparting an almost parlor-like atmosphere. The child is almost always accompanied by at least one adult, and this is often expanded to include both parents as well as siblings and other family members. Except for the most unusual circumstances, it is best to have the adults in the examining room with the child. Therefore, examination room seating should be available for three or four people at a minimum (Fig. 217–2). The ophthalmologist's attire is also important. It is often helpful to avoid white laboratory coats, which may elicit fear of injections or other painful procedures associated with physicians' offices and hospitals. A sport coat, smock, or a short pastel-colored laboratory coat is a pleasant alternative.

HISTORY

The child's history is essential in focusing subsequent steps of the ophthalmic examination. The inability of young and developmentally delayed children to respond reliably to subjective tests and the child's inability to concentrate for extended periods results in a greater dependency on historical information. Unfortunately, an accurate history often cannot be obtained from the child. The nonverbal child is unable to express the history, and the adult must therefore supply this information. Even in the older child, a great deal of historical information is provided by the parents. The indirect nature of the history creates a number of potential problems. Children will usually complain vigorously of painful symptoms but rarely report unilateral visual loss. Somewhat surprisingly, children also may have few complaints about painless, bilateral, slowly progressive visual loss, even when the reduction in acuity is quite severe. An example is bilateral visual loss resulting from chronic uveitis associated with juvenile rheumatoid arthritis. The remarkable adaptation abilities of children and the plasticity of the visual brain may contribute to the lack of complaints. In addition, children may not be forthcoming with important historical information, particularly with ocular injuries that occur as a result of a forbidden activity.

Ophthalmic disorders in young individuals are often congenital, and a number of congenital as well as acquired diseases are inherited. Individually, many of these disorders are rare, but collectively they constitute a significant percentage of ophthalmic diseases. Parents may recognize the familiar phenotypic characteristics of a well-known inherited disease and voluntarily report this to the examiner. More often, however, the ophthalmologist must seek out this information through well-directed and quite specific inquiries. Questions should be asked about other family members with ocular problems, such as blindness, poor vision, the need for thick glasses, difficulty ambulating in dim illumination, photophobia, color vision deficiencies, "lazy eye" or amblyopia, strabismus, nystagmus, leukocoria, or a history of eye surgery. The family history should also be pursued with respect to systemic disorders that may be associated with ocular abnormalities, because a wide variety of such disorders exist and may involve virtually any organ system. Examples include connective tissue and cardiovascular defects associated with Marfan's syndrome, midfacial hypoplasia and arthropathy associated with Stickler's syndrome, dental and umbilical abnormalities in Rieger's syndrome, urinary tract abnormalities in Lowe's syndrome, and neurologic and skin abnormalities in the phakomatoses. Therefore, a family history of systemic disease (particularly if early in onset), unusual physical traits, developmental delay, mental retardation, and early death may be important. Denial, illegitimacy, incest, paternal substitutions, and the natural variability in expression of inherited disorders make the process even more difficult. A standard pedigree diagram of the nuclear family can usually be obtained quickly and easily recorded in the record. An extended pedigree is often necessary with inherited disorders and may require a second visit or the assistance of a geneticist.

The prenatal and perinatal history is also important, and specific questions should be asked about the pregnancy, delivery, birth weight, gestational age, and neonatal health. Medications or illness during pregnancy

Table 217–1. GROSS MOTOR MILESTONES DURING INFANCY

Gross Motor Movement	Approximate Age (mo)
Rolls from prone to supine	4
Sits alone	6
Crawls	8
Walks	12

Modified from Capute AJ, Shapiro BK, Palmer FB, et al: Normal gross motor development: The influences of race, sex and socioeconomic status. Dev Med Child Neurol 27:6325, 1985.

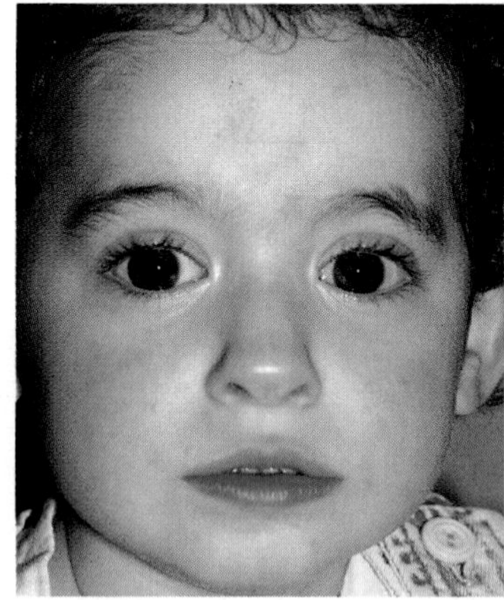

Figure 217–3. Observations should begin immediately upon introduction to the child and continue through the history-taking process, examination, and counseling period. This child's subtle left esodeviation and peripheral nasal leukokoria are manifestations of retinoblastoma.

may lead the examiner to search for particular abnormalities. Our evolving recognition of the teratogenic potential of medications and substances as common as ethyl alcohol make this information of great importance, particularly in infants or children with dysmorphic features. In addition, the relatively free passage of substances from the mother's circulation into breast milk provides the infant with yet another route of ingestion. The importance of prematurity and its relationship to retinopathy of prematurity is well recognized; however, parents may fail to mention prematurity once the child is discharged from the hospital and appears to be progressing satisfactorily.

Infant and early childhood development is profoundly influenced by the visual system. The ophthalmologist should be aware of the major gross motor and visual milestones that occur during infancy and early childhood (Tables 217–1 and 217–2).

COMPONENTS OF THE PEDIATRIC OPHTHALMIC EXAMINATION

The pediatric examination presents many challenges to the ophthalmologist. Subjective tests routinely employed in the adult examination may be impossible, difficult, or unreliable in children, resulting in a greater reliance on objective findings. The young child's ability to maintain concentration for only brief periods compounds the difficulties. In contrast, the elderly patient may enjoy a prolonged and detailed history followed by a meticulous and lengthy examination. The child quickly tires of repetitious or laborious tasks; it is therefore important to achieve speed during the examination without sacrificing accuracy. The various components of the examination are directed or focused at specific questions or issues, and the examiner quickly moves on to the next item in the examination sequence. This is greatly facilitated if the child's curiosity can be aroused and the examination is made interesting as well as fun.

It is helpful to begin observing various components of the examination while taking the history. The child's alertness and interaction with the parents should be evaluated, and other items such as head position, fixation and following ability, steadiness of gaze, and gross alignment of the eyes can usually also be observed (Fig. 217–3). It may be best to avoid a rigid examination sequence but rather to consider the examination as a dynamic process that is tailored to the child's unique situation. If the child or infant is on the verge of losing attention or crying, it is sometimes best to interrupt the history and begin the more entertaining aspects of the examination. Additional historical information can be obtained either during the examination or after the examination steps are completed.

Some maneuvers during the examination may interfere with subsequent steps. For instance, the strabismic deviation in a child with intermittent exotropia may be converted from a reasonably well-controlled exophoria to a constant exotropia after each eye is covered for visual acuity testing. All subsequent tests that require binocular interaction, such as stereopsis and the Worth four-dot test, may appear to be abnormal when the patient actually possesses excellent binocular capabilities.

Table 217–2. NORMAL HUMAN VISUAL DEVELOPMENT

Function	Age
Intermittent visual fixation present	Birth
Fixates well on nearby human face	2–3 mo
Smooth following movements on nearby objects	3 mo
Full accommodation possible	3–4 mo
Onset of stereopsis	3–5 mo
Fixates well on distant objects	6 mo
Subjective acuity possible	3 yr
Adult-type visual acuity testing possible	5–6 yr

SYSTEMIC ASPECTS AND EXTERNAL APPEARANCE

The comprehensive pediatric ophthalmic examination includes systemic as well as ophthalmic components. The child's general physical appearance should be noted, including alertness, overall size, weight, body structure, and interaction with the adults accompanying the child. In situations in which systemic disorders may be associated with ocular abnormalities, it is appropriate to undress the child and examine various areas such as the head and neck, integument, thorax, abdomen, genitalia, and skeletal structure using inspection, palpation, and auscultation, as indicated.

The child's head size and shape should be evaluated. Micro- and macrocephaly are commonly encountered in a referral population. Unusual skull contours, such as plagiocephaly, may be related to certain types of strabismus.[1] The position and size of the orbits should be observed, as should the relative position of the globes, which can usually be compared by looking down from over the child's forehead. When abnormalities are noted, exophthalmometry may be difficult or impossible using adult devices; however, globe position can often be measured monocularly, using a Luedde exophthalmometer or by marking a cotton-tipped applicator, which is held against the lateral orbital rim.

The palpebral fissures should be observed and compared with respect to contour, size, and location, as should the position and movement of the upper and lower eyelids and the presence of epicanthal folds. In appropriate situations, the intercanthal and interpupillary distances should be measured and can be compared with standard nomograms such as those listed in *Smith's Recognizable Patterns of Human Malformation*.[2] The lacrimal system should also be inspected with respect to the size of the tear meniscus, presence of epiphora, patency of the lacrimal puncta, and appearance of the areas overlying the lacrimal drainage system and the lacrimal gland. When appropriate, the orbital structures should be palpated and auscultated, emphasizing areas of special concern.

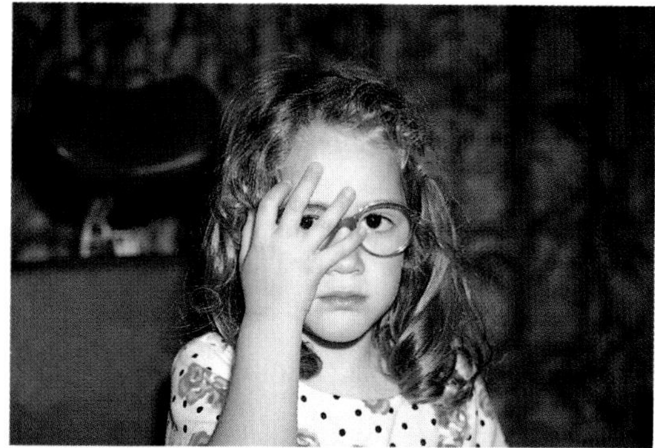

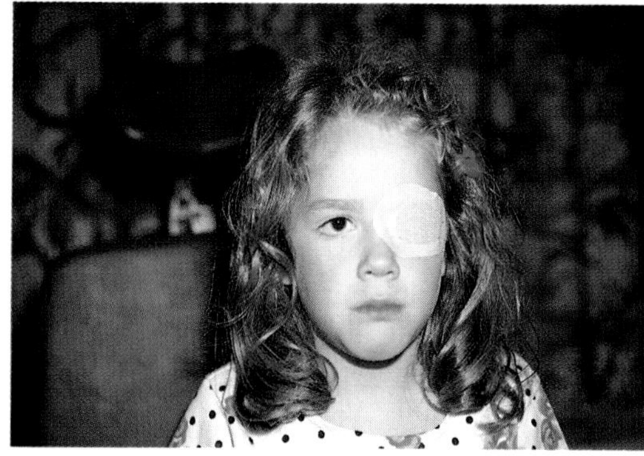

Figure 217–4. *A*, Peeking is a common source of error in visual acuity testing and can be eliminated by an occlusive patch (*B*) on the eye not being tested.

VISUAL FUNCTION

Visual function testing refers to a variety of studies that evaluate visual acuity, binocular interaction, color vision, and visual fields. The majority of these tests are subjective and therefore may be difficult or impossible to perform in young, developmentally delayed, or uncooperative children. In such instances, objective techniques must be employed. A thorough understanding of visual development and motor development is essential for meaningful and reproducible measurements.

Visual Acuity

Visual acuity testing in children is subject to many sources of error. Infants and young or developmentally delayed children are unable to identify figures or letters and their motor responses to visual stimulation are observed as a substitute for subjective acuity tests. Such clinical estimations of relative acuity, based on fixation preference, are crude, qualitative tests at best. Other problems in children exist as well. Sometimes the child may be so eager to please the examiner and parents that "peeking" occurs with the "occluded" eye, or portions of the test chart are memorized and recited. Peeking is also a common and natural process for the child with reduced acuity in one eye and is one of the most common sources of error in acuity testing. Peeking can be eliminated by placing an occlusive eye patch on the opposite eye when testing acuity (Fig. 217–4).

An incorrect response on acuity testing should generally not be acknowledged by the examiner or the parents because this may discourage a response at the next level of testing. Instead, the examiner plays the role of facilitator, often resembling a cheerleader, encouraging the hesitant child to provide an answer. This approach promotes guessing, and the examiner must evaluate enough responses to prevent chance from causing an overestimation of acuity.

Visual acuity testing in children varies greatly with age and mental status. Children with normal developmental milestones can generally be subdivided into three groups with respect to the techniques used for visual acuity testing: (1) birth to age 3 yr, (2) age 3 to 6 yr, and age 6 yr and older.

Visual Acuity Testing From Birth to Age 3 Yr

Infants and children up to the age of 2 1/2 to 3 yr are generally unable to accomplish subjective visual acuity tests. Older children with developmental delay and other disorders may also be unable to respond to subjective acuity testing. Visual acuity in these situations is evaluated using objective techniques, and such testing in the clinical office setting is usually performed by observing eye movements that are produced in response to visual stimulation. The ability to "fixate and follow" a target is the principal clinical acuity test used to assess central visual function in infants and young children.

Normal motor responses to visual stimulation in the child consist of fast, voluntary, refixation saccades as well as slow, smooth pursuit movements that occur as the eyes follow a moving target. Infants from birth to several months of age often show little or no response to inanimate targets or a flashlight. The light presents no discrete edges or lines and therefore is a poor stimulus for fixation and following in the immature visual system.[3, 4] The human face is generally the strongest visual stimulus for the young infant, and even newborn infants will intermittently attempt to fixate on a human face placed in close proximity.[5–8] The innate visual interest in the human face may well be related to infant-maternal bonding.[9] Visually induced motor response may be enhanced by holding the infant in a comfortable but upright position and placing the examiner's face close to the infant while the examiner slowly moves from side to side. If there is no reaction, the test should be repeated with the mother holding the child using her own face as the test stimulus while the examiner peers over her shoulder to observe the infant's eyes. It is important for the ophthalmologist to be aware that young infants are not capable of producing the normal slow, smooth pursuit movements seen in older children and adults. Instead, young infants display jerky, hypometric saccades in the same direction as the target moves.[10, 11] The examiner must also be careful not to rotate the infant during acuity testing, since rotation will induce the vestibuloocular reflex (VOR), which is a powerful nonvisual stimulus for eye movement.

The status of the visual motor system must be appropriately evaluated before concluding that the lack of eye movement responses by the infant signifies a reduction in visual acuity. The VOR can be quickly and easily elicited and serves as an excellent test of the integrity of the motor portion of the system and does not require any visual input. The infant is held facing the examiner at arms length with the head inclined 30 degrees forward. The examiner then slowly rotates in one direction while observing the infant's eyes. The normal response consists of true nystagmus with a slow tonic deviation in the direction toward which the examiner is turning, followed by a repetitive fast movement that shifts the eyes back toward the midline position. The response may be enhanced if the examiner's face is located slightly to the side, since visual fixation suppresses the VOR. An alternative technique is accomplished by placing the infant in an upright position in the mother's lap while the examination chair is rotated. Normal full-term infants beyond 1 wk of age generally will acquire a VOR. However, in neonates, the tonic phase predominates, whereas the fast component may be observed intermittently.[12–14] By 4 wk of age, both the slow and fast phases of vestibular nystagmus are easily elicited in almost all normal infants.[15] The young infant who appears to be blind but in whom a VOR fast phase also fails to develop may simply be unable to generate the normal hypometric, saccadic following movements in response to visual stimulation. This may occur in children with central nervous system damage, such as cerebral palsy, and may also be seen in rare conditions, such as congenital oculomotor apraxia.[9, 16, 17] The truly blind child will also fail to visually suppress the VOR in the usual 3 to 5 sec after the cessation of rotation. Instead, blind children may have nystagmus that persists for 15 to 30 sec.[9]

By 2 or 3 mo of age, most normal infants quite consistently fixate on and follow a nearby human face, as well as small toys such as finger puppets (Fig. 217–5). When possible, motor responses to visual stimulation should be evaluated at both near and distance. By 6 mo of age, most infants will fixate on moving toys or cartoons at the end of a 20-ft examining room. In the office setting, pediatric ophthalmologists commonly use a vertical array of two or three electrically operated mechanical toys located at the end of the examining room (Fig. 217–6). Each toy is individually illuminated and controlled by a foot pedal. The normal child will fixate on the toy that is illuminated and moving, and small vertical refixation saccades are easily observed as the child's attention is directed from one toy to another when the foot pedal is pressed. The noise generated by the toys is not sufficiently directional to elicit refixation saccades, since the toys are spaced about 1 ft apart.

The visual acuity using fixation responses is generally recorded using the *CSM method*. The *C* stands for

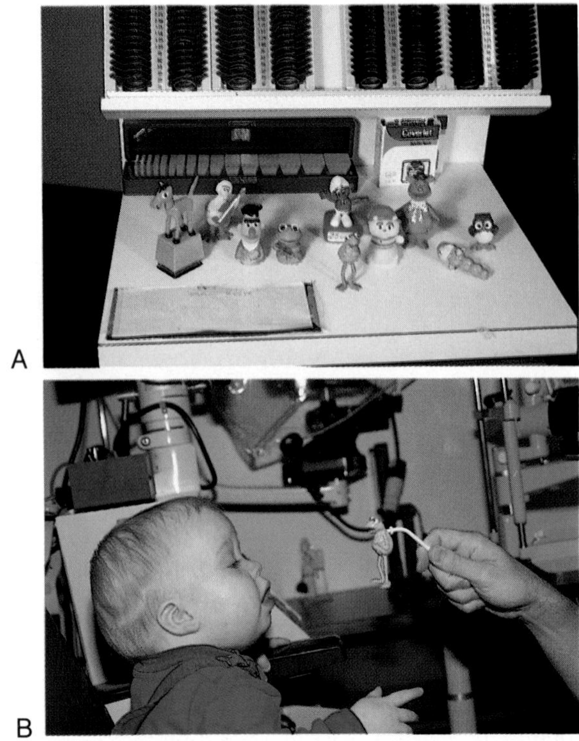

Figure 217–5. *A*, A collection of finger puppets and small toys provides fixation targets for infants and preverbal children. *B*, Fixation and following movements are observed and recorded using "CSM" notation.

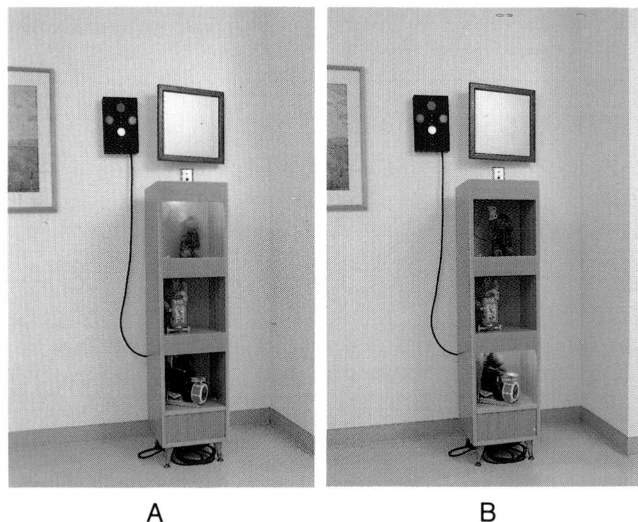

A B

Figure 217–6. A vertical array of three electrical toys is located at the end of the examining room. Each toy is individually controlled by a foot pedal. *A,* The upper toy is activated and illuminated, attracting the child's attention. *B,* The lower toys are then activated and illuminated, eliciting a small but easily observed vertical saccade as the child switches fixation from the upper to the lower toys.

central fixation, implying that fixation is foveal. The corneal light reflexes in each eye should be symmetrically located, allowing for the influence of angle kappa. The *S* stands for steady fixation, which means that the eye being tested is steadily fixating on a stationary or slowly moving target. Wandering eye movements or nystagmus indicate that fixation is not steady. The *M* conveys that the eye maintains fixation after the cover is removed from the opposite eye. Determining whether fixation is maintained in an eye requires strabismus to be present, either naturally occurring strabismus or a vertical deviation that is induced by a prism placed in front of one eye and then the other.[18]

For instance, the examiner notes that the right eye appears to be esotropic. A cover placed in front of the right eye confirms that the left eye is fixating centrally and steadily. When the left eye is covered, both eyes shift to the right, and the right eye takes up fixation, which the examiner notes is central and steady. However, when the cover is removed from in front of the left eye, both eyes quickly shift back to the left as the left eye takes up fixation. Each time the cover is removed from in front of the left eye, the left eye takes up fixation. The visual acuity would be recorded as follows:

VA O.D. = CS not M
VA O.S. = CSM

The CSM method may not adequately describe the reduced acuity in a child with a severe visual disability. In this situation, it may be appropriate to employ a narrative description of the level of visual responses, such as:

VA O.U. = No fixation or following efforts with human face, toys, or hand light at 1 ft distance. Mild photoaversion to bright halogen indirect ophthalmoscope light.

Visual Acuity Testing from Age 3 to 6 Yr

In developmentally normal children between the ages of 3 and 6 yr, a subjective acuity can usually be obtained. A wide variety of techniques are available for clinical office testing of recognition acuity using picture or letter optotypes at various distances. Distance acuity tests are generally preferred because they simulate the standard testing conditions used for adults and are not subject to significant angular size alteration if the child leans forward.

Many different optotypes have been developed for acuity testing in children and illiterate individuals. Picture optotypes, such as Allen figures, are inexpensive and widely used and at times are the only recognition optotype to which young children will respond.[19] However, the variable test distance employed with Allen figures and the lack of Snellen equivalency are two potential shortcomings of this technique. Letter optotypes, which resemble standard Snellen notation, are generally preferred, since the optotypes represent the most commonly used adult acuity test. Such tests include the Landolt C test, the HOTV test, and the "tumbling" or "illiterate" E test. The E test requires the patient to indicate the orientation of the optotype,[20] and young children may have difficulty distinguishing the left-right orientation of the letter.[21–25] Letter optotype tests have also been developed that avoid the left-right confusion of the E test. Such tests include the Sheridan STYCAR (Screening Tests for Young Children and Retardates) and a modification that uses only the letters H, O, T, and V. The HOTV acuity test requires the child to match the distance letter by pointing to the appropriate letter on a nearby key card that contains the letters H, O, T, and V (Fig. 217–7).

The crowding phenomenon should also be considered in children's visual acuity testing. Single letter acuity is often better than multiple letter acuity in children with amblyopia. This may relate to the size of the central receptive fields in amblyopia and the degree of lateral inhibition. As the threshold visual acuity is approached, it is preferable to present the child with a full line of optotypes, rather than single letters. If single letters are used, the visual acuity may be overestimated. In very young children, single optotype acuity may be all that is possible. As previously noted, an occlusive patch prevents peeking with the opposite eye during acuity testing. The testing technique should be indicated, as should the need for isolated optotype presentations. For instance:

VA sc O.D. = 20/40 HOTV, isolated letters
VA sc O.S. = 20/30 HOTV, isolated letters

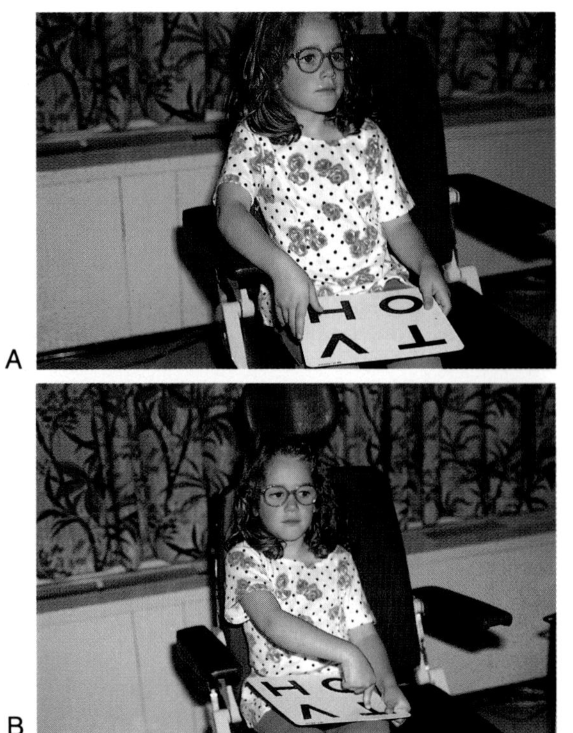

Figure 217–7. *A,* The letters HOTV of the Snellen chart can be presented at a distance while a card displaying the same letters rests in the child's lap. *B,* The child identifies the target optotype by pointing to the letter that "looks the same" on the card.

Visual Acuity Testing In Children Older Than 6 Yr of Age

Normal children beyond 6 yr of age can generally be tested using adult Snellen letter charts. Testing is accomplished at both near and distance using multiple letter presentation to uncover the crowding phenomenon. We also record the near point of accommodation, in centimeters, separately for each eye, as well as the near point of convergence on the initial examination.

Alternative Visual Acuity Testing Techniques

In preverbal children and infants, visual acuity is usually evaluated by fixation and following ability, as well as fixation preference when strabismus is present. Such methods are rapid and, for the most part, quite satisfactory. Quantitative techniques have recently been developed and have greatly enhanced our understanding of normal visual development. These same techniques are finding increasing uses in the clinical setting as well and are particularly helpful in comparing the relative acuity between the eyes.

The evolution of modern techniques for the quantitative measurement of visual acuity in preverbal children dates back to the 1957 study of optokinetic responses in newborn infants by Gorman and associates.[26] Preferential looking and visually evoked cortical potential were subsequently developed.

PREFERENTIAL LOOKING

Preferential looking is based on observations that infants are more interested in looking at patterns than at homogeneous fields.[27, 28] The infant is exposed to a pair of stimuli consisting of a field of black and white stripes of a specific spatial frequency and an identically sized gray field of equal luminance. An observer watches the infant's eyes and scores the number of times the infant fixates on each stimulus and the duration of fixation on each stimulus. Forced-choice preferential looking is a refinement in which the observer is not aware of which side the stripes are on but must make a commitment (forced choice) about which stimulus the infant is gazing at. The forced-choice technique removes some of the biases that were present in earlier preferential looking techniques.[29–32] The development of relatively simple, low-cost, rapid techniques allows testing to be completed in approximately 10 min in the clinical setting (Fig. 217–8).[33–35] Preferential looking is useful in the evaluation and follow-up of preverbal patients with disorders affecting visual acuity, particularly in situations in which it is important to compare the relative acuity between the two eyes.[36–39] The technique also is a useful method for vision screening in infants and young children.[38, 40–42]

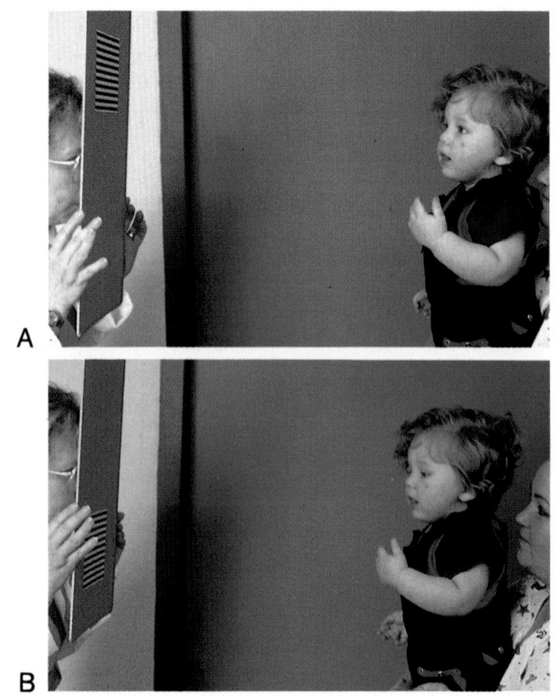

Figure 217–8. Preferential looking techniques present the infant or preverbal child with a grating of a particular spatial frequency and a homogeneous field of equal luminance. An observer, located behind the card, can see the child's eye's through a peep hole. The child's eyes can be seen to be directed (*A*) up at the grating and (*B*) down at the grating.

VISUALLY EVOKED CORTICAL POTENTIALS

Visual acuity in preverbal children can also be evaluated by measuring visually evoked cortical potentials. These techniques use checkerboard or striped gratings of various spatial frequencies and, unlike preferential looking, are not dependent upon eye movements.[43–46] The equipment used to measure visual evoked potentials is expensive and requires considerable expertise for its operation.

There are differences among the visual acuities measured by preferential looking, visually evoked cortical potentials, and subjective techniques, which probably relate to basic distinctions among psychophysical, electrophysiologic, and subjective testing. In addition, although preferential looking and visually evoked cortical potential acuities are often reported as Snellen fractions, these numbers should not be used to predict the child's future level of subjective acuity, which relies on recognition. However, comparison of visual acuity between the eyes, estimation of severe versus mild visual loss, and changes in acuity over time are probably valid.[47]

Tests of Binocular Function

STEREOPSIS TESTS

Stereopsis is the highest level of binocular interaction and requires, as prerequisites, good visual acuity in each eye, simultaneous perception, and fusion. The presence of excellent stereopsis implies a reasonably high level of visual acuity in each eye and the lack of a significant tropia. Stereopsis testing has been advocated as a means of screening both visual acuity and alignment.

Commercially produced clinical stereopsis tests use one of several haploscopic techniques, such as polarizing filters, red-green glasses and recently, goggles with electronically controlled liquid crystal windows that are synchronized with a television display. Some of these tests employ simple horizontal image disparity, whereas others use true random dot techniques.[48] The majority of these tests are performed near, although a few are designed for distance or variable distances.

The Titmus Stereo Test and the Randot Stereo Test (Stereo Optical, Chicago, Illinois) are commercially produced near stereopsis tests that require polarizing spectacles and are commonly used in the United States. The Titmus test has a large housefly with wings that present a test of gross stereopsis representing 3000 sec of arc. Nine sets of circles in the Titmus test provide horizontal disparity, ranging from 800 to 40 sec of arc. Three rows of animals in both these tests present horizontal disparities of 400, 200, and 100 sec of arc. There are 10 sets of circles in the Randot test ranging from 800 to 20 sec of arc. All of the images on the Titmus Stereo Test and some of the images on the Randot Stereo Test rely on horizontal image disparity of the full test object and may provide the opportunity for the patient to detect side shift rather than true stereopsis. However, the Randot Stereo Test also includes a second page of true random dot geometric figures representing 250 and 500 arc sec of stereopsis.

Several other stereopsis tests also present true random dot stereograms. The Random Dot E test (Stereo Optical, Chicago, Illinois) also requires polarizing spectacles and uses a single-sized test object, the letter E, at variable distances to determine the threshold level of stereopsis.[49, 50] The TNO Test employs a red-green haploscopic technique in a booklet format and requires the patient to wear red-green glasses. The Lang Test presents a random dot pattern using cylinder gratings to create separate images for each eye and therefore does not require the patient to wear special spectacles.[51]

Some individuals, who lack true stereopsis, are able to correctly identify a surprising number of the stereoscopic animals and circles on both the Titmus Stereo Test and Randot Stereo Test. This is probably because of the recognition of subtle horizontal image displacement of the full test target. Inversion of the test book makes the stereoscopic images look further away than the other targets, and the mature individual with true stereopsis quickly recognizes this phenomenon and reports it to the examiner. In addition, patients who lack true stereopsis are almost always unable to correctly identify the true random dot figures on the second page of the Randot Stereo Test, as well as on other true random dot stereograms.

There are two distance stereopsis tests in relatively common use in the United States. The first is the A-O Vectographic Project-O-Chart Slide (American Optical, Southbridge, Massachusetts), which is placed in a standard visual acuity projector and requires the patient to wear polarizing spectacles. Four rows of circles present stereoscopic horizontal image disparity ranging from 240 to 60 sec of arc. The second is the Mentor B-VAT II SG (Mentor O & O, Norwell, Massachusetts), which uses liquid crystal shutter goggles that are synchronized with a computer monitor. Using a remote hand control, the examiner can present either circles with horizontal image disparity or true random dot figures to the patient. Stereoscopic images can be presented from 240 to 15 sec of arc. The major amblyoscope can also be used to test stereopsis at optical infinity, and the arms can be adjusted to match the patient's angle of deviation if strabismus is present. Distance stereopsis tests may be useful in situations in which there is a difference in fusional status at near and distance. For instance, in patients with divergence excess-type intermittent exotropia, it is not uncommon to find normal stereopsis at near but no stereopsis at distance when the eyes are exophoric at near but exotropic at distance.

Stereopsis testing may occasionally be possible in 3-year-old children and is generally reliable in cooperative 5- and 6-year-old children (Fig. 217–9). All new pediatric ophthalmology patients receiving a comprehensive eye examination should have a baseline stereopsis test if age and level of development permit.

Fusion Tests

Fusion refers to the cortical unification of visual images from corresponding retinal elements; it has both

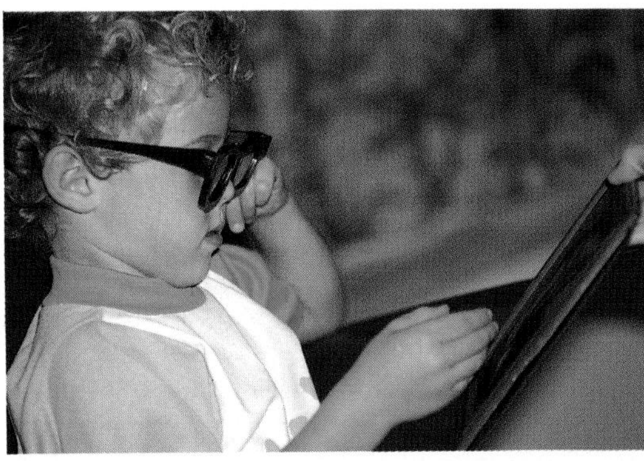

Figure 217–9. Stereopsis in this 3-year-old child is demonstrated by the elevated position of the fingers as he attempts to grasp the fly's wings on the Titmus stereo test.

sensory and motor components. Commonly used clinical tests of the sensory aspects of fusion include the Worth four-dot test, the red lens test, and Bagolini striated glasses. These tests can be employed in cooperative older children with suspected sensory or alignment defects. Fusion testing using the Worth four-dot test at near and distance is routinely performed on patients with reduced or absent stereopsis, the monofixation syndrome, and suspected intermittent or constant tropias. The test can detect and identify diplopic responses, suppression, and anomalous retinal correspondence.[52–54]

Color Vision Tests

Nearly 10 percent of otherwise normal males have color vision anomalies, making color vision defects the most common genetic eye disorder affecting males. All males mature enough to perform color vision testing should have their color vision evaluated as part of the initial comprehensive eye examination. The early detection of color vision anomalies may be important with respect to school performance and eventual choice of careers.

Commonly used clinical color vision tests include the full and concise editions of Ishihara's Tests for Colour-Blindness (Kanehara, Tokyo). For screening purposes, the concise edition is excellent (Fig. 217–10). Ishihara's plates detect red and green color vision defects. HRR (Hardy-Rand-Ritter) Pseudoisochromatic Plates are no longer commercially produced but are still available in many offices and institutions. These plates detect both red-green and blue-yellow deficiencies and qualitatively rate them as mild, moderate, or severe. In addition, the geometric figures used in the HRR test are excellent for children. Many other color vision tests are available.

Visual Field Tests

An assessment of confrontation visual fields should be included in the initial comprehensive eye examination. In young children and infants, this may be accomplished by attracting the child's attention straight ahead while bringing a small toy in from the temporal region. When the child detects the object approaching from the side there is usually an abrupt refixation saccade. If the child will tolerate monocular occlusion, the test can be accomplished monocularly in each of the quadrants. Visual field testing using Goldmann or automated techniques is not usually possible until the developmentally normal child is at least 7 or 8 yr of age.

Eye Movement and Alignment

Eye movement and alignment should be continually assessed during the examination, from the moment the child enters the examining room to the time the child leaves the office. An anomalous head position, eye movement abnormality, or problem with ocular alignment is sometimes easiest to detect when the child is in the waiting room or walking up the hall to the examining room.

Fast, refixation eye movements (saccades) and slow visual following movements (pursuit) should be observed in up, down, left, and right gaze. Optokinetic nystagmus (OKN) can be used to demonstrate both types of eye movements, using a rotating striped drum or an OKN tape. OKN testing may be particularly helpful in infants or children who appear to lack fixation and following movements, since it is a powerful visual stimulus causing a motor response that is difficult to suppress. If eye movements cannot be evoked by visual stimulation, vestibular nystagmus can be generated by holding the infant or young child at eye level, facing the examiner, and rotating the child. This elicits the VOR, which results in nystagmus through stimulation of the vestibular system. The lack of a motor response to visual stimulation with a normal VOR implies that the child has a visual abnormality.

The stability of fixation and the presence of nystagmus or nystagmoid eye movements should be noted when the infant or child is motionless. If nystagmus or nystagmoid eye movements are present, their direction, amplitude, frequency, and waveform should be recorded in primary as well as appropriate secondary and tertiary gaze positions.

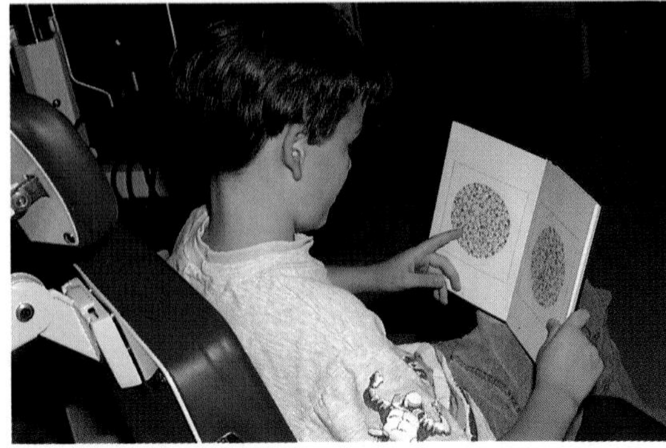

Figure 217–10. The concise edition of Ishihara's Test for Colour-Blindness can be used to screen for red-green color defects in males. Finger tracing can be used in nonverbal children.

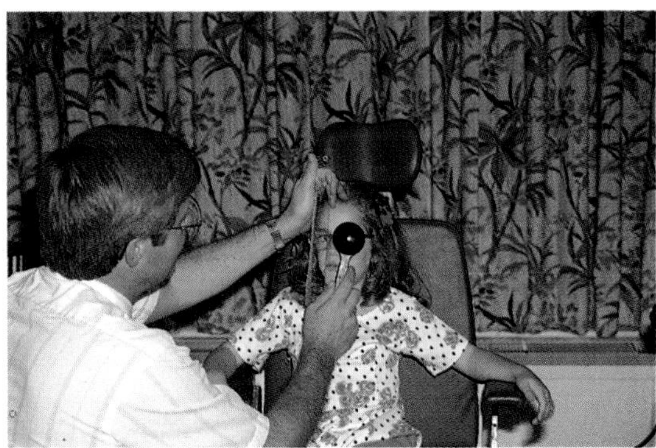

Figure 217–11. Cover testing is performed at distance and near with the appropriate correction in place.

Ocular alignment is qualitatively observed, along with monocular range of motion (ductions) and binocular conjugate eye movements (versions). Limitations in range of motion of one or both eyes, changes in palpebral fissure size, and apparent over- or underaction of the rectus or oblique muscles should be noted. Vergence movements are also evaluated, including the near point of convergence. Fusional vergence amplitudes should be measured in certain situations, particularly with symptoms or signs of convergence insufficiency.

Alignment is quantitatively evaluated using the light reflex test and cover testing. The position and symmetry of the corneal light reflex is compared between the two eyes, providing the examiner with a clinical estimation of angle kappa. At a minimum, cover testing should be performed in the primary gaze position at both distance and near on the initial comprehensive examination (Fig. 217–11). The alternate cover test may be a good screening technique because it elicits both phorias and tropias. Any ocular deviation detected on the alternate cover test should be identified as either a tropia or a phoria by employing the cover-uncover test. Quantitation of the phoria or tropia can be accomplished with prism and cover techniques.

Individuals with certain types of ocular misalignment may require detailed measurement of vertical and horizontal alignment in each of the nine diagnostic positions of gaze, as well as right and left head tilt and primary position at near. The monofixation syndrome is characterized by a small tropia that may be accompanied by a much larger phoria.[54] In this situation, the simultaneous prism and cover test is used to quantitate the small tropia, and alternate cover testing uncovers the larger phoria. Cranial nerve palsies affecting ocular motility, restrictive disorders, over- and underaction of the oblique muscles, and dissociated vertical deviation may result in unreliable alternate cover findings, and the prism under cover test may be useful in these situations. With the cover in place, the examiner peers around the edge of the cover and estimates the direction and magnitude of the ocular misalignment. An appropriate prism or prisms are placed under the cover, and the cover is moved to the opposite eye. The prisms are adjusted until movement of the covered eye is neutralized when the cover is shifted to the opposite eye.

The orientation in which the neutralizing prisms are held may affect the measured deviation. Stacking prisms with the bases in the same direction does not necessarily result in a prism effect that is equal to the sum of the two prism powers. Prism stacking should generally be avoided. However, the measurement of combined vertical and horizontal deviations using the prism under cover test may require the prisms to be stacked with the bases at right angles to one another.[55]

Pupils

Evaluation of the pupils should include size and shape in both ambient light and darkened room conditions to evaluate the status of the pupillary sphincter as well as the dilator muscles. In addition, the swinging light test should be employed to test for a relative afferent pupil defect. The swinging light test is often difficult to perform in children because the light commonly elicits convergence, accommodation, and miosis. It may be helpful to attract the child's attention at the end of the examining room. Other tests, such as the paradoxical pupillary response to darkness are evaluated when indicated.

Tension

The majority of pediatric ophthalmologists probably do not routinely check intraocular pressure in infants or young children unless there is a historical or examination finding to indicate the possibility of an elevation in pressure. In an otherwise normal infant or child, some pediatric ophthalmologists record that each eye is soft to palpation. Applanation pressures should be checked as part of the routine examination as soon as the child is old enough to cooperate with testing. The Perkins hand-held applanation tonometer is especially useful for testing acuity in reclining patients (Fig. 217–12).

The intraocular pressure must be measured in all infants and children in whom there is a reason to suspect an elevation in intraocular pressure. Indications may include a family history of congenital or pediatric glaucoma or the presence of a disorder known to be asso-

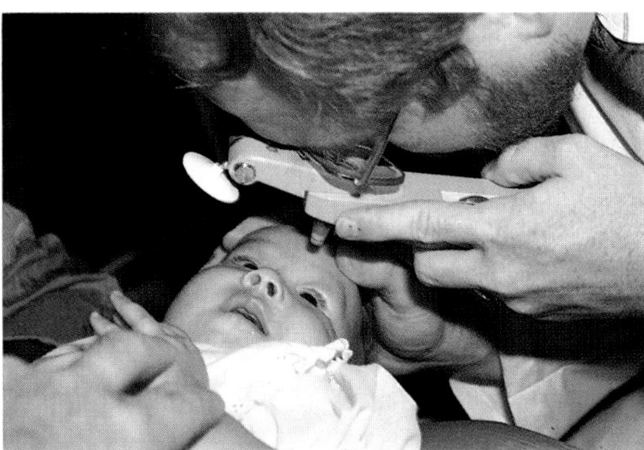

Figure 217–12. A Perkins hand-held applanation tonometer is used to check intraocular pressure in a reclining infant.

ciated with pediatric glaucoma. In addition, certain objective findings may indicate an increased risk of pressure elevation, such as photophobia, large or cloudy corneas, anterior segment anomalies, cataracts, uveitis, large cups, myopia, or asymmetric hyperopia. Intraocular pressure can be measured in some infants using the hand-held applanation tonometer. When intraocular pressure is to be determined, it is helpful if the infant is sleeping, which often occurs just after feeding. The infant's schedule can be used to advantage in these situations. If the pressure cannot be measured in the office, and clinical indications are sufficient, an examination in which sedation or anesthesia is used may be necessary.

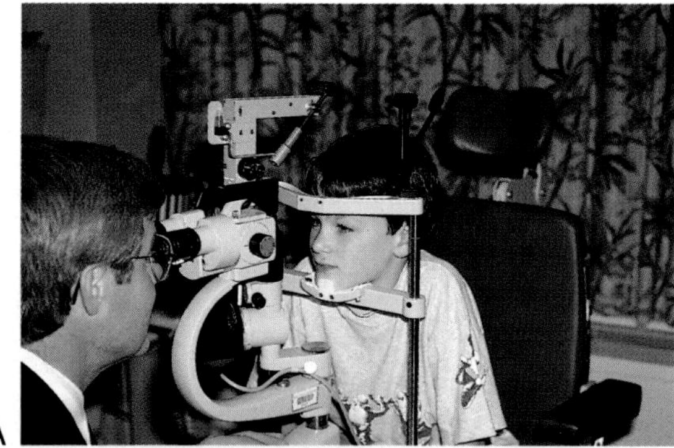

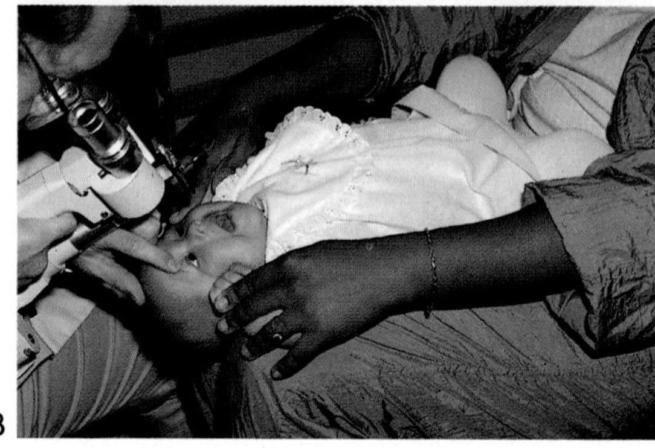

Figure 217–13. *A,* The older child sits comfortably at the standard, upright slit lamp, whereas infants (*B*) and very young children may require restraint and examination with a hand-held slit lamp.

Anterior Segment Examination

Infants and children can often be examined at a standard slit lamp. Young infants can usually be held in a prone position with the head slightly extended and advanced toward the slit lamp without difficulty. Sometimes a sheet is used to swaddle the infant. Older infants and very young children may approach the slit lamp with interest, whereas less cooperative infants and young children can be placed in a papoose board and held in front of the slit lamp, if necessary. A hand-held slit lamp is excellent for examination of the anterior segment in routine cases when it is difficult to get the child to the standard slit lamp.

Children from about the age 1 1/2 yr have a surprising level of interest in the slit lamp and are often quite cooperative if the device is presented in a relaxed way. Demonstrating how the face is placed in the chin rest is often helpful, as is pointing out that there is a "pretty light." A narrow slit helps reduce discomfort from the light source.

Uncooperative infants can be hugged against the mother or father with their legs around the parent's waist. The parent holds his or her knees together while the examiner faces the parent and places his or her own knees together, touching the parent's knees. The infant is then gently laid back so that the head is resting on the parent's or the examiner's legs, or on both. The baby's legs are pinned against the parent's waist by the parent's elbows, and both of the baby's arms are extended over the head and held in a position next to the baby's ears. These maneuvers place the baby in a reclining, face-up position while simultaneously immobilizing the legs, arms, and head without the need for extra personnel or special equipment (Fig. 217–13). The position is also quickly assumed so that the baby can be hugged by the parent between diagnostic maneuvers.

Fundus Examination

A dilated fundus examination with the binocular indirect ophthalmoscope is an essential component of the comprehensive pediatric ophthalmic examination. Problems with cooperation and unwanted eye movements are to be expected in children and certainly compromise the examination in comparison with the compliant adult patient. In spite of these limitations, a surprisingly good pediatric fundus examination can be accomplished in the office setting.

The eyes are fully dilated before the examination. The intensity of the light on the indirect ophthalmoscope is adjusted so that it is low but is adequate to view fundus details. The light must not be made so low that important findings are missed. Many children are interested in the bright light of the indirect ophthalmoscope and will fixate on it, providing an excellent view of the entire posterior pole region. An initial screening with a 28-D examining lens provides a broad overview extending well beyond the vascular arcades. This is followed by a 20-D lens, which has a narrower field of view but is brighter and enlarges the fundus details over that seen with the 28-D lens. Occasionally, a 14-D lens is also used to provide greater enlargement, particularly of the foveal area and optic nerve.

Older children will often voluntarily move their eyes in appropriate positions, allowing a view of the retinal periphery, whereas young children generally will not. The examiner may be able to view the retinal periphery in young children by either waiting for spontaneous movements in the appropriate direction or by abruptly changing the indirect ophthalmoscope angle and viewing the new area before the child again fixates on the light.

Infants and very young children with known or suspected retinal disease may require a restrained examination that sometimes includes topical anesthesia, an

A

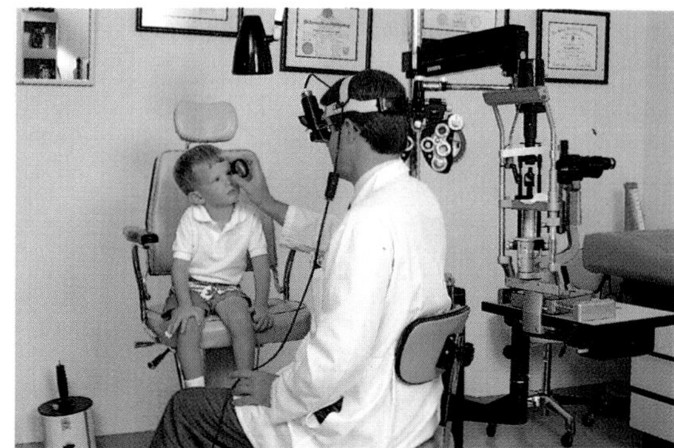

B

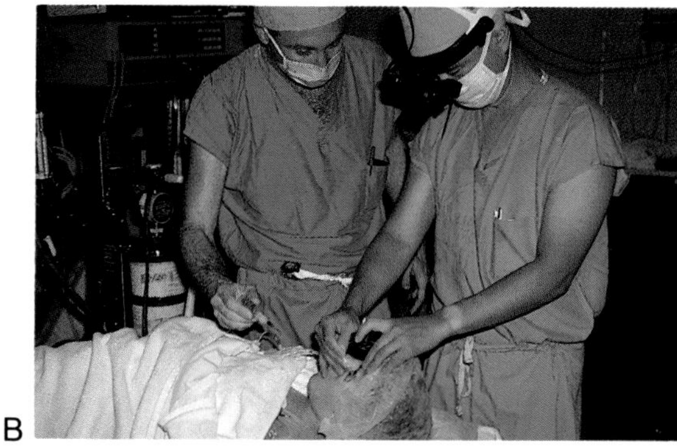

Figure 217–14. *A,* Indirect ophthalmoscopy is performed as part of the comprehensive pediatric ophthalmologic examination. *B,* Scleral depression is particularly difficult to accomplish in children, and examination under anesthesia may be necessary when the requirement for a detailed view of the fundus justifies the risk of anesthesia.

eyelid speculum, and scleral depression. This is a routine procedure in the neonatal nursery during examinations for retinopathy of prematurity. This type of examination can also be performed in the office on small infants using a papoose board or by swaddling the baby. The infant soon grows to a size that he or she is too strong for restraint and scleral depression, and a decision will need to be made regarding the need for an examination under general anesthesia (Fig. 217–14).

The ability of children to comply with fundus examination varies widely and even varies from visit to visit with the same child. A positive approach with encouragement and high expectations is often rewarded with a surprising level of compliance by the child. Generally, it is best to perform the least noxious portions of the examination first.

Cycloplegic Refraction

Cycloplegic refraction is an important component of the initial comprehensive pediatric ophthalmic examination. The tremendous accommodative abilities of infants and children and their inability to reliably respond to subjective refraction requires both cycloplegia and objective techniques. The relationship between horizontal strabismus and the refractive state is critical to accurate diagnosis and appropriate therapy. In the course of routine dilatation for the anterior segment and fundus examinations, appropriate agents for adequate cycloplegia should also be used.

Tropicamide alone does not provide adequate cycloplegia in children. Its cycloplegic effects are so brief that the many unexpected delays that occur in the average office may result in undetected resumption of accommodation. Atropine is the standard upon which all forms of cycloplegia are compared, but it suffers from a slow onset of effect and a prolonged duration of action. Several studies have compared cyclopentolate to atropine and found that cyclopentolate provides a short onset of action with an excellent cycloplegic effect of appropriate duration.

Atropine ointment can be used for cycloplegia as a 0.5 percent ointment in young infants and a 1 percent ointment after 3 mo of age. The ointment is usually instilled once or twice daily for 3 days prior to the examination. Atropine ointment is generally preferred to drops because the quantity instilled can be roughly monitored by the length of the cylinder of ointment placed on the eye, and systemic absorption is thought to be less. The onset of cycloplegia with atropine takes several hours, and the recovery of accommodation does not start until several days after the last instillation. Cycloplegic and mydriatic effects may last more than a week.

Cyclopentolate is preferable for routine cycloplegia in children because it is probably less toxic than some of the other agents, and its rapid onset of action allows the cycloplegic refraction and the examination under dilation to be performed at the time of the initial office visit.[56–58] Cyclopentolate provides a cycloplegic effect that is comparable to atropine. Atropine may uncover an additional 0.3 to 0.5 D of hyperopia in light, as well as deeply pigmented children with hyperopia[59] and white children with esotropia.[60]

Cyclopentolate is used as a 0.5 percent solution in the neonate and a 1 percent solution after the age of 3 mo. One drop is instilled into each eye twice, roughly 5 min apart, half an hour before retinoscopy. The cycloplegic effect achieves its maximal level within 30 min and returns to normal within 24 h. Cyclopentolate is less effective in dilating darkly pigmented irides. The dilation effect is enhanced with the addition of a drop of 2.5 percent phenylephrine in each eye to stimulate the pupillary dilator muscles.

Side effects of cycloplegic agents are usually due to topical sensitivity or parasympatholytic effects following systemic absorption. Higher doses increase the risk of dose-related systemic side effects. Children with Down's syndrome may be exceedingly sensitive to atropine. Systemic side effects include facial or generalized flushing from vasodilatation, elevated temperature, tachycardia, constipation, dry mouth, and transient central nervous system disturbances. More serious reactions are exceedingly rare. The side effects of phenylephrine include an elevation in systemic blood pressure from the α-adrenergic effect. This may be accompanied by a reduction in the pulse rate because of stimulation of baroreceptors by the elevated pressure.

Retinoscopy

Good quality cycloplegic retinoscopy can be obtained in the vast majority of infants and children on the initial visit. Occasionally, there are circumstances in which it may be helpful to have the child return for a dilated examination and retinoscopy; however, the delay in detecting possible intraocular abnormalities must be weighed against the reasons for the delay.

Retinoscopy should be performed in a setting in which the examiner, the child, and the parents are relaxed. With infants and very young children, it is often wise initially to perform retinoscopy for each eye using estimation techniques without the use of lenses held near the eye. It is a rare child who is not interested in looking at the retinoscope light, whereas many children strongly object to placing a cover over either eye or the use of trial lenses. Generally speaking, myopia, hyperopia, and the presence of significant astigmatism can be detected by simple estimation. Once estimation is completed, individual trial lenses or lens racks can be used for neutralization using plus or minus cylinder techniques. Lens racks are quick, but the vertex distance may be difficult to control. A cooperative child of about 2 1/2 yr or older can often use half-frame pediatric trial lens spectacles to hold the lenses at a constant vertex distance while retinoscopy is performed (Fig. 217–15).

It is helpful to occlude the opposite eye during retinoscopy while encouraging fixation on the light of the streak retinoscope with the uncovered eye. Occlusion of the opposite eye reduces the likelihood of accommodative stimulus from convergence and encourages on-axis retinoscopy in the uncovered eye in patients with strabismus. Off-axis retinoscopy should be avoided because inaccuracies result, particularly by the induction of false astigmatic errors.

It is generally better to perform retinoscopy prior to the slit-lamp examination and the fundus examination because retinoscopy is usually the least noxious.

Although an excellent fundus examination can be performed in the restrained, combative child, retinoscopy is far more accurate using more gentle techniques arousing the child's interest in the retinoscope light. Voluntary eyelid squeezing or the use of an eyelid speculum often results in distortion of corneal curvature and consequently induces continually changing irregularities in the streak reflex. Off-axis retinoscopy is also a problem in the restrained child and can be a significant problem under anesthesia as well.

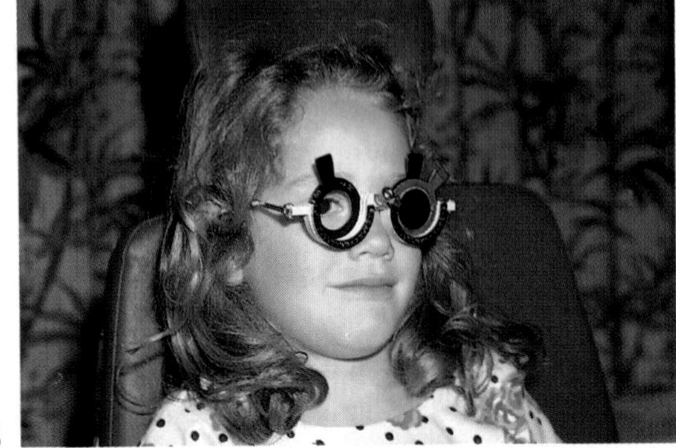

Figure 217–15. *A*, Cycloplegic retinoscopy is an important component of the comprehensive pediatric ophthalmologic examination. *B*, Half-frame trial lens spectacles control vertex distance and allow rapid lens changes. The opposite eye is occluded to encourage on-axis retinoscopy and to avoid convergence, which may induce accommodation.

CONCLUSIONS

The pediatric comprehensive ophthalmic examination includes the same individual components as the adult examination while emphasizing historical, ocular, and systemic aspects that are unique to children. There are significant differences with respect to examination techniques, level of cooperation, and ability of the child to respond to subjective testing, as well as with respect to the types of diseases encountered, their manifestations, and potential impact on the developing child. The pediatric examination can be a source of great enjoyment to the ophthalmologist and ideally should be an experience that is pleasant and long remembered by the child.

REFERENCES

1. Robb RM, Boger WP: Vertical strabismus associated with plagiocephaly. J Pediatr Ophthalmol Strabismus 20:58, 1983.
2. Jones KL: Smith's Recognizable Patterns of Human Malformation, 4th ed. Philadelphia, WB Saunders, 1988.
3. Hubel DH, Wiesel TN: Receptive fields, binocular interaction and functional architecture in the cat's visual cortex. J Physiol 160:106, 1962.
4. Hubel DH, Wiesel TN: Receptive fields and functional architecture of monkey striate cortex. J Physiol 195:215, 1968.
5. Goren CC, Sarty M, Wand-Wu PYK: Visual following and pattern discrimination of face-like stimuli by newborn infants. Pediatrics 56:544, 1975.
6. Hainline L: Developmental changes in visual scanning of face and nonface patterns by infants. J Exp Child Psychol 25:90, 1978.
7. Haith MM, Bergman T, Moore MH: Eye contact and face scanning in early infancy. Science 198:853, 1977.
8. Maurer D, Salapatek P: Developmental changes in the scanning of faces by young infants. Child Dev 47:523, 1976.
9. Hoyt CS, Nickel BL, Billson FA: Ophthalmological examination of the infant. Developmental aspects. Surv Ophthalmol 26:177, 1982.
10. Dayton GO, Jones MH: Analysis of characteristics of fixation reflex in infants by use of direct current electrooculography. Neurology NY 14:1152, 1964.
11. Dayton GO, Jones MH, Steele B, et al: Developmental study of coordinated eye movements in the human infant. II. An electrooculographic study of the fixation reflex in the newborn. Arch Ophthalmol 71:871, 1964.

12. Mitchell T, Cambon K: Vestibular response in the neonate and infant. Arch Otolaryngol 90:556, 1969.
13. Eviatar L, Eviatar A: Neurovestibular examination of infants and children. Adv Otorhinolaryngol 23:169, 1978.
14. Eviatar L, Miranda S, Eviatar A, et al: Development of nystagmus in response to vestibular stimulation in infants. Ann Neurol 5:508, 1979.
15. Archer SM, Helveston EM: Strabismus and eye movement disorders. *In* Isenberg SJ (ed): The Eye in Infancy. Chicago, Year Book Medical Publishers, 1989.
16. Cogan DG: A type of congenital motor apraxia presenting jerky head movements. Trans Am Acad Ophthalmol Otolaryngol 56:853, 1952.
17. Cogan DG: Congenital ocular motor apraxia. Can J Ophthalmol 1:253, 1966.
18. Wright KW, Edelman PM, Walonker F, et al: Reliability of fixation preference testing in diagnosing amblyopia. Arch Ophthalmol 104:549, 1986.
19. Allen HF: A new picture series for preschool vision testing. Am J Ophthalmol 44:38, 1957.
20. Committee on Vision, Assembly of Behavioral and Social Sciences, National Research Council, National Academy of Sciences: Recommended standard procedures for the clinical measurement and specification of visual acuity. Report of Working Group 39. Adv Ophthalmol 41:103, 1980.
21. Cairns NV, Steward MS: Young children's orientations of letters as a function of axis of symmetry and stimulus alignment. Child Dev 41:993, 1970.
22. Eldred CA: Judgements of right side up and figure rotation by young children. Child Dev 44:395, 1973.
23. Friendly DS: Preschool visual acuity screening tests. Trans Am Acad Ophthalmol 76:383, 1980.
24. Lippmann O: Vision screening of young children. Am J Public Health 61:1586, 1971.
25. Rudel HG, Teuber H: Discrimination of direction of line in children. J Comp Physiol Psychol 56:892, 1963.
26. Gorman JJ, Cogan DG, Gellis SS: An apparatus for grading the visual acuity of infants on the basis of opticokinetic nystagmus. Pediatrics 19:1088, 1957.
27. Fantz RL: Pattern vision in young infants. Psychol Rec 8:43, 1976.
28. Fantz RL, Ordy JM, Udelf MS: Maturation of pattern vision in infants during the first six months. J Comp Physiol Psychol 55:907, 1962.
29. Dobson V, Teller DY, Lee CP, Wade B: A behavioral method for efficient screening of visual acuity in young infants. I. Preliminary laboratory development. Invest Ophthalmol Vis Sci 17:1142, 1978.
30. Mayer DL, Fulton AB, Hansen RM: Preferential looking acuity obtained with a staircase procedure in pediatric patients. Invest Ophthalmol Vis Sci 23:538, 1982.
31. Held R, Gwiazda J, Brill S, et al: Infant visual acuity is underestimated because near threshold gratings are not preferentially fixated. Vision Res 19:1377, 1979.
32. Kessen W, Salapatek P, Haith M: The visual response of the human newborn to linear contour. J Exp Child Psychol 13:9, 1972.
33. Dobson V, Teller DY: Visual acuity in human infants: A review and comparison of behavioral and electrophysiological studies. Vision Res 18:1469, 1978.
34. Teller DY, McDonald M, Preston K, et al: Assessment of visual acuity in infants and children: The acuity card procedure. Dev Med Child Neurol 28:779, 1986.
35. Mayer DL, Dobson V: Assessment of vision in young children: A new operant approach yields estimates of acuity. Invest Ophthalmol Vis Sci 19:566, 1980.
36. Mohindra I, Jacobson SG, Held R: Development of visual acuity in infants with congenital cataracts. Invest Ophthalmol Vis Sci 19(Suppl):199, 1980.
37. Mohindra I, Jacobson S, Thomas J, Held R: Development of amblyopia in infants. Trans Ophthalmol Soc UK 99:334, 1979.
38. Fulton AB, Hansen RM, Manning KA: Measuring visual acuity in infants. Surv Ophthalmol 25:325, 1981.
39. Mayer DL, Moore B, Robb RM: Assessment of vision and amblyopia by preferential looking tests after early surgery for unilateral congenital cataracts. J Pediatr Ophthalmol Strabismus 26:61, 1989.
40. Mayer DL, Fulton AB, Rodier D: Grating and recognition acuities of pediatric patients. Ophthalmology 91:947, 1984.
41. Fulton AB, Manning KA, Dobson V: A behavioral method for efficient screening of visual acuity in young infants. II. Clinical application. Invest Ophthalmol Vis Sci 17:1151, 1975.
42. Fulton AB, Manning KA, Dobson V: Infant vision testing by a behavioral method. Ophthalmology 86:431, 1976.
43. Sokol S, Dobson V: Pattern reversal visually evoked potentials in infants. Invest Ophthalmol Vis Sci 15:58, 1976.
44. Sokol S: Measurement of infant visual acuity from pattern reversal evoked potentials. Vision Res 18:33, 1978.
45. Tyler C, Apkarian P, Levi D, Nakayama K: Rapid assessment of visual function: An electronic sweep technique for the pattern visual evoked potential. Invest Ophthalmol Vis Sci 18:703, 1979.
46. Norcia AM, Tyler CW, Hamer RD: Development of contrast sensitivity in the human infant. Vision Res 30:1475, 1990.
47. Day S: History, Examination and Further Investigation. *In* Taylor D (ed): Pediatric Ophthalmology. London, Blackwell, 1990.
48. Julesz B: Stereoscopic vision. Vision Res 26:1601, 1986.
49. Simons K, Reinecke RD: A reconsideration of amblyopia screening and stereopsis. Am J Ophthalmol 78:707, 1974.
50. Simons K, Reinecke RD: Amblyopia screening and stereopsis. *In* Symposium on Strabismus. Transactions of the New Orleans Academy of Ophthalmology. St Louis, CV Mosby, 1978.
51. Lang J: A new stereotest. J Pediatr Ophthalmol Strabismus 20:72, 1983.
52. Parks MM: Ocular Motility and Strabismus. Hagerstown, Harper & Row, 1975.
53. von Noorden GK: Binocular Vision and Ocular Motility, 4th ed. St. Louis, CV Mosby, 1990.
54. Parks MM: The monofixational syndrome. Trans Am Ophthalmol Soc 67:601, 1969.
55. Thompson JT, Guyton D: Ophthalmic prisms: Measurement errors and how to minimize them. Ophthalmology 90:204, 1983.
56. Bauer CR, Trottler MCT, Stern L: Systemic cyclopentolate (Cyclogyl) toxicity in the newborn infant. J Pediatr 82:501, 1973.
57. Praeger DL, Miller SN: Toxic effects of cyclopentolate. Am J Ophthalmol 58:1060, 1964.
58. Vale J, Cox B: Drugs and The Eye. London, Butterworth, 1978.
59. Robb RM, Petersen RA: Cycloplegic refractions in children. J Pediatr Ophthalmol 5:110, 1968.
60. Rosenbaum AL, Bateman JB, Bremer DL: Cycloplegic refraction in esotropic children. Ophthalmology 88:1031, 1981.

Chapter 218

Strabismus

Strabismus in Childhood

RICHARD M. ROBB

Strabismus is predominantly a disorder of childhood, and its management, particularly the treatment of strabismic amblyopia, is concentrated in the first decade. Early recognition of strabismus by pediatric practioners in this country has allowed occlusion therapy for amblyopia to be accomplished without delay, mostly before 4 years of age, when this therapy is most effective (Fig. 218–1).[1] Although continued monitoring of vision and periodic patching may be required through most of the first decade in patients with strabismus,[2] it is the early start of treatment that has reduced the prevalence of deep-seated amblyopia and eccentric fixation. Early efforts to realign eyes that are crossed in childhood are also advantageous. Prompt straightening of the eyes of a child with acquired strabismus may allow a return to normal binocular vision. Even approximate realignment of the eyes during childhood may allow the development of a stable small angle of deviation with sensory adaptations that may help to hold the eyes straight. Furthermore, children do not experience persistent diplopia at new angles of alignment as do many adults.

However, the manifestations of childhood strabismus do extend into the teenage and adult years, and there are some forms of strabismus that occur almost exclusively in adults, e.g., thyroid-related strabismus, misalignment associated with orbital floor fractures, and strabismus following retinal detachment surgery. Also, some treatment modalities, such as adjustable sutures for strabismus surgery, are mostly useful in older, cooperative patients.

The first section of this chapter therefore is arranged according to identifiable types of strabismus, classified partly according to the nature of the deviation and partly according to the age at which a particular type of strabismus is more frequently seen. There follows a discussion of anesthetic considerations in strabismus surgery and comments on general surgical techniques and some specific surgical procedures. Finally, there is a discussion of the relatively new use of botulinum toxin to effect changes in ocular alignment.

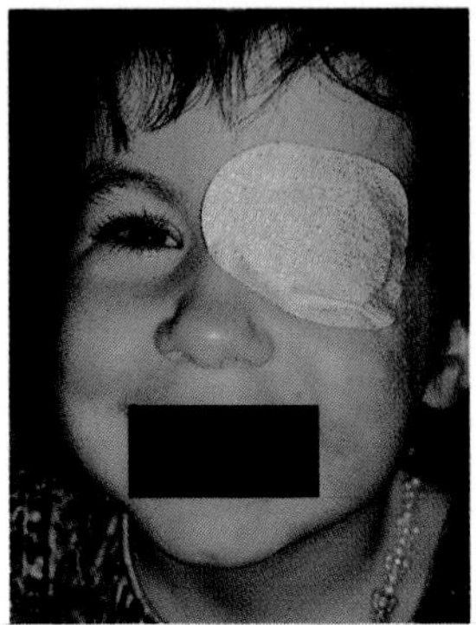

Figure 218–1. Occlusion therapy for strabismic amblyopia in the early years has reduced the prevalence of deep-seated amblyopia and eccentric fixation.

SPECIFIC TYPES OF STRABISMUS

Early Infantile Esotropia

The term *early infantile esotropia*,[3] or simply *infantile esotropia*,[4–6] is used to describe an esodeviation that is usually present by 6 mo of age (Fig. 218–2). Some ophthalmologists have preferred the term *congenital esotropia*,[7–10] but the deviation is not recognizable in many patients until 3 or 4 mo of age,[11] and certainly there is an evolution of the deviation during infancy.[3] The condition is probably heterogeneous,[5, 12] especially if patients with infantile esotropia and identifiable neurologic and systemic disorders are included. Patients with cerebral palsy have an increased prevalence of infantile esotropia along with their other motor problems.[6, 13, 14] On the other hand, most children with infantile esotropia do not have other recognizable neurologic disease.[3] Esotropic infants with generalized or ocular albinism (Fig. 218–3) have demonstrable abnormalities of their visual pathways,[15] whereas other patients with infantile esotropia do not.[16]

The characteristics of the deviation in infantile esotropia vary from patient to patient, but some features are frequent enough to be useful for descriptive purposes. The average deviation is 45 to 50 prism diopters (PD).[3, 17] There is often reluctance to abduct the eyes and increasing jerk nystagmus on attempted abduction. The fixation pattern may be monocular or alternating. When it is alternating, there is usually cross fixation; when it is monocular, the preferred eye often has better abduction than the squinting eye. The abduction difficulty improves with time and with strabismus surgery and is rarely noticed in older patients with a history of infantile esotropia. Refractive errors are not generally outside the usual range for infants, but significant hyperopia, myopia, and anisometropia may occur and may have an effect on the angle of deviation or the fixation

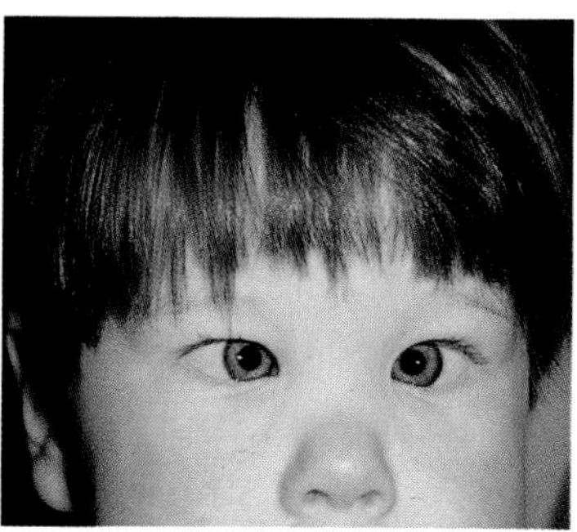

Figure 218–2. Infant with early onset esotropia. Although the term *congenital esotropia* is sometimes used, the deviation may not be apparent until 3 or 4 mo of age.

pattern. Latent or manifest latent nystagmus is present in some patients, and a dissociated vertical deviation is recognized sooner or later in about 40 percent of children with infantile esotropia.[3] Imbalance of the oblique muscles occurs in about one third of affected infants, the inferior oblique muscle being overactive much more often than the superior oblique (Fig. 218–4). The oblique muscle imbalance is not easily recognized on early examinations, perhaps because it does not develop until later, but also because the early reluctance of infants to abduct the eyes does not allow observation of the ocular versions in sufficient lateral gaze to make the imbalance obvious.

The management of early infantile esotropia requires most of the therapeutic modalities that are used to treat other forms of strabismus. Glass correction is required in 75 percent of patients at some time during the first decade to improve the ocular alignment or to provide clear focus.[3] It is important to check the refraction periodically, especially if there is a hyperopic error, since the hyperopia often increases between 2 and 5 yr of age and may become a factor in the esodeviation even if it did not appear to be so earlier.[18, 19] Occlusion therapy for strabismic amblyopia is required in approximately 60 percent of patients, and for half of these, the patching must be continued for extended periods of time.[3, 4] Opinions differ about the advantages of full-time versus part-time occlusion. If full-time occlusion is used in patients under 1 yr of age, careful monitoring is necessary to avoid a reversal of fixation and occlusional amblyopia in the patched eye.[20] Occlusion is usually continued until the fixation pattern becomes alternating. Preferential-looking tests have been used to monitor changes of visual acuity during occlusion therapy, but they appear to lack sensitivity in identifying strabismic amblyopia[21] and do not replace assessment of the fixation pattern.

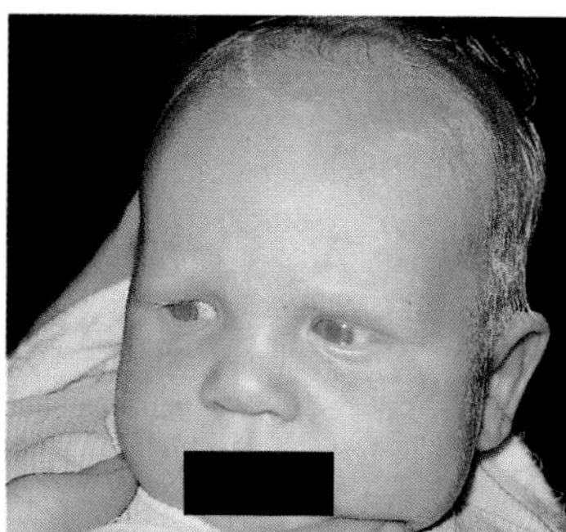

Figure 218–3. Infant with generalized albinism, in which there is a high incidence of strabismus and a deficiency of uncrossed fibers in the visual pathways.

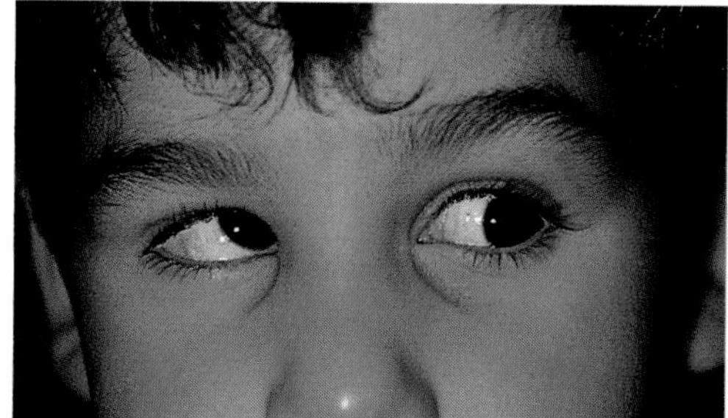

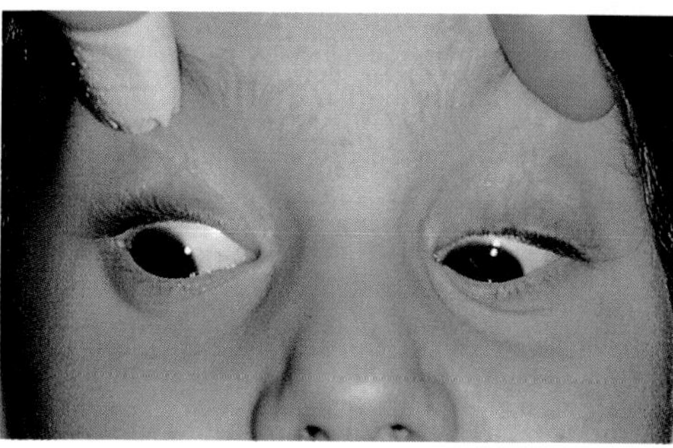

Figure 218–4. *A*, Child with overaction of the right inferior oblique muscle, which causes an upward drift in adduction. *B*, Child with overaction of the left superior oblique muscle, which causes downward deviation in adduction.

Surgery is often, but not always, required for ocular realignment. The eyes of between 15 and 25 percent of patients with infantile esotropia spontaneously diverge to an acceptable angle without surgery.[3, 4, 22, 23] For the remaining patients, either monocular or bilateral strabismus surgery may be employed. The best timing for surgery has been much discussed,[8, 9, 24–28] but there are still divergent opinions.[29, 30] It seems reasonable to proceed with surgery when the deviation has been characterized, amblyopia has been treated, and any accommodative factor has been corrected with glasses. There is some consensus that surgical realignment by 2 yr of age permits the development of binocular vision more often than alignment after that age,[9] but the cutoff is not sharp, and only a minority of patients achieve the partial binocularity that seems to be the best result obtainable with present techniques.[31] Several operations may be necessary to achieve satisfactory long-term alignment. Some surgeons actually prefer sequential operations to correct the larger deviations.[3, 8] Others chose to operate on three, four, or more muscles at one time to eliminate the deviation.[25] Because the traditional maximum 5-mm recession of both medial rectus muscles often undercorrects larger deviations, increasingly large medial rectus muscle recessions have been employed by some surgeons in recent years to improve the results of a two-muscle operation.[32] Long-term follow-up is not yet available to determine whether this approach will increase the number of late consecutive exotropias that are seen in any large group of children treated for infantile esotropia.[3, 33] If oblique muscle imbalance is recognized early, it may be corrected at the time of the initial horizontal muscle surgery; if the imbalance is later in onset, an additional operation is required. Consecutive exodeviations may also require reoperation. Continued observation and adjustment of therapy of all types is necessary throughout the first decade in order to obtain optimal results in patients with infantile esotropia.

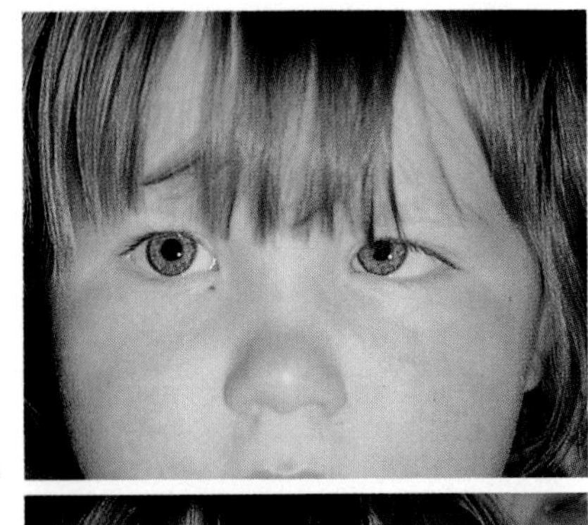

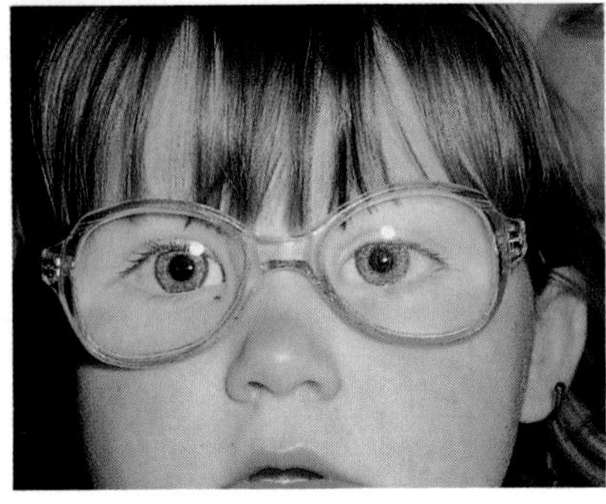

Figure 218–5. *A*, Child with acquired accommodative left esotropia. *B*, The deviation is eliminated by glasses to correct the child's full cycloplegic hyperopic error.

Acquired Accommodative and Nonaccommodative Esotropia

These forms of esotropia, being acquired after a child has experienced a period of single binocular vision, have a better prognosis for return to binocularity after treatment than does early infantile esotropia. The strabismus may be intermittent in onset. Sometimes parents can be quite accurate about the date the crossing first appeared, but often the time of the onset is known only approximately. Diplopia is rarely more than a fleeting symptom in childhood. If a monocular fixation pattern develops, amblyopia may ensue in the eye that is habitually suppressed.

If the esotropia develops in a child who is hyperopic, it may be partly or fully accommodative in nature. Parks[34] noted that there are two general categories of patients among those developing accommodative esotropia: those with high hyperopia, in the range of 4 diopters or more, with a normal accommodative convergence to accommodation (AC:A) ratio; and those with lesser amounts of hyperopia but a high AC:A ratio. Both are helped by glass correction to relieve the accommodative demand (Fig. 218–5). If the esotropia is fully accommodative, glasses to correct the full cycloplegic hyperopic error will allow the eyes to straighten and regain binocularity. Occasionally, the eyes are straight for distant fixation but crossed in the near range. In this case, bifocals may be helpful in controlling the near deviation.[35] It is not always necessary to use bifocals if the near deviation is intermittent and inapparent.[36] In either case, the bifocal is often removed in the teenage years, even if some near deviation remains. Glass correction for the hyperopia, on the other hand, cannot usually be discontinued unless the hyperopic error disappears with time,[37] and it is unwise to anticipate eventual removal of glasses in early discussions with patients or their parents. Contact lenses may be used to replace the distance glass correction in older children who are motivated.[38] Surgery is not a suitable alternative to the straightening effect of glasses in accommodative esotropia, and it is not recommended, even though parents often press for an operation, thinking it will eliminate the need for glasses.[39]

Patients with partly accommodative esotropia are improved by a full hyperopic glass correction but have a residual esotropia for distant and near fixation. The near deviation may be larger, but in this case, bifocals offer no additional advantage, since they do not reduce the near deviation enough to allow a return to binocular vision. If the residual distance deviation is sufficiently large (15 to 20 PD or more), surgical correction of the esotropia is appropriate, but glasses are continued postoperatively to control the accommodative element of the esotropia.

Acquired nonaccommodative esotropia is less common than the partly or fully accommodative variety, but the same potential for a return to binocular vision following amblyopia therapy and surgical realignment is present.[40] Glasses are not helpful except to sharpen the vision in one or both eyes. Recently, prism adaptation has been used preoperatively to bring out the full deviation and to estimate the fusional potential.[82] The possibility of an underlying lesion or malformation of the central nervous system should be kept in mind in these patients,[41, 42] and careful examination of the fundus for papilledema and optic atrophy is essential. Occasionally, this form of nonaccommodative esotropia occurs following temporary occlusion of one eye or in the course of treatment of nonstrabismic amblyopia.[43] At times it occurs spontaneously without an apparent precipitating factor.[44]

Intermittent Exotropia

The great majority of exodeviations seen in children are intermittent in nature (Fig. 218–6). They are more

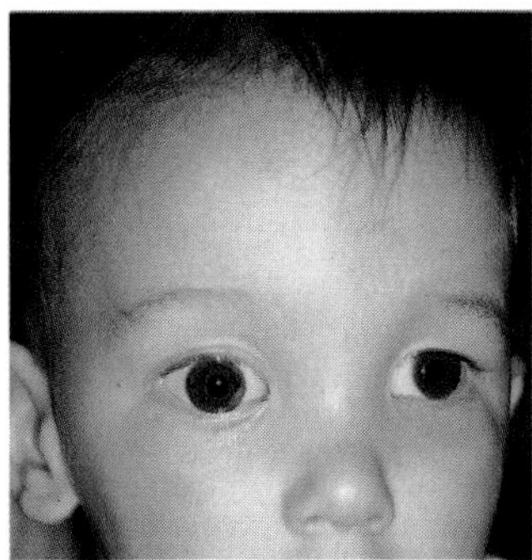

Figure 218–6. Child with left exotropia. Most exodeviations in childhood are intermittent in nature.

often manifest with distant than with near fixation,[45] and are more often noted by parents when the child is tired or ill. Squinting closed the eyelids of the deviating eye, especially in sunlight, is a characteristic feature of the condition, but it is not associated exclusively with exodeviations.[46] Control of the deviation in the near range allows binocular vision to be maintained at least part time, although in some patients this binocularity may be subnormal in quality.[47] The visual acuity is usually normal in both eyes unless refractive asymmetry is present. Refractive errors are similar to those in the general population.[48] Myopic refractive errors should be corrected to sharpen the retinal image at distance and to make use of induced accommodative convergence at near range. Some ophthalmologists have used deliberate overcorrection of myopia to control intermittent exotropia in the early years.[49] It should be noted, however, that the role of myopia in the etiology of exodeviations is less prominent than that of hypermetropia in esodeviations.[50]

Occasionally, intermittent exotropia becomes constant with time, but the great majority of exodeviations do not change dramatically in size or frequency over a period of years, and long-term follow-up has demonstrated remarkable stability of intermittent exodeviations of small to moderate size.[51] For this reason, surgical correction is often deferred until the patient has been followed for several years. There are advocates of early surgery,[52, 53] but others have pointed out the special disadvantages of surgical overcorrection of exotropia in young children: persistent small-angle deviations with amblyopia and loss of stereopsis.[54, 55] When surgery is performed after the age of 5 yr, temporary overcorrection of the exodeviation is desirable, since the effect of the surgery predictably diminishes with time.[56, 57] There are both proponents of bilateral surgery for exotropia[52, 53] and those who favor unilateral recess-resect procedures.[58] Recession of the lateral rectus muscles seems the more appropriate procedure when the exotropia is greater at distance than near, and a recess-resect operation is more satisfactory for those deviations that are the same at distance and near.[58] If a small surgical overcorrection is obtained, it is advisable to wait at least 6 mo before considering reoperation. Miotic therapy, plus lenses and alternate occlusion, may be helpful while waiting for the effect of the surgery to lessen. Base-out prisms have also been used to maintain binocularity during the period of overcorrection,[59] but it is not clear that the prisms change the ultimate outcome. A deliberate undercorrection of the deviation may actually be the preferred surgical result for older patients, who are intolerant of the diplopia that accompanies consecutive esotropia.[60]

Constant exotropia is uncommon in infancy and childhood. If strabismic amblyopia accompanies the deviation, it is managed in the usual way. When the deviation is stable and has been adequately characterized, surgical realignment is appropriate. Binocular vision is usually not obtained, unless it was present earlier at a time when the deviation was intermittent.

A and V Patterns

Any of the foregoing types of strabismus may exhibit a change in horizontal deviation in upward and downward gaze. If the deviation is more exotropic or less esotropic in upward gaze, the change is referred to as a V pattern (Fig. 218–7), if the deviation is more exotropic or less esotropic in downward gaze, the change is called an A pattern. By consensus the change from up- to downgaze must be at least 15 PDs in a V pattern and at least 10 PDs in an A pattern, although a difference of 20 PDs or more for each is more likely to be clinically significant.[61] A or V pattern occurs in from 15 to 25 percent of patients with horizontal strabismus.[62]

Although there is no clear understanding of the etiology of A and V patterns,[63] they are frequently associated with imbalance of the oblique muscles—A patterns with overaction of the superior oblique muscles and corresponding underaction of the inferior obliques, V patterns with overaction of the inferior oblique muscles and corresponding underaction of the superior obliques (see Fig. 218–7).[64] The oblique muscle imbalance does not appear to be due to paresis of the underacting muscles, since there is no change in vertical alignment with head tilt (Bielschowsky's head tilt test) as one would expect with an oblique muscle palsy. Nevertheless, there is a torsional change in eye position consistent with the oblique muscle imbalance evident on fundoscopy and demonstrable by heterotopia of the blind spots

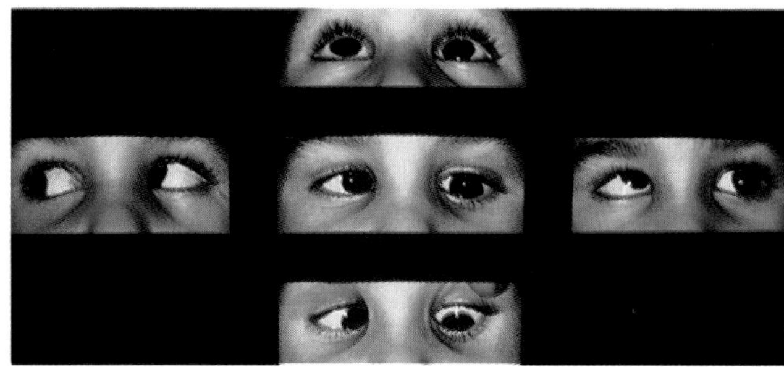

Figure 218–7. Patient with V-pattern esotropia. The deviation is more pronounced in down- than in upgaze. On lateral gaze, overaction of both inferior oblique muscles is evident.

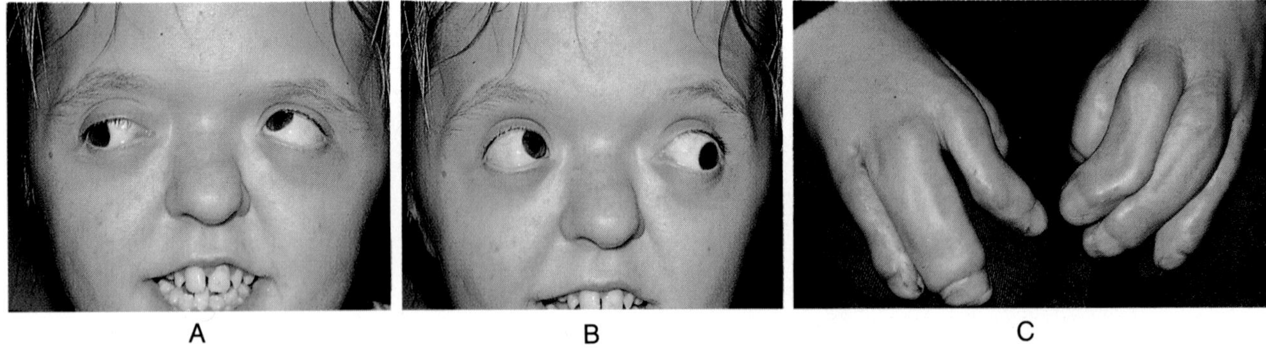

Figure 218–8. *A* and *B*, Overaction of inferior oblique muscles in a patient with Apert's syndrome, a variety of craniofacial dysostosis that is associated with syndactyly (*C*).

on visual field testing.[65] Weakening of the overacting oblique muscles collapses the A or V pattern, making the deviation more comitant in up- and downgaze.[64] There is relatively little change in the primary position alignment with bilateral inferior or superior oblique weakening procedures alone,[66, 67] so additional horizontal muscle surgery must be done to correct a significant deviation in the primary position.

There are a few special conditions in which oblique muscle imbalance similar to that seen in V patterns seems to be related to an abnormality of orbital anatomy. Patients with craniofacial dysostosis of the Crouzon or the Apert type frequently have overaction of the inferior oblique muscles and V pattern deviations (Fig. 218–8).[68, 69] Likewise, children with unilateral coronal synostosis and plagiocephaly frequently have hypertropia of the eye on the affected side with overaction of the inferior oblique muscle and underaction of the ipsilateral superior oblique (Fig. 218–9). The latter has been attributed to a change in the anatomy of the superior orbit and the position of the trochlea.[70, 71] However, most patients with A or V patterns do not have such obvious orbital malformation,[72] and an innervational etiology for the patterns must be assumed.

Rarely, patients with A or V pattern do not have obvious oblique muscle imbalance. In these patients, the change in horizontal deviation in upward and downward gaze can be neutralized by shifting the attachment of the horizontal rectus muscles up or down. This is often done at the time these muscles are recessed or resected to correct the associated horizontal strabismus.[61, 73, 74] The insertions of the horizontal recti are moved upward or downward in the direction one wishes to weaken their horizontal action. A similar effect can be obtained by monocular vertical displacement of the horizontal recti, moving one muscle up and its antagonist down according to the principle of displacing the muscle in the direction one wishes to weaken its horizontal action. Displacements of the horizontal recti are not effective in reducing A and V patterns if oblique muscle imbalance is present. For reasons that are not clear, surgical weakening of the inferior oblique muscle does not cause torsional symptoms, whereas tenotomy of the superior oblique muscle does induce a symptomatic torsional change.[75] Since adults have difficulty adjusting to changes in cyclotorsion, superior oblique weakening for A patterns in adults is not advisable.

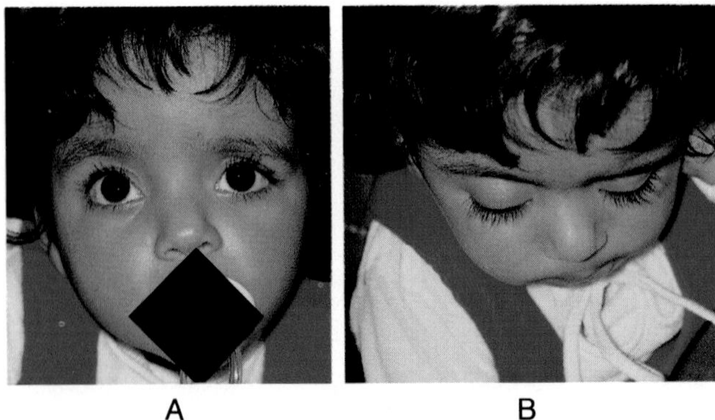

Figure 218–9. *A*, Right hypertropia in a patient with right coronal synostosis. *B*, View of the same patient from above, showing flattening of the right superior orbital rim and frontal bone.

Microtropia

Microtropia,[76, 77] or the monofixation syndrome,[78] refers to a type of strabismus in which the angle of deviation is small (from virtually undetectable to 8 to 10 PDs), and there is peripheral fusion with fusional vergences, coarse stereopsis, and a central scotoma in the nonfixating eye under conditions of binocular viewing. The scotoma is not present on monocular testing, but it can be demonstrated by binocular perimetry.[78] The scotoma is also reflected in abnormal responses to the 4-diopter prism test (Fig. 218–10),[79] the Worth 4-dot test, and polarized projected acuity charts.[78] The microtropia may be primary, or it may arise secondarily after surgical or nonsurgical treatment for a formerly larger angle of strabismus.[80] It is not infrequently the end result of surgical realignment of early infantile esotropia.[31] Anisometropia and amblyopia are often found, and eccentric fixation is present in some patients,[77] but these latter features are not considered essential for the diagnosis. Most of the microtropic deviations are esotropic deviations, but a few patients with microexotropia have been described.[81]

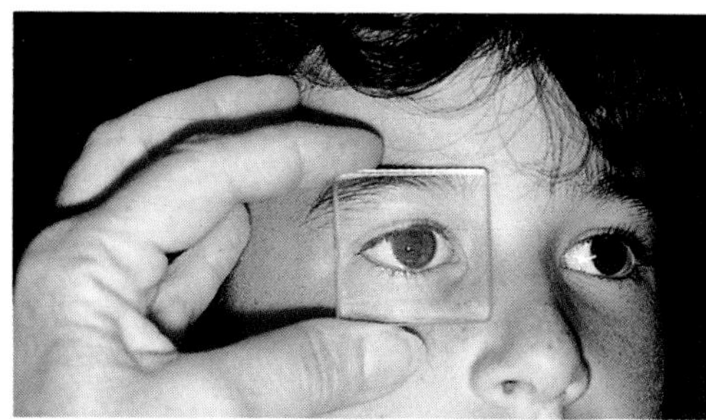

Figure 218–10. A 4-diopter prism test in a patient with small-angle right esotropia. The prism is placed base outward in front of the right eye while the eye is observed for a fusional movement. Absence of movement suggests a relative scotoma in the fixation area of the right eye. If the prism were placed in front of the fixing left eye, both eyes would shift slightly to the right.

From the standpoint of therapy, refractive errors should be corrected, and strabismic amblyopia can be treated. The scotoma present on binocular viewing has been resistant to therapy, and bifoveal fixation has not been achieved in these patients.[78] Their alignment is stable with time. Strabismus surgery is not indicated, unless the deviation exceeds the limits that can be controlled by peripheral fusion.

REFERENCES

1. Parks MM, Friendly DS: Treatment of eccentric fixation in children under four years of age. Am J Ophthalmol 61:395, 1966.
2. Ching FC, Parks MM, Friendly DS: Practical management of amblyopia. J Pediatr Ophthalmol Strabismus 23:12, 1986.
3. Robb RM, Rodier DW: The variable clinical characteristics and course of early infantile esotropia. J Pediatr Ophthalmol Strabismus 24:276, 1987.
4. Costenbader FD: Infantile esotropia. Trans Am Ophthalmol Soc 59:397, 1961.
5. Foster RS, Paul TO, Jampolsky A: Management of infantile esotropia. Am J Ophthalmol 82:291, 1976.
6. Friendly DS: Management of infantile esotropia. *In* Nelson LB, Wagner RS (eds): Strabismus Surgery. Int Ophthalmol Clin 25:37, 1985.
7. Taylor DM: Is congenital esotropia functionally curable? Trans Am Ophthalmol Soc 70:529, 1972.
8. Ing M, Costenbader FD, Parks MM, et al: Early surgery for congenital esotropia. Am J Ophthalmol 61:1419, 1966.
9. Ing MR: Early surgical alignment for congenital esotropia J Pediatr Ophthalmol Strabismus 20:11, 1983.
10. Nelson LB, Wagner RS, Simon JW, et al: Congenital esotropia. Surv Ophthalmol 31:363, 1987.
11. Nixon RB, Helveston EM, Miller K, et al: Incidence of strabismus in neonates. Am J Ophthalmol 100:798, 1985.
12. von Noorden GK: Infantile esotropia: a continuing riddle. Am Orthop J 34:52, 1984.
13. Seaber JH, Chandler AC Jr: A five-year study of patients with cerebral palsy and strabismus. *In* Moore S, Mein J, Stockbridge L (eds): Orthoptics: Past, Present, and Future. New York, Grune & Stratton, 1976, p 271.
14. Hiles DA: Results of strabismus therapy in cerebral palsied children. Am Orthop J 25:46, 1975.
15. Creel D, Witkop CJ Jr, King RA: Asymmetric visually evoked potentials in human albinos: Evidence for visual system anomalies. Invest Ophthalmol 13:430, 1974.
16. Hoyt CS, Coltrider N: Hemispheric visually evoked responses in congenital esotropia. J Pediatr Ophthalmol Strabismus 21:19, 1984.
17. Kraft SP, Scott WE: Surgery for congenital esotropia—an age comparison study. J Pediatr Ophthalmol Strabismus 21:57, 1984.
18. Rabb EL: Etiologic factors in accommodative esotropia. Trans Am Ophthalmol Soc 80:657, 1982.
19. Freeley DA, Nelson LB, Calhoun JH: Recurrent esotropia following early successful surgical correction of congenital esotropia. J Pediatr Ophthalmol Strabismus 20:68, 1983.
20. von Noorden GK: Binocular Vision and Ocular Motility, 4th ed. St. Louis, CV Mosby, 1990, p 467.
21. Mayer DL, Fulton AB, Rodier D: Grating and recognition acuities of pediatric patients. Ophthalmology 91:947, 1984.
22. Clarke WN, Noel LP: Vanishing infantile esotropia. Can J Ophthalmol 17:100, 1982.
23. Folk ER: Intermittent congenital esotropia. Ophthalmology 86:2107, 1979.
24. Taylor DM: How early is early surgery in the management of strabismus? Arch Ophthalmol 70:752, 1963.
25. Fisher NF, Flom MC, Jampolsky A: Early surgery of congenital esotropia. Am J Ophthalmol 65:439, 1968.
26. von Noorden GK, Isaza A, Parks MM: Surgical treatment of congenital esotropia. Trans Am Acad Ophthalmol Otolaryngol 76:1465, 1972.
27. Jampolsky A: When should one operate for congenital esotropia? *In* Brockhurst RJ, Boruchoff SA, Hutchinson BT, et al (eds): Controversy in Ophthalmology. Philadelphia, WB Saunders, 1977, p 416.
28. Parks MM: Operate early for congenital strabismus. *In* Brockhurst RJ, Boruchoff SA, Hutchinson BT, et al (eds): Controversy in Ophthalmology. Philadelphia, WB Saunders, 1977, p 432.
29. Lang J: The optimum time for surgical alignment in congenital esotropia. J Pediatr Ophthalmol Strabismus 21:74, 1984.
30. Ing MR: Surgical alignment for congenital esotropia. J Pediatr Ophthalmol Strabismus 21:76, 1984.
31. Botet RV, Calhoun JH, Harley RD: Development of monofixation syndrome in congenital esotropia. J Pediatr Ophthalmol Strabismus 18:49, 1981.
32. Mims JL III, Treff G, Kincaid M, et al: Quantitative surgical guidelines for bimedial recession in infantile esotropia. Binocular Vision 1:7, 1985.
33. Hiles DA, Watson BA, Biglan AW: Characteristics of infantile esotropia following early bimedial rectus recession. Arch Ophthalmol 98:697, 1980.
34. Parks MM: Abnormal accommodative convergence in squint. Arch Ophthalmol 59:364, 1958.
35. von Noorden GK, Morris J, Edelman P: Efficacy of bifocals in the treatment of accommodative esotropia. Am J Ophthalmol 85:830, 1978.
36. Albert DG, Lederman ME: Abnormal distance-near esotropia. Doc Ophthalmol 34:27, 1973.
37. Swan KC: Accommodative esotropia: Long-range follow-up. Ophthalmology 90:1141, 1983.
38. Sampson WG: Correction of refractive errors: effect on accommodation and convergence. Trans Am Acad Ophthalmol Otolaryngol 75:124, 1971.
39. von Noorden GK: Binocular Vision and Ocular Motility, 4th ed. St. Louis, CV Mosby, 1990, p 290.
40. Dankner SR, Mash AJ, Jampolsky A: Intentional surgical over correction of acquired esotropia. Arch Ophthalmol 96:1848, 1978.
41. Anderson WD, Lubow M: Astrocytoma of the corpus collosum presenting with acute comitant esotropia. Am J Ophthalmol 69:594, 1970.
42. Bixenman WW, Laguna JF: Acquired esotropia as initial manifestation of Arnold-Chiari malformation. J Pediatr Ophthalmol Strabismus 24:83, 1987.
43. Swan KC: Esotropia following occlusion. Arch Ophthalmol 37:444, 1947.
44. Burian HM: Sudden onset of concomitant convergent strabismus. Am J Ophthalmol 28:407, 1945.
45. Jampolsky A: Physiology of intermittent exotropia. Am Orthop J 13:5, 1963.
46. Wiggins RD, von Noorden GK: Monocular eye closure in sunlight. J Pediatr Ophthalmol Strabismus 27:16, 1990.
47. Baker JD, Davies GT: Monofixational intermittent exotropia. Arch Ophthalmol 97:93, 1979.
48. Burian HM, Smith DR: Comparative measurement of exodeviations at twenty and one hundred feet. Trans Am Ophthalmol Soc 69:188, 1971.

49. Coltrider N, Jampolsky A: Overcorrecting minus lens therapy for treatment of intermittent exotropia. Ophthalmology 90:1160, 1983.
50. von Noorden GK: Binocular Vision and Ocular Motility, 4th ed. St. Louis, CV Mosby, 1990, p 324.
51. Hiles DA, Davies FT, Costenbader FD: Long-term observations unoperated intermittent exotropia. Arch Ophthalmol 80:436, 1968.
52. Pratt-Johnson JA, Barlow JM, Tillson G: Early surgery in intermittent exotropia. Am J Ophthalmol 84:689, 1977.
53. Richard JM, Parks MM: Intermittent exotropia. Surgical results in different age groups. Ophthalmology 90:1172, 1983.
54. McDonald RJ: Secondary esotropia. Am Orthopt J 20:91, 1970.
55. Edelman PM, Brown MH, Murphree AL, et al: Consecutive esodeviation. . . . Then what? Am Orthop J 38:111, 1988.
56. Rabb EL, Parks MM: Recession of the lateral recti:early and late postoperative alignments. Arch Ophthalmol 82:203, 1969.
57. Keech RV, Stewart SA: The surgical overcorrection of intermittent exotropia. J Pediatr Ophthalmol Strabismus 27:218, 1990.
58. Burian HM, Spivey BE: The surgical management of exodeviations. Am J Ophthalmol 59:603, 1965.
59. Hardesty HH: Treatment of overcorrected intermittent exotropia. Am J Ophthalmol 66:80, 1968.
60. Schlossman, A, Muchnick RS, Stern KS: The surgical management of intermittent exotropia in adults. Ophthalmology 90:1166, 1983.
61. Knapp P: A and V patterns. *In* Symposium on Strabismus. Transactions of the New Orleans Academy of Ophthalmology. St. Louis, CV Mosby, 1971, p 242.
62. Costenbader FD: Symposium: The A and V patterns in strabismus. Introduction. Trans Am Acad Ophthalmol Otolaryngol 68:354, 1964.
63. von Noorden GK: Binocular Vision and Ocular Motility, 4th ed. St. Louis, CV Mosby, 1990, p 351.
64. Jampolsky A: Oblique muscle surgery of the A-V patterns. J Pediatr Ophthalmol 2:31, 1965.
65. Locke JC: Heterotropia of the blind spot in ocular vertical muscle imbalance. Am J Ophthalmol 65:362, 1968.
66. Stager DR, Parks MM: Inferior oblique weakening procedures. Effect on primary position horizontal alignment. Arch Ophthalmol 90:15, 1973.
67. Fierson WM, Boger WP III, Diorio PC, et al: The effect of bilateral superior oblique tenotomy on horizontal deviation in A pattern strabismus. J Pediatr Ophthalmol Strabismus 17:364, 1980.
68. Miller M, Folk E: Strabismus associated with craniofacial anomalies. Am Orthopt J 25:27, 1975.
69. Nelson LB, Ingoglia S, Breinin GM: Sensorimotor disturbances in craniostenosis. J Pediatr Ophthalmol Strabismus 18:32, 1981.
70. Bagolini B, Campos EC, Chiesi C: Plagiocephaly causing superior oblique deficiency and ocular torticollis. Arch Ophthalmol 100:1093, 1982.
71. Robb RM, Boger WP III: Vertical strabismus associated with plagiocephaly. J Pediatr Ophthalmol Strabismus 20:58, 1983.
72. Ruttum M, von Noorden GK: Orbital and facial anthropometry in A and V pattern strabismus. *In* Reinecke RD (ed): Strabismus II. Orlando, FL, Grune & Stratton, 1984, p 363.
73. Goldstein JH: Monocular vertical displacement of the horizontal rectus muscles in the A and V patterns. Am J Ophthalmol 64:265, 1967.
74. Metz HS, Schwartz L: The treatment of A and V patterns by monocular surgery. Arch Ophthalmol 95:251, 1977.
75. Jampolsky A: Vertical strabismus surgery. *In* Symposium on Strabismus. Transactions of the New Orleans Academy of Ophthalmology. St. Louis, CV Mosby, 1971, p 366.
76. Lang J: Microtropia. Arch Ophthalmol 81:758, 1969.
77. Helveston EM, von Noorden GK: Microtropia. A newly defined entity. Arch Ophthalmol 78:272, 1967.
78. Parks MM: The monofixation syndrome. Trans Am Ophthalmol Soc 67:609, 1969.
79. Jampolsky A: The prism test for strabismus screening. J Pediatr Ophthalmol 1:30, 1964.
80. Lang J: Lessons learned from microtropia. *In* Moore S, Mein J, Stockbridge L (eds): Orthoptics: Past, Present, Future. New York, Grune & Stratton, 1976, p 183.
81. Epstein DL, Tredici TJ: Use of four-diopter base-in prism test in microtropia. Am J Ophthalmol 74:340, 1972.
82. Prism Adaptation Study Research Group: Efficacy of prism adaptation in the surgical management of acquired esotropia. Arch Ophthalmol 108:1248, 1990.

Adult Strabismus

STEPHEN J. FRICKER

SPECIAL CONSIDERATIONS RELEVANT TO STRABISMUS IN ADULTS

Adult patients with strabismus have some problems in common with pediatric patients, but many adult cases are quite different in origin and treatment. Some adult patients may have undergone strabismus surgery when they were younger, and their histories may be readily available. However, many cases of adult strabismus are acquired in the adult years. Direct traumatic episodes are common, sometimes iatrogenic in nature, e.g. after retinal detachment repair or orbital surgery. Patients with primarily neurologic or medical problems may develop diplopia, either from their main problem or from their treatment. In general, such patients can be expected to have had previously unremarkable strabismus histories, but because of the incidence of childhood strabismus, a new adult strabismus problem can be superimposed on the residue of a childhood problem. This may be important, because one of the major features to be considered in dealing with adult strabismus cases is whether the patient has the capacity for fusion. If this is the case, then the goal of treatment is the elimination of diplopia and restoration of binocular vision, at least over a limited range of motion. If there is little or no apparent fusion potential, then improvement of the overall alignment of the eyes is the main objective. Thus it cannot be emphasized too strongly that obtaining a detailed history is most important in dealing with adult strabismus patients, although it should be remembered that histories are not always completely accurate.

For most adult patients with strabismus, there are only limited forms of nonsurgical therapy. For patients with small vertical deviations, it may be useful to prescribe small vertical prisms, approximately 5 diopters or less. Larger prisms rarely are helpful except in some cases of restrictive strabismus. Patients who have incomitant strabismus, with diplopia mainly in one field of gaze, may find partial occlusion of one lens acceptable, at least on a temporary basis. Although one rarely encounters a grossly undercorrected adult who is highly hyperopic with a developing strabismus problem, some patients with marginal complaints will benefit from an accurate refraction and prescription of the appropriate glasses.

When surgery is indicated, it is important to inform the patient preoperatively that although it usually is possible to obtain significant improvement, the results will not necessarily be perfect. Adequate preoperative discussion of this point prevents much misunderstanding and disappointment later on. The general risks of surgery, anesthetic reactions, and possible postoperative complications should also be discussed.

FURTHER SPECIFIC TYPES OF STRABISMUS

Paralytic Strabismus

With many cases of paralytic strabismus of recent onset, the patient either has had an intensive neurologic evaluation or should be scheduled for one. If the problem has obviously existed for a considerable time, the need for additional consultation or more investigative studies depends on how the patient and the strabismus surgeon evaluate the situation.[1] Sometimes the etiology of the problem is clear, but it frequently is not possible to pinpoint the source of the problem.[2, 3] With cases of recent onset, any spontaneous improvement may be expected to occur within approximately 6 mo. In any case, a period of watchful waiting is indicated. When there is little chance of further spontaneous improvement and the condition appears to be reasonably stable, the patient should be advised that a surgical approach may be in order. It is important to be conservative in making a prognosis. Patients accept the limitations of what can be achieved with more equanimity when they have not gained the impression that perfect results can be obtained.

THIRD NERVE PALSY

An individual who has severe acute third nerve palsy will have ptosis, exotropia, and, often, a small hypotropia of the affected eye (Fig. 218–11). The pupil may be dilated, and accommodation may be reduced or absent.[4] Intact sixth nerve function provides abduction of the globe, whereas intact fourth nerve function, innervating the superior oblique muscle, gives some incycloduction but only limited depression of the globe in its exotropic position. The use of botulinum in such patients appears to be limited but needs more investigation.[5]

Spontaneous resolution of the problem may first show with returning function of the levator, and diplopia may become troublesome as the ptosis improves. Later on, over a period of months, adduction may improve as the medial rectus regains function, but the vertical recti often do not share significantly in this improvement.

The best surgical approach depends on the extent of the residual problem. In general, if the patient can adduct the eye past the center line, a generous recess-resect procedure (perhaps with adjustable sutures) may suffice to obtain satisfactory horizontal alignment. Often, however, the patient cannot bring the abducted eye to the center line, and sometimes there appears to be practically no medial rectus function. Forced ductions can be informative, particularly if achieved with the patient awake and cooperative. In order to realign the eye, the abducting action of the lateral rectus muscle must be markedly decreased. Accomplishing a maximum resection of the paralytic medial rectus muscle does not usually help significantly, but it may occasionally be worthwhile, probably owing to unanticipated residual function of the muscle. Since the vertical recti usually have little if any function, either a Jensen procedure or a vertical recti transposition procedure has little to offer. Some surgeons advocate making use of the superior oblique muscle to provide some nasally directed restraining force.[6, 7] One method is to detach the superior oblique tendon from its insertion and then to attach the shortened tendon to the globe just anterior to or above the insertion of the medial rectus muscle. Other authors suggest first releasing the superior oblique tendon from the trochlea, so that the direction of the force exerted by the superior oblique muscle is better aligned with that normally provided by the medial rectus muscle. Sometimes the use of a traction suture combined with disconnection of the lateral rectus muscle is the best treatment that can be offered. In unilateral cases, some surgeons suggest that the uninvolved eye should be operated in order to obtain a better horizontal balance of the two eyes. This may involve a recession and/or a Faden procedure on the lateral rectus of the contralateral eye. It is difficult to estimate the possible

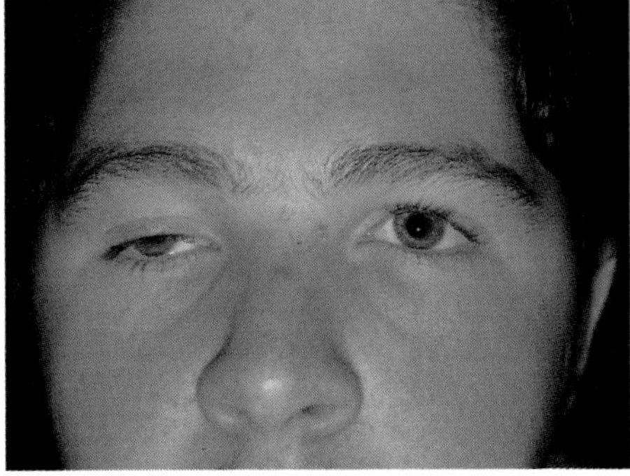
A

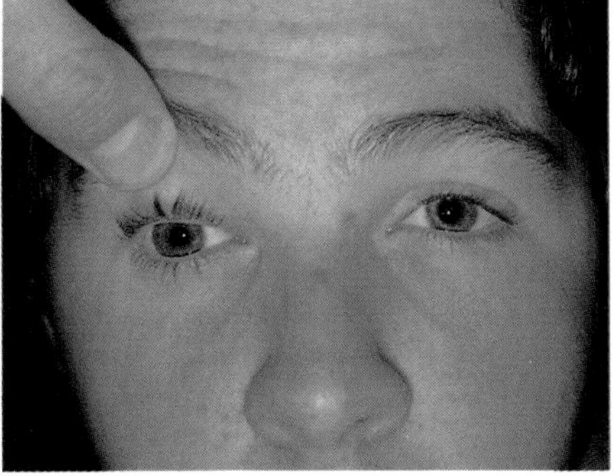
B

Figure 218–11. Patient with traumatic right third nerve palsy, showing ptosis of the right upper lid (*A*) and (*B* with lid elevated) exotropia and a small right hypotropia.

effectiveness of these procedures, and it is worth keeping in mind that some patients will not want to have surgery on their "good eye," regardless of the possible benefits that might be offered by such an approach. Furthermore, even if alignment of the two eyes is achieved over a restricted range, attempted motion beyond this range invariably results in misalignment and diplopia. Consequently, these patients almost always have to achieve some measure of suppression or learn to tolerate the diplopia. At times the ptosis accompanying third nerve weakness may concern patients more than the diplopia and the lack of motion of the eye. Occasionally, corneal exposure problems may exist, and the use of artificial tears and soft contact lenses may be helpful. Ptosis surgery, even of limited extent, can at times lead to severe corneal exposure problems. Patients may have limited appreciation of this possibility and may need a detailed discussion to understand the risks involved.

The effects of aberrant nerve regeneration may be seen after third nerve damage. Abnormal or inappropriate lid movements are most noticeable, but wide variations in function may be encountered. Suggestions have been made that in some cases of aberrant regeneration, operation on the appropriate muscle of the fellow eye might put to good use the aberrant nerve function. In general, such proposals have an air of unreality about them, and most strabismus surgeons probably have few occasions to seriously consider such procedures. In summary, it can be said that patients with severe third nerve problems offer major therapeutic challenges with results that often are not completely satisfactory.

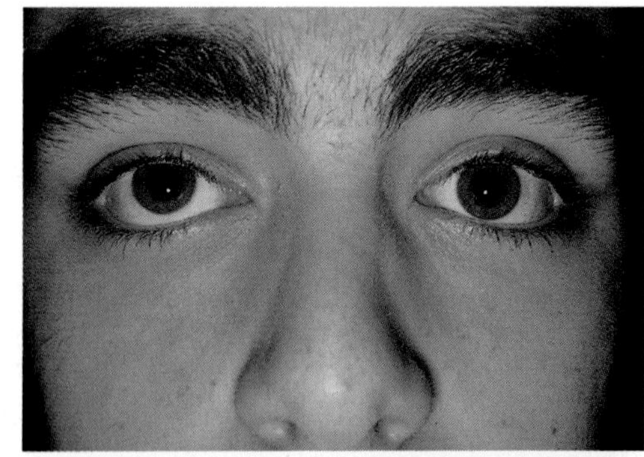
A

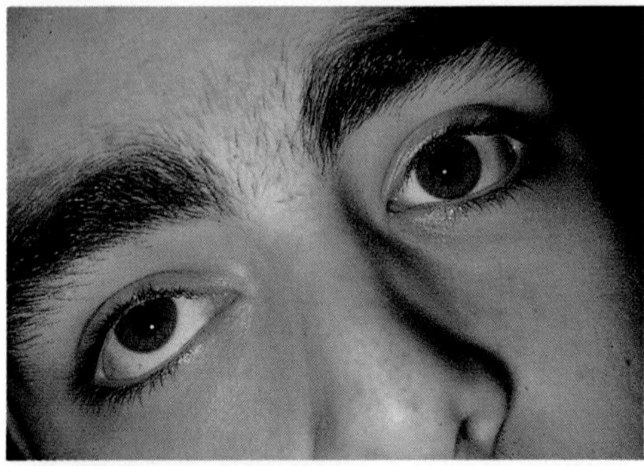
B

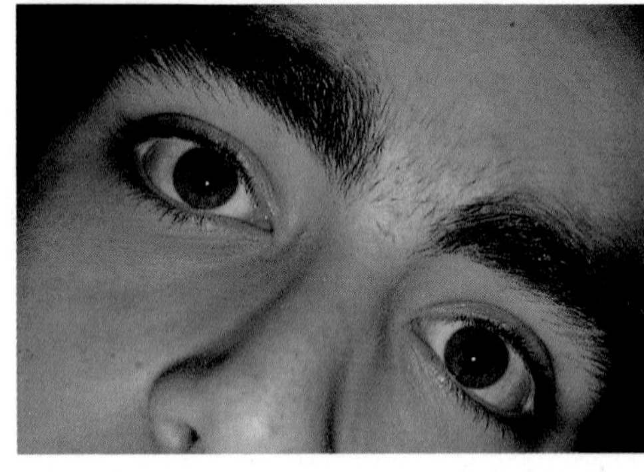
C

Figure 218–12. Patient with right fourth nerve palsy causing right hypertropia in the primary position (*A*). The Bielschowsky head tilt test reveals that the right hypertropia is increased on head tilt to the right (*B*) and decreased on tilt to the left (*C*), consistent with paresis of the right superior oblique muscle.

FOURTH NERVE PALSY

A patient with fourth nerve palsy usually has unilateral problems, but it should be kept in mind that bilateral cases do occur and often are quite asymmetric.[8–10] Many of these cases result from closed head trauma, or they may originate from orbital trauma or orbital or lid surgery.[11–13] A history of sinus problems may be pertinent. Often patients do not have a history of trauma, infection, surgery, or any other process. The patient may present with what appears to be a decompensating congenital fourth nerve weakness. As a head tilt often is one of the characteristic features of a fourth nerve problem, it is appropriate to question the patient and his or her family about this. Examination of old photographs of the patient can be rewarding in pointing to a long-standing problem.

A patient with a newly acquired unilateral fourth nerve palsy usually complains of vertical diplopia and may volunteer that there is a relative tilt to the two images. Usually, the patient adopts a head tilt away from the side of the affected eye and may have a chin down attitude, with the eyes directed up and away from the direction of action of the affected superior oblique muscle. The Bielschowsky response is positive (Fig. 218–12), and the three-step test can be applied readily. The rotational component of the misalignment can be measured, for example by using red and white Maddox rods in a trial frame (Fig. 218–13) to give the dissociated images an angular deviation that is then reduced by appropriate rotation of the Maddox rods. If there is bilateral involvement,[14] the relative vertical deviation is reduced, and the patient may adopt a chin-down, eyes up attitude. The angular displacement of the images can be a problem, but a significant head tilt may not be present in approximately symmetric cases, as the excycloduction of both eyes cannot be compensated simultaneously by tilting the head to one side.

When patients have superior oblique muscle problems that have existed for some time, there may be some elements of doubt about the diagnosis, since years of adjustment, possibly combined with some actual muscle changes, may result in eye movement abnormalities that cannot readily be categorized. Performing forced ductions may be helpful in determining if there is any restriction to motion in any field of gaze of either eye. Not all patients can be fitted into well-defined

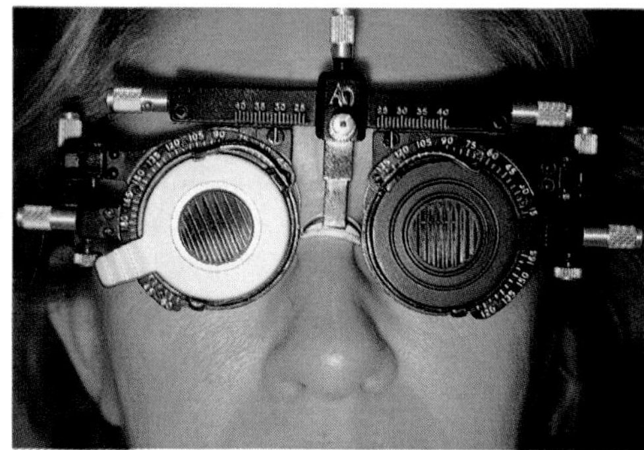

Figure 218–13. Red and white Maddox rods assessing torsional deviation of the eyes. The red Maddox rod has been rotated out to match the excyclotorsion of a patient with right fourth nerve palsy; in this position, the red and white lines would be seen as parallel.

subgroups, but Knapp has suggested a useful classification system.[8] Discussion of a slightly simplified version for unilateral cases of fourth nerve palsy follows.

For cases of recent onset, hypertropia is greatest when the affected eye is adducted. Knapp distinguished between class 1 and class 2 depending on whether the hyperdeviation is greatest in the field of action of the antagonist inferior oblique muscle or the weak superior oblique muscle. In the latter case, he recommends a tuck of the tendon of the weak superior oblique muscle, and possibly a recession of the contralateral inferior rectus muscle at a later time. Tucking the superior oblique tendon (discussed under Specific Surgical Techniques) helps to reduce rotational misalignment, but some surgeons find that only small amounts of vertical deviation are corrected, unless a large and possibly tight tuck is carried out. If the hypertropia in the primary position is less than approximately 15 diopters, weakening the antagonist inferior oblique muscle often provides satisfactory results with either category. If the deviation is larger than this, then in addition to weakening the ipsilateral inferior oblique muscle, a recession of the contralateral inferior rectus may be required. Tucking the affected superior oblique tendon is not always necessary. In a small percentage of patients, the involved eye may appear to have developed a tight superior rectus muscle. If this is the case this muscle needs to be recessed, but it is prudent to refrain from recessing the contralateral inferior rectus muscle at the same time, since the eventual vertical alignment cannot be predicted accurately. When possible, the use of adjustable sutures is worthwhile.

When the fourth nerve palsy is bilateral, a considerable degree of asymmetry may exist, and any surgery should be modified accordingly. More consideration may have to be given to treating the effects of residual bilateral excycloduction. Performing a tuck of the tendon of the superior oblique muscle of each eye will reduce the rotational misalignment, but the Harada-Ito procedure (see Specific Surgical Techniques) may be more effective in this respect.[15–18]

From the preceding remarks, it should be clear that satisfactory treatment of fourth nerve problems demands detailed consideration of the function of both eyes. The surgeon must be prepared to consider various alternatives and should make this clear to the patient before the operation. The patient should also be informed that although improvement can be offered in most cases, complete resolution of the problem will not necessarily be obtained and that more surgery may be needed.

SIXTH NERVE PALSY

An adult presenting with a sixth nerve palsy generally has diplopia, limitation of abduction, and sometimes a compensatory head turn. In a child, the diplopia is fleeting, and in addition to poor abduction an esotropia usually develops along with progressive contracture of the antagonist medial rectus muscle (Fig. 218–14). If there is no reliable history of trauma, one must consider the multitude of possible etiologies and must instigate the appropriate medical and neurologic evaluations. Cases have been reported as complications of lumbar puncture and myelography.[19, 20] The possibility that a tumor or an acute vascular problem may be responsible is the most immediate concern, and consultation should

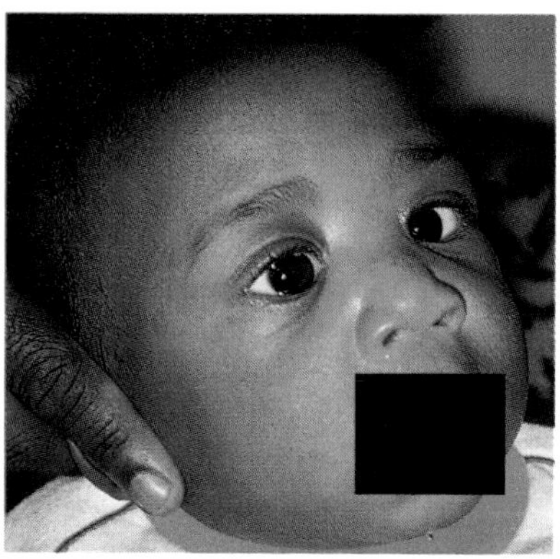

A

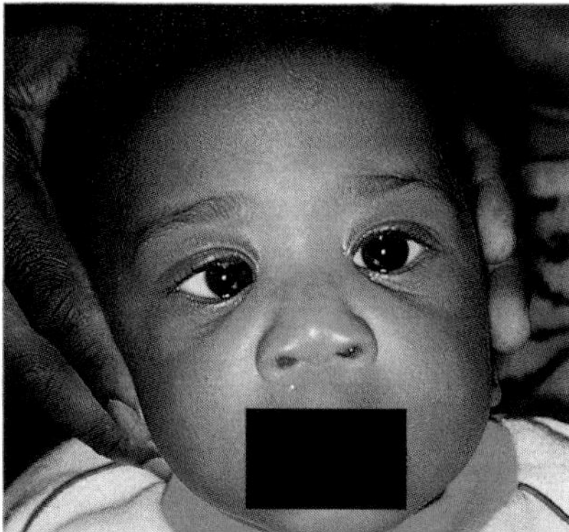

B

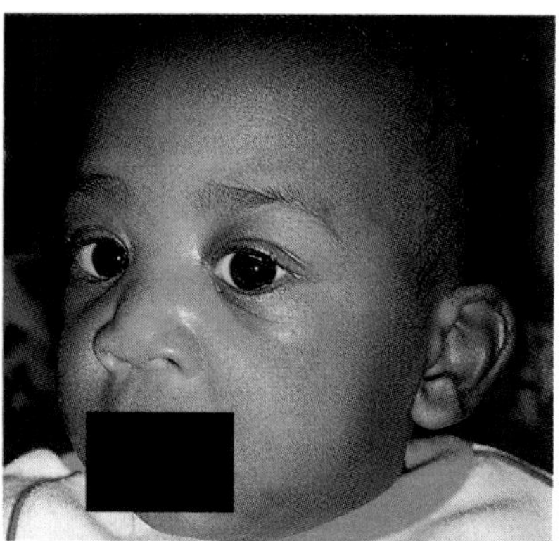

C

Figure 218–14. *A* to *C*, Child with right sixth nerve palsy secondary to middle ear infection (Gradenigo's syndrome). The right esotropia was associated with poor abduction.

be obtained promptly.[2, 3, 21–24] However, often no definite etiology can be established, even after extensive evaluation. Patience should be advised, as partial or complete recovery may ensue in the next three to six months. The usual questions arise concerning the possible development of contraction of the antagonist medial rectus muscle and whether botulinum injections should be used.[5, 25–28] Repeated measurements of the deviation document any improvement, and forced ductions give some indication of the extent of any contraction. Patients with bilateral sixth nerve problems often show an asymmetric recovery pattern. If recovery proceeds to the point at which binocular function is possible over a limited range, the patient should be encouraged to manage without patching one eye. At some stage, usually six months or so after the onset of the problem, a relatively stable condition will have been reached. If the residual deviation is minor in degree and diplopia is present only on almost full lateral gaze, most patients do not want anything done.

For patients with larger deviations but who are still able to move the eye past the center line, a recession-resection procedure may be effective in restoring more nearly normal function. Adjustable sutures can be used, and a slight initial overcorrection is desirable, since there is a tendency for the effect of the correction to decrease later. If the eye cannot be brought to the center line, there must be some combination of contraction of the antagonist medial rectus muscle and weakened lateral rectus muscle function. If forced ductions show that the medial rectus is tight as one attempts to abduct the eye, it will be essential to perform a generous recession of this muscle, approximately 7 to 8 mm. Usually, a transposition or a Jensen procedure (see Specific Surgical Techniques) will be necessary to bring the eye to an approximately midline position.[26, 29] If forced ductions are indicative of only moderate contraction of the medial rectus muscle and if the patient can move the eye approximately to the center line, there may be sufficient residual function of the lateral rectus muscle to justify first performing a large resection of the muscle, but often the long-term results are disappointing, and a transposition or a Jensen procedure will be needed later.

Strabismus After Cataract Surgery

Patients scheduled for cataract operations sometimes have long-standing strabismus problems, but because of some combination of suppression and poor visual acuity, they do not complain of diplopia. After operation there may be a period during which patients learn to adjust to their improved acuity. Occasionally, a preexisting strabismus problem diminishes after cataract surgery, and in such an event, the patient usually is not bothered by significant diplopia. On rare occasions after cataract surgery, patients complain of newly acquired diplopia, usually vertical in nature. Examination may show a problem that was not noted preoperatively.[30, 31] If the preoperative visual acuity had been extremely poor, it is possible that both the patient and the cataract surgeon might not have been aware of a small vertical imbalance. In most instances, however, one must conclude that something about the cataract operation produced a change in oculomotor function, either unmasking a previously tolerated problem or creating a new one.[32]

It is well recognized that some postoperative ptosis, presumably related to the combined effects of local injections, placement of stay sutures, and manipulation of the eye is relatively common after cataract surgery. Such ptosis often clears or regresses significantly in the postoperative period. The same factors could presumably account for the development of a postoperative, vertical tropia, but the frequency of occurrence of a persistent diplopia problem is low compared with the incidence of ptosis.[33, 34] In some instances, examination of the patient may show limitation of motion,[35] but usually this is not true. Moreover, the problem is not always attributable to a hypotropia of the eye that last underwent cataract surgery. It is unusual to find a new medical or neurologic problem. Initial treatment of the diplopia should be conservative. If the problem can be relieved by the use of small vertical prisms, the patient should be given the appropriate glasses. The patient should be followed for some months to determine the stability of the misalignment. In some patients, there may be indications that the diplopia is related to the unmasking of a fourth nerve problem or the beginning of an orbital problem, but often the patient is left with a persistent vertical tropia with no localizing signs. The surgeon is tempted to place the blame on a stretched or weakened superior rectus muscle and perhaps to consider a resection of the offending muscle. Although this may give satisfactory results in the primary position, any accompanying limitation of depression of the globe may cause the patient to experience diplopia when reading. Consequently, it may be preferable to carry out a recession of the inferior rectus muscle of a hypotropic eye,[36] using the adjustable suture technique if possible.

Strabismus After Surgery for Retinal Detachment

Surgery for treating retinal detachment often involves extensive dissection around the globe and muscles. Muscles are not disinserted as frequently now as in the past, but some muscle trauma can be caused by the use of traction sutures. Scleral flap dissection can inadvertently involve the insertion of the superior oblique tendon, and the use of plastic inserts can induce various mechanical effects. Thus it is surprising that there is not a greater incidence of strabismus problems after retinal surgery.[37–39] When a postoperative misalignment does occur, it may initially be masked by the poor acuity of the operated eye. When acuity improves, the patient may have a variable diplopia problem, but often this

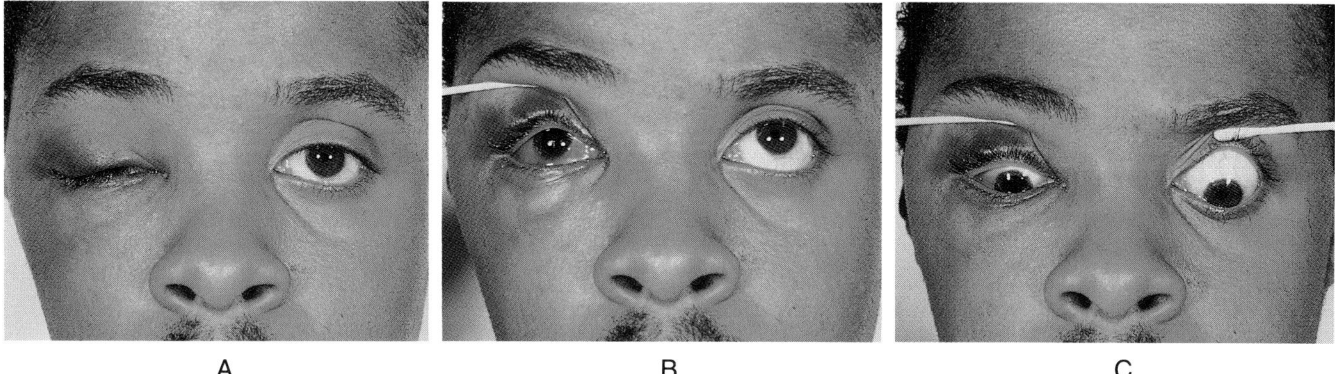

Figure 218–15. *A,* Patient with blowout fracture of the right orbital floor due to blunt trauma. *B,* The right eye exhibits restricted elevation because of entrapment of the inferior rectus muscle in the fracture line. Forced ductions would reveal a mechanical restriction of elevation in this eye. *C,* Downward movement of the right eye is also limited by the entrapment, but forced ductions would not show restricted movement in this direction.

improves spontaneously. When the problem persists, the strabismus surgeon has to estimate the possible relative contributions of weakened muscles, mechanical obstruction, and the effects of general scarring and adhesions.[40, 41] Knowledge of the details of the original operation can be helpful, but it often is difficult to determine the best course of action without exposing the muscles and any bands, inserts, sponges, and so on. This is best handled in close cooperation with a retinal surgeon, preferably the surgeon who originally repaired the retinal detachment. Sometimes the removal of external hardware will be enough to resolve the problem or at least to modify it significantly. Thus a two-stage approach may be best in some cases. It should be remembered that these cases can be technically challenging, and the strabismus surgeon must be prepared to modify his technique as the occasion demands.

Strabismus After Blowout Fracture

Usually, there is an adequate history for these cases, but for old problems the lack of a definite history may be misleading. Forced ductions can be helpful, and the use of modern imaging techniques often provides crucial information.[42] As a general rule, diplopia in the immediate postinjury period should not be taken to indicate the need for immediate surgery. Conditions often improve within 1 to 2 wk, and surgery may not be required. It should be remembered that blow-out fracture repair operations can be hazardous.[43] However, diplopia due to restricted upward and downward gaze suggests entrapment of the inferior rectus muscle in the fracture line (Fig. 218–15), and one should consider the optimal time for surgical intervention. Experience shows that if the orbital fracture is to be explored and repaired and trapped or damaged tissue is to be released, it is best to proceed with the surgery before significant fibrosis and adhesions have the chance to develop.

The strabismus surgeon may elect to work with a colleague specializing in orbital surgery or with an ear, nose and throat (ENT) surgeon if a Caldwell-Luc procedure is to be used. The initial object is to reduce the fracture, often with placement of a plastic implant,[44] and to release any tissue entrapment caused by the fracture. The results of such operations can be unpredictable as far as ocular alignment is concerned.[45] Sometimes reestablishment of a more normal orbital anatomy provides a surprising degree of improvement in oculomotor function and alignment, but often a significant misalignment persists (Fig. 218–16). One then has to consider the problem as one of muscle alignment. This is usually true when a patient with a healed blow-out fracture has a strabismus problem some months after the original injury, surgery, or both. In general, in relation to strabismus, there is nothing to be gained by revising the orbital repair provided that the state of the orbit is satisfactory. However, in some instances more orbital repair surgery may be planned, providing an opportunity to look at the surgical field and possibly to carry out forced ductions. Usually, it is best to wait several months after such surgery and then to examine the patient again to determine what strabismus surgery may be needed.

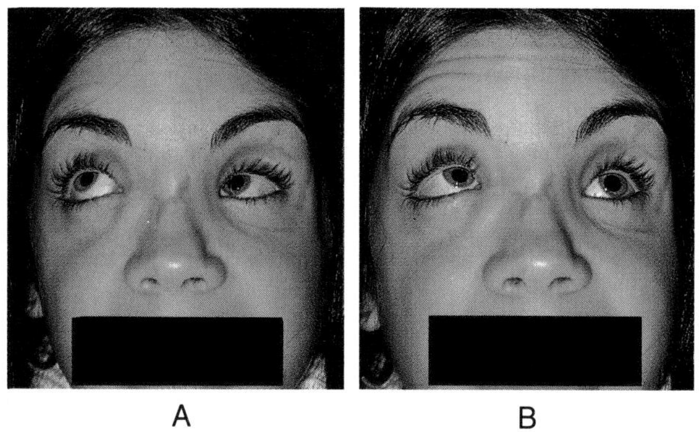

Figure 218–16. *A* and *B,* Patient with a history of trauma to the region of the midface and left orbit. Reconstruction of the orbit was performed, but the patient was left with enophthalmos and limitation of upward gaze in the left eye.

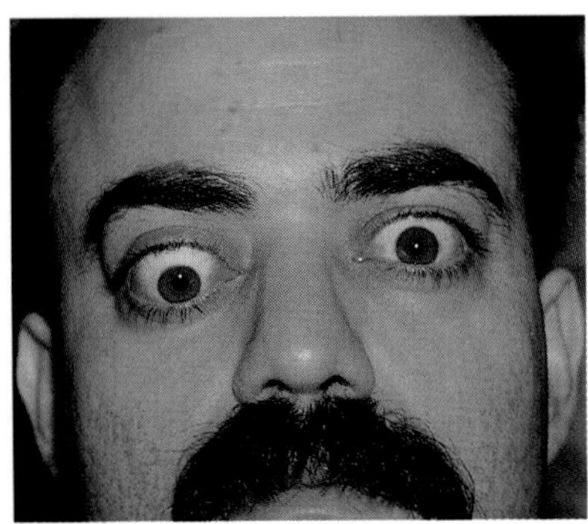

Figure 218–17. Patient with Graves' disease, exhibiting lid retraction, right hypotropia due to infiltration and restricted movement of right inferior rectus muscle, and injection over insertion of horizontal rectus muscles in both eyes.

If forced ductions continue to show restrictive limitations—for example, to elevation—recession of the affected muscle or muscles will be needed. If a muscle appears to have been weakened by the trauma or surgical repair, then recess-resect or even transposition procedures may be needed. The misalignment also can be affected by operating on the fellow eye—for example, by a recession or a Faden procedure on the yoke muscle, but as mentioned under third nerve problems, some patients refuse permission for operation on their good eye.

Strabismus Associated With Graves' Disease

Making the clinical diagnosis of Graves' disease usually presents no problem,[46–48] although occasionally a patient presents with a negative thyroid history and yet shows restrictive problems typical of Graves' disease. The proptosis and ocular misalignment secondary to Graves' disease can be distressing to patients (Fig. 218–17), but it is most important not to hurry with surgical correction of the diplopia. Other treatment may be necessary: systemic therapy with corticosteroids, radiation therapy, or orbital decompression. The results of decompressive surgery are important for strabismus, since regardless of the approach used to enlarge orbital volume, the secondary ocular misalignment effects can be significant.[49–51] Thus the correct sequence of operations is important: orbital surgery, if indicated, always should precede strabismus surgery. Because the involved muscles are always tight and firm to extension, the usual procedure is to perform muscle recessions or weakening procedures. Adjustable sutures (discussed later) have a definite place in this type of surgery.[52]

It is worth remembering that both orbits are usually involved, often to different degrees. For example, if a patient with a tight right inferior rectus muscle prefers to fix with the right eye, the left eye shows a large hypertropia. Surgery should primarily be directed to the right eye, involving a recession of the tight right inferior rectus muscle. However, some degree of tightness of the left superior rectus muscle may become evident either coincident with or following soon after the original surgery, and it may be necessary to recess this muscle too.

Duane's Retraction Syndrome

Most patients with Duane's syndrome (Fig. 218–18) have had the diagnosis made in their early years, particularly if they had a significant head turn or vertical eye motion abnormality.[53–56] Occasionally, Duane's syndrome appears to have been newly acquired.[57, 58] If the patient's head turn is minor and if the ocular alignment in approximately the primary position is satisfactory, no surgery is indicated. If there has been no treatment or ineffective treatment, a pronounced strabismus with head turn may still be evident in the adult patient.

In general, treatment involves muscle-weakening procedures, since resecting muscles will tend to make the retraction component worse. If there is obvious retraction of the globe or a significant vertical misalignment attempted adduction or abduction, it may be helpful to recess both the medial and lateral rectus muscles.[59–62] For example, for such a patient with type I Duane's

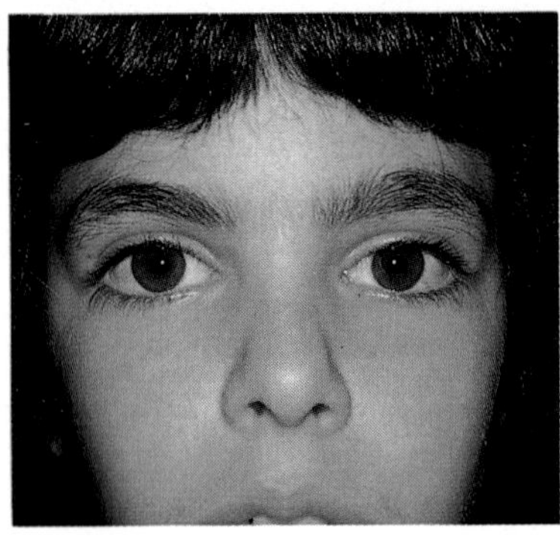

A

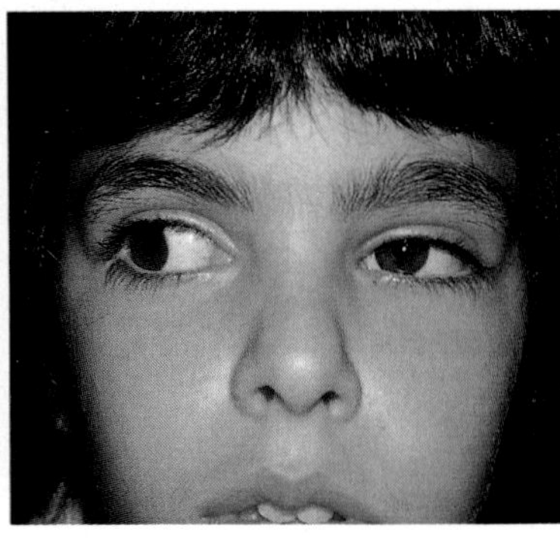

B

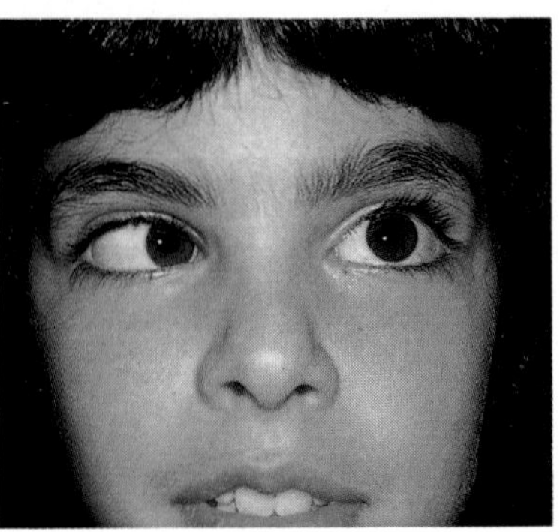

C

Figure 218–18. Patient with Duane's retraction syndrome in the left eye. The eyes are straight in the primary position (*A*), but an esotropia develops in left gaze (*B*), owing to the restricted abduction of the left eye. In right gaze (*C*), the left palpebral fissure narrows, owing to co-contraction of the left medial and lateral rectus muscles, causing retraction of the globe.

syndrome, the best initial procedure might be a generous recession of the medial rectus, up to 7 mm, and a smaller recession of the ipsilateral lateral rectus muscle. Other methods of controlling the secondary vertical deviation include using a posterior fixation suture,[60] or splitting the tendon of the tight horizontal muscle and transposing the halves vertically in opposite directions.[63] In the preceding example, if the patient had a major vertical shift of the eye on adduction, the tendon of the lateral rectus could be split, with the superior half moved up and the inferior half moved down relative to the original insertion.

Sometimes patients with Duane's syndrome have had previous surgery, but their condition has deteriorated with time. For such patients, further weakening procedures such as a Z-myotomy on the previously recessed muscle, can be tried. Because the vertical recti usually are functioning well, muscle transposition or a Jensen procedure may in some cases help to achieve better alignment in the primary position.[64]

Brown's Superior Oblique Tendon Sheath Syndrome

Congenital cases of Brown's superior oblique tendon sheath syndrome were probably diagnosed in early life (Fig. 218–19).[65] Minor cases may have escaped detection, but such cases presumably needed no treatment. Acquired cases of Brown's syndrome may result from trauma, orbital surgery or injections, orbital or sinus problems, or lid surgery.[66–73] Occasionally, a patient appears to develop a Brown's syndrome without obvious cause. The patient may be aware of some vague discomfort or noise on movement of the involved superior oblique tendon. Sometimes the examiner can palpate abnormalities of the superior oblique tendon, and imaging studies may be helpful. If an acute case is thought to be due to an inflammatory reaction, local injection of steroids can be tried,[66, 74] but this presents obvious risks. Usually treatment is surgical, but if the patient's eyes are satisfactorily aligned in the primary and reading positions, it is best to do nothing surgically. For a patient who has a significantly hypotropic eye, surgery is directed toward releasing the mechanically obstructed superior oblique tendon–trochlear mechanism, usually by a superior oblique tenectomy.[75–77] It is important to perform forced ductions repeatedly during operation to check that any restrictive effect is relieved. Some surgeons advocate a recession of the ipsilateral inferior oblique muscle at the same time, to avoid a secondary overaction of the inferior oblique.[78] In general, it would seem best to wait before doing this, to allow the results of the primary surgery to become apparent and stable. For the relatively unusual case in which the patient fixes with the involved eye, the contralateral eye may develop a secondary hypertropia. If surgery on the involved fixing eye does not improve the situation or is perhaps not permitted, a recession of the contralateral superior rectus muscle may offer some improvement.

Nystagmus and Abnormal Head Position

A patient with an abnormal head position may have nystagmus that varies in amplitude and frequency with direction of gaze. Visual function usually is best when

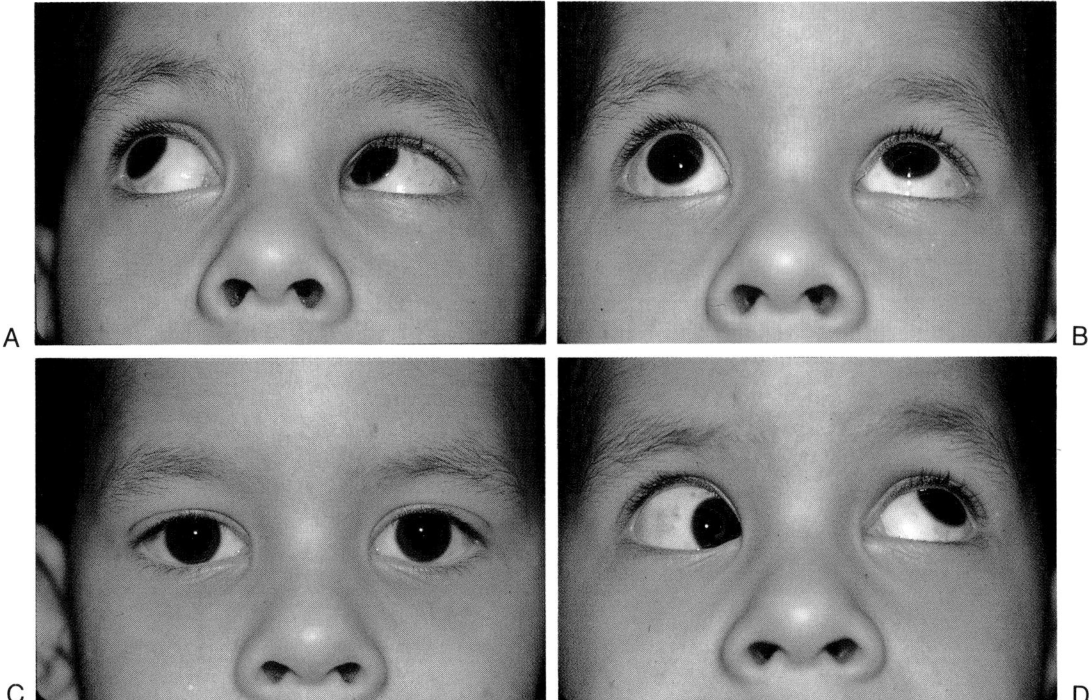

Figure 218–19. *A*, Patient with Brown's syndrome involving right superior oblique tendon. The eyes are straight in the primary position (*B*), but in upward gaze there is restriction of elevation in the adducted position (*C*). In abduction (*D*) the elevation is full.

the nystagmus is least; consequently, the patient may adopt a noncentered head-eye position. In some patients, the head turn may be small and may not be bothersome. Often, however, the nystagmus decreases only when the angle of gaze is far from the center line, resulting in the adoption of an abnormal head position. Most often this takes the form of a left or right head turn, but a chin-up or chin-down position is seen in some cases, and a definite head tilt is occasionally manifest. In addition, patients may have strabismus superimposed on the nystagmus and head turn, and they may have strabismic amblyopia as well as decreased visual acuity associated with the nystagmus. These patients need careful and repeated evaluation, since the nystagmus and abnormal head position are not always constant. Some patients may have two null positions for their nystagmus (e.g., on gaze left and on gaze right). Examination of old photographs can be useful, as mentioned earlier.

Various forms of treatment have been suggested and have been tried with varying degrees of success. An accurate refraction may help some patients but usually has little effect on even small head turns. The use of prisms should correct small angles of deviation, but patients rarely are concerned with deviations of only a few degrees. Prescribing large prisms is useless. Injection with botulinum may eventually have a place in the treatment of some patients, but at present there are no data to justify this as anything but an experimental approach.

For a patient with a significant head turn, usually horizontal, treatment is surgery on the appropriate muscles, usually referred to as a Kestenbaum or Kestenbach-Anderson procedure.[79–82] For example, consider a patient with an abnormal head position in the horizontal plane, such as a head turn to the right with eyes deviated to the left. One may avoid confusion by visualizing the Kestenbaum procedure as requiring disinsertion of the horizontal rectus muscles, rotation of the head to the left, followed by reattachment of the muscles. This particular example would require a recession of the left lateral rectus, a resection of the left medial rectus, a recession of the right medial rectus, and a resection of the right lateral rectus. The extent of muscle surgery has been the subject of discussion. Obviously, the amount of correction required depends to some extent on the magnitude of the eye-head turn, but because the purpose of operation is usually to correct a large angle of head turn, small variations in the scope of surgery are not very important. Most surgeons now would probably agree that the extent of recession-resection originally suggested by Kestenbaum is inadequate and should be enlarged.[81] Thus in the example cited, with the preferred gaze direction almost full left, the patient may require a 7-mm recession of the right medial rectus, an 8-mm resection of the left medial recuts, a 9-mm recession of the left lateral rectus, and a 10-mm resection of the right lateral rectus. Provided that one selects the correct muscles, the 7, 8, 9, 10–mm progression forms a useful reminder for the measurements involved. If an esotropia or exotropia is present in addition to the head turn, the surgeon may elect to correct this at a later time or may attempt to correct it during the original surgery by modifying these numbers. In effect, the extent of surgery needed for correction of the strabismic deviation can be added algebraically to the numbers selected for the Kestenbaum procedure. In the case cited here, if the patient had a predominantly left esotropia in addition to the head turn to the right, the left eye position would not need as much correction. The amounts of recession-resection suggested for the left eye would be reduced, depending upon the magnitude of the left esotropia compared with the amount of head turn. It is useful to review these numbers preoperatively several times and to have them available for reference in the operating room.

The results obtained with the Kestenbaum procedure can be impressive. Failure to achieve adequate correction of the head turn, or fairly rapid regression of an initial improvement is probably due to insufficient recession-resection. There is a tendency for the initial correction of head position to diminish with time.

GENERAL CONSIDERATIONS FOR STRABISMUS SURGERY

Anesthesia

General anesthesia is almost universally used for operations on infants, children, and most young adults. A first-rate anesthesia staff is an absolute requirement, and obviously the anesthetists should be experienced in handling small infants and children. For operations on cooperative adult patients, there is much to be said in favor of using local anesthesia. However, although it should be possible for most adult patients to be comfortable with local anesthesia, in practice many healthy adults do not appreciate this. Consequently, if there are any reservations about the possible effectiveness of local anesthesia, usually it is best to employ general anesthesia. Even when local anesthesia is used, it is appropriate to have the patient monitored by an anesthetist who is familiar with eye surgery.

For local anesthesia, a relatively short-acting agent may be used, such as 2 percent lidocaine HCl (Xylocaine). Some surgeons prefer to use a mixture that includes a longer-acting agent, such as 0.75 percent bupivacaine (Marcaine). Retrobulbar or peribulbar injections can be used, depending on the experience of the surgeon. Sometimes a patient with an apparently satisfactory local block reports discomfort when traction is applied to the ocular muscles. Such patients may require additional local injections of anesthetic agents in order to achieve a satisfactory level of anesthesia. Systemic medications can also be useful in such instances. Use of the longer-acting agents such as bupivacaine appears to provide longer postoperative periods of relative comfort, but individual reactions to this vary considerably.

Because most strabismus patients are basically healthy individuals, the overall anesthesia complication rate is low.[83-85] However, conditions can deteriorate rapidly and unexpectedly, cardiovascular crises can occur, and there is always the possibility of some unusual occurrence such as malignant hyperthermia.[86-89] This last is a hypermetabolic problem that may be triggered by anesthetic agents. Taking a complete and accurate history is most important in this respect, since the occurrence of any previous anesthetic problem with the patient or close relatives should raise the index of suspicion. However, it must also be recognized that susceptible patients can be given anesthetics uneventfully but develop malignant hyperthermia with the next anesthetic. Fortunately, treatment is available, so that with awareness of the potential problem on the part of all concerned, serious complications should be extremely unusual.

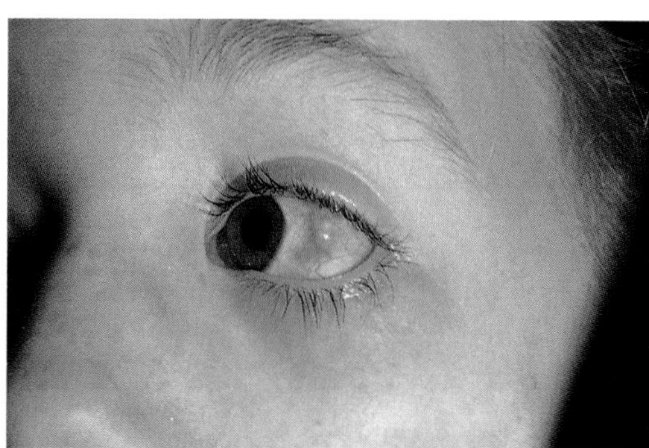

Figure 218–20. Suture granuloma at site of reattachment of lateral rectus muscle 1 mo after strabismus surgery in which gut sutures were used.

Surgical Considerations

The precise details of various surgical techniques are not discussed at length here. Many good sources, with photographs and drawings to illustrate various points, are available,[90-97] and video recordings allow a closer look at actual operations. Surgeons develop their own favorite methods of opening, performing the muscle surgery, and closing. The experienced surgeon will probably not change habits without good reason. The less experienced surgeon may wish to try different methods or perhaps to copy the techniques of a more senior associate. The overall aim should be to execute the proposed surgery accurately while minimizing the possibility of complications.

Stay sutures, in addition to providing traction, directly indicate the orientation of the globe; 6–0 silk sutures placed close to the limbus may be used, or in situations in which more traction is needed, 4–0 sutures may be placed around the muscles. The opening incision may be in the fornix,[98] postoperatively yielding a quiet-looking eye, but the exposure provided is sometimes limited. A limbal approach provides better exposure in general and heals in a satisfactory manner.[99] Dissection and exposure of the extraocular muscles should be carried out carefully, and unnecessary dissection should be avoided. Hemorrhage should be controlled with light cautery but preferably should be avoided in the first place.

The use of gut sutures for strabismus surgery has declined greatly with the introduction of synthetic absorbable sutures such as polyglactin 910 (Vicryl). Gut sutures often caused suture granulomas at the site of muscle reattachment (Fig. 218–20). Some surgeons use nonabsorbable sutures on the grounds of durability, lack of tissue reaction, and the like. These permanent sutures can be encountered many years after their placement, and there seems to be no overwhelming reason to use them except in particular situations such as a Jensen procedure. Spatula needles should be used in most cases.

It is good practice to be sure that the sutures are firmly attached to the muscle and that the muscle is anchored adequately to the globe. Lost or slipped muscles are complications best avoided in the first place. Various sutures can be used for closing the conjunctival flaps or incisions. Exposed Vicryl sutures can be irritating to the patient. Gut sutures are still used by some surgeons and in general are comfortable. Fine silk sutures (e.g., 7–0 black silk) are quite comfortable, and when tied tightly almost always fall out within approximately 2 wk.

Postoperative use of antibiotics and steroids depends on the surgeon's preference and on local practice. Experience shows that the incidence of postoperative infections is extremely low. Nevertheless, many surgeons feel more comfortable when patients postoperatively use local antibiotics for 1 to 2 wk. Whether using local steroids makes any significant difference is debatable.[100]

For each individual patient, the surgeon must estimate the extent of surgery required. Because of the many variables and unknown factors involved, generally it is futile to make specific recommendations for each case. The muscle surgery suitable for a 6-month-old esotropic infant will be less than that appropriate for an adult with high myopia and a large-angle deviation. However, some broad general limits are worth keeping in mind. For the horizontal rectus muscles, it is unusual to plan for less than 4 mm of recession or resection. For the vertical recti somewhat smaller lower limits are appropriate, approximately 3 mm, but it should be remembered that disinserting a muscle and placing sutures may introduce errors that can consume a large fraction of a nominal 3-mm adjustment.

The maximum amounts of surgery are more variable. For adults the medial rectus muscle can be recessed approximately 7 mm, although smaller recessions are more often used. The lateral rectus can be recessed a larger amount, to approximately 10 mm. For the vertical recti, smaller limits, approximately 5 mm for a recession, apply. The maximum amount a muscle can be resected depends to some extent on how much the surgeon is willing to risk some postoperative restriction of motion. For the lateral rectus, a resection of 8 to 10 mm is usually well tolerated. The length of medial rectus muscle available for resection is shorter, so that a limit of approximately 7 mm resection is appropriate. For the vertical recti, the usual upper limits for resection are smaller, approximately 5 mm, as is true for recessions of these muscles. When operating on infants and small children, the maximum amounts of muscle surgery described usually need to be reduced by approximately 30 percent or more in most conventional cases.

Sometimes previous surgery on an eye may have produced a later overcorrection, and a muscle that had been recessed is now required to be strengthened. This can be done by advancing the muscle from its recessed position to the original insertion site, and if indicated, by augmenting the effect with a simultaneous resection of the muscle.

The approximate limits discussed here should be viewed only as guidelines; they may need to be exceeded in special cases. Patients who have severe paralytic problems or restrictive myopathies often require larger amounts of surgery.

Surgical Complications

Penetration of the choroid and retina is a complication that probably was more common years ago.[101–104] Most strabismus surgeons at some time have likely wondered whether a needle was passed a little too deeply. Meticulous care in using needles is mandatory, and a conscious awareness should be maintained. If perforation is thought to have occurred, the pupil should be dilated and the retina examined. In many instances, the problem appears to be localized to the choroid, often without any significant hemorrhage. Treatment is somewhat controversial. Cryotherapy or diathermy can be applied, but many retinal surgeons advise only observation, which usually turns out to be appropriate. In any event, consultation with a retinal surgeon is advisable, and the patient obviously needs to be followed carefully in the postoperative period.

A different matter is that of the lost or slipped muscle.[105–107] If this problem is evident in the operating room, immediate repair should be attempted. Muscles do not simply disappear; often a muscle can be relocated by judicious probing in the region in which one would expect it to be found. It is more common to encounter this complication postoperatively, often on referral some time after the original operation. If the muscle is effectively disconnected from the globe, motion in the field of action of the muscle, apart from that due to the relaxation of its antagonist, will be almost nonexistent. Forced ductions can be most useful here, if they can be carried out with an awake and cooperative patient. However, complete disconnection of a muscle is less frequent than slippage with some residual muscle function. Usually, the etiology is not clear, although experience suggests that sometimes sutures may not have been securely attached to actual muscle but may have been placed in the muscle sheath or connective tissue. Also, very shallow placement of sutures in the sclera may result in the sutures pulling loose. If other procedures such as a scleral buckle[108] or orbital surgery have been performed, the situation may be more complicated. The surgeon should discuss the problem with the patient, pointing out the uncertain outcome of more surgery. Experience shows that it often is possible to improve matters considerably, even months or years after the development of the original problem, so that surgery can be offered with a reasonable expectation of achieving some improvement.

Significant postoperative complications are infrequent with strabismus patients. The appearance of the eye may worry the patient, and there may be concern about possible infection, but this fortunately is extremely rare.[109–112] The hallmarks of external infection are pain, lid edema, and chemosis, and if the orbit is more generally involved, there may be proptosis and significant limitation of motion. The time course of infection may vary considerably. Of most concern are the extremely unusual cases of suspected endophthalmitis, probably associated with globe perforation at surgery. With such cases, a few hours delay in diagnosis and treatment can be critical, but most strabismus surgeons do not encounter this complication during their professional lifetimes. However, if an infection of any sort is strongly suspected, appropriate and rapid treatment is indicated. Local and systemic antibiotics should be employed without delaying treatment for the results of cultures. For external infections, exploration and drainage may be necessary, but such procedures are uncommon. The strabismus surgeon is much more likely to receive patients' complaints of nonspecific eye pain without any obvious localizing or threatening signs. In such instances, routine postoperative care with close follow-up is often the best course.

Alterations in the local topography of the conjunctiva secondary to surgery sometimes lead to the occurrence of corneal changes, or dellen, owing to differences in the hydration of the cornea. Usually, the dellen are more apparent to the surgeon than to the patient. Prevention by making a smooth limbal closure and by avoiding the placement of large sutures at the limbus is the best approach. When they occur, dellen usually respond well to artificial tears, time, and sometimes a short period of firm patching.

Tissue reactions due to sutures were more common when gut sutures were used.[113] Now that most surgeons use absorbable synthetic sutures, the incidence of such reactions has decreased markedly, but they will still be encountered at times. In such patients, there is usually a modest inflammatory reaction that persists after the normal healing period. Sometimes suture ends may be evident on careful inspection, particularly if they are positioned so as to be approximately perpendicular to the ocular surface. Usually, it is best to treat these reactions with observation and mild steroid drops. In some patients, a cystic structure that does not shrink with time may develop. Aspiration can be tried, but it usually is necessary to excise a cystic lesion, taking care not to create a secondary strabismus problem. If the lesion is completely removed and light cautery is applied to the base area, recurrence is unusual.

Of particular interest to strabismus surgeons is an unusual but serious complication—anterior segment ischemia which is due to interference with the blood supply to the anterior segment of the eye.[114–120] The term *anterior segment ischemia* is more apt than the sometimes used *anterior segment necrosis*. Fortunately, massive necrosis usually is not encountered, but the effects of ischemia can be severe. The blood supply to the anterior segment of the eye largely depends on the integrity of the anterior ciliary arteries. When a rectus muscle is detached from the globe, for either a resection or a recession, there must necessarily be some degree of interference with the circulation to the anterior segment of the eye. Collateral circulation from untouched muscles usually provides an adequate blood supply, but occasionally this supply appears to fall short. Then, within hours after surgery, slit lamp examination will show evidence of corneal problems, with corneal haze and thickening, usually with abnormalities of Descemet's membrane. A significant anterior chamber reaction, often with an abnormal iris appearance and reaction, usually is present. Later, there may be marked iris atrophy, usually segmental in nature, and various degrees of cataract formation. This ischemic complication was formerly seen after some retinal detachment repairs, when muscles were detached to facilitate exposure and encircling bands were used.[121] Its occurrence following strabismus surgery is highly correlated with the number of muscles detached and with the general circulatory characteristics of the patient. Recent surveys have confirmed that the incidence of anterior segment ischemia is extremely low in young, healthy patients but increases with age and with the presence of circulatory problems. It should be remembered that there are reports of anterior ischemia following surgery on just two rectus muscles.[122] The lapse of time between successive operations on different muscles does not necessarily allow reestablishment of blood supply sufficient to protect the eye against the ischemic effects of later surgery. Thus when strabismus surgery is planned, it is wise not only to consider the blood supply changes directly related to the proposed surgery but also to remember that the risk of ischemia may be enhanced owing to previous surgery. Transposition procedures combined with the recession of an antagonist muscle obviously can give rise to such problems, particularly since these procedures are often performed on older patients.[123, 124] More is said on this subject later, in the discussion of the Jensen procedure.

There has been discussion about muscle surgery using microdissection of the major vessels, in order to avoid embarrassment of the anterior segment blood supply.[125] Although this is an appealing concept, it is not clear that it has major practical usefulness; indeed, the prolonged operative time and exposure could conceivably prove detrimental to patients.

In the unfortunate patients in whom anterior segment ischemia does occur, treatment should consist of the immediate use of local and systemic corticosteroids. When constrictive sutures are thought to contribute to the problem—for example, with the Jensen procedure—some surgeons advocate immediate release of the sutures. It is not clear that this really helps. Intensive treatment of the ischemic process fortunately appears to limit its progression in most cases, although later problems with cataract development, iris abnormalities, and posterior synechiae, are presumably related in some measure to interference with the blood supply to the anterior segment of the eye.

SPECIFIC SURGICAL TECHNIQUES

Exposure Problems

Operation on the lateral rectus muscle usually offers no problems with accessibility or exposure, but it should be remembered that the inferior oblique muscle may be encountered at the inferior aspect of the lateral rectus muscle. There may be a slightly more limited field when exposing the medial rectus muscle, depending on the patient's orbital and nasal anatomy. Also, when performing resections, the surgeon must be aware of the relatively limited amount of freely available medial rectus muscle—from 7 to 8 mm—and must not be tempted to dissect too far back, and to expose orbital fat. The ease of approach to the superior rectus muscle varies considerably from patient to patient. For individuals with deep-set globes and overhanging brows, the exposure and muscle surgery can be more demanding than with the horizontal muscles, requiring more use of retractors and careful placement of sutures. Strabismus operations on the superior rectus muscle are often limited in extent, so that usually the levator and the superior oblique tendon are not encountered, but excessive dissection of the superior rectus muscle and wide and deep sweeps with muscle hooks should be avoided when possible. When the inferior rectus is approached, the surgeon faces a potential problem arising from the proximity of the inferior oblique muscle. However, if only small amounts of surgery are involved, the procedure usually is straightforward. Some surgeons advocate extensive dissection of tissues surrounding the inferior rectus muscle to avoid causing postoperative problems with the position of the lower lid. This is useful when larger recessions are planned—for example, in patients with Graves' disease—but even then, lid repositioning procedures may be needed later. When extensive dissection is implemented, the possibility of causing damage to the innervation of the inferior oblique muscle is always present, but this fortunately seems to be a more theoretical than practical problem for the commoner strabismus procedures. The possibility of such damage obviously increases with cases involving orbital floor fractures, scleral buckling procedures, and orbital exploration.

Reoperations

The strabismus surgeon often must deal with patients who have had previous strabismus surgery, and instead of operating on previously untouched muscles, it may be necessary to reoperate on muscles that have undergone previous surgery. A previously recessed muscle may require tightening, so that some combination of advancement and resection of the muscle needs to be carried out. If the deviation is moderate in degree, only a small advancement of a previously recessed muscle may be needed. For a larger angle of deviation, the muscle may require resection and advancement to its original insertion site.

A further weakening or lengthening procedure may be indicated for a muscle that has already been recessed maximally. There has been some interest in the technique of lengthening a muscle by transplanting a segment that normally would be discarded, typically after a muscle has been resected.[126] Experience with this technique is limited, and it remains experimental. In practice one may perform a marginal myotomy (sometimes called a Z-myotomy),[127, 128] use a "hangback" suture,[129–133] or almost totally disconnect the muscle. The latter course is usually employed only in severe cases of paralytic strabismus. Since the postoperative position of a disinserted muscle is not known with any precision, residual attachments to the globe may still exist, and the outcome is somewhat uncertain.

Even when a muscle has been weakened to the point at which one would expect it to exert little force postoperatively, it sometimes may still function well enough so that strabismus may recur to a significant degree. When this problem is anticipated, it may be worthwhile to use stay or traction sutures in an attempt to forestall it.[134] One or two sutures (e.g., 5–0 Mersilene) are placed firmly in the sclera close to the muscle insertion or at the 6- and 12-o'clock positions. The sutures are passed out through the lid conjunctiva to exit on the skin surface and are tied over a small piece of silicone, or in some cases taped firmly to the skin. This is convenient when the sutures exit temporally, but when the eye has to be held adducted, it may be best to bring the sutures out through the nasal aspect of the upper lid and tape them to the forehead. Patients often find these sutures uncomfortable, and it is unusual for them to be left in place for more than 1 to 2 wk. After the stay sutures are removed, the eye sometimes has a distressing tendency to stray from its corrected position.

Closing the conjunctival flaps usually is straightforward in primary cases, although if the preoperative deviation was large, there may appear to be an excess of tissue on one side and a corresponding lack of tissue on the other side. When dealing with reoperations, the conjunctival flaps may be thickened and scarred. Excess fibrotic tissue can be excised, but the flap often retains some degree of inelasticity. A flap that appears to have excess tissue usually retracts and improves in appearance with time. A small section of the conjunctival edge of a flap may sometimes be removed to provide better approximation to the limbus. When a large exotropia is being corrected and the nasal flap is correspondingly full it may help to place an absorbable suture through the plica, back into the superficial aspect of the medial rectus muscle, and out again through the conjunctival flap. This suture is then tightened and tied to restore a more normal appearance of the nasal conjunctiva.

If the conjunctival flap on the side of the recessed muscle is stretched somewhat to make a limbal closure, it may exert sufficient tension to postoperatively affect the position of the eye (i.e., it may reduce the extent of the correction). For this reason, it sometimes is appropriate to reattach the flap to the sclera at a position recessed from the limbus, taking care that the flap covers the original muscle insertion (Fig. 218–21).[135]

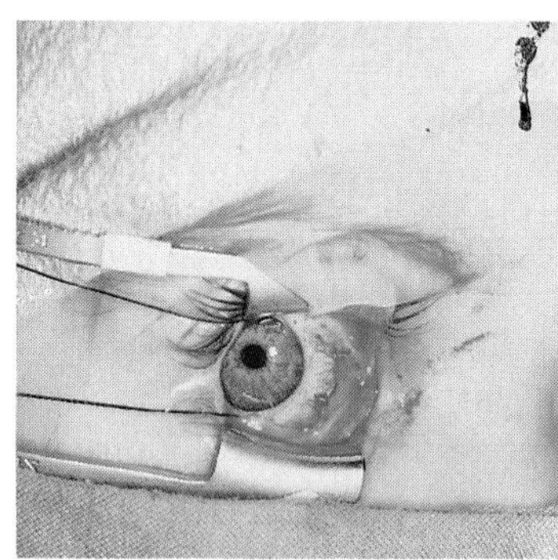

Figure 218–21. When closing a limbal incision, recession of the conjunctiva from the limbus is sometimes advisable to avoid traction that might otherwise limit the effect of a large rectus muscle recession.

Hangback Sutures

With this technique, the muscle to be further recessed is allowed to retract more by providing a suture extension of the muscle. Permanent sutures are attached firmly to the muscle, which is then dissected free from the globe. The sutures are placed in the sclera, but instead of attaching the muscle tightly to the globe the muscle is allowed to retract the estimated amount before the suture ends are tied. In general, it seems best to place the sutures so that minimum lengths are involved, thus limiting the distance the muscle can move from its intended position. Nevertheless, as with total disinsertion of a muscle, the final position of the muscle is not precisely predictable.

Marginal Myotomy (Z-Myotomy)

A marginal myotomy is accomplished by cutting some muscle fibers transversely in two positions on opposite sides of the muscle, separated by approximately one muscle width or more. The expanding incisions on opposite sides of the muscle allow the muscle to elongate, making this portion of the muscle resemble a capital Z lying on its side. This can be an effective weakening procedure, provided that attention is paid to details. Adequate exposure is essential. As the muscle almost always has been recessed at previous surgery, the posterior dissection of the muscle needs to be carried back further than usual to allow the posterior incision to be placed approximately one muscle width from the anterior incision. *Marginal myotomy* is not the most appropriate term, since it indicates one of the potential problems that may be encountered with this procedure, namely, the incisions across the muscle may be too limited in extent. In order to achieve significant lengthening and weakening of the muscle, it is essential that no intact muscle fibers should be left running the length of the muscle—i.e., that the incisions across the muscle must extend significantly beyond the approximate center line. It is best to make the posterior incision first, because retraction of the muscle after the initial incision makes exposure more difficult if the anterior incision is made first. To prevent hemorrhage, a small hemostat is clamped across most of the muscle width at the position of the incision. The hemostat is then removed, and the incision is made in the crushed area. The aim should be to transect approximately three fourths of the muscle. It may be helpful to carry out gentle probing with closed scissors to gauge the tension of the remaining muscle fibers. If only small incisions are made across the muscle, the procedure will not result in significant lengthening and weakening of the muscle.

Faden Procedure

This is an interesting technique for weakening muscle function.[136–140] The precise mechanism is subject to some question. If used with a patient who is essentially orthotropic in the primary position, the procedure usually has little effect on the primary position of the eye but will provide some limitation of movement in the field of action of the involved muscle.

The normal position of a rectus muscle on the globe allows the muscle a small arc of contact with the globe before it diverges from the globe. The Faden procedure extends this posterior arc of contact of the muscle with the globe by using nonabsorbable sutures to attach the muscle posteriorly to the globe. The geometry of the eye and of the rectus muscles in the orbit suggests that the procedure will have different results when applied to different muscles. It seems to be generally recognized that the procedure is most effective when employed with the medial rectus muscle and that when the lateral rectus muscle is involved, the sutures need to be placed considerably further back. In practice, this means that the fixation sutures should be placed approximately 10 to 15 mm behind the original insertion of the rectus muscle. Good exposure and illumination are necessary, and a headlight may be helpful. When working with the vertical rectus muscles, the positions of the vortex veins should be kept in mind, in order to reduce the risk of causing potentially troublesome hemorrhages. Also, there is an increased risk of scleral perforation with this technique.[103, 141]

In practice, the Faden procedure often is combined with a muscle recession. Even if a recession is not planned, disinsertion of the involved muscle may help provide better exposure of the posterior portion of the globe, where the sutures will be placed. The scleral positions for the posterior sutures are marked, and permanent sutures—for example, 5–0 Mersilene—are placed. The muscle is then positioned either in its recessed or its original position, and small bites with the preplaced posterior scleral sutures are taken through the corresponding positions on the muscle to attach it to the sclera. The muscle insertion is then reattached to the globe. It should be pointed out that in some instances, particularly when the superior rectus muscle is involved, implementing the Faden procedure can be more difficult than might be expected.

The effectiveness of the Faden procedure is open to question. Many surgeons feel that it works well and should be employed more often. Other surgeons are less enthusiastic, finding the results of limited usefulness.

Adjustable Sutures

It is clear to most strabismus surgeons that strabismus surgery is not an exact science. The amount of muscle that is recessed or the length of muscle resected is based partly on measurements, partly on experience, and partly on intuition. The surgeon is often left with considerable uncertainty about the amount of correction to be expected postoperatively. This can be a problem with patients who have had previous operations and for patients with orbital problems such as Graves' ophthalmopathy or traumatic problems. It was recognized years ago that some insurance against major over- and undercorrection could be obtained by using adjustable sutures. The procedure appeared to generate little interest and was not often used until Jampolsky emphasized its practical usefulness in selected patients.[142–151] The basic concept is that the sutures attached to the recessed or resected muscle are passed through their scleral anchoring points, but instead of tying them in position, a temporary tie is placed. After the patient has recovered from anesthesia, the alignment of the eyes is checked. The adjustable suture may then be tightened or loosened in order to improve the alignment. Surgeons often find that in practice the initial alignment is satisfactory, and the adjustable suture is simply tied in place. In patients in whom an adjustment is carried out, it is not always possible to be as specific as one would wish concerning the actual amount of adjustment, and there must always be questions about the future stability of the alignment.[152, 153]

It may sometimes be appropriate to use adjustable sutures on more than one muscle, although in the majority of instances, a single adjustable suture is employed. The technique can be used with either a recessed or a resected muscle. In many strabismus patients, a muscle has to be recessed or weakened substantially in order to allow the resected or advanced antagonist muscle or both to bring the eye into better alignment. The problem then is to decide how much resection to carry out without too much risk of overcorrection. In these instances, a somewhat larger than usual amount of muscle may be resected, advanced, or both, using an adjustable suture, and any significant overcorrection then can be reduced. Obviously, the choice of how to use adjustable sutures depends to a large extent on the surgeon's previous experience.

Adjustable sutures do not guarantee excellent results,

but they can be useful when more than the usual uncertainty exists about the expected degree of correction or when the patient has expressed definite opinions about the desired surgical outcome. A number of authors have described their experiences with adjustable sutures, but there have been no randomized prospective studies, and the reported results must be viewed with some degree of caution.

It is important to select carefully the patients with whom to employ this technique. Some authors report using adjustable sutures with young children or teenagers. Others point out that some patients are not suitable candidates for the manipulation involved in the adjustment process. It is clear that with children, the use of adjustable sutures is really a two-stage anesthesia procedure. The surgery is carried out, the child is awakened to some extent, and an estimate is made of the ocular alignment. Then, more anesthesia is given, to allow the suture to be adjusted and tied. This approach allows immediate correction of a major postoperative misalignment but usually is not suitable for more refined adjustment. The Q-Tips test may be useful in helping the surgeon select adult patients. This involves a moderately vigorous probing of the patient's eye with a cotton-tipped applicator. A stoical acceptance of this activity augers well for a relatively tranquil adjustment experience.

The actual technique is simple. The sutures should be firmly attached to the muscle and should be well placed in the sclera, so that there is little chance of the sutures being pulled loose. In addition, it is easier to hold the sutures temporarily in position if the scleral sutures are angled toward each other and placed so that the free ends of the sutures emerging from the sclera are in close apposition. Some surgeons advocate placing a slip knot for temporary fixation. This has the disadvantage that it may be difficult to know just where the muscle is when the adjustment is carried out. An alternative technique is to use a small loop of suture tied tightly around the main suture ends where they emerge from the sclera. This tight loop holds the sutures in position, but it can be moved along the free suture ends to more readily define the amount of adjustment. In either case, once the desired position is obtained, the suture ends are permanently tied, and the excess suture material is removed. A practical point concerns the need to move the patient's eye during the adjustment process. Even when topical anesthesia is used (e.g., 4 percent cocaine solution), the use of fixation forceps often is uncomfortable for the patient. A separate small loop suture (e.g., 5–0 Mersilene) may be placed in the sclera close to the limbus to provide a convenient and relatively painless way of controlling the position of the eye. The conjunctival flap can be left recessed to provide exposure for the suture adjustment, but this leaves the tied suture ends exposed. In general it would seem to be better practice and make the patient more comfortable to cover the suture ends with the conjunctival flap at the conclusion of the adjustment. This is readily achieved by placing the usual sutures for closing the conjunctival flap but leaving one or two sutures long and untied. When the adjustment is done, the loose portion of the flap is moved aside for exposure. After the muscle sutures have been tied and excess suture material has been removed, the conjunctival flap is brought back to its predetermined position and the preplaced conjunctival flap sutures are tied.

Weakening of Inferior Oblique Muscle

This procedure may be necessary in two main groups of patients: (1) a pediatric group with marked overaction of the inferior oblique muscles and (2) patients with superior oblique weakness. With pediatric patients who have only moderate overaction of the inferior oblique muscles, it probably is best not to operate on the inferior oblique muscles at an early age, since many of these patients appear to outgrow the problem. In some instances, as the patient grows, the overaction of the inferior oblique may persist or even appear to become worse, particularly if a dissociated vertical divergence problem becomes evident. These patients may benefit from surgery to reduce the action of the inferior oblique muscles.

Adult patients often present with more clearly defined cases of superior oblique weakness, sometimes congenital and sometimes acquired. These patients may need various types of eye muscle surgery, including weakening of the inferior oblique muscle.[154–157]

Various methods of weakening the inferior oblique muscle have been tried, each with its own advocates. The muscle may be disconnected, recessed, subjected to a myectomy on either the temporal or nasal side of the inferior rectus muscle, denervated, or extirpated. There are advantages and disadvantages to each technique. A method that has worked well over the years is that of a controlled recession. Stay sutures can be used to elevate and slightly adduct the eye, and the inferior oblique muscle is approached through the inferotemporal fornix. A retractor is used to expose the deeper portion of the incision, where the inferior oblique muscle can be picked up with a muscle hook. The muscle is then dissected from the surrounding tissue, and two closely spaced clamps are placed across the muscle toward the distal end. The muscle is severed between the clamps, cautery is applied to the ends of the muscle, and the distal clamp is released. A suture is tied to the end of the muscle just behind the proximal clamp, which is then also released. The suture is used to reattach the muscle to the sclera at a point generally located 2 to 3 mm laterally and approximately 5 to 6 mm posteriorly from the lateral edge of insertion of the inferior rectus muscle. The actual position of the scleral suture may vary somewhat, according to the degree of recession required. The suture should not be placed too far anteriorly, or the residual action of the muscle may cause it to act as a depressor. With extensive surgery the resulting scarring and fibrosis has been reported to result in the adherence syndrome in some cases.[158] Fortunately, this complication is unusual.

Superior Oblique Tendon Tucking

Superior oblique tendon tucking usually results in a relatively small correction of a vertical deviation and a rather variable amount of correction of excycloduction. The superior oblique tendon can be picked up on either side of the superior rectus muscle, but it is important to perform the tuck on the temporal side of the muscle, in order to reduce the chance of causing a postoperative Brown's syndrome.[8, 10, 11, 159] A tendon tucker may be used, with a 5–0 nonabsorbable suture tied across the bottom of the tuck. The size of tuck depends approximately on the desired correction. In general, one would not attempt a tuck of less than 5 to 6 mm, whereas the 10 to 12 mm maximum is usually limited by the tightness of the tendon. It is important to carry out forced ductions on the eye before closing in order to verify that no major restrictive limitation to elevation of the eye has been caused by the tuck.

Harada-Ito Procedure

A patient with a fourth nerve problem almost always has some degree of excycloduction of the eye, but the amount of this rotational misalignment varies considerably among patients. Fortunately, when the ipsilateral inferior oblique muscle is weakened, the rotational misalignment is often reduced to the point at which it does not bother the patient. In the relatively infrequent cases in which the patient continues to complain mainly of rotational problems, an alternative to the traditional tuck operation is the Harada-Ito procedure.[16, 149] In its basic form, this procedure involves first mobilizing the anterior portion of the superior oblique tendon by splitting it at its insertion. The anterior part of the split tendon is then moved to a new insertion point that is displaced temporally and slightly anteriorly. This can be achieved by tying a nonabsorbable suture to the anterior half of the split tendon a few millimeters from its original insertion and then suturing the tendon to the sclera at a point a few millimeters lateral to and anterior to the original insertion point. As a variation of this procedure, some surgeons prefer to disinsert the anterior half of the split tendon and to reattach it to the globe at approximately the upper edge of the insertion of the lateral rectus muscle. In effect this procedure can be regarded as a variant of the tuck, using a neater and less bulky mechanical arrangement for the tightened tendon. Adjustable sutures have been employed for this procedure.[160]

Transposition and Jensen Procedures

When there is almost complete paralysis of a muscle, forced ductions may indicate contraction of the antagonist muscle. The first and essential step in any correction procedure is to relieve the pull of the antagonist muscle by means of a large recession, or weakening procedure. This allows the eye to be moved to a more central position, but some restraining force is needed to keep the eye in position. In general, a large resection of an almost completely paralyzed muscle has at best only a transient effect. Stay sutures can be used postoperatively to hold the eye in position for some time, but this often is not satisfactory, since with time the eye may tend to drift. What is needed is an elastic restraining force provided by functioning muscles. In a patient with a paralytic lateral rectus muscle but with functioning superior and inferior rectus muscles, a transposition procedure of some sort is helpful. This technique was described by Hummelscheim, and there have been a number of variations.[161, 162] The basic procedure involves disinserting part or all of the superior and inferior rectus muscles and attaching these muscles, or parts of them, close to the insertion of the paralyzed lateral rectus muscle. Because this procedure has to be combined with a large recession or weakening of the antagonist medial rectus muscle, it is possible that anterior segment ischemia may develop.[115] The advantage of the Jensen procedure[163–165] is that this ischemic risk is reduced, since the insertions of the vertical rectus muscles are not detached.

To accomplish the Jensen procedure on an eye with a paralyzed lateral rectus muscle, the vertical rectus muscles are exposed and are split into approximate halves by blunt dissection with a small muscle hook but not disturbing the major vessels of the muscles. The lateral rectus muscle is split in a similar fashion. A nonabsorbable suture (e.g., 4–0 Mersilene) is placed around the lateral half of the superior rectus and the superior half of the lateral rectus muscle and tied loosely so that the muscle halves are brought together as the suture is moved posteriorly a centimeter or more. A similar procedure is carried out with the inferior half of the lateral rectus and the lateral half of the inferior rectus. It is important to emphasize that the suture should be quite loose, to leave between the muscle halves a gap approximately the same size as the enclosed muscle cross sections. This minimizes the risk of occluding the blood supply to the anterior segment[166, 167] and, in addition, makes it easier to move the suture back to a position approximately 10 to 15 mm from the muscle insertion. As noted in the section on postoperative complications, the possibility of anterior segment ischemia should be kept in mind, and the patient should be examined carefully for signs within 12 to 24 hr postoperatively.[114, 115]

The results obtained by the Jensen procedure combined with a large recession of the antagonistic muscle can be surprisingly good, although there usually is extremely limited motion postoperatively. In patients in whom slightly better postoperative motion is encountered, it seems most likely that it is due to less than complete paralysis of the affected muscle.

The procedure can be applied in other patients who have individual muscle weakness, such as a traumatic inferior rectus muscle problem. It may also be used in some unusual cases of Duane's syndrome when conventional measures have not been sufficient.

REFERENCES

1. Balkan R, Hoyt CS: Associated neurologic abnormalities in congenital third nerve palsies. Am J Ophthalmol 97:315, 1984.
2. Rush JA, Younge BR: Paralysis or cranial nerves III, IV, and VI: Cause and prognosis in 1000 cases. Arch Ophthalmol 99:76, 1981.
3. Rucker CW: Paralysis of the third, fourth, and sixth cranial nerves. Am J Ophthalmol 46: 787, 1985.
4. Elston JS: Traumatic third nerve palsy. Br J Ophthalmol 68: 538, 1984.
5. Metz HS, Mazow M: Botulinum toxin treatment of acute sixth and third nerve palsy. Graefes Arch Clin Exp Ophthalmol 226:141, 1988.
6. Metz HS, Yee D: Third nerve palsy: Superior oblique transposition surgery. Ann Ophthalmol 5:215, 1973.
7. Maruo T, Kubota N, Iwashige H: Transposition of the superior oblique tendon for paralytic exotropia in oculomotor palsy: Results in 20 cases. Binoc Vis Q 3:203, 1988.
8. Knapp P, Moore S: Diagnosis and surgical options in superior oblique surgery. Int Ophthalmol Clin 16: 137, 1976.
9. Hermann JS: Masked bilateral superior oblique paresis. J Pediatr Ophthalmol Strabismus 18:43, 1981.
10. von Noorden GK, Murray E, Wong SY: Superior oblique paralysis. A review of 270 cases. Arch Ophthalmol 104:1771, 1986.
11. Lavin PJ, Troost BT: Traumatic 4th nerve palsy. Arch Neurol 41:679, 1984.
12. Wesley RE, Pollard ZF, McCord CD Jr: Superior oblique paresis after blepharoplasty. Plast Reconstr Surg 66:283, 1980.
13. Couch JM, Somers ME, Gonzales C: Superior oblique muscle dysfunction following anterior ethmoidal artery ligation for epistaxis. Arch Ophthalmol 108:1110, 1990.
14. Kushner BJ: The diagnosis and treatment of bilateral masked superior oblique palsy. Am J Ophthalmol 105:186, 1988.
15. Kushner BJ: Surgery with respect to cyclotropia. Ocul Ther Surg 1:44, 1981.
16. Mitchell PR, Parks MM: Surgery for bilateral superior oblique palsy. Ophthalmology 89:484, 1982.
17. Pinchoff BS, Bergstrom TJ, Sandall GS: A combined surgical approach to bilateral superior oblique palsy. Ophthalmol Surg 13:1000, 1982.
18. Harada M, Ito Y: Surgical correction of cyclotropia. Jap J Ophthalmol 8:88, 1964.
19. Inset TR, Kakub NH, Risch SC et al: Abducens palsy after lumbar puncture [Letter]. N Engl J Med 303:703, 1980.
20. Miller EA, Savino PJ, Schatz NJ: Bilateral 6th nerve palsy: A rare complication of water-soluble contrast myelography. Arch Ophthalmol 100:603, 1982.
21. Savino PJ, Hilliker JK, Casell GH, et al: Chronic 6th nerve palsies: Are they really harbingers of serious intracranial disease? Arch Ophthalmol 100:1442, 1982.
22. Moster ML, Savino PJ, Sergott RL, et al: Isolated sixth nerve paresis in younger adults. Arch Ophthalmol 102:1328, 1984.
23. Arias MJ: Bilateral traumatic abducens nerve palsy without skull fracture and with cervical spine fracture. Neurosurgery 16:232, 1985.
24. Galetta SL, Smith JL: Chronic isolated sixth nerve palsies. Arch Neurol 46:79, 1989.
25. Fitzsimmons R, Lee JP, Elston J: Treatment of sixth nerve palsy in adults with combined botulinum toxin chemodenervation and surgery. Ophthalmology 95:1535, 1988.
26. Rosenbaum AL, Kushner BJ, Kirschen D: Vertical rectus muscle transposition and botulinum toxin (Oculinum) to medial rectus for abducens palsy. Arch Ophthalmol 107:820, 1989.
27. Wagner RS, Frohman LP: Long-term results: Botulinum for sixth nerve palsy. J Pediatr Ophthalmol Strabismus 26:106, 1989.
28. Fitzsimons R, Lee JP, Elston J: Treatment of sixth nerve palsy in adults with combined botulinum toxin chemodenervation and surgery. Ophthalmology 95:1535, 1988.
29. Frueh BR, Henderson JW: Rectus muscle union in sixth nerve paralysis. Arch Ophthalmol 85:191, 1971.
30. Hamed LM, Helveston EM, Ellis FD: Persistent binocular diplopia after cataract surgery. Am J Ophthalmol 103:741, 1979.
31. Hamed LM, Lingua RW: Thyroid eye disease presenting after cataract surgery. J Pediatr Ophthalmol Strabismus 27:10, 1990.
32. Kushner BJ: Ocular muscle fibrosis following cataract extraction. Arch Ophthalmol 106:18, 1988.
33. Rainin EA, Carlson BM: Postoperative diplopia and ptosis: a clinical hypothesis based on the myotoxicity of local anesthetics. Arch Ophthalmol 103:1337, 1985.
34. Catalano RA, Nelson LB, Calhoun JH, et al: Persistent strabismus presenting after cataract surgery. Ophthalmology 94:491, 1987.
35. Ong-Tone L, Pearce WG: Inferior rectus muscle restriction after retrobulbar anesthesia for cataract extraction. Can J Ophthalmol 24:162, 1989.
36. Burns CL, Seigel LA: Inferior rectus recession for vertical tropia after cataract surgery. Ophthalmology 95:1120, 1988.
37. Metz HS, Norris A: Cyclotorsional diplopia following retinal detachment surgery. J Pediatr Ophthalmol Strabismus 24:287, 1987.
38. Munoz M, Rosenbaum AL: Long-term strabismus complications following retinal detachment surgery. J Pediatr Ophthalmol Strabismus 24:309, 1987.
39. Smiddy WE, Loupe D, Michels RG, et al: Extraocular muscle imbalance after scleral buckling surgery. Ophthalmology 96:1485, 1989.
40. Wright KW: The fat adherence syndrome and strabismus after retina surgery. Ophthalmology 93:411, 1986.
41. Mallette RA, Kwon JY, Guyton DL: A technique for repairing strabismus after scleral buckling surgery. Am J Ophthalmol 106:364, 1988.
42. Wojno TH: The incidence of extraocular muscle and cranial nerve palsy in orbital floor blow-out fractures. Ophthalmology 94:682, 1987.
43. Nicholson DH, Guzak SV: Visual loss complicating repair of orbital floor fractures. Arch Ophthalmol 86:369, 1971.
44. Seiff SR: Cyanoacrylate fixed silicone sheet in medial blowout fracture repair. Ophthalmic Surg 20:674, 1989.
45. Emery JM, von Noorden GK, Schlernitzauer DA: Orbital floor fractures: long-term follow-up of cases with and without surgical repair. Trans Am Acad Ophthalmol Otolaryngol 75:802, 1972.
46. Scott WE, Thalacker JA: Diagnosis and treatment of thyroid myopathy. Ophthalmology 88:493, 1981.
47. Trobe JD: Graves' ophthalmopathy: A 1987 update. Am Orthopt J 38:151, 1988.
48. Char DH: Advances in the management of thyroid-related eye disease. Int Ophthalmol Clin 29:226, 1989.
49. Shorr N, Neuhaus RW, Baylis HI: Ocular motility problems after orbital decompression for dysthyroid ophthalmopathy. Ophthalmology 9:323, 1982.
50. Fells P: Orbital decompression for severe dysthyroid eye disease. Br J Ophthalmol 71:107, 1987.
51. Wulc AE, Popp JC, Bartlett SP: Lateral wall advancement in orbital decompression. Ophthalmology 97:1358, 1990.
52. Gardner TA, Kennerdell JS: Treatment of dysthyroid myopathy with adjustable suture recession. Ophthal Surg 21:519, 1990.
53. Duane A: Congenital deficiency of abduction associated with impairment of adduction, retraction movements, contraction of the palpebral fissure and oblique movements of the eye. Arch Ophthalmol 34:133, 1905.
54. Hotchkiss MG, Miller NR, Clark AW, et al: Bilateral Duane's retraction syndrome: A clinical-pathologic case report. Arch Ophthalmol 98:870, 1980.
55. Raab EL: Clinical features of Duane's syndrome. J Pediatr Ophthalmol Strabismus 23:64, 1986.
56. Miller NR, Kiel SM, Green WR, et al: Unilateral Duane's retraction syndrome (type I). Arch Ophthalmol 100:1468, 1982.
57. Baker RS, Robertson WC: Acquired Duane's retraction syndrome in a patient with rheumatoid arthritis. Ann Ophthalmol 12:269, 1980.
58. Osher R, Schatz NJ, Duane TD: Acquired orbital retraction syndrome. Arch Ophthalmol 98:1798, 1980.
59. Jampolsky A, Eisenbaum AM, Parks MM: A study of various surgical approaches to the leash effect in Duane's syndrome. Presented at the American Academy of Ophthalmology, Chicago, 1980.
60. von Noorden GK, Murray E: Up- and down-shoot in Duane's retraction syndrome. J Pediatr Ophthalmol Strabismus 23:212, 1986.
61. Pressman SH, Scott WE: Surgical treatment of Duane's syndrome. Ophthalmology 93:29, 1986.

62. Kraft SP: A surgical approach for Duane's syndrome I. J Pediatr Ophthalmol Strabismus 25:119, 1988.
63. Rogers GK, Bremer DL: Surgical treatment of the upshoot and downshoot in Duane's retraction syndrome. Ophthalmology 91:1380, 1984.
64. Molarte AB, Rosenbaum AL: Vertical rectus muscle transposition surgery for Duane's syndrome. J Pediatr Ophthalmol Strabismus 27:171, 1990.
65. Wilson ME, Eustis HS Jr, Parks MM: Brown's syndrome. Surv Ophthalmol 34:153, 1989.
66. Beck M, Hickling P: Treatment of bilateral superior oblique tendon sheath syndrome complicating rheumatoid arthritis. Br J Ophthalmol 64:358, 1980.
67. Wright KW, Silverstein D, Marrone AC, et al: Acquired inflammatory superior oblique tendon sheath syndrome: A clinicopathologic study. Arch Ophthalmol 100:1752, 1982.
68. Baker RS, Conklin JD: Acquired Brown's syndrome from blunt orbital trauma. J Pediatr Ophthalmol Strabismus 24:17, 1987.
69. Biedner B, Monos T, Frilling F, et al: Acquired Brown's syndrome caused by frontal sinus osteoma. J Pediatr Ophthalmol Strabismus 25:226, 1988.
70. Goldstein JH, Schneekloth BB, Babb J, et al: Acquired Brown's superior oblique tendon syndrome due to euthyroid Graves' disease ophthalmomyopathy. Binoc Vis Q 5:93, 1990.
71. Saunders RA, Stratas BA, Gordon RA, et al: Acute-onset Brown's syndrome associated with pansinusitis. Arch Ophthalmol 108:58, 1990.
72. Neely KA, Ernest JT, Mottier M: Combined superior oblique paresis and Brown's syndrome after blepharoplasty. Am J Ophthalmol 109:347, 1990.
73. Erie JC: Acquired Brown's syndrome after peribulbar anesthesia. Am J Ophthalmol 109:349, 1990.
74. Hermann JS: Acquired Brown's syndrome of inflammatory origin: response to locally injected steroids. Arch Ophthalmol 96:1228, 1978.
75. von Noorden GK, Oliver P: Superior oblique tenectomy in Brown's syndrome. Ophthalmology 89:303, 1982.
76. Crawford JS, Orton R, Labow-Daily L: Late results of superior oblique muscle tenotomy in true Brown's syndrome. Am J Ophthalmol 89:824, 1980.
77. Eustis HS, O'Reilly C, Crawford JS: Management of superior oblique palsy after surgery for true Brown's syndrome. J Pediatr Ophthalmol Strabismus 24:10, 1987.
78. Parks MM, Eustis HS: Simultaneous superior oblique tenotomy and inferior oblique recession in Brown's syndrome. Ophthalmology 94:1043, 1987.
79. Kestenbaum A: Nouvelle opération du nystagmus. Bull Soc Ophtalmol Fr 6:599, 1953.
80. Anderson JR: Causes and treatment of congenital eccentric nystagmus. Br J Ophthalmol 37:267, 1953.
81. Calhoun JH, Harley RD: Surgery for abnormal head position in congenital nystagmus. Trans Am Ophthalmol Soc 71:70, 1973.
82. Bérard PV, Mouillac N, Reydy R, et al: Surgical treatment of congenital nystagmus with horizontal torticollis. *In* Reinecke RD (ed): Strabismus. Proceedings of the Third Meeting of the International Strabismological Association. New York, Grune & Stratton 1978, p 169.
83. Cooper J, Medow N, Dibble C: Mortality rate in strabismus surgery. J Am Optom Assoc 52:391, 1982.
84. Isenberg SJ, Apt L, Yamada S: Overnight admission of outpatient strabismus patients. Ophthalmic Surg 21:540, 1990.
85. McCracken JS: Major ambulatory surgery of the ophthalmic patient. Surg Clin North Am 67:881, 1987.
86. Gronert G: Malignant hyperthermia. Anesthesiology 53:395, 1980.
87. McGoldrick KE: Malignant hyperthermia: a review. J Am Med Wom Assoc 35:95, 1980.
88. Negre F, Caujolle J, Ghenassia C, et al: Malignant hyperthermia in ophthalmologic surgery. J Fr Ophtalmol 11:53, 1988.
89. Marmor M: Malignant hyperthermia. *In* Sugar A (ed): Reviews in Medicine. Surv Ophthalmol 28:117, 1983.
90. Duke-Elder S, Wybar K: System of Ophthalmology. Vol 6: Ocular Motility and Strabismus. St. Louis, CV Mosby Co, 1973.
91. Parks MM: Atlas of Strabismus Surgery, Philadelphia, Harper & Row, 1983.
92. von Noorden GK: Atlas of Strabismus, 4th ed. St. Louis, CV Mosby, 1983.
93. Helveston EM: Atlas of Strabismus Surgery, 3rd ed. St. Louis, CV Mosby, 1985.
94. Nelson LB, Catalano RA: Atlas of Ocular Motility, Philadelphia, WB Saunders, 1989.
95. Parks MM, Mitchell PR: Cranial nerve palsies, *In* Tasman W, Jaeger EA (eds): Duane's Clinical Ophthalmology, rev. ed. Vol. 1. Philadelphia, JB Lippincott, 1989.
96. Reinecke RD: Muscle Surgery. *In* Tasman W, Jaeger EA (eds): Duane's Clinical Ophthalmology, rev. ed. Vol. 5. Philadelphia, JB Lippincott, 1989.
97. von Noorden GK: Binocular Vision and Ocular Motility, 4th ed. St. Louis, CV Mosby, 1990.
98. Parks MM: Fornix incision for horizontal rectus muscle surgery. Am J Ophthalmol 65:907, 1968.
99. von Noorden GK: Modification of the limbal approach to surgery of the rectus muscles. Arch Ophthalmol 82:349, 1969.
100. Wortham E, Anandakrishnan I, Kraft SP, et al: Are antibiotic-steroid drops necessary following strabismus surgery? A prospective, randomized, masked trial. J Pediatr Opthalmol Strabismus 27:205, 1990.
101. Gottlieb F, Castro JL: Perforation of the globe during strabismus surgery. Arch Ophthalmol 84:151, 1970.
102. Basmadjian G, LaSelle P, Dumas J: Retinal detachment after strabismus surgery. Am J Ophthalmol 79:305, 1975.
103. Alio JL, Faci A: Fundus changes following Faden operation. Arch Ophthalmol 102:211, 1984.
104. Apple DJ, Jones GR, Reidy JJ, et al: Ocular perforation and phthisis bulbi secondary to strabismus surgery. J Pediatr Ophthalmol Strabismus 22:184, 1985.
105. Rosenbaum A, Metz HS: Diagnosis of lost or slipped muscles by saccadic velocity measurements. Am J Ophthalmol 77:215, 1974.
106. Plager DA, Parks MM: Recognition and repair of slipped rectus muscle. J Pediatr Ophthalmol Strabismus 25:270, 1988.
107. Plager DA, Parks MM: Recognition and repair of the "lost" rectus muscle. Ophthalmology 97:131, 1990.
108. Hamlet YJ, Goldstein JH, Rosenbaum JD: Dehiscence of the lateral rectus muscle following intrascleral buckling procedure. Ann Ophthalmol 14:694, 1982.
109. von Noorden GK: Orbital cellulitis following extraocular muscle surgery. Am J Ophthalmol 74:627, 1972.
110. Wilson ME, Paul OT: Orbital cellulitis following strabismus surgery. Ophthalmic Surg 18:92, 1987.
111. Salamon SM, Friberg TR, Luxenburg MN: Endophthalmitis after strabismus surgery. Am J Ophthalmol 93:39, 1982.
112. Uniat LM, Olk JR, Kenneally CZ, et al: Endophthalmitis after strabismus surgery with a good visual result. Ophthalmic Surg 19:42, 1988.
113. Apt L, Costenbader FD, Parks MM, et al: Catgut allergy in eye muscle surgery. I: Correlation of eye reaction and skin test using plain catgut. Arch Ophthalmol 63:54, 1960.
114. von Noorden GK: Anterior segment ischemia following the Jensen procedure. Arch Ophthalmol 94:845, 1976
115. France TD, Simon JW: Anterior segment ischemia syndrome following muscle surgery: the AAPOS experience. J Pediatr Ophthalmol Strabismus 23:87, 1986.
116. Prakash R, Verma D, Menon V: Anterior segment ischemia following extraocular muscle surgery. Jpn J Ophthalmol 30:251, 1986.
117. Saunders R, Phillips MS: Anterior segment ischemia after three rectus muscle surgery. Ophthalmology 95:533, 1988.
118. Olver JM, Lee JP: The effects of strabismus surgery on anterior segment circulation. Eye 3(Pt 3):318, 1989.
119. George JL, Heymann V, Laroche P, et al: Ischemia of the anterior segment after surgery of strabismus: apropos of a case. Bull Soc Ophthalmol Fr 88(1):1403, 1988.
120. Lee JP, Olver JM: Anterior segment ischaemia. Eye 4(Pt 1):1, 1990.
121. Robertson DM: Anterior segment ischemia after segmental episcleral buckling and cryopexy. Am J Ophthalmol 78:871, 1975.
122. Raizman M, Beck RW: Iris ischemia following surgery on two rectus muscles [letter]. Arch Ophthalmol 103:1783, 1985.

123. Saunders RA, Sandall GS: Anterior segment ischemia syndrome following rectus muscle transposition. Am J Ophthalmol 93:34, 1982.
124. Keech RV, Morris FJ, Ruben JB, et al: Anterior segment ischemia following vertical muscle transposition and botulinum toxin injection. Arch Ophthalmol 108:176, 1990.
125. McKeown CA, Lambert HM, Shore JW: Preservation of the anterior ciliary vessels during extraocular muscle surgery. Ophthalmology 96:498, 1989.
126. Diamond GR: True transposition procedures. J Pediatr Ophthalmol Strabismus 27:153, 1990.
127. Helveston EM, Cofield DD: Indications for marginal myotomy technique. Am J Ophthalmol 70:574, 1970.
128. McPhee TJ, Dyer JA, Ilstrup DM: Marginal myotomy of the medial rectus with lateral rectus resection as a secondary procedure for esotropia. Graefes Arch Clin Exp Ophthalmol 226:197, 1988.
129. Clark DI, Markland S, Trimble RB: A study to assess the value of dacron slings in the management of squints which are not amenable to conventional surgery. Br J Ophthalmol 70:623, 1986.
130. Mills PV, Hyper TJ, Duff GR: Loop recession of the recti muscles. Eye 1:593, 1987.
131. Repka MX, Guyton DL: Comparison of hang-back medial rectus recession with conventional recession. Ophthalmology 95:782, 1988.
132. Capo H, Repka MX, Guyton DL: Hang-back lateral rectus recessions for exotropia. J Pediatr Ophthalmol Strabismus 26:31, 1989.
133. Potter WS, Nelson LB, Handa JT: Hemihang-back recession: description of the technique and review of the literature. Ophthalmol Surg 21:711, 1990.
134. Scott AB: Stay sutures to adjust strabismus surgery. Ann Ophthalmol 7:429, 1975.
135. Cole JG, Cole HG: Recession of the conjunctiva in complicated eye muscle operations. Am J Ophthalmol 53:618, 1962.
136. von Noorden GK: Indications of the posterior fixation operation in strabismus. Ophthalmology 85:512, 1978.
137. Shuckett EP, Hiles DA, Biglan AW, et al: Posterior fixation suture operation (fadenoperation). Ophthalmic Surg 12:578, 1981.
138. Guyton DL: The posterior fixation procedure: mechanism and indications. Int Ophthalmol Clin 25:79, 1985.
139. Buckley EG, Meekins BB: Fadenoperation for the management of complicated incomitant vertical strabismus. Am J Ophthalmol 105:304, 1988.
140. Paliaga GP, Braga M: Passive limitation of adduction after Cuppers' 'Fadenoperation' on medial recti. Br J Ophthalmol 73:633, 1989.
141. Lyons CJ, Fells P, Lee JP, et al: Chorioretinal scarring following the Faden operation: A retrospective study of 100 procedures. Eye 3(Pt 4):401, 1989.
142. Scott WE, Martin-Casals A, Jackson OB: Adjustable sutures in strabismus surgery. J Pediatr Ophthalmol Strabismus 14:71, 1977.
143. Jampolsky AL: Current techniques of adjustable strabismus surgery. Am J Ophthalmol 88:406 1979.
144. Rosenbaum AL, Metz HS, Carlson M, et al: Adjustable rectus muscle recession surgery. A follow-up study. Arch Ophthalmol 95:817, 1977.
145. Nelson LB, Wagner RS, Calhoun JH: The adjustable suture technique in strabismus surgery. Int Ophthalmol Clin 25:89, 1985.
146. Fells P: Adjustable sutures. Eye 2(Pt 1):33, 1988.
147. Franklin SR, Hiatt RL: Adjustable sutures in strabismus surgery. Ann Ophthalmol 21:285, 1989.
148. Kraft SP, Jacobson ME: Techniques of adjustable suture strabismus surgery. Ophthalmol Surg 21:633, 1990.
149. Elsas FJ: Vertical effect of the adjustable Harada-Ito procedure. J Pediatr Ophthalmol Strabismus 24:164, 1988.
150. Keech RV, Heckert RR: Adjustable suture strabismus surgery for acquired vertical deviations. J Pediatr Ophthalmol Strabismus 25:159, 1988.
151. Eustis HS: Syncopal episodes during postoperative suture adjustments in strabismus surgery: A survey. Binoc Vis Q 5:133, 1990.
152. Wisnicki HJ, Repka MX, Guyton DL: Reoperation rate in adjustable strabismus surgery. J Pediatr Ophthalmol Strabismus 25:112, 1988.
153. Chow PC: Stability of one-stage adjustable suture for the correction of horizontal strabismus. Br J Ophthalmol 73:541, 1989.
154. Parks MM: The weakening surgical procedures for eliminating overaction of the inferior oblique muscle. Am J Ophthalmol 73:107, 1972.
155. May MA, Beauchamp GR, Price RL: Recession and anterior transposition of the inferior oblique for treatment of superior oblique palsy. Graefes Arch Clin Exp Ophthalmol 226:407, 1988.
156. Hunter LR, Parks MM: Response of coexisting underacting superior oblique and overacting inferior oblique muscles to inferior oblique weakening. J Pediatr Ophthalmol Strabismus 27:74, 1990.
157. Gonzales C: Major review: Surgical anatomy, approach and exposure of the inferior oblique extraocular muscle. Binoc Vis Q 5:79, 1990.
158. Parks MM: The overacting inferior oblique muscle. Am J Ophthalmol 77:787, 1974.
159. Helveston EM, Ellis FD: Superior oblique tuck and superior oblique palsy. Aust J Ophalmol 11:215, 1983.
160. Metz HS, Lerner H: The adjustable Harada-Ito procedure. Arch Ophthalmol 99:624, 1981.
161. Hummelsheim E: Weitere Erfahrungen mit partieller Sehnenuberpflanzung an den Augenmuskeln. Arch Augenheilk 62:71, 1908–1909.
162. Helveston EM: Muscle transposition procedures. Surv Ophthalmol 16:92, 1971.
163. Jensen CDF: Rectus muscle union: a new operation for paralysis of the rectus muscle. Trans Pacif Coast Otoophthalmol Soc 45:359, 1964.
164. Selezinka W, Sandall GS, Henderson JW: Rectus muscle union in sixth nerve paralysis, Jensen rectus muscle union. Arch Ophthalmol 92:882, 1974.
165. Cline RA, Scott WE: Long-term follow-up of Jensen procedures. J Pediatr Ophthalmol Strabismus 25:264, 1988.
166. Romano PE: The unavoidable internal conflict of the surgeon [Editorial]. Binoc Vis Q 5:179, 1990.
167. Frey T: Anterior segment ischemia caused by Jensen's procedure. J Ocular Ther Surg 3:242, 1985.

Botulinum Toxin in the Management of Strabismus

ELBERT H. MAGOON

Alternatives to traditional incisional strabismus surgery have long been sought. In 1989, after more than 10 years of human research, botulinum toxin type A (BTX, Oculinum) was approved by the Food and Drug Administration (FDA) for strabismus and other indications for muscle relaxation.[1] For strabismus therapy, BTX can provide a temporary weakness of an overacting or tight muscle and thereby a long-term muscle lengthening that improves the eye alignment.

BACKGROUND AND MODE OF ACTION

BTX is a high molecular weight protein. It produces its muscle-relaxing effect by binding at receptor sites on motor nerve terminals and interfering with the release of acetylcholine. When injected into extraocular muscles for strabismus, only local effects, never systemic effects are seen. The duration and magnitude of the effect are dose-dependent, providing roughly 2 wk to 2 mo total extraocular muscle paralysis. There follows gradual recovery to normal muscle strength over a similar period of time. The drug exerts its permanent effect by permitting the relaxed muscle to be stretched by its unopposed antagonist. In this fashion, the length of the muscle is changed permanently, but the muscle strength recovers to its previous normal level in all cases.

It has long been known that patients with sixth nerve palsies who recover fully (determined by force measurements) nevertheless sometimes have a small esodeviation after that recovery. This circumstance has been presumed to be from the contracture of the unopposed medial rectus and the lengthening of the paralyzed lateral rectus. Imitation of this natural phenomenon with injection of BTX into a muscle which one desires to be longer or looser is the paradigm for the mechanism of strabismus treatment with BTX.

This mechanism of long-term effect is confirmed by the observation that when attempting to treat noncomitant paralytic strabismus, the drug provides a dramatic temporary change but little long-term effect. For comitant strabismus, which is nonparalytic and does not involve great amounts of contracture, BTX probably has its greatest effect.

The long-term effect of treatment is not dependent on binocular vision, since many blind eyes have been treated, with substantial long-term improvement; however, as with incisional surgery, the stability of effect is probably enhanced by binocular vision. Figure 218–22 shows a patient with poor vision in the right eye. She had an exotropia before injection of her right lateral rectus muscle. The bottom two photos show her improved alignment at 2 and 5 yr postinjection.

BTX is useful in acute paralytic strabismus to prevent contracture of the antagonist muscle and to help regain or even to test potential for binocular vision. Here the temporary nature of the paralytic effect and minimal long-term change are used to advantage with the expectation of spontaneous improvement of the acute paralytic strabismus.

Scott reported the grouped data from all patients in the study that led to FDA approval of botulinum in the treatment of strabismus.[2] Figure 218–23 shows the average initial and final deviations at a minimum of 6 mo after BTX injections in both children and adults.

It will be seen in Figure 218–23 that the results of treating children and adults are comparable and that smaller deviations are more likely to be treated with a result of less than 10 prism diopters (PD) posttreatment deviation than are moderate or large deviations. However, larger deviations have a greater total magnitude of improvement than do small deviations. Tables 218–1 and 218–2 show results of treatment in children and adults with the likelihood of successful treatment of less than 10 PD. If successful treatment is arbitrarily defined as 10 PD or less, more than 50 percent of patients achieve that improvement in most categories. Overcorrections are rare; the procedure routinely undercorrects.

For only a single injection, the results show 35 percent of adults and 38 percent of children with horizontal

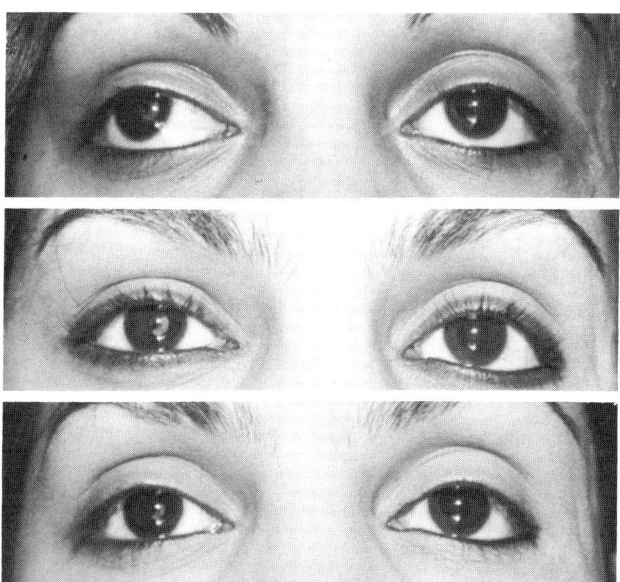

Figure 218–22. Patient with poorly seeing right eye and 40–prism diopter exotropia before treatment *(top)*, 2 yr after treatment *(center)*, and 5 years after treatment BTX *(bottom)*. (From Scott AB: Botulinum toxin treatment of strabismus. Focal Points: Clinical Modules for Ophthalmologists Vol. 7, Mod 12 [cover], 1989.)

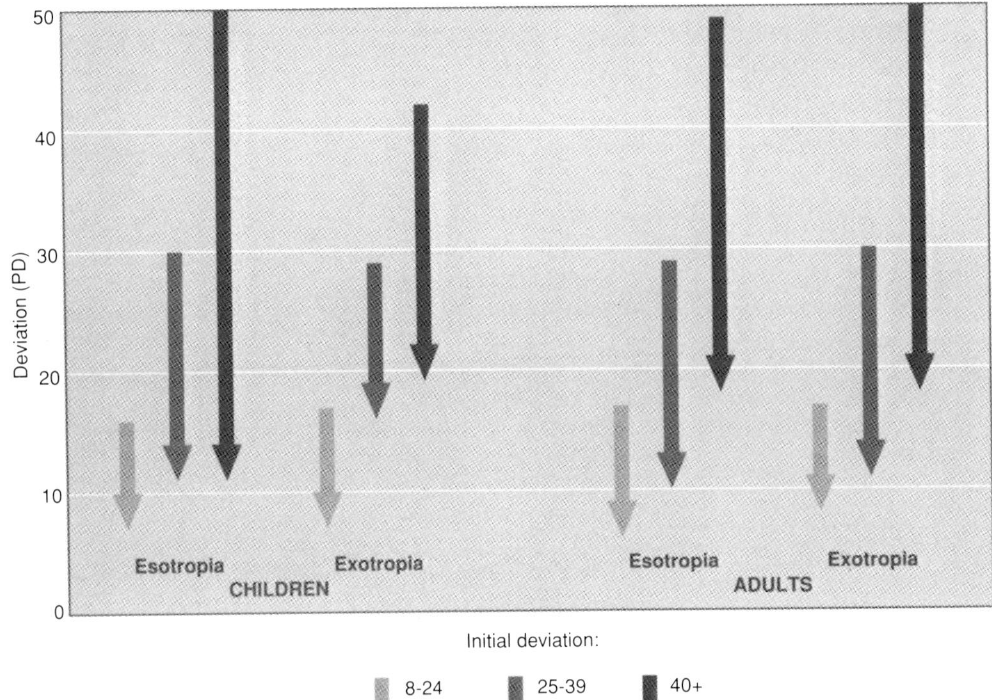

Figure 218–23. Initial and final deviation in children and adults a minimum of 6 mo after BTX injection. (From Scott AB: Botulinum toxin treatment of strabismus. Focal Points: Clinical Modules for Ophthalmologists 7(Mod 12):4, 1989.)

strabismus are corrected to within 10 PD of orthophoria. Biglan and associates found a 38 percent correction rate after an average of 1.3 injections in a similar mixed group of patients.[3]

It is expected that more than one injection will be needed for all but small deviations. Properly informed patients are happy to undergo multiple injections, but some choose surgery as being more likely to provide satisfactory treatment with one procedure. Lengthy discussion of expectations and possibilities for both treatment approaches is likely to yield satisfied patients, whatever they choose. Injection does not preclude later surgery. Surgery does not preclude later injection.

Most patients, in the author's experience, are satisfied with BTX treatment. Often a patient who has a residual deviation larger than the physician wishes is unwilling

Table 218–1. EFFECT OF BOTULINUM TOXIN INJECTION ON STRABISMUS IN CHILDREN

	Number of Patients	Average Deviation			Final Deviation ≤10 PD	
		Preinjection	*Postinjection*	*(%) Change*	*n*	*(%) Patients*
Esotropia						
By number of injections						
1 injection	146	28 PD	9 PD	68	101	68
>1 injection	115	35 PD	11 PD	69	77	67
All patients	261	31 PD	10 PD	68	178	68
By initial deviation						
8–24 PD	81	16 PD	7 PD	56	63	78
25–39 PD	108	30 PD	11 PD	63	68	63
40 + PD	72	50 PD	11 PD	78	47	65
All patients	261	31 PD	10 PD	68	178	68
Exotropia						
By number of injections						
1 injection	66	26 PD	12 PD	54	32	49
>1 injection	29	27 PD	15 PD	44	13	45
All patients	95	26 PD	13 PD	50	45	47
By initial deviation						
10–24 PD	43	17 PD	7 PD	59	29	67
25–39 PD	32	29 PD	16 PD	45	8	25
40 + PD	20	42 PD	19 PD	55	8	40
All patients	95	26 PD	13 PD	50	45	47

From Scott AB: Botulinum toxin treatment of strabismus. Focal Points: Clinical Modules for Ophthalmologists 7(Mod 12):3, 1989.

Results in 356 patients (ages 2 mo to 12 yr) with follow-up of 6 to 65 mo (average 27 mo). Reduction rate of strabismus is broken down by number of injections and initial deviation as measured in prism diopters (PD).

Table 218–2. EFFECT OF BOTULINUM TOXIN INJECTION ON STRABISMUS IN ADULTS

	Number of Patients	Average Deviation			Final Deviation ≤10 PD	
		Preinjection	*Postinjection*	*(%) Change*	*n*	*(%) Patients*
Esotropia						
By number of injections						
1 injection	225	28 PD	9 PD	69	151	67
>1 injection	159	32 PD	14 PD	58	68	43
All patients	384	30 PD	11 PD	65	219	57
By initial deviation						
0–10 PD	9	—	—	—	8	89
10–24 PD	132	17 PD	6 PD	62	95	72
25–39 PD	142	29 PD	10 PD	65	81	57
40 + PD	101	49 PD	18 PD	62	35	35
All patients	384	30 PD	11 PD	63	219	56
Exotropia						
By number of injections						
1 injection	139	28 PD	11 PD	61	83	60
>1 injection	154	34 PD	13 PD	61	72	47
All patients	293	31 PD	12 PD	61	155	53
By initial deviation						
0–10 PD	6	—	—	—	6	100
10–24 PD	93	17 PD	8 PD	53	62	67
25–39 PD	112	30 PD	11 PD	64	60	54
40 + PD	82	50 PD	18 PD	64	27	33
All patients	293	32 PD	12 PD	60	166	52

From Scott AB: Botulinum toxin treatment of strabismus. Focal Points: Clinical Modules for Ophthalmologists 7(Mod 12):3, 1989.

Results in 677 patients (ages 12 to 90 yr) with follow-up of 6 to 83 mo (average 17 mo). Reduction rate of strabismus is broken down by number of injections and initial deviation as measured in prism diopters (PD).

to undergo further treatment, because he or she is happy with the result. Remarkably few patients opt for subsequent surgical treatment rather than repeat injections. Some investigators contributing to the grouped data found that patients were undertreated because of inadequate delivery of the drug to the muscle; other investigators became discouraged with the treatment and recommended surgery after one injection. These considerations influence Scott's data and probably show the BTX treatment to be less effective than if more vigorous treatment had been employed.

As shown in Figure 218–2 and Tables 218–1 and 218–2, the results for childhood strabismus are comparable with those for adults. Magoon and Scott[4] reported 82 children, 85 percent of whom required more than one injection to achieve their final result. The average preinjection deviation of 31 PD was decreased to well under 10 PD. A study of BTX-treated children with a follow-up of 6 to 24 mo was compared with the same children whose follow-up was 2 to 5½ yr.[5] There was very little difference between the longer and shorter follow-up groups, indicating a fairly stable alignment over time. Scott and Colleagues[6] reported 356 children treated by four investigators with a follow-up of more than 6 mo. Two hundred twenty-three had correction within 10 PD of orthophoria and required an average 1.6 injections per patient. Surgery was required in 19 percent. Thirty-three percent had transient ptosis, but there was no amblyopia, visual loss, or globe perforation produced by injection in the series.

For vertical strabismus, treatment of an inferior rectus muscle can be effective. Exceedingly tight muscles, as can be found in Graves' disease, often yield a substantial acute response but a modest long-term response. Scott reported one series of 27 potential surgical candidates who had an inferior rectus injection. Eleven were adequately treated, usually by multiple injections, but 16 eventually required surgery.[2] He pointed out that treatment of the accompanying horizontal strabismus sometimes reduced the number of muscles requiring surgery. Magoon and Dakoske[7] reported good results with botulinum injection for vertical strabismus, but follow-up was short. Inferior oblique injections alone were only modestly effective. Treatment of the superior rectus muscle (often combined with inferior oblique injection) is effective but uniformly produces a profound ptosis lasting at least 1 mo.[8] In the future, treatment of the levator or other vertical muscles with antitoxin in conjunction with BTX treatment of a rectus muscle may increase the effectiveness of the injection treatment for vertical strabismus.

For paralytic strabismus, BTX injection of the antagonist can provide a temporary paralysis with minimal long-term alignment effect. In one series, 18 of 20 unilateral lateral rectus palsies recovered following injection of the medial rectus within 3 months of onset, whereas in an uninjected control group, 13 of 45 (29 percent) palsies recovered.[9] It is difficult to see how this treatment could contribute to recovery as might be inferred from this data, but there clearly is temporary improvement that provides eye alignment and an opportunity for fusion. Wagner and Frohman[10] show similar results in eight patients with unilateral sixth nerve palsy treated by injection.

A special indication for BTX treatment involves enhancement of vertical transposition surgery for complete palsies. In a sixth nerve palsy, for example, it is common to recess the medial rectus in association with a temporal transposition of the vertical muscles.[11] This probably involves increased risk of anterior segment ischemia and may not be necessary with the BTX injection of the medial rectus in association with the transposition surgery. We have used Oculinum to advantage in a limited number of third nerve palsies that required surgery and a few that did not. Metz and Mazow[9] found that nine acute third nerve palsies receiving a lateral rectus injection within 3 months of onset recovered horizontal alignment.

Patients diplopic after retinal detachment surgery constitute a special population with strabismus because they often have periocular foreign bodies, scarring, or high myopia which makes traditional surgical treatment less attractive. Scott reported 20 such patients with strabismus and diplopia treated with BTX. Twelve regained fusion with elimination of diplopia in primary gaze, three were partially helped, and five continued to have diplopia.[12]

Side effects of injection are always temporary but can be troublesome. It is fairly common to have a transient ptosis. Scott[2] reported partial ptosis to have occurred in 16 percent of adults and 25 percent of children. Complete ptosis was rare. It is much more common after medial rectus injection than after lateral rectus injection. It has even occurred after inferior rectus injection and is routine after superior rectus injection. No amblyopia from ptosis has been reported. It is recommended that the eye with better visual acuity be the treated eye, since the induced ptosis can be an advantage rather than a disadvantage for amblyopia therapy.

Diplopia is fairly common during the temporary overcorrection in the paralytic phase of treatment. It can be managed in teenagers and adults by patching. In children patching is often not necessary, but if used, it should be intermittent, alternate, or of the better eye. Children and adults can often turn the head to align the eyes and eliminate diplopia during the period of transient incomitant overcorrection.

Past pointing and spatial disorientation are seldom a substantial problem in BTX-treated children, even when the preferred eye is injected. In adults it can be a greater problem but usually resolves within a few days. When treating horizontal strabismus an induced vertical deviation is common as a transient effect but not as a permanent change. Scott[2] reports that vertical deviations occurred in 17 percent of both adults and children. Two percent of cases of induced vertical deviation of 2 PD or more persisted 6 mo or longer. The author's experience is that induced vertical deviations are less frequent.

Pupillary dilation occurred in 5 patients, possibly from ciliary ganglion trauma. Retrobulbar hemorrhage occurred in 16 patients and always cleared without residual, but one eye was decompressed when the surgeon believed the retinal circulation was compromised.[2]

Systemic effects are not seen with the doses used to treat strabismus. The estimated systemic toxic dose is in excess of 2000 to 3000 units for an adult. Since the usual treatment dose for strabismus is 1 to 5 (or occasionally up to 10) units, the therapeutic index reflects an extraordinarily high margin of drug safety, even when treating babies. Antibodies have not been detected in patients receiving small doses of BTX for strabismus, in spite of the fact that the drug is a good immunogen in larger doses.

Complications relate to incorrect needle placement. Scleral perforation has occurred in 9 of 8300 injections (0.11 percent).[2] These perforations occurred more commonly in myopic eyes and at prior surgical sites. No retinal detachment occurred in any case. Six perforations were untreated and three were treated by cryotherapy or laser. In one of the patients, a vitreous hemorrhage reduced vision for several months before clearing, and in another, a reduction of vision from 20/25 to 20/30 was reported. Injection of the wrong muscle is another complication that can recur, even with electromyographic control. Failure to place the BTX in the muscle is a common problem for investigators learning the technique and probably accounts for some of the undercorrections reported.

INDICATIONS

Indications for BTX treatment of strabismus are implied by the results described earlier. For horizontal strabismus, uncomplicated small deviations are most satisfactorily treated. Deviations of more than 40 PD are less likely to be effectively treated, but reasonable results can be achieved. Complex vertical and horizontal strabismus will probably require surgical intervention, but sometimes BTX can be used as an adjunct to decrease the number of muscles that require incisional surgery.

Vertical strabismus can be treated effectively with injection but is probably less suitable for treatment than is horizontal strabismus. Superior rectus injection should be undertaken only with the expectation of prolonged ptosis.

Patients with an unsuccessful result following strabismus surgery are often willing to have an injection to fine-tune the result but are sometimes unwilling to have a full-blown repeat surgical intervention.

In acute paralytic strabismus, treatment of the antagonist results in temporary improvement of eye alignment and opportunity for fusion with decreased contracture of the antagonist. BTX is not indicated for definitive treatment of chronic paralytic strabismus (unless a patient wishes repeated injections with full knowledge of the temporary nature of the treatment).

As an adjunct to surgery, the drug can be useful. Not only can it help to enhance a poor surgical result as described, but it can also assist as part of the surgical plan. For example, in paralytic strabismus requiring transposition procedure, the antagonist muscle that would normally be recessed can be injected instead, thereby decreasing the number of operated muscles.

Other special situations include such conditions as active Graves' disease with inflamed eyes, blind or prephthisical eyes, and diplopia from retinal detachment surgery as well as circumstances in which surgery is difficult owing to other factors, such as multiple prior strabismus operations or the presence of a filtering bleb.

Age of the patient is not shown to be a major factor in treatment results, although concern about amblyopia from transient ptosis in children is appropriate.

Fusional potential probably contributes to success with BTX treatment as it does with surgery, but it is not necessary for successful alignment improvement from BTX. Of course, a preservation or reestablishment of fusion is a critical indication for treatment intervention with either surgery or BTX. Fusion potential, even for patients with long-standing strabismus and amblyopia, has been demonstrated.[13]

Infantile esotropes represent a special situation. Esotropes treated with BTX before age 1 routinely show a head turn to align the eyes during the period of temporary overcorrection. For example, if a right medial rectus muscle is injected for infantile esotropia, the eye will typically be shown to turn out after 2 wk and cannot adduct beyond the midline. Very quickly the child learns to turn the face to the left to align the eyes in right gaze, since they are straight or even possibly still esotropic when looking at an object in right gaze but are grossly esotropic when looking at an object in primary position or leftgaze. Figure 218–24 shows an infant with esotropia before treatment, with exotropia 1 wk after treatment, and turning the head to fuse 2 wk after treatment. Ptosis or induced vertical deviation can interfere with this phenomenon, but it is a remarkably universal occurrence among adequately treated infants. This has led to speculation that the child's ability to align the eyes during this incomitant overcorrection might provide advantages during the early critical periods of sensory development.

Multiple studies are underway to determine optimal modes, doses, and timing of treatment for infantile esotropia and to compare results of surgery with those of injection. At this time, it can be stated that either BTX injection or surgery provides the potential for satisfactory treatment of infantile esotropia.

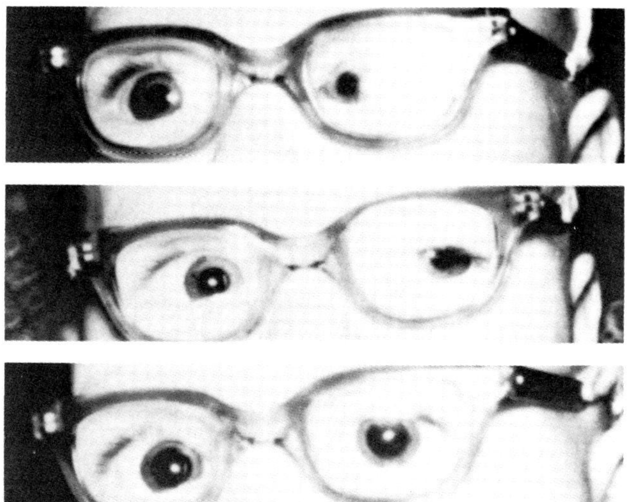

Figure 218–24. Infantile esotropia pretreatment *(top)*, exotropia 1 wk posttreatment *(center)*, and turning the head to fuse 2 weeks posttreatment *(bottom)*. (From Magoon EH: Botulinum toxin chemo-denervation for strabismus in infants and children. Pediatr Ophthalmol Strabismus 21:111, 1984.)

COMPARISON WITH SURGERY: ADVANTAGES AND DISADVANTAGES OF EACH

Surgery provides a reliable improvement for almost every form of strabismus. It usually is successful with just one procedure, but multiple operations are sometimes required. General anesthesia is traditionally used for children, but topical,[14, 15] peribulbar,[16] and retrobulbar blocks are being successfully employed in adults with greater frequency.

Advances in general anesthetic technique such as continuous blood oxygen monitoring and better management of malignant hyperthermia have decreased the risks of general anesthesia since BTX was first experimentally tested. Although it can usually be performed on an outpatient basis and recovery is quick, surgery is nevertheless as frightening for the patient with strabismus as it is routine for the strabismus surgeon. Parents and patients appreciate that the risks of anesthesia are small for strabismus surgery. Nevertheless, some believe that a lower risk of mortality and morbidity from injection makes it preferable to incisional surgery. Some patients and parents are simply unwilling to permit traditional surgery but will permit injection with BTX as an alternative. These people must be made aware of the disadvantages of BTX injection. As a practical consideration, the long-term undercorrection and need for reinjection is probably the most substantial problem. Another disadvantage of BTX treatment is the transient overcorrection that creates a problem for patients who appreciate diplopia, but most of them have previously been suffering from diplopia and can readily use a patch for the few weeks.

In children, the possibility of ptosis-induced amblyopia concerns many clinicians, but in practice it has not been a major problem. In 356 children, no ptosis-induced amblyopia was reported.[2] The injection of the preferred eye provides potential benefit to amblyopia therapy.

At the time of this writing, a major disadvantage of BTX therapy when compared with surgery is that it is not widely available, especially for children. All ophthalmologists have been trained in strabismus surgery and all pediatric ophthalmologists have had special training in surgical techniques and indications. A relatively small number of pediatric ophthalmologists have worked with Dr. Scott in his studies of BTX. All pediatric ophthalmologists feel comfortable with strabismus surgery, but not all have enough experience with BTX injection technique to feel comfortable with BTX injections. As clear-cut indications for injection (such as acute nerve palsy) emerge, perhaps more pediatric ophthalmologists and strabismologists will become proficient in the techniques of BTX injection.

Another disadvantage of BTX arises with a patient who has had BTX treatment but is about to undergo strabismus surgery. The surgeon may be uncertain of the basic alignment and therefore of the extent of modification required. Although no studies have been performed that specifically address this question, my data would indicate substantial stability of alignment 6 to 12 mo after injection.

Having discussed the disadvantages of BTX treatment, the advantages can be summarized: It is less painful than surgery, less costly, and generally causes less morbidity. There has been no mortality. These considerations all arise when BTX is an acceptable substitute for surgery. For some circumstances, there is no good surgical alternative to BTX. On the other hand, for some complicated types of strabismus, BTX does not constitute an acceptable substitute for surgery.

TECHNIQUE

Thorough understanding of the procedure is necessary for patient satisfaction, so informed consent is an important prerequisite. Topical proparacaine drops provide anesthesia, since the injection is not very painful. No other sedative or anesthetic is needed for older children and adults. A special needle electrode with an amplifier is used to provide auditory information to the surgeon from the electromyographic response of the muscle and gives the surgeon knowledge of the needle placement. The patient is asked to look away from the field of action of the muscle. The needle is inserted through the conjunctiva and Tenon's fascia tangential to the globe at a point between the fornix and muscle insertion. It is advanced posteriorly along the muscle. The needle is then angled into the muscle, using the electromyographic control for guidance. The electromyographic response of the muscle is activated by having the patient look into the field of action of the muscle. This also permits the surgeon to be certain the correct muscle is being injected. The procedure should be undertaken only by ophthalmologists familiar with eye muscle anatomy and physiology and by those who are experienced with strabismus therapy.

The drug is supplied freeze-dried and is reconstituted with unpreserved saline. It is extremely labile and is easily destroyed by heat, alcohol, or shaking. An appropriate dose of 1 to 10 units is delivered (the usual initial dose is 2.5 units). For children who are too young to cooperate, sedation can be provided with 0.5 to 1.0 mg/kg ketamine IV. This has been shown to be safe and quite effective. This produces enough sedation that the patient does not remember the procedure or move around much, but it is still appropriate to stabilize the head for the procedure. If the surgeon moves the head from side to side, the vestibuloocular response will move the eyes in an opposite direction, even with ketamine sedation. This can help the surgeon be certain the correct muscle is injected. Children who are less than 1 yr of age can generally be treated only with restraint and topical drop anesthesia, much as for an office tear duct probing.

REFERENCES

1. Scott AB: Botulinum toxin injection of eye muscles to correct strabismus. Trans Am Ophthalmol Soc 79: 734–770, 1981.
2. Scott AB: Botulinum toxin treatment of strabismus. Focal Points. Clinical Modules for Ophthalmologists. 7 Mod 12, 1989.
3. Biglan AW, Burnstine RA, Rogers GL, et al: Management of strabismus with botulinum A toxin. Ophthalmology 96:935–943, 1989.
4. Magoon EH, Scott AB: Botulinum toxin chemodenervation in infants and children: An alternative to incisional strabismus surgery. J Pediatr 110:719–722, 1987.
5. Magoon EH: Chemodenervation of strabismic children: A 2- to 5-year follow-up study compared with shorter follow-up. Ophthalmology 96:931–934, 1989.
6. Scott AB, Magoon EH, McNeer KW, et al: Botulinum treatment of strabismus in children. Trans Am Ophthalmol Soc 87:174–180, 1990.
7. Magoon EH, Dakoske C: Botulinum toxin injection for vertical strabismus. Am Orthop J 35:48–52, 1985.
8. McNeer KW: Botulinum toxin injection into the superior rectus muscle of the nondominant eye for dissociated vertical deviation. J Pediatr Ophthalmol Strabismus 26:162–164, 1989.
9. Metz HS, Mazow M: Botulinum toxin treatment of acute sixth and third nerve palsy. Graefes Arch Clin Exp Ophthalmol 226:141–144, 1988.
10. Wagner RS, Frohman LP: Long-term results: Botulinum for sixth nerve palsy. J Pediatr Ophthalmol Strabismus 26:106–108, 1989.
11. Fitzsimons R, Lee JP, Elston J: Treatment of sixth nerve palsy in adults with combined botulinum toxin chemodenervation and surgery. Ophthalmology 95:1535–1542, 1988.
12. Scott AB: Botulinum treatment of strabismus following retinal detachment surgery. Arch Ophthalmol 108:509–510, 1990.
13. Kushner BJ: Postoperative binocularity in adults with long-standing strabismus: Is surgery cosmetic only? Am Orthop J 40:64–67, 1990.
14. Thorson JC, Jampolsky A, Scott AB: Topical anesthesia for strabismus surgery. Trans Am Acad Ophthalmol Otolaryngol 70:968–972, 1966.
15. Diamond GR: Topical anesthesia for strabismus surgery. J Pediatr Ophthalmol Strabismus 26:86–90, 1989.
16. Sanders RJ, Nelson LB, Deutsch JA: Peribulbar anesthesia for strabismus surgery. Am J Ophthalmol 109:705–708, 1990.

Chapter 219

Congenital and Childhood Cataracts

RICHARD M. ROBB

DIFFERENCES BETWEEN CHILDHOOD AND ADULT CATARACTS

Differences in Surgery and Optical Rehabilitation

After Scheie reintroduced the aspiration technique for congenital and soft cataracts in 1960,[1] the surgical approach to cataract extraction in childhood gradually switched from needling[2] and linear extraction[3] to aspiration. In time, suction-cutting instruments were introduced to remove capsular or membranous material that could not be handled by aspiration alone.[4] In a child's eye, the entire lens nucleus and cortex can usually be aspirated through a 2-mm incision, whereas in the adult eye, the lens nucleus is usually too hard to be aspirated and must be extracted intact through an incision larger than that required for the aspirating instrument alone. This is not a major disadvantage in the adult eye, since optical rehabilitation is usually accomplished by means of an intraocular lens, the placement of which itself requires a larger incision. In children, however, intraocular lenses are seldom used, and a small incision that can be sutured securely with little risk of induced astigmatism is a decided advantage. Contact lenses are the preferred means of correcting pediatric aphakia (Fig. 219–1),[5] and these can be used as soon as the incision is healed well enough to allow the insertion and removal of the lens. Children's eyes also tolerate surgical removal of the posterior capsule of the lens better than do adult eyes.[6] Cystoid macular edema rarely follows opening of the posterior capsule in infancy,[7] and removal of the capsule obviates the problem of capsular opacification and reduces the incidence of postoperative membrane formation. A limited anterior vitrectomy at the time of posterior capsule removal helps to keep vitreous out of the anterior chamber and away from the wound, and this, too, seems to be well tolerated by a child's eye.

Amblyopia Associated With Childhood Cataracts

Amblyopia compounds the visual loss from many pediatric eye diseases, and childhood cataracts are no exception. The most profound amblyopia found in association with pediatric cataracts is deprivational amblyopia in eyes with unilateral congenital cataracts. It is now known that these eyes must be treated within the first several months of life if useful vision is to be obtained.[8, 9] Complete bilateral congenital cataracts may result in permanent bilateral amblyopia if they are not removed by approximately 7 yr of age,[10] a situation that fortunately is uncommon in the United States at this time. On the other hand, partial bilateral congenital cataracts of lamellar type are not associated with deprivational amblyopia, even if distance vision is demonstrably reduced by the lens opacities, and surgery can be delayed until the amount of reduction of vision is clearly defined.[11]

Strabismic amblyopia is also common in children with cataracts. Virtually all patients with visually significant unilateral congenital cataracts have strabismus, and the deviation persists even in patients who have had early cataract surgery and have undergone vigorous efforts to rehabilitate the affected eye.[8, 9] In children with bilateral cataracts, the prevalence of strabismus is high, in the range of 35 to 38 percent,[10, 12] and strabismic amblyopia may contribute to the visual disability.

Nystagmus Accompanying Congenital Cataracts

Congenital cataracts are frequently associated with nystagmus,[10, 11, 13] and the visual acuity in eyes with nystagmus is predictably poorer than in those without. Nystagmus is more common in patients with bilateral complete congenital cataracts and in eyes with small corneal diameters and poorly dilating pupils (personal

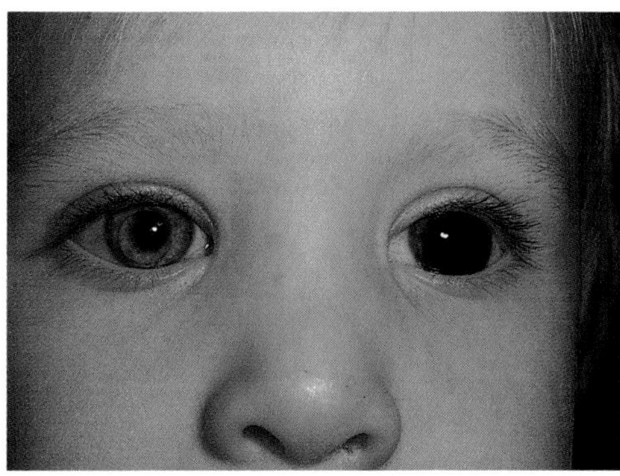

Figure 219–1. Infant with aphakic contact lens on the right eye and occluder contact lens on the left to encourage use of the right eye after cataract surgery.

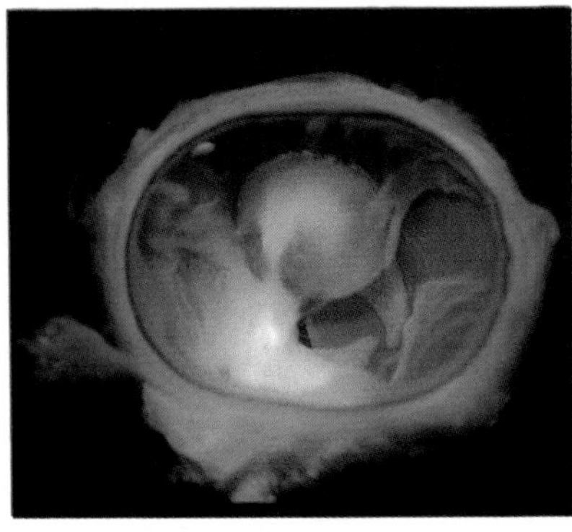

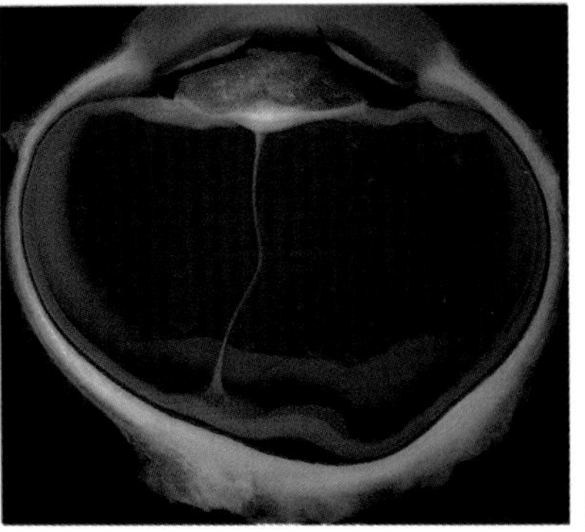

Figure 219–2. *A,* Eye of infant with 13 trisomy, showing displaced cataractous lens and malformed retina thrown into folds behind lens. *B,* Eye with a flattened cataract pushed forward by a persistent hyperplastic vitreous membrane. A hyaloid stalk extends from the membrane back to the optic disc.

observation).[14] It has been suggested that early surgery prevents the development of nystagmus,[15, 16] but this has yet to be confirmed in a large prospective series of patients. The nystagmus usually does not appear until 2 to 3 mo of age. It rarely develops in patients who acquire their cataracts after 6 mo of age.[13, 14]

Other Ocular Abnormalities With Pediatric Cataracts

Pediatric cataracts also differ from those of adults in their association with other ocular abnormalities. Striking examples are the cataracts found with trisomy of chromosome 13 and those associated with persistent hyperplastic primary vitreous (PHPV) (Fig. 219–2). The former are seldom operated on because of the limited life span of affected patients, but cataracts associated with PHPV frequently come to surgery, the results of which depend on the extent of the retrolenticular membrane and the presence of other posterior segment malformations.[17] Isolated posterior staphylomas may accompany congenital cataracts. They influence the postoperative refractive correction and may compromise macular function. Intrauterine infections such as toxoplasmosis and varicella cause chorioretinopathy in addition to cataracts,[18, 19] and significant retinal scarring and distortion can be anticipated when cataracts occur as a complication of the retinopathy of prematurity.[20] Retinal pigment epithelial changes in the congenital rubella syndrome, now fortunately a rarity in the United States because of a successful immunization program, do not in themselves have a major effect on visual acuity, but children with rubella cataracts seldom achieve good vision after cataract extraction because of their associated nystagmus, strabismus, microphthalmia, and pupillary membrane formation.[21]

IDENTIFIABLE TYPES OF CHILDHOOD CATARACTS

Although there are many identified causes of childhood cataracts and numerous diseases and syndromes in which cataracts are frequently or occasionally seen (Table 219–1), the largest categories are either dominantly inherited bilateral cataracts without systemic abnormalities or sporadic congenital cataracts, either unilateral or bilateral, for which no etiology can be found. (Table 219–2). Prior to the availability of rubella vaccine in 1979 cataracts associated with the congenital rubella syndrome were another important group,[21] but these are

Table 219–1. RECOGNIZED CAUSES OF CATARACTS IN CHILDHOOD

Inherited without systemic abnormalities
Autosomal dominant (varying types)[22] including anterior polar[23]
X-linked[24]
Autosomal recessive (rare)[25]
Chromosomal abnormalities
Trisomy 21 (Down's syndrome)[26]
Trisomy 13 (Patau's syndrome)[27]
Intrauterine infections
Rubella[21]
Varicella[19]
Herpes simplex[28]
Metabolic disorders
Galactosemia (transferase deficiency[29] and kinase deficiency[30])
Hypocalcemia[31, 32, 33]
Hypoglycemia[34]
Diabetes mellitus[35]
Fabry disease[36]
Mannosidosis[37, 38]
Zellweger syndrome[39]
Systemic syndromes and diseases
Hallerman-Streiff syndrome[40]
Conradi syndrome[41]
Oculocerebrorenal syndrome of Lowe[42]
Alport's syndrome[43]
Cockayne's syndrome[44]
Incontinentia pigmenti[45]
Rothmund-Thompson syndrome[46]
Werner's syndrome[47]
Atopic dermatitis[48]
Myotonic dystrophy[49]
Ectodermal dysplasia of Marshall[50]
LEOPARD syndrome[51]
Neurofibromatosis type 2[52]
Ocular diseases
Persistent hyperplastic primary vitreous[17]
Posterior lenticonus[53]
Retrolental fibroplasia[54]
Uveitis, especially associated with juvenile rheumatoid arthritis[55]
Congenital aniridia[56]
Retinal pigmentary degeneration[57]
Drugs and external agents
Systemic corticosteroids[58]
Radiation-induced[59]
Trauma[60]

Table 219–2. CATARACTS OF CHILDHOOD

Dominantly inherited	21
Idiopathic, bilateral	21
Idiopathic, unilateral	15
Posterior lenticonus	8
Persistent hyperplastic primary vitreous	5
Trauma	4
Radiation-induced	3
Congenital rubella	2
Infantile hypoglycemia	2
Idiopathic hypocalcemia	1
Progressive anterior polar	1
Uveitis	1
Alport's syndrome	1
Congenital sensory neuropathy	1
Familial intrahepatic cholestasis	1

From author's series of 87 patients coming to surgery from 1968 to 1987 at Children's Hospital, Boston.

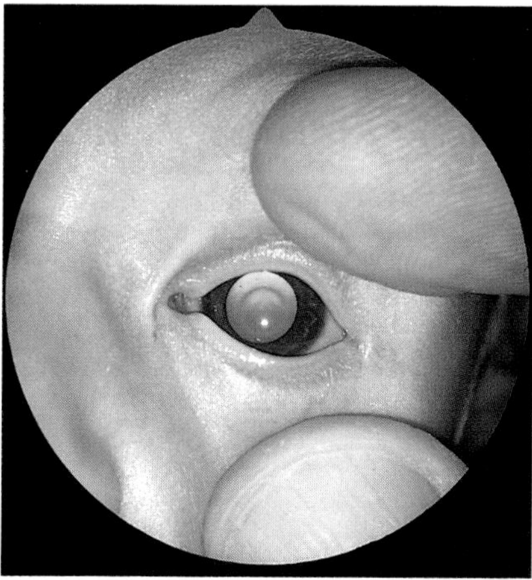

Figure 219–4. Oil droplet lens opacity in newborn infant with galactosemia due to galactose-1-phosphate transferase deficiency. Such an opacity would be expected to disappear when lactose was removed from infant's diet.

now seldom seen. Lens opacities associated with posterior lenticonus (Fig. 219–3) and with PHPV (see Fig. 219–2) are of moderate prevalence. They are important to identify because of the relatively favorable visual prognosis of the former[52] and the poor prognosis of the latter.[17] Those cataracts associated with systemic disease or recognizable syndromes are likely to be evident to an ophthalmologist and pediatrician working together to evaluate the patient.

In an apparently healthy child, only a few laboratory tests are useful in screening for hidden causes of cataract formation. Urine may be screened for reducing substances in both the galactokinase and galactose-1-phosphate transferase forms of galactosemia. In the more common transferase deficiency (Fig. 219–4), infants are usually sick from the time they start to drink whole milk,[29] but in the kinase deficiency they may be entirely well except for cataract formation.[30] Enzyme studies on erythrocytes will identify the kinase deficiency. A rubella antibody titer helps to recognize infants with the congenital rubella syndrome. Since maternal antibody is passed to the infant transplacentally, the mother's blood should also be tested. Passively transferred antibody in the infant declines during the first 6 mo, whereas infected infants maintain or increase their antibody levels. Hypocalcemia[31, 32, 33] and hypoglycemia[34] of infancy sufficient to cause cataracts are heralded by tetany or seizures in the neonatal period, and without this history,

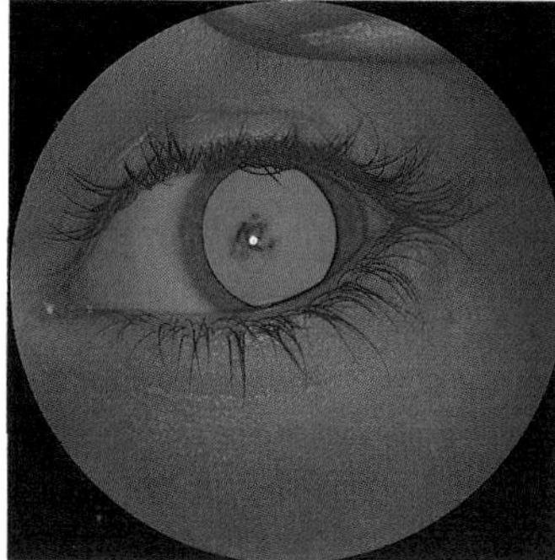

Figure 219–3. Cataract associated with posterior lenticonus seen against background of reflected fundus reflex.

routine testing of serum calcium and blood glucose is probably not warranted. Diabetes mellitus is an infrequent cause of childhood cataracts, and when lens opacities do occur in teenage diabetics, they are not the presenting signs of the disease.[35] Posterior subcapsular lens opacities due to systemic corticosteroid medication are usually distinctive in form and are evident from the history of steroid use.[58] Since the diseases for which steroid treatment is required are often prolonged and life-threatening, the medication can seldom be discontinued. Fortunately, steroid-induced cataracts have relatively little effect on vision and do not usually require surgery. Transient idiopathic cataracts have been described in premature infants, but they rarely persist or result in visually significant lens opacities.[61]

IMPORTANT ASPECTS OF THE NONSURGICAL MANAGEMENT OF CHILDHOOD CATARACTS

Early Detection of Childhood Cataracts

The detection of childhood cataracts is mainly done by pediatricians, who have become increasingly adept at recognizing lens opacities by examining the red reflex in the pupil with the direct ophthalmoscope. This can be done in the newborn nursery and at the time of routine follow-up examinations in the office. It is not necessary to dilate the pupil for this examination, although more of the lens can be seen through a larger pupil. Only anterior polar lens opacities (Fig. 219–5) and mature cataracts (Fig. 219–6) can be seen with diffuse external illumination, but virtually any visually significant cataract can be recognized with the direct ophthalmoscope as a shadow against the red reflex (Fig. 219–7). Nystagmus may occasionally be a secondary sign of bilateral cataracts, and strabismus may signal unilateral or asymmetrical lens opacities, but if deprivational amblyopia is to be avoided, it is preferable to identify

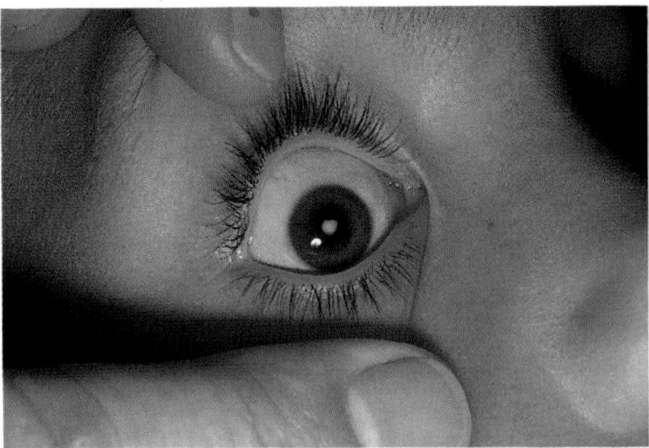

Figure 219–5. Anterior polar cataract located centrally in the pupillary space and evident on diffuse external illumination.

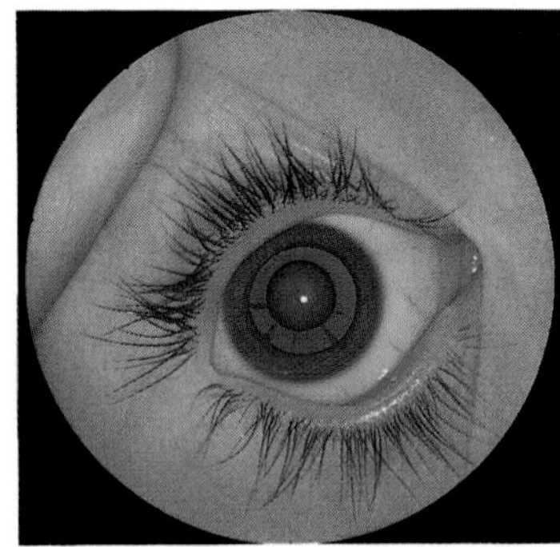

Figure 219–7. A lamellar cataract with several peripheral spoke opacities can be seen against fundus reflex as it would be with light from a direct ophthalmoscope.

pediatric cataracts before these secondary signs are present.

Assessment of Vision in Children With Lens Opacities

Assessment of the visual significance of lens opacities in preverbal children is based on the patient's visual behavior and on the density of the cataract as viewed with the direct ophthalmoscope. The density of the opacity seems to be more important than its size,[62] although both contribute to the visual disability. Fundus examination is often impaired with the direct ophthalmoscope, but many times it can be accomplished with the indirect ophthalmoscope through a dilated pupil. How well the pupil dilates should be noted, since a poorly dilating pupil may influence the later choice of surgical technique. When the fundus cannot be visualized, ultrasound examination with a contact scanner can be used to evaluate the posterior segment. It should be recognized, however, that a normal scan does not completely rule out significant fundus pathology. Although careful clinical examination is still the primary means of assessing the visual significance of pediatric cataracts, preferential-looking tests of visual acuity in preverbal infants are increasingly used (Fig. 219–8),[63] and pattern visual–evoked potentials are available in specialized centers.[64] In children with incomplete cataracts, especially bilateral lamellar opacities without nystagmus or strabismus, there is no harm in delaying cataract surgery

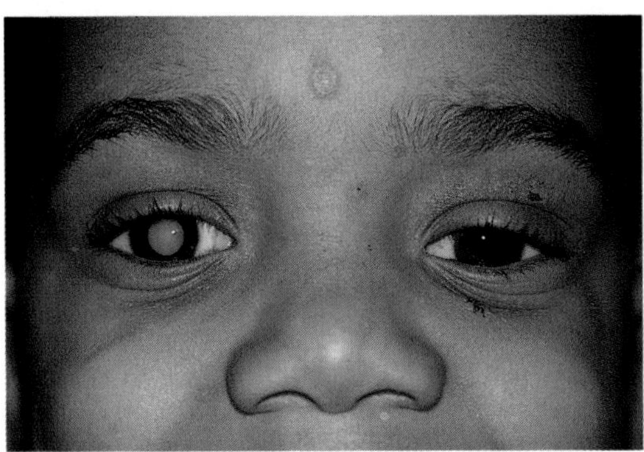

Figure 219–6. A mature cataract in this patient's right eye is visible with diffuse external illumination.

until it can be determined that visual acuity lags significantly behind normal levels for age.

Optical Correction of Pediatric Aphakia

After cataract surgery has been performed, the optical correction of aphakia in infants and children requires special consideration. Eyes with congenital cataracts often have unusually high degrees of aphakic hypermetropia. The average initial contact lens correction in infants with unilateral congenital cataracts is +30 diopters.[65] This ametropia decreases at a fairly predictable rate with increasing age, and the power of a corrective lens must be reduced accordingly. Contact lenses are now commonly used for the correction of pediatric aphakia in the early years (see Fig. 219–1). The lenses are well tolerated by infants and are available in the necessary strengths and sizes.[5] Aphakic spectacles are also useful, especially after bilateral cataract extractions and for children over 18 months of age. Although spectacle corrections introduce more image magnification than contact lenses and might therefore seem less attractive for unilateral aphakia, binocular vision is rare in children with unilateral cataracts, and a spectacle correction for the aphakic eye occasionally is quite useful if contact lenses are not well tolerated. Intraocular lenses have been used in infants by only a few surgeons.[66] They have failed to become more widely accepted because of the advantages of opening the posterior capsule at the time of initial surgery, the certainty of growth of the eye in the first 2 yr, the predictable change in refractive error with time, and the unknown long-term tolerance of the eye for an implanted lens. Epikeratophakia and secondary lens implants have also had limited use in infants, mostly in older infants who are contact lens–intolerant.[67] The disadvantage of both techniques is that amblyopia is usually deep and fixed by the time this intolerance is established.[75] Bifocal corrections are not required for children under the age of 3 or 4 yr.

Treatment of Amblyopia

The treatment of amblyopia can be a major challenge for children with unilateral aphakia or with strabismus

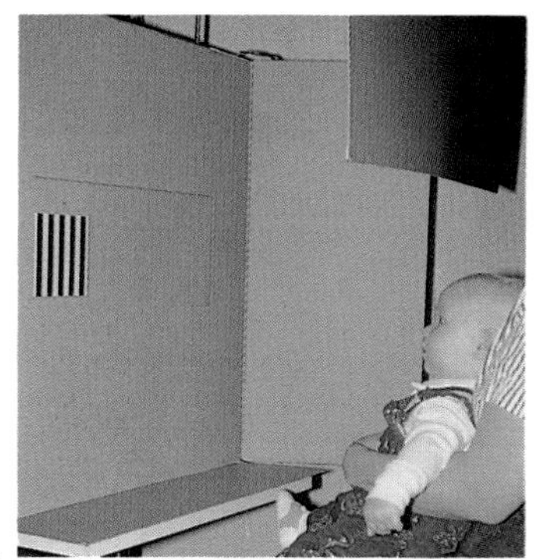

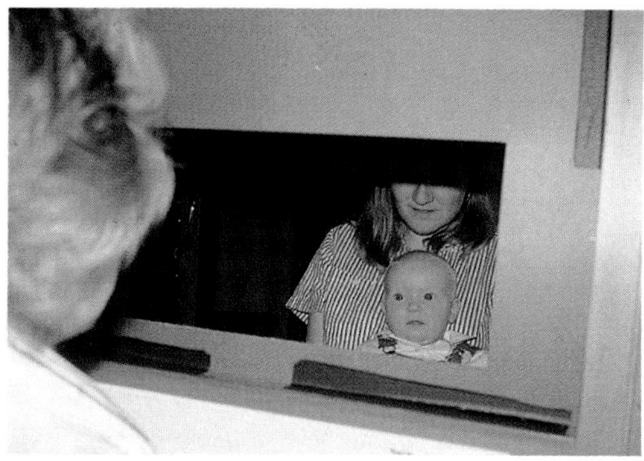

Figure 219–8. *A,* Infant being tested by preferential looking technique to determine visual acuity. Observer behind the screen judges infant's ability to fix on the striped pattern. *B,* View of infant and mother from observer's side of the screen after acuity card has been removed.

superimposed on bilateral aphakia. Occlusive patches are the mainstay of treatment, which must be pursued on a daily basis for a number of years. Sometimes children become intolerant of the adhesive patches. As an alternative, an occluder contact lens may be worn on the preferred eye (see Fig. 219–1). The opaqueness of the occluder lens must be sufficient to cause a switch in fixation to the amblyopic eye. In bilateral aphakia with strabismic amblyopia, the contact lens of the preferred eye can be removed for periods of time to induce this change in fixation pattern. As with most forms of functional amblyopia, the amblyopia that occurs in aphakic children owing to persistent monocular fixation must be followed and treated until 8 or 9 yr of age to obtain the best possible vision. When prolonged or intensive occlusion is being used, special care must be taken not to cause deprivation amblyopia in the occluded eye or to persist with patching when it is accompanied by reclusive behavior in the child. There certainly are times when the only reasonable choice is to forgo any further attempts at amblyopia therapy, and this decision should be shared by the ophthalmologist and the parents.

MONITORING VISUAL ACUITY AFTER CATARACT SURGERY

Monitoring visual acuity after cataract surgery in childhood is important in order to optimize the visual outcome. Serial measurements of visual acuity can help in adjusting patching programs for deprivational, refractive, or strabismic amblyopia. Acuity measurements also help to quantify the level of visual function in patients with nystagmus or other ocular abnormalities that complicate their aphakic condition. Vision testing in infancy has traditionally been done with fixation pattern and behavioral assessment. Preferential-looking tests with Teller acuity cards allow a more quantitative estimate and can easily be done in an office (see Fig. 219–8).[63, 68] Recognition acuities are not available for most children until after 3 yr of age; and linear Snellen acuities, not until 5 yr of age. It is well to remember that these various tests do not measure the same parameters of visual function, so they cannot simply be converted from one to the other as they become available, even though they are often expressed in the same Snellen notation. It is better to compare a patient's performance on a given test to the normal range of vision for that test at the age in question, since normal levels of visual acuity change throughout much of the period under consideration. In assessing amblyopia, the most useful comparison may be between the acuities of the two eyes of the same patient.[69]

LATE COMPLICATIONS OF PEDIATRIC CATARACT SURGERY

Beyond the issues of immediate postoperative management there are several longer-term matters of importance in following children who have had cataract surgery. First is the development of a secondary pupillary membrane. If the posterior capsule of the lens is left in place at the time of cataract surgery, in a child it virtually always thickens within months to years and must be opened or removed to clear the optical path. In infants, especially, having to deal with this secondary membrane may be an unwanted interruption of efforts to encourage the child to use the eye. Removal of the posterior capsule with a suction-cutting instrument at the time of initial surgery largely eliminates the problem of the secondary membrane[8] although a membrane does occasionally develop on the surface of the vitreous face.[70] Until recently most secondary membranes were incised with a knife or cut out with a suction-cutting instrument, but YAG lasers designed for pediatric use are now becoming available and allow the pupil to be cleared without an incision, as is commonly done after adult extracapsular cataract surgery.

The second issue to be kept in mind is the possibility of retinal detachment following childhood cataract surgery. This is not a frequent complication,[73, 74] but it may occur many years after the cataract surgery,[10] and current estimates may be low. In the author's experience, retinal detachments have occurred mainly in patients whose cataracts were associated with PHPV or with ocular trauma.[14]

Finally, it is necessary to be alert to the possible development of glaucoma in pediatric aphakic eyes. An incidence of between 6 and 11 percent has been reported.[73, 74] Angle-closure glaucoma secondary to pupillary block can be avoided by prolonged use of postoperative mydriatics.[11] It is less clear what the cause is or how to prevent late developing open-angle glaucoma, which may not appear for a number of years after cataract surgery.[10, 71–74] Treatment of this chronic glaucoma has been difficult. Medical therapy is customarily tried first, but cyclodestructive procedures or filtration may be required.

REFERENCES

1. Scheie HG: Aspiration of congenital or soft cataracts: a new technique. Am J Ophthalmol 50:1048, 1960.
2. Jones IS: The treatment of congenital cataracts by needling. Trans Am Ophthalmol Soc 58:188, 1960.
3. Cordes FC: Linear extraction in congenital cataract surgery. Trans Am Ophthalmol Soc 58:203, 1960.
4. Taylor D: Choice of surgical technique in the management of congenital cataract. Trans Ophthalmol Soc UK 101:114, 1981.
5. Hoyt CS: The optical correction of pediatric aphakia. Arch Ophthalmol 104:651, 1986.
6. Parks MM: Posterior lens capsulectomy during primary cataract surgery in children. Ophthalmology 90:344, 1983.
7. Pinchoff BS, Ellis FD, Helveston EM, et al: Cystoid macular edema in pediatric aphakia. J Pediatr Ophthalmol Strabismus 25:240, 1988.
8. Beller R, Hoyt CS, Marg E, et al: Good visual function after neonatal surgery for congenital monocular cataracts. Am J Ophthalmol 91:559, 1981.
9. Robb RM, Mayer DL, Moore BD: Results of early treatment of unilateral congenital cataracts. J Pediatr Ophthalmol Strabismus 24:178, 1987.
10. Francois J: Late results of congenital cataract surgery. Ophthalmology 86:1586, 1979.
11. Chandler PA: Surgery of the lens in infancy and childhood. Arch Ophthalmol 45:125, 1951.
12. Owens WC, Hughes WF Jr: Results of surgical treatment of congenital cataract. Arch Ophthalmol 39:339, 1948.
13. Taylor D: Amblyopia in bilateral infantile and juvenile cataract. Relationship to timing of treatment. Trans Ophthalmol Soc UK 99:170, 1970.
14. Robb R: Unpublished personal observation, 1991.
15. Gelbart SS, Hoyt CS, Jastrebski G, et al: Long-term visual results in bilateral congenital cataracts. Am J Ophthalmol 93:615, 1982.
16. Rogers GL, Tishler CL, Tsou BH, et al: Visual acuities in infants with congenital cataracts operated on prior to 6 months of age. Arch Ophthalmol 99:999, 1981.
17. Karr DJ, Scott WE: Visual acuity results following treatment of persistent hyperplastic primary vitreous. Arch Ophthalmol 104:662, 1986.
18. O'Connor GR: Manifestations and management of ocular toxoplasmosis. Bull NY Acad Med 50:192, 1974.
19. Lambert SR, Taylor D, Kriss A, et al: Ocular manifestations of the congenital varicella syndrome. Arch Ophthalmol 107:52, 1989.
20. Cohen J, Alfano JF, Boshes LD, et al: Clinical evaluation of school-age children with retrolental fibroplasia. Am J Ophthalmol 57:41, 1964.
21. Wolff, SM: The ocular manifestations of congenital rubella. A prospective study of 328 cases of congenital rubella. J Pediatr Ophthalmol 10:101, 1973.
22. Marner E: A family with eight generations of hereditary cataract. Acta Ophthalmol 27:537, 1949.
23. Jaafar MS, Robb RM: Congenital anterior polar cataract. A review of 63 cases. Ophthalmology 91:249, 1984.
24. Krill AE, Woodbury G, Bowman JE: X-chromosome–linked sutural cataracts. Am J Ophthalmol 68:867, 1969.
25. Saebo J: An investigation in the mode of heredity of congenital and juvenile cataracts. Br J Ophthalmol 33:601, 1949.
26. Ingersheimer J: The relationship of lenticular changes to mongolism. Trans Am Ophthalmol Soc 49:595, 1951.
27. Cogan DG, Kuwabara T: Ocular pathology of the 13–15 trisomy syndrome. Arch Ophthalmol 72:246, 1964.
28. Cibis A, Burde RM: Herpes simplex virus–induced congenital cataracts. Arch Ophthalmol 85:220, 1971.
29. Cordes FC: Galactosemia cataract: a review. Am J Ophthalmol 50:1151, 1960.
30. Beutler E, Matsumto F, Kuhl W, et al: Galactokinase deficiency as a cause of cataracts. N Engl J Med 288:1203, 1973.
31. Duke-Elder S: System of Ophthalmology, Vol. 11. Diseases of the Lens, Vitreous; Glaucoma and Hypotomy. St. Louis, CV Mosby, 1969, p 175.
32. Walsh FB, Murray RG: Ocular manifestations of disturbances in calcium metabolism. Am J Ophthalmol 36:1657, 1953.
33. Pohjola S: Ocular manifestations of idiopathic hypoparathyroidism. Acta Ophthalmol (Copenh) 40:255, 1962.
34. Merin S, Crawford JS: Hypoglycemia and infantile cataract. Arch Ophthalmol 86:495, 1971.
35. Duke-Elder S: System of Ophthalmology, Vol. 11. Diseases of the Lens, Vitreous; Glaucoma and Hypotony. St. Louis, CV Mosby, 1969, p 166.
36. Sher NA, Letson RD, Desnick RJ: The ocular manifestations in Fabry's disease. Arch Ophthalmol 97:671, 1979.
37. Arbisser AI, Murphree AL, Garcia CA, et al: Ocular findings in mannosidosis. Am J Ophthalmol 82:465, 1976.
38. Letson RD, Desnick RJ: Punctate lens opacities in type II mannosidosis. Am J Ophthalmol 85:218, 1978.
39. Haddad R, Font RL, Friendly DS: Cerebrohepatorenal syndrome of Zellweger. Ocular histopathologic findings. Arch Ophthalmol 94:1927, 1976.
40. Falls HF, Schull WJ: Hallerman-Streiff syndrome. A dyscephaly with congenital cataracts and hypotrichosis. Arch Ophthalmol 63:409, 1960.
41. Armaly MF: Ocular involvement in chondrodystrophia calcifans congenita punctata. Arch Ophthalmol 57:491, 1957.
42. Wilson WA, Richards W, Donnell GN: Oculo-cerebral-renal syndrome of Lowe. Arch Ophthalmol 70:5, 1963.
43. Nielson CE: Lenticonus anterior and Alport's syndrome. Acta Ophthalmol 56:518, 1978.
44. Pearce WG: Ocular and genetic features of Cockayne's syndrome. Can J Ophthalmol 7:435, 1972.
45. Scott JG, Friedman AI, Chitters M, et al: Ocular changes in the Block-Sulzburger syndrome (incontinentia pigmenti). Br J Ophthalmol 39:276, 1955.
46. Thannhauser SJ: Werner's syndrome and Rothmund's syndrome: two types of closely related heredofamilial atrophic dermatoses with juvenile cataracts and endocrine features. Ann Intern Med 23:559, 1945.
47. Petrohelos MA: Werner's syndrome. A survey of three cases, with review of literature. Am J Ophthalmol 56:941, 1963.
48. Cowan A, Klander JV: Frequency of ocurrence of cataract in atopic dermatitis. Arch Ophthalmol 43:759, 1950.
49. Burian HM, Burns CA: Ocular changes in myotonic dystrophy. Am J Ophthalmol 63:22, 1967.
50. Marshall D: Ectodermal dysplasia. Report of kindred with ocular abnormalities and hearing defect. Am J Ophthalmol 45:143, 1958.
51. Howard RO: Premature cataracts associated with generalized lentigo. Ophthalmology 87:234, 1980.
52. Kaiser-Kupfer MI, Freidlin V, Datiles MB, et al: The association of posterior capsular lens opacities with bilateral acoustic neuromas in patients with neurofibromatosis type 2. Arch Ophthalmol 107:541, 1989.
53. Crouch ER, Parks MM: Management of posterior lenticonus complicated by unilateral cataract. Am J Ophthalmol 85:503, 1978.
54. Cohen J, Alfano JE, Boshes LD, et al: Clinical evaluation of school-age children with retrolental fibroplasia. Am J Ophthalmol 57:41, 1964.
55. Chylack LT, Bienfang DC, Bellows AR, et al: Ocular manifestations of juvenile rheumatoid arthritis. Am J Ophthalmol 79:1026, 1975.
56. Lewallen WM: Aniridia and related iris defects. A report of twelve cases with bilateral cataract extraction and resulting good vision in one. Arch Ophthalmol 59:831, 1958.
57. Franceschetti A, Francois J, Babel J: Chorioretinal Heredodegenerations. Springfield, IL, Charles C Thomas, 1974, p 850.
58. Grant WM: Toxicology of the Eye, 2nd ed. Springfield, IL, Charles C Thomas, 1974, p 320.
59. Cogan DG: Lesions of the eye from radiant energy. JAMA 142:145, 1950.
60. Duke-Elder S, MacFaul PA: System of Ophthalmology, Vol. 14. Part 1. Mechanical Injuries. St. Louis, CV Mosby, 1972, p 121.
61. McCormick AQ: Transient cataracts in premature infants. A new clinical entity. Can J Ophthalmol 3:202, 1968.

62. Sheppard RW, Crawford JS: The treatment of congenital cataracts. Surv Ophthalmol 17:340, 1973.
63. Teller DY, McDonald M, Preston K, et al: Assessment of visual acuity in infants and children: the acuity card procedure. Dev Med Child Neurol 28:779, 1986.
64. Gottlob I, Fendick MG, Guo S, et al: Visual acuity measurements by swept spatial frequency visual-evoked cortical potentials (VECPs): clinical application in children with various visual disorders. J Pediatr Ophthalmol Strabismus 27:40, 1990.
65. Moore BD: Changes in the aphakic refraction of children with unilateral congenital cataracts. J Pediatr Ophthalmol Strabismus 26:290, 1989.
66. Hiles DA: Intraocular lens implantation in children with monocular cataracts, 1974–1983. Ophthalmology 91:1231, 1984.
67. Morgan KS, MacDonald MB, Hiles DA, et al: The nationwide study of epikeratophakia for aphakia in children. Am J Ophthalmol 103:366, 1987.
68. Catalano RA, Simon JW, Jenkins PL, et al: Preferential looking as a guide for amblyopia therapy in monocular infantile cataracts. J Pediatr Ophthalmol Strabismus 24:56, 1987.
69. Mayer DL, Moore B, Robb, RM: Assessment of vision and amblyopia by preferential looking tests after early surgery for unilateral congenital cataracts. J Pediatr Ophthalmol Strabismus 26:61, 1989.
70. Morgan KS, Karcioglu ZA: Secondary cataracts in infants after lensectomies. J Pediatr Ophthalmol Strabismus 24:45, 1987.
71. Phelps CD, Arafat NI: Open-angle glaucoma following surgery for congenital cataracts. Arch Ophthalmol 95:1985, 1977.
72. Boger WP: Late ocular complications in congenital rubella syndrome. Ophthalmology 87:1244, 1980.
73. Chrousos GA, Parks MM, O'Neill JF: Incidence of chronic glaucoma, retinal detachment and secondary membrane surgery in pediatric aphakic patients. Ophthalmology 91:1238, 1984.
74. Keech RV, Tongue AC, Scott WE: Complications after surgery for congenital and infantile cataracts. Am J Ophthalmol 108:136, 1989.
75. Elsas FJ: Visual acuity in monocular pediatric aphakia: Does epikeratophakia facilitate occlusion therapy in children of contact lens or spectacle wear? J Pediatr Ophthalmol Strabismus 27:304, 1990.

Chapter 220

Surgical Management of Pediatric Cataracts

DAVID S. WALTON

The need for and special characteristics of lensectomy in children has been discussed in the eye literature for more than 200 years. The modern era of this surgery was initiated by Scheie's paper, *Aspiration of Congenital or Soft Cataracts.*[1] In this paper, iridectomy, discission, linear extraction, intracapsular extraction, and aspiration techniques for pediatric cataracts are reviewed. His technique of lens removal by aspiration became universally adopted by pediatric surgeons, and aspiration of lens material has persisted as an important component of all pediatric lensectomy procedures performed today.

Contemporary pediatric lensectomy surgery now makes use of suction–vitreous cutting instrumentation, allowing both aspiration and cutting of intraocular tissue. Earlier techniques with aspiration alone, discission, or linear extraction did not provide the facility for handling vitreous tissue satisfactorily. The posterior capsule in these earlier operations was skillfully preserved as a barrier against vitreous presentation in order to facilitate lens removal and lessen the risk of secondary glaucoma or retinal detachment. If the posterior lens capsule was found opacified, it was often preserved for a necessary second operation, further delaying the goal of a clear pupil. The cutting mode in today's surgery has made possible safe removal of both the posterior lens capsule and anterior-directed vitreous and has enhanced the removal of lens cortex.

The indication for pediatric lensectomy is visual, refractive, medical, or cosmetic. Cataract removal is done not only to improve vision but also to facilitate the development of improved vision at an early age. Lens removal is also justified with subluxation of the lens that causes an excessive refractive impediment. When injured or displaced into the anterior chamber, early removal of the lens may be indicated for medical reasons. When desired, a lens may also be removed to restore darkness to the pupillary region for cosmetic reasons.

Now, use of a vitrectomy suction-cutting instrument is nearly universal, but other important decisions must be considered by the pediatric lens surgeon. Timing of surgery relative to the age of the patient and the visual requirements must be considered. To allow early initiation of visual development, infants are best operated on early but not necessarily in the first two weeks of life. The visual requirements of older children, taking into account their present function with cataracts versus the burdens of surgical aphakia, must be weighed. Family preparation for an important support role must be considered. Examination for evidence of ocular inflammation, such as conjunctivitis or nasolacrimal duct obstruction, and scrutiny of patients for other ocular defects is essential. Readiness for general anesthesia also must be determined.

SURGICAL CONSIDERATIONS

Mydriasis. Pediatric lensectomy has always been facilitated by a well-dilated pupil. Cyclopentolate and phenylephrine topically, and intracameral epinephrine when necessary, will produce and maintain maximum mydriasis. A preoperative topical prostaglandin inhibitor may also be helpful. Use of these agents is effective in producing and maintaining mydriasis and does not prevent acetylcholine-induced miosis at the end of this procedure.

Scleral Incision. The *size* of the scleral incision should allow entry of instruments and prevent excessive reflux of fluid. Too large an incision, resulting in excessive escape of fluid, can make maintenance of the anterior chamber difficult with the usual level of suction.

The *position* of the incision significantly determines the character of the surgery that follows. Limbal, pars plicata,[2] and pars plana approaches have been used. Fear of disturbing the vitreous base, if not the retina itself, by entry through the pars plana in eyes in which the pars plana is of variable width has made this entry site the least widely used.

Shifting of the entry site anteriorly, to the pars plicata, has been recommended and has been used successfully.[2, 3] Use of this site allows entrance to the posterior chamber without as much potential risk to the retina as the pars plana approach involves. Hemorrhage is infrequent. The inner tip of the suction-cutting instrument can be moved anteriorly into the lens with greater ease than is true in use of the pars plana entry.

The limbal entry site is used primarily for inserting instruments into the anterior chamber for surgery through the pupil. To operate on the lens successfully with this approach, a widely dilated pupil must be present, a condition not often present with infants even after maximum mydriatic medication. Limbal entry uniquely allows the surgeon to create a peripheral iridectomy, an important protection against the development of postoperative pupillary block. In the presence of a peripheral iridectomy, the suction-cutting instrument can also be introduced into the posterior chamber. Thus, adding an iridectomy to this surgery with a limbal entry also allows both access to the posterior chamber and a more anterior insertion, familiar to most anterior segment pediatric surgeons.

Excision of the Posterior Capsule. When lensectomy was performed by the linear extraction method and then by simple aspiration, successful surgery depended on preservation of the posterior capsule. Entry of vitreous could not be managed well by aspiration or other early instrumentation. Even after more complete removal of lens tissue by aspiration, opacification of the preserved posterior capsule occurred in the majority of patients. Reoperation to open the posterior capsule was then necessary for best visual results.

The development of the suction–vitreous cutting instrument made possible the successful management of vitreous in the anterior chamber. Vitreous removal prevented inappropriate adhesion to anterior segment structures and the surgical wound. Removal of the posterior capsule could now safely be added to the lensectomy procedure, dramatically decreasing the reccurrence of obstruction of the pupil by reforming lens tissue over an intact posterior capsule.

The more recent availability of the yttrium-aluminum-garnet (YAG) laser has provided an alternative method of managing posterior capsule opacification. When appropriate, the posterior capsule can be left in place, and opacification can be managed by use of this technology. Perforation of the posterior capsule by this method is usually associated, however, with entry of a significant amount of vitreous gel into the anterior chamber, where it may persist for many months or permanently. To have a peripheral iridectomy in place at this time is an important prophylaxis against the occurrence of pupillary block.

Lens Manipulation. The goal of the lensectomy procedure is removal of the displaced or opacified lens to clear the pupil without the subsequent occurrence of serious complications. Lensectomy in children has historically been significantly less successful than in adults, given the higher incidence of postoperative surgical complications. Disappointing results can also be related to poor postoperative vision related to preexistent occlusion amblyopia, associated ocular defects, or both.

Retinal detachment and glaucoma were historically the most serious and frequent postoperative complications after pediatric lensectomy.[4, 5] The use of aspiration and cutting instruments with improved management of vitreous and the use of microsurgical techniques have made the occurrence of retinal detachment now a rare occurrence.[6] Given the long life expectancy of patients after pediatric lens surgery, it will be reassuring with respect to retinal detachment if its occurrence remains rare with longer follow-up after surgery than present day results permit.

Glaucoma persists as a devastating complication of pediatric lens surgery with occurrence more frequent when surgery has been performed in the first year of life.[7] A much higher incidence of glaucoma followed lens needling and the linear extraction methods of lens removal.[5] This glaucoma typically followed the occurrence of pupillary block and was at first reduced in frequency by extensive iris surgery.[5] It was thereafter decreased dramatically in frequency by complete removal of lens and vitreous in the pupillary region.[6] Pupillary block and secondary glaucoma may, of course, still occur with use of aspiration-cutting instruments, but given the potential of these instruments to clear the pupillary region, it now happens less frequently.[7]

Without preceding pupillary block, the glaucoma that occurs following pediatric lensectomy appears to be associated with residual lens tissue and persistent inflammation following lens surgery. Characteristic gonioscopic abnormalities seen in the filtration angle are usually found in such instances. The trabecular meshwork shows increased opacification, and the peripheral iris is anteriorly drawn over the posterior trabecular meshwork, which is associated with the development of coarse synechiae from the iris root, first to the ciliary body band and then to the posterior trabecular meshwork. When the lens is removed more completely, by operating in the posterior chamber in very young patients with poor mydriasis or through the pupil with complete mydriasis, the postoperative inflammatory phase seen in the anterior chamber and iris after surgery is much less evident.[7] I am hopeful and encouraged by the results of surgery that this approach to the manipulation of the lens will also reduce further the risk of glaucoma following lensectomy in children.

REFERENCES

1. Scheie HG: Aspiration of congenital or soft cataracts: A new technique. Am J Ophthalmol 50:1048, 1960.
2. Peyman GA, Raichard M, Oesterle C, et al: Pars plicata lensectomy and vitrectomy in the management of congenital cataracts. Ophthalmology 88:37, 1981.
3. Green BF, Morin JD, Brent HP: Pars plicata lensectomy/vitrectomy for developmental cataract extraction: Surgical results. J Pediatr Ophthalmol Strabismus 27:229, 1990.
4. Cordes FC: Failure in congenital cataract surgery: A study of 56 enucleated eyes. Am J Ophthalmol 43:1–21, 1957
5. Chandler PA: Surgery for congenital cataract. Am J Ophthalmol 65:663, 1968.
6. Chrousos GA, Parks MM, O'Neill JF: Incidence of chronic glaucoma, retinal detachment and secondary membrane surgery in pediatric aphakic patients. Ophthalmology 9:1238, 1984.
7. Walton DS: Unpublished personal observation, 1987.

Chapter 221

Glaucoma in Childhood

DAVID S. WALTON

Glaucoma in childhood is infrequent but is caused by many different primary and secondary mechanisms (Table 221–1). It is necessary for ophthalmologists to be familiar with the conditions causing pediatric glaucomas and to be able to employ the appropriate examination techniques. Treatment of childhood glaucoma is a specialized division of pediatric and glaucoma care.

SIGNS AND SYMPTOMS

The signs and symptoms of childhood glaucoma vary greatly, depending on the age of the child, the cause of the glaucoma, and the suddenness and amount of the pressure elevation. Careful assessment of the anterior segment relative to the child's symptoms and for primary abnormalities and changes secondary to the eye pressure is helpful. Tonometry for children at all ages is an essential skill. Preparation for examination of children both in an office and in the operating room is appropriate.

In early infancy, the symptoms of glaucoma may be insignificant. Photophobia may be slight at first and may be misinterpreted as evidence of emotional insecurity. However, avoidance of light is usually progressive, causing a baby to protect its face with normal light exposure and to rub the eye frequently (Fig. 221–1). Associated epiphora may be misinterpreted as a tear duct obstruction. When an ocular discharge is also present, the possibility of both glaucoma and a tear duct obstruction should be considered. The onset of photophobia in infancy may also be sudden and intense, with equally rapid corneal opacification accompanied by an initial or new break in Descemet's membrane (Haab's striae). In older children, anterior segment symptoms are less frequent and play a less important role in the initial recognition of glaucoma. In these children, decreased visual acuity has frequently initiated an evaluation with recognition of glaucoma as its cause. Pain caused by glaucoma in childhood is experienced most frequently with the sudden pressure elevation accompanying a secondary glaucoma (e.g., pupillary-block glaucoma or traumatic glaucoma secondary to a hyphema).

Glaucoma in infancy produces important abnormalities that on examination are of diagnostic significance. Corneal opacification and enlargement are usually seen and may be present asymmetrically even with bilateral

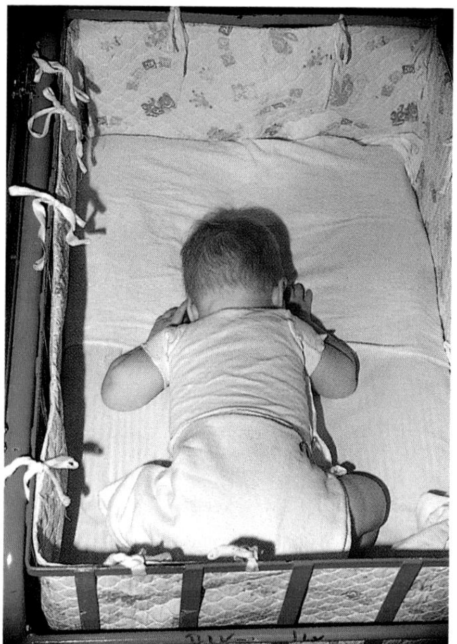

Figure 221–1. Glaucoma in infancy can cause extreme photophobia, causing infants to protect their eyes from even normal levels of light. This child can be seen blocking the entrance of side light with her hands clenched against her head.

Table 221–1. PRIMARY AND SECONDARY CHILDHOOD GLAUCOMAS

I. Primary (genetically determined) glaucomas
  A. Congenital open-angle glaucoma
    1. Infantile
    2. Late-recognized
  B. Juvenile glaucoma
  C. Primary angle-closure glaucoma
  D. Associated with systemic abnormalities
    1. Sturge-Weber syndrome
    2. Neurofibromatosis
    3. Stickler's syndrome
    4. Oculocerebrorenal (Lowe's) syndrome
    5. Rieger's syndrome
    6. Hepatocerebrorenal syndrome
    7. Marfan's syndrome
    8. Rubinstein-Taybi syndrome
    9. Infantile glaucoma associated with mental retardation and paralysis
    10. Oculodentodigital dysplasia
    11. Open-angle glaucoma associated with microcornea and absence of frontal sinuses
    12. Mucopolysaccharidosis
    13. Trisomy 13
    14. Cutis marmorata telangiectasia congenita
    15. Warburg's syndrome
    16. Kniest syndrome (skeletal dysplasia)
  E. Associated with ocular abnormalities
    1. Congenital glaucoma with iris and pupillary abnormalities
    2. Aniridia
      a. Congenital
      b. Acquired
    3. Congenital ocular melanosis
    4. Sclerocornea
    5. Familial hypoplasia of the iris
    6. Anterior chamber cleavage syndrome
    7. Iridotrabecular dysgenesis and ectropion uveae
    8. Posterior polymorphous dystrophy
    9. Idiopathic or familial elevated episcleral venous pressure
    10. Anterior corneal staphyloma

II. Secondary glaucoma
  A. Traumatic glaucoma
    1. Acute glaucoma
      a. Angle concussion
      b. Hyphema
      c. Ghost cell glaucoma
    2. Late-onset glaucoma with angle recession
    3. Arteriovenous fistula
  B. Secondary to intraocular neoplasm
    1. Retinoblastoma
    2. Juvenile xanthogranuloma
    3. Leukemia
    4. Melanoma
    5. Melanocytoma
    6. Iris rhabdomyosarcoma
  C. Secondary to uveitis
    1. Open-angle glaucoma
    2. Angle-blockage glaucoma
      a. Synechial angle closure
      b. Iris bombé with pupillary block
  D. Lens-induced glaucoma
    1. Subluxation-disclocation and pupillary block
      a. Marfan's syndrome
      b. Homocystinuria
    2. Spherophakia and pupillary block
    3. Phacolytic glaucoma
  E. Secondary to surgery for congenital cataract
    1. Lens material blockage of the trabecular meshwork (acute or subacute)
    2. Pupillary block
    3. Chronic open-angle glaucoma associated with angle defects
  F. Steroid-induced glaucoma
  G. Secondary to rubeosis
    1. Retinoblastoma
    2. Coats' disease
    3. Medulloepithelioma
    4. Familial exudative vitreoretinopathy
  H. Secondary angle-closure glaucoma
    1. Retinopathy of prematurity
    2. Microphthalmos
    3. Nanophthalmos
    4. Retinoblastoma
    5. Persistent hyperplastic primary vitreous
    6. Congenital pupillary iris-lens membrane
  I. Glaucoma associated with increased venous pressure
    1. Carotid or dural-venous fistula
    2. Orbital disease
  J. Secondary to maternal rubella
  K. Secondary to intraocular infection
    1. Acute recurrent toxoplasmosis
    2. Acute herpetic iritis

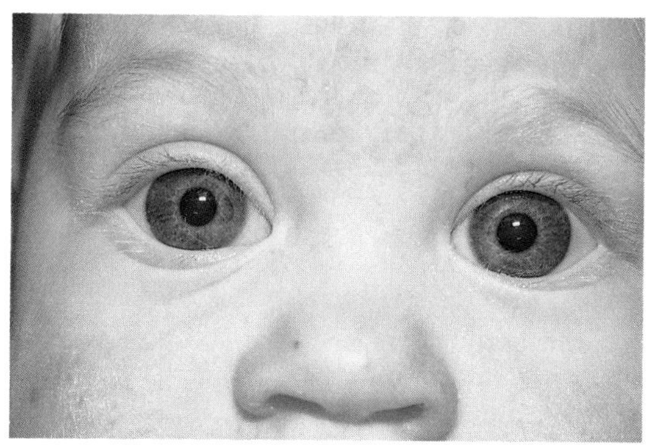

Figure 221–2. In this child with infantile glaucoma, bilateral corneal enlargement has occurred.

disease. Corneal and ocular enlargement is progressive early in life but is rarely seen in glaucoma beginning after 2 yr of age (Fig. 221–2). At birth an expected normal corneal diameter approximates 9.5 mm. With normal growth, a diameter of 11.5 to 12.0 mm is reached in the second year of life. Progressive corneal enlargement secondary to glaucoma exceeds normal measurements of diameter by 1.5 mm or more. Corneal opacification may be diffuse or localized and intense and may be related to epithelial edema or to profound stromal edema (Fig. 221–3). Corneal enlargement may occur with very little or any opacification. In the second year of life, opacification may lessen even without significant pressure control. Breaks in Descemet's membrane may be absent or may progress in number during the first 2 yr of life. Stromal and epithelial edema in proximity to a break in Descemet's membrane usually disappear, but the double curvilinear edges of the break remain as permanent stigmata of glaucoma early in life.

An additional nonspecific sign of glaucoma in early childhood includes a deep anterior chamber, especially with a primary glaucoma. Disc cupping also occurs and is variable; improvement with diminution of the cup size is usually seen accompanying successful glaucoma control.

In older children, assessment of the anterior segment is less important in recognition of glaucoma but is equally as important in determining its cause. Failure of a routine vision test may be caused by myopia or optic atrophy secondary to glaucoma. Visual field assessment usually becomes reliable in the second decade of life and plays an increasingly important role in glaucoma management. New field defects must be differentiated from newly recognized defects with adequate pressure control.

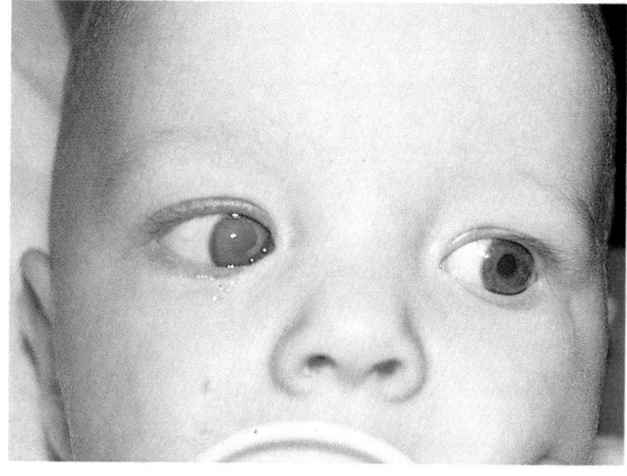

Figure 221–3. Acute, advanced corneal opacification occurred in the right eye of this child with infantile glaucoma. Bilateral corneal enlargement and opacification with a pressure of 38 mmHg were found in each eye; breaks in Descemet's membrane were present only on the right side.

PEDIATRIC GLAUCOMA EXAMINATION

The assessment of a child for glaucoma utilizes skills employed regularly for a complete pediatric ophthalmologic examination. However, in addition to recognition of glaucoma, determination of its cause, duration, severity, and appropriate treatment are goals of this examination.

Vision testing must be age-appropriate. In infants normal fixation, following, interest in toys, and the absence of nystagmus are evidence of good vision. After 3 yr of age, recognition acuity testing is important, and at approximately 10 yr of age, formal visual field testing can be done. Early refraction is important to determine early the need for occlusion therapy and optical correction to prevent suppression amblyopia.

Careful assessment of the ocular adnexa and *anterior segment* is important in care of both adult and pediatric glaucoma patients. The examiner should persist with this examination with young children. The information obtained will direct a future examination under anesthesia and will suggest what kind of treatment may be appropriate. Careful inspection of the cornea, anterior chamber, and iris, using a loupe and focused hand light and slit lamp often reveals a surprising amount of important information. This examination appropriately precedes gonioscopy, which can then be done with a Koeppe lens both in the office and later in the operating room (Fig. 221–4). Because of the magnification required, detailed gonioscopy is best done in young children under general anesthesia (Fig. 221–5). Older children, over 5 yr of age, often allow this to be done in the office. Careful, detailed recording of the pupil, iris, and filtration angle findings should always be done. This is both a challenging and a rewarding effort in children of all ages.

Tonometry should also be done in both the office and operating room when possible. Office measurements are uninfluenced by anesthesia and offer the opportunity for early confirmation of glaucoma. A hand-held applanation tonometer is a useful instrument for this purpose (Fig. 221–6). Operating room tonometry is also important. Unilateral glaucoma can be confirmed by the persistence of an asymmetric pressure measurement under anesthesia. The normal range of eye pressure in childhood is between 10 and 22 mm Hg.[1]

Funduscopy includes a complete fundus assessment but focuses especially on the optic disc. Associated choroidal abnormalities may be found (e.g., hemangioma in the Sturge-Weber syndrome). The cause of secondary glaucoma may be evident—for example, retinoblastoma, retinopathy of prematurity. Initial disc

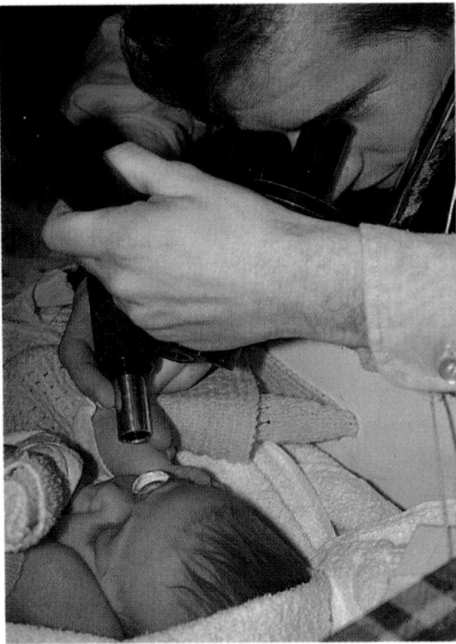

Figure 221–4. In preparation for a child's care in the operating room, Koeppe's gonioscopy in the office can supply useful preliminary information about the filtration angle.

findings must be carefully recorded for comparison with later observations to help appraise the success of glaucoma control.

DIFFERENTIAL DIAGNOSIS

It is important to establish the presence of glaucoma with certainty before a possibly unrewarding treatment for glaucoma is initiated. Persistent elevation of eye pressure is conclusive evidence for glaucoma; however, unreliable measurements while the patient is awake and acceptance of borderline measurements as abnormal when the patient is under general anesthesia may cause an erroneous diagnosis of glaucoma. The difficulty and importance of making an accurate diagnosis early in each child's care cannot be overstated. Even when the diagnosis of glaucoma in one eye is easily made, interpretation of findings in the fellow eye can be difficult. Tonometry in the office can be especially helpful for this and may be more useful than borderline findings at a future examination under general anesthesia.

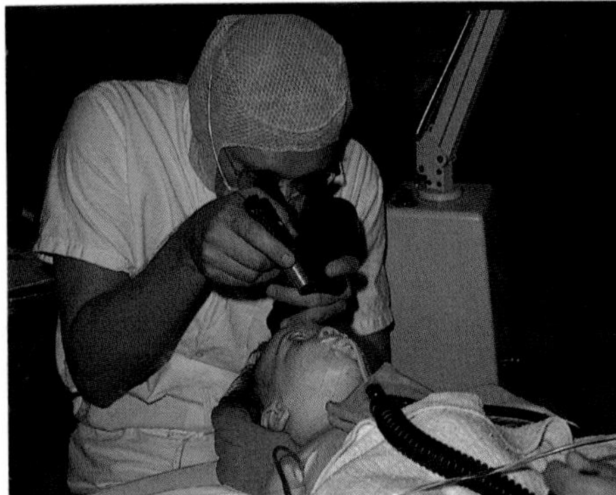

Figure 221–5. Operating room gonioscopy using a Koeppe lens and hand-held microscope supplies essential information for understanding the cause of childhood glaucoma and planning for its treatment.

Many eye conditions produce some of the signs and symptoms seen with childhood glaucoma. Like glaucoma, congenital punctal occlusion produces epiphora without discharge compared with the epiphora with discharge seen with nasolacrimal duct obstruction. Corneal edema associated with posterior polymorphous dystrophy may cause an acute onset of photophobia resembling the occurrence of a new break in Descemet's membrane secondary to glaucoma. Corneal enlargement may be present as a primary defect or may be suspected because of a microphthalmic fellow eye. Corneal epithelial opacification can be diffuse with storage diseases, resembling secondary corneal edema with glaucoma, and is seen early in mucolipidosis IV and later with stromal opacification in mucopolysaccharide (MPS) storage illnesses or Niemann-Pick disease. Trauma at birth may produce breaks in Descemet's membrane associated with corneal edema and photophobia. The history of difficult delivery, use of forceps, a cornea of normal size, a narrow rather than deep anterior chamber, and normal eye pressure help make a correct diagnosis.

One should be reminded also that one correct diagnosis does not rule out the additional presence of glaucoma as with iridocyclitis or retinoblastoma. Even storage illnesses may be complicated by glaucoma. After the diagnosis of glaucoma is made the clinical investigation is directed to determining its cause.

Table 221–1 outlines an array of varied causes of both primary and secondary glaucoma in children.

Primary Childhood Glaucoma

CONGENITAL OPEN-ANGLE GLAUCOMA[1, 2]

Congenital open-angle glaucoma is the most common primary glaucoma seen in childhood. Diagnosis is unu-

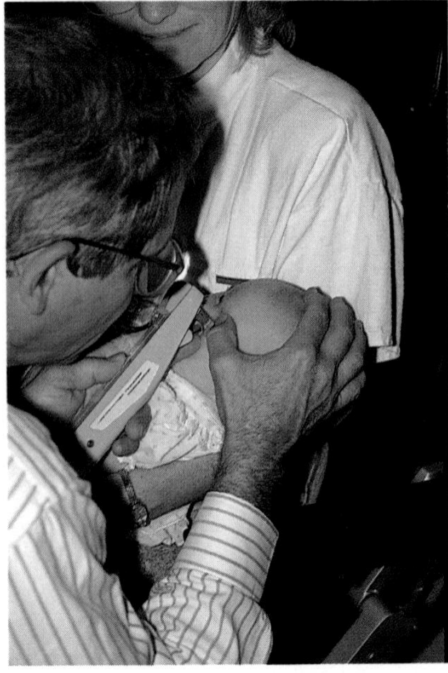

Figure 221–6. Measurement of the intraocular pressure is an important office skill and is best done with a hand-held applanation tonometer and with a parent's assistance.

sual in the neonatal period, recognition more often occurring between 3 and 9 mo of age. Late recognition during childhood also occurs in a small percentage of patients. Typically, signs and symptoms occur secondary to corneal abnormalities consisting of enlargement, edema, and breaks in Descemet's membrane. Accompanying photophobia can be severe.

Congenital open-angle glaucoma demonstrates polygenic or multifactorial inheritance, is often bilateral, and occurs slightly more frequently in males. Siblings and offspring are at approximately a 5 percent risk for this glaucoma.

The inherited defect seems to be confined to the filtration angle, causing impaired outflow of aqueous humor. The severity of the defect is quite variable, with also variable circumferential expression in the same eye and function typically more impaired in one eye than in the other such that eye pressure may remain within a normal range in one eye. Gonioscopy reveals decreased transparency of tissues at the level of the scleral spur and ciliary body band (Fig. 221–7). Severe cases suggest an anterior insertion of the peripheral iris with little evidence of scleral spur or ciliary body band. The peripheral iris frequently shows some thinning with exposure of the iris pigment epithelium, but the iris and pupil are normal in this disease. This type of primary glaucoma usually responds favorably to goniotomy or trabeculotomy, although either operation may have to be repeated to achieve satisfactory glaucoma control. This response to goniotomy is a special feature of this type of childhood glaucoma and regrettably is not a feature shared by many others.

JUVENILE OPEN-ANGLE GLAUCOMA

Juvenile open-angle glaucoma is much less frequent than congenital glaucoma and is acquired, with significant pressure elevation typically occurring by the end of the first decade. It is inherited as an autosomal dominant trait. Familial occurrences usually offer the opportunity to study and assist patients over a number of generations. Sporadic cases are more difficult to assign to this diagnosis. Involved patients are usually myopic. Gonioscopy can be expected to reveal no abnormality. Anterior chamber structures are normal. Goniotomy surgery may prove helpful and should be offered initially when glaucoma surgery must be considered.

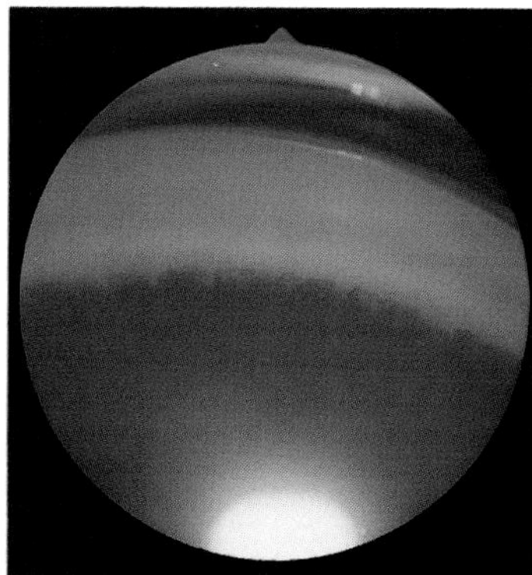

Figure 221–7. Gonioscopy in infantile glaucoma reveals a variable measure of forward insertion of the iris and opacification of tissue over the exposed ciliary body band.

PRIMARY GLAUCOMA ASSOCIATED WITH SYSTEMIC ABNORMALITIES

Sturge-Weber Syndrome. The Sturge-Weber syndrome is commonly complicated by glaucoma in association with an upper facial nevus flammeus and abnormal vascularity of the leptomeninges. The glaucoma is typically congenital but may be acquired at a later age. The occurrence of glaucoma is unilateral in 90 percent of patients. Abnormal tortuous conjunctival vessels, accompanied by a striking episcleral vascular net, are present circumferentially behind the limbus. The iris stroma may be more pigmented, and corneal changes secondary to glaucoma can be expected. Gonioscopy reveals filtration-angle abnormalities with a variable level of anterior insertion of the iris unaccompanied by a vasculature defect. Funduscopy usually reveals a low choroidal hemangioma. Medical treatment, including acetazolamide, may be helpful. Goniosurgery characteristically fails. A glaucoma implant and cyclodestructive surgery can also be helpful.

Neurofibromatosis. Neurofibromatosis is a common, autosomal dominant, inherited systemic disease. Neurofibromatosis has been subdivided into two types, NF-1 and NF-2. The more common and familial type, NF-1, is characterized by café-au-lait spots, frequent Lisch's nodules on the iris, and less frequent optic nerve glioma and plexiform neurofibroma of the eyelid. Congenital glaucoma is an infrequent occurrence in NF-1 but presents with distinctive abnormalities. It is almost always unilateral and is associated with a plexiform neurofibroma of the upper lid. Enlargement of the eye and cornea are usually striking and are abnormalities that may be seen in this setting even without glaucoma. Inspection of the anterior segment reveals an enlarged cornea, deep anterior chamber, and abnormal iris. Heterochromia may be present, and the pupil reveals an apparent ectropion uveae at its border. This latter defect is frequently progressive during the first 2 yr of life. Lisch's nodules develop less frequently in the eye involved with glaucoma. The lens is typically clear and the choroid is more heavily pigmented than that seen in the contralateral eye. Disc abnormalities secondary to glaucoma, myopia, or both are frequent. Successful glaucoma control is difficult. Goniosurgery is rarely helpful. Filtration surgery, cyclodestructive procedures, or both can be helpful.

Anterior Segment Dysgenesis. Anterior segment dysgenesis is represented by varied malformations of the anterior segment that have been nicely classified by Waring and colleagues.[3] Association with nonocular defects may occur. Isolated thickening and central displacement of Schwalbe's line (posterior embryotoxin) rarely causes a clinical problem. Associated or isolated processes from the peripheral iris to the trabecular meshwork or to a thickened Schwalbe's line (Axenfeld's anomaly) may be associated with glaucoma. When these defects are associated with iris defects (Rieger's anomaly), concern for glaucoma is justifiably increased. When these defects are stable, glaucoma probably occurs in a minority of children. A small percentage of patients with these angle and iris defects at birth show rapid changes during the first 5 to 7 yr of life. In these children, degeneration of the iris is associated with polycoria, corectopia, ectropion uveae, synechial angle closure, and near constant occurrence of glaucoma. This ocular syndrome may occur with and without systemic abnormalities of Rieger's syndrome.

Rieger's syndrome is an familial autosomal dominant disorder that typically reveals the ocular defects described above as Rieger's anomaly, associated with varied systemic abnormalities, including dental defects, ocular hypertelorism, dysplasia of the skull and skeleton, umbilical defects, and occasional endocrine defects (e.g., growth hormone deficiency).[4]

The treatment of childhood glaucoma complicating anterior segment dysgenesis is difficult. In the presence of synechia alone, goniotomy should be tried. Following complete obstruction of the angle, filtration surgery, implant surgery, and cycloablative procedures must be considered following appropriate trial of medical therapy.

PRIMARY GLAUCOMA ASSOCIATED WITH OCULAR ANOMALIES

Aniridia. Aniridia is a complex and poorly understood progressive eye disease with congenital anomalies consisting of small corneas, incomplete to near absence of the iris, frequent small lens opacities, macular hypoplasia, decreased vision, and sensory nystagmus. Congenital and infantile glaucoma are unusual. A variable occurrence of progressive corneal opacification, filtration-angle obstruction and glaucoma, and cataract formation occur in the first 10 to 15 yr of life with aniridia.

Aniridia has been subdivided into four types.[5] The relative risk of glaucoma in each type has not been determined but may be expected in at least 50 percent of patients in type I and much less frequently in type II. In type IV with a recognizable chromosomal defect (11p13), the manifestations of aniridia seem most severe with a high expectation of glaucoma and cataracts even in infancy.[5]

When aniridic glaucoma is congenital or begins in infancy, striking filtration-angle defects are already present. The periphery of the expected stump of iris may appear to insert anteriorly, and even where it is more open, the scleral spur and ciliary body band may be poorly defined. Surprisingly, goniosurgery has been very helpful with these young children but may be less successful when infantile glaucoma and aniridia are associated with a chromosomal defect.

Typically, aniridic glaucoma is acquired, with the progression of abnormal eye pressures occurring by the end of the first decade of life or early teenage years. This occurrence follows the progressive obstruction of the trabecular meshwork in most of these patients. Early in life, gonioscopy reveals a high, vascularized net over the posterior trabecular meshwork that is associated with fine, more posterior attachments to the peripheral iris. With time, the iris seems to be drawn anteriorly over the trabecular tissue, and the anterior net over the trabeculum becomes more homogeneous, with the simultaneous occurrence of glaucoma in most patients. Goniosurgery early in this course to prevent obstruction of the trabecular meshwork has produced promising results (Fig. 221–8).[6]

Treatment of established aniridic glaucoma is difficult. Goniosurgery is rarely helpful. Filtration surgery is highly problematic related to the unprotected lens. The role of implant surgery is not clear. Cycloablative surgery can be helpful. For most patients, medical treatment should be tried before surgery.

Familial Hypoplasia. Familial hypoplasia of the iris is a rare cause of childhood glaucoma. This condition is typically bilateral, inherited by autosomal dominant transmission, and characterized by the occurrence of glaucoma during the first decade of life. The iris stroma is thin, lacks normal crypts, and often appears dark owing to the visibility of the posterior iris pigment epithelium. Gonioscopy usually reveals abnormal tissue over the trabecular band and anterior insertion of the iris. Initial medical treatment is often helpful. Goniotomy is rarely successful. Standard filtration procedures should be helpful for older children and adolescents.

Peters' Anomaly. Peters' anomaly represents another variation of the anterior chamber cleavage syndrome, or anterior segment dysgenesis. The anomaly consists of a central corneal leucoma associated with absence of Descemet's membrane and attachments from the iris to the rim of the annular corneal defect. Corneolenticular attachments may also be present. The corneas are typically small, and this, combined with the corneal opacifications, makes gonioscopy difficult. Glaucoma certainly may complicate Peters' anomaly but occurs in a minority of affected eyes. Most patients do not have associated systemic defects. Familial occurrence is seen more often in siblings than in successive generations. It is usually bilateral and demonstrates a quite variable severity, one eye often being more severely affected.

Posterior Polymorphous Dystrophy. Posterior polymorphous dystrophy is an autosomal dominant familial ocular defect that is bilateral and may be asymptomatic, having very little effect on vision. A more severe expression of this disease is typically characterized by corneal

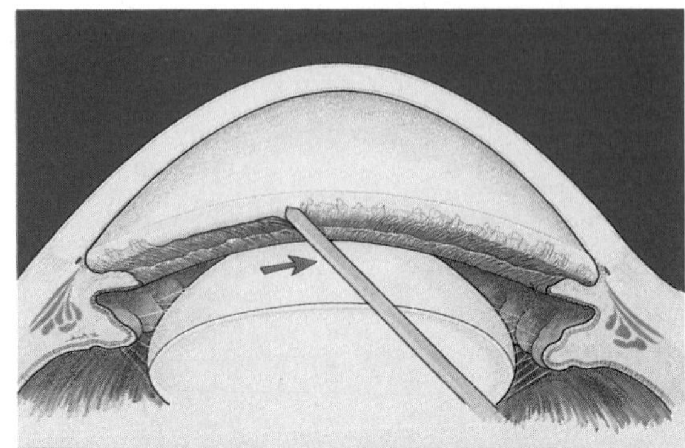

Figure 221–8. In aniridia, goniosurgery early in childhood can interrupt progressive blockage of the trabecular meshwork and may potentially delay or prevent complicating glaucoma.

opacification, with and without glaucoma, in infancy. Diffuse corneal stromal thickening occurs secondary to edema, and diffuse, irregular opacification of Descemet's membrane is seen. The acute onset of light sensitivity may occur without glaucoma. This circumstance strongly mimics the presentation of more common infantile glaucoma and may result in diagnostic uncertainty and unnecessary glaucoma surgery. Treatment of established glaucoma complicating polymorphous dystrophy is difficult. Medical treatment is helpful. Goniotomy surgery remains unproved.

Iridotrabecular Dysgenesis and Ectropion Uveae. Iridotrabecular dysgenesis and ectropion uveae is a cause of childhood unilateral glaucoma, glaucoma typically occurring in the first decade of life. On examination mild ptosis is common, and the anterior segment reveals a large ectropion uveae and an abnormal iris stroma that appears smooth and has been shown to possess a glassy anterior membrane. Gonioscopy reveals a conspicuously abnormal angle with absence of normal landmarks and anterior insertion of this iris. Goniotomy has not been helpful in this condition, but filtration procedures may work well.[7]

Secondary Childhood Glaucoma

Glaucoma may complicate many types of childhood eye diseases. These causes are tabulated in Table 221–1. When faced with a new occurrence of childhood glaucoma, the possibility of a secondary glaucoma must always be considered. Treatment usually involves both management of the glaucoma and treatment of the primary eye disease.

TRAUMA

Trauma to the anterior segment may result in both an immediate and a secondary (delayed) hemorrhage. Glaucoma most frequently complicates a secondary hemorrhage, occurring typically 1 to 4 days after the primary insult. Such patients are frequently treated with head elevation, bedrest, protective dressing, topical steroids, cycloplegics, and aminocaproic acid to lessen the risk of secondary bleeding. Acetylsalicylic acid by mouth may increase this risk and is contraindicated. Although specific components of this care remain controversial, the importance of managing the glaucoma is established. Medical glaucoma treatment utilizing acetazolamide and beta blockers topically and surgery, consisting of anterior chamber irrigation (washout) for persistent high pressure are important options to prevent further ocular damage caused by glaucoma.

The most frequent *neoplastic* cause of glaucoma in childhood is retinoblastoma, secondary to rubeosis or angle closure. Leukemia or lymphoma, as well as other rare ocular tumors (see Table 221–1), may also cause glaucoma early in life (Fig. 221–9).

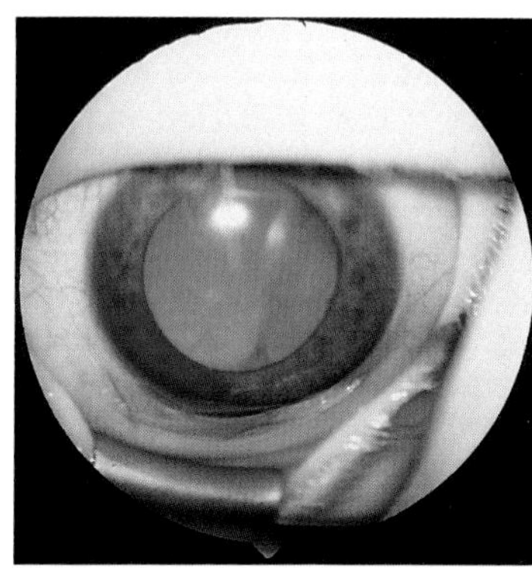

Figure 221–9. In this left eye of a young boy, glaucoma occurred secondary to rubeosis, complicating a cystic medulloepithelioma seen displacing the lens nasally.

JUVENILE XANTHOGRANULOMA

Juvenile xanthogranuloma typically is a skin condition of infancy that may occur infrequently with ocular lesions, alone or in association with the skin defects. The skin lesions consist of firm, yellow-to-orange, superficial nodules with a predilection for the head and upper body. Both skin and ocular lesions consist of a benign histiocytic infiltration. Iris lesions are extremely vascular, and spontaneous hyphemas typically occur with resultant secondary glaucoma. Gonioscopy reveals both blood and loose material from the histiocytic lesion against the filtration surface. Abnormal vessels may also be seen in the angle. Treatment is medical, consisting of acetazolamide and steroids for the histiocytic lesion. If recognized early and treated, involved eyes can usually be saved.

CHRONIC IRIDOCYCLITIS

Chronic iridocyclitis is a more common cause of childhood glaucoma than acute iritis and usually complicates juvenile rheumatoid arthritis or, less commonly, pars planitis. Affected eyes are usually receiving steroids topically, and the potentially adverse effect of this medication on the eye pressure must always be considered. In bilateral cases, the eye more resistant to anti-inflammatory treatment usually shows glaucoma sooner or more severely. This glaucoma is often asymptomatic. Gonioscopy reveals increased opacification of trabecular tissues and iris synechia to the ciliary body band and posterior trabecular meshwork. Continued medical treatment to control the inflammation and diminish further filtration-angle damage is imperative. Medical treatment of this glaucoma with beta blockers and acetazolamide is often helpful. Goniotomy for selected cases with open angles can be extremely helpful.[8]

LENS-INDUCED SECONDARY GLAUCOMA

Lens-induced secondary glaucoma typically occurs acutely, secondary to pupillary block and angle closure caused by the movement of a subluxed lens into the pupillary aperture, blocking the anterior flow of aqueous humor. This glaucoma is acute, painful, and associated with high ocular pressure. Treatment of this unique glaucoma consists of manual displacement of the lens posteriorly if possible, using a muscle hook against the cornea. If the lens is too firmly held in place by the iris, the pupillary block must be broken surgically by carefully drawing the iris to the periphery, using an iris spatula. With manual displacement of the lens behind the iris or after breaking of the pupillary block surgically, the aqueous humor will enter the anterior chamber. In acute cases, the angle will open spontaneously with relief of the glaucoma, but this occurrence must be established by gonioscopy.

GLAUCOMA FOLLOWING PEDIATRIC CATARACT SURGERY

Glaucoma following pediatric cataract surgery may occur shortly after surgery associated with pupillary block, but more typically occurs insidiously 1 to 3 yr following lens removal. Gonioscopy in such cases reveals an open angle with coarse synechia to the trabecular meshwork and forward attachment of the iris to the scleral spur and posterior trabecular meshwork regions. Successful treatment of this glaucoma is difficult. Efforts to prevent it by reducing postoperative inflammation and avoiding further lens surgery by complete lens removal appear to be rewarding.[8]

MISCELLANEOUS CAUSES

Miscellaneous causes of secondary childhood glaucoma are pupillary block glaucoma following retinopathy of prematurity (ROP) and with microphthalmia, glaucoma associated with maternal rubella infection and with carotid sinus fistula, or following topical systemic steroid administration.

Medical Treatment. When medical treatment for a pediatric glaucoma is indicated, miotics, adrenergic agents, and carbonic anhydrase agents may be used. The most effective of these is the carbonic anhydrase inhibitor acetazolamide (Diamox). A dose of 15 mg/kg/day by mouth is usually employed. Infants may experience secondary metabolic acidosis and may require supplementary sodium bicarbonate administration by mouth. A dose of 1 mEq/kg/day has proved helpful. Even when surgery is indicated as the primary treatment, acetazolamide may be helpful in clearing the cornea and controlling the pressure until the procedure is undertaken. The efficacy of β-adrenergic blocking agents is unclear, but they may be helpful, especially for glaucoma in older children.

Surgical Management. The primary objective of glaucoma surgery is to normalize and permanently control the intraocular pressure.

Goniotomy. The introduction of goniotomy by Barkan (1942) for congenital glaucoma represents the most significant single advance that has occurred in the surgical management of this condition.[9, 10] More than 80 percent of children may be cured by this procedure.

For this procedure, a goniotomy knife, operating goniolens, fixation forceps, magnification instrument, and illumination sources are used.

It is important that the angle be studied carefully before a goniotomy operation. This is done during an examination under anesthesia before the surgery. If significant corneal epithelial edema is present, so that the view is obstructed, the epithelium can be removed. When the angle can be viewed in greater detail, the surgery can be done with more confidence.

During the operation, satisfactory illumination can be supplied by a headlight or, alternatively, by an assistant holding a light as close to the surgeon's line of sight as possible. Magnification can be achieved by an operating loupe. An operating microscope may also be used when the cornea is clear.

Fixation of the globe is achieved by the use of locking fixation forceps. Forceps are usually placed on the superior and inferior rectus muscles when the eye is entered from above. The operating goniolens is applied to the cornea following fixation of the globe. The goniotomy knife is entered into the eye through clear cornea adjacent to the limbus and is passed across the anterior chamber to engage the trabecular meshwork in its anterior third. A circumferential cut is then made at approximately 5 hr of the angle circumference (Fig. 221–10). The knife is then withdrawn.

The results of goniotomy surgery are best in those patients with primary congenital open-angle glaucoma who possess a less severe angle anomaly and who are recognized during the first year of life. The results of goniotomy surgery in this group show control of pressure in more than 90 percent of patients. Newborn patients who are found to have glaucoma because of enlarged and cloudy corneas often possess a more severe angle defect and do significantly less well with goniotomy surgery. Patients found to have primary congenital open-angle glaucoma later in childhood also do less well with goniotomy, possibly as a result of damage to the filtration mechanism caused by the chronic elevation of pressure.

Various other procedures, also used in managing adult glaucoma, are utilized in children.

1. Trabeculotomy. The incision of the trabeculum by an external approach.
2. Trabeculectomy. The removal of a section of the trabeculum and adjacent Schlemm's canal.
3. Filtration procedures. The formation of a direct communication between the anterior chamber and subconjunctival space.

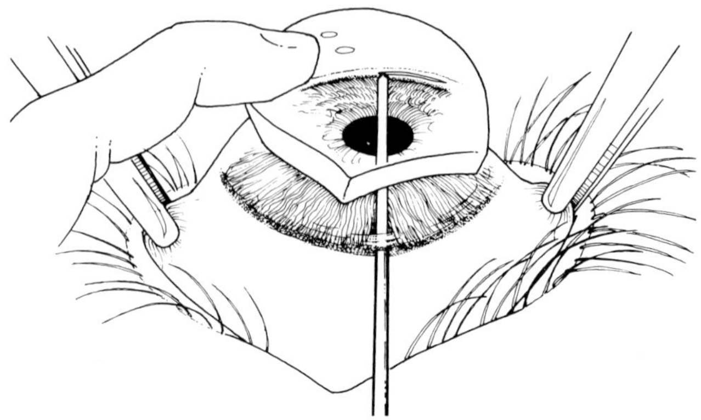

Figure 221–10. For a goniotomy, the knife is entered through the peripheral cornea to incise the midtrabeculum circumferentially.

4. Cyclodestructive treatment. The freezing or laser-induced destruction of the ciliary processes to injure the secretory ciliary epithelium and secondarily to decrease aqueous formation.

5. Implant surgery. The placement of a seton to facilitate drainage from the eye or the use of a drainage tube device, such as a Molteno implant, is representative of this type of glaucoma surgery. The use of the Molteno implant for resistant pediatric glaucoma cases has shown considerable promise but is associated with significant mechanical problems as well as the occurrence of chronic iritis.[11]

REFERENCES

1. Walton DS: Primary congenital open angle glaucoma: a study of the anterior segment abnormalities. Trans Am Ophthalmol Soc 77:746, 1979.
2. deLuise VP, Anderson DR: Primary infantile glaucoma (congenital glaucoma). Surv Ophthalmol 28:1, 1983.
3. Waring GO, Rodrigues MM, Laibson PR: Anterior chamber cleavage syndrome. A stepladder classification. Surv Ophthalmol 20:3, 1975.
4. Shields MB, Buckley E, Klintworth GK, Thresher R: Axenfeld-Rieger syndrome. A spectrum of developmental disorders. Surv Ophthalmol 29:387, 1985.
5. Elsas FJ, Maumenee IH, Kenyon KR, Yoder F: Familial aniridia with preserved ocular function. Am J Ophthalmol 83:718, 1977.
6. Walton DS. Aniridic glaucoma: the results of goniosurgery to prevent and treat this problem. Trans Am Ophthalmol Soc 84:59, 1986.
7. Dowling JL, Albert DM, Nelson LB, Walton DS: Primary glaucoma associated with iridotrabecular dysgenesis and ectropion uveae. Ophthalmology 92:912, 1985.
8. Walton DS. Unpublished personal observations.
9. Barkan O. Operation for congenital glaucoma. Am J Ophthalmol 25:552, 1942.
10. Barkan O: Techniques of goniotomy for congenital glaucoma. Arch Ophthalmol 4:65, 1949.
11. Billson F, Thomas R, Aylward W: The use of two-stage Molteno implants in developmental glaucoma. J Pediatr Ophthalmol Strabismus 26:3, 1989.

Chapter 222

Inherited Metabolic Disease With Pediatric Ocular Manifestations

LOIS HODGSON SMITH

Advances in molecular biology and genetics currently are changing the approach to treating inherited disease. The gene location has been identified in a number of diseases, including retinoblastoma and cystic fibrosis. This knowledge inevitably will lead to ways to identify disease antenatally and to treat it before a pathologic process begins. Therefore, it is important for physicians to identify those inherited diseases that are currently incurable, as well as those few that can be modified or treated, both for genetic counseling and for present and future treatment.

The phrase *inherited metabolic disease* can include almost every disease because all pathologic processes have a metabolic aspect; predisposition to many diseases has a genetic component. However, to be all-inclusive leads to confusion. Metabolic diseases can be grouped (and frequently are) by biochemical defect. However, these groupings are not practical. Therefore, in this chapter, metabolic diseases are grouped by clinical presentation—the way that is most useful to a practicing ophthalmologist.

The ophthalmologist encounters metabolic disease in two main contexts: first, as a consultant to a pediatrician or neurologist who has identified a neurologic deficit or physical finding such as hepatosplenomegaly and, second, as a physician examining a child who presents with abnormal ocular findings and then is found to have other systemic abnormalities.

This chapter is divided into groups of diseases with the following systemic findings: (1) neurologic degeneration of early, middle, and late onset with brief clinical descriptions to aid in diagnosis, (2) skeletal and facial abnormalities, (3) renal dysfunction, and (4) hepatosplenomegaly. It has been my experience that these are the most common physical findings that prompt a request for consultation. This chapter also contains discussions of disease based on the ocular findings. These discussions are not comprehensive but instead describe diseases that are prominently associated with specific ocular findings.

SYSTEMIC FINDINGS IN INHERITED METABOLIC DISEASES WITH PEDIATRIC OCULAR MANIFESTATIONS

Diseases Associated With Early-Onset Neurologic Dysfunction (0 to 12 Mo)

Canavan's Disease (Van Bogaert–Bertrand Disease).[1, 2] In children afflicted with Canavan's disease, or spongy degeneration of the nervous system, the neurologic developmental abnormalities are apparent by 3 mo of age. Clinical and ocular manifestations, including hypotonia and lack of movement, and the consistent findings of optic atrophy, blindness, and megaloencephaly without hydrocephalus occur as a result of demyelination and spongy changes in the cortex, perhaps caused by deficiencies of diphenylnitro-hydroazine and adenosine triphosphatase. Death usually ensues between the ages of 1 and 3 yr.

Farber's Lipogranulomatosis.[1,3] This autosomal recessive inherited disease, caused by ceramidase deficiency, is characterized by generalized swelling and infiltration of the joints and subcutaneous tissue by histiocytic granulomas, leading to severe arthropathy and a hoarse cry, severe malnutrition, severe psychomotor deterioration, and frequent febrile episodes. Ocular findings include grayness of the macula. Diffuse, fine pigmentary changes in the fundus have been reported but are not a prominent feature. Some cases of this disease are protracted and more benign. In the infantile form, onset is apparent during the first few weeks of life, and death usually occurs by 2 yr of age.

Gaucher's Disease (Type II, Infantile).[4,5] In children with Gaucher's disease (glucosylceramide lipidosis), caused by glucosylceramide-β-glucosidase (glucocerebrosidase) deficiency, psychomotor deterioration becomes apparent before 6 mo of age. The child presents with splenomegaly. Spasticity and dysphagia are characteristic, as is retroflexion of the neck. Gaucher's cells (histiocytes) are found in the bone marrow. Ocular manifestations include oculomotor paralysis and gaze palsies. The fundus appearance is normal. Death occurs before 2 yr of age.

GM_1 Gangliosidosis Type I.[6,7] This autosomal recessive inherited disorder of generalized gangliosidosis is caused by galactosidase deficiency. The defect has been localized to chromosome 3 (3p12–3p13). The onset, usually noted within the first few days of life, is characterized by severe progressive cerebral degeneration, dysmorphic facies, skeletal changes (Hurler-like), and hepatomegaly. A macular cherry-red spot is evident in 50 percent of cases, but its appearance may be delayed until 6 mo of age. Blindness and deafness occur later in the disease, prior to death before 2 yr of age.

GM_2 Gangliosidosis Type II: Tay-Sachs Disease.[6–9] Like GM_1 gangliosidosis, GM_2 gangliosidosis (Fig. 222–1) is also an autosomal recessive inherited trait. The disorder is caused by a deficiency of hexosaminidase A and has been localized to chromosome 15 (15q22–15q25.1). The patient presents with psychomotor deterioration beginning between 4 and 6 mo of age and visual loss starting as early as 4 mo of age. An abnormal acousticomotor reaction is a very early and characteristic

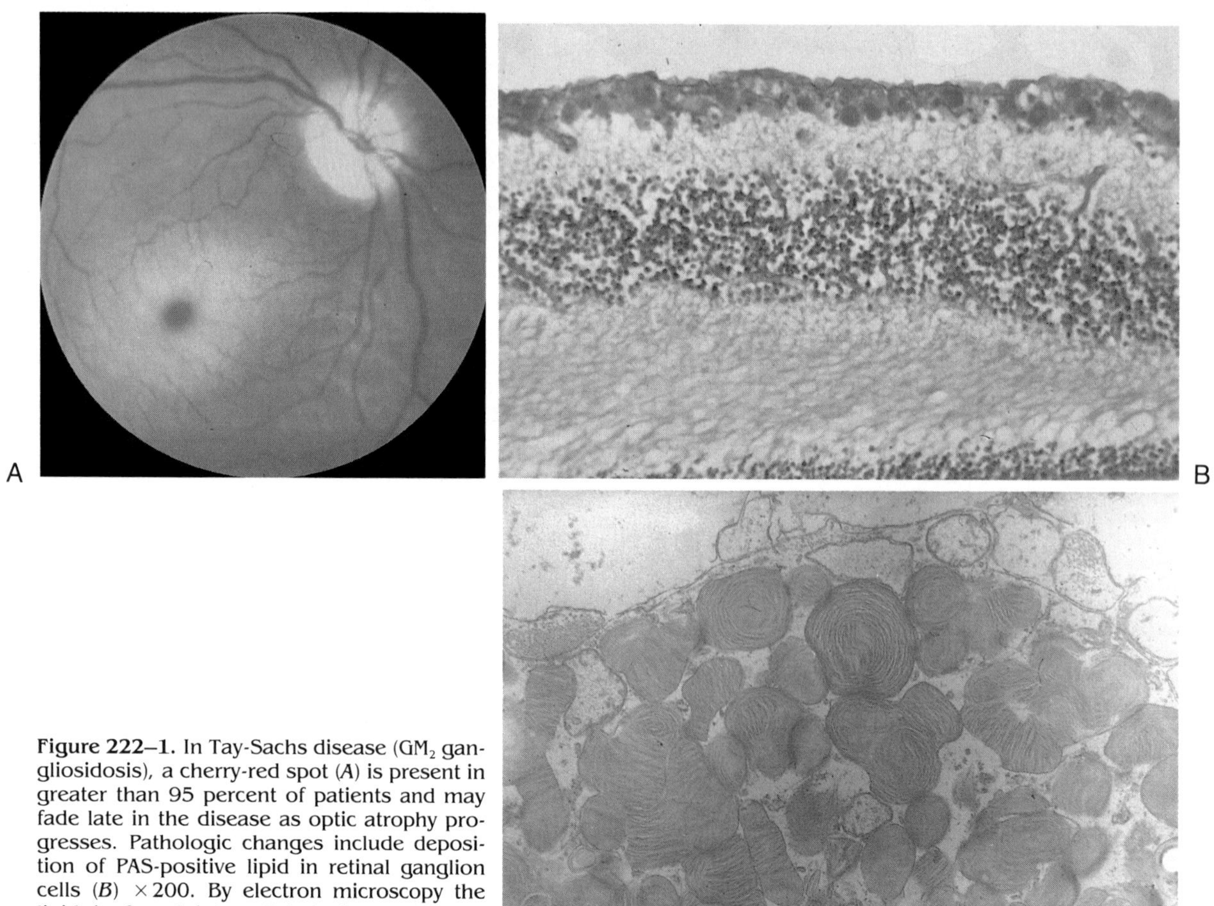

Figure 222–1. In Tay-Sachs disease (GM_2 gangliosidosis), a cherry-red spot (*A*) is present in greater than 95 percent of patients and may fade late in the disease as optic atrophy progresses. Pathologic changes include deposition of PAS-positive lipid in retinal ganglion cells (*B*) ×200. By electron microscopy the lipid is found intracellularly in membrane-bound lamellar inclusions (*C*) ×14,000.

sign of this disease. Hypotonia is a prominent feature. Ocular manifestations include a macular cherry-red spot (noted as early as 3 mo after birth) and late optic atrophy. Death occurs between the ages of 3 and 5 yr.

GM_2 Gangliosidosis Type II: Sandoff's Disease.[6, 7, 10] This disorder is clinically the same as Tay-Sachs disease, with variable hepatosplenomegaly. It is caused by a deficiency of hexosaminidases A and B, and the defect is localized to chromosome 5 (5q13). The macular cherry-red spot is a constant finding.

Krabbe's Infantile Leukodystrophy.[1, 11] The onset of this disease (before age 6 mo) is characterized by irritability. This autosomal recessive inherited disorder is caused by a deficiency of β-galactosidase. The child suffers late tonic spasms, spastic paralysis, seizures, and a rapid course of central nervous system deterioration, including optic atrophy with blindness and deafness. Autopsy reveals loss of myelin in the central nervous system with globoid cells in the area of demyelination. Death usually occurs between 1 and 2 yr of age.

Leigh's Disease.[1] This subacute necrotizing encephalomyelopathy is an autosomal recessive inherited disorder, with onset in the first 6 mo of life. It is caused by a deficiency of pyruvate carboxylase. Psychomotor regression usually appears during the first 6-mo period but may occur later (up to the second or third year of life). Intermittent abnormal respiratory rhythm is a constant and characteristic sign. The course of the disease is variable, and there are exacerbations with fever. Oculomotor and other cranial nerve palsies are characteristic, as are supranuclear gaze palsies, optic atrophy, and blindness. Death occurs between 2 and 10 yr of age. Autopsy reveals multifocal areas of spongy degeneration of the brainstem, spinal cord, and basal ganglia.

Lowe's Syndrome (Oculocerebral Syndrome).[12–15] This X-linked recessive inherited disorder (Fig. 222–2) is characterized by severe psychomotor retardation, hypotonia, and loss of deep tendon reflexes. The onset is apparent by age 6 mo. The characteristic appearance includes a prominent forehead, recessed globes, and flaring ears. Renal abnormalities are a prominent feature, with rickets, proteinuria, and renal tubular acidosis. Ocular findings include a very high incidence of congenital cataracts with small, thin lenses and glaucoma and miosis with poor pupillary dilatation.

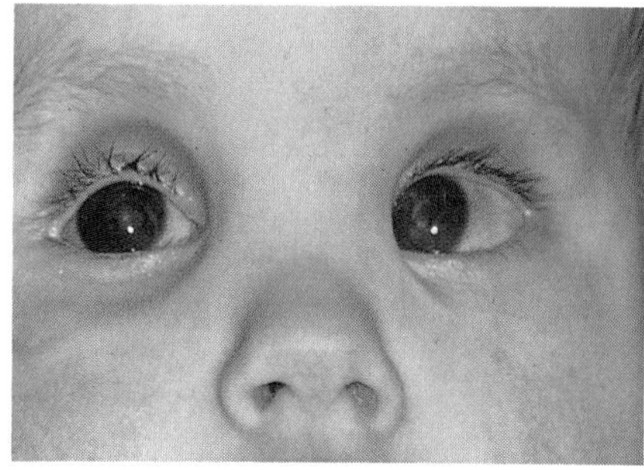

Figure 222–2. The oculocerebrorenal syndrome of Lowe is inherited in an X-linked manner. Affected males have cataracts, glaucoma, nystagmus, psychomotor retardation, aminoaciduria, and acidosis.

Niemann-Pick Disease (Infantile, Type A).[16–20] This autosomal recessive inherited disease (Fig. 222–3), characterized by progressive psychomotor deterioration, is caused by a deficiency of sphingomyelinase. Onset is between 6 mo and 1 yr of age. The patient presents with hepatomegaly and failure to thrive. Subtle corneal and lens opacities can be found. A macular cherry-red spot is characteristic in all cases in the early to middle stages of this disease. Death occurs between ages 2 and 3 yrs.

Pelizaeus-Merzbacher Disease.[1, 21] This disease, also called sudanophilic leukodystrophy, is an X-linked recessive disease. During the first month of the infant's life, irregular pendular nystagmus and head shaking become apparent. Choreiform movement of the arms appears later. Mental deterioration occurs only in the terminal stages of the disease. The most characteristic ocular finding is optic atrophy. Death occurs between ages 5 and 7 yr. Autopsy reveals patchy demyelination.

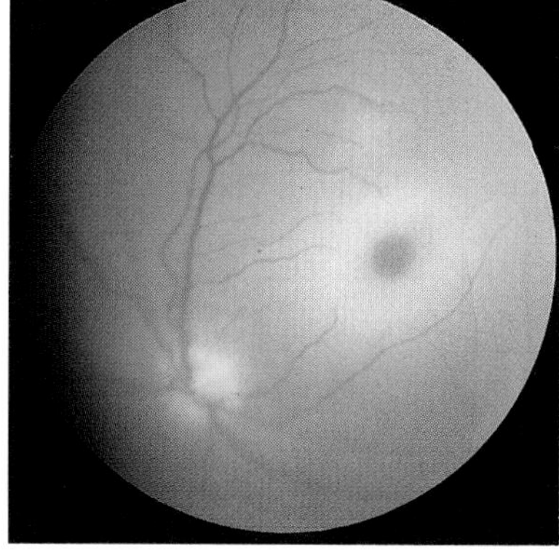

A

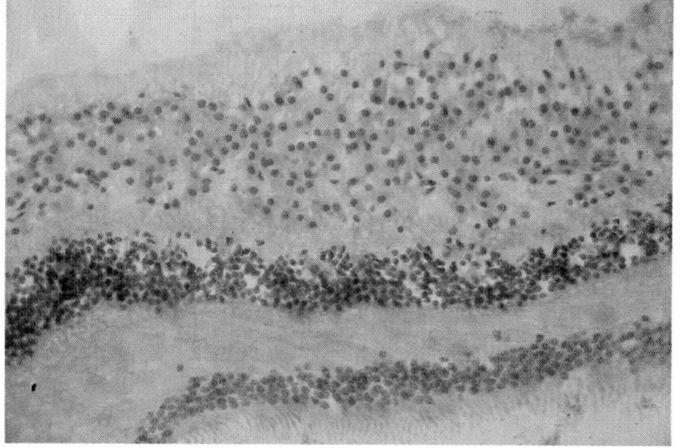

B

Figure 222–3. Niemann-Pick disease (type A or infantile form) is rapidly fatal with progressive loss of developmental milestones. A macular cherry-red spot (*A*) is characteristic, as are large, foamy, lipid-laden retinal ganglion cells (*B*) stained here with oil red O. ×250.

Zellweger's Cerebrohepatorenal Syndrome.[1, 12, 15, 19, 20, 22] This autosomal recessive inherited peroxisomal disorder (Fig. 222–4) is apparent at birth. The course of the disease is rapidly progressive, and death occurs within a few months. Severe hypotonia, lack of psychomotor development, abnormal facies, a high narrow forehead, wideset eyes, shallow supraorbital ridges, hepatomegaly and hepatic dysfunction, patellar calcifications, cerebral dysplasia, and cortical cyst of the kidneys are characteristic. Cataracts are present in 20 percent of cases, and glaucoma is present in 30 percent. Other findings include corneal opacities, retinal degeneration, and optic atrophy. Death usually occurs by 6 mo of age.

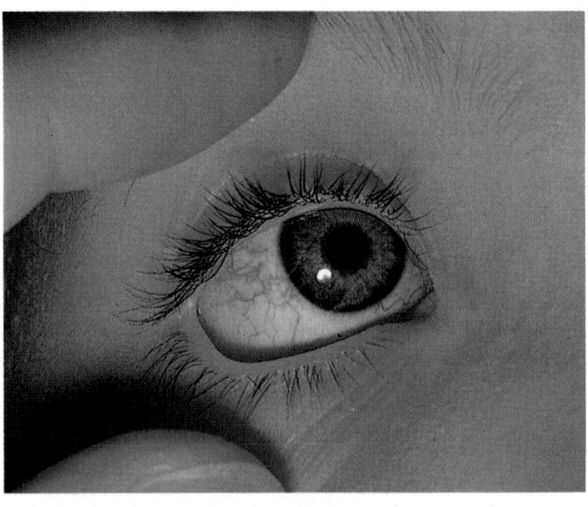

Figure 222–5. Ataxia-telangiectasia is a disease of abnormal DNA repair culminating in lymphatic malignancy. Tortuous conjunctival vessels are characteristic.

Diseases Associated With Middle-Onset Neurologic Dysfunction (1 to 4 Yr)

Ataxia-Telangectasia (Louis-Bar Syndrome).[23, 24] This autosomal recessive inherited neurologic disorder with onset in late infancy (Fig. 222–5) is characterized by severe progressive motor dysfunction, with ataxia, recurrent respiratory infections, and slow mental deterioration. Immunologic abnormalities include hypoplasia of the lymph nodes, tonsils, and adenoids. Oculomotor apraxia and incomplete convergence are seen in this disorder. Conjunctival telangectasia can occur between the ages of 4 and 6 yr. Death occurs during the second decade of life.

Cockayne's Syndrome.[1, 25] At birth, the infant with the autosomal recessive inherited trait appears to be normal in weight and length. The characteristics of dwarfism begin to appear during the second or third year of life. Progressive encephalopathy ensues; photosensitive dermatitis is a prominent feature. Characteristic facial features include sunken eyes, loss of subcutaneous fat, and microcephaly. Ocular findings include prominent retinal degeneration with extinction of the electroretinogram signal, late blindness, and cataracts. Nerve deafness is invariable. Death occurs in the second to third decade of life.

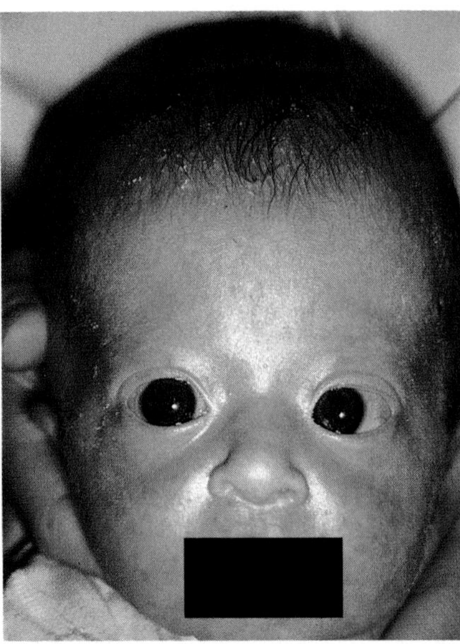

Figure 222–4. The facial features of cerebrohepatorenal syndrome (Zellweger's syndrome) include a long narrow head, a high forehead, and shallow supraorbital ridges.

Fucosidosis.[26] Signs of this autosomal recessive inherited disease, which is caused by a lysosomal α-fucosidase deficiency, appear during the first to third years of life. The defect has been localized to chromosome 1. Characteristics include psychomotor retardation and seizures, Hurler-like facial and skeletal changes, and angiokeratomas similar to those in Fabry's disease type 3 (with onset between the first and eighth years of life). Conjunctival and retinal vascular tortuosity is similar to that in Fabry's disease; diffuse corneal opacities are common.

Galactosemia.[27, 28] This disease is an autosomal recessive inherited disorder of galactose metabolism caused by a deficiency of the enzyme galactose-1-phosphate-uridyl transferase. It is characterized by vomiting and diarrhea in the newborn, as well as failure to thrive; hepatic dysfunction; mild mental retardation; and galactosuria. This defect has been localized to chromosome 9 (9p12–9p13). Placing the mother on a galactose-free diet, particularly during pregnancy, may prevent mental retardation. "Oil-drop" cataracts appear during the first year of life.

I-Cell Disease (Mucolipidosis Type II).[2, 13, 19, 24, 29] This autosomal recessive inherited disease, caused by the failure of acid hydrolase to be incorporated into the lysosomes, is characterized by early onset (during the first year of life) of rapidly progressive psychomotor retardation in a patient with a Hurler-like phenotype. In addition, the patient exhibits progressive facial and skeletal dysmorphism and prominent gingival hyperplasia. The funduscopic examination is normal; mild corneal opacification occurs late in the disease. Death usually occurs between 2 and 8 yr of life.

Mannosidosis.[13, 24, 30] A deficiency of lysosomal α-mannosidase is responsible for this autosomal recessive inherited disorder, which has been localized to chromosome 19 (19p–19q13). During the second or third year of life, the child begins to show signs of mental retardation. Gingival hyperplasia, recurrent respiratory infections, and mild Hurler-like facial and skeletal dysmorphism are other signs. Cataracts with spokelike posterior cortical opacification are common.

Metachromatic Leukodystrophy.[1, 31–33] This is an autosomal recessive inherited disorder caused by a deficiency of arylsulfatase A. Onset is usually characterized by difficulty walking at age 18 mo to 3 yr, progressing to dysarthria and dementia. Ocular findings are a slight perifoveal gray haze, simulating a cherry-red spot, and optic atrophy with resultant late blindness. Death occurs during the first decade of life.

Mucopolysaccharidosis Type I-H (Hurler's Syndrome).[5, 34–37] In this autosomal recessive inherited disorder (Fig. 222–6), caused by a deficiency of α-L-iduronidase, the child appears to be normal at birth but signs of progressive facial and skeletal dysmorphism and dwarfism become apparent starting in the first few months of life. Other characteristics include loss of developmental milestones, progressing to severe mental retardation, hepatosplenomegaly, hydrocephalus, and cardiac dysfunction. Progressive corneal clouding is an early and constant finding. Late pigmentary degeneration of the retina and optic atrophy may be seen. Death usually occurs by age 10 yr.

Mucopolysaccharidosis Type II (Hunter's Syndrome).[34–38] Progressive skeletal and facial dysplasia with dwarfism and stiff joints, as well as mild mental retardation, characterize this X-linked recessive inherited disease caused by a deficiency of iduronate sulfatase. The defect has been localized to the X chromosome (Xq26–27). Progressive deafness and hydrocephalus are common findings, with hepatosplenomegaly a constant finding. Cardiomyopathy can occur. Ocular features include some reports of cloudy corneas in later adulthood and possible pigmentary retinal degeneration. Death usually occurs between adolescence and adulthood.

Mucopolysaccharidosis Type III (Sanfilippo's Disease).[34–37] This disease is an autosomal recessive inherited disorder. Type A is caused by a heparan sulfatase deficiency; type B results from *N*-acetyl-αD-glucosaminidase deficiency. Characteristically, this is primarily a neurologic disease, with early marked mental deterioration starting at age 18 mo. There are minimal skeletal and facial abnormalities, but hepatomegaly is often present. The patient's corneas usually remain clear; however, retinal degeneration and optic atrophy may occur.

Mucopolysaccharidosis Type VII (Sly's Disease).[34–37] Another autosomal recessive inherited disease, mucopolysaccharidosis type VII is caused by a deficiency of β-glucuronidase and is characterized by hepatosplenomegaly, mental retardation, dystosis multiplex, and cloudy corneas.

Mucosulfatidosis.[1, 13] This disorder is similar to metachromatic leukodystrophy but also possesses features of the mucopolysaccharidoses. Multiple sulfatase deficiencies have been found responsible for this autosomal recessive inherited disorder. Onset is between 12 and 18 mo of life, with the child exhibiting difficulty walking. In addition, the patient has mild Hurler-like facial and skeletal abnormalities and hepatomegaly. Ichthyosis is present from the time of birth. Corneal opacities are lacking, but late optic atrophy and deafness develop. Quadriplegia and severe mental retardation ensue, and death occurs between the ages of 3 and 12 yr.

Mucolipidosis Type IV.[39] This is an autosomal recessive inherited disease in which psychomotor regression becomes apparent during the first year of life. There are no facial or skeletal changes. Cloudy corneas secondary to epithelial opacities are apparent during the first year of life.

Neuronal Ceroid Lipofuscinosis.[1, 40–42] This disease (Fig. 222–7) has three variants, all of which are autosomal recessive inherited traits: (1) polyunsaturated fatty acid lipidosis (infantile form, or Hagberg-Santavuori disease), (2) Batten-Bielschowsky-Jansky disease (late infantile form), and (3) Spielmeyer-Vogt disease (juvenile form).

Polyunsaturated fatty acid lipidosis has its onset at 12 to 18 mo of age, with rapid psychomotor deterioration and ataxia. By age 3 yr, the patient is unresponsive and has undergone decortication. Ocular manifestations include rapid loss of the electroretinogram and electroencephalogram signals. Retinal degeneration with narrowing of retinal vessels and late optic atrophy are apparent.

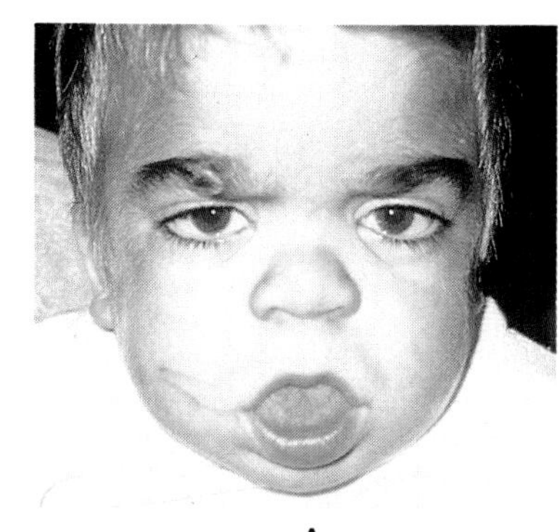

A

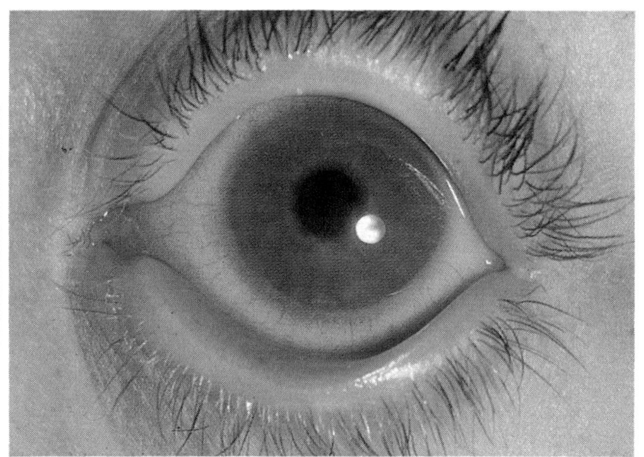

B

Figure 222–6. Hurler's syndrome (MPS I-H, or iduronidase deficiency, Hurler type) is the prototype of mucopolysaccharidoses. Patients are clinically normal at birth and deteriorate progressively, with dwarfism, coarse facial features (*A*), hepatosplenomegaly, mental retardation, stiff joints, and corneal clouding (*B*) increasing until death.

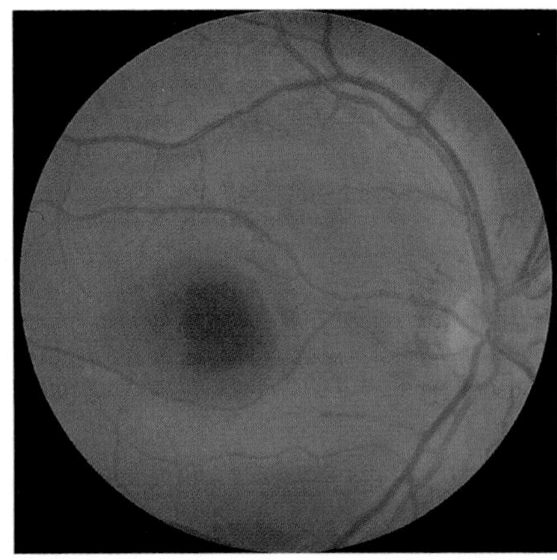

Figure 222–7. Batten's disease may have pigmentary macular changes as illustrated. These are different from a cherry-red spot because there is no gross deposition of lipid in the ganglion cells. The electroretinogram response is severely attenuated in Batten's disease.

Batten-Bielschowsky-Jansky disease has its onset at 2 to 4 yr of age with seizures followed by mental deterioration. As with polyunsaturated fatty acid lipidosis, the following are evident: retinal degeneration with narrowed retinal vessels and pigmentary changes, loss of the electroretinogram signal, and late optic atrophy.

Spielmeyer-Vogt disease has its onset between ages 5 and 12 yr with macular degeneration and a reduction in visual acuity. Seizures occur and are followed by psychomotor deterioration.

Niemann-Pick Variants.[16–18] These disorders are characterized by early hepatosplenomegaly. Neurologic degeneration occurs later, between the ages of 2 and 8 yr. The patient also suffers progressive dementia and cerebellar ataxia. Fundus examination is normal. Other ocular findings include supranuclear paralysis of the vertical gaze (often the presenting complaint is the inability to see low-placed objects), and oculogyric crisis.

Sialidosis (Goldberg's Syndrome). Caused by α-neuraminidase deficiency, this disease has a heterogeneous clinical picture. Early nonprogressive mental retardation becomes manifested by age 5 yr. Myoclonus and ataxia become apparent in early to late childhood. The macular cherry-red spot is a prominent feature in all cases. Corneal opacities are present but are seen only on slit-lamp examination.

Sulfite Oxidase Deficiency.[43] This autosomal recessive inherited disease is extremely rare. It is characterized by severe mental retardation and seizures, choreoathetosis, and early ectopia lentis.

Diseases Associated With Late-Onset Childhood Progressive Neurologic Disease (4 to 15 yr)

Abetalipoproteinemia (Bassen-Kornzweig Syndrome).[44] This autosomal recessive inherited disorder usually presents with ataxia and a neurologic syndrome similar to that in Friedreich's ataxia, with the following characteristics: low plasma cholesterol and triglyceride levels; lack of low-density lipoproteins, very low-density lipoproteins, and chylomicrons; intestinal fat malabsorption with poor absorption of vitamins A and E; and acanthocytosis and anemia. Onset occurs between the ages of 5 and 15 yr with ataxia, steatorrhea, hepatomegaly, and psychomotor retardation. Retinitis pigmentosa in adolescence is a prominent feature. The patient's dark adaptation may be restored with vitamin A supplementation.

Adrenoleukodystrophy.[1] This X-linked recessive inherited peroxisomal disorder of demyelinating brain lesions begins between the ages of 5 and 15 yr. The defect has been localized to the X chromosome in the glucose-6-phosphate dehydrogenase cluster. It is characterized by behavioral changes, hemiplegia, adrenal insufficiency secondary to adrenal atrophy, central deafness, optic atrophy, and central blindness and, frequently, homonymous hemianopia. The disease usually runs a 3- to 5-yr course before death occurs.

Fabry's Disease (Ceramide Trihexoside and Dihexoside Lipidosis).[45–48] Fabry's disease (Fig. 222–8) results from a deficiency of α-galactosidase A. Onset of this X-linked recessive inherited disease begins in early childhood to adolescence. The defect is localized to chromosome Xq22–24. Heterozygous females are mildly affected systemically, but all have subepithelial corneal

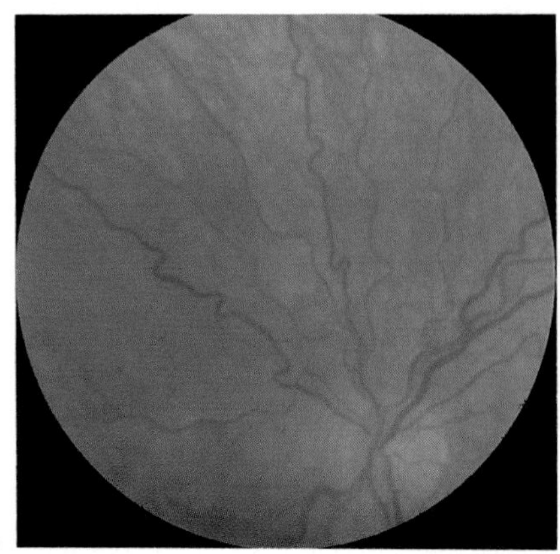

A

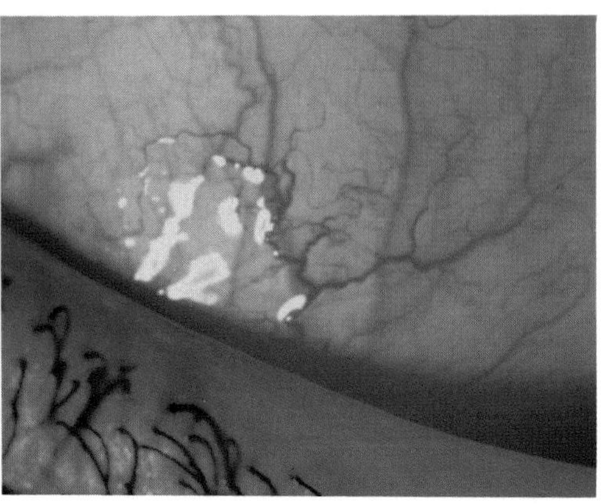

B

Figure 222–8. Galactosidase A deficiency or Farber's disease leads to systemic deposition of glycosphingolipids in viscera and in vascular endothelium. This results in pain in the extremities and vascular ectasia (angiokeratomas), as well as vascular tortuosity in retina (*A*) and conjunctiva (*B*). Subtle corneal opacities occur in a whorl pattern, and spokelike posterior lens opacities are characteristic.

changes. Affected males exhibit sausage-like tortuous vascular lesions in the conjunctiva and retina, corneal whorl-like opacities, posterior spokelike lens opacity or "Fabry cataract," angiokeratomas in "bathing suit distribution," recurrent burning pain in the extremities, and renal failure and stroke.

Friedreich's Ataxia.[1, 49] This autosomal recessive inherited disorder is caused by a disturbance of pyruvate metabolism, with onset between 10 and 20 yr of age. Characteristics include cerebellar ataxia, no tendon reflexes, and scoliosis. Ocular manifestations include vestibular nystagmus, variable optic atrophy and retinitis pigmentosa, and vertical gaze paresis. Cardiomyopathy is a prominent feature and is often the cause of death, which occurs during the third to fourth decades of life.

Neuronal Ceroid Lipofuscinosis (Spielmeyer-Vogt Disease).[1, 40, 41] Onset is between 5 and 10 yr of age. This autosomal recessive inherited disease is characterized by slow intellectual deterioration, myoclonic seizures, and dysartharia. Ocular signs include retinal degeneration, with loss of the electroretinogram signal progressing to total blindness, and gray macula. Death occurs after the patient has had the disease for 10 to 15 yr.

Refsum's Disease.[50] This autosomal recessive inherited disease is caused by a deficiency of phytanic acid hydroxylase. It is characterized by the onset of progressive polyneuropathy and may run a course marked by relapses and remissions in adolescence. Other features include elevated phytanic acid levels in the serum and urine, neurosensory deafness, retinal degeneration, and loss of vision. Night blindness may be a presenting complaint. The patient maintains normal intelligence.

Tangier Disease.[51] This disease is characterized by a deficiency of high-density lipoproteins in the plasma and low plasma cholesterol levels. The patient has normal intelligence. Other findings are cholesterol ester deposits in the tissue, yellow-orange tonsils, polyneuropathy (may be loss of pain fibers only), and fine dotted corneal stromal opacities seen only on slit-lamp examination. Normal vision is maintained.

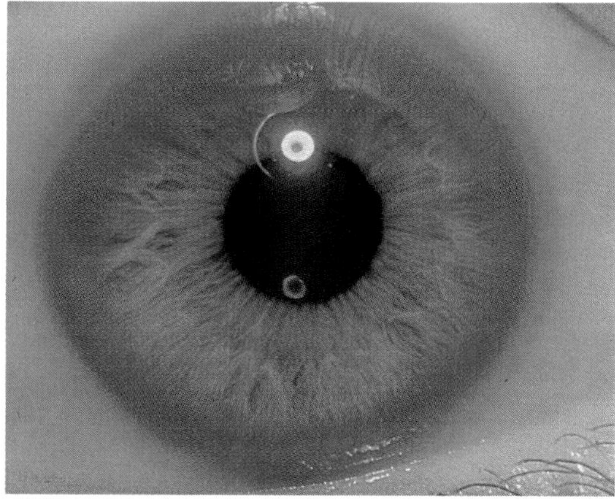

Figure 222–9. In Wilson's disease, abnormal copper metabolism results in accumulation of copper in the liver and other tissues. The copper deposition in Descemet's membrane in the peripheral cornea results in the classic Kayser-Fleischer ring, seen most densely at the upper and lower poles.

Wilson's Disease.[52–58] In this autosomal recessive inherited process (Fig. 222–9), the liver is the first organ affected, with resultant hepatic dysfunction and cirrhosis. Onset is during the second decade of life. Generalized rigidity and intention tremor are present if the disease goes untreated. Other findings include low serum ceruloplasmin levels, low serum copper levels, and high tissue copper levels. An early ocular manifestation is the Kayser-Fleischer ring in Descemet's membrane (generally considered pathognomonic). This ring is reversible when the patient is treated with penicillamine, a copper chelator. In addition, sunflower cataract is present in 20 percent of patients.

Other juvenile forms of Sandhoff's disease, Gaucher's disease, mucolipidosis type I, Krabbe's disease, Leigh's disease, and sulfatidosis may present in late childhood.

Inherited Metabolic Disease With Ocular Manifestations and Prominent Skeletal Changes and Facial Deformities

Diseases Causing Psychomotor Retardation. The ocular changes in the following inherited metabolic diseases have been discussed elsewhere in this chapter. In addition, there are prominent skeletal and facial changes. Patients with *Austin's disease*,[24] caused by multiple sulfatase deficiencies, exhibit mild Hurler-like skeletal changes and minimal Hurler-like facies. *Cockayne's syndrome*[25] is characterized by progressive dwarfism, a wizened appearance, microcephaly, thin atrophic skin, a prominent nose, and a sunken appearance of the eyes. *Fabry's disease*,[45–47] trihexoside and dihexoside ceramide lipidosis, results in arthritis of the distal interphalangeal joints and necrosis of the femoral heads. *Farber's lipogranulomatosis*[3] is characterized by granulomatous arthropathy of the limbs and larynx and juxtaarticular bone destruction. *Fucosidosis*[26, 59] causes minimal or marked Hurler-like skeletal changes and facies. *GM_1 gangliosidosis type I*,[6] generalized gangiosidosis (infantile), causes minimal Hurler-like skeletal changes and facies. *Homocystinuria*[60–63] is characterized by growth retardation, vertebral osteoporosis, radial and ulnar epiphyseal calcifications, and fractures. *I-cell disease*,[29] mucolipidosis type II, results in marked Hurler-like skeletal changes and facies.

Renal rickets with bone demineralization, a prominent forehead, recessed eyes, and large flaring ears are all signs of *Lowe's (oculocerebrorenal) syndrome* (see Fig. 222–2).[14] *Mannosidosis*[30] is characterized by minimal Hurler-like skeletal changes and facies. *Mucopolysaccharidosis type I-H*[35] (Hurler's disease) (see Fig. 222–6) results in dwarfism, claw-shaped hands, stubby fingers, chest deformity, kyphosis, and the characteristic coarse facial features, hirsutism, large skull, shallow orbits, and synostosis of the cranial sutures. *Mucopolysaccharidosis type II*[37] (Hunter's disease) is characterized by moderate Hurler-like skeletal and facial changes.

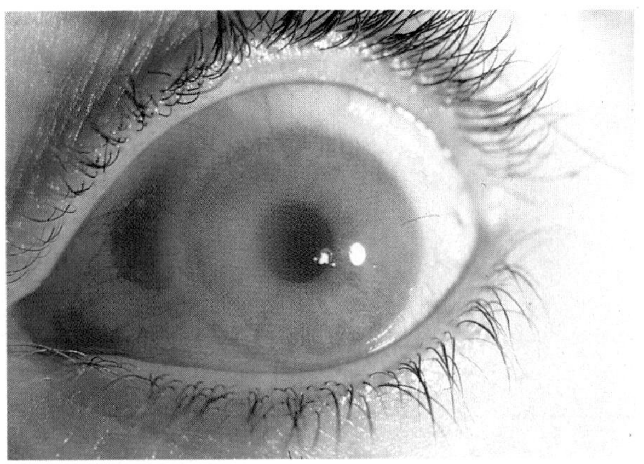

Figure 222–10. Scheie's syndrome (MPS I-S) is characterized by severe corneal clouding but normal intelligence and stature (unlike Hurler's syndrome, despite the same deficiency of α-iduronidase).

Mucopolysaccharidosis type III[37] (Sanfilippo's disease) causes very mild Hurler-like changes on x-ray film; vertebrae, femoral head, and acetabulum are abnormal. Minimal Hurler-like facies are also characteristic. *Pseudo-Hurler polydystrophy*,[64] mucolipidosis type III, results in short stature (Morquio-like). *Sialidosis*, mucolipidosis type I, exhibits inconsistent Hurler-like skeletal and facial changes. *Wilson's disease*[52–57] (Fig. 222–9) produces spontaneous fractures and arthropathy. *Zellweger's (cerebrohepatorenal) syndrome*[24] (see Fig. 222–4) is characterized by flexion contracture of the joints, patellar calcifications, and growth retardation. Facial characteristics include a high narrow forehead and flat supraorbital ridges.

Diseases in Which the Patient Has Normal Intelligence. *Conradi's syndrome*[15, 24] is characterized by stippled epiphyses and cataracts. In *mucopolysaccharidosis type I-S*[12, 24, 34] (Scheie's syndrome) (Fig. 222–10), the patient has mild skeletal abnormalities—i.e., mild Hurler's dysplasia, with stiff joints as a prominent feature. The facial changes are mild and Hurler-like. *Mucopolysaccharidosis type IV*[12, 24, 34] (Morquio's syndrome) (Fig. 222–11) is characterized by skeletal abnormalities, predominantly hypoplasia of the odontoid and compression of the spinal cord and roots. Minimal facial changes are seen. *Mucopolysaccharidosis type VI*[12, 24, 34] (Maroteaux-Lamy syndrome) (Fig. 222–12) is characterized by moderate skeletal dysplasia like Hurler's syndrome and marked Hurler-like facies. *Refsum's disease*,[50] a phytanic acid storage disorder, results in short metacarpal and metatarsal bones and epiphyseal dysplasia.

Table 222–1. INHERITED METABOLIC DISEASE WITH OCULAR MANIFESTATIONS AND WITH NEPHROPATHY AS A PROMINENT FEATURE

Disease	Cardinal Renal Features
Cystinosis (infantile)[64, 65]	Renal tubular acidosis
Fabry's disease[45–47]	Severe renal insufficiency, hypertension
Lowe's syndrome[14]	Tubular acidosis, aminoaciduria, proteinuria, rickets
Wilson's disease[52–57]	Nonspecific aminoaciduria, hematuria
Zellweger's syndrome[66]	Cystic dysplasia of kidneys, proteinuria

Inherited Metabolic Diseases With Ocular Manifestations and Nephropathy or Hepatomegaly-Splenomegaly As a Prominent Feature

These disorders are presented in tabular form in Tables 222–1 and 222–2.

OCULAR FINDINGS IN INHERITED METABOLIC DISEASES

Diseases Associated With Prominent Corneal Abnormalities

Disorders of Amino Acid Metabolism. *Alkaptonuria*,[67] an autosomal recessive inherited disorder caused by homogentisic acid oxidase deficiency, is manifested by spinal arthritis, darkening of the standing urine (early sign), and pigmentation in the interpalpebral fissure. *Cystinosis*,[64] a lysosomal storage disorder (Fig. 222–13)

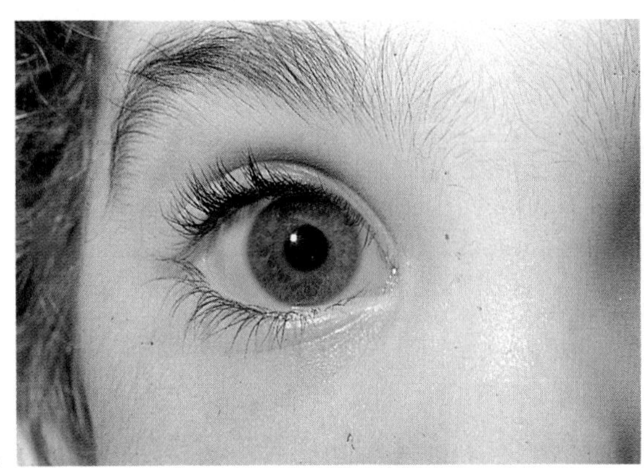

A

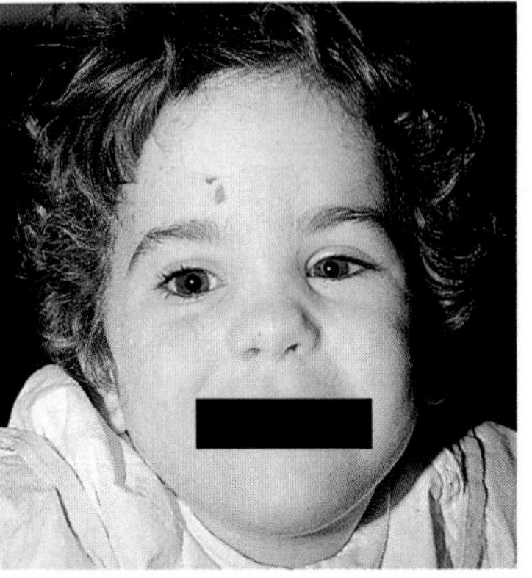

B

Figure 222–11. Morquio's syndrome (MPS IV) results from galactosamine-6-sulfate sulfatase deficiency (MPS IV-A) or β-galactosidase deficiency (MPS IV-B). The most prominent features are severe skeletal dysplasia, progressive deafness, mild late corneal clouding (*A*), and normal intelligence (*B*).

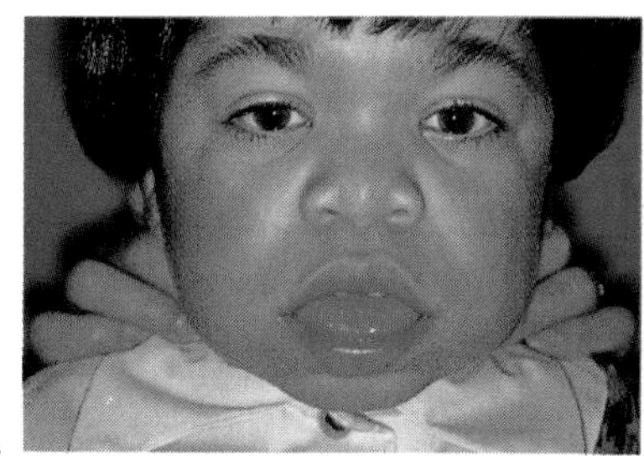
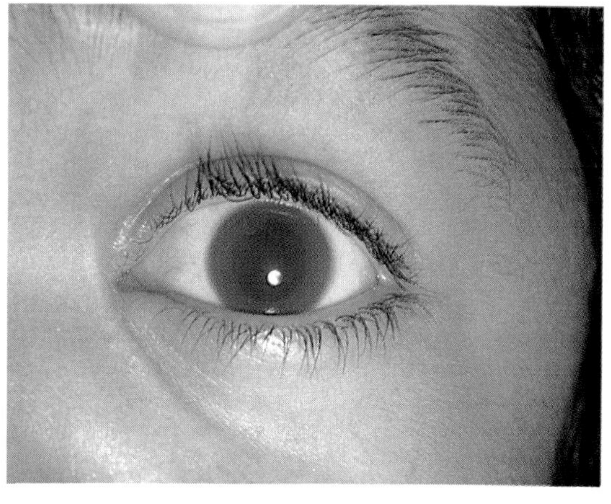

Figure 222–12. MPS VI or Maroteaux-Lamy syndrome is characterized by progressive dwarfism, coarse facial features (*A*), severe corneal clouding (*B*), and normal intelligence. It is a result of *N*-acetylgalactosamine-4-sulfatase (arylsulfatase B) deficiency.

marked by low plasma and high lysosomal cystine levels, is an autosomal recessive inherited disease with the following manifestations in its infantile form: severe renal tubular acidosis, rickets, short stature, hypopigmentation of the skin and hair, a consistent early finding of fine cystine crystals in the corneal stroma, and peripheral retinopathy in infants. *Familial dysautonomia* (Riley-Day syndrome),[68] an autosomal recessive inherited disorder caused by dopamine β-hydroxylase deficiency, has the following signs and symptoms: scoliosis, lack of lingual fungiform papillae, insensitivity to pain, emotional lability, cold hands and feet, vasomotor instability, recurrent gastrointestinal symptoms, impaired swallowing, lack of tearing, and corneal hypoesthesia with secondary ulcers. Patients with *Wilson's disease*,[52–57] an autosomal recessive inherited disorder (see Fig. 222–9) resulting in elevated tissue copper levels, show progressive liver disease and neurologic impairment presenting in adolescence. Ocular signs are the early appearance of the Kayser-Fleischer ring in the peripheral Descemet's membrane and sunflower cataracts in 20 percent of patients. Serum analysis shows low serum ceruloplasmin levels. Early treatment with penicillamine to promote elimination of tissue copper prevents and reverses the pathologic condition.

Disorders of Carbohydrate Metabolism (Mucopolysaccharidoses).[2, 19, 24, 34–37] *Mucopolysaccharidosis type I-H* (Hurler's syndrome) is an autosomal recessive inherited disorder caused by a deficiency of α-L-iduronidase. This disease is a prototype of the mucopolysaccharidoses. The infant appears normal at birth but exhibits severe, rapidly progressive skeletal dysplasia, hepatomegaly, cardiovascular disease, facial dysmorphism, and mental retardation. Death occurs by age 10 yr. Early progressive corneal clouding is evident in all cases. Late retinitis pigmentosa and optic atropy may be present. *Mucopolysaccharidosis type I-S* (Scheie's syndrome), like mucopolysaccharidosis type I-H, is also an autosomal recessive inherited disease caused by the same enzymatic defect as in Hurler's syndrome. However, the patient achieves normal stature and intelligence levels. Facies also are normal. Corneal clouding is a severe early ocular manifestation. *Mucopolysaccharidosis type IV* (Morquio's syndrome) is a disorder of marked skeletal abnormalities and characteristic facies with moderate and late corneal clouding. Mucopolysaccharidosis type IV is an autosomal recessive inherited

Table 222–2. INHERITED METABOLIC DISEASES WITH OCULAR MANIFESTATIONS AND HEPATOMEGALY AND/OR SPLENOMEGALY[1, 12, 15, 24]

Ceramide lactoside lipidosis
Chédiak-Higashi disease
Farber's disease
Fucosidosis
Galactosemia
Gaucher's disease—late infantile and juvenile
GM_1 gangliosidosis
Mucolipidosis II
Mucopolysaccharidoses I, II, III
Niemann-Pick disease
Tangier disease
Wilson's disease
Zellweger's syndrome

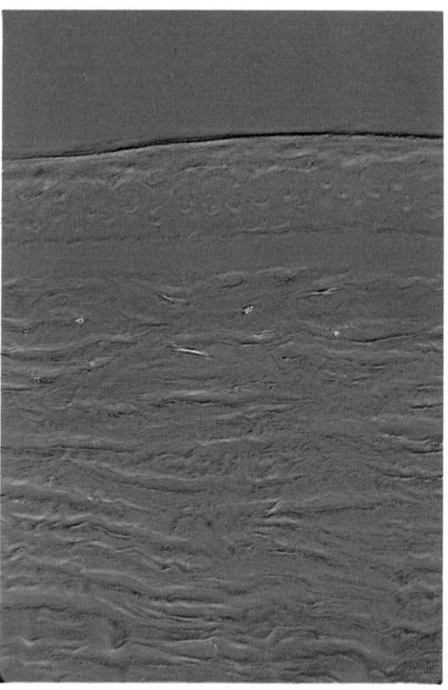

Figure 222–13. Birefringent crystals in cornea of patient with cystinosis. Findings are fair skin, small stature, and renal disease.

disorder that results from a deficiency of *N*-acetylgalactosamine 6-sulfate sulfatase. Intelligence levels are normal. In *mucopolysaccharidosis type VI* (Maroteaux-Lamy syndrome), the patient exhibits marked skeletal dysplasia, facial dysmorphism, and marked corneal opacification. This autosomal recessive inherited disorder results from a deficiency of aryl sulfatase B. The patient's intelligence is normal. *Mucopolysaccharidosis type VII* (Sly's syndrome) is an extremely rare autosomal recessive inherited disorder caused by a deficiency of β-glucuronidase. Skeletal dysplasia, mental retardation, and corneal clouding are reported findings.

Disorders of Lipid Metabolism. *Fabry's disease*[1, 2, 19, 24, 45–47, 51, 69, 70–81] is an X-linked recessive inherited disease (see Fig. 222–8) caused by a deficiency of ceramide α-trihexosidase. In males, there is burning pain in the extremities, progressive renal failure, hypertension, and stroke. Angiokeratoma corporis diffusum is seen in males in the bathing suit area. Carrier females and males have a subepithelial whorl pattern in the cornea and posterior spokelike cataracts. *Familial hyperlipoproteinemia* is an autosomal recessive inherited disorder. There are five distinct genetic types (I to V), all of which include elevated plasma lipid levels and can be distinguished by levels of chylomicrons, low-density lipoproteins, very low density lipoproteins, triglycerides, and cholesterol. Patients with types II and III may exhibit presenile corneal arcus during the first to third decades of life. Atherosclerotic heart disease is a common finding. Lipemia retinalis and xanthomas may be present. *Familial plasma cholesterol ester deficiency*, also an autosomal recessive inherited disorder, is caused by a deficiency of lecithin-cholesterol acyltransferase. Findings include high plasma lecithin and cholesterol levels, anemia, renal failure, and atherosclerotic vascular disease. In the eyes, corneal arcus and diffuse corneal opacities are present in all patients during the first decade of life. *Fish-eye disease* is an autosomal dominant disorder characterized by increasing corneal opacification in the second decade of life, normal high-density lipoprotein and normal lecithin-cholesterol acyltransferase levels, and elevated triglyceride levels. *Tangier disease*, with low plasma levels of high-density lipoprotein, is an autosomal recessive inherited trait characterized by low plasma and cholesterol levels, hepatosplenomegaly, hyperplastic orange tonsils, decreased high-density lipoprotein, hypercholesterolemias, and mild progressive corneal opacifications.

Disorders Affecting Both Lipid and Carbohydrate Metabolism.[2, 6, 19, 24, 29, 39, 82, 83] *GM_1 gangliosidosis type I* (generalized gangliosidosis, infantile type) is an autosomal recessive inherited disorder that has been localized to chromosome 3 (3p12–3q13). The following manifestations of the disease result from a lysosomal β-galactosidase deficiency: psychomotor retardation, hepatosplenomegaly, Hurler-like facies and skeletal abnormalities, a macular cherry-red spot, and corneal clouding in 50 percent of patients. Death occurs by age 2 yr. *I-cell disease* (mucolipidosis type II) is an autosomal recessive inherited disorder caused by the failure of acid hydrolase to be incorporated into the lysosomes. It is characterized by Hurler-like facies, psychomotor retardation, and mild corneal opacification. *Pseudo-Hurler polydystrophy* (mucolipidosis type III) is an autosomal recessive inherited trait that results from acid hydrolase occurring extracellularly, not in the lysosomes. This disorder is similar to Maroteaux-Lamy disease clinically. It is characterized by stiff joints, coarse facial features, and skeletal abnormalities. Peripheral corneal clouding by the first decade of life is a constant feature.

Tables 222–3 through 222–6 present metabolic diseases associated with prominent lenticular, retinal, and oculomotor abnormalities.

TREATABLE METABOLIC DISEASES

Abetalipoproteinemia.[44, 101, 102, 104] This disorder is characterized by steatorrhea, ataxia, retinitis pigmentosa, lack of β-lipoproteinemia in the serum, and low serum levels of cholesterol, triglycerides, carotene, and vitamins A and E. Treatment with vitamins A and E may improve dark adaptation but may not affect other aspects of retinitis pigmentosa.

Cystinosis.[64, 105, 106] The infantile form of this disorder (see Fig. 222–13) is characterized by short stature, fair complexion, rickets, and renal tubular acidosis. Other manifestations include cystine crystals in the corneal stroma, iris, and conjunctiva. Treatment consists of

A 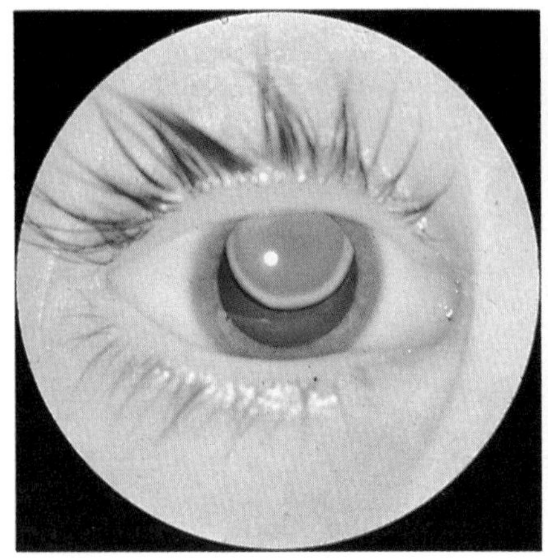

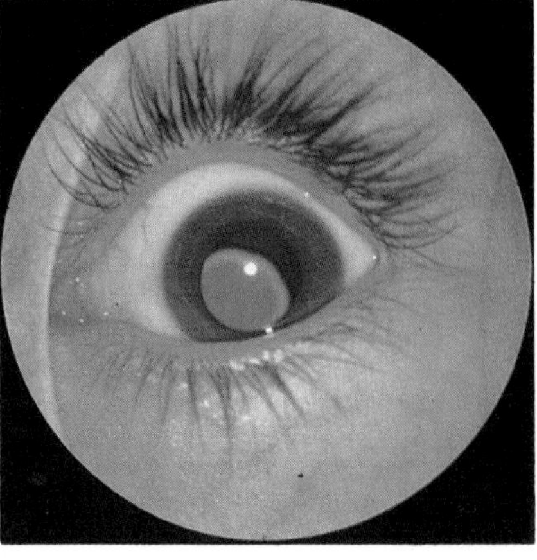 B

Figure 222–14. Ectopia lentis with superior displacement is more characteristic of Marfan's syndrome, which is also associated with arachnodactyly, cardiac abnormalities, and high myopia (*A*). Ectopia lentis with inferior displacement is more characteristic of homocystinuria (*B*).

Table 222–3. DISEASES ASSOCIATED WITH PROMINENT LENS ABNORMALITIES

Disease	Findings
Cataracts[84]	
Chromosomal disorders[85–87]	
Trisomy 13	Severe systemic abnormalities with cleft lip and palate; ocular malformation is prominent with microphthalmia, atypical colobomas and frequent cataracts
Trisomy 18	Failure to thrive; malformation of face and eyes with variable lens malformation
Trisomy 21	Acquired snowflake cataracts by second decade; other lens opacities can present at birth or in childhood
Abnormal carbohydrate metabolism[19, 24, 88]	
Diabetes mellitus	
Galactosemia	Mild mental retardation, failure to thrive, hepatosplenomegaly, "oil drop" cataracts in first year of life that may be reversible with early galactose restriction
Galactokinase deficiency	Congenital or infantile cataract only; no significant systemic manifestations
Hypoglycemia	Can be secondary to renal or hepatic diseases or other diseases such as Toni-Fanconi syndrome, hyperinsulinemia, and so on
Lysosomal storage disorders[30, 46, 47] (see Fig. 222–8)	
Fabry's disease	Angiokeratomas, tortuous retinal and conjunctival vessels; spokelike cataract in posterior cortex in both carrier females and homozygous males as well as whorl-like corneal opacity
Mannosidosis	Resembles Hurler's syndrome clinically; but also spokelike cataract in posterior cortex similar to that in Fabry's disease
Other inherited diseases with frequent cataract and unspecified metabolic deficit[14]	
Alport's syndrome	Congenital or early-onset (anterior lenticonus) cataracts; hemorrhagic nephritis; hearing loss
Conradi's syndrome	Stippled epiphyses and frequent cataracts
Lowe's syndrome	Congenital malformation of eye with congenital cataracts and infantile glaucoma; aminoaciduria, acidosis; severe psychomotor retardation (see Fig. 222–2)
Sjögren's syndrome	Ataxia; psychomotor regression; sometimes gaze and central nervous system palsies; progressive cataract onset at 2 to 3 yr of age
Zellweger's syndrome (peroxisomal disorder)	Congenital cataract, optic nerve hypoplasia, glaucoma, renal dysfunction
Lens dislocation[43, 60, 89–91] (Fig. 222–14)	
Homocystinuria	Mild mental retardation; homocystine in urine, positive nitroprusside test; thrombotic vascular occlusions; may be pyridoxine-responsive; lens dislocation in 90% (usually inferonasal)
Hyperlysinemia	Extremely rare; elevated plasma levels of lysine, questionable association with ectopia lentis
Marfan's syndrome	Aortic dilatation; aneurysms and floppy mitral valve; ectopia lentis in 50–80%, usually superotemporal; high myopia; arachnodactyly
Sulfite oxidase deficiency	Extremely rare disease; mental retardation and ectopia lentis
Weill-Marchesani syndrome	Short stature, short fingers, microspherophakia, and dislocated lens

Table 222–4. DISEASES ASSOCIATED WITH PROMINENT MACULAR CHANGES

Disease	Findings
Cherry-red spot in macula (Figs. 222–1 and 222–3)	
GM_1 gangliosidosis type I (generalized gangliosidosis)	Macular cherry-red spot in about 50% of cases; death by 2 yr of age
GM_2 gangliosidosis type II: Tay-Sachs disease	Cherry-red spot in 100% of cases; occurs early (usually within 3 mo)
GM_2 gangliosidosis type II: Sandhoff's disease	Cherry-red spot in most if not all cases; occurs early
Metachromatic leukodystrophy	Cherry-red spot occasionally reported; early death
Sphingomyelin-cholesterol lipidosis type A (infantile Niemann-Pick disease)	Cherry-red spot in all cases; death by 2 yr of age
Sialidosis (mucolipidosis type I)	Cherry-red spot in 100% of cases but later onset; Goldberg's syndrome is phenotypically the same
Other macular lesions	
Adult Niemann-Pick disease	Ring of perifoveal crystalloid deposits has been described
Farber's lipogranulomatosis (ceramide lipidosis)	Gray opacity in perifoveal area
Neuronal ceroid lipofuscinosis	Four clinical phenotypes; grayish pigmentary changes in macula are common; also progressive neurologic deterioration with seizures and loss of electroretinogram signal
Fucosidosis	A bull's-eye macular lesion has been reported
Lactosyl ceramidosis	One case reported with cherry-red spot
Sea blue histiocyte syndrome	One report of macular ring of granules
Von Gierke's disease	Yellow paramacular lesions

Table 222–5. DISEASES ASSOCIATED WITH RETINAL DEGENERATION—PIGMENTARY CHANGES*

Lipid-lipoprotein disorders
- Abetalipoproteinemia (Bassen-Kornzweig syndrome)
- Refsum's disease

Mucopolysaccharidoses
- Mucopolysaccharidosis type I-H (Hurler's syndrome)
- Mucopolysaccharidosis type I-S (Scheie's syndrome)
- Mucopolysaccharidosis type II (Hunter's syndrome)
- Mucopolysaccharidosis type III (Sanfilippo's disease)

Amino acid disorders
- Cystinosis
- Hyperornithinemia (gyrate atrophy)
- α-Amino butyric aciduria

Lysosomal enzyme disorders
- Neuronal ceroid lipofuscinosis
- Batten-Bielschowsky-Jansky disease
- Polyunsaturated fatty acid lipidosis or Hagberg-Santavuori disease
- Spielmeyer-Vogt disease

Other diseases with prominent retinal degeneration or retinal pigmentary changes
- Aicardi's syndrome
- Cockayne's syndrome
- Hallervorden-Spatz syndrome
- Hoof's syndrome
- Lawrence-Moon-Biedl syndrome
- Oxalosis
- Sjögren-Larsson syndrome
- Usher's syndrome

*See references 1, 2, 12, 19, 24, 34 to 37, 50, 64, 65, 94 to 100.

renal transplantation and oral and topical cystamine administration. The former corrects uremia, and the latter decreases the corneal crystals.

Familial Hyperlipoproteinemia, Types I to V. The five types of this disorder vary, but common signs and symptoms include atherosclerotic heart disease, xanthoma, pancreatitis, and abdominal pain. Ocular findings are lipemia retinalis and corneal arcus. Treatment includes institution of a low-fat diet and administration of nicotinic acid, clofibrate, and cholestyramine. Treatment, which varies with each type, may prevent and reverse vascular disease.

Galactokinase Deficiency. Treatment of this disorder consists of a galactose-free diet. Systemic findings of galactosemia are lacking. Cataracts are the only ocular finding that may be reversed with early treatment.

Galactosemia.[107, 108] This disorder, which is characterized by mental retardation, hepatosplenomegaly, and "oil drop" cataracts, is treated with a galactose-free diet—Nutraminagen, ProSobee. Galactose restriction early in pregnancy and infancy may reverse early cataracts and reduce the severity of central nervous system findings.

Gaucher's Disease (Infantile).[5, 109] Treatment consists of replacement of the deficient enzyme and bone marrow transplantation. Unpublished reports suggest successful prevention of the progression of symptoms.

Gyrate Atrophy.[110–112] Patients with this disorder present with retinal and choroidal atrophy. Treatment includes administration of pyridoxine (vitamin B_6) and a diet low in arginine. Treatment with pyridoxine improves ornithine excretion in the urine and may improve retinal function.

Homocystinuria.[104, 105, 113–115] Thromboembolism is the presenting sign. Mental retardation is another manifestation. A diet low in methionine and administration of pyridoxine (vitamin B_6) and vitamin B_{12} constitute the treatment of choice. Treatment with pyridoxine partially reverses homocystinuria in some cases.

Mucopolysaccharidosis Type I-H (Hurler's Disease).[5, 116, 117] Bone marrow transplantation may prevent some aspects of deterioration. No long-term follow-up data are currently available (see Fig. 222–6).

Refsum's Disease.[118–120] The patient presents with ataxia, peripheral neuropathy, and retinitis pigmentosa. Deafness is another sign. A diet restricting phytanic intake lowers phytanic acidemia and lessens the neurologic symptoms.

Tyrosinosis.[121] This disorder, characterized by renal tubular acidosis, corneal ulcers and cataracts, responds to a diet low in phenylalanine and tyrosine. As a result, renal function improves and corneal ulcers heal.

Wilson's Disease.[58, 122–126] The onset of this disease (see Fig. 222–9) begins in late childhood with liver dysfunction and neurologic degeneration, including tremors and ataxia. Other findings are low serum copper and high tissue copper levels, low serum ceruloplasmin levels, sunflower cataracts, and a Kayser-Fleischer ring in Descemet's membrane in the cornea. Treatment

Table 222–6. DISEASES ASSOCIATED WITH PROMINENT AND CHARACTERISTIC ABNORMALITIES OF OCULAR MOVEMENT[1, 12, 24]*

Disease	Findings
Abetalipoproteinemia	Supranuclear paralysis of lateral or vertical gaze
Ataxia-telangiectasia	Oculomotor apraxia; incomplete convergence
Friedreich's ataxia	Supranuclear paralysis of lateral or vertical gaze and vestibular nystagmus
Infantile Gaucher's disease	Nuclear ophthalmoplegia
Juvenile Gaucher's disease	Lateral gaze paralysis (supranuclear)
Kearns-Sayre disease	Progressive external ophthalmoplegia
Krabbe's disease	Sensory nystagmus may be seen before any other ocular findings
Leigh's disease	Supranuclear paralysis of lateral or vertical gaze; nuclear ophthalmoplegia and vestibular nystagmus
Metachromatic leukodystrophy	Sensory nystagmus may be seen before any other ocular findings
Late infantile or juvenile Niemann-Pick disease (neurovisceral storage disease with supranuclear vertical ophthalmoplegia)	Supranuclear paralysis of vertical gaze; often complaints of inability to see low-placed objects; oculogyric crises can occur
Pelizaeus-Merzbacher disease	Sensory nystagmus may be seen before any other ocular findings, with characteristic "eye rolling"

*Not included are metabolic ocular diseases with strabismus or nystagmus because these are often nonspecific findings.

includes D-penicillamine, zinc, and adherence to a diet low in copper. D-Penicillamine chelates copper in the tissue, prevents central nervous system symptoms, clears the Kayser-Fleischer ring, and improves tremor and mentation.

REFERENCES

1. Adams RD, Lyon G (eds): Neurology of Heritable Metabolic Diseases of Children. New York, McGraw-Hill, 1982.
2. Hogan GR, Richardson EP: Spongy degeneration of the nervous system (Canavan's disease). Report of a case in an Irish-American family. Pediatrics 35:284, 1965.
3. Cogan DG, Kuwabara T, Moser H, Hazard GW: Retinopathy in a case of Farber's lipogranulomatosis. Arch Ophthalmol 75:752, 1966.
4. Petrohelos M, Tricoulis D, Kotsiras I, Vouzoukos A: Ocular manifestations of Gaucher's disease. Am J Ophthalmol 80:1006, 1975.
5. Schaison G, Bordigoni P, Leverger G: Bone marrow transplantation for genetic and metabolic disorders. Nouv Rev Fr Hematol 31:119, 1989.
6. O'Brien JS: Five gangliosidoses. Lancet 2:805, 1969.
7. Godtfredsen E: New aspects of the classification and pathogenesis of lipidoses with neuro-ophthalmological manifestations. Acta Ophthalmol 49:489, 1971.
8. Brady RO: Tay-Sachs disease. N Engl J Med 281:1243, 1969.
9. Cotlier E: Tay-Sach's retina. Arch Ophthalmol 86:352, 1971.
10. Bronstein S, Carpenter S, Polomeno RC, Little JM: Sandhoff's disease (GM_2 gangliosidosis type II). Histopathology and ultrastructure of the eye. Arch Ophthalmol 98:1089, 1980.
11. Brownstein S, Meagher-Villemure K, Polomeno RC, Little JM: Optic nerve in globoid leukodystrophy (Krabbe's disease). Arch Ophthalmol 96:864, 1978.
12. Graymore CN, Hsia DY-Y: Inborn errors of metabolism affecting the eye. *In* Graymore CN (ed): Biochemistry of the Eye. London, Academic Press, 1970.
13. Goldberg MF (ed): Genetic and Metabolic Eye Disease. Boston, Little, Brown, 1986.
14. Curtin VT, Joyce EE, Ballin N: Ocular pathology in the oculocerebrorenal syndrome of Lowe. Am J Ophthalmol 64:533, 1967.
15. Duke-Elder S: Congenital deformities. *In* Duke-Elder S (ed): System of Ophthalmology, vol. 2. Part 2. St. Louis, CV Mosby, 1963.
16. Howes EL, Wood IS, Golbus M, Hogan ML: Ocular pathology of infantile Niemann-Pick disease. Arch Ophthalmol 93:494, 1975.
17. Libert J, Toussaint D, Guiselings R: Ocular findings in Niemann-Pick disease. Am J Ophthalmol 80:991, 1975.
18. Walton DS, Robb RM, Crocker AC: Ocular manifestations of Group A Niemann-Pick disease. Am J Ophthalmol 85:174, 1978.
19. Renic WA (ed): Goldberg's Genetic and Metabolic Eye Disease. Boston, Little, Brown, 1986.
20. Bondy PK (ed): Duncan's Diseases of Metabolism, 6th ed, vol. 1. Philadelphia, WB Saunders, 1969.
21. Rahn EK, Yanoff M, Tucker S: Neuroocular considerations in the Pelizaeus-Merzbacher syndrome. A clinicopathologic study. Am J Ophthalmol 66:1143, 1968.
22. Folz S-J, Trobe J-D: The peroxisome and the eye. Surv Ophthalmology 35:353, 1991.
23. Harley RD, Baird HW, Craven EM: Ataxia-telangiectasia. Arch Ophthalmol 77:582, 1967.
24. Punnet HH, Harley RD: Genetics in pediatric ophthalmology. *In* Harley RD (ed): Pediatric Ophthalmology. Philadelphia, WB Saunders, 1983, pp 28–80.
25. Coles WH: Ocular manifestations of Cockayne's syndrome. Am J Ophthalmol 67:762, 1969.
26. Snodgrass MB: Ocular findings in a case of fucosidosis. Br J Ophthalmol 60:508, 1976.
27. Benson PF, Brown SP, Cree J, et al: Phenotypic expression of galactokinase deficiency in heterozygous and homozygous subjects: In vivo and in vitro studies. *In* Bergsma D, Bron AJ, Cotlier E (eds): The Eye and Inborn Errors of Metabolism. New York, Alan R Liss, 1976, p 305.
28. Wilson WA, Donnell GN, Bergren WR: The dietary prophylaxis of cataracts in patients with galactosemia. *In* Bergsma D, Bron AJ, Cotlier E (eds): The Eye and Inborn Errors of Metabolism. New York, Alan R Liss, 1976, p 313.
29. Libert J, van Hoof F, Farriaux JP, Toussaint D: Ocular findings in I-cell disease (mucolipidosis type II). Am J Ophthalmol 83:617, 1977.
30. Arbisser AI, Murphree AL, Garcia CA, Howell R: Ocular findings in mannosidosis. Am J Ophthalmol 82:465, 1976.
31. Cogan DG, Kuwabara T, Moser H: Metachromatic leukodystrophy. Ophthalmologica 160:2, 1970.
32. Cogan DG, Kuwabara T, Richardson EP, Lyon G: Histochemistry of the eye in metachromatic leukoencephalopathy. Arch Ophthalmol 60:397, 1958.
33. Moser HW, Lees M: Sulfatide lipidosis: Metachromatic leukodystrophy. *In* Stanbury JB, Wyngaarden JB, Frederickson DS (eds): The Metabolic Basis of Inherited Disease, 2nd ed. New York, McGraw-Hill, 1966, pp 539–564.
34. Constantopoulos G, Dekabian AS, Sheie HG: Heterogeneity of disorders in patients with corneal clouding, normal intellect and mucopolysaccharidosis. Am J Ophthalmol 72:1106, 1971.
35. Gillis JP, Hobson R, Hanley B, McKusick VA: Electroretinography and fundus oculi findings in Hurler's disease and allied mucopolysaccharidosis. Arch Ophthalmol 74:596, 1965.
36. Goldberg MF, Maumanee AE, McKusick VA: Corneal dystrophies associated with abnormalities of mucopolysaccharide metabolism. Arch Ophthalmol 74:516, 1965.
37. McKusick VA: Heritable Disorders of Connective Tissue, 3rd ed. St Louis, CV Mosby, 1966, p 389.
38. Roberts SH, Upadhyaya M, Sararazi M, Harper PS: Further evidence localizing the gene for Hunter's syndrome to the distal region of the X chromosome long arm. J Med Genet 26:309, 1989.
39. Merin S, Livni N, Berman ER, Yatziv S: Mucolipidosis IV: Ocular, systemic and ultrastructural findings. Invest Ophthalmol 14:437, 1975.
40. Beckerman BL, Rapin I: Ceroid lipofuscinosis. Am J Ophthalmol 80:73, 1975.
41. Hittner HM, Zeller RS: Ceroid lipofuscinosis (Batten disease). Arch Ophthalmol 93:178, 1975.
42. Zeman W: Batten disease: Ocular features, differential diagnosis and diagnosis by enzyme analysis. *In* Bergsma D, Bron AJ, Cotlier E (eds): The Eye and Inborn Errors of Metabolism. New York, Alan R Liss, 1976, p 441.
43. Mudd SH, Irreverre F, Laster L: Sulfite oxidase deficiency in man: Demonstration of the enzymatic defect. Science 156:1599, 1967.
44. Bergsma D, Bron AJ, Cotlier E (eds): The Eye and Inborn Errors of Metabolism. New York, Alan R Liss, 1976, pp 385–399.
45. Christensen L, Heidensleben E, Larsen HW: The value of ocular findings in the diagnosis of angiokeratoma corporis diffusum (Fabry's disease). Acta Ophthalmol 48:1185, 1970.
46. Franceschetti AT: Fabry disease: Ocular manifestations. *In* Bergsma D, Bron AJ, Cotlier E (eds): The Eye and Inborn Errors of Metabolism. New York, Alan R Liss, 1976, p 195.
47. Spaeth GL, Frost P: Fabry's disease. Its ocular manifestations. Arch Ophthalmol 74:760, 1965.
48. Bishop DF, Calhoun DH, Bernstein HS, et al: Human-galactoside A: Nucleotide sequence of a cDNA clone encoding the mature enzyme. Proc Natl Acad Sci USA 83:4859, 1986.
49. Duke-Elder S, Scott GI: Neuroophthalmology. *In* Duke-Elder S (ed): System of Ophthalmology, vol. 12. St. Louis, CV Mosby, 1971, p 789.
50. Hansen E, Bachen NI, Flage T: Refsum's disease. Eye manifestations in a patient treated with low phytol, low phytanic acid diet. Acta Ophthalmol 57:899, 1979.
51. Clifton-Bligh P, Nestel PJ, Whyte HM: Tangier disease: Report of a case and studies of lipid metabolism. N Engl J Med 286:567, 1972.
52. Cairns JE, Williams HP, Walshe JM: "Sunflower cataract" in Wilson's disease. Br J Med 3:95, 1969.
53. Cartwright GE: Current concepts: The diagnosis of treatable Wilson's disease. N Engl J Med 298:1347, 1978.

54. Dingle J, Havener WH: Ophthalmoscopic changes in a patient with Wilson's disease during long-term penicillamine therapy. Ann Ophthalmol 10:1227, 1978.
55. Tso MOM, Fine BS, Thorpe HE: Kayser-Fleischer ring and associated cataract in Wilson's disease. Am J Ophthalmol 79:479, 1975.
56. Walshe JM: The eye in Wilson disease. *In* Bergsma D, Bron AJ, Cotlier E (eds): The Eye and Inborn Errors of Metabolism. New York, Alan R Liss, 1976, p 187.
57. Punnett HH, Kirkpatrick JA Jr: A syndrome of ocular abnormalities, calcification of cartilage and failure to thrive. J Pediatr 73:602, 1968.
58. Woods SE, Colon VF: Wilson's disease. Am Fam Physician 40:171, 1989.
59. Snyder RD, Carlow TJ, Ledman J, Wenger DA: Ocular findings in fucosidosis. *In* Bergsma D, Bron AJ, Cotlier E (eds): The Eye and Inborn Errors of Metabolism. New York, Alan R Liss, 1976, p 241.
60. Henkind P, Ashton N: Ocular pathology in homocystinuria. Trans Ophthalmol Soc UK 85:21, 1965.
61. Spaeth GL: Homocystinuria: The significance of a successful treatment. Trans Ophthalmol Soc UK: 88:47, 1968.
62. Spaeth GL: The usefulness of pyridoxine in the treatment of homocystinuria: A review of postulated mechanisms of action and a new hypothesis. *In* Bergsma D, Bron AJ, Cotlier E (eds): The Eye and Inborn Errors of Metabolism. New York, Alan R Liss, 1976, p 347.
63. Spaeth GL, Barber GW: Homocystinuria—Its ocular manifestations. J Pediatr Ophthalmol 3:42, 1966.
64. Kessing S: Infantile cystinosis. Acta Ophthalmol 45:491, 1971.
65. Wong VG: Ocular manifestations in cystinosis. *In* Bergsma D, Bron AJ, Cotlier E (eds): The Eye and Inborn Errors of Metabolism. New York, Alan R Liss, 1976, p 181.
66. Nissenson AR, Port FK: Outcome of end-stage renal disease in patients with rare causes of renal failure. I. Inherited and metabolic disorders. Q J Med 73:1055, 1989.
67. Wirtschafter JD: The eye in alkaptonuria. *In* Bergsma D, Bron AJ, Cotlier E (eds): The Eye and Inborn Errors of Metabolism. New York, Alan R Liss, 1976, pp 279–289.
68. Borochoff SA, Dohlman CH: The Riley-Day syndrome. Ocular manifestations in a 35-year-old patient. Am J Ophthalmol 63:523, 1967.
69. Carlson LA, Philipson B: Fish-eye disease: A new familial condition with massive corneal opacities and dyslipoproteinemia. Lancet 2:921, 1979.
70. Anderson B, Margolis G, Lynn WS: Ocular lesions related to disturbances in fat metabolism. Am J Ophthalmol 45:23, 1958.
71. Andrews JS: The lipids of arcus senilis. Arch Ophthalmol 68:264, 1962.
72. Blodi FC: Ocular manifestations of familial hypercholesterolemia. Trans Am Ophthalmol Soc 60:304, 1962.
73. Bron AJ: Dyslipoproteinemias and their ocular manifestations. *In* Bergsma D, Bron AJ, Cotlier E (eds): The Eye and Inborn Errors of Metabolism. New York, Alan R Liss, 1976, p 257.
74. Segall MM, Lloyd JK, Fosbrooke AS, Wolff OH: Treatment of familial hypercholesterolaemia in children. Lancet 1:641, 1970.
75. Spaeth GL: Ocular manifestations of lipoprotein disease. JCE Ophthalmol 41:11, 1979.
76. Stanbury JB, Wyngaarden JB, Fredrickson DS: The Metabolic Basis of Inherited Diseases. New York, McGraw-Hill, 1966, pp 429–485.
77. Varneck L, Schnohr P, Jensen G: Presenile corneal arcus in healthy persons: A possible cardiovascular risk indicator in younger adults. Acta Ophthalmol 57:755, 1979.
78. Gjone E, Bergaust B: Corneal opacity in familial plasma cholesterol ester deficiency. Acta Ophthalmol 47:222, 1969.
79. Horven I, Gjone E, Egge K: Ocular manifestations in familial ICAT deficiency. *In* Bergsma D, Bron AJ, Cotlier E (eds): The Eye and Inborn Errors of Metabolism. New York, Alan R Liss, 1976, p 271.
80. Yee RD, Herbert PN, Bergsma DR, Biemer JJ: Atypical retinitis pigmentosa in familial hypobetalipoproteinemia. Am J Ophthalmol 82:64, 1976.
81. Shirato S, Naito C: Lecithin-cholesterolacyltransferase deficiency (report of the first case in Japan). Metab Pediatr Ophthalmol 3:281, 1979.
82. Quigley HA, Goldberg MF: Conjunctival ultrastructure in mucolipidosis III (pseudo-Hurler polydystrophy). Invest Ophthalmol 10:568, 1971.
83. Goldberg MF, Cotlier E, Fichenscher LG, et al: Macular cherry-red spot, corneal clouding and B-galactosidase deficiency: Clinical, biochemical and electron microscopic study of new autosomal recessive storage disease. Arch Intern Med 128:387, 1971.
84. Endres W, Shin YS: Cataract and metabolic disease. J Inherited Metab Dis 13:509, 1990.
85. Ginsberg J, Perrin EV, Sueoka WT: Ocular manifestations of trisomy 18. Am J Ophthalmol 66:59, 1968.
86. Keith CG: The ocular findings in the trisomy syndromes. Proc R Soc Med 61:251, 1968.
87. Spaeth GL: Ocular teratology. *In* Jakobiec F (ed): Anatomy, Embryology and Teratology. New York, Harper & Row, 1982.
88. Merin S, Crawford JS: Hypoglycemia in infantile cataract. Arch Ophthalmol 86:495, 1971.
89. Harrett WH: Dislocation of the lens: A study of 166 hospitalized cases. Arch Ophthalmol 78:289, 1967.
90. Johnson V, Grayson M, Christian J: Dominant microspherophakia. Arch Ophthalmol 85:534, 1971.
91. Goldberg MF, Ryan SJ: Intercalary staphyloma in Marfan's syndrome. Am J Ophthalmol 67:329, 1969.
92. Dawson G, Stein AO: Lactosyl ceramidosis: Catabolic enzyme defect of glycosphingolipid metabolism. Science 170:556–558, 1970.
93. Cogan DG, Federman DD: Retinal involvement with reticuloendotheliosis of unclassified type. Arch Ophthalmol 71:489, 1964.
94. Tasman W: Retinal Diseases in Children. New York, Harper & Row, 1971, pp 71–104.
95. Carr RE: The night-blinding disorders. Int Ophthalmol Clin 9:971, 1969.
96. Duke-Elder S: Congenital deformities. *In* Duke-Elder S (ed): System of Ophthalmology, vol. 3. Part 2. St. Louis, CV Mosby, 1963, pp 619–623, 640–643.
97. Francosi J: Heredity in Ophthalmology. St. Louis, CV Mosby, 1961, p 692.
98. Inomata H, Arakawa T, Nishimura M, et al: Pigmentary retinal dystrophy in Hallervorden-Spatz disease: A clinico-pathological study. Jpn J Ophthalmol 22:155, 1978.
99. Hooft CP, de Laey J, Herpol J, et al: Familial hypolipidaemia and retarded development without steatorrhea. Another inborn error of metabolism. Helv Paediatr Acta 12:1, 1962.
100. Berson EL, Schmidt SY, Shih VE: Ocular and biochemical abnormalities in gyrate atrophy of the choroid and retina. Ophthalmology 85:1018, 1978.
101. Gouras P, Carr RE, Gunkel RD: Retinitis pigmentosa in abetalipoproteinemia: Effects of vitamin A. Invest Ophthalmol 10:784, 1971.
102. Carr RE: Abetalipoproteinemia and the eye. Birth Defects 12:385, 1976.
103. Spaeth GL, Barber GW: Homocystinuria in a mentally retarded child and her normal cousin. Trans Am Acad Ophthalmol Otolaryngol 69:912, 1965.
104. Sperling MA, Hiles DA, Kennerdell JS: Electroretinographic responses following vitamin A therapy in abetalipoproteinemia. Am J Ophthalmol 73:342, 1972.
105. Broyer M, Tete MJ: Treatment of cystinosis using cysteamine. Ann Pediatr (Paris) 37:91, 1990.
106. Jones NP, Postlethwaite JJ, Noble JL: Clearance of corneal crystals in nephropathic cystinosis by topical cysteamine 0.5%. Br J Ophthalmol 75:311, 1991.
107. Donnell GN, Koeh R, Bergren WR: Observation on results of management of galactosemic patients. *In* Hsia DYY (ed): Galactosemia. Springfield, Charles C Thomas, 1960.
108. Wilson WA, Donnell GM, Bergren AP: The dietary prophylaxis of cataracts in patients with galactosemia. Birth Defects 12:313, 1976.
109. Erikson A, Groth CG, Mansson JE, et al: Clinical and biochemical outcome of marrow transplantation for Gaucher disease of the Norrbottnian type. Acta Paediatr Scand 79:680, 1990.
110. Berson EL, Hanson AH III, Rosner B, Shih VE: A two-year trial of low protein, low arginine diets or vitamin B_6 for patients with gyrate atrophy. Birth Defects 18:209, 1982.
111. Kaiser-Kupfer MI, deMonasterio F, Valle D, et al: Visual results of a long-term trial of low-arginine diet in gyrate atrophy of choroid and retina. Ophthalmology 88:307, 1981.

112. Weleber RG, Wirta MK, Kennaway NG: Gyrate atrophy of the choroid and retina: Clinical and biochemical heterogeneity and responses to vitamin B_6. Birth Defects 18:219, 1982.
113. Bartholomew DW, Batshaw ML, Allen RH, et al: Therapeutic approaches to cobalamin-C methylmalonic acidemia and homocystinuria. J Pediatr 112:32, 1988.
114. Burke JP, O'Keefe M, Bowell R, Naughten ER: Ocular complications in homocystinuria—early and late treated. Br J Ophthalmol 73:427, 1989.
115. Holme E, Kjellman B, Ronge E: Betaine for treatment of homocystinuria caused by methylene tetrahydrofolate reductase deficiency. Arch Dis Child 64:1061, 1989.
116. Applegarth DA, Dimmick JE, Toone JR: Laboratory detection of metabolic disease. Pediatr Clin North Am 36:49, 1989.
117. Ortega-Aramburu JJ, Dominguez-Luengo C, Olive-Oliveras T: Bone marrow transplant in mucopolysaccharidosis Type I, Hurler-Scheie variety. Metabolic correction and clinical results. An Esp Pediatr 33:369, 1990.
118. Robertson EF, Poulos A, Sharp P, et al: Treatment of infantile phytanic acid storage disease: Clinical biochemical and ultrastructural findings in two children treated for 2 years. Eur J Pediatr 147:133, 1988.
119. Dickson N, Mortimer JG, Faed JM, et al: A child with Refsum's disease: Successful treatment with diet and plasma exchange. Dev Med Child Neurol 31:92, 1989.
120. Britton TC, Gibberd FB, Clemens ME, et al: The significance of plasma phytanic acid levels in adults. J Neurol Neurosurg Psychiatry 52:891, 1989.
121. Bienfang DG, Kuwabara T, Pueschel SM: The Richner-Hanhart syndrome. Arch Ophthalmol 94:1133, 1976.
122. Danks DM: Hereditary disorders of copper metabolism in Wilson's disease and Menkes' disease. *In* Stanbury JB, et al (eds): The Metabolic Basis of Inherited Disease, 5th ed. New York, McGraw-Hill, 1983.
123. Desnick RJ, Grabowski GA: Advances in the treatment of inherited metabolic disease. Adv Hum Genet 11:281, 1981.
124. Walshe JM: Wilson's disease presenting with features of hepatic dysfunction: A clinical analysis of eighty-seven patients. Q J Med 70:253, 1989.
125. Dastych M: Copper in the feces—A marker for the effectiveness of zinc in the treatment of Wilson's disease. Z Gastroenterol 28:389, 1991.
126. Schilsky ML, Scheinberg IH, Sternlieb I: Prognosis of wilsonian chronic active hepatitis. Gastroenterology 100:762, 1991.

Chapter 223

Developmental Abnormalities of the Eye Affecting Vision in the Pediatric Years

RICHARD M. ROBB

By virtue of the anatomic organization of other sections of this book, some congenital anomalies of the eye and adnexa are discussed elsewhere. In this chapter, several developmental abnormalities that may have an important effect on vision in the pediatric years are described. No uniform scheme of classification is satisfactory for these entities. Their causes are mostly unknown and are probably diverse.

INFANTILE HEMANGIOMAS

Infantile hemangiomas, sometimes descriptively called *strawberry hemangiomas*, are hamartomas—that is, benign tumor-like nodules composed of vascular elements that are normally found at the involved site but combined in proportions or configurations that are distinctly abnormal. They are often relatively inapparent at birth but undergo a period of early growth that brings them to medical attention in the first few months of life (Fig. 223–1). Their growth continues during the first 6 mo to 1 yr of life, after which they gradually recede over a period of years. These infantile hemangiomas may occur anywhere on the skin surface, but they most commonly are found in the head and neck region[1] and become important ophthalmologically when they involve the eyelids and orbit. Characteristically, there is no direct anatomic involvement of the eye, a feature that distinguishes these lesions from the congenital vascular port-wine stain of Sturge-Weber syndrome, which is often associated with episcleral vascular abnormalities, choroidal hemangioma, and ipsilateral glaucoma.[2] The ophthalmic consequences of infantile hemangiomas are secondary to occlusion of the visual axis or pressure on the globe that causes astigmatic refractive errors (Fig. 223–2).[3, 4] Smaller lesions that do not have these effects can be followed without intervention, as they wax and wane. Parental concern about cosmetic appearance must be dealt with. Generally, the final appearance is better if the temptation to irradiate, photocoagulate, or freeze the lesions is resisted.[5] Surgery is also usually of little help. Only occasionally is it possible to accomplish local excision of a hemangioma after its active growth has stopped (Fig. 223–3). More commonly, the lesion is too diffuse and extensive to allow surgical removal without undesirable sacrifice of normal structures. Very large lesions have been associated with platelet trapping and thrombocytopenia,[6] but this is an unlikely complication of periocular lesions.

In cases in which an actively growing hemangioma of the eyelids threatens to occlude the visual axis or appears to be responsible for the induction of asymmetric astig-

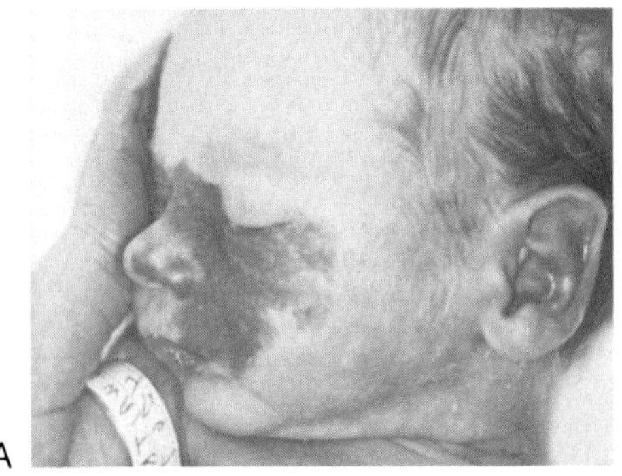

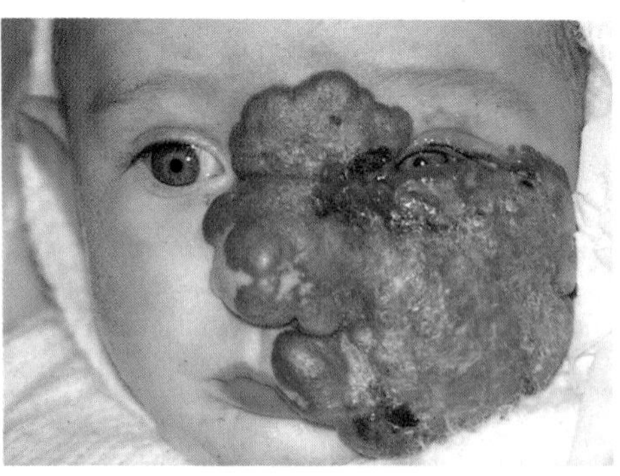

Figure 223–1. *A,* Newborn infant with flat hemangioma in left maxillary area and bridge of the nose. *B,* Same infant at 8 mo of age showing exuberant growth of hemangioma and involvement of entire left lower lid.

matism, treatment with local or systemic corticosteroids may limit or reverse the growth of the lesion (Fig. 223–4).[7, 8] The choice of the route of administration depends on the extent of the lesion, large hemangiomas being hard to treat effectively by injection. Systemic prednisone in doses of 1.5 to 2 mg/kg of body weight or intralesional injection of 40 mg of triamcinolone has been reported to be effective therapy.[7, 8] Not all corticosteroids have equal angiostatic properties, and a preparation's ability to inhibit angiogenesis does not necessarily parallel its glucocorticoid or mineralocorticoid activity.[9] A rebound of growth may occur when steroids are discontinued or after they have been absorbed from the injection site, so repeated treatment is sometimes necessary. Systemic side effects of the corticosteroids are dependent on the dose and duration of therapy. They are expected with systemic treatment but are also found after local injection.[10] Radiation therapy has been largely abandoned in the treatment of hemangiomas.[5] Although there were no endocrine complications attendant on this modality of therapy, cataracts did occur after relatively low doses of radiation to the eye,[11] and radiation effects in the skin gave less than optimal long-term results.[5]

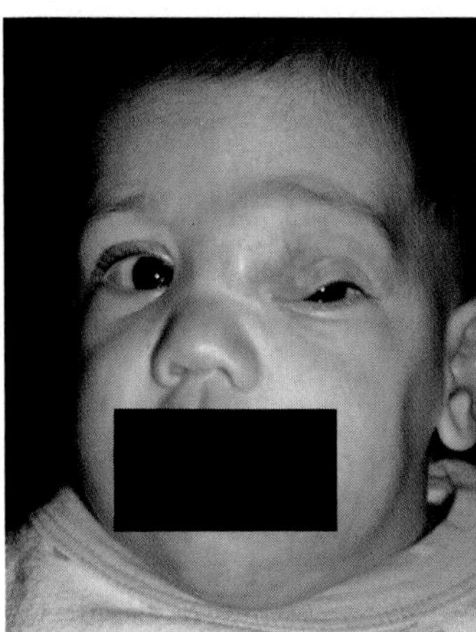

Figure 223–2. Five-month-old infant with hemangioma at inner aspect of left upper lid and brow. Lesions in this location are particularly apt to induce oblique astigmatism because of pressure on the cornea.

It is unusual to achieve complete resolution of any hemangioma with currently available treatment, so complications must be addressed. Eyeglasses may be necessary to treat induced refractive errors, and patching of the fellow eye may be required to reverse refractive or deprivational amblyopia. Parents of patients with infantile hemangiomas often need the emotional support and reassurance of an experienced physician as they deal with the slow resolution of a cosmetically disfiguring hemangioma, along with its ocular side effects.

OCULAR DERMOIDS

Congenital dermoids are choristomas, which are lesions composed of normal tissues, the elements of which are not normally found at the site of involvement. Ocular or epibulbar dermoids are distinguished here from the more common dermoid cysts that occur subcutaneously along the upper orbital margin, in the orbit itself, and in the scalp (Fig. 223–5). These dermoid cysts are usually isolated and unassociated with systemic disease and can be excised intact if care is used to dissect them from underlying periosteum and bone. Solid epibulbar dermoids are less common but more important from a visual standpoint. They occur either at the corneal limbus (Fig. 223–6) or at the lateral canthus (lipodermoid), extending subconjunctivally back over the lateral rectus muscle (Fig. 223–7). In the latter location, the lesions are relatively inconspicuous and are usually not approached surgically because of the scarring and altered ocular motility that can result from any extensive dissection in the area.[12] Limbal dermoids are more noticeable cosmetically, and they often induce oblique astigmatism with a plus cylinder axis in the meridian of the lesion. They can usually be shaved off the cornea and adjacent sclera to improve the appearance of the eye, even though a gray crescent of cornea always remains. Unfortunately, the associated astigmatism is not reliably improved by this surgery, and even astigmatic eyeglass correction may leave the patient with a degree of refractive amblyopia.

Epibulbar demoids are frequently associated with hemifacial microsomia[13] or its Goldenhar's syndrome variant.[14] Ipsilateral preauricular appendages, minimal

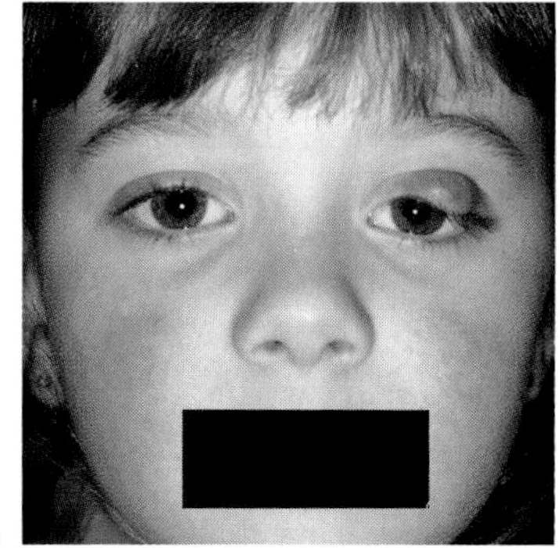
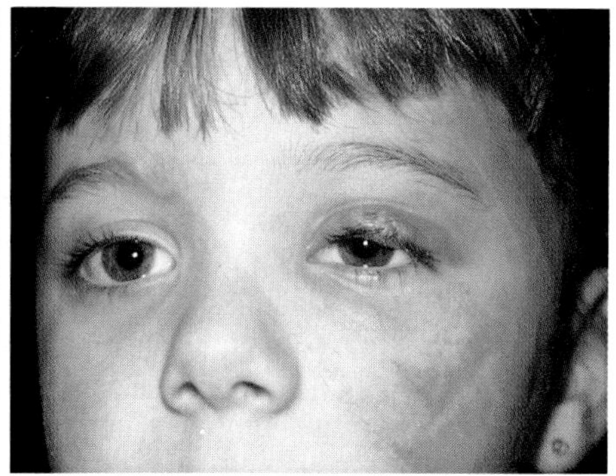

Figure 223–3. *A,* Three-year-old patient with pendulous hemangioma of left upper lid that was amenable to local excision after its active growth had stopped. *B,* Same patient 2 days after partial excision of hemangioma.

microtia, hearing loss, cleft lip or palate, and upper eyelid coloboma should therefore be looked for. Nearly all dermoids are located temporally on the globe. They are sporadic in occurrence, whether or not they are associated with other facial malformations, and chromosome studies have been normal when performed.

ANOMALIES OF WHOLE EYE FORMATION

Congenital anophthalmos and severe microphthalmos are clinically similar and are at the extreme end of a spectrum of ocular malformation in which the volume of the eye is reduced. The embryologic processes that determine the size of the eye are poorly understood. When an infant appears to be anophthalmic at birth (Fig. 223–8), a tiny rudiment of an eye can usually be found deep in the orbit. Small lid retractors may help to visualize the rudiment, and computed tomography scanning can identify the globe and any connection with the visual pathways (Fig. 223–9). Vision is lacking or limited to light perception. The defect can be unilateral or bilateral. At times, the severely microphthalmic eye is associated with a cyst that is located in the inferior portion of the orbit and communicates with the eye through an inferior coloboma. The cyst may be much larger than the eye, extending forward into the lower eyelid and obscuring the eye from view (Fig. 223–10). The cyst tends to enlarge with time and may have to be excised, along with the globe, to allow a prosthesis to be fitted. Otherwise the prosthesis can be placed directly over the ocular rudiment to help support the eyelids and improve the child's appearance.

Severe congenital microphthalmos may occur sporadically as an isolated event.[15] It may also be dominantly inherited with or without coloboma, and in this case, obtaining a family history or actually examining the parents may be helpful. Variable expressivity and incomplete penetrance have been observed, and thus individuals with minimal or no findings may carry the mutant gene.[16] Recessive modes of inheritance have also been described. Severe microphthalmos with coloboma may also occur with multisystem involvement in a variety of single-gene disorders,[17] chromosomal syndromes,[18] or nonrandom grouping of malformations (Table 223–1).[19] Evaluation of a patient should be interdisciplinary. If there is developmental delay and at least one other dysmorphic feature, a chromosomal analysis should be performed.

An additional, somewhat bizarre anomaly of whole eye formation, synophthalmos or cyclopia (Fig. 223–11), is a malformation invariably associated with structural abnormalities of the central nervous system that are not compatible with life. Chromosomal abnormalities may be found if they are looked for.[20]

COLOBOMATA

It is appropriate to discuss colobomata immediately after microphthalmos because the two are frequently (but not always) found together.[16] Typical colobomata result from failure of the embryonic fissure to close

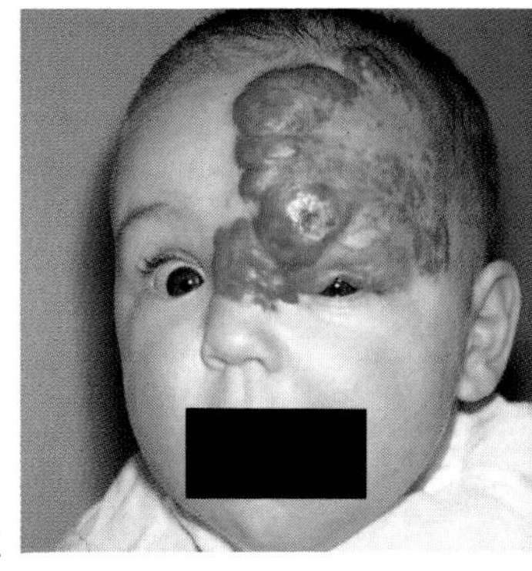
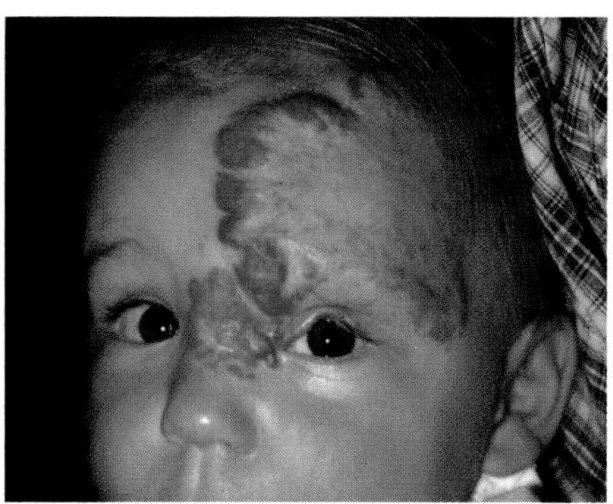

Figure 223–4. *A,* Five-month-old infant with hemangioma of left upper lid, brow, and forehead. Corticosteroids were injected into the upper lid and brow. *B,* Patient 6 mo after local steroid injection.

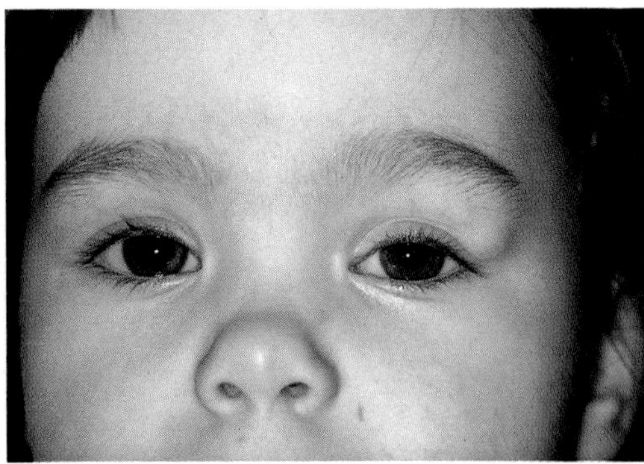

Figure 223–5. Child with dermoid cyst at temporal aspect of left upper lid near orbital margin.

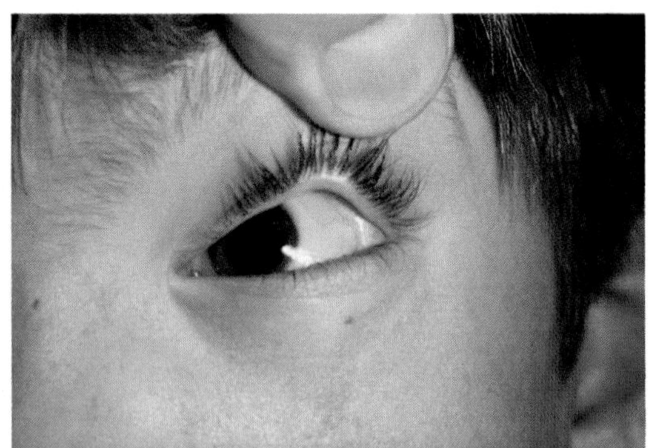

Figure 223–7. Lipodermoid at lateral canthus. These lesions extend subconjunctivally back into the orbit.

along the inferonasal aspect of the optic cup and stalk. In the normal eye, this fissure closes 33 to 40 days after conception.[21] When the retinal neurosensory elements and the retinal pigment epithelial precursors fail to become confluent, the underlying choroid fails to differentiate, and a bridge of bare sclera or a cyst is found (Fig. 223–12). Anteriorly, at the distal margin of the embryonic fissure, defects in the neuroectodermally derived iris pigment epithelium produce iris colobomata (Fig. 223–13). Posteriorly, the entire optic nerve head anlage may be involved in a colobomatous malformation (Fig. 223–14). There is evidence to support the possibility that optic nerve pits, the morning glory syndrome, and the congenital tilted disc syndrome are all variant products of the process that produces typical colobomata.[22] Colobomata can be unilateral or bilateral; when bilateral they are often asymmetric. The prognosis for vision depends on the amount of ocular malformation and the degree of microphthalmia. Coloboma of the optic nerve is usually associated with some decrease in visual acuity, even when the fovea is spared. Secondary retinal detachments may also cause a reduction in vision.[23]

Autosomal dominant inheritance of ocular coloboma as an isolated anomaly without other systemic malformations is well established.[24] Variable expression of the genetic trait encompasses the spectrum from iris coloboma to clinical anophthalmos, with various degrees of optic disc and chorioretinal coloboma as intermediate manifestations. Members of the same family may exhibit widely variable degrees of involvement,[25] making genetic counseling a more uncertain endeavor. A sporadic isolated coloboma with no other affected family member is common. Based on limited data, recurrence figures for the subsequent child of healthy unrelated parents have been estimated at 9 percent; for the childen of an affected person, these figures are as high as 46 percent.[25]

Ocular coloboma may be one aspect of a single-gene disorder with multisystem involvement (Table 223–1). Examples include the Lenz microphthalmia syndrome,[17] Goltz's focal dermal hypoplasia,[26] Meckel's syndrome,[27] and Warburg's syndrome.[28] Patients with Aicardi's syndrome may have optic disc colobomata as well as multiple lacunar defects in the retinal pigment epithelium (Fig. 223–15), no corpus callosum, infantile seizures, and mental retardation.[29] Because only affected females have been reported, the condition has been considered to be X-linked and lethal in males. Another multisystem disorder without known genetic cause is the CHARGE association of anomalies, which derives its acronym from the nonrandom grouping of a series of features: *c*olobomatous microphthalmos, *h*eart defects, choanal *a*tresia, *r*etarded growth, *g*enital anomalies, and *e*ar anomalies or deafness. At least three of the features are necessary for the diagnosis.[19] The phenotypes of some chromosomal syndromes, including trisomy 13 and trisomy 18, the 4p− syndrome, and the cat's eye syndrome, share some features with this association, so a

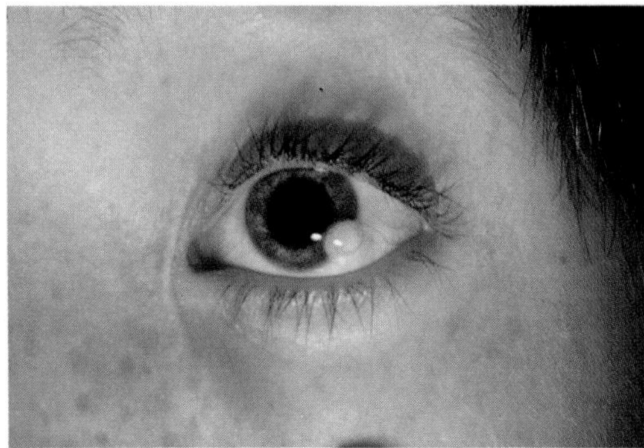

Figure 223–6. Epibulbar dermoid at inferotemporal limbus, at which 76 percent of such lesions occur.[13]

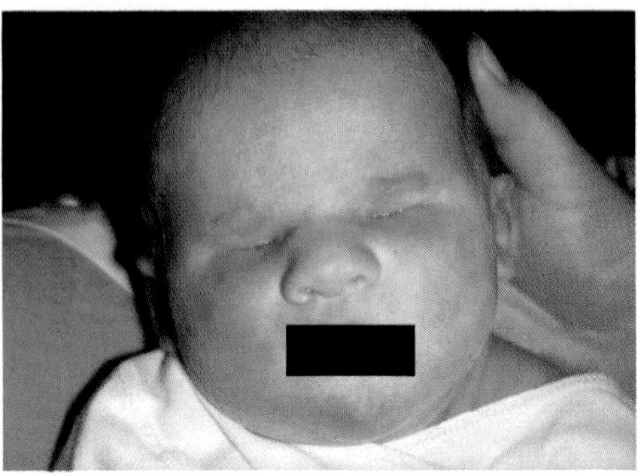

Figure 223–8. Infant with clinical anophthalmia at birth. Usually a tiny rudiment of an eye can be found deep in the orbit.

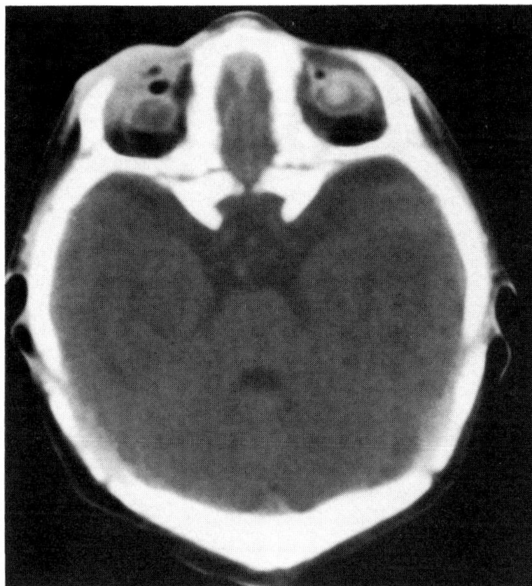

Figure 223–9. CT scan of the orbits of an infant with severe microphthalmia. Small globes containing lenses can be found on each side.

Table 223–1. VARIOUS SETTINGS FOR THE OCCURRENCE OF SEVERE MICROPHTHALMOS WITH COLOBOMA

Chromosomal abnormalities
Trisomy 13[18]
Cat eye syndrome[48]
4p− (Wolf-Hirschhorn) syndrome[49]
Single-gene disorders
Lenz's microphthalmia syndrome, X-linked recessive[17]
Goltz's focal dermal hypoplasia, X-linked dominant[26]
Meckel-Gruber syndrome, autosomal recessive[27]
Warburg's syndrome, autosomal recessive[28]
Aicardi's syndrome, X-linked dominant[29]
Multisystem syndrome of unknown cause
Goldenhar's syndrome[14]
Linear sebaceous nevus syndrome[45]
Rubinstein-Taybi syndrome[46]
Nonrandom grouping of anomalies of unknown cause
CHARGE association[19]
Teratogens
Thalidomide[47]
Isolated autosomal dominant inheritance[16]
Sporadic isolated colobomatous microphthalmos[15]

chromosomal analysis may be necessary to make the correct diagnosis.[16]

OPTIC NERVE HYPOPLASIA

Congenital optic nerve hypoplasia is, from a visual standpoint, one of the most important developmental abnormalities of the eye. First, it is a relatively common condition and second, it accounts for a significant reduction of vision in most cases.[30, 31] The diagnosis is made ophthalmoscopically by noting the small diameter of the optic nerve head, variable degrees of disc pallor, and abnormal termination of the retinal pigment epithelium at the disc border (Fig. 223–16). The perifoveal area may be somewhat flattened because of the reduced number of ganglion cells and nerve fibers, but the fovea is identifiable and distinct. The retinal vessels are normal, and the overall pigmentation of the fundus is unaffected. Optic nerve hypoplasia may be unilateral or bilateral. If unilateral, it usually presents as early-onset strabismus; if it is bilateral, the presenting signs are poor vision and nystagmus. The pupillary light reflex is usually present but is diminished in proportion to the degree of hypoplasia. In unilateral or markedly asymmetric cases, a relative afferent pupillary defect is found in the affected or more affected eye. Visual acuity and visual fields are reduced, sometimes to the level of light perception.

Since the poor vision of optic nerve hypoplasia is present from birth in children whose eyes may appear normal except for the optic disc changes, care must be taken to distinguish this entity from Leber's congenital amaurosis, another major ocular cause of poor vision in infants whose fundi may appear nearly normal.[32] In Leber's congenital amaurosis, the pathologic condition is an outer retinal degeneration of rods and cones,[33] and the electroretinogram signal is characteristically reduced, whereas in optic nerve hypoplasia, it is the retinal ganglion cells and their nerve fibers that are damaged, and the electroretinogram has been normal.[34] Conversely, in optic nerve hypoplasia, the visual evoked potential is severely affected.

It is important for the ophthalmologist to recognize that optic nerve hypoplasia may be associated with pathology in the central nervous system. Most of the pathologic specimens of hypoplastic optic nerves come from patients with anencephaly or hydranencephaly.[35]

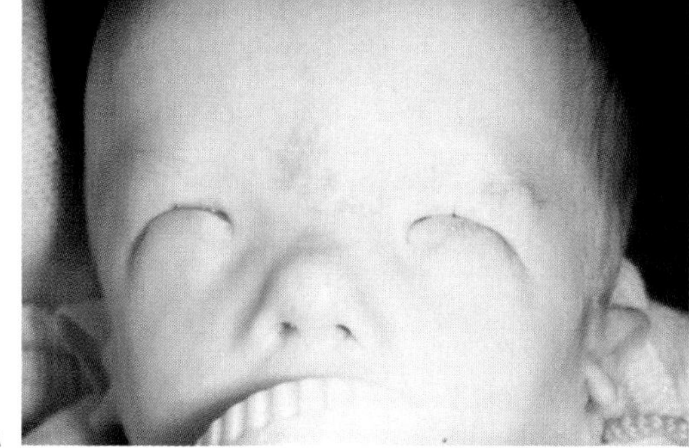

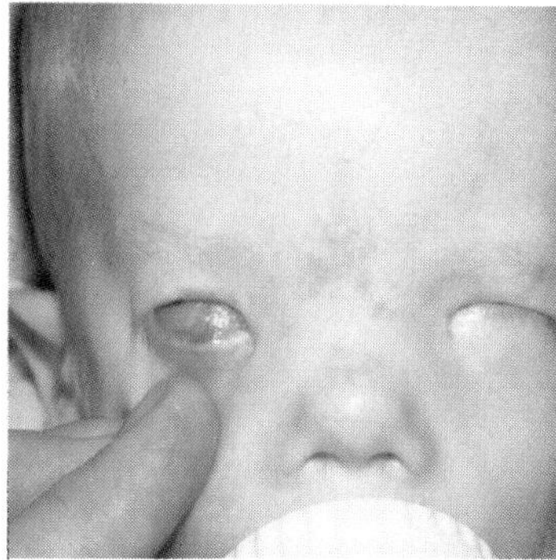

Figure 223–10. *A*, Patient with bilateral microphthalmos with cyst. *B*, The cyst extends forward into the lower eyelid, obscuring the rudimentary globe behind it.

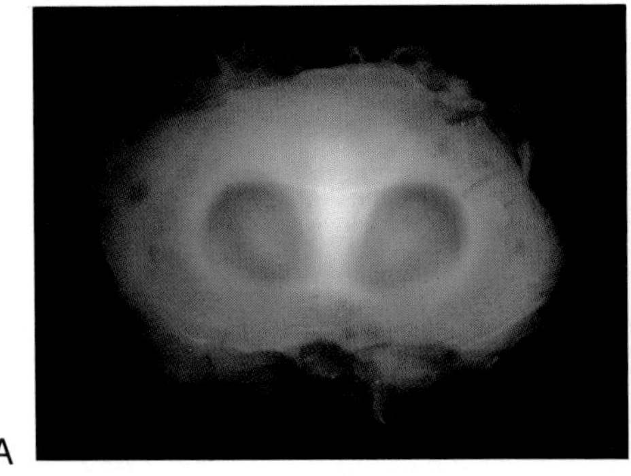

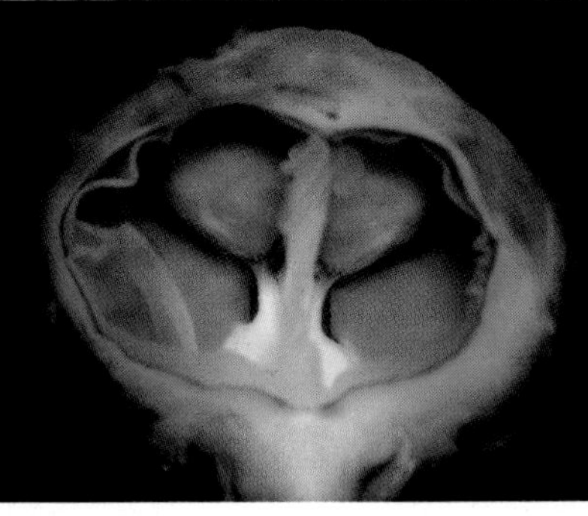

Figure 223–11. Enucleated synophthalmic eye. Two corneas can be seen, but the globes are fused medially. *B*, Same eye viewed from above after superior calotte has been removed. Two lenses and a medial partition can be seen.

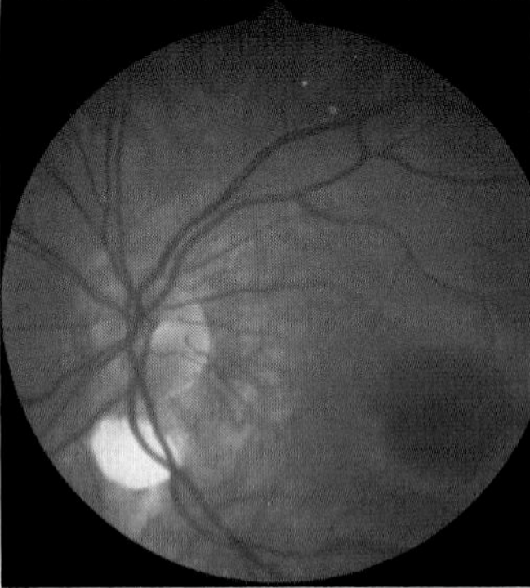

Figure 223–12. Chorioretinal coloboma situated below the optic disc. White sclera is visible at the point at which the retinal pigment epithelium and choroid have failed to develop.

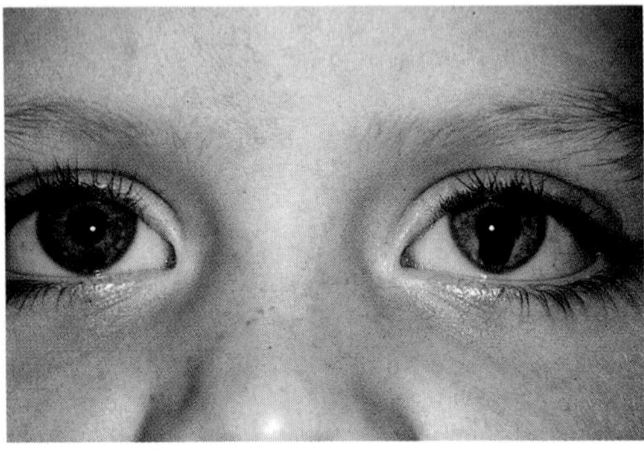

Figure 223–13. Patient with inferonasal iris coloboma in left eye.

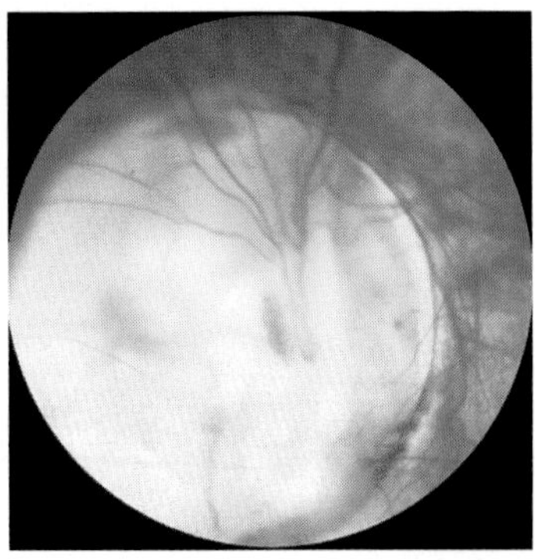

Figure 223–14. Coloboma of the optic disc. Retinal vessels can be seen coursing over the upper aspect of the coloboma.

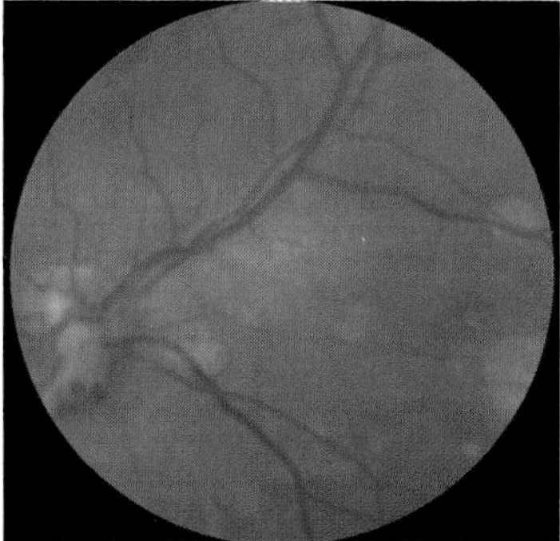

Figure 223–15. Fundus of a patient with Aicardi's syndrome showing lacunar defects in retinal pigment epithelium.

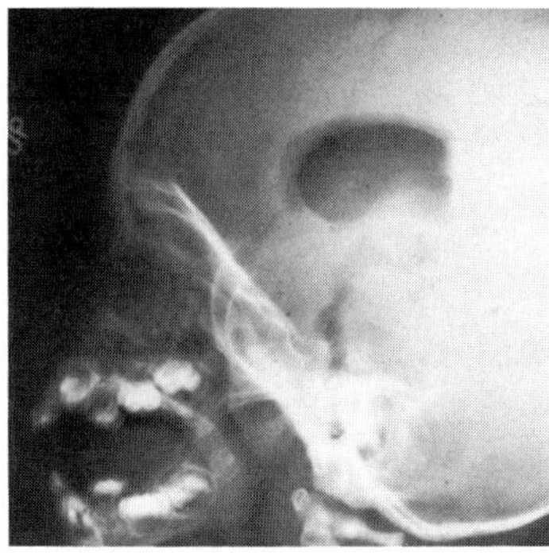

Figure 223–17. Pneumoencephalogram of patient with bilateral optic nerve hypoplasia, showing lack of septum pellucidum, an anatomic defect without known functional significance.

More important clinically is the association of optic nerve hypoplasia with midline cerebral defects, such as lack of the septum pellucidum (Fig. 223–17) and various pituitary abnormalities (dwarfism[36] and diabetes insipidus[37]). In contrast, review of large series of patients reveals that when strabismus and nystagmus are excluded, many children with optic nerve hypoplasia are otherwise normal.[30, 31, 38]

Optic nerve hypoplasia is sporadic in occurrence. A variant has been attributed to the use of quinine as an abortifacient.[39] A few familial cases have occurred in the offspring of diabetic mothers.[38] Originally, the abnormality was attributed to a defect in the formation of retinal ganglion cells early in gestation, but more recent evidence suggests that a later embryologic event may account for secondary degeneration and disappearance of ganglion cells from the retina, while the rest of the eye is left remarkably intact.[35] The condition is stationary and irremediable.

PERSISTENT HYPERPLASTIC PRIMARY VITREOUS

Persistent hyperplastic primary vitreous (PHPV) is included as the final developmental abnormality in this chapter, not only because of its impact on vision in the pediatric years but also because early surgical treatment has been recommended to avoid secondary glaucoma and intraocular hemorrhage.[40–42] PHPV is a distinctive anomaly occurring sporadically and, for the most part, unilaterally in full-term normal infants. The affected eye is variably microphthalmic with a shallow anterior chamber and a vascularized membrane behind the lens into which the ciliary processes are drawn (Fig. 223–18). The lens is often clear at first, but it develops a posterior opacity and swells, causing further shallowing of the anterior chamber and angle-closure glaucoma. Spontaneous intraocular hemorrhage presumably comes from the vascularized membrane or from hyaloid remnants that may be attached to its posterior surface (Fig. 223–19). PHPV can usually be distinguished from an uncomplicated unilateral congenital cataract by the presence of a shallow anterior chamber and the retrolenticular membrane. It is distinguished from retinopathy of prematurity by its unilaterality and occurrence in full-term infants and from retinoblastoma by its association with microphthalmos and the lack of intraocular calcification on computed tomography scanning. Rarely, these guides for differential diagnosis are insufficient, and a proper diagnosis can be made only by pathologic examination of an enucleated eye.[43]

If PHPV can be identified clinically, and the eye is not severely microphthalmic, extraction of the lens and retrolenticular membrane may be advisable to prevent

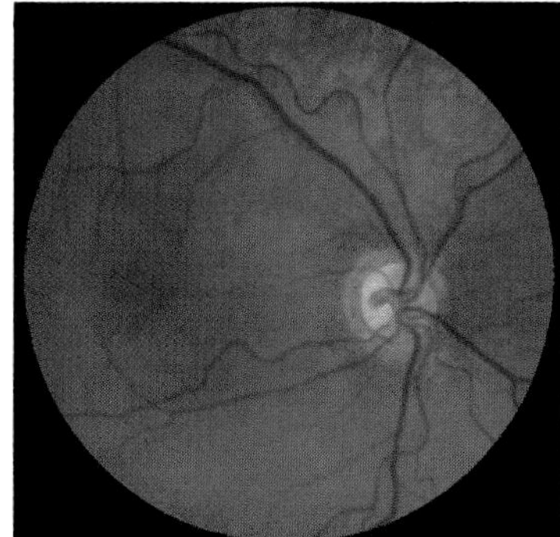

Figure 223–16. Optic nerve hypoplasia. Note small size of optic disc and irregular termination of retinal pigment epithelium at disc margin.

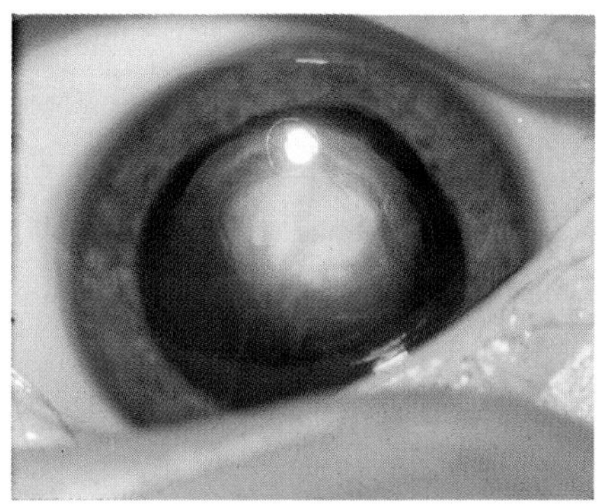

Figure 223–18. Retrolenticular membrane and posterior lens opacity in patient with persistent hyperplastic primary vitreous.

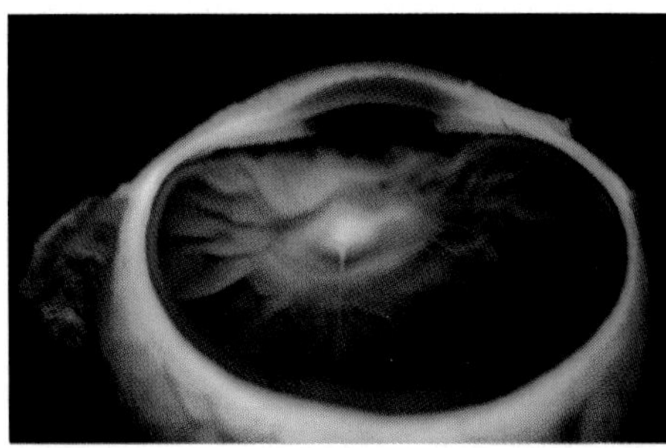

Figure 223–19. A hyaloid stalk extends back from the retrolenticular membrane in this enucleated eye with PHPV.

glaucoma and intraocular hemorrhage. Visual results of this kind of surgery have occasionally been good,[40–42] but more often, deprivation amblyopia and posterior segment abnormalities[44] have limited the development of central vision, and the justification for surgery has been retention of a viable eye with at least some peripheral vision. Retinal detachment and glaucoma have sometimes followed cataract and membrane removal in patients with PHPV,[41] so a guarded prognosis should be given at the outset of treatment.

REFERENCES

1. Mulliken JB: Cutaneous vascular lesions of children. *In* Serafin D, Georgiade N (eds): Pediatric Plastic Surgery. St. Louis, CV Mosby, 1984, p 137.
2. Dunphy EB: Glaucoma accompanying nevus flammeus. Trans Am Ophthalmol Soc 32:143, 1934.
3. Robb RM: Refractive errors associated with hemangiomas of the eyelids and orbit in infancy. Am J Ophthalmol 83:52, 1977.
4. Stigmar G, Crawford JS, Ward CM, et al: Ophthalmic sequelae of infantile hemangiomas of the eyelids and orbit. Am J Ophthalmol 85:806, 1978.
5. Walter J: On the treatment of cavernous hemangioma with special reference to spontaneous regression. J Faculty Radiol 5:134, 1953.
6. Katz HP, Asken J: Multiple hemangiomata with thrombopenia. Am J Dis Child 115:351, 1968.
7. Hiles DA, Pilchard WA: Corticosteroid control of neonatal hemangiomas of the orbit and ocular adnexa. Am J Ophthalmol 71:1003, 1971.
8. Kushner BJ: Local steroid therapy in adnexal hemangioma. Ann Ophthalmol 11:1005, 1979.
9. Folkman J, Ingber D: Angiostatic steroids: Method of discovery and mechanism of action. Ann Surg 206:374, 1987.
10. Weiss AH: Adrenal suppression after corticosteroid injection of periocular hemangiomas. Am J Ophthalmol 107:518, 1989.
11. Bek V, Zahn K: Cataract as a late sequel of contact roentgen therapy of angiomas in children. Acta Radiol 54:443, 1960.
12. Schultz GR, Wendler PF, Weseley AC: Ocular dermoids and auricular appendages. Am J Ophthalmol 63: 938, 1967.
13. Nevares RL, Mulliken JB, Robb RM: Ocular dermoids. Plast Reconstr Surg 82:959, 1988.
14. Baum JL, Feingold M: Ocular aspects of Goldenhar's syndrome. Am J Ophthalmol 75:250, 1973.
15. Fujiki K, Nakajima A, Yusuda N, et al: Genetic analysis of microphthalmos. Ophthamol Paediatr Genet 1:139, 1982.
16. Bateman JB: Microphthalmos. *In* Kivlin JD (ed): Developmental abnormalities of the eye. Int Ophthalmol Clin 24:87, 1984.
17. Goldberg MF, McKusick VA: X-linked colobomatous microphthalmos and other congenital anomalies. A disorder resembling Lenz's dysmorphogenetic syndrome. Am J Ophthalmol 71:1128, 1971.
18. Hoepner J, Yanoff ML: Ocular anomalies in trisomy 13-15: An analysis of 13 eyes with two new findings. Am J Ophthalmol 74:729, 1972.
19. Pagon RA, Graham JM Jr, Zonana J, et al: CHARGE association: coloboma, congenital heart disease, and choanal atresia with multiple anomalies. J Pediatr 99:223, 1981.
20. Howard RO: Chromosomal abnormalities associated with cyclopia and synophthalmia. Trans Am Ophthalmol Soc 74:505, 1977.
21. Mann I: The Development of The Human Eye. New York, Grune & Stratton, 1928, pp 1–29.
22. Apple DJ: New aspects of colobomas and optic nerve anomalies. *In* Kivlin J (ed): Developmental abnormalities of the eye. Int Ophthalmol Clin 24:109, 1984.
23. Jesberg DO, Schepens CL: Retinal detachment associated with coloboma of the choroid. Arch Ophthalmol 65:163, 1961.
24. Pagon RA: Ocular coloboma. Surv Ophthalmol 25:223, 1981.
25. Maumenee IH, Mitchell TN: Colobomatous malformations of the eye. Trans Am Ophthalmol Soc 88:123, 1990.
26. Warburg M: Focal dermal hypoplasia: Ocular and general manifestations with a survey of the literature. Acta Ophthalmol 48:525, 1970.
27. Fraser FC, Lytwyn A: Spectrum of anomalies in the Meckel syndrome. Am J Hum Genet 30: 102A, 1978.
28. Warburg M: Hydrocephaly, congenital retinal nonattachment, and congenital falciform fold. Am J Ophthalmol 85:88, 1978.
29. Denslow GT, Robb RM: Aicardi's syndrome: A report of four cases and review of the literature. J Pediatr Ophthalmol Strabismus 16:10, 1979.
30. Walton DS, Robb RM: Optic nerve hypoplasia. A report of 20 cases. Arch Ophthalmol 84:572, 1970.
31. Edwards WC, Layden WE: Optic nerve hypoplasia. Am J Ophthalmol 70:950, 1970.
32. Noble KG, Carr RE: Leber's congenital amaurosis. A retrospective study of 33 cases and a histopathological study of one case. Arch Ophthalmol 96:818, 1978.
33. Mizumo K, Takei Y, Sears ML, et al: Leber's congenital amaurosis. Am J Ophthalmol 83:32, 1977.
34. Brown G, Tasman W: Congenital Anomalies of the Optic Disc. New York, Grune & Stratton, 1983, p 202.
35. Mosier MA, Lieberman MF, Green WR, et al: Hypoplasia of the optic nerve. Arch Ophthalmol 96:1437, 1978.
36. Hoyt WF, Koplan SL, Grumbach MM, et al: Septo-optic dysplasia and pituitary dwarfism. Lancet 1:893, 1970.
37. Sheridan SJ, Robb RM: Optic nerve hypoplasia and diabetes insipidus. J Pediatr Ophthalmol 15:82, 1978.
38. Petersen RA, Walton DS: Optic nerve hypoplasia with good visual acuity and visual field defects. Arch Ophthalmol 95:254, 1977.
39. McKinna AJ: Quinine-induced hypoplasia of the optic nerve. Can J Ophthalmol 1:261, 1966.
40. Reese AB: Persistent hyperplastic primary vitreous. Am J Ophthalmol 40:317, 1955.
41. Smith RE, Maumenee AE: Persistent hyperplastic primary vitreous: Result of surgery. Trans Am Acad Ophthalmol Otolaryngol 78:911, 1974.
42. Nankin SJ, Scott WE: Persistent hyperplastic primary vitreous. Roto-extraction and other surgical experience. Arch Ophthalmol 95:240, 1977.
43. Irvine AR, Albert DM, Sang DN: Retinal neoplasia and dysplasia. II. Retinoblastoma occurring with persistence and hyperplasia of the primary vitreous. Invest Ophthalmol Vis Sci 16:403, 1977.
44. Pruett RC: The pleomorphism and complications of posterior hyperplastic primary vitreous. Am J Ophthalmol 80:625, 1975.
45. Marden PM, Venters HD: A new neurocutaneous syndrome. Am J Dis Child 112:79, 1966.
46. Rubinstein JH, Taybi H: Broad thumbs and toes and facial abnormalities. Am J Dis Child 105:88, 1963.
47. Cullen JG: Ocular defects in thalidomide babies. Br J Ophthalmol 48:151, 1964.
48. Schinzel A, Schmid W, Fraccaro M, et al: The "cat eye syndrome." Hum Genet 57:148, 1981.
49. Wolf U, Porsch R, Baitsch H, et al: Deletion of short arms of a B chromosome without "cri du chat" syndrome. Lancet 1:769, 1965.

Chapter 224

Retinopathy of Prematurity

ROBERT A. PETERSEN, DAVID G. HUNTER, and SHIZUO MUKAI

Retinopathy of prematurity (ROP) is one of the leading causes of childhood blindness in the developed countries. It was first described only 50 yr ago and became the leading cause of blindness in children within a few years. Our understanding of its causes has evolved and is still evolving. Attempts at prevention and treatment have similarly evolved, and there is hope that the more severe, blinding stages of the disease can be prevented or controlled.

HISTORICAL BACKGROUND

ROP was first described by Terry in 1942.[1] He described an abnormal growth of fibroblastic tissue and blood vessels behind the lens, causing bilateral blindness in premature infants. Many other reports of the disease soon followed, and in the 1940s and early 1950s, ROP, then called retrolental fibroplasia, had become the leading cause of childhood blindness in the developed countries. Before the introduction of the modern binocular indirect ophthalmoscope, only the more severe stages of the disease were recognized. Nevertheless, by the early 1950s, it was estimated that ten thousand infants were afflicted. Many theories were advanced as to the etiology of this new epidemic of blindness in infancy, including some that have recently regained currency. Factors associated with ROP in the early years included exposure to light, antenatal or postnatal viral infections, bacterial infection, anoxia, anemia, electrolyte imbalances, vitamin deficiency, hypervitaminosis, iron deficiency, substitution of cow's milk for breast milk, hormone deficiencies, and hypercapnea. Finally, the clinical reports of ROP occurring in conjunction with excessive oxygen use[2, 3, 4] and the experimental production by excessive oxygen in newborn experimental animals of vascular changes similar to ROP[5, 6, 7] led to a collaborative trial of oxygen restriction in the United States.

Two groups of premature infants were studied, one group receiving standard oxygen treatment, generally over 50 percent ambient oxygen concentration in the incubator, and the other group receiving no added oxygen or no more than 40 percent oxygen as indicated clinically. Seventy-two percent of the unrestricted group developed some ROP, whereas only 30 percent of those in the restricted group developed some stage of the disease.[8] Following this, the use of oxygen in premature infants was severely curtailed. The number of cases of severe ROP fell precipitously and remained relatively low until the early 1960s. At that time, reports of increased mortality[9] and morbidity[10] suggested that the reduction of ROP had been accompanied by increased deaths and neurologic damage in premature infants because of oxygen deprivation. This led to a liberalization of oxygen use in premature infants and a reemergence of ROP as an important blinding disease in infancy. In the 1960s, frequent blood gas determinations were routinely performed in premature infants who were undergoing oxygen therapy.[11] It was hoped that by controlling the arterial partial pressure of oxygen ($Pa{O_2}$), one would be able to provide the infant with sufficient oxygen and at the same time prevent excessive oxygen use causing the retinopathy. At this time also, frequent monitoring of the premature infants' retinal vasculature by an ophthalmologist was advocated in an attempt to identify those infants who were receiving excessive oxygen by observing the appearance of their retinal blood vessels.[12] The hope that ROP could be prevented by such careful monitoring was unfortunately not borne out. In the mid-1970s, a cooperative study involving a large number of newborn intensive care nurseries failed to correlate the $Pa{O_2}$ levels with the development of ROP. The duration of time in oxygen was correlated with the development of retinopathy, but neither levels nor fluctuations in the $Pa{O_2}$ could be correlated with the disease. The strongest correlations were with low birth weight and short gestational age.[13] Even with continuous transcutaneous monitoring of premature infants' oxygen, only very recently has some correlation been demonstrated between the patients' general state of oxygenation and the development of the disease.[14] The number of infants with serious vision loss due to ROP had increased by 1981,[15] probably because of the increased survival of very low birth weight infants.[16] The rest of the chapter deals with the continuing developments.

PATHOGENESIS

Understanding the *pathogenesis* of ROP depends on understanding the normal growth of retinal blood vessels in the human fetus. The normal retinal vasculature begins growing out of the optic nerve during the fourth month of gestation and reaches the ora serrata near term. Vascularization is probably complete some time between 38[18] and 40 wk,[19] although there is some evidence that remodeling may continue for several months post term.[20] The vessels grow by means of mesenchymal proliferation. In the most peripheral part of the wave of advancing vascularization, there are primitive spindle-shaped mesenchymal cells called the vanguard. Immediately behind the vanguard is a zone of mesenchymal cells that have differentiated into endothelial cells called the rearguard. These endothelial cells coalesce into solid cords that ultimately develop lumens, becoming a syncytium of primitive capillaries.[21] There is some controversy about whether the vanguard cells grow out from the optic disc or whether they are present throughout the primitive avascular retina as angioblasts.[22] The evidence for the latter view comes from experimental studies with beagle puppies,[22] but the authors draw parallels with human retinal angiogenesis.[23] Other investigators present evidence that these spindle cells, or vanguard cells, grow from the hyaloid artery and migrate outward.[19, 24] Since in humans the spindle cells reach the ora serrata by 29 wk of gestational age[24] and the mature blood vessels only reach the ora serrata near 40 weeks, it seems unlikely that preexisting angioblasts play a role in the development of human retinal vasculature.

When an infant is born prematurely, the blood vessels may continue to grow out normally as they would have in utero. In fact, in our group of 3400 high-risk premature infants (see later) examined since 1975 in the nurseries of the Joint Program in Neonatology at Harvard, 85 percent of the high-risk infants' retinas were vascularized normally on clinical examination. This agrees well with estimates of the cumulative incidence of acute ROP between 10 and 16 percent.[16, 25, 26]

Unfortunately, in many premature infants, the blood vessels do not continue growing normally but are arrested in their progress toward the peripheral retina. The vessels may then resume normal growth out to the periphery of the retina after a period of time, frequently leaving no sign of abnormality. Of the 11 percent of our patients in the Joint Program in Neonatology from 1975 to 1984 who had ROP, 62 percent experienced complete resolution with minimal or no signs of retinal abnormalities on follow-up (Table 224–1). The patients whose vascularization resumes in a normal fashion and are left with no permanent abnormalities are those who never progress beyond stage 1 or stage 2 ROP. The classification is later described in detail. The pattern of changes and regression were described and documented clinically by Flynn and associates in a seminal paper in 1977.[27] The authors described the changes in the progression of ROP as passing from the normal immature retina in which there is an almost imperceptible transition from vascularized to avascular peripheral retina through the early acute changes of ROP to ultimate spontaneous regression or progression to cicatricial ROP. The first sign of this disease the authors identified was the development of a sharp dividing line between the vascularized and avascular retina. Then, a widened and elevated structure between vascular and avascular retina, which they identified as an arteriovenous shunt, consisting of primitive vascular channels developed. They documented this shunting with fluorescein angiography. They hypothesized that mesenchyme of the advancing vascularization was piling up and that the vascular channels were lined with primitive endothelium, accounting for the leakage of fluorescein that the elevated tissue exhibited. They described an avascular zone just posterior to the shunt and dilatation and tortuosity of the arteries and veins connected to the shunt, suggesting that the shunt was of a high-flow type. Once the shunt was developed, either the vessels could bud off the anterior edge and normally vascularize the more peripheral retina, leading to regression, or cicatrization could occur. Their diagrammatic representation of these processes is reproduced in Figure 224–1. Associated with the acute changes of ROP may be small tufts of neovascularization and other microvascular abnormalities posterior to the elevated ridge. If a large amount of cicatricial tissue is formed, it exerts traction on the retina and, in the mildest degree, distorts the posterior retina somewhat or, in the worst case, progresses to retinal detachment and blindness. The section on classification, based on the stages in these abnormalities, follows later in the chapter. It presents changes in retinal blood vessel growth in more detail and puts them in clinical perspective.

As previously mentioned, innumerable *etiologic factors* have been proposed for the development of retinopathy in premature infants. This section highlights the currently known correlations between abnormalities occurring in these infants and the retinopathy as well as current hypotheses about its etiology. In our series of patients at the Harvard Joint Program in Neonatology, the only correlations that could be established with ROP were low birth weight, short gestational age, length of time in oxygen, and length of time on a mechanical ventilator (Table 224–2). No correlation could be established with levels of Pa_{O_2}, either when intermittent determinations were obtained in the early years of study or later when oxygen levels were measured by continuous transcutaneous monitoring. These findings agree with the large cooperative study reported in 1977 by Kinsey and colleagues.[13] Lucey and Dangman reviewed several cases of ROP developing in infants not exposed to supplemental oxygen and concluded that although

Table 224–1. RETINOPATHY OF PREMATURITY, JOINT PROGRAM IN NEONATOLOGY, HARVARD 1975–1990

	1975–1984	1985–1988	1989–1990	Total
Number of high-risk* infants examined	1998	981	439	3418
Number of infants with retinopathy of prematurity (ROP)	221	208	79	508
Percentage of high-risk infants developing ROP	11%	21%	18%	15%
ROP infants with complete follow-up	182	184	53	419
Unfavorable outcomes†	6	13	5	24
Percentage of ROP infants with unfavorable outcomes	3.6%	7.0%	9.4%	5.7%
Percentage of high-risk infants with unfavorable outcomes	0.3%	1.3%	1.1%	0.7%

*See text.
†Retinal detachment or retinal fold involving the macula.

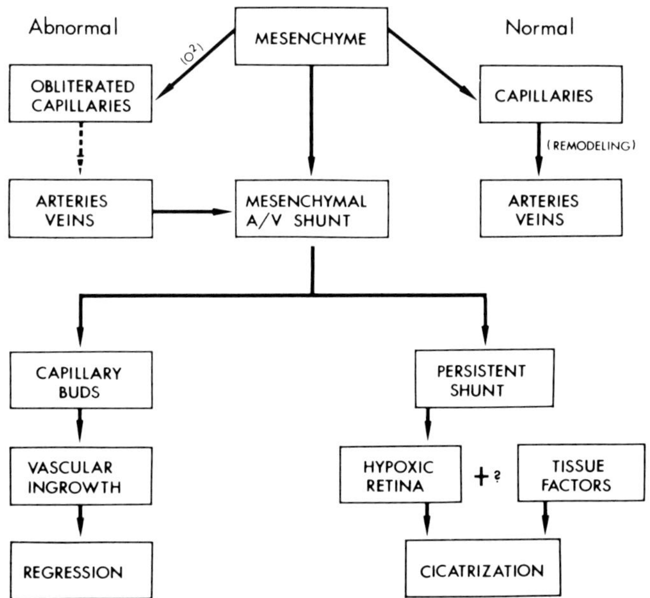

Figure 224–1. Diagrammatic representation of acute retinopathy of prematurity. (From Flynn, JT, O'Grady GE, Herrera J, et al: Retrolental fibroplasia. I: Clinical observations. Arch Ophthalmol 95:222, 1977. Copyright 1977, American Medical Association.)

oxygen and immaturity are important, other factors probably contribute to the development of this retinopathy.[28] Modern practice in newborn intensive care nurseries monitors and controls oxygen extremely carefully, and it seems unlikely that further attempts at reducing ROP by closer control of oxygen therapy will bear fruit.

Many other correlations with ROP have been reported, including hypoxia, hypoxia alternating with hyperoxia, transfusions, intraventricular hemorrhage, apnea, sepsis, hypercarbia and hypocarbia, patent ductus arteriosus, prostaglandin derangements, acidosis, xanthine administration, bronchopulmonary dysplasia, anemia, pneumothorax, perinatal asphyxia, and prolonged parenteral nutrition.[28–31] Since most of these factors are indicators of a very sick premature infant or are related to therapy for various abnormalities in the premature infant, it is tempting to suggest that since ROP occurs in sick premature infants, it is not surprising that changes associated with the severity of illness would also be associated with ROP and that there need not be a direct cause-and-effect relationship. An example of the difficulty in sorting out factors that might be responsible for this retinopathy is the role of methylated xanthines. Since aminophylline and theophylline are used to treat apnea and both the abnormality and the treatment are positively correlated with ROP, it is impossible to decide which, if either, may be an etiologic factor.[30] Another example is the occurrence of maternal bleeding at the time of birth, anemia, and blood transfusions; all three can be positively correlated with the development of ROP.[30] Since an infant who is born after a pregnancy complicated by blood loss, usually from placenta previa, is anemic and requires blood transfusions, it is impossible to decide which of these factors, if any, may be most important in causing ROP.

Two factors that have aroused great interest are vitamin E deficiency and excessive light exposure. These are examined in detail. Vitamin E was suggested as a way of preventing severe ROP in 1949.[32] Since shortly thereafter, it was thought that the problem of ROP had been solved by oxygen restriction, there was little further interest in the role of vitamin E. With the resurgence of the disease, interest in vitamin E revived and in 1981 Hittner and colleagues[33] presented the results of a masked controlled trial that demonstrated a statistically significant decrease in severe ROP in the treated infants as opposed to the controls. Kretzer, Hittner, and their coworkers have incorporated the role of vitamin E into a unified theory for the etiology of ROP.[24, 34, 35] According to their theory, as mentioned earlier in this section, the mesenchymal spindle cells grow out centripetally from the optic disc and gradually become differentiated into cords of endothelial cells that become canalized as blood vessels in the relatively hypoxic intrauterine environment. A sudden increase in tissue oxygen may damage the spindle cells, causing formation of extensive gap junctions between them and interfering with further migration and differentiation into endothelial cells. Vitamin E, by its antioxidant action, may remove the oxygen free radicals that are damaging the spindle cells. The damaged spindle cells may release humoral agents that stimulate neovascularization—that is, the fibrovascular growth of severe ROP, which might explain why retinal cryotherapy in the avascular zone is effective in reducing the severity of advanced ROP. This therapy is described in detail under Treatment.

Recent studies on the effect of excessive light in newborn nurseries have suggested that it may have a role in increasing the incidence of ROP.[36, 37] It is of note that serendipitously, because of the belief by our child development consultants that overstimulation of the premature infant is detrimental,[38] our nurseries in the Joint Program of Neonatology are dimly lighted. This is a possible explanation for our reduced incidence of

Table 224–2. RELATIONSHIP OF BIRTH WEIGHT, GESTATIONAL AGE, AND DURATION OF OXYGEN THERAPY AND MECHANICAL VENTILATION TO RETINOPATHY OF PREMATURITY

	Normal Eyes		All Infants With ROP	
	1975–88	*1989–90*	*1975–88*	*1989–90*
Birth weight (g)	1862	1172	1058	884
Gestational age (wk)	32.7	27.5	29	26
Duration of oxygen therapy (days)	12	22	64	55
Duration of mechanical ventilation (days)	6	14	38	34

ROP = retinopathy of prematurity.

unfavorable outcomes as compared with North America as a whole (see Table 224–1).[15] To date, we have not been able to identify other factors accounting for this difference.

EXAMINATION

Examination of the premature infant for ROP depends on an organized system so that information will be useful for follow-up examinations and for communication with other physicians about the findings. It is clearly a prerequisite for evaluation of any treatment that might be proposed. Reese and associates, in 1953, before the modern binocular indirect ophthalmoscope was in general use, developed a classification of retrolental fibroplasia.[39] As better examinations could be done, more useful classifications were proposed.[40–44] Because these classifications were not universally accepted and because they mostly described only the severity of the ROP and not its location or extent, an international committee of ophthalmologists interested in the disease met at the National Eye Institute in Bethesda, Maryland, and agreed on an international classification of ROP.[45, 46] Later, a similar committee met to subclassify the more advanced stages of ROP.[47]

In this classification, the stages of severity are *stage 1*, which consists of a distinct border between the vascularized retina and the peripheral avascular retina. In the normal premature retina, the vascular retina blends imperceptibly into the more peripheral avascular retina. The demarcation line found in stage 1 is illustrated in Figure 224–2. The character of the retina changes abruptly at this demarcation line from the pinkish, translucent vascularized retina to the whitish, grayish, more opaque peripheral retina.

In *stage 2*, a ridge that has volume develops at the demarcation line, so that one can clearly see both height and width on examination with the binocular indirect ophthalmoscope. This structure corresponds to the milder form of the "mesenchymal shelf" described earlier by Flynn.[27] Stage 2 is illustrated in Figure 224–3. At this point, there is no actual neovascularization in the area of the ridge, although innocuous neovascular tufts can be seen posterior to the ridge.

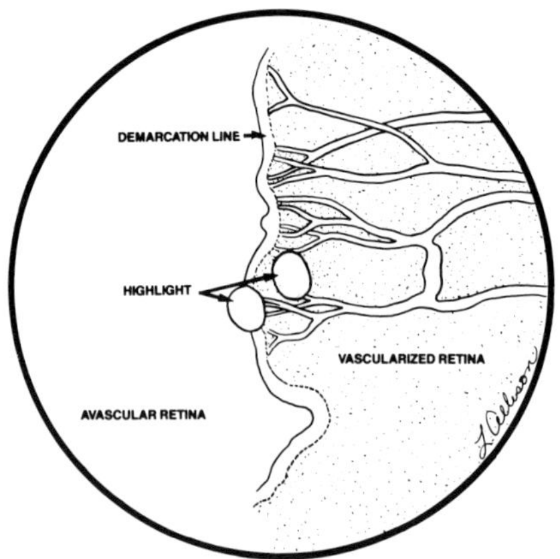

Figure 224–2. Stage 1 retinopathy of prematurity. (From The Committee for Classification of Retinopathy of Prematurity: An international classification of retinopathy of prematurity. Arch Ophthalmol 102:1131, 1984. Copyright 1984, American Medical Association.)

Stage 3 is characterized by extraretinal fibrovascular proliferation coming from the ridge. The first sign of this usually is a ragged or scalloped appearance of the posterior edge of the ridge rather than the smooth appearance seen in stage 2 (Fig. 224–4). As the extent of proliferation of extraretinal fibrovascular tissue increases, stage 3 may be subdivided into mild, moderate, and severe (Fig. 224–5). In most cases, all these stages of acute ROP are associated with excessive numbers of dilated peripheral retinal blood vessels just behind the line, or ridge. If dilatation and tortuosity of vessels in the posterior pole of the eye occurs, which is an indication of activity and possible progression, a *plus* is added to the number of the stage. As appears later, in Treatment, identification of the stage of disease, including any *plus* disease, is important in determining the indications for retinal cryotherapy. Up to this point, the retina has remained completely attached.

Stages 4 and 5 describe degrees of severity of retinal detachment.[47] *Stage 4A* describes a partial retinal detachment that does not involve the macula. This is usually a traction detachment that has a concave appearance in the periphery of the retina and may be limited to a small area or may involve the entire circumference of the retina. Figure 224–6 shows such a periph-

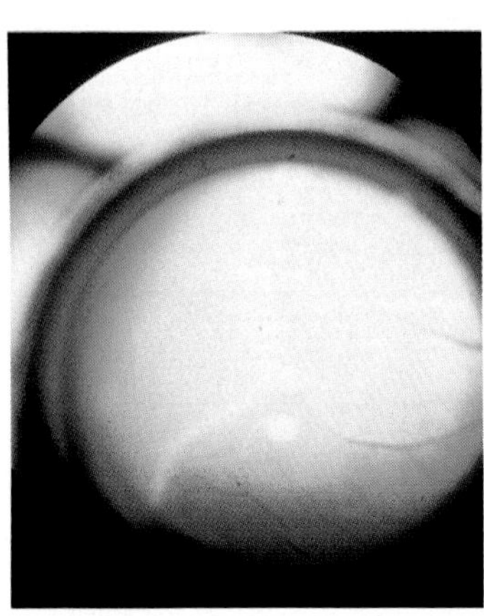

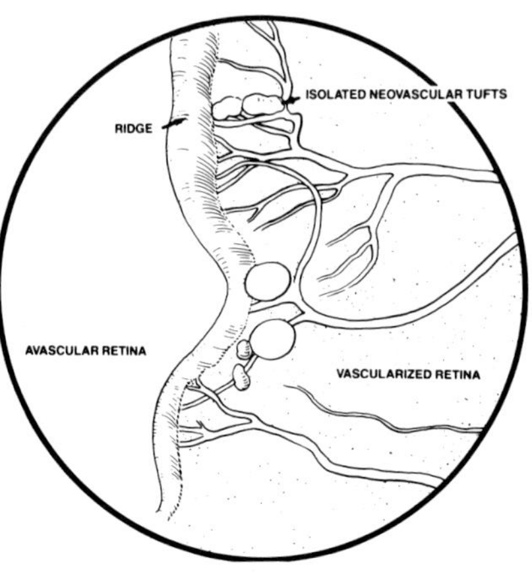

Figure 224–3. Stage 2 retinopathy of prematurity. (From The Committee for Classification of Retinopathy of Prematurity: An international classification of retinopathy of prematurity. Arch Ophthalmol 102:1131, 1984. Copyright 1984, American Medical Association.)

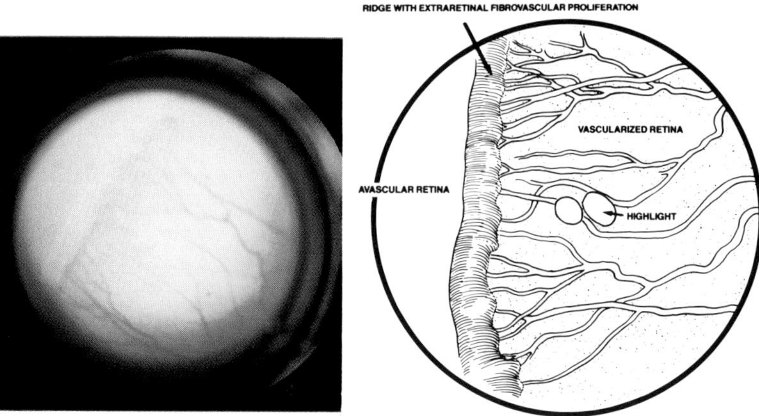

Figure 224–4. Stage 3 retinopathy of prematurity. (From The Committee for Classification of Retinopathy of Prematurity: An international classification of retinopathy of prematurity. Arch Ophthalmol 102:1132, 1984. Copyright 1984, American Medical Association.)

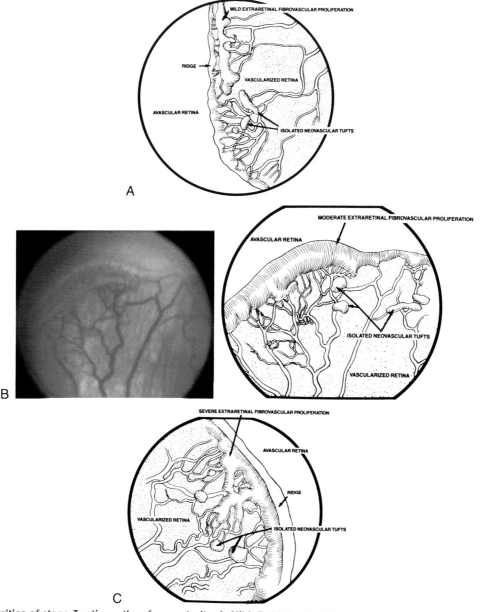

Figure 224–5. Severities of stage 3 retinopathy of prematurity: *A,* Mild; *B,* Moderate; *C,* Severe. (From The Committee for Classification of Retinopathy of Prematurity: An international classification of retinopathy of prematurity. Arch Ophthalmol 102:1134, 1984. Copyright 1984, American Medical Association.)

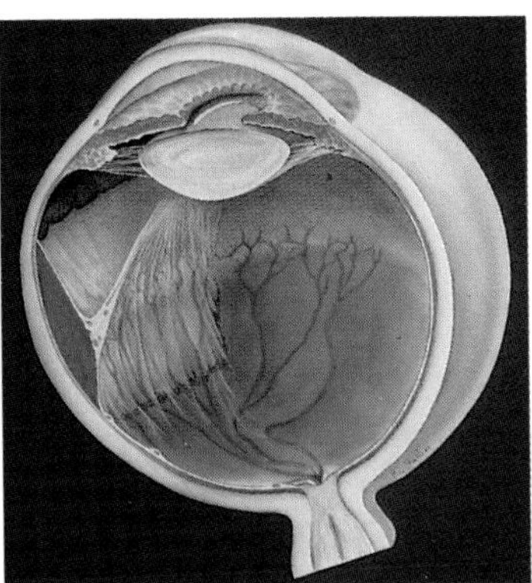

Figure 224–6. Peripheral retinal detachment in stage 4A retinopathy of prematurity. (From The International Committee for the Classification of the Late Stages of Retinopathy of Prematurity: An international classification of retinopathy of prematurity. II. The classification of retinal detachment. Arch Ophthalmol 105:906–912, 1987. Copyright 1987, American Medical Association.)

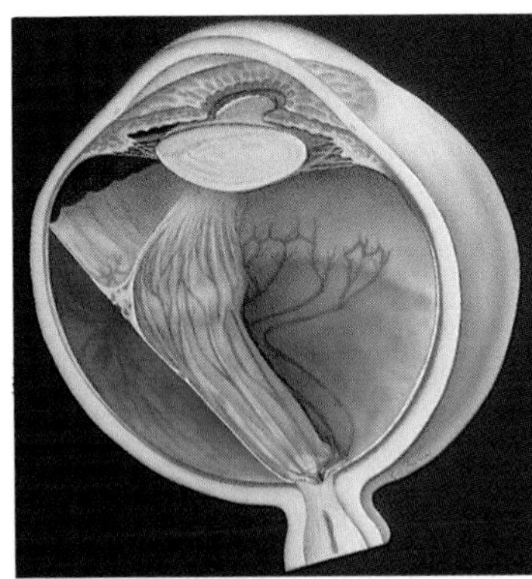

Figure 224–8. Partial retinal detachment involving the macula in stage 4B retinopathy of prematurity. (From The International Committee for the Classification of the Late Stages of Retinopathy of Prematurity: An international classification of retinopathy of prematurity. II. The classification of retinal detachment. Arch Ophthalmol 105:906–912, 1987. Copyright 1987, American Medical Association.)

eral retinal detachment. The traction may distort the posterior retina, leading to straightening and, usually, temporal displacement of the retinal vessels, and sometimes temporal displacement of the macula (Fig. 224–7). *Stage 4B* describes a partial retinal detachment involving the macula, demonstrated in Figure 224–8. Figure 224–9 shows the chronic appearance of a patient with stage 4B ROP. It can be seen that the final outcome of stage 4A may be favorable for vision, but this is not true for stage 4B when a retinal fold goes through the macula.

Stage 5 describes a total retinal detachment that forms a funnel-shaped structure, either open or closed (Fig. 224–10).[47, 48] These anatomic differences in the configuration of the retinal detachment are important from the point of view of treatment by vitreoretinal surgery (see Chap. 57).

It is important to recognize that ROP may regress at almost any stage in its development, although once retinal detachment has occurred, the prognosis for spontaneous regression with maintenance of good visual acuity is obviously reduced. We have seen two infants who had what appeared to be serous or exudative detachments. They were convex and bullous rather than concave, as are traction detachments, with fluid that shifted under the retina. Both detachments spontaneously reattached after several weeks, and both patients ended with abnormal retinal pigmentation but good visual acuity. One of them, now seventeen years old, has maintained visual acuity of 20/60 in her better eye with a correction for high myopia. The other was able to maintain steady fixation and following when, still a toddler, she was lost to follow-up.

The unique and extraordinarily useful aspect of the international classification of ROP is its ability to describe the location and extent of the disease. The retina is divided into three zones concentric with the disc. Zone 1 has a radius twice the distance from the disc to the macula. Zone 2 extends to the ora serrata nasally and just anterior to the equator on the temporal side. Zone 3 is a superior, temporal, and inferior crescent of the remaining retina. Each retina is also divided into clock hours. One can thus describe the location and extent of the disease on a simple diagram (Fig. 224–11). A more detailed examination record proposed by the committee for classification[47] is shown in Figure 224–12. As can be seen later under Treatment, the international classification of ROP was indispensible for determining the need for treatment, recording the treatment provided, and evaluating the effects of treatment in the study of cryotherapy for ROP.[49]

There are reports of patients who develop ROP earlier

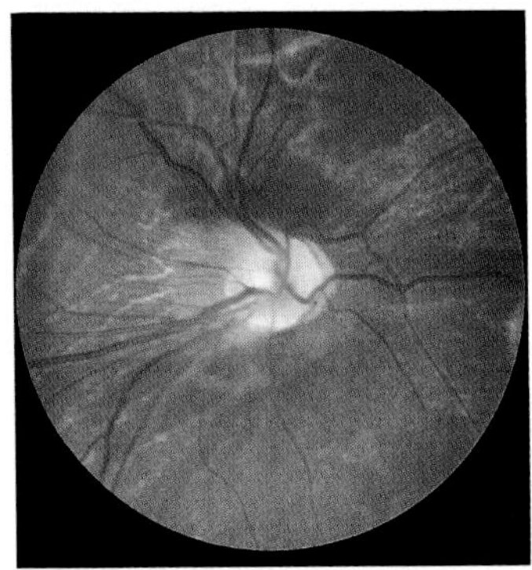

Figure 224–7. Temporal traction of retina in cicatricial retinopathy of prematurity.

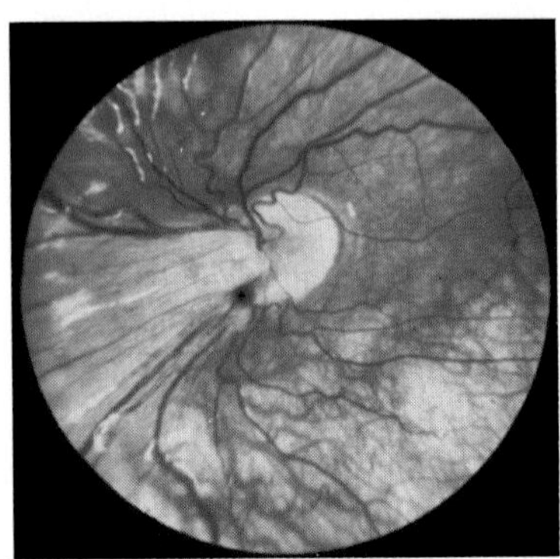

Figure 224–9. Fixed fold of detached retina in cicatricial stage 4B retinopathy of prematurity.

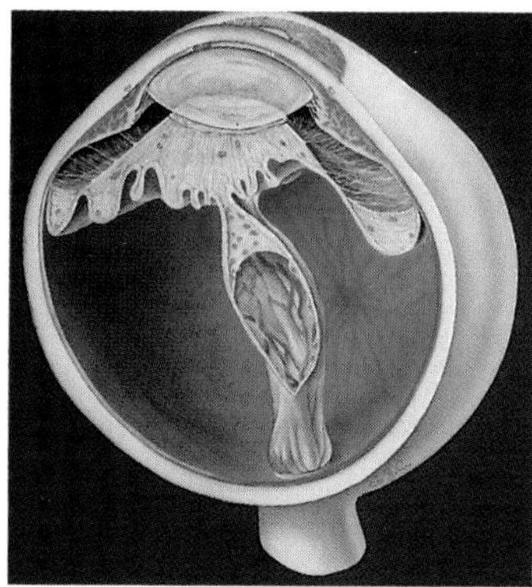

Figure 224–10. Stage 5 retinopathy of prematurity: closed funnel. (From Machemer R: Description and pathogenesis of late stage of retinopathy of prematurity. *In* Flynn JT, Phelps DL (eds): Retinopathy of Prematurity: Problem and Challenge. New York, Alan R. Liss, Inc, 1988, pp 275–280.)

than is typical (at age 3 to 5 wk). These patients have an extremely low birth weight (< 1000 g). Some of these patients progress rapidly to severe ROP and retinal detachment. This unusually aggressive pattern of ROP, usually occurring in zone 1, has been termed *rush disease*.[42, 50]

Since ROP occurs mainly in very premature infants, it is not necessary to examine all prematures. From 1975 through 1987, our criteria for examination included all infants with a birth weight of 1500 g or less, a gestational age of 32 wk or less, or those who had received oxygen or mechanical ventilation for four hours or longer. In 1988 because almost no infants in our nurseries who weighed more than 1250 g at birth had developed significant ROP, we began examining only infants who weighed less than 1250 g. Larger infants are examined if they have required oxygen or mechanical ventilation for more than 2 wk or if the neonatologists judge that they have been severely ill. Since 1988 we have seen one infant weighing 1300 g who developed stage 3+ ROP and required cryotherapy. All the others have weighed less than 1250 g. It must be pointed out that most centers use 1500 g birth weight as a cutoff for

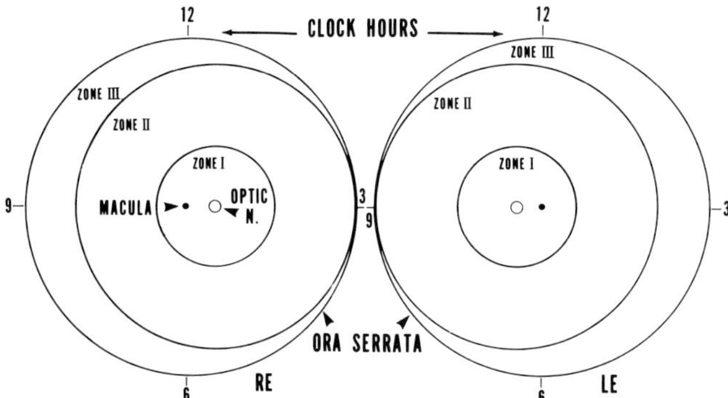

Figure 224–11. Retinal diagram for recording location and extent of retinopathy of prematurity. (From The Committee for Classification of Retinopathy of Prematurity: An international classification of retinopathy of prematurity. Arch Ophthalmol 102:1131, 1984. Copyright 1984, American Medical Association.)

examination. In a survey performed by Charles,[51] of 48 centers responding to his survey, 15 used 1500 g birth weight as the cutoff, and only two used 1250 g. Two centers actually examined all infants with birth weights of less than 2500 g. Thus although some centers routinely examine all infants who are born weighing 1500 g or less, it seems to us reasonable to use the 1250-g birth weight cutoff of the multicenter trial of cryotherapy for ROP,[49] which is discussed later in this chapter.

The criteria of the multicenter trial are appropriate for determining the timing and frequency of examination.[49] The first eye examination should be at age 4 to 5 wk if the infant is well enough to tolerate it, or as soon thereafter as possible. If no active retinopathy of prematurity is found, the infant should be examined every 2 to 3 wk until the retinal vessels reach the ora serrata. When ROP is present, follow-up examinations should be more frequent, consistent with the severity. If the retinopathy is resolving spontaneously, less frequent examinations may be indicated, with the caution that the disease may begin to worsen again. For the purposes of the study, regular examinations were continued on patients who never had ROP or in whom the disease had resolved completely spontaneously. This does not seem necessary in clinical practice, and our custom, once a completely normal eye examination has been obtained, is to have the patient return at 2 to 3 yr of age unless other ophthalmologic abnormalities are noted before then. More frequent follow-up is indicated if there are complications of ROP, such as myopia. The risk of late rhegmatogenous retinal detachment in patients with regressed ROP[52] mandates that patients be followed indefinitely if there are any cicatricial changes.

Patients with ROP, and, indeed all severely premature infants, should be followed ophthalmologically. Patients with regressed ROP as well as premature infants who never had any sign of the disease have a much higher incidence of ophthalmologic problems than the general population, although such problems seem to be more prevalent in patients with regressed ROP than in those without the disease. The ophthalmologic problems include strabismus, amblyopia, myopia and other refractive errors, and decreased visual acuity of unknown cause.[53–56] Sometimes macular distortion from peripheral retinal scarring reduces the visual acuity, but in some patients with macular ectopia from ROP the visual acuity is normal. Patients who have been successfully treated with cryotherapy for ROP without macular ectopia may suffer decreased visual acuity and structural changes in the macula visible both clinically and pathologically. Hittner and coworkers[57] have postulated that retinal cryotherapy stops the differentiation of the macula. Although the treatment may prevent the more devastating complications of advanced ROP, it may also prevent the macula from developing and thereby may adversely affect central vision. This is a problem especially in zone 1 ROP, as cryotherapy may be required before macular development is complete (see also Prognosis.)

Our examination technique is to dilate the infant's pupils beforehand and to examine the fundi out to the ends of the retinal blood vessels with a binocular indirect

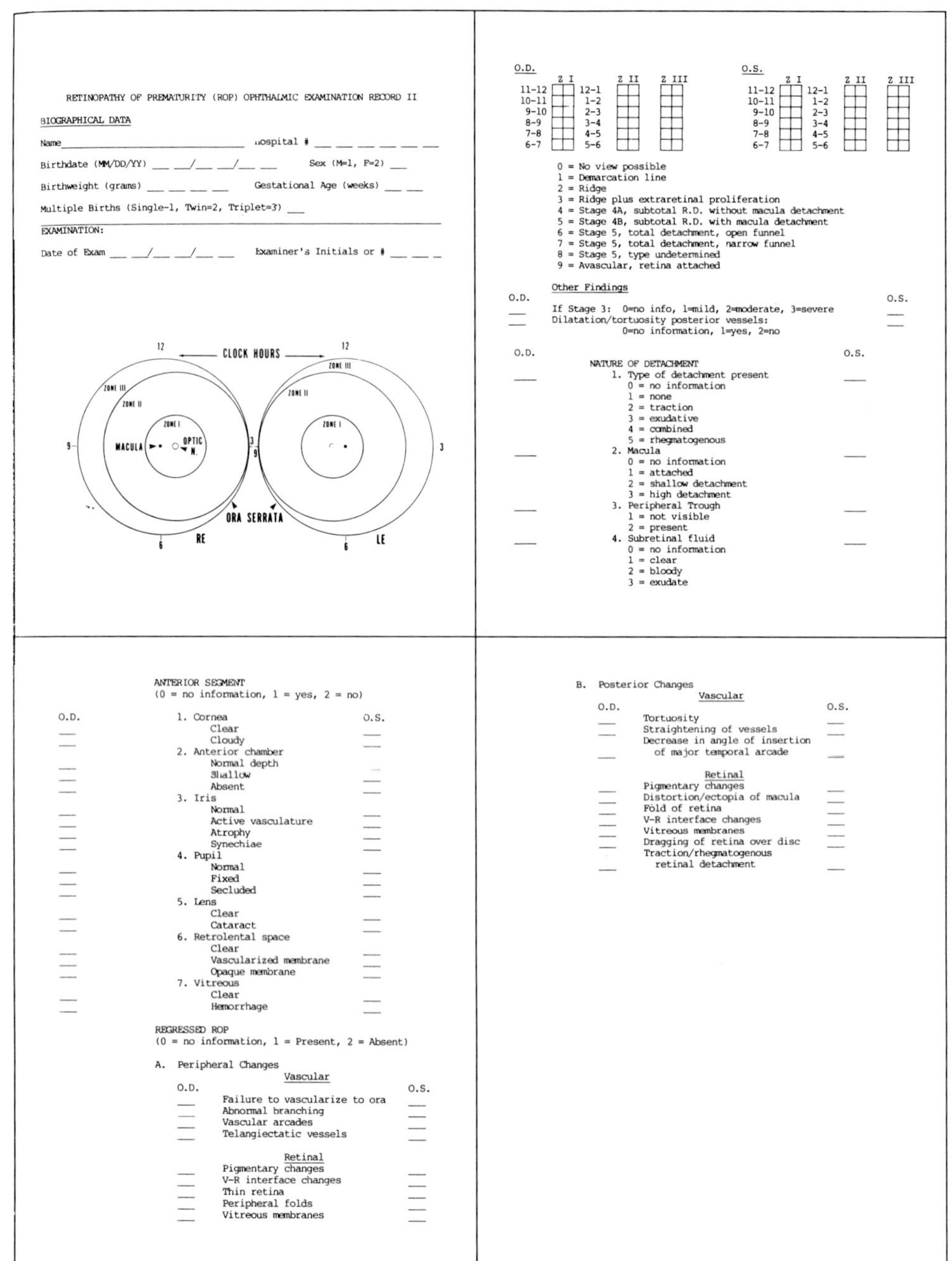

RETINOPATHY OF PREMATURITY (ROP) OPHTHALMIC EXAMINATION RECORD II

BIOGRAPHICAL DATA

Name ______________________ Hospital # __ __ __ __ __ __

Birthdate (MM/DD/YY) __ __/__ __/__ __ Sex (M=1, F=2) __

Birthweight (grams) __ __ __ __ Gestational Age (weeks) __ __

Multiple Births (Single-1, Twin=2, Triplet=3) __

EXAMINATION:

Date of Exam __ __/__ __/__ __ Examiner's Initials or # __ __ __

O.D.

	Z I		Z II	Z III
11-12	☐☐	12-1	☐☐	☐☐
10-11	☐☐	1-2	☐☐	☐☐
9-10	☐☐	2-3	☐☐	☐☐
8-9	☐☐	3-4	☐☐	☐☐
7-8	☐☐	4-5	☐☐	☐☐
6-7	☐☐	5-6	☐☐	☐☐

O.S.

	Z I		Z II	Z III
11-12	☐☐	12-1	☐☐	☐☐
10-11	☐☐	1-2	☐☐	☐☐
9-10	☐☐	2-3	☐☐	☐☐
8-9	☐☐	3-4	☐☐	☐☐
7-8	☐☐	4-5	☐☐	☐☐
6-7	☐☐	5-6	☐☐	☐☐

0 = No view possible
1 = Demarcation line
2 = Ridge
3 = Ridge plus extraretinal proliferation
4 = Stage 4A, subtotal R.D. without macula detachment
5 = Stage 4B, subtotal R.D. with macula detachment
6 = Stage 5, total detachment, open funnel
7 = Stage 5, total detachment, narrow funnel
8 = Stage 5, type undetermined
9 = Avascular, retina attached

Other Findings

O.D. / O.S.

__ If Stage 3: 0=no info, 1=mild, 2=moderate, 3=severe __
__ Dilatation/tortuosity posterior vessels: __
0=no information, 1=yes, 2=no

O.D. / O.S.

NATURE OF DETACHMENT

__ 1. Type of detachment present __
0 = no information
1 = none
2 = traction
3 = exudative
4 = combined
5 = rhegmatogenous

__ 2. Macula __
0 = no information
1 = attached
2 = shallow detachment
3 = high detachment

__ 3. Peripheral Trough __
1 = not visible
2 = present

__ 4. Subretinal fluid __
0 = no information
1 = clear
2 = bloody
3 = exudate

ANTERIOR SEGMENT
(0 = no information, 1 = yes, 2 = no)

O.D. / O.S.

1. Cornea
__ Clear __
__ Cloudy __
2. Anterior chamber
__ Normal depth __
__ Shallow __
__ Absent __
3. Iris
__ Normal __
__ Active vasculature __
__ Atrophy __
__ Synechiae __
4. Pupil
__ Normal __
__ Fixed __
__ Secluded __
5. Lens
__ Clear __
__ Cataract __
6. Retrolental space
__ Clear __
__ Vascularized membrane __
__ Opaque membrane __
7. Vitreous
__ Clear __
__ Hemorrhage __

REGRESSED ROP
(0 = no information, 1 = Present, 2 = Absent)

A. Peripheral Changes

Vascular

O.D. / O.S.

__ Failure to vascularize to ora __
__ Abnormal branching __
__ Vascular arcades __
__ Telangiectatic vessels __

Retinal

__ Pigmentary changes __
__ V-R interface changes __
__ Thin retina __
__ Peripheral folds __
__ Vitreous membranes __

B. Posterior Changes

Vascular

O.D. / O.S.

__ Tortuosity __
__ Straightening of vessels __
__ Decrease in angle of insertion of major temporal arcade __

Retinal

__ Pigmentary changes __
__ Distortion/ectopia of macula __
__ Fold of retina __
__ V-R interface changes __
__ Vitreous membranes __
__ Dragging of retina over disc __
__ Traction/rhegmatogenous retinal detachment __

Figure 224–12. Detailed examination record for retinopathy of prematurity. (From The International Committee for the Classification of the Late Stages of Retinopathy of Prematurity: An international classification of retinopathy of prematurity. II. The classification of retinal detachment. Arch Ophthalmol 105:906–912, 1987. Copyright 1987, American Medical Association.)

ophthalmoscope and a 20-diopter condensing lens. A lid speculum (Sauer, Stortz) is often necessary, and scleral depression is occasionally required. The patient's hands may be restrained by a nurse or by swaddling.

A word should be said about sporadic reports of toxicity from drops used to dilate the pupils.[58–60] One percent cyclopentolate (Cyclogyl) and 2.5 percent phenylephrine have both been implicated in toxicity. The 2.5 percent phenylephrine has been reported to have caused elevated blood pressure with the danger of intracranial hemorrhage,[58] and Cyclogyl is reported to have caused ileus with the possible consequence of necrotizing enterocolitis.[59] At the Joint Program in Neonatology, we use one drop of 1 percent Cyclogyl in each eye, repeated in 2 min, and use phenylephrine 2.5 percent only in those rare instances when the pupils are not adequately dilated with Cyclogyl alone. We have had no instance of toxicity from eye drops in examinations of more than 3400 infants, in many instances with repeated examinations. In our hands, Cyclomydril (0.1 percent cyclopentolate with 1 percent phenylephrine) has not reliably dilated premature infants' pupils.

TREATMENT

Until recently ROP was considered an untreatable disease. As mentioned earlier, its prevention was accomplished by severe restriction of oxygen therapy to premature infants. A large part of the success of this severe restriction of oxygen therapy was due to the increased mortality of infants who were at risk of developing ROP. The marked reduction in cases of severe ROP came at the expense of increased mortality and increased neurologic damage in prematures. By the time these problems were recognized, arterial blood gas determinations had become readily available, and it was hoped that by controlling PaO_2, the adverse effects of hypoxia could be avoided while also controlling the incidence of the disease. As we have seen earlier, this hope proved false. Other means of prevention or treatment seemed to be necessary.

Vitamin E

As already noted, there is evidence that vitamin E, given within the first day of life in dosage to bring blood levels to adult physiologic concentration, may reduce the severity of ROP.[33] The preterm infant is deficient in the antioxidant vitamin E at birth, with plasma levels of 0.4 mg/dl compared with 1 to 3 mg/dl in the adult. There is evidence that vitamin E supplementation might reduce the incidence of severe ROP. However, controversy over the efficacy of vitamin E supplementation has continued over the past decade.

In 1981 Hittner and colleagues[33] published a double-blind, controlled study that investigated the efficacy of vitamin E in preventing ROP in preterm infants. In that study, low doses or oral vitamin E brought the plasma level up to adult levels of 1.2 mg/dl. A statistically significant decrease in the incidence of severe ROP occurred in the treated infants. The study was supported by ultrastructural evidence that spindle cells in the retinas of treated infants did not develop the extensive gap junction linkages seen in eyes of the control group.[23, 61] Two other controlled clinical trials showed statistically significant efficacy of vitamin E in preventing ROP when given continuously from the first day of life.[62, 63] Finer and coworkers' study[62, 64] used oral and IM supplementation. The study by Johnson and associates[63] had a high target plasma level of 5 mg/dl and was thus complicated by evidence of vitamin E toxicity.

Three controlled clinical trials have failed to show efficacy of vitamin E, but each was flawed in its design or execution. In one study, the control group received supplemental vitamin E to a therapeutic level of 1.1 mg/dl.[65] In another, vitamin E was discontinued in the treated group after only 6 wk.[66] In the third study,[67] very high doses of vitamin E were given by rapid IV infusion, which increases the toxicity of the vitamin and delays the retinal uptake. Therapy was not continuous in many treated infants.[68]

Vitamin E does not eliminate ROP from the neonatal intensive care unit. However, a decrease in the incidence of severe cases has been observed in three properly conducted studies. In 1986 the Institute of Medicine of the National Academy of Sciences[69] concluded that there was no definite evidence of either benefit or harm from prophylaxis with vitamin E against ROP. They also concluded that the risks of giving vitamin E seemed minimal for premature infants as long as the blood concentration was kept below 3 mg/dl. As the controversy over vitamin E continues, multivitamin formulations in general use in neonatal intensive care units now contain sufficient vitamin E to maintain plasma levels close to the adult physiologic range. Combining these preparations with a single IM dose of 10 mg/kg α-tocopherol (in water) given within 24 hr of birth should be a safe and sufficient way to obtain the maximum benefit of vitamin E.[68, 70]

Control of Excessive Light

The suggestion that excessive light in the nurseries might cause ROP[36, 37] raises the possibility that the disease might be prevented by reducing the illumination in newborn intensive care nurseries. The common observation is that these nurseries are brightly illuminated day and night, presumably for the convenience of the staff and better observation of the infants.

Photocoagulation and Cryotherapy

Photocoagulation, and then cryotherapy, was first used to treat severe ROP in Japan beginning in the late 1960s.[71, 72] Because the media was frequently hazy in patients with this severe retinopathy, photocoagulation was difficult to perform, and cryotherapy seemed more effective. The initial intention was to close off the proliferating vessels in the fibrovascular tissue, but it was found that cryotherapy just anterior to the fibrovascular proliferation seemed more effective in controlling the disease. Ophthalmologists in Canada,[73, 74] Israel,[75] and Europe[76, 77] all reported good results from treating advanced ROP with cryotherapy. The experience in the United States was less favorable.[78, 79] All of these studies suffered from being anecdotal, poorly controlled, with inadequate sample sizes, or all three. In a disease that so commonly resolves spontaneously, only a well-controlled masked study with a large number of patients could demonstrate a statistical benefit from cryotherapy in severe ROP.

The *multicenter trial of cryotherapy* for ROP was begun in 1986. Twenty-three centers participated in the study. Premature infants weighing 1250 g or less who survived to 4 wk of age were invited to participate in the study. Initial examinations were done at 4 to 6 wk and then every 2 wk thereafter, unless the disease was extremely posterior or severe or was progressing, in which case these patients were examined more frequently. If ROP progressed to a threshold determined to be stage 3+ disease, which involved 5 contiguous clock hr or 8 intermittent clock hr, cryotherapy was offered to be given to one eye, determined by randomization if the disease was symmetrical. If only one eye reached threshold, then the patient was randomized either to treatment or to control group. Treatment consisted of contiguous single cryoapplications to the entire avascular zone of the retina of the treated eye. (Cryotherapy can usually be given transconjunctivally, but sometimes a conjunctival incision and isolation of extraocular muscles is necessary.) The fibrovascular ridge was not treated in order to avoid vitreous hemorrhage. The infants received a variety of anesthesias from topical to general. The patients were monitored continuously by a neonatologist or an anesthesiologist as was appropriate. The patients were reexamined a week after the cryotherapy, and if there were areas that had not received cryotherapy and the disease was progressing, further cryotherapy was used to fill in the untreated areas. At 3 mo after treatment, photographs of the posterior poles and anterior segments of both the control and the treated eye were sent to a reading center, where a masked observer looked for a retinal fold through the macula, a retinal detachment in the posterior pole, or retrolental tissue. It was statistically determined early in the study that there was a benefit from cryotherapy.[80] After 172 infants had completed the 3-mo evaluation following cryotherapy, it was found that there was approximately a 50 percent reduction in unfavorable outcomes—that is, 23.5% of the treated eyes had unfavorable outcomes as opposed to 45.6% of untreated eyes. The National Eye Institute sent a recommendation to all ophthalmologists likely to encounter premature infants that cryotherapy be offered to patients who had reached threshold disease, and publication of the preliminary results was expedited.[80] When a larger number of infants—260—could be evaluated at 3 mo, it was found that 31.1% of the treated eyes had unfavorable outcomes compared with 51.4% of untreated eyes.[49] The 1-yr follow-up of 246 patients who completed the 12-mo follow-up examination[81] indicated that this difference in outcomes was maintained and showed that 25.7% of treated eyes had an unfavorable outcome as opposed to 47.4% of untreated eyes. In addition, grating acuities, using the Teller acuity cards,[82] were obtained. These showed that treated eyes had an unfavorable visual outcome by this test in 35% of cases, whereas untreated eyes had an unfavorable visual outcome in 56% of cases. This demonstrates a striking benefit from cryotherapy in threshold ROP, even taking into account that the Teller acuity cards do not measure foveal visual acuity.[83] It should be mentioned that the threshold for cryotherapy for ROP used in the multicenter trial has been challenged[84] on the basis of more recent uncontrolled series of patients subjected to cryotherapy.[85–87] It has been advocated that patients with milder stage 3 disease should be treated and that better results are obtained when they are given such treatment. As mentioned before, in any disease subject to spontaneous remission, benefit from treatment must be demonstrated statistically in a controlled study. If one treats patients with milder ROP who would have regressed spontaneously, one is likely to increase the apparent cure rate. The milder the ROP, the better the outcome will be, either treated or untreated. The long-term effects of cryotherapy are not yet known, but already rhegmatogenous retinal detachments from tears at the edge of the cryotherapy scar have been reported.[88] It has been suggested that these tears may be due to the lack of adequate treatment up to the shunt to destroy myofibroblasts that subsequently induce traction.[89] Finally, eyes with zone 1 ROP that have reached threshold do not do well, with or without cryotherapy,[80, 90] and therefore the prognosis for such eyes should be extremely guarded. Unfortunately for our understanding of this problem, only 12 eyes (8%) in the multicenter cryotherapy trial had zone 1 ROP, and the zone 1 infants were grouped together with the larger number of zone 2 infants. Thus the decision about treating those infants cannot be based on current data. Until additional controlled studies are performed on zone 1 patients, the use of this form of treatment should be an individual decision made by the clinician and family.

When ROP progresses to stage 4 or 5, scleral buckling and vitrectomy may be of benefit. The treatment of retinal detachments in this disease is further discussed in the retina section (see Chap. 57).

The prognosis for vision in premature infants is generally good. Since 1975 at the Joint Program in Neonatology, 85% of high-risk infants have not developed any degree of ROP (see Table 224–1). Of those who developed the disease, the vast majority had good anatomic and presumably visual outcomes. Overall, 5 to 6 percent of the infants who developed ROP, or less than 1 percent of the high-risk infants who were examined, had unfavorable outcomes as defined by a retinal detachment or retinal fold involving the macula. Since 1985 the percentage of infants with unfavorable outcomes has increased slightly, so that in this period about 7 percent of patients who develop ROP, or a little over 1 percent of all high-risk infants, had unfavorable outcomes. There are two possible reasons for this increase. One is that smaller babies who are at risk of developing severe ROP are surviving in greater numbers now. In addition we reduced our criteria for examining babies from a birth weight of 1500 g or less to a birth weight of 1250 g or less in the beginning of 1989, so that we were examining babies at greater risk of developing ROP. Our experience over this 16-yr period is summarized in Table 224–2.

Fortunately, the vast majority of infants with ROP have mild disease that resolves spontaneously. Of 237 patients from 1985 to 1990 who had complete follow-up, 196 resolved completely to normal. Of these, 146 had never developed disease beyond stage 1. We began performing cryotherapy in 1988 after the results of the multicenter trial[80] had become known. Table 224–3 summarizes our experience during the period 1985 to 1990. It can be seen that even in the absence of treatment, most of the patients with severe ROP had a

Table 224–3. OUTCOME IN 237 PATIENTS WITH RETINOPATHY OF PREMATURITY WITH ADEQUATE FOLLOW-UP

	No Treatment			Cryotherapy (From 1988)
	Stage 1	*Stage 2*	*Stage 3 or 3+*	Stage 3+
Complete resolution	146	33	17	4
Peripheral scarring but favorable outcome,* both eyes	0	0	14	2
Favorable outcome,* one eye, poor† other eye	0	0	5	1
Poor outcome† both eyes	0	0	13	2

*Mild posterior pole distortion, myopia, or both but no retinal fold or detachment.
†Retinal fold or detachment involving the macula.

favorable outcome, although many have subnormal acuity with high myopia or mild posterior pole distortion. Since early 1988, all the patients who reached threshold for treatment[80] have been offered cryotherapy and all have accepted it and have elected to have both eyes treated. Our small experience (see Table 224–3) indicates a benefit from cryotherapy in agreement with the benefit in the multicenter trial.[80, 81] Only patients from our own nurseries are included in Table 224–3. We have not had as good results in the several patients who were referred to us from other intensive care nurseries. Most of them had extremely severe stage 3+, involving essentially the entire circumference of the retina by the time they arrived, and two even had retinal detachments by the time they were referred. The recommendations for frequent examinations with active ROP cannot be overemphasized.

PROGNOSIS AND COMPLICATIONS

Much of the emphasis on the morbidity of ROP is placed on the number of infants who are blind or suffer severe visual impairment. A much larger number of patients suffer less catastrophic complications that cause significant functional or cosmetic disability. Cats and Tan[53] found that 55 percent of patients with regressed ROP followed over 6 to 10 yr had ophthalmologic problems. These complications are not always considered in risk-benefit analyses when new treatments are introduced.[91] The most common nonneovascular complications are poor acuity, myopia, strabismus, and amblyopia.

Visual Acuity

Visual acuity is difficult to study in ROP because many years elapse between the time of disease onset and the time the child is mature enough for accurate measurement of vision. The refinement of acuity card procedures may allow earlier and more accurate assessment of visual acuity in these infants[82] Unfortunately, this procedure does not grade macular acuity.[83]

Children who have only moderate changes in the retinal periphery from ROP often have poor acuity. The mechanism behind this is not understood, although myopia appears to be associated with the poor vision. Biglan and coworkers[92] found that 33 percent of infants with advanced disease had less than 20/200 vision in their better eye. Twenty-six percent of stage 3 eyes had this level of acuity. Macular dragging was a frequent cause of decreased acuity.

Tasman and Brown[93] recently presented two disturbing cases of patients with mild to moderate sequelae of ROP who developed unexplained visual loss to 20/400 or worse years after the acute phase of the disease. Such case reports suggest that the long-term consequences of ROP may be underestimated.

Strabismus and Amblyopia

Strabismus and amblyopia are commonly observed residual complications of ROP. The reported incidence of strabismus ranges from 23 to 47 percent of infants with ROP, compared with 10 to 20 percent of premature infants who do not develop it.[53] Approximately one half of these patients are amblyopic.[92, 94] Management of these conditions is complicated by the asymmetric potential acuity of the two eyes, by nystagmus, and by very high refractive errors in some patients. When acuity remains asymmetric, any alignment achieved by surgery may be difficult to maintain.[95]

Dragging of the retina by peripheral proliferative tissue can lead to an ectopic location of the macula and resultant pseudostrabismus. This macular ectopia (or heterotopia) has been assigned the cumbersome eponym Annette von Droste–Hulshoff syndrome.[96] Retinopathy of prematurity is the most common cause of macular ectopia. In the study by Biglan and associates,[92] 18 percent of such patients had macular ectopia.

Myopia

Myopia is a frequent complication of ROP, occurring in up to 80 percent of patients with scarring sequelae.[97] If the disease regresses completely, there is no increase in refractive error.[98] However, if even minimal retinal sequelae such as peripheral vitreal changes are present, there is an increased risk of myopia, astigmatism, and anisometropia compared with other premature infants.[95] The anisometropia is of particular concern, since it can lead to amblyopia and visual loss in patients who had otherwise avoided significant anatomic damage.

The myopia is probably lenticular rather than axial in nature, although both mechanisms may contribute. Gordon and colleagues[99] found a statistically significant increase in lens power with a close correlation between lens power and degree of myopia in their patients. They noted a weaker correlation with keratometry readings and axial length. Lens power normally diminishes during development; thus the normal development of the lens may be arrested by the disease process. Unfortunately, the controls in the Gordon and coworkers' study were not premature infants and perhaps lenticular myopia is associated with prematurity alone.

GLAUCOMA

Narrow-angle glaucoma is becoming increasingly recognized as a complication of nonblinding forms of ROP.[100–102] The mechanism is usually pupillary block secondary to a large lens. As patients from the first epidemic of ROP reach their fourth decade, many more cases may occur. The glaucoma usually responds to iridotomy, but lensectomy may be necessary.[103, 104] In more severe cases, narrow angles develop earlier and usually require lensectomy for definitive treatment.

Other Late Complications

Other complications of mild to moderate ROP include nystagmus, cataract, peripheral retinal breaks, microcornea, and band keratopathy.

In Biglan and associates' study,[92] 80 percent of patients with stage 4 or 5 disease also had a seizure disorder, and 50 percent had other neurologic complications. Microcornea[105] was seen in 11 percent of cases. Only patients with stage 4 or 5 disease developed shallow anterior chambers. Optic atrophy was seen in 18 percent. Six percent of all eyes became phthisical.

SUPPORT FOR FAMILIES

It is important to provide continuing support to patients with ROP and their families. The sequelae of regressed ROP must be dealt with by the ophthalmologist in continuing close follow-up of the patients. It is obvious that refractive errors, strabismus, and amblyopia as well as the less common complications will require indefinite follow-up. In addition to ophthalmologic care, many patients will require referral for special educational services and early intervention programs. The ophthalmologist should be aware of the programs that are available in his or her region. Certainly every child who is legally blind should be referred to his or her state's Commission for the Blind. Parent support groups may be of great help to visually impaired children and their parents. Information about programs and parent support groups may be obtained from the International Institute for the Visually Impaired, 230 Central Street, Auburndale, Massachusetts 02166, telephone (617) 332-4014. This organization has also published books that are helpful to parents of visually impaired children. These books can be obtained directly from the Institute. Other books suitable for parents of visually impaired children are available as well.

REFERENCES

1. Terry TL: Extreme prematurity and fibroblastic overgrowth of persistent vascular sheath behind each crystalline lens. Am J Ophthalmol 25:203–204, 1942.
2. Campbell K: Intensive oxygen therapy as a possible cause of retrolental fibroplasia: A clinical approach. Med J Aust 2:48–50, 1951.
3. Crosse VM, Evans PJ: Prevention of retrolental fibroplasia. Arch Ophthalmol 48:83–87, 1952.
4. Patz A, Hoeck LE, DeLaCruz E: Studies on the effect of high oxygen administration in retrolental fibroplasia. I: Nursery observations. Am J Ophthalmol 35:1248–1252, 1952.
5. Patz A, Eastham A, Higginbotham DH, et al: Oxygen studies in retrolental fibroplasia. II. The production of the microscopic changes of retrolental fibroplasia in experimental animals. Am J Ophthalmol 36:1511–1522, 1953.
6. Ashton N: Animal experiments in retrolental fibroplasia. Trans Am Acad Ophthalmol Otolaryngol 58:51–54, 1954.
7. Gyllensten LJ, Hellstrom BE: Retrolental fibroplasia: Animal experiments. Acta Pediatr 41:577–582, 1952.
8. Kinsey V, Hemphill FM: Preliminary report of a cooperative study of retrolental fibroplasia. Am J Ophthalmol 40:166–174, 1955.
9. Avery ME, Oppenheimer EH: Recent increase in mortality from hyaline membrane disease. J Pediatr 57:553–559, 1960.
10. McDonald AD: Cerebral palsy in children of very low birth weight. Arch Dis Child 38:579–588, 1963.
11. Robertson NR, Gupta JM, Dallenburg GW, et al: Oxygen therapy in the newborn. Lancet 1:1323–1329, 1968.
12. Patz A: New role of the ophthalmologist in prevention of retrolental fibroplasia. Arch Ophthalmol 78:565–568, 1967.
13. Kinsey VE, Arnold HJ, Kalina RE, et al: Pa_{O_2} levels and retrolental fibroplasia: A report of the cooperative study. Pediatrics 60:655–668, 1977.
14. Flynn JT, Bancalari E, Snyder ES, et al: A cohort study of transcutaneous oxygen tension and the incidence and severity of retinopathy. N Engl J Med 326:1050–1054, 1992.
15. Phelps DL: Retinopathy of prematurity: An estimate of visual loss in the United States—1979. Pediatrics 67:924–926, 1981.
16. Flynn JT: Acute proliferative retrolental fibroplasia: Multivariate risk analysis. Trans Am Ophthalmol Soc 81:549–591, 1983.
17. Mann I: The Development of the Human Eye, 3rd ed. London, British Medical Association, 1964, pp 228–229.
18. Roth AM: Retinal vascular development in premature infants. Am J Ophthalmol 84:636–640, 1977.
19. Foos RY, Kopelow SM: Development of retinal vasculature in paranatal infants. Surv Ophthalmol 18:117–127, 1973.
20. Cogan DG: Development and senescence of the human retinal vasculature. Trans Ophthalmol Soc UK 83:465–489, 1963.
21. Foos, RY: Pathologic features of retinopathy of prematurity. *In* Flynn JT, Phelps DL (eds): Retinopathy of Prematurity: Problem and Challenge. New York, Alan R. Liss, 1988, pp 73–85.
22. Flower RW, McLeod DS, Lutty GA, et al: Postnatal retinal vascular development of the puppy. Invest Ophthalmol Vis Sci 26:957–968, 1985.
23. Ashton N: Retinal angiogenesis in the human embryo. Br Med Bull 26:103–106, 1970.
24. Kretzer FL, Mehta RS, Johnson AT, et al: Vitamin E protects against retinopathy of prematurity through action on spindle cells. Nature 309:793–795, 1984.
25. Kalina RE, Karr, DJ: Retrolental fibroplasia: Experience over two decades in one institution. Ophthalmology 89:91–95, 1982.
26. Purohit DM, Ellison RC, Zierler S, et al: Risk factors for retrolental fibroplasia: Experience with 3,025 premature infants. National Collaborative Study on Patent Ductus Arteriosus in Premature Infants. Pediatrics 76:339–344, 1985.
27. Flynn JT, O'Grady GE, Herrera J, et al: Retrolental fibroplasia. I. Clinical observations. Arch Ophthalmol 95:217–223, 1977.

28. Lucey JL, Dangman B: A re-examination of the role of oxygen in retrolental fibroplasia. Pediatrics 73:82–96, 1984.
29. Bossi E, Koehner F, Flury B, et al: Retinopathy of prematurity: A risk factor analysis with univariate and multivariate statistics. Helv Paediatr Acta 39:307–317, 1984.
30. Hamer ME, Mullen PW, Ferguson JG, et al: Logistic analysis of risk factors in acute retinopathy of prematurity. Am J Ophthalmol 102:1–6, 1986.
31. Shohet M, Reisner SH, Krikler R, et al: Retinopathy of prematurity: Incidence and risk factors. Pediatrics 72:159–163, 1983
32. Owens WC, Owens EU: Retrolental fibroplasia in premature infants. II. Studies on the prophylaxis of the disease: The use of alpha tocopheryl acetate. Am J Ophthalmol 32:1631–1637, 1949.
33. Hittner HM, Godio LB, Rudolph AJ, et al: Retrolental fibroplasia: Efficacy of vitamin E in a double-blind clinical study of preterm infants. N Engl J Med 305:1365–1371, 1981.
34. Hittner HM, Godio LB, Sper, ME, et al: Retrolental fibroplasia: Further clinical evidence and ultrastructural support for efficacy of vitamin E in the preterm infant. Pediatrics 71:423–432, 1983.
35. Kretzer FL, Hittner HM: Human retinal development: Relationship to the pathogenesis of retinopathy of prematurity. *In* McPherson AR, Hittner HM, Kretzer FL (eds): Retinopathy of Prematurity: Current Concepts and Controversies. Toronto, BC Decker, 1986, pp 27–52.
36. Glass P, Avery GB, Subramanian KN, et al: Effect of bright light in the hospital nursery on the incidence of retinopathy of prematurity. N Engl J Med 313:401–404, 1985.
37. Mosley MJ, Fielder AR: Light toxicity and the neonatal eye. Clin Vis Sci 3:75–82, 1988.
38. Als H, Lawhon G, Brown E, et al: Individualized behavioral and environmental care for the very low birth weight preterm infant at high risk for bronchopulmonary dysplasia: Neonatal intensive care unit and developmental outcome. Pediatrics 78:1123–1132, 1986.
39. Reese AB, King M, Owens WC: A classification of retrolental fibroplasia. Am J Ophthalmol 36:133–135, 1953.
40. McCormick AQ: Retinopathy of prematurity. Curr Prob Pediatr 7:3–28, 1977.
41. Kingham JD: Acute retrolental fibroplasia. Arch Ophthalmol 95:39–43, 1977.
42. Majima A: Studies on retinopathy of prematurity. 1. Statistical analysis of factors related to occurrence and progression in active phase. Jpn J Ophthalmol 21:404–420, 1977.
43. Cantolino SJ, Curran JS, Van Cader TC, et al: Acute retrolental fibroplasia: Classification and objective evaluation of incidence, natural history and resolution by fundus photography and intravenous fluorescein angiography. Perspect Ophthalmol 2:175–187, 1978.
44. Koerner F, Bossi E, Zulauf M: The significance of oxygen and other risk factors for predicting retinal risk in ROP. Presented at the Retinopathy of Prematurity Conference, Dec 4–6, 1981, Washington, DC, pp 414–423.
45. The Committee for the Classification of Retinopathy of Prematurity: An international classification of retinopathy of prematurity. Arch Ophthalmol 102:1130–1134, 1984.
46. An international classification of retinopathy of prematurity. Pediatrics 74:17–133, 1984.
47. The International Committee for the Classification of the Late Stages of Retinopathy of Prematurity: An international classification of retinopathy of prematurity. II. The classification of retinal detachment. Arch Ophthalmol 105:906–912, 1987.
48. Machemer R: Description and pathogenesis of late stage of retinopathy of prematurity. *In* Flynn JT, Phelps DL (eds): Retinopathy of Prematurity: Problem and Challenge. New York, Alan R. Liss, 1988, pp 275–280.
49. Cryotherapy for Retinopathy of Prematurity Cooperative Group: Multicenter trial of cryotherapy for retinopathy of prematurity. Three-month outcome. Arch Ophthalmol 108:195–204, 1990.
50. Nissenkorn I, Kremer I, Gilad E, et al: "Rush" type retinopathy of prematurity: Report of three cases. Br J Ophthalmol 71:559–562, 1987.
51. Charles S: Personal communication, 1989.
52. Faris BM, Brockhurst RJ: Retrolental fibroplasia in the cicatricial stage. The complication of rhegmatogenous retinal detachment. Arch Ophthalmol 82:60–65, 1969.
53. Cats BP, Tan KEWP: Prematures with and without regressed retinopathy of prematurity: comparison of long-term (6 to 10 years) ophthalmological morbidity. J Pediatric Ophthalmol Strabismus 26:271–275, 1989.
54. Biglan AW, Cheng KP, Brown OR: Update on retinopathy of prematurity. Int Ophthalmol Clin 29:2–9, 1989.
55. Kushner, BJ: Strabismus and amblyopia associated with regressed retinopathy of prematurity. Arch Ophthalmol 100:256–261, 1982.
56. Schaffer DB, Quinn GE, Johnson L: Sequelae of arrested mild retinopathy of prematurity. Arch Ophthalmol 102:373–376, 1984.
57. Hittner HM, Mehta RS, Brown ES, et al: Macular structure and fixation following surgical intervention for threshold retinopathy of prematurity. [Abstract] Invest Ophthalmol Vis Sci 30:317, 1989.
58. Lees BJ, Cabal LA: Increased blood pressure following pupillary dilation with 2.5% phenylephrine hydrochloride in preterm infants. Pediatrics 68:231–234, 1981.
59. Bauer, CR, Trottier MCT, Stern L: Systemic cyclopentolate (cyclogyl) toxicity in the newborn infant. Pediatr Pharmacol Ther 82:501–505, 1973.
60. Bates JH, Burnstine RA: Consequences of retinopathy of prematurity examinations. Case report. Arch Ophthalmol 105:618–619, 1987.
61. Johnson AT, Kretzer FL, Hittner HM, et al: Development of the subretinal space in the preterm eye: Ultrastructural and immunocytochemical studies. J Compar Neurol 233:497–505, 1984.
62. Finer NN, Grant G, Schindler RF, et al: Effect of intramuscular vitamin E on frequency and severity of retrolental fibroplasia: A controlled trial. Lancet 1:1087–1091, 1982.
63. Johnson L, Quinn GE, Abbasi S, et al: Effect of sustained pharmacologic vitamin E levels on incidence and severity of retinopathy of prematurity: A controlled clinical trial. J Pediatr 114:827–838, 1989.
64. Finer NN, Peters KL, Hayek Z, et al: Vitamin E and necrotizing enterocolitis. Pediatrics 73:387–393, 1984.
65. Puklin JE, Simon RM, Ehrenkranz RA: Influence on retrolental fibroplasia of intramuscular vitamin E administration during respiratory distress syndrome. Ophthalmology 89:96–102, 1982.
66. Milner RA, Bell E, Blanchette V, et al: Vitamin E supplement in under 1500-gram neonates. Presented at Retinopathy of Prematurity Conference, Washington, DC, Dec. 4–6, 1981, pp 703–716.
67. Phelps DL, Rosenbaum AL, Isenberg SJ, et al: Tocopherol efficacy and safety for preventing retinopathy of prematurity: A randomized, controlled, double-masked trial. Pediatrics 79:489–500, 1987.
68. Kretzer FL, Hittner HM: Retinopathy of prematurity: Clinical implications of retinal development. Arch Dis Child 63:1151–67, 1988.
69. Committee of the Institute of Medicine: Report of a study—vitamin E and retinopathy of prematurity. IOM 86–02. Washington, DC, National Academy Press, 1986.
70. Ehrenkranz RA: Vitamin E and retinopathy of prematurity: Still controversial. J Pediatr 114:801–803, 1989.
71. Nagata M, Yamagishi, N, Ikeda S. Summarized results of the treatment of acute proliferative retinopathy of prematurity during the past 15 years in Tenri Hospital. Acta Soc Ophthalmol Jpn 86:1236–1244, 1982.
72. Sasaki K, Yamashita Y, Maekawa T, et al: Treatment of retinopathy of prematurity in active stage by cryotherapy. Jpn J Ophthalmol 20:384–395, 1976.
73. Harris GS, McCormick AQ: The prophylactic treatment of retrolental fibroplasia. Mod Probl Ophthalmol 18:364–367, 1977.
74. Hindle NW: Cryotherapy for retinopathy of prematurity to prevent retrolental fibroplasia. Can J Ophthalmol 17:207–212, 1982.
75. Ben-Sira I, Nissenkorn I, Grunwald E, et al: Treatment of acute retrolental fibroplasia by cryopexy. Br J Ophthalmol 64:758–762, 1980.
76. Koerner FH: Retinopathy of prematurity. Natural course and management. Metabol Ophthalmol 2:325–329, 1978.
77. Keith CG: Visual outcome and effect of treatment in stage III developing retrolental fibroplasia. Br J Ophthalmol 66:446–449, 1982.

78. Kingham JD: Acute retrolental fibroplasia. Treatment by cryosurgery. Arch Ophthalmol 96:2049–2053, 1978.
79. Mousel DK, Hoyt CS: Cryotherapy for retinopathy of prematurity. Ophthalmology 87:1121–1127, 1980.
80. Cryotherapy for Retinopathy of Prematurity Cooperative Group: Multicenter trial of cryotherapy for retinopathy of prematurity: Preliminary results. Arch Ophthalmol 106:471–479, 1988.
81. Cryotherapy for Retinopathy of Prematurity Cooperative Group: Multicenter trial of cryotherapy for retinopathy of prematurity. One-year outcome—structure and function. Arch Ophthalmol 108:1408–1416, 1990.
82. Dobson, V, Quinn GE, Biglan AW, et al: Acuity card assessment of visual function in the cryotherapy for retinopathy of prematurity trial. Invest Ophthalmol Vis Sci 31:1702–1708, 1990.
83. Mayer DL, Fulton AB, Hansen, RM: Visual acuity of infants and children with retinal degenerations. Ophthalmic Paediatr Genet 5:51–56, 1985.
84. Hindle NW: Cryotherapy for retinopathy of prematurity: None, one, or both eyes. [Letter] Arch Ophthalmol 108:1375, 1990.
85. Nissenkorn I, Ben Sira I, Kremer I, et al: Eleven years' experience with retinopathy of prematurity: Visual results and contribution of cryoablation. Br J Ophthalmol 75:158–159, 1991.
86. Nagata M, Eguchi K, Majima A, et al: Multicenter prospective studies on retinopathy of prematurity. I: Incidence and results of treatment. Acta Ophthalmol Jpn 39:646–657, 1988.
87. Hindle NW: Critical mass retinopathy of prematurity: What is it and what can you do about it? Doc Ophthalmol 74:253–262, 1990.
88. Greven C, Tasman W: Scleral buckling in stages 4B and 5 retinopathy of prematurity. Ophthalmology 97:817–820, 1990.
89. Kretzer, FL, McPherson AR, Hittner HM: An interpretation of retinopathy of prematurity in terms of spindle cells: Relationship to vitamin E prophylaxis and cryotherapy. Graefes Arch Ophthalmol Clin Exp Ophthalmol 224:205–214, 1986.
90. Tasman W: Personal communication, 1989.
91. Phelps DL, Phelps CE: Cryotherapy in infants with retinopathy of prematurity. JAMA 261:1751–1756, 1989.
92. Biglan AW, Cheng KP, Brown DR: Update on retinopathy of prematurity. Int Ophthalmol Clin 29:2–9, 1989.
93. Tasman W, Brown GC: Progressive visual loss in adults with retinopathy of prematurity (ROP). Trans Am Ophthalmol Soc 86:367–379, 1989.
94. Snir M, Nissenkorn I, Sherf I, et al: Visual acuity, strabismus and amblyopia in premature babies without retinopathy of prematurity. Ann Ophthalmol 20:256–258, 1988.
95. Kushner BJ: The sequellae of regressed retinopathy of prematurity. *In* Silverman WA, Flynn JT (eds): Contemporary Issues in Fetal and Neonatal Medicine. 2. Retinopathy of Prematurity. Boston, Blackwell Scientific Publications, 1985, pp 239–248.
96. Alfieri MC, Magli A, Chiosi E, et al: The Annette von Droste-Hulshoff syndrome. Pseudostrabismus due to macular ectopia in retinopathy of prematurity. Ophthalmic Paediatr Genet 9:13–16, 1988.
97. Tasman W: Late complications of retrolental fibroplasia. Ophthalmology 86:1724–1740, 1979.
98. Schaffer DB, Quinn GE, Johnson L: Sequelae of arrested mild ROP. Arch Ophthalmol 102:373–376, 1984.
99. Gordon RA, Donzis PB: Myopia associated with retinopathy of prematurity. Ophthalmology 93:1593–1598, 1986.
100. Hittner HM, Rhodes LM, McPherson AR: Anterior segment abnormalities in cicatricial retinopathy of prematurity. Ophthalmology 86:803–818, 1979.
101. Pollard ZF: Secondary angle-closure glaucoma in cicatricial retrolental fibroplasia. Am J Ophthalmol 89:651–653, 1980.
102. Ueda N, Ogino N: Angle-closure glaucoma with pupillary block mechanism in cicatricial retinopathy of prematurity. Ophthalmologica 196:15–18, 1988.
103. Pollard ZF: Lensectomy for secondary angle-closure glaucoma in advanced cicatricial retrolental fibroplasia. Ophthalmology 91:396–398, 1984.
104. Smith J, Shivitz I: Angle-closure glaucoma in adults with cicatricial retinopathy of prematurity. Arch Ophthalmol 102:371–372, 1984.
105. Kelly SP, Fielder AR: Microcornea associated with retinopathy of prematurity. Br J Ophthalmol 71:201–203, 1987.

Chapter 225

Congenital Nasolacrimal Duct Obstruction

WILLIAM P. BOGER III

Congenital nasolacrimal duct obstruction is a common problem in the newborn period. Interest and debate concerning its treatment can regularly be generated among practicing physicians, and many of the lively discussions over the past century sound quite like those of today. Debate over deeply held convictions concerning the best timing for surgical intervention has often overshadowed the fact that there is much on which there is agreement. Often overlooked is the considerable anatomic literature documenting wide variations in the structure of the nasolacrimal duct and its entry into the nasal fossa. As one evaluates the options for therapeutic intervention, it is useful to consider that infants may vary considerably in their clinical symptoms: one child may have repeated infections despite the parents' best efforts, whereas with modest parental care, another infant of the same age may have little more than clear tearing aggravated by cold weather.

HISTORY: 1800s AND EARLY 1900s

Textbooks from the early 1800s devote considerable attention to the problems of nasolacrimal duct obstruction in adults. Repeated probings with metal probes and efforts to maintain the passageways with indwelling materials, including catgut, were documented by Mackenzie in 1830.[1] Late in the 1800s, the attention of clinicians was drawn to the frequent occurrence of nasolacrimal duct obstruction in the newborn period. In contrast to the frustratingly recurrent problems of the adult, the newborn situation quite often responded dramatically to a single probing of the nasolacrimal duct.

In 1879, Kipp[2] from Newark, New Jersey, commented on the scarcity of reference to this problem in the textbooks of his day. In his own practice over the preceding 2 yr, 3.6 percent of his patient population had suffered from diseases of the nasolacrimal drainage system, and 10 percent of these were under 1 yr of age. He compared his own experience with that expressed by the authors of the day. He recommended evacuation of the sac "by slight pressure." "If the disease does not get well under this simple treatment in the course of three or four weeks, I use Bowman's probes and injection of astringents in the same manner as in adults."[2]

In 1891 Peters[3] from Bonn articulated the mechanism of congenital nasolacrimal duct obstruction in terms that are now familiar. He quoted the findings of embryologists and anatomists:

> The lower end of the nasolacrimal duct in newborns has often been found totally covered by a layer of mucous membrane. When children grow this atrophies . . . it becomes clear why in newborns healing occurs after only a few probings. There is no stenosis, no disease of the mucous membranes, but drainage toward the nose [is obstructed only because of the persistence of the mucous membrane.][3]

In his report of 1891, Peters reviewed the already existing debate over the proper therapy for congenital nasolacrimal duct obstruction and offered his own recommendations. He had probed the first two patients but observed in other cases that newborns could be followed for a period of months without probing with eventual resolution of their symptoms. During the period of observation Peters recommended digital compression of the tear sac.

In 1892 Peters[4] readdressed the issue of nasolacrimal duct abnormalities in the newborn. He reported a 1-year-old youngster who responded well to a single probing of each eye. In response to Weiss' criticism of his digital compression of the sac, Peters clarified his own expectations of that maneuver. Although the membrane might actually rupture as a result of the digital compression in some cases, Peters felt that it was passage of time that allowed the membrane to perforate in the majority of cases.

> The reason for my previous report was not to completely reject the use of the probe in these cases—I even emphasized the justification for this treatment after persistence of the condition—but to give an explanation for either spontaneous healing or successful treatment after only one single probe treatment.[4]

From London in 1899, Stephenson[5] comments favorably on the use of careful digital pressure with a view:

> [1] to squeeze out secretion through the puncta lacrimalis and [2] to break down the obstruction that is present in the nasal duct. Indeed most of the cases make a speedy recovery under that simple maneuver, which succeeds in accordance with the care exercised in carrying it out. When compression fails we must clear away all obstruction by passing a small probe down the lacrimal duct. . . . As some little delicacy is called for to introduce the probe neatly, I always prefer to operate under a general anesthesia.[5]

Cutler (1903)[6] believed that most cases of nasolacrimal duct obstruction would clear spontaneously but was uncomfortable leaving a source of serious infection if the cornea were abraded. He also suggested that leaving the constant irritation to the nasolacrimal duct might "sow the seeds of more serious trouble in later life." He advocated, as had Jocqs of France, in 1899,[7] that forceful irrigation of fluid (syringing) rather than probing be used as the means of rupturing the membrane.

Weeks of New York, in 1904,[8] advocated waiting 2 mo, believing that patency of the passages would be established in the first 2 to 6 wk in most cases. On the other hand, in 1907 Jackson[7] from Denver "would not limit to two months, or even 6 months, the period in which it is proper to try milder measures, provided the symptoms are controlled by such treatments." In London in 1907, Parsons[9] recommended intervention by probing after a trial of lotions and lacrimal sac compression for a week or two, and in 1908 Zentmayer[10] from Philadelphia was so impressed with the parents' gratitude after his first case treated by probing that he recommended probing early for most cases.

In a discussion[10] of Zentmayer's 1908 paper, Kipp[10] reviewed his own experiences since his initial report 29 yr previously. "In all cases treated within the last 10 yr, I have used simply cleansing and pressure and have not had to use a probe in any case." Jackson[10] also commented on Zentmayer's paper of 1908 and summarized his own approach at that time:

> It is but right that the parents of an infant presenting this condition should be fully informed of the nature and probability of the case and allowed to choose whether or not any operative measure should be resorted to. At the same time, they should be informed that the condition could probably be relieved by a simple probing, and that complications might arise which would render operation urgent.[10]

In concluding the session, Zentmayer quotes Jackson as having stated that he "would treat a member of his own family in the expectant manner."[10] "So would I," says Zentmayer, "because I would have the patient under constant observation. In practice this is not possible, and if treatment is giving no result, the patient is apt to be neglected and serious trouble may supervene."[10]

In 1931 Woodruff[11] urged that infants with nasolacrimal duct obstruction be treated by probing before the condition became "seriously chronic." The average age of presentation was 6½ mo. Riser[12] (1935) emphasized the more favorable prognosis for those children with *congenital* nasolacrimal duct obstruction in contrast to those children with *acquired* forms of nasolacrimal duct obstruction. In 1941 Hardesty[13] alluded to some clinicians who advocated waiting 2 to 3 yr for spontaneous cures, but he suggested earlier surgical intervention. He found that irrigation of the sac could cure one third of his cases, whereas probing was used for the other two thirds. Simpson[14] in 1945 reported the use of oral sulfadiazine to treat dacryocystitis in the newborn period. Corner[15] (1946) pointed out that eye infections account for more than twice as many cases as any other single cause of neonatal infections.

FREQUENCY OF CONGENITAL NASOLACRIMAL DUCT OBSTRUCTION

It is remarkable how frequently the clinical signs of nasolacrimal duct obstruction manifest in the newborn period. Stephenson's report in 1899[5] remains vividly descriptive some 90 years later:

> A baby, generally aged less than 6 months, is brought with a statement that the eyes have been noticed to discharge either from or shortly after birth. . . . The amount of secretion is often said to vary from day to day without known reason. . . . On examination of the infant, a plug of mucus or mucopus can be seen lying at the inner canthus, gluing the lashes together. There is no swelling of the lids, and the baby is able to open his [or her] eyes freely; the eyeball is not bloodshot; the cornea is clear. . . . It is the exception for an obvious swelling to exist in the region of the lacrimal sac. . . . More commonly, there is a slight, ill-defined dullness of the region in question. When moderately firm pressure is made with the finger over the internal palpebral ligament, mucopus exudes from one or another punctum, and often a noteable quantity of discharge may in that way be squeezed into the conjunctival sinus. Compression over the sac less frequently gives rise to an escape of mucopus from the corresponding nostril. Most of the children appeared to enjoy excellent health. . . . Once a history was got of a similar condition having been present in two other children belonging to the same family. . . . It is not rare to find that both eyes were attacked to begin with, and while one was recovered with or without treatment, the other has not done so. . . . If the secretion expressed from the lacrimal sac be examined by means of cover glass preparations and cultures, it [will] be found to contain bacteria.[5]

Stephenson stated that among 1538 outpatients seen in the ophthalmic department, no less than 27, or 1.75 percent were affected. These figures, however, probably understate the frequency of the ailment.[5]

In 1948 Guerry and Kendig[16] examined 200 unselected, consecutive newborn infants and found 12 cases (6 percent) of congenital nasolacrimal duct obstruction as judged by tearing and presence of mucopus after pressure over the nasolacrimal sac. "In ten cases the epiphora appeared between the tenth and the twelfth day after birth, while in two cases tearing was delayed 3 and 4 wk respectively."[16] Cassady[17] in 1948 also reported that nasolacrimal duct obstruction occurred in 14 instances (5 percent) among a local series of 279 infants: "This latter figure probably is higher than usual because special inquiry was made by pediatricians and careful examination . . . was done in each of the 279 infants."

Clinical symptoms are seen in 5 to 6 percent of all infants, but anatomic studies suggest that persistence of a mucous membrane across the lower end of the nasolacrimal duct at birth is even more common than this. Vlacovich, in the late 1800s, is quoted[10, 12] as having performed autopsies on 18 newborn children and apparently found 4 cases in which the nasolacrimal duct was imperforate. Mayou (1908)[18] studied five full-term fetuses and concluded that at birth the nasolacrimal duct is either not patent at all or only partially so. Schwarz (1935)[19] found the opening of the nasolacrimal duct closed in 35 percent of late fetuses. Cassady[20] examined 15 full-term stillborn infants and concluded that in 73 percent the lumen of the lacrimal duct was not connected with the nasal cavity at birth. Busse and colleagues (1980)[21] performed postmortem investigations in 65 neonates: In 28 premature infants, a persistent membrane was present on one or both sides in 19 cases (68 percent); in 16 mature infants dying immediately post partum, 10 (63 percent) had a persistent membrane; and in 21 mature infants dying during the first month, 11 (52 percent) had a persistent membrane on one or both sides.

ANATOMIC VARIANTS

Anatomy and ophthalmology textbooks[22] generally present idealized versions of the nasolacrimal duct anatomy (e.g., Gerard, 1907,[23] Fig. 225–1). However, the actual internal anatomy of the nasolacrimal duct of a given individual is not available to inspection in the ordinary clinical setting. Information available from autopsy and radiographic studies suggests a high degree of individual variability in anatomic details that would have direct bearing on the clinical course of nasolacrimal duct obstruction and its therapy. Schematic representations of the nasolacrimal duct also tend to generalize from the configuration of the adult nasolacrimal duct rather than that of the newborn.

As early as 1899, Rochon-Duvigneaud[24] provided beautifully documented variations of nasolacrimal duct development (Fig. 225–2).

Schaeffer (1912[25] and 1920[26]) emphasized that irregularities in the nasolacrimal duct and diverticula are common congenital aberrations:

> Entirely apart from . . . minor irregularities, diverticula, or direct outpouchings of the nasolacrimal duct, are not uncommon. They vary from those of insignificant size to those of relatively large dimensions. In studying cross sections of the nasolacrimal duct, one is at times puzzled to explain what are apparently two ducts lying side by side. However, by following the sections serially one finds that one cavity sooner or later communicates with the other; i.e. one turns out to be the nasolacrimal duct proper and the other a diverticulum from it. These diverticula must be very important clinically since they are so located that they readily retain infectious material within their confines. Indeed, they may be important

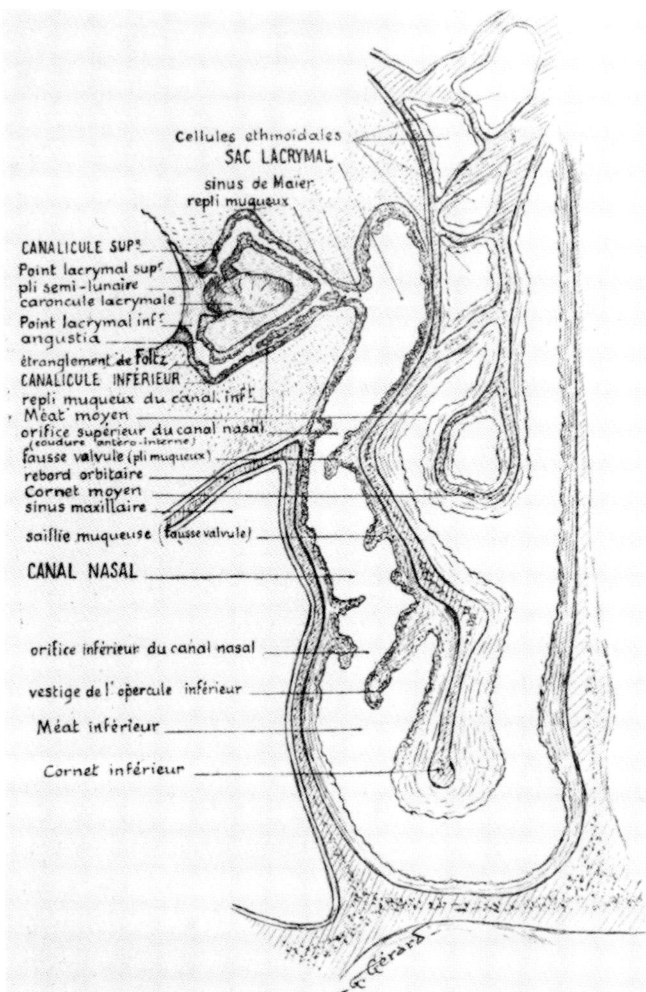

Figure 225–1. The nasolacrimal passages: the puncta, canaliculi, common canaliculus, nasolacrimal sac, and nasolacrimal duct, which enters the nasal fossa below the inferior turbinate. (From Gerard G: Des obstacles naturels capables de compliquer le catheterisme de vois lacrymoles. Ann d'Ocul 137:193, 1907.)

> factors in the chronicity of pathologic conditions of the nasolacrimal duct. . . . It must therefore be concluded from the evidence at hand that the diverticula from the nasolacrimal duct are of congenital origin and are not acquired in later life.

Schaeffer's emphasis on the congenital nature of diverticula is supported by subsequent workers, including Busse and colleagues.[21, 27]

Schaeffer[26] documents anomalous side-by-side union of the nasolacrimal duct with the lacrimal sac and points out that a probe would have difficulty following an appropriate channel in this situation (Fig. 225–3). Schaeffer's anatomic observations of the frequently anomalous development of the nasolacrimal system were confirmed radiologically with contrast techniques by Campbell and colleagues in 1922:[28] "There may be a side-to-side joining; we have seen several such cases in this series." Radiologic studies by other investigators[29–37] and specialized imaging studies[38–43] have added considerably to our understanding of the abnormalities that may occur in the nasolacrimal system, but without these special investigations, Schaeffer[26] summarizes the clinician's usual situation in daily practice: "Unfortunately, there is no way of knowing what type of duct confronts the operator."

Schaeffer[25, 26] also documents that the nasolacrimal duct may enter the nasal cavity in a variety of locations.

> The nasolacrimal ostium is usually a single opening. However, duplicate and triplicate communications between the inferior nasal meatus and the nasolacrimal duct are not infrequently met with. A study of a large series of specimens convinces the observer that there is no unvarying typical form of ostium but that several normal anatomic types are equally common. Indeed, it cannot be gainsaid that the notion of an ideal typical form must be abandoned more or less generally and in its place substituted the belief and knowledge of normal anatomic types. A reference to [Fig. 225–4] in which are represented actual delineations of human nasolacrimal ostia, will indicate a number of the fundamental anatomic types that are encountered. The belief that all nasolacrimal ostia are provided with a mucosal valve (plica lacrimalis), or the so-called valve of Hasner, must be abandoned. When the nasolacrimal duct terminates immediately caudal to the attached border of the inferior nasal concha, its ostium almost invariably stands permanently open, wide-mouthed and unguarded by a valvelike structure [see 1, 3, and 6 in Fig. 225–4]. In the type in which the nasolacrimal duct passed through the nasal mucous membrane rather obliquely, the ostium may be said to be guarded by a fold of mucous membrane, that is, a plica lacrimalis of Hasner [see Fig. 225–4, nos. 5 and 10]. Occasionally, the nasal end of the nasolacrimal duct pushes nipple-like into the inferior nasal meatus; surmounting the nipple is located the nasolacrimal ostium [see Fig. 225–4, no. 7]. At times the nasolacrimal ostium proper is more or less open and somewhat guarded by a plica lacrimalis. Extending from the ostium toward the floor of the nose is a fairly deep gutter-like groove, which tends to become deeper and deeper as one approaches its caudal limits. . . . It is the slitlike type of ostium located in the lateral wall of the inferior nasal meatus that is . . . readily compressed by enlargement of the inferior nasal concha, occluded by hypertrophy or congestion of the mucous membranes. Indeed in those cases of persistent nasolacrimal infection despite treatment, the type of nasolacrimal ostium may be an important factor in the chronicity of the ailment.

Busse and colleagues[21] and Grossmann and Putz[44] provide photographic documentation of these anatomic variations of the nasolacrimal duct's entry into the nasal cavity.

Larsson[45] and others[46–48] have emphasized the clinical and surgical importance of these particular anatomic variations at the nasal end of the nasolacrimal duct (Fig. 225–5).

Schaeffer[26] also points out:

> At best but papery laminae of bone intervene between the ethmoidal labyrinth and the orbit and between the ventral portion of the ethmoidal labyrinth and the lacrimal sac

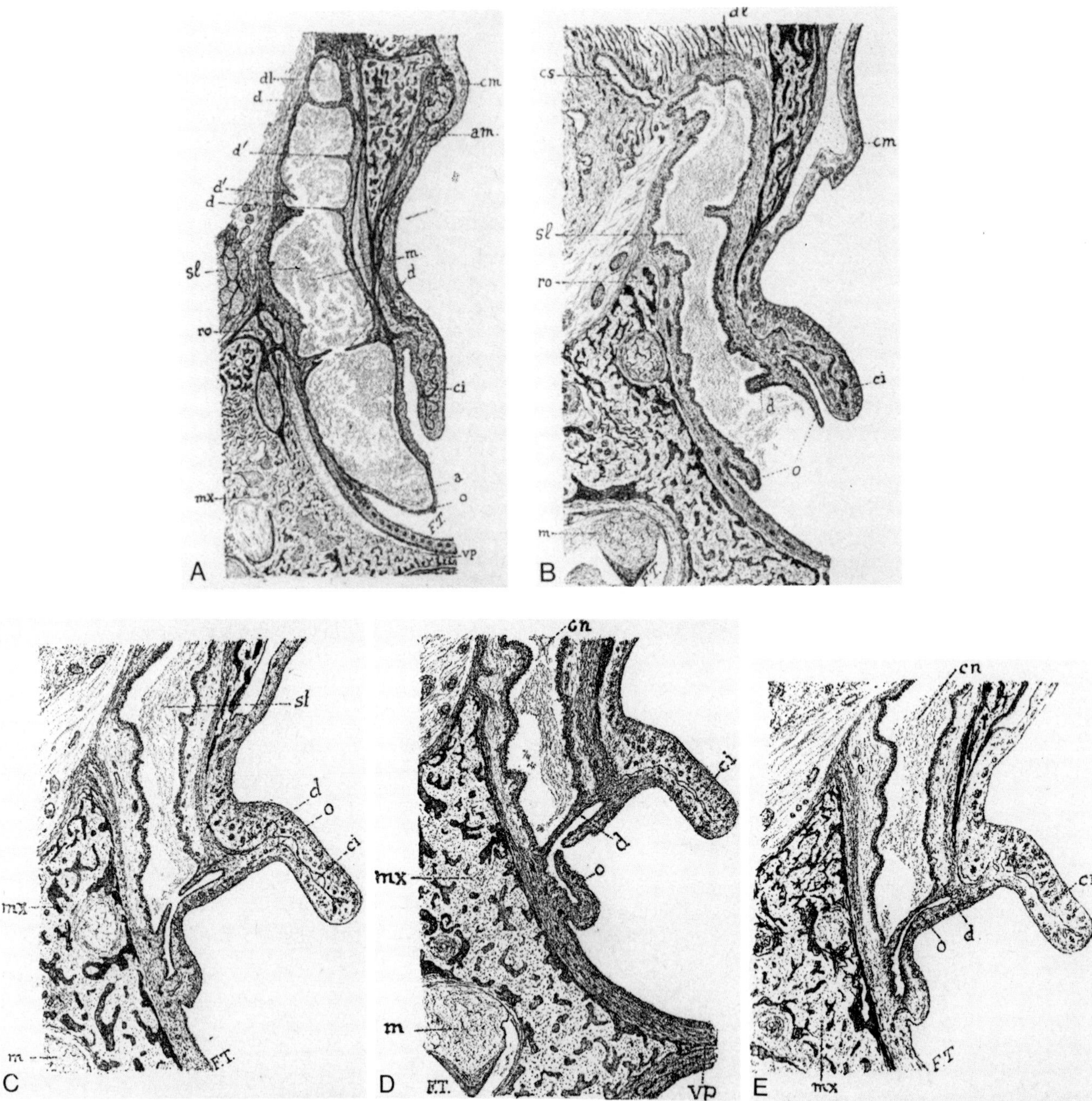

Figure 225–2. Detailed illustrations of the nasal end of the nasolacrimal duct in the fetus and newborn. *A,* The lacrimal sac and duct of a boy who lived 21 hr and was probably at term. The nasolacrimal duct is closed by a kind of operculum (o) that is very much distended. *B,* In a fetus of 7 mo gestation, the lower operculum (o) has ruptured. *C,* A male fetus between 6 and 7 mo gestation with diaphragms at the nasal end of the nasolacrimal duct similar in configuration to *A,* but the operculum (o) is less distended. *D,* The same nasolacrimal duct of the same fetus as C, but the section is slightly more anterior than in C. The section differs only in that the operculum (o) is perforated at its center, and the diaphragm (d) is continuous at this level. *E,* This section is slightly more anterior than that shown in *D.* At this level, the two diaphragms are both imperforate. (*A–E,* From Rochon-Duvigneaud: Dilatation of the tearducts in the fetus and newborn following perforation of the inferior cavity. Anatomical conditions which favor dacryocystitis. Arch d'Ophthalmologiques 19:81–89, 1899.)

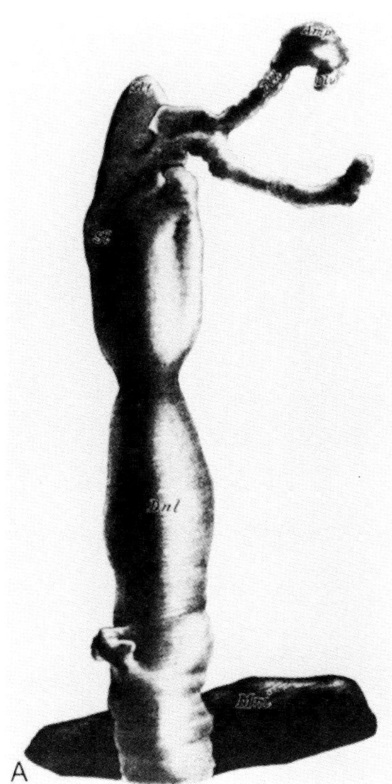

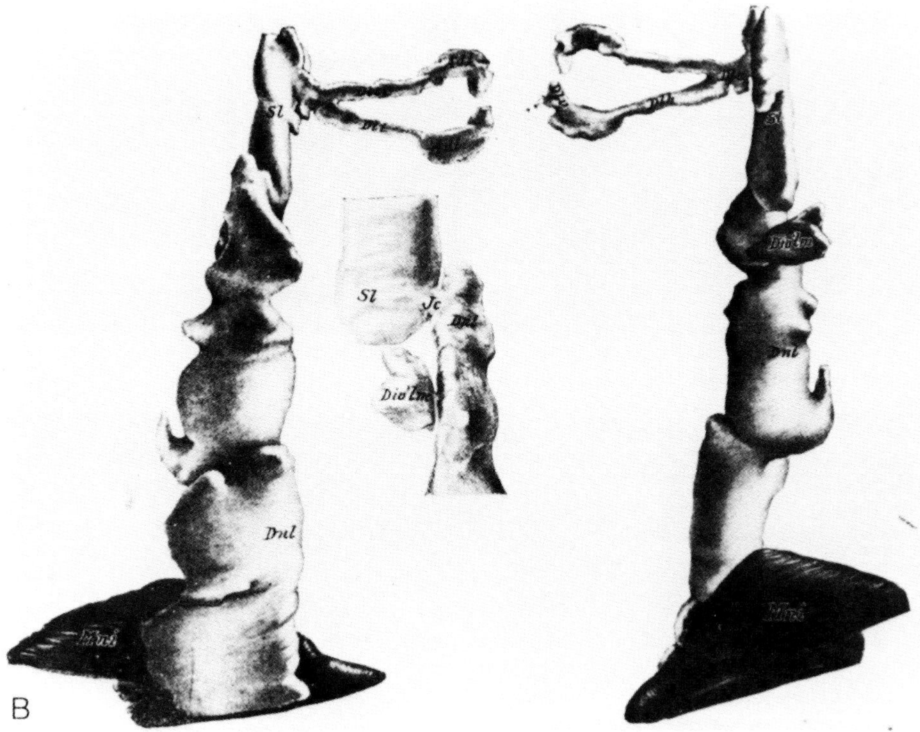

Figure 225–3. *A,* Reconstruction of the nasolacrimal passages of an adult aged 60 yr. Note particularly the regularity of the nasolacrimal duct in comparison with *B* and the straight union between the nasolacrimal sac and the nasolacrimal duct in comparison with the side-by-side union in *B*. The straight course of the lower aspect of the nasolacrimal duct that is so often presumed in diagrammatic representations of the nasolacrimal duct (for example, see Fig. 225–5) apparently is often not the case in the newborn period (see Fig. 225–7). *B,* Reconstruction of the nasolacrimal passageways of an adult aged 65 yr. The illustration on the left represents a medial view, and the one on the right, a lateral view of the model. Note especially the irregularity and diverticula of the nasolacrimal duct. Similar diverticula are not uncommon in newborn children and infants as congenital variations of development. The inset in the center shows the details of the side-by-side union of the lacrimal sac and the nasolacrimal duct (Jc) and in addition illustrates the large budlike diverticulum from the nasolacrimal duct (Div'lm). (*A* and *B* From Schaeffer JP: The Nose, Paranasal Sinuses, Nasolacrimal Passageways, and Olfactory Organ in Man. Philadelphia, P. Blakiston's, 1920.)

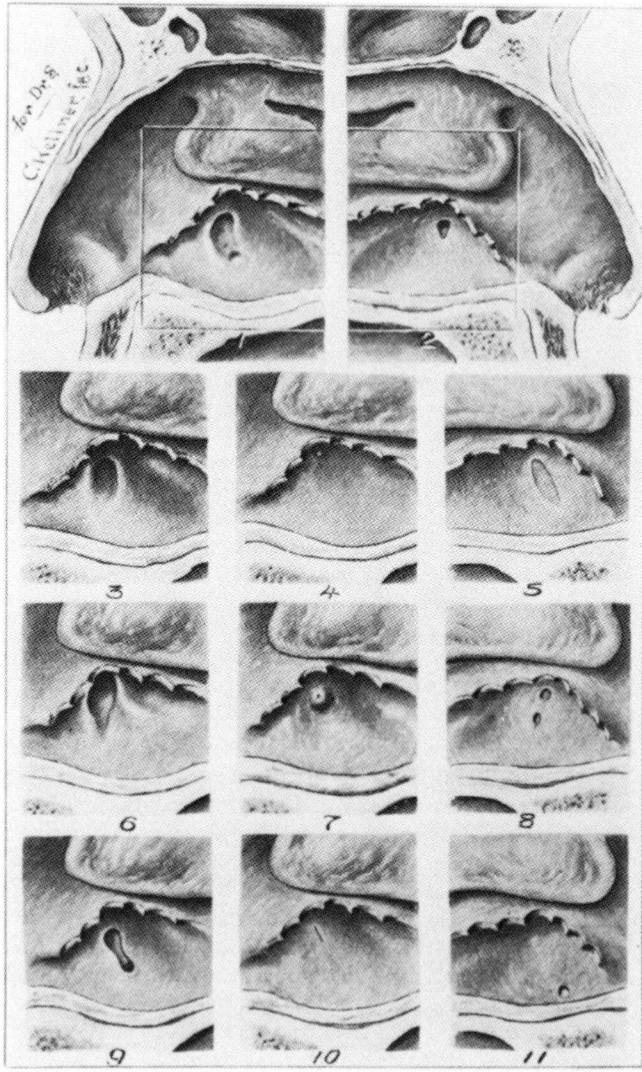

Figure 225–4. Drawings of actual dissections illustrating various types of ostia between the nasolacrimal duct and the nasal cavity. The inferior turbinate has been partly cut away to provide adequate exposure. (From Schaeffer JP: The Nose, Paranasal Sinuses, Nasolacrimal Passageways, and Olfactory Organ in Man. Philadelphia, P. Blakiston's, 1920.)

> and the nasolacrimal duct. . . . Indeed, congenital dehiscences in the bony "party-walls" are extremely commonplace.

It is notable that many authors who have carefully studied newborn anatomy express reservations about where the nasolacrimal Bowman's probe must be going. Jazbi and Cibis[49] reported their findings with a fiberoptic endoscope and fluoroscopy.

> Our experience with both endoscopy and dacryocystofluoroscopy reveals a previously unsuspected high incidence of false passages created by nasolacrimal duct probing—unsuspected in that these probings otherwise appeared clinically uncomplicated and were done by skilled experienced surgeons. Evidence of false passages were found in 15 of 56 probings for an incidence of 27%. The creation of false passages in our experience is therefore not the rare and isolated event the literature would lead one to believe. . . . In spite of the high incidence of false passages, our clinical success in curing the lacrimal obstruction is extremely high. Only three of the 56 cases needed repeat probing. Not every false passage therefore leads to a clinical failure (Fig. 225–6).

Even in 1909 Berry[46] stressed, "It should be remembered that the course of the canal in babyhood is quite irregular and radically different from that in the adult." Onodi[50] in 1913 provided meticulous measurements of the infant's nasolacrimal system. Woodruff[11] emphasized again in 1931 that the direction of the nasolacrimal duct in infancy "is quite different than it is later." After their postmortem study of 65 neonates, Busse and colleagues[21, 27] also put particular emphasis on the observation that in the newborn there frequently is a sharp angulation at the juncture between the nasolacrimal sac and the nasolacrimal duct and also that there is a deep bend in the nasolacrimal duct just before it enters the nasal passage. These characteristics make "it difficult to perforate a persisting Hasner's membrane by means of

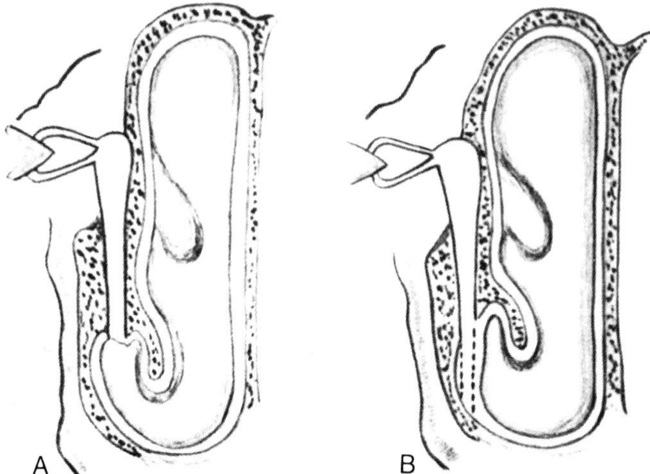

Figure 225–5. "It is well known that the nasolacrimal duct may be longer than the osseous canal containing it. In such cases the duct continues below the orifice of the bony canal, the medial wall of the duct being covered with nasal mucous membrane. In that case the normal opening of the duct sometimes forms a window on the medial wall and is located above the end of the duct. The sketches given above present a diagrammatic view of these conditions. [*A*] and [*B*]. If the course of the duct is as that in [*A*], it is evident that the probing must cause a radical opening of its lower end if this, owing to deficient canalization, is closed by a thin membrane. On the other hand, if the anatomical conditions are such as shown in [*B*], I deem it very plausible that probing need not necessarily bring about an opening of the duct. The probe introduced into a long duct of such location only proceeds to the floor of the nasal fossa without producing a perforation medially into the cavum nasi." (Note that this sketch, like many others in textbooks and original articles, presumes a straight course of the lacrimal sac into the nasolacrimal duct and of the nasolacrimal duct into the nasal cavity. See Figure 225–7 and corresponding text, documenting that this may well not be the case in many newborn children.) (From Larsson S: On the treatment of congenital atresia of the nasolacrimal duct. Acta Ophthalmol 16:271–278, 1938.)

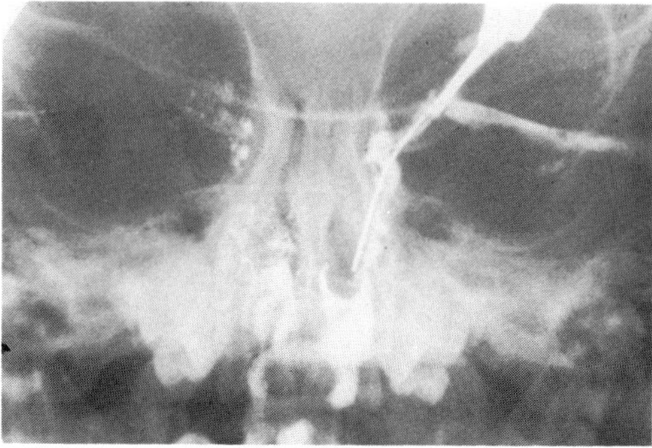

Figure 225–6. The probe is in a false passage. The dacryocystogram was performed by injecting contrast material through the lower canaliculus while the metallic probe was in place through the upper canaliculus. (From Jazbi BU, Cibis GW: Nasolacrimal duct probing in infants. Published courtesy of Ophthalmology 86:1488–91, 1979.)

a metal probe without creating a false passage" (Figs. 225–7 to 225–9).

Sevel[51, 52] expressed similar concerns in his discussion of the characteristic "give" at the conclusion of probing as the probe impinges against the distal angulated end of the bony wall of the nasolacrimal duct:

> A further obstacle to passing the probe is that the opening below the inferior concha enters the vestibule of the nose at approximately a 20-degree angle to the general direction of the bony canal. Therefore for the probe to enter the nose down the nasolacrimal duct, it would have to damage and tear the mucosa at this site. With probing, a typical resistance followed by a "give" is detected at the distal end of the nasolacrimal apparatus. As the flimsy membrane at the end of the nasolacrimal duct is composed of two layers of epithelium, it is unlikely that a metal probe, however gently passed, would detect a noticeable resistance. The most likely reason for this resistance is that the probe impinges against the distal-angled end of the bony wall of the nasolacrimal duct. The probe with extra pressure slips past the "give" and inevitably must traumatize the lining mucosa.[52]

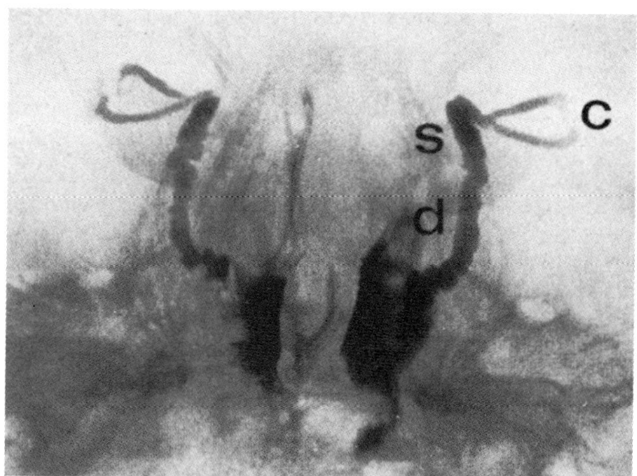

Figure 225–7. This postmortem dacryocystogram in a prematurely born infant (1800 g) shows distinct segmentation of the contrast column by transverse mucosal folds and deep inflexion of the nasolacrimal duct; C indicates canaliculi; S, nasolacrimal sac; and d, the nasolacrimal duct. (From Busse H, Muller KM, Kroll P: Radiological and histological findings of the lacrimal passages of newborns. Arch Ophthalmol 98:529–532. Copyright 1980, American Medical Association.)

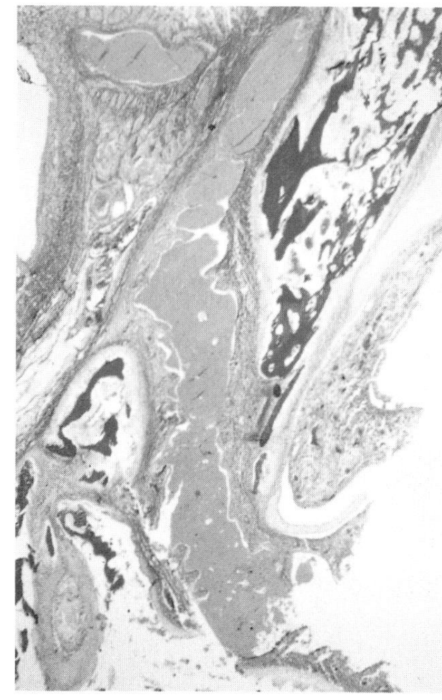

Figure 225–8. Right nasolacrimal duct with a perforated Hasner's membrane. This is from same 1800-g premature infant detailed in Figure 225–7. Van Gieson's stain, original magnification ×6. (From Busse H, Muller KM, Kroll P: Radiological and histological findings of the lacrimal passages of newborns. Arch Ophthalmol 98:529–532. Copyright 1980, American Medical Association.)

The inference from both Busse[21] and Sevel[51, 52] is that the angulations of the nasolacrimal duct are more marked in the newborn period in contrast to the more familiar adult configuration. Both authors worry about where a probe would actually pass, and they both suggest syringing rather than probing. Their observations might also be taken as reasons for delaying probing when it is practical.

DIGITAL COMPRESSION OF THE NASOLACRIMAL SAC

Kipp,[2, 10] Peters,[3, 4] and others[5, 7] discussed the role of nasolacrimal sac compression in the therapy of infants with nasolacrimal duct obstruction. Stephenson's observation[5] bears repetition: It is those physicians who give the most time and attention to the compression of the nasolacrimal sac and, in fact, those who perform the maneuver themselves during the office visits who will be most impressed with its helpfulness—not in all cases, but in sufficient number to be worthwhile. Crigler's report of 1923[53] is often quoted for its particular emphasis on nasolacrimal sac compression, but his implication that almost all cases could be relieved in this manner could well be considered overly optimistic. Crigler[53] was

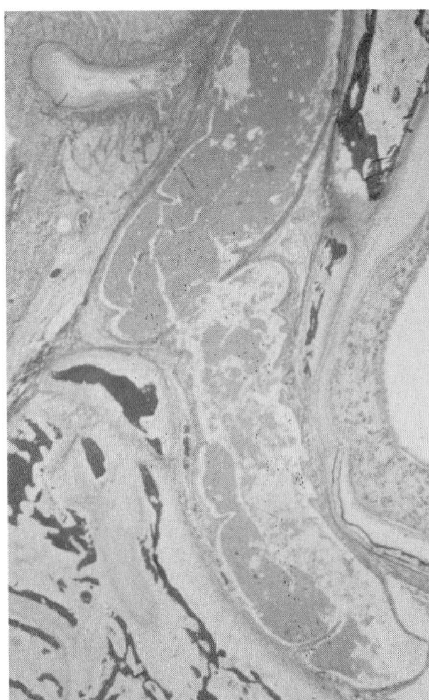

Figure 225–9. Right nasolacrimal duct from a 1850-g premature infant studied in the same fashion as the infant in Figures 225–7 and 225–8. Both postmortem dacryostography and histology demonstrate a persisting Hasner's membrane. Van Gieson's stain, original magnification ×6. (From Busse H, Muller KM, Kroll P: Radiological and histological findings of the lacrimal passages of newborns. Arch Ophthalmol 98:529–532. Copyright 1980, American Medical Association.)

preceded by Kipp[10] in both his enthusiasm for the maneuver and his overstatement of its efficacy. With this reservation about overstatement in mind, it must also be observed that those authors who conclude that nasolacrimal sac compression helps only rarely or is recommended principally to give the family a false sense of participation[54] may be underestimating a beneficial intervention.

According to Crigler[53]

> The salient points to remember are (1) pressure must be made over the sac only when it is extended; (2) care should be taken that the thumb is applied in such a way to prevent regurgitation in the conjunctival sac; and (3) sudden pressure over the sac causes the retained fluid to burst through the persistent fetal membrane which separates the mucous lining of the nose from that of the nasolacrimal duct.

In 1982 Kushner[55] conducted a prospective randomized study to evaluate the effectiveness of no massage at all versus simple massage versus specific attention to the detail of compression of the nasolacrimal duct in a manner that would increase the hydrostatic pressure within the nasolacrimal sac with the intent to rupture the membranous obstruction. The latter method of digital compression of the nasolacrimal sac was significantly more effective than simple massage or no massage at all. Kushner studied a total of 132 children with 175 affected eyes. The average age at the time of initial examination was approximately 7 mo for all three groups.

> Of the 58 eyes in the control group, four showed spontaneous resolution of symptoms and did not require probing. In the 58 eyes in the 44 infants in the simple massage group, five eyes had spontaneous improvement, which was not a statistically significant difference from the results in the control group. In the hydrostatic massage group, 18 of the 59 eyes showed spontaneous improvement. This finding represented a significant difference . . . when compared with results in the other two groups. Four parents with children in this last group indicated that they suddenly felt the obstruction "pop open" while they were in the process of massaging the nasolacrimal system and that this event was immediately followed by total cessation of epiphora and mattering.[55]

Frankel (1988)[56] reemphasized the importance of digital compression of the nasolacrimal sac in the therapy of nasolacrimal duct obstruction. Nucci and colleagues[57] in 1989 published a study of 59 children 1 to 24 mo of age with much the same conclusion.

> [The treatment employed in Nucci's study was] local hydrostatic massage and antibiotic eye drops. Children 1 to 12 months of age showed a cure rate of 93.3%; only two of them underwent nasolacrimal probing. Children 13 to 24 months of age had a cure rate of 79.3%, and six underwent probing. The initial probings were successful in both age groups.[57]

DOES TIMING OF PROBING OR SYRINGING AFFECT THE LONG-TERM OUTCOME?

In 1946 Price[58] raised the question whether pediatricians see a milder spectrum of clinical disease caused by nasolacrimal duct obstruction than do most ophthalmologists and thought, "Nature takes care of most of these cases of delayed development." Reviewing his records of 204 infants, Price had one case of true dacryocystitis that was referred directly to an ophthalmologist. Of the remaining 203 infants, 11 were eventually treated with probing. Of the 192 remaining infants, 149 (78 percent) were free of symptoms by 3 mo of age, 26 (14 percent) were free of symptoms by 6 mo of age, 12 more (6 percent) were clear by 1 yr, and 5 (3 percent) cleared during the second year. Contemporaneously, Cassady[17] in 1948 expressed his preference for probing "at once without a trial period of conservative treatment." Koke in 1950[59] also favored early probing if the symptoms had not cleared over a month. He reported a series of 116 infants of whom "88 were cured by a single probing, 11 by two or more probings, and 14 by irrigation, [whereas] three were not relieved by repeated probings."

Although many children with nasolacrimal duct obstruction are eventually relieved of their symptoms either as the result of time, digital compression, or surgical intervention with probing or syringing, it is important to note that this is not invariably so. Two of the areas of most lively current discussion center around these issues: (1) What procedure should be recommended for those difficult cases that do not respond to a series of probings and irrigations? and (2) Does the timing of probing or syringing influence the frequency of long-term cure?

Morgan (1938),[60] Redmond (1949),[61] Blankstein, (1952),[62] and Summerskill (1952),[63] reported on dacryocystorhinostomy procedures in children with chronic conditions for whom probings had failed, and many authors still recommend this approach.[54, 64] Dacryocystorhinostomy is the only option if one cannot pass a probe into the nose, but if symptoms persist, in spite of successful passage of a probe into the nose, many surgeons prefer to intubate the nasolacrimal passageways rather than to perform a dacryocystorhinostomy. Intubation of the nasolacrimal passages with a silk seton was described by Berry in a 5-year-old child as early as 1909.[46] Since the introduction of silastic tubing, an extensive literature and experience with intubation techniques has developed over recent decades[65–84] with some differences of opinion among authors as to how many "simple" probings to perform before introducing the indwelling plastic tubes and then how long to leave the tubing in place.[85, 86] Nordlow and Vennerholm (1953)[87] found that 14 percent of their infants failed to respond to 3 to 6 probings and recommended for this situation the surgical dislocation of the anterior part of the inferior turbinate along with the surgical removal of the nasal mucosa overlying the nasal end of the nasolacrimal duct. Infracturing of the inferior turbinate for resistant cases has been advocated by several authors as an alternative to dacryocystorhinostomy or silicone tube intubation or as adjunctive therapy to be used with silicone intubation in cases that have failed to respond to a series of probings.[46–48, 88–90]

It is evident in light of all this work on the complicated cases, that infants with nasolacrimal duct obstruction do not invariably get better with time alone or even with the assistance of probings and irrigations. All ophthalmologists agree on this fact and in general are more acutely aware of this problem than are pediatricians. A major difference of opinion among ophthalmologists is whether or not the existing data support the contention that the timing of probing influences the likelihood of a given individual's having a complicated course. Some authors have concluded that delay in probing might itself contribute to later problems because of secondary changes in the nasolacrimal drainage system consequent to chronic infection. Others conclude that the differences in outcome are more closely related to variations in the severity of congenital anatomic anomalies. Without direct access to the internal anatomy of the nasolacrimal duct over time in individual cases, it is difficult to put this discussion completely to rest.

Hurd (1955)[91] quoted Grantstrom that an infant had lost an eye "from this defection on more than one occasion. To be tolerant of such an infected pocket hardly seems sound if its elimination can be accomplished without complications by a relatively simple measure." Broggi (1959)[92] believed: "Damage occurs only as a result of temporizing or deferring probing rather than by early probing." Broggi strove to perform probing "as early as possible" after the diagnosis had been made and probed 30 infants between 3 and 4½ wk of age. He advocated probing both nasolacrimal ducts even in the absence of a diagnosis in the opposite eye. If these recommendations were generalized, 5 to 6 percent of all infants would be probed, and it would take quite a large series and lengthy follow-up to differentiate the benefit or harm of the probings relative to expected natural history. During the same decade, Evan (1956)[93] expressed the opinion, "Perhaps we interfere too early in the majority of cases."

Ffooks in 1961[94] provided a paper on dacryocystitis and observed that although the treatment of congenital nasolacrimal duct obstruction "has led to controversy for many years, its main complication, acute dacryocystitis with formation of lacrimal abscess, has received little attention." He suggested that acute dacryocystitis in infancy should be treated by early probing under cover of systemic antibiotics. In 1962 Ffooks[95] discussed nasolacrimal duct obstruction in general and noted the uncertainty of the result. Observing that Crigler[53] claimed to have no failures in 7 yr following a conservative regimen and that Nelson (1953),[96] who had advocated probing before the age of 2 mo, had also claimed to have no failures in 25 yr, Ffooks concluded: "Few surgeons nowadays would claim 100 percent success with either conservative or radical treatment, and it is well recognized that dacryocystorhinostomy is sometimes required, whatever method of treatment is employed." In his review of over 300 cases,[95] Ffooks also deliberated over the relatively large number of children who continued to have intermittent symptoms despite substantial improvement after one or more probings. He wondered if the timing of the probing affected the success of the procedure in eliminating the symptoms. "It is considered that no hard-and-fast rule can be given as to the duration of conservative treatment." Ffooks personally suggested probing between 3 to 4 mo of age. He believed his results indicated that "earlier probing does not have any greater success, nor does the cure rate from probing decrease markedly until after the age of 9 months."

Subsequent studies have not uniformly supported Ffooks' conclusion that probings after 9 mo of age have a lower success rate. Mittelman (1986)[97] thought his data suggested a threshold at 1 yr of age. Katowitz and Welsh (1987)[98] presented data on 572 eyes with a success rate of 97 percent with initial probing under 13 mo of age, compared with a mean success rate of 55 percent with intervention over 13 mo of age. El-Mansoury and colleagues (1986)[99] even reported a high success rate in 104 consecutive patients (138 eyes) with congenital nasolacrimal duct obstruction who were probed after the age of 13 months: "One hundred twenty-nine eyes (94 percent) were cured after the first probing."

Like Ffooks earlier, Katowitz and Welsh[98] specifically comment:

> It is of interest that most studies investigating the success of probing in congenital nasolacrimal duct obstruction eliminate acute dacryocystitis from the study. This is due

no doubt to the fact that this fortunately less common problem does not respond as well to our usual conservative medical or surgical efforts at management. It is important to recognize, however, that acute dacryocystitis can certainly result from congenital nasolacrimal duct obstruction and that it should not be completely disregarded as a concern.

Weil[54] concurs with the importance of dacryocystitis:

> In the series of infants studied at the Children's Hospital in Buenos Aires, a first probing was successful in 87.8 percent of cases. If such complications as a concurrent dacryocystitis were present, the success rate dropped to 71.1 percent. Under conditions in which there was no previous manipulation or trauma, no associated purulent dacryocystitis, and no associated congenital malformation, success rates in probing were 92.7 percent.

It may well be that, in some cases, dacryocystitis is alerting us to the presence of congenital aberrations like the diverticula described by Schaeffer[25, 26] and documented photographically by Busse and colleagues.[21] Bullock and Goldberg[100] provided an instructive dacryocystogram of a 6-month-old infant presenting with acute left periorbital cellulitis. Previous probing had demonstrated no obstruction to the nasolacrimal duct. The dacryocystogram showed multiple diverticula of the left lacrimal sac. The child's recurrent infections remitted after a left dacryocystorhinostomy with excision of the diverticula.

In helping a family weigh the merits of probing at different ages, it is useful to discuss the relative likelihood of resolution of symptoms over time. In 1978 Petersen and Robb[101] reported findings of a 5-yr study:

> Of 65 obstructed nasolacrimal ducts, 58 opened spontaneously and only seven required probing. Probing was successful on the first attempt in all seven. Spontaneous resolution occurred in the first few months of life in the majority of patients. Only a few obstructed nasolacrimal ducts opened spontaneously after the ninth month of life. However, one patient had a spontaneous resolution of his problem after he was 1 year of age. [In discussion they note that] it has been suggested that patients with congenital dacryostenosis who are not probed may develop obstruction later in life,[108] but if patency of the duct does develop spontaneously, it seems unlikely that probing would enhance the situation. There is, to our knowledge, no data to link congenital nasolacrimal duct obstruction with the kind of obstruction that develops later in life.

Paul (1985)[102] studied 55 infants who were diagnosed with congenital nasolacrimal duct obstruction by an ophthalmologist before the age of 3 mo:

> All were followed prospectively, primarily with medical management. Seven were treated surgically. In the 55 infants, there were 62 obstructed nasolacrimal ducts. Eighty-nine per cent (55 of 62) of the nasolacrimal ducts were opened with medical management only in the first 16 months of life. Of the nasolacrimal ducts that opened spontaneously, 15% (8 of 55) were open at 3 months, 45 percent (25 of 55) were open at 6 months, 71% (30 of 55) were open at 9 months and 93% (51 of 55) were open at 1 year. Based on this data one can advise the parents of infants with nasolacrimal duct obstruction what the odds of remission are without surgery by the twelfth month of age. Of the infants obstructed at 3 months of age, 80% were clear by the twelfth month. Of the infants obstructed at 6 months, 70% were clear by the twelfth month, and of those still obstructed at 9 months, 52% were clear by the twelfth month.

Paul himself interpreted these data as a reason for waiting a while before probing,[102] whereas Baker (1985)[103] uses similar numbers in his discussions with families before routinely probing as early as 3 mo of age and occasionally earlier:

> The parents are always explained the options of probing versus waiting. They are told that up to 80% of obstructed ducts may clear by age 8 months and that 60% may clear between 3 and 8 months of age. However, by the time the child is 4 to 6 months of age, most parents say they are tired of the situation and would like some definitive action taken.

Among all the many infants with clinical evidence of nasolacrimal duct obstruction (5 to 6 percent of all newborn children), only a small percentage go on to have tearing difficulties on a long-term basis despite a series of probings. Ophthalmologists remain divided with regard to the question of whether the timing of probing influences the long-term result in a percentage of infants with nasolacrimal duct obstruction. In either case, infection is undesirable. Even if low-grade infection were to cause only minimal damage to the nasolacrimal duct itself, an eye that chronically exudes pus presents an undesirable source of potential infection, be it dacryocystitis, preseptal or orbital cellulitis,[104] or endophthalmitis in the context of concurrent infantile cataract surgery.[105] There can be little doubt that the stagnant reservoir behind the blockage of a nasolacrimal duct obstruction can act as a source of infection. Schaeffer and colleagues (1990)[106] reported that a previously healthy patient became septic following a probing procedure. Stimulated by that observation they prospectively evaluated 12 patients and found that four of those children developed positive blood cultures after probing. The authors particularly emphasized that patients at risk to develop endocarditis should receive antibiotics prior to probing procedures.

Early probing offers the potential advantage of removing a source of chronic infection at the cost of a procedure that might not have been necessary if time, antibiotics, and digital compression of the lacrimal sac had been given a trial. The availability of antibiotics, both topically and systemically, has undoubtedly helped make most infections easier to control, and the risk of extremely serious infectious disease must be less than it was in the preantibiotic era.

CONGENITAL MUCOCELES

The term *mucocele* has been used for a noninflamed massive enlargement of the nasolacrimal sac (Fig. 225–10). The lower end of the nasolacrimal duct is obstructed

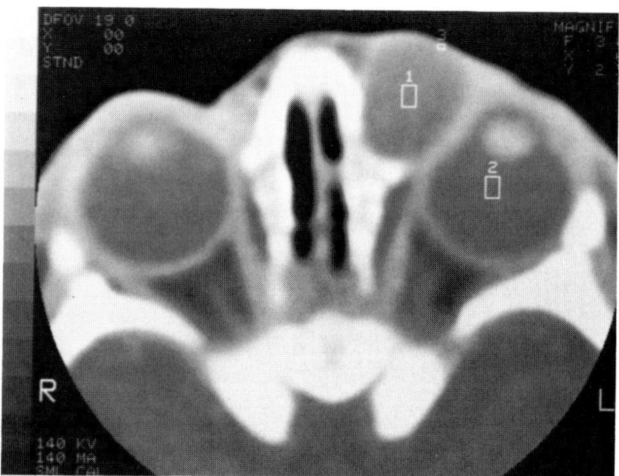

Figure 225–10. CT scan of an infant with a congenital mucocele. Note the massive enlargement of the nasolacrimal sac (1) in comparison to the size of the eye (2).

by a mucous membrane and there is at least a functional blockage in the upper portion of the lacrimal passageways that prevents spontaneous decompression through the canaliculi and puncta.

In 1900 Gunn[107] brought particular attention to the presentation of a mucocele:

> A lump in the region of the nasolacrimal sac is noticed soon or immediately after birth, but it does not inflame until a week or two later. . . . The condition, therefore, in so far as it is congenital, is one of mucocele, and not a dacryocystitis or abscess. . . . The most obvious explanation, then, of the presence of this cavity in some cases of congenital obstruction is that it represents a dilated duct, the dilation being brought about during fetal life by an obstruction at the lower end. . . . The rapid cure following the passage of a probe in some of the cases quoted points to the obstruction having been thin and membranous.

Gunn was subsequently quoted by Jackson (1907)[7] as reporting a case "in which the mucocele, after having persisted for 2 years, was cured by a single passage of the probe."

In 1938 Morgan[60] commented:

> In three cases . . . infants a few days old . . . developed a tense swelling of the lacrimal sac, which, on pressure, was slightly tender. No regurgitation of fluid could be produced either into the nose or into the conjunctival sac. I was tempted to pass a probe in the first case, but the lump suddenly disappeared, emptying presumably into the nose, and gave no further trouble. I used the same expectant treatment in the other two and they also cured themselves in the same way.

In discussion of Morgan's paper, Valentine reported his experience with two cases, each of which had responded well to a combined procedure involving a probing from above while "a rhinological colleague . . . passed a probe upward through the nose, which impinging on the lacrimal probe, made a perforation in the mucous membrane."

Jones and Wobig in 1977[108] proposed the term *congenital amniotocele*, presuming that "the tear sacs were distended with amniotic fluid at birth." Petersen and Robb in 1978[101] and Scott, and coworkers in 1979[109] preferred the term *congenital mucocele* and regarded it as one of the few indications for immediate lacrimal system probing in the newborn. Scott and colleagues expressed the opinion that the fluid within the mucocle was probably not amniotic but was rather normal secretion produced by the nasolacrimal system.

Jones and Wobig,[108] Levy,[110] Weinstein and associates[111] and Harris and DiClementi[112] confirmed Morgan's observation that congenital mucoceles sometimes resolve without surgical intervention, but in some of their patients, intervening dacryocystitis sometimes forced the decision to probe. Generally, the probing did resolve the problem. Wojno (1985)[113] described identical twins, both of whom were found to have unilateral congenital dacryoceles. Both were immediately probed, resulting in resolution in one twin and recurrence in the other. Weinstein and colleagues[111] emphasized that the differential diagnosis of swelling in the region of the lacrimal sac includes not only mucocele and dacryocystitis but also hemangioma and, of particular concern, encephalocele.

Cibis and colleagues (1986)[114] and Raflo and coworkers (1982)[115] used radiologic procedures to document remarkable enlargement of the lacrimal sac in the circumstance of congenital mucocele. With obstruction of the nasolacrimal passages both below and above, enlargement of the lacrimal sac can reach remarkable proportions. The pressure may not only distend the nasolacrimal sac, but may also cause distention of the mucous membrane at the lower end of the nasolacrimal duct to the point that the nasal cavity is obstructed. Indeed, Raflo and colleagues[115] reported that examination of the nose showed a large cystic structure totally occluding the right nostril. Surgical excision of the entire cyst was required to alleviate the patient's recurrent mucoceles of the lacrimal sac and epiphora. The need for nasal examination and more thorough evaluation in cases of recurrent obstruction was emphasized in evaluating patients with congenital obstruction of the nasolacrimal drainage system.

Divine and colleagues (1983)[116] reported "a newborn infant with bilateral mucoceles of the lacrimal sacs [who] also had submucosal masses along the floor of the nose, beneath the inferior turbinates, communicating with the mucoceles." Their treatment of this condition included "wide marsupialization of the nasal masses into the nose under direct visualization."

In the light of these reports of nasal masses, it is interesting to quote Peters[3] in 1891 referencing Coppez' case of congenital tear sac swelling, which was cleared by suctioning of the nose. Zentmayer[10] was apparently referring to the same early report by Coppez when he mentioned the historic report of a lacrimal tumor that had been "rapidly cured by the nurse applying suction to the nose of the infant."

CONCLUSIONS

The most important factor dictating the nature and timing of interventions for nasolacrimal duct obstruction is the frequency and severity of infections that occur in the presence of a stagnant reservoir of tears and mucus. An otherwise normal infant who has had a recurrently infected eye since birth is likely to improve following a probing of the nasolacrimal duct. In general there is little controversy within ophthalmologic circles with regard to the efficacy of probing, although anatomic studies have suggested that false passages are probably more common than realized, and some authors have advocated hydrostatic rupture of the membrane with saline or air under pressure rather than mechanical rupture with a metal probe. On the other hand, it has been documented that 80 to 90 percent of youngsters with nasolacrimal duct obstruction will experience a clearing of their symptoms during the first 9 to 12 mo of life if they are kept free of infection with topical antibiotics and if the nasolacrimal sac is decompressed manually to reduce stagnation.

There is considerable difference of opinion with regard to the timing of probing. Some ophthalmologists generally recommend probing after 3 to 4 mo,[95, 103, 117, 118] others after 6 mo of age,[119] some usually wait until approximately one year of age,[97, 120, 121] and some regularly wait until the second year of life.[57, 99, 122, 123] However, to qualify for this "timing" debate it is important that the infant's signs and symptoms of the nasolacrimal duct obstruction be reduced to clear tearing only, without evidence of chronic infection. Even an ophthalmologist who normally waits until 1 yr of age to recommend probing in the majority of instances may well recommend probing earlier if persistent infection is a problem in spite of the family's best efforts.

The parents should be taught to compress the lacrimal sac, and they should continue this treatment at home to keep the sac empty. When there is a thick discharge on the lashes in addition to clear tearing, it is best to prescribe an antibiotic ophthalmic ointment in addition to periodic direct compression of the lacrimal sac. The treatment objectives are to prevent infections and to minimize stagnation. Topical antibiotic therapy should be started at the first sign of infection (crusting or discharge on the lashes) without waiting for a secondary conjunctivitis or a dacryocystitis to develop.

Many parents find it easier to instill antibiotic drops than ointment, but the blinking mechanism is so vigorous and effective in young children that the antibiotic eye drop is quickly washed away. The half life of an eye drop is shorter in children than in adults. Eye ointments linger longer[124] and are generally more effective in this setting. Linn and Jones in 1968[125] demonstrated that petrolatum-based vehicles do not occlude the lacrimal excretory system. If discharge on the lashes cannot be controlled with a particular eye drop, consideration should be given to changing to an ophthalmic ointment as well as changing to an antibiotic with a different spectrum of activity. Culturing the discharge may be helpful if the infection is particularly severe or unusually persistent.

Issues relating to the timing of probing include not only the likelihood of resolution without probing but also anesthetic issues. Most ophthalmologists who recommend early probing (for example, up to 6 mo of age) tend to do them in the office. Youngsters at this age are smaller and weaker and require less restraint for probings done in the office. A general anesthesia is thus avoided, and despite the concerns raised about false passages by anatomic studies, the probing generally is successful in relieving the symptoms. Those ophthalmologists who wait until 1 to 2 yr of age before probing usually recommend that the procedure be done under a brief mask-inhalation anesthesia. Endotracheal intubation is not required. These ophthalmologists point out that far fewer probings are required with this strategy, and in general they feel that the brief anesthesia is an advantage rather than a disadvantage since the youngster is more relaxed and the procedure is less likely to cause inadvertent injury to the nasolacrimal system. Happily, most infants with nasolacrimal duct obstruction are symptomatically improved after the initial probing, but if tearing persists after the initial probing, another probing is indicated. If several probings have failed, more complex surgical procedures may be indicated.

REFERENCES

1. Mackenzie W: A Practical Treatise on the Diseases of the Eye. London, Longman, Rees, Orme, Brown, Green, 1830.
2. Kipp J: Dacryocystitis in nursing infants. Am Ophthalmol Soc Trans 12:537–538, 1879.
3. Peters A: On the so-called tear sac blennorrhea in newborns. Klin Monatsbl Augenheilkd 29:376–383, 1891.
4. Peters A: On the treatment of atresia of the lacrimal duct in newborns. Klin Monstsbl Augenheilkd 30:363–370, 1892.
5. Stephenson S: A preliminary communication on affections of the tear-passages in newly born children. Press Cir 68:103–104, 1899.
6. Cutler CW: Cases of delayed opening of the nasolachrymal septum in the new-born, with consequent dacryocystitis. Arch Ophthalmol 32:289–290, 1903.
7. Jackson E: Delayed development of the lacrimal-nasal duct. Ophthalmic Rec 16:321–324, 1907.
8. Weeks JE: Congenital occlusion of the lachrymal canal. JAMA 43:1760–1762, 1904.
9. Parsons JH: Symptoms and pathology lachrymal obstruction. Br Med 1:417–419, 1907.
10. Zentmayer W: Imperforation of the lachrymonasal duct in the new-born and its clinical manifestations. JAMA 51:188–191, 1908.
11. Woodruff HW: Congenital dacryocystitis. Ill Med 60:380–382, 1931.
12. Riser RO: Dacryostenosis in children. Am Ophthalmol 18:1116–1122, 1935.
13. Hardesty JF: Obstruction of the lacrimal passages in the newborn infant. J M Med Assoc 38:40–41, 1941.
14. Simpson GV: Sulfadiazine in treatment of dacryocystitis of the newborn. Arch Ophthalmol 33:62–66, 1945.
15. Corner B: Discussion of neonatal infections. Soc Med 39:383–388, 1946.
16. Guerry D III, Kendig EL: Congenital impatency of the nasolacrimal duct. Arch ophthalmol 39:193–204, 1948.
17. Cassady, JV: Dacryocystitis of infancy. Am Ophthalmol 31:773–780, 1948.
18. Mayou MS: Lachrymal abscess in the newborn. Lond Ophthalmic Hosp Rep 17:246–253, 1908.
19. Schwarz: Congenital atresia of the nasolacrimal canal. Arch Ophthalmol 13:301–302, 1935.
20. Cassady JV: Developmental anatomy of nasolacrimal duct. Arch Ophthalmol 47:141–158, 1952.

21. Busse H, Muller KM, Kroll P: Radiological and histological findings of the lacrimal passages of newborns. Arch Ophthalmol 98:528–532, 1980.
22. Whitnall SE: The Anatomy of the Human Orbit and Accessory Organs of Vision, 2nd ed. London, Humphrey Milford Oxford University Press, 1932.
23. Gerard G: Des obstacles naturels capables de compliquer le catheterisme des vois lacrymales. Ann d'Ocul 137:193, 1907.
24. Rochon-Duvigneaud: Dilation of the tearducts in the fetus and newborn following perforation of the inferior cavity. Anatomical conditions which favor dacryocystitis. Arch d'Ophthalmologiques 19:81–89, 1899.
25. Schaeffer JP: The genesis and development of the nasolacrimal passages in man. Anat 13:1–24, 1912.
26. Schaeffer JP: The Nose, Paranasal Sinuses, Nasolacrimal Passageways, and Olfactory Organ in Man. Philadelphia, P. Blakiston's, 1920.
27. Muller KM, Busse H, Osmers F: Anatomy of the nasolacrimal duct in newborns: therapeutic considerations. Eur J Pediatr, 129:83–92, 1978.
28. Campbell DM, Carter JM, Doub HP: Roentgen ray studies of the nasolacrimal passageways. Arch Ophthalmol 11:462–470, 1922.
29. Ewing AE: Roentgen ray demonstrations of the lacrimal abscess cavity. Ophthalmol 26:1–4, 1909.
30. Szily AV: The pathology of the tear sac and the ductus nasolacrimalis on the x-ray. Klin Monatsbl Augenheilkd 52:847–854, 1914.
31. Waldapfel R: Location of congenital dacryostenosis in children. Am J Ophthalmol 37:768–774, 1954.
32. Demorest BH, Milder B: Dacryocystography. Arch Ophthalmol 54:410–421, 1955.
33. Hurwitz JJ, Welham RA: The role of dacryocystography in the management of congenital nasolacrimal duct obstruction. Can J Ophthalmol 10:346–350, 1975.
34. Montanara A, Catalino P, Gualdi M: Improved radiological technique for evaluating the lacrimal pathways with special emphasis on functional disorders. Acta Ophthalmol 57:547–563, 1979.
35. Montanara A, Ciabattoni P, Rizzo P: Stenoses and functional disorders of the lacrimal drainage apparatus. Radiological examination. Surv Ophthalmol 23:249–258, 1979.
36. Montanara A, Mannino G, Contestabile MT: Macrodacryocystography and echography in diagnosis of disorders of the lacrimal pathways. Surv Ophthalmol 28:33–41, 1983.
37. Hurwitz JJ, Victor WH: The role of sophisticated radiological testing in the assessment and management of epiphora. Ophthalmology 92:407–413, 1985.
38. Rossomondo RM, Carlton WH, Trueblood JH, et al: A new method of evaluating lacrimal drainage. Arch Ophthalmol 88:523–525, 1972.
39. Amanat LA, Wraight EP, Watson PG, et al: Role of lacrimal scintigraphy and subtraction macrodacryocystography in the management of epiphora. Br J Ophthalmol 63:511–519, 1979.
40. Sorensen T, Jensen FT: Tear flow in normal human eyes. Determination by means of radioisotope and gamma camera. Acta Ophthalmol 57:564–581, 1979.
41. Raflo GT, Chart P, Hurwitz JJ: Thermographic evaluation of the human lacrimal drainage system. Ophthalmic Surg 13:119–124, 1982.
42. Doucet TW, Hurwitz JJ, Chin-Sang H: Lacrimal scintillography: advances and functional applications. Surv Ophthalmol 27:105–113, 1982.
43. White WL, Glover T, Buckner AB, et al: Relative canalicular tear flow as assessed by dacryoscintigraphy. Ophthalmology 96:167–169, 1988.
44. Grossman T, Putz, R: Uber die angelborene Travenganstenose der Neugeborenen, ihre anatomie, ihre Falgen und Behandlung. Klin Monatsbl Augenheilkd 160:563–572, 1972.
45. Larsson S: On the treatment of congenital atresia of the nasolacrimal duct. Acta Ophthalmol 16:271–278, 1938.
46. Berry JC: Treatment of obstruction of the lachrymal duct. Boston Med Surg J 160:541–544, 1909.
47. Wolter JR, Bogdasarian R: The management of persistent congenital occlusion of the nasolacrimal duct: after unsuccessful probing. Pediatr Ophthalmol 15:251–252; 1978.
48. Sterk CC: Probing in congenital dacryostenosis or atresia. Doc Ophthalmol 50:321–325, 1980.
49. Jazbi BU, Cibis GW: Nasolacrimal duct probing in infants. Ophthalmology 86:1488–1491, 1979.
50. Onodi A: The Relations of the Lachrymal Organs to the Nose and Nasal Accessory Sinuses, New York, William Wood, 1913.
51. Sevel D: Development and congenital abnormalities of the nasolacrimal apparatus. J Pediatr Ophthalmol 18:13–19, 1981.
52. Sevel D: Insufflation treatment of occluded nasolacrimal apparatus in the child. Ophthalmology 89:329–334, 1982.
53. Crigler LW: The treatment of congenital dacryocystitis. JAMA 81:23–24, 1923.
54. Milder B, Weil BA: The Lacrimal System. E. Norwalk, CT, Appleton-Century-Crofts, 1983, pp 102–103.
55. Kushner BJ: Congenital nasolacrimal system obstruction. Arch Ophthalmol 100:597–600, 1982.
56. Frankel CA: The treatment of dacryostenosis. JAMA 260:2666, 1988.
57. Nucci P, Capoferri P, Alfarano R, et al: Conservative management of congenital nasolacrimal duct obstruction. J Pediatr Ophthalmol Strabismus 26:39–43, 1989.
58. Price HW: Dacryostenosis. Pediat 30:302–305, 1947.
59. Koke MP: Treatment of occluded nasolacrimal ducts in infants. Arch Ophthalmol 43:750–754; 1950.
60. Morgan OG: Observations on the treatment of epiphora, with special reference to some cases treated by dacryocystorhinostomy. Trans Ophthalmol Soc UK 58:163–172, 1938.
61. Redmond KB: Dacryocysto-rhinostomy in an infant. Med J 1:462, 1949.
62. Blankstein SS: Dacryocystorhinostomy in infants and children. Arch Ophthalmol 48:322–327, 1952.
63. Summerskill WH: Dacryocystorhinostomy by intubation. Br J Ophthalmol 36:240–244, 1952.
64. Robb RM: Treatment of congenital nasolacrimal system obstruction. J Pediatr Ophthalmol Strabismus 22:36–37, 1985.
65. Keith CG: Intubation of the lacrimal passages. Am J Ophthalmol 65:70–75, 1968.
66. Christman EH: Adjuncts to tear duct probing. Eye Ear Nose Throat Mouth Ophthalmol 51:439–440, 1972.
67. Thornton SP: Nasolacrimal duct reconstruction with the nasolacrimal duct prosthesis; an alternative to standard dacryocystorhinostomy. Ann Ophthalmol 9:1575–1582, 1977.
68. Anderson RL, Edwards JJ: Indications, complications, and results with silicone stents. Ophthalmology 86:1474–1487, 1979.
69. Pashby RC, Rathbun JE: Silicone tube intubations of the lacrimal drainage system. Arch Ophthalmol 97:1318–1322, 1979.
70. Jackson ST: A new probe for silicone intubation of the lacrimal drainage system. Ophthalmic Surg 11:588–590, 1980.
71. Busse H, Junemann G, Kroll P: Simplified intubation technique in congenital dacryostenosis. Ocular Ther Surg 1:274–277, 1982.
72. Kraft SP, Crawford JS: Silicone tube intubation in disorders of the lacrimal system in children. Am J Ophthalmol 94:290–299, 1982.
73. Dortzbach RK, France TD, Kushner BJ, et al: Silicone intubation for obstruction of the nasolacrimal duct in children. Am J Ophthalmol 94:585–590, 1982.
74. Nagashima K: Silicone-octopus repair of lacrimal obstructions in children. Ophthalmic Surg 14:766–769, 1983.
75. Tse D, Anderson RL: A new modification of the standard lacrimal groove director for nasolacrimal intubation. Arch Ophthalmol 101:1938–1939, 1983.
76. Neuhaus RW, Shorr N: Modified lacrimal system intubation. Ophthalmic Surg 14:1026–1028, 1983.
77. Rutherford S, Crawford JS, Hurwitz JJ: Silicone tubing used in intubating the lacrimal system. Ophthalmology 91:963–965, 1984.
78. Dresner SC, Codere F, Brownstein S, et al: Lacrimal drainage system inflammatory masses from retained silicone tubing. Am J Ophthalmol 98:609–613, 1984.
79. Mader TH; Wells JR, Rockwell JC: A method of removing displaced silicone tubing from the nasolacrimal duct system. Am J Ophthalmol 99:730–731, 1985.
80. Jordan DR, Nerad JA, Tse DT: Complete canaliculuar erosion associated with silicone stents. Am J Ophthalmol 101:382–383, 1986.
81. Beyer RW, Levine MR, Sternberg I: A method for repositioning

or extraction of lacrimal system silicone tubes. Ophthalmic Surg 17:496–498, 1986.
82. Hedges CR: New techniques in suture-aided tear duct intubation. Ophthalmic Surg 18:45–46, 1987.
83. Crawford JS: Lacrimal intubation set with suture in the lumen. Ophthalmic Plast Reconstruc Surg 4:249–250, 1988.
84. Vila-Coro AA: Monocanalicular lacrimonasal intubations. J Pediatr Ophthalmol Strabismus. 25:301–303, 1988.
85. Migliore ME, Putterman AM: Silicone intubation for the treatment of congenital lacrimal duct obstruction: successful results removing the tubes after six weeks. Ophthalmology 95:792–795, 1988.
86. Welsh MG, Katowitz JA: Timing of Silastic tubing removal after intubation for congenital nasolacrimal duct obstruction. Ophthalmic Plas Reconstruc Surg 5:43–48, 1989.
87. Nordlow W, Vennerholm I: Congenital atresiae of the lacrimal passages: their occurrence and treatment. Acta Ophthalmol 31:367–371, 1953.
88. Havins WE, Wilkins RB: A useful alternative to silicone intubation in congenital nasolacrimal duct obstructions. Ophthalmic Surg 14:666–670, 1983.
89. Wesley RE: Inferior turbinate fracture in the treatment of congenital nasolacrimal duct obstruction and congenital nasolacrimal duct anomaly. Ophthalmic Surg 16:368–371, 1985.
90. Nagashima K: Diagnosis of inferior turbinate impaction. Arch Ophthalmol 106:1650, 1988.
91. Hurd AC: Congenital dacryostenosis. J Maine Med Assoc 46:12–14, 1955.
92. Broggi RJ: The treatment of congenital dacryostenosis. Arch Ophthalmol 61:30–36, 1959.
93. Evans PJ: Problems of lacrimal obstruction. Trans Ophthalmol Soc UK 76:343–353, 1956.
94. Ffooks OO: Lacrimal abscess in the newborn. A report of seven cases. Br J Ophthalmol 45:562–565, 1961.
95. Ffooks OO: Dacryocystitis in infancy. Br J Ophthalmol 46:422–434, 1962.
96. Nelson F: Management of congenital occlusion of the tear duct. Am J Ophthalmol 36:1587–1590, 1953.
97. Mittelman D: Probing and irrigation for congenital nasolacrimal duct obstruction. Arch Ophthalmol 104:1125, 1986.
98. Katowitz JA, Welsh MG: Timing of initial probing and irrigation in congenital nasolacrimal duct obstruction. Ophthalmology 94:698–705, 1987.
99. El-Mansoury J, Calhoun JH, Nelson LB, et al: Results of late probing for congenital nasolacrimal duct obstruction. Ophthalmology 93:1052–1054, 1986.
100. Bullock JD, Goldberg SH: Lacrimal sac diverticuli. Arch Ophthalmol 107:756, 1989.
101. Petersen RA, Robb R: The natural cause of congenital obstruction of the nasolacrimal duct. J Pediatr Ophthalmol Strabismus 15:246–250, 1978.
102. Paul TO: Medical management of congenital nasolacrimal duct obstruction. J Pediatr Ophthalmol Strabismus 22:68–70, 1985.
103. Baker JD: Treatment of congenital nasolacrimal system obstruction. J Pediatr Ophthalmol Strabismus 22:34–35, 1985.
104. Molarte AB, Isenberg SJ: Periorbital cellulitis in infancy. J Pediatr Ophthalmol Strabismus 26:232–235, 1989.
105. Good WV, Hing S, Irvine AR, et al: Postoperative endophthalmitis in children following cataract surgery. J Pediatr Ophthalmol 27:283–285, 1990.
106. Schaeffer AR, Gordon RA, Sood SK: Bacteremia following nasolacrimal duct probing. Poster No. 2987–34, ARVO Annual Meeting, Sarasota, FL, 1990. Invest Ophthalmol Vis Sci 31:610; 1990.
107. Gunn D: Lacrimal obstruction in the young. Ophthalmol Rev 19:31–48, 1900.
108. Jones LT, Wobig JL: Newer concepts of tear duct and eyelid anatomy and treatment. Trans Am Acad Ophthalmol Otolaryngol 83:603–616, 1977.
109. Scott WE, Fabre JA, Ossoinig KC: Congenital mucocele of the lacrimal sac. Arch Ophthalmol 97:1656–1658, 1979.
110. Levy NS: Conservative management of congenital amniotocele of the nasolacrimal sac. J Pediatr Ophthalmol Strabismus, 16:254–256, 1979.
111. Weinstein GS, Biglan AW, Patterson JH: Congenital lacrimal sac mucoceles. Ophthalmol 94:106–110, 1982.
112. Harris GJ, DiClementi D: Congenital dacryocystocele. Arch Ophthalmol 100:1763–1765, 1982.
113. Wojno TH: Congenital dacryocystocele in identical twins. Ophthalmic Plast Reconstr Surg 1:263–265, 1985.
114. Cibis GW, Spurney RO, Waeltermann J: Radiographic visualization of congenital lacrimal sac mucoceles. Ann Ophthalmol 18:68–69, 1986.
115. Raflo GT, Horton JA, Sprinkle PM: An unusual intranasal anomaly of the lacrimal drainage system. Ophthalmic Surg 13:741–744, 1982.
116. Divine RD, Anderson RL, Bumsted RM: Bilateral congenital lacrimal sac mucoceles with nasal extension and drainage. Arch Ophthalmol 101:246–248, 1983.
117. Veirs ER: The Lacrimal System. St Louis, CV Mosby, 1971.
118. Veirs ER: *Lacrimal Disorders: Diagnosis and Treatment.* St Louis, CV Mosby, 1976.
119. Pollard ZF: Tear duct obstruction in children. Clin Pediatr 8:487–490, 1979.
120. Robb RM: Treatment of congenital nasolacrimal system obstruction. J Pediatr Ophthalmol Strabismus 22:36–37, 1985.
121. Robb RM: Probing and irrigation for congenital nasolacrimal duct obstruction. Arch Ophthalmol 104:378–379, 1986.
122. Nelson LB, Calhoun JH, Menduke H: Medical management of congenital nasolacrimal duct obstruction. Ophthalmology 92:1187–1190, 1985.
123. Nelson LB, Calhoun JH, Menduke H: Medical management of congenital nasolacrimal duct obstruction. Pediatrics 76:172–175, 1985.
124. Hardberger R, Hanna C, Boyd CM: Effects of drug vehicles on ocular contact time. Arch Ophthalmol 93:42–45, 1975.
125. Linn ML, Jones LT: Rate of lacrimal excretion of ophthalmic vehicles. Am J Ophthalmol 65:76–78, 1968.

Chapter 226

Conjunctivitis and Orbital Cellulitis in Childhood

ANTHONY J. FRAIOLI

Neonatal Conjunctivitis

In 1881, Crede introduced the use of 2 percent silver nitrate drops for prophylaxis against gonococcal ophthalmia neonatorum.[1] Prior to that time, gonococcal conjunctivitis had an incidence of 10 percent and was a leading cause of blindness. Prophylaxis with silver nitrate and other agents has greatly reduced the incidence of gonococcal conjunctivitis (0.06 percent in one study),[2] and *Chlamydia trachomatis* is the organism that now is the leading cause of neonatal conjunctivitis in the United States. Despite prophylaxis, conjunctivitis remains the most common neonatal infection and has a much higher incidence in less-developed countries.[3] The ongoing epidemic of sexually transmitted disease and the association of serious systemic involvement with infection by these agents makes neonatal conjunctivitis a very active public health issue.

DEFINITION

Neonatal conjunctivitis is an inflammation of the conjunctiva in an infant less than 1 mo old. Edema and erythema of the eyelids is usually present, as is a purulent discharge. There is a significant association with serious systemic infection.

ETIOLOGY

Chemical conjunctivitis is caused by the use of prophylactic agents instilled in the eye of newborns and is classically associated with silver nitrate. Infectious agents that cause neonatal conjunctivitis include bacterial, chlamydial, and viral species. The infection is typically acquired during passage through the birth canal, though infection can also be transmitted soon after birth by handlers and caregivers. Disruption of the conjunctival epithelium by trauma facilitates the acquisition of infection.

The conjunctival flora of newborns reflects the exposure during the birthing process. Of infants delivered by cesarian section within 3 hr of membrane rupture, 80 percent had sterile conjunctivae.[4] Vaginally delivered infants have conjunctival flora similar to that of the female genital tract.[4, 5] This is of particular importance in regard to sexually transmitted diseases. In one American study, 2.7 percent of pregnant women had positive cervical cultures of *Neisseria gonorrhoeae* prenatally. The figure was 6.4 percent[6] for a study from Nairobi, Kenya. For *C. trachomatis*, the respective figures were 8 percent[3] and 22 percent.[6] The Kenyan study[6] also demonstrated that 42 percent of newborns exposed to *N. gonorrhoeae* and 31.1 percent of infants exposed to *C. trachomatis* experience conjunctivitis. Forty to 60 percent of newborns exposed to active genital herpes simplex virus (HSV), type 2 infections experience herpetic infection.[7] Many infected women shed HSV type 2 even without active genital lesions. Approximately one of five infants with congenital herpetic infection have ocular involvement.

CLINICAL CHARACTERISTICS

The conjuctivitis caused by *N. gonorrhoeae* is typically hyperacute, with eyelid swelling, chemosis, and marked purulence (Fig. 226–1). Symptoms begin 24 to 48 hr after birth, with inflammation, discharge, and eyelid swelling following a day later. Conjunctival membranes may form, and without treatment, the disease will progress to keratitis, corneal ulceration, and eventually perforation.

Chlamydial conjunctivitis has been classically described as beginning 5 to 14 days after birth. The difference in time of onset is not, however, a reliable discriminator from gonococcal infection. Chlamydial conjunctivitis can be quite variable in severity. It is characterized primarily by a discharge that is often thick and purulent. The disease is generally self-limited without sequelae, but corneal opacification has been described in late follow-up.[8]

Nongonoccocal bacterial conjunctivitis may result from a variety of organisms. Chief among these are *Staphylococcus aureus*, *S. epidermidis*, *Streptococcus pneumoniae*, *S. viridans*, *Haemophilus influenzae*, and *Escherichia coli*. Bacterial conjunctivitis typically begins on the fifth day after birth and may not be clinically distinguishable from gonococcal disease.

HSV neonatal conjunctivitis occurs within the first 2 wk after birth. Vesicular eyelid lesions may or may not be present. The conjunctiva is only moderately inflamed, and the discharge is serosanguineous. Corneal involve-

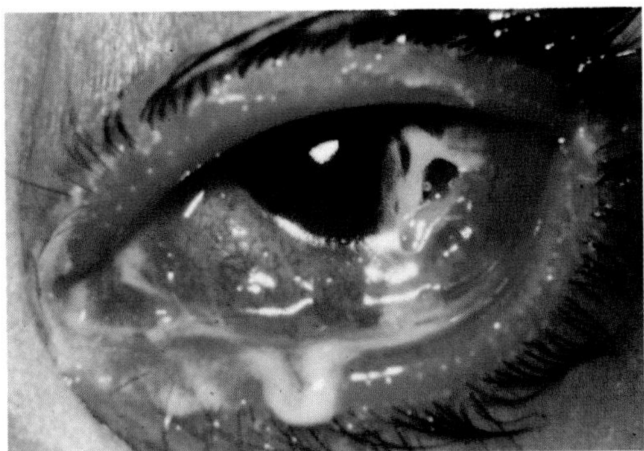

Figure 226–1. Hyperacute conjunctivitis of *N. gonorrhoeae*. Note the marked purulence and conjunctival chemosis.

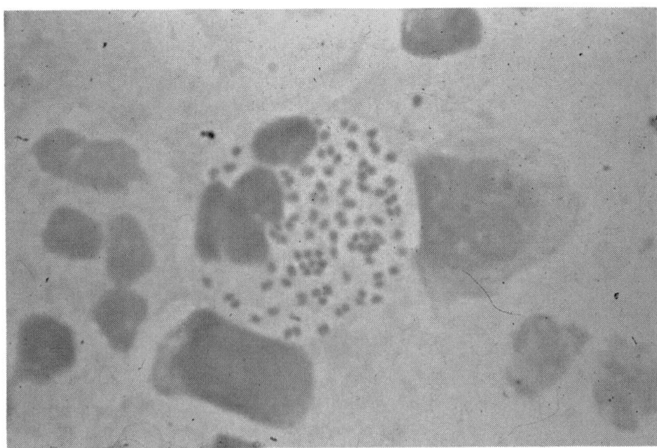

Figure 226–2. Gram stain showing intracellular gram-negative diplococci characteristic of *N. gonorrhoeae* infection.

ment is often not the usual herpetic dendrite seen in adult disease. Microdendrites and geographic ulcers are more typical in the neonatal form. Chorioretinitis and cataracts may also develop.[7]

SYSTEMIC COMPLICATIONS

Systemic complications from bacterial conjunctivitis are rare. However, infections with both gonococcus and *Pseudomonas* can progress to corneal ulcer, perforation, and endophthalmitis. Fatalities have been reported after *pseudomonas* endophthalmitis.

Twenty to 40 percent of newborns with chlamydial conjuctivitis experience chlamydial pneumonia by 90 days after birth.[9] Fourteen percent of these infants have rectal and vaginal cultures positive for *Chlamydia*.

Neonatal HSV infection can occur in a disseminated form, with an 85 percent mortality rate. Localized disease may involve the eyes, mouth, skin, or central nervous system. Infection of the central nervous system has a mortality rate of 50 percent. The ocular involvement may precede or follow disseminated disease.[10] Long-term survivors of neonatal HSV infections have a high rate of ocular sequelae,[9] including 37 percent with visual acuity less than 20/200.[11]

DIAGNOSTIC EVALUATION

Neonatal conjunctivitis is a potentially serious infection with systemic consequences and must be promptly and fully evaluated. A prenatal history must be taken, and cervical specimens should be taken from the mother for culture when appropriate. A full ocular and general physical examination should be performed to ascertain the extent of the disease.

Laboratory studies should include conjunctival scrapings for Gram and Giemsa staining. The cytologic findings of chemical conjunctivitis are characterized by the presence of neutrophils. In bacterial conjunctivitis, both neutrophils and bacteria are present. In gonococcal disease, the bacteria are seen as intracellular gram-negative diplococci present inside the neutrophils (Fig. 226–2). Giemsa staining of chlamydial conjunctivitis will demonstrate basophilic cytoplasmic inclusion bodies in epithelial cells in 50 to 90 percent of culture-proven cases (Fig. 226–3). Viral disease is characterized by a predominance of lymphocytes. Plasma cells and multinucleated giant cells may also be present.

Swabs of the conjunctiva should be planted on reduced blood agar and cooked meat or thioglycolate broth for bacterial cultures. Chocolate agar in a CO_2-enriched atmosphere or Thayer-Martin media should be used for gonococcal cultures.

McCoy cell cultures are the standard for culturing *Chlamydia*. There are two more rapid tests for chlamydial infection: an enzyme-linked immunoassay and a monoclonal antibody stain. The latter test has been found to have 100 percent sensitivity and 94 percent specificity when compared with the McCoy cell chlamydial culture.[12] Viral cultures are performed only when there are clinical indications of viral disease.

PROPHYLAXIS

Crede's use of silver nitrate and the resultant decrease in the incidence of blindness from gonococcal conjunc-

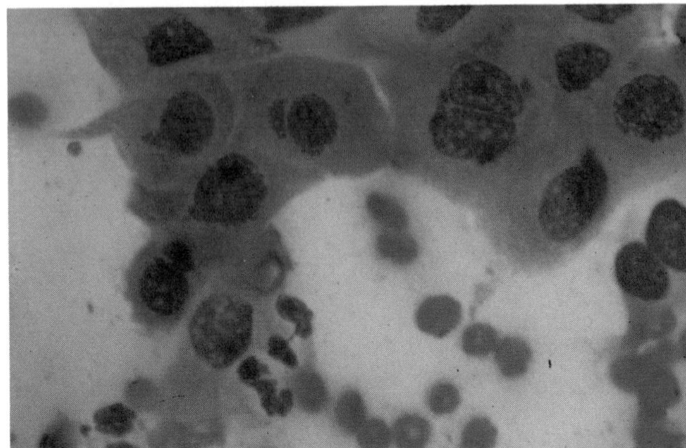

Figure 226–3. Giemsa stain showing basophilic, cytoplasmic inclusion bodies characteristic of *C. trachomatis*.

tivitis was one of the true triumphs of modern medicine. In recent years, however, the instillation of silver nitrate in the eyes of neonates has fallen into disfavor for two reasons. First, silver nitrate may cause a chemical conjunctivitis that may confuse the diagnosis. Second, with the declining incidence of gonococcal conjunctivitis in developed countries, *Chlamydia* has become the leading cause of neonatal conjunctivitis, and silver nitrate does not provide prophylaxis against *Chlamydia*.[2] In 1980 and again in 1986, the American Academy of Pediatrics endorsed the use of 1 percent tetracycline or 0.5 percent erythromycin ointment as prophylaxis against neonatal gonococcal conjunctivitis. Hammerschlag and associates[2] have demonstrated the equal effectiveness of silver nitrate drops, erythromycin ointment, and tetracycline ointment as prophylaxis against neonatal gonococcal ophthalmitis and the equal ineffectiveness of these same agents against *Chlamydia*. From Nairobi, Kenya, Laga and coworkers[6] demonstrated an 83 percent reduction in the incidence of gonococcal conjunctivitis with silver nitrate prophylaxis, whereas with tetracycline ointment, the reduction was 93 percent. For newborns exposed to *C. trachomatis* the reduction rates were 68 percent for silver nitrate and 77 percent for tetracycline.

Because of its potential for causing blindness, gonococcal disease should still be the chief target of prophylaxis. In patient populations in which careful prenatal care is routinely given, universal prophylaxis may not be necessary. (The United Kingdom and Sweden both have discontinued routine prophylaxis. In Sweden it is used only in cases in which prenatal care was not obtained.) In a large, diverse population such as that of the United States, however, and certainly in less-developed countries, it is not possible to identify the infants at risk. Therefore, prophylaxis with one of the three agents still seems appropriate.[13–15]

TREATMENT

The mainstay of treatment of gonococcal disease has been intravenous aqueous penicillin. In recent years, however, there has been a dramatic rise in the prevalence of penicillinase-producing strains of *N. gonorrhoeae*, especially in Africa and southeast Asia.[3, 16] Ceftriaxone and cefotaxime, third-generation cephalosporins, have been demonstrated in several studies to be safe in infants and effective against these strains. A single 125-mg intramuscular dose of ceftriaxone[17] or a 100 mg/kg intramuscular dose of cefotaxime[18] proved to be 100 percent curative against culture-proven gonococcal neonatal conjunctivitis. This treatment also eradicated *N. gonorrhoeae* from other mucosal sites and is now the treatment of choice. For penicillin-allergic patients, one dose of kanamycin, 75 mg intramuscularly, along with topically applied tetracycline, 1 percent ointment, instilled for 7 to 10 days is effective against gonococcal neonatal conjunctivitis but is less effective against nonocular infections.[19]

Treatment of conjunctivitis caused by *C. trachomatis* must also be systemically administered to target nasopharyngeal infection and possible pneumonia. The treatment is erythromycin syrup, 50 mg/kg/day P.O. in four divided doses for 14 days.[8, 20] Infection with *C. trachomatis* may coexist with that of *N. gonorrhoeae;* when this occurs both organisms must be treated simultaneously.

Herpes simplex conjunctivitis should probably be treated with topical 1 percent trifluridine solution, although the usefulness of the drug has not been well established in the absence of concomitant keratitis. HSV keratitis should be treated with 1 percent trifluridine drops every 2 hr for 7 days. Acyclovir, 10 mg/kg intravenously every 8 hr for 10 days, is used against systemic disease.

REFERENCES

1. Crede KSF. Die Verhütung der Augenentzündung der Neugeborenen. Arch Gynakol 17:50–53, 1881.
2. Hammerschlag MR, Cummings C, Roblin P, et al: Efficacy of neonatal ocular prophylaxis for the prevention of chlamydia and gonococcal conjunctivitis. N Engl J Med 320 (12):769–772, 1989.
3. Fransen L, Klauss V: Neonatal ophthalmia in the developing world. Epidemiology, etiology management and control. Int Ophthalmol 11:189–196, 1988.
4. Isenberg SJ, Apt L, Yoshimori R, et al: Source of the conjunctival bacterial flora at birth and implications for ophthalmia neonatorum prophylaxis. Am J Ophthalmol 106:458–462, 1988.
5. Isenberg SJ, Apt L, Yoshimori R, Alvarez S: Bacterial flora of the conjunctiva at birth. J Pediatr Opthalmol Strabismus 23:284–286, 1986.
6. Laga M, Plummer F, Piot P, et al: Prophylaxis of gonococcal and chlamydial ophthalmia neonatorum. N Engl J Med 318:653–657, 1988.
7. Nahmia AJ, Visintine AM, Coldwell DR, Wilson LA: Eye infections with herpes simplex viruses in neonates. Surv Ophthalmol 21:100–105, 1976.
8. Rotkis WM, Chandle JW: Neonatal conjunctivitis. *In* Tassman W, Jaeger E (eds): Duane's Clinical Ophthalmology, vol. 4. Philadelphia, JB Lippincott, 1987, pp 1–7.
9. Deschenes J, Scamone C, Baines M: The ocular manifestations of sexually transmitted diseases. Can J Ophthalmol 25:177–185, 1990.
10. Nahmias AJ, Hagler WS: Ocular manifestations of herpes simplex in the newborn (neonatal ocular herpes). Int Ophthalmol Clin 12:191–213, 1972.
11. el Azazl M, Malm G, Forsgren M: Late ophthalmologic manifestations of neonatal herpes simplex virus infection. Am J Ophthalmol 109:1–7, 1990.
12. Rapoza PA, Quinn TC, Kiessling LA, et al: Assessment of neonatal conjunctivitis with a direct immunofluorescent monoclonal antibody stain for *Chlamydia*. JAMA 255(24):3369–3373, 1986.
13. Chandler JW: Controversies in ocular prophylaxis of newborns. Arch Ophthalmol 107:814–815, 1989.
14. Hammerschlag MR: Neonatal ocular prophylaxis. Pediatr Infect Dis J 7:81–82, 1988.
15. Whitcher JP: Neonatal ophthalmia: Have we advanced in the last 20 years? Int Ophthalmol Clin 30:39–41, 1990.
16. Ullman S, Roussel TJ, Forster RK: Gonococcal keratoconjunctivitis. Surv Ophthamol:32:199–208, 1987.
17. Laga M, Naamara W, Brunham R, et al: Single-dose therapy of gonococcal ophthalmia neonatorum with ceftriaxone. N Engl J Med 315: 1382–1385. 1986.
18. Lepage P, Bogaerts J, Kestelyn P, Meheus A: Single-dose cefotaxime intramuscularly cures gonococcal ophthalmia neonatorum. Br J Ophthalmol 72:518–520, 1988.
19. Fransen L, Nsanze H, D'Costa L, et al: Single dose kanamycin therapy of gonococcal ophthalmia neonatorum. Lancet 2:1234–1237, 1984.
20. Schacter, J, Grossman M, Sweet RL, et al: Prospective study of perinatal transmission of *Chlamydia trachomatis*. JAMA 255: 3374–3377, 1986.

Preseptal and Orbital Cellulitis

Infection of the eyelids confined to the preseptal space (preseptal or periorbital cellulitis) is a relatively common but potentially serious infection of childhood. It is most common in childhood; 85 percent of patients in one series were less than 20 yr old, and 56 percent were younger than 5 yr of age.[1] True orbital infections are much less common but are potentially lethal. Although rare in children less than 5 yr of age,[2] 48 percent of patients in one series[3] were less than 20 yr of age, and in another,[4] 85 percent of all acute orbits (preseptal and orbital disease) were in patients younger than 20 yr.

In 1970, Chandler and associates[5] proposed a classification of the orbital complications of sinusitis. Because it is based on clear anatomic considerations, it has proved extremely useful and has been widely adopted and modified to describe orbital infections of all causes.[1, 3, 4, 6–12] It is not, however, intended to represent progressive or sequential stages of disease. Chandler's schema (expanded) is as follows:

Group 1: Preseptal (Periorbital) Cellulitis. The orbital septum is a fibrous connective tissue that extends vertically from the periosteum of the orbital rim to the tarsal plate of the upper and lower eyelids. Together with the tarsus, the septum constitutes the posterior border of the soft tissues of the eyelids, separating them from the orbit. Superiorly and inferiorly, fibrous bands from the skin to the orbital rim border the "preseptal space." Infection confined to this space is characterized primarily by inflammatory edema of the eyelids, with or without edema of orbital tissues (Fig. 226–4). Warmth and tenderness are also usually present. The septum is an effective barrier to posterior spread of infection, and therefore morbidity is low. An extensive system of valveless veins provides two-way communication between the face and the nasal cavity, paranasal sinuses, orbit, and ultimately the cavernous sinus. Orbital edema in preseptal cellullitis is usually secondary to venous congestion, but cavernous sinus thrombosis can follow facial infection. Such thrombosis has been extremely rare in the postantibiotic era.

Group 2: Orbital Cellulitis. Infiltration of the orbital tissues by bacteria and inflammatory cells results in edema of the orbital adipose and soft tissues. The edema results in proptosis, orbital discomfort, pain on attempted eye movement, and often ophthalmoplegia. Visual acuity may be impaired. Eyelid edema and erythema are present, as with preseptal cellulitis (Fig. 226–5). Conjunctival chemosis is frequently present, as are fever and leukocytosis. Orbital cellulitis is most commonly secondary to sinusitis[4, 5, 10, 13] (usually the ethmoid sinus) but may also be caused by trauma, surgery, or spread from other adnexal structures. The orbital periosteum and the very thin lamina papyracea form the medial wall of the orbit and separate it from the ethmoid sinus. These structures are penetrated by many neural and vascular foramina, thus explaining the access of purulent material from the ethmoid sinus to the orbit. The ethmoid and maxillary sinuses are well developed at birth, whereas the sphenoid sinus and frontal sinuses usually do not become clinically significant until 5 to 6 yr of age.

Group 3: Subperiosteal Abscess. The orbital periosteum (periorbita) may become stripped away from the bony orbital walls by purulent material extending from a paranasal sinus. Clinically, all the signs of preseptal and orbital cellulitis are present. The proptosis may be asymmetric (therefore, the eye is usually down and pointed in a lateral direction). Chemosis is often marked, and limitation of mobility is severe. There may be severe tenderness between the globe and the orbital rim. The abscess may extend and drain into the orbit or may drain anteriorly through the medial aspect of the lids. Visual loss is an ominous sign. Evaluation and management of this condition is still evolving and will be discussed later.

Group 4: Orbital Abscess. An abscess within the true

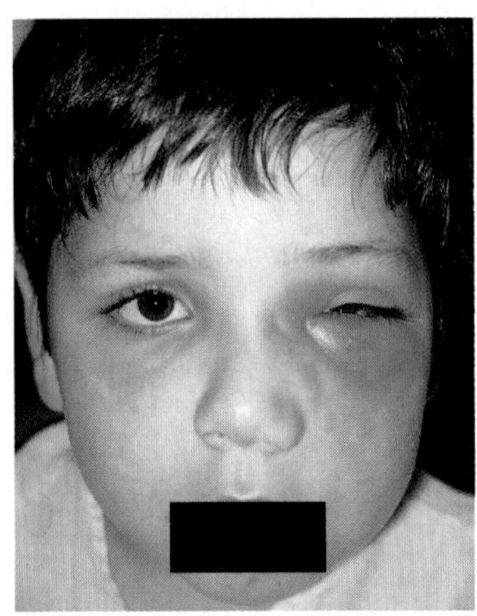

Figure 226–4. Preseptal cellulitis. There is edema and erythema of the eyelids without proptosis.

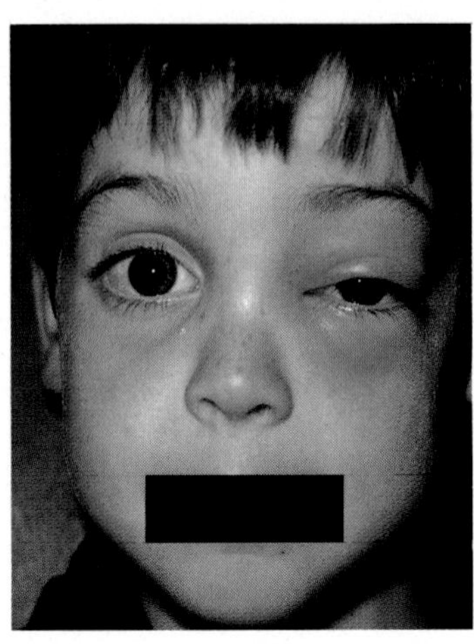

Figure 226–5. Orbital cellulitis. Eyelid edema and erythema are more severe. There is slight proptosis.

orbit (either within or out of the muscle cone) is fortunately rare. The signs of orbital cellulitis are present with variable severity, but typically proptosis, ophthalmoplegia, and visual loss are more severe and patients are more ill systemically. As with subperiosteal abscess, the abscess may extend anteriorly into the eyelids. Surgical drainage of these abscesses is usually indicated.

Group 5: Cavernous Sinus Thrombosis. As mentioned previously, the venous system of the orbits is devoid of valves and provides two-way communication between the face and the nasal cavities, paranasal sinuses, and the orbits and drains posteriorly into the cavernous sinus and inferiorly into the pterygoid plexus. Phlebitis migrating posteriorly into the cavernous sinus will result in a worsening of the symptoms of orbital cellulitis followed by extension of the same signs and symptoms contralaterally, resulting in bilateral disease. Patients have severe toxicity, and meningitis is common.

Clinically, it is most important to differentiate preseptal cellulitis from the other groups with true orbital involvement. Severe chemosis, proptosis, ophthalmoplegia, and visual loss are the most common signs of orbital involvement, and their presence should suggest a presumptive diagnosis of orbital cellulitis and trigger appropriate evaluation and management. Further discussion of the individual orbital infections follows.

PRESEPTAL CELLULITIS

Preseptal cellulitis is predominantly a pediatric infection. It occurs with much greater frequency than do orbital infections (70 to 94 percent of total cases).[1, 2, 14, 15] and constitutes almost 100 percent of cases in infancy.[16] Preseptal cellulitis is multifactorial and is commonly caused by trauma, external ocular infection, or spread of infection from the upper respiratory tract or middle ear, or both. The latter cause has been called nonsuppurative preseptal cellulitis.[17, 18] and is the most common form, encompassing 50 to 75 percent of pediatric cases.[1, 2] (including upper respiratory tract infection, sinusitis, and otitis) and 78 percent of infantile cases.[16] The infection is presumably spread via venous or lymphatic channels, and *H. influenzae* and *S. pneumoniae* are the most common offending pathogens.[1, 2, 15, 19, 20] Blood cultures are frequently positive,[2] and *H. influenzae* accounts for most of the positive cultures. Both of these organisms are encapsulated by a polysaccharide coat.[2, 21] The immune system of infants is deficient in its ability to respond to these antigens, putting them at risk for infection.[21] *H. influenzae*, type B can produce serious invasive disease in infants, with a predilection for the head and neck.[21] Facial cellulitis, epiglottitis, and meningitis are examples of serious invasive infection caused by *H. influenzae*. The peak incidence of *H. influenzae*, type B infections extends from 6 mo of age, when protection from maternal antibodies wanes, until 2 yr when natural antibodies begin to form.

An *H. influenzae*, type B vaccine (consisting of the purified capsular polysaccharide covalently linked to diphtheria toxoid) has been available since 1988 and is recommended for children at 18 mo of age. *H. influenzae*, type B was formerly uniformly sensitive to ampicillin, but 20 to 30 percent of strains now produce β-lactamase. Chloramphenicol has become the usual initial therapy until the β-lactamase status of the organism can be determined. Second- and third-generation cephalosporins are effective, and cefuroxime has been shown to be particularly useful for pediatric infections.[22]

Preseptal cellulitis caused by *H. influenzae*, type B is characterized by a violaceous discoloration of the eyelids. There is edema and erythema of the eyelids, but vision and extraocular motility are normal. Patients are febrile, with leukocytosis. Because of the risk of serious invasive disease, especially meningitis, patients should be hospitalized, but lumbar puncture is not necessary unless signs of meningeal irritation are present.[19] Cultures of the nose, throat, and nasopharynx are of little use because of high colonization rates, but blood cultures are useful. At present, the antibiotic of choice is intravenous cefuroxime (100 to 150 mg/kg/day), which is effective against *H. influenzae* and *S. pneumoniae* (as well as *S. aureus*). Sinus x-ray films are difficult to interpret in young children and seem to add little to management. A computed tomography (CT) scan is indicated if the infection does not respond to antibiotics or if signs of orbital extension develop.

Suppurative preseptal cellulitis is subdivided into (1) infections secondary to trauma and (2) spread of infection from other external ocular infection.

Preseptal cellulitis secondary to eyelid or eyebrow trauma is most commonly caused by *S. aureus* or *Streptococcus* spp.[21] Injury from human or animal bites raises the possibility of infection by anaerobic species indigenous to the oral cavity. Skin crepitation occurs with clostridial infection, which most likely occurs in wounds contaminated by soil. Blood cultures are usually negative, but percutaneous aspirates are frequently revealing.[2] Abscesses should be surgically drained, and abscess material should be submitted for Gram staining and culture. When possible, initial antibiotic therapy should be directed by Gram stain results and modified as culture results become available. Mild infections may be successfully treated on an outpatient basis with an oral penicillinase-resistant penicillin, such as cloxacillin or with a cephalosporin, such as cefaclor. Serious infections with signs of systemic toxicity require hospitalization and intravenous antibiotics until there is unequivocal clinical improvement (usually after 48 to 72 hr) at which time oral antibiotics may be substituted. Intravenous antibiotics should include a semisynthetic penicillin such as nafcillin for probable *Staphylococcus* or *Streptococcus* infection, and chloramphenicol should be added if anaerobic organisms or *H. influenzae* are suspected. Vancomycin or cephalosporins may be substituted (judiciously) for nafcillin in penicillin-allergic patients. A retained foreign body should be suspected if patients with a history of trauma do not respond promptly to intravenous antibiotics. A CT scan and possible surgical exploration is then indicated. A CT scan is also indicated in those children in whom orbital edema produces proptosis and raises suspicion of orbital cellulitis. Similarly, uncooperative children with significant eyelid edema in whom extraocular motility and proptosis cannot be evaluated should also have a CT scan.

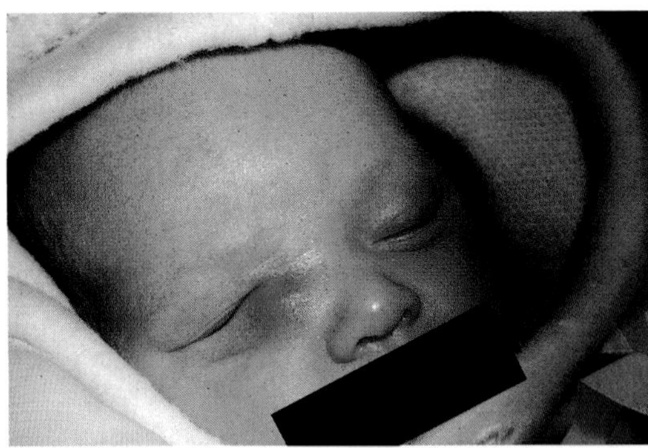

Figure 226–6. Dacryocystitis. Infection in the nasolacrimal sac is a common cause of suppurative preseptal cellulitis in infancy.

Suppurative preseptal cellulitis may also be secondary to external ocular infection. Neonatal conjunctivitis, dacryocystitis (Fig. 226–6), and ruptured dacryocystocele are the most common causes in neonates.[2, 16] Neonatal conjunctivitis and its treatment have been described previously. Dacryocystitis should be treated just as a traumatic eyelid abscess, namely, with hospitalization, surgical drainage of the abscess, and intravenous antibiotics. Probing and irrigation to provide patency of the lacrimal outflow system should follow resolution of the infection. Eyelid infections in older children are most commonly caused by an infected chalazion or hordeolum. Warm compresses, topical bacitracin ointment, and oral cloxacillin or cefaclor are effective treatments. Impetigo or secondary impetiginization of herpes simplex or chickenpox (varicella) lesions, usually caused by *S. aureus* or *Streptococcus* spp. are treated in a similar manner. Dermatitis caused by *S. pyogenes* (erysipelas) may cause systemic toxicity and signs of orbital involvement by producing toxins that diffuse across the orbital septum and induce aseptic orbital edema. Because of the signs and symptoms, hospitalization and CT scans, as with orbital cellulitis, are indicated. The dermatitis can be recognized by the sharply demarcated red plaque that the infection produces. It responds well to intravenous penicillin G.

ORBITAL CELLULITIS, SUBPERIOSTEAL ABSCESS, AND ORBITAL ABSCESS

True orbital infections are rare in childhood but are associated with serious morbidity. In the preantibiotic era, 20 percent of patients died of meningitis, brain abscess, or cavernous sinus thrombosis, and another 20 percent were left blind on the affected side. Causes of blindness include optic neuritis, central retinal artery occlusion, exposure keratitis, retinal and choroidal ischemia, and optic atrophy secondary to prolonged proptosis. The vast majority of cases are secondary to sinus infection (90 percent in one series[2]) but may also be secondary to trauma or ocular surgery[23, 24] spread from other adnexal structures or, rarely, hematogenous spread. Patients are typically older than 6 yr of age. They are usually febrile and generally unwell. The eyelids are reddened and swollen. Proptosis is present on the affected side. There is pain on attempted eye movement or frank ophthalmoplegia. Visual acuity may be depressed. Headache and rhinorrhea may also be present. Differential diagnoses include the idiopathic inflammation known collectively as orbital pseudotumor and rapidly growing orbital tumors (rhabdomyosarcoma, metablastic neuroblastoma, and leukemia).[18] The acute onset of pain, fever, and systemic illness, as well as radiologic findings, can usually distinguish true orbital cellulitis from these other causes of unilateral proptosis.

Bacterial orbital cellulitis is usually secondary to sinusitis. The common causative organisms are *S. aureus, S. pyogenes, S. pneumoniae*, and *H. influenzae*. Orbital cellulitis is rare in infancy, but when it occurs *H. influenzae* is the usual causative organism, and it is this group in which blood cultures are positive. Management of this condition requires hospitalization and consultation with ear, nose, and throat and pediatric infectious disease services. A complete eye examination and dental examination are mandatory. Sinus films are useful in children older than 2 yr of age, and all patients should have a CT scan with coronal as well as axial views for best imaging of the orbital apex. The case is made that CT scanning should be reserved for cases unresponsive to initial antibiotic treatment;[8, 13, 14] however, the earlier recognition of noninfectious causes and earlier detection of subperiosteal and true orbital abscesses afforded by CT scans should result in decreased morbidity and shorter hospital stays.[3, 7] The orbit is well imaged by CT scanning because the orbital fat is a low-density background for the other orbital structures.[25] The CT scan simultaneously images the orbit and its structures (extraocular muscles, optic nerve), the adjacent sinuses, orbital bones, and contiguous areas of the brain (Fig. 226–7). Obliteration of fat shadows in the orbit occurs in orbital cellulitis and can be used to differentiate it from preseptal disease.[26] An orbital abscess may appear as a ringlike, homogeneous, or heterogeneous mass on CT scan.[26, 27] An air-fluid level may be seen within the mass, and the walls may enhance with contrast. Subperiosteal inflammation can be detected by soft tissue swelling in the affected area. Thickening and displacement of the medial rectus muscle or displacement of the

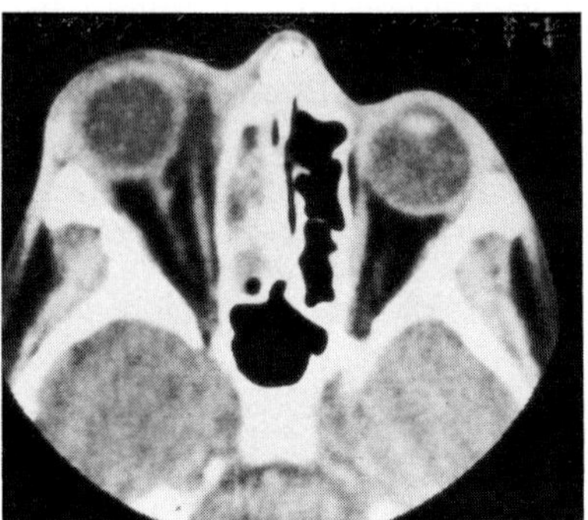

Figure 226–7. CT scan of the orbits demonstrates ethmoid cellulitis with spread into the orbit. The medial rectus is displaced and the anterior orbit is opacified. Note the marked proptosis.

globe, or both, can be seen. A mass confined by the periosteum is sharply delineated. CT scanning cannot, however, differentiate between a true subperiosteal abscess and a sterile collection of inflammatory edema.[8, 28] Orbital ultrasound can also reveal abscess formation but is inferior to CT scanning because of poor imaging of the orbital apex and of the adjacent structures (e.g., sinuses).

Blood should be drawn for culture in all patients, but they are infrequently positive. Conjunctival, nasal, and pharyngeal cultures rarely yield the causative agent. When available, aspirates from infected sinuses or from abscess cavities should yield the offending pathogen.

Initial treatment consists of aggressive broad-spectrum antibiotics. Cloxacillin or nafcillin (100 mg/kg/day) in combination with chloramphenicol, 75 mg/kg/day, provides coverage for the usual organisms encountered. Vancomycin, 30 mg/kg/day, is substituted for the penicillinase-resistant penicillin in allergic patients. Cefuroxime, 225 mg/kg/day, has been recommended as an effective alternative treatment for children younger than 6 yr of age.[8] Antibiotics should be adjusted as culture results become available. Clinical signs and symptoms such as fever, proptosis, ophthalmoplegia, pupillary signs, and visual activity should be monitored as often as every 2 hr. The fundus should be periodically evaluated for papilledema and congestion of retinal veins, as these may be early signs of cavernous sinus thrombosis. Presence of subperiosteal abscess on CT scanning is not by itself an indication for surgical drainage, as there are now many reports of successful resolution of this condition with medical treatment alone.[8, 11, 28, 29] Such patients should be monitored even more carefully and surgical drainage should be performed when there is any sign of a worsening clinical condition. Surgery is directed by the CT findings. It should be carried out in conjunction with an otorhinolaryngologist, and abscess drainage should probably be coupled with sinus drainage of the appropriate sinus cavities. In contradistinction to subperiosteal abscess, orbital abscess requires prompt surgical drainage, again with the aid of an otolaryngologist. Drainage material should, of course, be submitted for culture to direct further antibiotic therapy. Even without evidence of abscess by CT scanning, orbital decompression (with or without sinus drainage) should be performed when clinical signs are progressing, especially when there is visual loss or an afferent pupillary defect. In addition to blindness and cavernous sinus thrombosis, serious complications can include meningitis, brain abscess, and osteomyelitis. Serious complications, though much less frequent in the postantibiotic and post–CT scan era are still reported, underlining the serious nature of these infections.

CAVERNOUS SINUS THROMBOSIS

Prior to the introduction of antibiotics, cavernous sinus thrombosis was nearly uniformly fatal. It may be difficult to differentiate from orbital cellulitis but should be suspected whenever there is a worsening of clinical signs, especially marked systemic illness, afferent pupillary defect, anesthesia in the distribution of the fifth cranial nerve, engorgement of retinal veins, and optic disc swelling. The emergence of bilateral proptosis and other clinical signs solidifies the diagnosis. The management of this condition should be deferred to pediatric neurology and neurosurgical services.

ORBITAL CELLULITIS SECONDARY TO TRAUMA OR SURGERY

Orbital cellulitis after trauma is most often caused by *S. aureus*. Clostridial species, anaerobes, and polymicrobial infections are also common. CT scans are indicated to search both for abscess formation and for retained foreign bodies. Surgical exploration is indicated for both, and if any purulent material is obtained direct appropriate antibiotic treatment should be instituted. Broad-spectrum coverage for both gram-positive and gram-negative bacteria should be provided when definitive knowledge of the offending pathogen is lacking. Orbital cellulitis has been reported after a wide variety of surgical procedures but is extremely rare in childhood.[2] Of particular interest to pediatric ophthalmologists is the fact that only three cases of orbital cellulitis have been reported secondary to strabismus surgery since 1935.[23, 24] Blood cultures were negative in all three cases. One patient had a positive conjunctival culture for group A β-*Streptococcus*, a second patient had a positive conjunctival culture for *S. aureus*, and a third patient had no positive cultures. Intravenous antibiotics were sufficient treatment in all three cases.

ORBITAL CELLULITIS SECONDARY TO SPREAD FROM ADJACENT STRUCTURES

Orbital cellulitis may ensue after infection of structures other than the sinuses. Facial cellulitis, endophthalmitis, dacryocystitis, and dental infections may all result in orbital cellulitis. Dacryocystitis is most commonly due to *S. aureus, Streptococcus* spp., and *H. influenzae.* It occurs most commonly in young children, and cefuroxime is an appropriate antibiotic until culture results are available. Orbital cellulitis secondary to dental infections are rare in childhood but may be caused by anaerobes. Osteomyelitis of the superior maxilla is a condition of infancy that may present with the symptoms of orbital cellulitis.[30] It affects patients in the first few months of life. The infecting organism is usually *S. aureus* transferred from a mother with mastitis to the infant's gums and superior alveolar tooth buds. Central abscess formation in the superior maxilla may lead to proptosis and conjunctival chemosis. Edema of the palate and alveolus on the affected side will usually lead to the correct diagnosis. Surgical drainage of the abscess,

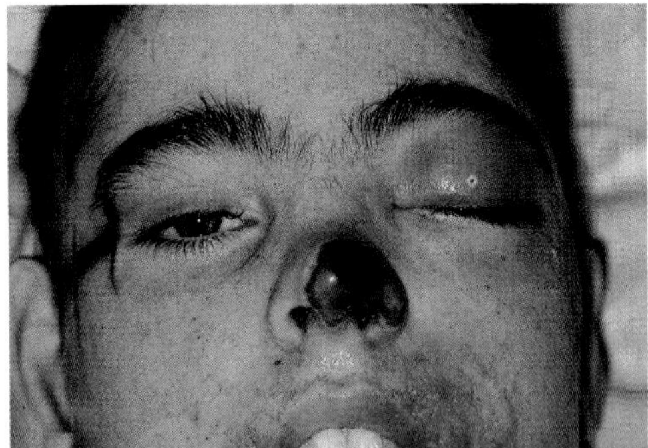

Figure 226–8. Mucormycosis of the orbit with ischemic necrosis of the nose.

preferably via the nose, by an otolaryngologist is indicated. Intravenous nafcillin or cloxacillin is the appropriate initial antibiotic until culture results are available.

ORBITAL MUCORMYCOSIS[31]

Fungal orbital cellulitis is extremely rare, but orbital mucormycosis (phycomycosis) can occur in childhood in one of three conditions. The most common condition is metabolic acidosis caused by the vomiting and diarrhea of gastroenteritis. Diabetic ketoacidosis and immunosuppression are the other two situations in which this fungal infection occurs. The organisms presumably gain access through the nose, and infection begins in the sinuses. The organism has a predilection for arteries, producing thrombosing vasculitis and ischemic necrosis of affected tissues (Fig. 226–8). The organism spreads hematogenously and may invade the orbit, the cavernous sinus, and intracranial vessels. Orbital involvement is demonstrated by eyelid edema, proptosis, and conjunctival chemosis, as well as significant periorbital pain. The orbital apex syndrome, with the resultant cranial nerve palsies, follows invasion of the orbital apex by the fungus. Optic neuropathy and central artery occlusion may occur (Fig. 226–9). Extension into the cavernous sinus carries a very poor prognosis. Diagnosis is made by recognition of the characteristic black ischemic lesions of affected tissues (palate, nasal mucosa). These

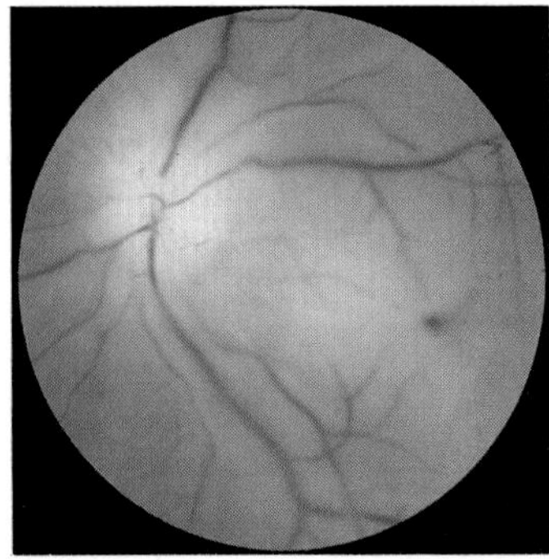

Figure 226–9. Same patient as in Figure 226–8. Central artery occlusion secondary to mucormycosis of the orbit.

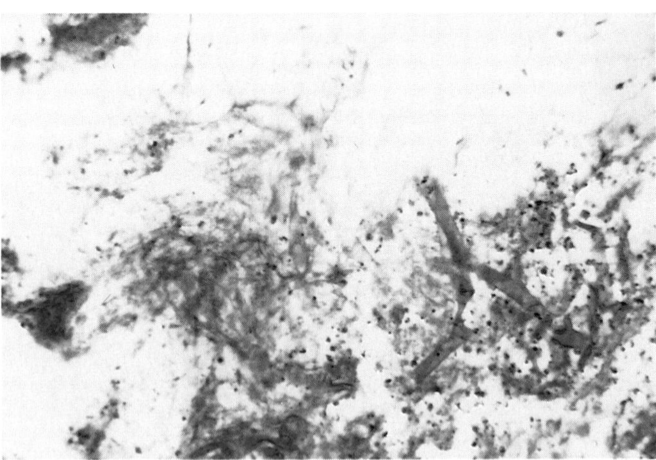

Figure 226–10. H&E stain of orbital tissue infected by *Zygomycetes.* Note the branching, nonseptate hyphae.

lesions should be biopsied and submitted for histologic sections. The presence of non-septate branching hyphae in these sections establishes the diagnosis (Fig. 226–10). Surgical debridement of affected tissues may require coordination among ophthalmologist, otolaryngologist, and neurosurgeon. Orbital exenteration may be necessary. Specific antifungal treatment with intravenous amphotericin B should be initiated. Renal function must be closely monitored because the drug is nephrotoxic. Attention must also be given to correcting the patient's underlying metabolic or immunologic abnormality.

REFERENCES

1. Jackson K, Baker S: Periorbital cellulitis. Head Neck Surg 9:227–234, 1987.
2. Weiss A, Friendly D, Eglin K, et al: Bacterial periorbital and orbital cellulitis in childhood. Ophthalmology 90:195–201, 1983.
3. Jackson K, Baker S: Clinical implications of orbital cellulitis. Laryngoscope 96:568–574, 1986.
4. Moloney JR, Badham NJ, McRae A: The acute orbit. Preseptal (periorbital) cellulitis, subperiosteal abscess and orbital cellulitis due to sinusitis. J Laryngol Otol 12:1–18 (Suppl), 1987.
5. Chandler JR, Langenbrunner DJ, Stevens ER: The pathogenesis of orbital complications in acute sinusitis. Laryngoscope. 80:1414–1428, 1970.
6. Schramm VL, Carter HD, Kennerdell JS: Evaluation of orbital cellulitis and results of treatment. Laryngoscope 92:732–738, 1982.
7. Hornblass A, Herschorn B, Stern K, et al: Orbital abscess. Surv Opthalmol 29:169–178, 1984.
8. Noël LP, Clarke WN, MacDonald N: Clinical management of orbital cellulitis in children. Can J. Ophthalmol 25:11–16, 1990.
9. Lawless M, Martin F: Orbital cellulitis and preseptal cellulitis in childhood. Aust NZ J Ophthalmol 14:211–219, 1986.
10. Goodwin WJ: Orbital complications of ethmoiditis. Otolaryngol Clin North Am 18:139–147, 1985.
11. Souliere CR Jr, Antoine GA, Martin MP, et al: Selective non-surgical management of subperiosteal abscess of the orbit: Computerized tomography and clinical course as indication for surgical drainage. Int J Pediatr Otorhinolaryngol 19:109–119, 1990.
12. Gutowski WM, Mulbury PE, Hengerer AS, et al: The role of CT scans in managing the orbital complications of ethmoiditis. Int J Pediatr Otorhinolaryngol 15:117–128, 1988.
13. Bergin DJ, Wright JE: Orbital cellulitis. Br J Ophthalmol 70:174–178, 1986.
14. Israele V, Nelson JD: Periorbital and orbital cellulitis. Pediatr Infect Dis 6:404–410, 1987.
15. Spires JR, Smith RJ: Bacterial infections of the orbital and

periorbital soft-tissues in children. Laryngoscope 96:763–767, 1986.
16. Molarte AB, Isenberg SJ: Periorbital cellulitis in infancy. J Pediatr Ophthalmol Strabismus 26:232–234, 1989.
17. Jones DB: Discussion of Weiss A, Friendly D, Eglin K, et al: Bacterial periorbital cellulitis and orbital cellulitis in childhood. Ophthalmology 90:201–203, 1983.
18. Steinkuller PG, Jones DB: Preseptal and orbital cellulitis and orbital abscess. *In* Linberg JV (ed): Oculoplastic and Orbital Emergencies. Norwalk, Conn, Appleton and Lange, 1990.
19. Antoine GA, Grundfast KM: Periorbital cellulitis. Int J Pediatr Otorhinolaryngol 13:273–278, 1987.
20. Weizman Z, Mussaffi H: Ethmoiditis-associated periorbital cellulitis. Int J Pediatr Otorhinolaryngol 11:147–151, 1986.
21. Halperin SA: Haemophilus influenzae type B and its role in diseases of the head and neck. J Otolaryngol 19:169–174, 1990.
22. Nelson JD: Cefuroxime: A cephalosporin with unique applicability to pediatric practice. Pediatr Infect Dis 2:394–396, 1983.
23. Von Noorden GK: Orbital cellulitis following extraocular muscle surgery. Am J Ophthalmol 74:627–629, 1972.
24. Wilson ME, Paul TO: Orbital cellulitis following strabismus surgery. Ophthalmic Surg 18:92–94, 1987.
25. Trokel SL: Computed tomographic scanning of orbital inflammations. Int Ophthalmol Clin 4:81–98, 1982.
26. Goldberg F, Berne AS, Oski FA: Differentiation of orbital cellulitis from preseptal cellulitis by computed tomography. Pediatrics 62:1000–1005, 1978.
27. Harr DL, Quencer RM, Abrams GW: Computed tomography and ultrasound in the evaluation of orbital infection and pseudotumor. Radiology 152:395–401, 1982.
28. Gold SC, Arrigg PG, Hedges TR III: Computerized tomography in the management of acute orbital cellulitis. Ophthalmic Surg 10:753–756, 1987.
29. Rubin SE, Slavin ML, Rubin LG: Eyelid swelling and erythema as the only signs of subperiosteal abscess. Br J Ophthalmol 73:576–578, 1989.
30. Cavenaugh F: Osteomyelitis of the superior maxilla in infants. Br Med J 1:468–472, 1960.
31. Schwartz JN, Donnelly EH, Klintworth GK: Ocular and orbital phycomycosis. Surv Ophthalmol 22:3–28, 1977.

Chapter 227

Delayed Visual Development, Early Retinal Degenerations, and Assessment of Retinal Function in Children

ANNE B. FULTON

Children who in early infancy are blind or visually inattentive fit into many diagnostic categories. Dependent on diagnosis and severity of involvement, their prospects for the future range from normal vision to blindness. Thus there is considerable obligation to secure a precise diagnosis as early as possible. However, given that development of the visual system, even of the abnormal visual system, continues after term,[1–3] it may not be possible to predict the visual capabilities of an individual.

For some of these infants the explanation for congenital blindness or visual impairment will become apparent on examination of their eyes. For example, developmental disorders of the posterior poles such as bilateral optic nerve hypoplasia[4] (Fig. 227–1) or choroidal colobomas involving the maculas are conspicuous ophthalmoscopically, and when present, account for the infant's visual behavior and foretell limited vision but not necessarily blindness.[3]

The visually inattentive or blind infant is unresponsive to smiles or familiar faces. Visual stimuli without auditory accompaniments fail to engage the infant's attention. Age-appropriate following of visual objects cannot be elicited. This describes the early infantile behavior not only of children with severe congenital malformations of the posterior pole structures but also of children with delayed visual maturation,[5–14] albinism,[15–23] achromatopsia,[24, 25] congenital retinal disorders[26–41] (sometimes classified as degenerations) such as Leber's congenital amaurosis,[33–41] and young patients with brain dysfunction.[42–49] These ophthalmic entities, in which visual development is delayed in the absence of major malformations of the ocular structures, are considered in the following pages along with evaluation of infant patients' retinal functions. A description of the development of normal retinal function can be found in *Principles and Practice of Ophthalmology: Basic Sciences,* Chapter 47 (hereinafter called *Basic Sciences*). Other aspects of infants' visual evaluation, such as acuity measures, are considered in *Basic Sciences,* Chapter 42.

DELAYED VISUAL MATURATION[5–14]

Delayed visual maturation of an infant who has normal eyes and brain can be considered a specific, albeit incompletely understood, entity. Typically, these infants behave as blind up to age 5 to 6 mo, despite good pupillary responses and normal fundi. There is a fre-

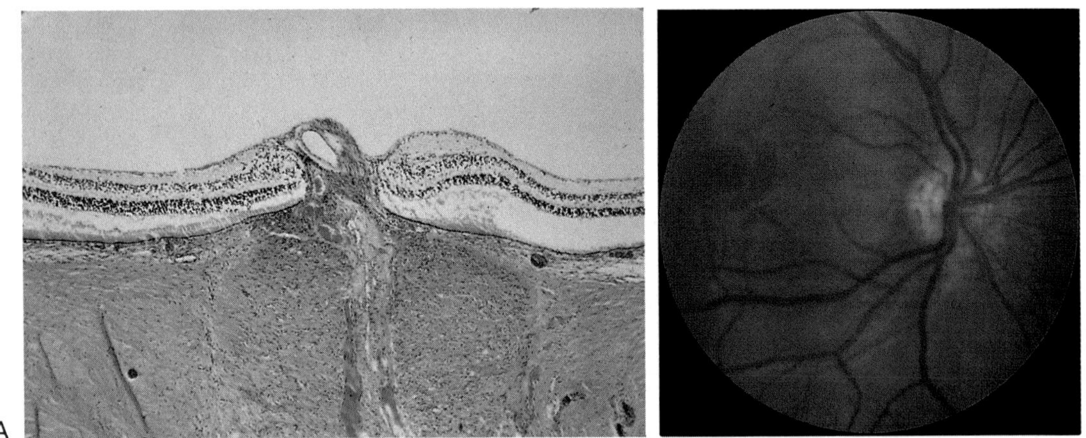

Figure 227–1. Optic nerve hypoplasia. *A* and *B*, An eye with marked optic nerve hypoplasia such as shown here is not expected to see well. Note that this small optic nerve lies within a hypopigmented annulus. Other features of the fundus, including the caliber and distribution of the retinal vasculature and the foveal reflex, are normal.

quent association of delayed visual maturation and premature birth, and some have remarked on the vulnerability of the visual cortex, lateral geniculate bodies, and oculomotor nuclei to damage in the perinatal period.[6] As parents often report, vision-mediated behavior characteristically turns on suddenly in these infants. The critical anatomic or molecular developments that underlie such a course remain to be identified.

ALBINISM[15–23]

Infants with albinism of all types are typically slow to see, often appearing blind in the early postnatal weeks. Mutations of the tyrosinase gene have been identified in some patients with oculocutaneous albinism.[20, 22] In the early weeks before the rhythmic movements of the nystagmus typical of albinos is manifest, wandering eye movements are seen. Irides that transilluminate light and the absence of a foveal reflex[18, 19, 21, 23] are diagnostic at this early age. In the normal eye, even at preterm ages, a foveal reflex is identifiable ophthalmoscopically.[50] The irides of a young, drowsy infant are easier to examine for transillumination defects than are those of an active toddler. The albino infants develop good grating acuity,[51] although optotype acuity is impaired to variable degrees.[23] The misrouting of the visual pathways characteristic of the hypopigmentation syndromes can be diagnosed using visually evoked potential techniques.[15–17] (See also *Basic Sciences,* Chapter 46.)

EARLY RETINAL DEGENERATIONS[26–41]

Leber's[37] congenital amaurosis (LCA), often classified with the retinal degenerations, may represent several different pathophysiologic disorders. The criteria adopted by many for a diagnosis of LCA include documented visual impairment before age 6 mo (in other words, "congenital"), poor pupillary reactions, and markedly attenuated or absent electroretinographic responses. Some infants with LCA have systemic abnormalities, including brain anomalies and mental retardation, but these complications are by no means part and parcel of LCA.[40, 41] Infants with LCA typically have wandering fixation, and visual attention is engaged only with difficulty, if at all. The pupillary reactions are sluggish or absent. Fundus appearance is extremely variable.[38, 39] It is often said that the fundus may show no lesions whatsoever.[36] However, at least subtle fundus abnormalities, such as mild attenuation of the retinal vasculature (Fig. 227–2) or a tiny clump of delicate bone spicules, are usually seen on adequate examination, which occasionally requires anesthesia. In early infancy, one should not expect to find the triad of pale discs, attenuated retinal vasculature, and pigmentary retinopathy that constitutes the ophthalmoscopic hallmarks of retinal degeneration in older patients.

For infants suspected of having LCA, electroretinographic (ERG) testing is the critical test. Because a young infant's ERG amplitudes and sensitivities[52] are less than those of adults, it is important that the infant's responses be compared with age-appropriate norms (see *Basic Sciences,* Chapter 47). Thus the young infant with achromatopsia, in whom pupillary responses are difficult to assess because of the photophobia and nystagmus, has small ERG responses compared with those of an adult but when the age-related norms are inspected can be seen to have normal scotopic amplitudes and absent photopic responses. Infants with other congenital anomalies of retinal function, such as congenital stationary night blindness,[53] have abnormal ERG responses and therefore are potentially confused with those having LCA. Almost all children with LCA, whether it is complicated or uncomplicated, are hyperopic.[33–35]

Other infantile conditions cause retinal degenerations and attenuation of ERG responses. These include neuronal ceroid fuscinosis,[32, 54] inborn errors of metabolism such as methylmalonic acidemia[27] that become apparent as the child's general medical problems are pursued, and syndromes such as Bardet-Biedl-Laurence-Moon[55–60]

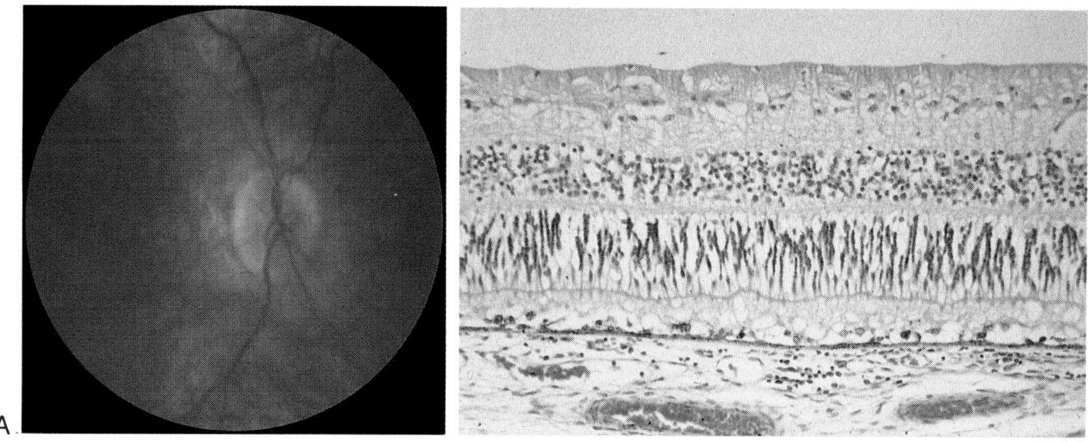

Figure 227–2. Leber's congenital amaurosis. *A* and *B,* One of many possible appearances of the posterior pole in Leber's congenital amaurosis is shown. The retinal vasculature of this patient is markedly attenuated, and the choroidal vasculature is visible throughout the pale extramacular fundus.

or Senior's syndromes,[28, 29] as well as early onset of the symptoms of retinitis pigmentosa.

ASSESSMENT OF INFANT'S RETINAL FUNCTION

Tests and procedures that have been invented to study the development of normal human retinal function[61–63] are also applied to the study of infant patients.[52, 54, 59, 64–66] Age-dependent variations in normal retinal function occur in infancy. Therefore the retinal responses of infant patients are interpretable only if compared with normal values for the age.[52] Mainstays in the testing of retinal function are ERG (see *Basic Sciences,* Chapter 47) and psychophysical measures of thresholds. Also useful in selected patients will be pupillographic assessment of rhodopsin regeneration[54, 61] and electrooculographic responses.[54, 63]

Indications for testing include visual deficits of infancy and childhood that cannot be explained by inspection of the eyes or to secure diagnosis of those entities described in the preceding paragraphs. Psychophysical assessment of retinal sensitivity becomes important if, for example, photoreceptor disease is sufficiently advanced to have extinguished ERG responses.

Techniques and protocols have been recently reviewed and summarized.[66] For the most part, the protocols for pediatric testing can and should be as complete as those recommended for adults. Successful application of such protocols to assessment of pediatric patients have been reported.[42, 43, 52, 54, 59, 64–66] The feasibility of child testing depends on the commitment of the laboratory to accomplish satisfactory recordings. Informed parents and a trusting parent-examiner partnership are unequivocally the most important factors for successful recordings of responses from awake infants and young children. Nearly all infants and children can be satisfactorily tested when awake.[66] In general, electrophysiologic recording artifacts are a greater problem in infants and children than in adults. Equipment should permit rejection of artifacts. Occasionally, off-line analysis, which permits inclusion and exclusion criteria to be applied to responses before averaging, has been used.

REFERENCES

1. Dubowitz LMS, Muskin J, Morante A, et al: The maturation of visual acuity in neurologically normal and abnormal newborn infants. Behav Brain Res 10:39, 1983.
2. Dubowitz LMSA, Mushin J, DeVries L, et al: Visual function in the newborn infant: Is it cortically mediated? Lancet 1:1139, 1986.
3. Fielder AR, Fulton AB, Mayer DL: The visual behavior of infants with severe ocular disorders. Ophthalmology 98:1306, 1991.
4. Lambert SR, Hoyt CS, Narahara MH: Optic nerve hypoplasia. Surv Ophthalmol 32:1, 1987.
5. Cole GF, Hungerford J, Jones RB: Delayed visual maturation. Arch Dis Child 59:107, 1984.
6. Editorial: Delayed visual maturation. Lancet 1:1158, 1984.
7. Fielder AR, Russell-Eggitt IR, Dodd KL, et al: Delayed visual maturation. Trans Ophthalmol Soc UK 104:653, 1985.
8. Harel S, Holtzman M, Feinsod M: Delayed visual maturation. Arch Dis Child 58:298, 1983.
9. Hoyt CS, Jastrzebski G, Marg E: Delayed visual maturation in infancy. Br J Ophthalmol 67:127, 1983.
10. Illingworth RS: Delayed visual maturation. Arch Dis Child 36:407:1961.
11. Lambert SE, Kriss A, Taylor D: Delayed visual maturation. Ophthalmology 96:524, 1989.
12. Mellor DH, Fielder AR: Dissociated visual development: electrodiagnostic studies in infants who are "slow to see." Dev Med Child Neurol 22:327, 1980.
13. Skarf B: Discussion of Lambert, Kriss, and Taylor's paper on delayed visual maturation. Ophthalmology 96:529, 1989.
14. Tresidder J, Fielder AR, Nicholson J: Delayed visual maturation: ophthalmic and neuro-developmental aspects. Devel Med Child Neurol 32:872, 1990.
15. Apkarian P, Reits D, Spekreijse H, et al: A decisive electrophysiological test for human albinism. Electroencephalogr Clin Neurophysiol 55:513, 1983.
16. Apkarian P, Reits D, Spekreijse H: Component specificity in albino VEP symmetry: maturation of the visual pathway anomaly. Exp Brain Res 53:285, 1984.
17. Creel D, Spekreijse H, Reits D: Visual evoked potential (VEP) methods of detecting misrouted optic projections. Doc Ophthalmol Proc Series 27:157, 1981.
18. Elschnig A: Zur Anatomie des Menschlichen Albinoauges. Graefes Arch 84:401, 1913.
19. Fulton AB, Albert DM, Craft JL: Human albinism. Arch Ophthalmol 96:305, 1978.
20. Giebel LB, Strunk KM, King RA, et al: A frequent tyrosinase

gene mutation in classic, tyrosinase-negative (type 1A) oculocutaneous albinism. Proc Natl Acad Sci 87:3255, 1990.
21. Naumann GOH, Lerch W, Schroeder W: Foveola Aplasia bei Tyrosinase-positivem oculocutanen Albinismus. Graefes Arch 200:39, 1976.
22. Spritz RA, Strunk KM, Giebel LB, et al: Detection of mutations in the tyrosinase gene in a patient with type 1A oculocutaneous albinism. N Engl J Med 322:1724, 1990.
23. Taylor WOG: Visual disabilities of oculocutaneous albinism and their alleviation. Trans Ophthalmol Soc UK 98:423, 1978.
24. Hagerstrom-Portnoy G, Freidman N, Adams AJ, et al: Vision function of rod monochromats. I. Advanced clinical measures. Non-invasive assessment of the visual system. Technical Digest Series, Opt Soc Am 3:13, 1988.
25. Sloan LL: Congenital achromatopsia: a report of 19 cases. J Opt Soc Am 44:117, 1954.
26. Heckenlively JR, Foxman SG: Congenital and early onset forms of retinitis pigmentosa. *In* Heckenlively JR (ed): Retinitis Pigmentosa. Philadelphia, JB Lippincott, 1988, pp 107–118.
27. Robb RM, Dowton SB, Fulton AB, et al: Retinal degeneration in B_{12} disorder associated with methylmalonic aciduria and sulfur amino acid abnormalities. Am J Ophthalmol 97:691, 1984.
28. Senior B, Friedman AI, Braudo JL: Juvenile familial nephropathy with tapetoretinal degeneration. Am J Ophthalmol 52:625, 1961.
29. Senior B: Familial-renal-retinal dystrophy. Am J Dis Child 125:442, 1973.
30. Stanescu B, Dralands L: Cerebro-hepatorenal (Zellweger's) syndrome: ocular involvement. Arch Ophthalmol 87:590, 1972.
31. Weleber RG, Tongue AC, Kennaway NG, et al: Ophthalmic manifestations of infantile phytanic acid storage disease. Arch Ophthalmol 102:1317, 1984.
32. Zeman W: Batten disease: ocular features, differential diagnosis and diagnosis by enzyme analysis. Birth Defects 12:441, 1976.
33. Dagi LR, Leys MJ, Hansen RM, et al: Hyperopia in complicated Leber's congenital amaurosis. Arch Ophthalmol 108:709, 1990.
34. Foxman SG, Heckenlively JR, Bateman JB, et al: Classification of congenital and early onset retinitis pigmentosa. Arch Ophthalmol 103:1502, 1985.
35. Karel I, Brachfield K, Styblova V, et al: Ophthalmological and general findings in congenital diffuse tapetoretinal degeneration. *In* Brunett JR, Barbeau A (eds): Progress in Neuro-ophthalmology. Princeton, NJ: Excerpta Medica 2:377, 1967.
36. Lambert SR, Taylor D, Kriss A: The infant with nystagmus, normal appearing fundi, but an abnormal ERG. Surv Ophthalmol 34:173, 1989.
37. Leber T: Ueber Retinitis pigmentosa und angeborene Amaurose. Graefes Arch Klin Exp Ophthalmol 15:1, 1869.
38. Margolis S, Scher BM, Carr RE: Macular colobomas in Leber's congenital amaurosis. Am J Ophthalmol 83:27, 1977.
39. Mizuno K, Takei Y, Sears ML, et al: Leber's congenital amaurosis. Am J Ophthalmol 83:32, 1977.
40. Nickel B, Hoyt CS: Leber's congenital amaurosis: Is mental retardation a frequent associated defect? Arch Ophthalmol 100:1089, 1982.
41. Noble KG, Carr RE: Leber's congenital amaurosis. Arch Ophthalmol 96:818, 1978.
42. Mayer DL, Fulton AB, Sossen PL: Preferential looking acuity of pediatric patients with developmental disabilities. Behav Brain Res 10:189, 1983.
43. Mayer DL, Fulton AB, Hansen RM: Visual acuity of infants and children with retinal degenerations. Ophthalmol Pediatr Genet 5:51, 1985.
44. McCulloch DL, Taylor MJ, Whyte HE: Visual evoked potentials and visual prognosis following perinatal asphyxia. Arch Ophthalmol 109:229, 1991.
45. Miranda SR, Hack M, Fantz RL, et al: Neonatal pattern vision: a predictor of future mental performance? J Pediatr 4:642, 1977.
46. Mohn G, van Hof–van Duin J: Behavioral and electrophysiological measures of visual functions in children with neurological disorders. Behav Brain Res 10:177, 1983.
47. Robertson R, Jan JE, Wong PKH: Electroencephalograms of children with permanent cortical visual impairment. Can J Neurol Sci 13:256, 1986.
48. Skarf B, Panton C: VEP testing in neurologically impaired and developmentally delayed infants and young children. Invest Ophthalmol Vis Sci 28(Suppl):302, 1987.
49. van Hof–van Duin J, Mohn G: Optokinetic and spontaneous nystagmus in children with neurological disorders. Behav Brain Res 10:163, 1983.
50. Isenberg S: Macular development in the premature infant. Am J Ophthalmol 101:74, 1986.
51. Mayer DL, Rodier DW, Fulton AB: Grating acuity differentiates good from poor prognosis for vision in infants with nystagmus. Invest Ophthalmol Vis Sci 29(Suppl):435, 1988.
52. Fulton AB, Hansen RM: Testing of the possibly blind child. *In* Isenberg S (ed): The Eye in Infancy. 2nd ed. Boston, Mosby-Year Book, in press.
53. Weleber RG, Tongue AC: Congenital stationary night blindness presenting as Leber's congenital amaurosis. Arch Ophthalmol 105:360, 1987.
54. Fulton AB, Hansen RM: Retinal adaptation in infants and children with retinal degenerations. Ophthalmic Pediatr Genet 2:69, 1983.
55. Campo RV, Aaberg TM: Ocular and systemic manifestations of the Bardet-Biedl syndrome. Am J Ophthalmol 94:750, 1982.
56. Green J, Parfrey PS, Harnett JD, et al: The cardinal manifestations of Bardet-Biedl syndrome, a form of Laurence-Moon-Biedl syndrome. N Engl J Med 321:1002, 1989.
57. Jacobson SG, Borruat F-X, Apathy MS: Patterns of rod and cone dysfunction in Bardet-Biedl syndrome. Am J Ophthalmol 109:676, 1990.
58. Katsumi O, Tanino T, Hirose T, et al: Laurence-Moon-Bardet-Biedl syndrome. Electrophysiological and psychophysical findings. Jpn J Ophthalmol 29:282, 1985.
59. Leys MJ, Schreiner LA, Hansen RM, et al: Visual acuities and dark adapted thresholds of children with Bardet-Biedl syndrome. Am J Ophthalmol 106:561, 1988.
60. Schachat AP, Maumenee IH: Bardet-Biedl syndrome and related disorders. Arch Ophthalmol 100:285, 1982.
61. Fulton AB, Hansen RM: The relation of retinal sensitivity and rhodopsin in human infants. Vision Res 27:697, 1987.
62. Fulton AB, Hansen RM, Yeh YL, et al: Temporal summation in 10-week old infants. Vision Res 31:1259, 1991.
63. Hansen RM, Fulton AB: Corneoretinal potentials in human infants. Doc Ophthalmol Proc Series 37:81, 1983.
64. Fulton AB, Hansen RM, Harris SJ: Retinal degeneration and brain abnormalities in infants and young children. Doc Ophthalmol 60:133, 1985.
65. Fulton AB, Mayer DL, Hansen RM, et al: Oscillatory potentials of visually inattentive children. Doc Ophthalmol 65:319, 1987.
66. Fulton AB, Hartmann EE, Hansen RM: Electrophysiologic testing techniques for children. Doc Ophthalmol 71:341, 1989.

Chapter 228

Congenital Ptosis

CARL CORDES JOHNSON

The gross anatomy of the orbit, lids, and ocular muscles is well described in many texts.[1,2]

The levator muscle arises with the other extraocular muscles at the orbital apex and fans out to insert anteriorly in the eyelid. It lies just dorsal to the superior rectus muscle and terminates in an ill-defined sheet of collagen fibers, an aponeurosis. The aponeurosis originates approximately 5 mm above the upper margin of the tarsus, with a gradual disappearance of the muscle fibers, and passes in front of the tarsus to insert chiefly in the septa that separate the bundles of the orbicularis muscle and those in the anterior surface of the tarsus (Fig. 228–1). The major insertion is into the septa of the lower half of the eyelid. Contrary to what has been generally claimed, we[5] found little evidence for insertion into the subepidermal portions of the eyelid. The major insertion is deeper, with an anatomic connection to the orbicularis. Its insertion produces the lid crease.

Müller's muscle arises from the belly of the levator, an unusual origin of smooth muscle from striated muscle. It arises abruptly from the underside of the levator just before or concomitant with the latter's transformation into its aponeurosis. So abrupt is the origin that smooth and striated muscle fibers may intermingle with each other for a short distance. This transitional area is unique in that it consists of irregularly grouped smooth muscle cells that intermingle with the thinning striated muscle fibers. Although cells of both types are frequently closely situated, there are no direct connections between them.

Müller's muscle fibers then descend toward the upper margin of the tarsus. In the adult, the muscle is 8 to 12 mm in length (5 mm in the 2-year-old). Its fibers do not comprise a distinct belly but are intermixed with connective tissue, fat, and blood vessels behind the aponeurosis of the levator muscle. They insert on the upper anterior surface of the tarsus, or, more correctly, they insert in dense connective tissue that separates the muscle fibers from the tarsus proper, with a few fibers inserting in the conjunctiva.

Histologic studies of the levator muscles in normal and pathologic conditions have not been pursued extensively. One of the difficulties in performing histologic studies of the pathologically affected muscles of the upper eyelid is that the surgically obtainable samples are crushed mechanically and consist mainly of connective tissue. Although the general construction of the normal eyelid and its muscles is well known,[1,2] only a few histopathologic studies of the eyelid muscles have been reported.[3,4] Electron-microscopic studies of the eyelid muscles, especially relationships between the striated levator muscles and Müller's smooth muscle cells, were first described in 1975.[5]

The most striking findings in ptosis cases, regardless of the cause, are the substantial reduction or absence of the striated levator muscles in the examined area, about 1 cm above the tarsus, where muscle cells are normally present. The area is occupied by connective tissue, including varying numbers of inflammatory cells. However, a few specimens of the belly portion of the levator muscles, which were obtained by deeper excisions, show various pathologic changes. Despite the striking disap-

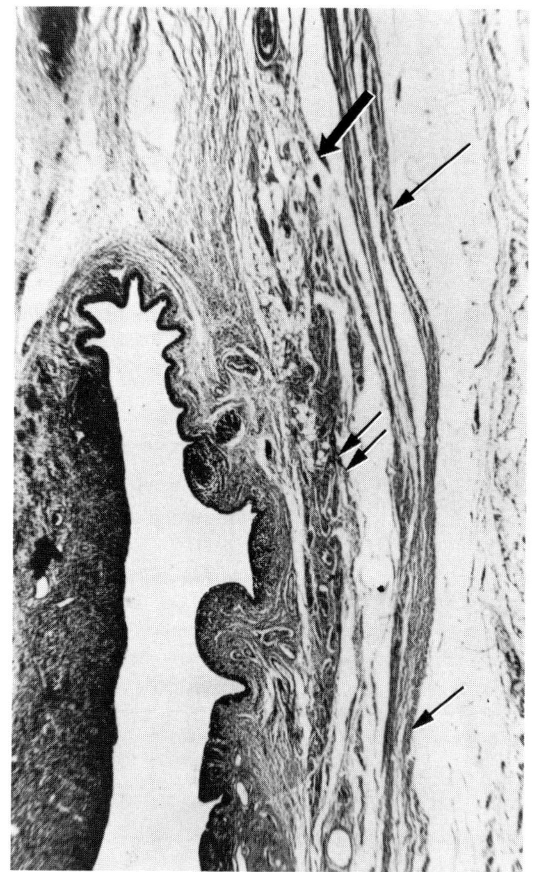

Figure 228–1. The upper inner portion of the human upper eyelid. The posterior portion of the levator muscle ends abruptly (*thick arrow*) and changes into Müller's smooth muscle (*double arrows*). The frontal half of the levator muscle becomes the aponeurosis, which extends toward the lid (*thin arrows*). This connective tissue does not attach to the tarsus but fans out into the orbicularis muscle. Celloidin section (H&E; original magnification ×32). (From Kuwabara T, Cogan OG, Johnson CC: Arch Opthalmol 93:1189. Copyright 1975, American Medical Association.)

pearance of the levator muscle cells, Müller smooth muscle cells are well preserved.

Congenital ptosis is usually unilateral (70 to 75 percent of patients) and nonhereditary, and the amount of levator function varies from none to good. Some cases of congenital ptosis are associated with weakness or paralysis of the superior rectus and some with paralysis of upward gaze. Others are due to a partial or complete third-nerve paralysis. Rare cases of congenital ptosis are due to a sympathetic paralysis (Horner's syndrome). In such patients, the iris of the affected eye is lighter in color than that of the other eye. Horner's syndrome may of course also be a cause of acquired ptosis, but in acquired cases, the irides of the two eyes are the same color.

Levator aponeurosis dehiscences and disinsertions are fairly common in acquired ptosis but rare in congenital ptosis and are quite possibly due to trauma during delivery.

Hereditary congenital ptosis is rare and is usually associated with other anomalies of the lids, such as epicanthus.

PREOPERATIVE INVESTIGATION

Investigation and Treatment of Associated Anomalies

Before surgical correction is attempted in a case of ptosis, the presence of associated anomalies should be determined.

First, abnormal motility of the other extraocular muscles may exist. There may be strabismus of any type with or without frank paralysis of the other extraocular muscles. The most commonly associated and most important anomaly is weakness of the superior rectus. It is important to know whether or not this muscle is functioning normally.

In addition, it is important to note whether or not the eyes roll up normally when the lids are *forcibly* closed (Bell's phenomenon). If Bell's phenomenon is not present, there is much greater postoperative danger of exposure keratitis, and the surgeon may have to be satisfied with an undercorrection of the ptosis. If, on the other hand, Bell's phenomenon is present, there is little danger of exposure keratitis, even if there is incomplete closure of the lids in sleep in young patients.

Paralysis of upward gaze and third-nerve paralysis, either complete or partial, may also be associated with ptosis.

If a horizontal strabismus is present, it may be corrected either before or after the ptosis is corrected, but vertical strabismus *must* be corrected before proceeding with the ptosis operation. It is impossible to repair the ptosis properly if the affected eye is lower than the other eye.

Second, amblyopia may be present in congenital ptosis, but except in cases due to lid or orbital tumors, it is almost always due either to a high astigmatism or an associated muscle imbalance, rather than to the ptosis

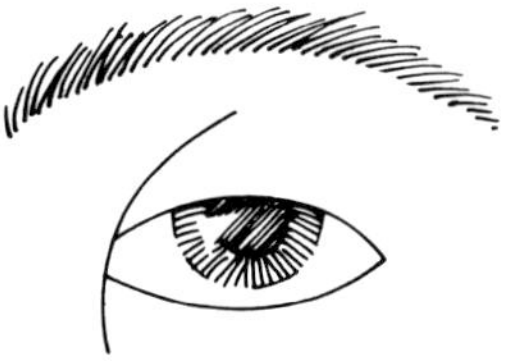

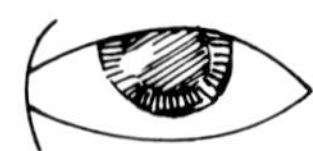

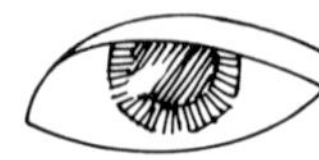

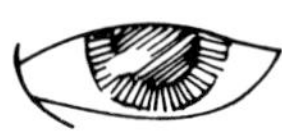

Figure 228–2. The four types of epicanthus. (From Johnson CC: Epicanthus and epiblepharon. Structure of the muscles of the upper eyelid. Arch Opthalmol 96:1030. Copyright 1978, American Medical Association.)

itself. Many of these children have an anisometropia and a high cylinder "with the rule" that must be corrected as early as possible.

Third, there may be associated abnormalities of the lids, such as epicanthus and blepharophimosis.

Duke-Elder[6] classifies epicanthus as follows (Fig. 228–2)

1. Epicanthus supraciliaris
2. Epicanthus palpebralis
3. Epicanthus tarsalis
4. Epicanthus inversus

Type I: *Epicanthus Supraciliaris.* In epicanthus supraciliaris, the epicanthal fold arises from the region of the eyebrow and runs toward the tear sac or nostrils. This type is extremely rare.

Type II: *Epicanthus Palpebralis.* In this type, the epicanthal fold arises from the upper lid, above the tarsal region, and extends to the lower margin of the orbit (Fig. 228–3).

Type III: *Epicanthus Tarsalis.* In epicanthus tarsalis,

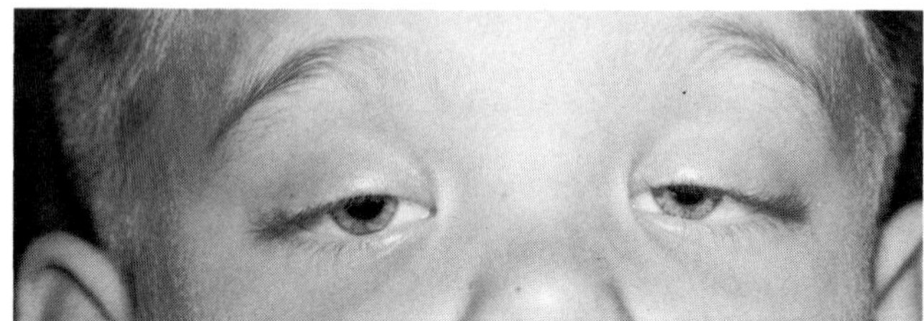

Figure 228–3. Epicanthus palpebralis. (From Johnson CC: Epicanthus and epiblepharon. Arch Ophthalmol 96:1031. Copyright 1978, American Medical Association.)

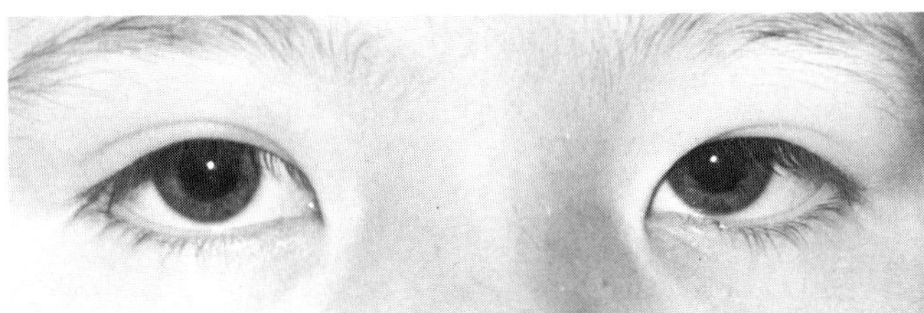

Figure 228–4. Epicanthus tarsalis. (From Johnson CC: Epicanthus and epiblepharon. Arch Ophthalmol 96:1031. Copyright 1978, American Medical Association.)

the epicanthal fold arises from the tarsal fold and loses itself in the skin close to the inner canthus (Fig. 228–4). Epicanthus tarsalis is important because it is closely allied to epiblepharon of the upper lid, the latter being essentially an exaggeration of the former.[7, 8]

An epicanthal fold is evident in all humans in the third to sixth mo of fetal life, usually disappearing before birth, but sometimes persisting into childhood in children of all races as epicanthus palpebralis or more often as epicanthus tarsalis. Epicanthus tarsalis persists as a normal finding in Asians. Johnson and Semple have found epicanthus tarsalis also in most Eskimo children and epiblepharon in a number of these.[9, 11]

Type IV: *Epicanthus Inversus.* This is sometimes called Waardenburg's type II syndrome (Fig. 228–5). In epicanthus inversus, the epicanthal fold is quite different from those in the other three types.

In this type, a small fold arises in the lower eyelid and extends upward, partially covering the inner canthus. It is associated always with some degree of blepharophimosis and with blepharoptosis, and there is rarely any appreciable levator function. Frequently, there is hypoplasia of the caruncle and semilunar folds; the inner canthi are displaced laterally owing to abnormally long medial canthal tendons, and the puncta are displaced laterally even more than would be expected because of the long medial canthal tendons. The margins of the upper lids usually have a slight S-shaped curve, and the lower lids frequently have an abnormal concavity downward. This concavity is greatest in the lateral half of the lid, and the lid frequently is separated from the globe, but without true ectropion. It is a dominant characteristic in many families (Fig. 228–6).

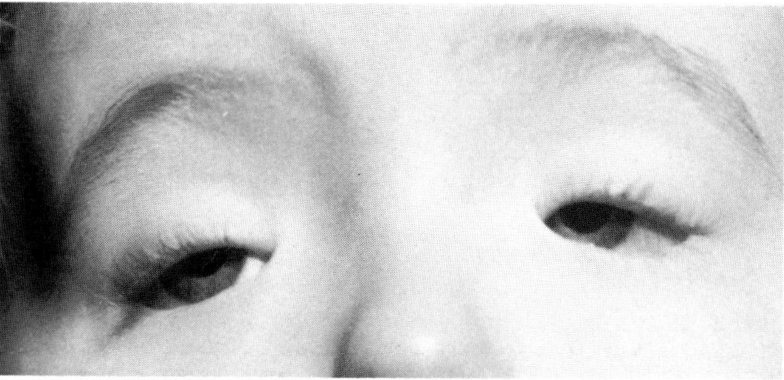

Figure 228–5. Epicanthus inversus. (From Johnson CC: Epicanthus. Am J Ophthalmol 66:939, 1968. Published with permission from The American Journal of Ophthalmology. Copyright by the Ophthalmic Publishing Company.)

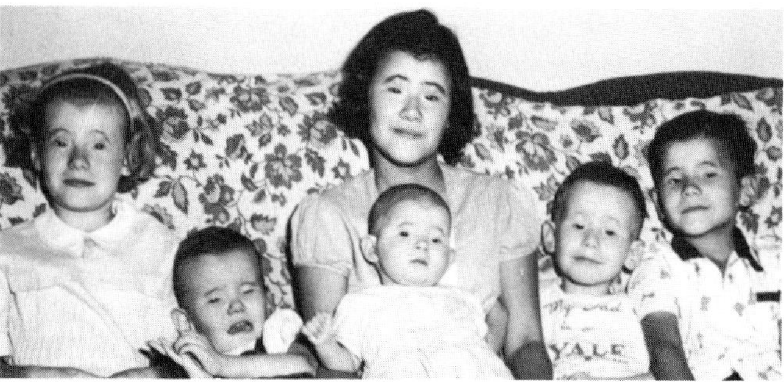

Figure 228–6. Epicanthus inversus in six of ten members of one generation. (From Johnson CC: Surgical repair of the syndrome of epicanthus inversus, blepharophimosis and ptosis. Arch Ophthalmol 71:510–516. Copyright 1964, American Medical Association.)

The term *telecanthus* was coined by Mustarde[10] and was defined as "an increased distance between the internal canthi." Some authors use the term in describing epicanthus inversus.[11]

Waardenburg[12] described type IV as "ptosis with blepharophimosis, often restricted epicanthus (epicanthus inversus), and dystopia lateroversa punctorum lacrimalium."

Waardenburg observed the dominant nature of the condition in many reported pedigrees. He stated that the ratio of affected to unaffected family members is extremely high (134:80), and that the male sex predominates. In one series he reviewed, the father transmitted the characteristic in 39 cases and the mother in seven. He pointed out that the syndrome shows a very high penetrance, seldom skipping a generation. He also noted that this condition, which he characterized as "stiff ptosis," had only rarely been noted in twins. In the author's series, epicanthus inversus is transmitted about five times as often by the father as by the mother. Apparently this is because many of these women are infertile.[13, 14] Waardenburg thought that the ocular defect represented a developmental fixation during the third mo of fetal development, which is a critical period in the development of the ovary and the initial formation of the uterus from müllerian duct fusion. The syndrome of epicanthus inversus, blepharophimosis, and ptosis occurs in about 3 percent of cases of congenital ptosis.

Despite Waardenburg's statement, it is important to note that the distance between the eyes and the interpupillary distance are almost always normal in patients with Waardenburg's syndrome[12, 20] and in those with epicanthus inversus, but the distance between inner canthi is increased owing to the long medial canthal tendons in epicanthus inversus.

Epicanthus inversus and Waardenburg's syndrome must not be confused with hypertelorism. In hypertelorism (Grieg's syndrome)[15, 16] there is an enlarged bony distance between the orbits.

Fox[17] states that most of the growth in fissure width (i.e., height) occurs in the first yr of life, but the 1- to 10-yr age group shows the rapid increase in palpebral fissure length (horizontal) during this period. There is very little increase in length from 10 to 60 yr. After age 60 yr there may be some decrease in fissure *width*.

The normal medial canthal tendons are about 8 to 9 mm long as measured from medial commisure to bony margins, whereas in epicanthus inversus the medial canthal tendons may be as long as 13 mm, even in young children. The taut lids rarely have any levator function, and there is always more or less blepharophimosis.

In normal individuals, the average fissure length is between 28 and 31 mm (26 to 32 in men, with an average of 31 mm; 24 to 31 in women, with an average of 28 mm). In epicanthus inversus, the fissure length is usually 20 to 22 mm and may be as short as 18 mm.

I find the intercanthal distance averages 32.6 mm in white men and 29.4 mm in white women. However, in small children with epicanthus inversus, it is greater, averaging 35 mm, with some being as great as 38 mm.

In addition, some of these children have an extremely high astigmatism and moderate amblyopia, sometimes with nystagmus. The astigmatism is frequently at an oblique axis.[18]

Unlike other types of epicanthus, epicanthus inversus tends to improve very little with age. Many surgeons, on first seeing infants with this condition, think that they must operate at once, because the palpebral fissures are so small that it seems impossible for such infants to see properly. When they start to walk, they tend to throw their heads back in order to see under the ptotic lids, with a resultant abnormal appearance. Early operation should however be avoided. A major reconstruction of the lids is imperative and, in my opinion, it is impossible to do this properly in very small children. I have not seen any spinal abnormalities in these children, so the position in which the head is held does not endanger future development of the spine. The larger and older the child, the better are the results. Incidentally, 50 percent of head growth occurs in the first 3 yr of life.

Of course, we almost always have to operate before such children go to school because psychological problems may arise if they are taunted by their peers. In the author's opinion, one cannot correct the ptosis properly until the epicanthus has been repaired and the vertical pull of the epicanthal fold has been relieved. In many instances, simply lengthening this abnormal fold reduces the amount of ptosis.[7, 8, 15, 19, 20]

Furthermore, the lid skin of these children is quite inelastic (stiff ptosis). As a matter of fact, it seems that they simply do not have enough skin to cover the underlying tissues properly. The upper lids are flat and foldless without the slightest sign of normal skin creases. The lower lid skin is tight, exemplified by the fact that the outer portions of the lids tend not to be in apposition to the globe, and when incised, the skin retracts.

Several surgical procedures may be utilized for the repair of epicanthus. In the first three types, repair is usually not necessary unless the epicanthus is accompanied by ptosis. Repair of the ptosis may exaggerate the epicanthus unless the ptosis operation is combined with repair of the epicanthus. As a matter of fact, the first three types of epicanthus usually disappear by the time the children are teen-aged.

In epicanthus palpebralis, a Y-V procedure can be done. In epicanthus tarsalis, a small V-Y can be done at the inner canthus. The Y-V of Verwey (Fig. 228–7)[21] as described by Hughes[22] and others[24] is satisfactory for the repair of epicanthus inversus, as are Mustarde's[9] rectangular flaps, or a W-type incision[23] (Figs. 228–8 and 228–9).

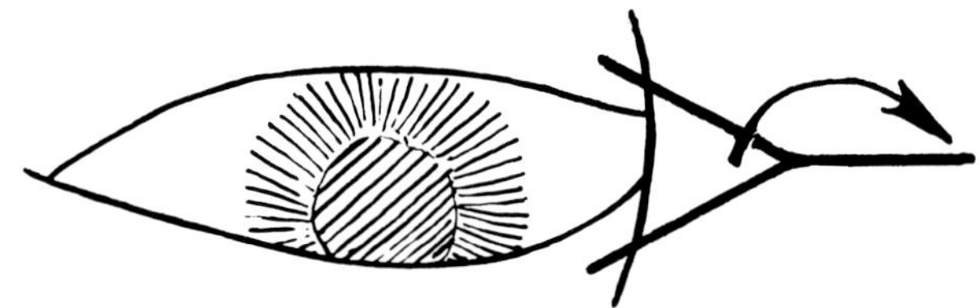

Figure 228–7. The Y-V of Verwey. (From Johnson CC: Epicanthus. Am J Ophthalmol 66:939, 1968. Published with permission from The American Journal of Ophthalmology. Copyright by the Ophthalmic Publishing Company.)

The Y-V plasty is the simplest procedure and will produce good results in milder cases of epicanthus inversus, but in more severe cases, a double Z at the inner canthus, combined with shortening of the medial canthal tendons and an external canthoplasty, will produce a better result. This has been modified from the original Blair procedure (Fig. 228–10, *A* and *B*).[7, 8, 15, 19, 20, 24]

It must be emphasized that in some cases hypertrophic scarring in the eyelid area can be alarming, but it usually reaches its height in about 6 wk and then subsides. Keloid is almost unknown in this area.

Epiblepharon is not often associated with ptosis but may be confused with it in severe cases. It is the height of the lid *margin* that is important in the diagnosis of ptosis, not abnormal lid folds such as epiblepharon and epicanthus.

Fourth, jaw-winking associated with congenital ptosis may be present. In 1883, Marcus Gunn described a case of congenital ptosis with peculiar associated movements of the affected lid.[25] This is now associated with his name and typically consists of a unilateral ptosis in which there is a retraction of the affected eyelid in conjunction with stimulation of the ipsilateral pterygoid muscle. It may also be set off by several other facial or tongue movements.[26]

The explanation as to the etiology is not clear. Some authors think that a branch of the fifth cranial nerve has been congenitally misdirected into the position of the third cranial nerve supplying the levator muscle.[27–29]

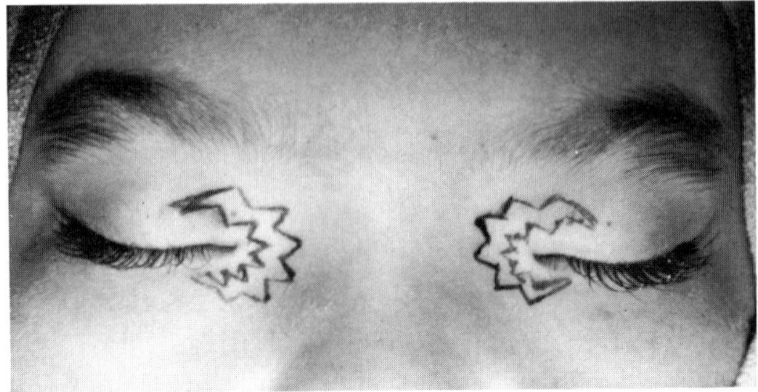

Figure 228–8. The W-type incision. (From Mullikan JB, Hoopes JE: W epicanthoplasty. Plast Reconstr Surg 55:435, 1975. © 1975, The Williams & Wilkins Company, Baltimore.)

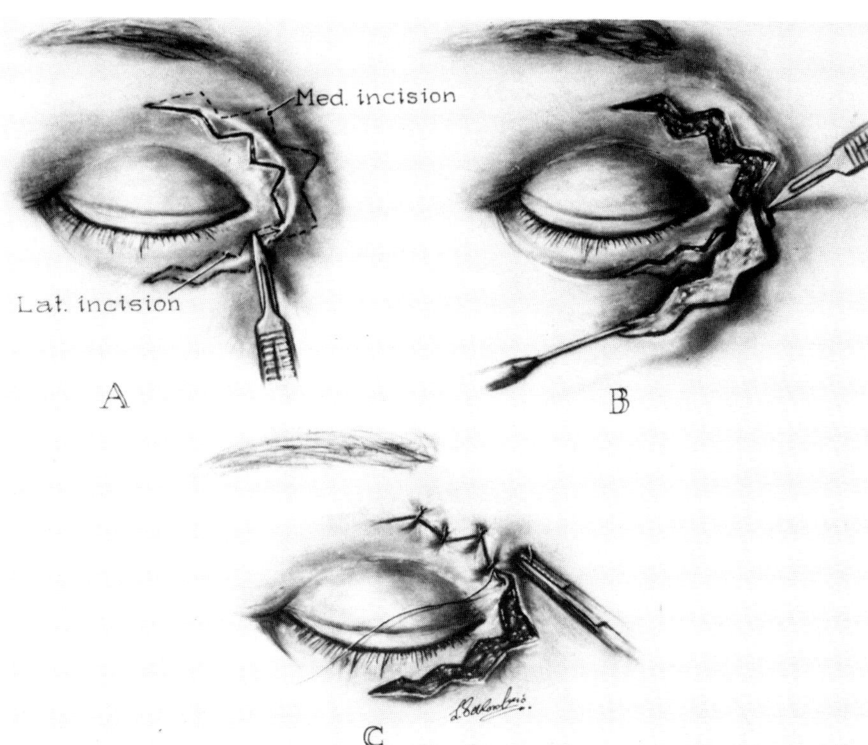

Figure 228–9. The W-type incision. (From Mullikan JB, Hoopes JE: W epicanthoplasty. Plast Reconstr Surg 55:435, 1975. © 1975, The Williams & Wilkins Company, Baltimore.)

Cogan[30] says that the cause is a "spread of stimulus" from the nucleus of the fifth cranial nerve to the nucleus of the third nerve.

Pratt and colleagues[26] at the Massachusetts Eye and Ear Infirmary reviewed 1376 consecutive cases of congenital ptosis that included 71 cases of jaw-winking, an incidence of 5 percent. Two cases had bilateral involvement. The authors recommended ipsilateral excision of the levator, patterned on resection of the levator in most cases with bilateral fascia lata–frontalis slings as described by Berke[31] and Iliff.[32]

Unilateral levator resections may be sufficient in cases with a minimal wink and minimal ptosis, but bilateral fascial slings produce consistently more uniform results.

As one would expect, there are more associated muscular imbalances associated with jaw-winking than with other types of congenital ptosis. The four most common ones in this study were amblyopia, double-elevator palsy, anisometropia, and superior rectus palsy.

Investigation of Ptosis Itself

After investigating associated anomalies and repairing those that require it, one then evaluates the ptosis itself.

Clinically, levator function is tested as follows: The patient's brow is held so that he cannot use the frontalis to help elevate the lid. A ruler is held alongside the lid and the patient is asked to look down and then up. The total excursion from maximum downgaze to maximum upgaze is measured on the ruler. Up to 2 to 3 mm is considered to be no function, as the lid will move this much simply owing to superior rectus attachment. The average normal levator excursion is 14 mm, but it may vary from 13 to as much as 16 mm; thus one can grade the excursion from 2 mm to 14 mm or more. Incidentally, in jaw-winking the extent of the "wink" is no indication of useful levator function. A much fancier method of testing is to use the Walter Reed blepharometer.[33]

The next step is to measure the amount, or degree, of ptosis. Finding a ptosis of 2, 3, or 4 mm is helpful only if the height of the other lid is known. Measuring the vertical fissure width is of little value (the normal is about 10 mm) because it does not take into account the level of the *lower* lid, which may be at, above, or below the lower limbus. If one describes the amount of ptosis by measuring the amount of corneal "overlap" in *each* eye, an accurate picture is obtained. The cornea may be

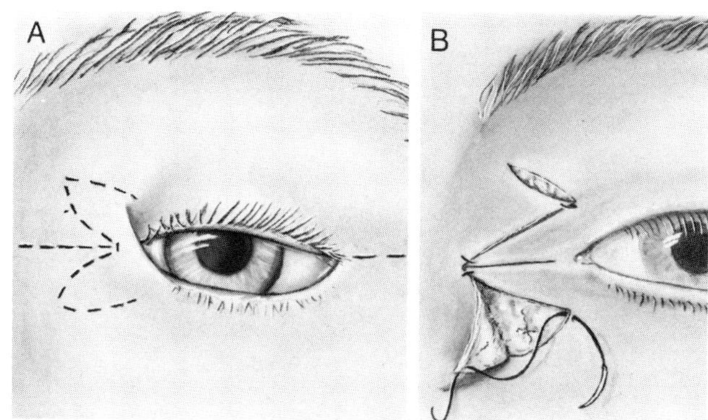

Figure 228–10. *A*, The double Z incision; *B*, the flaps transposed. (From Johnson CC: Epicanthus. Am J Ophthalmol 66:936, 1968. Published with permission from The American Journal of Ophthalmology. Copyright by the Ophthalmic Publishing Company.)

Table 228–1. PLACEMENT OF PTOTIC LID FOR VARIOUS AMOUNTS OF LEVATOR ACTION IN CONGENITAL MONOCULAR PTOSIS WHEN NORMAL LID COVERS CORNEA 2 TO 3 MM AND THE EXTERNAL APPROACH IS USED

Amount of Levator Action	Ptotic Lid Should Cover Cornea	Expected Lift	Postoperative Fall	Expected Overcorrection or Undercorrection	
2–3 mm	0 mm	0 mm	2–3 mm	Under	1–2 mm
4–5 mm	1–2 mm	0 mm	0–1 mm	Over	0–1 mm
6–7 mm	2–3 mm	0–1 mm	0 mm	Over	0–1 mm
8–9 mm	3–4 mm	2–3 mm	0 mm	Over	0–1 mm
10–11 mm	6 mm	4–5 mm	0 mm	Over	0–2 mm

considered, on average, to have a vertical diameter of 11 mm, therefore the center of the pupil is at 5.5 mm; the amount of overlap can be easily estimated from these figures. One must remember that in the case of unilateral ptosis the unaffected lid may be abnormally high (Hering's law), so it is helpful to occlude the affected eye for 30 min or so before making measurements.

The height of the lid crease in the normal lid must be noted so that the crease in the operated eye can be matched to it at operation. We take preoperative photographs in the primary position and with the patient looking up and down. Corneal sensitivity must be tested, as must the presence or absence of diplopia when the affected lid is raised.

SURGERY FOR CONGENITAL PTOSIS

There is still some disagreement among competent ptosis surgeons about whether to resect the levator from the skin surface or the conjunctival side, and a number of "simple" ptosis procedures have been proposed. The correction of ptosis is not a simple procedure and simple procedures are not necessarily good procedures.

In our opinion, levator resection through the skin surface is the preferred method when there is any appreciable levator function. This has been thoroughly described elsewhere,[34] has changed very little over the years, and is not discussed further here except to say that it is easier to resect through the skin surface and to grade the amount resected than to do so when operating on an everted lid.

Many years ago, Berke proposed a table that indicates where the margin of the upper lid should be placed at operation, depending upon the extent of levator excursion (Table 228–1).[35]

The Fasanella-Servat tarsoconjunctival resection[36–38] is indicated much less frequently than a levator resection in congenital ptosis but much more frequently in acquired ptosis. It may produce a good result if there is no more than 3 mm of ptosis and there is a levator excursion of at least 12 mm. Superior tarsal (Müller's muscle) resection produces comparable results.[39] Before either of these procedures, a 10 percent phenylephrin hydrochloride test should be done to ascertain that resection of Müller's muscle will produce a satisfactory result.

If there is minimal or no levator function in either unilateral or bilateral ptosis, a bilateral autogenous fascia lata–frontalis sling is indicated. The second-best material is preserved human fascia, but it should be used only if for some reason autogenous fascia is unobtainable. This limits the minimum age for correction, because the child's leg must be long enough to obtain sufficient fascia.

Synthetic materials are poor substitutes for human fascia, especially autogenous fascia. They tend to cut through the tissues, leading to a recurrence of the ptosis. In addition, there is a higher incidence of infection, possibly owing to the foreign material being in close proximity to the meibomian glands.

Autogenous fascia tends to maintain its normal structure when transplanted. We have had one case in which an autogenous fascial sling failed after 2 yr (done elsewhere, of course). The fascia was removed and compared with a fresh sample obtained from the patient. The pathologist was unable to find any microscopic difference in the two samples. A case has also been reported[40] in which autogenous fascia was removed after 42 yr. It remained viable both clinically and histologically.

We place the fascia in the shape of a trapezoid (not a rhomboid) beneath or deep in the orbicularis (Fig. 228–11).

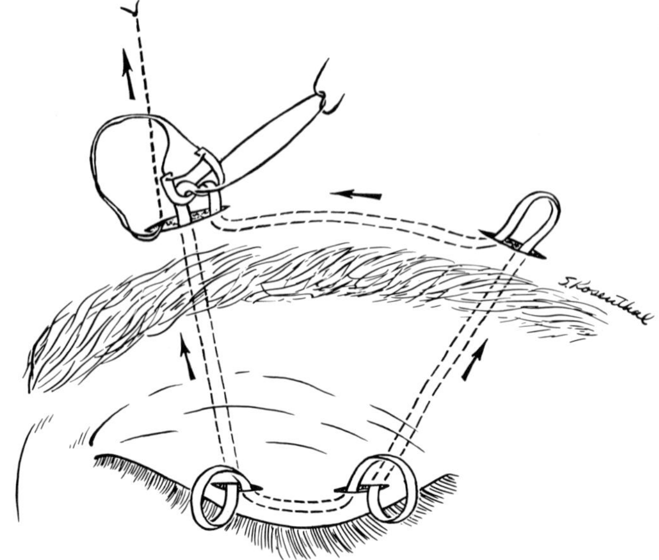

Figure 228–11. The fascial sling.

Complications of Ptosis Surgery

In anterior levator resections, if the initial skin incision is made too high it is easy to lower it at the end of the operation by resecting skin from the lower skin flap, but if it is made too low there is no recourse. In general, a lid crease that is slightly low always looks better than one that is too high.

The bulbs of the cilia may be damaged if the dissection is carried too close to the lid margin. The superior rectus can be damaged, but we have never encountered this problem. The same is true with the superior oblique. Buttonholing the levator can threaten the success of the operation, but this can usually be repaired easily. Buttonholing the conjunctiva is of no consequence. Injury to the lacrimal gland can occur.[41]

Prolapse of conjunctiva is usually easily controlled intraoperatively. If it occurs postoperatively, a pressure dressing will frequently take care of it; if not, sutures must be placed through the conjunctiva at the approximate location of the superior fornix and carried out through the skin.

Undercorrections in levator resections are a result either of inadequate resection of the levator muscle or of resecting in the presence of inadequate levator function, and they require an additional surgical procedure. If the excursion is 5 mm or more, another resection can be done; if less than this, *bilateral* fascia lata–frontalis slings should be performed.

Overcorrections are somewhat more difficult to handle. Usually, a levator tenotomy as advocated by Berke (Fig. 228–12)[42] is sufficient. An incision is made through the tarsus near its upper border and is extended deeply enough so that the wound can be opened approximately twice the amount of the overcorrection. A traction suture is placed, and the lid is pulled downward for a few days. The use of collagen film or other materials (sclera, fascia) has been suggested in cases with more severe overcorrections.[43, 44]

Exposure keratitis is not often a complication following levator resections, unless the operation is performed in the presence of inadequate levator function or inadequate tearing or, especially, if there is no Bell's phenomenon. Bell's phenomenon occurs on *forced* closure of the lids and is not usually present in sleep; nevertheless, it is a most effective protective mechanism.

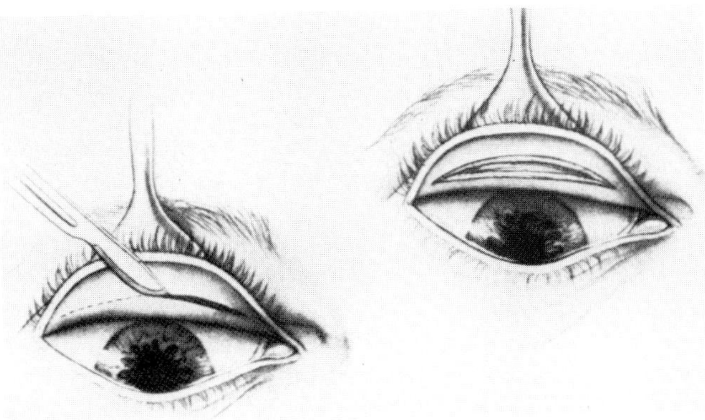

Figure 228–12. Berke's method of levator tenotomy.

Overcorrections and undercorrections in fascial slings should not occur if the lid height is properly adjusted intraoperatively. If they do occur, they are evident in the immediate postoperative period and can be repaired by opening the brow incision over the knot in the fascia and further shortening it in the case of undercorrection, or allowing the fascia to retract in the case of overcorrection.

REFERENCES

1. Whitnall SE: The Anatomy of the Human Orbit, and Accessory Organs of Vision, 2nd ed. Oxford, Humphry Milford, 1932.
2. Wolff E: Anatomy of the Eye and Orbit, 6th ed. Philadelphia, WB Saunders, 1968.
3. Berke RN, Wadsworth JAC: Histology of the levator muscle in congenital and acquired ptosis. Arch Ophthalmol 53:413, 1955.
4. Jones LT: The anatomy of the upper eyelid and its relation to ptosis surgery. Am J Ophthalmol 57:943, 1964.
5. Kuwabara T, Cogan DG, Johnson CC: Structure of the muscles of the upper eyelid. Arch Ophthalmol 93:1189, 1975.
6. Duke-Elder S (ed): System of Ophthalmology, Vol 3. London, Henry Kimpton, 1964, p 2.
7. Johnson CC: Epicanthus. Am J Ophthalmol 66:939, 1968.
8. Johnson CC: Epicanthus and epiblepharon. Arch Ophthalmol 96:1030, 1978.
9. Johnson GJ, Semple J: Epiblepharon in Labrador. Can J Ophthalmol 12:175, 1977.
10. Mustarde JC: Epicanthus and telecanthus. Br J Plast Surg 16:346, 1963.
11. Kohn R, Romano PE: Blepharoptosis, blepharophimosis, epicanthus inversus and telecanthus—a syndrome with no name. Am J Opthalmol 72:265, 1971.
12. Waardenburg PJ, Franceschetti A, Klein D: Genetics and Ophthalmology. Assn, Netherlands, Royal Van Gorcum, 1961, p 415.
13. Townes P, Muchler E: Blepharophimosis, ptosis, epicanthus inversus and primary amenorrhea, a dominant trait. Arch Ophthalmol 97:1664, 1979.
14. Zlotogora J, Sagi M, Cohen T: The blepharophimosis, ptosis and epicanthus inversus syndrome: delineation of five types. Am J Hum Genet 35:1020, 1983.
15. Johnson CC: Surgical repair of the syndrome of epicanthus inversus, blepharophimosis and ptosis. Arch Ophthalmol 71:510, 1964.
16. Blodi FC: Developmental anomalies of the skull affecting the eye. Arch Ophthalmol 57:593, 1957.
17. Fox SA: The palpebral fissure. Am J Ophthalmol 62:73, 1966.
18. Edmund J: The ocular function and motility in congenital blepharophimosis. Arch Ophthalmol 47:535, 1969.
19. Johnson CC: Operations for epicanthus and blepharophimosis. An evaluation and a method for shortening the medial canthal ligament. Am J Ophthalmol 41:71, 1956.
20. Johnson CC: Developmental abnormalities of the eyelids. The 1985 Wendell Hughes Lecture. Ophthalmol Plast Reconstr Surg 2:219, 1986.
21. Verwey A: Overhet. Maskergeloat en Zijn behandlung. Neth tij V gen 45:1956, 1909.
22. Hughes WL: Surgical treatment of congenital palpebral phimosis. Arch Ophthalmol 54:586, 1955.
23. Mullikan JB, Hoopes JE: W-epicanthoplasty. Plast Reconstr Surg 55:435, 1975.
24. Blair VP, Brown JB, Hamm WG: Correction of ptosis and epicanthus. Arch Ophthalmol 7:831, 1932.
25. Gunn RM: Congenital ptosis with peculiar associated movements of the affected lid. Trans Ophthalmol Soc UK 3:283, 1883.
26. Pratt SG, Beyer CK, Johnson CC: The Marcus Gunn phenomenon. Ophthalmology 91:27, 1984.
27. Beard C: Ptosis, 3rd ed. St. Louis, CV Mosby, 1981, pp 33–46.
28. Waller RR: Evaluation and management of the ptosis patient. *In*

McCord CD Jr (ed): Oculoplastic Surgery. New York, Raven Press, 1981, p 16.
29. Duke-Elder S (ed): System of Ophthalmology, Vol 3. Pt 2, Normal and Abnormal Development: Congenital Deformities. London, Henry Kimpton, 1964, p 900.
30. Cogan DG: Personal communication.
31. Berke RN: A simplified Blaskovics operation for blepharoptosis. Arch Opthalmol 48:460, 1952.
32. Iliff CE: A simplified ptosis operation. Am J Opthalmol 37:529, 1954.
33. La Plana FG, Przybyla VA Jr, Padgug L, et al: The Walter Reed blepharometer. Adv Ophthalmol Plast Reconstr Surg 1:3, 1982.
34. Johnson CC: Blepharoptosis. Selection of operation, operative techniques, complications. Arch Ophthalmol 66:793, 1961; Arch Ophthalmol 67:18, 1962.
35. Berke RN: Types of operation indicated for congenital and acquired ptosis. *In* Troutman RC, Converse JM, Smith B (eds): Plastic and Reconstructive Surgery of the Eye. Washington, Butterworths, 1962, p 125.
36. Fasanella RM, Servat J: Levator resection for minimal ptosis, another simplified operation. Arch Ophthalmol 65:493, 1961.
37. The Fasanella-Servat procedure: an update. Adv Ophthalmol Plast Reconstr Surg 1:95, 1982.
38. Servat J, Manrique A, Alaya H: The Fasanella-Servat operation: 1961–1981. Adv Ophthalmol Plast Reconstr Surg 1:99, 1982.
39. Dortzbach RK: Superior tarsal muscle resection to correct blepharoptosis. Ophthalmology 86:1883, 1979.
40. Orlando F, Weiss JS, Beyer-Machule CK, et al: Histopathologic condition of fascia lata implant 42 years after ptosis repair. Arch Ophthalmol 103:1518, 1985.
41. Beyer CK, Johnson CC: Anterior levator resection: problems and management. Trans Am Acad Ophthalmol Otolaryngol 79:687, 1975.
42. Berke RN: Complications in ptosis surgery. *In* Fasanella R (ed): Management of Complications in Ptosis Surgery. Philadelphia, WB Saunders, 1957.
43. Callahan A: Levator recession. Arch Ophthalmol 73:800, 1965.
44. Callahan A: Reconstructive Surgery of the Eyelids and Ocular Adnexa. Birmingham, AL, Aesculapius, 1966.

Index

Note: Page numbers in *italics* refer to illustrations; page numbers followed by t refer to tables.